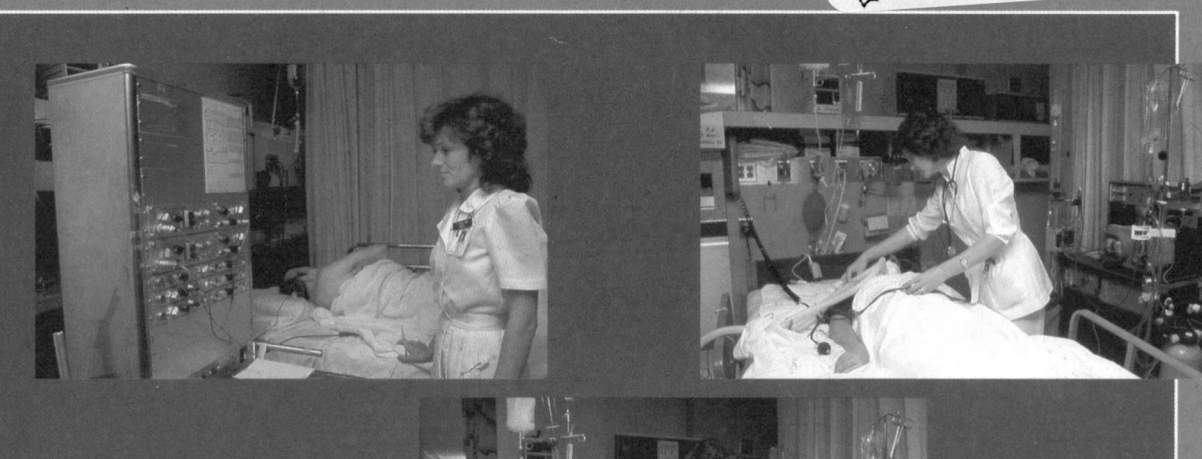

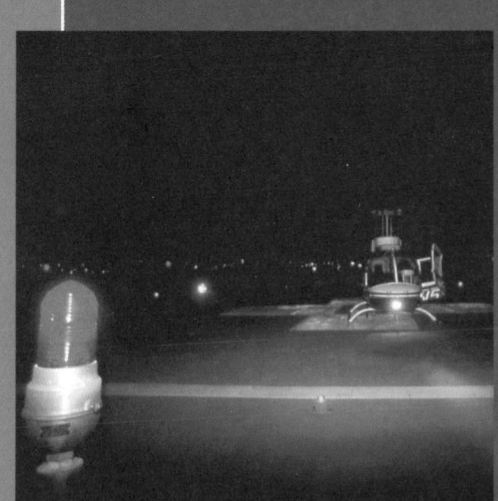

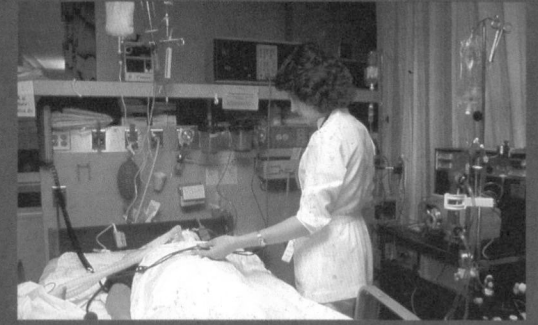

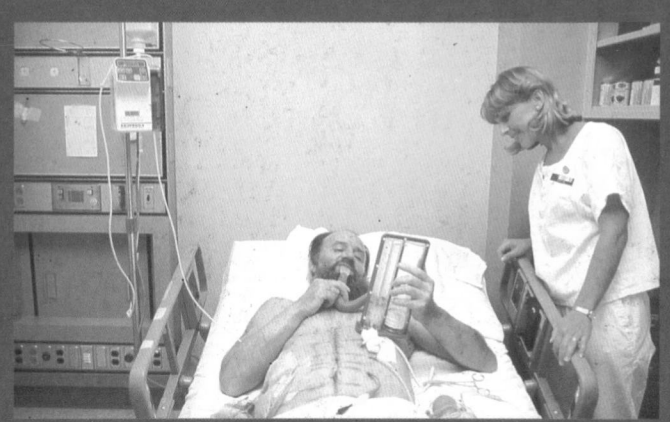

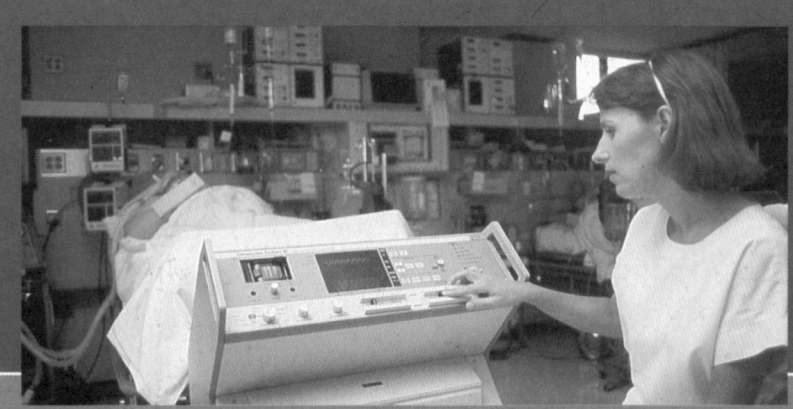

AACN's
Clinical Reference
for Critical-Care
Nursing

AACN'S Clinical Reference for Critical-Care Nursing

Marguerite Rodgers Kinney, R.N., D.N.Sc., F.A.A.N.

School of Nursing
University of Alabama at Birmingham
Birmingham, Alabama

Donna Rogers Packa, R.N., D.S.N.

School of Nursing
University of Alabama at Birmingham
Birmingham, Alabama

Sandra Byars Dunbar, R.N., D.S.N.

School of Nursing
University of Miami
Miami, Florida

McGraw-Hill Book Company

New York St. Louis San Francisco Auckland Bogotá Caracas
Colorado Springs Hamburg Lisbon London Madrid Mexico Milan
Montreal New Delhi Oklahoma City Panama Paris San Juan
São Paulo Singapore Sydney Tokyo Toronto

Notice

As new medical and nursing research and clinical experience broaden our knowledge, changes in treatment and drug therapy are required. The editors and the publisher of this work have made every effort to ensure that the drug dosage schedules herein are accurate and in accord with the standards accepted at the time of publication. Readers are advised, however, to check the product information sheet included in the package of each drug they plan to administer to be certain that changes have not been made in the recommended dose or in the contraindications for administration. This recommendation is of particular importance in regard to new or infrequently used drugs.

AACN'S CLINICAL REFERENCE FOR CRITICAL-CARE NURSING

1 2 3 4 5 6 7 8 9 0   RMTRMT   8 9 3 2 1 0 9 8

ISBN 0-07-034721-2

This book was set in Serif by the College Composition Unit in cooperation with Monotype Composition Company.
The editors were Sally J. Barhydt and James R. Belser; the designer was Caliber Design Planning, Inc.; the production supervisor was Denise L. Puryear.
Drawings were done by Caliber Design Planning, Inc.
Rand McNally & Company was printer and binder.

Library of Congress Cataloging-in-Publication Data

AACN's clinical reference for critical-care nursing.

   Includes index.
   1. Intensive care nursing.   I. Kinney, Marguerite
Rodgers.   II. Packa, Donna Rodgers.   III. Dunbar,
Sandra Byars.   IV. American Association of Critical-
Care Nurses.
RT120.I5A18   1988   610.73'61   87-17273
ISBN 0-07-034721-2

About the Editors

MARGUERITE KINNEY is professor and coordinator of cardiovascular nursing at the University of Alabama at Birmingham. She is a former president of the American Association of Critical-Care Nurses and is editor of *Focus on Critical Care,* an official publication of AACN. She is a fellow of the American Academy of Nursing and a member of Sigma Theta Tau, the international honor society in nursing.

Dr. Kinney was born in Tuscaloosa, Alabama, and has lived all her life in the South. She received both the bachelor of science and the master of science in nursing from the University of Alabama and the doctor of nursing science from the Catholic University of America. Her research has been in the area of patient teaching, energy expenditure, and nursing diagnosis.

DONNA PACKA received her bachelor of science in nursing from Murray State University in Murray, Kentucky. Her clinical practice included staff nursing and leadership in coronary care and medical intensive care units. She received the master of science in nursing and doctor of science in nursing degrees from the University of Alabama at Birmingham, where her doctoral studies focused on adult education with research related to the quality of life of heart transplant recipients. Dr. Packa is currently on the graduate faculty of the School of Nursing, the University of Alabama at Birmingham with responsibilities in both the master's and doctoral programs, and she is primarily involved in the cardiovascular clinical-nurse specialist major of the masters program. Dr. Packa has been a member of the American Association of Critical-Care Nurses since 1974 and has served on AACN's Technical Assistance Panel and on the Self-Assessment Task Force as both chairman and member. Dr. Packa has been a member of the editoral board of *Heart and Lung* since 1978.

SANDRA DUNBAR is associate professor of nursing at the University of Miami, Miami, Florida. Her responsibilities include classroom and clinical teaching at the graduate level and serving as co-director of the Transcultural Nursing Research Institute. She received her bachelor of science in nursing from the Florida State University in Tallahassee, master of nursing from the University of Florida, Gainesville, and was awarded the doctor of science in nursing from the University of Alabama at Birmingham. Her research has examined the effects of patient education after acute myocardial infarction, needs of families of critically ill patients, and timing of digoxin administration. Dr. Dunbar has served as president of the American Association of Critical-Care Nurses and is an active member of Sigma Theta Tau.

To our colleagues—those who have gone before and on whose shoulders we have stood; and those who came later and had the courage to soar toward enhanced visions; and those who will come to meet the new challenges and opportunities.

Contents

List of Contributors

Cathleen A. Acres, R.N., M.N.
Patient Representative
The New York Hospital/Cornell Medical Center
New York, New York

Judith Cook Albright, R.N., M.S.N.
(Former) Staff Nurse
New England Medical Center
Boston, Massachusetts

Charold Lee Baer, R.N., Ph.D.
Professor
Department of Adult Health and Illness
The Oregon Health Science Center
Portland, Oregon

Anne Elizabeth Belcher, R.N., Ph.D.
Director, Oncology Masters Program
Memorial Sloan-Kettering Cancer Center
    and
Associate Dean, Academic Affairs
Columbia University School of Nursing
New York, New York

Rochelle Logston Boggs, R.N., M.S.N., C.E.N.,
    CCRN.
Trauma/Critical-Care Clinical Nurse Specialist
Long Island College Hospital
Brooklyn, New York

Mary-Michael Brown, R.N., M.S.
Surgical Clinical Specialist
University Hospital at Boston University Medical
    Center
Boston, Massachusetts

Sheila M. Campbell, R.D., M.S.
Clinical Research Associate
Medical Nutritional Education
Ross Laboratories
Columbus, Ohio

Elizabeth A. Chaney, R.N., M.S.N., J.D.
Attorney and Counselor at Law
Monrovia, California

Susan B. Christoph, R.N., M.S.N., CCRN
Lt. Col., Army Nurse Corps
Chief Nurse, U.S. Army Research and
    Development Center
Fort Detrick, Frederick, Maryland

Frances L. Conrad, R.N., P.H.N.
Staff Nurse
Rocky Mountain Poison and Drug Center
Denver, Colorado

Diane M. Cooper, R.N., M.N.
Doctoral Candidate, School of Nursing
University of Pennsylvania
Philadelphia, Pennsylvania

Anne J. Davis, R.N., Ph.D., F.A.A.N.
Professor of Nursing
University of California—San Francisco
San Francisco, California

Richard A. de Asla, B.A.
Bioengineering Coordinator
Mount Sinai Medical Center
New York, New York

Mary Ann DiMola, R.N., M.A.
Director of Nursing Education and Research
St. Vincent's Medical Center
Jacksonville, Florida

Jeanne E. Doyle, R.N., B.S.
Nurse Consultant, Peripheral Vascular Surgery
University Hospital at Boston University Medical
    Center
Boston, Massachusetts

Sandra B. Dunbar, R.N., D.S.N.
Associate Professor of Nursing
University of Miami
Miami, Florida

Janet Eagan, R.N., M.S.
Head Nurse, Coronary Care Unit
University Hospital at Boston University Medical
    Center
Boston, Massachusetts

Reba Felks-McVay, R.N., M.S.N.
Formerly Cardiac Transplant Nurse Coordinator
    and Cardiovascular Clinical Nurse Specialist
University of Alabama Hospitals
Birmingham, Alabama

Sr. Mary Rebecca Fidler, Ph.D.
Provost and Dean of the Faculty
Salem College
Salem, West Virginia

Marsha D. M. Fowler, R.N., Ph.D.
Associate Professor of Nursing and Theology
Azusa Pacific University
Azusa, California

Sheila A. Glennon, R.N., M.A., CCRN
(Former) Chief, Critical-Care Nursing
Norwalk Hospital
Norwalk, Connecticut

Jonathan E. Gottlieb, M.D.
Director, Medical Respiratory Intensive Care Unit
Thomas Jefferson University Hospital
    and
Assistant Professor of Medicine
Jefferson Medical College
Philadelphia, Pennsylvania

Doris S. Greiner, R.N., M.S.N.
Associate Professor of Nursing
University of Alabama at Birmingham
Birmingham, Alabama

Eileen Lovett Griffin, R.N., M.A., M.Ed.
Head Nurse, Intensive Care Unit
St. Luke's Hospital
New York, New York

Jeanette Hartshorn, R.N., Ph.D., CCRN
Assistant Professor of Nursing
Medical University of South Carolina
Charleston, South Carolina

Cynthia A. Horvath, R.N., M.S.N.
Assistant Professor of Nursing
University of Alabama at Birmingham
Birmingham, Alabama

Brenda S. Jackson, R.N., Ph.D.
Associate Professor
Division of Nursing
Incarnate Word College
San Antonio, Texas

Molly Johantgen, R.N., M.S.N., CCRN
Critical-Care Clinical Specialist
Chrsit Hospital
Cincinnati, Ohio

Mary Brewer Jones, R.N., Ph.D.
Assistant Professor of Nursing
University of Texas Health Science Center at San
    Antonio
San Antonio, Texas

Patricia Kallweit Kaldor, R.N., M.S.N.
Assistant Director of Nursing, Critical Care
St. Joseph's Hospital
Milwaukee, Wisconsin

Mary Frances Keen, R.N., D.N.Sc.
Associate Professor and
Associate Dean, Undergraduate Programs
University of Miami
Miami, Florida

Marguerite R. Kinney, R.N., D.N.Sc., F.A.A.N.
Professor and Coordinator, Cardiovascular
  Nursing
University of Alabama at Birmingham
Birmingham, Alabama

Catherine Nuss Kotecki, R.N., M.S.
Education Instructor
West Jersey Health System
Voorhees, New Jersey

Diane Panton Lapsley, R.N., M.S., C.S.
Cardiovascular Clinical Nurse Specialist
West Roxbury Veterans Administration Medical
  Center
West Roxbury, Massachusetts

Beverly S. NcKenna, R.N., M.N.
Medical Surgical Clinical Nurse Specialist
Overlake Hospital Medical Center
Bellevue, Washington

Jane S. Martin, R.N., M.S.N.
Assistant Professor of Nursing
University of Alabama at Birmingham
Birmingham, Alabama

Vickie White Matus, R.N., M.S.N., CCRN, CNRN
Neurosurgical Nurse Clinician
Mt. Sinai Hospital
New York, New York

Linda J. Miers, R.N., M.S.N.
Assistant Professor of Nursing
University of Alabama at Birmingham
Birmingham, Alabama

Pamela H. Mitchell, R.N., M.S., F.A.A.N.
Professor of Nursing
University of Washington
Seattle, Washington

Marjorie Susan Morgan, Ph.D.
Chairperson, Health Sciences and
Associate Professor of Chemistry
Salem College
Salem, West Virginia

Donna R. Packa, R.N., D.S.N.
Assistant Professor of Nursing
University of Alabama at Birmingham
Birmingham, Alabama

Sarah J. Sanford, R.N., M.A.
Senior Vice President for Patient Care Services
Overlake Hospital Medical Center
Bellevue, Washington

Deborah L. Scherger, R.N., B.S.N.
Staff Nurse
Rocky Mountain Poison and Drug Center
Denver, Colorado

Dorothy M. Schulte, R.N., P.H.N.
Staff Nurse
Rocky Mountain Poison and Drug Center
Denver, Colorado

Rae Nadine Smith, R.N., M.S.
Clinical Nurse Specialist and
President, Medical Communicators and Associates,
  Inc.
Salt Lake City, Utah

Sr. Maurita Soukup, R.N., M.S.N. CCRN
Doctoral Student
School of Nursing
The Catholic University of America
Washington, D.C.

June L. Stark, R.N., B.S.N., CCRN
Critical-Care Instructor
New England Medical Center
Renal Nurse Consultant
Boston, Massachusetts

Susan Stewart, R.N., M.S., CCRN
Medical Cardiovascular Clinical Specialist
Albany Medical Center
Albany, New York

Elizabeth Trought, R.N., M.N.
Elizabeth Trought Consultants
Winterville, North Carolina

Nancie Urban, R.N., M.S.N., CCRN
Critical-Care Clinical Nurse Specialist
St. Luke's Samaritan Health Care, Inc.
Milwaukee, Wisconsin

Joan M. Vitello-Cicciu, R.N., M.S.N., CCRN, C.S.
Surgical Critical-Care Clinical Nurse Specialist
University Hospital at Boston University Medical
    Center
Boston, Massachusetts

Gayle R. Whitman, R.N., M.S.N., CCRN
Department Chairman for Cardiac Nursing
Cleveland Clinic Hospital
Cleveland, Ohio

Jacqueline A. Wilson, R.N., M.S.N.
(Former) Assistant Professor of Nursing
Wayne State University
    and
(Former) Chief, Critical-Care Nursing
Harper Grace Hospitals
Detroit, Michigan

Robert F. Wilson, M.D., F.A.C.S.
Professor of Surgery
Director of Thoracic and Cardiovascular Surgery
Wayne State University
    and
Chief of Surgery
Detroit Receiving Hospital
Detroit, Michigan

James B. Winkler, R.N., M.A.
Vice President for Nursing
University Hospital
Jacksonville, Florida

Kathleen M. Wruk, R.N., B.S.N.
Director of Professional Services
Rocky Mountain Poison and Drug Center
Denver, Colorado

Foreword

Recent changes in the economics of health care delivery in the United States have had a remarkable impact on patterns of hospitalization. With shorter hospital stays and increased outpatient services, hospitalized patients are more acutely ill and require more intensive nursing care than patients of a few years ago. Hospitals are evolving into giant-critical-care units.

Unfortunately, this spiraling patient acuity is now coupled with a shortage of critical-care nurses. Given the shrinking enrollments in schools of nursing across the United States over the past five years, it is unlikely that this shortage will be remedied in the near future.

These changes offer an unprecedented challenge to critical-care nursing as a specialty. At no time have critical-care nurses needed more—more education, more clinical expertise, more administrative support, more physical and financial resources. Clearly, this second edition of *AACN's Clinical Reference for Critical-Care Nursing* will meet some of these needs. It is a superb compendium of the latest findings and recommendations for nursing practice in the intensive care setting. The text also provides an excellent illustration of the value of collaboration between medicine and nursing, an approach that is an important part of the solution to today's crisis in critical care. The

authors have used the best of both disciplines in their discussion of various critical-care phenomena.

Nursing and medicine share the common goal of preserving and restoring health; however, physicians and nurses view the critically ill patient from somewhat different vantage points. While medicine focuses on the diagnosis and treatment of disease, nursing is concerned with disease prevention and the response of patients to illness, including emotional and social responses. These two points of view lead to the identification of correspondingly different problems in the same patient and emphasize the importance of collaboration to achieve optimal health care.

For many years, physicians and nurses functioned in a rigidly structured, hierarchical model of clinical practice. The team approach to patient care often translated to a team of physicians providing medical regimens that were implemented by a team of nurses, who in turn were assisted by a team of ancillary personnel. The patient was always the target of these team efforts (or, more accurately, these efforts of the teams), but clearly he or she resided on the bottom rung of the hierarchical ladder. Authority flowed from top to bottom and care was provided incrementally.

Even before the current crisis in critical care, many of the respective team members questioned the viability of the traditional practice model. The fragmentation of medicine and nursing into specialties and subspecialties, the increasing educational preparation of nurses, the explosion of patient-care technology, the patients' rights movement, and the changes in gender-role expectations that occurred in many societies all served as motivators to question the hierarchical model. Evidence of collaboration between nurses and physicians can be found in the National Joint Practice Commission's hospital demonstration projects, in the collaborative practice arrangements among physicians and nurses in private practice, and in the collaborative relationships within professional associations, such as the American Association of Critical-Care Nurses and the Society of Critical Care Medicine.

The collaborative practice model is based on a spirit of egalitarian cooperation in which both physicians and nurses assume full legal responsibility for their decisions and actions. The model also is based on the assumption that medicine and nursing are distinct but interdependent professions. In theory, the model benefits everyone. Patients receive care that is more personalized than in the traditional model. Services are more comprehensive because care is directed toward the multiple dimensions of a patient's illness, not just a physiological derangement. In may cases, care can be provided at a lower cost.

Physicians can be more productive because the collaborative model reduces those tasks that are superfluous to the practice of medicine. Moreover, in a system of equal accountability, the physician is no longer ultimately responsible for anything that happens or fails to happen to the patient (including inadequate nursing care). Job satisfaction may increase as physicians are freed from their supervisory functions to make decisions and perform tasks specific to medical practice.

Finally, nurses benefit when they experience an increase in autonomy and accountability. This increase is critical to the future of nursing. Many nurses and physicians have speculated that the declining enrollment documented by schools of nursing across the country is partially the result of other, traditionally male-dominated professions now being open to women. If nursing, an historically female profession, is to continue to attract intelligent, self-directed individuals into its ranks, it must be viewed as a fully autonomous and accountable profession that presents intellectual challenges to its members.

The editors and authors are to be commended for planning and writing a text that exemplifies the assumptions and characteristics of collaborative practice and that covers such a wide range of critical illnesses. Both the medical and nursing aspects of acute care are well described. This reference serves as an important addition to the critical-care nursing literature.

Kathleen Dracup, R.N., D.N.Sc.
Co-editor, *Heart & Lung:*
The Journal of Critical Care
Los Angeles, California

Preface

In an address given at the opening of the Bodley Shakespeare Exhibition in 1916, Sir William Osler, the eminent physician, remarked: "It is enough, as someone has said, if every book supplies its time with a good word." This is our hope for this text. *AACN's Clinical Reference for Critical-Care Nursing* is intended for use by practicing critical-care nurses, novices and experts alike, and by nursing students as they study critical-care nursing, a trend which we view with great optimism.

One of the words that seems always to come to mind as we turn our thoughts to critical-care nursing is *evolution.* Though young in years, critical-care nursing has come to occupy an established place on the landscape of health care in the modern world. Evolution seems a proper term to describe the current state of critical-care nursing because it connotes an unfolding: a process of change in a certain direction; a continuous change from a lower, simpler, or worse state to a higher, more complex, or better state; in a word, growth.

From simple beginnings, critical-care nursing has evolved into a complex process, demanding much of its practitioners. The complexity of practice in this specialty is evident when one considers that critical-care nursing is the diagnosis and treatment of human responses to life-threatening problems. Human responses take many forms, and the knowledge base required for diagnosis and treatment encompasses the biological and social sciences. The breadth and depth of knowledge required for practice is unmatched by any other nursing specialty and expands unabated in our technological world.

It is this expansion in the breadth and depth of knowledge required for critical-care nursing practice that stimulates the revision of this text. Scientific breakthroughs in our understanding of the human body and its response to disease and injury have spurred innovations in technology and therapeutics which require an updated, comprehensive reference. This has been our goal for the second edition.

The text has been reorganized to reflect the evolution in the conception of what critical-care nursing is all about. A presentation of conceptual foundations again sets the tone for succeeding chapters and can be found in Part 1. An important addition here is the discussion of ethical and legal issues which have so permeated practice in critical care. The critical-care environment influences all who are there and is described in Part 2. The reader will find a thorough discussion of the instrumentation so necessary in critical care as well as the needs for safety spawned by the technology. Moreover, because it is recognized that the environment itself can be a stressor, a chapter addressing responses to this environment has been added.

Although we still can only see through a glass

darkly, we are beginning to understand the phenomena that are of concern to nursing. No doubt other phenomena will be described as the evolution continues, but those common to critically ill patients are treated in depth in Part 3 of the text.

Various insults to the body cause an individual to require critical-care nursing. These assaults are presented through a systems approach as in the first edition. However, in this edition, Parts 4 through 12 present each system and include anatomy and physiology, data collection, medical and surgical therapeutics, and nursing therapies. This change is made to help the reader locate information needed to understand the assault and the therapy.

Critically ill patients present multisystem, complex problems that require a synthesis of the interrelation of the body's systems and responses to illness or injury. These problems are treated in Part 13 and are intended to provide information required for management of the complex assaults to the body. Finally, because pharmacologic therapy occupies such a prominent place in the offensive against the assaults with which we must deal, an appendix detailing drugs commonly used in treating the critically ill is included for quick reference.

Many have contributed to the development of this volume, and we know that our debt to others can never be repaid. We do, however inadequately, express our gratitude to those who have made the publication of this text possible. Foremost among the number is the American Association of Critical-Care Nurses for support and assistance wherever it was needed. A special word of thanks is given to Ellen French, Director of Communications, for her prompt attention to requests and solution of problems. This book is possible only because the contributors were willing to share their expertise, time, and talent, and we acknowledge their generosity. On occasion, new contributors built upon the works

of others in the previous edition, and these earlier authors are acknowledged as well: Joseph A. Albanese, Jerome B. Bart, Susan B. Biddle, Gail L. Bongiovanni, Debra C. Broadwell, Christopher W. Bryan-Brown, Mortimer J. Buckley, Carolyn B. Chalkley, A. Crane Charters, Ann Daly, Carol J. Dashiff, Cynthia B. Dear, Irving Feller, Gayle Ferguson, Penny J. Ford, Laura McHenry Fray, LaNelle E. Geddes, Vera M. Harmon, Betty Henderson, Billy M. Hightower, Theresa Holland, Claudella Archambeault-Jones, Joanne Lagerson, William C. McGarity, John A. Mantle, Michael J. Moran, Dorothy G. Moses, Scott M. Nadel, Silvio Papapietro, Helen F. Ptak, Charles E. Rackley, Cleo J. Richard, Marilyn M. Ricci, Sharon L. Roberts, William J. Rogers, Richard O. Russell, Jr., Nancy Stewart, Dorothy Voorman, Madeline M. Wake, Mary Webb Waldron, Lin C. Weeks, and Jeanne M. Wilson.

The photographs which grace the end papers were taken at University of Alabama Hospitals by Mr. Jim Willett, and we appreciate both the access to the facility and the talent of Mr. Willett.

The staff in the College Division at McGraw-Hill with whom we worked so closely assisted us in myriad ways. We particularly acknowledge the assistance of Sally Barhydt, Nursing Editor, and James R. Belser, Development Editor. Closer to home, the work would have been much more difficult without the cheery disposition and skillful assistance of June McKaig, Muriel Wright, Gloria Cooper, Sharon Simon, Ann Douglas, Linda J. Miers, Nancy O'Dell, and Shelia Small.

Finally, the editors thank their husbands, Bob, Joe, and David, for encouragement, patience, sometimes sacrifice, always love. Each has made a special contribution to our lives and to this book.

Marguerite Rodgers Kinney
Donna Rogers Packa
Sandra Byars Dunbar

AACN'S
Clinical Reference
for Critical-Care
Nursing

part 1

Conceptual Foundations for Critical-Care Nursing

1

The Practice of Critical-Care Nursing

Marguerite R. Kinney
Sandra B. Dunbar
Donna R. Packa

Introduction

Early observers of our profession viewed nursing as an art. Nightingale referred to nursing as "the finest of the fine arts" while Nutting wrote that nursing was "one of the most difficult of arts." Even today few would argue with the accuracy of these observations. Almost a century later, nursing began to be linked in the literature with science as nursing embraced the goal of developing a scientific base for practice.

Both science and art are difficult terms to define clearly and concisely, art perhaps more so than science. Webster's dictionary[1] requires considerable space to adequately treat the word "art," beginning with "the power of performing certain actions, especially as acquired by experience, study, or observation," and continuing with "a branch of learning." A number of synonyms are offered and have in common the notion of expert performance or execution of what is planned or devised.

The terms "art" and "nursing" go well together. Experience, observation, and study are all needed to provide care to the sick and injured, and a certain power is derived from the service, the power to make a difference in the lives of people who happen to become ill. Nursing and science are beginning to blend more smoothly as theory development and research expand within the profession. Research-based practice has moved from dream to reality, though much remains to be done.

The complexity of nursing is revealed in the American Nurses' Association definition of nursing as "...the diagnosis and treatment of human responses to actual or potential health problems."[2] Because human responses are so varied and relate to individual characteristics of the patient or family, it is clear that the practice of nursing requires depth and breadth in the knowledge base needed for practice. In 1986 a national panel noted that the diversity and complexity of nursing practice in the health care field require nurses who can think critically and creatively and have a sound education for practice.[3] Even in 1897, the noted physician Sir William Osler warned of "a thin veneer of knowledge."[4]

Scope of Critical-Care Nursing Practice

Critical-care nursing may be the most complex of all nursing specialties. The AACN defines critical-care nursing as "that specialty within nursing which deals with human responses to life threatening problems."[5] The scope of critical-care nursing is defined by the dynamic interaction of the critically ill patient, the critical-care nurse, and the critical-care environment (Fig. 1-1). Critical-care nursing is goal-directed and endeavors to ensure effective interaction of these three requisite elements to bring about competent nursing practice and optimal patient outcomes within an environment supportive of both. The framework within which critical-care nursing is practiced is based on a scientific body of knowledge, the application of that knowledge through the nursing process, and multidisciplinary collaboration in the care of the patient.

The Critically Ill Patient

The scope of critical-care nursing recognizes the centrality of the critically ill patient who has life-threatening problems or is at high risk for developing such problems. Because of the illness, the patient requires constant and intensive multidisciplinary assessment and intervention to restore sta-

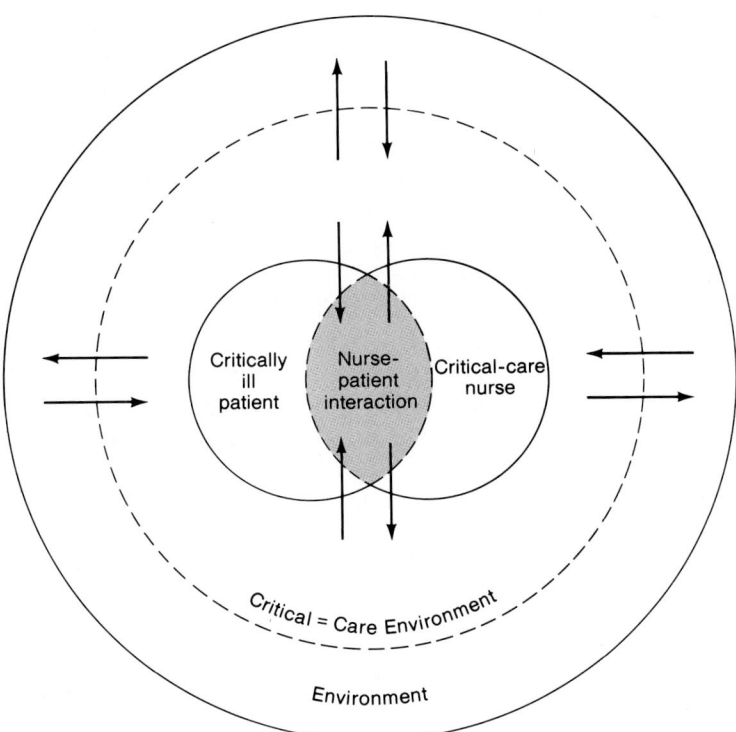

Figure 1-1 The scope of critical-care nursing.

bility, prevent complications, and achieve and maintain optimal responses.

In recognition of critically ill patients' primary need for restoration of physiologic stability, the critical-care nurse coordinates interventions directed at resolving life-threatening problems. Nursing activities also focus on support of the patient's adaptation, restoration of health, and preservation of the patient's rights, including the right to refuse treatment to the extent permitted by law, or to die. Inherent in the patient's response to critical illness is the need to maintain psychological, emotional, and social integrity. The familiarity, comfort, and support provided by social relationships can enhance effective coping. Therefore, the concept of the critically ill patient includes the interaction and influence of the patient's family and/or significant other(s).

The Critical-Care Nurse

The critical-care nurse is a licensed professional who is responsible for ensuring that all critically ill patients receive optimal care. Basic to accomplish-

ment of this goal is individual professional accountability through adherence to standards of nursing care of the critically ill and through a commitment to act in accordance with ethical principles.

Critical-care nursing practice encompasses the diagnosis and treatment of a patient's responses to life-threatening health problems. The critical-care nurse is the one constant in the critical-care environment and is responsible for coordination of the care delivered by various health care providers. With the nursing process as a framework, the critical-care nurse uses independent and collaborative interventions to restore stability, prevent complications, and achieve and maintain optimal patient responses. Independent nursing interventions are those actions which are in the unique realm of nursing and include manipulation of the environment, teaching, counseling, and initiating referrals. Collaborative nursing interventions are actions determined through multidisciplinary collaboration. Underlying the application of these interventions is a holistic approach that expresses human warmth and caring. This art, in conjunction with the science of critical-care nursing, is essential to the interaction between the critical-care nurse and critically ill patient in attaining optimal outcomes.

The critical-care environment is constantly changing. The critical-care nurse must respond effectively to the demands created by this environment for the broad application of knowledge. Essential for maintaining competency in critical-care nursing is a commitment to ongoing education concurrent with an expanding base of experience.

The Critical-Care Environment

The critical-care environment can be viewed from three perspectives. On one level the critical-care environment is defined by those conditions and circumstances surrounding the direct interaction between the critical-care nurse and the critically ill patient. The immediate environment must constantly support this interaction to achieve desired patient outcomes. Adequate resources, in the form of readily available emergency equipment, needed supplies, effective support systems for managing emergent patient situations, and measures for ensuring the patient's safety, are requisites. The framework for nursing practice in this setting is provided by standards for nursing care of the critically ill.

The institution or setting within which critically ill patients receive care represents another element of the critical-care environment. At this level, the critical-care management and administrative structure ensures effective care delivery systems for various populations of critically ill patients through provision of adequate human, material, and financial resources, through required quality systems, and through maintenance of standards of nursing care of the critically ill.

Additional elements contributing to effective care delivery include:

1. Participatory decision making whereby the critical-care nurse provides input into decisions affecting the nurse–patient interaction. The Joint Commission on Accreditation of Hospitals (JCAH) acknowledges the importance of participatory decision making by requiring a multidisciplinary approach with input from both nursing and medicine.[6] The National Commission on Nursing has supported collaboration by proposing that nurse-administrators have authority equal to that of medical leaders within institutions.[7] A consensus conference on critical-care medicine held at the National Institutes of Health in 1983 recommended that "organizational structures should promote and require that nurses and physicians work together as colleagues at all levels—especially the medical director and nursing director."[8] These groups based their recommendations for collaboration on demonstrated positive experiences and common sense.

2. A collaborative practice model that facilitates multidisciplinary problem solving and ethical decision making. An important study published in 1986 by Knaus and colleagues[9] of 5000 patients in 13 tertiary care facilities sought to determine factors which accounted for differences between predicted and actual death rates. Examination of the data revealed that differences could *not* be attributed to the patient's physiologic status, the degree of sophistication of available technology, or to whether or not the facility was a teaching institution. Rather, differences in patient outcome were related to the degree of interaction and communication between nurses and physicians. The researchers concluded that involvement and interaction of critical-care personnel can influence the outcome of critically ill patients. This study offers hard data in support of collaboration between physicians and nurses and should not be ignored.

3. Education of critical-care nurses consistent with standards for critical-care nursing education and practice. The AACN's *Education Standards for Critical-Care Nursing*[10] specifies goals for which to strive in providing high-quality critical-care education. The text includes structure standards, which identify those features which must be in place for a successful educational program or activity to occur as well as process standards, which include all stages of an educational program.

The broadest perspective of the environment encompasses a global view of those factors that have an impact on the provision of care to the critically ill patient. Monitoring of legal, regulatory, social, economic, and political trends is necessary to promote early recognition of the potential implications for critical-care nursing and to provide a basis for a timely response.

Domains of Nursing Practice

Benner[11] describes seven domains of nursing practice. All are present in critical-care nursing, although the priority and scope of the domain may vary depending upon the patient's situation.

The Helping Role

In the *helping role,* nurses provide different kinds of help for patients than is expected from or given by other helping professionals. This helping takes many forms and, in the critical-care environment, is often the establishment of a healing relationship or providing comfort measures and preserving personhood in the face of pain and extreme breakdown.

The Teaching and Coaching Function

In the *teaching and coaching function,* the critical-care nurse focuses on the patient's interpretation of his or her illness and assists in the integration of the implications of illness and recovery into the patient's and family's life-style.

The Diagnostic and Monitoring Function

A crucial domain in critical-care nursing is the *diagnostic and monitoring function.* Competence is required in all of the following aspects of this domain: detection and documentation of significant changes in a patient's condition, anticipating breakdown and deterioration prior to explicit confirmation, anticipating problems, anticipating the patient's care needs, and assessing the patient's potential for wellness and for responding to various treatment strategies.

Managing Rapidly Changing Situations

Nowhere is the need greater for a nurse who can *effectively manage rapidly changing situations* than in critical care. The competencies required in this domain include skilled performance in extreme life-threatening emergencies, rapid matching of demands and resources in emergency situations;

and identifying and managing a patient crisis until physician assistance is available. The very need for these competencies provided the impetus for the development of critical-care units and the need has escalated over time. Evidence abounds that these competencies will be in greater demand than ever in the hospital of tomorrow.

Administering and Monitoring Therapeutic Interventions and Regimens

Increasingly sophisticated technology and therapeutic regimens in critical care have highlighted this domain. Invasive equipment, potent and rapidly acting drugs, electrical and mechanical devices, all have been incorporated into the armamentarium of the critical-care nurse and require considerable skill and expertise.

Monitoring and Ensuring the Quality of Health Care Practices

Accompanying the growth of critical care has been a proliferation of members of the health care team. Professionals from a variety of disciplines and the technicians supporting their practice converge in the critical-care unit to meet the complex needs of patients.

The responsibility for monitoring and ensuring the quality of health care practices falls squarely on the shoulders of the critical-care nurse. As noted in the 1983 Consensus Conference on Critical Care Medicine sponsored by the National Institutes of Health, "nurses are the key element in critical care."[8] The nurse is also the designated professional who coordinates the activity of all other allied health personnel at the bedside.

Organizational and Work-Role Competencies

The final domain described by Benner is *organizational and work-role competencies.* Competencies included in this domain are setting priorities, building and maintaining a therapeutic team, and matching changing patient status with staff resources. The complex needs of the critically ill patient coupled with the need for highly specialized nurses create an unique challenge for managing this domain.

The competencies described are neither comprehensive nor exhaustive but serve to illustrate the complexities inherent in critical-care nursing practice. The demands and challenges *are* great, but the rewards and opportunities are also great. The journey from novice to expert in critical-care nursing is accomplished through commitment to a goal of excellence in *all* domains of practice with excellence as the yardstick by which the process is judged. Fortunately, the journey is never over as the rapidly occurring advances in science and technology and the expanding understanding of nursing as an art create a dynamic, ever-changing profession of critical-care nursing.

References

1. *Webster's Third New International Dictionary.* (1961). Springfield, MA: Merriam.
2. American Nurses Association. (1980). *Nursing: A social policy statement.* Kansas City: Author.
3. Hannah, J. (1986, November 18). Broader education needed to face rapid changes in nursing, study says. *The Birmingham News,* 5D.
4. Osler, W. (1897). *Essay on nurse and patient.* Johns Hopkins Hospital.
5. American Association of Critical-Care Nurses. (1984). *Definition of critical-care nursing.* Newport Beach, CA: Author.
6. Joint Commission on Accreditation of Hospitals. (1984). *Manual for Hospitals.* Chicago: JCAH.
7. National Commission on Nursing. (1983). Summary report and recommendation. Chicago: Author.
8. National Institutes of Health Consensus Conference. (1983). Critical Care Medicine. *Journal of the American Medical Association, 250,* 798–804.
9. Knaus, W, Draper, E, Wagner, D, & Zimmerman, J. (1986). An evaluation of outcome from intensive care in major medical centers. *Annals of Internal Medicine, 104,* 410–418.
10. Alspach, J. G., Bell, J, Canobbio, M. M., Christoph, S. B., Kuhn, R. C., Roberts, W. L., Turzan, L, & Wiencek, C. (Eds.). (1986). *Education standards for critical-care nurses.* St. Louis: Mosby.
11. Benner, P. (1984). *From Novice to Expert: Excellence and Power in Clinical Nursing Practice.* Menlo Park, CA: Addison-Wesley, 45–161.

2

Nursing Process in Critical Care

Donna R. Packa
Marguerite R.
Kinney
Sandra B. Dunbar

Introduction

The evolution of nursing is puncuated by attempts to articulate clearly what nursing is and how it is accomplished. As has often been the case in the helping professions, ideas generated by an early thinker lie dormant until given new life by someone else many years later. Such seems to be the case with the concept of nursing as a process. Though nursing was called a process for the first time in the mid-1950s by Lydia Hall and elaborated by Yura and Walsh in the decade of the seventies, Nightingale wrote in 1859 that nursing required "assessment and intervention according to a plan of care, followed by evaluation."[1]

Nursing as a process has been recognized by professional and legal bodies. In 1973, the American Nurses' Association (ANA) published generic *Standards of Nursing Practice*[2] followed by specialty standards. Each is based on the steps of the nursing process. The AACN's *Standards for Nursing Care of the Critically Ill*[3] also reflects the nursing process. The definition of nursing contained in the ANA's *Nursing: A Social Policy Statement*[4] refers directly to two steps in the nursing process: *diagnosis* and *intervention*. The AACN's definition of critical-care nursing reinforces this emphasis. Legal definitions of nursing in most states include the steps of the nursing process. Further, state boards of nursing require knowledge of the nursing process for licensure to practice as a registered nurse.

In 1986, Zeigler, Vaughan-Wrobel, and Erlen[5] elaborated on previous conceptualizations and described the *nursing process model,* which is based on the following assumptions:

1. The nursing process is the methodology of nursing practice; nursing diagnosis must be used within the nursing process.

2. Nursing includes independent and interdependent functions.
3. The nursing process consists of five steps: assessing, diagnosing, planning, implementing, and evaluating.
4. Each step is a process resulting in a product.
5. The nursing diagnosis is a statement of client response related to an etiology that the nurse can independently diagnose and treat.
6. The steps of the process are interrelated.
7. Knowledge is required to implement the steps of the nursing process.

Components of the Nursing Process

Assessment

As depicted in the nursing process model, *assessment* involves the systematic collection of data which are then organized in some predetermined manner. As proposed by Guzzetta and Kinney,[6] data collection must be consistent with nursing's view of health, guided by a holistic framework that addresses body, mind, and spirit. The product of data collection is the database, which should meet the needs of specific populations of patients who are the recipients of nursing care. In critical care, data arise from many sources, often requiring invasive devices and sophisticated technology. Data are also derived from astute observations by the critical-care nurse. Nightingale noted the significance of observation when she said, "In dwelling upon the vital importance of sound observation, it must not be lost sight of what observation is for. It is not for the sake of piling up miscellaneous information or curious facts, but for the sake of saving life and increasing health and comfort."[1]

A *diagnosis* is a conclusion reached following investigation or analysis of the cause or nature of a condition, situation, or problem.[7] In addition to data collection, Kelly describes the diagnostic process as incorporating data analysis and naming.[8] The diagnostician, Kelly says, must collect, sort, and organize cues in such a way that an accurate diagnosis emerges within the constraints of time. Disciplines differ according to the cues that are deemed important, the terms used to describe the cues, and diagnostic concepts used to organize, clarify, and explain the data.[9] Naming provides for a title or label to be given to the conclusion reached by analyzing the data. Kelly proposes that the nursing diagnosis should reflect a human response to an actual or potential health problem, including response to the internal environment, changes in activities of daily living, and alterations in life-style. The North American Nursing Diagnosis Association (NANDA) continues its efforts to standardize nursing diagnosis labels and develop a taxonomy of nursing diagnoses. Vaughan-Wrobel and Perkins[10] refer to the nursing diagnosis as the pivotal point of the nursing process because a diagnosis is required before care can be planned, implemented, or evaluated.

Planning and Intervention

Once the nursing diagnosis has been formulated, *goal(s)* are developed in direct relationship to the diagnostic statement of the problem, which identifies a positive change in the status of the patient and describes some degree of resolution of the problem. For example, a diagnosis of *alteration in comfort: Pain* may lead to a statement describing the absence of pain as the goal. The measures designed to alleviate the problem are referred to as *nursing interventions*. These interventions are specifically related to the etiological component of the diagnosis with the intention of alleviating the etiology of the problem and resolving the problem described in the diagnosis. In the absence of a diagnosis based on sound data, nursing interventions cannot be designed for problem resolution and become only technical functions based on intuition or policy.

Evaluation

The final phase of the nursing process, *evaluation,* is closely related to the diagnosis in that the degree

of goal attainment (and, therefore, problem resolution) is determined according to predefined criteria. Should the evaluation reveal failure to attain the specified goal, further data collection, as well as review of the diagnosis and goal for adequacy, accuracy, and appropriateness, is instituted. As a result of this analysis, modifications may be made in any aspect of the nursing process.

Conceptual Framework for Practice

An important consideration for the critical-care nurse in employing the nursing process in practice is the conceptual framework from which practice is derived. The purpose of the conceptual framework is to organize, use, and transmit knowledge that explains nursing and its goals.[11] Although a variety of frameworks have been proposed, critical-care nursing practice seems unique in relation to the difficulty experienced in use of these frameworks. Because the frameworks differ in regard to their approaches to humans, the environment, health, and nursing, use of a specific framework in practice creates diagnostic labels that are consistent with the constructs of each framework, but different from those labels generated by use of other frameworks. For example, nursing diagnostic labels generated by the nurse who uses Chrisman and Fowler's Systems-in-Change Model as a framework for practice may well include diagnostic labels consistent with those generated by NANDA. This model was conceived to articulate with the steps in the nursing process. The model is thus easily adapted for use in critical-care units which use the nursing process and diagnostic labels described by NANDA. However, nurses who use Roy's Adaptation Model or Orem's Self-Care Model as a framework for critical-care nursing practice generate nursing diagnoses consistent with the data collection, analysis, and constructs described in each of these models.

It is important for critical-care nurses to consider the framework or mosaic of frameworks from which practice is derived because practice is guided by these frameworks and the provision of holistic care is enhanced. Often the framework for practice exists but not at the conscious level of the nurse. Perhaps valuing of the conceptual framework as a way of developing uniqueness in provision of quality nursing care may encourage critical-care nurses to dissect practice in order to determine which frameworks underlie practice.

Nursing versus Medical Diagnosis

Once the conceptual phase of practice has been considered, other issues regarding use of nursing diagnosis in practice are apparent. One major concern is whether nurses should diagnose at all. Some nurses question whether by diagnosing a patient's responses to actual or potential health problems nursing is treading on medical turf. Gaines and McFarland[12] described the similarity between medical and nursing diagnosis in relation to the processes utilized to derive a diagnostic label. As they emphasize, an auto mechanic uses the same process of data collection and diagnosis of a problem (such as a dead battery) to arrive at an intervention deemed appropriate for resolution of the problem based on the knowledge and experience of the mechanic.

Andrews[13] describes the difference between medical and nursing diagnoses as relating to the nature and purpose of the diagnosis. The medical diagnosis is made to identify a specific pathophysiologic alteration (disease) encountered in a given patient, with the intent of prescribing treatment designed to cure the disease or reduce the somatic experience of the patient in regard to the disease or injury. There are 999 medical diagnoses listed in the *International Classification of Diseases*[14] that are accepted for use by physicians in diagnosing pathophysiologic patient problems.

The nursing diagnosis, on the other hand, may relate to the patient's and family's response to the disease or injury because it describes the effects of a patient's problems on the life-style of the patient and family. The patient who has a medical diagnosis of uncontrolled diabetes mellitus may have several related nursing diagnoses such as ineffective coping patterns related to individual and family denial of the presence of diabetes. In this instance, the medical diagnosis provides vital data for the nurse to assist the patient and family in adjusting to the presence of the disease so that management strategies can be effectively utilized by the patient and family.

The nursing diagnosis is not a restatement of the medical diagnosis because, although nurses in critical-care units may often have sufficient data and knowledge to make a medical diagnosis, the physician rather than the nurse is licensed and capable of treating pathophysiologic alterations in patients. Should the nurse have sufficient data to suggest a medical diagnosis, the data should be referred to the physician for treatment. Similarly, nursing diagnoses suggested by the data should be referred by physicians to nurses for management.

Kieffer[15] suggests that a broader conceptualization of nursing diagnosis compared to medical diagnosis is appropriate. Whereas medical diagnoses relate to pathophysiologic alterations in patients, nursing diagnoses identify alterations in emotional, cognitive, family, social, and cultural responses of patients to pathophysiologic processes described by medical diagnoses. The response of the patient to actual or potential health problems is of concern to the nurse. In addition to the biophysical response, the psychosociocultural response of the patient and family to a disease, illness, or injury is an important focus of nursing and is noted in the nursing diagnosis. The patient who is experiencing excruciating chest pain during an acute myocardial infarction needs nurses who are knowledgeable regarding the pathophysiologic processes involved and the appropriate actions to take in this regard. However, this patient also needs nurses who are knowledgeable regarding appropriate nursing diagnoses and interventions that might be useful in dealing with an alteration in comfort such as pain related to decreased myocardial tissue perfusion; anxiety related to an unfamiliar environment, equipment, procedures, and people; or perhaps fear of dying related to perceptions of the likelihood of death after a myocardial infarction. Having gathered the necessary data to support any or all of these diagnoses, the nurse can plan care for the patient in an organized, systematic fashion. This approach will provide continuity in managing the patient's problems, instead of isolated actions (such as administering morphine sulfate for pain without regard to the totality of the patient's problems and without collecting further data, which may indicate extension of the infarction).

As nurses in intensive care units, we have the responsibility for collecting data from patients and families who may be in crisis, and these data are imperative to plan care for the patient during the crisis and afterward. Often families are more verbal during a crisis situation and welcome an opportunity to talk to someone about their loved one. Gathering information regarding the patient can provide data that are useful in helping the critically ill patient come to grips with events and in decreasing the stressfulness of experiences. For patients who survive the initial crisis, data gathered in the critical-care environment are useful to nurses in the progressive unit, who can then provide continuity of care begun in the intensive care unit.

Use of Nursing Diagnosis

Classification

Although nursing diagnoses may be stated in a variety of ways, consistent use of terms by practitioners has been advocated by Andrews,[13] Kieffer,[15] Gebbie and Lavin,[16] Gordon,[17] Guzzetta,[18] and others. One concern cited by many nurses is that consistency is lost by use of a variety of terms to connote a patient's responses and communication of problems and intervention is hampered, which negates the value of nursing diagnosis altogether. It was from this perspective that Gebbie and Lavin called for the First National Conference on Nursing Diagnoses held in 1972. This conference and the ones that followed have provided an opportunity for sharing among nurses regarding use of diagnostic labels. Labels have been identified in each of the conferences and some have been accepted by the groups for testing. Unfortunately, there is a paucity of research support for all the diagnostic labels currently accepted for use. Research is sorely needed to determine the appropriateness of the labels and defining characteristics. However, some research regarding the diagnostic labels and defining characteristics is under way.

Some nurses fear that development and use of an accepted taxonomy of nursing diagnoses will cause rigidity in regard to use of accepted labels and in the practice of nursing. Use of a consistent vocabulary will allow accurate communication to occur among nurses in regard to patient problems. Some nurses find diagnostic labels awkward to use

but, like many other nursing activities, opportunities for practical use of the labels increases the comfort of nurses in accurately diagnosing patient responses. Once convinced of the utility of the labels, nurses often express wonder that they had refused previously to use the labels. Gebbie and Lavin[16] state that nurses cannot achieve a high level of professional effectiveness without a common vocabulary with which to communicate regarding patient problems.

The utility of a common vocabulary derived from a conceptual base for nursing practice in providing direction for nursing research, education, and management is evident. The medical diagnosis of a dissecting aortic aneurysm is understood by all those who interact to assist the patient in regard to this problem. How useful it would be to the profession of nursing if a nursing diagnostic label could relate information as clearly to nurses as does a medical diagnosis.

Usefulness of Nursing Diagnosis

Additional reasons for using nursing diagnoses were stated by Baer[19] when she said that diagnosis is advocated because it:

1. Assists in organizing, defining, and developing nursing knowledge
2. Aids in identifying and describing the domain and scope of nursing practice
3. Focuses nursing care on the patients' responses to problems
4. Prescribes diagnosis-specific nursing interventions that should increase the effectiveness of nursing care
5. Facilitates the evaluation of nursing practice
6. Provides a framework for testing the validity of nursing interventions
7. Provides a standardized vocabulary to enhance intra- and interprofessional communication
8. Prescribes the content of nursing curricula
9. Provides a framework for developing a system to direct third-party reimbursement for nursing services
10. Indicates a specific rationale for patient care based on nursing assessment
11. Leads to more comprehensive and individualized patient care.

Bruce sums up the vital nature of nursing diagnosis for the future of nursing practice when she says that it "may be the unifying link that will help nurses maintain their unique nursing identities and perspectives while they continue to alter roles and functions in response to the changing health care needs of society."[20]

Collaborative Problems

We in critical-care nursing, however, have a problem in the use of nursing diagnosis that is unique in nursing, in that much of the care provided to patients involves implementation of physician prescriptions related to altering pathophysiologic problems. None will argue the need for monitoring vital signs or titrating drug dosage rates for infusions in a patient with a medical diagnosis of hypertensive crisis. Yet, how can the nurse plan care for this patient when many of the nurse's functions are monitoring and surveillance and completing other actions prescribed by physicians? In response to this issue some have suggested that in critical situations as described above, the nurse should use the medical diagnosis to guide nursing care planning during the critical phase, and use nursing diagnosis at a later time. This approach negates the valuable input of nursing in the overall recovery of the patient.

An alternative for planning nursing care in the critical phase of the patient's illness is to develop what Carpenito[21] and Kim[22] call *collaborative problems*. These diagnoses require interventions from health professionals in addition to nursing for problem resolution. For patients who are critically ill, it is unlikely that either physicians or nurses alone can satisfactorily resolve the patient's problems, but by working together via medical and nursing interventions, problem resolution is expedited.

Carpenito[21] has pictorially described the interaction of medicine and nursing in relation to problem resolution. As noted in Fig. 2-1, there is an overlap of medical and nursing management of patient care problems which represents the area in which collaborative problems exist. Because of the nature of critical illness or injury, the overlap of medicine and nursing is likely to be substantially larger so that an increase in the number of collab-

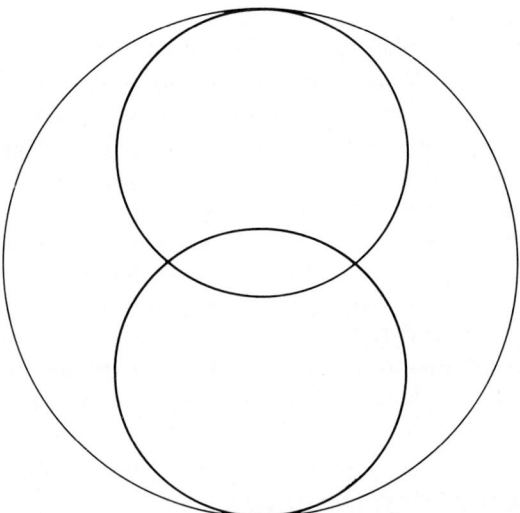

Figure 2-1 A model of interlocking circles which indicates in the common area those activities on which professionals collaborate. The remainder of the area indicates independent dimensions for which each professional is responsible. *(Used with permission of L. Carpenito, Nursing Diagnosis. Application to Clinical Practice, Lippincott, Philadelphia, 1983.)*

orative problems which require complex coordination of the two groups of health providers is expected. This overlap in medicine and nursing in the critical-care setting in diagrammed in Fig. 2-2.

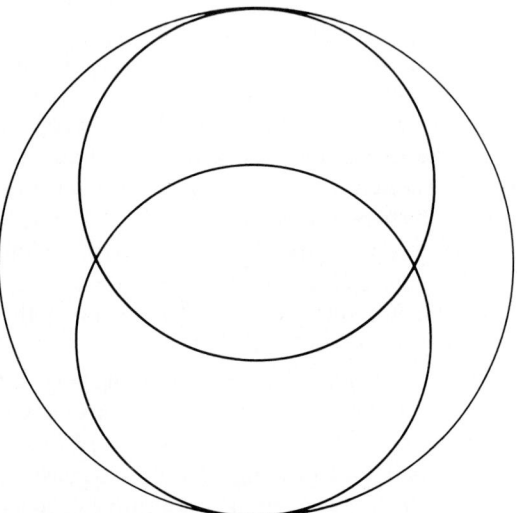

Figure 2-2 Adaptation of Fig. 2-1 which indicates the larger area of professional collaboration in critical care.

Summary

At this point in the development, utilization, and testing of nursing diagnoses it is reasonable to expect that differences in approaches to use of the labels and the process will exist among practitioners. Indeed, the reader of this text will find a variety of methods of stating nursing diagnoses and using the diagnostic label to plan nursing care. Because practitioners view the process differently, this variety is encouraged as development and testing of the labels continue. An attempt has been made, however, to use in the text whenever possible the diagnostic labels generated by the North American Nursing Diagnosis Association. Use of these labels brings at least some degree of structure to this component of practice about which so many differing views are held.

In critical-care nursing it is imperative that the critical problems of the patient be adequately managed because the patient can only respond to the threat to his or her very being in that crisis situation. Accuracy of nursing diagnoses is the key to provision of efficient, expert nursing care to the critically ill patient and family.

References

1. Nightingale, F. (1959). *Notes on nursing.* London: Harrison & Sons.
2. American Nurses' Association. (1973). *Standards of nursing practice.* Kansas City: The Association.
3. Thierer, J, Perhus, S, McCracken, M. L., Reynolds, M. A., Holmes, A. M., Turton, B., Berkowitz, D. S., & Disch, J. M. (Eds.). (1981). *Standards for nursing care of the critically ill.* Reston, VA: Reston.
4. American Nurses' Association. (1980). *Nursing: A social policy statement.* Kansas City: The Association.
5. Zeigler, S. M., Vaughan-Wrobel, B. C., & Erlen, J. A. (1986). *Nursing process, nursing diagnosis, nursing knowledge: Avenues to autonomy.* Norwalk, CT: Appleton-Century-Crofts.
6. Guzzetta, C. E., & Kinney, M. R. (1986). Mastering the transition from medical to nursing diagnosis. *Progress in Cardiovascular Nursing, 1*(1), 48–44.
7. *Webster's third new international dictionary.* (1986). Springfield, MA: Merriam.
8. Kelly, M. A. (1985). *Nursing diagnosis source book: Guidelines for clinical application.* Norwalk, CT: Appleton-Century Crofts.
9. Carnevali, D. L., Mitchell, P. H., Woods, N. F., & Tanner, C. A. (1984). *Diagnostic reasoning in nursing.* Philadelphia: Lippincott.
10. Vaughan-Wrobel, B. C., & Perkins, S. B. (1986). Nursing diagnosis: The pivotal point of the nursing process in cardiovascular nursing. *Cardiovascular Nursing, 22*(5), 25–29.
11. Ellis, R. (1986). Characteristics of significant theories. In L. Nichol (Ed.), *Perspectives on nursing theory.* Boston: Little, Brown.
12. Gaines, B., & McFarland, M. (1984). Nursing diagnosis: Its relationship to and use in nursing education. *Topics in Clinical Nursing, 5*(4), 39–49.
13. Andrews, P. (1982). Nursing diagnosis. In J. Griffith & P. Christensen (Eds.), *Nursing process: Application of theories, frameworks, and models.* St. Louis: Mosby.
14. Department of Health, Education, and Welfare. (1979). *International Classification of Diseases.* Washington, DC: National Center for Health Statistics.
15. Kieffer, J. (1984). Nursing diagnosis can make a critical difference. *Nursing Life, 4*(3), 18–21.
16. Gebbie, K., & Lavin, M. (1974). Classifying nursing diagnosis. *American Journal of Nursing, 74*(2), 250–253.
17. Gordon, M. (1983). Conceptual issues in nursing diagnosis. In N. Chaska (Ed.), *The nursing profession: A time to speak.* New York: McGraw-Hill.
18. Guzzetta, C. (1981). Nursing diagnosis. In *Proceedings of Eighth Annual National Teaching Institute of the American Association of Critical Care Nurses.* Irvine, CA: AACN.
19. Baer, C. (1984). Nursing diagnosis: A futuristic process for nursing process. *Topics in Clinical Nursing, 5*(4), 89–97.
20. Bruce, J. (1979). Implementation of nursing diagnosis. *14*(3), 509–515.
21. Carpenito, L. (1983). *Nursing diagnosis application to clinical practice.* Philadelphia: Lippincott.
22. Kim, M. (1983). Nursing diagnosis in critical care. *Dimensions of Critical Care Nursing, 2*(1), 5–6.

3

Ethics, Law, and Critical-Care Nursing

Marsha D. M.
Fowler
Elizabeth A.
Chaney
Anne J. Davis

Introduction

This chapter will examine selected ethical and legal duties of the critical-care nurse, using the *Code for Nurses*[1] as a framework for discussion. One could hardly find a more appropriate place to anchor a discussion than in the American Nurses' Association's (ANA's) *Code,* the official code of ethics of the profession. The moral tradition of nursing is long, distinguished, honorable, and truly worthy of pride of profession: That tradition finds its most public expression in "the *Code.*"

The *Code* is not a single document, chiseled in stone, for all eternity. It is a work, wrought with great care, which is neither static nor simple. It is not a "cookbook" set of prescribed rules. It is a dynamic and complex statement of the primary values and obligations of the profession, set within a social context which influences both its development and content.

The first code, *A Suggested Code* (1926), was never officially adopted. It was written in the genteel, flowery narrative style of the late 1800s and early 1900s. It did not, however, specify specific principles of ethics that many had sought. In 1940, *A Tentative Code* was proposed. It imported verbatim some of the content of the 1926 *Code,* and expanded it. The 1940 *Code* was never adopted. Instead, an entirely new code, in enumerated form, was prepared and officially adopted by the American Nurses' Association in 1950. In 1957, a single provision, on advertising, was revised. In 1960 and 1968, this code underwent more substantive revisions. The provisions of what is our current code were officially adopted in 1976. In 1985, though the provisions were left unchanged, the interpretive statements of the 1976 *Code* were revised.

In every revision, the *Code of Ethics* has become more specific to the particular social context of nursing, reflecting the dynamic nature of both society and nursing. Likewise, the law, though enduring, is not immutable.

From its inception in this country, nursing has been concerned with both ethics and law as they relate to practice and education. Nursing leaders clearly perceived the need to change the law and the necessity for nursing involvement in reshaping the laws affecting the profession. The adoption and implementation of a code of ethics for nursing was the first concern of nursing's foremothers, but they also recognized early on that a code could not be enacted until the laws regulating nursing practice were reformed.[2] Thus, work on the *Code* was set aside in favor of work on the law, specifically, laws concerning registration.

As the legal regulation of nursing practice and education and such issues as the grading of schools of nursing began to conform to nursing expectations (a process still going on), nursing attention turned toward the adoption of a code (1950) and toward an increasing concern for the law as it affects the practice of the individual nurse. A concern for both the ethical and legal obligations of the nurse is expressed in the present *Code.*

The *Code* forms something of a contract, even a covenant, which nursing makes with society; it is a unilateral, general pledge that the profession makes with regard to its duties and obligations in the exercise of its knowledge. As an expression, implicit or explicit, of the goals and values of the profession, it may also be used to define standards of legally competent nursing practice.

In light of this, a person considering a career in nursing would do well to examine the *Code* and to evaluate it for congruence with his or her personal goals. Those who feel that they cannot support the goals and values or live by the obligations and duties set forth in the *Code* should reconsider the personal cost of entering the profession.

The current *Code* is divided into 11 provisions, each of which addresses a distinctive concern of the profession. Collectively, the provisions deal with issues ranging from the treatment of individual patients, to social access to health care, to the advance of the knowledge and practice of the profession. Each provision is amplified by an "interpretive statement" which itself sets forth additional values and obligations related to the provision. The following sections will serve as a very brief introduction to *selected* ethical and legal concerns which fall within the scope of the individual provisions.

The Provisions

1. The nurse provides services with respect for human dignity and the uniqueness of the client, unrestricted by considerations of social or economic status, personal attributes, or the nature of the health problems.

Respect for human dignity is the overwhelming concern of the first provision. Respect for human dignity, i.e., respect for persons, is seen as the grounding for all other ethical principles and rules, including those of patients' rights to self-determination (autonomy), the nonprejudicial treatment of patients (justice as fairness), and the refusal to push intervention to excess, to the point of harm (nonmaleficence and beneficence). The primacy accorded human dignity in the *Code* reflects fundamental values set forth in the federal constitution and thus finds strong support in legislative, regulatory, and decisional law.

Respect for persons is often interpreted as respect for *autonomy,* sometimes called *self-determination.* A patient's autonomy can be difficult to ensure in the critical-care setting because autonomy is operationalized through the doctrine of informed consent.

In settings such as critical-care units, where patients are not always able to personally exercise their right to self-determination through the process of informed consent, ethics and the law recognize the use of surrogates such as designated persons acting under durable powers of attorney for health care, court-appointed conservators, or family members. A surrogate consents or refuses to consent by "standing in the shoes" of the patient and thereupon deciding as the surrogate believes the patient would decide if the patient were able to do so. The process of deciding is often referred to as the exercise of *substituted judgment.* Consistent with the notion of autonomy, the agent selected by the patient ordinarily supersedes even the family or a court-appointed conservator. A court-appointed conservator with authority to make medical decisions may supersede an agent and does supersede the family. To be legally and ethically valid, consent by even patients or surrogates must possess the qualities described in the following paragraphs.

Informed consent has two major components, capsulized as "full informedness" and "free consent." That is, the patient has sufficient and accurate information to make an informed choice, and is free of undue influence (internal or external) in making or acting upon that choice. The law adds a third element of *legal capacity.* To have legal capacity, the patient or surrogate must be of an age legally authorized to give consent *and* must have not been determined by a court to lack mental capacity for making decisions about medical care.

While no one can guarantee that a patient truly *understands* (intellectually or emotionally) information that is given, or even that the health professional truly *knows,* both ethics and law agree that it is more probable that patients will be "fully informed" when they receive information which is accurate, sufficient, and comprehensible.

"Accuracy" is interpreted to mean *complete,* without deception, and within the limits of what is currently known or believed to be true. The "gray areas" of scientific knowledge should be labeled as such and "opinion," even informed opinion, should be openly acknowledged. Accuracy encompasses a complete range of treatment options, including no treatment, and disclosure of the risks and benefits of each option.

There are two standards by which one can measure the sufficiency of information. The first is a professional-oriented position, which defines sufficiency in terms of what the *professional* feels the patient should know. As a patient-oriented profession, however, nursing would reject this position in favor of one which defines sufficiency from the patient's point of view.[3] The law also requires a patient-oriented measure of sufficiency.

For information to be sufficient, the patient or surrogate must be given all the material information a "reasonable person" would need to know in order to make a decision under similar circumstances.[4] The materiality standard is viewed, at law, as an objective test which is evaluated after the fact by a judge or jury. To meet the materiality standard, the professional must consider what a reasonable person with the characteristics of this particular patient would want and need to know in order to choose among the available treatment options. Thus, the patient or surrogate must be given all the material information made necessary by the patient's life situation or personal attributes (e.g., gender, age, or occupationally related data).

When professionals must consider the informational needs of persons who may seem less advantaged, as in the case of poor, elderly, or retarded persons, it is common to conclude that less information is desired or needed. Both ethics and law would caution against such a conclusion. The more invasive or risky the procedure, or the more affecting the consequences, the more important it can be ethically and legally to consult with others who can advise the professional of factors which may be material to decisions made by a patient possessing certain characteristics.

For a patient to be informed, he or she must comprehend the information. Information is comprehensible when it is conveyed in the language of the patient. The language of the patient may be aural or visual, English or foreign, well-educated or colloquial, medically technical or simple, or any combination of these. The vehicle used (e.g., one-to-one discussion, film, booklet, or group education) should be one customarily employed by the patient when seeking counsel or advice.[5]

When the patient is fully informed, but the pressure of the situation (whether personal or professional pressure) weighs heavily upon decision making, consent may not be considered to be "free," though in some instances it may be regarded as "implied." *Free consent* is consent which is not swayed by habit, impulse, irrationality, coercion, duress, fraud, deceit, or undue influence. It is not uncommon that the very mission of the critical-care unit leads patients and professionals alike toward preordained decisions, making consent a foregone conclusion. Thus, the critical-care unit may itself be a strong influence upon free consent.

There are two approaches to consent in critical care which merit attention here. Under the first, consent to all ordinary care within the unit is implied by the patient's presence. That is, a reasonable person is admitted to a critical-care unit to receive all the benefits the unit can offer, and there is no need to obtain a consent for procedures performed within the unit, unless the procedure is experimental or otherwise out of the ordinary. If consideration is given to withholding all or most medical treatment or to writing a "do not resuscitate" decision, then the patient should also be considered for transfer from the unit.

Under the second approach, the patient's presence in the critical-care unit is determined more by technology or convenience, and the patient's consent must be constantly reevaluated, with the help of surrogate decision makers if necessary. In this approach, decisions to withhold treatment, especially selected treatments, may or may not be accompanied by decisions to transfer the patient out of the unit. Transfer decisions may be made on the basis of factors such as cost reimbursement, physician preference, or bed space in the general duty area.

With increased concern for costly, nonconsensual treatment which is disproportionate in benefit to the patient, it is possible that, legally, consent in critical care will move toward a combination of the two approaches. That is, consent will be implied only in the standard imminent-threat-to-life emergency, where frequent consultation with surrogates will be required. Decisions to withhold all treatment or resuscitation will result in transfers to stepdown or general-care units. While such a move will make day-to-day decisions more complex, it may also contribute to improved morale among nurses who are discouraged by the loss of a patient's autonomy in critical-care units.

The issue of coercion, while important, is less a concern in critical care than is the patient's ability to make a rational choice when burdened by biological disequilibrium. Can the patient whose electrolytes are askew, whose body is wracked with pain, whose mentation is clouded by drugs truly give free consent? Our inclination is to say "no." "Maybe" is the better answer. However, pain, drugs, or physiological imbalance *do not automatically* preclude a patient from making a free decision. Knowledge of the patient and a thorough nursing assessment are keys to evaluating this. Thus, informed consent moves full circle. The professional must know the patient to know what information must be conveyed. The professional must know the patient in order to know if consent is free.

No discussion of informed consent is ever complete without discussion of who is legally accountable for informing the patient or surrogate about proposed medical or nursing interventions. The general rule at law is that the professional selecting the treatment option or intervention is the one who supplies the information and is accountable for accuracy, sufficiency, and comprehensibility of the information. If a physician attempts to inform a patient about nursing intervention options, the physician is accountable for knowing the current standards of nursing practice, the research findings, and the risks and benefits of each option. Similarly, nurses are held accountable for information possessed by the treating physician if the nurse takes on the duty of informing the patient about medical treatment options. It is consistent with respect for human dignity for nurses to insist upon the patient's right to receive information from the person who has control over the treatment option and access to the most complete information about that option.

This provision of the *Code* also focuses on the delivery of care with respect for human dignity, which is not to be defined in terms of personal attributes, socioeconomic status, or the nature of the illness. The implications of this position for critical-care nursing are profound. This provision would require that a criterion such as age, gender, wealth, religious beliefs, or the social unacceptability of a disease not become the determining factor in deciding between or among individuals vying for the same treatment. What this provision strives for is a genuine impartiality, equal respect for all persons, and a refusal to create a hierarchy of the worth of individuals.

Prejudicial treatment of persons on the basis of personal or other attributes constitutes a violation of another moral norm and ideal, precious to the profession for generations. Nursing places great, almost overriding, value upon affirming the worth of the patient, even when the patient becomes "unsalvageable."

But affirming worth does not mean that it is acceptable to treat a patient beyond the limits of his or her wishes, or beyond the point of benefit; that is a violation of a traditional moral norm of nursing. Ethically, to go beyond these limits constitutes *vitalism,*—the preservation of human biological life at any cost simply because it is human biological life. Vitalism is morally unacceptable in nursing as it is perceived as a violation of the dignity of the individual or, more succinctly, as harm.[6] In settings where an all-out effort is made to sustain life, professionals must not be swept along by their own capabilities into vitalism.

Recent court decisions have affirmed that the paramount value is to be placed on the patient's expressed desire regarding life-sustaining treatment[7] and that it is of great importance to provide comfort measures where all medical intervention is discontinued.[8] The *Code* underscores this point in its statement that:

> The measures nurses take to care for the dying client and the client's family emphasize human contact . . . they enable the client to live with as much physical, emotional, and spiritual comfort as possible, and they maximize the values the client has treasured in life.[4]

The values a patient has affirmed in life may include such values as what has been called "dying with dignity" (i.e., deciding to forgo life-sustaining treatment).

Failure to respect the patient's desire to have life-sustaining treatment withheld or withdrawn may result in liability for unconsented touching of the patient (battery), invasion of privacy, and/or failure to meet the standard of reasonably prudent, competent nursing practice (negligence). State statutes and regulations should also be consulted to determine whether the legislature or licensing agency has client advocacy as a criterion for competent nursing practice.

It is important, particularly for critical-care nurses, to note that there is no moral or legal distinction between the decision to forgo (withhold) life-sustaining treatment and the decision to withdraw from life-sustaining treatment; the difference between withholding and withdrawing such treatment is principally an emotional and psychological distinction. Justification which is adequate for withholding the initiation of life-sustaining treatment is also sufficient for withdrawing it.

The President's Commission on Bioethics has made it clear that, in its estimation, patients have a moral and a legal right to refuse either the initiation or continuation of life-sustaining treatment. The Commission writes:

> Neither criminal nor civil law—if properly interpreted and applied . . . forces patients to undergo procedures that will increase their suffering when they wish to avoid this by foregoing life-sustaining treatment.[4]

It further makes the following recommendations:

1. Provide respectful, responsive, supportive care when no further medical care is available or chosen.
2. Encourage institutions to establish procedures for decisionmaking, available to all patients.
3. Respect patient choices, even to forego life-sustaining treatment.
4. Provide mechanisms and guidelines for decisionmaking for patients who cannot decide for themselves.
5. When there is a question regarding what the patient would wish, presume in favor of life.[4]

There is a wealth of assistance to be found in the document which presents these guidelines; critical-care units should be encouraged to make a copy available as a reference for its professional personnel.

2. The nurse safeguards the client's right to privacy by judiciously protecting information of a confidential nature.

This provision goes directly to the heart of the nurse-patient relationship—trust—a moral trust which exceeds the lesser demands of the law. In the first provision, the patient must trust that the nurse will respect his or her right to participate in decision making with regard to health or illness care, even when that patient is unaware that such a right exists.

In this provision, the patient must be able to trust that both rules of confidentiality and privacy will be upheld. "Confidentiality" refers to the nondisclosure of information received from a patient. "Privacy" refers to a right to be left alone, a right, in a sense, to have secrets.[9] In health care, privacy incorporates the right to control who can invade one's body and to expose oneself to even medically prescribed display. The right to privacy includes the right to decide to withhold or discontinue life-sustaining measures in the presence of irreversibly fatal illness.

In the modern hospital, confidentiality often seems something of a technical fiction. If the patient is in a teaching hospital, in particular, or in a critical-care unit, especially, literally dozens of persons have legally accepted access to the patient's chart. First, a bevy of primary-care nurses and physicians scribble in the chart. Then comes a cloud of consultants, a clutch of medical and nursing students, a brace of initialed therapists, a gaggle of administrators and third-party insurers, a family of regulatory agencies, and a horde of clinical researchers. Confidentiality seems a myth, yet it remains an ideal which should be preserved as it serves to protect the patient.

In critical-care settings, confidentiality of medical information is commonly controlled by state statutes and administrative agency regulations. Typically, access to medical information is restricted to the patient and to categories of service providers who have a need for information in order to provide service or care to the patient. Disclosure in violation of a statute or regulation results in monetary fine, a charge of criminal misdemeanor, and/or civil liability for harm resulting from improper disclosure.

Neither marital, family, nor significant other relationships alone overcome the confidential nature of medical information. Thus, nurses are legally constrained in their communication with obviously intimate family or friends of the patient. During a period of patient vulnerability, the guarded nature of such communication often creates untrusting, adversarial relationships between the nurses and the patient's support system.

To avoid unnecessary tension and to promote effective relationships between nurses and the patient's support system, it is recommended that written consent to release information concerning medical and nursing care to specified family members and/or friends be obtained from the patient at the time of admission to the hospital or critical-care unit, or as soon thereafter as the patient can give consent.

Privacy, too, seems something of a fiction. In our contemporary health care system, it is cheaper to run a computerized panel of blood tests on a single specimen than it is to obtain by hand the single blood value needed. Collecting unnecessary data on a patient, whether by laboratory tests or by nursing assessment questions, ethically constitutes an invasion of privacy. In all instances, it is ethically desirable to keep data collection to the minimum necessary to deliver care that is both safe and effective.

At law, invasion of privacy requires crossing the threshold beyond which a reasonable person would find the invasion outrageously offensive, so as to be humiliating, degrading, or similarly injurious. Thus, requiring a patient to remain on a ventilator, in the face of irreversible and fatal illness, overriding his or her own written or verbal consent (or surrogate request) to have the ventilator withdrawn, would be viewed by many courts as an outrageously offensive act constituting an invasion of privacy. Overboard history taking or testing would be less likely to meet the legal test for privacy invasion, unless the plaintiff could make a showing of malicious intent to humiliate or embarrass.

In general, it is customary to find that law and ethics are mutually supportive.[10] There are some uncommon instances, however, when the demands of ethics exceed and conflict with the demands of the law. In such cases, the nurse must choose whether to violate legal or ethical precepts. Such decisions are not easily made. When one chooses in favor of ethical obligation over the obligation of the law, it should be done from an informed position. That is, the consequences of such an action should be known before the decision is made.

The notion of "privilege" (or privileged communication) presents precisely such a dilemma. Privilege is a corollary rule of confidentiality and serves to exempt certain categories of relationships from disclosure, even in a court of law. Privilege is not absolute; it can be overcome, as in situations involving child abuse, violent assault on adults, or serious threat of harm to another.

In the course of the discharge of their duties, priest—confessor, attorney–client, and physician–patient relationships are protected under the rule of privilege. There is evidence that early American nursing may have regarded nursing communication as existing under both a notion of confidentiality and privilege, particularly as nurses generally practiced their art in the home.[11]

Under the law, nurse–patient relationships are *not* considered privileged, even though the very nature of the nurse–patient relationship is such that nurses are privy to the most intimate, personal, and revealing information a patient could disclose. This is particularly the case in critical care where the nurse is present at the immediate bedside virtually 24 h a day.

It is possible that, in the course of care, the patient might reveal information of a sensitive nature which the law may subsequently demand that the nurse disclose. It is incumbent upon the nurse to make an ethical determination whether revealing that information would be injurious to the patient's best interests. That is, disclosure, even under court order, should not be automatic. The refusal to disclose could place the nurse in contempt of court and result in a jail sentence for so long as the nurse refused to comply with the court order.

3. The nurse acts to safeguard the client and the public when health care and safety are affected by incompetent, unethical, or illegal practice by any person.

To carry out this provision, the nurse must be able to make autonomous judgments about what is in the patient's best interests, based upon what he or she knows of the patient's interests and wishes, etc., and must take appropriate action upon these judgments. But, nursing autonomy is not sufficient. The nursing environment must be such that it supports the nurse who responds to this ethical duty, and there must be institutional mechanisms or processes for handling ethical and legal concerns.

For any setting, that would mean that there is a means of reporting which is both safe (from reprisal) and effective. For a critical-care unit in particular, that process must be expeditious. It is demoralizing to attempt to right a grievous or persistent wrong to a patient, only to face a cumbersome or obstructive process which impedes moral action.

Currently, an intrainstitutional ethics committee (IEC) is one of the most effective and potentially one of the most responsive vehicles for dealing with apparent moral violations, including morally wrong actions on the part of another. Unfortunately, hospitals have been slow to create and implement IECs, and they remain in something of a clinical trial stage.

Nursing has, however, been quick to see the advantages of the IEC in assuring reasoned and rapid means of dealing with ethical questions. Recently, the ANA Committee on Ethics prepared and published *Guidelines for Nurses' Participation and Leadership in Institutional Ethical Review Processes.*[12] These guidelines call for nurses to take a leadership role in participating in the development, implementation, and evaluation of formal mechanisms for multidisciplinary institutional ethical review such as institutional ethics committees. The IEC is a mechanism which will enable the critical-care nurse to forge ahead with all deliberate speed when an ethical wrong has been perpetrated, or when such behavior threatens a patient's well-being.

Two other points must be made here. First, the nurse must *act* upon his or her moral intuitions. Second, there will be times when the nurse will act on behalf of the patient, but to no avail. In instances where attempts to advocate for the patient have failed or have been obstructed, and all reasonable options have been tried, the nurse must not hold him or herself morally blameworthy. Ethics, though it aims toward the ideal, does not demand the impossible. In ethics, as in critical care, tragic failures are sometimes inescapable.

While institutional ethics committees address dilemmas and conflicts associated with treatment decisions, they are not an appropriate vehicle for taking action against all illegal, unethical, or incompetent practices by nurses or other members of the health team. Where patient safety is jeopardized by such conduct, the nurse is legally accountable for pursuing a remedy through the organizational hierarchy and, if there is no satisfactory resolution there, for going to outside agencies.

Many hospitals have implemented an internal "memorandum of concern" or incident report to encourage communication of specific problems with unsafe practice by physicians or others outside nursing administration's sphere of control. The internal memo of concern is forwarded to quality assurance, risk management, or medical practice committees as determined by hospital policy. Nurses may also initiate such memos by filing incident reports when telephone calls to a physician are not answered, are met with abusive language, or with other clinically hazardous behavior. It is important to keep copies of all incident reports and memoranda of concern in case the nurse needs to substantiate previous efforts to obtain a remedy within the organization.

An incident report or memorandum of concern can be viewed as a mechanism for alerting management to situations which are hazardous to patients' safety and therefore pose undue risks of lawsuit involving the hospital. Enlightened self-interest alone may motivate some managers to take action.

What if the threatened harm would be imminent and irreversible if no action were taken to stop the unsafe practice? The general rule is that one always gives the supervisor an opportunity to take appropriate action by letting the supervisor know immediately of the problem. If the supervisor will not or cannot act, then the nurse is justified in going beyond the supervisor to seek assistance. At this point, knowledge of the structure, function, and politics of the organization is critical as the nurse must then choose the person of power who is most likely to make an effective response, whether this is the chief of critical-care medicine, the chief of the medical staff, the nursing director, the hospital administrator, or another. The better-organized critical-care unit will anticipatorily address the issue of reporting and action by setting forth emergency procedures to follow when the nurse believes the patient has been placed in a position of imminent harm from unsafe practice.

Unsafe practice by nurse colleagues also requires attention. Suspected chemical abuse and inadequate knowledge or skill seem to be the more common problems and create more reporting difficulties than suspected patient abuse, hastening the death of a patient, or falsification of information about patient care. Perhaps the latter problems are so clearly criminal and so abhorrent to the values of nurses that appropriate action is more clear-cut to all involved. Again, the better-managed organization establishes clear lines for communicating concerns about nursing practice and obtaining feedback as to action taken.

In the absence of such operational policies, the process begins with reporting the observations to the immediate supervisor, requesting investigation of the problem. It is wise to work out a plan for safeguarding patients while the concerns are investigated. A time line should also be negotiated so that the nurse who reports the problem has some idea of when to expect feedback from the supervisor.

Depending on the track record nursing management has established for responding to nursing practice problems, the nurse may want to take the matter up the organizational ladder or go directly to an outside agency if the supervisor does not respond effectively.

Incident reports and memoranda of concern directed to the nursing supervisor, and successively responsible members of the nursing management team, are valuable methods of objectively setting forth the observable conduct which causes a nurse to be concerned about unsafe practice of a colleague. It is neither necessary nor desirable to label the conduct as "incompetent," "unethical," or "illegal." Describing the conduct is always preferable to any judgmental statements about "drug abuse," "negligence," or other similar opinions.

Where does the nurse take the problem of unsafe, incompetent, or illegal practice if there is no solution within the organization?

If the problem involves nurses, the outside agency is the state licensing board for nurses; if physicians, the state licensing board of medicine. If the problem is with overall management of the organization (e.g., unsafe staffing patterns, improper delegation of responsibilities to unlicensed personnel), the better resource is the state licensing agency which conducts periodic inspections.

It should be noted that there are some instances in which a particular action is *not legally actionable,* but *is morally actionable.* In these cases the nurse is enjoined in the *Code* to take action, though precisely what sort of action is not clearly specified. Further guidance for action on alleged

moral violations within the profession, particularly when a patient is involved, may be found in the American Nurses' Association publication, *Guidelines for Implementing the Code for Nurses.*[13] Though these *Guidelines* are rather problematic in their approach, they are a good starting point.

There is one caveat: The responsibility to assure patient safety does not make reporting a colleague any easier. Nearly all who seek to carry out that duty meet with varying degrees of criticism and discouragement. It is often helpful to obtain an outside opinion of the facts before proceeding. Anonymous consultation with practice consultants at the state licensing board for nursing, medicine, or health care facilities can be invaluable in assessing the facts and judging the course of action needed.

4. The nurse assumes responsibility and accountability for individual nursing judgments and actions.

The nurse who wishes to lay claim to independent, autonomous professional nursing judgment must then also embrace the rules of responsibility and accountability. Responsibility has been divided into four types.[14] *Causal responsibility* is assigned to persons, things, events, or processes that make something happen. *Role responsibility* refers to those sets of actions legally or morally expected of a person holding a particular social role—i.e., what one is supposed to do by virtue of holding a certain position, title, or relationship. *Capacity responsibility,* usually thought of in terms of *in*capacity, refers to those circumstances which can influence or obviate one's moral or legal responsibility. Examples here would include mental or emotional illness, duress or coercion (i.e., lack of free consent or true moral autonomy). Diminished capacity or coercion usually results in a judgment of diminished moral or legal responsibility. *Liability responsibility* involves judgments of blameworthiness or fault. The person who is to blame or is at fault (if in a negative sense) is then held accountable or answerable for the harm or wrong that has occurred.

The law holds the nurse personally liable for his or her nursing judgments and actions. The rule of personal liability prevents the nurse from shifting responsibility for negligent conduct to the physician, nursing supervisor, or other person who may have instructed the nurse to act in a particular manner. Personal liability also makes hollow those words often used by physicians or supervisors to cover a nurse's reluctance to act when she or he thinks it is unsafe: "Don't worry, you are practicing under my license." Each professional practices under her or his *own* license, and no other's.

Supervisors are personally liable for their actions as nursing supervisors. Thus, if a nursing supervisor orders a staff nurse to accept an assignment where the nurse is poorly prepared to carry out the duties or has a record of poor performance in the requisite skills or is objectively too inexperienced to handle the assignment, both the supervisor and the staff nurse will be individually accountable for their roles in any harm to patients that may result. The nursing supervisor can be found liable for assigning to a task or situation a nurse the supervisor knew or should have known lacked the knowledge or skill required in the situation. The staff nurse can be found separately liable for harm resulting from taking on an assignment for which she or he lacked the required knowledge or skill.

In many instances, a plaintiff may *choose* to shift liability to the employing hospital, alleging that the hospital is vicariously responsible for the wrongdoing of its agents and employees. But, shifting liability to the employer is a matter of efficiency and economics in malpractice litigation. The employer may, at its option, seek *contribution* from the nurse-employee for any damages awarded the plaintiff patient. The nurse's personal liability for professional judgments and actions makes legal action for contribution possible.

5. The nurse maintains competence in nursing. And,

6. The nurse exercises informed judgment and uses individual competency and qualifications as criteria in seeking consultation, accepting responsibilities, and delegating nursing activities.

Maintaining competence seems a self-evident component of ethical practice. But is it? What is competence in nursing? How does a nurse demonstrate competence?

Legally, the competent nurse is one who possesses that degree of knowledge and skill that would be possessed and used by a reasonably prudent nurse practicing under similar circumstances. Ethically, competence is both a virtue and a duty in nursing. As a duty, it can be seen as a derivative of professional autonomy, just as accountability and responsibility are linked to autonomy. As a duty, competence in nursing practice would entail that same prudent exercise of nursing knowledge and skill for the patient's good, as the law requires, but would also include knowledge and application of the *ethical standards* of the profession. As a virtue, competence is a habit of character which must be practiced, cultivated, and supported.

The nursing tradition seems to instill in all nurses a preconscious belief that a nurse who maintains competence never makes mistakes. Such a belief leads to the conclusion that nurses who make mistakes are incompetent. Error-free practice may be a legal and ethical ideal, but it is hardly within the realm of possibility in today's critical-care environment.

For many, economic pressures have produced increased patient care loads, unpredictable staffing patterns, and rapid movement of patients out of the unit. Nurses are "floated" from the unit with greater frequency. Meanwhile, technology continues to escalate and the half-life of nursing knowledge and skills plummets. Judgments in critical-care nursing become infinitely more complex and open to error. The number of opportunities for omission in performing a complex array of technical tasks grows constantly. Under similar circumstances, even exceptionally capable, prudent nurses make mistakes.

If error-free practice cannot be relied upon as a measure of competence, on what does the critical-care nurse rely? Reasonable standards of practice developed by peer groups are the primary resource. Such standards need to be subjected to rigorous review to ensure that they do not also reproduce the notion that competent nurses never err. Nurses also need to confront directly the error probability factor so as to provide a realistic basis for evaluating a nurse's performance against those standards. Similarly, nursing literature, hospital policies, and expert witnesses need to recognize the probability of error and the multiplicity of contributing factors in describing and discussing competent performance.

Competence in nursing is not maintained without significant support from the clinical environment. There are two aspects of the environment which are particularly important. First, the moral milieu of the unit must be such that it both fosters and facilitates *virtues,* habits of character necessary to do what is right.[15] That is, the critical-care unit must support, expect, and even reward such things as competence and skill, humility (not exceeding one's limits), compassion, knowledge, efficiency, respect for others (patients and peers), and honesty (openly dealing with mistakes).

Second, just as the moral milieu of the critical-care unit must foster the virtues nursing demands, so should it provide an environment which demands the virtue of excellence and the duty of self-improvement, a duty to oneself. Duties should not be interpreted as being entirely other-directed; nurses also have duties to themselves. These duties are both positive (e.g., self-improvement, maintaining personal health and well-being) as well as negative (e.g., preventing burnout, or preventing injury from a violent patient). The competent nurse directs concern to the good of the patient directly, through patient care, and indirectly through improvement of skill and knowledge as well as through a rational self-regard.

7. The nurse participates in activities that contribute to the ongoing development of the profession's body of knowledge.

There are many values which the profession of nursing holds dear. Many of these can be found embedded in such documents as *Nursing: A Social Policy Statement,* or in standards of practice adopted by nursing specialty organizations.[3] Nursing embraces values such as "human dignity," "health," "well-being," and the patient's "self-determination." Nursing must also, necessarily, value itself and its work, and strive to grow in its ability to serve those in need of nursing care. That is to say, nursing, as a profession, is a legitimate and valued end in itself.

But it must walk the picket fence, balancing serving the patient with serving the profession. That is, it is not concern for the profession but rather concern for the patient which is central to the profession. Concern for the profession itself is subsidiary to concern for the patient, and is legitimate only insofar as it is inextricably linked to it. For the advancement of the profession, the development or accrual of nursing knowledge, often involving research, must never be at the expense of the welfare or dignity of the patient. Critical-care

nurses who wish to advance nursing knowledge in their setting through research must ascertain that the research proposal is consistent with the values expressed in nursing generally, and in critical-care nursing as well. Some assistance in this endeavor can be found in position statements such as the American Association of Critical-Care Nurses' 1984 publication, *Ethics in Critical Care Research.*[16]

Human subject research is governed by myriad federal, state, and administrative agency regulations. Nurses must be assured of the protection of human subjects (whether patients, students, or peers) before agreeing to participate in or conduct a research project. Customarily this would entail strict adherence to human subjects regulations, protocols, and reviews. But the nurse must remember that the review conducted by any given institution (e.g., university, hospital, clinic) will reflect the values and obligations of that institution. It should *not* automatically be assumed that because one group approves of a research project, it will be consonant with nursing's ethics.

Informed consent is one vehicle for patient protection. There are some who argue that when a patient cannot give informed consent, if risks are held to a minimum, if the procedures are themselves ethically acceptable, and if the project would provide significant benefits to future patients, it could be morally permissible to include the patient in a research project, despite the nonconsent. Nursing would be hard pressed, given its traditional ethical climate, to adopt this position, even if an institution approved such a proposal.

8. The nurse participates in the profession's efforts to implement and improve standards of nursing.

Standards for a profession can be expressed in unwritten form, as through a tradition, or in written form, as in standards developed for various nursing specialties. The former is usually a statement of what the profession aspires to, i.e., an ideal. The latter can express either the minimum acceptable standard for behavior or practice or the direction a profession wishes to take (more concrete than an ideal). Most commonly, standards of practice set forth a minimum acceptable level of practice, generally for the patient's safety.

Minimum standards can be linked to more than one ethical rule or principle. On the one hand they can be tied to role responsibility and make explicit what is expected of every nurse who engages in practice; each nurse has the role responsibility to both implement and improve those standards. The nurse who fails to adhere to the standards set forth by the profession is morally, and sometimes legally, answerable to both society and the profession, *even when no harm has come to the patient*. On the other hand, minimum principles can reflect a concern for the welfare of the patient, and thus be bound to the principle of nonmaleficence, the noninfliction of harm.

The nurse who fails to observe minimum standards of practice is morally accountable whether or not a patient is harmed. Nurses have an obligation to avoid the infliction of harm and, when harm is inevitable (as with some therapeutic measures), to minimize that harm and ascertain that the benefit gained by the patient is "proportionate" to the harm incurred. That is to say, benefits should outweigh harms *from the perspective of the patient*. It is generally the intent of professional standards to assure that no harm comes to the patient because of lack of professional knowledge, skill, or commitment, and to provide a standard by which the public may judge nursing performance.

Maximal standards, the statement of an ideal, are not standards to which adherence can be demanded or expected. Generally, the nurse who consistently and selflessly lives out the ideals of the profession is considered to be morally praiseworthy, a nursing saint if you will. Beauchamp and Childress write:

> By comparison to ordinary duties, saintly and heroic actions conform to ideals. They transcend our duties and indicate higher possibilities, but we do not expect many persons to realize them. Indeed, they mark out optional but praiseworthy conduct.[17]

Critical-care nurses have both minimum standards and ideals for practice. Care must be taken so that the ideal in critical-care nursing practice is identified as an ideal, not as an expectation. Such an expectation would be neither healthy nor morally reasonable. Ethics does not expect the impossible, though it does reward it.

9. The nurse participates in the profession's efforts to establish and maintain conditions of employment conducive to high-quality nursing care.

Justice applies to the patient, particularly in terms of fair treatment and fair access to nursing care. Justice also applies to the nurse in terms of just compensation or recognition for services rendered and working conditions satisfactory to professional practice.

Early nursing ethics stressed the selflessness of the nurse—to a fault. The "angel of mercy" image was not an unfair portrayal of the almost totally other-regarding ethics of the early modern profession. But an ethic which is exclusively other-regarding will ultimately do a disservice to both the patient and the nurse. It was not until recent years that nursing began to realize that a lack of professional self-regard could bring about the demise of the profession or engender a situation in which adequately prepared nurses could not be recruited or retained for patient care. Nursing began to realize that it was worthy of the same regard that it demanded be accorded to the patient, and that working conditions and the economic and general welfare of the nurse was a *morally legitimate* concern of the profession and its individual members, if not an actual "duty to self."

Note again how concern for the patient is intertwined with concern for the profession or the individual nurse. This is not an attempt to "sanitize" self-interest in the *Code*. Rather, it is a demonstration of the interconnectedness of persons in the moral community, of the mutuality of human welfare, and of the application of the principle of justice (as the distribution of burdens and benefits in society) to both patient and nurse alike.

10. The nurse participates in the profession's effort to protect the public from misinformation and misrepresentation and to maintain the integrity of nursing.

Ethically, the *Code*'s declared obligation to protect the public from misinformation and misrepresentation may be more broadly understood as a concern for patient self-determination. This provision, derivative of the similar provisions in the 1950 and 1957 *Codes* which prohibited advertising, retained that flavor until the current (1985) revision. Prohibitions against advertising, though usually justified on the grounds of protecting the patient from false advertising, self-medication, and similar ills, can be linked to nursing's concern for its social standing as a profession. The current revision alters the overt and covert concerns, reshaping the provision as a prohibition against conflict of interest. This is, perhaps, a reflection of the contemporary marketplace where advertising health products has become rather lucrative. The critical-care nurse is not so much affected by warnings against advertising as he or she might be to the pressures of adopting products as a result of persuasive marketing. All sorts of vendors and drug companies advertise heavily in journals directed toward the critical-care nurse.

The focus on advertising, on using the title R.N., and on maintaining the integrity of nursing, which are found in the interpretive statement for this provision, are more than somewhat vestigial. Greater attention could have been paid to the responsibility of the nurse to educate the public in health care (and its moral basis), to instruct the individual patient, and to maintain the integrity of nursing (which is essential to the trust which must exist in the nurse–patient relationship).

11. The nurse collaborates with members of the health profession and other citizens in promoting community and national efforts to meet health needs of the public.

In the 1976 *Code,* the interpretive statement for this provision declared that "quality health care is mandated as a right to all citizens."[18] Yet that same *Code* stated that:

> The need for nursing care is universal . . . nursing care should be determined solely by human need, irrespective of background circumstances, or other indices of individual social and economic status.[18]

The new revision is clearer and more consistent: Nursing *and* health care should be made available to all in need and when all need cannot be met, access should be nonprejudicial and equitable.

An equally important thrust of the provision's interpretive statement is that nursing is not the sole provider of health care, and thus it has a responsibility to work both wisely and well in assuring that health care is made equally accessible. This, of course, entails a rather more activist and political notion of patient advocacy than nurses are accustomed to. Perhaps Freeman said it best when she called it "practice as protest."[19]

Practice as protest goes beyond the non-infliction of harm to positively benefiting others (beneficence). As a concept, Freeman intends that it be understood as an assertive beneficence through social action, meek or militant. This social action goes beyond the question of access alone, to include the relief of hunger, injustice, ignorance, and untimely death, as well as the achievement of self-respect and self-confidence among patients.

Nursing involvement in political and legislative health care issues of the day is essential to the welfare of present and future patients. Nursing, not just critical-care nursing, can ill afford to remain insular or parochial in its concerns. While moving toward enlarging the body of nursing knowledge, toward establishing work conditions conducive to high-quality nursing care, and toward establishing and enhancing the standards of professional practice, nursing must also move toward a stronger and unified voice in assuring fair access to critical care to all who need it, determining health care policy at a federal and state level, and toward correcting those social conditions which breed ill health.

Conclusion

"The purpose of the American Association of Critical-Care Nurses (AACN) is to promote the health and welfare of mankind by advancing the science and art of critical care nursing."[16]

This is a lofty ideal; its realization is made ever more difficult by contemporary economic pressures, technological complexity, and scientific advance. Yet, even in the face of these social forces, today's critical-care nurse practices in an exciting era. It is an era which promises meaningful life in the face of diseases, illnesses, trauma, or disability which formerly predestined us to a limited life span, debility, or certain death.

It is an era of promise. It is also an era of perplexity. Human life can be sustained beyond human sentience. DNA can be split and recombined. In vitro fertilization may eventually become in vitro gestation. Organs can be swapped, replumbed, or tuned up. ECGs can be bounced off satellites and read in distant cities. The potential for tampering, for good or for ill, is awesome in today's health care. It is hard to know what one "ought" to do when what "can" be done so staggers the imagination.

But in deciding what ought to be done, that is, what the legal and ethical duties necessary to practice are, the critical-care nurse has recourse to several sources. Chief among them is the *Code for Nurses*. Applying the *Code* is not without its problems; it is meant as a general statement of the ethical duties of the nurse and standards of practice, and is not a document specific to critical-care nursing. However, though critical-care nursing has its unique dilemmas, it is a member of a larger nursing community and thus shares the concerns of that community. This brief exposition of selected aspects of the provisions of the current code has been intended to demonstrate that the critical-care nurse shares in the basic values and obligations of nursing in general, yet the duties expressed in the *Code* can be applied to the special, unique context of critical-care nursing. Herein lies one of the chief values of the *Code* as a moral document; it is general enough that it can *both* speak for nursing as a profession, and speak to the particular needs of the critical-care nurse.

References

1. American Nurses' Association. (1985). *Code for nurses with interpretive statements*. Kansas City, MO: ANA, pp. 1–16.
2. Robb, I. H. A. (1898). Report of the committee on object, eligibility, officers. *Report of the first annual convention of the Associated Alumnae of Trained Nurses of the United States and Canada*. New York: O'Donnell Brothers, p. 22.
3. American Nurses' Association. (1980). *Nursing: A social policy statement*. Kansas City, MO: ANA, p. 5.
4. President's Commission for the Study of Ethical Problems in Medical and Biomedical and Behavioral Research. (1983). Deciding to forego life-sustaining treatment: Ethical, medical, and legal issues in treatment decisions. Washington, DC: USGPO, pp. 43–60.
5. Fowler, M. D. M. T'aint cricket: Ethical comments on patient informedness. *Heart & Lung,* 15, 414–415, 1986.
6. McCormick, R. A. (1974). To save or let die: The dilemma of modern medicine. *Journal of the American Medical Association, 229*(2), 172–176.
7. *Bartling v. Glendale Adventist Hospital,* Cal. App. 3d, 1985.
8. *Barber v. Superior Court,* Cal. App. 3d, 1983.
9. Oran, D. (1975). *Law dictionary for non-lawyers.* St. Paul, MN: West Publishing Co., pp. 72, 241.
10. Fowler, M. D. M., & Chaney, E. A. (1983). *Ethics and law in nursing: Reconcilable differences.* Prepublication manuscript.
11. Gretter, L. (1893). The Florence Nightingale pledge. Unpublished.
12. American Nurses' Association. (1985). *Guidelines for nurses' participation and leadership in institutional ethical review processes.* Kansas City, MO: ANA.
13. American Nurses' Association. (1980). *Guidelines for implementing the code for nurses.* Kansas City, MO: ANA.
14. Hart, H. L. A. *Punishment and responsibility.* (1968). New York: Oxford University Press.
15. Aquinas, St. Thomas. (1966). *Treatise on the virtues.* Translated by John A. Osterle. South Bend, Ind.: Notre Dame University Press, pp. 1–56.
16. American Association of Critical-Care Nurses. (1984). *Ethics in critical care research.* Newport Beach, CA: AACN.
17. Beauchamp, T., & Childress, J. (1979). *Principles in biomedical ethics.* New York: Oxford University Press, p. 230.
18. American Nurses' Association. (1976). *Code for nurses with interpretive statements.* Kansas City, MO: ANA.
19. Freeman, R. (1971). Practice as protest. *American Journal of Nursing,* 71, 918–921.

part 2

The Critical-Care Environment

4

Instrumentation

Rae Nadine
Smith
Richard A.
de Asla

Introduction

The modern critical-care environment is, in many ways, symbolic of the effect technology has had on our society. The development of modern mechanical, electromechanical, and electronic medical instrumentation has altered and shaped the way medical care is administered to the critically ill. Cardiac surgery as we know it today has been made possible by these developments. Specially designed instruments make possible the continuous monitoring of variables like arterial blood pressure, electrocardiograms (ECGs), pulse rate, and so on. The alarm functions contained in these instruments alert the staff to any deviation from a prescribed range. These and other features free the critical-care staff to perform true patient care. The proliferation of computers and computerized equipment into the critical-care environment promises to further enhance our capabilities.

Critical care might be defined as the management of patients with life-threatening physiologic derangements. Access to and understanding of multiple physiologic variables are intrinsic to this function. Since instrumentation must be used to acquire data with the frequency and accuracy needed, a basic understanding of the instrumentation is as important to the critical-care nurse as an understanding of the measured physiology.

Parameter Acquisition Instrumentation

Recording and Display

Oscilloscopes

The introduction of the oscilloscope into the clinical environment was the keystone of the modern intensive-care unit (ICU)–critical-care unit monitoring system. This device made it possible to continuously monitor a patient's electrocardiogram and thus to implement the basic principle of a critical-care unit. The advantages of having a real-time display of physiologic information, in addition to the electrocardiogram, were soon recognized; techniques such as the measurement of pulmonary capillary wedge pressure and intra-aortic balloon pumping require that the pertinent intravascular pressure be visible in order to make a proper interpretation and/or adjustment.

The "heart" of all oscilloscopes is the cathode-ray tube (CRT) (see Fig. 4-1). A simple CRT consists of:

1. A glass tube or envelope
2. A screen face made of some appropriate phosphor
3. A cathode and anode (anode not shown in Fig. 4-1)
4. A pair of horizontal deflection plates
5. A pair of vertical deflection plates

The principle of operation is as follows. A very large voltage difference is created between the anode and the cathode. (The anode is located near, but not on, the face of the screen.) When the cathode is heated, it emits a stream of electrons in the direction of the anode, i.e., in the general direction of the screen, because of the shape and construction of the CRT. The electron beam emitted from the cathode passes through two sets of deflection plates. When a voltage is applied to these sets of plates, it causes the electron beam to deflect vertically and horizontally, thus striking the phosphor screen. The phosphor deposited on the inside face of the screen has a special property that causes it to emit visible light when excited by an electron beam.

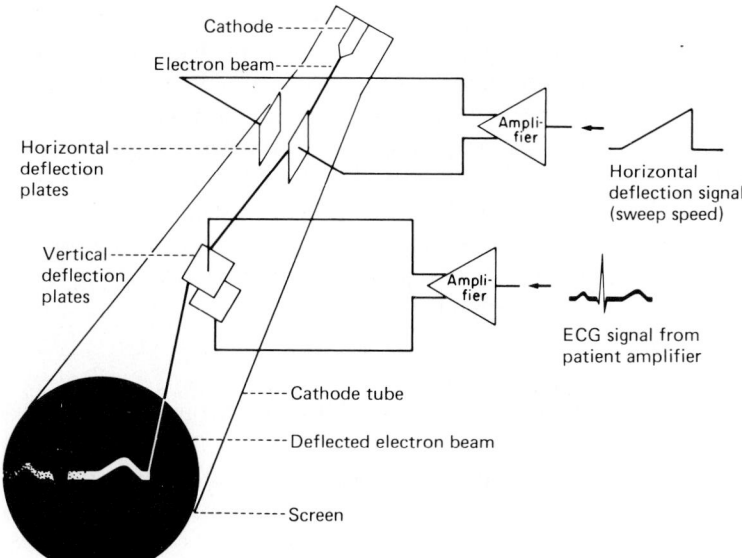

Figure 4-1 Cathode-ray tube (CRT) "scope" used for ECG monitoring.

Commercially manufactured oscilloscopes are available in a wide variety of configurations and have a multiplicity of features which include multiple channels, multiple sweep speeds, and a large variety of screen sizes. There are two different technologies used to generate the image, and thus the display, on the CRT. These warrant further discussion because it is important for the user to understand the advantages and disadvantages inherent in each. The two types are (1) the conventional oscilloscope, sometimes referred to as the "bouncing ball," and (2) the refreshed or "nonfade" display.

The conventional type of oscilloscope consists of a cathode-ray tube and internal horizontal and vertical amplifiers (Fig. 4-1). The input signal to the horizontal amplifier is the sweep signal which governs how fast the trace will move across the screen. Often the user can select the sweep speed with an external control. Most of the oscilloscopes designed for medical use have sweep speeds calibrated in millimeters per second; for example, the selection of a 25-mm/s sweep will render an image which has the same horizontal proportion as a standard electrocardiogram. The signal to be displayed is applied to the vertical amplifier, thus causing the electron beam to deflect along the vertical axis in direct proportion to the instantaneous voltage change of the electrocardiogram or other input signal. This type of oscilloscope utilizes a high-persistence phosphor which continues to emit light for a short period of time after excitation. Visual result of this system's operation is the writing of a slowly fading trace on the screen.

The refreshed-type medical oscilloscope utilizes an electronic memory to store the information displayed. This technique is termed *analog-to-digital* (A/D) conversion. The digitally stored signal is continually replayed on the oscilloscope screen, the last sample stored being the first to be read out. If the memorized signal were to be replayed exactly as stored, it would appear as a series of dots closely approximating the shape of the original signal (Fig. 4-2). In order to give this reconstructed signal greater fidelity, it is reproduced as a continuous line which connects all the sample points.

If the reader has found this explanation somewhat confusing, perhaps the following analogy may be helpful. Picture a clear tube into which a marble is being placed at the rate of one per second. Each marble has a number on it that represents the amplitude of the signal being monitored at the instant the marble is placed into the tube. When the tube is full, the addition of one marble will cause another one to fall out the other end. The tube represents the electronic memory, the marbles represent the digitized sample points. If we could, between each sample interval, plot the value of

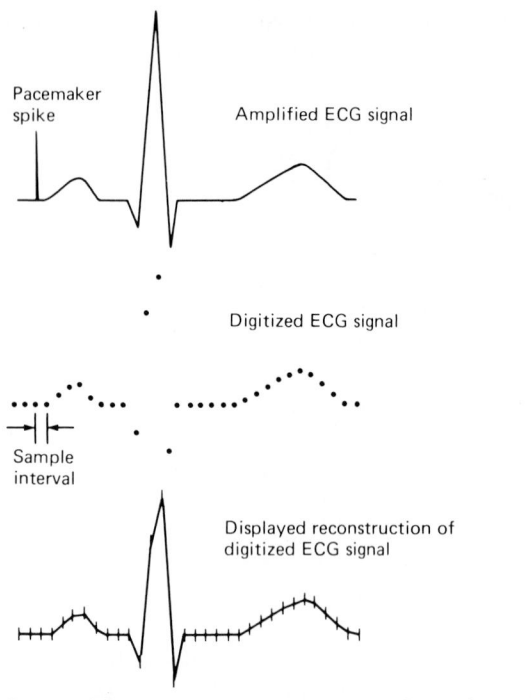

Figure 4-2 Graphic representation of signal processing for refreshed display "scopes."

each marble on the vertical axis of a graph and space them evenly on the horizontal axis in proportion to the sample interval, we would have a graphic representation of the input signal that would be updated each second. Of course, the electronic circuitry is capable of working at much higher speeds; in fact, it repeats this process 400 to 500 times per second.

The advantage of this somewhat complicated method of data display may now be appreciated. The trace on the oscilloscope screen does not fade but appears to move as if an ECG strip were being moved continuously behind the screen. Some instruments permit the user to "freeze" the display for further study, an obviously useful feature. The key point that must be remembered is that the displayed trace is a reconstruction from samples of the original, and that the fidelity of the reconstruction depends on the frequency with which the samples are taken.

For example, if an oscilloscope has a sample frequency of only 200 samples per second, the interval between samples would be 5 ms (0.005 s).

Consider that an external pacemaker has a pulse width of approximately 2 ms (implanted pacemakers often have shorter pulse widths). The pacemaker pulse is of shorter duration than the sample interval and could occur between sample periods; thus, if not sampled, it would appear to be absent on the oscilloscope display. A strip chart recorder that receives its input from the display oscilloscope memory can reproduce only what has appeared on the screen (Fig. 4-2).

Numeric Displays

There are a variety of ways to display numeric data at the bedside or central station. The two methods most commonly used in medical instrumentation are the analog meter and the digital display. Each method offers some advantages and disadvantages. The analog meter consists of an indicator needle mounted over a calibrated scale. Its major advantage is that an observer does not necessarily have to "read" it to obtain the desired information. For example, if we are monitoring a patient's heart rate on an analog meter whose scale reads from 0 to 200, a quick glance tells us the needle is slightly to the left or below center and the impression is one of normal range. It is not necessary to know that the heart rate is 87 beats per minute to reach that conclusion. Because it is possible to obtain a quick qualitative impression from this device, it is best suited for central station monitoring where the observer has to monitor data from several patients. The drawbacks of analog meters are that they are subject to mechanical drift, electrostatic interference, and interpolation error, and they tend to lack fine resolution.

Digital displays offer optimal resolution without risk of interpolation error. In addition, they have excellent readability at moderate distances. They must be "read," however, before an impression can be gained. In the opinion of the author, they are less suitable for central station monitoring but offer a superior choice at the bedside.

Paper Recorders

There are four types of paper recorders made for use in the clinical environment:

1. Photo-optical
2. Ink jet

3. Ink
4. Hot stylus

Optical recorders "write" on special photosensitive paper with a moving light beam. The paper is then either wet- or dry-developed. Their advantages include very fast paper speed (some as high as 4000 mm/s), high-frequency responses (as high as 5000 Hz), and full-trace overlap. This type of recorder is most often used in cardiac catheterization laboratories.

Ink jet recorders write by magnetically deflecting a stream of special ink. They have a frequency response of approximately 800 Hz and partial-trace overlap capability. These recorders are very flexible and thus are useful for many clinical and research applications.

Ink recorders utilize a hollow stylus to deposit ink on the moving paper. Their frequency response is approximately 100 Hz, with maximum paper speeds of approximately 200 mm/s. Some ink recorders, using a special paper, write dry, a useful feature in the patient-care environment. An advantage of ink over heated stylus recorders is that the trace thickness remains uniform regardless of paper speed or stylus motion.

Hot stylus recorders are the oldest and are most commonly used in the patient-care environment. They write with a heated edge on the end of a stylus. This heated edge melts the white coating on the paper, exposing the black underlayer. Newer chemically heat-sensitive papers are available for these machines. The advantage of this paper is that it can be handled and folded without smudging. The paper speed and frequency response of the heated stylus recorders are about the same as ink recorders.

Since recorder tracings are often used to make diagnoses, it is important that they undergo routine testing and calibration by qualified electronics personnel on a scheduled basis. Gain and paper speed errors may lead to false clinical impressions. For example, an ECG trace from a recorder with irregular paper speed may give the impression that an arrhythmia is present.

The commonly used paper speeds in the clinical environment are the following:

1. 0.1 to 1 mm/s for intracranial pressure
2. 5 mm/s for cardiac output recording
3. 25 mm/s for ECG and pressure
4. 50 mm/s for pediatric or adult tachycardia

Digital Recorders

Digital recorders combine new technologies to reproduce waveform images on paper. The waveform which is to be reproduced is digitized (sampled at regular time intervals; each sample is a number representing the amplitude of the waveform at that instant in time) and stored in a memory unit. This technology offers several unique features. Multiple copies of stored waveforms can be made. The time scale of the tracing can be altered to enhance the information. Likewise, the amplitude can also be altered. Multichannel digital recorders can display two or more waveforms at different time scales on the same record. A minor disadvantage is that it is usually not possible to see the waveform reproduced in real-time.

Invasive Measurements

Invasive Monitoring

For selected patients, the precise information needed to assist in diagnosis, to define therapy, and to evaluate the patient's response to the selected therapy is best obtained through continuous invasive monitoring. Physiological pressures that can be measured include arterial, venous, pulmonary artery, intracranial, spinal, gastrointestinal, urinary bladder, esophageal, intrauterine, intracompartmental, and interstitial pressures. Other parameters obtained via invasive measurements include blood gases and flow. Invasive monitoring indicates procedures which involve penetration of the skin, such as placement of an arterial cannula, a pulmonary artery catheter, or an intracranial pressure measurement device. The pressures measured, for example, pulmonary artery (PA), pulmonary capillary wedge (PCW), central venous (CVP), left atrial (LAP), intracranial (ICP), and mean arterial (MAP), are not readily detectable using noninvasive techniques.

The first report of direct arterial measurement was by Lambert and Wood in 1947. Ryder published on ICP monitoring in 1952, and in 1970 Swan and Ganz introduced the flow-directed, balloon-tipped pulmonary artery catheter. Invasive procedures have now become widely utilized to complement and supplement noninvasive forms of assessment, such as history taking, physical examination, and ECG monitoring. Invasive techniques provide the quickest, most accurate physiologic data. Eliminating the need for frequent, intermittent manual measurements, such as vital signs and blood gas samplings, permits increased time to be devoted to other aspects of caring for the critically ill patient. In the hands of skilled personnel, the insertion and maintenance of invasive lines to obtain accurate and continuous data provide less risk to the patient than the alternative of intermittent, estimated data. These procedures can be done with a high degree of safety and are well tolerated by the seriously ill patient.

Basic Pressure System   A frequently used system for the continuous measurement of physiologic pressure consists of a cannula or catheter connected to a transducer via a system of stopcocks and tubing. The area between the patient's blood or cerebral spinal fluid (CSF) and the diaphragm of the transducer is filled with solution to transmit the pressure from the patient to the monitor (Fig. 4-3).

Cannula→Stopcock→Pressure Tubing→
Transducer→Monitor

A variety of satisfactory techniques is in use to measure various pressures. An understanding of the basic principles of transducers and amplifiers will facilitate the setting up and use of any type of monitoring equipment for any type of pressure measurement (Fig. 4-4).

Transducers

A transducer is a device which converts one form of energy into another. It may be defined as a device used to change a varying pressure into a proportionately varying signal which can be displayed on an oscilloscope, meter, and/or recorder. The type of transducer discussed in this application is one which converts a physiologic pressure to an electric signal.

It is recommended that in a clinical setting only isolated transducers be used. The isolated transducer protects the patient against inadvertent shock and withstands the high voltage generated during electrocautery and defibrillation.

The following information is designed as a guide for the selection and use of reusable and disposable transducers in the critical-care environment (Fig. 4-5).

Reusable Transducers   A wide variety of reusable transducers is available. Solid-state technology has resulted in smaller, more durable transducers that can resist severe impact shock, electrical damage

Figure 4-3 Basic vascular pressure system.

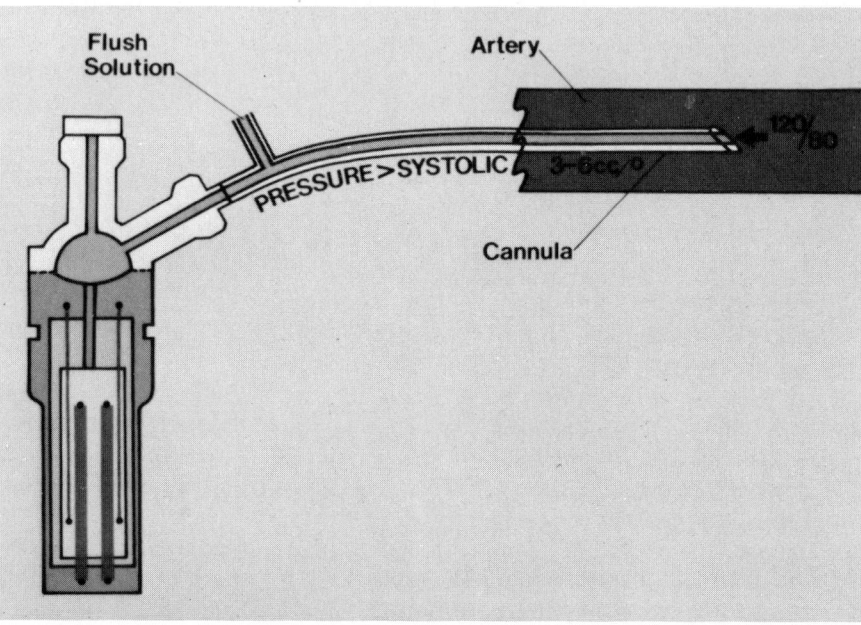

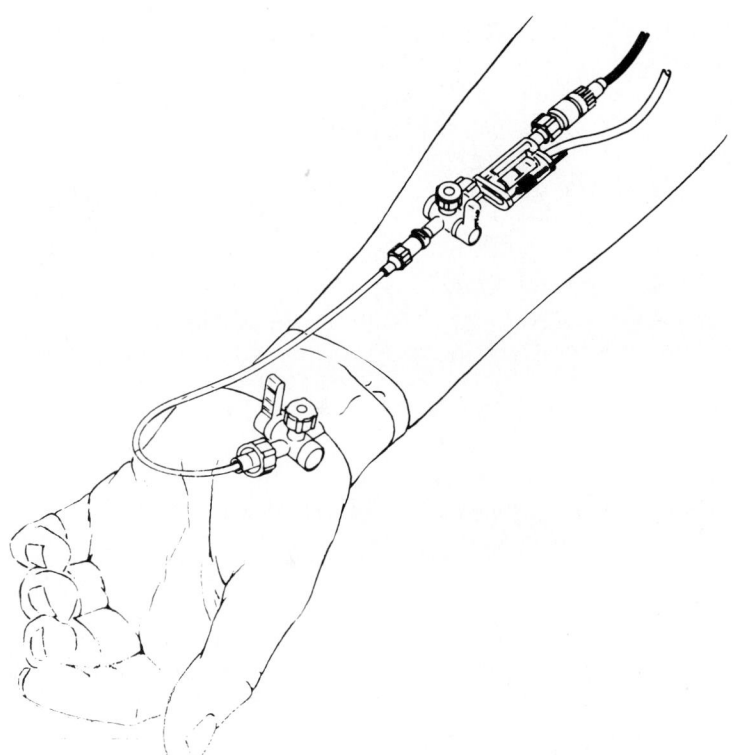

Figure 4-4   Basic set-up for a miniature-size transducer for a radial arterial line.

from electrocautery and defibrillation, and higher levels of overpressurization. These improvements have made transducers more compatible with the critical-care environment, in which transducers can be dropped, caught in siderails, overpressurized by syringes, or subjected to the high-voltage discharge of defibrillators and electrosurgical instruments. Reusable transducers are available with a variety of technologies, including unbonded strain gauges, semiconductors, differential transformers, and quartz. Standard-size and miniature reusable transducers are available.

The small, lightweight, solid-state miniature transducer, often having a shorter cable than is found in the standard-size transducers, is frequently preferred for direct patient mounting. Transducer holders designed for patient mounting, usually with Velcro straps, are available (Fig. 4-6).

Catheter-tip transducers provide high-fidelity measurements of pressure, sound, and velocity. Pressures and sounds associated with heart valve closure, swallowing, bladder function, and digestion can be recorded simultaneously. They are used primarily for research. Their major clinical application is in the cardiac catheterization laboratory. Catheter-tip pressure transducers are available in a variety of configurations, ranging in size from 4F to 8F, with one to six pressure sensors per catheter; velocity sensors; electrodes for stimulating, recording biopotentials, or measuring electrical impedance; and with various lumens for slow or high-speed injection, fluid sampling, and external pressure monitoring. Advancements in semiconductor technology have improved stability and durability of these highly specialized transducers. After careful cleaning, most reusable transducers may be sterilized with ethylene oxide gas or glutaraldehyde solution.

Disposable Transducers   A significant advancement in transducer technology has been the development of disposable transducers. These accurate, small, lightweight, rugged, and inexpensive transducers have eliminated many of the problems associated with transducer use in the critical-care setting. They are pretested, precalibrated, and pre-

Figure 4-5 Standard-size reusable transducer, miniature reusable transducer, and disposable transducer with integral flush system. (*Courtesy of Spectramed, Inc. formerly Gould Medical Products.*)

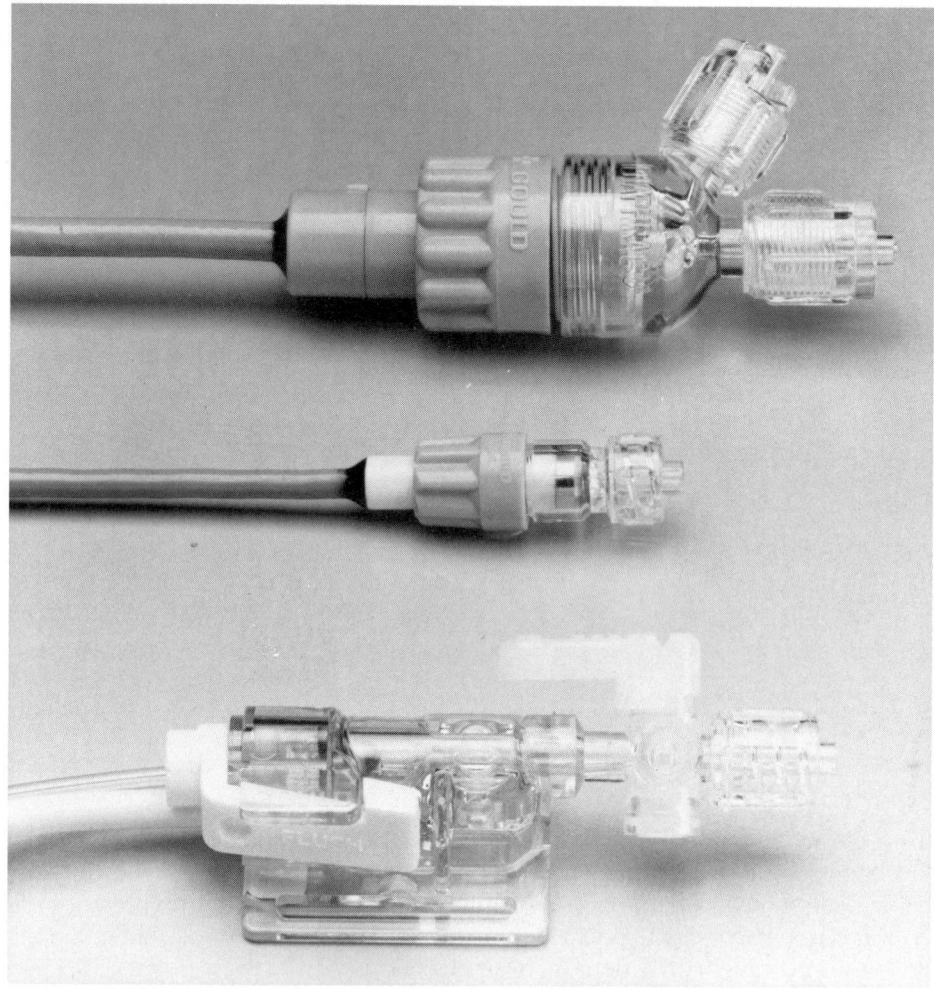

sterilized, minimizing the risk of cross-contamination. Preassembly reduces the risk of contamination associated with component assembly and saves valuable set-up time. Most disposable transducer set-ups are designed for either automatic self-filling or rapid manual filling. It is recommended that the disposable transducers be changed with the monitoring line, usually every 48 h. Patient transfer is facilitated by not having to keep track of the transducer or change transducers for monitoring compatibility. Since transducer cleaning, sterilization, repair, and replacement are eliminated, many hospitals find disposable transducers more cost-effective.

The majority of disposable transducers are based on semiconductor technology. The patient's physiologic pressure is transmitted to the external transducer sensor via a fluid-filled catheter system.

The most recent development in disposable transducer technology is the fiber-optic transducer. Since this transducer is at the tip of a catheter, the need for a fluid-filled catheter system is eliminated. Monitoring accessories such as pressure tubing, stopcock, flush devices, flush solution, pressure administration cuffs, and transducer holders are not utilized with this simplified set-up (Fig. 4-7).

The system consists of the fiber-optic transducer catheter and digital pressure monitor, which

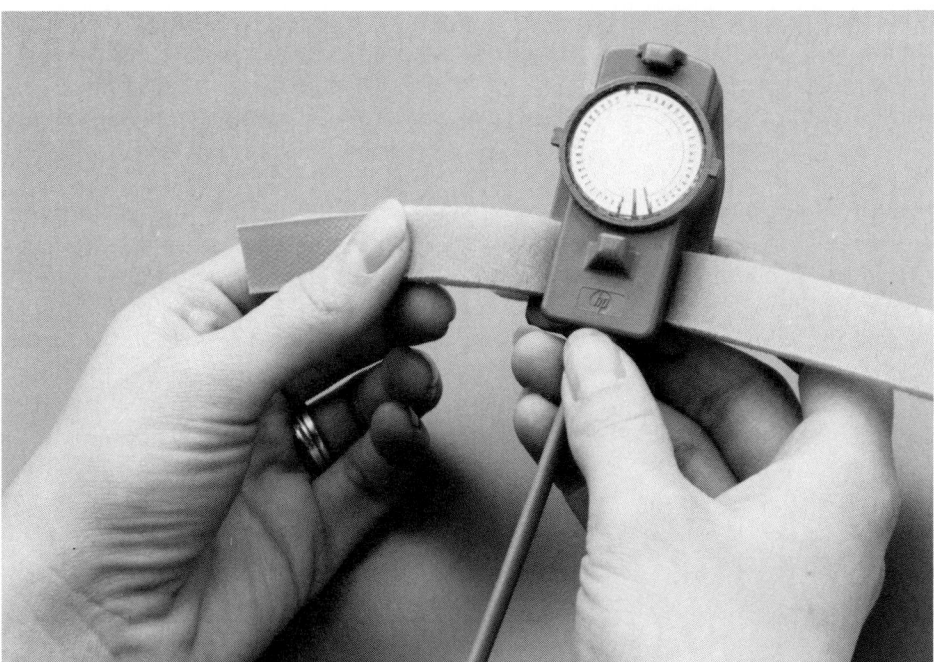

Figure 4-6   Quartz crystal transducer with disposable strap for arm mounting. (*Courtesy of Hewlett-Packard Company.*)

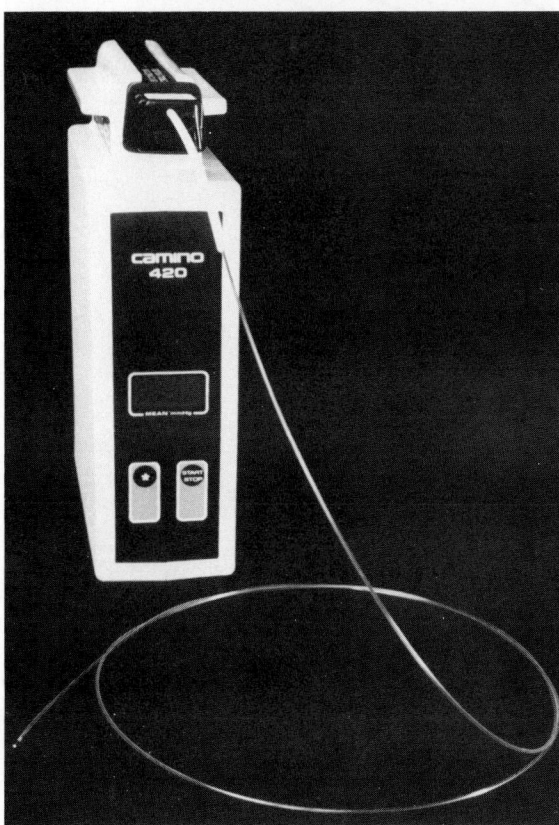

Figure 4-7   Fiber-optic transducer catheter and digital pressure monitor. (*Courtesy of Camino Laboratories.*)

is interfaced with standard hospital bedside monitors for waveform display. Fiber-optic catheters are available for obtaining intracranial pressures, vascular pressures, and cardiac output via the thermodilution technique (Fig. 4-8).

When selecting either a reusable or disposable transducer, manufacturer specifications should be reviewed for pressure ranges (usually −50 to 350 mmHg), overpressure tolerance, nonlinearity and hysteresis (accuracy), electrical isolation, thermal coefficients (temperature stability), light stability, and monitor compatibility.

Monitoring Kits   A wide variety of disposable presterilized, preassembled kits are available for both reusable and disposable transducers. They reduce the risk of contamination during assembly as well as set-up time. Kits should be evaluated for their effect on dynamic response as well as for safety characteristics of the connectors and continuous flush devices.

Domes   When the transducer is in use, the dome holds the solution which transmits the patient's pressure to the diaphragm, the sensing element of the transducer. When the transducer is not in use, the dome protects the transducer diaphragm from damage. On most disposable transducers, the dome is an integral part of the transducer. For reusable transducers, domes are available in a variety of configurations. From the standpoint of electrical safety, only plastic domes should be used in the

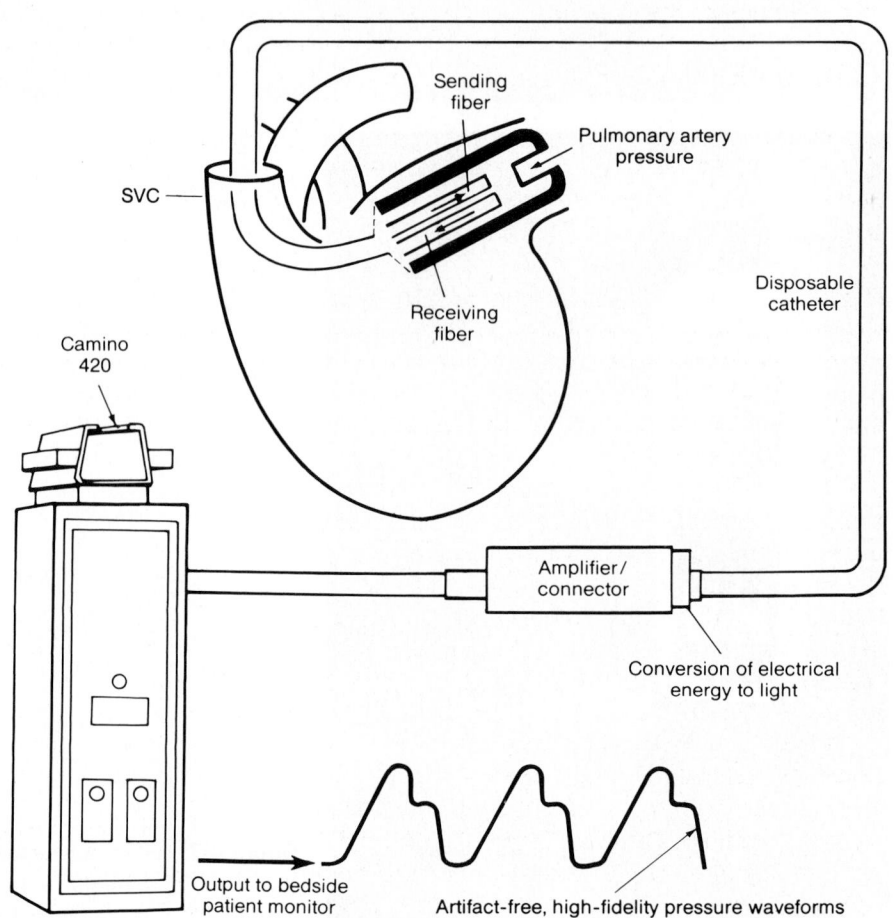

Figure 4-8   Fiber-optic transducer catheter system. (*Courtesy of Camino Laboratories.*)

critical-care area. All accessories such as stopcocks and tubing should also be plastic.

Several changes have been made in the domes available for reusable transducers. Diaphragm domes are available for both standard and miniature transducers. They contain a thin membrane or diaphragm which acts as a sterile barrier between the transducer and the sterile flush solution in direct contact with the patient. The need for sterilization of the transducer in most applications is reduced. The disposable diaphragm dome is strictly for one-patient usage. Episodes of sepsis secondary to resterilization of disposable diaphragm domes have been documented. Sterilizing agents may react with the thin dome diaphragm, causing it to develop small fissures, thereby eliminating the sterile barrier between the diaphragm of the dome and the diaphragm of the transducer. Domes are available with a built-in pressure relief valve to reduce transducer failure secondary to overpressurization, as well as with integral continuous flush devices.

Interface Adaptor Cables   All transducers require specific cables to make the monitor and the transducer compatible. With disposable transducers, the cable usually stays with the monitor when the transducer is disconnected. The cables should have labels indicating the name of the monitor manufacturer and model type. Active electronic cables provide monitor–transducer compatibility by compensating for the high-output impedance of the transducer element. Use of an incorrect cable can lead to errors in pressure readings.

Signal Conditioning Boxes   Selected transducers, usually of the disposable variety, require special signal conditioning boxes to interface between the transducer and bedside monitor. The cost and inconvenience of this interface box needs to be considered during selection of a pressure-monitoring system.

Dynamic Response Testing   Dynamic response is a significant factor in the accuracy of physiologic pressure readings. *Dynamic response* is the ability of a monitoring system to accurately reproduce the patient's pressure signal on the monitor. It is affected by the interdependent parameters of compliance or elasticity, fluid mass, and resistance or friction. To assess dynamic response, it is necessary to evaluate the natural frequency and damping coefficient. Although all components of a pressure-monitoring system affect response, in the clinical setting, the fluid-filled catheter system between the patient and the transducer is the aspect most likely to affect the accuracy of the pressure measurements. The presence and degree of pressure measurement distortion can be determined by dynamic response testing. In the critical-care setting, this is usually done with a continuous flush device and is often referred to as a "square-wave test." (See Fig. 4-9.) Activation of a fast flush valve provides an alteration in the pressure waveform trace which can be used to identify waveform distortion caused by over-damped and underdamped signals. Natural frequency and damping coefficients can be calculated. Measures, such as eliminating air bubbles and reducing the compliance of line components, can eliminate the false low systolic and false high diastolic pressure reading inaccuracies secondary to overdamping, while the use of variable damping devices can reduce the false high systolic readings associated with underdamping.

To optimize dynamic response, the monitoring system should be as simple as possible, contain the least compliant components available, have minimal connecting tubing, and be air-free. For accurate pressure measurement, the monitoring system should be periodically balanced and calibrated, with dynamic response testing utilized to ensure optimal dynamic response.

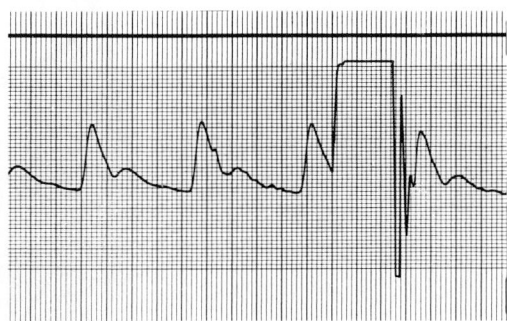

Figure 4-9   "Square-wave test" to assess dynamic response at the bedside.

Balancing and Calibration   All transducers must be balanced (zeroed) before and during pressure measurements. A balanced transducer gives a reading of zero (± 1 mmHg) (Fig. 4-10, Fig. 4-11). Since physiologic pressures are relative to atmospheric pressures, the transducer must be balanced at atmospheric pressure. This is done by referencing (venting) the diaphragm of the transducer to air while it is balanced via the amplifier. The level of the transducer system which is vented to air (e.g., stopcock port) should be at the patient's fourth intercostal midaxillary (right atrial) level. For every 1 in of discrepancy between heart level and transducer level, there will be an error of approximately 2 mmHg.

Prior to balancing, the transducer should be fluid-filled and attached to the monitor with the power turned on for the time recommended by the manufacturer, usually 1 to 5 min. Transducers in use for blood pressure measurement should be balanced approximately every 8 h. Transducers in use for low-range pressures, such as pulmonary artery and intracranial pressure, should be balanced approximately every 2 to 4 h. In addition, they should be rebalanced when they are repositioned, if the pressure reading is in question or if there is a loss of power. Some monitoring systems feature zero balancing storage, making it possible to hold the zero for a period of time after power loss.

Once the transducer is balanced, most systems require calibration. *Calibration* refers to adjusting the monitor to display the pressure being exerted on the transducer. The most accurate form of calibration is by mercury sphygmomanometer, and all systems should periodically be checked with this system (Fig. 4-12).

Pressure Amplifiers   The pressure amplifier or module in the monitor enlarges or amplifies the signal being transmitted from the patient via the transducer. Although widely diverse in appearance, all amplifiers perform the same basic functions. These consist of the following:

1. Display—Digital or analog meters display systolic, diastolic, and/or mean pressures, usually in millimeters of mercury.
2. Alarm controls—A means of selecting the highest and lowest acceptable range for the pressure being monitored.
3. Alarms—Audible and visual alarms indicate when a pressure change is above or below the range set on the meter.
4. Balance (zero) control—A means of adjusting the transducer to a zero reading at atmospheric pressure.
5. Calibration control—A means of adjusting the amplifier, oscilloscope, and/or recorder to read

Figure 4-10   Unbonded strain gauge illustrating concept of a balanced transducer in schematic on left.

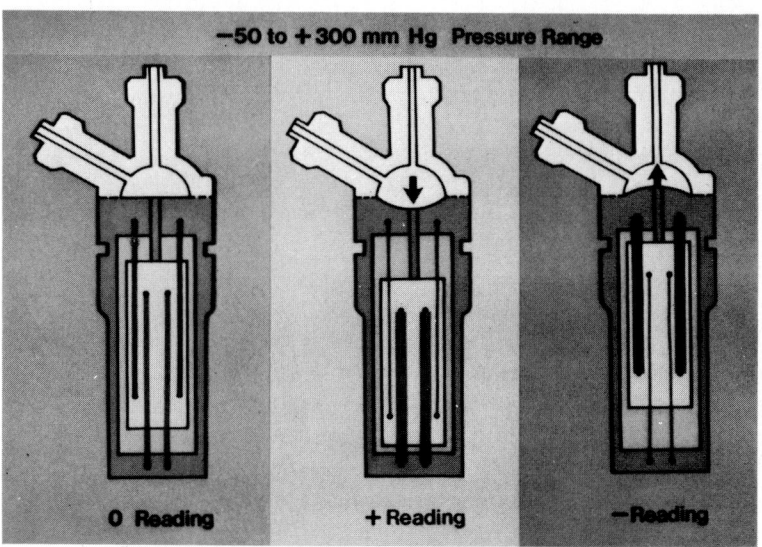

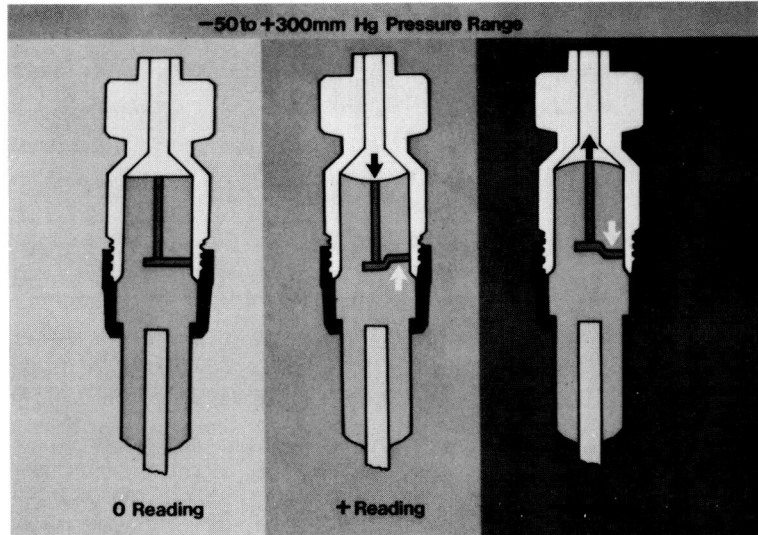

Figure 4-11 Semiconductor transducer illustrating concept of a balanced transducer in schematic on left.

the same pressure the transducer is receiving. Some monitors are precalibrated; others incorporate electronic calibration or calibration (cal) factors. Some older model amplifiers require direct pressure on the transducer via a mercury sphygmomanometer for calibration (Fig. 4-12).

6. Gain control (sensitivity)—A means of controlling the accuracy and size of the pressure displayed. For example, since pulmonary artery pressures are considerably lower than systemic arterial pressures, it is necessary to enlarge the waveform so that important waveform variations are easily visualized. This is done by changing the range switch on the amplifier to enlarge the signal being received. Frequently used gains are 0 to 250 or 300 mmHg for arterial blood pressure,

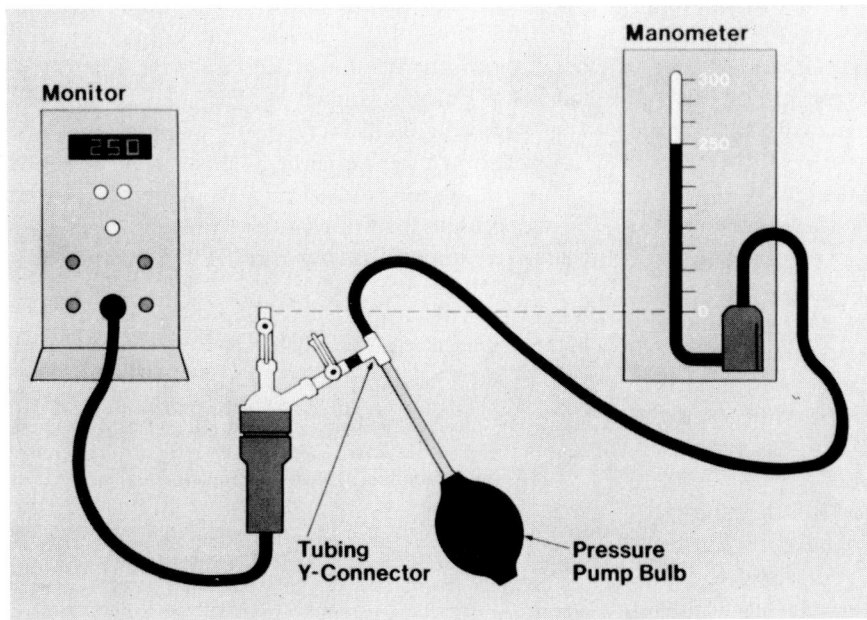

Figure 4-12 Mercury sphygmomanometer for calibration of transducer monitor system.

0 to 60 or 90 mmHg for pulmonary artery and intracranial pressures, and -5 to $+20$ or 30 mmHg for central venous pressures. Many monitors have an autoranging function which automatically selects the appropriate gain for the pressure being monitored.

7. Selector switch—A means of determining which pressure—systolic, diastolic, mean, or a combination of pressures—is to be displayed.

Systemic Arterial Blood Pressure

For the normotensive, noncritically ill patient, the indirect method of blood pressure measurement is usually satisfactory, since the inaccuracies inherent in the indirect or cuff method of measurement are not usually physiologically significant. In the critically ill, hypertensive, or hypotensive patient, however, alterations in cardiac output and peripheral vasoconstriction, combined with the inherent errors of the indirect method, cause measurement errors that could seriously distort blood pressure data. Such incorrect data could lead to inappropriate diagnosis and management. Indications for direct or invasive systemic arterial blood pressure monitoring include:

1. Hypotension—It is not always possible to obtain cuff or palpated pressures on a patient in shock. Obviously the patient still has a pressure at this critical stage, and it is very important to be able to accurately ascertain the pressure. When the patient has a low stroke volume and a low cardiac output with excessive peripheral vasoconstriction, Korotkoff sounds may not be heard at all.

2. Derived parameters—The combining of arterial blood pressure values with other bedside parameters to develop hemodynamic profiles facilitates optimal patient-specific, therapeutic intervention.

3. Vasoactive drug therapy—The administration of drugs which markedly lower or raise blood pressure, such as sodium nitroprusside or dopamine, requires continual monitoring of pressure for safe, effective regulation.

4. Blood sampling—The need for frequent blood samples for measurement of Pa_{O_2}, Pa_{CO_2}, pH, and other parameters is a major indication for an arterial line. The placement of an arterial cannula

leads to fewer complications than repeated needle punctures of an artery.

5. Neurologic conditions—In patients with increased intracranial pressure (IICP), or the potential to develop it, measures are taken to maintain cerebral perfusion pressures (mean arterial pressure minus mean intracranial pressure) of at least 50 mmHg. In the stroke patient, maintaining the mean arterial pressure at a level above 60 to 70 mmHg is believed to be helpful in preventing the loss of autoregulation mechanisms in areas of focal cerebral ischemia. Patients with acute cervical cord injuries are often hypotensive. An increase in blood pressure may be a sign that abnormal pressure is being exerted on the spinal cord. For example, a postoperative laminectomy patient may develop increased pressure on the cord from bleeding.

Catheter Insertion The direct measurement of systolic, diastolic, and mean arterial blood pressure is usually done by cannulating the radial, brachial, or femoral arteries. Ordinarily, after suitable preparation of the skin, the cannula is placed percutaneously and sutured in place. Occasionally an arterial cutdown is required. Systemic arterial pressure may also be obtained via catheterization of the central aorta or the axillary or superficial temporal arteries.

Although the radial artery is small and anatomically unstable, it usually has good collateral circulation. It is routinely used for short-term (less than 24 h) monitoring of cardiac surgery patients. The patient's palmar arch should be assessed prior to insertion of the radial line. This can be done by using the Allen test* and/or a Doppler ultrasound device. Prior to insertion of a radial line, the patient's wrist is restrained in a position of mild hyperex-

---

*Allen test: Simultaneously compress both the ulnar and radial arteries and open and close the hand to promote exsanguination. This takes approximately 1 min. Following release of one artery, usually the ulnar, there should be a blushing (reactive hyperemia) of the extended hand within 5 s. This reactive hyperemia due to capillary refilling indicates adequate circulation to the hand. If blanching occurs, it is evidence of inadequate palmar arch circulation. A radial artery cannula placed in such a patient could lead to the complication of ischemia of the hand. A false positive Allen test may occur with hyperextension of the fingers or wrist.

tension to avoid kinking the cannula. A kinked cannula interferes with infusion of the continual flush solution.

An alternative insertion site is the brachial artery. This vessel is larger and more anatomically stable than the radial, with less collateral circulation. For patients requiring long-term monitoring or for the restless patient, the femoral artery is frequently used. This is a large, anatomically stable artery with minimal collateral circulation. Location of the arterial cannula affects both contour and values of arterial pressures. For example, systolic pressure obtained in the femoral artery may be 25 to 50 mmHg higher than pressure in the radial or brachial arteries. Little variation occurs in diastolic pressures.

Waveform   A normal arterial waveform consists of a sharp ascent during systole with a gradual descent during diastole (Fig. 4-13). The downstroke has a dicrotic notch, indicating closure of the aortic valve. The more distal the cannula is from the aorta, the sharper the upstroke and the less defined the dicrotic notch. The ascent during systole correlates with electrical depolarization of the ventricles as demonstrated in the ECG by the QRS complex. Delay between the QRS and systolic ascent can be caused by many factors. One of these is the distance between the cannulated vessel and the left ventricle. For example, there will be more lag time noted between the QRS and the upstroke of the waveform if the cannula is in the femoral artery rather than in the central aorta. The dicrotic notch correlates with the T wave documenting the end of ventricular

repolarization (Fig. 4-14). Cardiac dysrhythmias can be reflected in alterations in the arterial pressure waveform (Fig. 4-15). Other causes of waveform variations are the patient's clinical state, certain drugs, cardiac output, and vascular resistance, as well as artificial pacemakers and artifacts in the monitoring system. Infrequently, inspirations and expirations will affect the overall waveform pattern, particularly in the dehydrated patient (Fig. 4-16).

Bedside Set-up for a Standard-size Transducer   A variety of satisfactory systems is available for doing direct blood pressure measurements. The various components are usually preassembled in a sterile kit. The use of a monitoring kit and premixed heparin flush solution reduces the risk of set-up contamination. The following procedure (and list of items necessary to carry it through) represents a frequently used system incorporating a continuous flush technique (Fig. 4-17).

Transducer

IV 500-mL bag of normal saline

IV heparin

Minidrop (microdrop) IV administration set (60 drops/mL)

Pressure tubing, male-female

Continuous flush device

Three-way stopcock (3)

Female cap or deadhead

Transducer holder

Pressure administration cuff

IV pole

1. Connect the transducer to the monitor with the power on so that the transducer will have at least 5 min to warm up.
2. Prepare a flush solution such as normal saline solution with 1000 units of aqueous heparin per 500 mL of solution.
3. Insert a minidrop (microdrop) infusion set (60 drops/mL) and place the solution in a pressure infusor bag. A syringe pump or roller pump may also be used.

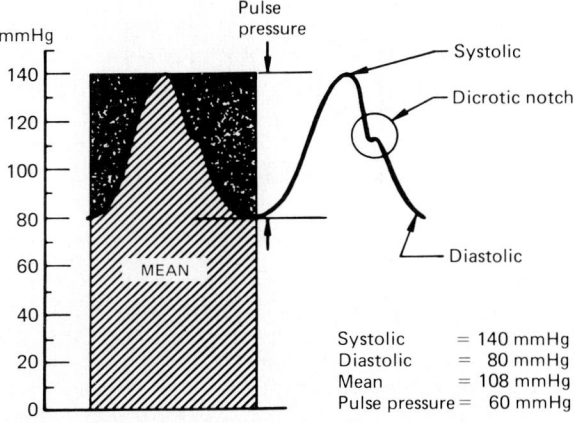

Figure 4-13   Typical arterial pressure waveform.

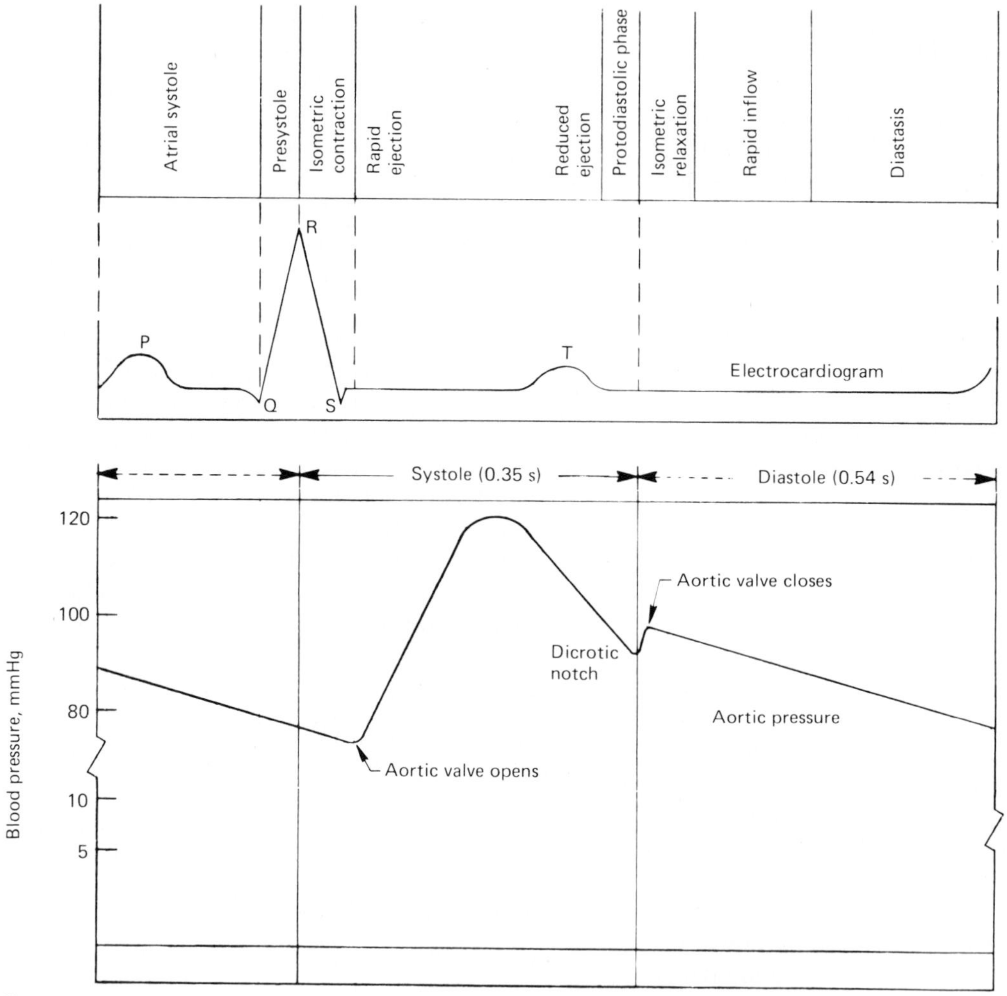

Atrial systole

Presystole

Isometric contraction

Rapid ejection

Reduced ejection

Protodiastolic phase

Isometric relaxation

Rapid inflow

Diastasis

R

P

Q S

T

Electrocardiogram

Systole (0.35 s) ———— Diastole (0.54 s)

120

100

Aortic valve closes

Dicrotic notch

80

Aortic valve opens

Aortic pressure

Blood pressure, mmHg

10

5

Figure 4-14 Correlation of arterial pressure waveform and ECG.

Figure 4-15 Effect of PVC on arterial pressure waveform demonstrating decreased stroke volume (paper speed 25 mm/s).

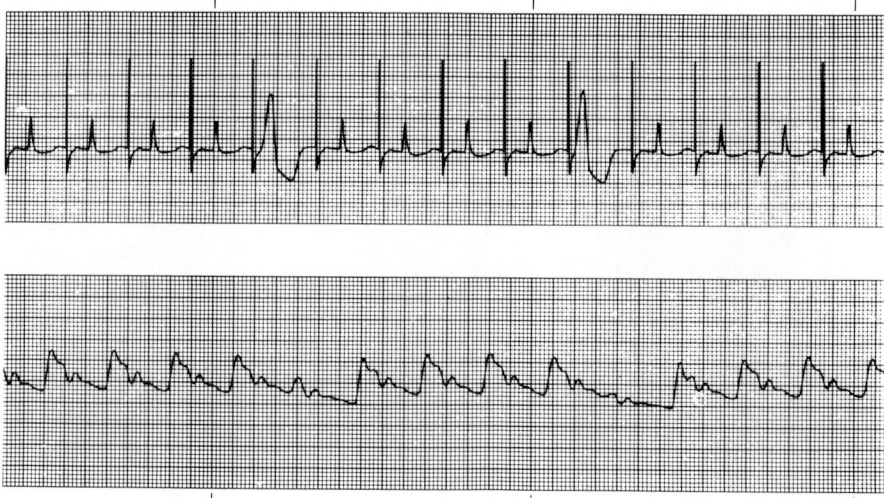

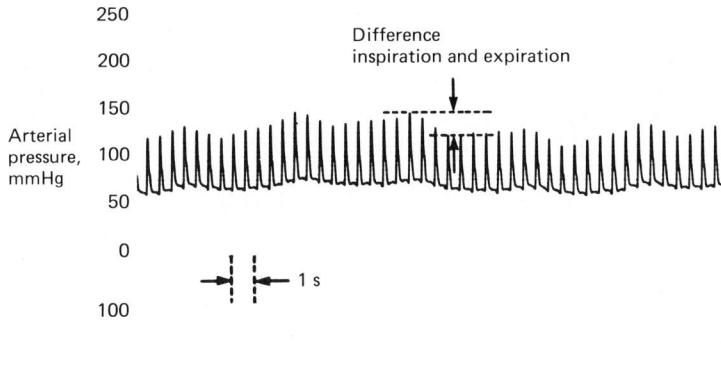

250
200
150
Arterial
pressure,   100
mmHg
50
0
100

Difference
inspiration and expiration

1 s

Airway
pressure,   50
cmH$_2$O
0

Figure 4-16   Effect of airway pressure on arterial pressure (paper speed 5 mm/s).

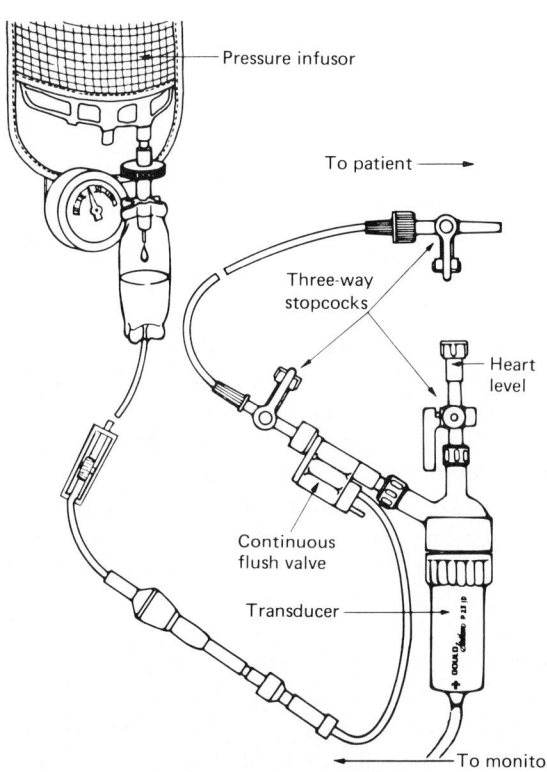

Pressure infusor

To patient →

Three-way
stopcocks

Heart
level

Continuous
flush valve

Transducer

To monitor

Figure 4-17   Bedside set-up for a standard-size transducer.

4. Inflate the pressure infusor bag to 300 mmHg and hang on an IV pole. Fill the IV tubing, making certain it is air-free.
5. Using sterile technique, fasten the continuous flush device to the side port of the transducer. Keep the cap on the unused port of the continuous flush device.
6. Connect the flush solution to the continuous flush device.
7. Activate the fast flush valve, filling the continuous flush device and the transducer dome. Make certain the continuous flush device and the area above the transducer diaphragm have no air bubbles.
8. Place a cap or stopcock on the vertical port of the transducer to close the system.
9. Connect a length of pressure tubing to the remaining port of the continuous flush device and fill the tubing with flush solution. A stopcock may be inserted between the pressure tubing and continuous flush device for the purpose of drawing blood samples.
10. Place the transducer in a holder at the bedside with the tip of the vertical port level with the patient's right atrium (approximately midaxillary).
11. With the vertical port vented to air, balance the transducer to zero, then calibrate as required.
12. Connect pressure tubing to the stopcock attached to the patient's cannula or catheter.

13. Flush by activating the fast flush valve, and check the waveform for any signs of damping. Check to be certain the minidrop rate is 3 to 6 drops per minute and the pressure infusor is at 300 mmHg (Fig. 4-17).

Central Venous Pressure

Central venous pressure (CVP) is the pressure of blood in the right atrium or vena cava. During opening of the tricuspid valve, right ventricular pressures are reflected. The CVP may be measured via the proximal port of a pulmonary artery catheter or via a catheter placed into the jugular, subclavian, antecubital vein (median basilic or lateral cephalic) and advanced into the vena cava or right atrium. Both percutaneous and cutdown insertion techniques are utilized.[1]

Central venous pressure measurements are useful for detecting changes in the right side of the heart. The CVP decreases when the volume of blood returning to the heart is reduced, as with bleeding, dehydration, drug-induced vasodilation, or vigorous diuresis. Elevated CVP may be seen with right ventricular failure, cardiac tamponade, a vasoconstrictive state, tricuspid stenosis and/or insufficiency, or a state of increased blood volume such as overtransfusion or overhydration. Used in conjunction with other clinical data, the CVP may provide important management information for the patient.

The right atrial waveform consists of A, C, and V waves, indicating atrial systole, valve closure, and ventricular systole, respectively. For continuous readings with a closed system, the CVP line may be set up the same as an arterial line.

Left Atrial Pressure (LAP)

This measurement is usually associated with cardiovascular surgery and requires surgical placement of the catheter directly into the left atrium. Left ventricular end diastolic pressure (LVEDP) is measured. Although it is important to keep air out of all vascular lines, this requirement is critical with the LAP line. Air on this side of the circulation may interrupt blood flow in the coronary arteries and cerebral vasculature.

The waveform consists of an A wave (atrial systole), a C wave (valvular closure), and a V wave (ventricular systole).

Pulmonary Artery and Pulmonary Capillary Wedge Pressures

Pressures within the pulmonary artery generated by contraction of the right ventricle to pump blood through the lungs reflect left ventricular function. Utilizing the Swan-Ganz technique, pulmonary artery (PA) and mean pulmonary capillary wedge (PCW) pressure may be obtained by inserting a flow-directed, balloon-tipped catheter via a large vein through the right side of the heart and into a branch of the pulmonary artery.

Prior to 1970, left heart function could be directly measured only in the cardiac catheterization laboratory. Use of the pulmonary artery catheter for diagnosis was supplemented by its use for monitoring as a result of the development of the flow-directed, balloon-tipped catheter by Drs. Swan and Ganz. Ordinarily, this procedure is now done without fluoroscopy at the bedside, with the position of the catheter being determined by the pressure waveforms.

Indications for pulmonary artery pressure measurements include:

1. Cardiac problems
2. Intravascular volume control
3. Pulmonary problems
4. Cardiac output determinations
5. Mixed venous blood samples
6. $S\bar{v}_{O_2}$ monitoring
7. Temporary pacing

Pulmonary artery catheters are available in a wide variety of configurations. Capabilities include direct-pressure monitoring from the right atrium, right ventricle, and pulmonary artery; cardiac output via thermodilution; continuous mixed venous oxygen saturation monitoring; and insertion of temporary pacing leads. The style and size of catheter used depend upon the type of patient being monitored. For the adult patient, the 4- or 5-lumen 7 or 8 French catheter is most frequently used. This enables the measurement of right atrial (CVP), PA, and PCW pressures with intermittent cardiac output determinations via thermodilution and continuous $S\bar{v}_{O_2}$.

Prior to insertion, the transducer system is set up as described under arterial blood pressure using as short a length of pressure tubing as possible. Using sterile technique, fill all pressure lumens with flush solution, usually mildly heparinized. The balloon is submerged in solution and inflated to test its symmetry and integrity. Tiny air bubbles can be detected if the balloon is defective.

The catheter is inserted via the internal or external jugular, subclavian, antecubital (median basilic or lateral cephalic), or femoral vein. The catheter is then advanced through the right atrium. Respiratory fluctuations in the waveform may be detected at this time. A large excursion in the right atrial waveform may be demonstrated by having the patient cough. The balloon may be inflated in the atrium (usually) or immediately after the flow of blood has propelled it through the tricuspid valve into the right ventricle. Although room air is usually used for balloon inflation, carbon dioxide should be used if a right-to-left shunt or septal defect is known or suspected. The solubility of carbon dioxide in blood minimizes the risk of air emboli entering the systemic circulation. As soon as the catheter enters the right ventricle, the balloon should be at full inflation to reduce stimulation of the ventricular wall during insertion. The circulation of blood through the heart will then float the catheter through the pulmonary valve into the pulmonary artery, advancing it until the balloon wedges in a distal branch of the pulmonary artery. Once it is determined that the catheter is correctly placed, an x-ray should be taken to confirm catheter-tip location, and the catheter should be sutured into place. As with an arterial line, the pulmonary artery line should be continually monitored.

It is very important that the critical-care nurse be very familiar with pulmonary artery pressure waveforms, since these waveforms are used to determine the positioning of the catheter in the heart (Fig. 4-18). It should be kept in mind that patients with chronic lung disease or ischemic heart disease often have pressures considerably higher than the normal range.

Right Atrial (RA) Pressure   Right atrial (RA) pressure reflects right ventricular (RV) pressure. It consists of three positive and three negative waves, or descents. The positive waves are A, C, and V. The A wave indicates right atrial systole. The C wave is caused by movement of the closed tricuspid valve during atrial diastole; the V wave is caused by atrial

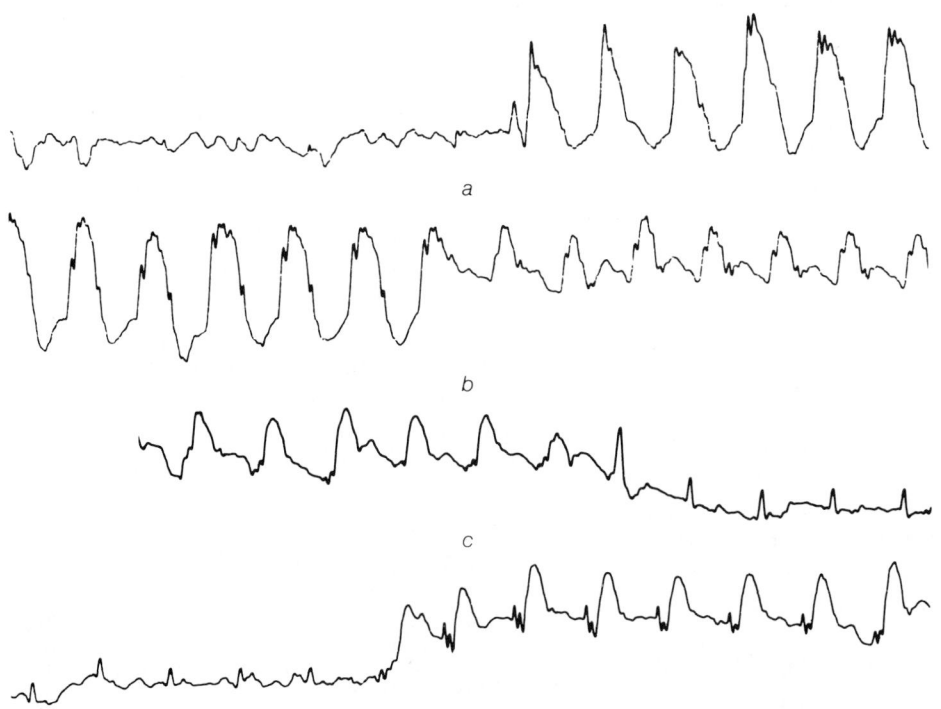

a

b

c

d

Figure 4-18 (A) Waveform during insertion of pulmonary artery catheter, right atrium to right ventricle. (B) Waveforms during insertion of pulmonary artery catheter, right ventricle to pulmonary artery. (C) Waveforms during insertion of pulmonary artery catheter, pulmonary artery to pulmonary capillary wedge. (D) Waveforms during insertion of pulmonary artery catheter, pulmonary capillary wedge to pulmonary artery.

diastole. The negative waves are X, X′, and Y, with the X indicating atrial relaxation, X′ atrioventricular movement, and Y passive right atrial emptying.

Right Ventricular (RV) Pressure   The ventricular waveform is demonstrated by a rapid rise representing isovolumetric contraction, followed by opening of the pulmonary valve with blood ejected from the RV into the pulmonary artery. With closure of the pulmonary valve, right ventricular pressure falls rapidly. The tricuspid valve opens with passive filling of the right ventricle from the right atrium.

Pulmonary Artery (PA) Pressure   Pulmonary artery (PA) systolic pressure represents right ventricular contraction; PA diastolic pressure reflects resistance to flow by small arterioles and pulmonary capillaries. When there is no pulmonary vascular obstruction, PA diastolic pressure is approximately the same as PCW pressure. A positive difference of 6 mmHg or more between PCW pressure and pulmonary diastolic pressure indicates the presence of obstructive vascular disease in the lungs, such as pulmonary fibrosis, pulmonary embolus, or cor pulmonale. Therefore, a patient's PCW and PA diastolic pressure need to be correlated before it can be assumed that the PA diastolic pressure is providing an accurate reflection of pulmonary venous pressure, PCW, LAP, or left ventricular end diastolic pressure (LVEDP). Pulmonary artery pressures are expressed in terms of systolic, diastolic, and mean pressures. A normal pulmonary artery pressure is 25/10 with a mean of 15 mmHg; a normal pulmonary capillary wedge pressure is in the range of 8 to 12 mmHg.

Pulmonary Capillary Wedge (PCW) Pressure   The pulmonary capillary wedge pressure obtained when the inflated catheter balloon occludes a branch of the pulmonary artery indicates (1) the presence and degree of pulmonary congestion, and (2) the performance of the left ventricle via mean left atrial and mean left ventricular diastolic pressure (in the absence of mitral valve disease). A normal PCW with a normal cardiac output indicates satisfactory ventricular performance.

The PCW waveform consists of A and V waves. The A wave indicates left atrial contraction during left ventricular relaxation. The V wave reflects left atrial relaxation during left ventricular contraction. A "giant V" wave can indicate mitral regurgitation. For maintenance of PA lines, it is essential to be able to differentiate between PA and PCW waveforms (Fig. 4-18).

Risks Associated with Vascular Lines

The three major risks associated with invasive vascular pressure monitoring are hemorrhage, thrombosis with emboli, and infections.[2] These complications can be kept to a minimum when patients are under the care of a skilled critical-care team with adequate instrumentation.

1. Bleeding back is the most obvious and most acute problem. The pressure of the systemic arterial system can cause rapid exsanguination through the 18- or 20-gauge cannula commonly used for arterial lines. Bleeding back is controlled by maintaining the flush solution in a closed system at a pressure greater than the patient's systolic pressure. Any leak within the system, such as tubing disconnecting or a stopcock in the wrong position, will cause bleeding back. It is essential that the alarm limits be set correctly and used to notify staff immediately of this complication.
2. Thrombus formation with the risk of emboli can be minimized by continuously flushing the vascular line with a mildly heparinized solution. The development of thrombus will cause damping of the waveform and initiate an alarm condition.
3. To prevent infection, sterile techniques must be utilized for the insertion and maintenance of invasive lines. When a reusable-type dome is used, both the dome and transducer must be sterilized since the flush solution in the dome is in direct contact with both the transducer and the patient. Disposable diaphragm domes are strictly for one-patient use. The resterilization and reuse of these disposable domes have resulted in death secondary to sepsis. The use of preassembled, sterile, disposable monitoring kits and premixed flush solution is recommended.
4. Insertion sites should be dressed daily. Evidence of infection at the cannulation site is an indication for cannula removal.

See Table 4-1.

Table 4-1 Troubleshooting Invasive Lines

Problem	Cause	Intervention
Overdamping of waveform (usually results in false low systolic and false high diastolic readings)		
A. Bleeding back	Patient's pressure has become higher than counteracting pressure of flush solution.	If continual flush device is being used, counteracting pressure (i.e., pressure bag) should be at 300 mmHg.
	Loose connection in the system.	Make certain dome is tightened securely on transducer. Check to see that all connections between patient and transducer are secure.
	Incorrect stopcock position.	Check stopcock positions. Flush line and check for a good waveform.
B. Air bubbles	Losse connection in system.	Check to be certain all connections are secure.
	Cracked stopcock, continuous flush device, or pressure tubing.	Change continuous flush device, pressure tubing, or stopcock with visible signs of damage.
	Pulling air into system during fast flushing with continuous flush device.	When using fast flush valve, watch drip chamber and control amount of valve pressure to prevent turbulence in drip chamber. Flush out all air bubbles between diaphragm of transducer and patient.
C. Clotting	Inadequate flush solution.	Adjust drip rate to 3 to 6 minidrops per minute (3 to 6 mL/h) of a mildly heparinized solution.
		Flush using fast flush valve of continuous flush device. (If waveform remains damped, aspirate with a syringe. Do not reinject any aspirated blood, since it may include clots.)
Transducer will not balance	Damaged transducer.	Try another transducer.
	Transducer may be connected to wrong amplifier.	Check the amplifier connection.
	Broken amplifier.	Change amplifiers.
Drifting	Insufficient warm-up time.	Allow recommended time for transducer warm-up with power on.
	Air vents in cable may be kinked or compressed.	Make certain cable is not compressed.
False low reading	Overdamped signal.	Eliminate air bubbles and compliant system components.
	Transducer not balanced correctly. Positioned above pressure source.	Place transducer at heart level for vascular pressures and level of foramen of Monro for ICP, and re-zero with transducer vented to air.
	Calibration incorrect.	Repeat balancing and calibration procedures.

(Continued)

Table 4-1 Troubleshooting Invasive Lines (Continued)

Problem	Cause	Intervention
False high reading	Underdamped signal.	Variable damping device.
	Transducer not balanced correctly. Positioned below pressure source.	Rebalance. For each foot of discrepancy between transducer and pressure source, there is an error of approximately 25 mmHg.
	Flush solution being administered too rapidly. A maximal continual flush during pressure measurement is 6 to 8 mL/h.	Slow continual flush to 3 to 6 mL/h.
	Air in the system.	Remove all air. At times, air in system will amplify pressure signal.
Cuff blood pressure different from direct blood pressure	Direct pressure is more accurate, particularly in hypotensive patients. Transducer pressure usually reads higher than cuff pressure.	None.
	Transducer measures systolic and diastolic from same heartbeat, whereas with cuff pressures systolic is taken from one beat and diastolic from another.	
	Low cardiac output and peripheral vasoconstriction make it difficult to hear indirect pressure.	
No waveform on oscilloscope	Transducer connected incorrectly.	Make certain transducer is securely connected and appropriate amplifier connector is used.
	Incorrect trace position.	Reposition trace.
	Cannula against vessel wall.	Reposition cannula.
	Incorrect gain setting.	Check to see that amplifier is not set on too low a gain.
	Damaged transducer.	Try another transducer.
	Broken amplifier.	Change amplifiers.
	Transducer not open to patient's pressure.	Check positions of stopcocks.
	Broken oscilloscope.	Replace oscilloscope.
Loss of ICP waveform	Occlusion of intracranial pressure measurement device.	Flush intracranial catheter or SA screw as directed by physician.
	Air between transducer diaphragm and pressure source.	Disconnect transducer and eliminate air from system.
Correlation of pressure readings taken with a water manometer to that taken with a transducer	Water manometers measure in cmH_2O, amplifiers usually display in mmHg.	Conversion: 1 mmHg = 1.36 cmH_2O.
Erratic or noisy traces	If a nonisolated transducer (exposed metal case) is in use, it may be secondary to electrical noise such as electrocautery.	Use an isolated transducer.

(Continued)

Table 4-1 Troubleshooting Invasive Lines (Continued)

Problem	Cause	Intervention
Erratic or noisy traces (continued)	If an isolated transducer is in use, it may mean that moisture has entered the back of the transducer via venting tubes in cable.	Use a different transducer on patient. Check cable for evidence of cracks. If cracked, have it repaired. Moisture may be removed from transducer by: a. Placing transducer through aeration cycle of a gas sterilizing chamber. b. Baking for 8 h at 150°F. c. Several days at room temperature (not in use).
	Patient's movement.	Limit patient's movement. Use solid-state transducers.
Leaky domes	All plastic (Lexan, polycarbonate) domes react to various sterilizing agents. After repeated sterilizations, they will become cloudy, warped, and cracked.	Discard dome and replace with sterile dome. Use disposable domes.
Frequent damping of waveform	The cannula may have lodged against a vessel wall.	A slight alteration in position of cannula will sometimes resolve this.
	A clot may be forming.	This may be indicated by the ability to flush but not aspirate the line.
	If a disposable diaphragm dome is in use, there may be air trapped between transducer diaphragm and dome diaphragm.	Follow manufacturer's instructions for dome application.

Risks associated with pulmonary artery pressure monitoring include thrombosis, emboli, perforation of the pulmonary artery, pulmonary infarction, intracardiac knotting of the catheter, ventricular arrhythmias, sepsis, and balloon rupture. The risk can be minimized by careful insertion and maintenance of the PA line.

Air emboli can result from the direct injection of air into the proximal or distal ports and/or balloon rupture. The latex balloon tends to absorb lipoprotein from the blood, causing it to lose elasticity, thereby increasing the risk of balloon rupture. Fragments of the balloon may become emboli. Ideally, the catheter should be removed from the patient and discarded after approximately 48 h.

PA catheters tend to be thrombinogenic. Continuous flushing of a heparinized solution through both distal and proximal lumens will aid in preventing thrombus formation. The development of thrombus at the lumens will be demonstrated as a damped waveform. Syringe flushing of the lumens may cause thrombotic emboli.

PA catheters may spontaneously advance into a wedge position without the balloon being inflated. If this occurs, it will be demonstrated on the monitor by a change in waveform from PA to wedge, a change in the mean pressure reading, and a drop in PA diastolic pressure. Leaving the balloon inflated for periods any longer than necessary for obtaining wedge readings may lead to pulmonary infarction.

Arrhythmias are often associated with catheter insertion and are resolved by correct placement or removal of the catheter. Should the catheter fall back into the right ventricle from the PA, ventricular tachycardia may occur. ECG should be monitored during insertion and maintenance of the line to indicate arrhythmias. Pneumothorax and damage to the brachial plexus by direct trauma or bleeding have been reported with catheter insertions via the subclavian or internal jugular veins.

The frequency of wedge measurement should be limited to avoid trauma to the pulmonary artery vessel wall. In addition, care should be taken not to "over-wedge" the catheter. During balloon inflation, the oscilloscope should be watched. As soon as the waveform converts from a PA to a PCW pattern, inflation should be stopped and the volume used to inflate the balloon noted. This minimizes trauma to the vessel and prevents false high or low pressure reading caused by overinflation of the balloon.

Cardiac Output/Cardiac Index (CO/CI)

Cardiac output, expressed in liters per minute, is the amount of blood pumped by the heart. It is the product of heart rate and stroke volume (the amount of blood ejected with each heartbeat). *Cardiac index* is the cardiac output per square meter of body surface area (height and weight). A small person requires less circulating blood and therefore less cardiac output than a larger person. By calculating the cardiac output and then computing the cardiac index according to the individual's height and weight, a more specific and useful measurement is available.

The intermittent measurement of cardiac output is essential to determine a patient's response to drugs which affect the heart and the blood vessels. With the aid of cardiac output measurements, a patient's poor response to a given therapeutic program can be recognized and alternative methods of therapy selected.

Techniques   A variety of invasive and noninvasive techniques is available for the measurement of cardiac output. These include Fick, dye, thermal, radioisotope, pulse contour, carbon dioxide rebreathing, and Doppler ultrasound methods.[3] The initial technique for cardiac output determination was introduced by Fick in 1870 and is still utilized widely in cardiac catheterization laboratories. To obtain accurate results with this procedure, the patient must be in a stable condition and be cooperative. Samples of expired oxygen and simultaneous venous and arterial blood are used to make the calculation. This procedure is impractical

for use on the critically ill patient because of the requirements for moving the patient to the equipment, for the patient to be in a stable condition, for highly trained technicians to perform the procedure, and for drawing arterial and venous blood samples.

The dye dilution technique requires the injection of dye, usually indocyanine green, into the patient's venous circulation. An arterial blood sample is withdrawn and passed through a densitometer to determine the degree to which the dye has been diluted by the blood. This technique has the disadvantage of requiring injecting into the patient a substance which recirculates many times before reabsorption, thereby interfering with repeated studies. Some patients have a serious allergic reaction to the dye. Dye dilution also requires blood withdrawal. For determination of certain types of shunts, however, it is the method of choice.

The most suitable procedure and the one most commonly utilized to determine cardiac output on the critically ill patient is thermodilution. The technique was introduced by Fegler in 1954 but did not become clinically applicable until the development of the balloon-tipped, flow-directed catheter by Swan and Ganz in 1970. The procedure is now routinely done at bedside by the critical-care nurse. A 4- or 5-lumen balloon-tipped catheter is placed in the patient's pulmonary artery. A bolus of cool solution, either D_5W or normal saline, is injected into the RA via the proximal port of the catheter. As venous mixing occurs, primarily in the right ventricle, the temperature of the injectate is altered. A thermistor bead (small thermometer) located near the tip of the catheter, which is in the pulmonary artery, measures the change in the temperature of the blood caused by the injection. A cardiac output computer, using the amount of temperature change that has occurred between the injection into the right atrium and the flow through the pulmonary artery, calculates the cardiac output in liters per minute. Using the patient's height and weight and cardiac output, the cardiac index is determined.

This procedure requires:

1. A flow-directed thermodilution catheter
2. A monitoring system
3. Injectate

4. Thermodilution cardiac output computer, preferably with recorder

A balloon-tipped, flow-directed catheter is prepared for insertion. This includes testing the integrity of the balloon under solution, testing the thermistor by attaching it to the cardiac output computer, filling both the proximal (CVP) and distal (PA) lumens with heparinized flush solution, and attaching the catheter to the monitoring system. The catheter must be kept sterile during these procedures.

The minimal requirements for a safe system for the insertion of the catheter into the pulmonary artery include a two-channel oscilloscope, ECG amplifier, and at least one pressure amplifier and transducer. The transducer set-up is similar to that of an arterial line. The only difference is that the catheter is attached to the transducer system and filled prior to insertion. In this way the pressure waveforms can be used to identify the location of the catheter tip within the heart.

With the later model cardiac output computers, cardiac output can usually be measured with room temperature injectate. Room temperature injectate is usually preferable to iced injectate. It provides more accurate cardiac output measurements because of less heat absorption during injection and it is easier to prepare with less risk of contamination. Because of the proximity of the pulmonary artery to the lungs, there are times when more temperature differential between the blood and injectate is necessary. Conditions which usually necessitate the use of iced injectate include cardiac output greater than 10 L/min, patients on respirators, and patients with erratic respiratory patterns such as Cheyne-Stokes.

A variety of injectate delivery systems is available. It has been noted that closed injectate systems are cost-effective and significantly decrease the incidence of contamination.[4-7]

Cardiac Output/Cardiac Index Computer Numerous computers are available. Current models incorporate catheters with thermistors which can measure the patient's body temperature directly from the pulmonary artery and have probes which measure the injectate temperature. The direct and continuous monitoring of the patient's temperature and the injectate temperature makes cardiac output/cardiac index measurement more accurate and simplifies the procedure. Ideally, the computer should be able to display cardiac output in liters per minute, and the temperature of the patient and the injectate in degrees Celsius or Fahrenheit.

The computer should have a test cycle so that the accuracy of the instrument can be verified before the procedure is begun on the patient. Alarms may indicate a low battery, faulty catheter, broken interface cable, or incorrect injectate temperature or volume.

The computer is corrected for the size of the catheter being used, the number of centimeters inserted, whether iced or room temperature injectate is used, and the warming of the injectate by the patient's body temperature (computation constant). Cardiac output/index monitors are now available for real-time measurement of stroke volume, cardiac contractility, heart rate, ventricular ejection time, and indexing, in addition to cardiac output. Bedside hemodynamic profile computers provide both hemodynamic and pulmonary derived parameters.

Thermal Curve Usually a 5 mm/s recorder is utilized to record the thermal curve. The curve is very useful in determining the accuracy of the cardiac output measurements. Many CO monitors now display the curve on the oscilloscope. Ordinarily, a series of four injections are done, with the first being discarded. If room temperature injectate is used, the bolus is injected into the proximal right atrial port at 1-min intervals. For iced injectate, 1½-min intervals are used. Three measurements are made to allow for normal variations in the patient's heart rate and stroke volume (Fig. 4-19). If one cardiac output value is significantly different from the others, the cause may be determined by evaluation of the thermal curve. An inverse correlation exists between the area under the curve and the

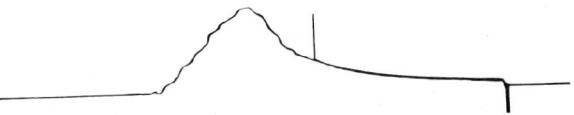

Figure 4-19 Thermal curve trace (paper speed 5 mm/s).

patient's cardiac output. In other words, the greater the area under the curve, the lower the cardiac output. Fluctuations in the baseline of the curve may be the result of respiratory irregularities (Fig. 4-19).

Guidelines

1. Prior to measurement, the position of the catheter in the pulmonary artery should be determined to ensure that the thermistor is not lodged against a vessel wall. This can be done by inflating the balloon and determining exactly the volume required to convert the PA waveform into a PCW. If less than 75 percent of maximum balloon volume is required, the catheter is too far advanced in the pulmonary artery for correct cardiac output determination, although it may be satisfactory for routine monitoring of PA and PCW.
2. Prior to the first measurement, flush the right atrial lumen with the same temperature and volume of injectate to be used for the following injections. Wait 1 min if using room temperature injectate and 1½ min after iced. The maximum injection volume for a 7 French catheter is 10 mL; for a 5 French, 5 mL.
3. Handle the syringes as little as possible so that the injectate temperature is not altered by your body temperature.
4. Make certain the volumes in the syringes are the same and inject as rapidly and smoothly as possible at the 1- or 1½-min intervals for a series of three measurements. Certain types of computers are injection-sensitive and may require the use of an automatic injector.
5. Low or erratic measurements may be due to lodging of the thermistor against a vessel wall or thrombus formation over the thermistor bead.
6. When possible, all IV solution should be reduced to keep open rates for 3 to 5 min prior to and during the cardiac output determinations.

Intracranial Pressure Monitoring

Intracranial pressure (ICP) is the pressure exerted by the brain constituents—blood, cerebrospinal fluid, and cerebral tissue—within the skull. Indications for intracranial pressure measurement include:

1. Increased volume of brain
2. Increased volume of blood
3. Increased volume of cerebrospinal fluid (CSF)
4. Lesions
5. Determination of cerebral perfusion pressure (mean arterial pressure minus mean intracranial pressure)

The three major techniques for monitoring intracranial pressure are intraventricular, subarachnoid, and epidural.

Intraventricular Technique   The intraventricular technique of ICP measurement was first reported in 1952 and consists of placing a catheter into the lateral ventricle. A twist drill hole is placed lateral to the midline at the level of the coronal suture, usually on the nondominant side. A catheter is placed through the cerebrum into the anterior horn of the lateral ventricle. On occasion, the occipital horn is used. Connected to the ventricular catheter via stopcock and/or pressure tubing is a pressure transducer (Fig. 4-20). Saline or Ringer's lactate solution provides the fluid column between the CSF and diaphragm of the transducer. A continuous flush system is not used.

1. Advantages:
   a. Direct measuring of pressure from the CSF
   b. Access for CSF drainage or sampling
   c. Access for determining volume-pressure responses

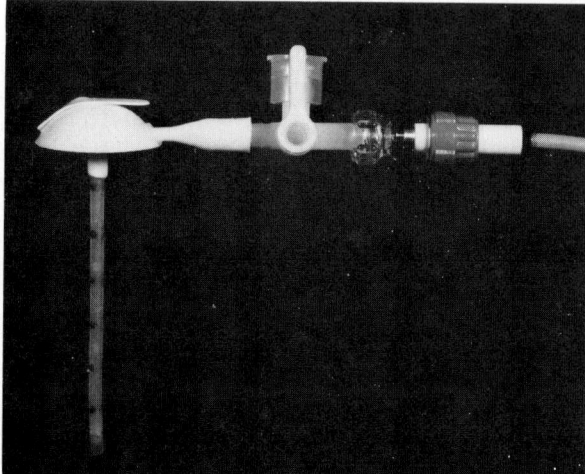

Figure 4-20   Intraventricular pressure cannula with miniature transducer.

2. Disadvantages:
   a. Risk of infection (Sundbarg et al.[8] documented a clinically apparent CNS infection rate of 1.1%.)
   b. Difficulty in locating the lateral ventricle following midline shifting of the ventricle, or collapse of the ventricle as a normal compensatory mechanism for increases in pressure

Subarachnoid Technique The measurement of ICP via a subarachnoid screw was first reported in 1973. The screw device is inserted via a twist drill hole and extends into the subdural or subarachnoid space. Although the cerebrum is not penetrated, pressures are measured directly from the CSF, as with the ventricular technique. A transducer filled with saline or Ringer's lactate solution may be fastened directly to the screw or connected via pressure tubing (Fig. 4-21). Volume-pressure responses have been determined using this technique.

1. Advantages:
   a. Direct pressure measurement from CSF
   b. Does not require penetration of cerebrum to locate ventricle
   c. Access for determining volume-pressure responses

d. Access for CSF drainage and sampling
   e. Ease of insertion
2. Disadvantages:
   a. Risk of infection comparable to intraventricular technique
   b. Requires closed skull
   c. Possible underestimation of elevated ICP

Epidural Technique This technique involves placing an epidural device such as a balloon with radioisotopes, a radio transmitter, a pneumatic device, or a fiber-optic transducer between the skull and the dura. Some researchers feel that dural compression and surface tension, as well as thickening of the dura during prolonged monitoring, tend to cause inaccuracies in the pressure readings. Although subarachnoid and intraventricular pressures correlate well with each other, there have been inconsistent correlations between direct CSF pressure and the various epidural techniques.

1. Advantages:
   a. Less invasive
   b. Anterior fontanelle monitoring is possible
2. Disadvantages:
   a. Questionable reflection of CSF pressure
   b. No route for CSF drainage and sampling
   c. Volume-pressure responses not feasible

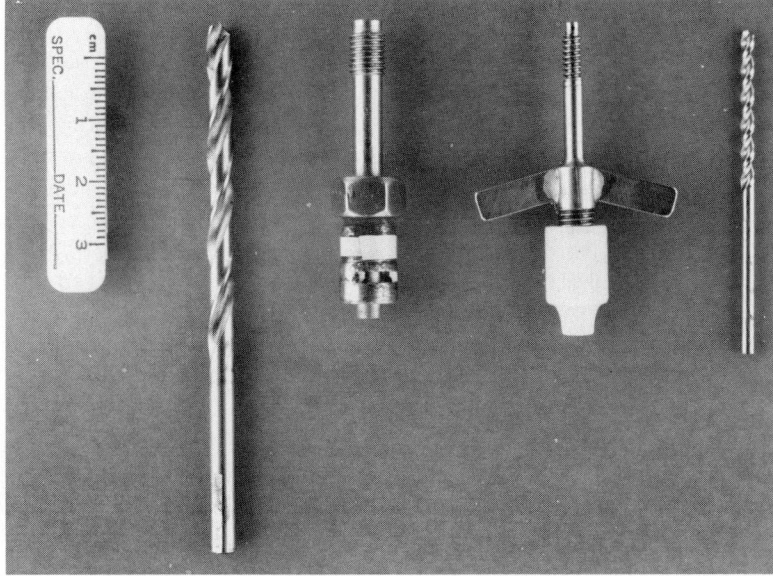

Figure 4-21   Subarachnoid ICP measurement devices. (*Courtesy of Camino Laboratories.*)

Telemetry Technique Telemetry systems are available for use with both epidural and intraventricular devices. They are designed for monitoring long-term patients such as those with hydrocephalus, those undergoing chemotherapy for brain tumors, and patients with some metabolic encephalopathies.[9]

Waveforms The type of pressure measurement technique will affect the waveform pattern. Hemodynamic and respiratory oscillations can be observed in the intracranial pressure traces. At times, the waveforms closely resemble arterial pressure waveforms (Fig. 4-22).

Certain patients exhibit a phenomenon know as *plateau waves*. These are exhibited as spontaneous, rapid increases in pressure to 50 to 115 mmHg and usually occur in patients with existing elevations of intracranial pressure. They last approximately 15 to 20 min and are usually accompanied by a temporary increase in neurologic deficits. Patients who sustain ICPs greater than 50 mmHg for periods longer than 20 min usually have a poor prognosis. Although the mechanisms of plateau waves (A waves) are not clear, they have been correlated with certain clinical conditions. An increased frequency of plateau waves in the patient with an aneurysm has been correlated with a tendency to rebleed. Although B and C waves have been described, these do not have the clinical significance of the A (plateau) wave.

Risks Associated with Intracranial Pressure Monitoring The complications associated with ICP monitoring are minimal. The infection rate in short-term monitoring (less than 5 days) using both the subarachnoid screw and intraventricular technique has been reported in the range of 0 to 1.1 percent.

Oxygen Monitoring

Adequate delivery and consumption of oxygen is necessary to maintain life. Deviations in oxygen delivery (D_{O_2}) may result from:

1. Changes in oxygen tension (Pa_{O_2}) and saturation (Sa_{O_2})
2. The amount of circulating hemoglobin
3. Cardiac output

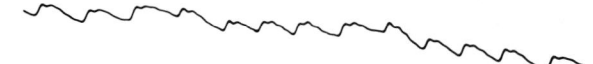

Figure 4-22 Intracranial pressure waveform.

Deviations in oxygen consumption ($\dot{V}_{O_2}$) may result from:

1. Changes in demand (e.g., shivering)
2. Impaired tissue oxygen extraction (e.g., sepsis)

These deviations in delivery and consumption may result in the failure of the oxygen supply to meet demand, leading to anaerobic metabolism, lactic acidosis, and ultimately death if not reversed.

A variety of invasive and noninvasive monitoring devices has been developed to assist in the detection of hypoxemic episodes, facilitating the initiation of treatment before complications develop. These include pulse oximeters, ear oximeters, continuous $S\bar{v}_{O_2}$ oximetry monitors, conjunctival oxygen tension monitors, and computer-processed EEG monitors. Some of the systems monitor oxygen saturation (Sa_{O_2}, $S\bar{v}_{O_2}$), the amount of oxygen attached to hemoglobin, and some of the systems measure oxygen tension or partial pressure, the amount of oxygen dissolved in the plasma (P_{O_2}). In arterial blood, approximately 97 percent of oxygen is attached to hemoglobin (Sa_{O_2}), while approximately 3 percent oxygen is dissolved in the plasma (Pa_{O_2}) (Fig. 4-23).

Oximetry is a method of estimating the oxygen saturation of the blood at various points in the oxygenation cycle (Fig. 4-24). Oximeters are devices which measure light absorption, providing a saturation reading based on the amount of hemoglobin and oxyhemoglobin in the blood (Fig. 4-25).

Pulse Oximetry

Pulse oximetry is a noninvasive optical method of measuring the oxygen saturation of arterial blood, Sa_{O_2}. Available in adult, pediatric, and neonatal models, it provides early warning of undetected hypoxemia via finger and nose sensors in the adult, and finger, toe, and foot sensors for pediatric and neonatal patients.[10]

In the adult patient, the finger sensor is most frequently used to provide continuous or intermittent real-time measurements of arterial oxygen saturation (Sa_{O_2}), pulse rate, and pulse amplitude

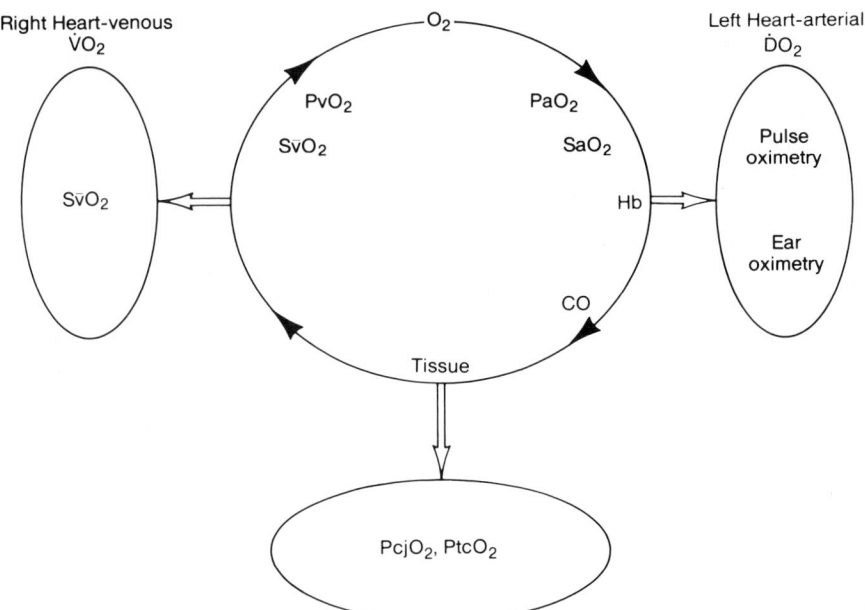

Figure 4-23   Oxygenation cycle.

with each heartbeat. The amount of arterial hemoglobin saturation is determined by beams of light passing through the tissue. The amount of color from the light absorbed by the "red" oxyhemoglobin and "blue" reduced hemoglobin in the pulsing arterial blood is determined by a photodetector and displayed as the percentage of arterial oxygen saturation. Systems are available with audible and visual alarms.

Advantages of pulse oximetry include minimal patient discomfort, patient safety, ease of use, and reliability. Limitations include error secondary to motion artifact, lack of pulse, severe anemia, presence of intravascular dyes, presence of pulsatile venous pressure as with severe right heart failure, high positive end-expiratory pressure, use of electrocautery devices, inability to measure from opaque surfaces such as synthetic fingernails, and failure to measure oxygen tension (P_{O_2}).

At this time, pulse oximeters are used most widely in operating rooms and on patients with limited movement in the ICU and recovery room.

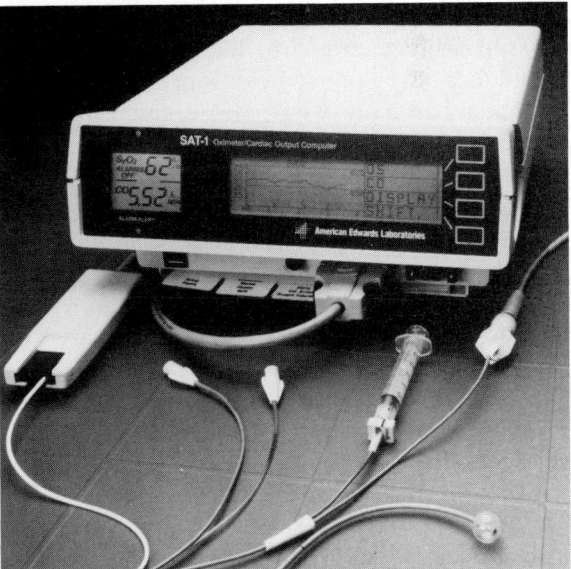

Figure 4-25   Swan-Ganz oximetry thermodilution system. (*Photograph courtesy of American Edwards Laboratories, American Hospital Supply Corporation.*)

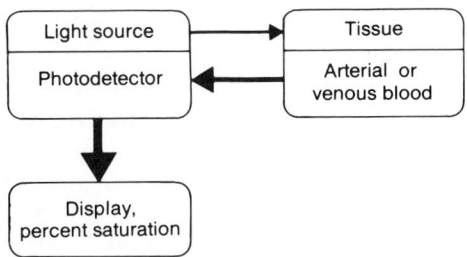

Figure 4-24   Oximetry.

Ear Oximetry

Ear oximetry is a noninvasive optical method of measuring the oxygen saturation of arterial blood (Sa_{O_2}), similar to pulse oximetry in many respects. Following placement of an earpiece on an arterialized ear, the pinna of the ear is penetrated by a light pulse passing from one fiber-optic bundle to another and then to a digital processor.

Ear and pulse oximetry are considered equally reliable indicators of alterations in arterial saturation. Pulse rate and amplitude are not available from ear oximetry.

Disadvantages of ear oximetry include site limitation and preparation, calibration requirements, patient discomfort, risk of burns from the internal heaters required for arterialization, and inaccuracy with peripheral vasoconstriction.

Pulmonary Artery Oximetry ($S\bar{v}_{O_2}$)

Pulmonary artery oximetry, most commonly referred to as mixed venous oxygen saturation (or continuous $S\bar{v}_{O_2}$) monitoring, is an invasive method of measuring the oxygen saturation of mixed venous blood. It reflects the overall tissue utilization of oxygen resulting from cardiorespiratory function and tissue perfusion. At this time, it is the most widely utilized oxygenation monitor in critical-care areas. It is used in conjunction with conventional hemodynamic monitoring such as pulmonary artery pressures, blood pressure, and cardiac output. In the adult, a fiber-optic catheter capable of obtaining pulmonary artery pressure measurements and cardiac output determinations via the thermodilution method and venous saturation via oximetry is placed into the pulmonary artery. Mixed venous oxygen saturation is determined via the technique of reflection spectrophotometry.

As with pulse oximetry, the technique involves the absorption of color from light, in this case from venous blood. The relative absorption of light by hemoglobin and oxyhemoglobin reflects the degree of deoxygenation of the mixed venous blood. Following processing by the photodetector, this light absorption is displayed as the percentage of mixed venous oxygen saturation. This provides a measure of the ability of the cardiac output and Sa_{O_2} to meet oxygen demand and consumption. Sixty to eighty percent is often used as the range

for normal, although clinically acceptable values are based on a variety of variables, including the patient's baseline values and pathophysiology. Systems are available with audible and visual alarms, and hard-copy printout.

Advantages of continuous $S\bar{v}_{O_2}$ monitoring include monitoring of the end result of delivery and consumption, consistent detection of hypoxemia and hypoxia, and accuracy during peripheral hypoperfusion.

The major limitations of continuous $S\bar{v}_{O_2}$ monitoring are the requirement for an indwelling vascular catheter with the risks inherent to any invasive vascular proceeding, and the complexity of the instrumentation and interpretation.

Continuous $S\bar{v}_{O_2}$ monitoring is widely used in operating rooms, recovery rooms, and intensive-care units. It has proven of value in the management of fluids, drugs, ventilators, and other therapeutic interventions[11] (Fig. 4-26).

Transcutaneous Monitoring

Transcutaneous or cutaneous (Pt_{CO_2}) monitoring is a noninvasive method of measuring oxygen and carbon dioxide tension (partial pressure) in both adults and neonates. Skin sensors which combine oxygen and carbon dioxide sensing elements or individual sensors are available.[10]

Advantages of noninvasive cutaneous gas monitoring include the ability to monitor P_{O_2} and P_{CO_2} from one site, patient safety, minimal patient discomfort, and ease of use and reliability.

Disadvantages include the requirements for sensor placement on flat, wrinkle-free skin with high capillary density, and inaccuracy during peripheral hypoperfusion.

Conjunctival Monitoring

Conjunctival monitoring is a noninvasive method of measuring oxygen tension from the conjunctiva, providing an indication of alterations in tissue perfusion secondary to arterial circulation.[12]

A miniature Clark-type electrode located in a conjunctival sensor monitors conjunctival oxygen tension (Pcj_{O_2}) from the eyelid of either the right or left eye. This method is based on the conjunctiva being highly vascularized tissue with the capillary bed in close proximity to the surface. Blood flow

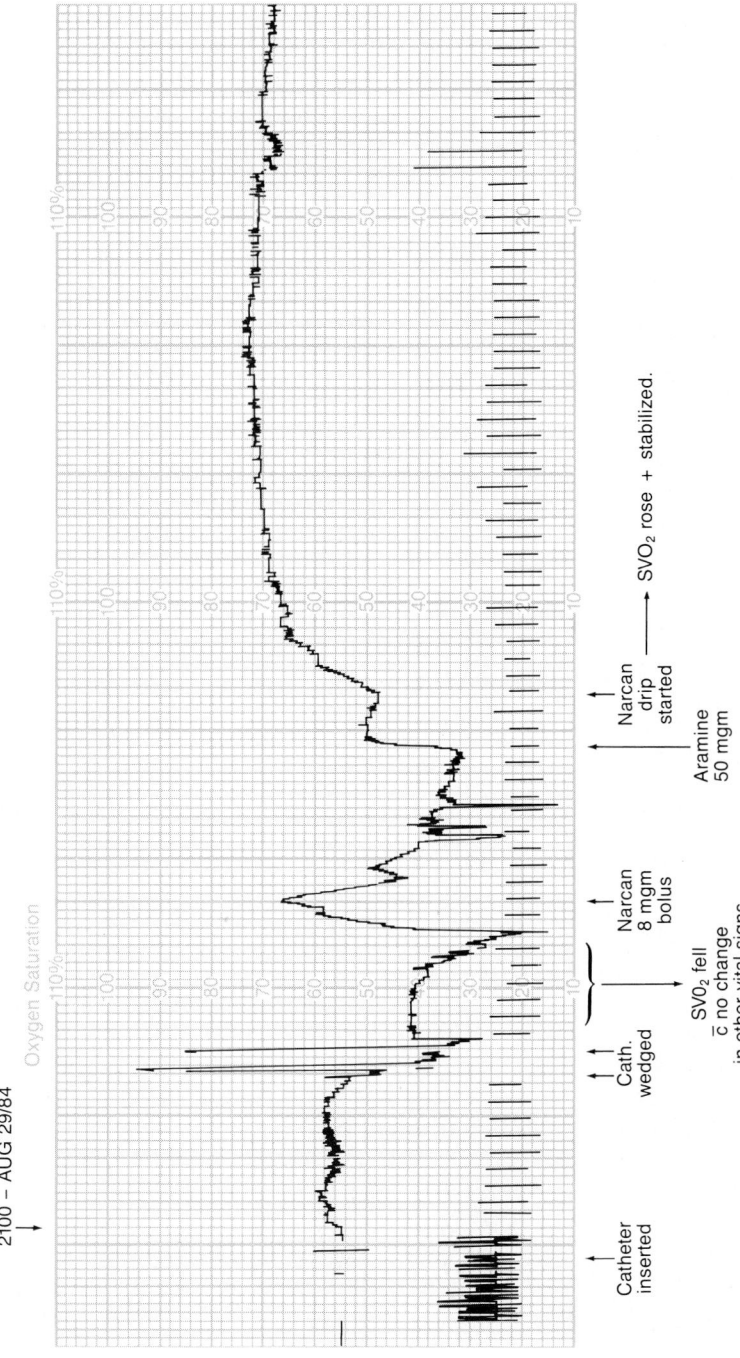

Figure 4-26 $S\bar{v}_{O_2}$ monitoring strips illustrating changes in mixed venous oxygen saturation associated with clinical interventions and patient activity. (*Courtesy of P. Preston, R. N., Hamilton General Hospital.*)

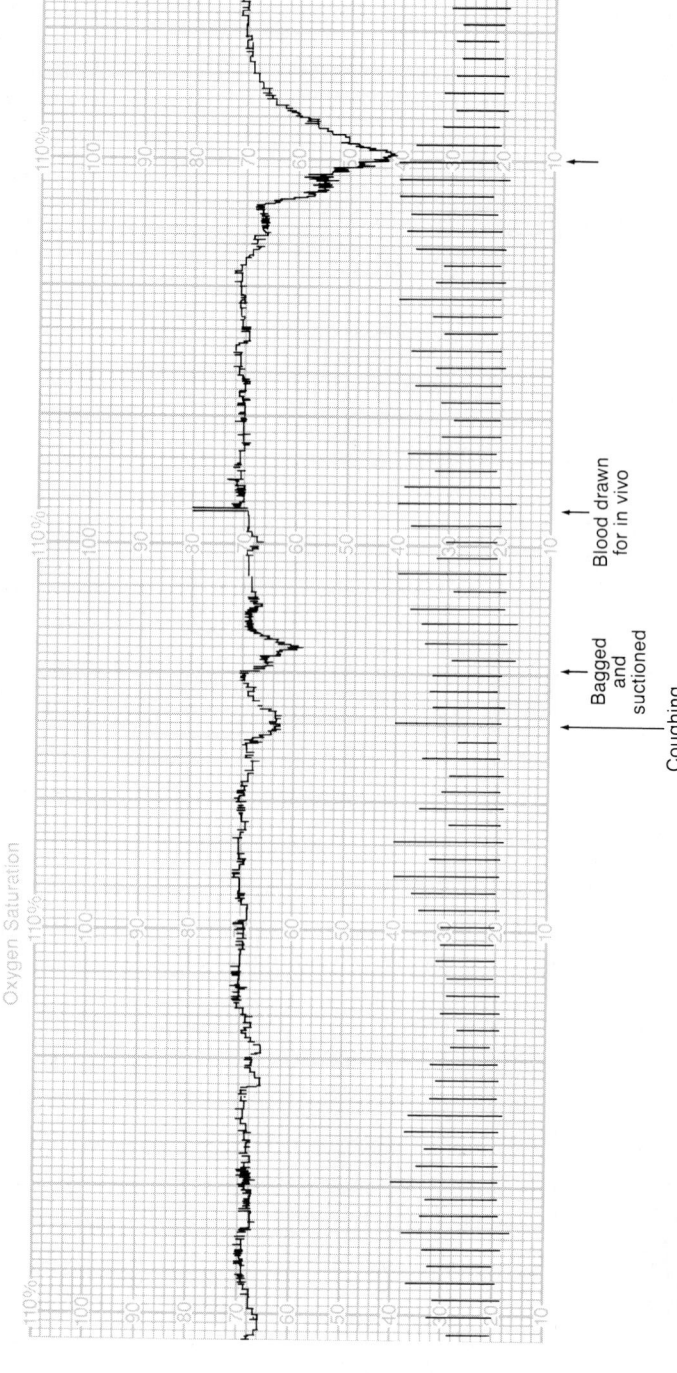

Figure 4-26 S̄v̄o₂ monitoring strips illustrating changes in mixed venous oxygen saturation associated with clinical interventions and patient activity. (*Courtesy of P. Preston, R. N., Hamilton General Hospital.*)

to the conjunctiva is primarily from the internal carotid artery. With a Pa_{O_2} of 100 mmHg, a normal Pcj_{O_2} is usually considered in the range of 60 to 70 mmHg.

Advantages of noninvasive conjunctival oxygen monitoring include the ease of sensor placement and sensitivity to changes in perfusion.

Disadvantages of conjunctival monitoring include the inability to place sensors in the presence of certain eye diseases or eye abnormalities, the inability to monitor accurately during peripheral hypoperfusion, and dislodging of the sensor by the patient's activity.

Conjunctival oxygen tension monitoring is most widely used in the emergency room, with some application in operating rooms and intensive-care units.

As with all oxygen and carbon dioxide monitoring devices, blood gas samples are used to determine accuracy and make any adjustments or calibrations necessary in the continuous monitoring equipment.

Computer-Processed EEG Monitoring

Computer-processed EEG monitoring is a noninvasive method of continuously measuring the adequacy of cerebral blood flow (CBF). Unlike conventional EEG monitoring, this new technology is relatively easy to set up and use. Raw EEG data are processed, compressed, and displayed in a format that makes significant trends in the oxygenation and perfusion of the patient's brain easy to detect. Interpretation by neurologists or EEG technicians is seldom, if ever, necessary.

These portable EEG systems have proven useful in operating rooms, recovery rooms, and for selected ICU patients. In the operating room, EEG monitors are used to show changes in the EEG caused by anesthetic agents. In the ICU, continuous EEG monitoring has been used to monitor brain activity during barbiturate coma, to document seizure activity, and to assist in prognosis. Ischemic episodes are indicated by a decrease in high-frequency activity followed by a loss of power and amplitude in the EEG signal. Most EEG monitors provide a printed copy of the trends displayed on the screen. Some have the capability of concurrent analysis and display of somatosensory-evoked potentials.

During the last few years, application of the various techniques for monitoring oxygenation have proved valuable in managing critically ill patients. The availability of early and continuous monitoring as an adjunct to arterial blood gases has proved helpful during use of vasoactive drugs, fluid administration, ventilator adjustments, and routine patient care. The obtaining of arterial blood gases, venous blood samples, and cardiac output measurements can be timed for optimal effectiveness. In selected patients, the use of oxygen and carbon dioxide monitoring devices may contribute to decreasing morbidity and mortality, as well as decreasing cost of care (Fig. 4-27).

Noninvasive Measurements

The Electrocardiogram (ECG)

The electrocardiogram is probably the most commonly monitored physiologic signal in the critical-care environment. From this signal, information can be derived about cardiac rhythm, atrial-ventricular conduction, ischemia, infarction, and so on. The clinical significance derived from the interpretation of the electrocardiogram will not be discussed in this section but rather a description of the techniques and technology attendant on its acquisition will be presented.

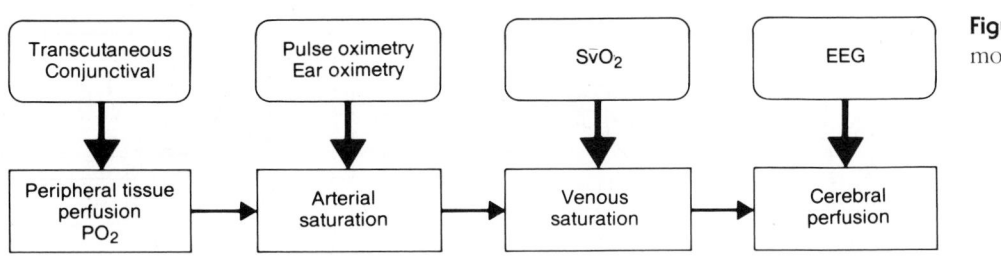

Figure 4-27 Oxygen monitoring techniques.

As can be seen in Fig. 4-28, a basic ECG monitor consists of four elements:

1. Electrodes
2. Cable
3. Amplifier
4. Display oscilloscope

Electrodes In critical-care units where reliable monitoring of the electrocardiogram for extended periods of time is required, it is particularly important that special attention be given to both the type of electrode used and the site and nature of attachment. Poor quality and/or attachment of electrodes is the single most common cause of a poor-quality signal. Although it is true that properly trained and experienced personnel are usually able to discriminate artifact and thus not be misled by it, the same is not so of the tachycardiographs (heart rate monitors) which are often part of the monitoring system. Artifact-riddled signals will often give false tachycardia alarms, and if a patient-monitoring system is given to frequent alarms, its utility will be discredited.

The electrodes commonly used in the critical-care environment are the pregelled adhesive type. The best-quality recordings are obtained when the electrode skin contact impedance is low and as stable as possible. Contact impedance for the individual electrodes should be as equal as possible; also, any potential difference provided across the electrode–skin interface should also be as small as possible and should differ little from one electrode to the other. To ensure this, the skin should be prepped by mild abrasion. Silver–silver chloride electrodes are considered best for long-term mon-

itoring applications. A chest lead system that approximates leads V_2 and V_6 was suggested by Marriott[13] (Fig. 4-29).

Cable A discontinuity in the cable which interfaces the patient's electrodes to the amplifier is probably the second most common cause of failure in an ECG monitoring system. At times a cable break may behave in an intermittent fashion, thus making troubleshooting an exasperating experience. Troubleshooting by switching cable sets is the easiest and quickest way to find this problem.

In addition to providing an interface, cables often contain resistance elements for the purpose of limiting current flow when a patient is defibrillated. Since this and other features may be included in the cable by the monitor manufacturer, using cables other than those supplied. is not recommended unless the user is infor.ned as to the special features that may or may not be required.

Amplifiers The type of amplifier used not only in electrocardiography but in the measurement of most bioelectric signals is called a *differential amplifier*. An in-depth description of this device is beyond the intended scope of this chapter. However, an understanding of its principle of operation can be very helpful to clinical personnel in quickly making the diagnosis between an external (i.e., electrode or cable) or an internal (i.e., electronic) malfunction.

A differential amplifier as used in electrocardiography is an electronic device that amplifies the instantaneous difference between the electric signals present and its two inputs. This is one of the features that makes this device suitable for the

Figure 4-28 The elements of a basic ECG monitor.

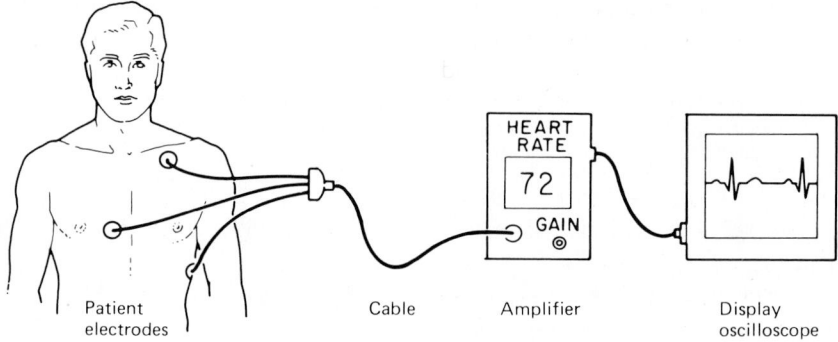

Patient electrodes   Cable   Amplifier   Display oscilloscope

HEART RATE

72

GAIN

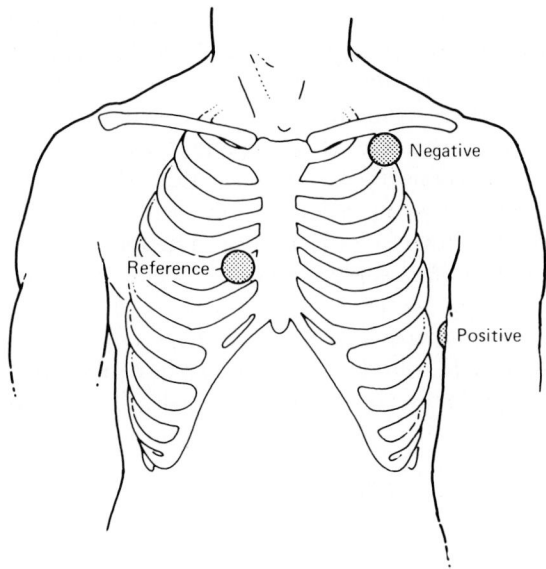

Figure 4-29   Chest lead placement. *(After Marriott, 1983.)*

amplification of electrocardiograms. Since the frontal plane representation of the electrical axis of the heart is a two-dimensional vector, the difference between two of the three basic limb leads yields a time variant signal with the dimensional component of that vector. When augmented or chest leads are monitored, a resistive network is used to sum the signals from two or more limb leads as one input; the second input is then the lead of interest. For example, *AVR* is the differential input between the sum of the left arm and left leg and the right arm. A second useful feature of the differential amplifier is the ability to cancel out signals simultaneously common to both inputs. This feature is commonly referred to as the amplifier's common-mode rejection; i.e., an amplifier with good (the higher the number the better) common-mode rejection will be less affected by 60-cycle interference.

The last feature of an ECG amplifier to be discussed is the gain or degree of amplification of which it is capable. Instruments used for the recording of diagnostic electrocardiograms have fixed gains since the amplitude of the recorded signal has diagnostic significance. In contrast, ECG amplifiers used for monitoring have either an automatic

gain control (AGC) or a variable gain control. The requirement for this seemingly nonstandard feature is mandated by the fact that these monitors often are equipped with some kind of rate indicator. Functionally these devices detect the QRS, and then the lengths of the RR intervals are used to calculate the heart rate. Because of the variety of monitoring leads used in addition to the variable effects of pathology, it is necessary for a *tachycardiograph* to have some threshold for QRS detection. The satisfaction of these threshold requirements can be met either automatically with an automatic gain control or manually by operator adjustment. It should be borne in mind that the gain needed for QRS detection is independent of, and usually not the same as, the gain required for a diagnostic electrocardiogram.

Display Oscilloscopes   Oscilloscopes are discussed in this chapter under "Recording and Display."

ECG Telemetry   The monitoring of ambulatory patients' electrocardiograms can be accomplished with the use of an appropriately designed radio transmitting and receiving system. All the factors discussed in the previous paragraphs relative to the acquisition and display of an electrocardiogram apply to a telemetry system. However, the fact that the ECG signal from the patient's amplifier to the display is now accomplished via a radio link introduces yet another dimension that may deleteriously affect the electrocardiographic signal. Most modern commercially available telemetry systems are designed so that they are unlikely to be affected by, or interfere with, other types of radio frequency. However, they are affected by environmental factors that attenuate the received signal. These factors are:

1. The distance between the transmitter and the receiver
2. The structure within which they must operate

These factors singularly or in combination can create "dead spots" from which the transmitted signal is too weak to be received properly. The staff of a telemetry-equipped unit should be made aware of any dead spots that may be present in an ambulatory patient's environment.

Pulse

In situations where it is not possible to obtain a clear ECG or when the QRS amplitude is insufficient to trigger a cardiotachometer, monitoring the pulse will provide an indication of heart rate. The device used to obtain the pulse signal from the patient is called a photoplethysmograph. This instrument contains a light source and photosensor. When the light source is directed into the skin, the blood flowing through the capillary bed, driven by the pulse pressure, will transiently make the skin more opaque, thus modulating the light received by the photosensor. This signal, when received by an appropriately designed amplifier, can be used to calculate the heart rate. The major limitation of this method is that it will not function in the presence of vasoconstriction. The usual sites of attachment for photoplethysmographs are the fingers or ears.

When the intra-arterial pressure waveform is available, some commercially available monitors are able to use this signal to derive and display the heart rate.

Indirect Pressure Measurement

In the contemporary clinical environment, the arterial pressure is probably one of the most measured and treated of physiologic parameters. In spite of the emphasis given the interpretation and management of central arterial pressure, often there is insufficient attention given to the technical details of its acquisition. Since the topic of this chapter is instrumentation, it seems logical to subdivide the topic according to the technique of measurement used, hence indirect versus direct methods.[14] It is certainly accurate to state that virtually all nursing personnel are trained and skilled in the standard method of indirect pressure measurement, i.e., the use of a sphygmomanometer and stethoscope. However, it is probably equally accurate to state that not all the users of these instruments are aware of their limitations and of all the factors that affect their accuracy. Riva-Rocci reported on the first clinically acceptable sphygmomanometer before the Italian Congress of Medicine in 1896. He occluded the upper arm with an inflatable rubber cuff until it obliterated the brachial artery pulse, thus obtaining the systolic pressure. In 1901 von Recklinghausen increased the width of the cuff from 5 to 11 to 13 cm for greater accuracy, and in 1905

Korotkoff introduced the auscultatory method for measuring the systolic and diastolic brachial artery pressures. Since that time many studies have been published regarding the accuracy, instrumentation, and techniques relevant to this method.

A discussion of the origin of Korotkoff sounds is beyond the intended scope of this chapter; however, if the reader is interested in doing further research on this subject, Geddes[15] offers an excellent synoptic review.

Goodman and Howell recognized five phases of Korotkoff sounds. Their description has stood the test of time. In their own words, they are as follows:

Phase I–A loud clear-cut snapping tone

Phase II–A succession of murmurs

Phase III–The disappearance of the murmurs and the appearance of a tone resembling to a degree the first phase but less well marked

Phase IV–Becomes less clear in quality or dull

Phase V–The disappearance of all sounds[16]

Noninvasive Automatic Arterial Pressure Measurement   *Noninvasive automatic arterial pressure measurement* is most often used in situations where the need for frequent determinations is expected to be relatively brief and the need for arterial blood sampling is very limited or absent.

There are many automatic or semiautomatic noninvasive arterial pressure measurement instruments available on the market (Fig. 4-30). They all have in common the use of an occlusive cuff; therefore, the previous discussions pertaining to cuff size and applications are relevant to these instruments. The system used to detect the systolic and diastolic pressure is either acoustic, ultrasonic, or oscillometric. The acoustic systems utilize a microphone located under the occlusive cuff to detect the Korotkoff sounds. Specially designed circuitry then determines and displays the measured systolic and diastolic pressures. The ultrasonic systems utilize an ultrasonic beam to detect the artery wall motion beneath the cuff, and from this motion information the systolic and diastolic points are determined. The oscillometric method of determination is accomplished by a sensitive transducer

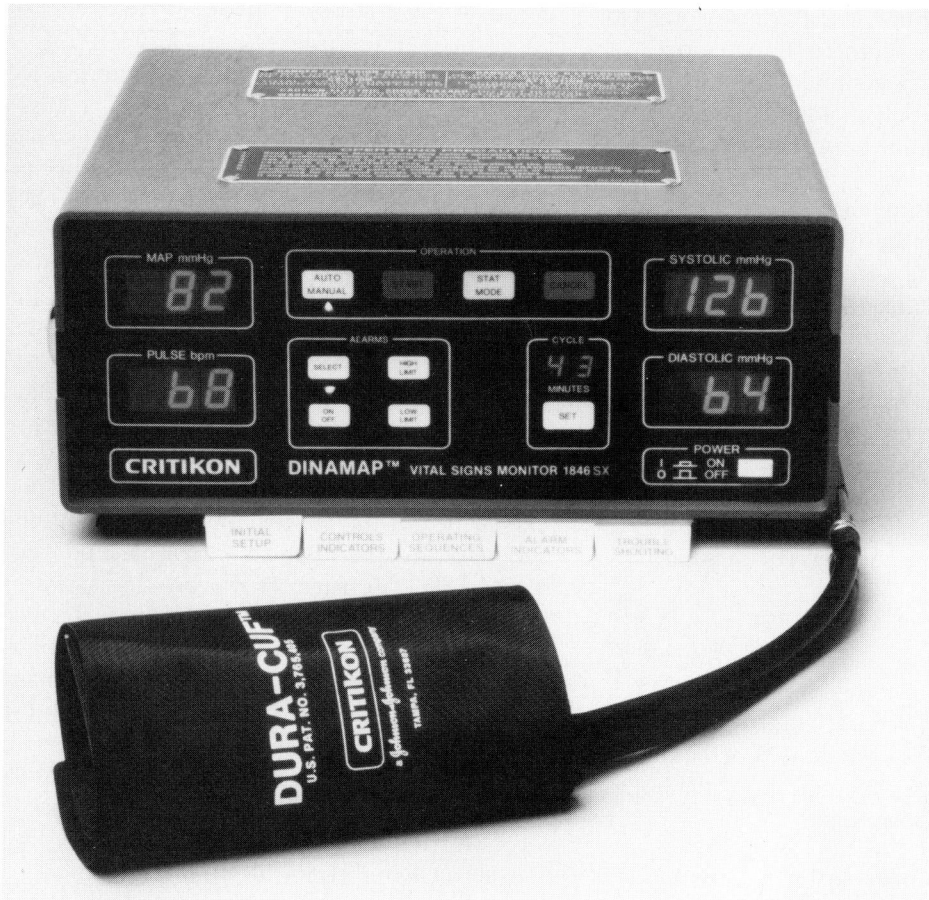

Figure 4-30   Noninvasive blood pressure monitor. (*Courtesy of Critikon.*)

which not only measures the cuff pressure, but also the minute pressure oscillations within the cuff. This method has the advantage of being able to measure the mean pressure in addition to the systolic and diastolic pressure.

These types of automated noninvasive systems make it possible to take more frequent measurements at regular intervals than would otherwise be practical. The obvious advantage of noninvasive measurement is offset by some disadvantages. The principal disadvantage of these systems is that they are sensitive to the patient's motion, and therefore, motion artifact can cause erroneous readings. In addition, if very frequent measurements are needed, i.e., once a minute, the patient's discomfort may alter the physiologic variable we are attempting to record.

The two elements that determine the accuracy of these methods are the cuff and the technique used.

Cuff Size   One of the most important factors that influence the accuracy of the occlusive cuff method is the length of the arterial segment which is compressed. This is determined by the width of the occluding cuff relative to the size of the limb on which it is applied. If the cuff is too narrow, the indirect pressure will be read higher than actual. Conversely, if the cuff is too wide, the pressure will read lower. From von Recklinghausen (1901) to the present, investigators have studied the relationship of cuff width to limb diameter in terms of its effect on accuracy.[16] The presently accepted recommendation is that the cuff should be 20 percent wider than the diameter of the arm. Because commercially available cuffs are often sized by age range (i.e., adult, child, and so on), it should be remembered that this is intended only as a guide and that the width of the cuff should be appropriate for the size of the limb to which it is applied. Circumference, being easier to measure than diameter, can be used as a determinator by using a cuff width about 40 percent of the limb circumference.

Whether the inflatable bladder within the cuff should be long enough to surround the extremity or half encircle it is not certain. In 1967 the American Heart Association Committee reported: "The inflatable bag should be long enough to go halfway round the limb if care is taken to put it directly over the compressible artery. A bag 30 cm in length which nearly (or completely) encircles the limb obviates any risk of misapplication."[17] This standard is still accepted today.

Technique   There are four factors attendant to the technique of indirect arterial pressure measurement that influence its accuracy and reproducibility. They are: (1) cuff placement, (2) deflation rate, (3) systolic and diastolic identification points, and (4) the auscultatory apparatus.

1. Cuff placement—The inflatable bladder within the cuff should be placed directly over the artery to be compressed. Failure to do so will cause the measured pressure to be higher than it actually is.
2. Deflation rate—Since the technique of listening to Korotkoff sounds is a time-sampling process, the rate of deflation relative to the heart rate will influence the resolution of the method. For example, a measurement is being made on a patient with a systolic pressure of 100 mmHg and a heart rate of 50 beats per minute. In addition, the cuff is being deflated at a rate of 10 mm/s. Will the measurement error be acceptable? Let us assume that when the cuff pressure is at 101 mmHg, and systole occurs, it will not be recorded. When the next systole occurs, the cuff pressure recorded will be 89 mmHg, an error of more than 10 percent. A deflation rate of 2 to 3 mmHg per heartbeat is recommended to accommodate both slow and

fast heart rates and to avoid unnecessary venous congestion in the distal bed.
3. Systolic and diastolic points—The criterion for identifying the systolic pressure has not changed since it was suggested by Korotkoff. Systolic pressure is recorded when the first sound appears during deflation of the cuff. Some have suggested that the systolic pressure be checked by palpation, and if higher, it be reported. The criterion for diastolic pressure has been, and may still be considered to be, controversial. Should the diastolic pressure be recorded when the Korotkoff sounds become dull and muffled or when the sounds disappear? After an extensive review of the literature, Geddes wrote: "In view of all this evidence and in the opinion and experience of the author, the point of muffling should be accepted as the most constant indicator of diastolic pressure. However, this point is known to occur at a cuff pressure above the true diastolic pressure. Nonetheless, its reliability argues in favor of its use because, in the many instances, sounds often persist well below the true diastolic pressure."[15]
4. Auscultatory apparatus—The observer's auditory system and a stethoscope constitute the auscultatory apparatus. Since Korotkoff sounds are low-frequency sounds just above the normal hearing threshold, it is obvious that normal hearing is a prerequisite for the observer. A good quality stethoscope with an intact diaphragm and ear pieces that effect a good seal is equally important in ensuring an accurate measurement.

Temperature

Continuous temperature monitoring should be, and usually is, the simplest and most trouble-free of measurements. One simply places the thermistor probe in the desired location (skin, esophagus, tympanic membrane, and rectum are the most common sites), plugs the other end into the electronic thermometer, and that's it! Actually, nothing is that simple. There are some pitfalls.

1. The cleaning solutions used on temperature probes may tend to corrode the surface of the plug which goes to the electronic thermometer. The corroded surface (not always obvious) causes

an increased resistance at the plug connection. Since the electronic thermometer determines the temperature by measuring the thermistor resistance, and the plug is in series with that resistance, the indicated temperature may be erroneously low (as much as 2°C in the authors' experience).

2. Not all temperature probes are interchangeable. Unfortunately, this is most often the case with instruments that use temperature as a control input, i.e., radiant infant warmers, warming and cooling blanket units, and so on. The user must pay careful attention that the probe being used is the one specified by the instrument's manufacturer. To restate, although all or most of the probes seem to have the same size phone plug, the thermistor in the probe may be very different. It must be checked. The normal failure mode of thermistor temperature probes is a short or open wire in the probe cable. Fortunately, this is very easy to diagnose; the temperature reading will be unrealistically high or low if one of these conditions is present. The more sophisticated electronic thermometers usually have a feature that will directly indicate a fault in the probe.

Variations in temperature occur according to the technique employed in measurement. Usually, rectal temperatures are approximately 1°F higher than oral temperatures (normal 98.6°F, 37°C); axillary temperatures, 1°F lower. Most pulmonary artery catheters contain thermistors which measure the pulmonary artery temperature and display it on a cardiac output/index computer. Since pulmonary artery temperatures are core temperatures taken directly from pulmonary artery blood, they may be higher than rectal temperatures. Because skin temperature is a function of peripheral circulation, skin probes (banjo type) are affected by changes in peripheral vascular tone.

A relatively unique method of measuring skin temperature is the use of "liquid crystals." These are commercially available as adhesive strips that change color at different temperatures.

Respiratory Parameters

Respiratory Rate   Respiratory rate may be continuously monitored utilizing the principle of impedance pneumography. Two electrodes are placed on the patient's chest, approximately midaxillary at the level of maximal chest excursion. An ECG signal may also be obtained. A respiratory amplifier displays the respiratory rate, and a respiratory waveform may be displayed on an oscilloscope and/or recorder. Amplifiers are available which indicate periods of apnea as well as respiratory rate. Apnea monitors are particularly valuable for infants.

This type of respiratory monitoring is based upon the relationship between the tidal volume and thoracic electrical impedance. As the patient breathes, the changing volume of air in the lungs alters the thoracic impedance (resistance to the electrical signal through the thorax). Thoracic impedance increases during inhalation and decreases during exhalation.

Technique and location of electrode placement are very important. Many monitors indicate if the electrodes have been adequately applied for respiratory rate monitoring. Frequently, when a patient goes on or off a respirator, the level of the electrodes must be changed. The sensitivity of the amplifier may need to be adjusted if the depth of the patient's respirations vary.

Wright Respirometer   The Wright respirometer is a low-resistance, mechanical, hand spirometer. It consists of low inertia miniature air tubing responding to airflow in only one direction. The number of liters of gas which have passed through the respirometer between two successive readings is shown on a dial. It is useful in bedside measurements of the patient's tidal and minute volumes. It is also used to monitor tidal volumes delivered by respirators. It underreads low flows and overreads high flows.[18] The respirometer may be attached directly to a tracheostomy tube via an adapter and is often used as an indicator of the patient's tolerance to ventilator weaning.

Capnometer   The *capnometer* is an instrument for determining Pa_{CO_2} with minimal discomfort to the patient. It is a carbon dioxide analyzer used on adults and infants to determine the volume percent CO_2 in expired gases. A range of 0 to 10 volume percent CO_2 can be measured. A pulmonary recorder may be attached.

The capnometer is utilized in detecting chronic hyperventilation, hypoventilation, and other similar ventilatory disorders. The instrument may be used during anesthesia and in the critical-care area for regulating ventilators to control the patient's P_{CO_2}. This limits the frequency of arterial blood gas determinations. In the neurosurgical unit, P_{CO_2} measurements are made on patients with increased intracranial pressure. An increase in Pa_{CO_2} in such patients promotes cerebral vasodilation with further intracranial pressure increases.

Most, if not all, capnometers designed for clinical use operate on the principle of absorption of infrared radiation by carbon dioxide. The radiation intensity transmitted across a sample chamber is inversely proportional to the concentration of carbon dioxide. There are two types of capnometers available; those with the sample chamber incorporated into the airway and those that draw a small portion of the airway gas through a sample chamber that is not a part of the airway (Fig. 4-31).

The sampling type of instrument, i.e., those that withdraw a portion of the airway gas for analysis, tend to be the least expensive. However, they have two minor drawbacks: (1) they are susceptible to clogging from airway secretions, and (2) they create a "controlled leak" in the airway, which may be significant in a ventilated patient if the sample volume is more than 5 to 10 percent of the minute volume. The in-line analyzers seem to be better suited to the ICU environment because they are less likely to be affected by secretions, and they require that no gas be taken from the airway. In addition, at least one of these units is designed with a built-in calibration capability which is a significant convenience, since it eliminates the need to order special calibration gases.

Mass Spectrometer   These instruments are used for the continuous or intermittent monitoring of airway, tissue, and blood gases. In respiratory monitoring, gas is withdrawn from the airway by the instrument's vacuum system. Blood gas monitoring is done via the use of special catheters that have semipermeable membranes. These catheters permit dissolved gases in the plasma to be withdrawn for analysis. Mass spectrometers have rapid response times, which make them suitable for breath-by-breath respiratory analysis. There are two types of mass spectrometers available. Magnetic mass spectrometers are capable of measuring multiple gases (up to eight); however, installation and/or modification to obtain different gases require internal alterations. The main advantage of the magnetic mass spectrometer is that it requires little operator intervention after the critical set-up. With Quadrapole mass spectrometers, the operator can tune the instrument to sample any gas or gases (up to eight) desired; however, this device requires significant operator intervention and is probably best suited for use in a pulmonary laboratory rather than at a patient's bedside.

Respiratory Waveforms   A mechanical ventilator's airway pressure and volume measurement apparatus are, in most institutions, used to monitor respiratory function. The information yielded is mainly quantitative rather then qualitative. The acquisition and monitoring of qualitative parameters require the acquisition of respiratory waveforms.

Figure 4-32 (see page 74) shows the variables acquired by a computerized respiratory monitoring system developed by Dr. John Osborn.[19] From these four variables can be calculated the following parameters: respiration rate, tidal volume in, tidal volume out, minute volume, inspiratory/expiratory ratio, maximum inspiratory pressure, compliance, resistance, work of inspiration, fraction of inspired oxygen, fraction of expired oxygen, end-tidal CO_2, oxygen uptake, CO_2 production, and the respiratory quotient. Although this is an exceptional example, it serves to illustrate how much information can be obtained by having respiratory waveforms available. Several recently introduced volume ventilators generate airway pressure and flow signals internally. These are available for recording and computational purposes. The airway pressure signal shown in Fig. 4-33 (see page 74) can be used to calculate not only the positive end-expiratory pressure (PEEP) level but also system resistance and total chest compliance when the tidal volume is known. The availability of respiratory waveforms offers the additional advantage of providing the ability to more rapidly and accurately diagnose subtle ventilator malfunctions.

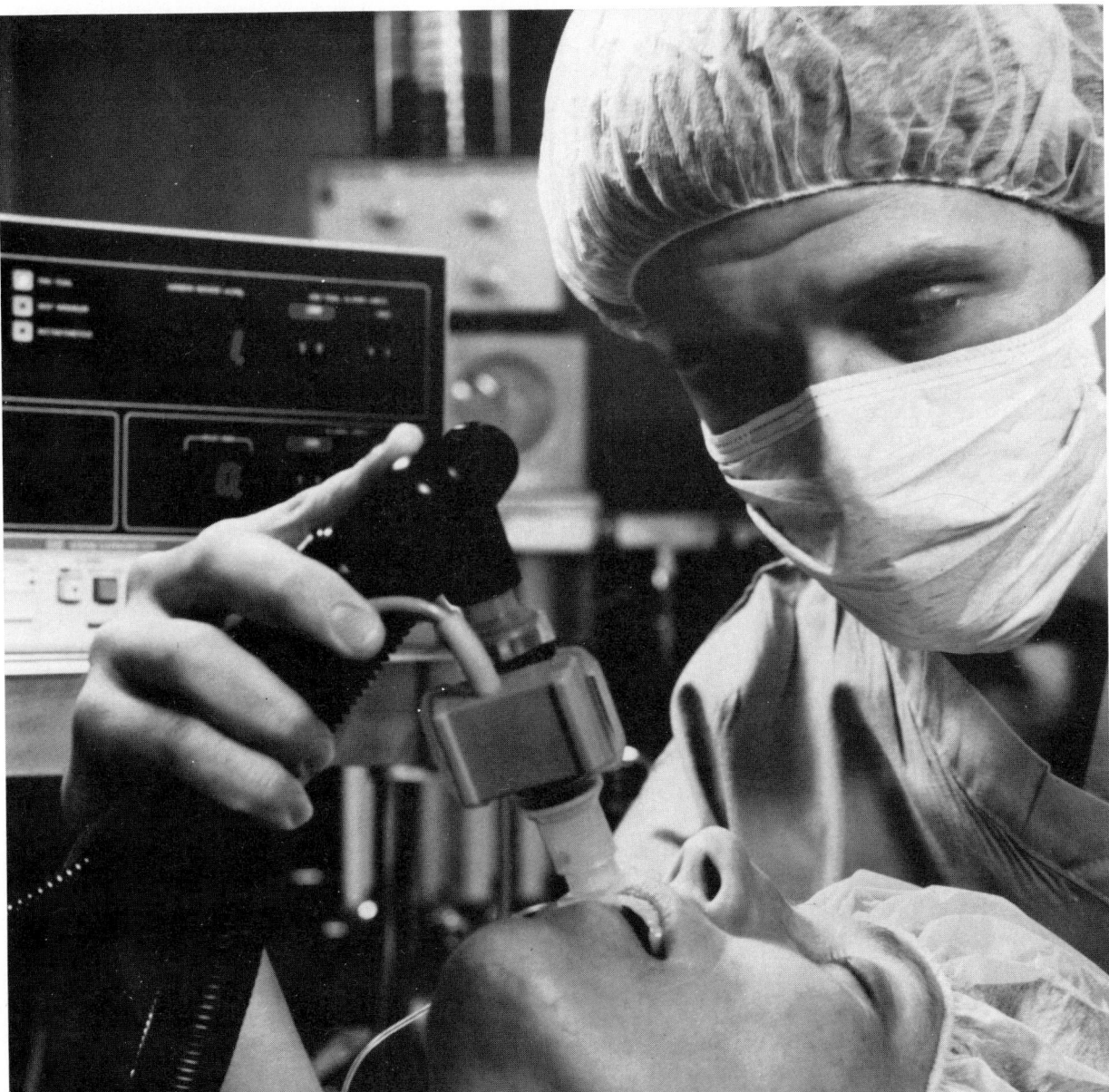

Figure 4-31 An airway-mounted carbon dioxide analyzer is shown mounted between the "Y" piece and the endotracheal tube of a ventilator circuit. (*Courtesy of Hewlett-Packard Company.*)

Therapeutic Instrumentation

Defibrillators

After its development in 1962 by Dr. Bernard Lown, the direct current (dc) defibrillator rapidly became a fundamental necessity in the critical-care environment. Defibrillators, relative to most other medical instruments, are internally rather simple. They function by first charging a large capacitor to a high voltage. When triggered by the operator, or if synchronized by the ECG, the capacitor is dis-

Figure 4-32 Computer-acquired respiratory wave-forms.

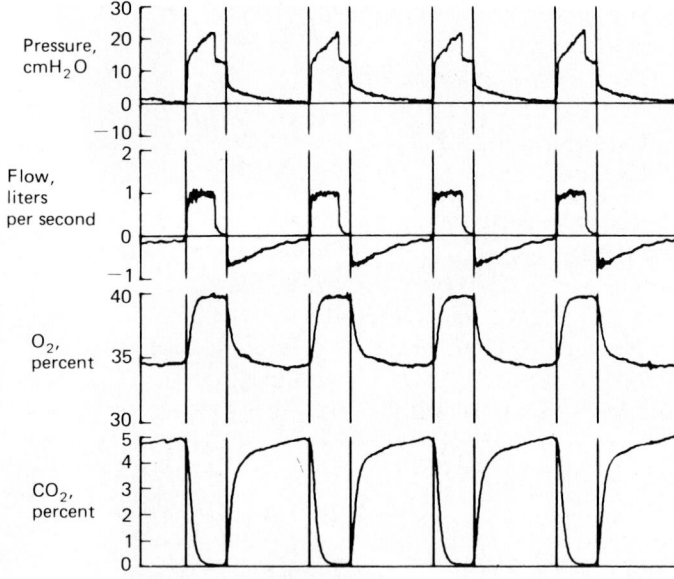

charged within a few milliseconds across the patient's chest. An inductor, in series with the capacitor, is used to damp the output waveform and thus eliminate a sharp current spike that would otherwise occur at the beginning of discharge.

In spite of their simplicity, defibrillators, like all other machines, are subject to failure. It is imperative that these instruments undergo frequent functional checks. There are three levels of testing that can be applied to defibrillators. All involve discharging the device into a simulated patient load (50 Ω) and obtaining some indication of its output. The simplest test uses a neon bulb to indicate that some threshold, commonly 75 to 100 W·s, has been met or exceeded. Although these test devices are built into many defibrillators, they provide only minimal information as to the unit's function. The second level requires the use of a calibrated defibrillator tester. This instrument has a readout that

records the energy output of the defibrillator in watt-seconds or joules. The third level requires that the discharge voltage waveform be displayed for analysis. It is the only way to recognize certain faults, such as transient spikes, that may occur in an apparently functional unit. The last two tests are best done by qualified electronic personnel.

The preceding functional tests help ensure that patients will be properly served. Visual inspection of the paddle insulators and cables for cracks and for fraying is equally necessary to protect the clinical staff.

Successful electroversion requires that sufficient electric energy to depolarize a critical mass of myocardial cells be passed through the heart. This is a deceptively simple concept in patients with an intact chest. The principal factors that influence how much energy passes through the myocardium are the following:

Figure 4-33 Airway pressure with PEEP.

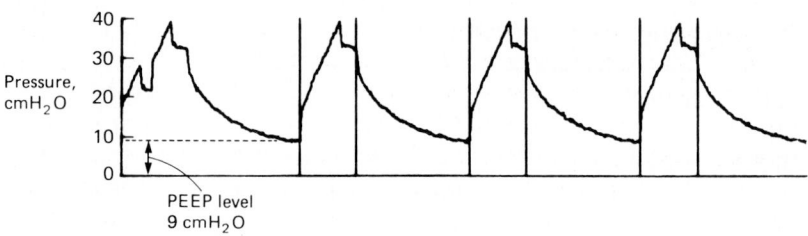

1. The power stored in the defibrillator at the time of discharge
2. The location of the paddles
3. The size of the paddles
4. The electrical properties of the coupling paste
5. The pressure applied to the paddles

The last three factors determine what the paddles' impedance will be, and this influences how the stored charge will be transferred to the patient.

Current will follow the path of least resistance. To be sure that the heart is a major part of the current path, for anterior placement one paddle electrode should be placed over the cardiac apex, the other at the right upper sternal border. The optimal location for the second paddle, whether anterior or posterior, has not been conclusively determined. However, there does seem to be some advantage in using the large (12.8-cm-diameter) posterior paddle because it presents a lower impedance. Despite the defibrillator's universal acceptance, there still remain certain unanswered questions pertaining to its optimal use. For example, we do not know how to calculate the optimal dose for a given patient or what the toxic dose will be for that patient. We do not know whether energy or peak current is clinically the most relevant way to measure dose. Energy is presently used, probably because it is technically easier and cheaper to measure. More research must be done before definitive answers to these questions are found.

External Pacemakers

External pacemakers contain circuitry for generating stimulating pulses at adjustable rates and for controlling their current or voltage intensity. The electric pulses applied to the heart are generally in the range of 5 to 15 V, or up to 20 mA, and have a duration of 1.5 to 2.5 ms.

Pacemakers are connected by wires that are attached directly to the surface of the heart (surgically implanted) or by catheter electrodes that are introduced transvenously into the right ventricle. There are various types and manufacturers of external pacemakers. These instruments have a wide variety of special features. The most common feature is *sensing,* i.e., the ability to sense an R wave and inhibit the pacemaker output. Usually the R wave is sensed through the pacing wires or catheter

so that no additional connections are required. Other features may include output rates to 800 pulses per minute, used for suppression of atrial arrhythmias, and dual outputs for sequential atrial and ventricular pacing.

It is incumbent on the clinical staff to become familiar with *all* the operating characteristics of pacemakers used on their patients. In the authors' experience, the manufacturers' support literature concerning the operation and clinical use of these instruments is excellent.

Infusion Pumps

There are generally two classes of infusion pumps available today. One class is categorized as volumetric, the other as rate controllers. The volumetric type, as the name implies, functions on the principle of direct volume displacement at a controlled rate. This class of pump is the most accurate, both in terms of volume infused and minimal variation in the rate of infusion. Because of their superior accuracy, it is recommended that volumetric pumps be used to infuse potent pharmacologic agents such as sodium nitroprusside and all intravenous medications for infants and neonates. The rate controllers use drops as their measure of volume, and they control the drop rate by either pumping or restricting the flow of fluid to the patient.

The mechanical designs used to implement these classes of infusion pumps are as varied as the number of manufacturers. Choosing a particular make and model is sometimes difficult. The following guidelines may be useful:

1. Choose a pump that will handle a variety of infusion needs, i.e., hyperalimentation, IV medications, blood, etc.
2. Calculate the disposable cost. Since most volumetrics require the use of a disposable appliance, the cost of the pump over a period of time may be insignificant compared with the cost of the disposables.
3. Air emboli detectors are a must for these units.
4. Last and most important, obtain a trial before purchasing.

Due to the wide variety of configurations and features, the set-up time and ease of use of these pumps vary.

Closed-Loop Control

A closed-loop control system can be defined as one in which a monitored parameter is driven to, or held within, a specified range. An example of the most basic type of controller is the thermostat which can be found in a refrigerator. When set to a temperature this thermostat will turn on the cooling mechanism (compressor) whenever the temperature goes above the set point. When the temperature reaches some level below the set point the cooling device is turned off. This type of controller is said to be the most simple because the controlling action can only be turned on or off at two fixed points. A more sophisticated controller would, for example, cool at different rates depending on how close or far from the set point the temperature was.

Examples of some of the most sophisticated control systems can be found in human physiology. The control of cardiac output and temperature are excellent examples of systems that are not only individually complex, but also interrelated. Applications of closed-loop systems in the clinical environment are simplistic by physiologic standards. In the clinical environment, closed-loop control has been applied to the maintenance of circulating volume, mechanical ventilation, maintenance anesthesia, and the control of acute hypertension. It has been shown, for example, that an appropriately designed control program can usually control a hypertensive patient's arterial pressure with less error than can the clinical staff.[20] Closed-loop control has the potential to improve a patient's care by adding greater precision while freeing staff for more important tasks.

Autotransfusion

Autotransfusion is the collection, filtration, and reinfusion of the patient's own (autologous) blood. A variety of autotransfusion devices is available for use in emergency rooms, operating rooms, and intensive-care units. Autotransfusion devices intended for use in the emergency room and intensive-care unit are usually designed for the reinfusion of whole blood, whereas operating room devices may be designed for either whole blood or blood component (washed blood) reinfusion.

The use of autotransfusion is usually contraindicated in the presence of contamination by bacteria, bile, urine, malignant cells, amniotic fluid, or gastrointestinal contents; or in the presence of a substance not intended for intravenous use (e.g., topical hemostatic agents); and in coagulopathies and excessive hemolysis, such as that found in injuries more than 6 h old.

Advantages of autologous blood include elimination of disease transmission, elimination of transfusion reaction, reduction of religious objections, cost-effectiveness, availability, and superior blood quality. Autotransfused red blood cells have a near-normal survival time. Autologous blood contains viable platelets and normal levels of 2,3-DPG (diphosphoglycerate), essential to adequate tissue oxygenation. In contrast, platelets in homologous (bank) blood become nonviable within 24 h and there is a total loss of 2,3-DPG within 10 days. In addition, unlike bank blood, various clotting factors remain near normal in autologous blood.

Indications for emergency autotransfusion include hemothorax (most common application) and primary injuries of the lungs, liver, chest wall, heart, pulmonary vessels, spleen, kidneys, inferior vena cava, and iliac, portal, and subclavian veins.

Preoperative autotransfusion is used primarily for patients with rare blood types, for procedures where massive blood loss is anticipated, for patients in whom isoimmunization may present a complication, and for patients who refuse homologous blood.

Intraoperative autotransfusion has been used most frequently during thoracic and cardiovascular procedures. It has also been used for orthopedic, gynecologic, general, and neurosurgical procedures. A cell washer-processor is often used to reduce anticoagulated whole blood to washed red blood cells for reinfusion.

Postoperative autotransfusion is used to collect shed mediastinal blood via chest tubes after cardiac surgery.

Although various techniques have proved safe and effective, there are certain risks associated with autotransfusion procedures. These include hemolysis, sepsis, air and particulate emboli, coagulation, thrombocytopenia, and citrate toxicity. At this time, no major complications have been reported with equipment currently on the market.[21]

Computers

Introduction

Before beginning the discussion of computer applications, it might be helpful to present some very basic concepts concerning the nature of computers.

A computer can be thought of as a functional unit or device capable of performing computations and logic operations. This device can be made up of one or more components that function together; this is what is commonly referred to as the *hardware*. However, the hardware is incapable of doing anything useful by itself. It is a little like a phonograph without a record. The phonograph has the potential to play music, but to do so it requires the information contained on the record. Like the phonograph, the computer also needs information. The information needed by the computer is a series of instructions that completely control its function. A group of instructions that control the execution of one or more tasks is called a program, also referred to as *software*.

Microprocessors are computers whose functional elements have been greatly reduced in size. In addition to their small size, the technology used to manufacture microprocessors lends itself to high-volume mass production. This has lowered the cost of these devices dramatically. Some of these so-called computers on a chip can be purchased for less than 10 dollars. The use of microprocessors has changed the way in which new equipment is designed. The computerization of what now appears to be the majority of biomedical equipment has led to increased complexity and flexibility. At the same time, the reliability of most biomedical equipment is improving. The fact that a particular piece of equipment contains a microcomputer may not be obvious to the user.

Although it is helpful to have some understanding of how computers work, it is far more important that potential clinical users have a grasp of the functional strengths and limitations of these machines.

Strengths and Weaknesses

Several benefits of computers in critical care include the following strengths:

1. Awesome computational capabilities (by human standards).
2. Able to store large amounts of data, both text and numeric.
3. Stored data can be manipulated in many useful ways.

Computers, however, have no intuitive sense or what is often referred to as common sense. A computer responds to inputs only in ways that it has been programmed to. A simple example illustrates this point. The computer is expecting a numeric entry. The operator mistakenly includes an alpha character (letter) in the entry. If the programmer did not anticipate this error at this time and had not added error-trapping capability to the program, this input would cause the computer to stop because it would not know how to deal with this input.

Even though computers have perfect recall, getting information in and out can be awkward for their human operators. Voice entry, where the operator speaks to the computer directly, is in limited use today, mainly in industrial applications. Some experts predict that the technical limitations of voice entry will be overcome by the mid-1990s. Although advances continue to be made in natural language input and voice output, these technologies are still not sufficiently mature for use in the clinical environment.

A "paperless environment" is one of the promises of computer technology. Although this goal is attractive to most of us, it must remain a goal and not a reality for the near future. If we examine superficially the path which information follows we will gain some insight into the advantages and disadvantages of computer data management. The "data circle" consists of the acquisition, storage, and retrieval of data. Acquisition simply involves getting the information. In the clinical environment there are commonly two methods of data acquisition, automatic and manual. As the names imply, one method requires no operator action while the other does (i.e., a patient's temperature can be acquired automatically by connecting a temperature measuring device directly to the computer). The technical details of automatic data acquisition are not trivial, but given sufficient resources most data can be automatically acquired.

The decision to automatically acquire data should normally be made based on a cost/benefit ratio. A good rule to follow is to evaluate a parameter in terms of how often it should be measured in order to provide the most meaningful representation of the patient's condition. For example, weighing a patient every minute is not likely to provide more useful information than if the patient were weighed every 4 h. On the other hand, measuring the arterial blood pressure every minute might give a clearer picture of an unstable patient's condition.

Applications

Bedside monitors now are available with sufficient memory to store the trends of monitored param-eters for from 8 to 24 h. In addition, some of these units have built-in calculators for drug, cardiac output, and other calculations (Fig. 4-34).

Today's technology also permits all bedside monitors in a critical-care unit to be connected not only to a central station but also to each other. This interconnection system or network allows alarm and other information to be forwarded from one bed to another. This feature can be useful if more than one patient is under the care of a single nurse. Networks also facilitate the remote access of a patient's data by one or more remote computers. This in turn enables staff to review a patient's data, permits generation of unit-wide reports, and facil-itates remote acquisition of clinical data for research purposes (Fig. 4-35).

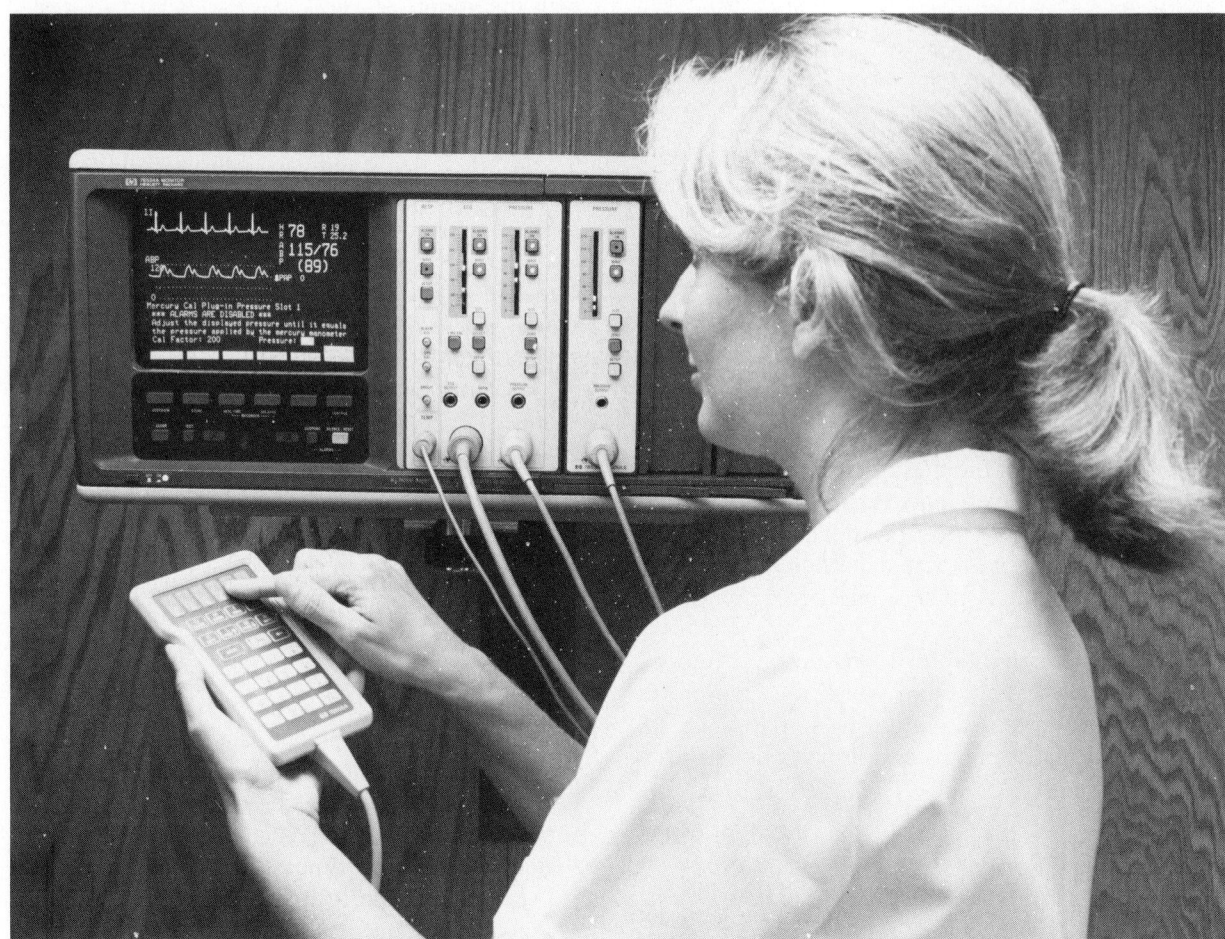

Figure 4-34   Bedside monitor with terminal capabilities. (*Courtesy of Hewlett-Packard Company.*)

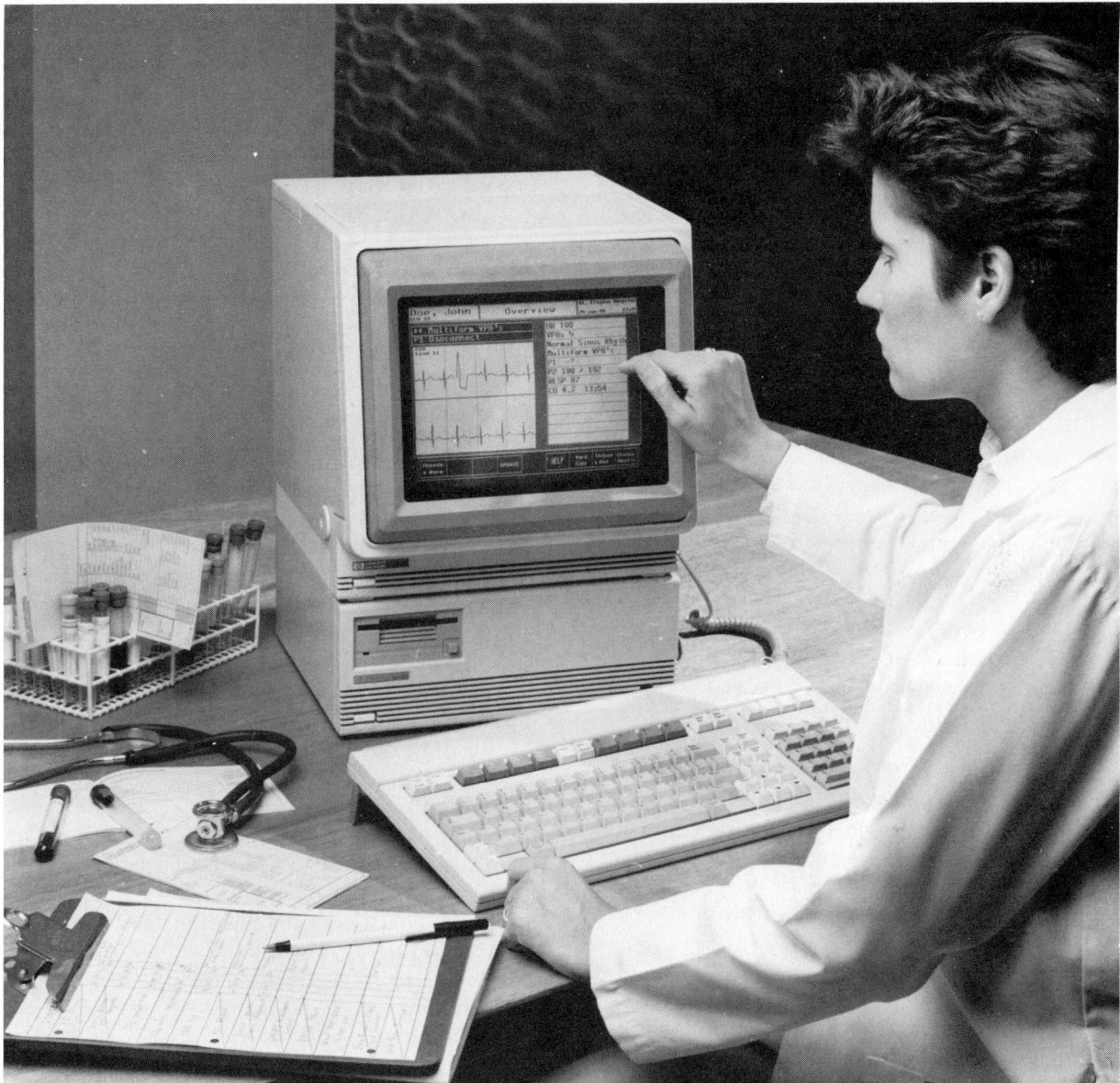

Figure 4-35   Desktop personal computer shown displaying real-time patient data sent over a network from the bedside monitor. (*Courtesy of Hewlett-Packard Company.*)

It is also possible to have bedside monitors behave as computer terminals, capable of gaining access to information from remote computers. This remote access can be used to deliver laboratory results to the bedside or to access more complex programs than can be contained in the bedside monitor (e.g., a drug interaction program).[22]

Glossary

Aerobic   Requiring oxygen in the atmosphere.

Amplifier   An electronic device which increases the gain (size) of the signal being received, such as blood pressure or ECG.

Anaerobic   Without oxygen.

Analog   A readout of a parameter, such as blood pressure, on a meter as distinguished from an oscilloscope or digital readout.

Balancing   Term used to indicate a zero output from a Wheatstone bridge; for example, balancing a transducer to read zero at room air.

Blood Oxygen Content   Whole-blood oxygen content is the combined volume of two components, oxyhemoglobin and dissolved oxygen.

Bridge   Abbreviation of Wheatstone bridge. An electric circuit useful in measuring small changes in resistance; for example, the sensitive electric circuit of a transducer which can be broken by overpressurizing the diaphragm of the transducer.

Ca_{O_2}   Arterial oxygen content. The amount of oxygen bound to hemoglobin and dissolved in the arterial blood. See blood oxygen content. Determined primarily by hemoglobin and Sa_{O_2}.

$C\bar{v}_{O_2}$ Venous oxygen content. The amount of oxygen bound to hemoglobin and dissolved in venous blood. See blood oxygen content. Determined by Sa_{O_2}, CO, hemoglobin, and $\dot{V}_{O_2}$.

Calibration   Checking output against a known value.

Cannula, Arterial   A length of Teflon or polyethylene tubing, usually 2½ to 6 in long and 16- or 18-gauge, which is placed in the patient's artery (radial, brachial, femoral) for the purpose of monitoring pressure and/or obtaining blood samples.

Capacitance   That property which permits the storage of electrically separated charges when potential differences exist between conductors. It is measured in farads.

Capacitor   A device that stores electric energy as a result of its capacitance.

Cardiac Output (CO)   The amount of blood pumped by a ventricle during 1 min. It is determined by stroke volume and heart rate. Normal range = 4–8 L/min.

Cerebral Perfusion Pressure (CPP)   Mean arterial pressure minus mean intracranial pressure, usually measured in millimeters of mercury.

Current   The movement of electrons through a conductor; measured in amperes.

Damping or Damped   Distortion of the waveform; e.g., an arterial waveform without a dicrotic notch.

Dome   The disposable plastic (Lexan) or permanent epoxy reservoir that holds the fluid connecting the patient to the transducer.

Drift   A shift in the position of the zero baseline with time.

Frequency Response   The portion of the frequency spectrum which can be reproduced by a device within specified limits of amplitude error.

Gain   An increase in size (power) when a signal is transmitted through an amplifying device.

Gauge   Same as transducer.

Gradicule   Lines applied to the face of an oscilloscope to visually indicate levels of pressure waveform, usually in millimeters of mercury. Same as grid.

Hz   Abbreviation for "hertz," cycles per second.

Hemoglobin, Hb   Hemoglobin is a combination of iron (heme) and a complex protein (globin). Oxygen can attach or bind at four different sites on each hemoglobin molecule and is measured as oxygen saturation (Sa_{O_2}). At 100% saturation, each gram of hemoglobin carries approximately 1.34 mL O_2. Therefore, at a normal hemoglobin of 15 g/100 mL of blood, the O_2 capacity of the blood is approximately 20 mL/100 mL of blood (15 × 1.34).

Hypoxemia   Inadequate blood oxygen level. A decrease in Pa_{O_2} resulting in arterial hypoxia.

Hypoxia   Tissue oxygen deficiency.

Impedance   The total opposition (i.e., resistance and reactance) a circuit offers to the flow of alternating current. It is measured in ohms.

Inductance   The property which opposes any change in existing current. Inductance is present only when the current is changing.

Inductor   A conductor used for introducing inductance into an electric circuit.

Interpolation   The estimation of a value based between two known values.

Joule   The unit of work and energy in the MKSA system. It is equal to 1 W·s (watt-second).

Lactic Acidosis   The result of oxygen demand and consumption exceeding oxygen delivery at the tissue level. An $S\bar{v}_{O_2}$ of less than 60% indicates an imbalance between oxygen supply and overall oxygen demand which may result in lactic acidosis.

Line (Arterial, PA, LAP, or Venous)   The system of a cannula in either the artery or vein which is fastened via stopcocks or by some other method to the transducer.

Linearity   Constant gain ratio between input and output through its specified range.

Manifold   A device which contains a series of stopcocks, often used for setting up two or more transducers.

Millisecond   One thousandth of a second.

Mixed Venous Oxygen Saturation   See $S\bar{v}_{O_2}$.

Module   An individual component, such as an amplifier

of a monitoring system; e.g., a blood pressure module.

Noise   An alteration of waveform and readout caused by electrical disturbance or mechanical vibration.

Ohm   A unit of resistance. One ohm is the value of resistance through which a potential difference of 1 V will maintain a current of 1 A.

Overpressurization   Application of pressure in excess of what the transducer is designed to tolerate; results in breaking of bridge of the transducer.

Oximeter   A device to continuously measure and record oxygen saturation in vivo, utilizing fiber-optic reflectance.

Oxygen Consumption $\dot{V}_{O_2}$ The volume of oxygen consumed each minute at the tissue level. It is the product of cardiac output and A-V$_{O_2}$ content difference. Normal range = 225–275 mL/min in resting adult.

Oxygen Delivery $\dot{D}_{O_2}$ The volume of oxygen delivered each minute at the tissue level. It is the product of CO and arterial oxygen content. Normal range = 900–1100 mL/min in a resting adult.

Oxygen Transport   Oxygen transport is the process of delivering sufficient oxygen at the tissue level to meet metabolic demands.

Oxygenation   The process of transmitting atmospheric oxygen to the tissue level.

Oxyhemoglobin, Hb-O$_2$ Approximately 97 percent of oxygen is bonded to hemoglobin to form oxyhemoglobin. The oxygen-carrying capacity of hemoglobin equals 1.34 mL O$_2$/g Hb.

Pcj_{O_2}   The partial pressure of conjunctival tissue oxygen. Normal range = 60–70 mmHg (Pa_{O_2} 100 mmHg).

P_{O_2}   The partial pressure of oxygen dissolved in blood plasma. Oxygen tension.

Pv_{O_2}   Mixed venous oxygen tension. Normal range = 40 mmHg.

Parameter   Commonly used to mean variables measured; e.g., pulse, blood pressure, central venous pressure, temperature, pulmonary artery pressure, intracranial pressure.

Pulse Pressure   Systolic pressure minus diastolic pressure.

Resistance   The opposition which a material offers to current. It is measured in ohms.

Sa$_{O_2}$ Arterial oxygen saturation. The oxyhemoglobin saturation of arterial blood. Normal range = 95–97.5%.

S$\bar{v}_{O_2}$ Mixed venous oxygen saturation. Measured in the pulmonary artery, S$\bar{v}_{O_2}$ is a reflection of overall tissue utilization of oxygen. It is the net result of overall cardiorespiratory function and tissue perfusion. It is determined by Sa$_{O_2}$, CO, hemoglobin, and oxygen consumption. Normal range = 60–80%.

Sensitivity   The function is the same as gain.

Servo   A device that delivers power to move a controller.

Thermistor   A solid-state semiconducting device, the electrical resistance of which varies with temperature; e.g., the thermistor bead in a cardiac output catheter.

Voltage   The force which causes current to flow through an electrical conductor. It is measured in volts.

Watt   Unit of electric power required to do work. It is the power expended when 1 A of direct current flows through a resistance of 1 Ω.

Watt-second   The amount of energy corresponding to 1 W acting for 1 s. It is equal to 1 J.

Zeroing   Same as balancing.

References

1. Verweij, Jaap, et al. (1986). Comparison of three methods for measuring central venous pressure. *Critical Care Medicine, 14* (4), 288–290.

2. Damen, J. (1986). The microbiological risk of invasive hemodynamic monitoring in adults undergoing cardiac valve replacement. *Journal of Clinical Monitoring, 2* (2), 87–94.

3. Vandenbogaerde, Johan F., et al. (1986). Comparison between ultrasonic and thermodilution cardiac output measurements in intensive care patients. *Critical Care Medicine, 14* (4), 294–297.

4. Burke, Kathleen G., et al. (1986). Evaluation of the sterility of thermodilution room-temperature injectate preparations. *Critical Care Medicine, 14* (5), 503–504.

5. Nelson, Loren D., et al. (1986). Incidence of microbial colonization in open versus closed delivery systems for thermodilution injectate. *Critical Care Medicine, 14* (4), 291–293.

6. Barcelona, Marlene, et al. (1985). Cardiac output determination by the thermodilution method: Comparison of ice-temperature injectate versus room-temperature injectate contained in prefilled syringes of a closed injectate delivery system. *Heart & Lung, 14* (3), 232–235.

7. Ricard, Pauline, et al. (1985). Protection of indwelling vascular catheters: Incidence of bacterial contamination and catheter-related sepsis. *Critical Care Medicine, 13* (7), 541–543.

8. Sundberg, G. et al. (1973). Complications due to prolonged ventricular fluid pressure recording in clinical practice, in M. Brock & Dietz (Eds.), *Intracranial pressure,* New York: Springer-Verlag.

9. Smith, Rae N. (1986). Invasive neurologic assessment techniques. In C. Hudak, B. Gallo, & T. Lohr (Eds.), *Critical care nursing: A holistic approach.* Philadelphia: Lippincott, pp. 452–464.

10. New, William. (1985). Pulse oximetry versus measurement of transcutaneous oxygen. *Journal of Clinical Monitoring, 1* (2), 126–129.

11. Davidson, Lynda J., & Brown, Sherry. (1986). Continuous S$\bar{v}$O$_2$ monitoring: A tool for analyzing hemodynamic status. *Heart & Lung, 15* (3), 287–292.

12. Chapman, K. R., et al. (1985). Conjunctival oxygen tension and its relationship to arterial oxygen tension. *Journal of Clinical Monitoring, 2* (2), 100–104.

13. Marriott, H. (1983). *Practical Electrocardiology,* 7th ed. William & Wilkin, Co.

14. Venus, Bahman, et al. (1985). Direct versus indirect blood pressure measurements in critically ill patients. *Heart & Lung, 14* (3), 228–231.

15. Geddes, L. A. (1970). *The direct and indirect measurement of blood pressure.* Chicago: Year Book.

16. Goodman, E. H., & Howell, A. A. (1911). Further clinical studies in the auscultatory method of determining blood pressure. *American Journal of Medical Science, 142,* 334–352.

17. Kirkendal, W., et al. (1967). The American Heart Association recommendations for human blood pressure determination by sphygomomanometer. *Circulation, 36,* 980–988.

18. Hill, D. W., & Dolan, A. M. (1976). *Intensive care instrumentation.* New York: Grune & Stratton.

19. Osborn, J. J., et al. (1968). Measurement and monitoring of acutely ill patients by digital computer. *Surgery, 64,* 1057.

20. de Asla, R. A., et al. (1985). Management of postcardiotomy hypertension by microcomputer controlled administration of sodium nitroprusside. *Journal of Thoracic Cardiovascular Surgery, 89,* 115–120.

21. Smith, Rae N. (1986). Autotransfusion. In C. Hudak, B. Gallo, & T. Lohr (Eds.), *Critical care nursing: A holistic approach.* Philadelphia: Lippincott, pp. 201–207.

22. Jurado, R. A., Fitzel, H. L., de Asla, R., et al. (1977). Reduction of unexpected life-threatening events in post-operative cardiac surgical patients: the role of computerized surveillance. *Circulation, 56* (3), supplement.

5

Safety

Elizabeth A.
Trought

Introduction

The words *critical-care environment* will bring many mental images to mind. What is the critical-care environment? For many it is the large, open, surgical critical-care unit with monitors buzzing, ventilators flowing, lights flashing, people shouting, and unconscious patients tied to many lines and connected to all varieties of devices. To others, the critical-care environment is the private, quiet area of the coronary care unit. Here the patient is connected to some equipment, but there is a hushed tone to both the technology and the physical environment. Between these two mental images are the many other critical-care units such as the emergency room, recovery room, medical intensive care, and so on, which are combinations of the hushed and highly stimulating extremes found in critical care.

Does the critical-care environment hold unique dangers for patients and staff? Are there any standards which should define the dimensions, shape, and design of the critical-care environment? What are the hazards associated with the critical-care environment? Are there any guidelines for nursing staff to follow for safely and effectively working within this unique environment? This chapter will attempt to provide the reader with an appreciation for and at least some preliminary answers to the questions raised above.

The critical-care environment is a complex area where new technology and techniques of patient care abound. Innovation is the rule rather than the exception. Application of electronics and physics to enhance techniques of patient care has led to improved capabilities of diagnosis and therapy. Along with these benefits have come hazards associated with equipment and the critical-care environment itself.

A *hazard* is a possible source of danger. It may threaten or involve a patient, nurse, or any other member of the health care team. For a device, support system, or procedure to be labeled hazardous, no actual injury need occur. Even a reasonable probability of injury justifies the label "hazardous."

Nurses and other health professionals frequently and unknowingly aid in developing a hazardous care environment by their attitude of acceptance and enthusiasm for all that is "new technology." The lack of critical acceptance of new devices and support systems contributes to the problems associated with managing patients in a critical-care environment. Institutions frequently buy medical devices or build in specified "necessary" support systems for critical-care units on the advice of health professionals. Nurses involved in these decisions frequently speak not from knowledge, but on the basis of brochures read or a sales representative's statements about safety and performance. Careful evaluation and clinical analysis of safety and performance should not be replaced by enthusiasm for new technology. Qualified engineering advice should be sought in environmental design and device selection, either through in-house experts or special consultants. Most new equipment should be used and evaluated by clinical staff prior to final selection of a vendor. The first step in providing a safe critical-care environment is adequate design and critical purchase of safe and effective technology.

Hazards may be inadvertently designed into health technology or may develop after installation and use. This implies a responsibility to the purchaser to incorporate safety checks prior to use and evaluation of equipment periodically thereafter. Institutions which have developed such safety programs have frequently found support systems and medical devices that simply do not operate according to their specifications upon delivery or installation. They have also found that the ability to identify problems with periodic checks has prevented some hazardous situations. It is obvious that an institution which is going to offer critical-care services must have not only specially trained health professionals and quality technology, but also an adequate engineering support service.

The density of technology in use in most critical-care units causes some common hazards revolving around the use of electricity and the devices themselves. These hazards will be explored in an effort to provide background information and some basic methods for preventing and safely handling these problems. Then issues relating to the unique clustering of vulnerable patients requiring complex procedures will be explored, with recommendations on how to protect patients and staff from the hazards inherent in these situations.

Potential for Injury to Staff and Patients

Electrical Safety

In considering the issue of electrical safety, it is necessary to put it into perspective. Electrical hazards in hospitals have received a great deal of publicity. The Food and Drug Administration (FDA) has estimated that more than 1600 injuries and 100 deaths are caused by electrical equipment annually. Hazards associated with the use of electronics include electric shock, fire, and explosion. Sparking and overheating of electrical equipment are documented causes of hospital accidents. In critical-care units these events become particularly important since the frequent use of oxygen provides an environment which more readily supports fire.[1] Some authorities think the FDA estimated injuries and deaths are exaggerated; nevertheless, the possibility of electrical hazards must be acknowledged, and prevention of injury to both patients and staff must be a realistic goal for every health care institution.[2]

To attain the goal of prevention of electrical hazards, it is necessary for the health care team at the bedside to participate in an active program of electrical safety. Nurses must understand some basic principles of electricity and acquire safety habits in surveying the critical-care environment and handling equipment to participate responsibly in this program.

To understand electricity and how it works in the environment, it is necessary to master a new vocabulary. Many texts and monographs are available which provide in-depth discussions of electricity for those who would like to pursue this interest. The following discussion reflects the belief that nurses need no more than a cursory knowledge of electricity to perform safely in a critical-care environment, if they follow electrical safety guidelines.

The Basics of Electricity

Electricity is simply a form of energy which has magnitude (force) and travels in a certain direction. Conceptually, consider that the world is made of atoms. Each atom consists of a central nucleus and rings of particles called *electrons*. The electrons in the rings farthest from the nucleus have the ability to move to the rings of an adjacent atom. The movement of electrons from atom to atom is the flow of electricity. The directed movement of electrons is electricity and is commonly called *electric current* (Fig. 5-1).

Voltage is the pressure needed to force electrons to move from atom to atom. Voltage is necessary for electrons to flow, and, therefore, for electric current to flow. A *volt* (V) is the unit of measurement for this pressure or electrical potential. Generally, voltage comes through power lines and in the United States is around 110 to 120 V, except for specially wired areas which receive 220 to 240 V to provide electric current for particular appliances such as stoves, air conditioners, x-ray equipment, and so on.

There is also a unit of measurement for how much current is flowing. An *ampere* (A) reflects the

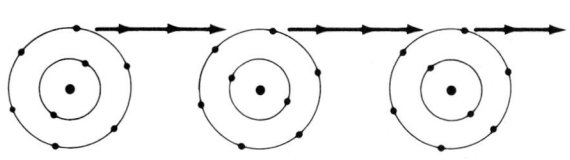

Figure 5-1   Electric current. The arrows indicate the movement of electrons from atom to atom.

number of electrons passing a given point per second. The materials which carry electricity in homes and hospitals typically have an electric current capacity of 15 A.

Different materials either enhance or restrict the flow of electrons or the flow of electric current. An *ohm* (Ω) is a unit of measurement which indicates a level of resistance to electric flow. The factors which influence the amount of resistance in any material are numerous, but generally are (1) the individual components of the material, and (2) the diameter of the material. Individual components of material allow their classification as either conductors or insulators. *Conductors* are materials which permit the easy flow of electricity. All metals are conductors, but some of the best are copper, silver, gold, aluminum, nickel, iron, and zinc. Copper wire is the most widely used conductor of electricity.

The diameter of a material also affects the flow of electricity. The thicker the diameter of a conductor, the more current can flow; therefore, large-diameter conductors offer less resistance than thin, smaller-diameter conductors.

Insulators are the opposite of conductors. *Insulators* are highly resistant to the flow of electrons. That is, they do not allow an electric current to flow through them. Some examples of widely used insulators are rubber, mica, porcelain, glass, plastic, cotton, and ceramics.

A final unit of electrical measurement is the watt. A *watt* (W) is a unit of electric power and reflects the rate at which energy is used. Different electric devices consume different amounts of power. For example, a small light bulb uses only 10 W of power, while an electric toaster uses approximately 1000 W. This is because more electrons are needed to heat the large heating elements in the toaster as compared to the small filament in a light bulb.

To harness the energy of electricity to perform work, the electric circuit is used. An electric circuit always has a certain configuration. It begins with a power source of electrons. A power source may be a battery which supplies electrons because of internal chemical reactions or an electric power generating station which supplies electrons by mechanical means.

The electric current flows on a lead wire (conductor) which is surrounded by a layer of insulation. The insulation restricts the flow of electrons to the conductor. The flow of electric current is initially from the power source, via the lead wire, to the device which uses electricity. From the device, the current then flows along a second wire, the return wire, back to the power source via a connection to a physical ground. For any circuit to be complete so that current may flow, all four components must be intact. Generally the lead wire of the circuit is called the *hot wire* and the return wire is called *neutral* (Fig. 5-2).

Switches function to control the current flow through the circuit. When an electric switch is off, the continuity of the circuit is broken so electric current cannot flow. When the electric switch is on, the continuity of all four parts of the circuit is reestablished and the current can flow. Fuses and

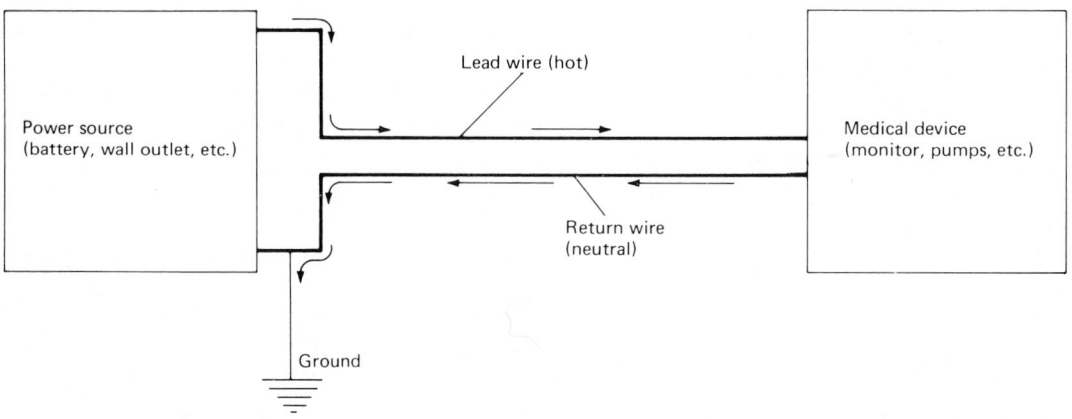

Figure 5-2   Electric circuit. The arrows indicate the movement of electrons through the circuit.

circuit breakers are only protective switches which will interrupt the continuity of the circuit if the electric current level becomes too high. The only difference between a fuse and a circuit breaker is that a fuse must be replaced to reestablish the circuit, whereas a circuit breaker needs only to be reset.

In summary, electricity can be channeled to do work whenever an electric circuit is intact. In a hospital all that is needed to power most electric devices is an electric system which has a lead wire (hot wire) connected to a power source and a return wire (neutral wire) connected to a ground. A device is then attached to this electric system by a plug which connects lead wires and return wires. When the device is switched on, the electric current will flow through the circuit, causing the device to become operational.

Safety

For safety reasons, a third wire has been added to the electric system in all patient-care areas and in most other areas of institutions as well. This third wire, or ground wire, is a conductive low-resistance connection to a physical ground. It connects to the metal frame or chassis of an electric device and provides a pathway for any stray current which might be on the chassis to return to ground safely.

To understand how a grounding system provides a safer electrical environment, it is important to remember that the return wire (neutral wire) of any electric circuit is merely a means of returning the flowing electrons to the physical earth where they can be returned to a source. Therefore, anything which would allow the flow of electrons (electric current) back to the physical ground, when brought into contact with a lead wire, will complete a circuit. People standing on floors in buildings with metal frames which connect to the earth could allow such a flow when brought into contact with a source of electric current. This generally does not happen because electricity follows the path of least resistance, and the human body, though a conductor, is higher in resistance than the return wire. However, if the return wire is broken or if current inadvertently comes into contact with metal not attached to the return wire (a fault), then it is possible for an individual to complete a circuit (Fig. 5-3). The grounding system serves to prevent this accident from occurring by providing a backup low-resistance pathway for any current to follow which contacts the chassis of a device.

Electric systems in critical-care environments must be designed not only to protect personnel and patients from the obvious hazard of becoming part of a circuit when a fault develops, but also to protect patients from small amounts of current called leakage current. *Leakage current* is the loss from the electric circuit of minute numbers of electrons onto the metal frame or chassis of an electric device. These currents are typically small in comparison to the current which flows through the device in operation and usually present no hazard to a normal person. However, these leakage

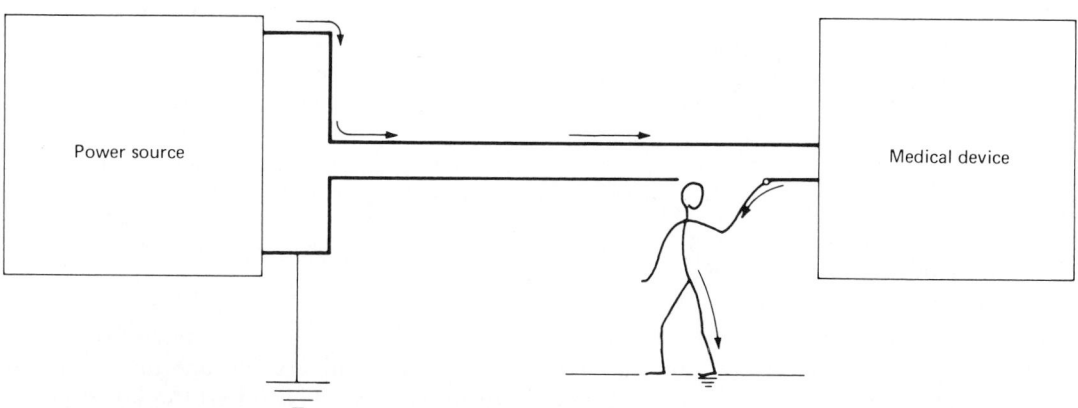

Figure 5-3   The stick figure represents a human who is completing a faulty circuit. This hazard can be prevented by properly grounding the electric circuit.

currents are hazardous to patients who have direct connection, or current pathways, to the heart. Transvenous and transthoracic pacemakers, pulmonary artery lines, and such, all effectively bypass the patient's skin and provide direct pathways to the heart. Patients with such devices in place are termed *electrically sensitive* or *electrically susceptible* because leakage currents, though very small, can disrupt the normal electrical function of the heart when introduced to the heart via a current pathway. The possibility of this occurrence is frequently termed *microshock hazard.* Most critical-care units today are designed to prevent this occurrence by providing effective grounding equipment so all leakage current bypasses patients. Also, special electrical isolation systems have been added to most monitoring systems as well as other devices which prevent patients from inadvertently becoming alternative ground pathways for electric currents if the ground system fails.

Nurses can greatly enhance safe patient care by following the steps for electrical safety given in Table 5-1. The point of a grounding system most susceptible to damage is the plug and the line cord of an electric device; therefore, they must be handled particularly carefully. A routine electrical safety program should be carried out by the hospital engineering department or service consultant. This should include examination of all new devices for electrical safety prior to use, and periodic checking of outlets and devices for intact wiring on a routine basis.

Technological Safety

The recognition of the electrical safety problem in critical-care units has led to a proliferation of information concerning that issue. This has frequently resulted in an overemphasis on the electrical safety problems in critical-care units and has caused practitioners to forget that all devices and support systems have other hazards inherent in their use. It is important to remember that a functional failure of any device or support system can be just as lethal as an electric shock and is perhaps more likely to occur in a critical-care unit.

Examples of nonelectrical hazards associated with critical-care technology are not uncommon and represent almost every class of equipment

Table 5-1 Three Steps to Electrical Safety

1. Handle equipment with care.

   Do not step on or roll equipment over plugs or line cords.

   Do not remove a plug from an outlet by pulling on the line cord itself.

   Do not use any piece of equipment which has a damaged plug or line.
   Inspect all cords for cracked or frayed insulation. Always coil line cords properly to avoid kinks. Keep line cords out of traffic paths and away from sources of heat (radiators). Have the hospital engineering staff replace all damaged plugs and line cords.

2. Be alert to signs of trouble.

   Report all outlets which do not firmly hold a plug. A plug that is loose in an outlet indicates that the outlet must be replaced.

   Report all complaints of shock, even if a slight tingle is felt.
   Realize that a small amount of electric current through the body is not harmful, but may be sufficient to cause fibrillation if it flows through a patient's heart.

   Report anything suspicious immediately. Unplug equipment that is giving off smoke, sparks, or strange noises. Place a prominent warning sign on any faulty equipment that reads, "Do Not Use," and call the hospital engineering department immediately.

3. Follow electrical safety guidelines.

   Never use equipment with two-wire cords and plugs in the vicinity of patient. Have the hospital engineering staff rewire all two-wire equipment with three-wire cords and plugs.

   Never use a "cheater" adaptor to connect a three-wire plug to a two-wire outlet. Have the hospital engineering staff replace all two-wire outlets with three-wire outlets.

   Never break off the third prong (ground) of a plug or use a plug with this prong broken off. Have the hospital engineering staff replace all damaged plugs.

   Never use two-wire extension cords to connect electrical equipment. Extension cords should be avoided, but if used, must have three wires and be as heavy duty as the line cord of the equipment.

used. Not too many years ago, bag-mask resuscitators were available in critical-care units without nonrebreathing valves or standard 15-mm adaptors. Nurses, respiratory therapists, and physicians used this equipment, accepting without criticism design faults which essentially provided recycled CO_2 to patients rather than oxygen, and wasted precious minutes during crises while staff tried to identify and attach various-size adaptors.

Examples

Every critical-care nurse can cite examples of devices with manufacturing defects which have seriously endangered patients. The list of examples could be enormous; a few which serve to illustrate this point are the following:

The pulmonary artery catheter with a defective balloon which no one discovered prior to insertion, therefore requiring repetition of a serious procedure

The endotracheal tube whose balloon slips down during inflation, thus obstructing the patient's airway

The intravenous infusion regulator which allowed excess volume to be flushed into a patient with tenuous cardiac function

Gas systems are used in all critical-care units to drive ventilators, provide oxygen, and apply suction. There is nothing more frustrating and dangerous than the situation where an unconscious patient vomits and the wall suction is not functioning with a high enough flow to remove the vomitus quickly.

Another example of a hazard associated with pneumatic systems is the inadequate functioning of a ventilator in providing respiratory support because of changing pressures in the gas system. The maintenance of gas systems is essential to effectively run supporting equipment. Critical-care nurses should be alert to malfunction of these systems which may directly compromise patients or indirectly cause other equipment to malfunction. Pneumatic systems should be routinely checked to be sure that the correct pressure and flows are in fact being maintained.

All devices have evolved to perform a specific function. A device may be hazardous if it does not perform its functions adequately. For example, a defibrillator which delivers substantially less than the indicated voltage may be ineffective in converting ventricular fibrillation. This may directly contribute to the patient's death. A suction machine which does not function to adequately aspirate secretions because of inadequate airflow or other malfunctions may directly contribute to a patient's developing further physiological complications. This category of performance-related hazards has been the least explored in the literature but is perhaps the most dangerous and common in the critical-care environment.

Equipment Precautions

These examples serve to illustrate that critical-care nurses must be aware not only of the electrical safety issue, but also of how equipment and support systems should operate and therefore how they may malfunction. Nurses do not have to understand the internal workings of all equipment, and they should not be required to provide engineering evaluations. However, it is a nurse's professional responsibility to understand the actions of the technology in use and the principles of how it functions, just as one would strive to understand the actions, methods of action, and adverse effects of any drug prescribed for a patient. Understanding increases the practitioner's sensitivity to possible problems so that they can be detected early, thus avoiding harm to patients and personnel.

Common sense is the most important factor in detecting malfunction. When a device is not functioning as anticipated and one has progressed through all the troubleshooting maneuvers, the device should be replaced with another which is functioning appropriately. When a support system, e.g., gas, humidity, or temperature, is suspected of not functioning adequately, it should be reported repetitively until measures are instituted to maintain its effectiveness or alternative arrangements are provided for the support needed.

Malfunctioning equipment or support systems should be referred to an engineering support department (e.g., biomedical engineering) for repair. It is impossible to maintain a safe critical-care environment without adequate engineering support which routinely checks equipment and support systems to determine their ability to function safely and which is available for repairs when malfunctions occur.[3-4]

When a class of devices repeatedly malfunctions or a serious device-related incident occurs which may indicate poor design or manufacturing defects, these should be reported to an appropriate agency. The FDA maintains a hazardous-device reporting system, administered by the U.S. Pharmacopeia, which routinely sends reporting forms to selected critical-care and other specialty nurses. If the form is unavailable, telephone (800) 638-6725, or send reports to: Medical Device and Laboratory Product Problem Reporting Program, U.S. Pharmacopeia, 12601 Twinbrook Parkway, Rockville, Maryland 20852.

Some professionals or their employing agencies are hesitant to contact a governmental agency to report technology problems, suspicious devices, or incidents. An alternative is to report problems to the nonprofit consumer organization, E.C.R.I., which publishes *Health Devices*. Over 2000 hospitals in the United States subscribe to *Health Devices*, a comprehensive medical device safety publication and service which both alerts health professionals and agencies to hazards and evaluates the safety and effectiveness of equipment. The nursing staff should determine if its hospital subscribes to *Health Devices*, report suspected hazards on the hazard forms provided, and routinely review the publication for product evaluations and hazard alerts.[5]

Nosocomial Infection

A constant hazard to the critically ill patient is *nosocomial infection*. Infections acquired during a critical illness at least complicate a patient's recovery, and often contribute to or cause a patient's demise.[6-8] Prolonged stays within the critical-care environment and hospital due to infection have become even more problematic with prospective reimbursement programs.

Patients in a critical-care environment are more susceptible to pathogens for several reasons. First, their level of illness is associated with a lowering of their normal body defenses. Second, frequently prolonged care, with invasive devices and decreasing nutritional status, contributes to lowered resistance.

Sources

There are three possible sources of infection: autogenous, environmental, or cross infection.[9-10] Frequently, the single origin of an infection cannot be identified with certainty or the infection is found to have many sources. Many studies have shown that patients who become infected may do so from organisms found in their own intestinal and/or respiratory tracts (autogenous source).

Common nursing procedures can reduce the problem of autogenous sources of infection by reducing the numbers of organisms and/or preventing them from contaminating a susceptible site for pathogenic growth. One example is meticulous oral hygiene to prevent contamination of endotracheal tubes and subsequent respiratory complications. Another common example is a patient's touching of invasive devices with hands that have not been cleaned after elimination. The patient's hygiene is within the nurse's realm of responsibility, and it should be attended to seriously.

Environmental sources found within critical-care units are multiple. Generally, the environmental sources which most support the growth of organisms are those which provide a warm, humid environment. Some examples of frequently encountered sources within the critical-care unit are sinks, ventilators, humidifiers, suction apparatus, tubes of lubricating jelly, and stock bottles of various solutions. It is obvious that the potential sources of infection in a critical-care unit are almost infinite.

Cross infection is another source of infection which occurs when an organism travels from one human source to another. Usually, the source of the organism is another patient, and the transporter is a nurse or other health professional; however, it is not unknown for an unsuspecting member of the staff to function as a source.

Various methods have been devised to protect patients in critical-care units from nosocomial infection. Some units have tried to protect the patient by refusing admission of any infected patients to the area. This is usually not successful for several reasons: (1) The patient may be admitted prior to detection of the infection and therefore be a source of contamination to other patients, (2) the noninfected patient may become infected while being cared for in the critical-care unit, and (3) patients with sepsis must often be admitted to critical-care units for various political and/or administrative reasons. The reality exists that there may be no other nursing area that can provide the level of care the critically ill infected patient requires. Even if the infected patient could be eliminated from the critical-care environment, a poorly designed facility will frequently serve as a source of contamination to patients in the critical-care unit.

Protective Measures

Generally, infection can be controlled in the critical-care unit by the staff. The first rule should be absolute cleanliness within the unit. The physical environment should be designed to allow periodic cleaning with a liquid germicide. Sinks should be immediately available for personnel to wash hands frequently. Critical-care units should set up systems to monitor the obvious sources of environmental infection.[11] Most units have guidelines requiring respiratory equipment to be sterilized at least between patients' usage and frequently periodically during use. They also require bacteriologic testing of respiratory devices several times a week during use on an individual patient. All ventilator, oxygen, and suction tubing should be replaced periodically. Some units choose to change these as frequently as every 24 h.

Invasive devices and their attachments should be considered sources of infection. Many units change all IV tubing every 24 h, though a study by the IV team at Duke University Medical Center indicates that every 48 h may actually be preferred.[12] Transducers and other devices directly attached to invasive systems should be sterilized on a scheduled basis. Other common sources of infection within the environment, such as sinks, overflows, and water taps, should have routine bacteriologic monitoring.

The critical-care unit should be air-conditioned and its temperature maintained at approximately 75°F, with a relative humidity of close to 50 percent. A slight positive pressure relative to the outside corridor should be maintained to prevent infiltration of contaminating air. At least 12 air changes per hour are needed, and higher rates of ventilation will reduce the concentration of contaminants. The ventilation system should be independent of other areas of the hospital, preferably with no recirculation. Ideally, each room and cubicle in the critical-care unit should have an independent air inlet and exhaust, with the system balanced for equal pressure in bed areas and elsewhere in the unit.

Nurses can best protect patients from infections by washing their hands between patient contacts. Staffing should be maintained so that nurses may work at a steady pace which allows time for frequent hand washing. Remember, not only hands but frequently the tools used at the bedside (e.g., stethoscope) come in contact with a variety of patients, one of whom may be a source of infection. Equipment used on one patient should never be used on another without decontamination.

Programs for comprehensive infection surveillance should be developed in all critical-care units. Assistance in development of specific criteria is available through review of material published by the U.S. Department of Health and Human Services, Public Health Service, and the Centers for Disease Control. Consultation is available through the Centers for Disease Control in Atlanta to obtain answers to specific questions. Other important resources include the hospital infection control nurse and the infection committee.

Radiation Exposure

Exposure to radiation is a hazard both to patients and employees. Carrier and Martel[13] state that

> . . . radiation presents two basic risks. The first is somatic in nature, that is, the more a population receives radiation, the more likely it is to develop cancer. The second is genetic. The more a population receives radiation, the more likely it is to induce weakness in the next generation.

Although the development of modern radiologic equipment has reduced the degree of radiation exposure, thereby decreasing the potential for harm, danger still exists during unique situations (early stages of pregnancy) or prolonged exposure. Radiation dosage is felt to be cumulative and therefore repeated high exposures, particularly over short periods of time, could produce deleterious health effects.[14]

The use of radiographic techniques for diagnosis and treatment of critically ill patients is usually necessary for a successful outcome. Although some procedures could probably be safely eliminated and the numbers of other procedures reduced, there is no way to totally eliminate either an individual patient's or the staff's exposure. Therefore, the objective must be to reduce the amount of exposure whenever possible. There are several factors which influence the amount of radiation exposure, but the more important are exposure time, shielding, and, particularly for staff, distance from the patient. These factors can be used to develop strategies to reduce radiation exposure.

Exposure time can be decreased by the optimal utilization of the fastest film/screen combination to obtain a diagnostically satisfactory radiograph. Use of newer mobile diagnostic x-ray equipment also should accomplish this goal. However, this should be confirmed with the radiology department. Mobile fluoroscopy is frequently used during the positioning of pacemakers and central vascular catheters. The physicians who perform these procedures may not be versed in the hazards of radiation, and the procedures themselves often require prolonged time to be successfully completed. Consequently, the time of fluoroscopic exposure is sometimes prolonged. The nursing staff should be aware of this added risk and implement prevention strategies to reduce personal exposure for everyone involved.

Protective Measures

One significant method of reducing exposure is shielding. If one must provide direct care to a patient being exposed to radiation, the use of a barrier shield or a lead apron is necessary. A lead apron will reduce the amount of scattered radiation to the trunk by a factor of at least 100. Aprons should be used by nurses, physicians, and other personnel involved in lengthy procedures. Lead aprons should be kept in every critical-care unit for staff use. Each mobile diagnostic x-ray unit should carry at least one apron for use by personnel who must hold or stay in close proximity to a patient being examined. This protective strategy is also effective for the uniquely vulnerable patient and should be used more frequently. For example, with young women, where the possibility of pregnancy exists, covering the lower abdomen during x-ray examinations with a lead apron provides some protection to the developing fetus. In general, gonadal shielding should be used whenever practical.

Increasing distance is the easiest and most effective means of decreasing exposure for staff.

Remember that staff exposure comes from radiation scattered from the exposed patient. The amount of scattered radiation is reduced by the inverse square law as distance from the patient is increased. That is, if one stands twice as far away, the radiation exposure is reduced to one-fourth. Prudently locating oneself, other personnel, and students can reduce exposure to insignificant levels. If one can't leave the room, standing directly behind the mobile radiographic unit is safest.

How much exposure does staff receive in caring for patients in the critical-care setting? Herman, Patrick, and Tabrisky[15] found that maximum exposure at a nurses' station was approximately 0.05 mR to 0.2 mR per week. Their observations were made in an open four-bed surgical intensive-care unit and were based upon 20 exposures per bed per week. The beds were located 11 to 17 ft away from the nursing station. This exposure level is well below the maximal permissible dose of 10 mR per week for nonoccupational workers. Another study of CCU nurses found that measurable exposure levels were associated with length of working time in the CCU.[16] However, all exposure values were well below the recommended safety limits. Some hospitals use x-ray badges to try to monitor staff exposure, but have not found the results very meaningful as normal routine frequently finds staff members covering badges (e.g., apron covering badge while holding patient), or staff members inconsistently wearing badges. Where badges are available, staff members should cooperate fully by wearing their badges consistently.

A balance must be struck between the practice of unnecessary exposure and the inordinate fear of radiation resulting in the abandonment of patients requiring acute care during radiographic procedures. The prudent combination of distance, location, and shielding should reduce personnel exposure to insignificant levels while allowing for safe patient care. The nursing staff should have inservice instruction by the hospital radiation safety officer or consultant which includes strategies for protection for both patients and staff.

Fire

The threat of fire is one every nurse has been educated to respond to since the early days of nursing education. However, it is a threat which can become too familiar since most nurses will never see a hospital fire during their careers though they will certainly participate in many fire drills. Critical-care nurses frequently only participate in a marginal manner in fire drills, since the patient's requirements prevent interruption of care routines for the traditional simulations most hospitals go through during these drills.

Critical-care units are prime targets for fire because of their oxygen-enriched environment. Add to this the large number of specialized devices in use which can produce overheating or sparking to initiate a fire, and the staff must be prepared to deal with fires within the unit.[17] Nurse managers can ask their staff the following questions: "What would you do if you saw what appeared to be a minor explosion during an attempted defibrillation and then smoke and flames on the patient's bed? Would you use a pitcher of water to extinguish the flame or run for a fire extinguisher? Do you know where the fire extinguisher is and how to use it? Should you pull the patient out of the bed or try to extinguish the flames with the bed sheets?" These are multiple questions which require rapid evaluation and decision making in the event of a real accident. Simulation of fire emergencies are well worth reflection before they occur, with in-service time provided for training.[18]

Recent literature on actual hospital fires points out the willingness of the nursing staff to follow direction and face personal risk to ensure their patients' safety, but the need for rapid and correct responses by nurses without knowledgeable supervision emphasizes the responsibility of each nurse to become familiar with alternative actions and hospital protocols.[19] The nursing staff should know the hospital fire plan, practice fire prevention guidelines, and actively participate in mock simulations of both in-unit fire emergencies and evacuation procedures.[20] Evacuation of any bedridden patient is difficult, particularly down several flights of stairs. Plans to transport the most clinically dependent, unstable patient and life support equipment must be thought out in advance. What would you take with you to maintain the patient in the evacuation area?

Hospital fires are rare but they do happen. The critical-care nurses' knowledge may not only save patients assigned to their care but also their own lives. A review of the unit and hospital fire plan should be routinely discussed at staff meetings. Fire drills where the doors are closed and staff goes on with the routines of the shift will not help during a real emergency. A real fire will come without warning and demand more than a closed door—critical-care nurses must be prepared to respond competently.

Employee Health

Nurses employed in critical-care units are subject to most of the same environmental hazards discussed in relation to patients. Just as the nurse must protect patients, families, and other employees from radiation, infection, electric shocks, etc., the obligation exists to protect oneself. Nurses are not infrequently victims of these environmental hazards causing personal illness, disability, and occasionally even death. Nurses must become more aware of the environment within which they work, not only for the patients' protection, but for the protection of themselves and their families. The dangers are not only somatic but as with patients include risk of psychological hazards.[21] Most studies find stress inherent in nursing and prevalent in the critical-care setting. In a study on causes of death in registered nurses, Katz found an elevated risk of death from suicide for R.N.s.[22] Studies of alcohol and drug abuse also point to nursing as a profession with high prevalence. Ability to successfully cope with the stress of critical-care nursing varies with individual personality, life situation, and particular working environment. Most nurses will need assistance at some point in their professional careers to overcome particular stress problems.

Who helps the critical-care nurse control the hazards of the critical-care environment? Obviously, some other organizational components of the hospital should share in these complex responsibilities. Hospitals have traditionally left the physical safety issues discussed in this chapter to the safety committee, infection committee, and the medical staff critical-care committees to recognize and solve. These committees, required by the Joint Commission on Accreditation of Hospitals (JCAH) and usually primarily focused on patients' risks, have not had a history of marked effectiveness for employee occupational safety. No component of traditional hospital organizations (except some pastoral service departments) deal with the well-documented need of emotional support for patients and staff. Recently, some institutions have shown progress by linking an effective employee health service to existing committees and thus realizing enormous benefits for both the institution and staff.

Eliopoulos explored the benefits of a comprehensive employee health service and stresses the need for immediate development of this concept to maintain productivity and reduce personnel costs in hospitals.[23] Critical-care nurses should be in the forefront in requiring such comprehensive services from their employers. Where such services exist, nurses should develop positive communication with the health service staff, helping to educate them on the hazards of the critical-care workplace and in return drawing on their resources to prevent and solve problems.

The employee health service should provide pre-employment physicals, first aid, routine health assessments, counseling, and health and occupational safety education to employees, regardless of the shift to which they are assigned. The employee health service should be the place where staff members can go to get questions answered and confidential assistance for problems affecting their work. The following questions are examples of many that an informed critical-care nurse may encounter and need assistance in resolving:

"Are you a young male or female thinking of having a child? What about cytomegalovirus (CMV) and how it could affect the fetus? Should you continue working in NICU or MICU during this stage of life? What about a transplant unit?"

This decision is personal, yet will have major professional implications for you and perhaps your employer. Such decisions require that the most current research data be made available and reviewed with the employee. This is a unique occupational hazard whose personal implications cannot be effectively dealt with in hallway consultations, and therefore requires an informed and effective employee health service.

Critical-care nurses have the same responsibility as all nurses to continually expand their knowledge so they can provide safe and effective care to patients and protect themselves, as well. However, with the deluge of information flooding them, most nurses seem to focus on the patient's needs and forget themselves. This is unfortunate since nurses cannot continue to provide effective service when they themselves may be victims. A comprehensive employee health service can go a long way in helping staff members care for themselves so they can continue to provide safe and effective care to patients.

Summary

The critical-care environment is complex and may provide more hazards to patients and staff than initially recognized. Knowledge of the technology used within this setting provides a base for establishing methods of control which can substantially reduce the potential for adverse effects.

Regardless of the particular critical-care environment in which one works, a nurse functioning within the framework of the following principles will protect patient, family, and personnel.

1. Be assured of a safe physical environment. If a routine preventive maintenance system does not exist, ask for one. Keep in contact with the biomedical engineering department or your hospital's biomedical consultant and use them to help acquire new equipment and supplies.
2. Follow the three steps to electrical safety (Table 5-1). Vigilance may prevent a needless accident.
3. Treat equipment with care. Know manufacturers' recommended routines for cleaning and general maintenance of each device in the unit. Follow the guidelines carefully at regular prespecified intervals.
4. Be alert to defective equipment and supplies. Even manufacturers with excellent quality control systems make mistakes. Early detection of defects saves time and protects both patients and employees.
5. Actively participate in in-unit and hospital fire training exercises. Think ahead to those worst-case scenarios and decide what to do before they happen.
6. Use the resources available in the hospital such as safety and infection control committees and the employee health service to stay current with

newly identified hazards to nurses or patients, and participate in activities to prevent hazard occurrence.

References

1. Brooks, C. G. (1984). Warning: Oxygen in use. *Critical Care Nurse, 4*(2), 42, 44.

2. Friedlander, C. D. (1971, Sept.). Electricity in hospitals—elimination of lethal hazards. *IEEE Spectrum.*

3. Hill, D. W., & Dolan, A. M. (1982). *Intensive care instrumentation* (2d ed.). New York: Grune & Stratton.

4. Spooner, R. B. (Ed.). (1977). *Hospital instrumentation, care and servicing for critical care units.* Pittsburgh: Instrument Society of America.

5. *Health Devices.* E.C.R.I., 5200 Butler Pike, Plymouth Meeting, PA. 19462.

6. Baltimore, R. S. (1984). Nosocomial infections in pediatric intensive care unit. *Yale Journal of Biology on a Medicine, 57*(2), 185–197.

7. Craig, C. P., et al. (1984). Effect of intensive care unit nosocomial pneumonia on duration of stay and mortality. *American Journal of Infection Control, 12*(4), 233–238.

8. Larson, E. (1985). Infection control issues in critical care. *Heart & Lung, 14*(2), 149–156.

9. Kottra, C. J. (1983). Infection in the compromised host—an overview. *Heart & Lung. 12*(10), 10–14.

10. Levenson, S. M., & Laufman, H. (1977). Infection hazards of surgical intensive care. In L. Levenson and C. W. Thomson (Eds.), *Manual of surgical intensive care,* Philadelphia: Saunders, 157–160.

11. Tafuro, P., et al. (1984). Recognition and control of outbreaks of nosocomial infections in the intensive care setting. *Heart & Lung, 13*(5), 486–495.

12. Hope, A., Personal Communication, Durham: Duke University Medical Center.

13. Carrier, R., & Martel, G. (1985, October). Working with radiation: Reducing the risks. *The Canadian Nurse, 81* (9), 19.

14. Wagner, H. N., & Stolz, K. V. (1983). Symposium on the perception of the risk of radiation. *American Journal of Radiology. 140,* 595–603.

15. Herman, M. W., Patrick, J., Tabrisky, J. (1980). A comparative study of scattered radiation levels from 80-kVp and 240-kVp x-rays in the surgical intensive care unit. *Radiology, 137,* 552.

16. Jankowski, C. B. (1984). Radiation exposure of nurses in a coronary care unit. *Heart & Lung, 13*(1), 55–58.

17. Brooks, C. G. (1984). Warning: Oxygen in use. *Critical Care Nurse, 4*(2), 42, 44.

18. Costello, M., & Habel, M. (1984). Teaching fire safety: Practice beats preaching. *Nursing Management, 15*(8), 11–12.

19. Scanlon, J. (1983). F-I-R-E! Evacuating St. Joseph's. *Dimensions in Health Services, 60*(5), 18–19.

20. Wyatt, D. M. (1985). Are you prepared for a hospital fire? *Nursing 85, 15*(2), 51.

21. Cohen, H. H., & Lin, L. (1984, January). Hospital employee safety and health: Current problems and practices. *Professional Safety,* pp. 32–35.

22. Katz, R. M. (1983) Causes of death among registered nurses. *Journal of Occupational Medicine, 25*(10), 760–762.

23. Eliopoulos, C. (1984, October). Employee health services: A mutually beneficial program for facility and staff. *The Health Care Supervisor,* pp. 37–47.

6

Responses to the Environment

Nancie Urban

Introduction

The critical-care environment is notorious for its extremes of technology. Indeed, few other specialties within the health care system impose as much "high-tech" as the intensive care unit. While this technology provides innumerable advantages in the treatment of disease and the saving of lives, it has also been the focus of criticism. Dehumanization, especially of patients, may be the most noted of these criticisms.

The many machines, devices, and interventions inherent in the critical-care unit are the obvious source of claims that critical care is technical to the point of being dehumanizing. The highly technological aspects of critical care include the personnel as well as the machinery. Nurses in particular must direct a great deal of attention to the machinery, devices, and complex treatment protocols required in the care of the critically ill. In addition, multiple care givers, specialists, and technicians may cause fragmented care which further compounds the potentially dehumanizing nature of critical care. As a result, the technology of the critical-care unit includes both the machines and the personnel. Since the machines are unable to alter their function based on the individual patient's needs, the critical-care personnel, specifically critical-care nurses, become the essential force in integrating the technology with preservation of the humanity of the patient.

The presence of high technology without compensatory "high-touch" has been associated with rejection of technology.[1] Unfortunately, rejection of technology is not an easy option in the critical-care unit. While some patients may choose to refuse life-supporting technology, many find themselves recipients of all the critical-care unit has to offer before their options are considered.

Cessation of technological support, once initiated, poses many legal and ethical problems. The addition of personnel who are perceived by patients and families to be cold and efficient rather than warm and caring increases the tension and desire to reject the care now available. The critical-care nurse plays the essential role in providing the "high-touch" that can balance the "high-tech" of the critical-care environment.

This chapter will describe the effects of the critical-care environment on patients, their families, and the staff. Beginning with a discussion of communication as the core of sound management of the critical-care environment, each subsequent section will review major problems, effects, and nursing interventions.

Communication

In many ways, communication may be viewed as the essential ingredient in both efficient and compassionate management of the critical-care environment. Communication with patients and their families or significant others is as important as communication with other members of the health care team. Due to the unpredictable and often life-threatening nature of critical illness, communication with physicians and other care providers is often given priority over discussion with patient or family. While seemingly understandable, the highly interrelated nature of communication in the critical-care environment must be appreciated and supported to provide the patient and family the necessary attention (see Fig. 6-1).

Communication between members of the health care team may also present special problems. While considered a priority, communication may be hindered by interpersonal conflicts to the point

Critical-Care Environment

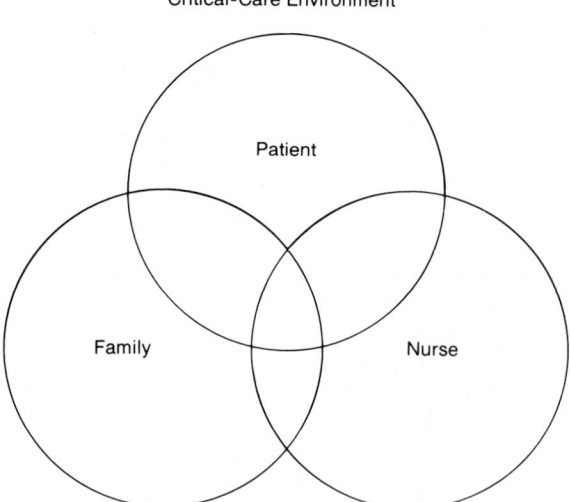

Figure 6-1   Interrelated nature of communication in the critical-care environment.

of jeopardizing patient care. Failure to confront issues out of fear of reprisal, passive-aggressive behavior, and scapegoating are only a few of the negative results of poor communication among the personnel of the critical-care environment. Furthermore, patients and their families are not oblivious to staff conflict. Their personal concerns make them especially sensitive to any indication that there is division within the health care team. Perceptions of conflict serve only to increase anxiety for all involved. Anxious patients and families make extra demands on the staff; an anxious nursing staff makes extra demands on physicians and each other; and anxious physicians make extra demands on the staff. The result can be a vicious cycle of distrust, conflict, and less than optimal care.

Open communication based on mutual respect and trust can preserve quality care under the most difficult conditions. Consideration of the effects of the critical-care environment on patients, their families, and the staff provides insights that may make an essential difference in maintaining optimum nursing care.

The Patient

Introduction to the health care system can be an intimidating experience for an individual. Consider

the effect of entering an unfamiliar building that was designed for efficiency rather than comfort. Add to this the removal of clothing and personal valuables, endless repetition of questions, many of which are of a highly personal nature, and severely limited contact with familiar persons and objects. Under such circumstances claims of dehumanization and feelings of threatened personal dignity are not surprising.

Needs of the Critically Ill

Human needs have been defined as conditions to be fulfilled to maintain life or well-being that encompass physical, psychological, and sociocultural aspects.[2] Human needs may change with the person or the situation, but always involve all three components in a highly integrated fashion. In addition, these needs are based on the needs of the individual patient, the family, and society as a whole.

The critically ill patient may be thought of as having dual needs consisting of physical needs and "person" or human needs (Fig. 6-2). Critically ill persons have physical needs, first of all, to survive and recover. They also express the need to recover with a minimum of suffering.[2] The person needs include the need to be seen as an individual, to be respected, to be provided information, to be involved in decision making regarding care, and to receive emotional support. All of these needs must be considered in terms of the sociocultural needs of patients and their families as well. A highly

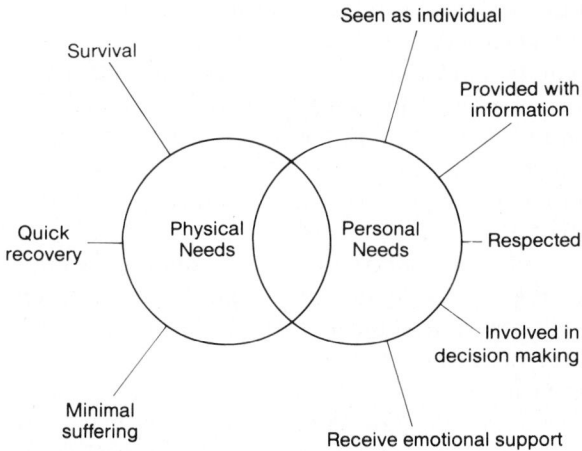

Figure 6-2   Dual needs of the critically ill.

interactive process between patient, family, and staff is required for successful fulfillment of the dual needs of the critically ill. Without full attention to both sets of needs, critically ill patients are placed at a disadvantage.

The critically ill are often viewed as being highly dependent due to the unstable nature of their situation. In addition, life-threatening illness may prompt a focus on physical needs to the exclusion of other needs. Often comatose, heavily medicated, or otherwise unable to directly participate in decision making regarding their care, the critically ill may be at higher risk of having their person needs overlooked. Such an imbalance between the physical and person needs has been associated with the traditional medical model of health care.[3] While successful in the basic treatment of diseases, the mind-body dualism of this approach is often dissatisfying to the patient. The holistic approach of treating both the physical and person needs is not only more satisfying to the patient, but may yield greater success in the overall recovery.[4] As a result, putting the person needs of the patient aside is not only discourteous but may be unethical and even unscientific.

Impact of the Critical-Care Environment

The tremendously technical nature of the critical-care environment exposes the patient to a great deal of abnormal stimuli. At the center of this situation is the potential for almost total loss of privacy and very little preservation of the patient's dignity unless explicit plans are implemented to preserve both. Critical-care units with rarely drawn curtains between the beds, coupled with assessments and treatments that often involve exposing the bodies of patients, set the stage for loss of privacy that would be considered unbelievable in other contexts. Along with many other aspects of the physical structure of the critical-care unit, experiences such as these have both psychological and physical influences on patients. Table 6-1 summarizes these influences.

Physical Environment

Most critical-care units have an element of crowding. Open-style units with only curtains between the

Table 6-1 Physical and Psychological Impact of the Critical-Care Environment on the Critically Ill Patient

Physical Impact	Psychological Impact
Crowding	Lack of privacy
Lighting	Sensory overload
Odors	Sensory monotony
Noise	Sensory deprivation
Painful touch	Isolation
	Sleep deprivation

beds often appear crowded, especially as additional equipment is brought in. Even in units with individual cubicles, however, crowding can be a problem. Supplemental equipment and lack of windows, regardless of the basic design of the unit, can result in a sense of being crowded for the patient, family, and staff. The result is a violation of territoriality based on the need of all individuals for a personally determined minimum amount of space between themselves and others or objects around them. Violation of that space causes a magnification effect on the stress perceived by patients.[5] In an already stressful environment with physical stressors also at play, aspects such as crowding compound the negative effect of the critical-care environment.

Lighting is another major factor in promoting adverse patient responses. Bright overhead lights, necessary for procedures and assessments, can have a deleterious effect on the patient. Bright lights shining directly overhead may actually be painful to patients. In addition, constant lighting around the clock interrupts natural sleep/wake cycles and contributes to sleep deprivation in critically ill patients. Appropriate amounts of uninterrupted sleep are necessary to preserve psychological integrity.[6] Sleep has also been shown to influence ability to respond to physical stressors in an adaptive way and to promote healing.[7]

Odors are another element of the critical-care environment that may distress patients, especially if the odors are coming from themselves. In studies done to determine patient stressors related to the critical-care environment, the issue of odors has been cited frequently.[7] Aside from the unpleasant nature of many odors, some odors may be a source of fear more than embarrassment to patients such as when the odor cannot be identified or is related to pathology rather than normal body functions.

Noise is one of the most significant problems in the critical-care environment. Noise levels measured at less than 40 dB permit rest and sleep. Noise levels in the average critical-care unit range from 45 to 85 dB.[8] Considering that those who are ill are less tolerant of any noise, these elevated levels of noise take on even greater significance. In the many studies done on the level of noise from various types of machinery and activity in critical-care units, several interesting findings emerge. The constant low, rhythmic noise from a ventilator, for example, has been found to be less bothersome to patients than was anticipated.[7] In fact, constant low-pitched noise that becomes part of the background may have a soothing or filtering effect, screening patients from more bothersome sounds. The noises that have been reported to be most disturbing to patients are high-pitched, loud, unexpected noises.[7] Another unpleasant quality is noise that increases in intensity or is likely to persist rather than noise that decreases in intensity or is of very short duration.[7] Most significant, however, is the finding that the noises that are perceived as most disturbing to patients are those that are produced by the staff. Conversation and loud laughter is more disturbing to patients as it causes them to worry that they are the focus of staff comments.[9]

Touch is another reality of the critical-care unit that can be perceived negatively. In this context, touch that results in pain or an invasion of privacy is the issue. Indeed, the critically ill must be touched in ways that could be perceived as unpleasant or threatening in an effort to provide them with needed intervention and care. Even the simple act of turning a patient may cause pain in certain situations. While the need to touch patients in performing procedures cannot be avoided, such touching need not occur without warning or lack appropriate prior explanation.

Psychological Environment

A complex psychological environment also exists within the critical-care unit that, related to the physical environment, has a major impact on patients, families, and staff. The illness of the patient alone may provoke severe psychological demands. In addition, the invasion of privacy discussed earlier as an element of the physical environment may also impair patients psychologically by threatening their dignity, self-esteem, and self-concept. Preservation of these factors is as necessary to the well-being of the patient as is the patient's physical recovery.

Sensory overload of abnormal stimuli is prevalent in critical-care units. Disturbances such as beeping monitors, alarms, ringing telephones, suction equipment, ventilators, and constant interruptions combine to constantly bombard patients with stimuli that are quite unlike what they are accustomed to. Coupled with a lowered ability to tolerate stressors brought about by the illness itself, an overload of abnormal stimuli can overwhelm patients. In addition, the repetitive nature of many of these stimuli may lead to sensory monotony. The result may be an environment that begins to assume a reality all its own for patients.

Sensory deprivation of familiar stimuli serves as the alternate to sensory overload in the psychological environment of the critical-care unit. Sometimes overridden by technological overload and other times simply absent, familiar sights, sounds, and smells may become distant memories to the critically ill. In addition, the extensive monitoring that may result in almost total restraint of the patient compounds the overwhelming psychological impact of the critical-care environment.

Similar to sensory deprivation, isolation presents a serious situation in critical care. One might wonder how anyone could feel isolated in a critical-care unit that normally bustles with activity and patient interruptions 24 hours a day. The isolation, however, is a product of separation from family, familiar surroundings, and social activity as well as the physical illness, pain, and alien environment. There can be little wonder that patients may begin to feel cast adrift in a terrible nightmare.

Sleep deprivation is another aspect of the psychological environment of the critical-care unit that has been studied and reported extensively in the literature. Associated with both physical and psychological well-being and recovery, adequate uninterrupted sleep is essential to healthy individuals and is especially important to the critically ill.[10] Ability to cope with and recover from critical illness may be severely compromised by sleep deprivation.[11] Yet environmental conditions in the critical-care unit often impose a degree of sleep deprivation that is unequalled by any other area in the health care system. While understandable in terms of the amount of continuous care that critically ill patients require, sleep deprivation must be avoided in order to preserve the mind and spirit of the patient as well as to promote physical healing.

Patient Responses

Many critically ill patients appear to tolerate the critical-care experience remarkably well. Other patients, however, may experience suffering that transcends that caused by their illness alone. Table 6-2 outlines the following discussion of patients' responses to the critical-care environment.

A common response to the critical-care experience is *fear* and *anxiety*. Fear may be of death, pain, or potential disability. Fear of the critical-care environment in combination with fear related to the illness is a frequent source of anxiety. While patients may feel offended by the invasion of privacy, painful procedures, restraints, and the like, they also have an acute sense of their need for the care givers. The dichotomy of feeling anger or fear about the care that is being provided, yet at the same time recognizing the need for the care and the care providers establishes the foundation for the anxiety so many critically ill patients experience.

Behaviorally, it is not uncommon to observe varying degrees of *annoyance* in patients. Unannounced intrusions, lack of consultation with the patient regarding delivery of care, and physical discomfort are only a few good reasons for patients to become annoyed with the care they are receiving or with those who are delivering that care. Noise is another factor that has been directly related to causing significant annoyance in critically ill patients.[7] As noted earlier, conversation among staff has been cited as most annoying. In addition, loud,

Table 6-2 Patient Responses to the Critical-Care Environment

Fear
Anxiety
Annoyance
Depression
Powerlessness
Spiritual distress
Pain intolerance
ICU psychosis
Transfer anxiety

high-pitched, unexpected noises that persist over time also provoke feelings of annoyance in patients. While there are many individual and cultural variables that influence the readiness with which patients may become annoyed by the critical-care environment, the behavioral demonstration of this emotion must be placed in appropriate context so that the patient's care may be maintained at an optimal level.

More worrisome than annoyance, *depression* is an all too common response to the critical-care experience. Behaviors including lack of motivation, withdrawal, tearfulness, and avoidance of eye contact may signal a patient who has become depressed as a response to the situation. Patients who are depressed may also become anorexic, further complicating their recovery due to inadequate nutrition. Sleep disturbances, either insomnia or increased sleep and lethargy, may also be symptoms of depression. Feelings of worthlessness, helplessness, despair, or threatened self-esteem may further complicate the problem. Finally, depression may be accompanied by dependency behavior that can frustrate the most dedicated efforts to rehabilitate the patient.

Powerlessness and *spiritual distress* may be the focus of a patient's responses to critical care. These responses may be similar to depression in some of their behavioral manifestations but are actually distinctly different. Powerlessness is a particularly difficult problem. When patients determine that there is nothing they can do to influence the outcome of their situation, powerlessness exists.[12] Powerlessness is associated with disinterest in events and activities associated with care, extreme lack of motivation, and an "I don't care" attitude that may severely hinder recovery and rehabilitation. Individuals who normally are in control or power positions in their daily lives may be at special risk for powerlessness when placed in the extremely dependent role of the critically ill patient. Anyone, however, can develop a sense of being out of control when subjected to the exceptionally structured environment of the critical-care unit and the extremely competent, "in charge" personnel.

Spiritual distress is the other problem often associated with depression. Considered the "neglected crisis" by some practitioners, this problem may be avoided or misinterpreted by staff.[13] Critical illness may certainly provoke spiritual questioning and conflict in patients and their families. Spiritual distress may be based on formal religious beliefs or on more general value system beliefs. In any case, unless the staff is secure in their personal beliefs and values, recognizing and dealing with this response can be difficult. Spiritual distress must be clarified, however, so that appropriate interventions may be instituted. Referral to another member of the staff, a consultant, or chaplain is recommended in situations where the primary care givers are uncomfortable or have insufficient time to devote to resolving this serious psychological problem. Lack of specific attention to this response may complicate the patient's ability to cope with the experiences in the critical-care unit.

Pain is often a major problem for both patients and staff in the critical-care unit. Research has demonstrated that patients in critical-care units appear to have heightened pain perception.[7] This increased perception of pain is associated with anxiety and environmental stressors such as noise. In any case, pain management becomes an essential priority in critical care. A component of such pain management may include environmental alterations such as noise control and measures to reduce fear and anxiety.

ICU Psychosis

ICU psychosis deserves special attention in any discussion of a patient's responses to critical care. Influenced by both the illness and the environment, an episode of psychosis is a distressing occurrence for the patient, family, and staff.[14] Identifying the specific cause of ICU psychosis is very difficult as it includes both physical and psychological factors. The illness itself may be a major factor. In addition, factors such as electrolyte imbalance, oxygenation deficits, fever, and pain will influence the patient's perceptions and behavior. The alien and unfamiliar nature of the environment with its seemingly bizarre machines and noises also serves as a cause. The need for physical restraint may further provoke paranoid feelings. The culmination of all the sensory overload coupled with sleep deprivation often results in overtly psychotic reactions in patients.

Signs and symptoms of ICU psychosis often begin with perceptual distortions which are very patient-specific. Examples of such distortions include perceiving a speckled pattern on ceiling tiles as insects, interpreting the blowing sounds of an airflow system as rain or running water, or mistaking an intraaortic balloon pump positioned at the foot of a bed for an animal.

Disorientation, especially to time and place, commonly occurs. Day and night quickly blend and blur as lights remain on and procedures are carried out at regular intervals 24 h a day. In addition, units without windows compound the inability of patients to maintain orientation to time. Disorientation to place is also common. When asked where they are, disoriented patients may been heard to reply "home," perhaps out of wishful thinking; "here with you," perhaps as a means to avoid admitting they really cannot recall where they are; or "hell," perhaps the most accurate description of what their experience must seem to be.

Actual hallucinations may also occur with ICU psychosis. Ranging from amusing to terrorizing, hallucinations warrant careful assessment. At times, patients may realize that what they see is not actually there. Unfortunately, this realization may not dispel the hallucination. More often, patients believe their hallucinations to be real. When of a frightening nature, swift intervention is especially important.

Overt paranoia further complicates the problem of ICU psychosis. Many of the procedures and activities that are necessary in the care of the critically ill may provide a fertile basis for paranoid thoughts, which only add to the difficulty in correcting this problem. Paranoia may also be directed at family members or patients may involve family members in their paranoid behavior. This situation requires extremely sensitive intervention in order to protect patients and their family members from feelings of guilt or distrust of the staff.

Restlessness and outright combativeness are frequent behavioral components of ICU psychosis. Combativeness may require the use of restraints to protect both the patient and the staff. Use of restraints, however, may accent the already paranoid fears of the patient. Sedation is usually necessary. The best treatment, of course, is to institute interventions that serve to prevent the psychosis from occurring in the first place. The nursing interventions that will be discussed in context with general patient responses to the critical-care environment apply to the problem of ICU psychosis as well.

Essential interventions, however, include fostering adequate sleep, providing structured contact with familiar stimuli such as family members or favorite television programs, and controlling pain.

Nursing Interventions

Protecting patients from ill effects of the critical-care environment is a significant responsibility of the nurse. Who is better able to manage this important aspect of a patient's care than the health care professional who is at the bedside 24 hours a day? Accomplishing this worthy goal presents many difficult challenges. Many interventions, however, are really quite simple (see Table 6-3).

First, and perhaps foremost, patients should be treated with the respect due any individual. Addressing patients by their appropriate title and family name, especially when the patient is an adult, is important. Many individuals consider a stranger addressing them by their first name disrespectful, even when that familiarity is intended to put them at ease. These same individuals as a patients may not state that they do not wish to be addressed by their first name. In fact, when asked if their first name may be used, they may say yes out of fear that they will alienate the nurse if they refuse. An unsolicited invitation to use the patient's first name is the best indication that a first-name basis is acceptable to the patient. Exceptions to this include patients who may be comatose or otherwise neurologically impaired and who, as a result, may be more inclined to respond to their more familiar first name rather than their family name. Another exception is the patient who is a child or a very young adult who may be uncomfortable with the more formal style of address.

Another primary aspect of nursing intervention is to preserve a patient's privacy and dignity. Such intervention may present a difficult challenge in the critical-care unit, especially when the patient requires extensive monitoring and support. Suddenly appearing at the bedside may startle a patient and may certainly be viewed as an invasion of basic privacy. Strategies to optimize a patient's privacy include knocking before entering the patient's room or cubicle. Where there is nothing to knock on, an announcement of one's presence may be substituted. Also, assessments and procedures can be conducted so that as little of the patient's body is exposed as possible, and judicious use of curtains and doors should become commonplace. Keeping the patient informed of all activities, regardless of how minor they may be, also adds to a patient's respect and privacy.

Conversation that does not include the patient should be strictly avoided at the bedside. Whether such conversation is related to the patient or simply personal exchange between care givers, it is inappropriate. Such conversation serves to reduce the status of the patient to that of an object. It is rude at the very least and may contribute to paranoia or feelings of worthlessness and powerlessness at the worst. This is not to say that personal conversation should never occur at the bedside. When the patient is included, general conversation may provide a pleasant distraction from the otherwise stressful environment of the critical-care unit. Conversation is certainly easier to control among the nursing staff than among other members of the health care team. A tactful reminder properly placed usually serves to keep everyone on track with relatively consistent success.

Offering patients choices, no matter how minor, helps them maintain a sense of control and may be instrumental in preventing powerlessness. Encouraging participation in decision making and care as much as is realistic based on the patient's ability is another strategy. Critically ill patients are very sensitive to the preferences of their care givers. Dependency is fostered in patients in subtle as well as direct ways.[15] Involving patients in their own care as much as possible serves to minimize this effect.

Table 6-3 Nursing Interventions for Patient Responses to the Critical-Care Environment

Address respectfully
Preserve privacy
Control bedside conversation
Offer choices
Encourage participation
Maintain independent identity
Control noise
Allow adequate sleep
Structure activities
Use comforting touch liberally
Facilitate family contact

In a somewhat similar vein, helping the patient maintain a sense of identity separate from the critical-care unit may also have empowering value. Adoption of the sick role can be especially dangerous for the patient who becomes a long-term resident in the critical-care unit. Directing the family to bring in personal items from home such as family photographs, pictures drawn by young members of the family, or a favorite pillow help to maintain a sense of connection to home for the patient. In addition, coordinating care so that the patient may be taken outside the unit for a short time may yield extremely positive results. Strategies such as these also help patients to maintain a sense of hope that they are still a part of the world and that they may yet recover. Any intervention that supports a sense of hope in the patient is worth whatever effort is required because, without hope, recovery may be impossible.[16]

Controlling noise is another environmental intervention that can yield important results. Minimizing the amount of equipment in the patient's room will help reduce noise. This intervention will also help reduce the sense of crowding and violated personal territory that patients often experience in critical care. If there are doors to each patient's area, keeping them closed whenever possible is an important intervention. Carpeting in the corridors also helps reduce the noise of unit traffic. Turning off all equipment that is not in use (especially suction equipment, which can be particularly noisy) is another successful strategy. Making sure that patients have been oriented to the various sounds, especially alarms, is important so that they are not unnecessarily frightened by them. Turning the audio pulse monitors down, if not off, positioning ventilators so that the exit valve points away from the patient's head, and refilling infusion pumps before they alarm are just a few additional interventions that can be accomplished with relative ease if planned for in advance.

Providing adequate opportunities for uninterrupted sleep is also an essential nursing intervention (see Chap. 14). Control of noise and lights is usually an essential aspect of this intervention. Sleep research unanimously supports the conclusion that adequate sleep is essential for physical and psychological survival.[17] The minimum amount of time needed to complete a sleep cycle is 90 min to 2 h. Planning care to allow 2-h periods of uninterrupted sleep, especially during the night hours, can have a remarkable effect on preventing ICU psychosis and promoting a patient's recovery.

Structuring most of the activity in the critical-care unit may aid in protecting patients from the critical-care environment. Scheduling therapeutic activities such as assessments, bathing, physical therapy, and treatments so that adequate rest can be obtained by patients is an important component of such structure. Use of radio and television, a common intervention to help patients maintain a sense of connection to the outside world, is also best used in a structured manner. Most important, music and program selections must be based on a patient's preferences rather than those of the care providers. In addition, avoiding continuous playing of the radio or television 24 hours a day is needed so that day–night orientation is not compromised.

Touch may also be used as a nursing intervention to manage a patient's responses to the critical-care environment. When critically ill and extensively monitored, patients may begin to feel like an untouchable object. The need to touch patients for the purpose of assessments and procedures may compound their feelings of dehumanization. A gentle touch, intended to provide comfort rather than specific therapy, reinforces patients' sense of themselves as worthy of human attention and concern.[18] Families should also be encouraged to touch the patient regardless of the amount of technological intervention that may be involved in the patient's care. Lowering the side rails so that family members can reach the patient, offering a chair so that they can make themselves more comfortable, and giving permission for them to touch the patient are simple yet effective methods for facilitating the positive use of touch by the patient's family. The many tubes, wires, and machines may intimidate family members and cause them to hesitate to touch the patient. Clearing a path to the patient and encouraging physical contact between family and patient provide a source of touch that may become the patient's primary tie to a sense of humanity.

Maintaining relationships between patients and their families is a final area of nursing intervention designed to help patients weather the critical-care experience. Touch, as just discussed, is an important component of this intervention. In addition, visiting opportunities need to be individualized to accommodate familial and cultural variances as well as the clinical situation. Contact with family provides a source of normal stimuli, support, and comfort. Facilitating family visitation may be the key intervention in preventing the feeling of isolation that critically ill patients may develop. Social isolation may be a component of responses such as feelings of hopelessness, worthlessness, despair, powerlessness, or depression. As a result, maintaining family relationships is a priority intervention.

Nursing interventions to minimize adverse patient responses to the critical-care environment involve both awareness of those responses and a willingness to take necessary action.[19] Passive acceptance of the potentially dehumanizing aspects of the critical-care environment is not acceptable. Such acceptance may also have ethical and legal implications considering the detrimental effects that an uncontrolled critical-care experience could have on a patient. Nurses must be willing to alter the "routines" on behalf of the patient when appropriate. Rigid focus on routines or retreat behind the outdated nurse's role of silent emissary of the medical plan of care does a great disservice to the patient. At times, active advocacy on behalf of the patient may be required to protect the patient from unnecessary physical and psychological strain from the critical-care environment. These goals certainly may be difficult to achieve, especially when the patient is extremely unstable and requires extraordinary physical support. The benefits of successful implementation of a plan of care that meets both the physical and psychological needs of the patient, however, are quality nursing care and optimum patient outcomes.

Transfer Anxiety

In spite of the unpleasant nature of being hospitalized in the critical-care unit, many patients are anxious and even fearful about being transferred from the area. The constant monitoring and presence of the staff may result in a sense of security. Also, the extremely intensive nature of care in the critical-care unit often facilitates a high level of trust in the nurse–patient relationship. Transfer to the stepdown unit means less supervision and the need to get to know new staff. Both of these factors may diminish the trust of the patient in the staff during the initial transfer period. In addition, the time of transfer may be the first time that family members consider it safe enough to leave the hospital for a short time. The result is depletion of the patient's support system at a sensitive time.[20]

Nursing interventions that prevent, control, or reduce transfer anxiety begin with the awareness that transfer is a time of stress for the patient. Studied in coronary care patients, the stress of transfer has been noted to have adverse physiological effects such as increased heart rate, increased blood pressure, and increased risk to cardiac dysrhythmias.[21] Preparation for transfer is most successful when it is structured and includes the following: allowing patients opportunities to ventilate their feelings, portraying the transfer as a positive sign of recovery, identifying the patient's individual learning needs regarding the transfer, preparing the patient in advance of the transfer so that it does not come as a surprise, and showing trust in the expertise of the nurses on the transfer unit.[22] Facilitation of the transfer process requires a skillful approach that is carefully structured so that the patient can be separated from the intense environment of the critical-care unit without unnecessary concern or anxiety.

Summary

Overall, a confident and caring approach to the patient serves to temper the "high-tech" of the critical-care unit. Such an approach provides the "high-touch" that is essential to what is also described as humane care.[23] Many of the adverse responses to the critical-care environment may be the only way a patient can reject the high-tech nature of the critical-care unit. Interventions that address the impact of the critical-care environment by modifying that environment, countering what cannot be modified with caring and humane approaches, and preparing the patient to progress and transfer from the critical-care unit with confidence are needed to preserve the patient as both a physical and human being.

The Family

Family members of critically ill patients are also affected by the critical-care environment. The stress induced by the environment may aggravate family members' ability to cope with the critical illness of a loved one. The technology, bright lights, crowding, and odors are experienced by the family as well as by the patient. While the family members may not experience the full impact of the high-tech nature of the critical-care unit, as does the patient, they cannot help but recognize the overwhelming nature of the patient's circumstances as they are exposed to an overview of all that the critical-care unit imposes. In addition, families are also influenced by the psychological environment of the critical-care unit, including factors such as lack of privacy, threat to personal dignity, and sensory overload.

While it is appropriate that the patient be the first priority of the nurse, it is also appropriate to keep in mind that patients are members of families. It is possible that a patient's recovery may actually be enhanced or hindered by the family. From admission through rehabilitation and discharge, the family is an integral part of "total" patient care.[24]

Critical illness has also been suggested as carrying the potential of placing the entire family in crisis.[25] Such an occurrence is not just a problem for the family. The nurse may find that families can become quite disruptive to a patient's care when they become dysfunctional. In the interest of patient care, as well as out of concern for the family, consideration of the effect of the critical-care experience on all concerned is indicated.

Family Responses

Family responses to the critical illness of a loved one and the critical-care environment, summarized in Table 6-4, present many challenges to the nurse. Fear and anxiety are common reactions in family

Table 6-4 Family Responses to the Critical-Care Environment

Fear
Anxiety
Helplessness
Anger
Hostility
Guilt
Grief
Disruptive behavior
Withdrawal

members. Critical illness may occur suddenly and unexpectedly as in an accident or acute myocardial infarction. Even when the patient has been ill for a period of time before requiring critical care, family members may express feelings of shock and disbelief that the situation could have accelerated to the point of critical illness. The use of mechanical support and extensive monitoring equipment may look more harmful than helpful to family members who typically have never seen the inside of a critical-care unit before. In addition, misconceptions of what many of the machines and interventions mean may exist as a result of information gleaned from the media or stories heard from others in the community.

Not only may family members be fearful of losing the patient as a result of the illness, they may also fear touching the patient out of concern that they might disrupt the medical support being provided. Touch between the patient and family members may be the only link that the patient has with a more normal and "human" view of self. Touch may also be the only means by which the family can feel that they are contributing to the patient's care in a positive way. In addition, it may be the last contact family members have with the patient before his or her death. As a result, families who are so overwhelmed and fearful of the critical-care environment that they cannot seem to make even simple contact with the patient need the support, encouragement, and, often, permission of the nurse to maintain this essential link with the patient.

Helplessness is another common reaction of the family to the critical-care environment. The machinery, tubes, and wires can be extremely intimidating to anyone who does not work with them regularly. Serious illness itself places family members who desperately want to help in a very helpless position. As they stand by and witness all that is being done, much of which may involve considerable suffering on the part of the patient, they struggle with feelings of inadequacy and helplessness.

Reactions to the environment, or to initial feelings of fear or helplessness, may include expressions of anger and hostility. Often considered highly problematic, these reactions may actually be considered healthy. Anger and hostility are visible attempts of the family to fight back under difficult circumstances. While such reactions require great diplomacy and care, it is far better to have the family's feelings out in the open where they can be identified and addressed. It is essential that the nurse not respond in a way that implies intimidation. It is equally important that responses to family anger not provoke a power struggle in which the patient inevitability loses the most.

Guilt on the part of family members may severely complicate a patient's care. Motivated by interpersonal conflicts within the family unit prior to the illness or as a result of the events and experiences within the critical-care unit, guilt feelings in family members are best handled when they can be identified in terms of their cause. Guilt is especially problematic in situations where difficult decisions must be made about persisting in a line of therapy or providing comfort measures only. While family members are feeling guilty, they generally will be unwilling to discuss care alternatives and hold to the "do everything possible" position regardless of probable outcome or patient suffering.

Grief is also seen as a response to critical illness that may be compounded by the stressors of the critical-care environment. Fearing loss of the patient or feeling helpless to alleviate his or her suffering, family members may grieve for the patient and themselves. Tearfulness, sadness, and other grief behaviors may be seen. Appropriately placed support is indicated.

Disruptive behavior or demands may be the result of a family having difficulty coping with the critical-care experience. Constant and repetitive questioning of the staff, disregard for visiting regulations, and threats of legal action if demands are not met are only a few examples of disruptive behavior that may be rooted in the overwhelming nature of the critical-care situation. Violent behavior may also erupt, especially in response to bad news. On the other hand, cultural variables may be the foundation for what is deemed disruptive behavior by the staff. While it may be difficult to negotiate with the family for more acceptable behavior, the line must be drawn if and when family behavior compromises a patient's care. Most family members will be willing to compromise to at least a partial degree if they can be made to appreciate how their behavior hinders the patient's care. Cultivating a trusting relationship with the family is a necessary adjunct to successful resolution of disruptive family behavior. Deferring to the family whenever possible, especially when cultural differences are the basis for the conflict, is a fairly successful method for initiating a trusting relationship. Once such a relationship is established, family behavior is likely to be at least relatively more negotiable.

Withdrawal is a far more problematic reaction of the family to the critical-care experience. Potentially caused by the threatening appearance of the critical-care environment and intense fear for the survival of the patient, family members may respond with withdrawal behavior. Such behavior may present as reluctance to touch the patient, difficulty remaining at the bedside for more than the briefest of moments, or avoidance of visiting altogether. When present, family members may avoid eye contact with the patient and staff, deny questions, and resist efforts to discuss their feelings and fears. Withdrawal may also hamper the ability of the family to engage in decision making if and when patients are not able to take responsibility for this action on their own. Maintenance of the family as a support system for the patient and the family unit itself is essential to safe and optimal patient care.

Family Needs

Consideration of the stated needs of families, as well as their responses to the critical-care environment, is an important aspect of preparing to provide comprehensive care. Nursing research has specified the most significant needs of family members of critically ill patients.[26] Identified by family members themselves, the needs of family members change somewhat from the time of admission to the time the immediate crisis has passed (see Table 6-5).

At the time of admission and during the first several days, family members state that their greatest need is to feel that the highest quality care is being delivered to the patient. The basis of this concern is that the staff is competent and that they care about the patient in a personal way. Families also have identified immediate needs for concrete information, estimation of probable outcome, honesty, to feel confident that they would be contacted if there were any changes in the patient's condition, and hope for a positive outcome. Basic explanations of what the machines and tubes are and what they

Table 6-5 Immediate, Delayed, and Ongoing Needs of Families of the Critically Ill

Immediate	Delayed	Ongoing
Quality care	Visitation	Caring
Concrete information	Involvement	Honesty
Estimation of outcome	Telephone availability	Updates
Honesty	Comfort	Hope
Updates	Discussion	
Continuity	Privacy	

do to help the patient should be included in the information provided the family. Unit routines and communication systems are also important information items. Updates regarding the medical and nursing plans of care have also been identified as important.

Another interesting finding, singled out in the study by Bouman, is that families find talking with the same nurse every day particularly reassuring.[26] Continuity of care givers is clearly considered an advantage by family members. Perhaps such continuity supports the development of a trusting relationship or is related to inability to tolerate frequent changes of any kind when stressed. Interestingly, families related a willingness to forgo frequent visitation and efforts to provide for their personal comfort as long as these priority needs were met.

Once the initial crisis is passed, the needs of family members change. Now the opportunity to visit more often becomes more important. In addition, families greatly appreciate the opportunity to participate in the patient's care at this point. Availability of a telephone and a comfortable place to wait near the patient are also more important once the initial crisis has passed. Evidently, once their worry about the patient stabilizes, family members become more aware of their personal needs. The need to talk about their feelings and fears may also become more important once the initial scare has dissipated. Such talk may center on the events preceding or precipitating the critical illness, the extent of the interventions being administered to the patient, or the possibility of the death of the patient. On the other hand, some family members relate the need to have a place within the hospital where they can be alone.

Regardless of the timing, families require several essential aspects of care. A caring attitude from the staff is always perceived as a need. While initially considered a priority for the patient, families eventually look for caring behaviors to include them as well. Honesty, frequent updates regarding the status and progress of the patient, and hope are additional ongoing needs for families. Regardless of the probable outcome for the patient, family members express a strong need for being allowed even a small measure of hope at all times.

Nursing Interventions

A primary aspect of intervening on behalf of family members of a critically ill patient is to begin with a careful, formal family assessment.[27] Such an assessment provides information to enable the nurse to meet the family's needs both effectively and efficiently. The time-saving aspect of a preliminary assessment is significant in light of the often hectic nature of caring for the critically ill. Establishment of a baseline of information regarding the patient's family is well worth the initial investment of time if it results in the ability of the nurse to provide ongoing care to the family with a minimum of conflict with providing patient care.

The essential elements of a family assessment (see Table 6-6) include the following:

1. Demographic data, including a description of the family constellation and their availability to the patient and each other.
2. Description of the role of each family member and the patient in the family unit. When the patient is the primary decision maker for the family, it is important to identify who will assume this responsibility and how the family will interact to make needed decisions in the interim. Determination of a single family spokesperson who will have open privileges to call the unit

Table 6-6 Outline for Family Assessment

1. Demographic data
    Family constellation
    Availability
2. Family roles
    Decision maker
    Spokesperson
3. Economic and social resources
4. Family perceptions/coping styles
5. Health maintenance activities
    Eating habits
    Sleeping habits
    Medications

for information and then serve as the source of information for the rest of the family may facilitate meeting a family's need for information without placing an inordinate burden on the nurse.

3. Identification of economic and social resources at the family's disposal.

4. Assessment of family perceptions of the illness of the patient and the coping styles of family members. Such information becomes extremely valuable when deciding how to structure visiting, when to provide ancillary support such as a chaplain or social worker, or when the services of a clinical nurse specialist may be indicated.

5. Identification of the family members' personal health maintenance activities. Ensuring that family members are eating, sleeping, and taking their own medications when necessary helps them to maintain their personal health and may prevent noncoping behavior on their part in the future.

With the many psychological stressors that the critical illness of the patient and the critical-care environment present to the family, avoidance of physical stressors may prevent the family from becoming overwhelmed by the experience. The family assessment also provides an opportunity to establish rapport with the family, and the information obtained provides the basis for family intervention.

In addition to the assessment, there are a number of general interventions that are useful in the care of family members (see Table 6-7). A caring approach is essential in meeting family needs and establishing trust. Verbal and nonverbal behavior that indicates sincere concern for the family as well

as the patient may be the single most successful strategy in caring for families of the critically ill.

Honesty is another key ingredient in family care. Family members are usually very sensitive to the nonverbal messages sent by care givers. Any discrepancy between the information provided and the nonverbal messages simultaneously delivered will be noticed by the family. As a result, honesty is the only safe and ethical approach. Such honesty is best coupled with care and concern, however, especially when the news is bad.

Providing information frequently and consistently is also important. Families should be provided with information about the critical-care unit environment, routines, and visiting regulations as soon as possible. Information must be provided in terms the family can understand. The amount and detail of the information must be gauged on an individual basis. It is also useful to offer information updates rather than waiting for the family to ask. This is especially important as it relates to the critical-care environment, since family members may be too overwhelmed by the technology to know what to ask. Another strategy is to encourage the family to keep a list of questions as they occur to them. Such a list helps family members obtain answers to all of their questions in a more timely fashion and without the additional stress of trying to remember everything when an opportunity to discuss the patient's care arises.

Allowing family members to express their feelings is another essential nursing intervention. Fear, guilt, anger, and other feelings are easier to deal with if they can be identified and discussed openly. A nonjudgmental atmosphere of trust will facilitate expression of feelings by family members. A quiet area that is separated from the bedside but close to the critical-care unit may also provide an

Table 6-7 Nursing Interventions for Family Responses to the Critical-Care Environment

Caring approach
Family assessment
Honesty
Volunteer information
Allow expression of feelings
Flexible visitation
Involve family in care
Grant permission for family self-care
Allow hope

advantage in discussing family members' feelings. The machines and noises of the critical-care environment or reluctance to talk in the presence of the patient may distract or inhibit open discussion of feelings within the family. Privacy is especially important when dealing with hostile or potentially violent family members. The added stressors inherent in the critical-care environment may aggravate an already unstable situation. A quiet area where attention may be focused on the distress of the family is most helpful in quelling potential outbursts. In the face of hostility, it is advisable to modify the approaches used to demonstrate care and concern for the family. Touch, for example, is often used with great success in demonstrating to family members that their well-being is a priority. However, an attempt to touch an angry or hostile family member may be interpreted as an aggressive or intrusive action.[28] A quiet, calm approach that acknowledges the family member's feelings, yet places them in context with the situation is advisable. When family anger is justified, acknowledgment and apology is in order. Developing a plan for future care or communication may also help dispel the current situation and prevent recurrence.

Including the family in both patient education and decision making also enhances family care. In many instances, the family may need to carry the responsibility for both aspects. Involving the family enables them to provide appropriate support for the patient and each other. Families also appreciate the opportunity to be involved in the direct care of the patient. Such involvement helps forestall feelings of helplessness. In addition, providing family members with constructive outlets for their feelings and concerns may be instrumental in preventing more disruptive behavior on their parts. Even in the most critical of patient situations, some small aspect of patient care can usually be found in which the family can participate.

Permission may need to be granted by the nurse for the family to meet their personal needs. At the bedside, it is not uncommon that the family must be encouraged to touch their loved one. Preparing the family for what to expect to see and hear at the bedside, lowering the bed and side rail, pulling up a chair, and inviting the family member to sit down and hold the patient's hand or talk to the patient may need to be formally done before the family will feel free to make direct contact with the patient. Clearing at least some small area of the patient of tubes, wires, and machines is also helpful as a means to facilitate contact between family and patient. Away from the bedside, families may need to be given permission to leave the hospital to tend to personal needs. Reassurance of immediate notice of any changes and expression of concern for the welfare of the family are often necessary before family members will be willing to risk leaving the hospital.

Visitation is an issue that often becomes a power struggle between staff and families. The extensive care needs of critically ill patients, the technology that must be monitored and adjusted, and the demands of coordinating multiple care givers creates an understandable need for time that must be dedicated solely to the care of the patient. In addition, some interventions may be difficult for family members to observe. On the other hand, patients and their families have need of one another. An overly rigid set of rules that severely limits visiting invites friction and additional stress for all concerned. Visitation may be used to the best advantage of all. Negotiating adequate time to complete patient care, allowing visiting time in accordance with patient and family preferences whenever possible, and imposing limitations on visiting to provide rest for both patient and family are ways in which to effectively meet the needs of all concerned. While easier to discuss than implement at times, a flexible attitude toward visitation generally yields significantly more positive results than adding prolonged separation and isolation to the stressors already at play in the critical-care environment.

Hope is as important for the family as it is for the patient. Family members may have to struggle to maintain a sense of hope as they view the extensive technology applied to care for the patient. They require simple explanations of what is routine and a means of support for the patient so that they do not inaccurately perceive the significance of what they see and hear. At other times, the condition of the patient may offer little hope of recovery. Regardless of the severity of the illness or in spite of possible decisions for no further resuscitation, families still must be allowed to cling to some shred of hope no matter how small. At times, families may appear to be unrealistic in their hope. Before pressing the hard realities, a gentle investigation of their understanding of the probable outcome may often reveal that they do not lack understanding but choose to hope for a "miracle." As long as their hope does not interfere with the patient's care, allowing the family this coping choice should be accepted. Such acceptance is not allowing or encouraging false hope. Instead, it represents willingness to meet the individual needs of both patient and family. Of all the nursing interventions to assist families to cope with the critical-care environment, the concern and caring demonstrated by allowing even a small measure of hope is, perhaps, the most significant and compassionate of all.

The Staff

The staff of the critical-care unit is also bombarded with the technology, noises, and other stimuli of the critical-care environment. In addition, the multidisciplinary nature of the average critical-care staff increases the complexity of the environment with which each staff member must deal. Along with the physical stressors, the staff must also confront the psychological stress of rapid changes and life and death decision making. This incredible combination of stimuli presents special challenges to the staff.

The critical-care nurse must command an extraordinary blend of skills. Knowledge of complex physiology, pathology, medical treatment, and pharmacology represents just one component. The constant advances in technology and the introduction of computers places another set of knowledge and skill requirements on the nurse. The ongoing care and evaluation of highly unstable individuals, integration of their physical and psychosocial needs, and incorporation of the patients' families' needs is a third area of expertise required. All of these skills are combined in the formulation of nursing diagnoses and truly individualized, total patient care.

Knowledge, application of the nursing process, and communication are the cornerstones of critical-care nursing practice. Yet, in spite of the best skill in these areas, nursing practice in the critical-care unit has its hazards. The constant fast pace combined with extremes in patient acuity and high death rates take their toll on the nurse. The exceptional complexity and constant demands of the environment and the potential for communication problems also contribute to staff strain.

Staff responses to the stressors of the critical-care environment may include tension, short temper, rigid adherence to rules and procedures, unwillingness to accept help, and passive-agressive behavior. Anger is another reaction not often admitted or discussed. Anger, however, is not a surprising response when patient census and acuity levels soar, staffing is marginal, personalities of the health care team clash, and administration seems too far away to understand or provide relief. In combination with a nursing staff truly dedicated to providing quality patient care, these conflicts may easily result in feelings of anger. The ultimate result of uncontrolled negative responses to the critical-care environment has been referred to as *burnout.*

Communication may be the key to maintaining the balance between quality nursing care and nurse burnout. Communication lines must be kept open at all times with patients, families, other members of the health care team, and administration. Patient and family communication based on honesty and concern offers a strong probability of success. Communication with other members of the health care team is also best served if it remains honest, straightforward, and based on respect for self and others. Utilization of the administrative structure may facilitate communication at this level. Staff meetings can be used as a forum to openly discuss staff concerns and brainstorm solutions. Working through the committee structure of the organization can be an effective way to realize productive changes in policy and practice. The key to communicating concerns to administration is to do so in the spirit of seeking to improve patient care in responsible, cost-effective ways. Offer suggestions rather than complaints, and use the system to your advantage.

In addition to good communication, staff members must take care of themselves as well. Working together to provide opportunities to obtain breaks is important. Furthermore, taking breaks away from the unit whenever possible is strongly advised so that one may better relax. The ability to say no at times without feeling guilty is a skill that critical-care nurses may need as much as their clinical skills. Some method of personal stress management is also a valuable tool in coping with the stressors of the critical-care unit. Burnout need not be an inevitable consequence of critical-care practice.

Summary

The critical-care environment has an impact on patients, families, and staff. Physical and psychological stressors bombard all who provide or receive care in this high-tech area of health care. The stress and anxiety that too often occur as a result of the high-tech nature of the critical-care environment are best managed by high-touch interventions. A caring approach to all—patients, families, and staff—is the foundation for optimal care and survival in the critical-care environment. Critical-care nurses are exceptional in their ability to provide this type of tender, yet competent care.

References

1. Naisbitt, J. (1982). *Megatrends,* New York: Warner Books.
2. Bergman, R. (1983). Understanding the patient in all his human needs. *Journal of Advanced Nursing, 8,* 185–190.
3. Garrett, S., & Garrett, B. (1982). Humaneness and health. *Topics in Clinical Nursing, 3*(1), 7–12.
4. Friedman, H., & DiMatteo, M. (1979). Health care as an interpersonal process. *Journal of Social Issues, 35*(1), 1–11.
5. Gowan, N. (1979). The perceptual world of the intensive care unit: An overview of some environmental considerations in the helping relationship. *Heart and Lung, 8*(2), 340–344.
6. Helton, M., Gordon, S., & Nunnery, S. (1980). The correlation between sleep deprivation and intensive care unit syndrome. *Heart and Lung, 9*(3), 464–468.
7. Baker, C. (1983). Sensory overload and noise in the ICU: Sources of environmental stress. *Critical Care Quarterly, 6*(1), 66–80.
8. Hilton, A. (1985). Noise in acute patient care areas. *Research in Nursing and Health, 8,* 283–291.
9. Hansell, H. (1984). The behavioral effects of noise on man: The patient with intensive care unit psychosis. *Heart and Lung, 13*(1), 59–65.
10. Brewer, M. (1986). To sleep or not to sleep: The consequences of sleep deprivation. *Critical Care Nurse, 5*(6), 35–40.
11. Beglinger, J. (1983). Coping tasks in critical care. *Dimensions of Critical Care Nursing, 2*(2), 80–89.
12. Miller, J. (1983). *Coping with chronic illness: Overcoming powerlessness.* Philadelphia: F. A. Davis.
13. Ryan, J. (1984). The neglected crisis. *American Journal of Nursing, 84,* 1257–1258.
14. Kleck, H. (1983). ICU syndrome: Onset, manifestations, treatment, stressors, and prevention. *Critical Care Quarterly, 6*(1), 21–28.
15. Griffin, J. (1982). Forced dependency in the critically ill. *Dimensions of Critical Care Nursing, 1*(6), 350–352.
16. Ramlow, M. (1984). Hope. *FOCUS on Critical Care, 9*(5), 10.
17. Fisher, M., & Moxham, P. (1979). ICU syndrome. *Critical Care Nurse, 4*(3), 39–45.
18. McGuire, M. (1983). A touch in the dark. *Critical Care Nurse, 3*(5), 53–56.
19. Carter, S. (1983). Rehumanizing the nursing role: A question of love. *Topics in Clinical Nursing, 5*(10), 11–17.
20. Schwartz, L., & Brenner, Z. (1979). Critical care unit transfer: Reducing patient stress through nursing interventions. *Heart and Lung, 8*(3), 540–546.
21. Toth, J. (1980). Effect of structured preparation for transfer on patient anxiety on leaving coronary care unit. *Nursing Research, 29*(1), 28–34.
22. Poe, C. (1982). Minimizing stress of transfer responses. *Dimensions of Critical Care Nursing, 1*(6), 364–374.
23. Curtin, L. (1984). Nursing: High-touch in a high-tech world. *Nursing Management, 15*(7), 7–8.
24. Daley, L. (1984). The perceived immediate needs of families with relatives in the intensive care setting. *Heart and Lung, 13*(3), 231–237.
25. Lust, B. (1984). The patient in the ICU: A family experience. *Critical Care Quarterly, 6*(4), 49–57.
26. Bouman, C. (1984). Identifying priority concerns of families of ICU patients. *Dimensions of Critical Care Nursing, 3*(5), 314–319.
27. Jillings, C. (1981). Nursing intervention with the family of the critically ill patient. *Critical Care Nurse, 1*(5), 27–31.
28. Poster, E., & Betz, C. (1984). When the patient dies: Dealing with the family's anger. *Dimensions of Critical Care Nursing, 3*(6), 372–377.

part 3

Phenomena of Concern in Critical-Care Nursing

7

Tissue Perfusion

Gayle R.
Whitman

Introduction

Relevance to Critical-Care Setting

Maintenance of adequate tissue perfusion is a basic and essential function for the survival of any living cell, organ, or system. In the critical-care setting maintaining this basic function frequently becomes the major activity and primary goal. Inadequate tissue perfusion is often blatant, as in cases of severe cardiogenic shock or hemorrhage. On the other hand, it can also be a less obvious or silent process, such as is seen in early septic shock. Therapy to maintain tissue perfusion may be singular, involving only volume replacement; or complex, involving volume replacement, pharmacologic manipulation, and mechanical supports. In all these instances the role of the critical-care nurse is paramount. As the consistent presence at the patient's bedside, the critical-care nurse will most frequently identify subtle or acutely blatant assessment parameters which indicate inadequate perfusion. In addition, the nurse plans, implements, and evaluates appropriate nursing interventions to limit the effects of inadequate perfusion while concurrently collabo-

rating with the physician in implementing medical therapies to reverse the inadequate perfusion state. To effectively perform these functions it is essential that the critical-care nurse be cognizant of and knowledgeable about these various processes. This chapter will describe the alterations which occur in inadequate perfusion, from the cellular to the system level, and will delineate the various appropriate interventions utilized to prevent, limit, or reverse inadequate perfusion.

Cellular and Subcellular Anatomy and Physiology

While all cells are not exactly alike in structure and function, they all possess to varying degrees some similarities. Typically, a cell consists of two major components: the nucleus and the cytoplasm (Fig. 7-1). The *nucleus* is the control center of the cell and is responsible for cell reproduction and for controlling the many chemical reactions which occur throughout the cell. The nucleus is situated in the middle of the cell, surrounded by cytoplasm and encapsulated by the nuclear membrane. This

Figure 7-1 Schematic representation of a typical cell and its organelles. Section of the cell membrane (lower left) depicting protein and carbohydrate portions which extend from the membrane and serve as receptor sites for various agents.

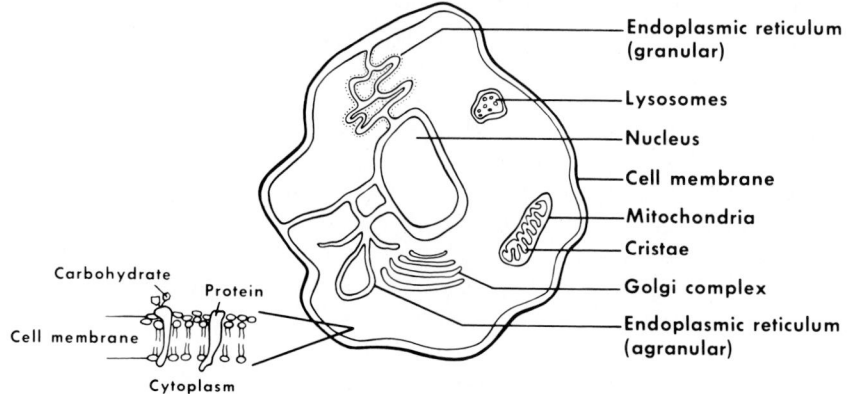

nuclear membrane consists of two layers made of lipids, carbohydrates, and proteins, and is characterized by having large pores which facilitate the flux of fluid and particles between the nucleus and the cytoplasm. The nucleus contains large amounts of deoxyribonucleic acid (DNA) in the form of genes. The genes determine the function and activities which occur in the cytoplasm of the cell and actively engage in replication.

Surrounding the nucleus floats the *cytoplasm*. Within the cytoplasm there are numerous highly organized physical structures called *organelles*. The major organelles of the cell include the mitochondria, the endoplasmic reticulum, the Golgi complex, and the lysosomes. The *mitochondria* are considered the powerhouses of the cell since they are responsible for producing energy from the nutrients and oxygen that the cell receives from the capillary circulation. The number of mitochondria per cell varies from cell to cell, depending upon the amount of energy each cell needs. Under normal circumstances, the mitochondria can produce 95 percent of the body's energy needs via aerobic metabolism. The mitochondria accomplish this by converting glucose into energy via the process of glycolysis. With this process 1 mol of glucose in the presence of oxygen can synthesize 36 mol of adenosine triphosphate (ATP) (Fig. 7-2). Adenosine triphosphate is a high-energy phosphate which readily releases a phosphate radical and then forms adenosine diphosphate (ADP). During this process, it also releases energy, and it is this energy which drives the numerous cellular processes. Conversely, ADP can easily recombine with a phosphate group to form another ATP so that constant energy sources are available. Under anaerobic conditions, that is, without oxygen, 1 mol of glucose can only synthesize 3 mol of ATP. Therefore, any process which limits cellular oxygen delivery will have an impact on energy production.

Structurally, the mitochondrial walls consist of an outer and an inner membrane. On the inner membrane are numerous infoldings which form shelves, or cristae, where oxidative enzymes responsible for ATP production are stored.

Another organelle, the *endoplasmic reticulum* (ER), is a network of tubular structures which connects with the nuclear membrane and then extends into the cytoplasm. The ER transports

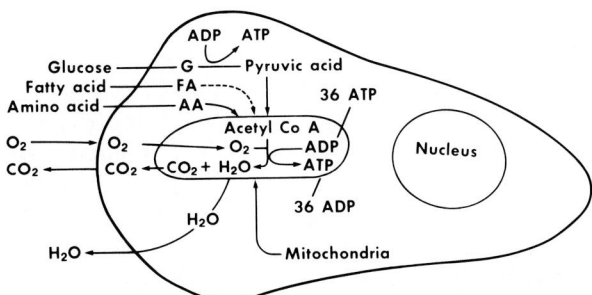

Figure 7-2 Formation by the mitochondria of adenosine triphosphate. (*Adapted from Guyton, A. Textbook of medical physiology. Philadelphia: Saunders, 1981, 21.*)

substances from one part of the cell to another. Portions of the ER which have ribosomes attached to them appear granular and are referred to as the *granular endoplasmic reticulum*. The ribosomes contain ribonucleic acid (RNA) and play a major function in the synthesis of protein. The portion of the ER without attached ribosomes is called the *smooth* or *agranular ER*. This structure plays a role in lipid synthesis. The smooth ER can also control glycogen breakdown when glycogen is used for energy, and can detoxify substances such as drugs, since it also stores enzymes.

The *Golgi complex* appears similar to the agranular ER. It consists of four or more stacked layers of flat, thin vesicles near the nucleus. This complex works closely with the ER, processing substances such as proteins after the ER synthesizes them. These processed substances then are packaged in vesicles which are released from the Golgi complex. They either extrude their protein contents outside the cell or they fuse their contents to structures inside the cell. Many vesicles fuse with the cell membranes or walls of the mitochondria and thereby replenish those structures with new proteins.

In addition, the Golgi complex synthesizes fructose and galactose and causes saccharide polymers such as hyaluronic acid and chondroctin sulfate to be formed. These latter substances are major components of the interstitial spaces where they serve as filler or gel between collagen fibers and the cells.

Finally, the last major structure to be considered is the *lysosome,* which serves as an intracellular digestive system. The lysosome has a double lipid membrane which encapsulates various hydrolytic enzymes. These enzymes are capable of splitting an organic compound into two or more parts. Normally, the lysosomes engulf unwanted substances such as dead cells or damaged substances and their enzymes digest and thereby remove them. Lysosomes also contain bactericidal agents that can kill phagocytized bacteria before they cause cellular damage. Specifically, these agents include *lysozyme,* which dissolves bacterial membranes; *lysoferrin,* which binds iron and other metals needed for bacterial growth; and acids with a pH less than 4.0. Lysosomes also contain hydrogen peroxide, which can poison bacterial metabolic systems, and which has also recently been shown to have a direct effect on the functioning and activity of the excitation/contraction coupling system in the cardiac muscle.[1] While these lysosomes are an effective and remarkable asset to the cell when the cell is functioning optimally, under certain pathologic conditions they can rupture their membranes and spill these same contents internally. Internal cellular destruction then ensues and the cell autolyses.

All these organelles and the cytoplasm are also encapsulated by a bilayer cellular membrane consisting of lipids, proteins, and carbohydrates (Fig. 7-1). The lipid components of the cell membrane are arranged in two straight rows on top of each other and allow the cell to be almost impermeable to water and to water-soluble substances such as glucose, ions, urea, and others. On the other hand, fat-soluble substances such as oxygen and carbon dioxide can penetrate this portion of the membrane.

The proteins in the membrane are intermittently scattered throughout the lipids and largely serve two functions. First, because they are wedged between the lipids, they can provide structural pathways or pores through which water and water-soluble substances, especially ions, can diffuse between intracellular and extracellular fluids. In addition, some reside entirely on the inside of the membrane and act almost exclusively as enzymes. The carbohydrates are most often found on the outside of the membrane. There they play a role in the immune system and serve as receptor substances for hormones such as epinephrine and norepinephrine.

In order for the cell to live and grow, it must be able to bring nutrients and oxygen through the cell membrane. The two major processes by which this is accomplished are *diffusion* and *active transport.* Diffusion is the movement of particles from the side of the membrane where its concentration is high, to the side where it is low. As previously mentioned, some particles can diffuse through the pores or pathways created by the wedged proteins in the cellular membrane and some easily diffuse through the lipid portions. Another method of diffusion is *facilitated diffusion.* In this instance, a particle diffuses or moves through the lipid portion of the cell membrane by combining first with a carrier substance. In tandem, the carrier substance and the particle cross the membrane and enter the cell. This is the mechanism by which glucose enters the cell.

Active transport similarly involves moving a particle attached to a carrier from one side of the membrane to the other. Active transport, however, occurs from an area of low concentration to an area of high concentration. Facilitated diffusion can move particles only in the direction of higher to lower concentrations. In active transport, this uphill action is powered by energy in the form of adenosine triphosphate (ATP). This energy is delivered to the cell membrane from the cytoplasm of the cell. There are various substances which use this method of entry into the cell. The most common are sodium, potassium, calcium, hydrogen, urate and chloride ions, amino acids, and various sugars.

The most important ionic active transport system is the sodium-potassium pump (Na^+/K^+ pump) or sodium pump. Present in all cells, the sodium pump serves to pump sodium out of the cell and into the extracellular fluid and to bring potassium from the extracellular fluid into the intracellular fluid. The carrier substance for this activity is sodium-potassium ATPase. This ATPase has the ability to bind sodium and potassium and to split ATP molecules to use their energy for active transport. The active transport process is initiated inside the cell and requires intracellular ATP to carry out its actions. Therefore, any deficit in cellular ATP production will seriously affect this ionic pump as well as many others.

Another process that can serve to transport particles into the cell is the process of *endocytosis.*

With endocytosis the cellular membrane actually engulfs the extracellular fluid and its contents or a particulate. Once inside the cell, the materials are digested and destroyed. Both *phagocytosis* and *pinocytosis* are mechanisms of endocytosis. Phagocytosis is the process where large particles, bacteria, and other cells or particles of degenerating tissue are removed. *Pinocytosis* is the ingestion of minute quantities of extracellular fluid and dissolved substances. Phagocytosis will occur when objects which have an electropositive charge contact the cell membrane. Most natural substances in the extracellular fluid are negatively charged. Foreign material and damaged tissues are specially prepared by antibodies via a process of *opsonization* so that they are positively charged, making them ideal candidates for phagocytosis. Pinocytosis occurs in the same manner when substances such as electrolytes and proteins contact the membrane. Once inside the cell, lysosomes attach to the substances and begin to hydrolyze them into amino acids, glucose, fatty acids, phosphates, etc.

In addition to these various transport functions, the cell membrane plays an important role in many chemical pathways. One that becomes particularly important in shock is the process related to adrenergic receptor reactions. Figure 7-3 schematically depicts the series of reactions which, originating at the cell membrane level, cascade into the cell and lead to enhanced myocardial contractility. On the surface of cell membranes are various receptor sites which can ultimately elicit various responses. In this situation, the receptor site is an alpha 1 receptor site which, once activated, should

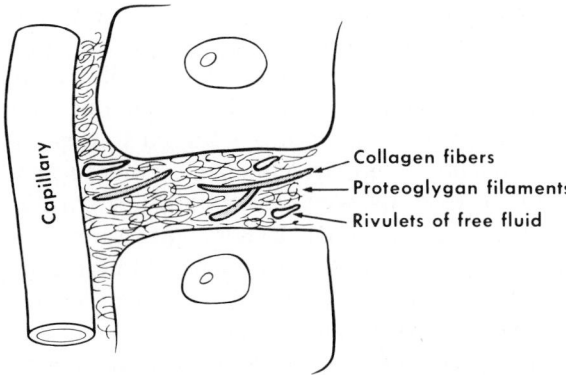

Figure 7-4   Structure of the interstitium, consisting of proteoglycan filaments and collagen bundles. (*Adapted from Guyton, A. Textbook of medical physiology. Philadelphia: Saunders, 1981, p. 362.*)

improve muscle contraction. Once an agonist (a substance which elicits a response) binds with this site, adenyl cyclase is activated. Adenyl cyclase is an enzyme embedded in the cellular membrane. It is theorized that there is also a coupling factor present in the cell membrane which facilitates the interaction between the agonist and adenyl cyclase. Once adenyl cyclase is activated, ATP in the presence of magnesium is converted to 3',5-cyclic adenosine monophosphate (cAMP). Cyclic AMP can be deactivated by an enzyme called phosphodiesterase or it can remain active and convert inactive protein kinase into active protein kinase. This ultimately leads to an enhancement of a number of calcium-dependent processes which improve muscle contraction. While this mechanism will be discussed later in the chapter, it is highlighted here to illustrate another major function of the cell membrane. Integrity of the cell membrane is of *paramount* importance in order to maintain structural and metabolic functions of the cell.

The interstitium provides a connection between the cells. Totally, one-sixth of the body's tissue is interstitium. The interstitium consists of two major solid structures: *collagen fiber bundles* and *proteoglycan filaments* (Fig. 7-4). These proteoglycan filaments synthesized from products made in the Golgi complex are very thin and when combined with the interstitial fluid form a gel between the cells. It is the formation of this gel which prevents fluid in the body from rapidly

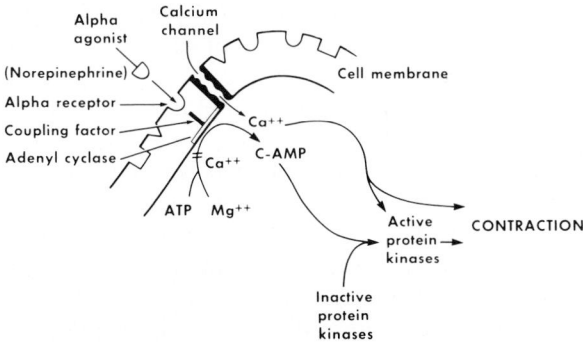

Figure 7-3   Triggering of the contraction process by an alpha-agonist via a cell membrane receptor site.

moving to dependent segments following any position change, and it is also this gel which assists in preventing microorganisms from rapidly gaining access to the body. Fluid moves through this interstitium mostly by diffusion. Scattered throughout the interstitium are rivulets of free fluid. As fluid accumulates in the interstitial bed it first expands the gel 30 to 50 percent. Further expansion beyond this point is not possible; excess fluid then accumulates in the rivulets. Once in the rivulets the fluid is very mobile. Clinically, this results in pitting edema. Pitting edema can be elicited by pressing on an edematous area for a few seconds and seeing the creation of an indentation in the skin. This indentation usually disappears a few seconds later. This indentation and subsequent disappearance reflects the mobility of the fluid in the rivulets.

Capillary and Fluid Dynamics

As was mentioned earlier, oxygen and nutrients make their way to the cells via the capillary system. The capillary system is so extensive that cells are generally no further away from a capillary than 30 θm. The structure of a typical capillary network is depicted in Fig. 7-5. Arterioles continuously surrounded by smooth muscle fibers gradually develop into metarterioles which are only intermittently surrounded by smooth muscle fibers. The smooth muscle fibers are responsible for the expansion and contraction of the diameter of these vessels

and are controlled by the sympathetic nervous system. Sympathetic stimulation will cause vasoconstriction and thereby alter the volume of these vessels and thus the volume of blood in the peripheral circulation. Due to the amount of smooth muscle encapsulating the arteriole, the diameter of the arteriole can be altered to a greater extent than the metarteriole, and therefore arteriolar vasoconstriction has a greater impact on the circulatory status.

Between the metarterioles and the capillaries there is a junction known as the *precapillary sphincter.* This sphincter consists of a band of smooth muscle fibers surrounding the capillary which regulates the flow of blood to the capillary. Neither the capillaries nor sphincters have sympathetic fibers attached to them to assist them in constricting; however, under normal circumstances these sphincters and the smooth muscle of the metarteriole intermittently contract and relax on their own 5 to 10 times a minute. This opening and closing of the sphincters is referred to as *vasomotion.* This process is controlled by autoregulation. That is, when the tissue oxygenation level is low, the sphincter relaxes and blood flow enters the capillary. As that area becomes adequately oxygenated, that sphincter will close and another will open in an area of inadequate oxygenation. Blood flow to the capillaries then is not continuous but rather intermittent. There are two types of capillaries, the *preferential channels,* which are somewhat large, and the *true capillaries,* which are small. The walls of the capillaries themselves consist of only one layer of endothelial cells. Small intercellular clefts or slitlike pores lie between adjacent endothelial cells. In addition, some have *fenestrae,* large openings in the middle. Substances can pass back and forth between the capillary and the interstitium, either through the capillary membrane via diffusion or pinocytosis, or across the intercellular clefts or fenestrae via diffusion.

Finally, as blood flow exits the capillaries, it returns to the venules. As can be seen by the diagram, the venules also are surrounded intermittently by smooth muscle fiber. This muscle allows them also to contract. Even though there is less smooth muscle available on the venules for contraction, contraction can be quite strong, since the pressure the venules are working against, the

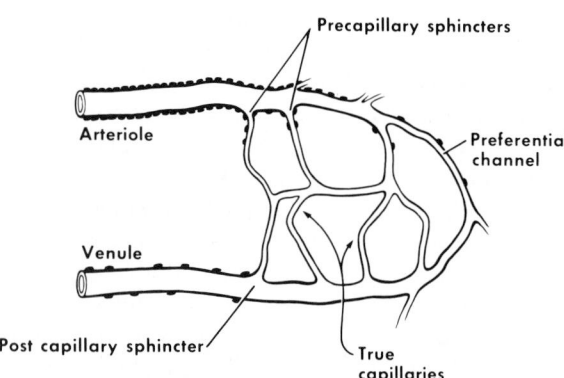

Figure 7-5   Typical capillary network depicting arterioles, metarterioles, capillaries, venules, and veins. (*Adapted from Guyton, A. Textbook of medical physiology. Philadelphia: Saunders, 1981, p. 233.*)

venous pressure, is lower than the arteriolar pressure.

In addition to their role of carriers of nutrients and oxygen, the capillaries play a major role in maintaining a balanced movement of fluid between themselves and the interstitial spaces. While the movement of this fluid is accomplished by the process of diffusion, this movement is controlled by various forces inside the capillary and in the interstitial spaces. These forces and their relationship to each other are illustrated in the following equation and in Fig. 7-6.

$$Qf = K(Pmv - Pi) - K\sigma\ (\pi mv - \pi i)$$

in which

 Qf = Net transvascular flow of fluid through the vessel.

 K = Capillary filtration coefficient. This value varies from one type of tissue to another and refers to that tissue's particular permeability. The permeability of brain tissue, for example, is significantly less than that in the intestine, and therefore movement of substances across the capillaries in the brain is limited.

Pmv = Microvascular or capillary hydrostatic pressure. This is the water pressure in the capillary which favors outward flow of fluid across the capillary membrane.

 Pi = Interstitial hydrostatic pressure. This refers to water pressure in the interstitium which favors movement of water into the capillary and out of the interstitium.

 σ = Protein reflection coefficient. This coefficient relates to the size of protein molecules which would be able to sieve through the membrane.

πmv = Serum protein osmotic pressure. This force tends to draw fluid into the capillary and out of the interstitium.

 πi = Interstitial protein osmotic pressure. This refers to the pressure which favors movement of fluid out of the capillary and into the interstitium.

Under normal circumstances, there is a tremendous amount of movement and flux of fluid and substances across the capillary membrane. However, with these forces operating, normally

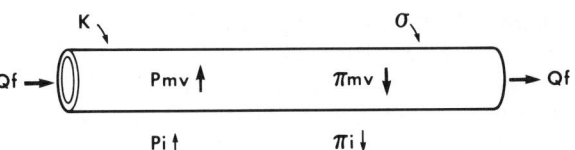

Figure 7-6 Starling's equation governing the effect of forces on the capillary.

there is little net difference in movement of fluid in and out of the capillary. Any net increase in movement out of the capillary and into the interstitium is then removed from the interstitium by the lymphatic system and is ultimately returned to the vascular bed. As will be seen later in the chapter, major alteration of any of these forces or alteration in capillary wall integrity, such as occurs in permeability leaks, can lead to significant symptoms.

Definition of Shock

Generally, shock has been defined as a state which develops when there is inadequate tissue perfusion. And certainly in the case of cardiogenic shock or hemorrhagic shock, this has been true. However, in hyperdynamic stages of septic shock, xenon studies have shown that the blood flow to the capillaries may be greater than normal.[2] The major problem in this situation appears to be an inability of the cell to appropriately extract and utilize substrates and oxygen from that delivered blood. Therefore, shock more appropriately should be considered as a pathophysiologic abnormality in which there is inadequate blood flow to vital organs and/or the inability of the tissues or individual cell to metabolize nutrients normally. The clinical syndrome of shock and its sequelae result from sustained, inadequate tissue perfusion and utilization which then leads to alterations in tissue metabolism, structure, and function at the subcellular, cellular, and systems level.[3–5]

Cycle of Cellular Deterioration in Shock

The general sequence of events which occurs in the cell during shock is well documented[3,6,7] and is depicted in Fig. 7-7. The decrease in oxygenation causes the cell membrane potential to decrease and

Figure 7-7 Effects of inadequate perfusion at the cellular level. (*Adapted from Chaudry, I. D. Cellular mechanisms in shock and ischemia and their correction. Am. J. Physiol., 1983, 245, R117–R134.*)

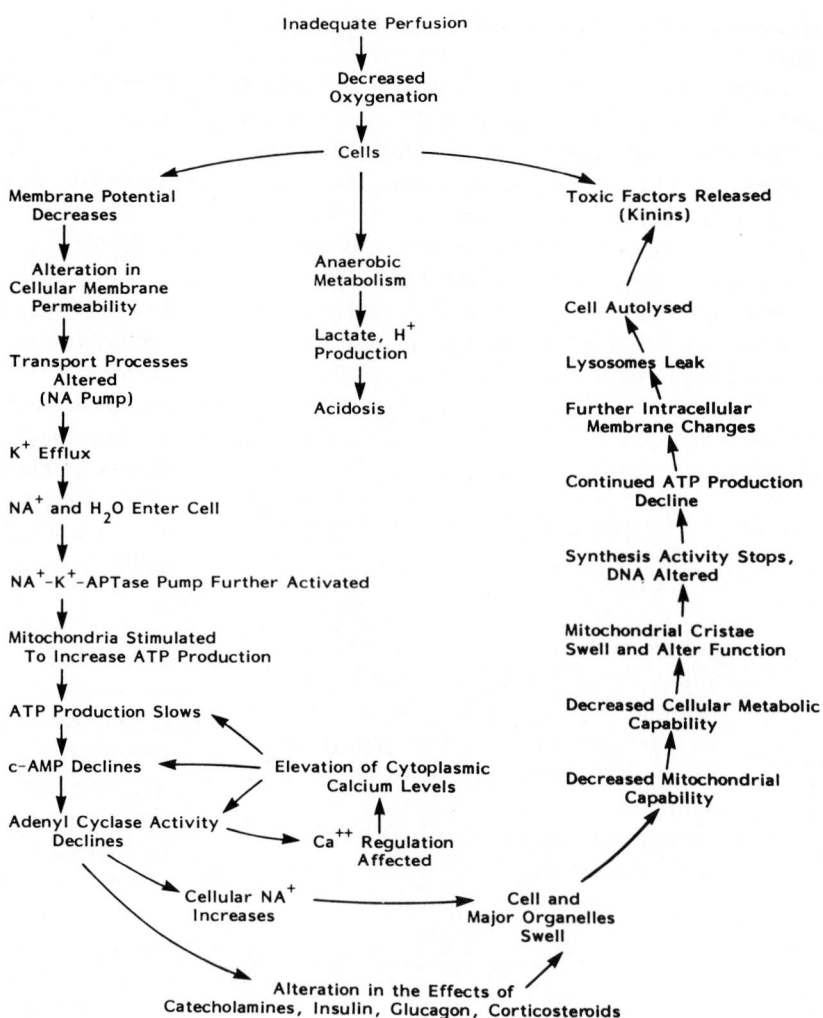

membrane permeability to alter. Consequently, both structural and metabolic processes are affected. The sodium pump begins to fail, thus altering transport processes and potassium effluxes out of the cell, and intracellular sodium and water increase. As sodium accumulates in the cell, the Na^+/K^+-ATPase pump is stimulated to work faster. This causes an increased consumption of ATP and forces the mitochondria to increase production. However, with inadequate oxygen delivery, this production quickly slows. As ATP production decreases and damage to the cell membrane occurs, cAMP production declines. As indicated earlier, cAMP plays a crucial role in catecholamine function, calcium regulation, and numerous other cellular processes. In order

to form, cAMP needs the presence of ATP and adenyl cyclase. Normally, adenyl cyclase is attached to the cell membrane, readily available to assist in the transformation of cAMP. With loss of ATP and the breakdown in the cellular wall, cAMP is decreased, and the reactions it initiates are diminished.

Calcium fluxes develop, and calcium regulation is compromised. Normally the mitochondria contain significant supplies of calcium. As ATP continues to convert to ADP, free phosphates accumulate in the cytoplasm. This causes the mitochondria to lose their calcium supply. Also, with impairment of the cell membrane, calcium leaves the extracellular fluid and enters the cell. All these actions create an elevation of the cytoplasmic Ca^{2+}

levels and this appears to inhibit the mitochondria from releasing ATP into the cytoplasm. High cytoplasmic calcium also interferes with the adenyl cyclase in the cell membrane, thereby decreasing the production of cAMP. As mentioned earlier, this affects the cell's response to adrenergic agents.

At this stage, not only does the cell itself swell but the major organelles such as the ER, the mitochondria, and the cell membrane also swell. Protein synthesis and ion pumps begin to halt their actions. As the cristae and the inner mitochondrial membranes swell, only minimal ATP synthesis can occur since now the structures responsible for production are destroyed. At this point, if perfusion is reinstituted the cell can still recover; however, if not halted at this point, anaerobic glycolysis continues to completely take over and lactic and pyruvic acid production will continue to increase. Ultimate cellular survival becomes less and less likely.

At this point the lysosomes begin to leak and release their hydrolases which initiate internal digestion of the remaining cellular contents. Ultimately these enzymes will assist in the destruction of neighboring cells. The proteolytic enzymes from the lysosomes are particularly active and can convert inactive kininogens into active kinins. One of these kinins is *bradykinin,* which is a potent vasodilator responsible for skin flushing, which can develop particularly in septic shock. Bradykinin is also linked with the ability to increase capillary permeability.

The rate of progression through this entire series of events varies from cell to cell. Skeletal muscle cells and smooth cells move very slowly through this process. This perhaps could be due to the fact that these cells have a high capacity for anaerobic metabolism. Even if circulation is reestablished before the cell autolyses, the cells do not immediately return to their correct size. It takes time for the edema to resolve and, consequently, further damage, injury, and perhaps death can result from the ischemia which is induced by the edematous environment.

Systemic Responses to Shock

In the previous section the sequential responses of individual cells to inadequate perfusion were described. As inadequate perfusion persists and significant numbers of cells are affected, organ systems begin to malfunction and clinically perceptible signs and symptoms begin to appear. At this point hypoxemia, hypotension, and acidosis begin to activate some of the body's compensatory mechanisms.

One of the first mechanisms to be activated is the sympathetic nervous system. Falls in arterial pressure are quickly sensed by the baroreceptors in the aorta and the carotid sinus. Once stimulated, these receptors send impulses to the vasomotor center in the medulla. Consequently, the vasomotor center signals the sympathetic nerve fibers throughout the body to discharge norepinephrine from their endings. This discharge will create vasoconstriction of the arteriolar beds, which will assist in raising arterial pressure. In addition, the adrenal medulla will also be sympathetically stimulated by the vasomotor center and will release both epinephrine and norepinephrine into the bloodstream. In this manner, even cells not attached to sympathetic fibers, such as the metarterioles, are exposed to the vasoconstrictor effects of these hormones.

In early stages of shock, blood is shunted away from organs that tolerate ischemia well, such as the skeletal muscles, fat, and skin. In these areas, arterioles contract and shunt blood away from the capillaries and through arteriovenous fistulas into the venous system. In organs which cannot tolerate lack of oxygen, such as the heart and brain, the arterioles remain open and the true capillaries still receive their blood flow.[8] As shock progresses this mechanism fails. Arteriolar and precapillary sphincter constriction requires sufficient energy in the form of ATP to maintain a vasoconstrictive state. As energy dissipates, the sphincters relax and blood then flows into these organs and sequesters. Sludging of the blood in these capillary beds occurs and the microcirculation becomes blocked. Metabolic waste products, microaggregates of platelets, white blood cells, and clots accumulate, further enhancing sludging and contributing to the development of metabolic acidosis. Arachidonic acid metabolites such as thromboxane A_2 and prostacylin might also play an important role in the events which occur in the microcirculation. Thromboxane A_2 and prostacyclin experience high serum levels in severe shock. Thromboxane A_2 is produced by white blood cells and platelets and is a potent platelet aggregator and a vasoconstrictor. Prostacyclin is produced by the vascular endothelium and is a potent antiplatelet aggregator and a vasodilator. These two substances normally counterbalance each other and maintain homeostasis. However, in severe hypovolemic and septic shock the actions of thromboxane A_2 seem to dominate. This might contribute significantly to the clotting and sludging in the microcirculation which appear in these states.[9–12]

As was noted above, epinephrine plays an important role in the body's response to shock. In addition to its effect on the vascular bed it also plays a role in enhancing myocardial contractility and increasing blood levels of glucose. It accomplishes the latter by increasing the breakdown of glycogen, by increasing gluconeogenesis from amino acids and lactate, and by inhibiting the secretion of insulin. Epinephrine also increases serum levels of free fatty acids by stimulating lipolysis. All these activities are aimed at supplying the body with readily available energy sources to assist in maintaining metabolic functions. Serum levels of the glucocorticoids, cortisone and cortisol, also rise in early stages of shock. They, as epinephrine, play a role in producing glucose and free fatty acids. Additionally, glucocorticoids have a mild inotropic effect on the myocardium and may assist in stabilizing subcellular, cellular, and endothelial membranes.

A fall in arterial pressure near the aortic and carotid bodies can also initiate a respiratory compensatory response. If the fall in arterial pressure creates a decrease in oxygen concentration to the receptors, an increase in respiratory rate will occur. This is an attempt by the body to increase oxygenation.

Another compensatory mechanism is the formation of angiotensin, another powerful vasoconstrictor. When the juxtaglomerular apparatus in the nephron senses a fall in arterial pressure or sodium concentration, it releases renin. Renin stimulates the release of angiotensin I. Angiotensin I is converted into angiotensin II in the lungs, and this stimulates the adrenal cortex to synthesize and release aldosterone. Aldosterone allows the kidney to save sodium and water and to excrete potassium and hydrogen. This provides the body with a mechanism to maintain or retain volume. In addition, angiotensin II causes marked vasoconstriction of the peripheral arterioles and a moderate con-

striction of the veins, thus assisting in increasing systemic blood pressure.

The formation of *antidiuretic hormone* (ADH) or *vasopressin* is also a component of the body's compensatory plan. Vasopressin is the body's most potent vasoconstrictor substance. It is formed in the hypothalamus and secreted by the posterior pituitary in response to a decreased blood pressure and an increased osmolality. Vasopressin is released as early as 15 min following an insult.[13] The fall in blood pressure activates the baroreceptors which stimulate the hypothalamus and posterior pituitary to synthesize and release ADH. The osmolality directly affects the hypothalamus. If the osmoreceptors detect a dilute osmolality, then ADH is inhibited; if the osmolality is high, then ADH is secreted. Also, in shock states a loss of 10 percent of the person's blood volume can create a moderate release in ADH. Loss of blood volume is detected by low-pressure receptors in the atria. Other factors responsible for an increase in ADH production are trauma, pain, anxiety, morphine, tranquilizers, and some anesthetic agents. The action of ADH is on the distal renal tubules so that water is reabsorbed. This mechanism further augments venous return and improves cardiac output.

The reverse stress relaxation response of the circulatory system also plays a compensatory role. This is a mechanism which allows blood vessels, once volume has been lost, to constrict around the remaining blood volume so that the volume left will more adequately fill the circulation. This mechanism assists in returning blood to the myocardium. Other mechanisms which assist in returning volume to the vascular bed and then ultimately to the myocardium include the absorption of fluid from the intestines and from the interstitium.

All the previously identified mechanisms were initiated at the peripheral level either via baroreceptors, chemoreceptors, or low-pressure receptors. One last powerful response remains in the central nervous system and this is referred to as the *CNS ischemic response*. This response is elicited when the vasomotor cells begin to experience ischemia, high carbon dioxide, and lactic acid levels, usually when arterial pressure falls below 50 mmHg. This stimulation elicits a sympathetic drive which can raise the arterial pressure by 15 to 20 mmHg.

Associated Problems

As the effects of shock persist, specific organ systems begin to develop clinical syndromes in response to their ischemic states. Inadequate perfusion will lead to a decreased removal of waste products and metabolites in the cell's immediate environment, since the normal function of circulation is not only to perfuse and bring in oxygen and nutrients, but also to carry away metabolic waste products. As these waste products accumulate they can cause depression of the reticuloendothelial system (RES). Under normal circumstances this system plays an important role in phagocytosis and removal of waste products. The exact cause of RES dysfunction is not known; however, it has been reported that it may be associated with dysfunction of the opsonization process. As stated earlier, this is a process whereby foreign or waste materials are acted upon by antibodies which make them positively charged. Positively charged materials are targets for phagocytosis, and without this marking process these substances will not be identified as removable.[14] There is a strong correlation between the degree of RES dysfunction and mortality.[15]

The pulmonary system can be affected tremendously by shock. Pulmonary edema states can develop as the forces in the capillary fluid dynamics equation are altered. In patients with cardiogenic shock, a cardiac or hydrostatic pulmonary edema can develop. In this situation, as the left ventricle fails and left ventricular volumes and pressures rise, this creates an elevation in pulmonary pressures. This increase leads to an increased capillary or microvascular hydrostatic pressure in the lung, and fluid begins to leak out into the interstitial spaces. If it is only a moderate increase, the lymphatics will drain the excess fluid. However, as transudation of this fluid approaches 200 mL per hour, the lymphatics will no longer be able to keep pace with the fluid removal, and interstitial pulmonary edema will develop[16] (Fig. 7-8A). As the capillary hydrostatic pressure increases further, fluid will begin to accumulate in the alveoli, leading to the development of alveolar edema (Fig. 7-8B). The mainstay of therapy for these types of pulmonary edema is aimed at fluid removal, either with diuretics or by improving myocardial contractility.

Another type of pulmonary sequela which can develop in shock states is permeability pulmonary edema. There are generally two types of this pulmonary edema. The first, *noncardiac edema* (NCE), develops when there is damage to the capillary endothelium (Fig. 7-8C). This damage allows colloid to leak across the capillary and lie in the interstitium. In this fashion, the interstitial protein osmotic pressure is altered, thus favoring fluid sequestering in the interstitium. The precipitating factors in this endothelial damage can be ischemic damage to the lung parenchyma itself or due to the effects of toxic factors. Noncardiac permeability pulmonary edema develops into adult respiratory distress syndrome (ARDS) when the permeability damage involves both capillary endothelium and alveolar epithelial structures (Fig. 7-8D). In this situation, the leak and cellular disruption is so great that colloid leaks into both the interstitium and the alveolus. This tremendously alters the normal fluid equation and favors fluid accumulation in both the interstitium and alveolus. Adult respiratory distress syndrome develops when there is a massive insult to the cells, either from severe ischemic insult from low-flow states or more commonly from exposure to toxic substances which are released in septic shock.

Disseminated intravascular coagulopathy (DIC) is another associated problem which can develop as a consequence of inadequate perfusion states. Under normal circumstances the processes of thrombosis (clot formation) and fibrinolysis (clot digestion) occur at a localized site of an injury and ultimately prevent hemorrhage. In DIC, these processes occur generally throughout the microcirculation and result in extensive hemorrhage. In the setting of inadequate tissue perfusion, DIC is most likely to be triggered by infectious agents, massive tissue trauma, or burns.[17] These processes serve as the initiators of this clot formation and clot digestion cycle. In the clot formation process thrombin is generated from prothrombin. In the circulation, thrombin cleaves fibrinogen to form insoluble fibrin clots. These fibrin clots deposited in the microcirculation lead to tissue ischemia and contribute to the consumption of platelets and other clotting factors such as fibrinogen, prothrombin, and factors V, VIII, and XIII. The clot dissolution or fibrinolysis process digests fibrinogen, fibrin, and

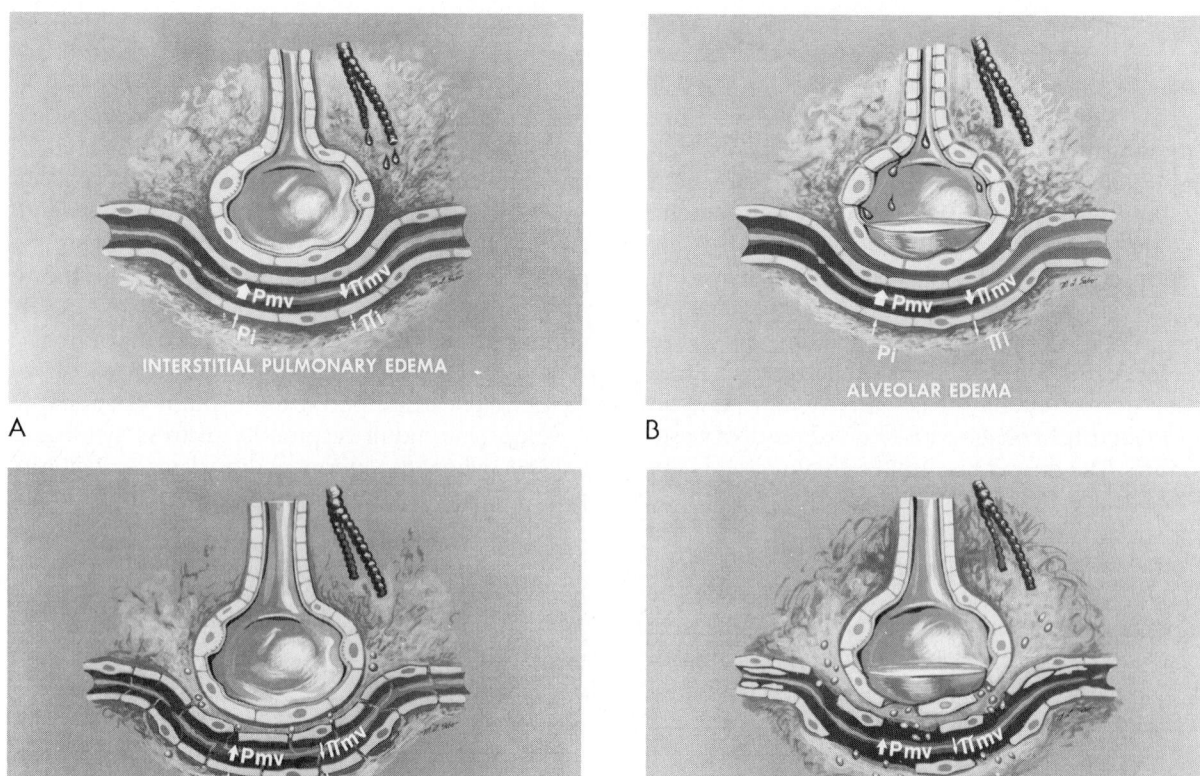

Figure 7-8   *A.*   Alveolar and pulmonary capillary changes associated with interstitial pulmonary edema. The lymphatics can no longer remove fluid rapidly enough and it accumulates in the interstitial space. *B.* Alveolar and capillary changes with alveolar edema. Fluid is now sequestering in both the interstitium and the alveoli. *C.* Alveolar and capillary changes seen in noncardiac edema. Capillary endothelial cells are disrupted. *D.* Alveolar and capillary changes seen in adult respiratory distress syndrome. Alveolar epithelial and capillary endothelial cells are disrupted.

factors II, V, VIII, and XIII. In addition, fibrin degradation products are formed after fibrinogen and the newly formed fibrin monomers are split by plasmin. These fibrin degradation products are potent anticoagulants. These factors—the consumption or digestion of platelets and clotting factors, the fibrinolytic or clot dissolution activity of plasmin, and the anticoagulant properties of fibrin degradation products—contribute to the systemic bleeding and hemorrhage problems seen clinically with DIC.

Treatment of DIC involves treating and correcting the underlying triggering event, replace-

ment of clotting factors, and heparin therapy[18,19] (Chap. 43). Replacement component therapy generally includes platelet units to replace platelets; fresh frozen plasma to replace factors V, VIII, and XIII; and cryoprecipitate to replace fibrinogen and factor VIII. The use of heparin therapy remains controversial as there exist no controlled studies which support its efficacy.[20]

Prerenal and acute renal failure are common sequelae of shock states. With slight or moderate decrease in cardiac output the kidney compensates as discussed earlier by conserving sodium and water and by shunting its blood flow from the cortical nephrons to the sodium-saving juxtaglomerular ones. Urine produced during this stage is low in volume and is concentrated. With the restoration of perfusion, the kidney will most often quickly resume normal functioning. However, with severe and prolonged falls in cardiac output the renal parenchymal cells become damaged and acute tubular necrosis develops. It should also be pointed out that, in addition to ischemia, other factors also contribute to the development of acute renal failure. Some of these factors playing a role include: tubular obstruction, glomerular ultrafiltration back diffusion, decreased glomerular permeability coefficient, persistent fibrin deposits in the glomerular capillary, and changes in intracellular biochemistry.[21,22]

Hepatic complications seen in hypoperfusion states include centrolobular necrosis, enlarged Kupffer cells, and fatty infiltrates. These processes lead to alterations in hepatic functions such that transaminase levels rise and albumin and prothrombin production fall. Gastrointestinal problems also develop as erosions and ulcerations in the stomach and enteritis develop. These alterations are believed to be caused by back diffusion of hydrogen ions across the mucosa and maldistribution of blood flow to the mucosa due to low flow. The mucosa is primarily affected since it performs most of the work for the gastrointestinal system and therefore is a high consumer of oxygen. Additionally, Mallory-Weiss syndrome can be produced by shock. This syndrome consists of longitudinal lacerations of the gastric mucosa below the esophagus and is frequently associated with hemorrhage. Major bleeding from these areas can be avoided by increasing the gastric pH with antacids or drugs.[23]

Generally, the last organ to be damaged by the shock state is the brain. Protected by various cerebral compensatory mechanisms, blood flow to the brain is preserved when all other vessels are constricted. However, ultimately persistent low flow does lead to damage, and EEG changes develop. Clinically the patient gradually progresses from restless and agitated states to somnolence and coma. Evaluation of the extent of permanent CNS damage may be difficult to ascertain since other depressive factors such as acidosis and other metabolic derangements may be present concurrently.

Stages of Shock

In general, shock can be divided into two stages: *compensated shock* and *decompensated shock*.[15,24] *Compensated shock* refers to that stage during which the severity of the shock itself and the intensity of the compensatory mechanisms are such that the vital organs have continued to be adequately perfused. *Decompensated shock* refers to that stage during which the severity of the shock itself or the inadequacy or failure of the compensatory mechanisms are such that the vital organs are hypoperfused. In hypovolemic shock, for example, a moderate loss of blood volume from an external hemorrhage may trigger the previously described compensatory mechanism, and adequate perfusion to vital organs is maintained. If, however, volume loss continues without replacement, the patient might additionally develop myocardial ischemia from poor coronary artery filling, leading to eventual decompensation. Effective treatment modalities would be aimed at supporting the compensatory mechanisms and remedying the underlying problem.

Etiologies of Altered Tissue Perfusion

Generally, there are four major types of shock: *hypovolemic, cardiogenic, distributive,* and *obstructive*. Each of these types has specific mechanisms whereby tissue perfusion is altered. In hypovolemic shock, inadequate volume causes a decrease in tissue perfusion, while in cardiogenic shock an inadequate pump causes a decrease in tissue perfusion. Maldistribution of the circulation and obstruction to the distribution of the circulation are the major factors interfering with tissue perfusion in distributive and obstructive shock. The next section will describe in detail the specific etiologies which create these shock stages and the accompanying pathophysiologic changes.

Hypovolemic Shock

Hypovolemic shock develops when there is inadequate blood volume to fill the intravascular space.[25]

This occurs in states where there are obvious or direct volume losses and in states where there are indirect volume losses. Direct losses occur with external hemorrhage, diarrhea, vomiting, massive diuresis, and loss of plasma from skin lesions or exposed burn areas. Direct losses are for the most part easily identifiable and can to some extent be quantified. Indirect losses are less measurable and can be caused by situations where there is a sequestering of fluids in third spaces. This can be seen in patients with cirrhosis who sequester fluid in the peritoneal cavity. Interstitial tissue spaces can also serve as reservoirs of fluid, particularly when there is an alteration in capillary permeability or when there is a fall in colloidal osmotic pressure. In intestinal obstruction there is a tendency for fluid to mobilize from the intestinal capillaries and fill the lumen of the intestine, thereby creating an intravascular deficit. Internal hemorrhages such as a hemothorax, hemorrhagic pancreatitis, a ruptured spleen, or long bone fractures also lead to hypovolemic shock. Lastly, severe salt depletion, Addisonian crisis, and hypopituitarism can also serve as causes of hypovolemic shock.[26,27]

Generally, there are three stages of hypovolemic shock: mild, moderate, and severe.[28] Depending on the severity and the rate of the volume loss, the patient may progress through these stages very slowly or very rapidly. In the mild stage, the patient generally experiences a blood volume deficit ranging from 0 to 10 percent or approximately 500 mL.

This volume deficit creates a reduction in venous return and cardiac output which is sensed by the baroreceptors. The autonomic nervous system is activated and the subsequent increase in sympathetic constriction of the vasculature and the increase in myocardial contractility serve to maintain arterial pressure and cardiac output. Secretion of antidiuretic hormone, renin, and aldosterone also begins at this point. Blood flow is shunted away from the skin, fat, and skeletal tissues and the patient may begin to appear pale. The first phase of the transcapillary refill mechanism becomes activated when the sympathetic nervous system constricts the precapillary sphincters, the postcapillary sphincters, and the small veins.[21,29,30] With this, the capillary hydrostatic pressure decreases and fluid moves from the interstitium into the

capillary. The ultimate rate of transcapillary refill can be as high as 1 L an hour.[31] Since the large fenestrae in the capillary are normally closed at this time, minimal protein moves into the circulation with this volume.[32] Because of the activation of all these mechanisms the patient remains relatively if not totally asymptomatic during this mild stage of hypovolemic shock. In general, the relationship between cardiac output and acute volume loss is not a straight line but rather a curved one (Fig. 7-9). The curved portion represents the protective effects of the compensatory mechanisms. Major deteriorations in cardiac output normally occur with volume losses exceeding 25 to 30 percent.

Almost concurrently, as the first stage is activated, the second phase of transcapillary refill begins to additionally assist in volume restoration.[33] In the initial phase, fluid moved from the interstitium into the intravascular compartment. This created an increase in capillary hydrostatic pressure and a subsequent dilution in plasma protein concentration. The falling interstitial hydrostatic pressure and the rising interstitial oncotic pressure allow protein to mobilize from the interstitium and invade the vascular space. In addition, the elevated interstitial oncotic pressure facilitates movement of fluid from intracellular sites to interstitial lodgings.[34] The end result is continued restitution of volume losses. Albumin synthesis has been reported to increase by 12 to 75 percent after hemorrhage.[35] However, the magnitude of protein returned to the

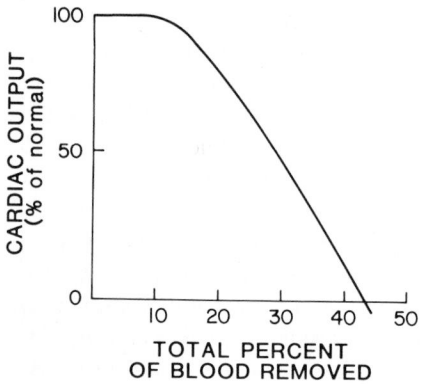

Figure 7-9 The effect of blood volume removal on cardiac output.

vascular bed shortly after the onset of hemorrhage indicates that the source of albumin is more likely to be preformed albumin mobilized from the interstitium,[36] rather than newly formed albumin.

In moderate hypovolemic shock, there is a marked reduction in cardiac output and arterial pressure, and a 15 to 20 percent reduction in blood volume is experienced. There is intense arteriolar vasoconstriction and diminished blood flow to the liver, pancreas, kidney, and gastrointestinal tract. In this stage there is also a general venoconstriction which assists in increasing venous return to the general circulation. The intense adrenergic discharge which occurs results in tachycardia, tachypnea, cutaneous vasoconstriction, pallor, diaphoresis, piloerection, apprehension, and restlessness. Synthesis of replacement blood components occurs. However, synthesis cannot keep pace with massive losses. Platelets and polymorphonuclear leukocytes are the elements most quickly mobilized. Plasma proteins are restored at various rates and red cells take the longest to form.

In severe hypovolemic shock, the blood volume deficit exceeds 25 percent, and small additional losses create major falls in cardiac output, blood pressure, and tissue perfusion. At this point, all the compensatory mechanisms are functioning at maximum capacity, and even the brain and the myocardium now are subject to a fall in perfusion. The patient becomes confused, anxious, agitated, obtunded, and comatose. Metabolic alterations now become very evident. Hyperglycemia develops as glucose is mobilized. Lipids are also mobilized, and lactate levels rise. Severe lactic acidosis and oliguria develop, and mixed venous oxygen tension is low.

At this point, the precapillary sphincters may lose their spasm while the postcapillary sphincters remain constricted. This allows capillary hydrostatic pressure to elevate and facilitates loss of volume and protein into the interstitial spaces.[8] If the shock state persists, cellular death from severe organ vasoconstriction occurs.

The goal of therapy in hypovolemic shock is to restore adequate intravascular volume as quickly as possible. This can be accomplished most readily by the infusion of various replacement solutions and by the use of various external devices. These therapies will be discussed in detail in a later section.

Cardiogenic Shock

Cardiogenic shock occurs when there is an inability of the myocardium to function as a pump to maintain adequate tissue perfusion. This results directly from a severe impairment of ventricular pumping function. However, other mechanisms such as hypovolemia and vasomotor, metabolic, or microcirculatory dysfunction may contribute to progressive cardiovascular deterioration. The highest incidence of cardiogenic shock occurs in patients who have atherosclerotic heart disease in which either a massive singular myocardial infarction or multiple small myocardial infarctions have destroyed 40 to 50 percent of the left ventricular myocardium.[37,38] Cardiogenic shock can also develop if the infarction creates mechanical problems such as mitral regurgitation from a papillary muscle rupture or if a ventricular septal defect due to an intraventricular septal infarction is created. Additionally, patients with end-stage cardiomyopathies can also develop cardiogenic shock.

A transient cardiogenic shock can develop following cardiac surgery in which the myocardium is depressed following hypothermia, cardioplegic arrest, and surgical incisions. And lastly, arrhythmias can be responsible for this shock state. A listing of etiologies of cardiogenic shock is given in Table 7-1. Regardless of the etiology, the end result is a

Table 7-1 Etiologies of Cardiogenic Shock

Acute myocardial infarction
  Loss of 40–50% of critical myocardial mass
  Mechanical complications
    Perforated intraventricular septum
    Papillary muscle rupture or dysfunction
    Cardiac rupture
    Ventricular aneurysm

Cardiomyopathies (end stage)
  Congestive
    Alcoholic, hypertensive, ischemic, myocarditis,
      amyloid, idiopathic
  Hypertrophic
  Restrictive

Valvular heart disease
  Severe valvular stenosis
  Acute valvular regurgitation

Postoperative low cardiac output syndrome

Dysrhythmias

cardiac output insufficient to meet tissue needs. As stated above, the initial problem is an impairment of ventricular pumping action. This creates a reduction in stroke volume and cardiac output. If this fall in cardiac output is not compensated by an increase in vascular resistance, the mean arterial pressure will fall. This will further compromise the ventricle since coronary artery blood flow is in part determined by aortic pressure. A fall in aortic root diastolic pressure will lead to a fall in coronary artery blood flow. If the compensatory mechanisms are working, the systemic vascular resistance will become elevated in an attempt to maintain mean arterial pressure. Simultaneously, the sympathetic nervous system activates catecholamine release. This could also be detrimental and potentiate low cardiac output since this increases the afterload or the resistance against which the ventricle must contract in order to eject volume. In addition, the sympathetic drive will increase ventricular contractility which might also potentiate myocardial ischemia and, hence, failure.

The left ventricular end-diastolic volume and pressure continue to increase as long as the ventricle fails to successfully eject adequate volumes. This leads to distention of the ventricular cavity, which further increases afterload and also can serve to limit filling of endocardial coronary arteries, thereby creating endocardial ischemia. The elevated left ventricular end-diastolic pressure is passively transmitted to the pulmonary veins and the pulmonary bed. The increase in pulmonary venous pressure can lead to the development of pulmonary edema. Arterial hypoxemia is related to this pulmonary venous congestion. Pulmonary artery pressures become elevated due to this hypoxia and concurrent acidosis. Right ventricular failure can also develop from this volume load and this pulmonary hypertension. Additionally, a right ventricular infarction can occur isolated from this left ventricular event due to right ventricular coronary artery disease.

While the hypovolemic patient is best described in phases, hemodynamic subset classifications are most commonly used to describe a patient's progressing into or recovering from cardiogenic shock. Figure 7-10 depicts a hemodynamic subset classification in which the cardiac index is compared to the pulmonary capillary

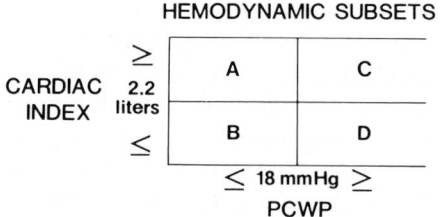

Figure 7-10 Hemodynamic subset classification.

wedge pressure (PCWP). In class A, patients have a cardiac index greater than 2.2 L/min per m² and normal to low pulmonary capillary wedge pressures. This class is generally reflective of patients who have experienced small myocardial infarcts. Mortality in this group is generally 10 percent. Class B is characterized by patients with a cardiac index less than 2.2 L/min per m² and pulmonary capillary wedge pressures less than 18 mmHg. This class represents patients who are relatively hypovolemic. Mortality in this group is usually 30 to 50 percent. In class C, cardiac indexes are greater than 2.2 L/min per m² and the wedge pressures are elevated. This group is generally hypervolemic and also experiences a mortality of 30 to 50 percent. Finally, class D patients present with a cardiac index less than 2.2 L/min per m² and elevated filling pressures. Mortality in this group can be as high as 90 percent as the patient moves to the lower right portion of that class. The majority of patients with cardiogenic shock can be categorized as class D.

A cardiac index less than 1.8 L/min per m² in an adequately volume-loaded patient is generally the agreed-upon definition for cardiogenic shock. Therefore, if the cardiac index is less than 1.8 and the PCWP is less than 18 mmHg, the etiology of the shock state is perhaps more hypovolemic than cardiogenic. Using this method of classification as a background, therapeutic modalities for the cardiogenic shock patient can be sequentially delineated for the classes (Fig. 7-11). The specific therapeutic modalities will be discussed in further detail later in the chapter.

Obstructive Shock

Obstructive shock develops when there is a physical obstruction to flow somewhere in the circulatory system. This can develop with pulmonary embo-

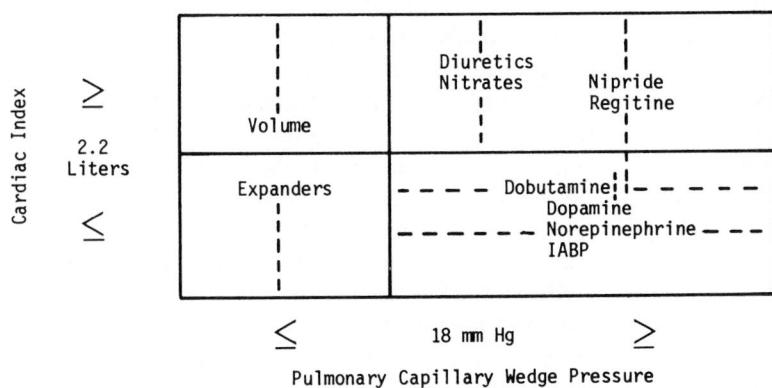

TREATMENT MODALITIES BASED ON
HEMODYNAMIC SUBSETS

Figure 7-11 Treatment modalities commonly associated with the hemodynamic subset classifications.

lisms, dissecting aortic aneurysms, pericardial tamponade, atrial myxoma, tension pneumothorax, or a ruptured hemidiaphragm with evisceration of abdominal contents into the thoracic cavity. These events will impair venous return because of the high pressures surrounding the right atrium. With the tension pneumothorax and the ruptured hemidiaphragm, venous return is impaired because the great veins are compressed as they enter the chest. Clinically, with the exception of the distended neck veins, these patients resemble those in hypovolemic shock. Ultimate treatment modalities for these patients are largely surgical in nature.

Distributive Shock

Distributive shock refers to states where there is an abnormal distribution of the intravascular volume. Septic, anaphylactic, and neurogenic shock all fall in this classification. In septic shock, the abnormal distribution of intravascular volume is due to the massive vasodilation which develops related to microorganisms and their by-products. Before describing the specific pathophysiologic changes associated with septic shock, it is helpful to view septic shock from the perspective of a clinical continuum which gradually progresses through the stages of septicemia—preshock, hyperdynamic shock, hypodynamic shock, and multiple system organ failure.[39] The progression through these phases depends on the types and number of organisms, the treatment-related factors to which

the host is exposed, and the risk factors inherent in the host.[39,40] Chapter 58 provides an in-depth discussion of these factors.

Inherent risk factors for sepsis within the host include chronic diseases such as cardiac, pulmonary, renal, or hepatic disease; diabetes mellitus or alcoholism; malnutrition; debilitation; pregnancy; or extremes of age. Inadequate myocardial, respiratory, endocrine, or renal function limits the host's ability to cope with the numerous stresses associated with septic shock. In hepatic disease, the ability of the host's Kupffer cells to phagocytize bacteria is altered. This factor is also present in hosts with a history of alcoholism. In addition, these patients are also generally malnourished. The risk of a ruptured ectopic pregnancy or an incomplete septic abortion serves to make pregnancy a risk factor. And age extremes, hosts under the age of 1 and over 65 years of age, are also placed at high risk due to developmental changes in immune systems.

Treatment-related factors associated with a high risk of septic shock are also quite numerous. The presence of invasive devices, such as intravascular or intracavity catheters or drains, serve as ideal portals for microorganisms to gain access to a host. Some surgical procedures, such as genitourinary procedures, place the host at a higher risk due to the likelihood of introducing microorganisms. Also, in recent years immunosuppression has developed into a significant risk factor. Use of irradiation or cytotoxic drug therapy for neoplastic disease and the growing use of immunosuppressive agents in transplant patient populations have generated a whole new group of patients whose immune systems have been iatrogenically suppressed. These hosts are susceptible not only to typically virulent bacteria but also to many normal flora. Finally, widespread use of antibiotics has led to the development of multiresistant organisms, organisms resistant to currently available antibiotics. The major causative organisms in septic shock are gram-negative bacteria, which are responsible for two-thirds of all cases of septic shock.[41] Additionally, gram-positive bacteria, viruses, fungi, and rickettsiae are also causative agents.

When bacteria invade an organism and die, they release substances embedded in their walls. These substances have varying deleterious effects on specific tissues and organs. Gram-positive bacteria release substances known as exotoxins which have minimal effects on tissues. Gram-negative bacteria, on the other hand, release substances known as endotoxins. Septic shock resulting from gram-negative organisms is also known as endotoxic shock. Endotoxins are lipopolysaccharides embedded in the cell walls of gram-negative bacteria, which, when released in the circulation, have the ability to activate numerous protein systems and other chemical mediators which can create major deleterious effects.[42]

The specific protein systems which are activated are the complement, clotting, kinin, and renin-angiotensin systems. The specific initiators of these systems are not known yet. However, the microorganism itself, certain immune cells, or a leukocyte endogenous mediator (LEM) which is released after phagocytosis of the organism have all been considered initiators. Under normal situations the complement system, a system of nine different enzyme precursors, serves to attack invading agents and initiates local tissue reactions which provide protection against damage by the microorganism. Usually a protective mechanism, complement effects are so systemic and widespread that major problems develop in the septic shock situation. Specifically, activation of complement increases release of C5a and C3a, proteins known as anaphylatoxins. Neutrophil aggregation is enhanced by C5a. This aggregation can lead to microembolization and ultimately tissue ischemia. Additionally, as neutrophils aggregate they can cause endothelial cell damage

which can lead to peripheral vascular insufficiency. Activation of complement also leads to increased production of platelets, leukocytes, and mast cells, which creates release of histamine, prostaglandins, bradykinin, and serotonin, all vasoactive mediators. Again, under normal circumstances and on small levels, these substances cause a beneficial vasodilation and increased capillary permeability. This vasodilation increases blood flow to locally damaged tissue and assists in fighting the infection. The increased capillary permeability allows the area to wall itself off from the rest of the tissue so that microorganisms do not travel as far.[43] In sepsis, however, this process is occurring throughout the body, and massive vasodilation and widespread capillary permeability can be disastrous. The last sequela of complement system activation is that of myocardial depression. This is largely seen in the hypodynamic stage of septic shock.

The clotting system is also activated by endotoxin which stimulates Hageman factor (factor XII). This initiates the development of multiple fibrin clots, which impair blood flow and consequently perfusion. This inappropriate clotting and resultant consumption of clotting factors can result in disseminated intravascular coagulation (DIC) (Chap. 43). Factor XII also stimulates the conversion of inactive kinins to active kinins, specifically, bradykinin and serotonin, all of which are potent vasodilators which can also tremendously alter capillary permeability.

The production of renin and consequently angiotensin is mediated by microorganisms. This creates the release of epinephrine, norephinephrine, and aldosterone; consequently, sympathetic drive is increased, myocardial contractility improved, and sodium and water retained.

Other chemical mediators which are activated by various stimuli include histamine, prostaglandins, myocardial depressant factor (MDF), and leuckocyte endogenous mediator (LEM).[44] Histamine, released by the mast cells, causes capillary permeability, vasodilation, and myocardial depression. The prostaglandin thromboxane A_2, produced by platelets, is a potent platelet aggregator. The prostaglandin F_2 is also released in septic shock and is associated with pulmonary vasoconstriction in animals in septic shock.[4]2 Prostacyclin (PGI_2), another prostaglandin, decreases in septic shock.

Lack of PGI_2 leads to thrombogenesis and peripheral vascular insufficiency since its normal role is as a vasodilator and an antiplatelet aggregator. Myocardial depressant factor (MDF) is released from the pancreas following periods of hypoperfusion in animals.[45] While its presence in humans has not been clearly delineated, its actions are to serve as a negative inotrope which can severely alter myocardial contractility. Myocardial depressant factor also inhibits phagocytosis and causes splanchnic vasoconstriction.[46]

The last chain of events which is activated by microorganisms is the leukocyte endogenous mediator system. In conjunction with endogenous pyrogen and lymphocyte activating factor, LEM creates the following effects: endorphin release, an increase in protein catabolism of skeletal muscle, glucagon and insulin release from the pancreas, an alteration in heat regulation by the hypothalamus, increased amino acid uptake, and hepatic synthesis of acute phase reactants such as the alpha and beta globulins, fibrinogen, and polysaccharides, and increased neutrophil release from the bone marrow. Endorphins are suspect in creating hypotension and myocardial depression in septic shock and hemorrhagic shock.

As indicated earlier, the stages of septic shock include septicemia, preshock, hyperdynamic and hypodynamic shock, and multisystem organ failure. In the first stage, septicemia, the host reactions and system changes described above are initiated. The sympathetic nervous system is activated, and the patient experiences tachycardia, an increased cardiac output, and an increased respiratory rate. In the preshock phase, the patient's systemic vascular resistance is decreased, the cardiac index is increased, and the mean arterial pressure remains somewhat normal. As the patient proceeds to the next stage, there is a hypotensive event which is triggered by a fall in the cardiac index to normal values and a decrease in systemic vascular resistance. The myocardium fails to compensate for the fall in systemic vascular resistance. After that, return of the cardiac index to higher levels and significant increases in systemic vascular resistance only achieve minor arterial pressure elevations.[47,48] This hypotensive event initiates the hyperdynamic stage. In this stage there is significant peripheral vasodilation, a low systemic vascular resistance, and increased

or normal cardiac output/cardiac index and hypotension. The next phase is the hypodynamic phase in which the cardiac output and index are very low, the systemic vascular resistance is elevated, and there is inadequate tissue perfusion and profound hypotension. The contractility of the myocardium is directly affected further by MDF, hypoxemia, acidosis, and endotoxins, resulting in an even greater fall in cardiac output. The sympathetic nervous system activates, and tremendous vasoconstriction develops in an attempt to maintain perfusion. However, tissue ischemia becomes increased. Vasoconstriction coupled with the previous and concurrent vasodilation create a capillary environment where there is slow, sluggish flow and inadequate oxygenation. Sludging of blood in such an environment is conducive to microemboli formation and clotting malfunctions, and thus DIC.

The patient gradually slips into the next and last stage, multisystem organ failure. Mizock[40] details three phases to this stage. In phase one, the patient experiences septicemia, respiratory failure, and hypoxemia. Hepatic dysfunction begins to manifest itself in phase two and the patient experiences a reduced serum albumin and is jaundiced. Mizock also states that coma, anemia, stress ulcers, inadequate wound healing, and anergy to skin test antigens are present. Finally, in phase three, the patient proceeds to biventricular failure, pulmonary edema, atelectasis, and pneumonia. If treatment is not successful, the patient then finally expires with coagulopathy, refractory hypotension, and asystole. Treatment modalities for septic shock can include volume replacement, pharmacologic therapy, and mechanical assistance (Chap. 58).

Neurogenic shock is also a form of distributive shock. As with septic shock, the physiologic change is due to abnormal distribution of volume due to vasodilation. The major cause of neurogenic shock is loss of vasomotor tone. This can develop following deep general anesthesia or spinal anesthesia, especially when spinal anesthesia extends up the spinal column. Brain damage of the basal regions or prolonged medullary ischemia can also cause vasomotor collapse.

In *anaphylactic shock,* another type of distributive shock, an antigen-antibody reaction is the initiating event. This reaction can cause direct damage to the adjacent vascular walls and also cause cells throughout the body to release histamine and histamine-like substances. This results in tremendous vasodilation with resultant hypotension and increased capillary permeability with loss of fluid into the interstitial space (Chap. 47).

Assessment of Tissue Perfusion and Alterations

As was stated in the beginning of this chapter, it is frequently the critical-care nurse's responsibility to constantly assess and identify the subtle and blatant findings and parameter changes indicative of inadequate tissue perfusion. Both subjective and objective data should be gathered and analyzed. Some findings will be consistently present regardless of the etiology of inadequate perfusion. However, in some instances assessment parameters are quite helpful in establishing a diagnosis, as their values vary depending on the etiology of inadequate perfusion. The following section will describe such assessment parameters and Table 7-2 will summarize assessment findings which can vary with different etiologies and stages of shock.

Table 7-2 Assessment Parameters for Various Stages and Types of Shock

	Cardiogenic		Hypovolemic		Distributive		Obstructive	
	Compensated	Decompensated	Compensated	Decompensated	Early	Late	Compensated	Decompensated
Subjective								
Thirst	↑		↑					
Nausea	↑		↑					
Anxiety	↑		↑		↑		↑	
Objective								
Heart rate	↑/↑	↑↓	↑	↑	↑	↑↓	↑	↑
Arrhythmias	↑↑	↑↑↑	—	↑	—	↑	—	↑
Temperature								
Core	↑	↑	—	—	↑↑↑	↑↑	—	—
Skin	↓	↓	—	↑	↑	↓	—	↓
Blood pressure								
Mean arterial pressure	—	↓	—	↓	↑/—	↓	—	↓
Pulse pressure	↓	—	↓	—	—	↓	↓	—
Diastolic	—	↓	—	↓	↓	↓/—	—	↓
Systolic	↓	↓	↓	↓	↓	↓	↓	↓
Hemodynamic parameters								
Right atrial pressure	↑/—	↑↑	↓	↓↓	↓	↑	↑	↑↑
PAP	↑	↑↑	↓	↓↓	↓	↑	↑/—	↑/—
PCWP	↑	↑↑	↓	↑↑	↓	↑↑	↓	↓
SVR	↑	↑↑↑	—	↑	↓	↑↑↑	—	↑
CO/CI	↓	↑↑↑	↓	↑↑↑	↑↑	↓↓↓	↓	↓↓↓
Respiratory parameters								
Tachypnea	↓	↑↑	↑	↑	↑	↑↑	↑	↑
Rales/rhonchi	↑	↑↑	—	—	↑	↑↑	↑/—	↑/—
Chest X-ray changes	↑	↑↑	—	—	↑	↑↑	↑/—	↑/—
Acid-base findings								
Respiratory alkalosis	↑		↑		↑		↑	
Metabolic acidosis		↑		↑		↑↑		↑

Subjective Data

In the early stages of shock the patient may be adequately alert and awake to report various symptoms which are significant. *Thirst,* a conscious desire for water, is a common complaint, both for patients in hypovolemic and cardiogenic shock. In hypovolemic patients thirst is usually expressed when there has been a 10 percent loss of blood volume. Patients with a low cardiac output from congestive heart failure also develop an intense thirst. It is theorized that this thirst is created by the presence of excessive amounts of angiotensin II which stimulates a neural center under the third ventricle of the brain.[43]

Nausea, the conscious recognition of a subconscious excitation of the medulla close to the vomiting center, is another subjective symptom. Sequestering of fluid in the gastrointestinal tract as is seen in some types of hypovolemic and cardiogenic shock can cause an irritative impulse to be transmitted to the medulla. *Apprehension, anxiety,* and *fear* are also described by patients in early shock stages and are related to elevated serum levels of catecholamines and hypoxemia. Initial peripheral vasoconstriction will also lead to subjective symptoms of being *cold.* Finally, *syncope* upon changing positions, particularly from supine to upright positions, may be a reflection of a hypovolemic state.

Objective Data

Heart Rate

Generally, patients will experience a sinus tachycardia of 110 to 120 beats per minute as the myocardium attempts to compensate for the low cardiac output through a rate increase. One exception to this may occur in patients with cardiogenic shock secondary to an inferior or posterior wall myocardial infarction. In this situation, ischemic stimulation of cholinergic ganglia at the posterior margin of the AV node may reflexly produce sinus bradycardia or heart block. Excessively high heart rates (greater than 150 beats per minute) can lead to a fall in cardiac output and a higher incidence of ischemic dysrhythmias. Dysrhythmias, such as conduction defects or supraventricular or ventricular dysrhythmias, are most commonly seen in patients experiencing cardiogenic shock; however, in the presence of severe acidosis or hypoxia, premature ventricular contractions (PVCs) may be commonplace. Additionally, the release of histamine in septic shock has been demonstrated to cause AV conduction abnormalities and ventricular arrhythmias.[49] S_3 and/or S_4 heart sounds will develop as the myocardium itself fails. This occurs most frequently in cardiogenic shock but can also develop in the end stages of distributive shock. In cardiogenic shock, cardiac murmurs such as the holosystolic murmur of a ventricular septal defect or mitral regurgitation may develop in the presence of these structural abnormalities. A transient functional mitral regurgitant murmur can similarly develop with excessive volume loading.

Ischemic changes on the electrocardiogram can occur, particularly in patients with underlying coronary artery disease. However, S-T segment elevations and subendocardial ischemic changes have been documented in patients without ischemic heart disease during both septic and hemorrhagic shock. These were presumably caused by severe anemia or by a decrease in coronary perfusion pressure.[50]

Skin Color and Temperature

Due to the extensive vasoconstriction associated with inadequate perfusion, the patient's skin color is generally pale, except in the hyperdynamic septic state where it is generally reddened and moist. As perfusion becomes tremendously compromised, mottling and cyanosis develop. Piloerection (goose bumps) occurs as a method of avoiding loss of body heat. The skin temperature is cool to the touch.

In recent years, the measurement of the temperature gradient between the great toe and ambient room temperature has demonstrated that parameter to be a good predictor of survival or mortality in patients in circulatory shock. Specifically, studies demonstrate that patients who survived circulatory shock had increases in the toe minus ambient room temperature gradient of more than 4°C. Patients with a gradient less than 3°C for a 12-h period generally expired due to their low-flow state. Monitoring the toe temperature and toe gradient difference to room air can help in quantifying the subjective assessment of skin temperature, and also for assessing the value of the various therapeutic actions undertaken.[51]

Rectal, oral, and core temperatures are generally within normal limits. Exceptions to this occur in sepsis where, particularly with gram-negative endotoxin release, the hypothalamus is stimulated and temperatures can rise to the 101-to-105°F levels. Slight temperature elevations can develop in cardiogenic shock. This is a consequence of the tissue damage associated with myocardial infarction. Mild hypothermia may develop in some cases of distributive shock, particularly in the presence of gram-positive organisms.

Blood Pressure

Monitoring blood pressures in these patients is a critical activity. Cuff blood pressures are generally inadequate due to the severe vasoconstriction and low stroke volumes these patients generate. For these reasons, the Korotkoff sounds are barely audible and difficult to discern. Cuff blood pressures can underestimate the true arterial pressure by an average of 15 mmHg and occasionally by as much as 100 mmHg.[52] Therefore, intraarterial pressure monitoring is required.

There are three components of the arterial pressure which should be monitored and evaluated: the pulse pressure, the diastolic pressure, and the systolic pressure. The pulse pressure is the difference between the systolic and diastolic pressures and primarily reflects the stroke volume and resistance to blood flow in the aorta and its major branches. Changes in the pulse pressure reflect stroke volume changes. For example, if a blood pressure changes from 100/60 to 90/70, and thus the pulse pressure falls from 40 to 20 mmHg, the stroke volume will be decreased by 50%.[5] Diastolic pressure is most reflective of the amount of vasoconstriction present, particularly in the arterioles. And, finally, systolic pressure is determined by these other two pressures. In all cases of shock, the mean arterial pressure falls either slowly or precipitously. However, the pattern of alterations viewed in these other three components varies, based upon the etiology of the inadequate perfusion state.

In the compensated stages of cardiogenic or hypovolemic shock the systolic pressure may fall slightly, but the diastolic pressure will remain constant or perhaps increased due to vasoconstric-

tion. This allows the pulse pressure to narrow, and this may be the first significant change that occurs in the blood pressure measurement. As the patient moves into the decompensated stage, both systolic and diastolic pressures will fall, and the pulse pressure will then remain constant. In distributive shock another pattern develops. With vasodilation, both systolic and diastolic pressures fall, and thus the pulse pressure remains constant. During late stages when vasoconstriction develops, the diastolic pressure is affected slightly and may remain constant or slow its decline. This then allows the pulse pressure to narrow slightly.

Hemodynamic Parameters

Monitoring of hemodynamic parameters is essential for the accurate diagnosis and treatment of shock states. Commonly monitored parameters include the central venous pressure (CVP), the pulmonary artery pressure (PAP), and the pulmonary capillary wedge pressure (PCWP).

Normal values for these parameters are as follows:

CVP	3–11 mmHg
PAP	
Pulmonary artery systolic pressure (PAS)	20–30 mmHg
Pulmonary artery diastolic pressure (PAD)	10–15 mmHg
Pulmonary artery mean pressure (PAM)	10–20 mmHg
PCWP	4–12 mmHg

In addition, derived parameters such as the systemic vascular resistance (SVR), the pulmonary vascular resistance (PVR), and the cardiac index (CI) are also monitored. Normal values for these parameters are as follows:

SVR	800–1300 dyn/s/cm^{-5}
PVR	80–240 dyn/s/cm^{-5}
CO	5–8 L/min
CI	2.5–3.5 L/min per m^2

In cardiogenic shock, the majority of the hemodynamic alterations are manifested by the parameters which reflect the function of the left ventricle. Specifically, the PCWP becomes elevated as the left ventricle loses its contractility and blood sequesters in the left ventricle, left atrium, and then passively fills the pulmonary tree. Since most infarctions involve the left ventricle as opposed to the right ventricle, the CVP, the main indicator of right heart function, is not affected. If, however, right heart failure or biventricular failure develops, hen the CVP becomes elevated. Pulmonary artery systolic and diastolic pressures generally remain in their normal ranges. Cardiac output/cardiac index is diminished, and SVR is elevated due to the sympathetic drive which develops. PVR is generally unaffected until significant pulmonary changes develop.

In hypovolemic shock, all parameters are diminished. The CVP is low due to inadequate filling of the right heart. Additionally, the PCWP and PAP pressures are low due to inadequate volume. The cardiac output and CI are less than normal ranges, and the SVR remains normal or slightly elevated due to vasconstriction.

With distributive shock various changes develop. In the hyperdynamic state, since the patient is experiencing vasodilation and fluid is sequestering peripherally, the filling pressures are initially low. The SVR is low also due to the massive vasodilation the patient experiences. Cardiac output is exceptionally elevated, perhaps as a compensatory response to deliver blood to a peripheral bed where there is diffuse shunting. As hypodynamic shock develops, the cardiac output and index fall and the SVR elevates as the patient suffers vasoconstriction. The right and left heart filling pressures now rise as the vascular bed constricts and the myocardium fails. With obstructive shock, the cardiac output is low since blood cannot pass easily into the left heart due to obstruction in the pulmonary bed or the right-sided inflow tracts. The CVP is elevated due to this obstruction while the PCWP is normal or in lower ranges.

Respiratory Changes

As with other organs, the rate and intensity of respiratory changes a patient experiences in a shock state vary with the severity of that state. For example, in cardiogenic shock following a massive myocardial infarction the respiratory alterations which develop are rapid and acute. For slowly evolving poor perfusion states the symptoms will also evolve slowly. Earlier, the physiologic changes associated with interstitial and alveolar pulmonary edema were described. Generally, it is these two types of pulmonary problems which the patient in cardiogenic shock develops. With interstitial edema the patient develops dyspnea and tachypnea. The tidal volume remains the same, but the minute ventilation increases. Slight wheezing may develop, and fine to

moderate moist rales can be auscultated. The chest film generally demonstrates some lymphatic enlargement, and Kerley B lines are present. Arterial blood gases generally exhibit slight respiratory alkalosis and slight arterial hypoxemia.

These above symptoms reflect the accumulation of fluid in the interstitial spaces between the alveoli and therefore are not dramatic clinical signs and symptoms. However, once alveolar edema develops dramatic signs and symptoms appear. Severe dyspnea and shortness of breath develop as the fluid in the alveoli serves to inhibit gas exchange. Intubation and mechanical ventilation are generally required at this point. Coarse rales, rhonchi, and wheezing are heard throughout the chest. The chest x-ray is characterized by diffuse haziness. Blood-tinged sputum is present. This sputum has a low protein content; specifically, less than 60 percent of the plasma protein concentration. This last finding can be important when a differential diagnosis between hydrostatic edema and permeability edema is necessary. In permeability edema the ratio is greater than 60 percent. That is, pulmonary secretions approach serum plasma composition. Therefore, a permeability leak must be present in the alveoli to allow this admixture. In alveolar edema, the alveolus is intact and there is no sieving of protein into the sputum.[53,54]

In distributive shock, particularly septic, in which the initiating problem is not volume but rather toxic substances, the clinical picture of permeability edema is more likely to arise. With this entity, tachypnea and increased minute ventilation develop. Sequestering of fluids in the interstitium and alveoli is generally not present so that rales and rhonchi may or may not be significant. However, as capillary endothelial and alveolar epithelial cell damage develop, hypoxemia develops rapidly, and mechanical assistance is required. Refractory hypoxemia is frequently present with ARDS. Refractory hypoxemia refers to the inability to improve arterial oxygenation despite increases in the percentage of delivered inspired oxygen. Lung compliance is decreased. Chest x-ray findings demonstrate diffuse haziness and the cardiac silhouette is normal. The edema fluid/plasma protein ratio, as mentioned earlier, is usually greater than 60 percent.

Physical respiratory findings in hypovolemic and obstructive shock are generally nonspecific since the pulmonary bed is not generally a major focus in their etiologies.

Arterial Blood Gases and Acid-Base Changes

Due to the previously mentioned hyperventilation, blood gases obtained in early stages of shock generally reflect adequate arterial oxygenation and a respiratory alkalosis. As the shock progresses, a slight to moderate arterial hypoxemia develops as oxygen delivery begins to fall. The exception to this occurs in hypovolemic shock where the arterial oxygenation may remain within the normal limits. This occurs as a result of a decreased amount of blood in the lung. In this case the ventilation/perfusion ratio increases, and thus better pulmonary compliance and function are present.

As lactate and hydrogen ions accumulate in shock, a metabolic acidosis develops. This causes the patient to hyperventilate further as a compensatory measure. If the Pa_{CO_2} is driven below 25 mmHg this severe hypocapnea may itself cause hemodynamic impairment.

Metabolic alkalosis generally does not occur in patients in shock. However, on occasion it may develop in patients receiving high doses of antacids or in those undergoing removal of large quantities of gastric secretions. When metabolic alkalosis is present the degree of metabolic acidosis present is masked and underappreciated. This may later prove problematic as the severe acidosis may become almost refractory to treatment.

If the shock state is not improved the metabolic acidosis will increase. Additionally, a respiratory acidosis will develop as the patient gradually loses the ability to excrete carbon dioxide as the number of functional pulmonary capillaries decreases. Gradually the Pa_{CO_2} rises and reaches levels above normal. In the final stages of shock the blood gases demonstrate a combined metabolic and respiratory acidosis with an elevated Pa_{CO_2}, a low bicarbonate, and a very low pH.[55]

Serum Lactate Levels

Measurement of arterial lactate levels has recently become a common practice in caring for shock patients. An indicator of anaerobic metabolism, it has been demonstrated that levels higher than 4.4 nmol/L are associated with a high mortality. Trends in these levels, however, are perhaps more bene-

ficial than isolated values.[56–59] Falling lactate values indicate an improvement in perfusion.

Urine Output and Composition

Within the context of shock states the renal system is not viewed as a vital organ but rather a peripheral organ. Therefore, regardless of the type of shock, the kidney is immediately affected by hypoperfusion and provides signs and symptoms as to the severity of the hypoperfusion. Generally there is a good correlation between the amount of renal blood flow and the amount of urine output. Since renal blood flow depends on cardiac output, any alterations in cardiac output greatly influence urinary output. Therefore, if cardiac output falls precipitously, there is a concurrent precipitous fall in urine output. With a moderate or gradual fall in cardiac output the composition of the urine output may change prior to changes in urinary volume, and alterations in various serum and urine laboratory values will occur. With a moderate fall in cardiac output the renal arterioles constrict and blood flow is shunted from the cortical nephrons of the kidney to the juxtaglomerular nephrons. Juxtaglomerular nephrons have the ability to conserve more sodium than the cortical nephrons. In addition, the renin-angiotensin-aldosterone system discussed earlier is activated. This system also allows the body to conserve sodium.

The end result of these effects is sodium retention assisting in volume conservation, a process which the body views as the mechanism to increase its currently low cardiac output. Consequently, the volume of urine produced may fall slightly and its composition will change. In relation to the volume, the kidney will still produce volumes greater than 400 mL a day. Volumes less than this amount or less than 0.5 mL per kilogram per hour are generally considered oliguric levels. However, the urine composition will be low in sodium, generally less than 20 meq/L. Additionally, the specific gravity will be greater than 1.015 and the urine/serum osmolality ratio will be greater than 1.5.

All these values indicate that the nephrons are still functional and are trying to compensate for the inadequate perfusion. Serum levels of urea nitrogen rise during this stage due to its back diffusion across the nephron; however, serum creatinine levels remain within normal ranges since the nephron still remains capable of clearing this metabolic end product. The end result is a blood urea nitrogen/creatinine ratio of greater than 10:1. This state is generally referred to as a prerenal state or a prerenal failure state.

As the fall in perfusion to the kidney persists, and the renal parenchyma itself becomes damaged, acute tubular necrosis ensues. In this state, urine output falls to anuric levels. Because the nephron can no longer continue with its functions, urine sodium levels rise to levels greater than 30 meq/L as sodium traverses the nephron untouched, and specific gravities fall to levels equal to 1.010. This latter value reflects the kidney's inability to concentrate urine. Additionally, the urine/serum osmolality ratio approaches a level less than 1:5. Blood urea nitrogen (BUN) and creatinine ratios remain in a 10:1 ratio since urea nitrogen continues to be reabsorbed and creatinine is no longer cleared.[5,60]

Level of Consciousness

The patient's level of consciousness can range from mildly confused to comatose. Initially, anxious behavior may be present due to slight hypoxemia and the catecholamine drive the patient experiences. Gradually, as cardiac output and cerebral perfusion fall, lethargy and confusion develop. With severe hypoperfusion and metabolic alterations, unresponsiveness and coma develop.

Gastrointestinal Findings

As cardiac output falls, blood flow is gradually shunted to areas of high priority and away from other organs. The gastrointestinal system falls into the category of non-highly prioritized systems and as such can become ischemic. Due to the low flow initial changes in gastrointestinal function consist of hypoactivity of the GI tract. If alert, the patient may complain of nausea. Bowel sounds become hypoactive and the abdomen may become distended, particularly if third spacing is occurring in this area. It may be necessary for a nasogastric tube to be inserted to assist in the removal of gastric secretions which are unable to adequately move through the intestinal system. Ulcerations may develop and Hematest-positive gastric contents may be present. If this inadequate perfusion persists, an ischemic gut can develop. This can further compound the shock state as fluid sequesters in the area and the metabolic acidosis worsens.

Treatment Modalities

Position

In all types of shock positioning the patient to facilitate ventilation and to prevent skin breakdown is vital. Optimally, this involves having the patient sit in an upright position which allows the diaphragm to fall and the chest to expand maximally. In addition, frequent position changes to avoid pressure ulcers from developing would be desirable. However, most often due to the patient's tenuous hemodynamic status these positions are unachievable and the supine position with the head of the bed elevated 20 to 30° is perhaps the most optimal position the patient can tolerate. In this event, turning the patient from side to side is also desirable. If a full side-lying position cannot be achieved, even slight elevation of the shoulders or rotation of the hip with a single pillow will assist in some improvement in local tissue perfusion. Heel and elbow protectors are also beneficial.

The idea of altering a patient's position to improve hemodynamic values remains a controversial issue. Placing a patient in Trendelenburg's position with the legs elevated higher than the torso probably does little to improve cardiac output in the shock state. This elevation may elevate the pressure in the veins and venules but does so at the expense of the myocardium, which now experiences an increase in afterload.[61] However, in a hypovolemic patient with a healthy myocardium, this maneuver may be transiently beneficial until volume replacement is accomplished.

Positioning a patient in obstructive shock can be very critical. An atrial myxoma, for example, while partially attached to the atrial wall, may also have a portion which is mobile and can move to obstruct either the pulmonary veins or the mitral valve orifice. When this occurs, immediate cardiac decompensation occurs. In this situation, the nurse at the bedside needs to be aware that this phenomenon can occur and then must decide which position provides the patient with the best hemodynamic response.

MAST (Military Antishock Trouser)

The MAST suit is an inflatable trouser consisting of an abdominal compartment and two separate lower-extremity compartments. Each compartment has its own inflating and pressure-relief valve. The suit produces titratable external pressure on the abdomen and lower extremities. The external counterpulsation created by inflation has several beneficial effects. The redistribution of venous blood flow from the abdomen and lower extremities to organs above the diaphragm creates an autotransfusion effect, and a redistribution of 750 to 100 mL can be appreciated. Autotransfusion is accompanied by an increase in central venous pressure, an increase in both aortic and carotid flow and pressure with a concomitant decrease in femoral flow and pressure. Systemic vascular resistance, arterial blood pressure, and stroke volume is increased. However, cardiac output is unchanged due to the consequent decrease in heart rate which occurs. The bradycardia is a result of depressor reflex stimulation secondary to increased aorta and carotid sinus arterial pressures. Other concomitant physiologic effects include an increased venous return to the lungs with a corresponding increase in pulmonary wedge pressure and also mild lactic acidosis. Acidosis results from the decrease in lower extremity blood flow. A decrease in respiratory excursion due to abdominal compression may also create acidosis.

Clinical indications for use of MAST include treatment of hypovolemic and neurogenic shock, intraabdominal hemorrhage, hemorrhage of any portion of the body encircled by the device, and femoral and pelvic fracture splinting. Bleeding is decreased through an external tamponade effect from the direct pressure being exerted and through internal pressure. The external compression is transmitted to the internal vasculature with a resulting increase in intraperitoneal pressure.

Nursing care of the patient includes vigilance both to hemodynamic changes related to volume needs and to the pressure readings of the suit compartments. The latter are assessed to ensure adequate suit inflation. As the suit may depress respiratory excursion, continued respiratory assessment, including monitoring of breath patterns, arterial blood gases, tidal volume, and vital capacity,

is essential. Pressure on the abdominal organs may cause emesis as well as defecation and/or urination, and therefore a nasogastric tube and Foley catheter should be in place.

Removal of the suit is determined by the attainment of a normovolemic and hemodynamic state. Deflation is achieved gradually, 5 mmHg at a time. Venous access and on-site volume replacement must be present. A drop in systolic blood pressure stops the deflation process until restoration of blood pressure is achieved and sustained. After successful deflation the suit should be left in place for at least 12 h before it is removed.[62–64]

Volume Replacement

Volume replacement to some extent is essential in any type of shock. Generally, this procedure is carried out to correct relative or absolute hypovolemia and restore an adequate intravascular volume to establish hemodynamic stability necessary for optimum tissue perfusion, and to maintain the oxygen-carrying capacity of the intravascular volume.[65] The amount of volume replaced is individually determined; however, some general rules of thumb exist. Table 7-3 describes steps that Weil and Rackow recommend for volume resuscitation.[66] The needed type of volume is related to the type of intravascular deficit the patient experiences. Specific replacement fluids are described in the next section and in Table 7-4.

Crystalloids

Crystalloids are those solutions which consist of dextrose in water or electrolytes dissolved in water. Since electrolytes are freely permeable to the vascular membrane, infusion of electrolytes assists in both plasma fluid volume expansion and interstitial fluid volume expansion. It is this latter attribute, that of interstitial volume expansion, which can be a disadvantage in clinical situations in which intravascular fluid volume expansion is the primary need. Specifically, an approximate amount of only one-fourth of infused saline solutions remains in the vascular space. The other 75 percent rapidly diffuses into the interstitial space. Therefore, a patient may have double or triple the amount of crystalloids infused as compared to colloids in order to obtain the same degree of plasma expansion.[67]

Table 7-3 Fluid Challenge Protocol

Step I

Observe baseline readings of CVP or PCWP for 10 min

Step II

If CVP value	Then rate of fluid infusion
Less than 12 cmH$_2$O	20 mL/h
Between 12–18 cmH$_2$O	10 mL/h
Greater than 18 cm H$_2$O	5 mL/h

If PCWP value	Then rate of fluid infusion
Less than 12 mmHg	20 mL/h
Between 12–18 mmHg	10 mL/h
Greater than 18 mmHg	5 mL/h

Step III

Infuse fluid for 10 min	
If CVP increases more than 5 cmH$_2$O	Stop infusion
If PCWP increases more than 7 mmHg	

Step IV

At end of 10 min	
If CVP increases by 2 cmH$_2$O or less	Repeat challenge
If PCWP increases by 3 mmHg or less	
If CVP increases by 2–5 cmH$_2$O	Discontinue infusion
If PCWP increases by 3–7 mmHg	

Step V

Observe patient for 10 min	
If CVP falls to within 2 cmH$_2$O of initial value	Resume challenge
If PCWP falls to within 3 mmHg of initial value	
If CVP does not fall to within 2 cmH$_2$O of initial value	Discontinue challenge
If PCWP does not fall to within 3 mmHg of initial value	

Adapted from Weil, M. H., & Rackow, E.C. A guide to volume repletion. *Emerg. Med.*, 1984, *16*, 101–110.

In patients with altered capillary permeability this leakage into the interstitial space is even greater. Therefore, crystalloids are not the agent of choice when permeability problems are suspected or present. Another disadvantage associated with crystalloids is that patients given crystalloid fluids tend to easily and perhaps prematurely develop peripheral edema. This peripheral edema is frequently identified as an indication of fluid overload and consequently crystalloid resuscitation is halted before adequate vascular volume is actually achieved.[68]

Normal saline, as an isotonic solution, is an excellent solution to replace extracellular body fluid. It increases plasma volume but it can dilute extracellular calcium and potassium, causing hypokalemia, hypernatremia, and metabolic acidosis. Serum electrolyte values should be checked frequently during saline infusion. Normal saline solution is an ideal solution to use in patients with hypovolemic shock when the red blood cell mass is adequate. It is generally not used in patients with cardiogenic shock for volume loading due to its high sodium content.

Lactated Ringer's solution is also used to replace body fluid and in addition serves to buffer acidosis since the lactate it contains is converted to bicarbonate in the liver. Also used in hypovolemic states, this fluid is avoided in cardiac patients due to the sodium load. In addition, it should be used carefully in low-flow states since it can increase lactic acidosis. Simple Ringer's solution, however, can be given to patients with hypoperfusion since it contains no lactate. It also replaces body fluid and electrolytes but should be used cautiously in cardiogenic shock patients.

Half normal saline or 0.45% saline solution is also used to raise total fluid volume. Its infusion serves to dilute plasma proteins and electrolytes, and it readily moves into the interstitial and intracellular areas and leads to edema. However, this solution and dextrose and 0.2 percent sodium chloride are perhaps the best agents for volume replacement in patients with significant cardiac problems due to their relatively low sodium content. Dextrose 5% and water (D$_5$W), also referred to as free water, evenly distributes itself throughout the entire body. For this reason, it is an excellent agent to use for the treatment of dehydration. Caution needs to be used in administration of D$_5$W since it will also dilute the serum levels of electrolytes when given in sufficient quantities.

Colloids

In contrast to crystalloids, colloids are relatively impermeable to the vascular membrane. They determine the oncotic or colloid osmotic pressure

Table 7-4 Volume Replacement Solutions and Their Ingredients

Crystalloids

Normal saline	0.9% sodium chloride in water	Sodium	154 meq/L
		Chloride	154 meq/L
		Osmolality	308 meq/L
Lactated Ringer's	0.9% sodium chloride in water with electrolytes and buffers	Sodium	130 meq/L
		Potassium	4 meq/L
		Calcium	2.7 meq/L
		Chloride	107 meq/L
		Lactate	27 meq/L
		pH	6.5
Ringer's solution	0.9% sodium chloride in water with potassium and calcium	Sodium	147 meq/L
		Potassium	4 meq/L
		Calcium	5 meq/L
		Chloride	156 meq/L
Half normal saline	0.45% sodium chloride in water	Sodium	77 meq/L
		Chloride	77 meq/L
5% Dextrose in water (D_5W)	5% dextrose		

Colloids

5% Albumin (Albumisol)	Aqueous fraction of pooled plasma prepared from whole blood in buffered normal saline.	Albumin	50 g/L
		Sodium	130–160 meq/L
		Potassium	300 mOsm/L
	250- and 500-mL bottles	Osmolality	
		Osmotic pressure	20 mmHg
		pH	6.4–7.4
25% Albumin (salt poor)	25, 50, and 100-mL bottles	Albumin	240 g/L
		Globulins	10 g/L
		Sodium	130–160 meq/L
		Osmolality	1500 mOsm/L
		pH	6.4–7.4
Dextran Low-molecular-weight dextran (LMWD)	500-mL bottles, 10% dextran in normal saline or D_5M	Glucose polysaccharide molecules with an average molecular weight of 40,000	
High-molecular-weight dextran (HMWD)	500-mL bottles, 6% dextran in normal saline or D_5M	Glucose polysaccharide molecules with an average molecular weight of 70,000	
Hetastarch	500-mL bottles, 6% solution of a synthetic polymer of hydroxyethyl starch in normal saline	Branched chain hydroxyethyl starch prepared from amylopectin.	
		Sodium	154 meq/L
		Chloride	154 meq/L
		Osmolality	310 mOsm/L
		Colloid osmotic pressure	30–35 mmHg

which maintains the balance of water between the interstitial spaces and the intravascular space. Both natural and synthetic colloids are commercially available. The most abundant natural colloid is albumin. Normally, albumin plays a principal role in the retention of fluid in the vascular space. With a molecular weight of 68,000, albumin is primarily responsible for the plasma oncotic pressure. Commercially, albumin is available in 5% and 25% solutions. It is an excellent agent to give when the goal is to increase the plasma colloid osmotic pressure and thus plasma volume. It is particularly useful in hypovolemic shock with protein losses as is seen following burns. For every milliliter of 5%

albumin infused, the plasma volume expands 1 mL.[65] And for every 25 g of 25% albumin infused, the plasma volume increases by 400 mL.[69]

In hypovolemic states, albumin infusions have also demonstrated their ability to bring serum albumin to normal levels. However, while serum albumin levels have returned to normal, some studies have indicated that albumin resuscitation can decrease the other plasma proteins such as immunoglobulins. The clinical significance of these data is as yet unclear.[70,71]

Dextran is a synthetic agent which consists of various sizes of linear glucose polymers. Dextran is fractionated into low-molecular-weight dextran (LMWD) and high-molecular-weight dextran (HMWD). LMWD has a molecular weight around 40,000, making it similar in that respect to albumin. Its half-life is approximately 2 h and it has plasma-expanding capabilities of 1.5 times its volume. High-molecular-weight dextran has a molecular weight of 70,000 and a half-life of 12 h. Both agents are useful when there is a need to rapidly expand the plasma volume. Both agents are also associated with coagulation problems and may cause bleeding in patients as they decrease platelet adhesiveness and dilute clotting factors such as fibrinogen. Therefore, dextran may not be the ideal replacement fluid in hemorrhage since it may exacerbate the problem. Dextrans can also interfere with blood grouping when administered in large volumes.

Hetastarch is a hydroxethyl starch which has an average molecular weight of 69,000. Since it is similar to albumin in molecular weight it has generally the same volume-expansion characteristics of albumin. However, its effects can last up to 36 h. Recent studies have demonstrated it to be as effective in increasing blood pressure, cardiac output, and tissue perfusion as 5% albumin.[72,73] In addition, it can increase colloidal osmotic pressure to levels three times higher in hypovolemic patients than 5% albumin or normal saline solution.[74] Hetastarch has been shown to increase serum amylase levels since it combines with amylase during the degradation process. Since the half-life of hetastarch is so long, the attached amylase also develops elevated levels. Glucose levels also rise following infusion of hetastarch because glucose is a by-product of hetastarch's degradation process. If dilution of clotting factors occurs due to excessive infusion of hetastarch, clotting parameters such as the prothrombin time, partial thromboplastin time, and platelet count will be affected.

Blood and Blood Products

The use of whole blood as a replacement agent is generally restricted to hypovolemic shock states associated with hemorrhage or in situations where the hemoglobin is less than 12 g/100 mL and the hematocrit is less than 30 percent.[65] Whole blood less than 24 h old is preferable since older stored blood contains less clotting factors and more cellular debris, potassium, citrate, and other waste products. Additionally, stored blood is deficient in 2,3-diphosphoglycerate (2,3-DPG) and this deficiency enhances the affinity of hemoglobin for oxygen and consequently decreases oxygen release to the tissues. If banked blood is given, calcium also needs to be administered since the citrate in banked blood binds with calcium and thereby decreases circulating levels. With massive transfusion, this loss of ionized calcium can seriously affect myocardial contractility. All efforts are made to cross-match the recipient and donor blood prior to transfusion. However, in the severely hypovolemic trauma patient when time is limited, it has been demonstrated that type-specific uncross-matched blood is safe to administer and more rapidly available.[75]

Packed red cells are also used as replacement agents when the hematocrit is less than 30 percent and the red cell mass needs to be increased to improve the oxygen-carrying capacity of the blood. The advantage of packed cells over whole blood is that less infused volume is required to deliver the red cell mass, and less metabolic waste products are infused. This makes packed cell infusion an attractive alternative for cardiogenic shock patients. Disadvantages center on the high viscosity of the cells, which makes them difficult to infuse, and their lack of coagulation factors so that other blood components may be necessary to replace those components. Fresh frozen plasma contains plasma proteins, clotting factors, and plasma and is used to replace clotting factors and restore plasma volume in hypovolemic shock.

The need for fresh frozen plasma can be assessed by the results of the prothrombin time (PT), partial thromboplastin time (PTT), and fibrinogen levels. The PTT is a measure of the intrinsic pathway while the PT measures the extrinsic pathway. If either is abnormal, fresh frozen plasma is indicated. Plasma needs to be administered as soon as it is thawed so that deterioriation of its clotting factors is limited. Plasma does not contain platelets, so that if thrombocytopenia is identified as the cause of hemorrhage, platelet units need to be transfused.

Cryoprecipitate is another blood component which can be used to control coagulopathies. It contains all the clotting elements of fresh frozen plasma except platelets. Its advantage is that it requires only 20 mL of volume to deliver equivalent factors compared to fresh frozen plasma's 200 mL of volume. Therefore, cryoprecipitate is ideal for patients in congestive heart failure. It is also especially rich in factor VIII and fibrinogen and is most frequently given following fluid resuscitation in which a dilutional coagulopathy has developed. Recent studies have also demonstrated that cryoprecipitate may assist in restoring opsonic activity after injury and may play an important role in septic shock.[76]

Artificial Blood

In this category there are generally three different types of agents, all of which are currently undergoing investigation and are as yet not part of conventional volume replacement therapies. These three agents are *perfluorochemicals, stroma-free hemoglobin,* and *chelating agents.* Perfluorochemicals (Fluosol) have the ability to transport oxygen to the tissues, and in anemic states in which whole blood is not used for either religious or availability reasons, Fluosol could be an alternative. Initial studies have demonstrated Fluosol to be effective as an oxygen carrier. Side effects at this point seem to include liver and kidney damage and possibly carcinogenic effects. Stroma-free hemoglobin is hemoglobin stripped of all its cell membrane elements. It is obtained from outdated human red blood cells and also has a significant capacity for carrying oxygen. And lastly, oxygen-binding chelates are also being developed. These are substances that act like hemoglobin and bind substances such as oxygen to themselves for transport.[77–79] Again, while currently not part of the conventional treatment

plan these agents hold considerable promise and advantages for the future.

Pharmacologic Agents

For the most part the goals of pharmacologic therapy in shock are the same regardless of the type of shock. In all types of shock there is first a need to increase perfusion to vital organs, to limit or decrease the amount of myocardial demand this vital organ perfusion requires, and to decrease pulmonary congestion. In addition, increasing peripheral organ perfusion is also a goal.[80] In cardiogenic shock, these goals are achieved by surgical, mechanical, or pharmacologic support. In hypovolemic shock, these goals are achieved by volume replacement for the most part, but in severe states or in end stages, pharmacologic support is necessary. And in septic shock, volume manipulation and pharmacologic agents are the major therapies. The next section will briefly describe various agents used in shock.

Vasopressors and Inotropes

There are numerous vasopressors and inotropes which can be utilized to improve blood flow to vital organs. While they most often accomplish this by their beta-adrenergic activity which increases myocardial contractility, and their alpha-adrenergic effects, which allow them to vasoconstrict peripheral organs, other pathways for their effects also exist. These effects are summarized in Table 7-5. Whatever the mechanism of action, the end result of these effects is improved flow to vital organs, decreased flow to peripheral organs, and an increase in myocardial workload and hence oxygen consumption due to the increased contractility and increase in afterload. In the shock state, these effects may be briefly appropriate but peripheral organ ischemia needs to be reversed as soon as possible.

Dopamine hydrochloride (Intropin) is perhaps the most common vasopressor. As an inotrope, it increases cardiac contractility through its beta-adrenergic receptor activity. However, in addition, at low doses of 1 to 2 μg per kilogram per minute, its actions are exerted on the peripheral bed dopaminergic receptor sites in the renal and mesenteric areas. Dopamine's action is to selectively

Table 7-5 Relative Mechanisms of Action and Effects of Commonly Used Vasopressors and Inotropes

	Mechanism of Action			Effects		
	Alpha	Beta$_1$	Other	Cardiac Output	Heart Rate	Systemic Vascular Resistance
Dopamine	+ + +	+ + +		+ + +	+ +	+
Dobutamine	+	+ + +		+ + +	+ (+ + +)	+
Isoproterenol	−	+ + +		+ + +	+ + +	− −
Norepinephrine	+ + +	+ + +		+ + +	+ +	+ + +
Epinephrine	+ + +	−		+ + +	+ +	+ + +
Amrinone	−	−	? cAmp	+ + +	+	− −
Neo-Synephrine	+ + +	−		+ + +	+	+ + +
Methoxamine	+ + +	−		+ + +	+	+ + +
Glucagon	−	−	Adenyl cyclase activator			
Salbutamol	−	+		+	+	−
Prenalterol		+ +		+ +	+	−

dilate these vessels to assist in improving blood flow to them despite the low cardiac output. In shock states this role is very critical as the renal beds become constricted early in shock since they are viewed as nonvital organs. Dopamine continues to serve as a vasodilator to the peripheral beds when the dose is increased to 2 to 4 μg per kilogram per minute. However, as doses exceed 6 μg per kilogram per minute its effects on the peripheral beds become progressively more vaso-constrictive as both arterioles and veins constrict. At these doses dopamine is similar to other vaso-pressors.[81,82]

Dobutamine hydrochloride (Dobutrex) is a synthetic catecholamine which acts on the beta-adrenergic receptors and thus enhances contractility. It is an ideal agent to use in any stage of cardiogenic shock and in late distributive shock. When administered in doses greater than 10 to 15 μg per kilogram per minute tachycardia may become a problem. This may create myocardial ischemia in patients with failing ventricles and may necessitate a change in vasopressors or additional lowering of systemic vascular resistance.[83]

Isoproterenol hydrochloride (Isuprel) is a beta agonist which can enhance contractility but also serves as a chronotropic agent. It is useful in shock states where bradycardia is present or in situations where pulmonary vascular resistance is elevated since it can lower this resistance. The major disadvantage of this drug centers on its tendency to create supraventricular and ventricular tachyarrhythmias. In cardiogenic shock this could facilitate the extension of a myocardial infarction.

Norepinephrine (Levophed) in doses less than 0.02 to 0.2 μg per kilogram per minute creates a moderate yet significant increase in contractility due to its beta-adrenergic receptor effects. At doses exceeding 0.3 μg per kilogram per minute it becomes a strong peripheral arteriolar and venous constrictor due to its alpha effects and is an ideal agent for severe shock in which significant peripheral vasodilatation is present. The increase in systemic vascular resistance which Levophed creates, however, can severely impair left ventricular ejection, particularly in cardiogenic or septic shock patients where the myocardium is already failing dramatically. Careful titration to avoid this effect is essential.

While in theory Levophed is an ideal agent to administer in late stages of septic shock, where the goal is to increase systemic vascular resistance, in the clinical setting Levophed is frequently ineffective in this endeavor as are other alpha agents. Chernow[84] has recently demonstrated that, in sepsis, it appears as if the number of alpha receptors which would normally elicit constriction of the vascular beds are down-regulated or decreased. In addition, as Fig. 7-12 illustrates, there is evidence that in sepsis the calcium channel in the cell closes, and the other receptors inhibit the alpha receptors from functioning. Specifically, high prostacyclin levels activate the PGI_2 receptors and turn off the alpha receptors, and the circulating endorphins activate their receptors, turning off more alpha receptors. These cellular events then lead to the clinical situation where massive doses of Levophed or other catcholamines are infused and the systemic vascular resistance remains static. However, Chernow has also demonstrated that infusion of an experimental calcium agonist can open the calcium channel and can improve blood pressure by bypassing the adrenergic pathway and working directly on the cellular contractile process. While this is currently a laboratory finding, this has tremendous relevance for future investigations and explains the present ineffectiveness of some protocols in septic shock.

Epinephrine as a beta-adrenergic agent also elicits a strong inotropic response. In low doses it decreases systemic vascular resistance and in high doses increases vascular resistance. As with some of the other agents above, the positive inotropic effects of this agent are negated once systemic vascular resistance becomes elevated enough to stress or impede left ventricular function. Once this occurs the shock state worsens. Therefore, most of these agents are used concurrently with vasodilators in order to achieve the optimum hemodynamic effects.

Neo-Synephrine (phenylephrine hydrochloride) is a pressor agent which accomplishes its effects without any beta-adrenergic effects. It is a pure alpha-adrenergic drug and consequently increases blood pressure by vasoconstricting the peripheral beds. Methoxamine hydrochloride or Vasoxyl is also an alpha-adrenergic stimulator which causes significant vasoconstriction.[85]

Amrinone lactate, a new clinically available agent, is a nonglycoside, nonadrenergic cardiotonic agent. It is a positive inotrope and a vasodilator. Amrinone's exact mechanism of action is unknown but it also seems able to directly stimulate cellular processes without utilization of the adrenergic receptor sites. Specifically, amrinone appears to have an ability to stimulate cyclicAMP, which then proceeds to produce an increase in contractility.[86]

In addition to these commonly used agents there are other inotropes which can be used to increase contractility. Hypertonic solutions of glucose, insulin, and potassium (GIK) have been shown to improve hemodynamic parameters in bacterial shock. While the exact mechanism for this outcome is not known, it is believed that the result is related to the ability of the solution to decrease myocardial cellular edema, enhance the excitation-contraction coupling process, and improve the energy balance, particularly in depressed left ventricles.[87–89]

Salbutamol, a beta agonist which also dilates coronary arteries, has been shown to have weak inotropic effects. Its use is generally limited to early stages of cardiogenic shock since it has much less stimulant action on the heart than other catecholamines.[90,91]

Glucagon is another weak inotropic agent which has some limited usage. Glucagon activates adenyl cyclase without using the beta receptor, and via this mechanism can increase contractility. Because of this, glucagon has been found to be effective in shock states where beta-adrenergic blockade is present.[90,92]

Prenalterol is another new inotropic drug. It is a beta agonist agent with selective inotropic effects, less chronotropic effects, and minimal pe-

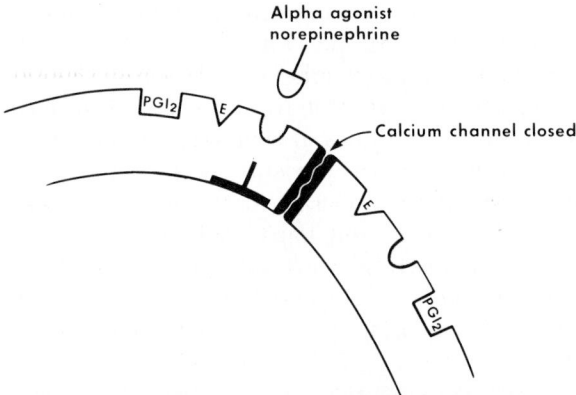

Figure 7-12 Blockade of various receptor sites in endotoxic shock with consequent disruption of the metabolic pathways which produce muscle contraction.

ripheral actions. Currently, it has shown some effectiveness in the treatment of patients with cardiogenic shock following an acute myocardial infarction.[90]

Calcium was identified earlier in this chapter as a critical element in the excitation-contraction mechanism of the myocardium and other muscles. Because of this inotropic effect, replacement and administration of calcium during treatment of the shock patient is essential. Particularly, following infusion of whole blood, calcium may need to be administered since the citrate in banked blood binds with calcium. This makes calcium unavailable for metabolic processes such as contraction. Additionally, administration of calcium may be necessary following hemorrhagic and septic shock, as recent evidence indicates that there is a fall in ionized calcium levels with these entities.[93–95]

Vasodilators

In the previous section it was stated that the primary goal of pharmacologic therapy was to increase vital organ perfusion and to concurrently limit or decrease the myocardium's workload as much as possible and limit pulmonary congestion. It is these latter two effects which vasodilators are responsible for producing. Vasodilators accomplish these effects by dilating the veins and arterioles to various extents. By dilating the veins and venules, venous capacitance is increased, and this decreases preload, which diminishes pulmonary congestion. By dilating the arterioles, the systemic vascular resistance is lowered, and this decreases impedance to left ventricular ejection. Consequently, myocardial oxygen consumption is lessened. In addition, coronary artery dilators can be administered which can assist in increasing the supply of oxygen to the myocardium. Specific agents responsible for these actions include nitroprusside (Nipride), phentolamine (Regitine), and nitroglycerin (Tridel).

Nitroprusside is a potent, rapidly reversible peripheral vasodilator which creates a rapid reduction in systemic vascular resistance by its actions on both the peripheral venous and arterial bed. It is administered via a continuous infusion, and therefore its effects can be titrated and controlled. Phentolamine is a alpha-adrenergic blocking agent which also serves as a direct vascular smooth muscle relaxer. It reduces preload and afterload by relaxing

both the arterial and venous beds; however, its actions are more predominantly arterial in nature. Nitroglycerin primarily acts as a venous dilator. It increases venous capacitance but has also been demonstrated to be able to increase blood flow in the coronary artery collateral vessels.[96,97] Morphine sulfate can also be used as a vasodilator. As a powerful venodilator, it can reduce preload and can also reduce myocardial oxygen consumption. Morphine can also block sympathetic stimulation and this assists in decreasing afterload.

These above agents, while not always used in shock, serve as excellent adjunct agents to assist in decreasing elevated vascular resistances and preloads. Most commonly, they are employed in cardiogenic and late-stage septic shock.

Antiarrhythmic Agents

Particularly in cardiogenic and septic shock, dysrhythmia management may become necessary. Dysrhythmias generally develop from injury to the myocardium as can be seen in acute infarctions, or develop in response to hypoxia and acidosis. The first hallmark, then, of dysrhythmia management dictates that adequate oxygenation and acid-base balance be present. With that present, then various other agents may be effective (see also chap. 11 and the Appendix). For treatment of bradycardia, atropine or isoproterenol can be used. Insertion of a temporary transvenous pacemaker may also be required to treat a persistent bradycardia. Supraventricular tachydysrhythmias also develop, particularly when the atria become distended with excessive volume. Atrial fibrillations, flutters, and tachycardias can be treated with digoxin, verapamil, or propranolol. These agents are used with caution in cardiogenic or late-stage septic shock since they accomplish their intended effects by depressing contractility or increasing myocardial oxygen demand. Ventricular tachydysrhythmias and premature beats can be treated with lidocaine, procainamide, or bretylium. Both lidocaine and procainamide may also depress contractility and bretylium may potentiate the hypotension of shock, so caution should also be used with these agents.

Beta-adrenergic blocking agents, such as propranolol, have been shown to be effective in preventing myocardial hypoxic damage and limiting the effects of ischemia which develop from sympathetic drive. It has also been suggested that they can prevent myocardial necrosis in some patients who would have otherwise developed an infarction.[98,99] These agents should not be administered to prevent infarct extension if bradycardia or hypotension exist as these agents will only exacerbate these problems and cardiogenic shock will develop.[100]

Corticosteroids

The use of steroids in septic shock still remains controversial. However, for those investigators who advocate the use of steroids, the recommendation is to administer them early in the treatment of gram-negative shock rather than as an end-stage therapy.[101–103] It is felt that the beneficial effects of steroid therapy are derived from the ability of steroids to reduce capillary permeability, to stabilize lysosomal membranes, and to inhibit the release of chemical mediators in the septic process.

Diuretics

Diuretics are also valuable adjunctive agents to use in shock states. They are particularly helpful in maintaining patency of the renal tubules and reducing preload, which assists in diminishing pulmonary congestion. Caution should be used in their administration since they can be nephrotoxic and can produce acute tubular necrosis. This usually occurs when they are administered during episodes of low cardiac output where they then have a long residence time in the nephron. In this situation, they are chemically irritating to renal cells and cause disruption. Commonly used agents include furosemide (Lasix), bumetadine (Bumex), and ethacrynic acid (Edecrin). Mannitol, an osmotic diuretic, can also be used.

More recently, the utilization of hemofiltration has been demonstrated to be an effective, hemodynamically stable method of removing excessive fluid in oliguric patients.[104,105] Figure 7-13 depicts a hemofiltration system. The system consists of a small ultrafiltration membrane which is attached to a vascular access site such as a shunt. Blood flows through the arterial portion of the shunt where it is heparinized to prevent clotting. As it passes through the ultrafiltration membrane, plasma water or ultrafiltrate is removed at a rate determined by the attached infusion pump. The rate of fluid

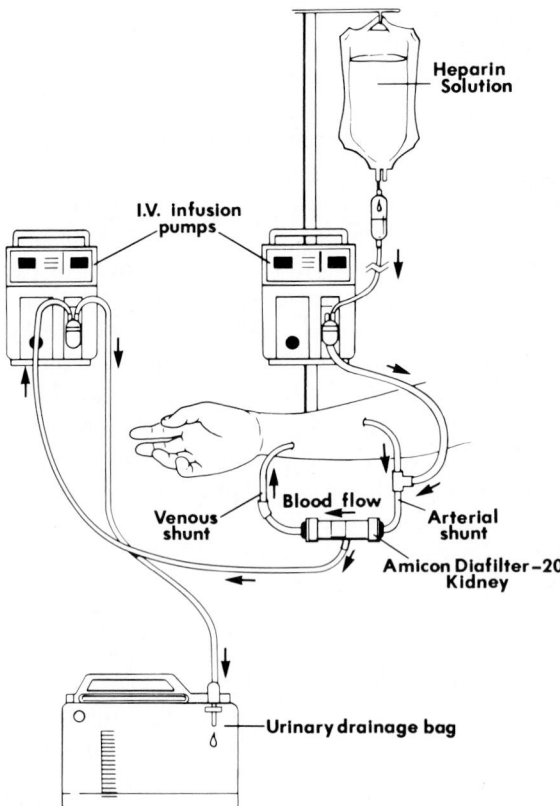

Figure 7-13   Schematic representation of the ultrafiltration system used for fluid removal in oliguric renal failure.

removal is determined by the patient's individual status but is generally 100 to 200 mL per hour. The remaining components of the blood do not sieve out of the membrane but rather stay in the circuit and return via the venous portion of the shunt. This form of continuous slow fluid removal can continue for days to weeks at a time and allows large volumes of vasoactive agents to be infused without worsening the patient's volume status.

Antibiotics

Ideally, antibiotic therapy should not be prescribed until the infecting organisms have been identified. However, in severe cases of septic shock antibiotics can be prescribed based on the most likely infecting organisms. For example, if the infection is felt to be hospital-acquired and occurs in a nonimmunosuppressed patient (neutrophil count greater than 1000 per mm^3) an aminoglycoside and a cephalosporin are recommended. If, however, the patient is immunosuppressed (neutrophil count less than 1000 per mm³) then an aminoglycoside and piperacillin or ticarcillin are recommended.[41]

Heparin

Heparin therapy may be required in patients who develop disseminated intravascular coagulation as a consequence of septic shock. Indications for the use of heparin are generally quite limited and include deep venous thrombosis, pulmonary embolism, or other arterial thrombosis. If heparin is administered, concurrent replacement with fibrinogen, clotting factors, and platelets also needs to occur so that a major hemorrhage does not ensue due to the heparin therapy.[106]

Other Agents

More recently, other therapeutic avenues for the treatment of shock have been addressed. In the fluid of septic shock, the use of a human antiserum to the endotoxin core of gram-negative bacteria has demonstrated that this can improve survival in gram-negative bacteremia.[107] It has been mentioned previously that thromboxane A₂ is implicated in the genesis of endotoxic shock. Recent investigations with dazoxiben, a thromboxane synthetase inhibitor, indicate that it has the ability to lower plasma thromboxane levels in patients with sepsis and adult respiratory distress syndrome. However, while it lowered thromboxane levels, dazoxiben did not alter the clinical course in the patients studied.[108]

Naloxone hydrochloride (Narcan) has also recently entered the arena of controversial drugs used to treat shock. An opiate receptor antagonist, naloxone has been shown in some cases to reverse the hypotension in hypovolemic, endotoxemic, and spinal shock caused by endorphins and other endogenous opiates.[109,110] However, not all investigators achieved the same positive results with naloxone and further studies are needed to determine its ultimate efficacy.[111,112]

Diphenhydramine (Benadryl) can also be given to patients in septic shock. When given at the beginning of the hyperdynamic phase, it can block histamine release. And, in addition, aspirin and indomethacin (Indocin) can be given to block the synthesis of one of the prostaglandins. This helps diminish pulmonary vasconstriction.

Correction of Acid-Base Abnormalities

The majority of acid-base abnormalities which develop in shock will improve spontaneously once adequate ventilation and perfusion are achieved. In hypovolemic shock, however, there may be a transient increase in acidosis following initial volume resuscitation. This develops due to the washout of lactic acid from the tissues which occurs when perfusion dramatically improves as it frequently does in hypovolemic shock. If severe metabolic acidosis persists, then therapy should be initiated to reverse the imbalance. Some investigators suggest that acidosis can go uncorrected until it reaches a pH of 7.2 or less since evidence indicates that myocardial depression does not develop until the pH is 6.9.[113,114] Once correction is required, the agent of choice is sodium bicarbonate. Overcorrection should be avoided as there is an increase in the incidence of supraventricular tachycardia with a pH higher than 7.5.[115]

Circulatory Assist Devices

There are currently a few circulatory assist devices available which can be utilized to stabilize patients in shock. They are the external counterpulsation device, the intraaortic balloon pump (IABP), and the external right and left ventricular assist devices (RVAD, LVAD). The external counterpulsation system is similar to the military antishock trouser. The difference lies in the fact that with external counterpulsation, the suit will inflate and deflate in conjunction with the cardiac cycle. Specifically, during diastole the system is pressurized, thereby increasing coronary blood flow. During systole, it deflates to avoid increasing afterload. It is usually only placed on the patient four times daily for 50 to 120 min. Its efficacy is best seen in patients with cardiogenic shock in class A or B of the hemodynamic subset classification.[116–118]

The intraaortic balloon pump (IABP) is a sausage-shaped balloon mounted on a catheter which is inserted most often through the femoral artery and is then placed distal to the left subclavian artery in the descending thoracic aorta. The action of the balloon is to inflate during systole (Fig. 7-14). Inflation allows blood to be pushed retrograde into the aortic root. This increases coronary artery blood supply and hence oxygenation. Deflation of the balloon just prior to systolic ejection creates a negative intraaortic pressure and therefore decreases afterload. By these actions of increasing coronary artery blood flow and decreasing afterload, the total work of the heart is reduced. Intraaortic balloon pumping is most commonly used in patients with cardiogenic shock. However, it can also assist in the hypodynamic stage of septic shock to support a failing myocardium while antibiotics and other activities are attempting to control the sepsis.[119,120]

The last type of circulatory assist device is the external ventricular assist device. These devices are indicated for use in patients with markedly impaired ventricular failure unresponsive to pharmacologic or IABP support. They could also be patients with end-stage cardiac disease who are waiting transplantation and who are deteriorating. While these devices vary in their specific designs, their techniques generally consist of removing blood via cannulas from the left atrium or ventricle and reinfusing it into the aortic root, or removing blood from the right atrium or ventricle and infusing it into the pulmonary artery. This technique bypasses the ventricle and consequently requires no ventricular contraction. Blood flow in these systems can be either pulsatile or nonpulsatile and is maintained by roller, centrifugal, or pneumatically powered drive systems.[121,122]

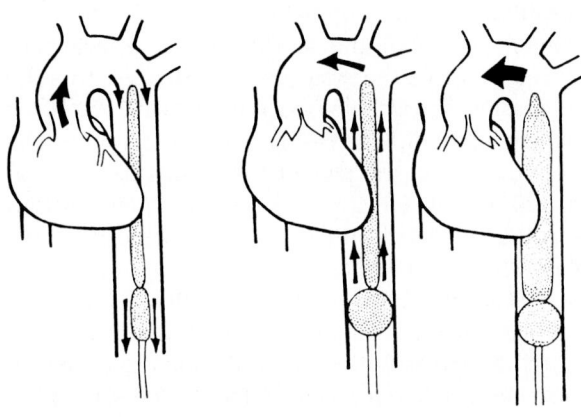

SYSTOLE   **DIASTOLE**

Figure 7-14 Schematic representation of the intraaortic balloon catheter in systole and diastole.

All these above systems are temporary in nature and are discontinued or weaned from the patient as improvement is noted.

Case Presentation

Mrs. W. is a 54-year-old white female who, while attending her daughter's wedding reception, developed shortness of breath and left-sided shoulder and chest discomfort. Upon arrival in the emergency room her cuff blood pressure was 80/58; heart rate was sinus tachycardia at 120 beats per minute; respiratory rate was 34 breaths per minute; S_3 and S_4 heart sounds were heard; the ECG showed S-T changes in leads I and aVL; the chest film revealed a normal cardiac silhouette and clear lung fields; and fine moist rales were present in the lower lobes. Arterial blood gases were pH = 7.50, Pa_{O_2} = 85, Pa_{CO_2} = 30. Her skin was cool and clammy and peripheral pulses were weak.

An initial diagnosis of a lateral wall myocardial infarction was established, and Mrs. W. was transferred to the coronary care unit, where a pulmonary artery flow-directed catheter was inserted. The thermodilution cardiac output was 4.5 L/min with a cardiac index of 2.2 L/min per m². Pulmonary capillary wedge pressure was 14 mmHg and right atrial pressure was 9 mmHg. Systemic vascular resistance was 1500 dyn/s/cm^{-5}. An indwelling Foley catheter was inserted and the hourly urine output was 20 mL per hour. Concurrent therapy with supplemental oxygen administration, volume loading, dobutamine, nitroglycerine, and Nipride infusions were initiated and over the next hour the cardiac index rose to 2.5 L/min per m²; the PCWP rose to 16 mmHg; the right atrial pressure to 12 mmHg; and the systemic vascular resistance fell to 1280 dyn/s/cm^{-5}. Urine output increased to 50 mL per hour. Appropriate patient problems and specific interventions for Mrs. W. at this point are described below.

Selected Problems for a Patient in Cardiogenic Shock

Nursing Diagnoses

I. Alteration in cardiac output related to:
   A. Decreased contractility from myocardial infarction

B. Myocardial structure abnormalities

C. Conduction system disturbances and dysrhythmias

II. Impaired gas exchange related to acute alterations in tissue perfusion

Goals

I. The patient will exhibit signs of adequate cardiacoutput and contractility as evidenced by:

A. Normal CO/CI: CO = 5L/min, CI = 2.5–3.5 L/min per m²

B. Warm vasodilated extremities

C. Adequate peripheral pulses

D. Adequate urinary output: 0.5 mL per kilogram per hour

E. Absence of further ECG changes

F. Absence of dysrhythmias or presence of a hemodynamically stable dysrhythmia

G. Normal sensorium

II. Patient will exhibit signs and symptoms of adequate gas exchange evidenced by:

A. Adequate respiratory rate and rhythm

B. Adequate color

C. Absence of adventitious sounds

D. Presence of normal breath sounds

E. Normal chest x-ray

F. Adequate arterial blood gas values:

1. Pa_{O_2} 85–100 mmHg with $F_{I_{O_2}}$ at 0.40

2. Pa_{CO_2} 35–45 mmHg

3. pH 7.35–7.45

G. Adequate neurologic status

Interventions

I. Identify and describe factors which can further alter contractility after a myocardial infarction (see Table 7-1 for etiologies of cardiogenic shock). Specifically, in this patient with a lateral wall infarction rupture or dysfunction of the chordae tendineae or the papillary muscle can develop, creating mitral regurgitation. Premature ventricular contractions or other ventricular dysrhythmias may develop and further limit cardiac output since damage is located in the ventricle. Atrial dysrhythmias are less likely to occur but may develop, particularly following mitral regurgitation as the left atrium is stretched from the regurgitant flow.

II. Monitor, assess, and record signs and symptoms of decreased contractility and increased cardiogenic shock.

A. Decreased CO/CI: CO less than 5 L/min or CI less than 2.2 L/min per m².

B. Hypotension: Systolic blood pressure less than 80 mmHg and/or MAP less than 60 mmHg.

C. Elevated SVR: SVR greater than 1300 dyn/s/cm⁻⁵.

D. Elevated left ventricular filling pressures: PCWP greater than 18 mmHg.

E. Urinary output less than 30 mL/h or less than 0.5 mL per kilogram per hour.

F. Presence or development of S_3 and S_4 heart sounds.

G. Presence or development of a new murmur. With lateral wall infarction, papillary muscle rupture is common, thereby creating mitral regurgitation and consequently a holosystolic murmur develops.

H. Jugular venous distention. This will develop when biventricular failure occurs.

I. Increase in quality and extent of rales. This can indicate a worsening pulmonary function and development of pulmonary edema.

J. Tachycardia. Heart rate greater than 110 beats per minute.

K. Cold, clammy skin.

L. Decreased peripheral pulses.

M. Decreased level of consciousness.

N. Presence of a pulsus alternans on the arterial tracing. This is a pattern of alternating high and low arterial pressure waves. It is a classic sign of left ventricular failure and reflects a myocardium which has limited reserve and hence alternating capabilities for contraction.

O. Hypoxemia and acidosis.

P. Presence of new ECG changes or development of dysrhythmias.

III. Implement strategies according to either the physician's prescriptions or standing unit policies to improve myocardial contractility.

A. Identify commonly used pharmacologic drugs which improve contractility. Identify their routes of administration, actions, and dosages. These drugs can include:

1. Dopamine

2. Dobutamine

3. Isoproterenol
4. Norepinephrine
5. Epinephrine
6. Digoxin
7. Glucagon
8. Calcium chloride
9. Oxygen
10. Sodium bicarbonate

B. Administer above pharmacologic agents at doses specified by physician's prescriptions and titrate them when appropriate to achieve parameters determined by physician. Usual parameters might include a MAP greater than 60 mmHg and/or a CI greater than 2.5 L/min/per m². During administration of these vasopressors and inotropic agents the nurse should perform the following:

1. Observe MAP every 2–3 min when active titration of vasoactive drugs is being done.
2. Record MAP every 15 min or more frequently to adequately reflect patient's clinical course.
3. Observe for new or increased dysrhythmias or ECG changes that might indicate further myocardial ischemia from too much inotropic drive.
4. Monitor filling pressures for hypervolemic parameters. The presence of v waves on the PCWP tracing could indicate regurgitant blood flow back across mitral valve. This regurgitant flow can occur following rupture of papillary muscle or can develop if ventricle is distended sufficiently to prevent mitral valve cusps from approximating during closure and consequently regurgitation occurs.
5. Obtain CO/CI parameters per physician order or unit routines.

IV. Implement strategies according to either physician's prescriptions or standing unit policies to decrease afterload or reverse systemic vasoconstriction.

A. Identify commonly used pharmacologic drugs which decrease vasoconstriction. Identify their routes of administration, actions, and dosages. These drugs can include:

1. Sodium nitroprusside

2. Phentolamine
3. Nitroglycerine

B. Administer above pharmacologic agents at dosages specified by physician's prescriptions and titrate them when appropriate to achieve parameters determined by physician. Usual parameters might include: lower the SVR to levels less than 1300 dyn/s/cm^{-5} and maintain MAP greater than 80 mmHg.

1. Observe MAP every 2 to 3 min during active titration of these agents.
2. Record MAP every 15 min to provide a record which adequately reflects patient's response to these therapies.
3. Observe the monitored filling pressures every 2 to 3 min, i.e., right atrial pressure or pulmonary artery diastolic pressure.
4. Record filling pressures every 15 min to adequately capture patient's responses. Observe for hypovolemia due to vasodilator effects of drugs.
5. If severe hypovolemia and hypotension develop, immediately decrease or discontinue vasodilator.
6. Avoid MAP pressures less than 60 mmHg since at levels lower than this coronary blood supply can become diminished and further ischemia or infarction could ensue.

V. Identify and describe mechanisms or factors that contribute to impairment of gas exchange in association with inadequate tissue perfusion states (see Associated Problems section). Hydrostatic pulmonary edema such as interstitial or alveolar edema are most likely to occur after a myocardial infarction or in cardiogenic shock. These edemas develop due to inadequacy of left ventricle to maintain adequate stroke volumes. Consequently, left ventricular end-diastolic pressure and volume rise, creating fluid sequestration in pulmonary bed.

VI. Monitor, assess, and record signs and symptoms of hydrostatic edema.

A. Inadequate rate, rhythm, and depth of respiration.
B. Inadequate arterial blood gases, particularly mild to moderate hypoxemia and respiratory alkalosis.

C. Presence of abnormal breath sounds, particularly rales or wheezes, as fluid entrapment narrows airways and causes wheezes and accumulation in alveoli of fluid precipitates.

D. Abnormal chest film, specifically lymphatic enlargement, presence of Kerley B lines, and diffuse haziness.

E. Presence of excessive bronchial secretions with low protein-to-serum protein ratios.

VII. Implement strategies according to either physician's prescriptions or standing unit policies to maintain adequate gas exchange.

A. Position patient to facilitate optimum expansion of lungs. Most frequently this is achieved in upright, supine position so that diaphragm is lowered. However, frequently severe hypotension prevents this position and a 30–40° supine head elevation is all that can be achieved. If patient is intubated, lateral recumbent positions can be used. Repositioning every hour is advisable to prevent atelectasis and areas of poor ventilation from developing.

B. Assist with maintaining or initiating adequate oxygenation therapies, i.e., nasal oxygen to endotracheal intubation.

C. Perform suctioning procedures as necessary. In patients with known coronary artery ischemia constant observation of ECG is essential to assure rapid identification of abnormalities with subsequent immediate discontinuation of suctioning and reoxygenation.

D. Provide information and care to reduce patient's anxiety and fear.

E. Frequently remind patient that ventilator has taken over the work of breathing but that this is only temporary.

F. Provide patient with a method of communicating, i.e., paper and pencil, alphabet board, etc.

G. If patient is on controlled ventilation, assess if patient is out of phase with ventilator and supply reassurance and sedation as necessary. Breathing against or out of phase with ventilator can increase myocardial workload and jeopardize a recovering myocardium.

Over the next 4 h, Mrs. W. became progressively more short of breath and again experienced chest discomfort. Her rales became progressively more coarse and a v wave was discerned on her PCWP tracing. A holosystolic murmur was heard over her apex and she began to have frequent premature ventricular contractions. Arterial blood gases now were pH = 7.59, Pa_{O_2} = 65, Pa_{CO_2} = 25. She was intubated and placed on mechanical ventilation. The cardiac index was 1.9 L/min per m², the systemic vascular resistance was 1800 dyn/s/cm^{-5}, and the PCWP was 32 mmHg. Vasoactive drugs were appropriately increased, and Mrs. W. was taken to the cardiac catheterization laboratory. A left-sided catheterization study was performed, which revealed mitral regurgitation, 80 percent occlusion of the left anterior descending artery, total occlusion of the high lateral circumflex vessel, and 50 percent occlusion of the low lateral circumflex artery. The right coronary artery was open and the ventriculogram demonstrated hypokinesis of the anterior and lateral walls. No dyskinetic or akinetic areas were found. The patient was taken to the operating room where a mitral valve replacement was performed and myocardial revascularization was performed on the left anterior descending and lower circumflex vessel. Her postoperative course was unremarkable except for occasional premature ventricular contractions for which she was placed on procainamide. She was discharged 10 days after surgery.

Approximately 4 weeks later, Mrs. W. was brought to the emergency room by her son, who stated that she had had a seizure at home that morning and ever since was confused and lethargic. On admission her temperature was 105°F, she was experiencing shaking chills, cuff blood pressure was 106/60, heart rate was 120 beats per minute, surgical incisions were intact and revealed no obvious sites of infection, and valve sounds were clear and intact. She was admitted to the critical-care unit and a pulmonary artery flow-directed catheter was inserted. Specific values were as follows: RAP = 3 mmHg; PAS = 25 mmHg; PAD = 8 mmHg; PCWP = 7 mmHg; CO = 9 L per minute; CI = 3.6 L/min per m²; and SVR = 800 dyn/s/cm^{-5}. An arterial line was inserted and MAP was 62 mmHg. At this point, admission laboratory data returned to reveal her hemoglobin and hematocrit to be 12.0

g/100 mL and 34 percent and the WBC to be 500 per milliliter. It was felt that her leukopenia was related to her procainamide therapy. Blood, sputum, and urine cultures were obtained and Mrs. W. was placed in reverse isolation and the procainamide was discontinued. Due to the low filling and arterial pressures, volume replacement was initiated with crystalloid and colloid solutions. Within a 2-h period the RAP was 7 mmHg and the PCWP was 10 mmHg. The MAP remained at 60 mmHg and the CI fell to 2.5 L/min per m². Dobutamine was initiated for inotropic support and low-dose dopamine was started when the urinary output fell to 20 mL per hour. Intubation and mechanical ventilation were instituted as the patient continued to be tachypneic and arterial blood gases demonstrated a Pa_{O_2} of 69 with a non-rebreathing mask on with an oxygen flow of 60 percent. The MAP continued to fall to 50 mmHg, the cardiac index fell to 1.9 L/min per m², and the SVR rose to 1800 dyn/s/cm⁻⁵. The rate of the dobutamine infusion was increased and shortly after, an infusion of norepinephrine was initiated when no response was achieved. A small-dose infusion of phentolamine was also started in an attempt to decrease the systemic vascular resistance and facilitate cardiac output. Specific culture reports were as yet not available so broad-spectrum antibiotics were started. Appropriate patient problems and actions are listed below.

Selected Problems for a Patient in Septic Shock

Nursing Diagnoses
I. Actual fluid volume deficit related to massive vasodilation

Goals

I. Patient will exhibit signs and symptoms of adequate volume status as evidenced by:
   A. Adequate CO/CI: CO = 5L/min, CI = 2.5–3.5 L/min per m²
   B. Adequate filling pressures: RAP = 0.7 mmHg, PCWP = 10–12 mmHg
   C. Normotension
   D. Absence of physical signs and symptoms of hypovolemia or hypervolemia
   E. Adequate electrolyte, hematologic, and coagulation profiles
   F. Adequate urinary output: 0.5 mL per kilogram per hour

Interventions

I. Identify and describe factors of mechanisms that contribute to alterations in volume status associated with shock. In hyperdynamic stages of septic shock significant vasodilation develops and a relative hypovolemia appears. This is treated with aggressive volume replacement. Careful assessment must take place during replacement process since if sepsis continues and worsens, patient will gradually or abruptly develop vasoconstriction. Consequently, within 1 h the nurse may be dealing with a hypovolemic patient and then a hypervolemic patient.
II. Monitor, assess, and record signs and symptoms of hypovolemia and hypervolemia:
   A. CO/CI outside normal parameters.
   B. Filling pressures above or below normal parameters.
   C. Alterations in hemodynamic wave configurations. In hypovolemic patients fluctuations in baseline of right atrial pressure occurs with inspiration and expiration. Also, in hypovolemic states the arterial wave configuration is characterized by a slow upstroke, a prolonged peak, and a dicrotic notch that is less than one-third of the height of the curve. (In hypervolemic patients a *v* wave on the PCWP trace indicates regurgitant flow across mitral valve. This can occur with structural damage to mitral valve or as a functional consequence in which excessive dilation of ventricle from volume overload causes mitral valve cusps to fail to approximate and hence there is regurgitation. Since in this case the patient has had a valve replacement, these above factors do not apply. However, in sepsis there is always a concern that valvular endocarditis can occur, which creates the possibility of erosion around the valve ring which can produce regurgitation.)
   D. Alterations in skin turgor. In hypervolemic patients pitting edema develops, while in hypovolemic situations skin turgor is diminished and tenting occurs. *Tenting* refers

to the ability to pinch the skin upwards and have it remain in that position for a few seconds.

E. Tachycardia. Tachycardia occurs in both hypo- and hypervolemic states.

F. Alterations in peripheral pulses. In hypovolemia, weak, thready, easily obliterated pulses are present, while in hypervolemia full and bounding pulses are the rule.

G. Alterations in breath sounds. Hydrostatic pulmonary edema can commonly occur with overaggressive volume replacement.

III. Implement strategies according to either physician's prescriptions or standing unit policies to assist in controlling volume status.

A. Identify therapies and agents commonly used to control volume status. Recognize specific side effects and specific administration procedures which need to be used to administer these agents.
   1. Crystalloid solutions
   2. Colloids
   3. Blood products

B. Administer preceding agents per physician's prescriptions or unit routines. During administration observe for signs of hypovolemia or hypervolemia and perform the following:
   1. Monitor MAP and heart rate consistently and record every 15 min. Observe for signs of myocardial ischemia.
   2. Monitor filling pressures consistently. The pulmonary artery systolic and pulmonary artery diastolic pressures can be constantly displayed since volume is not given through these lines. Their values should be documented every 15 min during periods of aggressive fluid replacement. If the right atrial port is not used for fluid administration it should also be monitored constantly. If it is used for volume infusion, parameter recordings should still be obtained every 30 min. In patients with known poor left ventricular function, values should be obtained between each 100–200 mL of volume infused.
   3. Obtain CO/CI as needed.
   4. Monitor and assess for signs of hypovolemia and hypervolemia.
   5. Monitor and assess electrolyte, hematologic, and coagulation parameters.
   6. Carefully label, verify, and record all fluid administered.
   7. Observe for development of adverse reactions and record appropriately.
   8. Monitor and record hourly urinary outputs, nasogastric drainage, or any other measurable output loss.
   9. Calculate and record fluid intake as a cumulative and ongoing process following infusion of every 100–200 mL of volume.

The pH was progressively becoming more acidotic and sodium bicarbonate was given. Ventilation was increased and a Fi_{O_2} of 100% with 10 cm of PEEP was required to maintain a Pa_{O_2} of 75 mmHg. An infusion of epinephrine was added and the MAP continued to fall to 39 mmHg; the cardiac index was 0.9 L/min per m^2 and the systemic vascular resistance was 2300 dyn/s/cm^{-5}. A percutaneous intraaortic balloon pump catheter was inserted and pumping was initiated. The patient stabilized with a MAP of 40 mmHg and a cardiac index of 1.0 L/min per m^2 for the next 30 min. Gradually over the next 8 h her MAP returned to 70 mmHg; CI increased to 2.4 L/min per m^2 and SVR returned to 1700 dyn/s/cm^{-5}. Now established, an extensive physical examination revealed a small perirectal abscess from a hemorrhoid. Within 72 h the intraaortic balloon and the vasoactive pharmacologic support were discontinued. Mrs. W.'s pulmonary function gradually improved and she was extubated 1 week later. Discharge from the hospital occurred 2 weeks later.

References

1. Manson, N. H., & Hess, M. L. (1983). Interaction of oxygen free radicals and cardiac sarcoplasmic reticulum: Proposed role in the pathogenesis of endotoxin shock. *Circulatory Shock, 10,* 205–213.

2. Duff, J. H. (1976). Cardiovascular changes in sepsis. *Heart & Lung, 5,* 722.

3. Chaudry, I. (1983). Cellular mechanisms in shock and ischemia and their correction. *American Journal of Physiology, 245,* R112–R134.

4. MacLean, L. D. (1985). Shock. A century of progress. *Annals of Surgery, 201,* 407–414.

5. Wilson, R. F. (1980). The pathophysiology of shock. *Intensive Care Medicine, 6,* 89–100.

6. Rush, B. F. (1980). Shock and the sick cell. *The American Surgeon, 100,* 6–13.

7. Chaudry, I., Ohkawa, M., Clemens, M. G., & Baue, A. E. (1983). Alterations in electron transport and cellular metabolism with shock and trauma. In Lefler, A., and Schumer, W. (Eds.), *Molecular & cellular aspects of shock & trauma.* New York: Alan R. Liss, Inc.

8. Holcroft, J. W. (1982). Impairment of venous return on hemorrhagic shock. *Surgical Clinics of North America, 62,* 17–29.

9. Demling, R. H., Duy, N., & Manohar, M. (1980). Comparison between lung fluid filtration rate and measured Starling forces after hemorrhagic and endotoxic shock. *Journal of Trauma, 20,* 856.

10. Harlan, J. M., & Harker, L. A. (1981). Hemostasis, thrombosis and thromboembolic disorders: The role of arachidonic acid metabolites in platelet-vessel wall interactions. *Medical Clinics of North America, 65,* 855.

11. Kuehl, F. A., & Egan, R. W. (1980). Prostaglandins, arachidonic acid and inflammation. *Science, 210,* 978.

12. Moncado, S., & Vane, J. R. (1979). Arachidonic acid metabolites and interaction between platelets and blood vessel walls. *New England Journal of Medicine, 300,* 1142.

13. Wilson, M. F., Brachett, D. J., Tompkins, P., Benjamin, B., Archer, L. T., & Henshaw, L. B. (1981). Elevated plasma vasopressor during endotoxin and *E. coli* shock. *Advances in Shock Research, 6,* 15–26.

14. Saba, T. M., & Jaffe, E. (1980). Plasma fibronectin opsonic glycoprotein: Its synthesis by vascular endothelial cells and role in cardiopulmonary integrity after trauma as related to RES function. *American Journal of Medicine, 68,* 577–594.

15. Altura, B. (1980). Reticuloendothelial system and neuro-endocrine stimulation in shock therapy. *Advances in Shock Research, 3,* 3–25.

16. Staub, N. C. (1974). Pulmonary edema. *Physiology Review, 54,* 3–25.

17. Sharp, A. A. (1972). Diagnosis and management of disseminated intravascular coagulation. *British Medical Bulletin, 33,* 265–272.

18. Carter, A. J. (1985-1986). Disseminated intravascular coagulation. In Brain, M. C., and McCullock (Eds.), *Current therapy in hematology oncology.* St. Louis: Mosby.

19. Snyder, E. L. (Ed.) (1983). *Blood transfusion therapy. A physicians handbook.* Arlington, VA: American Association of Blood Banks.

20. Feinstein, D. I. (1982). Diagnosis and management of disseminated intravascular coagulation: The role of heparin therapy. *Blood, 60,* 284–287.

21. Offenstadt, G., & Pinta, P. (1982). Hemorrhagic shock. *Resuscitation, 10,* 1–11.

22. Reubi, F. C., & Vorburger, C. (1976). Renal hemodynamics in acute renal failure after shock in man. *Kidney International, 10,* 137–143.

23. Riede, V., Sandritter, W., & Mittermayer, C. (1981). Circulatory shock: A review. *Pathology, 13,* 299–311.

24. Wells, S. (1982). Nursing care of patients in shock: Part 3: Evaluating the patient. *American Journal of Nursing, 82,* 1723–1746.

25. Perry, A. C., & Potter, P. A. (1983). *Shock, comprehensive nursing management.* St. Louis: Mosby.

26. Shumer, W. (1979). Hypovolemic shock. *Journal of the American Medical Association, 24,* 615–616.

27. Houston, M. C., Thompson, W. L., & Robertson, D. (1984). Shock: Diagnosis and management. *Archives of Internal Medicine, 144,* 1433–1439.

28. Collins, J. (1982). The pathophysiology of hemorrhagic shock. In Collins, J. (Ed.), *Massive transfusion in surgery and trauma.* New York: Alan R. Liss, pp. 5–29.

29. Jakschik, B. A. (1974). Profile of circulating vasoactive substance in hemorrhagic shock and their pharmacologic manipulation. *Journal of Clinical Investigation, 54,* 842.

30. Watkins, G. M. (1974). Bodily changes in repeated hemorrhage. *Surgery, Gynecology and Obstetrics, 139,* 161.

31. Moss, G. S., & Saletta, J. D. (1974). Traumatic shock in man. *New England Journal of Medicine, 290,* 724–726.

32. Casley-Smith, J. R. (1976). The functioning and interrelationship of blood capillaries and lymphatics. *Experientia, 32,* 1–12.

33. Drucker, W. R., Christopher, D. J., Chadwick, M. D., & Gann, D. S. (1981). Transcapillary refill in hemorrhage and shock. *Archives of Surgery, 116,* 1344–1353.

34. Pirkle, J. C., & Gann, D. S. (1976). Expansion of interstitial fluid is required for full restitution of blood volume after hemorrhage. *Journal of Trauma, 16,* 937–947.

35. Grossman, J., Yalow, A. A., & Wiston, R. E. (1960). Albumin degradation and synthesis influenced by hydrocortisone, corticotropin and infection. *Surgical Forum, 9,* 528–550.

36. Skillman, J. J., Awwad, H. K., & Moore, F. D. (1967). Plasma protein kinetics of the early transcapillary refill after hemorrhage in man. *Surgery, Gynecology and Obstetrics, 125,* 983–996.

37. Page, D. L., Caulfied, J. B., Kastol, J. A., DeSanetes, R. W. & Sander, C. A. (1971). Myocardial changes associated with cardiogenic shock. *New England Journal of Medicine, 285,* 133.

38. Alonso, D. R., Scheidt, S., Post, M., & Killip, T. (1973). Pathophysiology of cardiogenic shock, quantification of myocardial necrosis, clinical, pathologic and electrocardiographic correlations. *Circulation, 48,* 588.

39. Rice, V. (1984). The clinical continuum of septic shock. *Critical Care Nurse, 4,* 85–109.

40. Mizock, B. (1983). Septic shock, a metabolic perspective. *Archives of Internal Medicine, 144,* 579–585.

41. Cowley, R. A., & Trump, B. F. (1982). *Pathophysiology of shock, anoxia and ischemia.* Baltimore: Williams & Wilkins.

42. Parker, M. M., & Parillo, J. E. (1983). Septic shock: hemodynamics and pathogenesis. *Journal of the American Medical Association, 250,* 3324–3327.

43. Guyton, A. C. (1981). *Textbook of medical physiology.* Philadelphia: Saunders.

44. Wilson, M. F., & Brackett, D. J. (1983). Release of vasoactive hormones and circulatory changes in shock. *Circulatory Shock, 11,* 225–234.

45. Lefer, A. M., & Martin, J. (1970). Origin of myocardial depressant factor in shock. *American Journal of Physiology, 218,* 1423–1427.

46. DeSantes, D., Phillips, P., Spath, M. A., & Lefer, A. M. (1981). Delayed appearance of a circulating myocardial depressant factor in burn patients. *Annals of Emergency Medicine, 10,* 22–24.

47. Abraham, E., & Schoemaker, W. C. (1983). Sequential cardiopulmonary patterns in septic shock. *Critical Care Medicine, 11,* 799–803.

48. Abraham, E., Bland, R., & Cobo, J. (1984). Sequential cardiorespiratory patterns associated with outcome in septic shock. *Chest, 85,* 75–79.

49. Trzeciakowski, J. P., & Leu, R. (1982). Reduction of ventricular fibrillation threshold by histamine: Resolution into separate H1 and H2 components. *Journal of Pharmacology and Experimental Therapies, 223,* 774–783.

50. Terradellas, J. B., Bellot, J. F., Saris, A. B., Gel, C. L., Torrallar-dono, A. T., & Garriga, J. R. (1982). Acute and transient ST segment elevation during bacterial shock in seven patients without apparent heart disease. *Chest, 81,* 444–448.

51. Henning, R. J., Weiner, F., Valdes, S., & Weil, M. H. (1979). Measurement of toe temperature for assessing the severity of acute circulatory failure. *Surgery, Gynecology and Obstetrics, 149,* 1–7.

52. Cohn, J. N. (1967). Blood pressure measurement in shock: Mechanisms of inaccuracy in auscultatory and palpatory methods. *Journal of the American Medical Association, 199,* 198–222.

53. Carlson, R. W., Schaeffer, R. C., Michaels, S. G., & Weil, M. H. (1979). Pulmonary edema fluid. *Circulation, 50,* 1161–1166.

54. Fein, A., Grossman, R. F., & Jones, J. G. (1979). The value of edema fluid protein measured in patients with pulmonary edema. *American Journal of Medicine, 67,* 32–37.

55. Wilson, R. F., & Krome, R. (1969). Factors affecting prognosis in clinical shock. *Annals of Surgery, 169,* 93–105.

56. Peretz, D. I., Scott, H. M., & Duff, J. (1965). The significance of lactic acidemia in the shock syndrome. *Annals of the New York Academy of Science, 119,* 1133–1135.

57. Broder, G., & Weil, M. H. (1964). Excess lactate: An index of reversibility of shock in human patients. *Science, 143,* 1459–1461.

58. Vincent, J. L., & DuFaye, P. (1983). Serial lactate determination during circulatory shock. *Critical Care Medicine, 11,* 449–451.

59. Carey, L. C., Lowery, B. D., & Cloutur, C. T. (1971). Hemorrhagic shock. *Current Problems in Surgery, 6,* 1–48.

60. Lucas, C. E., Rector, F. E., Werner, M., & Rosenberg, T. K. (1973). Altered renal homeostasis with acute sepsis. *Archives of Surgery, 106,* 444–449.

61. Sibbald, W. J. (1979). The Trendelenburg position: Hemodynamic effects in hypotensive and normotensive patients. *Critical Care Medicine, 7,* 218–228.

62. Hoffman, J. R. (1980). External counterpressure and the MAST suit: Current and future roles. *Annals of Emergency Medicine, 9,* 420–425.

63. Carter, J. L., & Smith, B. L. (1982). Use of military antishock trousers: Nursing Implications. *Heart & Lung, 11,* 422–425.

64. Alfaro, R. (1982). Pneumatic antishock suits: When and how to use them. *Dimensions of Critical Care Nursing, 1,* 9–16.

65. Rice, V. (1984). Shock management. Part I. Fluid volume replacement. *Critical Care Nurse, 4,* 69–82.

66. Weil, M. H., & Rackow, E. C. (1984). A guide to volume repletion. *Emergency Medicine, 16,* 101–110.

67. Ross, A. D., & Angaram, D. M. (1984). Colloids versus crystalloids—a continuing controversy. *Drug Intelligence and Clinical Pharmacy, 18,* 202–212.

68. Shine, K. I., Kuhn, M., Young, L. S., & Tillisch, J. H. (1980). Aspects of the management of shock. *Annals of Internal Medicine, 93,* 723–734.

69. Collins, J. A., Murawski, K., & Shafer, A. W. (1982). Massive transfusion in surgery and trauma. *Progress in Clinical and Biological Research, 108.*

70. Lucas, C. E., Bouwman, D. L., & Ledgerwood, A. M. (1980). Differential serum protein changes following supplemental albumin resuscitation for hypovolemic shock. *Journal of Trauma, 20,* 47–51.

71. Faillace, D. F., Ledgerwood, A. M., & Lucas, C. E. (1982). Immunoglobulin changes after varied resuscitation regimens. *Journal of Trauma, 22,* 1–5.

72. Puri, V. K. (1983). Resuscitation in hypovolemia and shock: A prospective study of hydroxyethyl starch and albumin. *Critical Care Medicine, 11,* 518–523.

73. Puri, V. K., Paidipaty, B., & White, L. (1981). Hydroxyethyl starch for resuscitation of patients with hypovolemia and shock. *Critical Care Medicine, 9,* 833–837.

74. Haupt, M. T. & Rackow, E. C. (1982). Colloid osmotic pressure and fluid resuscitation with hetastarch, albumin and saline solutions. *Critical Care Medicine, 10,* 159–162.

75. Gerven, A. S., & Fischer, R. P. (1984). Resuscitation of trauma patients with type-specific uncross-matched blood. *Journal of Trauma, 24,* 327–329.

76. Saba, T. M., & Jaffe, E. (1980). Plasma fibronectin opsonic glycoprotein: Its synthesis by vascular endothelial cells and role in cardiopulmonary integrity after trauma as related to the reticuloendothelial system. *American Journal of Medicine, 68,* 577–594.

77. Nishimura, N., & Takahiro, S. (1984). Changes of hemodynamics and O_2 transport associated with the perfluorochemical blood substitute-fluorol-DA. *Critical Care Medicine, 11,* 943–945.

78. Schwartz, T. (1982). It's not artificial blood—but it can do the work of RBC's. *RN, 45,* 38–43.

79. Smith, S. (1984). Perfluorochemicals: Artificial blood. *Dimensions in Critical Care Nursing, 3,* 198–206.

80. Wells, S. (1982). Nursing care of patients in shock. Part I: Pharmacotherapy. *American Journal of Nursing, 82,* 943–964.

81. Barrows, J. J. (1982). Shock demands drugs. *Nursing '82, 12,* 34–41.

82. Richard, C., Recome, J. L., & Remalko, A. (1983). Combined hemodynamic effects of dopamine and dobutamine in cardiogenic shock. *Circulation, 67,* 620–626.

83. Rackow, E. C. (1984). Of shock and vasoactive drugs. *Emergency Medicine, 8,* 115–123.

84. Chernow, B., & Roth, B. L. (1986). Pharmacologic manipulation of the peripheral vasculature in shock: Clinical and experimental approaches. *Medicine, 13,* 566–570.

85. Rice, V. (1985). Shock management. Part II. Pharmacologic intervention. *Critical Care Nurse, 5,* 42–57.

86. LeJemtel, T. H., Keung, E., Sonnenblick, E. H., & Ribner, H. S. (1979). Amrinone: A new non-glycosidic, non-adrenergic cardiotonic agent effective in the treatment of intractable myocardial failure in man. *Circulation, 59,* 1098–1104.

87. Vincent, J. L., Dufaye, P., & Berre, J. (1981). Infusion of glucose and insulin in circulatory shock. *Critical Care Medicine, 9,* 209–216.

88. Archer, L. T., Beller, B. K., & Drake, J. K. (1976). Reversal of myocardial dysfunction in endotoxin shock with insulin. *Canadian Journal of Physiology and Pharmacology, 216,* 898–914.

89. Bronsveld, W., Van den Bos, G. C., & Thijs, L. G. (1985). Use of glucose-insulin-potassium (GIK) in human septic shock. *Critical Care Medicine, 13,* 566–570.

90. Herbert, P., & Tinker, J. (1980). Inotropic drugs in acute circulatory failure. *Intensive Care Medicine, 6,* 101–111.

91. Dawson, J. R., & Poole-Wilson, P. A. (1980). Salbutamol in cardiogenic shock complicating acute myocardial infarction. *British Heart Journal, 43,* 523–526.

92. Modlen, I. M., & Jaffe, B. M. (1980). Clinical usefulness of glucagon. *Surgery, 87,* 470–472.

93. Trunkey, D. D., Holcroft, J. W., & Carpenters, M. A. (1976). Calcium flux during hemorrhagic shock in baboons. *Journal of Trauma, 16,* 633–643.

94. Woo, P., Carpenter, M. A., & Trunkey, D. D. (1979). Ionized calcium: The effect of septic shock in the human. *Journal of Surgical Research, 26,* 605–611.

95. Harrigan, C., Lucas, C. E., & Ledgewood, A. M. (1983). Significance of hypocalcemia following hypovolemic shock. *Journal of Trauma, 23,* 488–493.

96. Chiariello, M. (1976). Comparison between the effects of nitroprusside and nitroglycerin on ischemic injury during acute myocardial infarction. *Circulation, 54,* 766–772.

97. Goldstein, R. E. (1974). Intraoperative coronary collateral function in patients with coronary occlusion disease: Nitroglycerin responsiveness and angiographic correlation. *Circulation, 49,* 298–304.

98. Peter, T., Norris, R. M., Clark, E. D., & Heng, M. K. (1978). Reduction of enzyme levels by propranolol after acute myocardial infarction. *Circulation, 57,* 1091–1099.

99. Rasmussen, M. N., Reimer, K. A., Kloner, R. A., & Jennings, R. B. (1977). Infarct size reduction by propranolol before and after coronary ligation in dogs. *Circulation, 56,* 794–799.

100. Geddes, J. S., Adgey, A. A., & Pantridge, J. F. (1980). Prevention of cardiogenic shock. *American Heart Journal, 99,* 243–254.

101. Sprung, C. L., Coralis, P. V., Marcial, E. H., & Pierce, M. (1984). The effects of high-dose corticosteroids in patients with septic shock. *New England Journal of Medicine, 311,* 1137–1143.

102. Lucas, C. E., & Ledgerwood, A. M. (1984). The cardiopulmonary response to massive doses of steroids in patients with septic shock. *Archives of Surgery, 119,* 537–541.

103. Nicholson, D. P. (1983). Corticosteroids in the treatment of septic shock and the adult respiratory distress syndrome. *Medical Clinics of North American, 67,* 717–724.

104. Ossenkoppele, G. J., Van der Meulen, J., Bronsveld, W., & Thijs, L. G. (1985). Continuous arteriovenous hemofiltration as an adjunctive therapy for septic shock. *Critical Care Medicine, 13,* 102–104.

105. Paganini, E. P. (1986). *Acute continuous renal replacement therapy.* Boston: Martinus Nijhoff.

106. Corrigan, J. J., & Jordan, C. M. (1970). Heparin therapy in septicemia with disseminated intravascular coagulation: Effect on mortality and correction of hemostatic defects. *New England Journal of Medicine, 283,* 778–785.

107. Ziegler, E. J., McCutchan, J. A., Fierer, J., Glauser, M. P., & Sadoff, J. C. (1982). Treatment of gram-negative bacteremia in shock with human antiserum to a mutant *Escherichia coli. New England Journal of Medicine, 307,* 1225–1230.

108. Reines, H. D., Halushka, P. V., Olanoff, L. S., & Hunt, P. S. (1985). Dazoxiben in human sepsis and adult respiratory distress syndrome. *Clinical Pharmacology Therapy, 37,* 391–396.

109. Groeger, J. S., Carlon, G. C., & Howland, W. S. (1983). Naloxone in septic shock. *Critical Care Medicine, 11,* 650–654.

110. Faden, A. I. (1984). Opiate antagonists and thyrotropin-releasing hormone. *Journal of the American Medical Association, 252,* 1177–1180.

111. Chen, H. L. (1984). Naloxone in shock and toxic coma. *American Journal of Emergency Medicine, 2,* 444–452.

112. Rock, P., Silverman, H., Plump, D., & Kecala, Z. (1985). Efficacy and safety of naloxone in septic shock. *Critical Care Medicine, 13,* 28–33.

113. Wildenthal, K., Mierzweak, D. S., & Myers, R. W. (1968). Effects of acute lactic acidosis on left ventricular performance. *American Journal of Physiology, 136,* 421–426.

114. Siegel, H. W., & Downing, S. E. (1970). Reduction of left ventricular contractility during acute hemorrhagic shock. *American Journal of Physiology, 218,* 772–782.

115. Ream, A. K., & Fogdall, R. P. (1982). *Acute cardiovascular management: Anesthesia and intensive care.* Philadelphia: Lippincott.

116. Soroff, H. S. (1974), External counterpulsation: Management of cardiogenic shock after myocardial infarction. *Journal of the American Medical Association, 229,* 1441–1445.

117. Amsterdam, E. A. (1980). Clinical assessment of external pressure circulatory assistance in acute myocardial infarction. *American Journal of Cardiology, 45,* 349–353.

118. Cohen, L. S. (1974). Hemodynamic studies of sequenced and nonsequenced external counterpulsation. *American Journal of Cardiology, 33,* 131–137.

119. Pierce, W. S., Parr, G. V., Myers, J. L., & Pae, W. E. (1981). Ventricular-assist pumping in patients with cardiogenic shock after cardiac operations. *New England Journal of Medicine, 305,* 1606–1610.

120. Pennington, D. G., Mirjavy, J. P., & Swartz, M. T. (1985). The importance of biventricular failure in patients with postoperative cardiogenic shock. *Annals of Thoracic Surgery, 39,* 16–26.

121. Orlando, R., & Drezner, A. D. (1983). Intra-aortic balloon counterpulsation in blunt cardiac injury. *Journal of Trauma, 23,* 424–427.

122. DeWood, M. A., Notske, R. N., Hensley, G. R., & Shields, J. P. (1980). Intra aortic balloon counterpulsation with and without reperfusion for myocardial infarction shock. *Circulation, 61,* 1105–1112.

8

Breathing and Gas Exchange

Jonathan E.
Gottlieb

Introduction

As life evolved from simple single-celled organisms, the problem of gas exchange became increasingly complex. Whereas in an aqueous environment oxygen could diffuse into, and carbon dioxide diffuse out of, the organism, the addition of subsequent layers of cells to form tissues increased the distance between the aqueous environment and the centers of gas exchange. It soon became imperative that some method of gas transport occur to permit atmospheric oxygen to reach and carbon dioxide to leave the internal milieu of the organism. The process of gas exchange in the human being is marvelously complex; we may begin to gain an understanding of its perturbations by examining the process from both anatomic and physiologic standpoints.

Anatomy of Respiration

Growth and Development

The human lung can first be recognized as a pouch from the primitive foregut as early as the third week of embryologic development. Although the entire bronchial tree may be developed by 4 months gestational age, the lung continues to develop until age 8 or 10 years. Further growth in size of airways (but not in number) may continue until after puberty.

Upper Airway

Assuming a normal tidal volume of 500 to 700 mL and a normal respiratory rate of 15 per minute, approximately 10,000 L of air each day must pass in and out of the lungs; this same volume first is modified as it enters the nose and mouth. As air passes into the nose, it divides through the left and right nasal passages separated by the nasal septum. At the back of the nasopharynx these two passages merge into one. Within the nasal passages are the turbinates, which have a rich blood supply and may swell or shrink as environmental conditions dictate. The airway is lined with ciliated epithelium and mucous glands which help to trap particles and contaminants in the air.

The major functions of the nasal mucosa are to modify the atmospheric air. This process includes heating, absorption of noxious gases, humidification, and filtration. By the time the air has reached the posterior nasopharynx, it is within a few degrees of body temperature and saturated with water vapor. Water-soluble gases such as sulfur dioxide are readily absorbed in the nasopharynx, and many large particles are filtered within the passage. Thus, the initial few centimeters of the respiratory tree are responsible for the majority of cleaning, humidification, and warming of air that reaches the lungs.

As air passes through the pharynx it enters the larynx and from there the trachea. It should be noted that the entire upper airway may contribute at different points to resistance in airflow because of variability in diameter. For example, because of the high collapsibility of the nasopharynx, inspiratory airflow is limited to a maximum of approximately 2 L per second through the nose; this is in contrast to maximum inspiratory flows of about 10 L per second through the mouth. Constriction in the airway may also occur in the oral pharynx when obstructed by the base of the tongue as in obstructive sleep apnea, or in the larynx from vocal cord paralysis.

Tracheobronchial Tree

Air passes through the nose and mouth into the oral phayrnx, through the larynx, and into the trachea, the largest of the *conducting airways*. These include the trachea which bifurcates into two mainstem bronchi, which in turn divide into approximately seven divisions of smaller bronchi. These bronchi lose their cartilage as they branch into bronchioles. After about 20 divisions, respiratory bronchioles can be identified along whose circumference are situated the sites of gas exchange. Alveolar ducts are noted after 23 divisions from the trachea; these lead directly into the alveoli, whose major function is that of gas exchange.

As each airway branches from the trachea to the smallest terminal bronchioles, the diameter of each division becomes progressively smaller. However, the total cross-sectional area at each division increases, so that the velocity of gas decreases as the airstream moves to the periphery of the lung.

The conducting airways do much more than simply conduct air from the outside world to the interior; they are lined with cells which may secrete mucus, immunoglobulins, and other substances, and they may dilate and contract in response to the tone of the smooth muscle contained in their walls.

At the very end of the conducting airways distal to the end of a terminal bronchiole lies the *terminal respiratory unit*. This may consist of an *alveolar duct* with one or more *alveolar sacs* containing individual *alveoli*.

The alveolus may be thought of as the final respiratory chamber. It is typically 250 μm in size, and each person may have 300 million alveoli. The total surface area of alveoli is approximately 80 m², of which the great majority (about 80 percent) is covered with pulmonary capillaries. The surface area exposed to the atmosphere within the lung is 40 times as great as the surface area of the skin, so that the lung provides us with our greatest area of direct contact with the atmosphere.

The surface of the alveolus is where the exchange of gases takes place between the environment and the organism. The epithelium of the alveolus consists of *type I* cells or *squamous pneumocytes,* and *type II* cells or *granular pneumocytes*. It is believed that the type II cells are responsible for secretion of *surfactant*, which is a lipoprotein material vital in maintaining the lung in an uncollapsed state. The alveolar surface abuts directly on the capillary surface to provide a region over which oxygen and carbon dioxide can pass to and from the blood through capillary and alveolar endothelium, alveolar airspace, and atmosphere.

In summary, as the flow of gas moves from the atmosphere into the lung, it passes through the nasal and oral pharynx, past the larynx into the trachea, down the left and right mainstem bronchi, through seven divisions of cartilaginous bronchi, through a dozen more divisions of noncartilaginous conducting airways, into the terminal respiratory units which contain respiratory bronchioles, alveolar ducts, and alveoli. Gas can then move from the alveolus across the epithelium and into the pulmonary capillary where it may be carried throughout the body.

Pulmonary Vasculature

There are two circulations to the lungs; the *pulmonary circulation* is by far more important than the *bronchial circulation*. The main pulmonary artery arises from the outflow tract of the right ventricle and divides into the left pulmonary artery which runs posteriorly, and the right pulmonary artery which runs anteriorly. The pulmonary arteries, which carry unoxygenated blood from the body to the lungs, generally follow the route of the tracheobronchial tree. The proximal pulmonary arteries are primarily elastic, whereas the smaller arteries which accompany the bronchioles have a thin muscular coat. The *pulmonary arterioles* are the smallest branches of the pulmonary arterial system; these arterioles lead directly into the *pulmonary capillaries*. As blood emerges from these pulmonary capillaries, it enters the *pulmonary veins* which eventually merge into several main pulmonary veins to return oxygenated blood to the left atrium. The major function of the pulmonary veins is to serve as a reservoir of blood for the left atrium and the left ventricle.

In contrast to the pulmonary arterial circulation, the bronchial circulation supplies the lungs with oxygenated blood for nutrition of the pulmonary nerves and ganglia, arteries and veins, pleura and connective tissue. The right lung is supplied by a right intercostal artery which originates from the right subclavian or internal mammary artery; the bronchial supply to the left lung originates from the aorta. Unlike the pulmonary arterial circulation which receives the entire cardiac output, only 1 or 2 percent of the cardiac output is distributed to the lung via the bronchial circulation.

Lymphatic Vessels

As blood flows through the pulmonary capillaries, some of the plasma is filtered into the interstitium of the lung, where it is collected into lymphatic channels and ultimately returned to the general circulation. Most authorities believe that the major function of the pulmonary lymphatics is the removal of interstitial fluid and the prevention of pulmonary edema. Although most of the filtered fluid returns through lymphatics that run through the lung parenchyma, another set of lymphatic vessels returns lymph over the surface of the lung within the pleura. When interstitial lymphatic vessels become enlarged through increased fluid filtration such as may occur with pulmonary edema, they may be identified as horizontal linear opacities (Kerley B lines) on the plain chest radiograph. Normal lymph flow has been estimated in humans at 20 mL per hour, increasing to 200 mL per hour during pulmonary edema. In conditions where the major lymphatic drainage through the thoracic duct is blocked, lymph may back up through the lymphatics to form a pleural effusion composed of lymph; this is called a *chylous* effusion.

Nerve Supply to the Lung

The major nerve supplies to the lung are carried by the vagus nerve and by thoracic sympathetic ganglia. The vagus returns information to the central nervous system from several receptors within the lung, including stretch receptors, irritant receptors, and J receptors.

Stretch receptors may respond to lung inflation or increased lung volume with bronchodilatation, tachycardia, and decreased systemic vascular resistance. *Irritant receptors* may be responsible for wheezing, bronchoconstriction, and cough after being stimulated by pulmonary edema and chemical or mechanical irritation. *J receptors* are believed to result in laryngeal constriction, hypotension, and bradycardia when stimulated by embolism or pulmonary edema.

Other responses of the lung such as pulmonary hypertension from hypoxia or bronchoconstriction may occur in the absence of any nervous system input, and probably are caused by local responses of the lung to a variety of stimuli.

Lung parenchyma contains no pain fibers, and procedures such as transbronchial biopsy need no anesthetic. However, blood vessels and pleura are pain-sensitive, and pathways involve predominantly intercostal nerves and thoracic ganglia.

Muscles of Respiration

When there is no muscular activity of the respiratory system or when the patient is completely paralyzed, the thorax is in the position of passive end-expiration, and the lung volume is said to be at *functional residual capacity* (FRC). Anything which changes the volume of the lungs or thorax from this position must result from active contraction of the respiratory muscles.

The *diaphragm* is the major muscle of respiration. It is shaped like a dome and contracts in a downward and forward position, pulling the lungs open and increasing their volume. As inspiration proceeds, the volume in the thorax increases and the abdomen appears to enlarge in an anteroposterior dimension, because the abdominal contents are compressed by the diaphragm. Additional inspiratory muscles include the *scaleni*, the *sternocleidomastoideus*, and the *external intercostals*, all of which help to pull the ribs upward to increase the volume of the thorax.

Normally, expiration is passive. In other words, no active muscle contraction is needed to expel air from the lungs. Rather, the elastic recoil of the lung returns the lung to its original volume after cessation of inspiratory muscle activity. Expiration may be aided by active contraction of the *rectus abdominis, iliocostalis lumborum,* and *intercostales interni,* all of which may aid in depressing the ribs to decrease the volume of the thorax, and contracting the abdominal wall to press the abdominal contents back up into the chest.

The diaphragm receives its nerve supply from the phrenic nerves which arise from the third, fourth, and fifth cervical segments of the spinal cord. Most of the other accessory respiratory muscles are innervated from thoracic and lumbar segments. For this reason, lower cervical or thoracic injuries may completely paralyze the accessory muscles, while action of the diaphragm is preserved.

Physiology of Respiration

Ventilation and Mechanics of Breathing

Lung Volumes

In order to understand how the anatomic components of the respiratory system interact in health and disease, it is important to be familiar with the physiologic concepts applied to breathing. As mentioned in the previous section, the column of air from atmosphere to alveolus is continuous; however, for conceptual purposes it is helpful to divide this air into different compartments.

Total lung capacity (TLC) is the total volume of gas contained in the respiratory system, including gas contained in the upper airway, conducting airways, and alveoli. In order to measure TLC directly, it would be necessary to completely empty all the gas from the respiratory system. Since this is not possible in humans, a method is employed which introduces a known quantity of gas such as helium. By allowing the helium to equilibrate throughout the respiratory system, one can then measure the concentration of helium in an expired sample and calculate the total quantity of gas that must be present to produce this final concentration.

If one takes a deep breath and inhales maximally to TLC, the total amount of gas that is expelled on a forced expiration is termed the forced *vital capacity* (VC). This can be measured by exhaling into a calibrated spirometer which measures the amount of gas exhaled. The amount of gas that remains in the respiratory system after a vital capacity maneuver is the *residual volume* (RV). Normally, we do not breathe from total lung capacity to residual volume; instead we take a submaximal inspiration and submaximal exhalation. This amount of air, which is normally inhaled and exhaled during quiet breathing, is called the *tidal volume* (V_T). This, too, can be measured spirometrically. The amount of gas remaining in the respiratory system at the end of a quiet exhalation is called the *functional residual capacity*.

If one accumulates the tidal volume for 1 min the result is the *minute ventilation* (V_E); this is the total amount of gas that passes in and out of the lungs in 1 min. Alternatively, one may measure the minute ventilation and then divide by the respiratory frequency (F) to obtain the tidal volume.

Alveolar Ventilation and Dead Space

Just as the structure of the respiratory tract changes from upper airway to the alveoli, so does its function. One way to describe these differences in function is to separate the tidal volume into portions which are involved in gas exchange (*alveolar ventilation*, or V_A), and those areas which serve merely to conduct the air but are not involved in gas exchange (*dead space*, or V_D).

$$V_T = V_D + V_A$$

It is easy to envision the upper airway, trachea, major bronchi, and smaller conducting bronchioles as contributing to *anatomic dead space*, whereas respiratory bronchioles and alveoli all contribute to the alveolar ventilation. Normally, approximately 150 mL, or about one-third of the tidal volume, occupies dead space and does not participate in gas exchange. In diseased states, however, not all of the anatomic gas-exchanging units may be functioning; for example, emphysema or obliterative vascular disease may result in loss of the ability of respiratory bronchioles to exchange gas. Under these conditions, those structures which would normally participate in alveolar ventilation contribute functionally to dead space; their volume is referred to as *physiologic dead space*.

Physiologic dead space in normal subjects is usually very close to anatomic dead space and is frequently expressed as the ratio of dead space to tidal volume (V_D/V_T). Normal values for V_D/V_T are about 0.33 (one-third of the tidal volume).

In practice, the physiologic dead space-to-tidal volume ratio may be measured simply by drawing a sample of arterial blood and measuring the P_{CO_2}, and by collecting the patient's expired gas in a Douglas bag or other similar device for several minutes. By withdrawing a sample of mixed expired air in the bag and obtaining the partial pressure of carbon dioxide, one can calculate the dead space-to-tidal volume ratio in the following manner:

$$V_D/V_T = (Pa_{CO_2} - PE_{CO_2})/Pa_{CO_2}$$

where $P_{E_{CO_2}}$ equals the partial pressure of carbon dioxide in the mixed expired air.

Resistance and Compliance

With an appreciation of how the respiratory muscles inflate the lung, it is also important to understand the factors which impede air movement. *Elastic resistance* is the tendency of the lungs to oppose stretching because of frictional and elastic properties of the connective tissue of the lung. Abnormalities of the chest wall or abdominal cavity such as ascites or bony deformity may also oppose inflation of the lung.

An additional form of resistance to airflow is offered by *airway resistance*. When gas flow through the airways is strictly laminar, the resistance of the airways is expressed by Poiseuille's law:

$$R = \frac{8nl}{\pi r^4}$$

This law demonstrates that the major components of resistance to airflow are the radius of the airway (r), the length of the airway (l), and the viscosity of the gas (n). In most clinical situations (during laminar flow) the major determinants of resistance are airway caliber and length. Since resistance is a function of the radius to the fourth power, airway caliber is more important than length. For example, halving of the radius will increase the resistance by 16 times. High peak pressures seen on a ventilator during inspiration may result from bronchospasm, mucous plugging, or airway edema, all of which increase airway resistance. The airway resistance (R) may be roughly estimated by dividing the change in pressure between peak (P_{max}) and pause (P_{plat}) values by the airflow (Q) at that point:

$$R = \frac{P_{max} - P_{plat}}{Q}$$

Airflow may be determined by reading the value set on the ventilator (MA-1, Bear) or by dividing the delivered tidal volume by the inspiratory time (Servo). In general, the greater the difference between peak and pause pressure, the greater the airway resistance. The less the difference between peak and pause pressure, the greater is the share of compliance in accounting for pressures observed during mechanical ventilation.

The resistance to inflation under conditions of no airflow is described by the concept of *compliance*. Compliance refers to the distensibility of a structure in terms of its volume and pressure. For example, a patient with highly compliant lungs will be able to take a large breath without developing high pressures across the lung. In contrast, a patient who may have low compliance from ARDS or pulmonary edema will require much higher pressures to distend the lung to the same degree. Changes in compliance may be demonstrated clinically by determining the static pressures on the ventilator at the end of an inspiration in relation to the volume of inspired gas. *Static compliance* (C_{stat}) of the respiratory system may be calculated by dividing the change in volume (ΔV) by the change in pressure (ΔP):

$$C_{stat} = \frac{\Delta V}{\Delta P} = \frac{\text{Tidal volume}}{P_{plat} - P_{end\text{-}expiration}}$$

The change in volume may be obtained by knowing the tidal volume set on a respirator; the change in pressure may be obtained by subtracting starting pressure ($P_{end\text{-}expiration}$; usually zero or atmospheric, but may be more when the patient is receiving positive end-expiratory pressure) from the pause pressure at the end of an inspiration (P_{plat}). Note that airway resistance is a factor only during airflow, and when there is no flow, then none of the airway pressure results from resistance. Compliance, on the other hand, has nothing to do with flow, or how fast the volume is changed, but rather describes how "stretchable" the respiratory system is. Clearly, in critically ill patients both resistance and compliance play a role in ventilator management.

Distribution of Gas within the Lungs

As air moves into the respiratory system, it must all pass through the trachea. The velocity of gas moving in and out of the trachea is relatively great; as the conducting airways branch through subsequent divisions, the total cross-sectional area gradually increases. At first, this might seem surprising, since the airways become progressively narrower. However, even though the airways narrow, there are more of them so that the total area increases. As a result, the velocity of gas moving at any point in the respiratory system decreases from the trachea toward the alveoli. Near the alveoli, the velocity of gas approaches zero; in fact, at the level of the alveoli there is really no mass movement of gas in and out. Instead, diffusion of gas in the alveoli accounts for exchange of oxygen and carbon dioxide.

The distribution of gas to all parts of the lung is not uniform, because of the gravitational and anatomic forces. In an upright position, the alveoli in the apices of the lung are relatively open and distended; since pressure changes during breathing are smallest in that portion of the lung, there is relatively little ventilation distributed to the upper regions. In contrast, near the bases of the lung, the alveoli are subject to greater changes in pressure; most of the ventilation is distributed to the bases. Most critically ill patients are supine, so that the situation is somewhat different, but the same general principles apply: The anterior or uppermost portions of both lungs are not as well ventilated as are the posterior or dependent portions.

Small airways are very flexible, and some of them may collapse as lung volume decreases while gas still remains in the alveoli. The lung volume at which a significant portion of alveoli contain trapped air is known as the *closing volume*. In normal persons, this occurs well below functional residual capacity, so that all the alveoli remain open during quiet breathing. In diseased states such as obesity, obstructive lung disease, or adult respiratory distress syndrome (ARDS), these alveoli may tend to close more readily so that some air trapping may occur even during normal breathing. For this reason, the semi-Fowler's position may be beneficial for the obese patient with respiratory difficulty. The closing volume may be measured in the pulmonary function laboratory with the single-breath nitrogen test; this is not widely available, and is not practical in critically ill patients.

Regulation of Ventilation

Of all the muscular functions which are vital to life, two of the most critical are the beat-to-beat contraction of the heart and the regular rhythm of the respiratory muscles. Of course, the automatic contraction of muscles throughout the body is necessary for maintenance of basic functions, including contraction of smooth muscle in the vessels to maintain vascular tone, action of the muscles within the GI

tract to aid digestion, contraction of the bladder to facilitate micturition, and the regular contraction of smooth muscle in lymphatic channels to propel lymph. Among all these examples, the respiratory system is unique; the muscles of respiration are entirely composed of voluntary, striated muscle, yet their control is automatic.

The regulation of ventilation cannot be explained by a single mechanism. Rather, many different mechanisms may come into play at different times to exert influence on breathing. Unfortunately, we do not yet have a complete understanding of this complex and multifaceted system. Some of the major components which contribute to the regulation of breathing include:

1. The integrity of neurons in the medulla
2. Reciprocal innervation between inspiratory and expiratory neurons in the pons
3. Acid-base status of the organism
4. The state of wakefulness

Many texts describe the apneustic and pneumotaxic pontine respiratory centers, which control the innate respiratory rhythm and inhibition of inspiration. However, the nervous control of respiration is considerably more complex, and not simply the result of interaction of two discrete centers in the brainstem. Nevertheless, the central nervous system controls the basic rate and rhythm of regular breathing. This basic rhythm may be influenced by a variety of voluntary and involuntary factors.

Modification and fine-tuning is achieved in large part by peripheral and central chemoreceptors. The *peripheral chemoreceptors* monitor arterial oxygen, carbon dioxide, and hydrogen ion concentration. The *carotid bodies* are the peripheral chemoreceptors which exert the major influence on the respiratory system. They receive a tremendous blood flow relative to their weight, and are capable of responding to changes in arterial blood-gas tension within several seconds. Discharge from their afferent nerves (which follow the glossopharyngeal nerve) may occur with a decrease of arterial P_{O_2} below about 60 mmHg. The carotid bodies may also respond to a decrease in pH, an increase in temperature, low perfusion, or chemical stimulation by substances such as nicotine, cyanide, or carbon monoxide.

The *central chemoreceptors* are found in the medulla although their precise location is unknown. They are stimulated by increases in P_{CO_2} or decreases in pH, with an uncertain response to bicarbonate. It should be noted that hypoxia, which stimulates the carotid body, may have no effect on central chemoreceptors, or may even depress respiratory rate and volume.

Other factors which can affect the pattern and extent of ventilation include pulmonary stretch reflexes, the inflation reflex, and the cough reflex. Additionally, baroreceptors in the carotid sinus and aortic arch may respond to a drop in blood pressure by signaling an increase in rate and depth of respiration. This reflex may be clinically evident in patients in shock who hyperventilate in response to low cardiac output.

In critically ill patients an additional factor must be considered: the effect of drugs on the control of ventilation. Commonly used stimulant drugs include aminophylline, which causes an increased sensitivity to p_{CO_2} and may induce hyperventilation. Large doses of barbiturates may depress the ventilatory response, and opiates are well known to cause severe respiratory depression in both volume and frequency.

Pulmonary Blood Flow

The lungs are the only organs in the body that receive the entire cardiac output. Venous blood which drains the lower portions of the body returns via the inferior vena cava, and blood which drains the upper portions of the body returns via the superior vena cava into the right atrium. During diastole, blood flows from the right atrium through the tricuspid valve into the right ventricle. As systole begins, blood moves from the right ventricle through the pulmonic valve into the main pulmonary trunk. Since there is no net gain or loss of blood volume from the pulmonary or systemic circulation, the blood flow through the pulmonary artery must be the same as the blood flow through the aorta. Interestingly, the pressures in the pulmonary circulation are much lower than in the systemic circulation, even though the blood flows are equal. This is because the pulmonary circulation offers a much lower resistance to blood flow than does the systemic circulation.

The concept of *pulmonary vascular resistance* is analogous to the concept of airway resistance; the major determinants of vascular resistance include vessel length, radius to the fourth power, and viscosity. Just as in the airways, the caliber of the blood vessels is the major determinant of resistance. In the circulation, however, viscosity may also play a role, such as when the hematocrit is high from chronic hypoxemia. In this condition, the elevated hematocrit causes greater resistance in the pulmonary circulation, and pulmonary vascular pressures may be increased.

The factors that determine pulmonary vascular caliber are complex, but several of them may be considered separately. First, the level of perfusion of the pulmonary vascular system may affect its resistance. For example, under conditions when blood volume is very low, such as in hemorrhagic shock, the pulmonary vascular system may not be distended enough to open all the pulmonary capillaries. Those pulmonary capillaries which do not participate in blood flow remain closed, and thereby decrease the total cross-sectional area of the pulmonary vascular tree. As blood volume is replaced and cardiac output increases, more of these pulmonary capillaries will open and begin to participate in blood flow through the lungs. This concept of opening pulmonary capillaries by increasing blood flow is called *recruitment*.

Increasing pulmonary blood volume may lower pulmonary resistance in another way. As blood volume and cardiac output increase, pulmonary capillaries may distend with blood, resulting in a larger radius. Since resistance falls as a function of increasing radius, distending pulmonary capillaries will cause a decrease in pulmonary vascular resistance. Although most physiologists believe that recruitment is the major process of decreasing pulmonary vascular resistance with increasing flow, *distention* may also be an important factor.

Second, the state of lung inflation may affect the caliber of pulmonary capillaries. As the lung is progressively inflated, it enlarges in all dimensions. This results in a stretching of pulmonary capillaries along their length. More importantly, it results in a squeezing of the pulmonary capillaries between inflated alveoli. As the lung is inflated and as alveolar pressure increases, the pulmonary capillaries are progressively squeezed so that their radius decreases. Thus, high levels of lung inflation are associated with an increased pulmonary vascular resistance, wheras lower lung volumes are associated with lower pulmonary vascular resistance.

Third, the pulmonary vessels may respond with active constriction to a variety of stimuli. In humans, the most potent stimulus for pulmonary vasoconstriction is hypoxia. This is usually evident at a p_{O_2} of less than 60 mmHg. *Hypoxic pulmonary vasoconstriction* is an important factor in many disease processes, including pulmonary hypertension from chronic obstructive lung disease and high-altitude pulmonary edema. In addition to hypoxia, acidosis may cause elevated pulmonary artery pressures from pulmonary vasoconstriction.

Fourth, other factors may influence the caliber of pulmonary capillaries. For example, pulmonary edema may result in the accumulation of fluid in the interstitium. Fluid accumulation may increase so that pulmonary capillaries are compressed, thereby increasing pulmonary vascular resistance.

Finally, a variety of destructive and obliterative disease processes may increase pulmonary vascular resistance. These include pulmonary embolism, which decreases the total cross-sectional area of the pulmonary vascular tree by occluding several of its major branches; and emphysema, which increases pulmonary vascular resistance in large part by reducing the number of available pulmonary capillaries.

Pulmonary vascular resistance may be calculated in a manner entirely analogous to that for airway resistance. Since resistance is a function of pressure and flow, a pulmonary artery catheter provides the means for estimating pulmonary vascular resistance. Flow may be determined from obtaining a cardiac output (CO) by thermodilution; pressure may be determined by subtracting the pulmonary capillary wedge pressure (PCWP) from the mean pulmonary artery pressure (PAP):

$$\text{Pulmonary vascular resistance} = \frac{\text{PAP} - \text{PCWP}}{\text{Cardiac output}}$$

Mean pulmonary artery pressure may be estimated by adding one-third of the pulmonary artery systolic pressure to two-thirds of the pulmonary artery diastolic pressure.

Pulmonary blood flow is influenced by several factors, including the amount of blood that is returned to the heart (venous return), the function of the heart, and pulmonary vascular resistance. These are similar to the factors of preload, contractility, and afterload, respectively, that are applied to the study of left ventricular physiology.

The distribution of blood to the lungs is not uniform; the effects of gravity cause increased blood flow in the lower portions of the lung relative to the upper portions. In an upright person, this means that there may be little or no pulmonary blood flow to the apices of the lung, with most of the blood flow going to the bases. Most critically ill patients are in the supine position, so that the blood flow to the apical region is similar to that to the bases of the lungs. However, the lowest portions of the lung, that is, the dependent or posterior regions of the lung, receive more blood flow than the anterior portions, because of the effects of gravity.

Matching of Ventilation and Perfusion

From the foregoing discussion it is evident that neither ventilation nor blood flow is distributed uniformly throughout the lung; rather, different parts of the lung receive different amounts of ventilation and blood flow.

In areas of the lung which receive similar amounts of blood flow and ventilation, we say that there is good *ventilation-perfusion matching.* In such areas of the lung, gas exchange is most efficient, since carbon dioxide diffuses out of pulmonary arterial blood to the alveolus, and oxygen brought in from the atmosphere diffuses into the blood with ease. Other areas of the lung, however, may demonstrate *ventilation-perfusion inequality,* resulting in less efficient gas exchange.

At one extreme, we may imagine the situation where ventilation is maintained to alveoli, but no blood flow passes through the pulmonary capillaries. This may result from vascular occlusion with pulmonary emboli, low cardiac output, hypoxic vasoconstriction, or gravity. Under these conditions, ventilation is wasted, since it does not allow exchange of gases through the pulmonary vasculature. You will recall that this concept of wasted ventilation was referred to as physiologic dead space. In fact, physiologic dead space represents one extreme of ventilation-perfusion inequality; when the ratio of ventilation to perfusion is extremely high, physiologic dead space is the result.

At the other end of the spectrum are lung units with low ventilation-perfusion ratios. Clinical examples of this situation include mucous plugging or obstruction of a bronchus by a tumor or foreign body. Under this condition, pulmonary arterial blood, which contains low levels of oxygen and high levels of carbon dioxide, is exposed to poorly ventilated alveolar air containing low P_{O_2} and high P_{CO_2}. Thus, hypoxemic and hypercarbic blood is returned to the left side of the heart for distribution to the systemic arterial circulation. When blood perfuses an area of lung with essentially no ventilation, we say the blood is "shunted" past the lung.

The approximate fraction of shunted blood relative to total blood flow ($\bar{Q}_S/\bar{Q}_T$) may be estimated from the following formula:

$$\bar{Q}_S/\bar{Q}_T = \frac{(Cc_{O_2} - Ca_{O_2})}{(Cc_{O_2} - C\bar{v}_{O_2})}$$

where $\bar{Q}_S$ equals the flow of shunted blood, $\bar{Q}_T$ equals the total cardiac output, Cc_{O_2} equals the oxygen content in capillary blood, Ca_{O_2} equals the oxygen content in arterial blood, and $C\bar{v}_{O_2}$ equals the oxygen content in mixed venous blood. Arterial and venous oxygen contents may be calculated by measuring the hemoglobin and obtaining blood gas samples from a peripheral artery and from the pulmonary artery through a Swan-Ganz catheter.

Pulmonary capillary oxygen content may be calculated by assuming that pulmonary capillary blood becomes perfectly equilibrated with alveolar air; to calculate the oxygen content, one uses the alveolar P_{O_2} calculated from the alveolar air equation (see below). In normal persons, approximately 2 percent of the total cardiac output is shunted. Patients with the most severe form of ARDS may show shunt fractions of 50 percent.

Between these two extremes a wide spectrum of ventilation-perfusion inequality may occur, resulting in intermediate problems in gas exchange. Thus, the pulmonary venous blood which returns to the left atrium is a mixture of blood from different areas of the lungs with differing ventilation-perfusion ratios. When we obtain a sample of arterial blood for oxygen and carbon dioxide analysis, we measure the overall function of the lung, and the arterial value represents a kind of average of the gas-exchanging function of the lung as a whole. The concept of ventilation-perfusion imbalance in diseased states will be discussed in a subsequent section.

Another important concept in ventilation-perfusion ratios concerns the zones of the lung (Fig. 8-1). In a normal upright individual, pulmonary arterial pressure may be insufficient to reach the very top of the lungs; thus, no blood flow is distributed to these areas. The result is physiologic dead space. This is referred to as *zone 1*. Just below

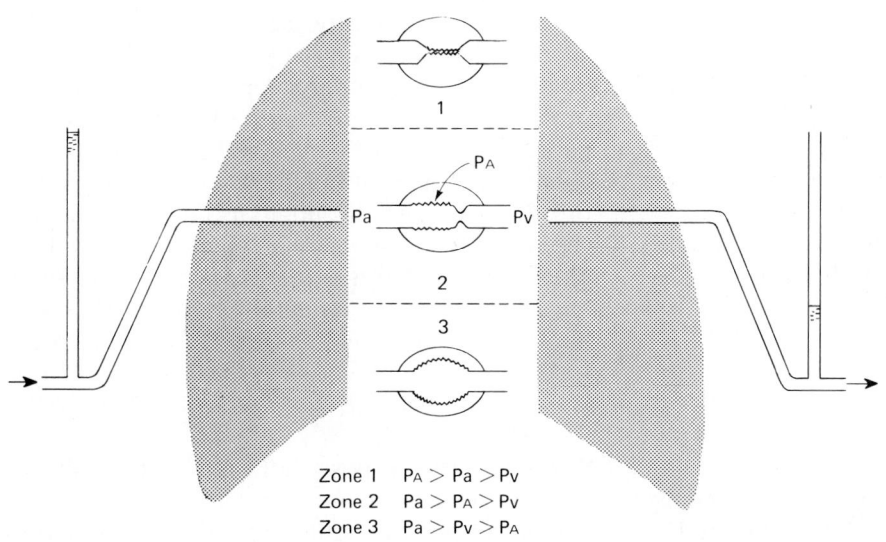

Zone 1 $P_A > P_a > P_v$
Zone 2 $P_a > P_A > P_v$
Zone 3 $P_a > P_v > P_A$

Figure 8-1   Model to explain the distribution of pulmonary blood flow based on pressures affecting the capillaries. The lung is divided into three zones depending on the magnitude of the pulmonary arterial, alveolar, and venous pressures. The lines separating the zones are not topographically precise. *(From John B. West, The use of radioactive materials in the study of lung function. In Alfred P. Fishman, ed., Pulmonary Diseases and Disorders. New York: McGraw-Hill, 1980. Used by permission of the publisher.)*

zone 1, pulmonary artery pressure may be high enough to perfuse pulmonary capillaries. However, alveolar pressure is high enough to cause partial collapse of the pulmonary capillaries, because alveolar pressure is higher than pulmonary venous (or left atrial) pressure. In this condition, it is the relationship between pulmonary artery pressure and alveolar pressure that determines how much blood flow will be delivered to that lung segment. This condition is called *zone 2*. Below zone 2, pulmonary venous pressure is increased because of gravity, and will be greater than alveolar pressure. Here the difference in pressure between pulmonary artery and pulmonary vein (or left atrium) will determine how much blood flow is delivered. This condition is known as *zone 3*.

In the supine patient, zone 1 is normally not encountered, because pulmonary artery pressure is sufficient to perfuse all areas of the lung. The use of positive end-expiratory pressure (PEEP) in critically ill patients, however, may result in alveolar pressures that are sufficiently high to collapse pulmonary capillaries and prevent perfusion of certain segments of the lung. In actual practice, positive end-expiratory pressure is well known to increase the physiologic dead space in the lung by this mechanism.

Exchange and Transport of Oxygen and Carbon Dioxide

Review of Gas Laws

A basic understanding of the physical behavior of gases is necessary to understand the normal and altered physiology of the respiratory system. The ideal gas law states that pressure, volume, and temperature have fixed relationships. What this means is that one cannot change one of these factors without altering the other in a predictable way. The quantitative relationships between volume, pressure, and temperature have been defined by basic gas laws.

Boyle's Law

$$P_1 \times V_1 = P_2 \times V_2 \text{ (at constant temperature)}$$

Since the product of pressure and volume is constant, then an increase in pressure must be accompanied by a decrease in volume. Similarly, if one increases the volume of a gas, then the pressure must decrease.

Charles' Law

$$\frac{V_1}{T_1} = \frac{V_2}{T_2}$$

An increase in temperature must be accompanied by an increase in volume. Alternatively, if the volume of a gas is to increase, then the temperature must rise.

By combining the above equations we obtain the general gas law:

$$P \times V = R \times T$$

where R is a constant. These equations are used to correct the volume of gas collected under one set of conditions but measured under another. For example, lung volumes are reported at body temperature, but the spirometer which measures the gas is at room temperature. To correct, we may use Charles' law to multiply the volume in the spirometer (V_1) by the ratio of body temperature (T_2) to ambient temperature (T_1) (in degrees Kelvin):

$$V_2 = V_1 \times \frac{T_2}{T_1}$$

Dalton's Law of Partial Pressure

This law states that the total pressure of a volume of gas equals the sum of the *partial pressures* of each individual gas in the gas mixture. For example, room air at sea level has a pressure of 760 mmHg (about 30 in of mercury, or about 1000 cm of water), and contains 21 percent oxygen and 79 percent nitrogen (carbon dioxide and water vapor contents are negligible). To determine the partial pressure of oxygen, we multiply the concentration (frequently expressed as $F_{I_{O_2}}$) by the total pressure. Thus, the partial pressure of oxygen in room air at sea level is 760 mmHg times 21 percent, or 158 mmHg. *Tension* is another word for partial pressure.

Henry's Law

When gases are exposed to a liquid, some of the gas will dissolve in the liquid. The amount of gas that moves into the liquid depends on two factors:

the partial pressure of the gas over the liquid, and the solubility of the gas in the liquid. The solubility of the gas in the liquid is determined by the chemical composition of the particular gas and the liquid; the partial pressure may be determined by the total pressure and the concentration of the gas (Fig. 8-2).

A common example of Henry's law is demonstrated when a bottle of carbonated beverage is opened. Before the cap is removed, a relatively large quantity of carbon dioxide is dissolved in the liquid because the pressure within the bottle is high. When the cap is removed, the pressure falls to atmospheric, and dissolved gas from the liquid moves out into the atmosphere. It is this partial pressure of gas moving out of a liquid phase that is measured when one obtains a sample of blood for blood gas analysis. The results are written as Pa_{O_2} for the arterial partial pressure of oxygen, and Pa_{CO_2} for that of carbon dioxide.

Diffusion of Gases

Diffusion of gas refers to the transfer of molecules of gas from an area of high partial pressure to an area of lower partial pressure. Unlike other examples of gas movement which we have considered up to this point, there is no bulk movement of gas. Rather, there is random movement of molecules,

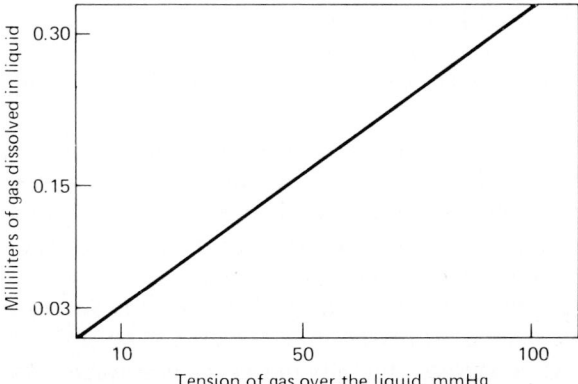

Figure 8-2   Henry's law. Henry's law states that the solubility of a gas in a liquid is proportional to the tension of the gas over the liquid. But O_2 is not very soluble in plasma, so only a small amount is dissolved in the blood. *[From Mary W. Waldron, Oxygen transport. Am. J. Nurs., 9 (2):272–275, 1979.]*

without a total pressure gradient between one area of diffusion and another. For example, if we were to open a bottle of 100 percent oxygen in room air, the total pressure inside the bottle and outside the bottle would each be 760 mmHg. However, because the partial pressure of oxygen inside the bottle (760 mmHg) is higher than the partial pressure outside the bottle (158 mmHg, or 760×0.21), the gas in the bottle diffuses out of the mouth of the bottle by random movement of the molecules. Diffusion will continue to occur until the partial pressure of oxygen inside the bottle is equal to that outside the bottle. It should be noted that there is another gradient for diffusion, namely the diffusion of nitrogen from outside the bottle to inside the bottle. Here, the relevant partial pressures are 602 mmHg outside ($760 \text{ mmHg} \times 0.79$) to 0 mmHg inside the bottle.

Quantitative aspects of diffusion are demonstrated by a modification of Fick's law:

$$\text{Diffusion} = \frac{A}{T} \times D \times (P_1 - P_2)$$

where A is the total area over which the gas diffuses, T is the thickness of the area over which the gas diffuses, P_1 and P_2 are the partial pressures of the gas on the two sides, and D is a diffusion constant which is related to the solubility and molecular weight of the gas. From simple inspection of this equation, it can be seen that increases in area, decreases in thickness, and increase in pressure difference between the two sides will all increase diffusion.

In the alveoli, fresh gas from the atmosphere mixes by diffusion with venous gas coming into the alveolus from the pulmonary capillaries. The gas then must diffuse through a pathway which includes the alveolar epithelium and basement membrane, the pulmonary interstitium, which includes collagenous and elastic fibers, and the pulmonary capillary endothelium and basement membrane; the total thickness is about 0.5 μm. Once the gas has reached the capillary, it has a very short distance to travel before reaching the red blood cell, because the diameter of the capillary is very narrow, and the red blood cell must squeeze through it in order to pass. Thus, the red cell surface is almost in contact with the pulmonary capillary wall. The final pathway of diffusion into the blood includes the distance from the periphery to the interior of the red blood cell, which is about 2.5 μm.

Under normal circumstances, the diffusion of oxygen and carbon dioxide is accomplished very rapidly. It takes only a fraction of a second for the partial pressures of oxygen and carbon dioxide to become nearly equal in the capillary and alveolus. This is important because, at rest, blood moves through the capillary at a fixed rate, and there must be sufficient time for diffusion to occur before the red blood cell leaves the pulmonary capillary. The red blood cell spends an average of 0.75 s within the pulmonary capillary, and diffusion is nearly complete by about 0.25 s. Under certain conditions, discussed below, abnormalities of the diffusion process may prevent the red blood cell from reaching equilibrium with alveolar gas by the time it leaves the capillary.

Transport of Oxygen and Carbon Dioxide in the Blood

With an understanding of the behavior of gases according to physical gas laws, we must now consider the unique property of hemoglobin in its relationship to the oxygen-carrying capacity of blood.

Hemoglobin is a molecule comprised of a ferrichrome and a globin or protein portion. Each hemoglobin molecule can bind four atoms of oxygen near its iron-containing ring. This unique property of hemoglobin allows much more oxygen to be carried in a given volume of blood than could be carried by dissolved oxygen alone. To gain an appreciation for the enormous capacity of hemoglobin to carry oxygen, we may perform some simple arithmetic estimates of the *oxygen content* of blood with and without hemoglobin.

The amount of oxygen dissolved in blood, as described by Henry's law, is a function of the partial pressure of oxygen and the solubility of oxygen. To calculate the amount of dissolved oxygen, we can multiply the factor 0.0031 by the partial pressure of oxygen in millimeters of mercury. For example, with a P_{O_2} of 100 mmHg, the amount of dissolved oxygen would equal 0.0031 × 100, or 0.3 mL of oxygen for every 100 mL of blood. This quantity of oxygen is insufficient to sustain life.

Each gram of hemoglobin, when fully saturated with oxygen, can carry 1.34 mL of oxygen. To calculate the oxygen-carrying capacity of 100 mL of

blood one needs to know how much hemoglobin is present and how saturated it is with oxygen. The concentration of hemoglobin (in grams per 100 mL) is multiplied by 1.34, and that number is multiplied by the percent saturation. For example, in someone with a hemoglobin concentration of 10 g/100 mL and fully saturated hemoglobin, the amount of oxygen carried by the hemoglobin would be equal to 1.34 × 10, or 13.4 mL of oxygen per 100 mL of blood. Clearly, the amount of oxygen carried by fully saturated hemoglobin at a P_{O_2} of 100 mmHg is over 30 times the amount carried in the dissolved form. The total amount of oxygen carried by a quantity of blood is known as the *oxygen content,* and is the sum of the dissolved and hemoglobin-bound oxygen. The factors which affect the oxygen content include the P_{O_2} in the blood, the hemoglobin concentration, and the percent saturation of hemoglobin (Hb):

$$O_2 \text{ content} = (\text{Hb in grams} \times 1.34 \times \% \text{ sat}) + (0.0031 \times P_{O_2})$$

As one might imagine, when the P_{O_2} is extremely high (above about 150 mmHg), then the hemoglobin is completely saturated with oxygen; in other words, all four binding sites on each hemoglobin molecule are occupied with an atom of oxygen. When the P_{O_2} is very low, then many of the binding sites on the hemoglobin will be unoccupied. The precise relationship between partial pressure of oxygen (P_{O_2}) and the number of binding sites occupied by oxygen atoms is described by the *oxygen-hemoglobin dissociation curve.* This is not a simple relationship, but follows a sigmoid shape as shown in Fig. 8-3.

Several aspects should be emphasized regarding the relationship between the partial pressure of oxygen and the percent saturation of hemoglobin. First, at partial pressures of oxygen above about 60 mmHg, the hemoglobin is more than 90 percent saturated with oxygen. This means that even large increases in P_{O_2} will not be able to further increase the amount of oxygen carried by hemoglobin, because all the binding sites are already occupied. The amount of dissolved oxygen, however, will increase as a function of increasing the P_{O_2} as described earlier (Fig. 8-4).

Second, once the P_{O_2} falls below 60, the amount of oxygen carried by the blood decreases significantly. For example, when the P_{O_2} falls from

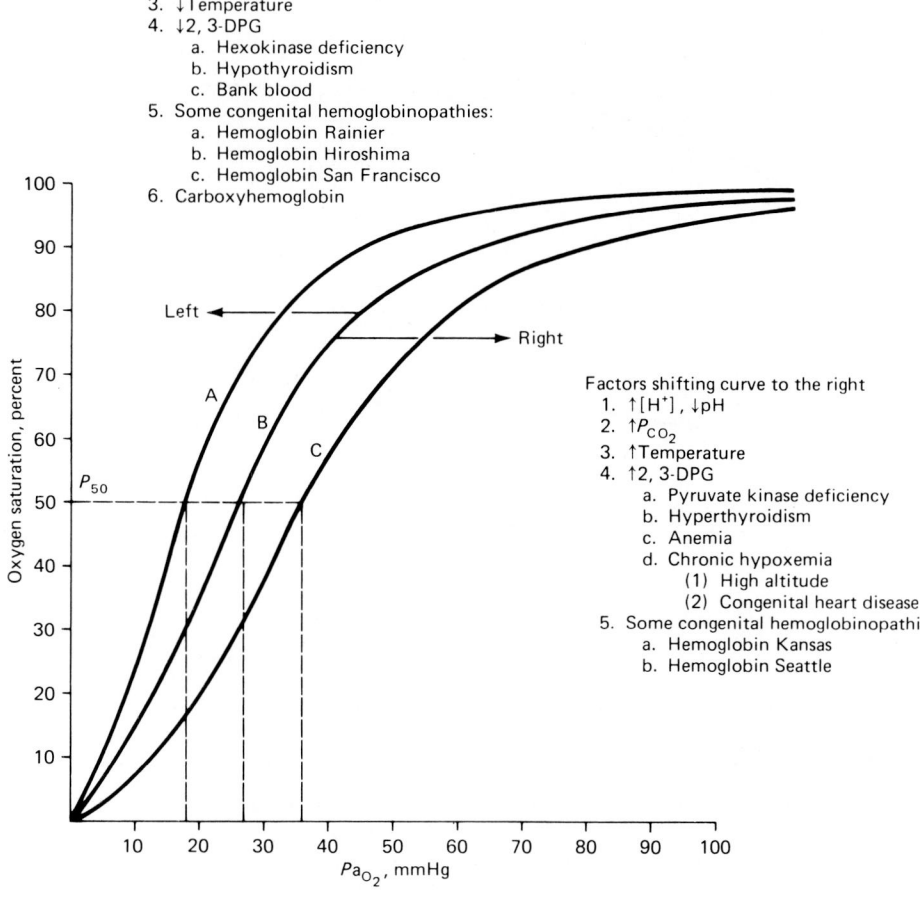

Factors shifting curve to the left
1. $\downarrow[H^+]$, $\uparrow pH$
2. $\downarrow P_{CO_2}$
3. $\downarrow$Temperature
4. $\downarrow$2, 3-DPG
   a. Hexokinase deficiency
   b. Hypothyroidism
   c. Bank blood
5. Some congenital hemoglobinopathies:
   a. Hemoglobin Rainier
   b. Hemoglobin Hiroshima
   c. Hemoglobin San Francisco
6. Carboxyhemoglobin

Factors shifting curve to the right
1. $\uparrow[H^+]$, $\downarrow pH$
2. $\uparrow P_{CO_2}$
3. $\uparrow$Temperature
4. $\uparrow$2, 3-DPG
   a. Pyruvate kinase deficiency
   b. Hyperthyroidism
   c. Anemia
   d. Chronic hypoxemia
     (1) High altitude
     (2) Congenital heart disease
5. Some congenital hemoglobinopathies:
   a. Hemoglobin Kansas
   b. Hemoglobin Seattle

Figure 8-3 Factors affecting hemoglobin's affinity for oxygen. Curve B is the standard oxyhemoglobin dissociation curve. Factors that result in a shifting of this curve either to the left or to the right are represented by curves A and C, respectively.

60 mmHg to 40 mmHg, the saturation of hemoglobin may fall from 90 percent to 75 percent. By substituting into the equation for oxygen content above, one can see that this represents a decrease in oxygen content of about 15 percent.

Third, the relationship between P_{O_2} and hemoglobin saturation is not absolute, and may be affected by several common clinical conditions. Factors which are said to decrease the affinity of hemoglobin for oxygen (shift the hemoglobin-oxygen dissociation curve to the right) include fever, acidosis, elevated P_{CO_2}, and elevated 2,3-diphosphoglycerate (2,3-DPG). Factors which tend to increase the affinity of hemoglobin for oxygen (shift the hemoglobin-oxygen dissociation curve to the left) include hypothermia, alkalosis, low P_{CO_2}, and decreased 2,3-DPG.

Carbon dioxide is transported differently from oxygen in the blood. It may be found in three forms: in the form of *bicarbonate,* in a *dissolved* form, and in *combination with proteins.* Dissolved carbon dioxide behaves very much like dissolved oxygen, except that carbon dioxide is 20 times more soluble in blood than is oxygen. As a result, almost 10 percent of the entire carbon dioxide content in the blood is carried in the dissolved form.

Bicarbonate is formed by the combination of carbon dioxide with water to form carbonic acid, H_2CO_3. In plasma, carbon dioxide and water combine very slowly, but in the red blood cell the presence of the enzyme *carbonic anhydrase* speeds the reaction considerably (Fig. 8-5). Carbonic acid then dissociates to hydrogen ion, H^+, and bicar-

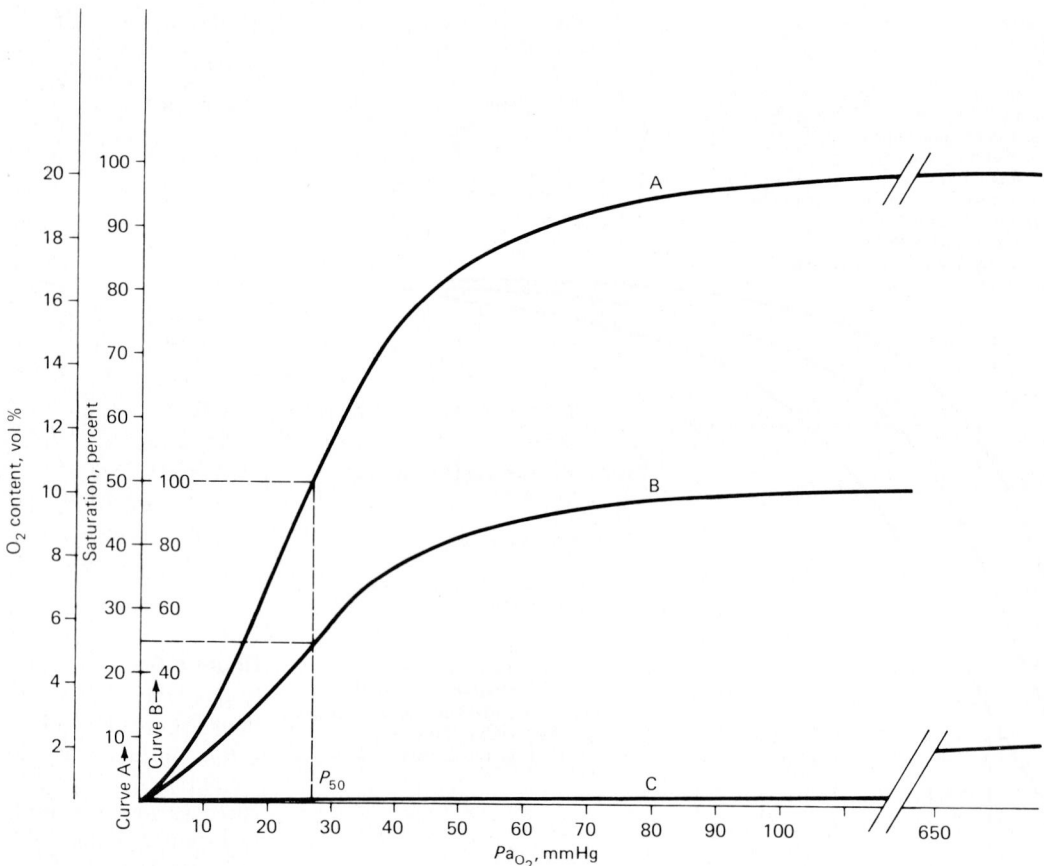

Figure 8-4   The oxyhemoglobin dissociation curve. Curve A shows the standard oxyhemoglobin dissociation curve formed when hemoglobin is exposed to air containing increasing amounts of oxygen. Plotted on the ordinate are both percent saturation of hemoglobin and hemoglobin oxygen content (15 g Hb per 100 mL of blood). The abscissa is the PaO$_2$ value. Curve B is a similar plot for a patient with anemia (7.5 g Hb per 100 mL of blood). Notice how the sigmoid shape, percent saturation, and the P_{50} value are unchanged; but the maximum oxygen content is one-half of the normal situation. Line C represents the dissolved oxygen. Note that oxygen content increases linearly with increasing oxygen tensions, but that the total amount is very small compared with the oxygen carried by hemoglobin.

bonate ion, HCO_3^-. Because of the permeability characteristics of the cell membrane, HCO_3 may diffuse out but H^+ remains within the cell. To maintain electrical neutrality, chloride diffuses into the cell from the plasma. Some of the hydrogen ion produced from the dissociation of carbonic acid combines with reduced hemoglobin; oxygenated hemoglobin is less able to combine with hydrogen ion. This increased ability of deoxygenated blood to help with CO_2 transport is known as the Haldane effect.

Carbon dioxide may combine with proteins to form carbamino compounds. The most important protein which combines with carbon dioxide is hemoglobin. Of note, unoxygenated hemoglobin is capable of binding more carbon dioxide than is fully saturated hemoglobin. Thus, consumption of oxygen in the periphery and unloading of oxygen atoms from the hemoglobin molecule increase the ability of hemoglobin to combine with carbon dioxide for removal to the lungs.

In arterial blood, 90 percent of the total carbon dioxide content is carried in the form of bicarbonate. Only about 5 percent is carried in the form of carbamino compounds and another 5 percent as dissolved CO_2.

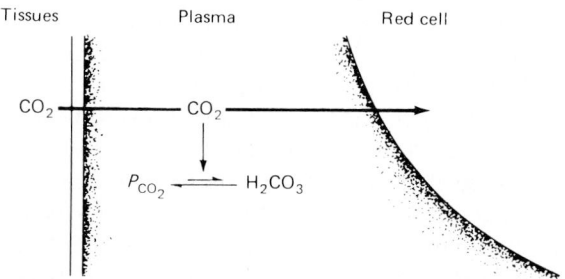

Figure 8-5   Carbon dioxide–carbonic acid relationship in plasma; 5 percent of the CO_2 entering the blood remains in plasma. Most of this exists as dissolved CO_2 since the chemical reaction $H_2O + CO_2 \rightarrow H_2CO_3$ is very slow; therefore, measuring P_{CO_2} is equivalent to measuring H_2CO_3 concentration. *(From Barry Shapiro, Clinical application of blood gases. Chicago: Yearbook, 1979.)*

You will recall that the relationship between oxygen content (expressed as hemoglobin saturation) and the partial pressure of oxygen was described by the sigmoid relationship of the oxygen hemoglobin dissociation curve. In a similar manner, we can portray the relationship between carbon dioxide content and partial pressure of CO_2 by utilizing the CO_2 content curve. Unlike the sigmoid hemoglobin-oxygen dissociation curve, the CO_2 content curve is linear over the entire physiologic range. What this means is that increases in partial pressure of CO_2 will increase the total CO_2 content. This is not the case with oxygen content, where increasing P_{O_2} above 60 mmHg has little effect on increasing the content of oxygen.

The normal mixed venous P_{CO_2} is about 45 mmHg, in contrast to the normal arterial P_{CO_2} of 40 mmHg. The increased carbon dioxide which results from cellular metabolism is returned to the lungs in mixed venous blood, where it is removed by alveolar ventilation. Approximately 10,000 meq of carbonic acid are excreted every day through the lungs.

Oxygen Delivery

Even a very high oxygen content will be of no help to the patient if sufficient delivery of that oxygen to the tissues is not accomplished. Of course, the way in which oxygen is transported is through the

systemic circulation. *Oxygen delivery* may be calculated according to the following equation:

$$O_2 \text{ delivery} = O_2 \text{ content} \times \text{cardiac output}$$

From inspection of this equation, we can see that oxygen delivery may be increased either by increasing the oxygen content or by increasing the blood flow, or both. Conversely, it should be recognized that oxygen delivery may be severely compromised by an inadequate cardiac output, even though the O_2 content may be completely normal.

When cardiac output falls, as in cardiogenic shock, several internal regulatory mechanisms are called into play to protect vulnerable organs, including regulation of the distribution of blood flow. In shock states, blood flow to less vital areas such as the skin and gut is decreased to maintain blood flow to more vital structures such as the brain and heart.

Oxygen Consumption

Teleologically, the major purpose of the respiratory and cardiovascular systems is the transport of gases to and from the atmosphere and tissues for energy production. As oxygenated blood moves through the arterial tree, it does so in arteries and arterioles of successively decreasing caliber, finally entering the systemic capillaries which supply oxygenated blood to the tissues. The various tissues and organs of the body may differ very widely in their demands for oxygen (Table 8-1). For example, the heart and brain require high amounts of oxygen for normal functioning, whereas the kidney and skin require very little. To some degree, this is accounted for

Table 8-1   Oxygen Extraction by Various Organs and Their Characteristic Venous Oxygen Tensions

Organ	Arteriovenous Oxygen Content Differences, vol %	$P\bar{V}_{O_2}$, mmHg
Heart	11.4	23
Muscle	8.4	34
Brain	6.3	33
Splanchnic	4.1	43
Kidney	1.3	56
Skin	1.0	60

Adapted from C. A. Finch and C. Lenfant, Oxygen transport in man. *N. Engl. J. Med.*, 1972, 286, 407.

by internal regulation of blood flow to specific areas as their needs for oxygen dictate. However, regional differences in blood flow do not entirely meet the demands of individual organs. Thus, some tissues extract more oxygen over a period of time than do others since they require more oxygen.

If oxygen is delivered to a tissue at a certain rate (oxygen delivery), and oxygen is extracted from the blood supply at a constant rate (oxygen consumption), then by simple arithmetic a certain amount of oxygen will remain in the venous blood. This relationship may be expressed by the Fick equation:

O_2 consumption

  = O_2 delivered − O_2 remaining

  = cardiac output × arterial O_2 content

  − cardiac output × venous O_2 content

The two commonly performed measurements of oxygen in the venous blood are the mixed venous oxygen saturation and the mixed venous P_{O_2}. Unfortunately, we are unable to measure the individual oxygen consumption of different tissues; this would require a sampling of venous blood draining each of the tissues in which we were interested. However, we may measure the venous oxygen tension of the entire patient.

The measurement of mixed venous P_{O_2}, or mixed venous oxygen saturation, is commonly performed by placing a catheter in the pulmonary artery. Since the blood in the pulmonary artery is a mixture of the venous blood draining all the tissues, it is an indication of the overall state of oxygen extraction of the patient. The mixed venous P_{O_2} thus reflects the balance between overall oxygen delivery and oxygen extraction. Areas or organs that have relatively greater proportion of delivery, or relatively greater oxygen extraction, will contribute a greater portion to the mixed venous P_{O_2}.

In general, a mixed venous P_{O_2} of 40 mmHg is normal, and values less than 40 may be due to a limited number of factors. We may rewrite the Fick equation to better examine those factors that influence the mixed venous O_2 content (or mixed venous P_{O_2}):

Mixed venous O_2 content

$$= \text{arterial } O_2 \text{ content} - \frac{O_2 \text{ consumption}}{\text{Cardiac output}}$$

First, the overall oxygen consumption may be increased. This is seen during generalized hypermetabolic states such as hyperthyroidism, fever, seizures, trauma, etc. Second, a low mixed venous P_{O_2} may result from inadequate arterial oxygen content, such as during hypoxia from a variety of causes, anemia, or shift in the hemoglobin-oxygen saturation curve. Third, low mixed venous O_2 may occur from decreased cardiac output. This is because less O_2 is delivered over a period of time when the cardiac output is low, so that less O_2 will remain in the venous blood if O_2 consumption does not change.

Cellular Respiration

One of the most important aspects of respiration is also one of the most poorly understood, in part because of its inaccessibility: the uptake of oxygen by tissues and cells. The final pathway for oxygen is the diffusion out of the capillary into the tissues, cells, and organelles. Estimates of the P_{O_2} necessary to maintain cellular energy stores within mitochondria are as low as 1 mmHg!

Although the basic processes which govern diffusion of oxygen into and diffusion of carbon dioxide out of tissues are no different from those described above, we are somewhat hampered in our further understanding by our inability to measure tissue or cellular P_{O_2}. Factors which may influence the diffusion of oxygen from capillaries into the tissues include the density of capillaries in a given tissue, the blood flow through the capillaries, and the oxygen extraction by the tissues. It may be that these are the various factors which are most disturbed in clinical examples of sepsis, shock, and ischemia. Unfortunately, it is at the tissue and cellular level that we are least successful in our therapy. Thus, most therapeutic efforts are aimed at increasing total oxygen delivery either through increasing cardiac output or oxygen content.

Blood Gas Analysis

When a sample of blood is sent to the laboratory for blood gas analysis, the partial pressures of oxygen and carbon dioxide are measured by exposing the sample to oxygen and CO_2 electrodes. Actually, the electrode is separated by a thin membrane from the blood itself, so that the oxygen diffuses from the blood into the solution surrounding the electrode. The amount of current passed across the electrode is proportional to the P_{O_2}.

Carbon dioxide tension is measured somewhat differently. The CO_2 electrode is in reality a pH electrode which is surrounded by a bicarbonate buffer separated from the blood. As CO_2 diffuses from the blood into the buffer around the electrode, the pH of the buffer changes. This is measured by the electrode and the results are reported as P_{CO_2}.

It is important to remember that blood gas analysis can tell us only the partial pressures of the gases within the blood sample, and may not reflect the oxygen content. You will remember that oxygen content is a function not only of the partial pressure of oxygen, but of the hemoglobin concentration and the affinity of that hemoglobin for oxygen as well (saturation).

Normal oxygen tensions are dependent upon the age of the patient. In general, normal oxygen tensions are between 80 and 100 mmHg; normal P_{CO_2} lies between 35 and 45 mmHg. Normal pH values range from 7.35 to 7.45. When submitting a sample of blood for blood gas analysis, it is important also to record the patient's temperature. You will recall that an increase in temperature will shift the hemoglobin dissociation curve to the right, while a decrease may shift it to the left. Calculations of hemoglobin saturation are available on most blood gas machines, and take into account the normal position of the oxygen-hemoglobin dissociation curve, with subsequent corrections for the patient's temperature, pH, and P_{CO_2}.

Mixed venous blood is often sent for blood gas analysis as well. Normal mixed venous blood has a P_{O_2} of about 40 mmHg, and a P_{CO_2} of 45 mmHg.

Abnormalities of Gas Exchange

The process of normal gas exchange depends on the coordination and interaction of many factors, as can be appreciated from the foregoing sections. In this section, we will examine in detail abnormalities of gas exchange. These will include problems in oxygenation and problems with carbon dioxide.

It is important to clarify certain terms. *Hypoxia* is the condition of insufficient oxygen availability for normal function of the patient. *Hypoxemia* may be defined as an abnormally low partial pressure of oxygen. *Ischemia* refers to inadequate oxygenation because of insufficient flow of oxygen-containing blood to a local area; when blood flow is inadequate for the entire patient, this is sometimes referred to as circulatory hypoxia. *Hypercarbia* refers to elevated partial pressure of carbon dioxide.

Hypoxia

Before explaining each type of hypoxia in more detail, it is important to make some remarks about hypoxia in general.

The body's oxygen stores are small, and everyone is dependent upon a continuing and virtually uninterrupted supply of oxygen, since only about a 5-min supply exists. The organs, however, vary as to their susceptibility to sustained hypoxia, with the brain being one of the most sensitive structures. As mentioned previously, tissue oxygen tensions cannot be measured directly, and therefore indirect methods of assessing the state of tissue oxygenation must be used. In the absence of an adequate mitochondrial oxygen supply, metabolic activity through the usual aerobic pathway ceases, and the less efficient anaerobic pathway is utilized. This pathway produces lactic acid as a metabolic end product and yields a metabolic acidosis that can be identified by a large anion gap and an elevated blood lactate level. Therefore, lactic acidosis is presumptive evidence of tissue hypoxia. Table 8-2 shows some of the parameters commonly evaluated in the assessment of tissue hypoxia.

Hypoxemic Hypoxia

Hypoxemic hypoxia is, in essence, inadequate tissue oxygenation (hypoxia) that is caused by a decreased arterial blood oxygen tension (hypoxemia). The decreased Pa_{O_2} may come from one or more of the abnormalities in the process of respiration, and is one of the most common causes of tissue hypoxia encountered in clinical practice. A detailed discussion is presented in the next section.

Anemic Hypoxia

Anemic hypoxia is deficient tissue oxygenation resulting from a decrease in arterial blood oxygen

Table 8-2 Assessment of Tissue Hypoxia

1. Evidence of anaerobic metabolism:
   Lactic acidosis
2. Evidence of altered perfusion:
   Tachycardia
   Hypotension
   Changes in skin color and temperature
   Changes in capillary filling
3. Evidence of organ dysfunction:
   Brain: altered sensorium
   Myocardial: low cardiac output
   Renal: decreased urine output
4. Assessment of oxygen delivery:
   Pa_{O_2}
   Hemoglobin concentration
   Arterial blood oxygen content
   Oxyhemoglobin dissociation curve
   Cardiac output
   Regional blood flow characteristics
5. Invasive parameters:
   Mixed venous oxygen tension ($P\bar{V}_{O_2}$)
   Arteriovenous oxygen content difference

content. This deficiency may result either from a decrease in the amount of hemoglobin present (i.e., anemia) or from a decrease in the ability of hemoglobin to hold oxygen (e.g., carboxyhemoglobin, methemoglobin). Recall this equation:

$$\text{Oxygen content} = \text{oxygen combined with Hb} + \text{oxygen dissolved in plasma}$$

$$\text{Oxygen content} = (\text{hemoglobin} \times 1.34 \times \text{(vol \%)} \% \text{ saturation}) + (Pa_{O_2} \times 0.003)$$

As previously discussed, the amount of oxygen dissolved in the blood is small, owing to the low solubility of oxygen (solubility coefficient = 0.003 vol %/mmHg). Even with a patient breathing 100% oxygen (which at sea level would produce a maximum Pa_{O_2} of 650 mmHg), the total contribution from dissolved oxygen is less than 2 vol % (i.e., 650 × 0.003).

Hemoglobin, on the other hand, is responsible for the majority of the oxygen carried by the blood. The oxygen-carrying capacity of 15 g of hemoglobin is 20.1 mL. This value must be multiplied by the hemoglobin saturation to get the actual amount of oxygen combined with hemoglobin.

In Table 8-3, notice that the total oxygen content of the blood in a normal person with a hemoglobin concentration of 15 g/100 mL (and a saturation of 97.5 percent) equals 19.9 vol %, of which 19.6 vol % is oxygen carried by hemoglobin and only 0.3 vol % is dissolved oxygen.

In the anemic patient (with a hemoglobin concentration of 7.5 g/100 mL), the oxygen content is decreased to 10.1 vol %, of which 9.8 vol % is oxygen combined with hemoglobin. If the anemia is severe enough to result in an inadequate supply of oxygen to the tissues (relative to oxygen demand), then anemic hypoxia results. In clinical practice this seldom occurs, since the body will respond to a severe anemia by increasing the cardiac output, thereby increasing tissue oxygen delivery per unit of time. If this is still not adequate to meet the oxygen demand, then "high output failure" supervenes. It is therefore more common to see anemia contributing to overall hypoxia, as in a setting that combines anemia with hypoxemia, low arterial saturation, and a low cardiac output from congestive heart failure.

Table 8-3 Calculation of Oxygen Content

| Patient | Measured Values | | | Calculated Values (vol %) | | | |
	Hb, g/100 mL	Pa_{O_2} mmHg	O_2 Saturation, %	O_2 Capacity of HB*	O_2 Combined with Hb†	Dissolved O_2‡	Total O_2 Content§
Normal	15.0	100	97.5	20.10	19.6	0.30	19.9
Anemia	7.5	100	97.5	10.05	9.80	0.30	10.1
Hypoxemia	15.0	50	83.5	20.10	16.79	0.15	16.94

* Step 1: Oxygen capacity of Hb (vol %) = Hb (g/100 mL) × (1.34 mL O_2/g Hb).
† Step 2: Oxygen combined with Hb (vol %) = Hb (g/100 mL) × 1.34 (mL O_2/g Hb) × saturation (%).
‡ Step 3: Oxygen dissovled in plasma (vol %) = Pa_{O_2} (mmHg) × 0.003 (vol %/mmHg).
§ Step 4: Total oxygen content (vol %) = Step 2 + Step 3.

Carbon Monoxide   Another type of "anemic" hypoxia results from the inactivation of hemoglobin by carbon monoxide. Carbon monoxide and oxygen bind to hemoglobin at exactly the same site; the two molecules are, in effect, in competition for these hemoglobin-binding sites. However, since carbon monoxide has a much stronger affinity for hemoglobin (some 210 times stronger), it is bound more avidly and held tighter. To use the magnet analogy, hemoglobin is not only an oxygen magnet but a carbon monoxide magnet as well. In fact, it is a much stronger carbon monoxide magnet, and if given a choice between the two molecules, it will combine with carbon monoxide every time. In this way, carbon monoxide produces a "functional" anemia, since it occupies potential oxygen-binding sites. It is convenient to discuss carbon monoxide's effect on hemoglobin as the equivalent reduction in the amount of hemoglobin that is available to combine with oxygen. Therefore, a carboxyhemoglobin level of 10 percent means there is 10 percent less hemoglobin available to combine with oxygen.

While the ambient levels of carbon monoxide are usually quite low, tobacco smokers and people in some urban environments may develop high levels of carbon monoxide in the blood. For example, heavy cigarette smokers may achieve carboxyhemoglobin levels as high as 15 percent; and cases of carbon monoxide poisoning (accidental or otherwise) attain levels that are much higher.

The danger level of carbon monoxide in the blood depends to a certain extent on the individual. A normal person may tolerate levels as high as 40 percent with only a headache, nausea, and vomiting; but above 50 percent, seizures and coma appear. The lethal level of carbon monoxide is usually between 67 and 70 percent. However, a patient with severely compromised cardiac function could experience more difficulty with lower levels of carbon monoxide in the blood; a 20 percent carboxyhemoglobin level may prove fatal. In each case, tissue hypoxia resulting from a decreased oxygen content of the blood is the mechanism whereby carbon monoxide produces its ill effects.

Circulatory Hypoxia

Circulatory hypoxia is an example of deficient tissue oxygenation that results from a decrease in blood supply. As noted earlier, oxygen delivery is a function of both oxygen content and blood flow. Blood flow may be generally decreased (i.e., decreased cardiac output), or it may be deficient in one region. Examples of the latter include local obstructions to arterial blood flow, as in peripheral arterial lesions from advanced arteriosclerotic disease or from direct arteriovenous connections that bypass the systemic capillary bed, and therefore result in a decrease in tissue capillary blood flow. Note that circulatory hypoxia is strictly a cardiovascular phenomenon and need not be accompanied by arterial hypoxemia or a decrease in blood oxygen content.

Lowered cardiac output is perhaps the most common cause of tissue hypoxia, and may be due to numerous conditions. Therapy is aimed at the underlying cause and the cardiac hemodynamics. Oxygen therapy would be expected to have only minimal benefit if the arterial blood oxygen content were otherwise normal, since the problem is in the delivery of that oxygen.

The effect of regional blood flow abnormalities depends upon the severity of the ischemia and the particular vascular bed involved. In this way, a decrease in blood flow to a small portion of the brain (as may result from an intracerebral thrombosis or hemorrhage) may lead to severe consequences, and similarly from a relatively small vascular thrombosis in a major coronary artery. Prolonged hypoxia in these circumstances may lead to actual cell death and necrosis (infarction).

Finally, various types of direct arteriovenous (A-V) communications may occur and lead to tissue hypoxia by diverting blood away from the capillary bed. Examples include deliberate production of A-V fistulas in patients with renal disease undergoing hemodialysis; patients with cirrhosis of the liver who have abnormal A-V communications in the skin and viscera (including the lung); fistulas that form as a result of trauma or infections; and rare inherited or congenital lesions as in the Osler-Weber-Rendu syndrome. This type of regional blood flow abnormality only rarely results in clinically significant tissue hypoxia.

Hypoxia from Increased Hemoglobin Affinity for Oxygen

Tissue hypoxia may occur despite a normal Pa_{O_2}, adequate arterial oxygen content, adequate cardiac output, and sufficient local vascular perfusion. In this instance, enough oxygen is delivered to the tissues; but because of an increase in hemoglobin's affinity for oxygen, the O_2 is more tightly bound and therefore released more reluctantly in the tissues. This was previously described as a shift to the left in the oxyhemoglobin dissociation curve, and Fig. 8-3 lists some of the possible causes. It is noted that while the basic mechanism is a decrease in oxygen delivery to the tissues, there are fundamental differences that allow for a clear separation between this phenomenon and the other causes of decreased oxygen delivery: hypoxemic hypoxia, anemic hypoxia, and circulatory hypoxia.

Clinically, this mechanism should be kept in mind when dealing with patients who have undergone massive transfusions with old bank blood [with depleted supplies of 2,3-diphosphoglycerate (2,3-DPG)]. Various congenital hemoglobinopathies may result in a left-shifted oxyhemoglobin dissociation curve, but these are not compatible with life if they lead to significant tissue hypoxia.

Histotoxic Hypoxia

Histotoxic hypoxia refers to hypoxia that occurs as a result of the inability of the tissues to utilize oxygen. As in the case of hypoxia from increased hemoglobin affinity for oxygen, the parameters of tissue oxygen delivery are all normal; the abnormality is in oxygen utilization. The classic example of this type of hypoxia is cyanide poisoning. Detailed investigations of these patients will reveal a decrease in oxygen consumption, an increased mixed venous oxygen tension, and a decreased arteriovenous oxygen content difference.

Table 8-4 is a quantitative comparison between the four classic types of hypoxia. The values presented are only approximate and are rounded off for illustrative purposes. In the normal situation, note the parameters of oxygen delivery (arterial blood oxygen capacity, saturation, content, and tension; and cardiac output) and oxygen utilization (oxygen consumption; mixed venous blood, oxygen saturation, content, and tension; and arteriovenous oxygen content difference). In hypoxemic hypoxia, the *primary abnormality* is a decreased Pa_{O_2} which results in a decreased hemoglobin saturation and O_2 content; but O_2 capacity and O_2 consumption are normal. Cardiac output is increased to assure adequate oxygen delivery. Values in venous blood are decreased in proportion to the arterial hypoxemia, and the A-V oxygen content difference is near normal. In anemic hypoxia, the primary abnormality is a decrease in O_2 capacity, with a normal Pa_{O_2}. Note the compensatory increase in cardiac output (which is necessary if O_2 delivery is to remain normal in the face of a decreased arterial blood O_2 content). Circulatory hypoxia, in the example shown, has a decrease in cardiac output as the primary abnormality responsible for the hypoxia. Note that the arterial blood values are all normal, but the mixed venous blood reflects the effects of increased oxygen extraction and the A-V oxygen content difference is widened. Finally, histotoxic hypoxia has as its primary insult a decreased oxygen consumption. Therefore, starting with normal arterial blood parameters, the mixed venous blood reflects this lack of oxygen extraction, and the A-V oxygen content difference is narrowed.

Table 8-4 A Quantitative Comparison between the Four Classic Types of Hypoxia

	Arterial				Venous			A–V O_2 Content, Difference, vol %	O_2 Consumption, cm³/min	Cardiac Output, L/min
	O_2 Capacity, vol %	Hb Saturation, %	O_2 Content, vol %	Pa_{O_2}, mmHg	Hb Saturation, %	O_2 Content, vol %	$P\bar{V}_{O_2}$, mmHg			
Normal	20	95	19	100	70	14	40	5	250	5.0
Hypoxemic hypoxia	20	75	15	*50*	55	11	30	4	250	7.0
Anemic hypoxia	*10*	95	9.5	100	65	6.5	35	3	250	9.3
Circulatory hypoxia	20		19	100	50	10	27	9	225	*2.5*
Histotoxic hypoxia	20	95	19	100	85	17	60	2	*150*	7.5

Hypoxemia

The Oxygen Cascade

The concept of the oxygen cascade is helpful in differentiating many of the causes of hypoxemia. It is referred to as a *cascade*, because at each successive step along the pathway of movement of oxygen from atmosphere to the blood, the P_{O_2} falls in steps (Fig. 8-6). To begin, we may calculate the partial pressure of oxygen in room air according to Dalton's Law:

$$(P_{B_{O_2}}) = Pb \text{ (barometric pressure)} \times F_{I_{O_2}}$$

where $F_{I_{O_2}}$ is equal to the fraction of inspired

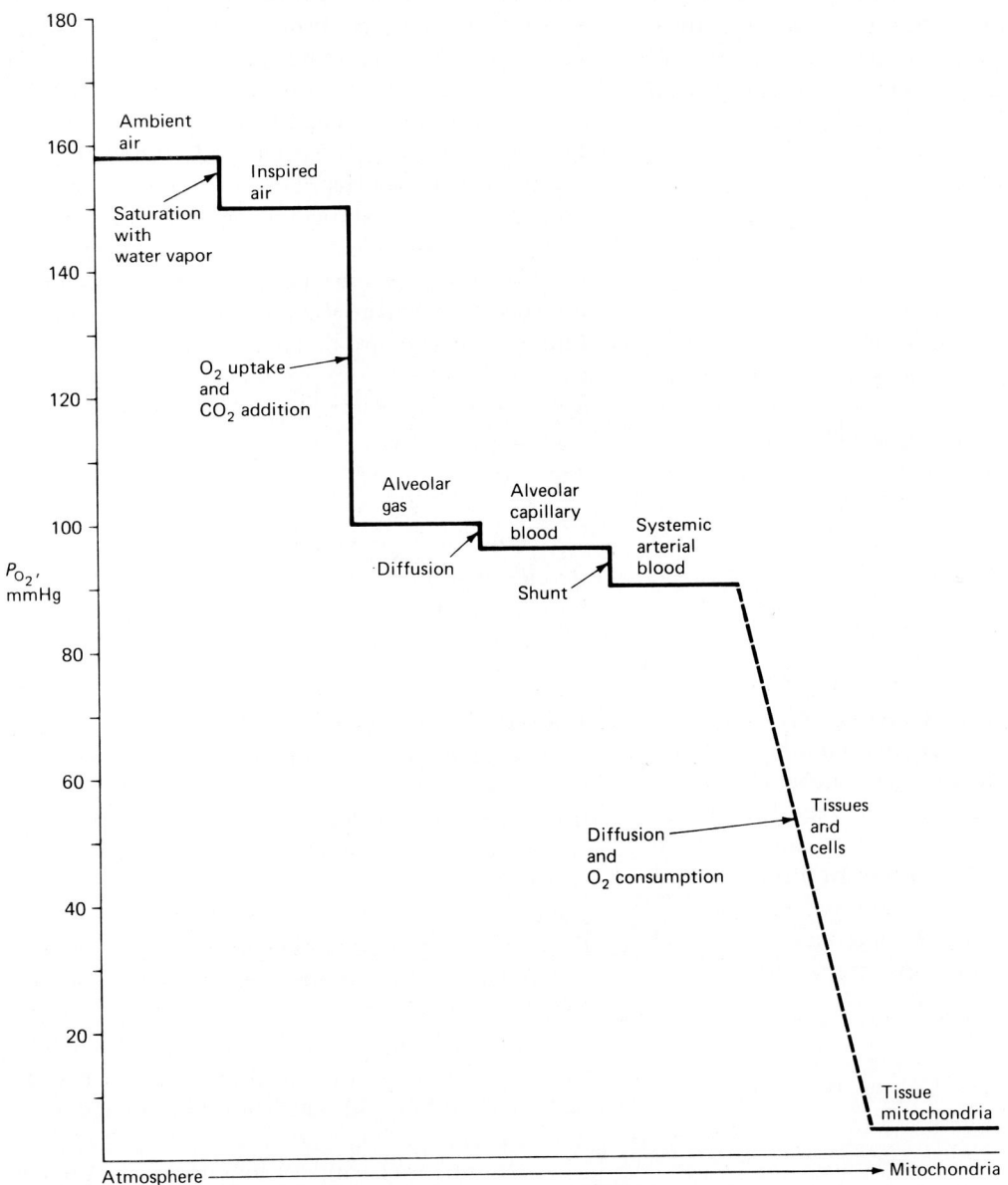

Figure 8-6   The oxygen cascade—a stepwise change in oxygen tension occurs as oxygen moves from the atmosphere to the mitochondria. See text for explanation. (*Adapted from J. B. West, Respiratory physiology. Baltimore: Williams & Wilkins, 1974.*)

oxygen, and $P_{B_{O_2}}$ is the partial pressure of oxygen in the atmosphere. Substituting normal values:

$$P_{B_{O_2}} = 760 \times 0.21$$

$$= 158\ mmHg$$

When room air enters the airway, it is humidified with water vapor. This gas has a partial pressure of 47 mmHg at body temperature. Since we must now account for this additional gas added to the total mixture at barometric pressure, we must subtract this value from barometric pressure and recalculate our partial pressure of oxygen within the airway:

$$P_{O_2} = (760 - 47) \times 0.21$$

$$P_{O_2} = 713 \times 0.21$$

$$P_{O_2} = 150\ mmHg$$

As saturated air moves into the alveolus, it encounters an additional gas: carbon dioxide, which is produced by the body and added to alveolar air. Thus, our first approximation of alveolar P_{O_2} ($P_{A_{O_2}}$) can be represented by:

$$P_{A_{O_2}} = P_{i_{O_2}} - P_{A_{CO_2}}$$

$$P_{A_{O_2}} = 150 - 40$$

$$P_{A_{O_2}} = 110\ mmHg$$

This equation is not entirely accurate because oxygen and carbon dioxide pressures are not static in the alveolus. Instead, oxygen is continually being taken up by the capillaries and carbon dioxide is continually being delivered into the alveolar air. For this reason, we include a factor known as the respiratory quotient, R, to correct for this decreased pressure of oxygen and increased pressure of CO_2. This is practically done by assuming a normal respiratory quotient of 0.8 for average conditions:

$$P_{A_{O_2}} = P_{i_{O_2}} - \frac{P_{A_{CO_2}}}{R}$$

$$= 150 - \frac{40}{0.8}$$

$$= 150 - 50$$

$$= 100\ mmHg$$

This is a simplified form of the *alveolar air equation*. Note that at a constant $P_{i_{O_2}}$, increases in carbon dioxide tension would lower the $P_{A_{O_2}}$: decreases in carbon dioxide tension will increase the $P_{A_{O_2}}$. This reciprocal relationship will be discussed in a subsequent section under causes of hypoxemia.

Once we know the tension of oxygen within the alveolus, we may next want to consider the tension of oxygen in pulmonary arterial blood. The concept of the *alveolar-arterial O_2 difference* has frequently been employed to describe the imperfect transfer of gas from alveolus to artery. Although several factors may impede perfect equilibration between the alveolar oxygen and arterial oxygen, the most common one is ventilation-perfusion inequality. In normal people breathing room air, about 10 mmHg is lost in transferring oxygen from the alveolus to the artery. Thus, we can write an equation to calculate the arterial P_{O_2} ($P_{a_{O_2}}$), taking into account the alveolar-arterial O_2 difference:

$$P_{a_{O_2}} = P_{A_{O_2}} - (\text{A-a})O_2\ \text{difference}$$

$$= 100 - 10$$

$$= 90\ mmHg$$

From inspection of this equation, one can deduce that an increase in the (A-a)O_2 difference will lead to a decrease in arterial P_{O_2}, but P_{CO_2} and inspired oxygen may be completely normal.

Adequacy of Oxygenation

Even though a young person may have a predicted P_{O_2} of 90 mmHg, a measured P_{O_2} of 80 mmHg may not reflect any serious underlying disorder (of course, even a mildly abnormal test may indicate subclinical disease and may need to be investigated). In terms of actual oxygenation, however, there is little difference between a P_{O_2} of 80 and 90 mmHg. This is because, as you will recall, the oxygen content is not very different in blood that has a P_{O_2} of 80 from that with a P_{O_2} of 90 mmHg, since the amount of dissolved oxygen is nearly the same and because the saturation of hemoglobin is not different.

On the other hand, even a normal or greater than normal P_{O_2} may be present in light of severely impaired oxygenation. This is because, once again, the oxygen delivery must be considered. For example, in a severely anemic patient, the P_{O_2} may be normal, but because there may be only half the hemoglobin normally available, there will only be half the oxygen content normally available. Similarly, a patient with severe cardiac failure may have a normal hemoglobin and a normal P_{O_2}, but a marked reduction in oxygen delivery because of the low cardiac output. In this situation, oxygenation of the tissues could be severely impaired even though oxygen content is normal.

Thus, the question of adequate oxygenation needs to be answered in light of adequate oxygen supply to meet the body's demands. Assessing the adequacy of oxygen supply remains a pressing problem in critical-care medicine. The best overall method to judge the adequacy of oxygen delivery is to observe the function of the various organ systems (Table 8-2).

Abnormal mentation, confusion, sleepiness, hallucinations, and other signs of CNS dysfunction may result from inadequate oxygen delivery to the brain. The brain is very intolerant of hypoxia, and may sustain irreversible neuronal damage within minutes of interruption of oxygen supply. Evidence of inadequate oxygen supply to the heart is suggested by angina pectoris, congestive heart failure, papillary muscle dysfunction, and arrhythmias or even myocardial infarction. Abnormal oxygen delivery to the skin can be seen in livedo reticularis, a condition in which the skin is mottled with a blue or purple discoloration from ischemia. The liver may show evidence of insufficient oxygenation in a variety of ways, the most serious of which is the picture of "shock liver," in which serum transaminases are markedly elevated; global liver dysfunction may be present with elevated bilirubin, alkaline phosphatase, and depressed synthetic function demonstrated by prolonged partial thromboplastin and prothrombin times, and decreased serum albumin. The mesenteric circulation may be impaired during severe hypoxia or ischemia, resulting in abdominal pain or bowel infarction. Renal and endocrine manifestations of hypoxia include decreased glomerular filtration rate and increased secretion of antidiuretic hormone and hyponatremia.

In the critically ill patient, additional methods are employed to assess overall oxygenation. One of these is the measurement of the serum lactate.

Under hypoxic conditions, cellular metabolism results in an accumulation of lactic acid, which is then released into the blood. One example of lactate accumulation which does not indicate disease is severe exercise. During exercise to near exhaustion, blood flow to the working muscles is insufficient to keep up with energy production, so that the muscle turns to anaerobic metabolism and lactate production to meet its energy needs; this is an example of local ischemia resulting in lactate production. When oxygen delivery to the entire patient is depressed, lactate may accumulate and be measured in the blood. Lactate levels greater than approximately 2 mmol per liter suggest inadequate oxygen delivery, and lactate levels greater than 20 mmol per liter may imply poor chance of recovery.

The mixed venous P_{O_2} is also used as an indicator of adequate oxygen delivery. A normal person will consume 250 mL of oxygen per minute, corresponding to a difference between arterial and venous oxygen contents of 5 mL of oxygen per 100 mL of blood. If the oxygen demand remains constant and oxygen consumption does not change, then a decrease in oxygen delivery will result in a decreased venous content. Normal mixed venous P_{O_2} is about 40 mmHg, corresponding to a saturation of approximately 75 percent. A mixed venous P_{O_2} of 30 to 40 mmHg suggests inadequate oxygen delivery, and a mixed venous P_{O_2} below 30 mmHg suggests severe depression in oxygen delivery.

It should be emphasized that although it is a laudable goal to maximize oxygen delivery, we still have much to learn about the interpretation of mixed venous P_{O_2} and the relationship between oxygen delivery and oxygen consumption. For example, it has been suggested that in septic shock, tissue extraction of oxygen might be impaired; since less oxygen is extracted by tissues, the mixed venous P_{O_2} will be increased. In this situation, the mixed venous P_{O_2} may be a better indicator of oxygen utilization than oxygen delivery. Additionally, some investigators have suggested that in diseases such as adult respiratory distress syndrome (ARDS), oxygen consumption may increase as oxygen delivery is increased; this makes interpretation of the mixed venous P_{O_2} more difficult. At the present time, it is this author's belief that the mixed venous P_{O_2} may serve as a useful adjunct to other clinical estimates of adequacy of oxygenation.

Mechanisms of Hypoxemia

Aerohypoxia   Aerohypoxia may be defined as a low arterial P_{O_2} which results from a decreased partial pressure of oxygen in the inspired gas mixture. This situation is most frequently encountered during travel to high altitude, since barometric pressure decreases as one ascends. For example, barometric pressure at the top of Mount Everest (where the altitude is 29,000 ft) is 235 mmHg. Therefore, the partial pressure of oxygen in the atmosphere on the top of Mount Everest is 235 × 0.21 = 49 mmHg; this is in contrast to the partial pressure of oxygen at sea level, which is approximately 160 mmHg.

Another example of decreased barometric pressure is travel in commercial airliners. Cabins of these aircraft may be pressurized to only about 7000 ft, corresponding to a barometric pressure of somewhere around 600 mmHg; the inspired partial pressure of oxygen would be correspondingly reduced. One other situation which is fortunately quite rare, but which may account for aerohypoxia, is the inadvertent substitution of inappropriate gas mixtures in a controlled setting, such as during anesthesia or mechanical ventilation. Administration of nitrous oxide instead of oxygen, for example, may result in aerohypoxia by decreasing the fractional concentration of inspired oxygen.

The treatment of aerohypoxia is straightforward: Increasing the concentration of oxygen will correct the difficulty.

Hypoventilation   We have previously described minute ventilation as the total amount of gas that moves in and out of the lungs in 1 min; reduction in this minute ventilation may have predictable results. First, since oxygen is continually removed from the alveoli into the blood, insufficient oxygen from the atmosphere will be delivered to renew the gas being absorbed in the alveoli, so that the partial pressure of oxygen within the alveoli will decrease. Secondly, carbon dioxide, which is normally removed from the alveolus by ventilation, will continue to accumulate (Fig. 8-7). The hallmark of hypoxemia resulting from hypoventilation, then, is an elevated partial pressure of carbon dioxide. In fact, an elevated partial pressure of carbon dioxide may be used to define hypoventilation (Table 8-5).

A common clinical problem is presented by the patient who develops hypoxemia and an elevated P_{CO_2}. The question arises: Is this patient's hypoxemia all attributable to hypoventilation? To answer this question, one has simply to use the alveolar air equation.

As we have seen, aerohypoxia results from a decreased $P_{I_{O_2}}$; hypoxemia from hypoventilation results from an increased P_{CO_2}. Other causes of hypoxemia result from an increase in the alveolar-arterial O_2 difference. A clinical example may illustrate this point.

Suppose a patient has blood gases which show a P_{O_2} of 65 mmHg and a P_{CO_2} of 60 mmHg while breathing room air. We wish to know if the hypoventilation, that is, the elevated P_{CO_2}, alone may account for his low P_{O_2}. To answer this question, we substitute into the alveolar air equation:

$$Pa_{O_2} = P_{I_{O_2}} - \frac{Pa_{CO_2}}{R} - (\text{A-a})O_2 \text{ difference}$$

We know that the $P_{I_{O_2}}$ is approximately 150 mmHg, and we assume that the $(\text{A-a})O_2$ difference is normal, that is, about 10 mmHg. Substituting into the equation:

$$Pa_{O_2} = 150 - \frac{60}{0.8} - 10$$

$$Pa_{O_2} = 150 - 75 - 10$$

$$Pa_{O_2} = 65$$

Thus, we would predict that with a normal $(\text{A-a})O_2$ difference and a normal inspired oxygen tension, an elevation in the P_{CO_2} to 60 mmHg would result in a P_{O_2} of 65 mmHg. We conclude that hypoventilation alone accounts for the observed blood gases.

Hypoventilation most often occurs in the setting of chronic obstructive pulmonary disease. Patients with bronchitis are especially prone to elevated P_{CO_2} from a variety of causes. First, because of increased airway resistance, they must work harder to maintain an adequate minute ventilation; if they cannot sustain the increased work of breathing, then they lower their minute ventilation, resulting in CO_2 retention. Second, the increased work of breathing may cause the respiratory muscles to produce increased quantities of CO_2, placing a greater demand on the minute ventilation. Finally,

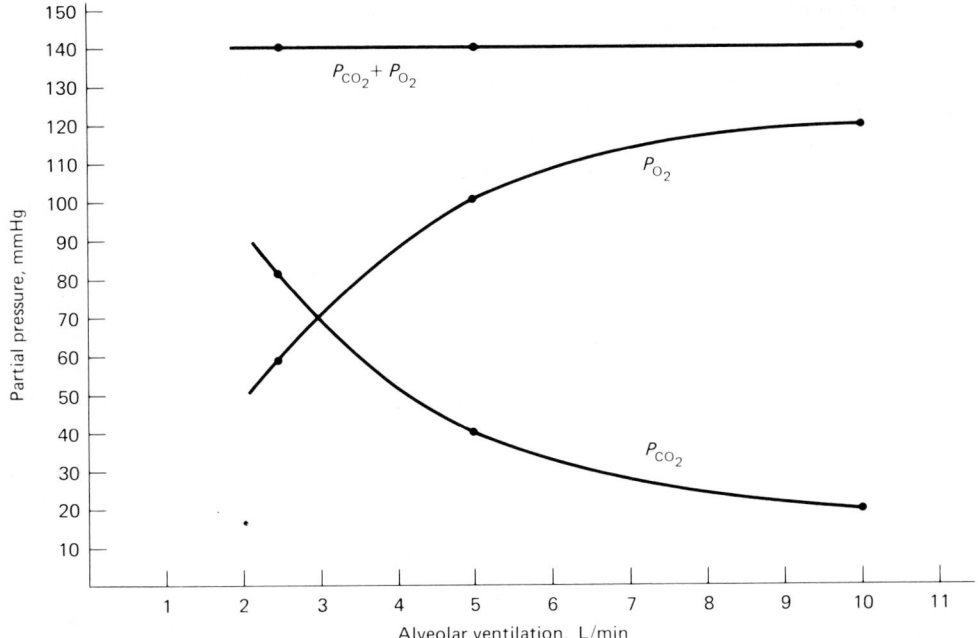

Figure 8-7 Normal alveolar ventilation. $\dot{V}A$ is approximately 5 L/min and corresponds to a P_{CO_2} of 40 mmHg (the P_{CO_2} here may be either PA_{CO_2} or Pa_{CO_2}, since carbon dioxide is readily soluble). Under these conditions, the normal P_{O_2} is approximately 100 mmHG (the P_{O_2} here is the PA_{O_2}, as Pa_{CO_2} is expected to be slightly lower, owing to the $D(A=a)O_2$ and oxygen's low solubility). Note that by halving $\dot{V}A$, the P_{CO_2} doubles and the P_{O_2} falls accordingly; but the P_{CO_2} and P_{O_2} total remains close to 140 mmHg. Similarly, by increasing $\dot{V}A$, P_{CO_2} falls and P_{O_2} rises, but the total remains close to 140 mmHg. Hypoxemia due solely to hypoventilation displays this feature. If other mechanisms of hypoxemia are operative, then the P_{CO_2} and Pa_{O_2} total will be less than the predicted 140 mmHg. (Compare this approximation to the $D(A-a)O_2$ calculation.)

patients with a variety of lung diseases have an increased dead space-to-tidal volume ratio (VD/VT), leaving less available tidal volume for alveolar ventilation. Since a greater part of each breath ventilates dead space, there is less opportunity for CO_2 to be removed from the alveolus.

A diagnosis of hypoxemia from hypoventilation may indicate some problem other than intrinsic lung disease. In other words, there may be no problem in gas exchange of the lung, but rather a problem in regulating ventilation to remove carbon dioxide. The therapy of hypoxemia from hypoventilation is to correct the cause of the hypoventilation. In practice, this may involve reversal of sedative drugs, stimulation of respiration, or mechanical ventilatory support.

Abnormalities of Diffusion Although the process of diffusion is an important part of gas exchange within the lungs, it is unlikely that a simple derangement in the pathway for diffusion of oxygen is responsible for most instances of clinical hypoxemia. One of the reasons for this is that the lung has much reserve with respect to diffusion. Under normal conditions diffusion is complete by about 0.25 s, but the red blood cell spends another 0.5 s (0.75 s total) within the pulmonary capillary. In addition, the pathway for diffusion involving the alveolar–capillary interface is relatively short in the overall pathway, which includes the alveolar air space, endothelial and epithelial membranes, capillary plasma, and the interior of the red blood cell. In general, it is safe to say that diffusion impairment

Table 8-5 Hypoxemia Due to Hypoventilation

I. Pathophysiology:
   Hypoxemia always accompanied by hypercarbia ($\uparrow Pa_{CO_2}$)

II. Etiology:
   A. Hypoventilation with normal lungs:
      1. Damage to or depression of the brain's respiratory center:
         Head trauma
         Strokes
         CNS depressant drugs
      2. Neuromuscular defects in the respiratory apparatus:
         Myasthenia gravis
         Guillain-Barré syndrome
         Polio
         Spinal cord injuries
         Botulism
         Tetanus
         Neuromuscular blocking drugs
   B. Hypoventilation with abnormal lungs:
      1. Obstructive airways disease (asthma, chronic bronchitis, and emphysema)
      2. Loss of elasticity of pulmonary parenchyma (emphysema)
      3. Restrictive lung diseases (e.g., kyphoscoliosis, morbid obesity)

III. Diagnosis:
   By arterial blood gases
   Hypoxemia with a $\uparrow Pa_{CO_2}$ and a normal $D_{(A-a)}O_2$

IV. Therapy:
   Improve oxygenation by increasing alveolar ventilation
   Specific therapy depending upon the specific etiology

alone (as measured by the diffusing capacity for carbon monoxide) is of little significance in the hypoxemic, critically ill patient.

There are several conditions, however, under which diffusion impairment may significantly contribute to hypoxemia (Table 8-6). One of these is exercise. During exercise cardiac output is greatly increased, so that the velocity of blood traversing the pulmonary capillaries is increased; therefore, the amount of time spent in a pulmonary capillary by each red blood cell is shortened. If some abnormality of diffusion is already present, then increases in cardiac output might result in insufficient time for equilibration within the pulmonary capillary (Fig. 8-8). In fact, this is commonly seen when one performs measurements of arterial oxygen tension in patients with interstitial lung disease

during exercise. Other causes of local increases in blood flow could also cause hypoxemia in the setting of a diffusion impairment, such as a pulmonary embolus. One might imagine that a pulmonary embolism in one portion of the lung might divert blood to another, resulting in a local increase in velocity of blood and insufficient time for equilibration.

Another situation in which diffusion impairment may play a role in clinically observed hypoxemia is in aerohypoxia. When inspired oxygen tensions are decreased, such as at high altitude or in a pressurized airplane cabin, then the gradient for gas diffusion may be decreased; the result would be a prolongation of the time needed to reach equilibrium within the pulmonary capillary, and hypoxemia due to a diffusion problem.

More commonly, processes which result in marked diffusion abnormalities and thickening of the alveolar-capillary membrane also result in widespread ventilation-perfusion inequality. Most of the hypoxemia observed in these conditions, which include sarcoidosis, interstitial fibrosis, collagen vascular diseases of the lung, including scleroderma and lupus erythematosis, and other similar disorders, results from uneven distribution of ventilation and perfusion. The decreased diffusion capacity seen in emphysema may be a result of destruction of functioning alveoli, so that the interface between the alveolar and the pulmonary capillary surface is disrupted. This may be thought of as a decrease in the total area over which diffusion may occur. Nevertheless, hypoxemia in patients with emphysema is more a result of ventilation-perfusion inequality than diffusion problems.

Because it is technically difficult to measure the diffusing capacity for oxygen, clinical pulmonary function laboratories measure the diffusing capacity for carbon monoxide. In addition to the length and cross-sectional area, the pulmonary blood volume is another important factor which may affect the diffusing capacity for carbon monoxide. In fact, conditions which cause a high pulmonary blood volume result in a measurably increased diffusion capacity; conditions which cause a decreased pulmonary blood volume result in a decreased diffusing capacity. Furthermore, the hemoglobin concentration may also affect diffusing capacity. Elevation in hemoglobin results in an increased diffusing

Table 8-6 Hypoxemia Due to Diffusion Abnormalities

I. Pathophysiology:
   A. Increased diffusion pathway—prevents equilibrium between alveolar oxygen and pulmonary capillary blood, so that the blood exiting the capillary is hypoxemic
   B. Decreased diffusion area—destruction of membrane surface area available for diffusion and loss of pulmonary capillary bed
II. Etiology:
   A. Increased diffusion pathway:
      1. Accumulation of fluid—e.g., congestive heart failure and pulmonary edema
      2. Accumulation of collagen in the pulmonary interstitium—e.g., idiopathic pulmonary fibrosis, sarcoidosis, and collagen-vascular disease
   B. Decreased diffusion area:
      1. Pulmonary resection
      2. Destructive lung diseases—e.g., emphysema and obliterative pulmonary vascular diseases
III. Diagnosis:
   A. History and physical findings compatible with the primary diagnosis
   B. Laboratory:
      1. PFTs reveal decreased DL_{CO}, exercise arterial blood gas measurements reveal arterial desaturation
      2. Chest x-ray compatible with interstitial fibrosis, emphysema, etc.
IV. Treatment:
   A. Oxygen administration
   B. Evaluation of need for home oxygen therapy

capacity, whereas anemia may result in a decreased diffusing capacity.

Hypoxemia due to impairment in diffusing capacity may be readily corrected by administration of 100 percent oxygen. This is because when pure oxygen is administered, the P_{O_2} in the alveolus rises to very high levels. Since one of the factors which determines diffusion is the partial pressure gradient, diffusion is greatly facilitated by increasing the

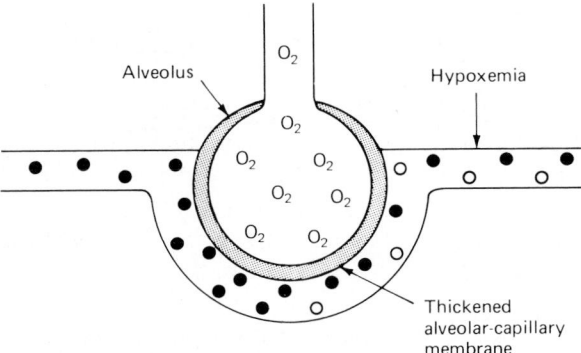

Figure 8-8   Schematic representation of a diffusion defect. Note the marked thickening of the alveolar-capillary membrane. Hypoxemia results because a red blood cell traversing this capillary does not have sufficient time to establish equilibrium with the alveolar oxygen.

partial pressure of oxygen in the alveolus to very high levels.

Ventilation-Perfusion Imbalance   This is the most common cause of hypoxemia, and is the main mechanism accounting for hypoxemia occurring in such diverse conditions as pulmonary embolism, chronic obstructive lung disease, pneumonia, and interstitial lung disease (Table 8-7).

For the entire lung, the overall ventilation-perfusion ratio is about 0.8. This is because normal alveolar ventilation is approximately 4 L per minute, and normal pulmonary blood flow (cardiac output) is about 5 L per minute; thus, the ratio of ventilation to perfusion is 4 to 5, or 0.8. In order to reach this average, it is clear that the average ventilation-perfusion ratio for each of the lungs' 300 million alveoli is 0.8. In actuality, however, some alveoli have ventilation-perfusion ratios that are greater, and some have ventilation-perfusion ratios smaller than 0.8.

As you will recall from preceding sections, there is greater blood flow to the lung bases primarily because of the effect of gravity. Similarly, the greater proportion of ventilation is to the bases of the lungs. Figure 8-9 portrays this relationship and emphasizes another fact: Blood flow increases out of proportion to the increase in ventilation as

Table 8-7 Hypoxemia Due to V̇/Q̇ Mismatching

I. Pathophysiology:
    A. Low V̇/Q̇ units, with perfusion in excess of ventilation, result in hypoxemia because the blood traversing these units is not fully oxygenated.
    B. Low V̇/Q̇ units may result from partial obstruction of airways by foreign bodies, secretions, edema, inflammation, bronchospasm, etc.

III. Etiology:
    A. Obstructive airway disease:
        Chronic bronchitis
        Emphysema
        Asthma
    B. Restrictive lung disease:
        Obesity
        Kyphoscoliosis
        Interstitial lung disease
    C. Pulmonary vascular disease

III. Diagnosis:
    A. History—look for clues to the above diagnoses.
    B. Physical exam—abnormal chest wall motion, abnormal distribution of breath sounds, bronchospasm.
    C. Laboratory data—arterial blood gases with hypoxemia and a widened $D(A-a)O_2$; characteristic change on CXR, PFTs, and V̇/Q̇ scan.

IV. Treatment:
    A. Administer supplemental oxygen.
    B. Identify the underlying cause.
    C. Specific therapy varies depending upon the specific etiology.

Figure 8-9   The relationship between ventilation and perfusion in different lung zones. Notice how both V̇ and Q̇ increase toward the base of the lung; but since perfusion shows a proportionately greater increase, the V̇/Q̇ ratio decreases. *(Adapted from R. M. Cherniack et al., Respiration in health and disease, 2d ed. Philadelphia: Saunders, 1972.)*

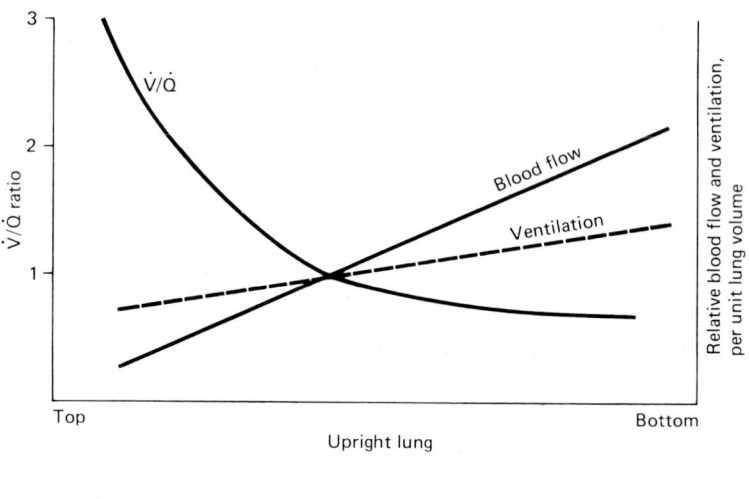

Lung zone	Top	Middle	Bottom
Ventilation (V̇), L/min	0.6	1.0	2.4
Perfusion (Q̇) L/min	0.2	1.0	3.8
V̇/Q̇	3.0	1.0	0.65

one moves toward the dependent portions of the lung, so that the ventilation-perfusion ratio decreases at the lung bases.

Lung units with high ventilation-perfusion ratios are normally found at the apex of the lung; this is because blood flow is relatively low or even absent in the upright position at the apex of the lungs, whereas ventilation is only modestly reduced compared to the bases. Pulmonary capillary blood returning from apical portions of the lung has a high P_{O_2} and low P_{CO_2}. However, such units have little effect on the arterial blood gas findings, since blood flow is so low that they contribute a relatively small volume of blood toward the final composition of mixed arterial blood. In areas where ventilation is extremely high in proportion to blood flow, or where blood flow is practically zero, physiologic dead space is the result.

Figure 8-10 demonstrates the effect of units with high and low ventilation-perfusion ratios on the mixed arterial blood oxygen tension. Figure 8-10a portrays the normal situation in which ventilation and perfusion are matched. Figure 8-10b demonstrates a unit with a high ventilation-perfusion ratio resulting from a decreasing blood flow. Although this ventilation contributes to dead space ventilation, there is little effect on the arterial blood gas tension, because there is little blood flow from such units. Figure 8-10c demonstrates a unit with a low ventilation-perfusion ratio because of partial collapse of the airway. In this example, unoxygenated mixed venous blood enters the unit from the pulmonary artery and passes through the capillary without becoming saturated with oxygen. The result is that relatively unoxygenated blood from this low ventilation-perfusion unit mixes with the blood from the remainder of the lung, resulting in hypoxemia.

Abnormalities in ventilation-perfusion matching may occur from a variety of pulmonary diseases. Airway secretions, edema, or inflammation such as are seen in bronchitis or asthma will cause the alveoli distal to those airways to be underventilated. Interstitial lung diseases, including idiopathic pulmonary fibrosis, may be characterized by unevenness in ventilation-perfusion matching, resulting in hypoxemia.

Hypoxemia is a common finding in acute pulmonary embolism, and usually results from

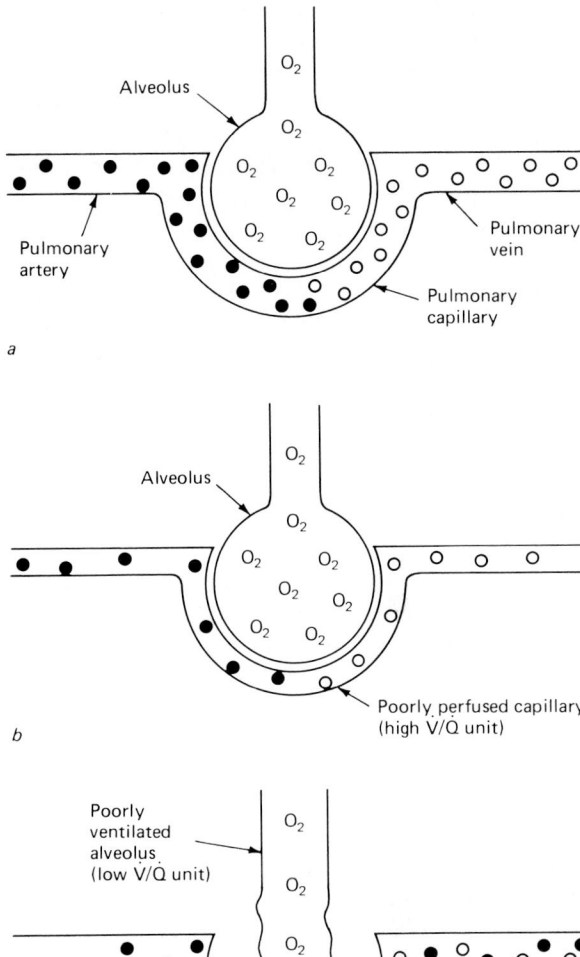

Figure 8-10   Schematic representation of a normal alveolar-capillary unit (*a*), a high $\dot{V}/\dot{Q}$ unit (*b*), and a low $\dot{V}/\dot{Q}$ unit (*c*). See text for explanation. The illustration depicts oxygen (O_2) in the airways and the ventilated alveoli; deoxygenated venous blood in the pulmonary artery entering the alveolar-capillary unit (represented by the solid circles); and oxygenated blood (represented by the open circles) emerging from the alveolar-capillary unit and entering the pulmonary vein on the way back to the left side of the heart. Notice how low $\dot{V}/\dot{Q}$ units cause hypoxemia by failing to normally oxygenate all the blood that flows through these areas.

ventilation-perfusion inequality. As one envisions an embolism lodged in a pulmonary artery, blood flow would be interrupted but ventilation would be maintained to that area of the lung. The result would seem to be an area of dead space. However, blood flow would now be directed away from one portion of the lung into another, with a reduction in the ventilation-perfusion ratio. Furthermore, the elaboration by the embolus of chemical mediators may result in changes in ventilation and perfusion ratios in the embolized areas of the lung.

If one analyzes the problem of hypoxemia in a patient with ventilation-perfusion imbalance by using the alveolar air equation, the result is that the A-a gradient is increased. Ventilation-perfusion abnormalities are the second of three causes of increased A-a gradients.

The treatment of hypoxemia from ventilation-perfusion inequality is the administration of oxygen. Since, by definition, there is still some ventilation present to areas of low ventilation-perfusion ratios, increasing the inspired oxygen tension will result in an increased partial pressure of oxygen in the alveolus. Thus, an improvement in oxygenation to the blood perfusing these units will be the result. Returning to Fig. 8-10c, we can see that if the partially collapsed alveolus were filled with a large number of O_2 molecules, then the unoxygenated blood entering this unit would become normally oxygenated, with relief of the hypoxemia.

Shunting We have previously referred to shunting as one extreme of ventilation-perfusion imbalance, that is, the extreme where ventilation is zero. Thus, mixed venous blood is shunted past the lung without becoming oxygenated and is returned directly to the heart for mixing in the arterial tree, resulting in hypoxemia (Table 8-8).

Shunts may be divided into *anatomic* and *physiologic* types (Fig. 8-11). An anatomic shunt is present in normal persons, comprising approximately 2 percent of the cardiac output. It is the result of the blood flow through bronchial, pleural, and thebesian veins that drain directly into the arterial circulation. Their presence is part of the reason that the alveolar-arterial oxygen gradient exists in normal subjects.

Pathologic anatomic shunts may occur as congenital arteriovenous fistulas, from trauma, from cirrhosis of the liver, or in the heart. Tetralogy of Fallot or Eisenmenger's syndrome are examples of right-to-left shunting through the heart. Perhaps a more common form of intracardiac shunting may be observed in patients with high pulmonry artery pressures, in whom the foramen ovale may become patent and allow right atrial blood to pass directly into the left atrium, bypassing the lungs.

Physiologic shunts occur at the alveolar level. They may occur, for example, as the result of total alveolar collapse in association with atelectasis, obstruction from a tumor, or from a pneumothorax

Table 8-8 Hypoxemia Due to Shunting (R → L)

I. Pathophysiology:
    A. Hypoxemia results from venous admixture when deoxygenated, mixed venous blood bypasses functional alveolar-capillary units and mixes with normally oxygenated blood in the systemic circulation.
    B. Shunts may be either anatomic or physiologic.
II. Etiology:
    A. Anatomic shunts: blood bypasses the alveolar-capillary unit
        1. Normal anatomic shunts—bronchial, pleural, thebesian veins
        2. Intrapulmonary shunts—e.g., pulmonary A-V fistulas
        3. Intracardiac shunts—e.g., tetralogy of Fallot, Eisenmenger's syndrome
        4. Other pathologic shunts—e.g., shunts associated with neoplasms
    B. Physiologic shunts: blood shunted through nonfunctional alveolar-capillary units
        1. Alveolar collapse—e.g., atelectasis, pneumothorax, hemothorax, pleural effusion
        2. Alveoli filled with a foreign material—e.g., pulmonary edema, pneumonias, ARDS
III. Diagnosis:
    A. Hypoxemia with a normal or decreased Pa_{CO_2} and a widened $D(A\text{-}a)O_2$
    B. 100% O_2 test: widened $D(A\text{-}a)O_2$ persists, shunt may be estimated
IV. Treatment:
    A. Oxygen administration has little effect.
    B. Proper therapy depends upon the specific etiology.

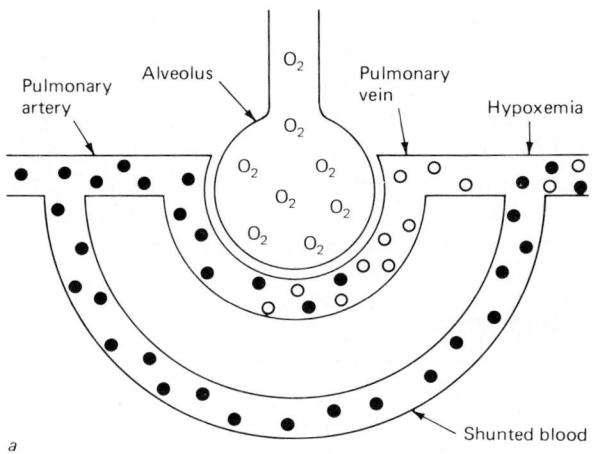

a

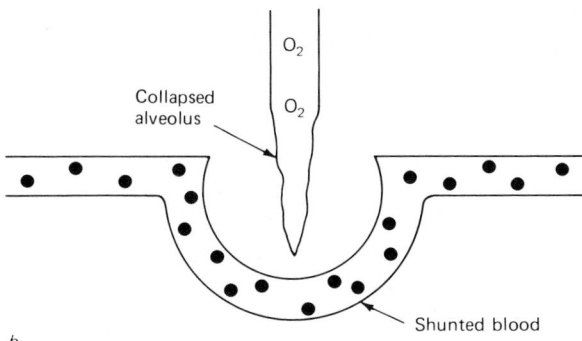

b

Figure 8-11 Schematic representation of the two main types of shunts. An example (*a*) of an anatomic shunt, illustrated as an anomalous communication between a pulmonary artery and a pulmonary vein. These shunts occur normally in the chest (bronchial, pleural, and thebesian veins), and are seen in a variety of pathologic conditions. A physiologic shunt (*b*) caused by $\dot{V}/\dot{Q}$ unit with intact blood flow but no ventilation because of a totally collapsed alveolus ($\dot{V}/\dot{Q}$ ratio of zero). In both instances the shunted blood is not exposed to oxygen and therefore emerges from the lung as unaltered venous blood.

or pleural effusion. Additionally, physiologic shunting may occur in alveoli which are open, but which are filled with fluid as in pulmonary edema. Pneumonia represents a condition in which alveolar spaces may be filled with inflammatory exudate, and ARDS may result in alveoli filled with proteinaceous material.

The degree of hypoxemia that results from a shunt depends upon two factors: the severity or degree of shunt (usually expressed as a percentage of the total cardiac output) and the oxygen content of the shunted blood. This latter point should be stressed further.

Let us take the example of a patient with pneumonia and sepsis. Because of the pneumonia, our patient has a 10 percent shunt. The following day, it is noted that the patient's cardiac output has fallen dramatically, and that her arterial hypoxemia has worsened even though there is no change on the x-ray and no change in administered oxygen. The explanation may be that, because of a decreased cardiac output, decreased oxygen has been delivered to the tissues. Since the oxygen consumption has remained the same, there is less oxygen remaining in the blood after consumption by the body; the result is a decreased mixed venous P_{O_2}. As this mixed venous P_{O_2} with a lower oxygen tension and lower oxygen content moves through the 10 percent shunt, it mixes with arterial blood and worsens the degree of hypoxemia. In other words, even though the degree of shunt has not changed, the composition of the blood passing through the shunt has changed, resulting in altered arterial oxygen tension.

The shunt equation has been previously discussed, and may be utilized to calculate the degree of shunt. One needs to know the oxygen content of mixed venous blood, the oxygen content of arterial blood, and oxygen content of pulmonary capillary blood (one assumes that capillary P_{O_2} equals alveolar P_{O_2}; the alveolar oxygen tension must be calculated from the alveolar air equation). A rough estimate of degree of shunt is provided by the following rule: With a patient breathing 100 percent oxygen for 15 min, an arterial blood gas sample is drawn and the P_{O_2} in the sample is compared to the normal value of 650 mmHg. For every 50 mmHg that the patient's arterial P_{O_2} falls below the normal value of 650, a 2.5 percent shunt is present. For example, if the observed P_{O_2} under such conditions is 450 mmHg, then this represents 4 decrements of 50 mm below the target value of 650, corresponding to a 4 × 2.5 or 10 percent shunt.

Unlike diffusion abnormalities and ventilation-perfusion imbalances, the administration of oxygen would be expected to have no effect on shunt. This is because the shunted blood has no opportunity to come into contact with gas-exchanging tissues. Thus, although the administration of high oxygen levels would be expected to increase alveolar P_{O_2}, shunted blood would be unaffected. Although increasing alveolar P_{O_2} may increase the saturation in blood draining normal units, there will be little overall effect on the arterial blood, since the blood is already 95 percent saturated with oxygen. Thus, the lack of response to administration of 100 percent oxygen defines the presence of anatomic or physiologic shunt.

Since administration of oxygen has little effect on hypoxemia resulting from shunt, one must look to other methods for treating pulmonary shunts. The treatment of shunts lies in the treatment of their underlying causes. Thus, attention must be focused on proper treatment of pneumonia, pul-monary embolism, ARDS, or some other primary etiologic factor. Additionally, the effect of a shunt, though not the magnitude, may be decreased by ensuring adequate cardiac output and thereby preventing a decrease in the mixed venous P_{O_2}. Positive end-expiratory pressure may also decrease the shunt by increasing lung volume and recruiting additional alveoli for gas exchange.

Bibliography

Murray, J. F. (1986). *The normal lung*, 2d ed. Philadelphia: Saunders.

Nunn, J. F. (1977). *Applied respirtory physiology*. London: Butterworths.

West, J. B. (1979). *Respiratory physiology—the essentials*. Baltimore: Williams & Wilkins.

9

Charold L. Baer

Regulation and Assessment of Fluid and Electrolyte Balance

Introduction

The life of every individual depends on the maintenance of a stable internal environment. That internal environment is composed of water, electrolytes, and metabolic end products. In a normal, healthy person, the internal environment is regulated and maintained by a variety of physiologic functions. However, when a person suffers a critical illness due to acute or chronic pathology, the normal homeostatic mechanisms of the body are often not sufficient to maintain a stable internal environment. As a result, alterations in the internal environment occur and directly affect the individual's physiologic functioning, physical appearance, and behavior. Indeed, these alterations may be severe enough to precipitate the individual's demise. Therefore, it is essential that the patient receive support from the health care team during this period of instability.

While it is true that all health care team members play an important supportive role in the patient's care during this time, much of the responsibility resides with the nurse because of proximity and the amount of time spent with the individual. Because the nurse has the most frequent, consistent, and extensive contact with the patient, he or she can easily detect changes in patterns of function or behavior. The nurse's responsibilities in relation to alterations in a patient's internal environment include (1) monitoring, (2) interpreting, (3) reporting and recording, (4) intervening, and (5) evaluating. Figure 9-1 illustrates this relationship.

As depicted in Fig. 9-1, the nurse's responsibilities are implemented in response to the external manifestations exhibited by the individual because of the alterations in the internal environment. The nurse functions in a systematic manner that begins with *monitoring*. This includes observing the patient as well as assessing all laboratory and technological data. Monitoring is followed by *interpreting*, which involves using one's knowledge of the individual's history, physiology, and pathophysiology to determine if the information gained from monitoring is normal or abnormal for the patient and to what degree. Then the information is *reported* and *recorded*. This responsibility is important because in order to provide quality care, periodic assessments of the patient must be documented as well as conveyed to the physician.

The next responsibility of the nurse is *intervening*. Intervening is the essence of health care, whether it is based on nursing or medical prescriptions. Intervening means *action,* and it is action that makes the impact on the individual's health state. A nurse could monitor, interpret, report, and record forever, but unless there is action taken based on those functions, the patient's condition may continue to deteriorate. All action, however, must be based on sufficient data because to intervene inappropriately could also threaten the individual's stability.

The final responsibility of the nurse is to *evaluate* the results of the intervention based on the desired patient outcomes, or, in other words, to find out if the actions taken changed the individual's health state.

These five responsibilities or functions, performed at periodic intervals as determined by the health state of the patient, provide the framework for delivering nursing care.

The implementation of these nursing responsibilities has a significant impact on the care of the patient with an altered internal environment. To perform these responsibilities, the nurse must have a basic comprehension of the components of the internal environment. This discussion is designed

194

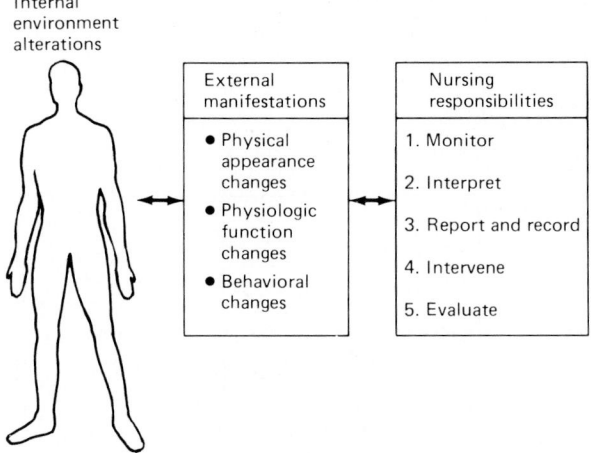

Figure 9-1   Nursing responsibilities related to alterations in an individual's internal environment.

to provide information prerequisite to that understanding.

Amount and Distribution of Body Fluids

Total Body Water

The total body water of a person is approximately 60 percent of the total body weight in kilograms. This percentage varies according to the muscle mass, amount of body fat, and age of the individual. Since muscles contain a high proportion of water, someone with a large muscle mass would have a higher percentage of total body water than someone with less muscle mass. Fat contains less water than lean tissues, so individuals with more body fat tend to have a lower percentage of total body water. These two facts explain why females have lower percentages of total body water than males. Age also affects the percent of total body water. As a person ages, the percent of total body water decreases. Therefore, a lean, young adult male would theoretically have the highest percentage of total body water, while an obese, elderly female would have the lowest.

Amounts and Distribution

The total body water of an individual is distributed into several different compartments. The two pri-

mary compartments are the intracellular and extracellular fluid spaces. The intracellular fluid space includes all the water contained within the cells, including the red blood cells, which are also designated as part of the intravascular fluid. The extracellular fluid space includes the water contained in several smaller fluid compartments. Among these compartments are the interstitial, plasma, transcellular, bone, and connective tissue spaces. Of these fluid spaces, the interstitial and plasma spaces contain functional extracellular fluid, while the transcellular (pleural, peritoneal, joint, and cerebrospinal fluid spaces), bone, and connective tissue spaces contain nonfunctional extracellular fluid. Each of these fluid compartments or spaces contains a percentage of the individual's total body water. Figure 9-2 illustrates the distribution of the total body water throughout the compartments by percent of body weight for a normal, healthy adult male. It also indicates that there is an additional fluid compartment, the intravascular space, that contains both extracellular and intracellular fluid. The percentages of body water shown in Fig. 9-2 are translated into liter volumes for a normal, healthy 70-kg male and 60-kg female in Table 9-1.

Electrolyte Composition of Body Fluids

A person's internal environment does not consist merely of water; it also has numerous electrolytes. These electrolytes are essential to a variety of physiologic functions. The specific physiologic functions in which each electrolyte participates will be enumerated in the discussion of each electrolyte later in this chapter. The electrolytes are present in different amounts in the major fluid compartments of the body. Table 9-2 presents the approximate amount of each of the electrolytes in the various major fluid compartments.

Osmolality, Osmolarity, and Tonicity

The distribution of body fluids in the various compartments depends primarily on the osmotic pressure that exists in those spaces. This osmotic pressure is referred to as the osmolality, osmolarity, or tonicity of the fluid in the space.

Figure 9-2 The distribution of total body water by compartment according to the percent of body weight for a normal healthy adult male.

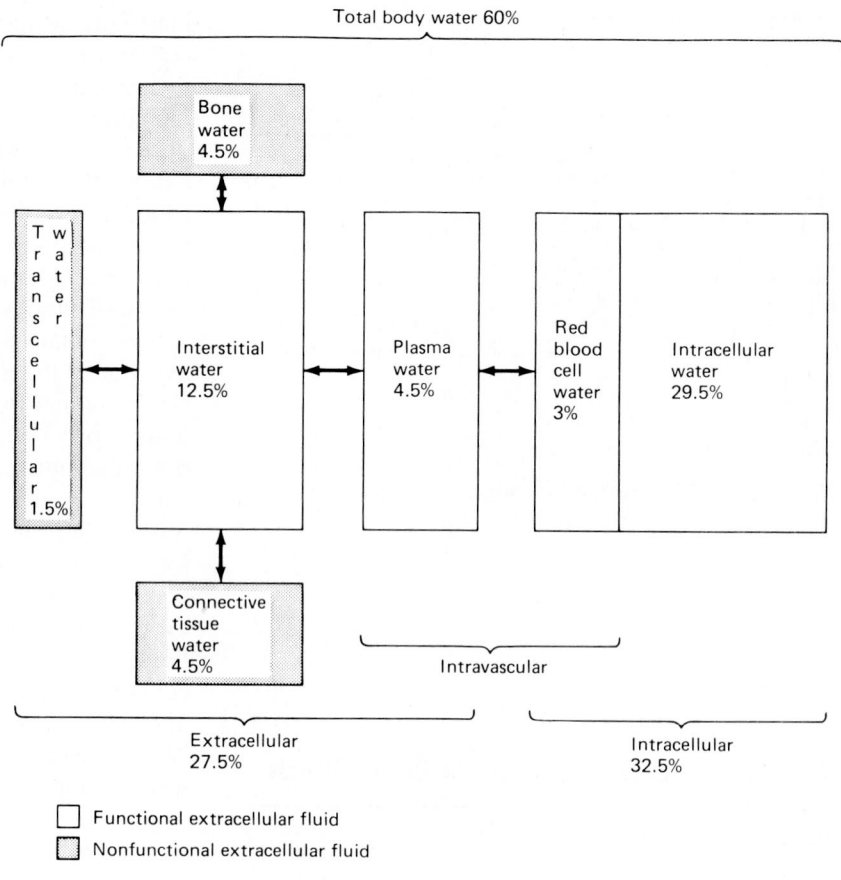

Functional extracellular fluid

Nonfunctional extracellular fluid

Table 9-1 Distribution of Total Body Water per Compartment in Percent of Body Weight and Liter Volume for a Normal, Healthy Adult Male and Female

	70-kg Male		60-kg Female	
Compartment	% Body Weight	Volume, L	% Body Weight	Volume, L
Intracellular	32.5	23	27.5	17
Red blood cells	3	2	3	2
Other cells	29.5	21	24.5	15
Extracellular	27.5	19	27.5	17
Interstitial	12.5	9	12.5	7
Plasma	4.5	3	4.5	3
Transcellular	1.5	1	1.5	1
Bone	4.5	3	4.5	3
Connective tissue	4.5	3	4.5	3
Intravascular*	7.5	5	7.5	5
Red blood cells	3	2	3	2
Plasma	4.5	3	4.5	3

* Combination of intracellular and extracellular fluid.

Table 9-2 Approximate Electrolyte Composition of the Major Fluid Compartments of the Body in Milliequivalents per Liter

Ions	Plasma	Interstitial Fluid	Intra-cellular Fluid
Cations			
Na	142	145	10
K	4.5	4	135
Ca	5	3	10
Mg	2.5	2	25
Totals	154	154	180
Anions			
Cl	104	115	5
HCO_3	24	27	10
HPO_4	2	2	100
SO_4	1	1	5
Organic acid	6	7	10
Protein	17	2	50
Totals	154	154	180

Definitions

Osmolality is the concentration of solute, expressed in terms of the number of particles per liter of *solvent. Osmolarity* is the concentration of solute, expressed in terms of the number of particles per liter of *solution. Tonicity* describes the comparison of the osmolality or osmolarity of one solution to another. If solution A had a higher osmolality than solution B, solution A would be described as being hypertonic to solution B. Solution B, on the other hand, would be hypotonic to solution A, because solution B had a lower osmolality. If both solutions were of equal osmolality, they would be described as being isotonic to each other. Such is the case with the body fluids of the normal individual.

Osmolality and osmolarity concentration measurements are so similar in dilute solutions, such as the body fluids, that they are often used interchangeably. However, the two measurements are not obtained by the same method, and the laboratory should specify which measurement is being reported. In most cases, the laboratories use a freezing-point method of determining concentration that measures osmolality. Hence the term *osmolality* tends to be used more frequently when discussing the concentration of body fluids.

Osmolality and osmolarity are both measured in milliosmoles. A milliosmole is $\frac{1}{1000}$ of an osmole.

An osmole, the unit for measuring osmotic pressure, is equal to the number of particles in 1 g molecular weight of a dissolved, nondiffusible, nonionizable substance. The normal osmolality of extracellular and intracellular body fluids is approximately 280 to 295 mosmol/L.

Regulation

The osmolality of body fluids is regulated by the osmoreceptor–antidiuretic hormone system and thirst. The osmoreceptor–antidiuretic hormone system involves the functions of the hypothalamus, neurohypophysis, antidiuretic hormone, and renal tubules, while thirst is primarily associated with the hypothalamus.

The Osmoreceptor–Antidiuretic Hormone System

The osmoreceptor–antidiuretic hormone system responds to alterations in the osmolality of the body fluids of as little as 1 to 2 percent. The response begins with the osmoreceptors that regulate the release of antidiuretic hormone. The osmoreceptors are specialized neurons located in or near the supraoptic nuclei of the anterior hypothalamus. These neurons contain fluid chambers filled with intracellular fluid that continuously emit nerve impulses. The fluid chambers respond specifically to changes in the extracellular fluid concentration, with sodium being the most effective stimulant. When the osmolality of the extracellular fluid decreases, making it hypotonic to the fluid in the chambers, water enters the fluid chambers in an attempt to establish equilibrium between the two fluids. The influx of water forces the fluid chambers to swell, which results in a decreased rate of impulse discharge. This means that fewer impulses are transmitted from the osmoreceptors in the supraoptic nuclei through the pituitary stalk to the neurohypophysis to promote the release of antidiuretic hormone. Thus, as illustrated in Fig. 9-3, less antidiuretic hormone is secreted.

When the extracellular fluid osmolality increases, the reverse of the process occurs. The increase in osmolality creates extracellular fluid that is hypertonic to the fluid in the chambers. Water then leaves the fluid chambers and flows into the extracellular fluid, shifting the system

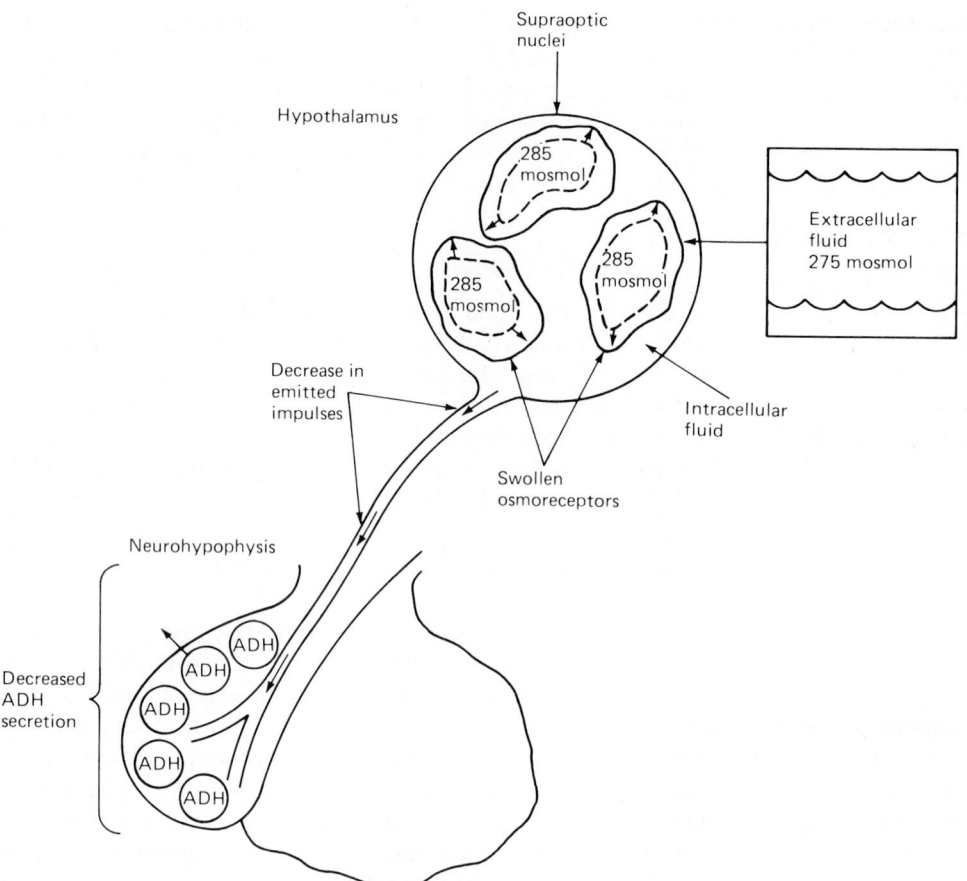

Figure 9-3   The osmoreceptor-antidiuretic hormone system response to decreased extracellular fluid osmolality.

toward equilibrium. This outflow of water results in a shrinking of the fluid chambers and an increase in the rate of impulse discharge to the neurohypophysis. The net effect, as shown in Fig. 9-4, is an increased secretion of antidiuretic hormone.

Antidiuretic hormone is synthesized in the supraoptic and paraventricular nuclei of the hypothalamus and stored as granules in the posterior pituitary. It is secreted into the blood according to the rate of impulses transmitted from the osmoreceptors to the neurohypophysis. Once it is in the blood, it circulates to the kidneys and acts on the distal tubules and collecting ducts to increase water reabsorption. Thus, the more antidiuretic hormone secreted, the more water reabsorbed.

In summary, the osmoreceptor–antidiuretic hormone system responds to a decrease in extracellular fluid osmolality by decreasing the secretion of antidiuretic hormone, resulting in less water reabsorption, more water excretion, and a return of the osmolality to normal. Conversely, the system reacts to an increase in extracellular fluid osmolality by increasing the secretion of antidiuretic hormone, resulting in more water reabsorption, less water excretion, and a return of the osmolality to normal.

Thirst

Thirst is also an important mechanism in regulating the osmolality of body fluids, because it is the primary regulator of water intake. There is a thirst center located in the hypothalamus that slightly overlaps the osmoreceptor area. Thirst is stimulated by the effect of intracellular dehydration on the neurons in the thirst center. It is inhibited by the act of drinking and the fullness of the gastrointestinal tract. These two states excite peripheral sensory receptors that transmit impulses to the thirst center to decrease the thirst. Thus, the thirst mechanism is actually inhibited *before* the intracellular dehydration is alleviated. This is a protective feedback mechanism to prevent voluntary water intoxication.

Calculating Osmolality Values

The most accurate method for determining osmolality is to measure it directly. Plasma osmolality can be quickly and accurately measured by determining its freezing point, since the freezing point of a solution decreases in direct proportion to its osmolality. If the plasma osmolality has not been measured, however, it can still be calculated or estimated using other serum laboratory values. It has been found that in normal plasma, the osmotic coefficients and other solute concentrations cancel each other in such a manner that the sodium concentration multiplied by two equals the plasma osmolality. The plasma osmolality, however, is also significantly influenced by glucose and urea, so they must be included in the calculation. In order to include glucose and urea in a formula for determining plasma osmolality, their values must be converted to milliosmoles. A simplified formula for including sodium, glucose, and urea in the calculation of plasma osmolality is:

$$2\,\text{Na}\,(\text{meq/L}) + \frac{\text{Glucose}\,(\text{mg/100 mL})}{18}$$

$$+ \frac{\text{BUN}\,(\text{mg/100 mL})}{3}$$

$$= \text{serum osmolality}\,(\text{mosmol/L})$$

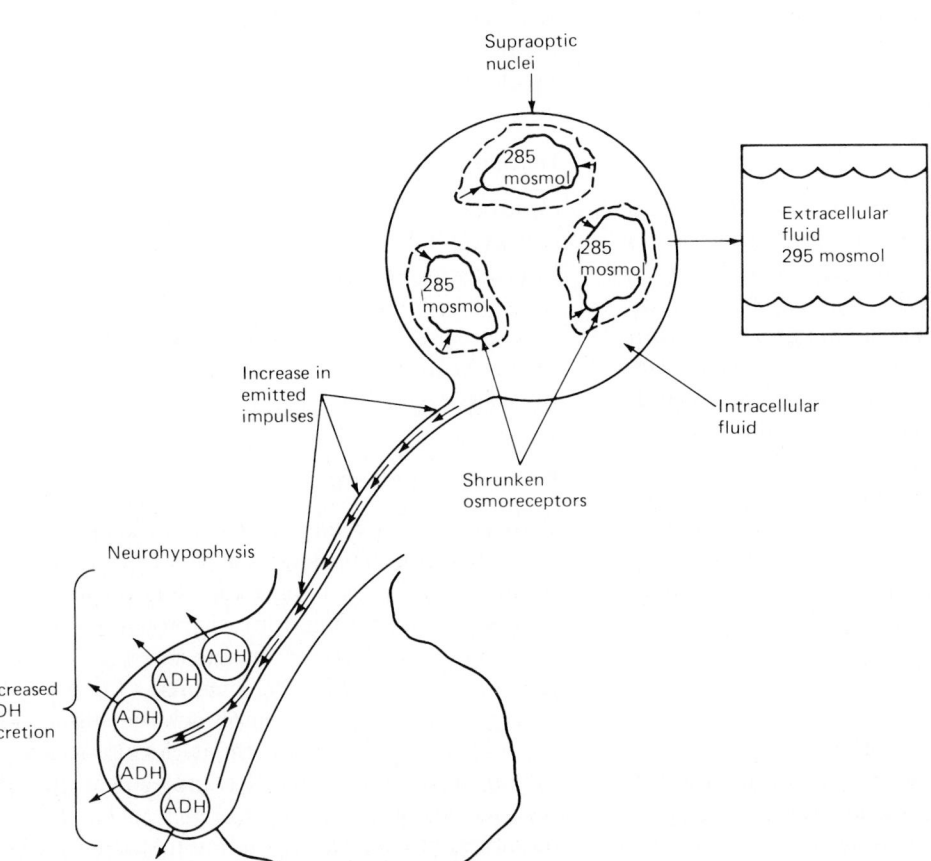

Figure 9-4   The osmoreceptor-antidiuretic hormone response to increased extracellular fluid osmolality.

The formula would be applied in the following manner:

Individual's serum laboratory values:

Na = 140 meq/L
Glucose = 90 mg/100 mL
BUN = 18 mg/100 mL

$$2(140) + \frac{90}{18} + \frac{18}{3} = \text{serum osmolality (mosmol/L)}$$

$$280 + 5 + 6 = 291 \text{ mosmol/L}$$

This calculated value would provide a close approximation of the actual serum osmolality.

Fluid and Electrolyte Transport

The processes involved in the transport of fluids and electrolytes include osmosis, diffusion, active transport, filtration, pinocytosis, and phagocytosis. Each of these processes affects the movement of fluids and electrolytes in a specific way.

Osmosis

Osmosis is a process that results from the kinetic motion of molecules in solution on either side of a semipermeable membrane. The motion of the molecules is such that water will pass through the membrane to the side that has the greater concentration of nondiffusible substances. This process results in a movement toward establishing equilibrium between the concentration of the solutions on either side of the membrane.

Osmosis can be negated by applying a pressure gradient across the semipermeable membrane in a direction opposite to that of the water flow. The amount of pressure required to negate osmosis is called the *osmotic pressure* of the solution.

Diffusion

Diffusion is the net movement of a given substance from one point to another due to the random kinetic motions of its molecules. Molecules diffuse from areas of higher concentration to areas of lower concentration. The net effect of this continuous kinetic movement is the establishment of an equal concentration of the substance throughout the medium, be it liquid, solid, or gas.

The rate at which diffusion occurs is determined by (1) the concentration gradient, (2) the cross-sectional area of the container or chamber, (3) the temperature of the solution, (4) the molecular weight of the molecules, and (5) the distance the molecules have to travel. The greater the concentration gradient, cross-sectional area, and temperature, the greater the diffusion rate. The greater the molecular weight and distance, the less the diffusion rate.

Active Transport

The process of moving a substance against a concentration, electrical, or pressure gradient is called *active transport.* In active transport, energy must be expended to move the substance against the gradient across the cell membrane. The energy that is expended probably comes from the adenosine triphosphate that is available in large quantities just inside the cell membrane.

Filtration

Filtration is the process of moving water and dissolved substances through a permeable membrane from an area of higher pressure to an area of lower pressure. Filtration results from the hydrostatic pressure produced by the pumping action of the heart. Filtration is opposed by the oncotic pressure created by proteins in the solution.

Pinocytosis and Phagocytosis

Pinocytosis and *phagocytosis* are transport processes that move substances across cell membranes by invagination and ingestion. Pinocytosis is the process of transporting primarily proteins and strong electrolyte solutions by invagination. Invagination functions in the following manner: (1) Molecules in the extracellular fluid approach the surface of a cell. (2) Absorption causes the molecules to adhere to the cell surface. (3) The molecules alter the surface tension of the cell membrane. (4) The cell membrane folds inward, pulling the adhering molecules with it. (5) The outer edges of the cell membrane then rejoin to form a continuous cell wall. (6) The result is a cell with a pinocytotic vesicle incorporated within its walls. Pinocytosis seems to be the only way of transporting proteins through the cell membrane.

Phagocytosis is the process of transporting large particles of selected matter by cell ingestion. Ingestion occurs in the same sequence of steps as invagination. The only difference is that a phagocytic vesicle is formed rather than a pinocytic vesicle. Phagocytosis is an efficient method of eradicating selected matter such as bacteria, other cells, and degenerating tissue. In order for matter to be selected for phagocytosis, it must have the following characteristics: (1) a rough, irregular surface; (2) an electropositive surface charge; and (3) the ability to adhere to the phagocytic cell. This third characteristic is enhanced by antibodies called *opsonins* that combine with the particles.

Fluid and Electrolyte Requirements

In discussing the daily fluid and electrolyte requirements for the normal adult, the following must be considered: (1) the average daily fluid intake and output, and (2) the composition of specific body fluids.

Average Daily Fluid Intake and Output

The average daily fluid intake and output volumes are reflections of the net fluid gains and losses of the body from all sources. Table 9-3 provides a list of the sources and ranges of the volumes for those

gains and losses. It is significant to note that in the healthy adult who is in a state of dynamic equilibrium, the volumes of the gains and losses are equal.

Composition of Specific Body Fluids

Each of the specific fluids in the body has its own composition. Table 9-4 presents an analysis of the various body fluids in terms of their major cations, anions, and water composition.

Alterations in Fluid and Electrolyte Requirements

Healthy adults deal with alterations in the water and electrolyte composition of their body fluids by the normal process of ingestion. They eat and drink the appropriate foods and fluids to maintain the equilibrium of their internal environment. However, when adults suffer dysfunction, they often cannot cope with the alterations in their internal environment and require professional assistance. In the process of receiving this assistance, they often develop additional changes in the water and electrolyte composition of their body fluids. As a result, they may experience a variety of undesirable physiologic, psychologic, and behavioral changes due to the alterations.

The alterations individuals experience are due to varying levels of the following substances in the body: water, sodium, potassium, calcium, magnesium, chloride, phosphates, sulfates, proteins, and organic acids. The remainder of this chapter will discuss the functions, regulation, and variances of

Table 9-3 Average Adult Daily Fluid Intake and Output

Intake		Output	
Source	Volume, mL	Source	Volume, mL
Water from fluids	500– 1700	Urine	800– 1600
Water from food	800– 1000	Vapor from lungs and skin	600– 1200
Water from oxidation	200– 300	Feces	100– 200
Total	1500– 3000	Total	1500– 3000

Table 9-4 Water and Electrolyte Composition of Various Body Fluids

Body fluid	Na, meq/L	K, meq/L	Cl, meq/L	HCO₃, meq/L	Water, mL/day
Cerebrospinal fluid	140	3.3	130	24	500
Sweat	45	5	60	—	500
Saliva	40	20	30	30	1500
Gastric juice	60	10	85	—	2500
Bile	150	5	100	40	500
Pancreatic juice	140	5	75	120	700
Small bowel fluid	110	5	105	20	3000
Normal feces	10	10	15	—	100
Loose feces	80	30	60	—	3000 +
Urine	90	80	90	—	1500

each of these substances. The variances for most of the substances will be presented in terms of the following: definition, etiology, clinical assessment parameters, laboratory assessment data, clinical and nursing implications, and treatment.

Water

Functions

The functions of water in the body are (1) to provide the internal medium for cell metabolism, (2) to transport nutrients and waste products, (3) to participate in chemical and metabolic processes, (4) to provide a lubricant for moving parts, and (5) to participate in the regulation of body heat.

Regulation

The regulation of body water is accomplished by the complex action and interaction of the following: the renal concentration and dilution of urine, circulating angiotensin II, antidiuretic hormone, and thirst.

Renal Concentration of Urine
The kidneys produce a concentrated urine by conserving body water while excreting solute. The concentration process occurs primarily as a result of the countercurrent mechanism which takes place within the renal medullary interstitium. It is composed of two processes: countercurrent multiplication and countercurrent exchange.

The countercurrent multiplication process occurs in the loop of Henle and is the mechanism that enables the body to excrete urine that has an osmolality higher than that of serum. The process facilitates this phenomenon by creating hypertonic medullary interstitial fluid from the generation of multiplying osmotic gradients through the active transport of sodium chloride from the impermeable ascending limb of the loop of Henle.

The countercurrent exchange process is the maintenance component of the countercurrent mechanism. This process involves the vasa recta or blood vessels that are looped around the tubules in the renal medullary interstitium. The vasa recta minimize the loss of solute from the interstitium by passive diffusion, thus maintaining the osmotic gradients necessary for the countercurrent multiplication process.

Both of these processes involved in the countercurrent mechanism are significantly affected by the secretion of antidiuretic hormone. Antidiuretic hormone increases the permeability of the renal collecting ducts to water, which assists in producing an osmotically concentrated urine. Antidiuretic hormone also assists in maintaining the hypertonic medullary interstitium by decreasing the rate of blood flow through the vasa recta of the medulla.

Renal Dilution of Urine
The ability of the kidney to affect body water by excreting excessive water in a dilute urine is dependent upon two mechanisms. The first mechanism is the active transport of sodium chloride from the impermeable ascending limb of the loop

of Henle. This mechanism results in a glomerular filtrate that is hypotonic to the plasma. The second mechanism is the decreased reabsorption of water that occurs at the collecting ducts due to their low permeability. The result of this mechanism is that the filtrate remains hypotonic and a dilute urine is excreted.

Circulating Angiotensin II

Circulating angiotensin II affects body water by increasing the passive reabsorption of water to increase the total volume. Angiotensin II is the potent vasoconstrictor produced via the renin-angiotensin system in response to a real or perceived decrease in arterial pressure or extracellular fluid volume, or an alteration in the renal intratubular sodium load. Angiotensin II not only promotes vasoconstriction but also stimulates the suprarenal cortex to secrete aldosterone. Aldosterone facilitates the active reabsorption of sodium, passive reabsorption of water, and active secretion of potassium at the renal tubules. The net effect of these processes is an increase in body water.

Antidiuretic Hormone and Thirst

The effects of antidiuretic hormone and thirst on body water are to conserve and replace it. The mechanisms by which antidiuretic hormone and thirst achieve their results were outlined previously in the discussion of osmolality.

Variances

The variances or imbalances associated with body water are hypervolemia and hypovolemia. While these labels indicate expansion and contraction of body water, they do not indicate what type of expansion or contraction has occurred. In order to provide that information, the expansion or contraction would need to be further categorized as isosmotic, hyperosmotic, or hyposmotic in relation to normal plasma. This additional categorization would assist the health care personnel in understanding the imbalance more completely. For example, an isosmotic contraction would indicate that the individual had lost equal amounts of solute and water. A hyposmotic expansion would indicate that the individual had gained more water than solute in the process of achieving the imbalance. Obviously, applying this additional classification to the

individual's health state necessitates understanding the etiology of the existing imbalance.

Hypervolemia

Definition

Hypervolemia is an excess in extracellular fluid volume.

Etiology

Excessive extracellular fluid volume can have many specific causes. However, the following three general factors seem to be common to all: (1) increased sodium and water amounts due to retention and/or excessive intake, (2) decreased renal excretion of water and sodium, and (3) decreased mobilization of fluid within the intravascular space.

Some specific causes of an excess in extracellular fluid volume are excessive ingestion or intravenous infusion of sodium chloride, renal dysfunction, inappropriate secretion of antidiuretic hormone, excessive use of adrenal cortical hormone therapy, hyperaldosteronism, hypoproteinemia, cirrhosis, and cardiac dysfunction.

Clinical Assessment Parameters

Clinically, an individual experiencing hypervolemia might exhibit any combination of the following signs and symptoms: acute weight gain, usually in excess of 5 percent of the total body weight; systemic, peripheral edema that may be pitting in nature; puffy eyelids; ascites; increased central venous pressure; hypertension; bounding pulse; dyspnea; and moist rales in the lungs.

Based on the above signs and symptoms, the nurse would focus on the following clinical parameters in order to assess an individual for the presence of hypervolemia: body weight, skin turgor and elasticity, central venous pressure, blood pressure, pulse, respiratory patterns, lung auscultation, cardiac auscultation, and in some cases abdominal girth and neck vein distention.

Laboratory Assessment Data

Data obtained from laboratory testing of blood and urine samples can provide the nurse with valuable information in assessing an individual's internal environment. To interpret the data reported, the nurse must know the normal values for those items tested. While it is true that each institution has its own set of standardized normal values that have been calibrated and calculated according to the specific equipment used, in most cases the normal values tend to be very similar. Table 9-5 presents the normal values for selected substances commonly tested for in the blood, and Table 9-6 presents those values for selected substances commonly tested for in the urine.

Laboratory assessment data may be of dubious assistance in determining the presence of excessive extracellular fluid volume, particularly if it is an isotonic imbalance. However, the following changes are often present: decreased serum values for hematocrit, hemoglobin, and red blood cell counts; and decreased urine values for sodium and specific gravity. Depending upon the etiology of the imbalance, there may also be an increase or decrease in the serum sodium and an increase in the serum blood urea nitrogen and creatinine values.

Clinical and Nursing Implications

The primary clinical implication of hypervolemia for the individual is that it could result in pulmonary edema, a life-threatening complication.

The nursing implications of hypervolemia include performing both monitoring functions and therapeutic interventions. Monitoring functions are (1) to measure all intake and output precisely; (2) to maintain accurate records of all intake and output; (3) to obtain accurate daily weights; (4) to monitor

Table 9-5 Normal Values for Common Blood Laboratory Tests

Item	Normal Values*
Sodium	136–146 meq/L
Potassium	3.5–5.5 meq/L
Chloride	96–106 meq/L
BUN	9–20 mg/100 mL
Creatinine	0.7–1.5 mg/100 mL
Calcium	8.5–10.5 mg/100 mL
Phosphorus	2.0–4.5 mg/100 mL
Carbon dioxide combining power	24–28 meq/L
Magnesium	1.6–2.2 meq/L
Osmolality	280–295 mosmol/kg H_2O
Hematocrit	40–50%
Hemoglobin	12–16 g/100 mL

*Values given are eclectic and for adults.

Table 9-6 Normal Values for Common Urine Laboratory Tests

Item	Normal Values*
Amount	1200–1500 mL
Specific gravity	1.003–1.030
pH	5.0–8.0
Creatinine	1.0–1.6 g/24-h period
Osmolality	50–1200 mosmol/kg H_2O
Sodium	50–130 meq/L
Potassium	20–70 meq/L
Chloride	50–130 meq/L
Calcium	5–12 meq/L
Phosphorus	1 g/24-h period
Magnesium	2–18 meq/L

*Values given are eclectic and for adults.

all vital signs closely; and (5) to observe for peripheral dependent, systemic, and pulmonary edema.

Therapeutic interventions include (1) providing only those fluids and foods that are consistent with the restrictions; (2) administering prescribed diuretics appropriately; and (3) infusing intravenous fluids (if prescribed) at a constant, appropriate rate.

Treatment

Excessive extracellular fluid volume is usually treated by eradicating or dealing therapeutically with the causative factors and decreasing the excess volume. Decreasing the excess volume often involves using diuretics, fluid and sodium restrictions, and in some cases, dialysis therapy.

Edema

Edema is often associated with hypervolemia. However, edema can, and does, accompany other imbalances as well as many pathological conditions. Indeed, edema is such a common occurrence that it warrants further discussion.

Definition

Edema is an excessive accumulation of interstitial fluid. It may be either localized or generalized in nature. Localized edema results from either the activation of the inflammatory process or the decreased physiologic ability to remove interstitial fluid from a specific area of the body. Generalized edema results from clinical dysfunction in a primary body system responsible for transporting and/or regulating fluids and electrolytes. Such body systems include the cardiovascular, renal, lymphatic, endocrine, and hepatic systems.

Etiology

Edema can result from a variety of causes. However, each cause seems to have its origin in one or more of the six influencing factors listed in Table 9-7.

Clinical Assessment Parameters

Clinically, assessment of an edematous individual focuses on the following parameters: (1) the presence and degree of edema; (2) the location and distribution of edema; (3) the color, integrity, turgor, elasticity, sensitivity, and temperature of the skin; (4) the presence and degree of neck vein distention; (5) body weight; (6) vital signs; and (7) the presence and degree of discomfort (particularly in dependent body parts).

Laboratory Assessment Data

Laboratory data most helpful in assessing an individual in terms of edema are serum and urine protein and sodium values. The amounts of these substances vary according to the cause of the edema, but the common pattern seen is that of hypoproteinemia, hypoalbuminemia, proteinuria, albuminuria, and hyponaturia. The serum sodium level varies so greatly depending on the cause that it is difficult to identify any common pattern in edema. It is accurate to say, however, that in some cases of edema, the serum sodium is altered significantly enough to require close monitoring.

Clinical and Nursing Implications

Edema can have several clinical implications for an individual, some of which are very hazardous to well-being. The significance of edema is dependent upon its location, severity, and mobility. Certainly severe, painful edema of dependent extremities is significant, but not as significant as mild or moderate cerebral or pulmonary edema. Generalized edema can pose problems, but those problems can be vastly intensified if the edema is mobilized and large shifts of fluid from the interstitial to the intravascular space occur.

Many of the nursing implications associated with edema are similar to those previously discussed in relation to hypervolemia, especially the monitoring functions. Included in those monitoring functions are (1) monitoring and recording intake and output accurately, (2) assessing the status of edematous tissues, (3) obtaining precise measurements of daily weights, (4) monitoring vital signs and laboratory data periodically, and (5) assessing for changes in venous pressure.

Therapeutic nursing interventions that might be used with an individual with edema include (1) providing only fluids and foods consistent with the prescribed restrictions; (2) administering diuretics and other medications as prescribed; (3) providing meticulous skin care to prevent the breakdown of edematous tissues; (4) maintaining bed rest or a decreased level of activity appropriate to the degree of edema; and (5) promoting comfort in edematous extremities by elevating them, repositioning them carefully and frequently, and ensuring the appropriate use of constrictive and nonconstrictive clothing, coverings, or bandages on them.

Treatment

The treatment of edema is based on four general principles. Those principles are (1) to treat the underlying primary disease or pathology responsible for the edema, (2) to restrict the amount of salt and water intake based on the needs of the patient, (3) to promote the mobilization of edema fluid, and (4) to promote the excretion of edema fluid. Adherence to these treatment principles usu-

Table 9-7 Factors Influencing Edema Formation

Factor	Clinical Examples
Sustained increase in capillary pressure	Dependent venous stasis Thrombophlebitis
Decreased plasma oncotic pressure	Starvation-catabolic states Nephrotic syndrome
Decreased tissue pressure	Malnutrition Glucocorticosteroid therapy
Increased capillary permeability	Burns Infection
Lymphatic obstruction	Neoplasms Burns
Dilation of precapillary sphincters	Insect toxins Inflammation

ally results in a decrease in, if not total resolution of, the edema.

Hypovolemia

Definition
Hypovolemia is a deficit in extracellular fluid volume.

Etiology
Extracellular fluid volume deficit occurs as a result of any one of the following three abnormal physiologic processes: (1) excessive loss of fluids and electrolytes, (2) decreased intake of fluids and electrolytes, and (3) shifts of fluids and electrolytes into nonaccessible areas such as third spaces.

The process of losing excessive amounts of fluids and electrolytes seems to be the underlying mechanism in most etiologies of hypovolemia. The most common reasons for such losses are vomiting, gastrointestinal suction, diarrhea, draining fistulas or wounds, systemic infection, profuse diaphoresis, burns, and excessive use of diuretics.

The two causes of hypovolemia due to a decreased intake of fluids and electrolytes are (1) coma, an inability to swallow, or any other state in which it is physically impossible for the individual to ingest substances; and (2) the absence or unavailability of fluids and electrolytes.

The process of "third spacing," or the shifting of extracellular fluid into cavities where it accumulates and is physiologically inaccessible for use by the body, is another underlying mechanism for hypovolemia. Clinical examples of third spacing include ascites, peritonitis, intestinal obstruction, burns, and pancreatitis.

Clinical Assessment Parameters
An individual with an extracellular fluid volume deficit will exhibit any number of the following clinical signs and symptoms: acute weight loss, usually in excess of 5 percent of the total body weight; dry skin and mucous membranes; decreased skin turgor and elasticity; longitudinal wrinkling or furrows of the tongue; subnormal body temperature; lassitude or fatigue; oliguria or in a few cases anuria; thirst; decreased postural systolic blood pressure; decreased tension or turgor of the eyeball; decreased venous pressure; increased pulse rate;

and decreased perspiration. Of all these parameters, body weight is considered by many to be the most important indicator of a person's fluid balance. In fact, body weight has been used to roughly categorize degrees of extracellular fluid volume deficit. Table 9-8 presents one such categorization.

Laboratory Assessment Data
The laboratory data that are the most useful in assessing an individual for hypovolemia include serum hemoglobin, hematocrit, red blood cell count, and BUN levels; and urine sodium, chloride, and specific gravity values. The urine-to-serum osmolality ratio also provides valuable assessment data, as can the serum sodium if the cause of the imbalance is considered. The pattern of these values exhibited by an individual experiencing hypovolemia includes increased serum values for hematocrit, hemoglobin, red blood cell count, and blood urea nitrogen; decreased urine values for sodium and chloride; increased urinary specific gravity; increased urine-to-serum osmolality ratio; and variable serum sodium values depending on the etiology of the imbalance.

The importance of including urine values in an assessment of an individual for hypovolemia should be emphasized. Many clinicians feel that the urine values may provide the earliest signs of hypovolemia. The parameters most frequently cited as guidelines for determining if the specific urine values are indicative of hypovolemia are a sodium content less than 20 meq/L, a specific gravity greater than 1.026, and a urine-to-serum osmolality ratio greater than 2.

Clinical and Nursing Implications
The clinical significance of hypovolemia for a patient is that there are insufficient body fluids to carry out

Table 9-8 Degrees of Extracellular Fluid Volume Deficit According to Percent Loss of Total Body Weight

Degree of Extracellular Fluid Volume Deficit	Loss of Total Body Weight, Percent
Mild	2–5
Moderate	6–10
Severe	11–15
Fatal	> 15

the normal physiologic and metabolic processes necessary to sustain life. Of course, the more severe the imbalance the greater the threat to the patient's well-being.

Nursing monitoring functions related to hypovolemia include (1) obtaining accurate daily weights; (2) measuring and recording *all* intake and output accurately; (3) assessing vital signs, venous pressure, and laboratory data periodically; (4) measuring expanded third-space areas, such as the abdomen, frequently; (5) assessing the status of the skin and mucous membranes periodically; and (6) continuously evaluating the individual's overall energy level.

Nursing interventions used with an individual with hypovolemia are (1) to administer intravenous replacement fluids precisely at a constant rate; (2) to ensure that all fluids administered to the individual, including irrigation solutions, are of the appropriate electrolyte balance; (3) to provide frequent oral hygiene to maintain the integrity and hydration state of the mucous membranes; and (4) to provide skin care to decrease breakdown and promote integrity.

Treatment

The treatment of hypovolemia has two components. The first component is to treat or correct the primary cause of the imbalance. The second component is to replace lost fluids and electrolytes.

Replacement therapy is usually instituted according to a tri-level approach. The first level is based on an assessment of the individual's renal status. If there is a question as to the adequacy of the individual's renal function, a hydrating solution is given to challenge the renal system and promote function. This hydrating solution is usually composed of water, carbohydrate (in the form of 5% dextrose), sodium, and chloride. Once adequate renal function has been established, replacement therapy moves to the second level.

The second level of replacement therapy can be initiated as soon as it has been determined that renal function is adequate. Thus, in some cases, the first-level replacement can be deleted and replacement therapy actually begins with second-level solutions. Second-level solutions are balanced solutions designed to supply water, calories, and electrolytes in sufficient quantities to meet the maintenance needs of the body as well as to correct existing deficits. These solutions are composed of physiologic proportionate amounts of water, carbohydrate, sodium, potassium, magnesium, chloride, phosphate, and lactate. These balanced solutions are often called *all-purpose* solutions and are utilized frequently in fluid replacement therapy.

Third-level replacement therapy is aimed at replacing specific, concurrent, or ongoing water and electrolyte losses. This level of therapy involves using solutions individually mixed to replace specific fluid and electrolyte losses, such as those created by gastrointestinal suction or fistula drainage. These solutions are composed of water, carbohydrate, and varying amounts of specific electrolytes selected to meet the needs of the patient. It is not uncommon in replacement therapy to see both balanced solutions and specifically created solutions used simultaneously to achieve and maintain proper balance.

Sodium

Functions

Sodium, the major cation of extracellular fluid, has four general functions in the body. Those functions are (1) to promote the normal distribution and volume of fluids in the body by creating and maintaining the normal osmolality of those fluids; (2) to enhance the transcellular movement of substances by altering cell permeability; (3) to promote normal neuromuscular irritability by enhancing the conduction and transmission of electrochemical impulses; and (4) to contribute to the regulation of acid-base balance by exchanging with selected cations such as potassium and hydrogen, and combining with certain anions such as chloride and bicarbonate.

Regulation

The renal system, in concert with other mechanisms, has primary responsibility for regulating the reabsorption and excretion of sodium. Approximately 99 percent of the total filtered load of sodium is reabsorbed by various parts of the nephron, leaving only about 1 percent to be excreted in the urine.

Of the 99 percent that is reabsorbed, about 70 percent is actively reabsorbed in the proximal tubule, 20 percent is passively reabsorbed in the loop of Henle, 8 percent is actively reabsorbed in the distal tubule, and about 1 percent is actively reabsorbed in the collecting duct. This reabsorption and excretion of sodium is influenced by several factors, many of which are related to maintaining an effective arterial blood volume. Those influencing factors include glomerulotubular balance, aldosterone, third factor, the redistribution of renal blood flow, peritubular capillary oncotic pressure, the serum sodium concentration, catecholamines, and prostaglandins.

Glomerulotubular Balance

Glomerulotubular balance is the phenomenon of having the rate of tubular sodium reabsorption change in the same direction as the filtered load of sodium because of alterations in the glomerular filtration rate. This mechanism prevents the loss of large amounts of sodium that would result from increases in the glomerular filtration rate.

Aldosterone

Aldosterone is a mineralocorticoid hormone that is secreted through the activation of the renin-angiotensin system in response to a real or perceived decrease in effective arterial volume. Aldosterone acts on the distal renal tubule to promote increased sodium and water reabsorption and potassium excretion.

Third Factor

"Third factor" is thought to be a natriuretic regulatory mechanism that increases the renal excretion of sodium in the presence of saline volume expansion. The factor is thought to function independently of aldosterone and glomerular filtration rate in regulating sodium excretion. Research continues to be conducted on third factor to determine its precise physiologic nature and composition.

Redistribution of Renal Blood Flow

The redistribution of renal blood flow occurs as a result of a reduction in effective arterial volume sufficient enough to decrease the total blood flow to the kidneys. In such a situation, blood is shunted from the cortical nephrons to the juxtamedullary nephrons. The juxtamedullary nephrons, with their long loops of Henle, tend to retain more sodium for reabsorption than do the cortical nephrons. Thus, this selective perfusion of the juxtamedullary nephrons promotes the increased reabsorption of sodium.

Peritubular Capillary Oncotic Pressure

The peritubular capillaries regulate sodium reabsorption and excretion according to the amount of oncotic pressure in them. An increased protein concentration (usually resulting from a volume and/or sodium deficit), which increases the oncotic pressure, promotes the reabsorption of sodium and water from the nephron. This process assists in returning the peritubular capillary oncotic pressure to normal.

Serum Sodium Concentration

Serum sodium levels seem to have an influence on sodium reabsorption and excretion, but the exact mechanism for this influence is not known. However, it is known that hyponatremia promotes, and hypernatremia inhibits, sodium reabsorption by the renal tubules.

Catecholamines

Catecholamines are thought to enhance sodium reabsorption, but again, the mechanism for this action is not clearly understood. There seem to be differing opinions as to whether the effect of the catecholamines is direct or indirect in relation to sodium reabsorption.

Prostaglandins

The role of prostaglandins in the regulation of sodium is controversial at this time. It seems that certain prostaglandins may have a natriuretic effect, but the mechanism for that effect is not at all clear. Further research is required on prostaglandins, as well as other factors, before all of the mechanisms involved in sodium regulation are precisely comprehended.

Variances

The variances or imbalances related to sodium are hypernatremia and hyponatremia. It should be noted, however, that serum sodium levels cannot be assessed in isolation. For when serum sodium levels are assessed, it is sodium concentration that is being assessed and concentration should not be evaluated without considering fluid volume. Indeed, the variances in serum sodium can occur in conjunction with euvolemia, hypovolemia, or hypervolemia. Thus, serum sodium and fluid volume should be assessed concurrently. Such an assessment, then, makes it possible to determine, for example, if an increased serum sodium level is actually due to hypernatremia, or if it is merely a reflection of hypovolemia. In the latter instance, the serum sodium level is not indicative of total body sodium, which might be normal. Rather, it is indicative of having the same amount of sodium present in less fluid volume. With this caution in mind, the discussion concerning hypernatremia and hyponatremia can proceed.

Hypernatremia

Definition
Hypernatremia is an excess of sodium in the extracellular fluid.

Etiology
Hypernatremia can result from two types of causes: (1) those that promote either the loss of water in excess of sodium loss or the inadequate replacement of water; and (2) those that foster sodium retention or excess. Examples of the first type are decreased water intake, the inability to swallow, unconsciousness, the unavailability of fluids, vomiting, diarrhea, diabetes insipidus, osmotic diuresis, fever, heat stroke, high environmental temperatures, hyperventilation, and dialysis therapy. Examples of the second type are excessive ingestion or infusion of sodium chloride, ingestion of seawater, acidosis, renal dysfunction, primary hyperaldosteronism, excessive use of corticosteroid therapy, and neurological lesions.

Clinical Assessment Parameters
The hypernatremic individual usually exhibits many of the following signs and symptoms: dry, sticky mucous membranes; a rough, dry tongue; flushed, dry skin; increased tissue turgor; thirst; decreased lacrimation; elevated body temperature; tachycardia; oliguria; lethargy; central nervous system irritability; muscular rigidity and weakness; tremors; seizures; and coma.

Laboratory Assessment Data
The laboratory values that provide the most data for assessing a patient for hypernatremia are serum sodium and chloride, and urine sodium, chloride, osmolality, and specific gravity. The levels of those values that provide a general pattern consistent with hypernatremia are the following: a serum sodium greater than 146 meq/L, a serum chloride greater than 106 meq/L, a urine sodium less than 50 meq/L, a urine chloride less than 50 meq/L, a urine osmolality of greater than 800 mosmol/L, and a urine specific gravity greater than 1.030.

Clinical and Nursing Implications
Hypernatremia can result in serious clinical difficulties for an individual. Probably the most significant problems are those related to the central nervous system and neuromuscular functioning. Certainly it is easy to visualize the effects of muscular hyperirritability, seizures, and coma on one's health state. Such problems are definitely a threat to well-being and necessitate appropriate nursing support.

The nursing support related to hypernatremia includes the following monitoring functions: (1) assessing the skin turgor, temperature, color, and moisture; (2) assessing the moisture of the tongue and mucous membranes; (3) obtaining precise daily weights; (4) measuring and recording intake and output accurately; (5) monitoring vital signs and laboratory values periodically; (6) assessing muscle movement; and probably the most important function, (7) assessing the neurological status and level of consciousness frequently.

Nursing interventions that provide support for the hypernatremic patient are: (1) providing fluids and foods consistent with the prescribed restrictions; (2) maintaining skin integrity through the use of meticulous hygienic measures, moisturizing agents, and frequent repositioning; (3) maintaining the integrity of the oral cavity with frequent oral care employing a variety of nondehydrating agents; (4) promoting comfort by decreasing thirst using a variety of creative measures; (5) instituting seizure precautions; and (6) providing for the patient's general, overall environmental safety.

Treatment

The treatment for hypernatremia revolves around treating the cause and correcting the imbalance. The ideal form of treatment is to treat the primary disorder that perpetuates the imbalance, and whenever possible, this is done. The second part of the treatment, correcting the imbalance, is based on the nature of the etiology. The general parameters for therapeutic intervention are: (1) if the imbalance is due to a loss of extracellular fluid, intravenous isotonic saline solution will be administered to correct the imbalance; and (2) if the imbalance is due to a sodium excess, the individual's daily sodium intake will be restricted to anywhere from 0.5 g to 2 g, and intravenous 5% dextrose and water will be given to replace the intracellular fluid deficit created by the hypernatremia. More specific therapeutic guidelines are presented in Table 9-9.

Hyponatremia

Definition

Hyponatremia is a deficit of sodium in the extracellular fluid.

Etiology

Hyponatremia has two types of causes: (1) those that produce dilutional extracellular fluid expansion, and (2) those that result in a deficit of sodium. The causes of dilutional hyponatremia are excessive ingestion or infusion of electrolyte-free solutions, excessive use of tap water enemas, irrigation of gastrointestinal tubes with electrolyte-free solutions, renal dysfunction, inappropriate secretion of antidiuretic hormone, cirrhosis, congestive heart failure, and hyperglycemia. (In the case of hyperglycemia, it has been estimated that each 100 mg/100 mL increase in the glucose concentration above normal results in sufficient extracellular fluid volume expansion to decrease the serum sodium concentration by about 1.6 meq/L.)

A deficit of sodium is caused by inadequate ingestion of dietary sodium, infusions of solutions that are sodium-deficient, salt-wasting renal dysfunction, potent diuretic therapy, adrenal insufficiency, severe vomiting, severe diarrhea, excessive perspiration, gastrointestinal suction, potassium depletion, burns, "third spacing," and severe malnutrition.

Clinical Assessment Parameters

An individual experiencing hyponatremia may exhibit any combination of the following signs and symptoms: fatigue, muscle weakness, lethargy, confusion, headache, tremors, hyperreflexia, convulsions, coma, apprehension, anorexia, nausea, vomiting, abdominal cramps, diarrhea, and oliguria. As with hypernatremia, the neurological signs and symptoms of hyponatremia seem to be the most clinically significant. However, because the neuro-

Table 9-9 Guidelines for Treating Hypernatremia

Volume Status	Urine Osmolality	Urine Na+	Treatment
Hypovolemia	Hypertonic	<10 meq/L	Isotonic saline IV followed by hypotonic saline IV or oral water
Hypovolemia or euvolemia	Isotonic or hypotonic	>20 meq/L	Isotonic saline IV followed by hypotonic saline IV or oral water
Hypovolemia or euvolemia	Hypotonic, isotonic, or hypertonic	Variable (usually >20 meq/L)	Water replacement as hypotonic IV fluid or oral water
Hypovolemia or euvolemia	Hypertonic	Variable (usually >20 meq/L)	Water replacement as hypotonic IV fluid or oral water
Hypervolemia or euvolemia	Isotonic or hypertonic	>20 meq/L (usually much greater)	Water replacement as hypotonic IV fluid or oral water and diuretics

logical signs and symptoms are so similar in the two conditions, they offer little help in differentiating between the two states. Therefore, the gastrointestinal signs and symptoms may be more discriminating, even if clinically less significant, in identifying hyponatremia.

Laboratory Assessment Data

Hyponatremia can be identified from an assessment of the following laboratory data: serum sodium and chloride, and urine sodium, osmolality, and specific gravity. The general pattern characteristic of hyponatremia is a serum sodium less than 136 meq/L, a serum chloride less than 96 meq/L, a variable urine sodium, usually less than 20 meq/L, a urine osmolality less than 300 mosmol/L, and a urine specific gravity less than 1.010.

Clinical and Nursing Implications

Clinically, hyponatremia can be a life-threatening imbalance, depending on its severity. The hazards to the patient stem from the effects of the imbalance on the central nervous system. These effects, ranging anywhere from mere confusion to convulsions and coma, certainly represent a threat to the individual's health state. These effects, however, usually do not occur unless the serum sodium falls to less than 120 meq/L.

Nursing monitoring functions that are performed in relation to hyponatremia include (1) assessing levels of consciousness and central nervous system functioning frequently, (2) assessing muscle strength and energy levels periodically, (3) obtaining precise daily weights, (4) measuring and recording intake and output accurately, and (5) monitoring vital signs and laboratory data at intervals.

Nursing interventions that would be performed with an individual with hyponatremia are (1) giving foods and fluids high in sodium content as prescribed; (2) maintaining fluid restrictions as prescribed (interventions 1 and 2 are *not* done in concert, since the first aims at replacement therapy and the second at returning a diluted, expanded extracellular fluid volume to normal); (3) instituting seizure precautions; (4) promoting the conservation of energy by limiting activity; (5) establishing a physical environment conducive to maintaining the individual's safety and orientation; and (6) promoting overall comfort by using creative pain-relieving methods and administering medications as prescribed.

Treatment

The treatment of hyponatremia depends, of course, on its etiology. The first goal of therapy is to treat the cause or primary disorder responsible for producing the imbalance. The second goal is to treat the imbalance. The general parameters for therapeutic intervention are: (1) if the imbalance is the result of a dilutional expansion of the extracellular fluid, treatment will consist of restricting the fluid intake (and in some cases administering diuretics); and (2) if the imbalance is due to sodium loss, replacement therapy in the form of oral preparations, dietary provisions, or hypertonic or isotonic saline infusions will be instituted. More specific therapeutic guidelines are presented in Table 9-10.

Table 9-10 Guidelines for Treating Hyponatremia

Volume Status	Urine Osmolality	Urine Na⁺	Treatment
Hypovolemia	Hypertonic	<10 meq/L	Isotonic saline IV
Hypovolemia	Hypotonic, isotonic, or hypertonic	>20 meq/L	Isotonic saline IV, possibly accompanied by moderate water restriction
Euvolemia	Hypertonic	>20 meq/L	Fluid restriction, possibly accompanied by salt replacement and/or diuretics
Hypervolemia	Hypertonic	<10 meq/L	Fluid restriction
Hypervolemia	Isotonic or hypertonic	>20 meq/L	Fluid restriction

Potassium

Functions

Potassium, the major cation of the intracellular fluid, has several important physiologic functions that it performs in the body. Those functions include (1) creating and maintaining the osmotic pressure of the intracellular fluid, (2) maintaining the transmembrane electrical potential difference between the extracellular and intracellular spaces that regulates neuromuscular excitability and is necessary for muscle contraction, (3) participating in the maintenance of acid-base balance, (4) enhancing the synthesis of protein, and (5) participating in the metabolism of carbohydrates and synthesis of glycogen.

Regulation

Potassium is regulated primarily by the renal system. Although some potassium is lost in perspiration and the feces, the kidneys remain the foremost organs for the excretion and reabsorption of potassium. The renal handling of potassium begins at the glomerulus where it is filtered. Of that filtered load of potassium, about 70 percent is actively reabsorbed in the proximal tubule, 20 percent is passively reabsorbed in the loop of Henle, and the remaining 10 percent is delivered to the distal tubule. Further active reabsorption can occur in the distal tubule and collecting duct, depending on the level of potassium in the body. The *principal* activity of the distal tubule, however, is the active or passive secretion of potassium. This distal tubular secretion, the main regulator of renal potassium excretion, is influenced by the following factors: aldosterone, the amount of sodium delivered to the distal tubule, hydrogen ion secretion, the presence of nonreabsorbable anions, urine flow rates, potassium intake, and diuretic therapy.

Aldosterone

Aldosterone, a mineralocorticoid hormone, increases potassium excretion through two very interrelated mechanisms. The first mechanism is related to the increased permeability of the distal tubular luminal membrane to potassium and sodium that is produced by aldosterone. This change

in permeability enhances the diffusion of potassium out of the tubular cell into the lumen where it can be excreted. It also enhances the entry of sodium from the lumen into the tubular cell which facilitates active sodium reabsorption. The increase in sodium reabsorption increases the transmembrane potential difference in the distal tubule, which facilitates the passive diffusion of potassium into the lumen for excretion.

The second mechanism is related to the increased concentration of potassium in the tubular cell that is produced by aldosterone. Aldosterone stimulates the peritubular uptake of potassium, thus increasing the concentration in the tubular cell. This increase in concentration enhances the passive diffusion of potassium into the lumen where it can be excreted.

Sodium Delivery to the Distal Tubule

The effect of the concentration of distal tubular sodium on potassium excretion has been mentioned in the previous discussion on aldosterone. When increased concentrations of sodium are delivered to the distal tubule, the amount of sodium that is reabsorbed is increased. The increased reabsorption of sodium creates an increase in the transmembrane potential difference which facilitates the passive diffusion of potassium into the tubular lumen where it can be excreted. Thus, the end result is an increase in urinary potassium excretion.

Hydrogen Ion Secretion

The secretion of distal tubular potassium is influenced by the rate of hydrogen ion secretion. In acute acidotic conditions, there is an extracellular to intracellular shift of hydrogen ions and an intracellular to extracellular shift of potassium. The lower intracellular concentration of potassium in the distal tubular cells decreases the electrical and chemical gradients that enhance the passive secretion of potassium into the lumen. This results in a decreased renal secretion and excretion of potassium, accompanied by a preferential obligatory secretion of hydrogen ions that is facilitated by the increase in the intracellular concentration of hydrogen ions. Of course, the reverse of this process occurs in alkalotic states, and there is an increased urinary excretion of potassium.

Nonreabsorbable Anions

Nonreabsorbable anions, such as phosphate, sulfate, and bicarbonate, are those anions that cannot accompany reabsorbed sodium as easily as chloride does. When there are increased amounts of these anions in the distal tubular fluid, the negative transmembrane electrical gradient is increased as sodium is reabsorbed, resulting in an increased diffusion of potassium into the lumen. Thus, this mechanism increases the urinary excretion of potassium.

Urine Flow Rates

Urine flow rates seem to have some correlation with urinary potassium secretion and excretion rates. When urine flow increases, so does potassium secretion and excretion. Likewise, when urine flow decreases, there is also a decrease in the urinary secretion and excretion of potassium. The mechanisms responsible for these variations seem to be the increased sodium concentration that accompanies the urine flow to the distal tubule and the decreased reabsorption of potassium that results from the low potassium concentration of the luminal fluid. Both of these factors contribute to the increased urinary excretion rates of potassium in the presence of high urine flow rates.

. Potassium Intake

An increase in the extracellular concentration of potassium due to increased intake increases the urinary secretion and excretion rate of potassium. The effect of an increased extracellular potassium concentration on the rate of urinary secretion and excretion of potassium results from its participation in the following processes: (1) the production of a higher tubular luminal concentration of potassium, (2) the stimulation of increased aldosterone secretion, (3) the production of an increased transmembrane potential difference at the distal tubular cell, and (4) the stimulation of sodium-potassium-adenosine triphosphatase which increases the rate of potassium flow across the peritubular cell membranes.

Diuretic Therapy

Most of the pharmacologic agents that produce diuresis are kaliuretic in nature and result in increased urinary losses of potassium. The mechanisms by which they produce this effect vary according to the specific diuretic employed. However, most of them function by either increasing the urinary flow rate, decreasing potassium reabsorption, increasing sodium delivery to the distal tubule, or altering the transmembrane potential.

Variances

The variances associated with potassium are hyperkalemia and hypokalemia.

Hyperkalemia

Definition

Hyperkalemia is an excess of potassium in the extracellular fluid.

Etiology

The etiologies of hyperkalemia can be classified into three general categories based on the mechanism by which they produce the excess in potassium. Those categories are decreased renal excretion, translocation from the cells, and increased intake. Those etiologies that result in hyperkalemia because of a decreased renal excretion include renal dysfunction, adrenocortical insufficiencies such as Addison's disease and hyporeninemic hypoaldosteronism, and the use of potassium-sparing diuretics such as spironolactone or triamterene.

Those etiologies that result in hyperkalemia because of the translocation of potassium from the intracellular to the extracellular fluid space include severe catabolism, burns, rhabdomyolysis, acute acidosis, intravascular hemolysis, and hyperkalemic familial periodic paralysis.

Hyperkalemia can also be caused by the excessive intake of potassium, usually in the form of intravenous infusions or the oral ingestion of medications or food substances that are high in potassium. This etiology, however, is rarely the cause of hyperkalemia if the individual has normal renal function. This is because in most instances it is difficult to exceed the renal capacity for excreting potassium, so even additional loads of potassium are easily excreted. The renal excretion capacity can be exceeded, however, by large bolus intravenous infusions of potassium.

In addition to all the above causes of hyperkalemia, there are other changes that occur in the body that produce a false hyperkalemia. Pseudo-hyperkalemia can result from the following: increased leukocyte or thrombocyte counts, the hemolysis of drawn blood samples, and using a tourniquet to assist in drawing blood samples.

Clinical Assessment Parameters

Most of the clinical signs and symptoms of hyperkalemia are related to the neuromuscular, cardiac, and gastrointestinal systems. Those signs and symptoms as exhibited by the hyperkalemic individual include mental confusion, neuromuscular hyperexcitability, weakness, paresthesia, ascending flaccid paralysis, cardiac dysfunction (as described below), cardiac arrest, abdominal distention, diarrhea, intestinal colic, and oliguria (which is more a reflection of the etiology than an effect of the imbalance).

The cardiac dysfunction that occurs in response to hyperkalemia seems to follow a distinct pattern. The earliest signs of dysfunction are seen on the electrocardiogram in the form of tall, peaked, tented T waves and a depressed ST segment. As the imbalance progresses, the P waves decrease in amplitude and the P-R interval is prolonged. Then atrial asystole occurs with a widened QRS complex that eventually merges with the T wave forming the sine wave characteristic of hyperkalemia. Dysrhythmia, fibrillation, and cardiac arrest can occur at any time during the above sequence of events, depending on the severity and rate of progression of the hyperkalemia.

Laboratory Assessment Data

The laboratory value that provides the most data in assessing an individual for hyperkalemia is the serum potassium. A serum potassium level greater than 5.5 meq/L is indicative of hyperkalemia.

The urinary potassium value may provide additional data. However, this value will vary depending on the etiology of the imbalance and thus may be more reflective of the specific etiology than of the existence or magnitude of the imbalance.

Clinical and Nursing Implications

The clinical significance of hyperkalemia is based on its profound effect on the neuromuscular and cardiac systems. Certainly nothing could be worse for a patient than paralysis or cardiac arrest.

The nursing implications associated with hyperkalemia include monitoring or assessing the following: (1) rate, rhythm, and characteristics of the pulse (with or without a cardiac monitor); (2) level of consciousness and orientation; (3) muscle strength, sensation, and movement; (4) characteristics of the abdomen; (5) characteristics of the feces; (6) laboratory values; and (7) urinary output.

Also included in the nursing implications of hyperkalemia are the following interventions: (1) providing only those foods and fluids that are consistent with the prescribed potassium restriction; (2) administering medications as prescribed; (3) establishing a safe physical environment for the individual; (4) providing stimuli appropriate for enhancing orientation; (5) instituting limited active or passive range of motion exercises; (6) assisting with the normal activities of daily living; and (7) providing meticulous skin care at the rectal orifice.

Treatment

The treatment of hyperkalemia focuses on eliminating the primary cause and correcting the imbalance. Measures for correcting the imbalance are aimed at (1) reducing potassium intake, (2) antagonizing the membrane effect of hyperkalemia, (3) shifting the potassium intracellularly, and (4) increasing the excretion of potassium.

Reducing the potassium intake is accomplished by restricting the amounts of potassium ingested in dietary substances or medications and/or infused in intravenous solutions. The usual daily restriction of potassium is about 40 meq, but this amount can vary according to the specific needs of the individual.

The agents most frequently used to antagonize the effect of hyperkalemia on the cell membrane are calcium salts, such as calcium chloride, or hypertonic sodium salts, such as sodium chloride or sodium bicarbonate. While these agents may be very successful in treating severe cases of hyperkalemia quickly (because they are effective within 1 to 5 min after administration), they are also therapeutically very transient and last only 30 min. Furthermore, they have no effect on either serum or total body potassium levels.

Infusions of glucose and insulin or sodium bicarbonate will correct hyperkalemia by facilitating the shift of potassium into the cell. For example, when 1 g of glucose is converted to glycogen, approximately 3.6 meq/L of potassium are retained intracellularly. The glucose and insulin therapy becomes effective about 10 to 15 min after infusion, but the sodium bicarbonate requires about an hour. Both agents produce only a temporary correction of the imbalance that is perhaps 2 to 4 h in duration. Both agents will decrease the serum potassium level but have no effect on total body potassium.

The increased excretion of potassium is effected through the use of sodium chloride infusions, cation exchange resins, diuretics, and dialysis. Sodium chloride infusions are effective within 1 h but do not last very long. The infusions are effective in reducing the serum potassium level but have only a slight effect on the total body potassium. Cation exchange resins, diuretics, and dialysis are effective within minutes to hours and last longer than the other types of therapies mentioned. All these methods are effective in decreasing both the serum and total body potassium levels.

Hypokalemia

Definition
Hypokalemia is a deficit of potassium in the extracellular fluid.

Etiology
Hypokalemia results from the following five categories of causes: (1) an increased intracellular shift of potassium, (2) decreased potassium intake, (3) increased gastrointestinal potassium loss, (4) excessive renal potassium loss, and (5) excessive integumentary potassium loss.

Specific etiologies that cause hypokalemia by enhancing the intracellular shift of potassium are acute alkalosis, the intravenous infusion of glucose and insulin, and familial hypokalemic periodic paralysis.

The etiologies that produce hypokalemia as a result of decreased intake are the inability to physically ingest fluids or foods, the unavailability of food or fluids, the infusion of large quantities of potassium-free intravenous solutions, and the prolonged ingestion of diets deficient in potassium.

Increasing the gastrointestinal loss of potassium is the mechanism by which the following etiologies cause hypokalemia: vomiting, fistulas, malabsorption, diarrhea, inflammatory bowel disease, laxative abuse, and ureterosigmoidostomies.

Etiologies that produce hypokalemia by increasing the renal excretion of potassium include diuretic therapy, renal tubular acidosis, chronic interstitial nephritis, primary and secondary hyperaldosteronism, Cushing's syndrome, adrenal steroid therapy, the excessive ingestion of mineralocorticoid-like substances such as licorice, and diabetic ketoacidosis.

The loss of potassium through the integument in the form of excessive perspiration also causes hypokalemia. This etiology is most frequently observed in individuals who exercise or work intensely in hot climates.

Clinical Assessment Parameters
The clinical manifestations of hypokalemia are evident in almost every system of the body. This imbalance seems to produce signs and symptoms in the neuromuscular, cardiovascular, respiratory, gastrointestinal, endocrine, and renal systems. Table 9-11 summarizes the signs and symptoms of hypokalemia that are observed in those body systems.

Table 9-11 Signs and Symptoms of Hypokalemia According to Body Systems

System	Signs and Symptoms
Neuromuscular	Drowsiness, confusion, apathy, irritability, coma, muscle weaknesses, paresthesias, muscle pain, muscle cramps, muscle tenderness, hyporeflexia, tetany, paralysis
Cardiovascular	Weak pulse; bradycardia; ECG changes, including a depressed S-T segment; flattened, inverted T waves; and U waves
Respiratory	Muscle weakness, hypoventilation
Gastrointestinal	Nausea, vomiting, anorexia, abdominal distention, abdominal cramps, paralytic ileus
Endocrine	Polydipsia, hyperglycemia, and in some cases negative nitrogen balance
Renal	Polyuria, nocturia

Laboratory Assessment Data

The most significant laboratory values used in assessing an individual for hypokalemia are the serum values for potassium, bicarbonate, and pH. A serum potassium of less than 3.5 meq/L and an increased plasma bicarbonate and pH are indicative of hypokalemia.

Other laboratory values that provide additional information in assessing for hypokalemia are the following: urine osmolality, pH, potassium, and phosphate. The levels of those urine values that are consistent with hypokalemia are a decreased osmolality, a decreased pH, a normal potassium (within the first 3 weeks of the imbalance, then it decreases), and an increased phosphate.

Clinical and Nursing Implications

Hypokalemia presents many clinical problems for the individual. The most significant of those problems are the apnea, cardiac dysrhythmias, muscle paralysis, and paralytic ileus that may develop as the hypokalemia progresses in severity. With the possibility of such severe alterations occurring, the implications for nursing support are crucial.

Nursing support includes the following monitoring functions: (1) assessing the rate, rhythm, and characteristics of the respirations and the pulse (with or without a cardiac monitor); (2) monitoring all other vital signs; (3) assessing the level of consciousness frequently; (4) evaluating muscle strength, movement, and sensation; (5) assessing the characteristics of the abdomen; (6) monitoring bowel sounds; (7) measuring and recording intake and output accurately; and (8) monitoring the appropriate laboratory values.

Nursing support for the patient with hypokalemia also includes the following interventions: (1) administering oral or intravenous potassium preparations carefully and as prescribed; (2) positioning the individual to facilitate adequate respirations; (3) providing appropriate stimuli to promote orientation; (4) establishing a safe physical environment for the individual; (5) providing creative comfort measures; and (6) assisting the individual with the normal activities of daily living.

Treatment

The treatment of hypokalemia involves eliminating the cause, if possible, and correcting the imbalance.

The preferred method for correcting hypokalemia is to replace the deficit orally with high-potassium foods or potassium supplements. (When liquid potassium preparations are given, they should be well diluted to decrease gastrointestinal irritation.) Using this method of replacement therapy decreases the likelihood of creating a rebound hyperkalemia.

Intravenous potassium chloride is usually used to replace acute potassium deficits. The potassium chloride is generally infused into a peripheral vein at a rate of 10 to 20 meq/h using a concentration of 40 meq/L. This rate and concentration ensures that the deficit will be slowly but adequately corrected with minimum risk to the individual.

Calcium

Functions

Calcium, an important, abundant cation in the body, is involved in a variety of physiologic functions. Included among those functions are the following: (1) participating in bone formation and metabolism; (2) influencing neural transmission and function; (3) initiating muscle contraction; (4) participating as a coenzyme in blood coagulation and activation of the complement system; (5) influencing cardiac action potential; (6) participating in the regulation of many enzyme systems; (7) influencing the secretion of blood exocrine and endocrine glands; and (8) preserving the functional integrity of cellular membranes.

Regulation

Serum calcium is regulated primarily by exchange between the extracellular fluid and the intestines, bones, and kidneys. Figure 9-5 illustrates these regulatory relationships and indicates their relative importance by the size of the arrows. These exchanges, or relationships, are influenced by a variety of hormonal and other factors as summarized in Table 9-12.

Intestines

The intestines absorb from 25 to 70 percent of the dietary calcium ingested. The efficiency of this absorption seems to vary inversely with the amount of calcium ingested. The absorption process is

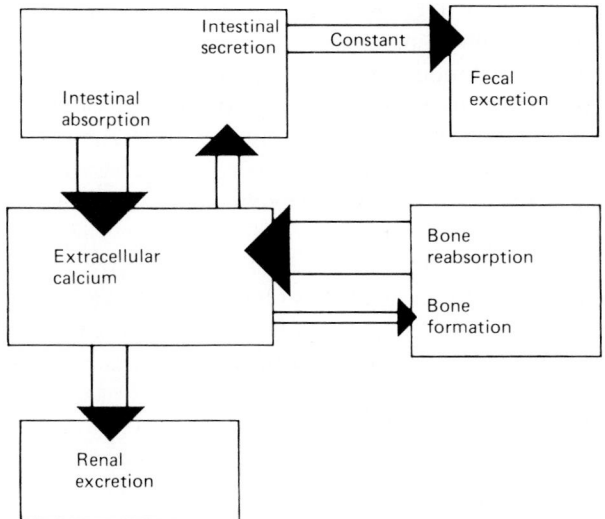

Figure 9-5   Mechanisms for regulating extracellular calcium (arrow size indicates relative importance).

of amount and is not dependent upon the quantity ingested.

Bones

The movement of calcium to and from the bones contributes significantly to maintaining a normal extracellular ionized calcium concentration. While it seems that the rates of bone formation (calcium deposition) and bone resorption (calcium release) participate in the exchange process equally, that is not the case. Bone resorption appears to be the principal process involved in the exchange and thus compensates for lowered serum calcium levels. Bone resorption is stimulated by vitamin D, parathyroid hormone, thyroid hormone, prostaglandins, and acidosis. It is inhibited by thyrocalcitonin, glucocorticoid hormones, androgen, estrogen, hyperphosphatemia, and alkalosis.

Kidneys

The renal system regulates calcium by maintaining a balance between intake and output. The renal regulation of calcium is mainly excretory in nature and varies according to dietary intake. Of the filtered calcium load, about 55 percent is reabsorbed in the proximal tubule, about 30 percent is reabsorbed in the loop of Henle, and about 12 percent is reabsorbed in the distal tubule. The remaining 3

enhanced by vitamin D, parathyroid hormone, and growth hormone. It is inhibited by thyrocalcitonin and glucocorticoid hormones.

In addition to supplying the body with essential calcium by the absorption process, the intestines also secrete calcium, which is excreted (along with the unabsorbed calcium) in the feces. The intestinal secretion of calcium seems to be constant in terms

Table 9-12 Factors Influencing Calcium Regulation

Regulating System	Stimulating Factor	Inhibiting Factor
Intestinal (absorption)	Vitamin D Parathyroid hormone Growth hormone	Thyrocalcitonin Glucocorticoid hormones
Skeletal (bone resorption)	Vitamin D Parathyroid hormone Thyroid hormone Prostaglandins Acidosis	Thyrocalcitonin Glucocorticoid hormones Androgen Estrogen Hyperphosphatemia Alkalosis
Renal (excretion)	Increased arterial pressure Most diuretics Hypercalcemia Hypophosphatemia Thyrocalcitonin Growth hormone Thyroid hormone Glucocorticoid hormones Acidosis	Decreased arterial pressure Thiazide diuretics Hypocalcemia Hyperphosphatemia Vitamin D Parathyroid hormone Alkalosis

percent is excreted by the kidneys. The renal excretion of calcium is increased by the following: increased effective arterial pressure, most diuretics, hypercalcemia, hypophosphatemia, thyrocalcitonin, growth hormone, thyroid hormone, glucocorticoids, and acidosis. Those factors that decrease the renal excretion of calcium include decreased effective arterial volume, thiazide diuretics, hypocalcemia, hyperphosphatemia, vitamin D, parathyroid hormone, and alkalosis.

Variances

The variances associated with calcium are hypercalcemia and hypocalcemia.

Hypercalcemia

Definition

Hypercalcemia is an excess of calcium in the extracellular fluid.

Etiology

Hypercalcemia can be caused by a variety of etiologies, the most common of which is malignant tumors. Other causes are vitamin D intoxication, hyperparathyroidism, hypophosphatasia, hyperproteinemia, hyperthyroidism, adrenal insufficiency, renal dysfunction, immobilization, thiazide diuretics, milk–alkali syndrome, sarcoidosis, tuberculosis, idiopathic infantile hypercalcemia, and vitamin A intoxication.

Clinical Assessment Parameters

The clinical signs and symptoms that may accompany hypercalcemia include fatigue, muscle weakness, muscle hypotonicity, drowsiness, lethargy, disorientation, loss of memory, depression, stupor, coma, deep bone pain, anorexia, nausea, vomiting, constipation, thirst, polyuria, renal stones, and cardiac dysrhythmia, which can progress to cardiac arrest. (Hypercalcemia is evidenced on the electrocardiogram by a shortened Q-T interval.)

Laboratory Assessment Data

In assessing an individual for hypercalcemia, the following values provide important data: serum calcium, urine calcium, urine osmolality, and urine specific gravity. The pattern characteristic of hypercalcemia is a serum calcium greater than 10.5 mg/100 mL, an increased urine calcium, a decreased urine osmolality, and a decreased urine specific gravity. Remember that serum calcium must be evaluated in terms of serum albumin, and for every 1.0 mg/100 mL change in albumin from the norm of 4.0 mg/100 mL, there is a corresponding change of 0.8 mg/100 mL in the serum calcium.

Clinical and Nursing Implications

The clinical implications of hypercalcemia are very significant for the individual. Not only can this imbalance cause cardiac arrest, but it can also lead to renal dysfunction, central nervous system depression, pain, and pathologic fractures.

The implications for nursing include performing the following monitoring functions: (1) assessing the rate, rhythm, and characteristics of the pulse; (2) evaluating the level of consciousness frequently; (3) monitoring muscle movement, strength, and tone; (4) assessing bowel sounds; (5) measuring and recording intake and output accurately; (6) obtaining a daily weight; (7) straining and monitoring the urine for stones; and (8) monitoring all appropriate laboratory data.

Nursing interventions performed with a hypercalcemic individual are (1) to encourage frequent ambulation whenever appropriate; (2) to institute active and passive range of motion exercises; (3) to provide appropriate stimuli to increase the patient's level of orientation; (4) to provide a safe physical environment for the individual; (5) to encourage acid-ash fluids such as cranberry or prune juice; (6) to encourage an increased oral intake of fluids; (7) to administer medications as prescribed; (8) to provide foods and fluids that are consistent with the dietary restrictions, if any are prescribed; and (9) to institute extra safety precautions and provide for gentle movement of the individual.

Treatment

As with all other types of imbalances, the treatment of hypercalcemia involves treating the underlying cause and correcting the imbalance. Thus, whenever possible, an attempt is made to deal with the etiology as soon as it is feasible.

Hypercalcemia can be corrected by a variety of therapeutic methods. One of the first methods employed is the administration of saline infusions.

These infusions not only hydrate the individual but also dilute the extracellular calcium concentration and increase the renal excretion of calcium through the sodium diuresis. Diuretics are also given to increase the renal excretion of calcium. Other forms of treatment include administering the following: sodium bicarbonate to induce alkalosis and reduce the ionized calcium fraction; phosphate to inhibit the resorption of bone; glucocorticoids to inhibit calcium absorption and shift the extracellular calcium intracellularly; mithramycin, indomethacin, or calcitonin to decrease bone resorption; ethyl-ene-diaminetetraacetic acid (EDTA) to lower the serum calcium by chelation; and dialysis therapy to deplete the serum calcium.

Hypocalcemia

Definition

Hypocalcemia is a deficit of calcium in the extra-cellular fluid.

Etiology

Hypocalcemia is caused by the following: hypoproteinemia; idiopathic, surgical, or pseudohypoparathyroidism; renal dysfunction; hyperphosphatemia; vitamin D deficiency; magnesium deficiency; acute pancreatitis; inadequate dietary intake; intestinal malabsorption; alkalosis; excessive administration of citrated blood; massive subcutaneous infections; osteomalacia; and malignant neoplasms, especially those with bone metastases.

Clinical Assessment Parameters

The person experiencing hypocalcemia exhibits a variety of signs and symptoms, the majority of which are neuromuscular in nature. Clinical signs and symptoms of hypocalcemia include numbness and tingling of the extremities, circumoral tingling, muscle cramps, tetany, positive Chvostek's and Trousseau's signs, epileptiform seizures, laryngeal stridor, carpopedal spasms, hyperreflexia, mental depression, psychoses, cardiac arrest, abdominal cramps, nausea and vomiting, diarrhea, cataracts, keratitis, dry skin, brittle nails, alopecia, coagulation dysfunction (rarely occurs), and pathologic fractures. If the individual is being assessed using a cardiac monitor, the electrocardiogram will reflect a lengthened S-T segment and a prolonged Q-T interval, which are characteristic of hypocalcemia.

Laboratory Assessment Data

The serum calcium is the most helpful of all the laboratory data for determining hypocalcemia. A serum calcium value less than 8.5 mg/100 mL is indicative of hypocalcemia.

Clinical and Nursing Implications

Clinically, hypocalcemia presents many hazards to the patient's health state and normal ability to function. The neuromuscular effects of hypocalcemia alone constitute major problems for the individual. Add to those effects the cardiovascular and gastrointestinal effects, and the patient, indeed, becomes severely compromised and in need of supportive care from the nurse.

Supportive nursing care for an individual experiencing hypocalcemia includes performing the following monitoring functions: (1) assessing neuromuscular function frequently; (2) monitoring the rate, rhythm, and characteristics of the pulse; (3) evaluating the rate, pattern, and characteristics of the respirations; (4) checking Chvostek's sign periodically (this involves percussing the facial nerve in the area of the face just anterior to the ear. If this percussion elicits a unilateral twitching of the facial muscles, including the eyelid and lips, it indicates hypocalcemia.); (5) testing Trousseau's sign periodically (this involves occluding the blood supply to an extremity to produce ischemia. Usually this sign is tested by applying a tourniquet, or inflating a blood pressure cuff around the upper extremity for 3 or 4 min. If the induced ischemia precipitates carpopedal spasms, it indicates hypocalcemia.); (6) assessing the individual's mental status; (7) monitoring the characteristics of the feces; (8) assessing visual acuity and the characteristics of the eyeballs; (9) evaluating the intactness of the skeletal system; (10) assessing the characteristics of the skin, nails, and hair; and (11) monitoring the serum calcium values and the electrocardiograms.

The intervening functions that are performed with the hypocalcemic individual are (1) providing a safe physical environment for the patient; (2) instituting seizure precautions; (3) providing an environment with decreased, but appropriate amounts of stimuli; (4) administering prescribed medications appropriately; (5) providing foods that are high in calcium and low in phosphorus, if prescribed; (6) providing meticulous hygienic care for the skin, nails, and hair; and (7) implementing a variety of nursing comfort measures to deal with the gastrointestinal effects.

Treatment

Hypocalcemia is treated by dealing with the underlying cause, if possible, and correcting the imbalance. The therapy used to correct the imbalance differs, depending on whether it is an acute or chronic imbalance. Acute hypocalcemic imbalances are usually treated with intravenous infusions of calcium chloride, calcium gluconate, or calcium gluceptate. (The digitalized individual is monitored extremely closely during these infusions because calcium increases the sensitivity of the heart to digitalis and thus may precipitate digitalis toxicity.)

Chronic calcium depletion is effectively treated by the following methods: administering daily doses of oral calcium preparations, such as calcium lactate, calcium gluconate, or calcium carbonate; administering daily doses of oral vitamin D preparations; increasing the dietary intake of calcium through the use of foods high in calcium content; and restricting the dietary intake of foods high in phosphorus content.

Magnesium

Functions

The functions of magnesium in the physiologic processes of the body include the following: participating as a coenzyme in transphosphorylation reactions that result in a release of energy; activating other enzyme systems and thus influencing carbohydrate metabolism, protein synthesis, and nucleic acid synthesis and metabolism; acting as a mediator at the myoneural junction; activating adenosine triphosphatase; acting as a mediator of neural transmission in the central nervous system; influencing the transport of sodium and potassium across cell membranes; acting as a structural element of the bone; and influencing the secretion of parathyroid hormone.

Regulation

The extracellular concentration of magnesium is regulated by intestinal absorption and secretion, an exchange process between bone and the extracellular fluid, and renal excretion.

Intestinal Absorption and Secretion

Approximately 30 to 40 percent of the magnesium ingested is absorbed by the intestines, primarily the small intestines. The efficiency of this absorption varies inversely with the amount of dietary magnesium ingested. The absorption process seems to be enhanced by parathyroid hormone and vitamin D and inhibited by thyrocalcitonin.

There appears to be some intestinal secretion of magnesium, but it is minimal.

Exchange between Bone and Extracellular Fluid

The exchange of magnesium between bone and the extracellular fluid seems to contribute minimally to the regulation of extracellular magnesium concentration. The factors that govern this exchange process are elusive and have yet to be defined.

Renal Excretion

The renal excretion of magnesium is the primary determinant of magnesium balance in the body. Reabsorption of magnesium occurs in all parts of the tubule but more so in the ascending limb of the loop of Henle. This reabsorption is regulated by the tubular maximal capacity which seems to be equal to the filtered load of magnesium that is present at normal plasma concentrations of magnesium. Therefore, even small increases in extracellular magnesium surpass the tubular maximal reabsorption capacity and increase the renal excretion of magnesium. Factors other than hypermagnesemia that increase the renal excretion of magnesium include extracellular fluid volume expansion, especially with saline solutions; diuretic agents including osmotic diuretics; renal vasodilatation; hypercalcemia and hypercalciuria; thyrocalcitonin; alcohol ingestion; thyroid hormone; growth hormone; increased sodium intake; acute metabolic acidosis; chronic mineralocorticoid effect; and phosphate depletion. Factors that decrease the renal excretion of magnesium are hypomagnesemia, parathyroid hormone, and decreased extracellular fluid volume.

Variances

The variances associated with magnesium balance are hypermagnesemia and hypomagnesemia.

Hypermagnesemia

Definition

Hypermagnesemia is an excess of magnesium in the extracellular fluid.

Etiology

Hypermagnesemia occurs rather infrequently because of the renal system's capacity to excrete large quantities in excess of normal. Therefore, the primary etiology of hypermagnesemia is renal failure. Other factors that can also result in hypermagnesemia include adrenal insufficiency, shock, hypothermia, and an increased intake of magnesium. An increased intake of magnesium may result from excesses in any of the following: infusions of intravenous solutions containing magnesium, intramuscular injections of magnesium, oral laxatives containing magnesium, and enemas containing magnesium.

Clinical Assessment Parameters

The clinical signs and symptoms of hypermagnesemia are exhibited by the patient based on the severity of the imbalance. The individual seems to tolerate instances of mild hypermagnesemia without displaying clinically observable signs and symptoms. As the hypermagnesemia increases, however, the individual exhibits many signs and symptoms. These signs and symptoms increase in severity in accordance with the increased serum magnesium levels. Table 9-13 presents a correlation of the serum magnesium level with the signs and symptoms exhibited by the individual according to body system.

Laboratory Assessment Data

The serum magnesium level is the most significant laboratory value used in assessing an individual for

Table 9-13 Signs and Symptoms of Varying Levels of Hypermagnesemia According to Body System

Serum Magnesium Level, meq/L	Body System	Signs and Symptoms
2.2–3.0	None	None
3.1–5.0	Vascular Gastrointestinal	Hypotension Nausea Vomiting Thirst
	Nervous Integumentary	Depressed deep tendon reflexes Flushing
5.1–7.0	Nervous	Drowsiness Depression
7.1–10.0	Nervous Muscular Cardiac	Loss of deep tendon reflexes Weakness Sinus bradycardia Prolonged P-R interval Prolonged Q-T interval
10.1–15.0	Respiratory Muscular Nervous	Hypoventilation Paralysis Coma
15.1–20.0	Cardiac Respiratory	Arrest Apnea

hypermagnesemia. A serum magnesium value greater than 2.2 meq/L indicates hypermagnesemia.

Clinical and Nursing Implications

Clinically, the effects of hypermagnesemia are not hazardous to the individual until the serum magnesium level is increased to four or five times its normal value. At that point, the increase in serum magnesium not only threatens the patient's ability to function, but even the ability to survive.

The nursing care of the individual experiencing hypermagnesemia includes the following monitoring functions: (1) assessing the rate, rhythm or pattern, and characteristics of all vital signs; (2) assessing the level of consciousness frequently; (3) evaluating muscular strength and function periodically; (4) monitoring neurological responses; (5) monitoring renal output frequently; (6) assessing gastrointestinal function; and (7) monitoring serum magnesium values and the electrocardiogram.

Nursing interventions performed with the hypermagnesemic patient are (1) administering the prescribed medications appropriately; (2) providing a safe physical environment for the individual; (3) providing appropriate stimuli for maintaining orientation; (4) positioning the person appropriately to facilitate adequate respirations; (5) maintaining bed rest and a decreased activity level as appropriate; (6) instituting active and passive range of motion exercises; and (7) providing nursing comfort measures appropriate for dealing with the gastrointestinal signs and symptoms.

Treatment

Goals for the treatment of hypermagnesemia are to correct the underlying disorder, counteract its harmful effects, and increase renal excretion. Correcting the underlying disorder is easy if the hypermagnesemia is due to excessive intake. However, it may be impossible to treat or stop the underlying cause if it is due to renal failure.

The harmful effects of hypermagnesemia can be effectively counteracted by infusing intravenous calcium preparations because the calcium ion antagonizes the action of the magnesium ion on the neuromuscular junction.

Increasing the renal excretion of magnesium can be accomplished in the presence of normal renal function by expanding the extracellular fluid volume with saline solution and/or administering diuretics. If renal dysfunction is present, dialysis therapy will effectively remove the increased serum levels of magnesium.

Hypomagnesemia

Definition

Hypomagnesemia is a deficit of magnesium in the extracellular fluid.

Etiology

The etiologies of hypomagnesemia can be classified according to the following five categories: (1) decreased intake, (2) decreased intestinal absorption, (3) excessive loss of body fluids, (4) excessive loss in the urine, and (5) miscellaneous factors.

Those etiologies of hypomagnesemia that are included in the category of decreased intake are prolonged intravenous therapy using magnesium-free solutions, protein-calorie malnutrition, and starvation.

The category of etiologies that result in hypomagnesemia due to decreased intestinal absorption include malabsorption syndrome such as nontropical sprue, surgical resection of the small bowel, and hereditary intestinal defects in magnesium absorption.

The etiologies of hypomagnesemia that are classified in the category of excessive loss of body fluids are intestinal and biliary fistulas, enema and nonmagnesium laxative abuse, prolonged use of nasogastric suctioning, and severe diarrhea, such as that which accompanies ulcerative colitis.

The category of etiologies that produce hypomagnesemia due to excessive magnesium loss in the urine include chronic alcoholism; diuretic therapy; primary hyperaldosteronism; the diuretic phase of acute renal failure; hypercalcemia, particularly in association with primary hyperparathyroidism, malignancies, and vitamin D intoxication; hyperthyroidism; phosphate deficiency; renal tubular acidosis; diabetic ketoacidosis; chronic renal failure with magnesium wasting; idiopathic renal magnesium wasting; cardiac glycosides; and aminoglycosides.

The last category of etiologies of hypomagnesemia is the group of miscellaneous causes that include acute pancreatitis, hypoparathyroidism, idiopathic hypomagnesemia, inappropriate secretion of antidiuretic hormone, burns, and multiple transfusions with citrated blood.

Clinical Assessment Parameters

The clinical signs and symptoms of hypomagnesemia are very similar to those seen with hypocalcemia. The hypomagnesemic individual will exhibit any combination of the following signs and symptoms: muscle fasciculation; muscle weakness; coarse, flapping tremors; ataxia; vertigo; paresthesias; positive Chvostek's and Trousseau's signs; generalized tetany; generalized muscle spasticity; spontaneous carpopedal spasms; seizures; apathy; confusion; irritability; psychoses; depression; nystagmus; hypertension; cardiac dysfunction; dysphagia; anorexia; and nausea.

If the patient is being assessed using a cardiac monitor, the electrocardiogram will reflect the following changes: a prolonged Q-T interval, broadened T waves of decreased amplitude, and an occasional shortened S-T segment.

Laboratory Assessment Data

The laboratory values used to assess an individual for hypomagnesemia are the serum magnesium, calcium, and potassium, and the urine magnesium and calcium. The levels of these values that are characteristic of hypomagnesemia are a serum magnesium of less than 1.6 meq/L, a decreased serum calcium and potassium, and a decreased urine magnesium and calcium.

Clinical and Nursing Implications

The clinical implications of hypomagnesemia are significant because of the extensive involvement of the neuromuscular system. Having that particular body system so compromised certainly places the patient's well-being at risk.

The implications of hypomagnesemia on the nursing care of the individual require that the following monitoring functions be performed: (1) assess neurologic function frequently; (2) monitor the level of consciousness periodically; (3) assess muscle strength and movement; (4) check Chvostek's and Trousseau's signs; (5) assess gastrointestinal function; (6) monitor the rate, rhythm, and characteristics of the pulse; (7) monitor all other

vital signs; and (8) assess the appropriate laboratory values periodically.

The nursing interventions performed with the hypomagnesemic patient include (1) instituting seizure precautions, (2) providing a safe physical environment for the individual, (3) maintaining bed rest or limited activity as appropriate, (4) instituting active and passive range of motion exercises as appropriate, (5) providing appropriate stimuli for maintaining orientation, and (6) providing nursing comfort measures to deal with the gastrointestinal effects.

Treatment

As with all the other imbalances, treatment of hypomagnesemia is aimed at halting the primary cause and correcting the imbalance. The imbalance is usually corrected by administering either intravenous infusions of magnesium sulfate or magnesium chloride, or intramuscular injections of magnesium sulfate. The replacement therapy usually consists of administering 10 to 40 meq of magnesium daily until the serum magnesium level returns to normal. Dietary substances and oral magnesium preparations can also be used as replacement therapy, particularly in cases of mild hypomagnesemia. It should be noted, however, that intestinal absorption of oral magnesium preparations is extremely variable, thus necessitating continuous, close monitoring of the individual's serum magnesium level.

Chloride

Functions

The functions of chloride in the body are to assist in maintaining the osmotic pressure of the extracellular fluid, to participate in maintaining water balance, to participate in normal gastric digestion by providing an acid medium through the production of hydrochloric acid, and to assist in maintaining acid-base balance.

Regulation

Extracellular chloride concentration is regulated primarily by the renal system. This regulation is dependent upon the acid-base balance of the body fluids and aldosterone secretion.

In general, the renal handling of chloride is very similar to that of sodium, primarily because the two ions are coupled in many of the reabsorption, secretion, and transport processes, thus maintaining electrical neutrality. In most instances, then, chloride ion movement is passive and depends on active sodium transport. There are, however, two sites in the tubular system where this dependent relationship does not exist. The first site is the proximal tubule, where chloride reabsorption and excretion are dependent upon hydrogen ion secretion rather than on sodium transport. Thus, the degree of proximal tubular acidification determines the amount of chloride that is reabsorbed and excreted. The nature of this relationship is such that an increase in hydrogen ion secretion in the proximal tubule results in a compensatory increase in chloride excretion in response to an increase in bicarbonate reabsorption.

The second site is in the loop of Henle where chloride ion transport may be more active than passive. Consequently, chloride movement is less dependent on sodium transport in this portion of the tubule.

The influence of aldosterone in the regulation of chloride is secondary to its effect on sodium and water reabsorption. As was previously discussed, aldosterone acts on the distal tubule and collecting duct to increase the reabsorption of sodium. As the sodium is actively reabsorbed, water and chloride are passively reabsorbed along with it. Thus there is increased reabsorption of sodium, chloride, and water.

Variances

The variances in the balance of extracellular chloride are hyperchloremia and hypochloremia.

Hyperchloremia

Definition

Hyperchloremia is an excess of chloride in the extracellular fluid.

Etiology

Hyperchloremia is caused by the following: excessive intake of chloride, usually in the form of medications; renal tubular acidosis; ureterosigmoidostomy; and increased sodium intake, especially if there is an associated decrease in the extracellular fluid volume.

If the chloride increase is not accompanied by a proportional increase in sodium, hyperchloremic acidosis can result because of decreased hydrogen ion secretion in the proximal tubule.

Clinical Assessment Parameters

The individual experiencing hyperchloremia that is disproportionate to the hypernatremia exhibits the following signs and symptoms: muscle weakness, decreased level of consciousness, and deep, rapid respirations. The person experiencing hyperchloremia that is proportionate to the hypernatremia will exhibit signs and symptoms that are reflective of either the increased sodium concentration or the decreased fluid volume. (The signs and symptoms of both of those imbalances have been previously delineated.)

Laboratory Assessment Data

The laboratory values that provide the most data for assessing a patient in terms of hyperchloremia include the following: serum chloride, sodium, bicarbonate, and pH; and urine pH and specific gravity. The pattern of these values that is consistent with hyperchloremia is a serum chloride greater than 106 meq/L, an increased serum sodium, a decreased serum bicarbonate and pH, an increased urine pH, and a decreased urine specific gravity. The changes in serum pH and bicarbonate and urine pH are reflective, of course, of the hyperchloremic acidosis rather than hyperchloremia accompanied by a proportionate hypernatremia.

Clinical and Nursing Implications

The clinical implications of hyperchloremia are related to the acidotic, hypernatremic, and hypovolemic conditions that may accompany it. This array of imbalances, which will significantly interfere with internal physiologic processes, will create threats to the individual's well-being.

The implications of hyperchloremia for providing nursing care for the individual include monitoring and intervening functions related to all the mentioned imbalances. Since the nursing behaviors related to the hypovolemic and hypernatremic individual have been previously delineated, they will not be repeated. However, those actions specific for caring for the patient's hyperchloremic imbalance will be discussed.

Monitoring functions performed with individuals experiencing hyperchloremia include (1) assessing the level of consciousness frequently; (2) monitoring the rate, rhythm, and characteristics of the respirations; (3) evaluating muscle strength; (4) monitoring appropriate laboratory values; and (5) monitoring all other vital signs.

The intervening nursing functions performed with hyperchloremic individuals are (1) to provide a safe physical environment for the patient; (2) to position the individual appropriately to facilitate adequate respirations; (3) to provide adequate, appropriate stimuli to promote orientation; (4) to maintain an activity level consistent with his or her muscle strength; (5) to administer fluids and/or medications as prescribed by the physician; and (6) to restrict chloride intake if consistent with the medical plan of care.

Treatment

The treatment of hyperchloremia usually involves a combination of the following therapies: treating the primary underlying cause; administering or encouraging fluids to dilute the serum chloride; administering sodium bicarbonate; and, in some cases, administering diuretics.

Hypochloremia

Definition

Hypochloremia is a deficit of chloride in the extracellular fluid.

Etiology

Hypochloremia is caused by the following: excessive loss of gastric secretions, usually due to vomiting or nasogastric suctioning; excessive secretion or administration of adrenocorticoid hormones; decreased intake, usually seen with severely salt-restricted diets; and, in some cases, rigorous use of diuretic therapy.

Hypochloremia is usually associated with hyponatremia, and if the loss of the two ions is proportional, the serum pH will remain virtually unchanged. However, if the chloride loss is dispro-

portionately higher than the sodium loss, a hypochloremic alkalosis may result.

Clinical Assessment Parameters

The hypochloremic individual with a chloride loss disproportionate to the sodium loss exhibits the following signs and symptoms: muscle weakness; tetany; agitation; irritability; and slow, shallow respirations. An individual with hypochloremia that has resulted from proportionate losses of chloride and sodium exhibits the signs and symptoms characteristic of hyponatremia and/or hypervolemia. Those signs and symptoms have been previously discussed.

Laboratory Assessment Data

The laboratory values that provide the most data in determining hypochloremia in the individual are the following: serum chloride, sodium, bicarbonate, and pH. The pattern characteristic of hypochloremia is a serum chloride less than 96 meq/L, a decreased serum sodium, and increased serum bicarbonate and pH values.

Clinical and Nursing Implications

The clinical implications for the hypochloremic patient are definitely related to the alkalosis, hyponatremia, and hypervolemia that may accompany the hypochloremia. The interrelationship of those imbalances in an individual indeed jeopardizes well-being and it requires supportive nursing measures.

The monitoring and intervening nursing behaviors implemented with individuals experiencing hyponatremia and hypervolemia have been previously discussed. Therefore, only those nursing behaviors that directly relate to the care of the hypochloremic individual are discussed at this time.

Monitoring functions performed in caring for an individual experiencing hypochloremia include (1) assessing the level of consciousness; (2) monitoring the rate, rhythm, and characteristics of the respirations; (3) evaluating all other vital signs; (4) assessing muscle strength and movement; (5) measuring and recording intake and output accurately; and (6) monitoring appropriate laboratory values.

Intervening functions performed with the hypochloremic patient are (1) to provide a safe physical environment for the individual; (2) to provide a quiet environment with decreased stimuli to minimize agitation; (3) to limit activity in accordance with muscle strength; (4) to provide foods and fluids high in chloride if appropriate; and (5) to administer prescribed medications correctly.

Treatment

The treatment of hypochloremia includes treating the primary underlying cause and correcting the imbalance. The imbalance is usually corrected by replacing the lost chloride with sodium chloride, potassium chloride, or ammonium chloride. Replacement therapy usually involves replacing three-fourths of the imbalance with sodium chloride and one-fourth with potassium chloride. Ammonium chloride is used in place of potassium chloride if the serum potassium concentration is already elevated.

Phosphate

Functions

The functions of the anion phosphate in the body are (1) participating as a structural element of the bone; (2) influencing the production of energy sources by the red blood cells that are necessary for oxygen delivery; (3) participating in the metabolism of carbohydrates, lipids, and nucleic acids; (4) acting as the major urinary buffer in the formation of titratable acid; (5) participating in oxidative phosphorylation; (6) influencing the absorption of glucose and glycerol in the intestines; and (7) maintaining the structural integrity of the cell wall.

Regulation

The extracellular concentration of phosphate is regulated by the following four mechanisms: intestinal absorption, exchanges between the bone and extracellular fluid, exchanges between the intracellular and extracellular fluid, and renal excretion.

Intestinal Absorption

Of all the dietary phosphate ingested, approximately 70 percent is absorbed in the jejunum and the remaining 30 percent is excreted in the feces. The

intestinal absorption of phosphate is increased by parathyroid hormone and vitamin D and decreased by thyrocalcitonin and binding by calcium or antacids.

Bone and Extracellular Fluid Exchange

The regulation of extracellular phosphate by exchange between the bone and extracellular fluid depends primarily upon a similar exchange process that occurs as part of calcium homeostasis. When calcium is resorbed or released from the bone, phosphate accompanies it. Likewise, when calcium is deposited in the bone, phosphate is also deposited. The more active of the two exchange processes in regulating extracellular phosphate concentration is bone resorption. Bone resorption is increased by parathyroid hormone and vitamin D and decreased by thyrocalcitonin.

Intracellular and Extracellular Fluid Exchange

The concentration of phosphate in the extracellular fluid is also influenced by the exchange of phosphate ions between the intracellular and extracellular fluids. The rate of this exchange is dependent upon the rate of glycolysis that occurs in the cell. When glycolysis occurs, phosphate shifts into the cell. Thus, an increase in glycolysis would increase the phosphate shift into the cell, and a decrease in glycolysis would increase the shift of phosphate out of the cell. Those factors which would facilitate glycolysis and thus a phosphate shift into the cell include acute alkalosis and the administration of glucose, insulin, or epinephrine. Acute acidosis is one factor that would increase the shift of phosphate out of the cell, probably due to tissue hypoxia with its accompanying increase in ATP degradation.

Renal Excretion

The renal regulation of phosphate is excretory in nature. The renal excretion of phosphate is dependent primarily upon the serum phosphate concentration and parathyroid hormone. These two factors affect renal excretion by determining the amount and rate at which phosphate can be reabsorbed by the kidney.

Seventy percent of the filtered phosphate is reabsorbed in the proximal tubule and 25 percent in the distal tubule. This reabsorption is dependent on the tubular maximal reabsorptive capacity that is established by parathyroid hormone.

The renal excretion of phosphate is increased by the following factors: parathyroid hormone, acute fluid volume expansion, hyperphosphatemia, thyrocalcitonin, metabolic acidosis, hypokalemia, and diuretics that function by acting on the proximal tubule. The renal excretion of phosphate is decreased by vitamin D, growth hormone, hypophosphatemia, and a decrease in fluid volume.

Variances

The variances or imbalances that occur in relation to phosphate are hyperphosphatemia and hypophosphatemia.

Hyperphosphatemia

Definition

Hyperphosphatemia is an excess of phosphate in the extracellular fluid.

Etiology

Hyperphosphatemia is caused by the following: renal dysfunction (probably the most common cause), hypoparathyroidism, pseudohypoparathyroidism, hyperthyroidism, excessive ingestion or infusion of phosphate salts, catabolic states, neoplastic diseases, and overingestion of vitamin D metabolites.

Clinical Assessment Parameters

An inverse relationship exists between phosphate and calcium in the extracellular fluid. Therefore, a hyperphosphatemic condition also results in hypocalcemia. This relationship accounts for the fact that the clinical signs and symptoms of the hyperphosphatemic individual are indeed the same as those seen in the hypocalcemic individual. Those signs and symptoms have been previously delineated and will not be repeated. It should be noted, however, that the primary effect of hypocalcemia on the individual was in relation to the neuromuscular system.

Laboratory Assessment Data

Laboratory values used to assess the individual in relation to hyperphosphatemia are the serum phosphorus and calcium values. The pattern characteristic of hyperphosphatemia is a serum phosphorus greater than 4.5 mg/100 mL and a decreased serum calcium.

Clinical and Nursing Implications

Since the clinical manifestations of hyperphosphatemia are the same as those accompanying hypocalcemia, it is logical that the clinical implications and nursing behaviors are also the same. Those implications and behaviors have been previously discussed in relation to hypocalcemia.

Treatment

The treatment of hyperphosphatemia is aimed at eliminating the cause and correcting the imbalance. Correcting the imbalance can be accomplished by the following methods: restricting the intake of phosphate; administering intestinal phosphate-binding agents, such as aluminum hydroxide gel; administering diuretics, if renal function is present; and implementing dialysis therapy if renal dysfunction is present.

Hypophosphatemia

Definition

Hypophosphatemia is a deficit of phosphate in the extracellular fluid.

Etiology

The following are causes of hypophosphatemia: primary and secondary hyperparathyroidism; primary renal tubular defects in phosphate reabsorption; states of chronic metabolic acidosis, as seen with renal tubular acidosis and ureterosigmoidostomies; hypokalemia; extracellular fluid volume expansion; administration of phosphate binders; vomiting; malabsorption; starvation; prolonged use of phosphate-free intravenous solutions; abnormalities in vitamin D metabolism, as in vitamin D-associated rickets; alcohol withdrawal; the recovery phase of diabetic ketoacidosis; the administration of agents designed to increase glycolysis; severe burns; and the recovery phase of malnutrition.

Clinical Assessment Parameters

The clinical signs and symptoms exhibited by a hypophosphatemic individual are, of course, direct manifestations of the biochemical changes produced by the imbalance. Those biochemical changes are significant, not only to the individual's functioning but also to the nurse's understanding of the associated clinical signs and symptoms. Therefore, those biochemical changes are summarized according to body system in Table 9-14.

The resulting clinical signs and symptoms exhibited by the hypophosphatemic patient are: irritability, confusion, disorientation, seizures, coma, anisocoria, ptosis, nystagmus, muscle weakness, paresthesias, tremors, ataxia, ballism, dysrhythmia, hyperventilation, anorexia, nausea, vomiting, bruising, bone pain, pathologic fractures, and arthralgias. If the imbalance is prolonged, there may be addi-

tional clinical signs and symptoms exhibited in relation to platelet dysfunction and decreased white blood cell phagocytic activity.

Laboratory Assessment Data

The most significant laboratory value used in assessing an individual for hypophosphatemia is the serum phosphorus. A serum phosphorus less than 2 mg/100 mL is consistent with hypophosphatemia. Urine laboratory values may provide additional assessment data because hypophosphatemia seems to result in: hypercalciuria, hypophosphaturia, bicarbonaturia, and decreased hydrogen ion excretion.

Table 9-14 The Biochemical Changes Accompanying Hypophosphatemia Summarized According to Body System

Body System				
Central Nervous	Neuromuscular	Hematologic	Cardiovascular	Respiratory
Hypoxia	Rhabdomyolysis	Red cell rigidity	Decreased electrical conduction	Decreased ATP, creating fatique
Abnormal conduction velocity	Increased CPK	Hemolysis		
	Decreased transmembrane resting potential gradient	Decreased 2,3,-DPG resulting in tissue hypoxia	Decreased mechanical function	
		Decreased phagocytosis		
		Decreased chemotaxis		
		Platelet destruction		
		Shift of the hemoglobin dissociation curve		

Body System			
Gastrointestinal	Hepatic	Skeletal	Renal
Increased calcium absorption	Hepatic dysfunction due to decreased oxygen	Increased calcium resorption	Hypercalciuria
			Hypophosphaturia
		Decreased osteoid calcification	Decreased H$^+$ ion excretion
			Decreased tubular reabsorption of HCO$_3$ and glucose
			Increased systhesis of vitamin D
			Bicarbonaturia

Clinical and Nursing Implications

The clinical implications of hypophosphatemia for the individual are certainly threatening to well-being. The most significant implications of hypophosphatemia for the patient seem to be related to its effects on the central nervous and neuromuscular systems. These effects decrease the individual's ability to carry out the activities of daily living, as well as to participate in health care. Thus, he or she requires nursing support.

Monitoring functions that are a part of nursing support include (1) assessing muscle strength, (2) evaluating the individual's level of consciousness, (3) monitoring for signs of associated hypercalcemia, (4) assessing the individual's comfort level, (5) observing for signs of decreased clotting or decreased inflammatory response, (6) monitoring intake, (7) monitoring all vital signs, and (8) monitoring appropriate laboratory values.

The following intervening functions are performed with the hypophosphatemic patient: (1) assisting with the activities of daily living; (2) providing activity in accordance with muscle strength; (3) instituting active and passive range of motion exercises; (4) providing stimuli appropriate for maintaining orientation; (5) establishing a safe physical environment for the individual; (6) providing food and fluids high in phosphate, if appropriate; (7) presenting small amounts of food and fluids at intervals in an appetizing manner; (8) providing nursing comfort measures; and (9) administering medications as prescribed.

Treatment

Hypophosphatemia is usually treated by dealing with the primary underlying cause and replacing the lost phosphate. The replacement therapy may be implemented using either oral or intravenous phosphate preparations or, in cases of mild imbalance, dietary substances.

Sulfate

Functions

The functions of sulfate in the body are to participate in the synthesis of sulfated mucopolysaccharides for the cartilage and bone matrix, to influence the synthesis of heparin and the mucoprotein secretions of the gastrointestinal tract, and to detoxify drugs and foreign compounds in the liver.

Regulation

The concentration of sulfate in the extracellular fluid seems to be regulated by intake, the rate of release by metabolic degradation, and renal excretion. The exact mechanisms for these regulating processes are not known.

Variances

The variances in sulfate balance in the body seem to be clinically insignificant.

Protein

Functions

The primary functions of protein in the body are (1) to provide colloid osmotic pressure for regulating fluid volume, (2) to participate in enzyme processes, (3) to influence the development of natural and acquired immunity, (4) to participate in the regulation of acid-base balance, (5) to participate in blood coagulation, and (6) to influence the production of hormones and some vitamins.

Regulation

The concentration of extracellular protein is regulated by the following factors: dietary intake, the rate of formation by the liver, and the rate of use by the tissues.

Variance

The variance in protein balance that has clinical significance for the individual is hypoproteinemia.

Hypoproteinemia

Definition

Hypoproteinemia is a deficit of protein in the extracellular fluid.

Etiology

Hypoproteinemia is caused by the following: inadequate dietary intake; hemorrhage; severe prolonged infection; gastrointestinal pathology that inhibits absorption, such as obstruction or fistulas; fractures; medical pathology and surgical procedures that produce catabolic states; hypokalemia; and prolonged illness, especially when accompanied by fluid imbalances.

Clinical Assessment Parameters

The individual experiencing hypoproteinemia exhibits the following signs and symptoms: weight loss, muscle wasting, decreased muscle tone, fatigue, mental and emotional depression, anorexia, nausea, vomiting, decreased wound healing, decreased immunity or resistance to infection, and edema.

Laboratory Assessment Data

The laboratory value that provides the most significant data for assessing an individual in relation to hypoproteinemia is the serum albumin. A serum albumin value of less than 4 g/100 mL is consistent with hypoproteinemia. Other laboratory values that may provide additional data, if iron intake has been adequate, are hemoglobin, hematocrit, and red blood cell count. Decreased values for these three items, in the presence of adequate iron intake, are consistent with hypoproteinemia.

Clinical and Nursing Implications

The clinical implications of hypoproteinemia for the individual are very significant. Without adequate protein, the individual does not heal or resist infection well. Thus, he or she is predisposed to developing life-threatening complications such as septicemia.

The implications of hypoproteinemia for providing nursing care for the patient indicate that the following monitoring behaviors be performed: (1) monitoring protein intake closely; (2) obtaining precise daily weights; (3) assessing muscle strength and movement; (4) assessing level of consciousness periodically; (5) monitoring gastrointestinal functioning; (6) assessing skin integrity, texture, and turgor; (7) monitoring vital signs; and (8) monitoring appropriate laboratory values.

Intervening behaviors performed with a hypoproteinemic individual are (1) providing a physical environment that decreases exposure to bacterial contamination, (2) maintaining a limited activity level consistent with the person's muscle strength, (3) instituting active and passive range of motion exercises, (4) assisting with the activities of daily living, (5) providing stimuli appropriate to maintain orientation, (6) providing meticulous skin care, (7) instituting nursing comfort measures to deal with gastrointestinal effects, (8) using creative nursing measures to decrease mental depression, and (9) providing high-protein foods and fluids as prescribed.

Treatment

Hypoproteinemia is treated by dealing with the underlying cause and correcting the imbalance. The imbalance is usually corrected by providing a high-protein diet balanced with adequate calories, vitamins, and minerals; using high-protein oral supplements; or infusing proteins and amino acids parenterally. In some cases, the high-protein oral intake is given via a nasogastric tube if the individual has difficulty taking nourishment.

Organic Acids

Organic acids, such as pyruvic acid and lactic acid, which are produced as a result of carbohydrate metabolism, are present in small amounts in the extracellular fluid. Normally, these fixed, nonvolatile acids are clinically not significant for the individual because they are buffered and excreted by the kidneys. When they are produced in abnormal quantities, they result in a change in the acid-base balance of the body. Thus, the clinical significance of having abnormal quantities of organic acids in the extracellular fluid will be discussed in Chapter 10.

Clinical Application

All the previous information regarding fluid and electrolyte balances and imbalances is essential for the clinician in providing quality patient care. The nurse must be able to accurately assess the individual's internal environment to determine appropriate strategies for care. One example of how a clinician would apply such information is depicted in the following case study and its associated discussion.

Case Study

R. M. is a 38-year-old Caucasian male who is admitted to the hospital. His chief complaint is general weakness and malaise due to "flu-like" symptoms. He states that he has been nauseated and vomiting for the past five days and has been unable to tolerate any type of food or liquid. He also states that he has lost approximately 10 lb this past week and is down to about 170 lb right now. In addition, he says that he is very thirsty but every time he drinks any kind of liquid he regurgitates it.

R. M. is noted to have dry, wrinkled skin; dry mucous membranes; and a furrowed tongue. His admission vital signs are: blood pressure, 108/66; pulse, 112; respirations, 28; and oral temperature, 99.6°. His laboratory values are:

addition, his urine laboratory values reveal oliguria, increased density, alkalinity, normal glucose, normal protein, normal creatinine, normal osmolality, hyponaturia, normal potassium, hypochloruria, hypocalciuria, and hypophosphaturia. These values are also consistent with hypovolemia. Based on these assessment data, the nurse would formulate a plan of care to assist R. M. in coping with a decreased fluid volume. Such a plan would include the following continuous monitoring functions: (1) obtaining precise daily weights, (2) measuring all secretions and accurately recording all intake and output, (3) assessing all vital signs and appropriate laboratory values, (4) evaluating the patient's energy level, and (5) assessing the status of the skin and mucous membranes. In addition, the following intervening functions would also be implemented: (1) administering appropriate intravenous replacement fluids precisely and at a constant rate, as prescribed; (2) providing frequent oral hygiene; (3) providing meticulous skin care to maintain integrity; (4) assisting with activities of daily living; and (5) administering medications as prescribed to assist in treating the etiology. This combination of

Serum Values		Urine Values	
Sodium	149 meq/L	Amount	600 mL/24°
Potassium	6 meq/L	Specific gravity	1.031
Chloride	108 meq/L	pH	7.0
BUN	60 mg/100 mL	Glucose	negative
Creatinine	5 mg/100 mL	Protein	negative
Calcium	7.5 mg/100 mL	Creatinine	1000 mg/100 mL
Phosphorus	5.5 mg/100mL	Osmolality	800 mOsm/kg H_2O
CO_2 combining power	18 meq/L	Sodium	16 meq/L
Magnesium	1.8 meq/L	Potassium	20 meq/L
Osmolality	318 mOsm/kg H_2O	Chloride	20 meq/L
Hematocrit	55%	Calcium	4 meq/L
Hemoglobin	20 g/100 mL	Phosphorus	300 mg/24°

Discussion

R. M.'s clinical signs and symptoms and history suggest that he is experiencing hypovolemia. His serum laboratory values indicate the following imbalances: hypernatremia, hyperkalemia, hyperchloremia, azotemia, hypocalcemia, hyperphosphatemia, metabolic acidosis, normomagenesemia, hyperosmolality, and hemoconcentration. All these imbalances are consistent with hypovolemia. In

nursing functions will assist R. M. in maintaining optimum function during the therapeutic process of reestablishing an adequate fluid volume and stable internal environment.

This case study is only a brief example of how a clinician uses the information about fluid and electrolyte balances and imbalances to formulate plans for care. In actuality, a clinician may encounter five or six or even more individuals with the same types of imbalances during an 8-h time span. In addition, some patients may develop two or more imbalances within that same time. Thus, the clinician frequently needs to use the knowledge base related to such imbalances several times a day.

Summary

This chapter has discussed the regulation and assessment of fluid and electrolyte balance. The critical-care nurse is constantly making decisions about patient care based on the utilization of this information. In conducting an assessment of a patient, the critical-care nurse proceeds by beginning with the highest priority substance for the individual. In general, the critical-care nurse would assess the patient in the following manner: fluid volume, acid-base balance, potassium, calcium, sodium, chloride, magnesium, and phosphate. Certainly, this order might change depending on the specific history and presenting behaviors of the individual, but all areas would be included in the assessment. To assist the critical-care nurse in performing this assessment, the signs and symptoms of each imbalance have been summarized according to body systems in Table 9-15.

Table 9-15 Summary of the Signs and Symptoms of Fluid and Electrolyte and Acid-Base Imbalances According to Body Systems

Imbalance	Central Nervous	Neuro-muscular	Cardio-vascular	Respiratory	Gastro-intestinal	Integu-mentary	Skeletal	Renal
Hypervolemia			Weight gain Systemic edema Ascites ↑ CVP Hypertension Bounding pulse	Dyspnea Moist rales		Puffy eyelids		
Hypovolemia	Lassitude	Fatigue	Weight loss ↓ Postural BP ↑ Pulse ↓ Venous pressure		Thirst	Dry skin Dry mucous membranes ↓ Skin turgor ↓ Elasticity Furrowed tongue ↓ Temperature ↓ Eyeball turgor ↓ Perspiration		Oliguria
Metabolic acidosis	Headache Drowsiness ↓ Mentation Confusion Coma Seizures	Fatigue	Hypotension Hypoxia Dysrhythmia	Kussmaul respirations	Anorexia Nausea Vomiting	Tissue hypoxia		
Metabolic alkalosis	Seizures Belligerence Confusion Stupor Coma	Irritability Tetany	Dysrhythmia	Hypoventilation	Nausea Vomiting Diarrhea			

Body System (spanning header above: Central Nervous, Neuro-muscular, Cardio-vascular, Respiratory, Gastro-intestinal, Integu-mentary, Skeletal, Renal)

Table 9-15 Summary of the Signs and Symptoms of Fluid and Electrolyte and Acid-Base Imbalances According to Body Systems (Continued)

Imbalance	Body System							
	Central Nervous	Neuro-muscular	Cardio-vascular	Respiratory	Gastro-intestinal	Integu-mentary	Skeletal	Renal
Respiratory acidosis	↓ Mentation Apprehension Restlessness Headache Drowsiness Disorientation Coma	Fatigue Muscle weakness Flapping tremors Uncoordination ↓ Reflexes	Tachycardia	Hypoven-tilation Dyspnea		Cyanosis		
Respiratory alkalosis	Vertigo Syncope Nervousness Seizures ↓ Mentation Confusion Anxiety	Paresthesias Muscle cramps Tetany ↓ Psychomotor function	Dysrhythmia Hypotension	Dyspnea Hyperven-tilation		Perioral paresthesia		
Hyperkalemia	Confusion	Hyperexcitability Muscle weakness Paresthesias Flaccid paralysis	Dysfunction Arrest		Distention Diarrhea Intestinal colic			
Hypokalemia	Drowsiness Confusion Apathy Coma	Irritability Muscle weakness Paresthesias Muscle pain Muscle cramps Muscle tender-ness Hyporeflexia Tetany Paralysis	Weak pulse Bradycardia	Weakness Hypoven-tilation	Nausea Vomiting Anorexia Distention Cramps Paralytic ileus Poly-dipsia Hyper-gly-cemia Negative nitrogen balance			Polyuria Noc-turia
Hypercalcemia	Drowsiness Lethargy Disorientation Loss of mem-ory Depression Stupor Coma	Fatigue Muscle weakness Hypotonicity	Dysrhythmia Arrest		Anorexia Nausea Vomiting Consti-pation Thirst		Deep bone pain	Polyuria Calculi
Hypocalcemia	Seizures Depression Psychoses	Paresthesias Muscle cramps Tetany Positive Chvos-tek's Positive Trous-seau's Carpopedal spasms Hyperreflexia	Arrest	Laryngeal stridor	Cramps Nausea Vomiting Diarrhea	Circumoral pares-thesia Cataracts Keratitis Dry skin Brittle nails Alopecia	Pathologic fractures	
Hypernatremia	Lethargy Irritability Seizures Coma	Muscular rigidity Muscular weak-ness Tremors	Tachycardia		Thirst	Dry, sticky mucous mem-branes		Oliguria

(Continued)

Table 9-15 Summary of the Signs and Symptoms of Fluid and Electrolyte and Acid-Base Imbalances According to Body Systems (Continued)

	Body System							
Imbalance	Central Nervous	Neuro-muscular	Cardio-vascular	Respiratory	Gastro-intestinal	Integu-mentary	Skeletal	Renal
						Rough, dry tongue Flushed, dry skin ↑ Turgor ↓ Lacrima-tion ↑ Temper-ature		
Hyponatremia	Lethargy Confusion Headache Seizures Coma Apprehension	Fatigue Muscle weakness Tremors Hyperreflexia			Anorexia Nausea Vomiting Cramps Diarrhea			Oliguria
Hyperchlore-mia	↓ Level of conscious-ness	Muscle weakness		Deep and rapid res-pirations				
Hypochloremia	Agitation Irritability	Muscle weakness Tetany		Slow and shallow respira-tions				
Hypermag-nesemia	Drowsiness Depression Coma	↓ Deep reflexes Loss of deep re-flexes Muscle weakness Paralysis	Hypotension Bradycardia Arrest	Hypoven-tilation Apnea	Nausea Vomiting Thirst	Flushing		
Hypomag-nesemia	Seizures Apathy Confusion Irritability Psychoses Depression	Muscle fascicula-tion Muscle weakness Flapping tremors Positive Chvos-tek's Positive Trou-seau's Tetany Muscle spasticity Carpopedal spasms Nystagmus Paresthesias	Hyperten-sion Dysfunction		Anorexia Nausea Dys-phagia			
Hyperphos-phatemia	Seizures Depression Psychoses	Paresthesias Muscle cramps Tetany Positive Chvos-tek's Positive Trou-seau's Carpopedal spasms Hyperreflexia	Arrest	Laryngeal stridor	Cramps Nausea Vomiting Diarrhea	Circumoral pares-thesia Cataracts Keratitis Dry skin Brittle nails Alopecia	Pathologic fractures	
Hypophos-phatemia	Irritability Confusion Disorientation Seizures Coma Anisocoria Ptosis Nystagmus	Muscle weakness Paresthesias Tremors Ataxia Ballism	Dysrhythmia	Hyperven-tilation	Anorexia Nausea Vomiting	Bruising	Bone pain Pathologic fractures Arthralgias	

Bibliography

Aberman, A. (1982). The ins and outs of fluids and electrolytes. *Emergency Medicine, 14,* 121, 123–124, 127.

Anderson, R. J., & Schrier, R. W. (1978). Physiology of renal water excretion. *Contributions to Nephrolology, 14,* 50–63.

Andersson, B. (1978). Regulation of water intake. *Physiological Reviews,* 58, 582–602.

Arieff, A. I., & DeFronzo, R. A. (1985). *Fluid, electrolyte and acid-base disorders* (vol. 1). New York: Churchill Livingstone.

Burgess, A. (1979). *The nurse's guide to fluid and electrolyte balance* (2d ed.). New York: McGraw-Hill.

Carroll, H. J., & Oh, M. S. (1978). *Water, electrolyte and acid-base metabolism: Diagnosis and management.* Philadelphia: Lippincott.

Catchpole, M. (1982). Electrolytes, their physiological action and interaction: A review. *Journal of the American Association of Nurse Anesthetists, 50*(5), 476–481.

Collins, R. D. (1983). *Illustrated manual of fluids and electrolyte disorders* (2d ed.). Philadelphia: Lippincott.

Conner, C. S. (1984). Hypophosphatemia, *Drug Intelligence and Clinical Pharmacy, 18*(7/8), 595.

DeRubertis, F. R. (1984). Hypercalcemia and hypocalcemia. *Topics in Emergency Medicine, 5*(4), 64–73.

Felver, L. (1980). Understanding the electrolyte maze. *American Journal of Nursing, 80,* 1591–1595.

Folk-Lighty, M. (1984). Solving the puzzles of patient's fluid imbalances. *Nursing 84, 14*(2), 39–41.

Geiderman, J. M., Goodman, S. L., & Cohen, D. B. (1979). Magnesium—the forgotten electrolyte. *JACEP, 8*(5), 204–208.

Guyton, A. C. (1986). *Textbook of medical physiology* (7th ed.). Philadelphia: Saunders.

Hays, R. M. (1978). Principles of ion and water transport in the kidney. *Hospital Practice, 13*(9), 79–88.

Humes, H. D., Narins, R. G., & Brenner, B. M. (1979). Disorders of water balance. *Hospital Practice, 4*(3), 133–145.

Janson, C., Birnbaum, G., & Baker, F. J., II. (1983). Hypophosphatemia. *Annals of Emergency Medicine 12*(2), 107–116.

Kee, J. L. (1979). Clinical implications of laboratory studies in critical care. *Critical Care Quarterly, 2*(3), 1–17.

Keithley, J. K., & Fraulini, K. E. (1982). What's behind that I. V. line? *Nursing 82, 12*(3), 33–42.

Keyes, J. L. (1985). *Fluid, electrolyte, and acid base regulation.* Monterey: Wadsworth Health Sciences Division.

Klahr, S. (1978). *Differential diagnosis: Renal and electrolyte disorders.* New York: Arco.

Martof, M. (1985). Part II—Electrolyte balance. *Journal of Nephrology Nursing, 2*(2), 49–54.

Massry, S. G. (1978). The clinical pathophysiology of magnesium. *Contributions to Nephrology, 14,* 64–73.

Maxwell, M. H., & Kleeman, C. R. (1980). *Clinical disorders of fluid and electrolyte metabolism* (3d ed.). New York: McGraw-Hill.

McFadden, E. A., & Zaloga, G. P. (1983). Calcium regulation. *Critical Care Quarterly, 6*(3), 12–21.

McGeown, M. G. (1983). *Clinical management of electrolyte disorders.* Boston: Martinus Nijhoff.

Menzel, L. K. (1980). Clinical problems of electrolyte balance. *Nursing Clinics of North America, 15*(3), 559–576.

———. (1980). Clinical problems of fluid balance. *Nursing Clinics of North America, 15*(3), 549–558.

Metheny, N., & Snively, W. D. (1983). *Nurses handbook of fluid balance* (4th ed.). Philadelphia: Lippincott.

Narins, R. G. (1979). A practical approach to managing hyponatremia. *Consultant, 19*(2), 25–29, 34–35.

Otrakji, J. (1983). Disorders of potassium metabolism. *Topics in Emergency Medicine, 5*(2), 53–57.

Quinlan, M. (1983). Would you recognize this dangerous electrolyte imbalance? *RN, 46*(3), 50–55.

Rice, V. (1983). Magnesium, calcium, and phosphate imbalances; their clinical significance. *Critical Care Nurse, 3*(3), 90–112.

———. (1984). Shock management, part 1. fluid volume replacement. *Critical Care Nurse, 4*(6), 69–82.

Ross, A. D., & Angaram, D. M. (1984). Colloids vs. crystalloids—a continuing controversy. *Drug Intelligence and Clinical Pharmacy, 18*(3), 202–212.

Schrier, R. (1986). *Renal and electrolyte disorders* (3d ed.). Boston: Little, Brown.

Sneid, D. (1983). Hypercalcemia, *Topics in Emergency Medicine, 5*(2), 8–17.

Stein, J. H., & Reineck, H. J. (1978). Regulation of sodium balance in normal and edematous states. *Contributions to Nephrology, 14,* 25–49.

Thomas, A. G. (1983). Disorders of sodium metabolism. *Topics in Emergency Medicine, 5*(2), 46–52.

Valtin, H. (1979). *Renal dysfunction: Mechanisms involved in fluid and solute imbalance.* Boston: Little, Brown.

Vander, A. J. (1985). *Renal physiology* (3d ed.). New York: McGraw-Hill.

Verbalis, J. G., & Robinson, A. G. (1984). Hypernatremia and hyponatremia. *Topics in Emergency Medicine, 5*(4), 79–89.

Weil, M. H., & Rackow, E. C. (1984). A guide to volume repletion. *Emergency Medicine, 16*(8), 100–105, 108–110.

Zaloga, G. P., & Chernow, B. (1983). Magnesium metabolism in critical illness. *Critical Care Quarterly, 6*(3), 22–27.

Zeluff, G. W., Suki, W. N., & Jackson, D. (1980). Hypercalcemia—etiology, manifestations, and management. *Heart & Lung, 9*(1), 146–151.

Zeluff, G. W., Suki, W. N., & Jackson, D. (1978). Hypokalemia—cause and treatment. *Heart & Lung, 7*(5), 854–860.

10

Charold L. Baer

Regulation and Assessment of Acid-Base Balance

Introduction

Acids and bases are essential to the body not only for their participation in the physiologic processes, but also for helping to maintain a stable environment to facilitate those processes. The physiologic processes and associated chemical reactions of the body occur in a stable, slightly alkaline environment. When the normal balance of that environment is disturbed through an increase or decrease in hydrogen ions, those processes and reactions may be accelerated, deterred, or totally inhibited. Thus, a change in the pH of the internal environment can affect the entire body. As a result, the individual will require nursing and medical support during the period of instability to sustain life and regain normal function. Appropriate nursing support cannot be provided unless the nurse is able to accurately assess, plan, implement, and evaluate care for the patient. This discussion provides information basic to the nurse's comprehension of the components of acid-base balance and imbalance in order to facilitate the provision of appropriate nursing support for the individual.

Functions

The acid-base balance of body fluids or, more specifically, the pH of the internal environment, is an essential component of metabolism. Variations in pH will produce significant deviations in metabolic function by altering blood flow, secondary messengers and/or cellular structure, electrolytes, proteins, and gradients. For example, an increase in pH will result in the following metabolic changes: (1) increased lactate production; (2) increased insulin-induced glycolysis; (3) decreased Krebs cycle oxidations in the muscles and renal cortex; (4) decreased gluconeogenesis in the renal cortex; (5) a decreased 2,3-diphosphoglycerate concentration in the red blood cell, with a corresponding left shift in the oxyhemoglobin dissociation curve; (6) decreased vascular tone; and (7) increased effectiveness of circulating catecholamines. A decrease in pH will create the following changes: (1) decreased lactate production; (2) decreased conversion of inactive phosphorylase B to active phosphorylase A; (3) decreased quantities of liver glycogen; (4) increased Krebs cycle oxidations in the muscles and renal cortex; (5) increased gluconeogenesis in the renal cortex; (6) decreased glycolysis; (7) decreased lipolysis; (8) increased pulmonary vascular resistance; (9) increased pulmonary blood flow; (10) decreased threshold levels for ventricular fibrillation; (11) decreased cardiac sensitivity to catecholamines; (12) an increased 2,3-diphosphoglycerate concentration in the red blood cell, with a corresponding right shift in the oxyhemoglobin dissociation curve; (13) decreased peripheral resistance; (14) decreased mesenteric blood flow; (15) decreased pulmonary macrophage function; (16) decreased granulocyte function; (17) decreased immune responses; (18) decreased insulin secretion and binding to receptors; and (19) decreased pancreatic amylase secretion. In addition, variations in pH will also influence the transmembrane movement of various substrates such as serine and alanine, and hepatic processes such as acetate oxidation, glycogen synthesis, and glutamine metabolism.

Regulation

The hydrogen ion concentration, or pH, of body fluids is maintained and regulated by the following three mechanisms: the body fluid buffers, the respiratory system, and the renal system. These mechanisms act by buffering hydrogen ions to prevent not only increases in hydrogen ion concentration, which would result in acidosis, but also decreases in hydrogen ion concentration, which would result in alkalosis.

Body Fluid Buffer System

The body fluid buffer system is composed of buffer pairs consisting of a weak acid and its conjugate base, a salt of that weak acid. Table 10-1 presents the composition and approximate amounts of those buffer pairs in the body. As is depicted in Table 10-1, the carbonic acid-sodium bicarbonate pair is the primary constituent of the body fluid buffer system. Figure 10-1 uses the carbonic acid-bicarbonate buffer pair to illustrate how the body fluid buffer system functions.

The body fluid buffer system reacts within a fraction of a second to prevent changes in hydrogen ion concentration in the body fluids. Because of its fast action, it is often called the first line of defense against acid-base imbalances.

Respiratory System

The respiratory system regulates hydrogen ion concentration in the body fluids by altering the amount of carbon dioxide available for forming carbonic acid. This alteration in the amount of available carbon dioxide is governed by the respiratory control center in the medulla which varies the rate and depth of ventilation according to the carbon dioxide concentration. An increase in carbon dioxide concentration is responded to by an increase in the rate and depth of ventilation. Thus, the carbon dioxide concentration in the alveoli is decreased and less is available for forming carbonic acid. The reciprocal of this process occurs when there is a decrease in carbon dioxide concentration in the alveoli. Figure 10-2 illustrates these respiratory processes for regulating hydrogen ion concentration in the body fluids.

The respiratory system usually responds to changes in hydrogen ion concentration within 1 to 3 min to prevent imbalances from occurring.

Renal System

The renal system regulates hydrogen ion concentration in body fluids through the following five processes: (1) hydrogen ion secretion; (2) sodium reabsorption; (3) bicarbonate reabsorption; (4) excretion of titratable acids, or acidification of phosphate salts; and (5) ammonia synthesis. Figure 10-3 depicts these processes.

The renal system requires hours to days to respond to changes in hydrogen ion concentration and thus is the slowest, but most effective, regulatory method.

Variances

The variances or imbalances associated with acid-base changes are metabolic acidosis, metabolic

Table 10-1 Composition of the Body Fluid Buffer System

Buffer Pairs		Percent Contributed to Total Buffering
Weak Acid	Conjugate Base	
Carbonic acid (H_2CO_3)	Sodium bicarbonate ($NaHCO_3$)	53
Hemoglobin (Hb)	Potassium hemoglobinate (KHb)	35
Oxyhemoglobin ($HHbO_2$)	Potassium oxyhemoglobinate ($KHbO_2$)	
Plasma protein (HPr)	Proteinate (NaPr)	7
Acid organic phosphate ($NaRHPO_4$)	Alkaline organic phosphate (Na_2RPO_4)	3
Acid inorganic phosphate (NaH_2PO_4)	Alkaline inorganic phosphate (Na_2HPO_4)	2

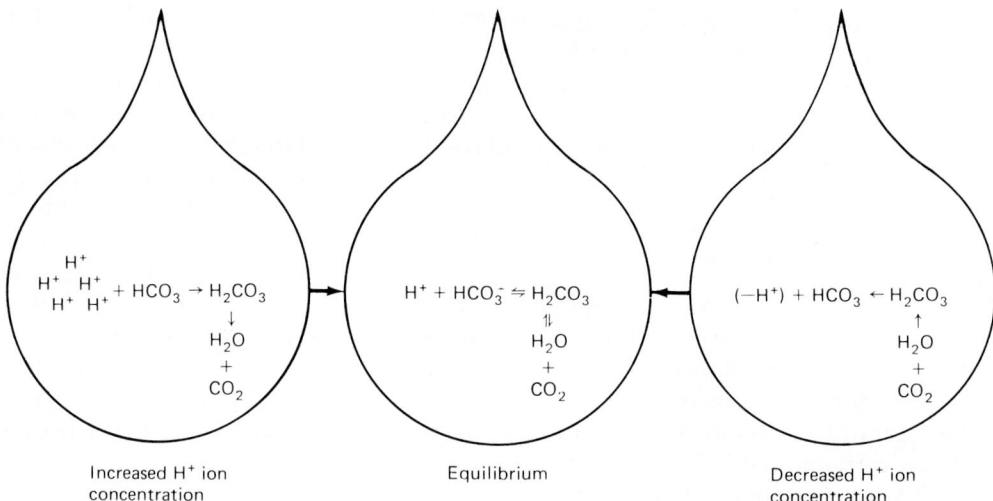

Figure 10-1   Regulation of hydrogen ion concentration by the body fluid buffer system using the carbonic acid–bicarbonate pair.

alkalosis, respiratory acidosis, and respiratory alkalosis.

Metabolic Acidosis

Definition

Metabolic acidosis is a deficit of bicarbonate in the extracellular fluid.

Etiology

Metabolic acidosis results from two categories of etiologies. It occurs either from causes that produce a loss of bicarbonate from the body, or from causes that produce increased amounts of nonvolatile acids in the body.

Those etiologies that produce a loss of bicarbonate from the body result in hyperchloremic acidosis with a normal anion gap. That means that

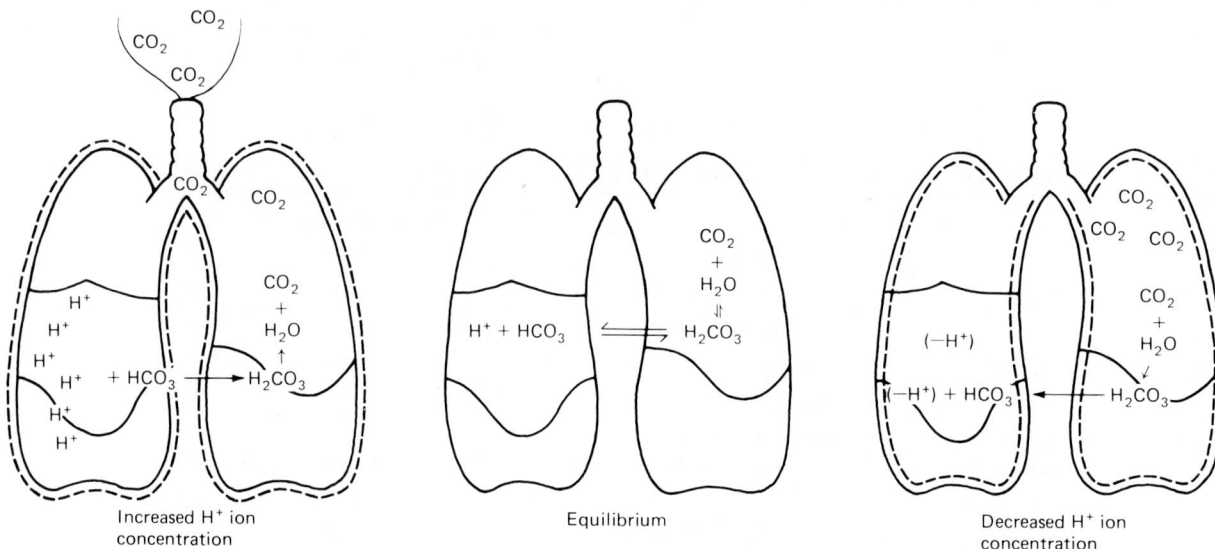

Figure 10-2   Regulation of hydrogen ion concentration by the respiratory system.

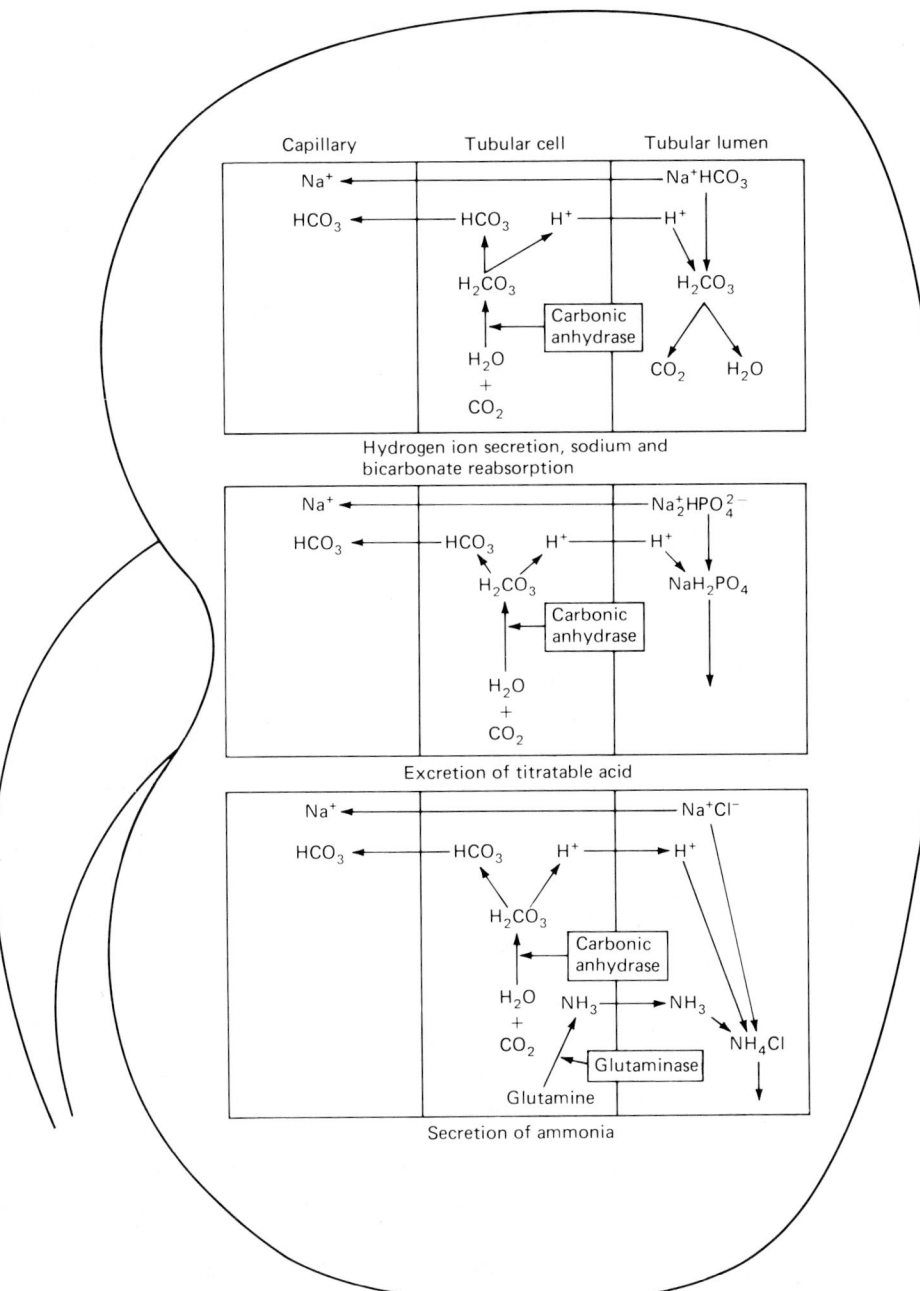

Figure 10-3   Regulation of hydrogen ion concentration by the renal system.

the individual's serum sodium value minus the sum of the chloride and bicarbonate values equals a value that falls within the normal range for the anion gap of 8 to 16 meq/L. In other words, the formula for calculating the anion gap is:

$$\text{Anion gap} = Na^+ - (Cl^- + HCO_3)$$

When the formula is applied to those etiologies that produce increased amounts of nonvolatile acids in the body, the result is an increase in the anion gap.

Those etiologies that produce a loss of bicarbonate from the body include renal tubular acidosis; use of carbonic anhydrase inhibitors; extracellular fluid volume expansion; hyperalimentation; administration of chloride-containing acids, such as hydrochloric acid or ammonium chloride; diarrhea; pancreatic or small bowel draining fistulas; ureterosigmoidostomy; ileal conduit; and the use of anion exchange resins, such as cholestyramine.

Those etiologies that produce metabolic acidosis by increasing the amount of acid in the body, creating a normochloremic acidosis, are renal failure, diabetic ketoacidosis, lactic acidosis, starvation, ethanol intoxication, tissue hypoxia, paraldehyde intoxication, salicylate intoxication, methanol intoxication, and high-fat diets.

Clinical Assessment Parameters

The individual experiencing metabolic acidosis exhibits a combination of the following signs and symptoms: headache, fatigue, drowsiness, decreased mental function, confusion, coma, seizures, hypotension, tissue hypoxia, cardiac dysrhythmia, Kussmaul respirations, anorexia, nausea, and vomiting.

Laboratory Assessment Data

The laboratory values that provide the most significant data for assessing the acid-base balance of an individual are the blood gas values. Table 10-2 presents the normal values for both arterial and mixed venous blood gas samples. In addition to the blood gas values, selected serum and urine values also provide significant assessment data.

The pattern of laboratory values that is characteristic of metabolic acidosis is a pH less than 7.37, a bicarbonate less than 22 meq/L, a base excess

Table 10-2 Normal Blood Gas Values

Substance Measured	Arterial Blood	Mixed Venous Blood
pH	7.37–7.43 (7.35–7.45)*	7.33–7.39 (7.31–7.41)*
P_{O_2}	80–100 mmHg	35–40 mmHg
O_2 saturation	95–97%	70–75%
P_{CO_2}	37–43 mmHg (35–45 mmHg)*	41–51 mmHg
HCO_3	22–26 meq/L	22–26 meq/L
BE (base excess)	+2 to −2	+2 to −2

*The more liberal range is gaining wider acceptance as being the norm.

less than −2, a decreased P_{CO_2}, an increased serum potassium; and usually a decreased urine pH that may vary depending on the etiology.

Clinical and Nursing Implications

The clinical implications of metabolic acidosis for the patient are significant because the body does not tolerate changes in hydrogen ion concentration in the internal environment very well. Such changes will accelerate, deter, or inhibit various metabolic processes, creating greater hazards to the individual's health state. However, the most threatening change that occurs with severe acidosis is cardiovascular collapse due to arteriolar dilation and decreased cardiac contractility. This change obviously can result in the patient's death.

The nursing monitoring functions performed with the individual experiencing metabolic acidosis include (1) assessing the level of consciousness periodically; (2) evaluating overall muscle strength; (3) assessing the rate, rhythm, pattern, and characteristics of all vital signs, especially the pulse and respirations; (4) monitoring the color and temperature of the skin as a means of determining tissue perfusion status; (5) assessing gastrointestinal functioning; (6) measuring and recording intake and output meticulously; (7) obtaining accurate daily weights; (8) assessing the comfort level frequently; (9) assessing for signs of hyperkalemia; and (10) monitoring appropriate laboratory values periodically.

Nursing interventions that are performed with the patient with metabolic acidosis are (1) administering fluids and medications as prescribed, (2) instituting seizure precautions, (3) maintaining bed rest and instituting active and passive range of motion exercises, (4) assisting the individual in assuming a position to facilitate respirations, (5) providing stimuli appropriate to maintaining orientation, (6) providing nursing comfort measures to deal with the gastrointestinal effects, (7) providing frequent oral hygiene using nondrying agents, and (8) establishing a safe physical environment for the individual.

Treatment

The treatment of metabolic acidosis is aimed at dealing with the underlying cause. Thus, the therapy used will vary according to the etiology. However, if the acidosis is severe, it is important to replace the lost bicarbonate simultaneously while treating the underlying cause. The general rule is to replace the bicarbonate loss slowly with an appropriate alkali over several hours. It is also suggested in this case that a slight undercorrection be achieved to prevent a rebound metabolic alkalosis from occurring.

Metabolic Alkalosis

Definition

Metabolic alkalosis is an excess of bicarbonate in the extracellular fluid.

Etiology

Metabolic alkalosis is caused by the following: vomiting; gastrointestinal suctioning; diarrhea (if it has a high chloride content); diuretic therapy; laxative abuse; cystic fibrosis; primary and secondary hyperaldosteronism; Cushing's syndrome; licorice abuse; excessive ingestion of bicarbonate, or other alkalinizing salts; hypokalemia; and hypercalcemia.

Clinical Assessment Parameters

Metabolic alkalosis is exhibited clinically in an individual by a combination of the following signs and symptoms: increased neuromuscular irritabil-

ity, tetany, seizures, belligerence, confusion, stupor, coma, hypoventilation, cardiac dysrhythmia, nausea, vomiting, and diarrhea.

Laboratory Assessment Data

The laboratory data used to assess an individual for metabolic alkalosis are provided primarily by the blood gas values, but selected serum and urine values can also be of assistance. The pattern of laboratory values characteristic of metabolic alkalosis is a pH greater than 7.43; a bicarbonate greater than 26 meq/L; a base excess greater than $+2$; an increased P_{CO_2}; a decreased serum chloride; a decreased serum potassium; a decreased serum calcium; and a decreased urine chloride, the degree of which depends on the etiology. If the etiology of the metabolic alkalosis is associated with extracellular fluid volume depletion, the patient exhibits a urinary chloride of less than 10 meq/L. If the etiology is related to extracellular fluid volume expansion, the urinary chloride is greater than 20 meq/L.

Clinical and Nursing Implications

The clinical significance of metabolic alkalosis for a patient is related to the neuromuscular and respiratory effects of the imbalance. The hyperirritability of the central nervous system and the compensatory hypoventilation represent definite risks to a person's well-being.

The nursing monitoring functions performed with the individual experiencing metabolic alkalosis include (1) assessing the level of consciousness; (2) evaluating neuromuscular function periodically; (3) monitoring muscle strength and movement; (4) assessing the rate, rhythm, pattern, and characteristics of all vital signs, especially respirations; (5) measuring and recording intake and output accurately; (6) obtaining precise measurement of daily weights; (7) assessing the characteristics of the feces; (8) monitoring Chvostek's and Trousseau's signs for hypocalcemia; and (9) monitoring appropriate laboratory values periodically.

The intervening functions that are part of the nursing care performed with patients with metabolic alkalosis are (1) establishing a safe physical environment, (2) instituting seizure precautions, (3) providing stimuli appropriate to maintaining orientation, (4) assisting the individual with the activities of daily living, (5) providing nursing comfort measures to deal with the gastrointestinal effects of the imbalance, and (6) administering fluids and medications as prescribed.

Treatment

The treatment of metabolic alkalosis involves eliminating the primary cause and correcting the imbalance. Correcting the imbalance is accomplished by a four-level therapeutic approach. This therapeutic approach includes (1) replacing any extracellular fluid volume deficit with saline; (2) administering chloride (in the form of ammonium chloride or arginine hydrochloride if the sodium chloride in the saline solution is not sufficient to replace the lost anion); (3) correcting the potassium depletion with potassium chloride; and (4) increasing the excretion of bicarbonate by using carbonic anhydrase-inhibiting diuretics, or, in instances of renal dysfunction, by dialysis therapy.

Respiratory Acidosis

Definition

Respiratory acidosis is an excess of carbonic acid in the extracellular fluid.

Etiology

Respiratory acidosis is caused by etiologies that create hypoventilation and result in the retention of carbon dioxide in the body. Those etiologies are categorized according to the mechanisms responsible for creating the hypoventilation. There are five categories of etiologies that result in respiratory acidosis: (1) airway obstructions, (2) depressants of the respiratory center, (3) defects in the nerves and muscles of respiration, (4) lung diseases, and (5) thoracic cage disorders. Table 10-3 presents specific examples for each of the categories of etiologies of respiratory acidosis.

Clinical Assessment Parameters

The person experiencing respiratory acidosis exhibits many of the following signs and symptoms:

Table 10-3 Specific Etiologies of Respiratory Acidosis

Category	Examples
Airway obstructions	Aspiration
	Foreign bodies
	Pulmonary embolus
	Severe bronchospasms
	Pulmonary edema
	Laryngeal edema
Depressants of the respiratory center	Sedatives
	Chronic narcotic abuse
	Metabolic alkalosis
	General anesthesia
	Increased intracranial pressure
	Medullary tumors
	Meningitis
	Vertebral artery embolism or thrombosis
Defects in the nerves and muscles of respiration	Myasthenia gravis
	Guillain-Barré syndrome
	Poliomyelitis
	Botulism
	Spinal cord injury
	Paralysis associated with hypo- or hyperkalemia
Lung diseases	Chronic obstructive pulmonary disease
	Smoke inhalation
	Pneumonia
	Atelectasis
	Asthma
	Interstitial lung disease
	Bronchitis
	Bronchiectasis
Thoracic cage disorders	Flail chest
	Pneumothorax
	Pickwickian syndrome
	Ankylosing spondylitis

dull, slow mental responses; apprehension; restlessness; headache; drowsiness; disorientation; coma; tachycardia; hypoventilation; dyspnea; fatigue; weakness; flapping tremors; uncoordination; and decreased reflexes. Cyanosis due to hypoxia is also present as a *very late* sign of respiratory acidosis.

Laboratory Assessment Data

The blood gas values provide the most significant laboratory data for assessing an individual for respiratory acidosis. However, there are some serum and urine values that can provide additional assessment data. The characteristic pattern of values exhibited by patients experiencing respiratory acidosis is a pH less than 7.37, a P_{CO_2} greater than 43 to 45 mmHg, a normal to increased bicarbonate, a normal to decreased P_{O_2}, a normal to increased serum potassium, and a decreased urine pH.

Clinical and Nursing Implications

The clinical significance of respiratory acidosis for a patient is related not only to the effects of the acidosis on the body, but also to the effects of the accompanying hypoxia. Without sufficient oxygen, the human organism cannot survive. Thus this imbalance indeed represents a crisis and requires nursing support in the form of monitoring and intervening functions.

The monitoring functions performed with a patient experiencing respiratory acidosis include (1) assessing skin color, temperature, and moistness for signs of hypoxia; (2) monitoring the rate, rhythm, pattern, and characteristics of all vital signs; (3) assessing the level of consciousness frequently; (4) evaluating muscle strength, coordination, and movement; (5) assessing the individual's comfort level; and (6) monitoring all appropriate laboratory values at intervals.

The intervening functions performed with the individual with respiratory acidosis are (1) providing a safe physical environment for the person, (2) maintaining a decreased activity level consistent with the level of hypoxia, (3) assisting the patient with all activities of daily living, (4) providing a quiet environment with enough stimuli to maintain orientation, (5) providing emotional support and reassurance, (6) assisting the individual to assume a position that facilitates adequate respirations, (7) instituting preventive pulmonary maintenance therapies to increase the removal of carbon dioxide by the lungs (turning, coughing, deep breathing, suctioning, resistance breathing), (8) administering oxygen when appropriate and as prescribed, and (9) administering fluids and medications if prescribed.

Treatment

The goal for treating respiratory acidosis is to reestablish effective ventilation for the individual. In some instances this may require creating an artificial airway and/or using mechanical ventilation until the primary etiology can be treated. Bicarbonate and oxygen may be administered concurrently with efforts to treat the cause in an attempt to correct or lessen the immediate effects of the imbalance.

Respiratory Alkalosis

Definition

Respiratory alkalosis is a deficit of carbonic acid in the extracellular fluid.

Etiology

Respiratory alkalosis is caused by etiologies that produce hyperventilation and a decrease of carbon dioxide in the body. Those etiologies include alcoholic intoxication, anemia, gram-negative sepsis, meningitis, encephalitis, head trauma, brain lesions, congestive heart failure, exercise, fever, cirrhosis, paraldehyde intoxication, pulmonary fibrosis; hypoxia, thyrotoxicosis, mechanical hyperventilation, salicylate intoxication, anxiety, hysteria, and voluntary hyperpnea.

Clinical Assessment Parameters

The individual experiencing respiratory alkalosis exhibits a combination of the following signs and symptoms: breathlessness, vertigo, syncope, nervousness, paresthesias of the extremities, perioral paresthesia, muscle cramps and tetany, seizures, decreased mentation, confusion, decreased psychomotor performance, anxiety, hyperventilation, cardiac dysrhythmia, and hypotension.

Laboratory Assessment Data

The blood gas values are the most significant laboratory data used in assessing an individual for respiratory alkalosis. The characteristic pattern is a pH greater than 7.43, a P_{CO_2} less than 37 mmHg, and a decreased bicarbonate.

Clinical and Nursing Implications

The clinical significance of respiratory alkalosis for a patient is related to the neuromuscular effects it produces. Those effects make it impossible for a person to function and carry out the normal activities of daily living. The individual may also develop life-threatening seizures as a result of the respiratory alkalosis.

The nursing monitoring functions performed with a patient experiencing respiratory alkalosis include (1) assessing the level of consciousness frequently; (2) monitoring the rate, rhythm, pattern, and characteristics of all vital signs; (3) monitoring sensation in the extremities and perioral area; (4) assessing muscle movement and strength; and (5) monitoring all appropriate laboratory data.

The intervening functions performed with an individual experiencing respiratory alkalosis are (1) establishing a safe physical environment for the individual; (2) maintaining an activity level appropriate to the degree of weakness, vertigo, and syncope; (3) instituting seizure precautions; (4) providing sufficient stimuli to maintain orientation; (5) assisting the individual in performing activities of daily living; (6) providing emotional support and reassurance; (7) instituting nursing measures to assist in decreasing hyperventilation and increasing carbon dioxide (such as teaching breathing exercises or having the individual breathe in and out of a paper bag, thus rebreathing carbon dioxide); and (8) administering medications as prescribed.

Treatment

The treatment of respiratory alkalosis is aimed at dealing with the underlying cause. However, when it is not possible to eradicate the cause, sedation, administration of 3 to 5 percent carbon dioxide, and breathing exercises are used to correct the imbalance.

Clinical Application

The pH of a person's internal environment can be significantly altered by varying types of pathophysiologies, thus creating an unstable state. As a result, the individual requires nursing and medical support to maintain and regain appropriate physiologic functioning. To provide appropriate nursing support, the nurse must be able to comprehend and apply the previously discussed information regarding acid-base balances and imbalances to formulate a plan of care. The following is an example of how such information might be utilized in the clinical setting.

Case Study

J. W. is a 24-year-old Caucasian male admitted to the hospital with an initial diagnosis of septicemia incurred as a result of drug abuse. He states that he has developed a fever and has had nausea, vomiting, shaking chills, and decreased urinary output over the last 4 or 5 days.

Upon admission he is noted to be an emaciated, pale, drowsy individual with moderate peripheral edema. He also has stomatitis; halitosis; warm, dry, needle-tracked skin; and mild tremors of all extremities. His vital signs are: blood pressure, 148/98; pulse, 104; respirations, 30; and oral temperature, 103°. His laboratory values are:

Serum Values		Urine Values		Blood Gas Values	
Sodium	138 meq/L	Amount	288 mL/24°	pH	7.21
Potassium	7.2 meq/L	Specific gravity	1.010	P_{CO_2}	24 mmHg
Chloride	99 meq/L	pH	8	HCO_3	12.5 meq/L
BUN	80 mg/100 mL	Glucose	negative	P_{O_2}	91 mmHg
Creatinine	8 mg/100 mL	Protein	negative	O_2 sat	90%
Calcium	7 mg/100 mL	Creatinine	120 mg/100 mL		
Phosphorus	6 mg/100 mL	Osmolality	280 mOsm/kg H_2O		
C_{O_2} combining		Sodium	40 meq/L		
power	12 meq/L	Potassium	10 meq/L		
Magnesium	2 meq/L	Chloride	40 meq/L		
Osmolality	307 mOsm/kg H_2O	Calcium	3 meq/L		
Hematocrit	30%	Phosphorus	200 mg/24°		
Hemoglobin	10 g/100 mL				

Discussion

The nursing care planning for J. W. begins with a total assessment, which will of course include his clinical signs and symptoms and an interpretation of his laboratory values. J. W.'s clinical signs and symptoms are consistent with a diagnosis of septicemia, but they also suggest malnutrition; potential renal dysfunction; and several fluid, electrolyte, and acid-base imbalances. An interpretation of his laboratory values will assist in further delineating his needs.

The nurse would probably elect to begin by interpreting J. W.'s blood gas values. In this process, the steps listed in Table 10-4 would be employed. Thus, the nurse would: (1) assess the pH, determine that it was decreased and that acidosis was the imbalance; (2) assess the P_{CO_2} and decide that it was decreased; (3) assess the HCO_3 and decide that it was decreased; (4) note that a decreased P_{CO_2} (which is the acid, respiratory component of acid-base balance) will not create acidosis in the body, but that a decreased HCO_3, (which is the base, metabolic component of acid-base balance), will create acidosis, and thus determine that this imbalance is metabolic acidosis and that the decreased P_{CO_2} reflects partial respiratory compensation; and (5) assess the P_{O_2} and O_2 saturation and determine that they are both normal. The nurse would then continue to assess J. W.'s other laboratory values before formulating a plan of care.

An interpretation of the other serum laboratory values reveals that J. W. also has normonatremia, hyperkalemia, normochloremia, uremia, hypocal-

cemia, hyperphosphatemia, acidosis, normomagnesemia, hyperosmolality, and anemia. In addition, he has an increased anion gap of about 26 meq/L. His urine values indicate oliguria, a fixed density, alkaline urine, normal glucose, normal protein, hypocreatininuria, hypoosmolality, hyponatruria, hypokaluria, hypochloruria, hypocalciuria, and hypophosphaturia. These values are all consistent with a diagnosis of septicemia accompanied by acute renal failure.

Based on these assessment data, the nurse would formulate a plan of care that would encompass the following continuous monitoring functions: (1) assessing the level of consciousness; (2) evaluating overall muscle strength; (3) assessing the rate, rhythm, pattern, and characteristics of all vital signs; (4) monitoring skin color and temperature; (5) meticulously monitoring and recording intake and output measurements; (6) obtaining accurate daily weights; (7) assessing gastrointestinal functioning; (8) assessing comfort level; and (9) monitoring appropriate laboratory values.

Such a plan of care would also include the following intervening functions: (1) administering medications as prescribed; (2) instituting seizure precautions; (3) assisting the individual in assuming a position to facilitate respirations; (4) providing stimuli appropriate for maintaining orientation; (5) providing adequate calories and nutrition consistent with fluid, sodium, potassium, and protein restrictions; (6) establishing a safe physical environment for the individual; (7) maintaining bed rest and instituting active and passive range of motion exercises; (8) providing comfort measures to deal with the gastrointestinal effects; (9) providing frequent oral hygiene using nondrying agents; (10) instituting positive preventative pulmonary maintenance therapies; (11) avoiding instrumentation and manipulation whenever possible; (12) providing meticulous skin care and daily hygiene; and (13) preparing the individual for or implementing dialysis therapy as prescribed.

The clinician engages in the process illustrated by the above example numerous times during every clinical or working day. Such activities are integral components of the systematic process of delivering quality patient care. Thus, this process and its essential underlying content comprise one of the major accoutrements of professional clinical nursing.

Table 10-4 Steps for Interpreting Blood Gas Values

1. Assess the pH and determine if it is increased, indicating alkalosis; decreased, indicating acidosis; or normal, indicating no imbalance.
2. Assess the P_{CO_2} and decide if it is increased, decreased, or normal.
3. Assess the HCO_3 and decide if it is increased, decreased, or normal.
4. If there is an imbalance, determine whether it is respiratory or metabolic. Remember the P_{CO_2} is the acid, respiratory component of acid-base balance and HCO_3 is the base, metabolic component.
5. Assess the P_{O_2} and O_2 saturation and determine if they are increased, decreased, or normal.
6. Determine the type of nursing interventions necessary to assit the patient in coping with the acid-base imbalance.

Summary

This chapter has discussed the regulation and assessment of acid-base balance. The information contained in this chapter is continuously utilized by clinicians as they make decisions regarding patient care. Because of the importance of acid-base balance in maintaining a stable internal environment for the individual, the content of this discussion assumes high priority for the critical-care nurse. In fact, acid-base balance is second only to fluid balance in priority in relation to patient care. Thus, the critical-care nurse must be well acquainted with this information and ready to apply it in all instances. To assist the nurse in making such applications, the signs and symptoms of each acid-base imbalance have been summarized according to body systems in Table 9-15. The acid-base imbalances appear in priority order in Table 9-15 and follow the fluid volume imbalances.

Bibliography

Aberman, A. (1984). An update on diabetic ketoacidosis. *Emergency Medicine, 16*(3), 90, 92–93, 97–98.

Arieff, A. I., & DeFronzo, R. A. (1978). *Fluid, electrolyte and acid-base metabolism: Diagnosis and management.* Philadelphia: Lippincott.

Clausen, J. L., & Murray, K. M. (1985). Clinical applications of arterial blood gases: How much accuracy do we need? *Journal of Medical Technology, 2*(1), 19–21.

Cohen, J. J., & Kassirer, J. P. (1982). *Acid-base.* Boston: Little, Brown.

Cohen, S. (1978). Metabolic acid-base disorders. Pt. 1. Chemistry and physiology—programmed instruction. *American Journal of Nursing, 78*(3), 1–16.

Done, A. K. (1981, Oct. 15). The toxic emergency. Acid-base disturbances: Aids to differential diagnosis. *Emergency Medicine 13,* 68, 73–76, 79, 83–84.

———. (1981, Sept. 15). The toxic emergency. Acid-base disturbances: Aids to evaluation. *Emergency Medicine 13,* 159–161, 165–166, 168–171.

Flenly, D. C. (1982). Blood gas and acid-base interpretation. *Respiratory Care, 27*(3), 311–317.

Flomenbaum, N. (1984). Acid-base disturbances. *Emergency Medicine 16*(3), 59–61, 65–66, 71–72, 77–78, 81–86, 88–89.

Glass, L. B., & Jenkins, C. A. (1983). The ups and downs of serum pH. *Nursing 83, 13*(9), 34–41.

Greenberg, A. (1984). Common emergencies of acid-base balance. *Topics in Emergency Medicine, 5*(4), 1–16.

Green, D. A. (1984). Diabetic ketoacidosis. *Topics in Emergency Medicine, 5*(4), 17–32.

Guyton, A. C. (1986). *Textbook of medical physiology* (7th ed.). Philadelphia: Saunders.

Hricik, D. E., & Kassirer, J. P. (1983). Understanding and using the anion gap. *Consultant, 23*(7), 130–134, 143.

Janusek, L. W. (1984). Metabolic acidosis: Physiology, signs and symptoms. *Nursing 84, 14*(7), 44–45.

Keyes, J. L. (1985). *Fluid, electrolyte, and acid-base regulation.* Monterey: Wadsworth Health Sciences Division.

Klahr, S. (1978). *Differential diagnosis: Renal and electrolyte disorders.* New York: Arco.

Kurtzman, N. A., Arruda, J. A. L., & Westenfelder, C. (1978). Renal regulation of acid-base homeostasis. *Contributions to Nephrology, 14,* 1–13.

Maxwell, M. H., & Kleeman, C. R. (1980). *Clinical disorders of fluid and electrolyte metabolism* (3d ed.), New York: McGraw-Hill.

Miller, W. C. (1984). The ABCs of blood gases. *Emergency Medicine, 16*(3), 37–38, 43–45, 48, 51–52, 54–56.

Moore, V. B. (1979). Analyzing the ABG analysis. *Nursing 79, 9*(9), 28–33.

Neff, J. A. (1984). Acid-base balance: A tool for rapid evaluation. *Journal of Emergency Nursing, 10*(6), 322–324.

Perkins, C., & Bralley, H. K. (1983). Metabolic alkalosis. *Nursing 83, 13*(1), 57.

Porter, R., & Lawrenson, G. (1982). *Ciba Foundation symposium 87—Metabolic acidosis.* London: Pitman.

Randall, H. T. (1976). Fluid, electrolyte, and acid-base balance. *Surgical Clinics of North America, 56*(5), 1019–1058.

Ryou, K. (1981). Interpretation of acid-base status. *Journal of the American Medical Technologists, 43,* 61–65.

Schrier, R. (1986). *Renal and electrolyte disorders* (3d ed.). Boston: Little, Brown.

Shapiro, B. A. (1979). *Clinical application of respiratory care* (2d ed.). Chicago: Year Book.

Taylor, D. L. (1984). Respiratory acidosis—physiology, signs, and symptoms. *Nursing 84, 14*(10), 44–45.

Valtin, H. (1979). *Renal dysfunction: Mechanisms involved in fluid and solute imbalance.* Boston: Little, Brown.

Vander, A. J. (1985). *Renal physiology* (2d ed.). New York: McGraw-Hill.

11

Cardiac Electrical Activity

Linda J. Miers

Function of the heart muscle is dependent on an interaction between an electrical stimulus and a mechanical response. The importance of the electrical activity of the heart, therefore, cannot be overstated. This chapter is devoted to describing the propagation of the electrical stimulus; explaining the measurement of the cardiac electrical activity in the clinical setting; and discussing the cause, identification, and treatment of common electrical abnormalities.

Electrophysiology

Transmembrane Potential

Within intracellular and extracellular fluids are concentrations of electrolytes normally totaling about 155 meq per liter of positively charged ions (cations) and negatively charged ions (anions). Usually, excess numbers of cations accumulate along the outside surface of the membrane, while excess numbers of anions accumulate along the inside of the membrane, resulting in a *transmembrane potential*. When the internal environment of the atrial and ventricular myocardial cells is electrically measured, it is found to have about -90 millivolts (mV) with respect to the outside. The cell is said to be *polarized* when the internal environment is negative with respect to the outside.

Development of Potential

The two electrolytes most involved in the physics of transmembrane potentials are sodium and potassium. The intracellular concentration of potassium is approximately 140 meq, while the extracellular concentration normally ranges between 3.5 and 4.5 meq/L. Conversely, the intracellular sodium concentration is approximately 10 meq/L; the ex-

tracellular sodium concentration is approximately 140 meq/L. The concentration gradient for potassium favors movement from the inside to the outside of the cell. Sodium is favored to move intracellularly along its concentration gradient.

Calculation of the resting transmembrane potential is based on the potential for diffusion across the cell membrane as a result of concentration and electrical gradients. As potassium diffuses out of the cell along its concentration gradient, it leaves behind large numbers of negatively charged proteins, organic phosphates, and other anions which are too large to diffuse through the cell membrane. The internal concentration of nondiffusible anions is approximately 150 meq/L; the external concentration is approximately 5 meq/L. Thus, the internal environment of the cell becomes increasingly negative, while the extracellular environment becomes increasingly positive. The positive charges line up outside the cell membrane, attracted by the internal negativity. A balance is reached when the concentration gradient for potassium efflux is equalized by the internal attraction of the negative ions for those remaining positive ions. The actual calculation of -90 mV is based on the Nernst equation, which states that a cation gradient favoring outward movement causes internal negativity, while an anion gradient in the reverse direction also causes internal electronegativity.

When the extracellular potassium concentration increases, the resting transmembrane potential can become more negative. The electrical gradient remains unchanged, but the concentration gradient for potassium diminishes; therefore, the transmembrane potential could exceed the normal negativity of -90 mV (hyperpolarization).

The role of other ions in the development of transmembrane potential is a relatively passive one.

The next most abundant anion is chloride, which has an extracellular concentration of approximately 100 meq/L and an intracellular concentration of about 4 meq/L. This distribution is maintained by the electrical gradient within the cell which repels the negative chloride ion. Magnesium, a cation with an intracellular concentration of 58 meq/L and a very low extracellular concentration, follows a diffusion pattern similar to that of potassium, while calcium has a relatively low concentration both intra- and extracellularly. The major role of calcium and magnesium is thought to be the alteration of membrane permeability to other ions.

The Action Potential

Any stimulus which increases the permeability of the membrane to sodium so that a critical threshold is reached will generate an *action potential*. The cardiac action potential is a graphic representation of the rapid and abrupt pulselike changes in the membrane potential (Fig. 11-1). The electrical potential, measured in mV, is indicated along the vertical axis of the graph. Time, measured in milliseconds (ms), is indicated along the horizontal axis. The action potential consists of three to five phases, labeled as phase 0 through phase 4. Each phase represents a particular electrical event or combination of electrical events. The events, the duration of the events and action potential, and the transmembrane potential vary with the type of cardiac cell being measured. Figure 11-1A is an action potential representative of a normal ventricular muscle cell. The cardiac action potential of the sinus node is illustrated in Fig. 11-1B.

Depolarization

Once the internal negativity decreases from its resting potential of approximately −90 mV to −60 mV or the threshold potential (TP in Fig. 11-1A), a very rapid loss of negativity and positive overshoot to about +30 mV occurs and the fiber is *depolarized*. This rapid change in potential is identified as *phase 0* on the cardiac action potential.

The basis for the very rapid change in the permeability of the membrane is unknown. Guyton postulated that certain channels or pores exist for the passage of sodium which, during resting potential, are obstructed through calcium binding to

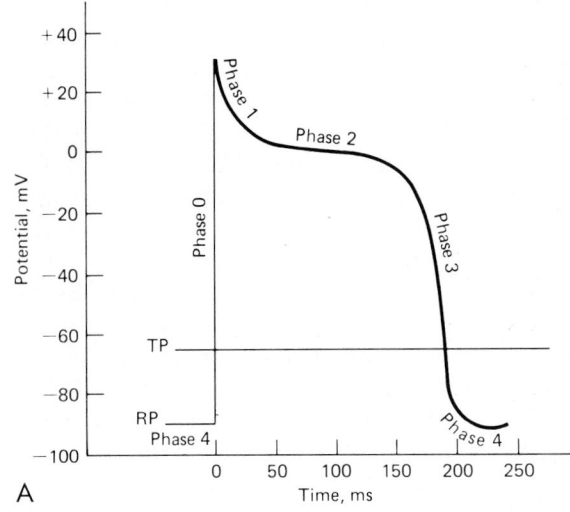

A

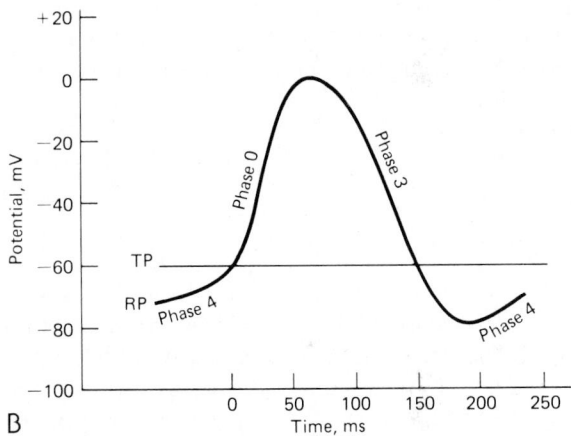

B

Figure 11-1   Transmembrane potentials (TMP) from two types of cells. *A.* TMP from ordinary myocardial muscle fibers. *B.* TMP from the SA node which is representative of myocardial cells capable of automaticity. See text for discussion. *(From J. W. Hurst, R. B. Logue, R. C. Schlant, and N. K. Wenger, eds., The heart, arteries, and veins, McGraw-Hill, New York, 1978, p. 639. Copyright 1978 by McGraw-Hill Book Company. Adapted by permission.)*

proteins in the membrane.[1] Because calcium is a cation, sodium is repelled and cannot pass through. Following excitation of the membrane, the calcium ions are somehow dislodged from their binding sites and sodium rapidly diffuses into the cell. Others have theorized the existence of actual activation gates which open to allow sodium passage during phase 0 of the action potential, and inactivation gates which inhibit the fast sodium current later on in the depolarization of the muscle fiber.

The resting membrane potential is a critical determinant in depolarization. A less negative resting potential can lead to inexcitability of the fiber even if the concentration for sodium is normal. The inactivation process for the sodium channels, then, is extremely important because the fast sodium channels are not thought to function properly unless the membrane is returned to the normal resting potential. Once an action potential has been generated, the fast sodium channels cannot be activated again until the membrane has been returned to near resting potential, thus preventing sustained muscle contraction.

Once the peak of the positive overshoot is approached within the membrane, the rapid sodium influx has diminished considerably. This happens for at least two reasons: (1) The increase in positivity inside the membrane begins to repel further influx of sodium; and (2) the inactivation process blocks the fast sodium channels, perhaps through binding with calcium or by means of the inactivation gates.

Early Repolarization

Once rapid sodium influx is terminated, a brief phase of repolarization occurs. This early repolarization is identified as *phase 1* and results from a rapid, but brief, influx of the anion chloride and an efflux of potassium. During this phase the transmembrane potential is reduced to approximately 0 mV.

The Plateau

In myocardial cells there is a period of sustained contraction known as the *plateau (phase 2)*. There seems to be a slow inward sodium current which is different from the rapid influx of sodium during phase 0. In addition, there is a slow calcium inward current which is instrumental in myocardial contractility. Apparently, both ions are carried by the same inward channel.

The concentration gradient is unchanged for potassium, thereby promoting an outward current of potassium which would bring about rapid repolarization of the fiber. During phase 2, however, the permeability of the membrane for potassium decreases, thereby decreasing potassium conduct-

ance (anomalous rectification). Consequently, the fiber is able to sustain contraction.

Repolarization

Return of the membrane to resting potential in *phase 3 (repolarization)* is accomplished almost entirely by potassium efflux along its concentration gradient. Also, the slow inward currents of sodium and potassium are inactivated. With the rapid outward movement of potassium, the cell becomes increasingly negative until resting potential is restored.

Active Transport of Sodium and Potassium

Maintenance of the resting potential is clearly dependent on potassium. However, sodium has a concentration gradient favoring inward movement. During the resting state (*phase 4 of the action potential*) the membrane is 50 to 100 times less permeable to sodium than to potassium. Even so, some sodium does leak into the cell during the resting state. Were the sodium allowed to build up within the cell, resting potential would soon be dissipated. The sodium pump is in constant operation in order to actively transport sodium to the extracellular fluid against its concentration gradient. An active transport pump also functions to bring potassium into the cell against its concentration gradient. The sodium and potassium pumps require energy to function and can become inhibited by medication such as digitalis and perhaps also by ischemia. The effect of inhibition of the potassium pump is the same as inhibition of the sodium active transport mechanism: loss of internal electronegativity.

Excitability

When cardiac tissue is capable of being depolarized by a stimulus it is said to be *excitable*. While the degree of excitability depends on many factors, at any given physiologic state it is related to the phase of the cardiac cycle. During phase 4 the excitability of the cardiac cell is at a maximum. Beginning at phase 0 and continuing to approximately the midpoint of phase 3, the cell is in a period of *absolute* or *effective refractoriness,* and excitability is zero (ARP, ERP on Fig. 11-2). No stimulus, regardless of

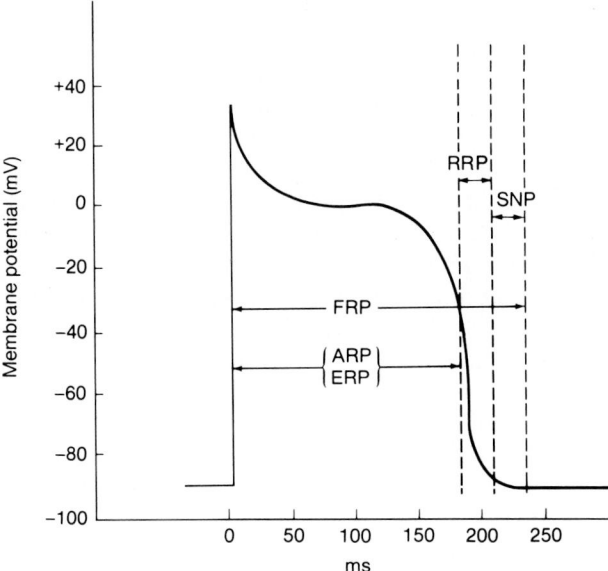

Figure 11-2 Excitability during the cardiac action potential. See text for discussion.

magnitude, will produce a response. The period from the midpoint of phase 3 extending to just before the beginning of phase 4 is known as the *relative refractory period* (RRP on Fig. 11-2). The fiber is capable of generating an action potential, but only if the stimulus is stronger than that which would be required during phase 4. During a brief period following phase 3 and ending when the fiber returns to its resting potential, known as the *supernormal period* and shown as SNP on Fig. 11-2, a stimulus slightly less than normal can cause a propagated action potential. Generally, the later in phase 3 that stimulation occurs, the greater the amplitude and velocity of conduction. However, the action potential that results from excitation during the supernormal period is not unusually large; rather, the action potential is usually reduced in amplitude due to the slow recovery of the sodium channels.

The basis for the refractory periods probably resides with the inactivation of the fast sodium currents occurring in repolarization; thus, the closer the membrane is to resting potential when excited, the more fast sodium channels will be reactivated. The duration of the refractory period varies according to the type of action potential, whether a fast or slow response, and probably according to other factors as well. In cells characterized by the slow response, the effective refractory periods are longer than in the normal myocardial fiber. The absolute refractory periods can continue well beyond phase 3, and the relative refractory period continues into phase 4. Impulses which arrive somewhat early in phase 4 are conducted very slowly, even though the membrane is at resting potential and fully repolarized.

Automaticity

Certain specialized fibers within the myocardium possess the property of *automaticity*; that is, they attain threshold in the absence of any external stimulus. These automatic, or pacemaker, cells lie primarily within the sinoatrial (SA) node, the atrioventricular (AV) junction, and the Purkinje network of the cardiac conduction system. A comparison of the action potential of an automatic myocardial fiber (Fig. 11-1*B*) with that of a normal ventricular myocardial fiber (Fig. 11-1*A*) shows the following: The resting potential of the sinus node automatic cells can be seen to be much slower and less negative; the phase 0 upstroke is more sluggish; and the amplitude of the action potential is not as great as that of a ventricular myocardial fiber—there is little or no positive overshoot within the action potential of the automatic cell. In addition, the automatic cell is capable of diastolic depolarization. During phase 4 of the sinoatrial (SA) node fiber, the membrane does not maintain a constant resting potential as do ventricular myocardial fibers, and diastolic depolarization brings the membrane to threshold, eliciting an action potential. Generally, these properties are limited to automatic cells; however, under certain conditions such as ischemia, the action potential of other cells may shift to assume some of the properties of the pacemaker or "slow" action potential by a rise in threshold potential from -90 mV to levels of approximately -60 mV. It is apparent that conduction in tissue responding with a "slow" action potential would be characterized by a decreased conduction velocity, a property which can increase the potential for conduction block.

The ionic basis of the slow-response action potential parallels phase 2 of the ventricular myocardial fiber or fast-response cell. The positive overshoot does not occur within the slow-response cell, presumably because there is no rapid influx of sodium. For all practical purposes, then, there is no corollary of phase 1 or phase 2 within the slow-response cell; the slow inward currents for sodium and calcium account for the slow positive upstroke of phase 0 in Fig. 11-1*B*.

Propagation of the Action Potential

Since the myocardium is surrounded by intracellular and extracellular fluids which are replete with electrolytes, the myocardial fibers are surrounded by excellent conductors of electricity. With stimulation of the fiber, the positive charges flow inward, thus attracting negative ions to the external surface. Because current flows from higher to lower potential, the external flow is in the direction of right to left (from positive to negative), while intracellularly it flows from left to right (Fig. 11-3). At any given point in the process of activation there is a boundary which separates the depolarized and polarized zones. It is these differences in potential which are measured by the lead systems of the electrocardiogram. During the period in which depolarization has been completed and the muscle sustains activation, there is no difference in electrical potential and, therefore, no current to be measured by the electrocardiogram.

The velocity of the conduction across the muscle is dependent on the difference in potential between the activated and resting muscle. The greater the magnitude of the action potential and the faster the positive overshoot occurs, the more rapidly conduction occurs. When the resting potential becomes more positive, such as in ischemic tissue or in premature beats, the velocity of conduction diminishes.

The impulse, once initiated, is propagated in all directions until depolarization of the entire myocardium has been effected. Known as the "all-or-nothing law," the impulse spreads from one muscle fiber to the next with no additional stimulation until the wave of excitation reaches a point where there is insufficient voltage to attain threshold potential. The heart behaves as a single cell, a functional syncytium.

Automatic pacemaker cells, or those cells which are characterized by the slow response, possess a much slower speed of conduction. The greater vulnerability of the slow-response fibers to block has already been mentioned. In addition, these fibers are unable to conduct at rapid rates. The velocity of conduction may differ according to the direction of conduction (whether antegrade or retrograde) in the slow-response fibers. The basis of reentry exists in the frequency with which a slow-response fiber can conduct an impulse in one direction but block it in the opposite direction.

Normal Electrical Conduction

The SA Node

At the junction of the superior vena cava and the right atrium lies the normal pacemaker of the heart, the *sinoatrial (SA) node*. The node is approximately 10 to 20 mm long, 3 to 4 mm wide, and 2 mm thick. The functional organization of the sinus node is probably such that several groups of sinus node cells undergo pacemaker activity simultaneously and without interference from each other. The obvious benefit is that in the event of failure in the excitation of one group of cells, another is available with little change in rate. Pathology involving the SA node is frequently a result of its anatomic position or blood supply. Because the node is superficial, lying scarcely a millimeter beneath the

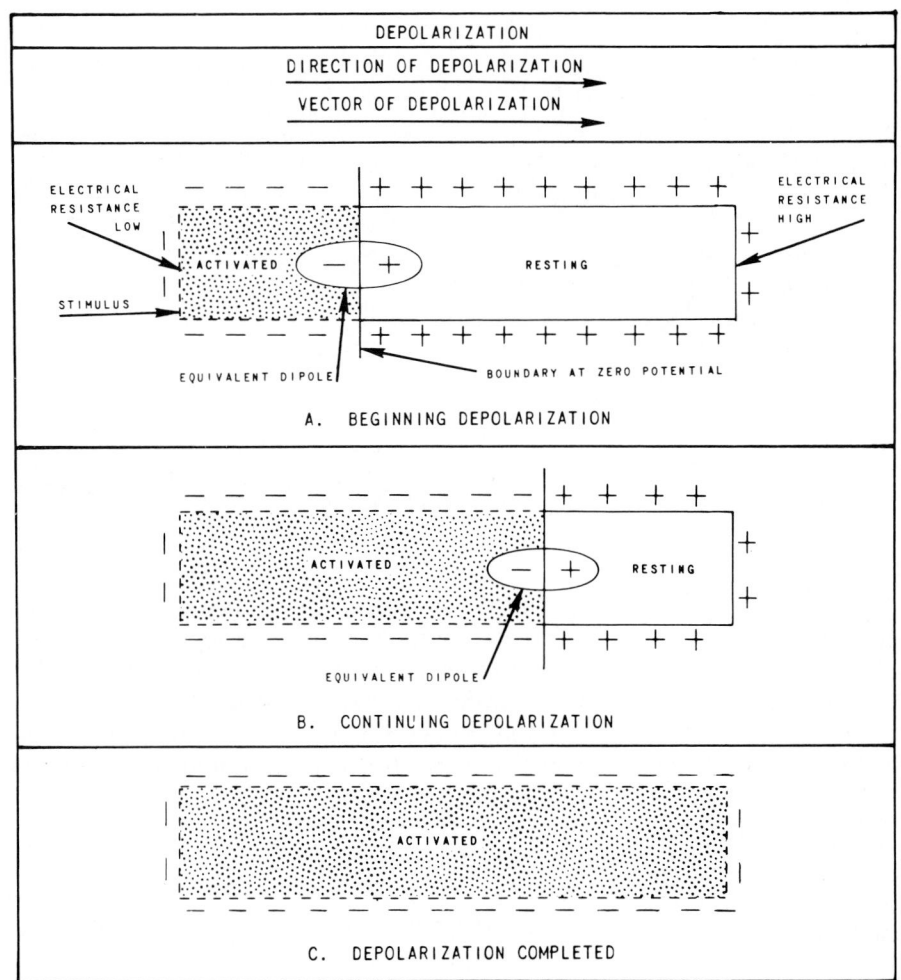

Figure 11-3 Depolarization of the muscle fiber. See text for description. *(From H. H. Friedman, Diagnostic electrocardiography and vectorcardiography, McGraw-Hill, New York, 1985, p. 2. Copyright 1985 by McGraw-Hill Book Company. Reprinted by permission.)*

pericardium, it is subject to diseases affecting the superficial tissues, for example, pericarditis.

Because the major function of the SA node is to serve as pacemaker of the heart, its action potential is typical of a slow-response cell (Fig. 11-4). The property which determines this role as pacemaker is that of diastolic depolarization. In addition, the SA node has a low resting membrane potential in comparison to other myocardial fibers. The cause of the low resting potential is thought to be a very high sodium conductance within the sinus membranes. Inactivation of the potassium current during phase 4, together with early opening of the slow sodium and calcium channels, is presumably the basis of diastolic depolarization.

The frequency of discharge of the SA node is ordinarily determined through control of the sympathetic and parasympathetic nervous systems. With an increase in sympathetic stimulation, norepinephrine is released from the nerve endings to increase the heart rate as well as to increase cardiac excitability and contractility. The effect of norepinephrine lies in its ability to increase membrane permeability to sodium which, in the sinus node, causes an increase in the velocity of reduction in membrane potential to threshold, thus increasing the heart rate. Stimulation of the parasympathetic system causes release of acetylcholine at the vagal nerve endings. Acetylcholine produces the opposite effect of norepinephrine on the heart: It decreases

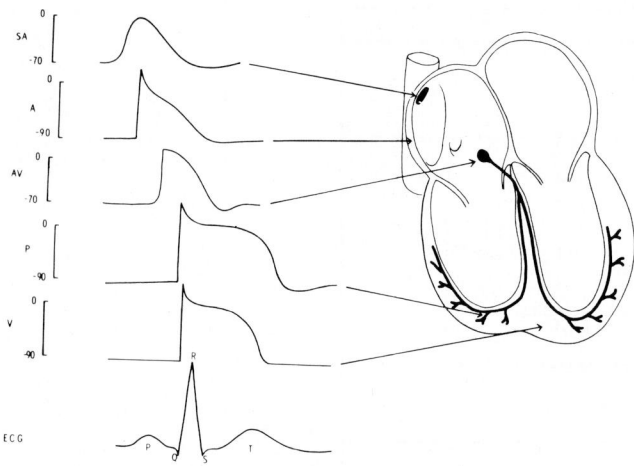

Figure 11-4 Comparison of action potentials in differing myocardial tissue. Sinoatrial (SA) pacemaker cells possess phase 4 spontaneous depolarization, a slow upstroke in phase 0, poorly differentiated phases 1 and 2, and a well-developed repolarization in phase 3. Atrial muscle cells (A) are characterized by a rapid upstroke in phase 1, with a well-developed positive overshoot and a relatively long phase 3. Phases 2 and 3 are difficult to differentiate. Atrioventricular cells (AV) may possess a period of hyperpolarization at the end of phase 3 and do not appear to possess true phase 4 diastolic depolarization. The Purkinje cells (P) possess an extremely rapid upstroke in phase 1 and a lengthy phase 2, and they appear to demonstrate phase 4 depolarization. Ventricular cells (V) have a much shorter repolarization phase (phase 2) than Purkinje cells and do not possess diastolic depolarization *(From J. W. Hurst, R. B. Logue, R. C. Schlant, and N. K. Wenger, eds., The heart, arteries, and veins, McGraw-Hill, New York, 1978, Copyright 1978 by McGraw-Hill Book Company. Reprinted by permission.)*

the rate of discharge at the SA node and decreases the rate of conduction of the impulse from the atria to the ventricles. When stimulated by acetylcholine, the cardiac fibers become extremely permeable to potassium so that very rapid efflux of potassium occurs within the cell. This results in hyperpolarization of the fiber because its resting potential is more negative than normal and, therefore, less excitable.

Another effect of vagal stimulation on the SA node, and resulting from the decrease in rate, can be escape beats from lower pacemakers within the conduction system; if the reduction in sinus discharge continues, the lower pacemaker takes over at a slower rate than that of the sinus node. Normally the intrinsic rate of sinus discharge is between 60 and 100 impulses per minute, with a minimum range of 40 to 50 and a maximum of 200 to 220 impulses per minute.

Atrial Conduction

From the SA node, the impulse is immediately conducted through the atria and to the AV node via the internodal pathways. The sinus node fibers are continuous with the atrial fibers; thus the impulse spreads in a wavelike pattern in all directions, reaching the distal portions of the atria in about 0.08 s. The atrial action potential is illustrated in Fig. 11-4. It is difficult to differentiate phase 2 from phase 3; repolarization (phase 3) is also prolonged.

AV Conduction

The action potential within the AV node region (N) is similar to that of the SA node (Fig. 11-4). The resting potential is less than in the ordinary myocardial fiber, and the refractory period extends beyond phase 4. There may be a period of hyperpolarization at the end of phase 3, followed by a return to a stable resting potential. Cells within this area are not thought to demonstrate true diastolic depolarization. The AV node exhibits the property of decremental conduction; that is, impulses are blocked that would be conducted in other areas of the heart, and should the atria depolarize at a high rate, only a portion of the impulses are normally conducted through the AV node. The major goal of decremental conduction is to prevent the ventricles from contracting before adequate filling occurs.

The effects of norepinephrine and sympathetic stimulation upon the AV node is one of increasing excitability within the potential pacemakers of the AV junction as well as increasing conduction time. Parasympathetic stimulation, as previously mentioned, can either lengthen conduction time from the node to the ventricle, or cause partial or even complete blockage of atrial impulses within the node and result in junctional escape rhythms. The intrinsic rate within the junction is approximately 40 to 60 impulses per minute.

Transmission through Purkinje System

The *Purkinje system* has the major task of rapidly and synchronously conducting the wave of excitation to the ventricular myocardial fibers. As noted in Fig. 11-4, the action potential of the Purkinje fiber has a very rapid upstroke as well as a prolonged plateau phase (phase 2). In addition, the Purkinje action potential demonstrates spontaneous diastolic depolarization.

In addition to its primary function as an extremely rapid conductor of the atrial impulse to the ventricles, the Purkinje system has two other fundamental properties. The first relates to the very long repolarization phase mentioned above. Figure 11-5 compares the refractory periods of the specialized conducting system. The shaded areas at the bottom represent refractory periods; it is apparent that the areas with the greatest refractory periods are the AV node and the distal Purkinje fibers (DPF). The DPF are also called *gate cells* in deference to their role in protecting the ventricles from premature beats which may be conducted by the AV node but are blocked by the gate cells because of their long refractory period. This mechanism is especially effective at slow heart rates. As the heart rate increases, the refractory period within the gate cells decreases. Within the AV node, however, the absolute refractory period remains unchanged and can even increase with very rapid rates; thus the AV node assumes the role of the Purkinje gate cells in tachycardia.

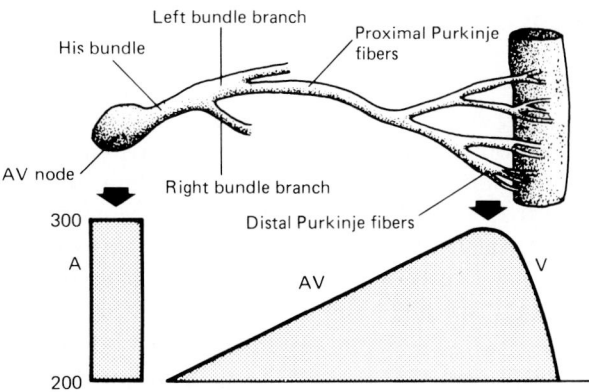

Figure 11-5   Refractory periods within the heart. Represented in the upper diagram is the conduction system: the AV node, His bundle, left and right bundle branches, and the conduction tissue connecting junctional and ventricular conducting tissue, which is divided into the proximal Purkinje fibers and distal Purkinje fibers. The shaded areas are representative of refractory periods, the ordinate being 200 to 300 ms. The arrows emphasize peak refractory periods in the AV node and distal Purkinje network. See text for further details.

The second function of the Purkinje system is that of pacemaker. Though the action potential does not exhibit the classic slow response of the other automatic cells, the pacemaker function of the Purkinje fibers is evident through diastolic depolarization and can become manifest through escape rhythms or in assumption of the role of pacemaker of the heart in severe conduction disturbances, as in complete heart block. The intrinsic rate of the Purkinje system is less than 40 impulses per minute.

Electrocardiography

Purpose

The electrocardiogram gives essential information regarding variations in rate and rhythm of the heart, effects of altered electrolyte concentrations, the electrical orientation of the heart as influenced by anatomic factors, and the influence of certain drugs such as digitalis. The electrocardiogram gives no direct information regarding the contractile state or mechanical performance of the heart.

Basis of Lead System

An electrocardiograph is essentially a modification of the galvanometer, in that there are two terminals: one connected to a positive electrode and one connected to a negative electrode. When the two electrodes are placed at different points in an electrical field, a lead is formed; the axis of that lead is described by joining the two sites with a hypothetical line.

Bipolar leads record the potential between a positive and a negative electrode which are placed within the area of electrical potential. A unipolar lead gives information about the variation in potential taking place underneath a single exploring electrode. It records the difference between an indifferent electrode (which is at zero potential) and the exploring electrode (positive).

Figure 11-6 represents a ventricular muscle strip which is connected to a unipolar lead. Exploring electrodes, which are attached to a recorder, are placed at three points on the muscle strip: on the endocardium, on the epicardium, and at the midportion of the strip. The direction of depolarization in the normal ventricle extends from endocardium to epicardium; the reverse is true for the direction of repolarization.

In the polarized or resting state, depicted in section *A* of Fig. 11-6, there is no difference in potential and, therefore, no activity to be measured. With excitation, the epicardial lead inscribes an upstroke because it faces the positive side of the advancing electric charge. As a wave of depolarization arrives at the electrode, depicted in sections *C* and *D*, the peak of the deflection occurs and the muscle strip is completely depolarized; the deflection then returns very suddenly to baseline. The conventional description of the first positive deflection in ventricular activation is the *R wave*. Briefly following the R wave is a short period in which the muscle remains activated and at the same potential. This period in which no change in potential occurs (isoelectric period) is called the *S-T segment*. With repolarization, the negative charge

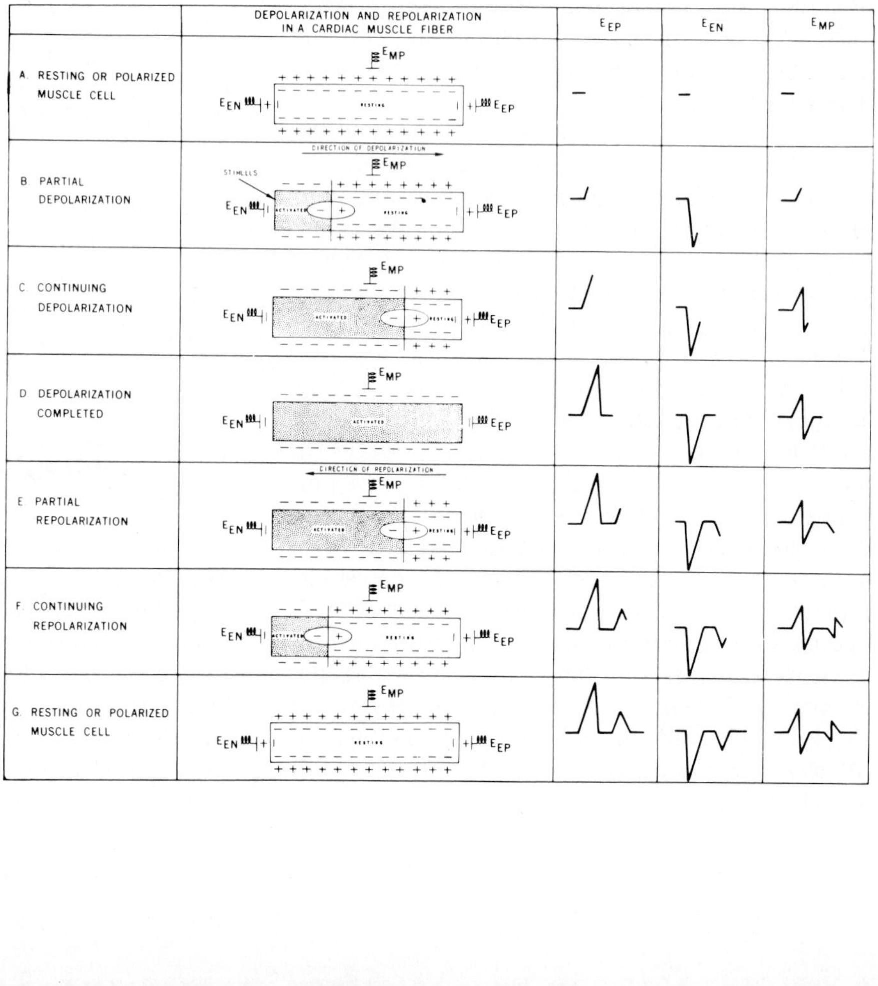

Figure 11-6 The potentials recorded by unipolar leads during depolarization and repolarization of a cardiac muscle fiber. E_{EP}, epicardial lead; E_{EN}, endocardial lead; E_{MP}, a lead at the midpoint of the muscle strip. See text for further description. *(From H. H. Friedman, Diagnostic electrocardiography and vectorcardiography, New York, McGraw-Hill, 1985, p. 7. Copyright 1985 by McGraw-Hill Book Company. Reprinted by permission.)*

precedes the positive and travels to the endocardial end of the muscle. Because the charge faces the positive exploring electrode, an upright deflection, the *T wave,* is inscribed. As long as polarization and depolarization take place in opposite directions, the R and T waves are recorded in the same direction.

In the endocardial lead, the electrode faces the negative side of the charges; therefore, a negative deflection, the *Q wave,* is inscribed. The peak of the activation occurs rapidly and closer to the beginning of the wave of current where the electrode is closest to the negative charge. As the wave moves away from the electrode to complete activation of the muscle, the deflection returns gradually to the baseline. This ventricular deflection is termed the *QS complex.* Because repolarization occurs in the reverse direction and the negative charge faces the electrode, an inverted T wave is recorded.

When the exploring electrode is equidistant from the ends of the muscle, first a positive deflection occurs; as the wave of excitation passes the electrode (Fig. 11-6C), maximum amplitude is reached and the deflection becomes negative as the charge moves away from the electrode. A biphasic complex, which is termed an *RS waveform,* is recorded. The T wave produced is also biphasic.

Relationship between Lead Axis and Amplitude

The magnitude of the waveforms is greatest when the direction of electrical forces lies parallel to the lead axis. This is shown in Fig. 11-7 in which various leads are noted with broken lines in a hexaxial reference system. Note that when electrical forces are parallel to a lead (in this case the horizontal lead), the deflection is of greatest magnitude (Fig. 11-7, arrow A). If the forces are directed toward, but not parallel to, the lead, the deflection diminishes in magnitude (Fig. 11-7, arrows B and C). Finally, if the direction of the forces is perpendicular to the lead axis, the deflection may be small, isoelectric, or equiphasic (Fig. 11-7, arrow D). When forces are directed away from the positive electrode of a lead, the deflection is negative; however, the relationship regarding magnitude remains the same (Fig. 11-7, arrow E).

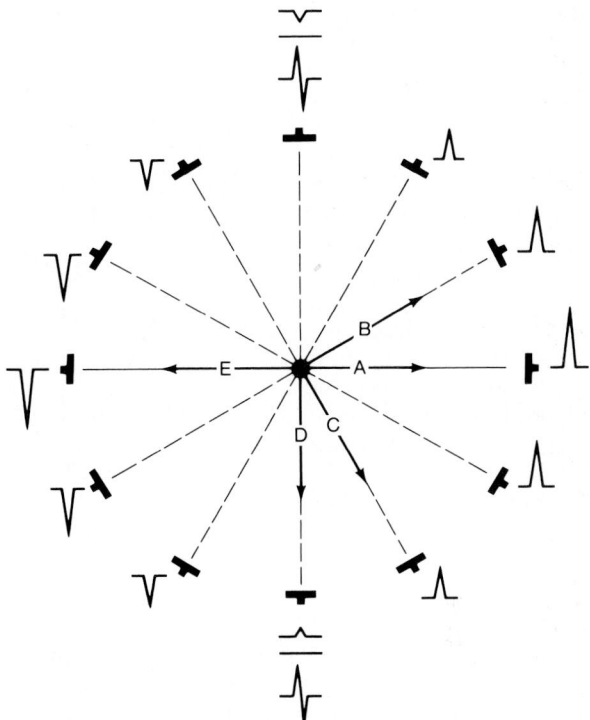

Figure 11-7 Various QRS complexes during depolarization of a muscle strip plotted in a hexaxial reference frame. See text for discussion. *(From E. K. Chung, Electrocardiography. Practical applications with vectorial principles, Appleton-Century-Crofts, Norwalk, CT, 1985, p. 18. Copyright 1985 by Appleton-Century-Crofts. Adapted by permission.)*

Einthoven Triangle

The basis of modern electrocardiography resides in the system devised by William Einthoven. His hypothesis assumes that the heart lies in the center of an equilateral triangle, the apices of which are the right and left shoulders and pubic region; and that the body fluids act as a volume conductor so that the standard limb leads record differences in potential between the apices of the triangle. The conventional limb leads are (1) *lead I,* recording the differences in potential between the negative right (RA) and positive left (LA) arms; (2) *lead II,* recording the differences between the negative RA and positive left leg (LL); and (3) *lead III,* measuring the variations between the left arm (negative) and left leg (positive) (Fig. 11-8A). The standard limb

Figure 11-8 Einthoven's triangle and hexaxial reference system. *A.* Einthoven's equilateral triangle showing the axes of bipolar standard limb leads I, II, and III. Superimposed on the triangle are the axes of the unipolar limb leads. The heart is at the center or zero point. *B.* The axes of the standard and augmented limb leads are combined to form the hexaxial reference system, a modified version of Einthoven's triangle. See text for a more detailed description.

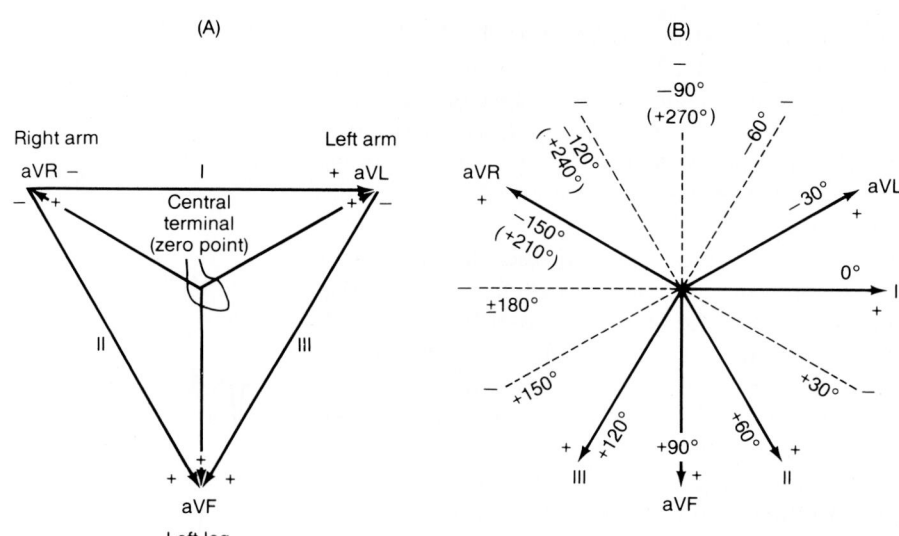

leads are such that in most persons the electrical recordings of the three leads produce positive deflections.

Unipolar leads recorded from the right arm (VR), left arm (VL), and left leg (VF) are based on the theory that the indifferent electrode located at the central terminal maintains zero potential throughout the cardiac cycle (Fig. 11-8A). By comparing the potential of an exploring electrode with that of the central terminal, it is evident that only the variation of potential under the exploring electrode is recorded. Because the deflections which are measured are very small, augmentation of their amplitude is performed so that these leads are designated as *aVR, aVL,* and *aVF.* These leads together with the three bipolar leads describe the electrical forces along the frontal plane.

Modification of Einthoven's triangle such that the center point of the three bipolar leads is superimposed on the central terminal of the three unipolar leads produces a hexaxial reference system (Fig. 11-8B). The lines of the reference system create 12 30° angles which together total 360° or a full circle. The angles above the lead I axis or the horizontal axis are identified with minus signs, that is, −30° to −150°, and the angles below the lead I axis are labeled with positive signs (+30° to +150°). The positive and negative ends of the lead I axis are labeled as 0° and ±180° respectively. The hexaxial reference system is more useful than

Einthoven's triangle in determining the electrical axis of depolarization and repolarization forces.

Precordial Leads

There are six precordial leads identified on the electrocardiogram as V_1 through V_6. These leads are unipolar in that they utilize a positive electrode and an indifferent electrode with zero potential. By convention the six precordial electrodes are placed as noted in Table 11-1. Occasionally, additional precordial leads are recorded from the right precordium. A common example is V_3R which provides another viewpoint over the right chest. These chest leads all depict the electrical forces of the heart in the horizontal or transverse plane.

When looking at the deflections of the QRS complexes in the precordial leads, the observer will note that the magnitude of the R wave progresses from V_1 to V_6 (Fig. 11-9). This normal occurrence is due to the way the ventricles are depolarized. The papillary muscles and interventricular septum are activated first, except for a small section near the base of the septum (Fig. 11-9, phase 1). Because the initial wave of depolarization is oriented to the right and superiorly, a small R wave is recorded in the right precordial leads (V_1 and V_2) and a small Q wave is recorded from the left precordium (V_5 and V_6).

The activation spreads from endocardium to epicardium and over both the right and left ventricle

Table 11-1 Placement of Positive and Negative Electrodes for Each of the 12 Leads of an Electrocardiogram

Lead	+ Electrode	− Electrode
I	Left arm	Right arm
II	Left leg	Right arm
III	Left leg	Left arm
aVR	Right arm	
aVL	Left arm	
aVF	Left leg	
V_1	4th ICS,[a] RSB[b]	
V_2	4th ICS, LSB[c]	
V_3	Midway between V_2 and V_4	
V_4	5th ICS, MCL[d]	
V_5	5th ICS, AAL[e]	
V_6	5th ICS, MAL[f]	

[a] ICS = intercostal space
[b] RSB = right sternal border
[c] LSB = left sternal border
[d] MCL = midclavicular line
[e] AAL = anterior axillary line
[f] MAL = midaxillary line

(Fig. 11-9, phase 2). Because the left ventricle is greater in mass and, therefore, greater in electrical potential, it determines the direction, polarity, and magnitude (vector) of the QRS as anterior and leftward and inscribes a positive R wave in all leads. During the third phase, most of both ventricles are depolarized and again the left ventricle overpowers the right ventricular waveform. Because this phase has considerable amplitude and is oriented leftward and posteriorly, a deep S wave is recorded in the right precordial leads, while tall R waves are recorded in the left precordial leads. Activation of the posterobasal region of the left ventricle, the base of the septum, and the base of the right ventricle occurs during phase 4. The upstroke of the S wave in the right precordial leads (V_1 and V_2) and the downstroke of the R wave and a small S wave in the left precordial leads (V_4 through V_6) are inscribed on the electrocardiogram.

Monitoring Leads

At the bedside it is not practical to attach electrodes to the arms and legs of the patient in order to obtain routine and continuous recordings of the heart's electrical activity. Consequently, modifications of the standard limb and precordial leads are utilized. Electrode placement for the monitor limb leads is similar to the standard placement except that the left and right shoulder or subclavicular areas and the lower left quadrant of the abdomen are used for electrode placement (Fig. 11-10A).

Monitor lead II is a commonly used lead in many critical-care units. In other units, particularly coronary or cardiovascular care units, a modified CL (MCL) monitoring system is used. In the case of MCL_1, the precordial V_1 lead is simulated by placing the positive electrode in the standard V_1 position, the negative electrode just below the left midclavicle, and the ground electrode below the right midclavicle (Fig. 11-10B). Other precordial leads can be simulated in a similar manner; MCL_6 is the most common and has the positive electrode placed in the standard V_6 position.

Waves, Complexes, and Intervals

The electrical activity of the entire heart is inscribed on the electrocardiogram (ECG) as a series of waveforms, each of which represents a particular electrical event in the cardiac cycle. The waveforms are identified by the letters P, Q, R, S, T, and U (Fig. 11-11).

P Wave

Atrial depolarization is represented on the ECG by the *P wave*. The duration of atrial depolarization is less than 0.11 s in normal hearts. The height of the P wave is normally less than 3 mm. The waveform

Figure 11-9 Schematic representation of ventricular depolarization in the normal heart. See text for description. *(From H. H. Friedman, Diagnostic electrocardiography and vectorcardiography, McGraw-Hill, New York, 1985, p. 54. Copyright 1985 by McGraw-Hill Book Company. Reprinted by permission.)*

VENTRICULAR DEPOLARIZATION IN THE NORMAL HEART

SEQUENCE OF VENTRICULAR ACTIVATION

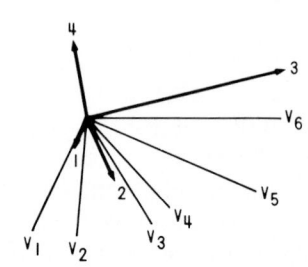

PHASE 1   INITIAL SEPTAL ACTIVATION. (0.01 SEC)

PHASE 2   CONTINUED ACTIVATION OF SEPTUM AND ACTIVATION OF APICO-ANTERIOR PORTIONS OF RIGHT AND LEFT VENTRICLES. (0.02 SEC)

PHASE 3   COMPLETION OF SEPTAL ACTIVATION AND ACTIVATION OF MOST, IF NOT ALL, OF RIGHT VENTRICLE AND MOST OF LEFT VENTRICLE. (0.04-0.06 SEC)

PHASE 4   ACTIVATION OF POSTEROBASAL REGION OF LEFT VENTRICLE, BASE OF SEPTUM AND BASE OF RIGHT VENTRICLE. (0.06-0.08 SEC)

VENTRICULAR ACTIVATION VECTORS IN THE TRANSVERSE PLANE

QRS COMPLEXES IN THE PRECORDIAL LEADS

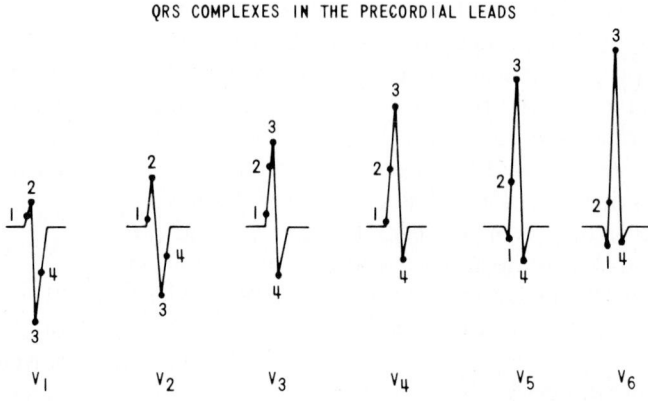

should be upright and symmetrically rounded in leads I, II, aVF, and V_4 through V_6 (Fig. 11-11) and inverted in lead aVR. It may be diphasic, flat, or inverted in leads III, V_1, and V_2, but the negative component should not be excessively deep or wide. If the P wave is peaked or notched it is abnormal and indicates abnormal depolarization of one or both atria secondary to chamber enlargement or conduction defect.

QRS Complex

The *QRS complex* represents ventricular depolarization. The *Q wave* is the first negative deflection after the P wave and it may or may not appear,

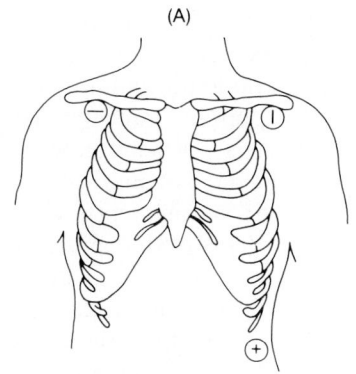

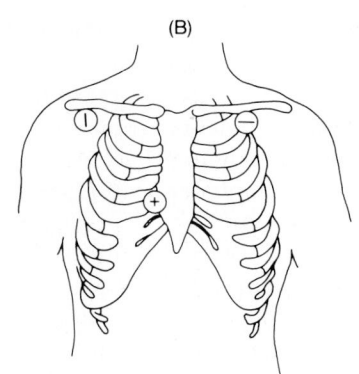

— = Negative electrode

+ = Positive electrode

I = Indifferent or ground electrode

Figure 11-10 Electrode placement for routine monitoring. *A.* Electrode placement for monitoring lead II. *B.* Electrode placement for MCL₁.

depending on the given lead being monitored. The *R wave* is the first positive deflection after the P wave. The negative deflection after the R wave is the *S wave* (Fig. 11-11). While this complex is by convention identified with all three letters, it is possible that more or less of the waveforms will be inscribed. For example, when no positive deflection occurs, a QS exists. If more than one R or S is inscribed, the second is indicated by a prime (′) and is called R prime (R′) or S prime (S′). When

it is necessary to specifically describe each portion of the complex, lower- and uppercase letters are used to denote the relative sizes of the components, that is q or Q, r or R, and s or S.

S-T Segment

The isoelectric line following the QRS complex and ending with the start of the T wave is the *S-T segment* (Fig. 11-11). As noted earlier, this represents the period after ventricular depolarization

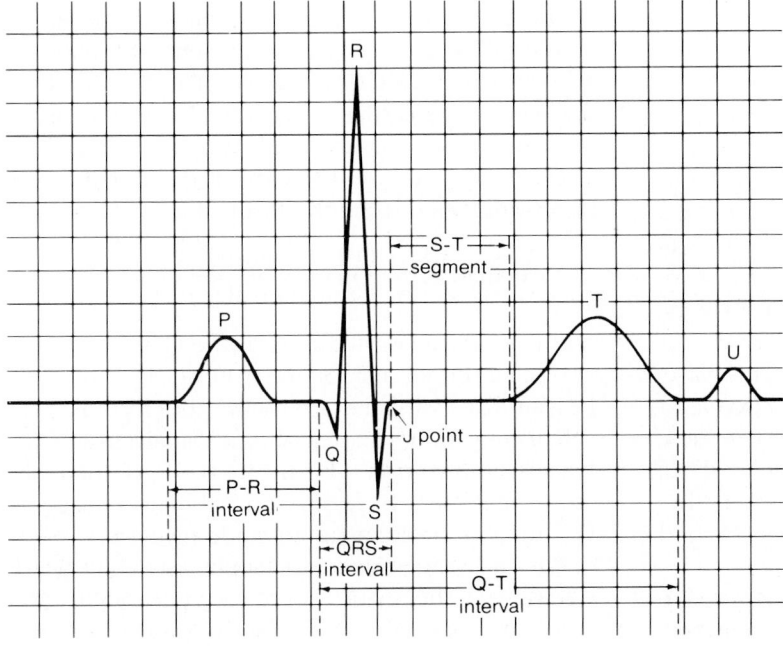

Figure 11-11 Electrocardiographic complexes and intervals representative of lead II.

when there is no change in electrical potential. The junction between the end of the QRS complex and the beginning of the S-T segment is referred to as the *J point* (Fig. 11-11). Normally the S-T segment begins flat on the baseline (isoelectric) and curves gently and imperceptibly into the proximal limb of the T wave. However, it may be elevated up to 1 mm in the limb leads or 2 mm in some precordial leads. It is normally not depressed more than 0.50 mm. If it is excessively elevated or depressed, pathological conditions such as myocardial ischemia or injury are indicated.

T Wave

The *T wave* represents the recovery phase after ventricular depolarization (Fig. 11-11). This deflection should be upright in leads I, II, and V_3 to V_6 and inverted in lead aVR. In leads III, aVL, V_1, and V_2 the direction of the deflection is variable. The T wave is normally slightly rounded and slightly asymmetrical. Sharply pointed or grossly notched T waves should be considered suspicious. The height of the T wave is normally less than 5 mm in the limb leads and less than 10 mm in the precordial leads. Waves may be depressed, elevated, or inverted due to drugs, ischemia, or injury. The last one-half to one-third of the T wave is often referred to as the vulnerable period. An electrical stimulus during this portion of the T wave may precipitate a serious ventricular arrhythmia.

U Wave

A small and usually positive deflection immediately following the T wave and preceding the P wave is the *U wave* (Fig. 11-11). The exact cause of this deflection is unknown but is thought to be the result of the slow repolarization of the intraventricular conduction system. Frequently the U wave is so small that it is unidentifiable. It may be visualized best in lead V_3. If a prominent U wave is noted, one should suspect hypokalemia. This waveform may be inverted with myocardial ischemia or left ventricular overload. It is of interest to note that most ventricular extrasystoles occur at about the same time as the U wave in the cardiac cycle.

P-R Interval

The period from the beginning of the P wave to the beginning of the QRS complex is the *P-R interval* (Fig. 11-11). This portion of the cardiac cycle represents the time required for the original impulse to travel from the SA node through the atria and the AV node to the bundle branches. The duration of the P-R interval is normally between 0.12 and 0.20 s. A delay in the P-R interval (P-R greater than 0.20 s) indicates a conduction delay through the AV node or depressed conduction secondary to drug therapy such as digitalis. A shortened P-R interval indicates an abnormal conduction pathway which allows the impulse to bypass the AV node and stimulate the ventricles early.

QRS Interval

The *QRS interval* is that period of time required to fully depolarize the ventricles (Fig. 11-11). Normally this interval is between 0.06 and 0.10 s. Prolongation up to 0.12 s indicates an incomplete conduction defect and prolongation equal to or greater than 0.12 s is indicative of a complete conduction defect. Consequently, the ventricles are depolarized abnormally. Causes of a prolonged QRS interval are ischemia or injury of the conduction system, premature systoles from the atria which depolarize aberrantly through the ventricles, and ventricular extrasystoles.

Q-T Interval

Measuring from the beginning of the QRS complex to the end of the T wave one obtains the duration of the *Q-T interval,* which represents the entirety of ventricular electrical systole (Fig. 11-11). This portion of the cardiac cycle varies with the heart rate, being shorter in rapid rates and longer in slower heart rates. Calculation of the Q-T interval is accomplished using the formula

$$\text{Q-T calculation} = \frac{\text{Q-T (measured)}}{\sqrt{\text{R-R interval (s)}}}$$

and is indicated on the ECG as the Q-T$_c$.

It is important for the critical-care nurse to be familiar with and to utilize the formula for calculating the Q-T interval when analyzing ECGs because individuals with prolonged Q-T intervals are predisposed to reentry arrhythmias. Causes of Q-T interval prolongation include myocarditis secondary to congestive heart failure, ischemic heart disease, or rheumatic fever; cerebrovascular disease; and electrolyte disturbance, particularly hypocalcemia. Drug therapy with quinidine and amiodarone may prolong the Q-T interval as may hypothermia or stringent dieting. Any Q-T interval greater than one-half of the preceding R-R interval or a Q-T$_c$ greater than 0.42 s is considered to be abnormally long.

The Q-T interval may also be abnormally short. Digitalis therapy, hypercalcemia, and potassium intoxication may be causes of short intervals. Unfortunately though, the lower limit of normal for the Q-T interval is not well defined. Therefore, it is more difficult to determine when the Q-T interval is abnormally short.

Heart Rate and Rhythm Determination

Standard ECG paper is made up of a series of 1-mm squares from which both voltage and time can be measured (Fig. 11-12). Each group of five small squares is marked by a darker line. Voltage is measured along the vertical axis of the graph. At normal standardization, every 10 mm of stylus excursion is equal to 1 mV (1 mm = 0.1 mV). Time is measured along the horizontal axis and, at normal recording speed of 25 mm/s, each millimeter equals 0.04 s (40 ms) and 5 mm or one large square equals 0.20 (200 ms). Thus, at the normal speed, 1500

small and 300 large squares pass through the recorder each minute.

Calculation of Heart Rate

There are a number of methods available for calculating the heart rate on the ECG. However, two methods are used most often and will be described here. The first method is used for regular rhythms and the second should be used when the cardiac rhythm is irregular, but it can also be used for regular rhythms.

If the cardiac rhythm is regular, that is, the R-R interval is constant, the heart rate can be determined rapidly and quite accurately by dividing the number of large squares per minute, 300, by the number of large squares between two consecutive R waves. For example, if the R-R interval is three large squares, the heart rate is 100 (300 ÷ 3 = 100). Figure 11-13*A* illustrates this method of heart rate determination and gives the heart rate for six different R-R intervals.

Unfortunately, not all R-R intervals can be measured by whole large squares. Frequently, the R-R interval is composed of a number of both large and small squares. Figure 11-13*B* illustrates such a circumstance. In this example the R-R interval is composed of four large and two small squares and

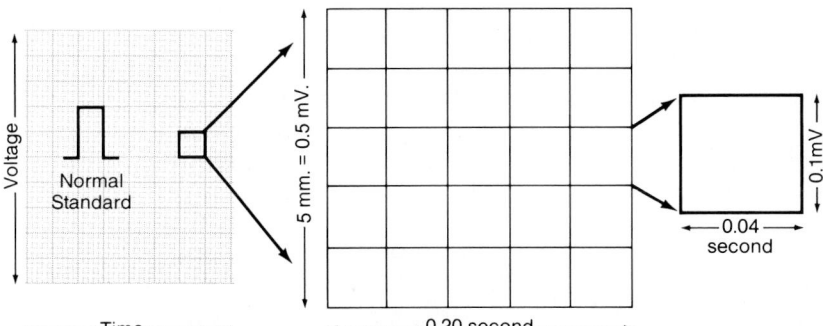

Figure 11-12   Standard ECG paper. ECG paper is a graph divided into millimeter squares. Time is measured on the horizontal axis with each small square equal to 0.04 (at 25 mm/s paper speed) and each large square equal to 0.20 s. Note the time markers at the top of the paper indicating a 3-s interval. Markers are usually located at 2- or 3-s intervals. Voltage is measured on the vertical axis of the graph. At normal standardization (1 mV) each small square is equal to 0.1 mV.

Figure 11-13   Rapid heart rate determination. *A.* Divide 300 by the number of large squares between R waves. In this example the rate is about 100. Rates for six R-R intervals are shown. *B.* When the R-R interval is not equal to a large square interval but falls between the large square markers, the rate can be calculated as described in the text. The rate for this rhythm strip is 69. Values for small squares between various large square markers are shown.

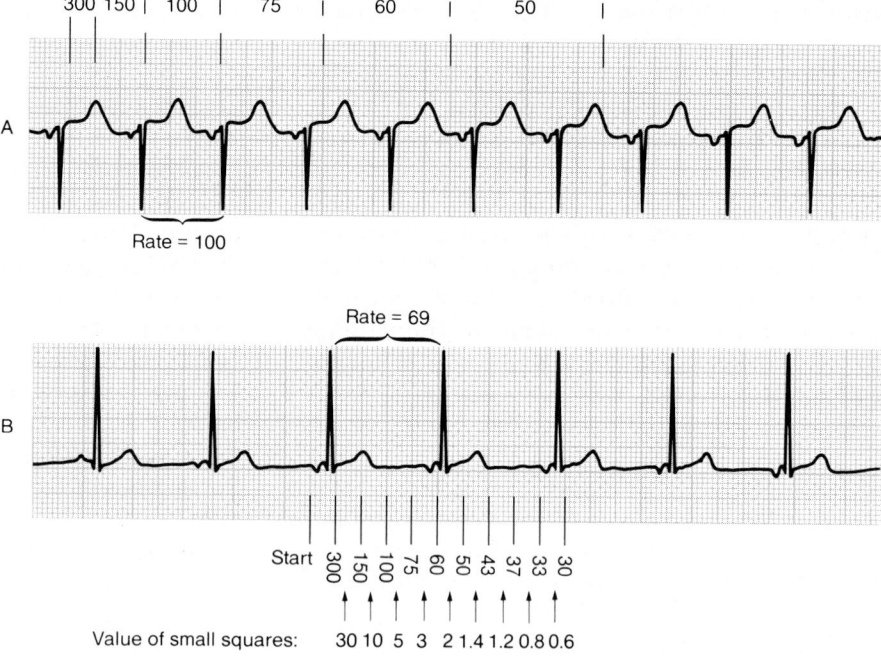

the heart rate is 69 beats per minute. This rate is determined by subtracting the numerical value for each small square from the rate for an R-R interval of four large squares [75 − (2 × 3) = 69]. In this instance the small square value is three and is calculated by subtracting 60 from 75 and dividing that number by 5 (75 − 60 = 15; 15 ÷ 5 = 3). The numbers 75 and 60 are used because they represent what the rate would have been had the R-R interval been four or five large squares. The numerical value for small squares varies and the different values are shown on Fig. 11-13*B*.

When the heart rate is irregular the first method described does not yield an accurate rate.

Consequently, the second method for heart rate calculation must be utilized. In this method, which may also be used with regular rhythms, the number of cardiac cycles (R-R intervals) in a 6-s period (30 large squares = 6 s) is counted and multiplied by 10. This method is made easier because ECG paper is marked off in either 2- or 3-s sections by a vertical line at the top of the paper. Figure 11-14 illustrates this method of calculating heart rate.

Determination of Rhythm

The regularity of the cardiac rhythm is important to assess because it provides information regarding the site of the electrical stimulus, the function of

Figure 11-14   Measurement of heart rate per minute by counting number of cardiac cycles in a 6-s interval and multiplying by 10. In this example there are 10 cycles per 6 s, resulting in a rate of 100 (10 × 10 = 100).

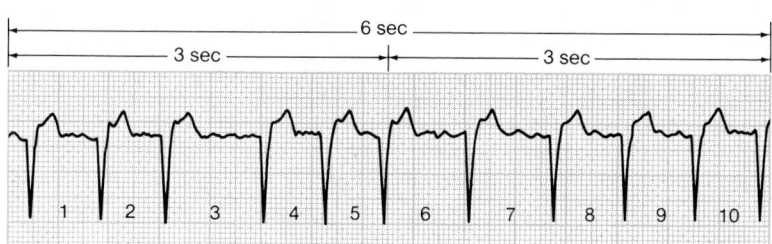

that site, and whether more than one site is influencing the cardiac cycle. The easiest way to make this assessment is to measure the R-R (or P-P) intervals and determine if they are constant in length. This can be done with calipers or with marks made on a piece of paper. The rhythm is said to be regular if the length of the shortest and longest R-R (or P-P) intervals varies by less than 0.16 s. If the intervals vary by more than 0.16 s the rhythm is irregular and should be further assessed to determine if there is any kind of pattern to the irregularity. The rhythm may be regularly irregular, thus showing a definite pattern, or it may be totally erratic.

Electrical Axis Determination

The axis of a lead can be divided into a positive and negative portion by a perpendicular line through its center. Figure 11-8*B* illustrates the axis in degrees and the positive and negative poles of the frontal plane bipolar and unipolar leads. The frontal plane is defined by two axes, the left and right axis, or lead I, and the superior and inferior axis, or lead aVF. Leads I and aVF divide the frontal plane into four quadrants (Fig. 11-15). The *left superior* quad-

rant is circumscribed by the negative pole of lead aVF and the positive pole of lead I whereas the *left inferior* quadrant is circumscribed by the positive pole of both leads I and aVF. The positive pole of lead aVF and the negative pole of lead I are the borders for the *right inferior* quadrant. The *right superior* quadrant is bordered by the negative pole of leads I and aVF.

When determining the electrical axis in the frontal plane, one identifies the direction of the sum of the electrical forces (vectors) of one cardiac cycle. Two rules, the *quadrant rule* and the *perpendicular rule,* assist in identifying the electrical axis of the P wave, the QRS complex, and the T wave. For the purposes of this discussion, the determination of only the QRS axis will be described. The axis of the P and T waves are determined following the same format.

The *quadrant rule* localizes the mean QRS vector to one of the four frontal plane quadrants. The specific quadrant is identified by looking at the direction of the QRS deflections in leads I and aVF. If the QRS in lead I is predominantly positive, but in lead aVF it is predominantly negative, the mean vector points somewhere in the left superior quadrant, or 0° to −90°. If, however, the QRS deflection is positive in both leads I and aVF, the mean vector lies within the left inferior quadrant, or 0° to +90°. When the QRS deflection is negative in lead I and positive in aVF, the mean vector is directed toward the right inferior quadrant, or −90° to ±180°. The right superior quadrant, −90° to ±180°, is the location of the mean vector when the QRS deflection is negative in leads I and aVF.

The *perpendicular rule* localizes the mean QRS vector in degrees. This rule states that the mean QRS vector lies perpendicular to the axis of the lead with the most equiphasic complex and in the previously identified quadrant. Therefore, to determine the degree of the QRS axis, the lead with the most equiphasic or isoelectric QRS is identified. Next, the lead perpendicular to the first lead is identified. (It is useful to note that leads perpendicular to each other are I and aVF, II and aVL, and III and aVR.) Finally, note the degrees of the axis of the perpendicular lead in the quadrant selected with the quadrant rule.

The steps to follow, then, for determining the electrical axis of the QRS are:

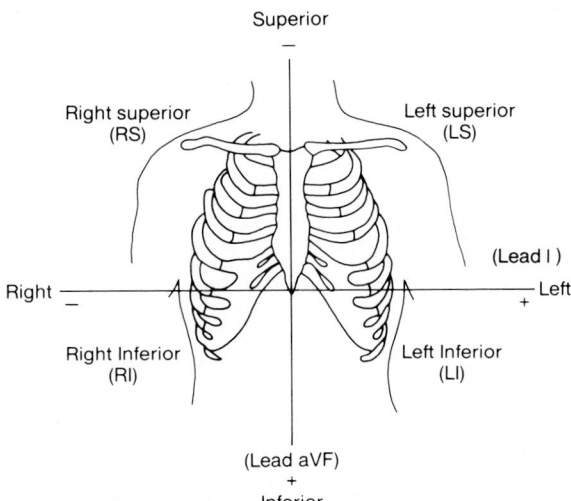

Figure 11-15 Quadrants of the frontal plane. Leads I and aVF divide the frontal plane into four quadrants: left superior (LS), left inferior (LI), right inferior (RI), and right superior (RS). See text for further discussion.

1. Examine lead I and determine if the forces are directed to the right or to the left. If the QRS in lead I is positive, the vector is to the left. If the QRS in lead I is negative, the vector is to the right.
2. Examine lead aVF and determine if the forces are directed inferiorly or superiorly. The QRS in lead aVF will be positive if the vector is inferior, and negative if the vector is superior.
3. From the information gained in steps 1 and 2, identify the quadrant toward which the vector is directed.
4. Locate the most equiphasic or isoelectric QRS from leads I through aVF and identify that lead.
5. Identify the lead perpendicular to the lead selected in step 4. This lead should have the greatest amplitude. If it does not, repeat the steps to ensure correct lead identification.
6. Identify the degrees of the axis of the lead in step 5. Remember to select the pole of the lead which is in the quadrant identified in step 3.

Review Fig. 11-16 for an example of how these steps are used to identify the QRS axis for the frontal plane leads of the ECG.

In a normal ECG, the electrical axis of the QRS in the frontal plane leads should be between $-30°$ and $+100°$. The mean QRS vector normally shifts leftward as an individual ages. If the axis falls outside the boundaries of normal it is said to have rotated or deviated to the right (clockwise shift) or to the left (counterclockwise shift).

Left axis deviation (LAD) exists when the frontal plane QRS axis is $-30°$ or more superior. A number of clinical conditions or circumstances may cause this deviation. Some of the causes include: (1) mechanical shifts secondary to respiratory expiration or a high diaphragm from pregnancy, ascites, or abdominal tumors; (2) left anterior hemiblock; (3) left bundle branch block; (4) congenital lesions such as endocardial cushion defect and several other cyanotic and acyanotic defects; (5) Wolff-Parkinson-White syndrome; (6) emphysema; (7) hyperkalemia; and (8) ventricular ectopic rhythms.[2] *Extreme* or *marked left axis deviation* exists when the QRS axis is $-45°$ or more superior. Usually, marked LAD is due to left anterior hemiblock but pure inferior wall myocardial infarction without left anterior hemiblock may also be a cause.

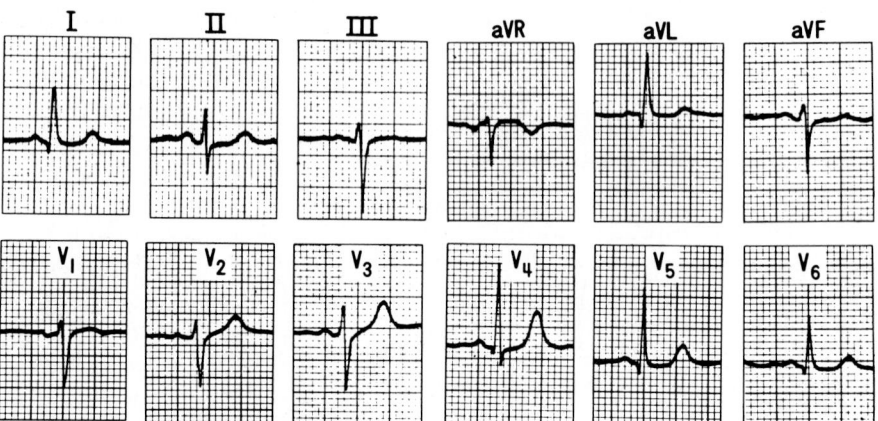

Figure 11-16 A normal electrocardiogram from an elderly woman. The QRS in lead I is positively deflected, indicating the forces are directed to the left. The electrical forces in aVF are directed superiorly (the QRS is a negative deflection). Therefore, the mean axis is in the left superior quadrant. The QRS in lead II is the most equiphasic, indicating that the mean forces are directed parallel to lead aVL, the lead perpendicular to lead II. Lead II in the left superior quadrant is at $-30°$. Consequently, the mean QRS axis for this ECG is $-30°$. *(From H. H. Friedman, Diagnostic electrocardiography and vectorcardiography, McGraw-Hill, New York, 1985, p. 99. Copyright 1985 by McGraw-Hill Book Company. Reprinted by permission.)*

When the QRS axis is rotated clockwise to +100° or more, *right axis deviation* (RAD) exists. Causes of RAD include: (1) mechanical shifts secondary to inspiration or emphysema, (2) right ventricular hypertrophy, (3) right bundle branch block, (4) left posterior hemiblock, (5) dextrocardia, (6) ventricular ectopic rhythms, and (7) Wolff-Parkinson-White syndrome.[2]

When the electrical axis falls within the right superior quadrant the frontal axis is said to be *indeterminant.* The reason for this is that without a vectorcardiogram, it is impossible to know whether the forces were directed to this area by extreme right axis deviation or extreme left axis deviation. The clinical situation may provide some clues.

It should be noted that it is possible to determine the mean vector in the horizontal plane. In this situation a different hexaxial reference system, the precordial hexaxial system, is used. Directions on this reference system are right, left, anterior, and posterior. A discussion of the methodology for determining the horizontal QRS axis is beyond the scope of this chapter.

Normal 12-Lead Electrocardiogram

Systematic Review of the ECG

To determine if the ECG is normal or abnormal it is recommended that a systematic format for review be followed. A number of formats are available and one should be selected and used for all ECG analyses. The format suggested by Marriott is used in this chapter.[2]

The first step in ECG analysis involves assessment of the rhythm. Examine both the P-P and R-R intervals for regularity. If one or both are irregular, is there a pattern to the rhythm or is it completely erratic? Is there a relationship between the two rhythms? Next, the rate of both atrial and ventricular depolarization are determined. Two methods for determining rate were discussed previously.

Once the rhythm and rate have been determined, close inspection of each wave, complex, and interval should follow. Begin by inspecting each P wave, noting the direction of the deflection, the amplitude, the width, whether it is diphasic, and the presence or absence of notching and peaking. Of course it is also important to note the

absence of any P waves. The axis of the P wave may also be identified.

Follow P wave inspection with measurement of the P-R interval. Consider if all intervals are the same or if they vary. Also note if the measurement obtained is short of or exceeds the limits for normal. Proceed to the measurement of the QRS interval. Again note if the value obtained exceeds the normal limits. Next, measure the Q-T interval, taking care not to measure a Q-U interval by mistake. Calculate the Q-T$_c$.

After measuring the P-R, QRS, and Q-T intervals, analyze the QRS complex. First, measure the amplitude in the various leads, noting excessive or low voltage. Then examine the Q waves. Note the leads in which they are present or absent. Measure the depth and width. Determine the frontal plane electrical axis for the QRS. Note whether there is deviation to either the right or the left. Next, look at the relative prominence of the component waves in the precordial leads. Is there R wave progression or is it absent? In which lead does the deflection of the complex pass through transition (change from a predominantly negative to a predominantly positive waveform)? While examining the precordial leads note the timing of the *intrinsicoid deflection.* This deflection is measured from the beginning of the QRS complex to the point on the isoelectric line which would be intersected by an imaginary perpendicular line from the peak of the R wave (Fig. 11-17). A delay in the intrinsicoid deflection generally indicates ventricular enlargement or blockage in the ventricular conduction system. Lastly, examine the general configuration of the total complex, noting the presence and location of any slurs or notches.

After the examination of the QRS, assess the S-T segment for any elevation or depression and note the leads where any changes are observed. Look for any abnormal sharp angles or notches.

The direction, shape, and height of the T wave are assessed next. Remember that sharply pointed or grossly notched T waves are abnormal and should be further assessed for the possible cause. The mean vector of the T wave may be identified if desired. Look for the U wave next. Lead V$_3$ may provide the best view.

Once the ECG has been examined and information analyzed, various interpretations may be

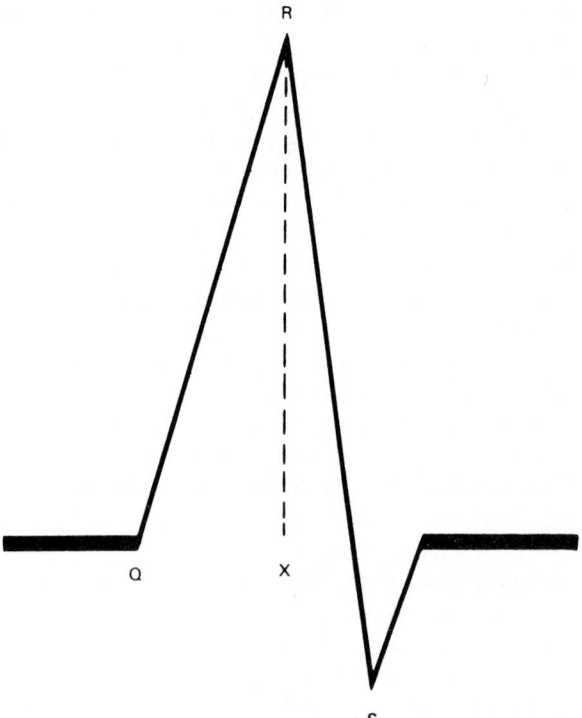

Figure 11-17 The intrinsicoid deflection (line connecting R and S). The time required from the beginning of the QRS complex to the peak of the R wave is measured horizontally (Q-X). *(From E. K. Chung, Electrocardiography. Practical applications with vectorial principles, Appleton-Century-Crofts, Norwalk, CT, 1985, p. 38. Copyright 1985 by Appleton-Century-Crofts. Reprinted by permission.)*

made. The cause of abnormalities can be identified many times by comparing findings to the ECG criteria for specific clinical situations. The critical-care nurse must know which ECG findings to report and when to report that information.

Criteria for a Normal ECG

Table 11-2 lists the criteria which need to be present for an ECG to be interpreted as normal. Figure 11-18 is an example of a normal ECG.

Abnormalities of Electrical Activity

The electrocardiogram may be altered by a number of anatomical and physiological conditions including electrolyte imbalance, ischemia, and chamber enlargement. In addition, effects of drug therapy may alter the ECG. Changes in the ECG which these conditions create may include alterations in voltage, electrical axis, rate, rhythm, and timing of intervals. Following is a discussion of some of the more common abnormalities of electrical activity.

Dysrhythmias

When considering cardiac rhythm disturbances (dysrhythmias) it is important to bear in mind the relationship between heart rate and cardiac output. Stroke volume (SV) and heart rate (HR) determine cardiac output. Consequently, if the heart rate is depressed for some reason, the cardiac output will be reduced unless there is a sufficient increase in stroke volume to offset the effect. Conversely, if the heart rate is enhanced, cardiac output will rise, assuming there is not a concurrent drop in stroke volume. At very rapid rates it is likely that cardiac output will suffer because the ventricular diastolic filling time is reduced, thereby reducing the stroke volume. Therefore, monitoring for and understanding cardiac rhythm disturbances is crucial in the critical-care environment.

Genesis of Dysrhythmias

Abnormalities in cardiac rhythm are a consequence of disturbances in electrical impulse formation, impulse conduction, or a combination of formation and conduction. Three mechanisms may cause disturbance in impulse formation. They are (1) normal automaticity, (2) abnormal automaticity, and (3) triggered activity. Mechanisms which cause disturbances in impulse conduction include (1) decremental conduction, (2) inhomogeneous conduction, (3) supernormal conduction, (4) concealed conduction, and (5) unidirectional block with or without reentry. A brief discussion of some of these mechanisms is warranted. However, for a more in-depth presentation of the genesis of arrhythmias the reader is directed to current electrocardiography texts.

Normal Automaticity The mechanism of automaticity was described earlier in this chapter. The sinus node normally controls the cardiac rhythm because its cells spontaneously depolarize and reach threshold potential faster than do the pacemaker cells of other areas of the heart. The rate of

Table 11-2 Criteria for a Normal Electrocardiogram

Component	Criteria
Rhythm	Atrial and ventricular rhythms are the same.
	R-R and P-P intervals vary less than 0.16 s.
Rate	Atrial and ventricular rates are equal and between 60 and 100 cycles per minute.
P Wave	Present; only one P for every QRS.
Direction of deflection	Upright in leads I, II, aVF, and V_{4-6}; inverted in aVR; and diphasic, flat, or inverted in leads III, V_1, and V_2.
Amplitude	< 3.0 mm.
Width	1.5 to 2.5 mm (0.06 to 0.10 s).
Shape	Gently rounded without notches or peaks.
Axis	$0°$ to $+90°$.
P-R interval	0.12 to 0.20 s (adults); 0.11 to 0.18 s (infants and children).
QRS interval	0.06 to 0.10 s.
Q-T interval	$<$ half the preceding R-R interval in normal rates.
	$Q\text{-}T_c \leqq 0.39$ s in males and 0.42 s in females.
QRS Complex	Follows each P wave.
Q waves	Width: $\leqq 0.039$ s.
	Depth: 1–2 mm in I, aVL, aVF, V_5, and V_6. Deep QS or Qr in aVR and possibly in III, V_1, and V_2.
Amplitude	>5 mm and < 25 mm in limb leads; 5 to 30 mm in V_1 and V_6; 7 to 30 mm in V_2 and V_5; 9 to 30 mm in V_3 and V_4.
R progression	Progressive rise in R wave amplitude from V_1 and V_6.
Axis	$-30°$ to $+100°$ in frontal plane.
Transition	V_3 or V_4.
Intrinsicoid deflection	$\leqq 0.02$ s in V_1; $\leqq 0.04$ s in V_6.
S-T segment	Isoelectric, but may be elevated $\leqq 1$ mm in limb leads and $\leqq 2$ mm in some precordial leads.
	Not depressed more than 0.05 mm.
	Curves gently into proximal limb of T wave.
T wave	
Direction	Upright in I, II, and V_{3-6}; inverted in aVR; and varies in III, aVL, aVF, V_1, and V_2.
Shape	Slightly rounded and asymmetrical.
Height	$\leqq 5$ mm in limb leads; $\leqq 10$ mm in precordial leads.
Axis	Left and inferior.
U wave	
Direction	Upright.
Amplitude	0.33 mm in precordial leads (average); 2.5 mm (maximum).
Width	$\leqq 0.24$ s.

Figure 11-18 A normal electrocardiogram. Follow the format discussed in the text to systematically interpret the ECG. *(From H. H. Friedman, Diagnostic electrocardiography and vectorcardiography, McGraw-Hill, New York, 1985, p. 98. Copyright 1985 by McGraw-Hill Book Company. Reprinted by permission.)*

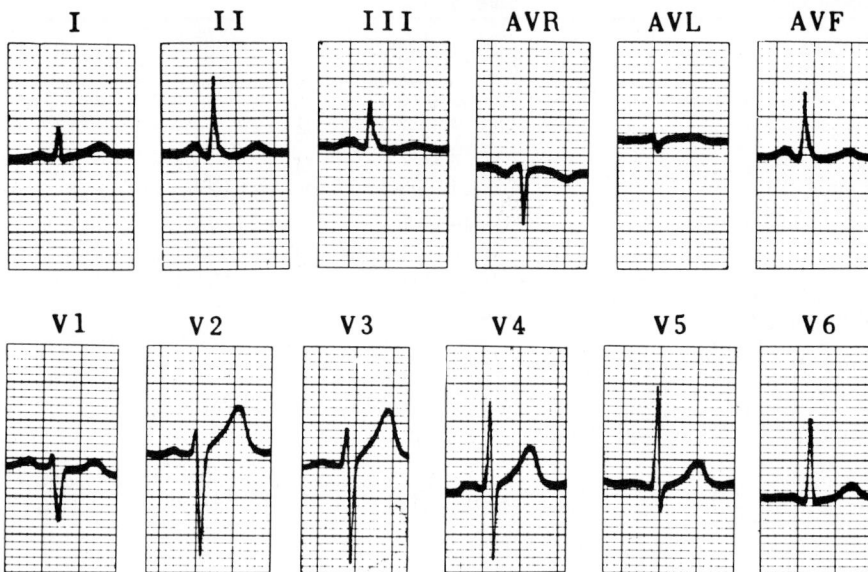

spontaneous depolarization in the sinus node is influenced by the balance between the sympathetic and parasympathetic autonomic effects, temperature and metabolic activity of the pacemaker cells, and the effect of electrolyte and pH changes on the heart. Consequently, if the autonomic balance or the environment of the sinus node cells is altered, the rate of impulse formation is changed. If the rate of phase 4 depolarization is increased in pacemaker cells other than those in the sinus node, for example the junction or ventricles, the automaticity of those sites is said to be *enhanced.* Extrasystoles or tachycardic rhythms may result. Conversely, if the rate of spontaneous depolarization of the sinus node is decreased, bradycardic or escape rhythms result.

Abnormal Automaticity When conditions are suitable, cells which do not normally possess automaticity may become capable of depolarizing spontaneously during phase 4. The automaticity in these sites may be depressed by acetylcholine and hastened by catecholamines. The abnormal automaticity may not necessarily suppress faster pacemakers, and may in fact be accelerated by overdrive pacing.

Triggered Activity Triggered activity refers to ectopic firing, often repetitive, which occurs in the absence of enhanced automaticity and is not sus-

tained by reentrant conduction. It results from afterdepolarizations, either early or late, which are of a magnitude great enough to reach threshold potential. The role of this mechanism in the creation of clinically observed dysrhythmias is unclear at this time.

Unidirectional Block with Reentry Reentry circuits or loops may be established when an initiating impulse, from either the SA node or an ectopic site, encounters an area of slow conduction which is long enough to delay the impulse passing through until the rest of the myocardium is nonrefractory, and an area of unidirectional conduction which inhibits or blocks impulse propagation in one direction but permits the impulse to pass through from the opposite direction, allowing it to restimulate the repolarized tissue. Figure 11-19 illustrates a reentrant loop which in this instance is located in the Purkinje fibers of the ventricles. However, reentrant circuits with one-way block may appear in the SA node, the atria, the AV junction, and the ventricles. Accessory pathways may serve as one branch of a reentry loop.

Classification of Dysrhythmias

There are a variety of ways to classify cardiac dysrhythmias. From an electrophysiologic viewpoint it is useful to classify them according to

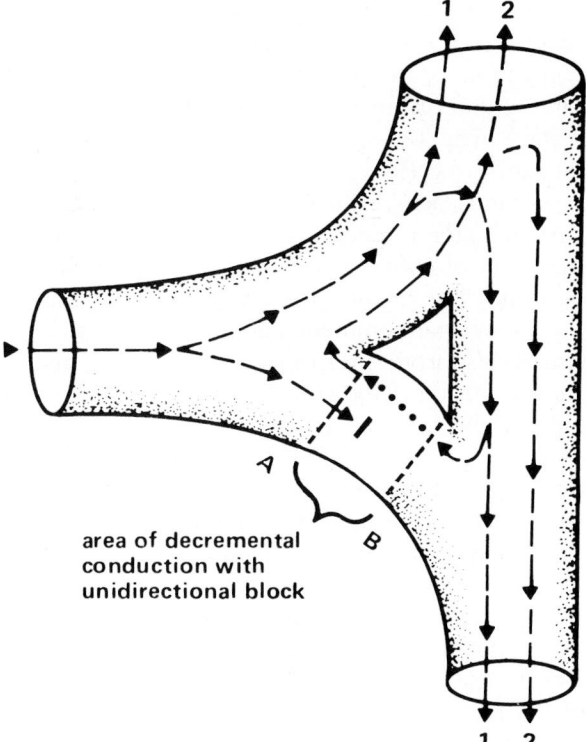

Figure 11-19 Reentry at the point of impingement of a Purkinje fiber on the ventricular myocardium. A region of decremental conduction with unidirectional block (A-B) blocks antegrade conduction of the normal impulse (1) but allows this impulse to traverse the depressed region in the retrograde direction (dotted line) after a delay. This retrograde impulse reenters the myocardium proximal to the region of decremental conduction after the proximal tissue has recovered from the normal impulse, thereby allowing the retrograde impulse to initiate a premature systole (2). *(From A. M. Katz, Physiology of the heart, Raven Press, New York, 1977, p. 330. Copyright 1977 by Raven Press Books, Ltd. Reprinted by permission.)*

(within figure: area of decremental conduction with unidirectional block)

whether they result from disturbances in impulse formation, impulse conduction, or a combination of these. However, in the clinical setting arrhythmias are more commonly classified by rate (tachyrhythms or bradyrhythms), by site of origin (sinus node, atria, junction, or ventricles), or by a combination of systems. For the purposes of this text, a combination of systems is utilized but the site of origin is the predominant classifying characteristic.

Sinus Node Dysrhythmias

Disturbances in either impulse formation or impulse conduction in the SA node result in sinus node dysrhythmias. These rhythm disturbances are characterized by a P wave of sinus origin and a constant and normal P-R interval. However, the configuration of the P wave, the rate of impulse formation, and the regularity of the cycle may be abnormal depending upon the given rhythm disturbance. Following is a discussion of the sinus dysrhythmias of sinus bradycardia, sinus tachycardia, sinus arrhythmia, wandering sinus pacemaker, sinus arrest, and sinoatrial block.

Sinus Bradycardia *Sinus bradycardia* is a rhythm originating in the sinus node but at a slower than normal rate (less than 60 beats per minute). Figure 11-20 is a rhythm strip depicting sinus bradycardia. Note that all aspects of the electrocardiographic recording are normal except for the rate. The usual rate of sinus bradycardia is from 45 to 59 beats per minute but may be as low as 35 beats per minute.

Sinus bradycardia may coexist with sinus arrhythmia but does not always do so. The rhythm must be distinguished from sinus arrest, SA block, AV junctional escape rhythm, idioventricular rhythm, and atrial fibrillation or flutter with AV block. If the

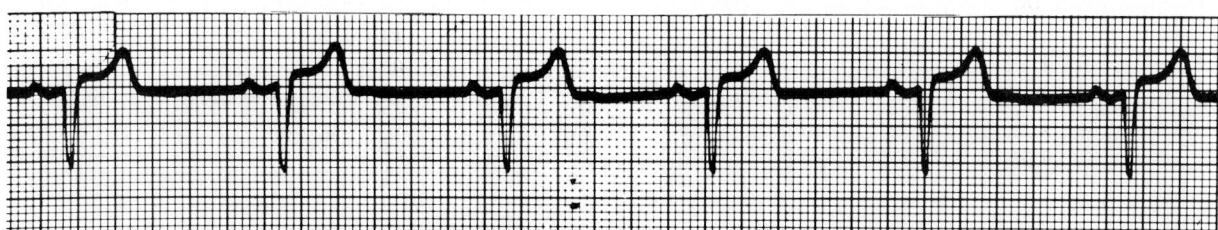

Figure 11-20 Sinus bradycardia. This rhythm strip was recorded from lead MCL₁. The heart rate is 52 beats per minute. The P-R, the QRS, and the Q-T intervals are normal. The configuration of the QRS complex, the S-T segment, and the T wave are abnormal for this lead.

sinus rate is equal to or less than that of the AV junctional rate, the the sinus rate is equal to or less than that of the AV junctional rate, the the sinus rate is equal to or less than that of the AV junctional rate, the junction may assume control of the ventricles, creating a dissociation between atrial and ventricular electrical activity.

Sinus bradycardia is common in healthy young adults, especially those with well-conditioned cardiovascular systems, and in the elderly, particularly during periods of sleep or immediately upon awakening. Altered automaticity secondary to increased parasympathetic influence is the usual cause of spontaneous sinus bradycardia. Factors which increase the sympathetic tone increase the rate. Various pharmacologic agents, such as reserpine, methyldopa, guanethidine, digitalis, and beta blockers, may cause a slowing of the sinus rate.

Symptoms from sinus bradycardia generally do not occur unless the rate is very slow or unless the rhythm appears in the presence of cardiac disease. Generally this rhythm disturbance requires no therapy; however, if the rate is markedly low, creating a reduction in cardiac output, sympathomimetic drugs such as atropine, isoproterenol, and ephedrine sulfate may be administered. If the rhythm fails to respond to drug treatment, pacemaker therapy may be instituted.

Sinus Tachycardia   A sinus rhythm with a rate in excess of 100 beats per minute is characteristic of *sinus tachycardia*. Rates between 101 and 160 beats per minute are usual but rates up to 180 beats per minute may be found in young adults during exercise. All other criteria for normal sinus rhythm are present (Fig. 11-21). However, with the increase in rate may come other electrocardiographic changes, such as S-T segment depression, altered T wave configuration, and prominent or inverted U waves. The P-R interval may be shortened and the P wave voltage may be increased. Occasionally the P-R interval is increased.

Sinus tachycardia is often observed in healthy persons after physical exercise; emotional stress; ingestion of coffee, tea, or alcohol; or smoking a cigarette. The rhythm may result from administration of sympathomimetic agents such as epinephrine and isoproterenol, or parasympatholytic agents such as atropine. Individuals with congestive heart failure, shock, acute rheumatic fever, pulmonary embolism, acute myocardial infarction, malignancy, or chronic lung diseases may exhibit an associated sinus tachycardia. It is also likely to be noted in individuals with an elevated temperature. The clinical significance of sinus tachycardia, then, is dependent upon the underlying cause of the rhythm.

This dysrhythmia generally does not produce symptoms. However, some individuals may complain of palpitations, restlessness, and anxiety while the rhythm is occurring, particularly if it is very rapid and persists for a long period of time. Frequently, a functional systolic murmur is heard at either the base or apex of the heart during a rapid sinus tachycardia, especially when the rhythm is secondary to a high cardiac output state.

Treatment for sinus tachycardia is generally not necessary except when the rhythm is associated with a disease process. In these instances, treatment of the underlying disease usually takes care of the dysrhythmia. Of course, the patient's hemodynamic status should be monitored to detect early signs of cardiac output deficits secondary to the tachy-

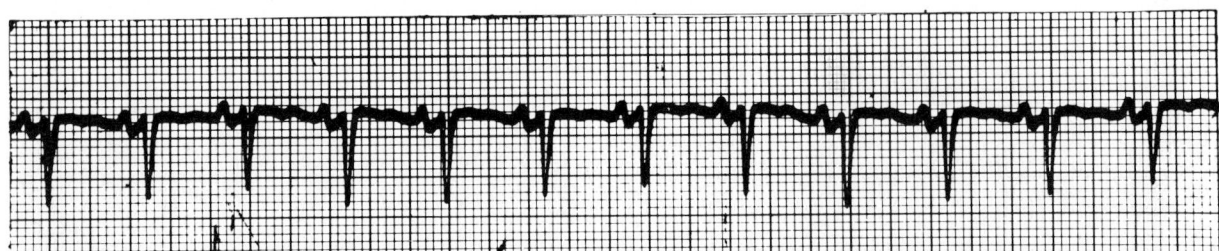

Figure 11-21   Sinus tachycardia. The heart rate of this rhythm strip, recorded from lead MCL₁, is 120 beats per minute. Other measurements are normal for a sinus rhythm.

rhythm. In healthy individuals the rhythm generally returns to normal without therapy once the causative factor is eliminated.

Sinus Arrhythmia   When the P-P (or R-R) cycles of a sinus rhythm vary by 0.16 s or more the disturbance is identified as *sinus arrhythmia* (Fig. 11-22). As with sinus bradycardia and sinus tachycardia, all other features of the rhythm usually meet the criteria for a normal sinus rhythm, although frequently the rate may be less than 60 beats per minute or greater than 100 beats per minute.

Sinus arrhythmia may be divided into two types. The first type, known as *respiratory sinus arrhythmia,* is produced by variations in vagal tone during the respiratory cycle. The second type of sinus arrhythmia is cyclic but not in relation to the respiratory pattern. It is, therefore, known as *nonrespiratory sinus arrhythmia*. It may also be called *idiopathic sinus arrhythmia* if the etiology is not known, or *pernicious sinus arrhythmia* if the rhythm is associated with cardiac disease.

If the sinus rate slows to an extent that causes it to be equal to or less than the intrinsic rate of the AV junction, the junctional pacemaker may assume control of the ventricles, resulting in AV dissociation. Sinus arrhythmia needs to be distinguished from sinus arrest; SA block; AV block, particularly 1° AV block; atrial premature complexes; and atrial flutter or fibrillation with a high degree of AV block.

Healthy children, young adults, and elderly individuals commonly exhibit respiratory sinus arrhythmia. People with cardiac disease also may experience this rhythm but more commonly exhibit nonrespiratory sinus arrhythmia. This rhythm is very common during the first 24 to 72 h after an acute inferior wall myocardial infarction. Sinus arrhythmia may be observed in patients with increased intracranial pressure from a variety of causes. Digitalis, morphine, and factors which increase parasympathetic tone may also cause sinus arrhythmia.

Respiratory sinus arrhythmia is generally not associated with symptoms unless the rate is especially slow (below 40 beats per minute). The patient may complain of palpitations and dizziness and may faint. Symptoms occur more frequently with nonrespiratory sinus arrhythmia and are generally dependent on the underlying cause of the dysrhythmia.

Treatment for respiratory sinus arrhythmia is generally not indicated unless the rhythm is particularly slow and producing symptoms. Atropine may be given under these circumstances to increase the heart rate. Nonrespiratory sinus arrhythmia-producing symptoms is treated by treating the underlying heart disease or other cause.

Wandering Sinus Pacemaker   A variant form of sinus arrhythmia in which the pacemaker shifts from site to site within the sinus node is known as *wandering sinus pacemaker*. This rhythm rarely exists in the absence of an associated sinus arrhythmia and can be recognized on the ECG when the P wave of sinus origin varies in configuration from beat to beat in each given lead, the P-R interval is within normal limits and relatively constant, the P-P cycle is slightly irregular, and the rate is between 45 and 100 beats per minute. It is important to note that the configuration of the P wave may vary slightly or markedly but remains positive in lead II and

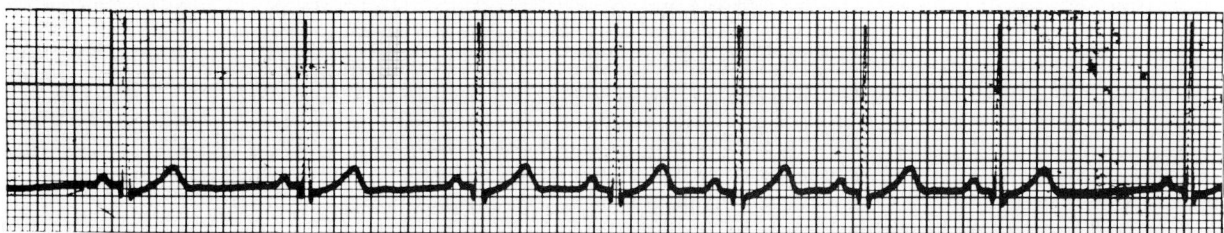

Figure 11-22   Sinus arrhythmia. The rhythm is irregular but all other criteria are normal for a sinus rhythm. A longer strip would demonstrate the cyclic nature of the irregular rhythm. The strip was recorded from lead II.

inverted in aVR and is generally altered greatly when wandering sinus pacemaker coexists with sinus arrhythmia. During rapid rates the P wave is taller and the P-R interval is longer, whereas during slower rates the reverse is found.

Wandering sinus pacemaker is considered clinically to be very similar to sinus arrhythmia. It may be found in healthy individuals, especially when sinus arrhythmia and sinus bradycardia exist simultaneously. The rhythm may be induced by digitalis. If wandering sinus pacemaker occurs spontaneously and persists, it may be an early indication of sick sinus syndrome.

Sinus Arrest   When impulse formation within the sinus node fails entirely, the node is said to *arrest* (Fig. 11-23). The electrocardiographic consequence is the absence of a P wave as well as the QRS complex and T wave. Because the absence of a complete electrical cycle results in a pause in the rhythm, sinus arrest is also sometimes known as *sinus pause* or *sinus standstill.*

When sinus arrest occurs, the subsidiary pacemaker sites within the junction or the ventricles may assume control of ventricular electrical activity. Commonly, an AV junctional escape rhythm appears because of its faster inherent rate of automaticity, but occasionally an idioventricular escape rhythm must assume control. Obviously, if both alternate pacemaker sites fail to take over the pacing responsibility of the heart during a prolonged sinus arrest, cardiac standstill will result.

Sinus arrest is differentiated from sinoatrial block when the pause is *not* an exact multiple of the basic cycle length. With sinus arrest the P-P cycle length of the pause bears no relationship to the normal P-P cycle; however, in sinoatrial block the P-P cycle length for the pause is an exact multiple of the basic P-P cycle or exhibits a regular irregularity. Sinus arrest must also be distinguished from marked sinus arrhythmia, second- or third-degree AV block, and nonconducted premature atrial complexes.

Normal individuals with an increased vagal tone or a hypersensitive carotid sinus may experience sinus arrest. Generally the rhythm is associated with a marked sinus arrhythmia but it may also occur without sinus arrhythmia as a result of quinidine or digitalis overdose or on a reflex basis. Other causes of sinus arrest include acute myocarditis, acute myocardial infarction with sinus node involvement, and administration of parasympathetic agents or potassium. Carotid sinus stimulation of the patient with digitalis intoxication also may result in sinus arrest. Frequent occurrence of sinus arrest with long duration is commonly caused by advanced sick sinus syndrome.

The underlying cause and cardiac status greatly influence the treatment of sinus arrest. The rhythm may be treated successfully by removing the etiologic factor. If the patient is asymptomatic and the heart rate is greater than 45 beats per minute, therapy may not be warranted. However, if the patient is symptomatic, atropine, ephedrine sulfate, an artificial pacemaker, and/or cardiopulmonary resuscitation may be required.

Sinoatrial (SA) Block   Blockage of sinus impulse conduction at the sinoatrial junction is generally thought to be the mechanism resulting in SA block. This rhythm disturbance can be classified into three degrees similar to those of AV block. *First-degree*

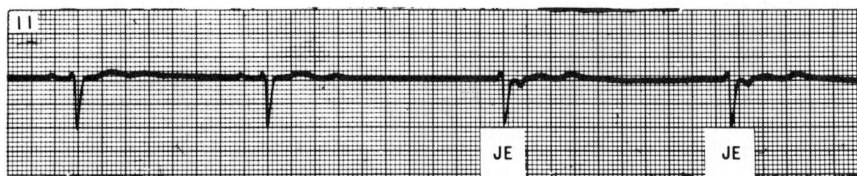

Figure 11-23 Sinus arrest. After two normal beats, a sinus impulse fails to appear. During the pause, two AV junctional escape beats (JE) occur. Each junctional beat is followed by a retrograde P wave. *(From H. H. Friedman, Diagnostic electrocardiography and vectorcardiography, McGraw-Hill, New York, 1985, p. 456. Copyright 1985 by McGraw-Hill Book Company. Reprinted by permission.)*

SA block probably occurs theoretically, but it is impossible to diagnose electrocardiographically because the ECG does not record sinus activity and consequently, actual sinoatrial conduction time is not known. *Second-degree SA block* can be divided into a *Mobitz type I* and a *Mobitz type II* SA block. The latter is the more common variety of the two types, and both can be identified on the ECG. *Third-degree SA block,* however, cannot be diagnosed on the ECG due to the absence of the P, QRS, and T complexes for indefinite periods.

SA block should be distinguished from SA arrest, AV block, and sinus arrhythmia. Mobitz type II SA block (Fig. 11-24) is recognized on the electrocardiogram when there is an occasional absence of one or more complete electrical cycles (including P, QRS, and T waves) and when the P-P cycle of the SA block is exactly or almost exactly a multiple of the basic P-P cycle. In other words, the P-P interval including the SA block is frequently three or four times the basic P-P interval. If a 2:1 SA block occurs consecutively, it may appear as a slow sinus bradycardia. If it occurs repeatedly for three, four, or more impulses, cardiac standstill results for that period of time unless a subsidiary pacemaker activates the atria and ventricles.

Mobitz type I SA block (Fig. 11-25) is difficult to differentiate from sinus arrest because the long P-P interval of the block is *not* a multiple of the basic P-P cycle. This rhythm can only be diagnosed when the Wenckebach pattern of the block can be identified. In this instance the P-P intervals prior to the long pause become progressively shorter until an entire cycle is dropped. As with Mobitz type II

SA block, the AV junction may escape for one or more impulses to control the ventricles.

SA block is usually a transient rhythm but may continue for a long period of time. Like sinus arrest it may be found in healthy individuals with increased vagal tone or a hypersensitive carotid sinus, as well as in individuals suffering from myocarditis or acute inferior wall myocardial infarction. Quinidine or digitalis toxicity and hyperkalemia may induce SA block. If the rhythm is not drug induced and if it occurs frequently, sick sinus syndrome may be implicated.

Generally a transient SA block produces no symptoms and requires no treatment. However, when the block persists and no subsidiary pacemaker escapes to control the ventricles or an escape rhythm produces a particularly slow ventricular rhythm, the patient may experience dizziness or perhaps fainting episodes. Therapy in these instances depends on the underlying cause and the underlying cardiac status. Therapeutic methods are those used for sinus arrest.

Sick Sinus Syndrome   Brief mention should be made regarding *sick sinus syndrome.* This syndrome is manifested by a variety of sinus impulse formation and conduction disturbances. The ECG of sick sinus syndrome may exhibit marked sinus bradycardia, sinus arrest, and SA block. Episodes of atrial tachyarrhythmias may coexist with episodes of bradyarrhythmias resulting in a brady–tachyarrhythmia syndrome which is a common manifestation of sick sinus syndrome. These ECG findings are *not* drug induced.

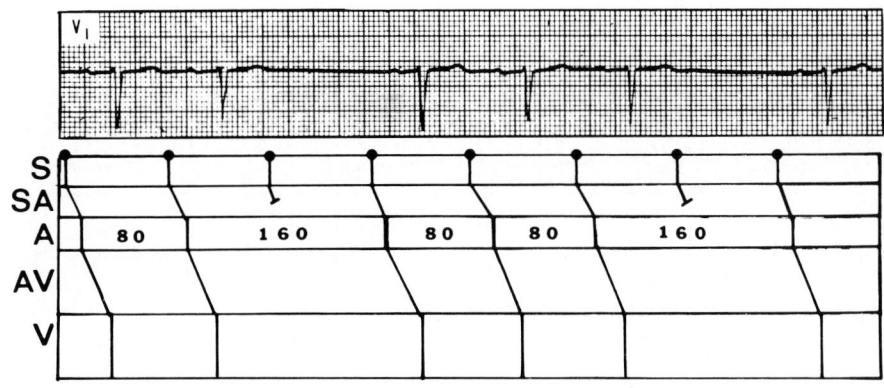

Figure 11-24   Type II SA block. The pauses equal two cycle lengths. The time intervals are shown in hundredths of a second. *(From H. H. Friedman, Diagnostic electrocardiography and vectorcardiography, McGraw-Hill, New York, 1985, p. 581. Copyright 1985 by McGraw-Hill Book Company. Reprinted by permission.)*

Figure 11-25 Type I (Wenckebach) 4:3 SA block. *(From H. H. Friedman, Diagnostic electrocardiography and vectorcardiography, McGraw-Hill, New York, 1985, p. 580. Copyright 1985 by McGraw-Hill Book Company. Reprinted by permission.)*

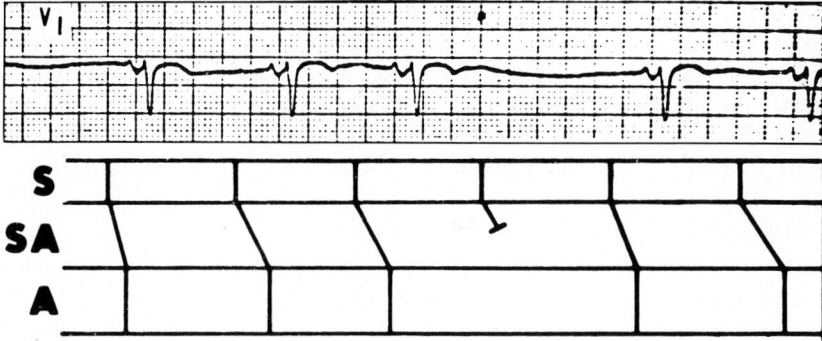

Clinical significance and treatment of sick sinus syndrome depends on the severity of the sinus node dysfunction and the symptoms experienced. Treatment is directed at the symptoms the rhythm disturbance produces.

Atrial Dysrhythmias

Rhythm disturbances of atrial origin may be initiated from any site within the atria other than in the SA node. Atrial dysrhythmias are almost always produced by active impulse formation and, therefore, almost always appear as some form of an atrial tachyarrhythmia. The rhythm disturbances of atrial premature complex, atrial tachycardia, multifocal atrial tachycardia, atrial flutter, and atrial fibrillation will be discussed in this section.

Atrial Premature Complex   Premature impulse formation from within the atria but outside the SA node results in what is known as *atrial premature complex (APC)*. The most obvious diagnostic feature of this rhythm disturbance is the premature occurrence of the complex (Fig. 11-26). Other ECG findings which assist in the diagnosis include: (1)

a P wave configuration which differs from the P wave of the sinus-originated complexes and which varies, depending on the site of the ectopic focus; (2) P-R intervals of variable duration but frequently within the normal range; however, they may be abnormally short or abnormally long; (3) a postectopic pause which is usually not fully compensatory (the interval between the normal complex preceding the premature complex and the normal complex after the APC is not two times the normal P-P cycle); and (4) the interval from the ectopic P to the preceding P wave of the basic rhythm (coupling interval) is usually constant. The configuration of the QRS following the premature P wave is somewhat dependent on the degree of prematurity of the extrasystole and may be normal due to normal ventricular conduction, abnormal due to aberrant ventricular conduction, or absent (termed *nonconducted APC*) due to the refractory state of the ventricular myocardium (Fig. 11-27). APCs may occur as a single event or they may occur more frequently. If they alternate with the basic cycle the rhythm is identified as *atrial bigeminy*. They also may occur every third complex (*atrial trigeminy*)

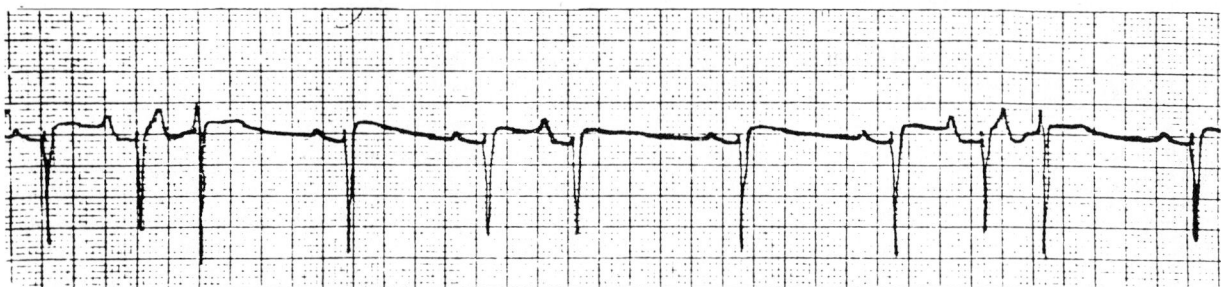

Figure 11-26 Atrial premature complexes. The second, third, sixth, ninth, and tenth P waves are premature. The third and tenth QRS complexes are slightly aberrant.

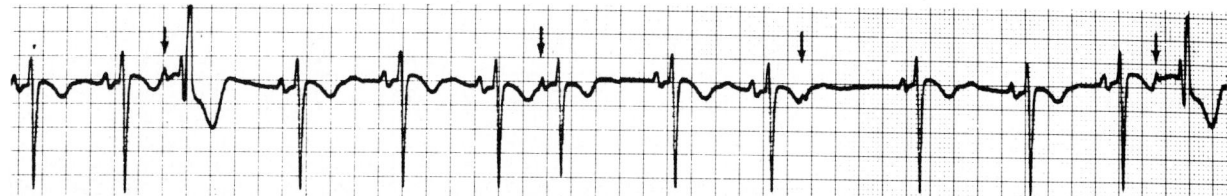

Figure 11-27 Atrial premature complexes. The first APC (P′) is aberrantly conducted, the second is conducted normally, and the third is not conducted (nonconducted APC). Note the P-P′ coupling intervals. The third premature P wave occurs much earlier than the others and finds the ventricles refractory. The first premature P wave finds the ventricles partially refractory, causing the conduction to be aberrant. The least premature P wave is the second one and it conducts normally. *(From A. E. Lindsay and A. Budkin, The cardiac arrhythmias, second edition, Year Book, Chicago, 1975, p. 12. Copyright 1975 by Year Book Medical Publishers, Inc. Reprinted by permission.)*

or every fourth complex (*atrial quadrageminy*). The extrasystoles may occur consecutively in pairs or triplets. If six or more occur consecutively the rhythm disturbance is labeled *atrial tachycardia.*

The arrhythmogenic mechanism of atrial premature complexes is likely to be either reentry or enhanced focal excitability. This rhythm disturbance is often observed in healthy individuals without organic heart disease. In these people the arrhythmia may be related to emotional stress, physical or mental fatigue, excessive smoking, or ingestion of coffee or alcohol. Atrial premature complexes are more frequent, however, in people with heart disease, particularly those with atrial disease or atrial enlargement. Mitral stenosis and cor pulmonale are two conditions in which one would expect to observe frequent APCs that often lead to atrial flutter or atrial fibrillation.

Infrequent APCs are generally clinically insignificant. However, when atrial premature complexes are more frequent, occurring every sixth complex or more often, they may cause the individual to experience palpitations. Only if the symptoms of APCs are significant is there a need to treat the rhythm disturbance. Quinidine may be the drug of choice; however, other oral antiarrhythmic agents may be prescribed.

Atrial Tachycardia *Atrial tachycardia* (AT) is generally defined as six or more consecutive atrial extrasystoles (Fig. 11-28); however, some may consider atrial tachycardia to be present when as few as three consecutive APCs occur. As with other atrial dysrhythmias, this rhythm disturbance originates within the atria but outside the SA node. The

entire atria, including the SA node, are activated by the ectopic rhythm. Consequently, the pacemaking ability of the SA node is suppressed for the duration of the rhythm. When the episode of atrial tachycardia terminates, it is followed by a long pause until the pacemaking function of the sinus node is restored.

In addition to the appearance of consecutive atrial extrasystoles, other ECG findings may be helpful for the recognition of atrial tachycardia. The P wave configuration of the ectopic complexes is different from that of the sinus P wave. While the specific configuration is variable based on the site of the ectopic focus, the extrasystolic P waves have a common morphology and are generally upright in lead II and inverted in aVR. The P waves may appear to be absent but are probably superimposed on the preceding QRS complex, S-T segment, T wave, or U wave. The atrial rate is usually between 160 and 250 beats per minute but may be as low as 120 beats per minute. The ventricular rate is equal to the atrial rate when atrial tachycardia is uncomplicated and the rate is less than 200 beats per minute. However, when the atrial rate is very rapid (greater than 200 beats per minute) the AV junction may be physiologically refractory, allowing only every other impulse to conduct to the ventricles. In this instance the ventricular rate will be half the atrial rate. The P-R interval in atrial tachycardia is determined by the status of the AV conduction system and the atrial rate. Generally, the P-R interval is within normal limits in uncomplicated atrial tachycardia.

Atrial tachycardia is usually initiated by a single APC and ends abruptly in a paroxysmal form. As noted previously, when the tachycardic rhythm ends

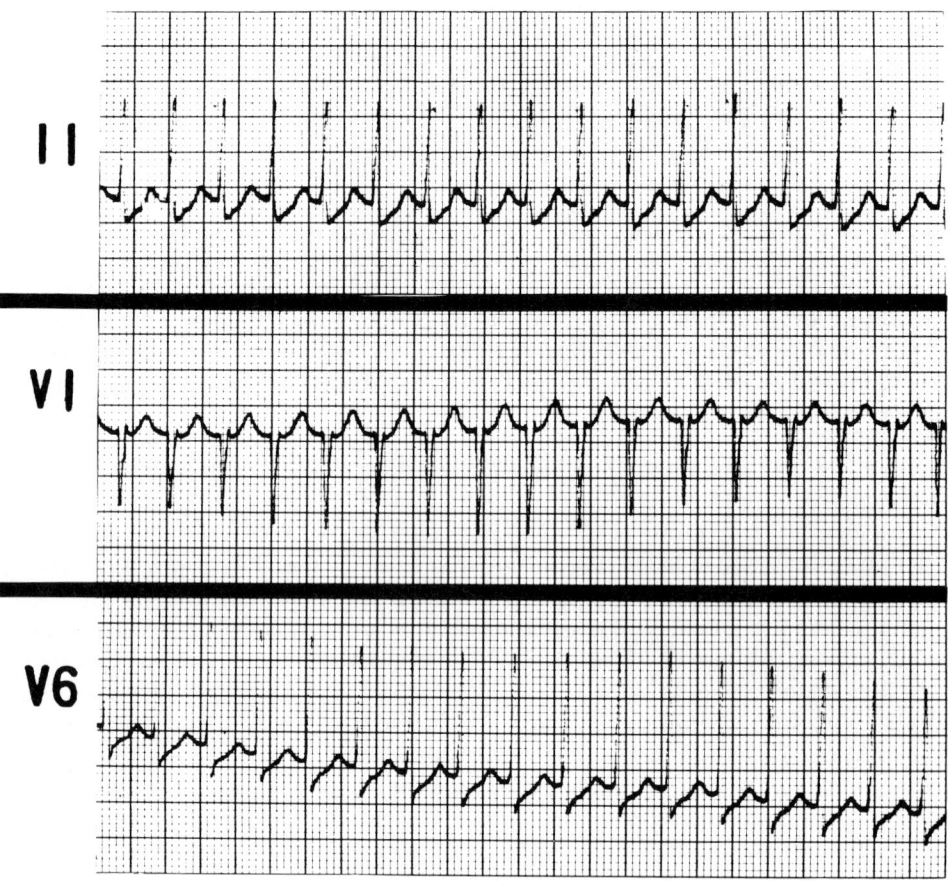

Figure 11-28 Atrial tachycardia. The rate is about 200 beats per minute. P′ waves are difficult to identify but are probably hidden in the previous S-T segment or T wave. *(From N. K. Wenger, J. W. Hurst, and M. C. McIntyre, Cardiology for nurses, McGraw-Hill, New York, 1980, p. 294. Copyright 1980 by McGraw-Hill Book Company. Reprinted by permission.)*

it is followed by a pause which is longer than the basic P-P cycle and is due to the reestablishment of the pacing function of the sinus node. This rhythm often becomes chronic in diseased hearts.

Precisely regular P-P and R-R cycles are usual in uncomplicated atrial tachycardia, but these cycles may be irregular. The configuration of the QRS complex, as with APCs, may be wide and bizarre due to abnormal conduction. This is particularly true in very rapid rates due to the partially refractory state of the ventricular conduction system. In these instances, and particularly when the P wave cannot be seen, atrial tachycardia may resemble ventricular tachycardia. Care in the diagnosis of this rhythm is, therefore, very important.

The arrhythmogenic mechanism of atrial tachycardia is usually the same as that for a single APC. The rhythm can be found in healthy individuals and in those with heart disease. Rheumatic and coronary heart disease, particularly acute myocardial infarction, are the two disease processes most often associated with atrial tachycardia. This rhythm disturbance may also be associated with digitalis intoxication, in which case it coexists with AV block, and with a number of other cardiovascular disease processes.

The occurrence of symptoms due to atrial tachycardia is dependent on the disease state of the individual and the rate of the rhythm. Healthy people can tolerate paroxysmal atrial tachycardia for long periods of time if the rate is not too rapid (not greater than 180 beats per minute). In diseased hearts, though, even slow ventricular rates may cause or aggravate congestive heart failure or angina pectoris. Symptoms produced by atrial tachycardia include palpitations, chest pain, weakness, dizziness, anxiety, apprehension, and feelings of impending doom.

Medical management of atrial tachycardia may include withdrawal of the etiologic factor when possible; Class IA, II, III, or IV antiarrhythmic agents (see Appendix A); digitalis, if it is not the cause of the rhythm disturbance; carotid sinus stimulation; overdrive pacing; and direct current (dc) shock. Sedation in conjunction with other therapeutic measures may be beneficial.

Multifocal Atrial Tachycardia   Atrial tachycardia with variable P wave morphology and irregular ectopic P-P cycles, a rate between 100 and 250 beats per minute, an isoelectric line between P-P intervals, and varying P-R intervals with AV block of varying degrees is identified as *multifocal atrial tachycardia (MAT)* (Fig. 11-29). Other terms used to describe this electrocardiographic pattern are *chaotic atrial tachycardia, repetitive multifocal paroxysmal atrial tachycardia,* and *wandering atrial pacemaker.*

Multifocal atrial tachycardia differs from unifocal atrial tachycardia in that it does not usually appear in paroxysmal form and frequently produces a slower atrial as well as ventricular rate. The ventricular rate may be as slow as 50 to 60 beats per minute but usually exceeds 100 beats per minute. This rhythm disorder may be mistaken for sinus arrhythmia, wandering sinus pacemaker, atrial flutter, or atrial fibrillation. When the multifocal P waves conduct through the ventricles in an aberrant fashion, the rhythm may be misidentified as ventricular tachycardia or ventricular fibrillation.

This rhythm disturbance is usually seen in seriously ill elderly patients with acute and chronic lung disease. It is also seen frequently in patients who have hypertensive or valvular heart disease. Digitalis intoxication may or may not be associated with MAT but probably is not a cause of the dysrhythmia. Infrequently, MAT may be identified in individuals with electrolyte imbalance, particularly hypokalemia. The mechanism of this rhythm disturbance is probably enhanced automaticity.

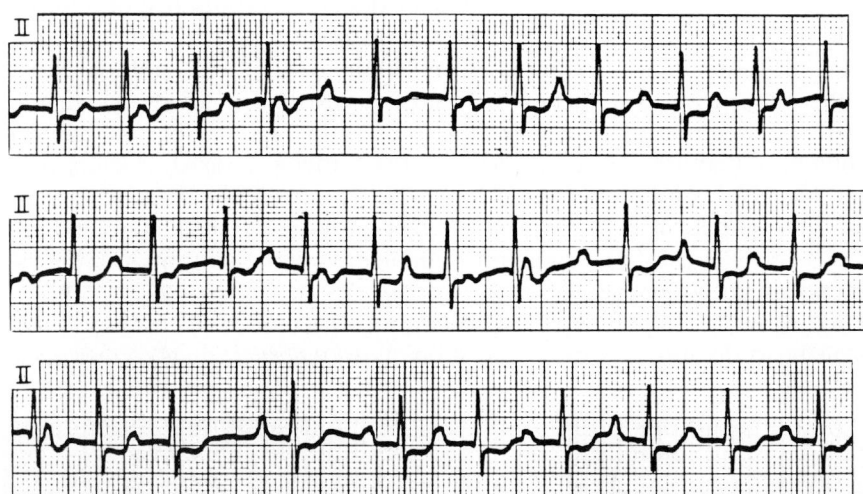

Figure 11-29   Multifocal atrial tachycardia. The tracings are not continuous but were taken from a longer recording. The morphology of the P′ waves is variable. The P-P′ intervals are irregular. AV conduction varies from beat to beat. Although the S-T, T changes are the result of digitalis effect, the arrhythmia was not produced by digitalis toxicity. *(From H. H. Friedman, Diagnostic electrocardiography and vectorcardiography, McGraw-Hill, New York, 1985, p. 464. Copyright 1985 by McGraw-Hill Book Company. Reprinted by permission.)*

Antiarrhythmic drug therapy is not generally useful in treating MAT. It is usually more beneficial to treat the dysrhythmia by treating the underlying disease process.

Atrial Flutter   Rapid regular atrial deflections (F waves) which characteristically have a sawtooth appearance are the electrocardiographic hallmark of *atrial flutter* (Fig. 11-30). Other features are (1) an atrial rate that is usually between 250 and 350 beats per minute, (2) a variable rate and rhythm of ventricular depolarization which is dependent on the atrial rate and the status of AV conduction, and (3) a QRS configuration which may be either normal or abnormal, depending on the conduction status of the ventricles.

One group of researchers[3] has identified two types of atrial flutter, which are categorized by the atrial rate. Type I had a rate of 240 to 338 beats per minute and Type II had a rate of 340 to 433 beats per minute. In the clinical setting an atrial electrogram is used to assist with the identification of these two types. The clinical significance of the two types seems to rest with their response to rapid atrial pacing. Type I can be influenced by rapid atrial pacing from the high right atrium but type II cannot.

The arrhythmogenic mechanism of atrial flutter is unclear. However, four theories continue to be considered and tested. The theories include circus movement, multiple reentry phenomenon, unifocal impulse formation, and multifocal impulse formation. Atrial flutter may occur transiently and intermittently or it may persist in a chronic form for months and years.

This arrhythmia is less common than atrial fibrillation and atrial tachycardia and is seen most often in elderly patients with organic heart disease.

Common etiologies are coronary artery disease; rheumatic heart disease, particularly mitral stenosis; and hypertensive heart disease. Atrial flutter often develops after cardiac surgery. Less commonly it is associated with thyrotoxicosis, cardiomyopathy, acute and chronic cor pulmonale, pulmonary diseases, and pericarditis. Digitalis intoxication is rarely a cause of the arrhythmia. Infrequently, atrial flutter is identified in healthy individuals without heart disease.

Signs and symptoms of atrial flutter are dependent on a variety of factors but particularly on the nature of the underlying heart disease, the ventricular rate, and the duration of the rhythm disturbance. When the ventricular rate is slow, symptoms are absent. With rapid ventricular rates and in elderly individuals with advanced cardiac disease, congestive heart failure (CHF) is likely to occur. Patients may experience palpitations, chest pain, and symptoms of reduced cardiac output including increased fatigability, shortness of breath, and mental confusion. These patients should be assessed for signs and symptoms of pulmonary and systemic thromboemboli secondary to atrial hemostasis.

Therapy for atrial flutter is dependent on the underlying heart disease, the presence or absence of CHF, metabolic disorders, and drug toxicity. Transient forms of the rhythm with short durations generally require no treatment. Acute and chronic forms resulting in symptoms may be treated with antiarrhythmic drug therapy, rapid atrial pacing, and/or (dc) shock. The particular form of therapy selected depends on the clinical situation and the urgency for elimination of the rhythm disturbance.

Atrial Fibrillation   The mechanism responsible for the creation of *atrial fibrillation* is controversial

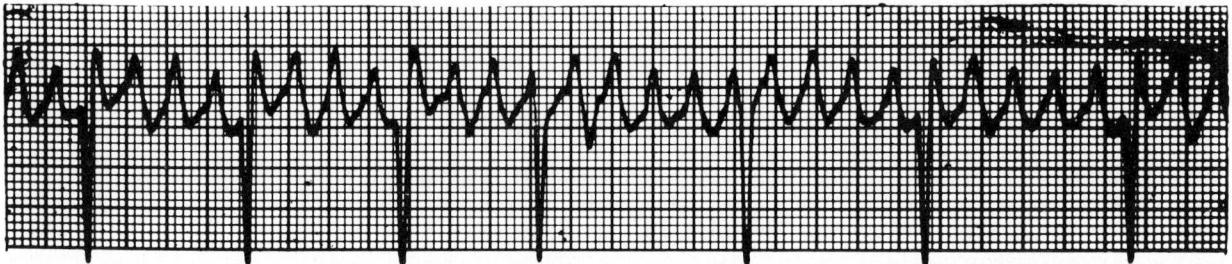

Figure 11-30   Atrial flutter. The A-V conduction is variable. Note the sawtooth appearance of the "F waves."

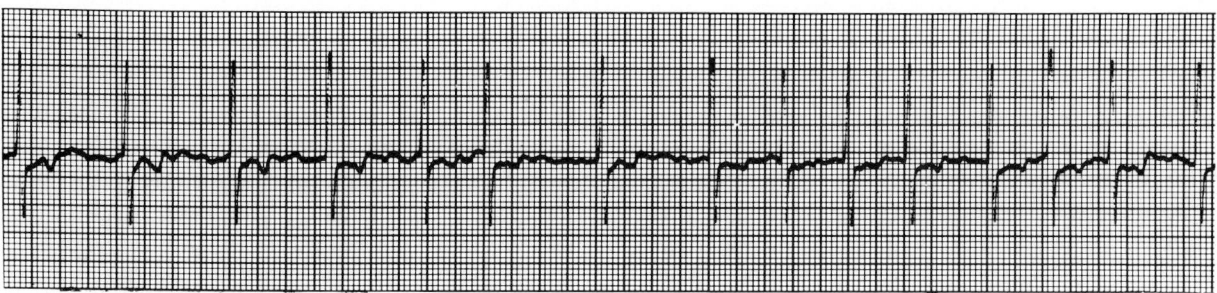

Figure 11-31 Atrial fibrillation.

but is theorized to be one of the four mechanisms mentioned in the discussion of atrial flutter. The ECG findings of this rhythm disturbance include atrial activity represented by fibrillatory (f) waves which replace the P wave and ventricular activity which is totally irregular (Fig. 11-31). Note that in the presence of AV block, though, the ventricular rhythm may be regular. The f waves exhibit a varying amplitude, duration, and morphology, causing the baseline to oscillate randomly. The QRS configuration may be altered by (1) the superimposition of f waves on a portion of the QRS complex, (2) aberrant conduction secondary to varying degrees of refractoriness of the myocardial cells, or (3) ventricular preexcitation.

Frequently the atrial rate in atrial fibrillation cannot be determined. Probable rates range from 450 to 650 beats per minute with the slower rates occurring in coarse atrial fibrillation and the faster in fine atrial fibrillation. The distinction between coarse and fine fibrillation rests with the size and amplitude of the f waves. The ventricular rate is generally quite rapid, between 120 and 200 beats per minute in untreated cases of atrial fibrillation. Slower rates are possible when there is a coexisting AV conduction abnormality. Complete AV block is suggested when there is a slow ventricular rhythm (25 to 40 beats per minute) and a regular R-R interval. The escape pacemaker site is either the AV junction or the His-Purkinje system.

Wells and associates[4] identified four types of atrial fibrillation in postoperative cardiac surgery patients. Recording of bipolar epicardial atrial electrograms (AEG) revealed atrial fibrillatory waves of varying sizes, shapes, polarities, amplitudes, and beat-to-beat intervals. Type I was characterized by discrete AEG complexes separated by an isoelectric baseline free of disturbance. Type II had discrete AEG complexes but with perturbations of the baseline between complexes. AEGs which failed to demonstrate either discrete complexes or isoelectric intervals were identified as Type III. Type IV atrial fibrillation was characterized on the AEG by alternating periods of Type I and Type II patterns. The ability to distinguish between the types of atrial fibrillation may lead to more effective treatment of the arryhthmia.

Atrial fibrillation is a very common arrhythmia and is the usual underlying rhythm in patients with CHF. It is frequently associated with Wolff-Parkinson-White syndrome in adults. Like atrial flutter, atrial fibrillation is associated with rheumatic, coronary, and hypertensive heart diseases and with hyperthyroidism. Coarse atrial fibrillation is almost always due to rheumatic heart disease but may be found in thyrotoxicosis. Fine atrial fibrillation is almost always found in coronary or hypertensive disease. When an underlying heart disease is present, both coarse and fine atrial fibrillation generally become chronic.

Less common causes of atrial fibrillation include cardiomyopathy, acute myocarditis, acute pericarditis, and chest trauma. It is rarely observed in digitalis intoxication. Healthy individuals may exhibit atrial fibrillation as a result of heavy smoking; excessive ingestion of alcohol, coffee, or tea; and sudden emotional excitement.

Symptoms resulting from atrial fibrillation vary with the presence or absence and nature of the heart disease, the presence or absence and degree of CHF, the ventricular rate, and the duration of the rhythm. Patients with transient atrial fibrillation may be symptom-free. Those with CHF may have mild symptoms of palpitations, anxiety, a fluttering or pounding feeling, and the sensation of skipped heart beats, or they may experience more severe symptoms including worsening CHF, syncope, angina, and a feeling of impending death.

The treatment of choice for atrial fibrillation with rapid ventricular rates, either in the presence or absence of CHF, is digitalis. This drug is most effective when significant CHF exists. Other methods for treating atrial fibrillation include antiarrhythmic agents and dc shock. Withdrawal of precipitating factors such as alcohol is also an important therapeutic intervention.

AV Junctional Dysrhythmias

Cardiac rhythms in which the site of impulse formation is within the AV junction are identified as *AV junctional dysrhythmias*. The actual site of the pacemaker is difficult to locate from the surface ECG but may be from low atrial foci, the coronary sinus ostium, the bundle of His, the node–His (N–H) region of the AV node, and possibly the atrionodal (AN) region of the AV node. Impulse formation does not originate in the nodal (N) region of the AV node. Rhythm disturbances may not originate in the nodal (N) region of the AV node. Rhythm disturbances may be due to an escape mechanism secondary to depression of SA node function, SA block, or AV block or to enhanced automaticity of the AV junctional pacemaker. In the first case (escape mechanisms) the heart rate is 40 and 60 beats per minute and in the latter (enhanced automaticity), rates are usually faster than 60 beats per minute.

The electrocardiographic features of all AV junctional dysrhythmias are similar, differing only in their effect on the cardiac rhythm and the time of onset in the cardiac cycle. Because the atria must be stimulated in a retrograde fashion, the junctional P wave (when present) is inverted in leads II, III, and aVF, and upright in aVR. It is also upright in leads I and V_6. The P wave may occur prior to the QRS, indicating that the atria depolarized before the ventricles; or after the QRS, indicating initial ventricular depolarization which is followed by atrial depolarization. The junctional P wave is superimposed on the QRS if the atria and ventricles depolarize simultaneously and, therefore, is not visible on the ECG. If the junctional pacemaker is blocked from conducting antegrade to the ventricles, the P wave will appear without a QRS complex. If it is blocked from conducting retrograde to the atria, no P wave will appear. The contour of the P wave is generally abnormal.

The P-R interval (or R-P interval) for AV junctional complexes varies according to the location of the ectopic focus within the junction and the condition of antegrade and retrograde conduction. Generally the P-R interval is equal to or less than 0.12 s and the R-P interval is between 0.10 and 0.20 s. The configuration of the QRS complex of AV junctional complexes, either escape beats or extrasystoles, is often normal but it may be wide and bizarre due to either aberrant or preexisting ventricular conduction abnormalities.

In this section the dysrhythmias of AV junctional beats (or rhythm), AV junctional premature complex, nonparoxysmal AV junctional tachycardia, paroxysmal AV junctional tachycardia, and paroxysmal supraventricular tachycardia are discussed.

AV Junctional Beats (Rhythm) An *AV junctional beat* or *rhythm* occurs as a physiologically passive escape mechanism when the SA node fails to function or is blocked from stimulating the AV junction or ventricles. The junction may escape for a single beat or for multiple consecutive beats and is usually a transitory event. Six or more consecutive junctional escape beats constitute an AV junctional rhythm (Fig. 11-32).

The rate of impulse formation for AV junctional rhythm ranges from 40 to 60 beats per minute but may rarely be as low as 30 beats per minute. The R-R intervals are almost always precisely regular and seldom vary by more than 0.04 s. The P wave configuration varies, depending on the activation site for the atria. If the sinus node activates the atria, the P wave will be normal in appearance, but will not be associated with ventricular activation (AV dissociation). If both the sinus node and the AV junction activate the atria, atrial fusion beats result and the P configuration varies with the degree of fusion between the two impulses. When the atria are activated by retrograde conduction from the AV junction, the P wave is inverted in leads II, III, and aVF, and upright in lead aVR.

The appearance of an occasional and intermittent AV junctional beat or rhythm is clinically insignificant in healthy individuals or those with

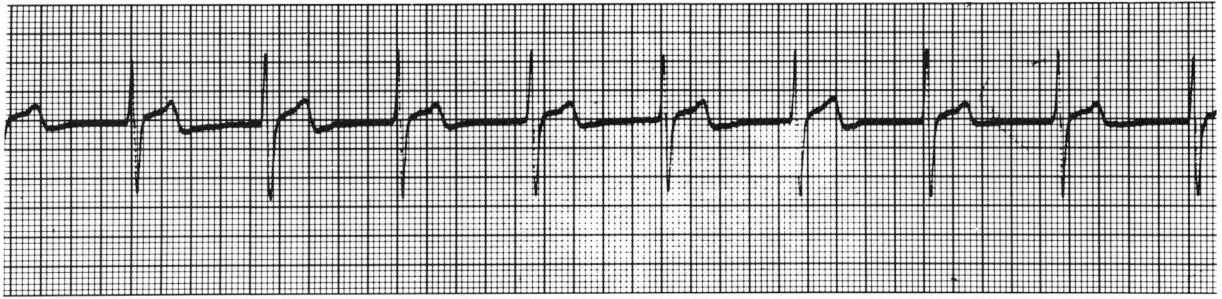

Figure 11-32 AV junctional rhythm. No P waves are evident, indicating that the atria and ventricles are activated simultaneously or that retrograde conduction to the atria is blocked.

diseased hearts if the beat or rhythm follows a postectopic pause, sinus bradycardia, sinus arrest, or SA block of short duration. An individual is often symptomatic, however, when the escape beat or rhythm occurs secondary to complete AV block, sinus arrest, or SA block of long duration, and especially in the presence of serious heart disease or drug intoxication. Symptoms are generally dependent on the ventricular rate. If it is particularly slow, the patient will likely experience dizziness, mental confusion, and Adams-Stokes syndrome due to reduced cerebral blood flow and may experience angina pectoris due to reduced coronary blood flow. Congestive heart failure may develop in patients whose AV junctional rhythm is secondary to complete AV block.

Treatment of AV junctional beats or rhythm is unnecessary unless it occurs secondary to com-plete AV block. Treatment in this situation is dependent on the ventricular rate. If the rate is relatively rapid (40 to 60 beats per minute) it may not be treated. However, if the ventricular rate is quite slow, a permanent artificial pacemaker may be required.

AV Junctional Premature Complex   The electro-cardiographic features of *AV junctional premature complex* (Fig. 11-33) are: (1) a premature complex in relation to the basic cycle, (2) a P wave config-uration characteristic of an AV junctional beat, (3) a coupling interval that is usually constant, and (4) a postectopic pause which is usually not fully compensatory. Like atrial premature complexes, junctional premature complexes (JPC) may occur in pairs, or in bigeminal, trigeminal, or quadragem-inal frequencies. A JPC must be differentiated on

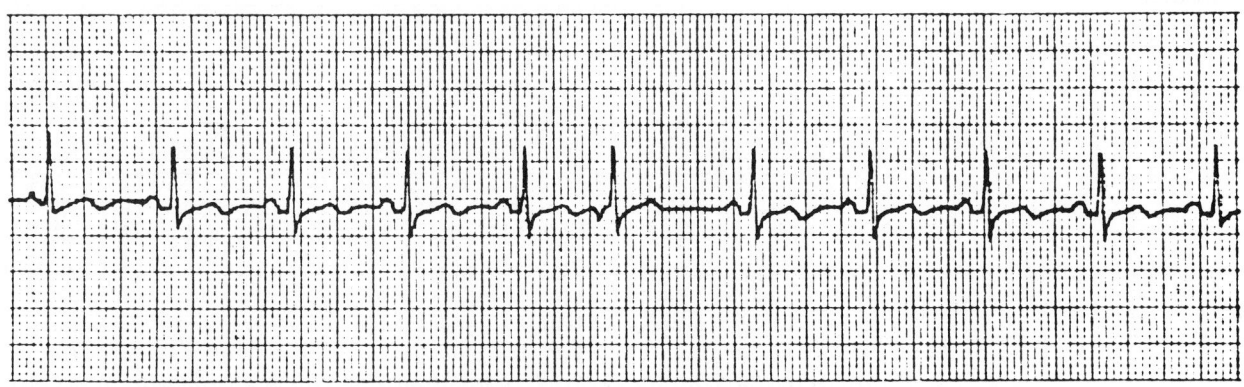

Figure 11-33 Junctional premature complex.

the ECG from APCs and ventricular premature complexes (VPC).

As with other premature complexes, the mechanism responsible for generating a JPC is likely to be either reentry or enhanced focal excitability. Junctional premature complexes may occur infrequently when compared to atrial and ventricular premature complexes. They may be observed on the ECG of a healthy individual or an individual with heart disease, and they may be induced by digitalis therapy.

Occasional JPCs are generally clinically insignificant and, therefore, require no therapy. If they occur every sixth beat or more frequently, if they occur in groups, or if they produce irritating symptoms, therapy may be required to prevent an AV junctional tachycardia. When JPCs occur secondary to CHF, digitalization may eliminate the dysrhythmia. Obviously, if digitalis is the suspected cause of the rhythm disturbance the drug may need to be discontinued. Other therapies include quinidine, propranolol, and other antiarrhythmic agents used for supraventricular tachyarrhythmias.

Nonparoxysmal AV Junctional Tachycardia   A junctional rhythm with a rate within the range of sinus rhythm and sinus tachycardia (65 to 130 beats per minute) is identified as *nonparoxysmal AV*

junctional tachycardia (NJT). The rhythm may also be known as *accelerated AV junctional rhythm.* The ECG characteristics of this dysrhythmia are generally those of a junctional rhythm except for the more rapid rate (Fig. 11-34). As in atrial tachycardia, the QRS complex in NJT may be wide and bizarre if there is aberrant ventricular conduction, but aberrancy in this rhythm rarely occurs. Nonparoxysmal junctional tachycardia is usually the result of enhanced automaticity of the AV junction. Consequently, the rhythm is not initiated by a premature complex and is without the sudden onset and termination of paroxysmal tachycardia.

Digitalis intoxication, acute myocardial infarction, intracardiac surgery, or myocarditis are the most common causes of NJT. It is more often associated with inferior than anterior myocardial infarction and is considered a poor prognostic sign when observed in the latter. The underlying rhythm is often chronic atrial fibrillation when the rhythm disturbance is the result of digitalis intoxication. Patients with NJT often experience the various signs and symptoms of CHF or digitalis intoxication.

The key to therapy for NJT is to remove the cause when possible. Treatment of the cause when it cannot be eliminated is equally important. Drugs used to treat NJT include quinidine and propranolol as well as other agents known for their antiar-

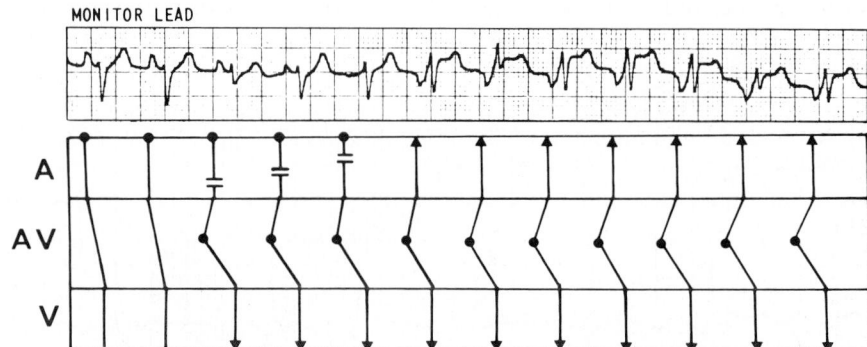

Figure 11-34   Nonparoxysmal AV junctional tachycardia. After two sinus beats, an AV junctional tachycardia at a rate of 107 beats per minute takes over control of the heart. The third, fourth, and fifth P waves are atrial fusion beats. *(From H. H. Friedman, Diagnostic electrocardiography and vectorcardiography, McGraw-Hill, New York, 1985, p. 499. Copyright 1985 by McGraw-Hill Book Company. Reprinted by permission.)*

rhythmic effect on supraventricular tachyarrhythmias.

Paroxysmal AV Junctional Tachycardia   AV junctional rates ranging from 140 to 250 beats per minute characterize *paroxysmal AV junctional tachycardia* (PJT) (Fig. 11-35). Unlike NJT, this rhythm is usually initiated by a premature complex and has an abrupt onset and termination. There may be a brief, irregular, initial "warm-up" period if the mechanism is enhanced automaticity; otherwise, the R-R cycles are perfectly regular. The initiating beat and all subsequent R-R cycles are perfectly regular. The initiating beat and all subsequent beats are morphologically the same. The last complex of the paroxysm is followed by a brief pause until the original rhythm is reestablished. The configuration of the P wave varies, depending on the activation site for the atria, and the appearance is that described earlier in this chapter for AV junctional beats. The QRS may be normal or aberrant depending on the status of the ventricular conduction system.

The mechanism responsible for initiating PJT is either AV nodal reentry or enhanced focal excitability or automaticity. Reentry is the most common mechanism of action. Like PAT, PJT may occur in healthy individuals as well as in those with coronary artery disease, hypertension, rheumatic heart disease, and hyperthyroidism. It may also be associated with digitalis intoxication. Patients may complain of a variety of symptoms including palpitations, chest tightness or pain, weakness, dizziness, anxiety, apprehension, or perhaps a feeling of impending death.

If the rhythm can be terminated by vagal stimulation, the mechanism is most likely a reentrant one. When the mechanism is enhanced excitability or automaticity, vagal stimulation may slow the rate temporarily but the rhythm resumes its previous rate after termination of the stimulation. Treatment regimens for PJT are those used for other supraventricular tachyrhythms.

Paroxysmal Supraventricular Tachycardia   *Paroxysmal supraventricular tachycardia* (PSVT) is a term used to describe the arrhythmias paroxysmal atrial and paroxysmal AV junctional tachycardia. The term is particularly useful when the particular type of paroxysmal supraventricular tachycardia is difficult to identify from the surface ECG. As previously indicated in the discussions specific to the two tachycardia sites, the mechanisms recognized as being responsible for the genesis of PSVT are reentry and abnormal automaticity. The rhythm may be the result of sinus node reentry, intraatrial reentry, AV nodal reentry, reentry using an accessory pathway, reentry using a concealed AV bypass tract, enhanced automaticity of an atrial focus, or enhanced automaticity of an AV junctional focus.[5] Electrophysiological studies (EPS) are often necessary for correct identification of the cause of PSVT. Treatment depends on the specific cause but generally PSVT secondary to sinus and AV nodal reentry can be effectively terminated with vagal stimulation, whereas the other forms cannot.

Ventricular Dysrhythmias

Rhythm disorders in which the pacemaker site is from within the ventricles are termed *ventricular dysrhythmias*. The mechanism of action generating ventricular rhythm disturbances may be either enhanced automaticity, reentry, or a combination of

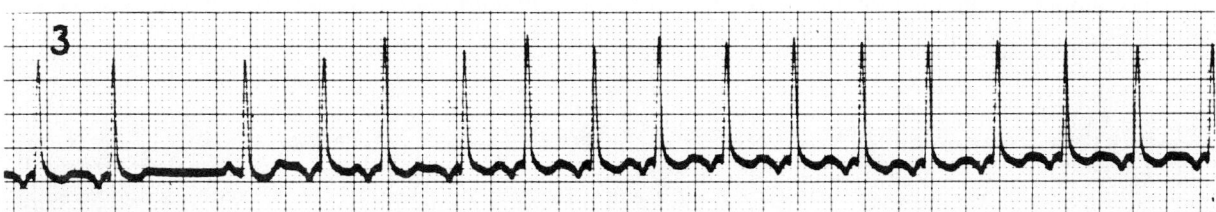

Figure 11-35   Paroxysmal AV junctional tachycardia with initial retrograde atrial activation. *(From A. E. Lindsay and A. Budkin, The Cardiac arrhythmias, second edition, Year Book, Chicago, 1975, p. 58. Copyright 1975 by Year Book Medical Publishers, Inc. Reprinted by permission.)*

both. If a higher pacemaker site, the sinus node or AV junction, fails to produce a stimulus, a ventricular escape beat or an idioventricular rhythm must assume the role of pacemaker to prevent cardiac standstill. In contrast, ventricular extrasystoles may occur due to an active mechanism of enhanced automaticity or reentry. The ventricular focus may produce a ventricular premature complex, ventricular tachycardia, ventricular flutter, or ventricular fibrillation.

Regardless of the mechanism, ventricular dysrhythmias may originate from any location within the ventricles. If the ectopic focus is in the septum near the His bundle, the QRS may be almost normal and resemble a sinus-initiated complex. However, the lower the pacemaker site within the septum the wider and more bizarre the complex becomes. Impulses originating from the fascicles of the left bundle branch generally produce a narrow QRS complex with a right bundle branch block (RBBB) pattern (see "Ventricular Conduction Abnormalities" in this chapter). Sites from the left ventricle produce positive QRS complexes in the right precordial leads and negative complexes in the left precordial leads. The converse is true if the ectopic site is right ventricular; the right precordial leads exhibit generally negative QRS complexes and the left precordial leads exhibit predominantly positive QRS complexes. The QRS duration may be fairly normal but is generally wide, being 0.12 s or more. This reflects the additional time required to depolarize the ventricles through an abnormal conduction pathway.

In this portion of the chapter the arrhythmias of idioventricular escape beats and rhythm, ventricular standstill (VS), ventricular premature complex, accelerated ventricular rhythm (AVR), paroxysmal ventricular tachycardia (PVT), torsades de pointes, and ventricular fibrillation will be discussed.

Idioventricular Escape Beats and Rhythm   If a faster pacemaker site fails to stimulate the ventricles or if the stimulus from those sites is for some reason slower than the inherent rate of a ventricular pacemaker, the ventricles passively assume the role of pacemaker for the heart. This control by the ventricular focus may occur for a single *idioventricular beat* or consecutively in groups of beats. When six or more consecutive idioventricular escape beats appear, an *idioventricular escape rhythm* (IVR) exists (Fig. 11-36).

The ECG features of either idioventricular escape beats or IVR are a QRS configuration and duration which vary according to the site of the ectopic ventricular focus; an irregular R-R cycle, although less commonly it may be regular; a ventricular rate which is usually between 30 and 40 beats per minute, but which may be as low as 15 beats per minute or slightly faster than 40 beats per minute; and independent atrial and ventricular activation. In the dying heart atrial activity may be nonexistent (atrial standstill) or may be exhibited as a fine undulation which may or may not be due to a fine atrial fibrillation. Under these circumstances the undulating baseline may represent independent ventricular activity.

The underlying rhythm disturbance which allows the ventricular pacemaker to escape is almost always complete AV block. Occasionally, though,

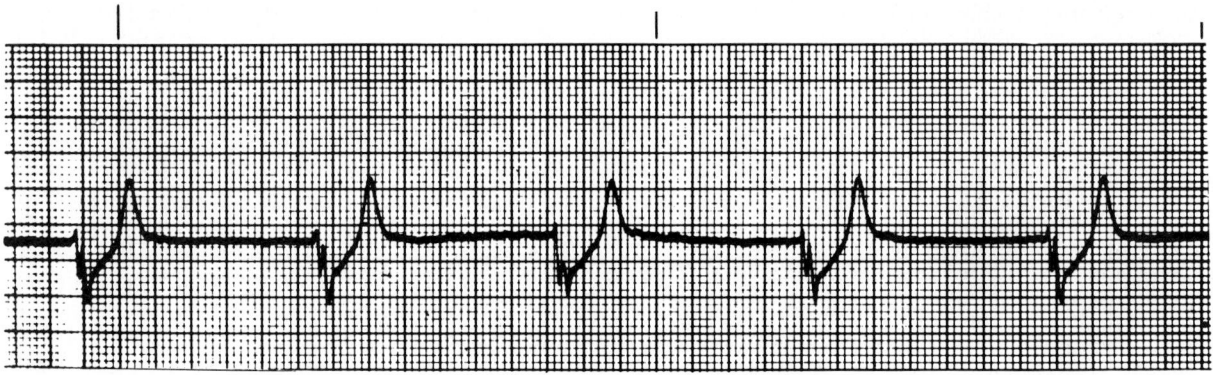

Figure 11-36   Idioventricular rhythm.

this escape mechanism may appear secondary to sinus arrest or SA block when the junctional pacemaker fails to initiate an escape impulse.

Therapeutic measures utilized for treating patients with an idioventricular rhythm are often dependent on the nature of the underlying heart disease and the severity of the problem. Frequently, a permanent artificial cardiac pacemaker is necessary to maintain life.

Ventricular Standstill When both the junction and ventricle fail to produce a QRS complex for either a few seconds or a longer period, the heart is said to be in *ventricular standstill* or *arrest* (Fig. 11-37). Ventricular standstill may occur in the presence or absence of atrial activity. It almost always is the consequence of another cardiac arrhythmia, for example sinus arrest, SA block, ventricular tachycardia, or ventricular fibrillation. It may occur during carotid sinus stimulation when this intervention is used to treat supraventricular tachyarrhythmias. The mechanism of action is depressed automaticity of the subsidiary pacemaker sites.

The significance of this rhythm disorder rests with the duration of the VS and the nature and severity of the underlying cardiac rhythm and heart disease. If the pause is of short duration, such as that which may occur following ectopic tachycardia, the VS is probably insignificant. However, a VS of longer duration can be terminal if an effective cardiac rhythm is not established by cardiopulmo-

nary resuscitation (CPR) and implantation of an artificial cardiac pacemaker. Ventricular standstill is most commonly observed in patients with acute myocardial infarction and in those with digitalis intoxication.

Ventricular Premature Complex The most commonly occurring arrhythmia is the *ventricular premature complex*. This rhythm disturbance is characterized on the ECG by a wide (equal to or greater than 0.12 s) and bizarre QRS complex which is premature but rarely preceded by a premature P wave and which is almost always followed by a full compensatory pause (Fig. 11-38). The premature QRS complex is accompanied by secondary S-T and T wave changes; that is, the direction of the S-T segment and T wave are opposite to those of the QRS. The VPC may be followed by a retrograde P wave if the ectopic impulse is able to conduct to the atria. The configuration of the QRS may be uniform (Fig. 11-38) or multiform (Fig. 11-39). Multiform VPCs may be initiated from a single focus or multiple foci within the ventricles. The coupling interval for unifocal VPCs is usually constant but varies when there are VPCs arising from multiple foci. When the coupling interval is very short the QRS morphology is more bizarre. If the coupling interval is quite long (termed a late diastolic VPC) a ventricular fusion beat may result. This is due to the fusion of the ventricular premature impulse with the sinus impulse somewhere in the ventricles.

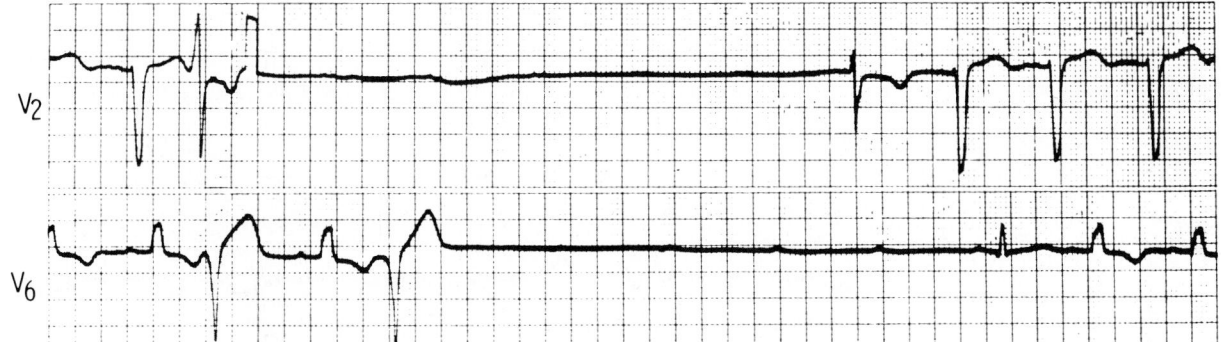

Figure 11-37 Ventricular standstill. The basic rhythm is sinus (atrial rate: 72 beats per minute) with left bundle branch block. Note a long ventricular standstill (5.8 s in lead V₂ and 4.74 s in lead V₆) initiated by a ventricular premature complex. After the long ventricular pause, a normally conducted sinus beat is observed. *(From E. K. Chung and D. K. Chung, ECG diagnosis: Self assessment, Harper & Row, New York, 1972, p. 128. Copyright 1972 by Harper & Row, Publishers, Inc. Reprinted by permission.)*

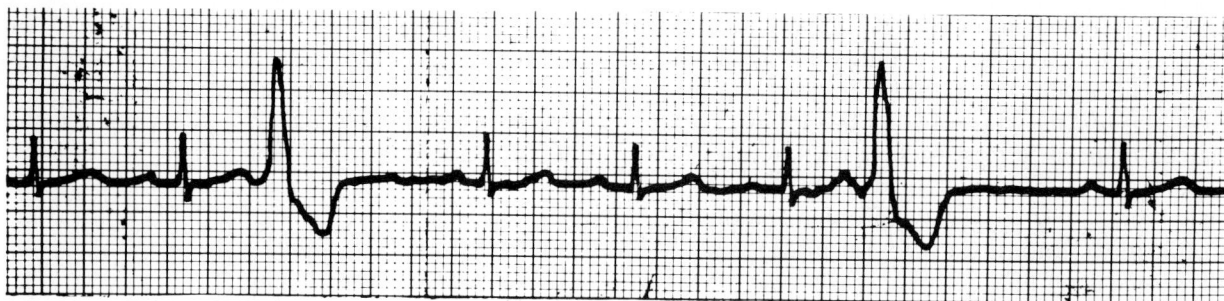

Figure 11-38 Ventricular premature complexes. Note the full compensatory pause after the first PVC.

The frequency of VPCs may be bigeminal, trigeminal, quadrageminal, or consecutive in couplets or triplets. Varying definitions of VT exist,[5-7] but it is defined here as six or more consecutive VPCs. Consecutive VPCs in groups of three, four, or five complexes are termed ventricular *salvos*. Occasionally, a single VPC may occur between two sequential normal beats without disturbing the underlying rhythm. This occurrence is identified as an *interpolated VPC* and happens when the sinus rate is slow and the VPC is particularly early.

The mechanism responsible for generating VPCs is generally thought to be either reentry or enhanced focal excitability. Ventricular premature complexes probably occur in all healthy individuals at some time or other during their lifetime. The incidence of VPCs increases with age. Predisposing factors include excessive ingestion of beverages containing caffeine, heavy smoking, and emotional stress. Ventricular premature complexes also occur in the presence of organic heart disease and drug intoxication. Digitalis intoxication should be suspected when ventricular bigeminy occurs during digitalization and most especially when the bige-

miny is in the presence of atrial fibrillation with AV junctional escape rhythm or nonparoxysmal junctional tachycardia. Ventricular premature complexes are also a common occurrence in patients with mitral valve prolapse syndrome. Frequent VPCs and those which occur early in the cardiac cycle are common phenomena during the first 48 to 72 h after an acute myocardial infarction. Ventricular premature complexes which are superimposed on the preceding T wave (R on T phenomenon) and group beats may initiate ventricular tachycardia or fibrillation (Fig. 11-40). Consequently, the occurrence of VPCs under these circumstances is considered to be potentially lethal and, therefore, warrants early and effective treatment.

Therapy for VPCs is dependent on the cause and severity of the arrhythmia. The occasional VPC occurring in the healthy individual is generally not treated. However, the precipitating cause (such as caffeine) should be eliminated if the incidence of the arrhythmia is frequent. Class IA, B, or C antiarrhythmic agents may be prescribed if the arrhythmia persists. Frequent (greater than six VPCs per minute), multiform, or repetitive VPCs or those occur-

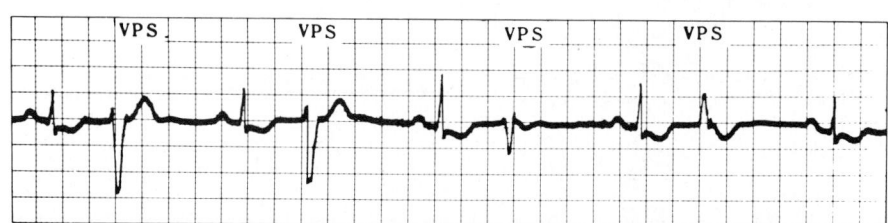

Figure 11-39 Multiform ventricular complexes with bigeminy due to digitalis intoxication. *(From H. H. Friedman, Diagnostic electrocardiography and vectorcardiography, McGraw-Hill, New York, 1985, p. 433. Copyright 1985 by McGraw-Hill Book Company. Reprinted by permission.)*

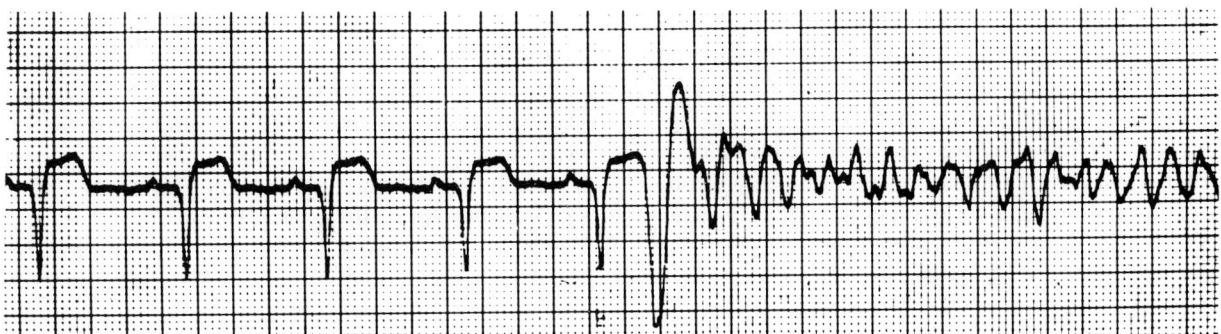

Figure 11-40 Ventricular premature complex on a T wave (R on T) initiating ventricular fibrillation in a patient with an anterior wall myocardial infarction. The rhythm was recorded from lead MCL₁.

ring on or near the preceding T wave in the patient with an acute myocardial infarction should be treated with an intravenous injection of lidocaine followed by a slow continuous infusion of the drug. Digitalis should be withheld immediately if it is suspected to be the cause of the arrhythmia. Dilantin and potassium may also be useful in treating digitalis-induced VPCs. Propranolol is useful as the therapeutic agent in catecholamine-induced VPCs and in those associated with mitral valve prolapse syndrome.

Accelerated Ventricular Rhythm (Idioventricular Tachycardia)   One form of ventricular tachycardia is known as *accelerated ventricular rhythm, nonparoxysmal ventricular tachycardia,* or *idioventricular tachycardia* (Fig. 11-41). Using the strict definition for tachycardia in the adult (that is, a heart rate greater than 100 beats per minute), the latter two labels are misnomers because the ventricular rate of this rhythm disturbance is between 60 and 100 beats per minute. However, this rate is tachycardic for an idioventricular pacemaker and this fact has led some to use these labels to describe

the rhythm. The preferred and less confusing term, though, is *accelerated ventricular rhythm.*

In addition to the rate in the range of that for normal sinus rhythm, other ECG criteria for an AVR include (1) wide and bizarre QRS and T complexes which occur in regular rhythm; (2) brief, transient episodes of the rhythm which last only a few seconds or minutes; (3) initiating beats which occur late in diastole and are fused with a sinus conducted beat; and (4) frequent ventricular capture and fusion beats. Frequently, this rhythm is accompanied by a generally independent atrial rhythm resulting in AV dissociation. Accelerated ventricular rhythm is often replaced by a sinus rhythm when the sinus rate is increased to a rate fast enough to suppress the ventricular pacemaker.

Accelerated ventricular rhythm must be differentiated from nonparoxysmal AV junctional tachycardia. These two rhythms may be very similar in appearance if the NJT occurs in the presence of a preexisting intraventricular conduction defect. The ventricular capture and fusion beats of AVR may serve as useful clues in the differentiation process.

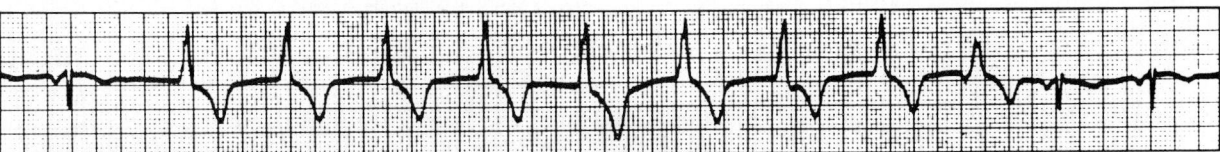

Figure 11-41 Accelerated ventricular rhythm recorded from a monitor lead. The nine-beat run of idioventricular tachycardia begins as an escape rhythm. The last beat of the tachycardia is a ventricular fusion beat. *(From H. H. Friedman, Diagnostic electrocardiography and vectorcardiography, McGraw-Hill, New York, 1985, p. 507. Copyright 1985 by McGraw-Hill Book Company. Reprinted by permission.)*

An AVR may be observed in patients experiencing either acute inferior or anterior myocardial infarctions. It may also be frequently observed following reperfusion of the coronary arteries through the use of thrombolytic agents such as streptokinase. Other forms of heart disease, including hypertensive, rheumatic, and congenital, may also be associated with this dysrhythmia. Occasionally the rhythm may be caused by digitalis. In all instances, the mechanism of action is likely to be enhanced automaticity or focal excitability of the ventricular pacemaker, which allows that pacemaker to suppress or override the slower sinus pacemaker. Often this occurs when the rate of impulse formation of the sinus node is in the bradycardic range.

Patients with AVR generally experience no symptoms or negative effects from this rhythm disturbance. This is due to the relatively normal rate of the cardiac rhythm. The rhythm, therefore, may not require therapy. However, if treatment is necessary, therapeutic measures are directed at increasing the rate of impulse formation of the sinus node. Pharmacologic agents generally used for other forms of ventricular tachycardia are usually not warranted and in fact may do more harm than good if they suppress the ventricular pacemaker when there is no other pacemaker.

Paroxysmal Ventricular Tachycardia Another form of ventricular tachycardia is *paroxysmal ventricular tachycardia,* which exists when six or more ventricular ectopic beats occur in rapid succession (Fig. 11-42). This rhythm is said to be sustained if it lasts longer than 30 s or nonsustained if the duration of the paroxysm is less than 30 s. The ventricular rate

for this rhythm is usually between 140 and 200 beats per minute but may be slightly slower or faster. A ventricular premature complex initiates the paroxysm and the abrupt termination of the tachycardia is followed by a postectopic pause. Frequently the initiating complex falls on the T wave of the preceding complex (R on T phenomenon) but late diastolic VPCs may also initiate the tachyrhythm. The QRS complex of ventricular tachycardia is wide, being 0.12 s or more, and bizarre. The T wave is also abnormal and has a vector opposite to that of the QRS. The rhythm is generally regular but might appear slightly irregular with variations of the R-R cycle of up to 0.03 s. Occasionally dissociated P waves may be seen but more frequently they are "lost" in the ventricular complexes. In approximately 50 percent of the cases of paroxysmal ventricular tachycardia, the ventricular impulse conducts retrograde to the atria. In these cases the associated P wave follows the QRS and is inverted in leads II, III, and aVF, and upright in aVR. Ventricular capture and ventricular fusion beats (Dressler beats) may occur when the rate of the ventricular rhythm is less than 150 beats per minute but these are rare occurrences.

The same mechanisms which are responsible for ventricular premature complexes are also thought to be responsible for PVT. The setting for the mechanisms of reentry and enhanced excitability to produce ventricular tachycardia is almost always that of advanced organic heart disease. The most common disease process causing the rhythm is ischemic or coronary heart disease resulting in acute myocardial infarction. Digitalis intoxication is also a common cause of ventricular tachycardia.

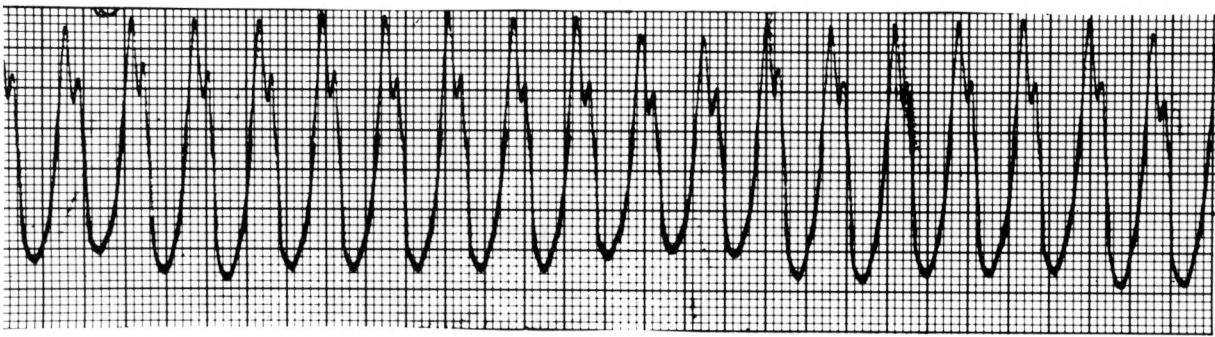

Figure 11-42 Paroxysmal ventricular tachycardia.

Less frequently, the rhythm disturbance is seen in patients with hypertensive or rheumatic heart disease, cardiomyopathy, and mitral valve prolapse. Only rarely does paroxysmal ventricular tachycardia occur in healthy individuals without heart disease.

When ventricular tachycardia occurs in patients with CHF, the failure can be aggravated by the tachyrhythm. In addition, the condition of CHF is a prime situation for the induction of ventricular tachycardia. The failure may further induce cardiac ischemia, thus changing the cell environment and promoting ventricular extrasystoles. The tachycardia then promotes further failure, and consequently ischemia, by decreasing the diastolic filling time. The resulting reduction in cardiac output may produce syncopal episodes.

Patients who experience ventricular tachycardia may suffer from a wide range of signs and symptoms. Depending upon the underlying heart disease and the rate of the ventricular tachycardia, the patient may be relatively free of symptoms or may be severely symptomatic and near death. Acute myocardial infarction, CHF, and digitalis intoxication generally complicate the clinical manifestations of ventricular tachycardia.

A variety of therapeutic interventions may be used to treat PVT. The therapy of choice will depend upon the specific cause of the arrhythmia as well as the severity of symptoms. Lidocaine injection followed by a continuous infusion of the drug is the preferred therapeutic intervention when the PVT is associated with acute myocardial infarction. However, if the patient is severely unstable hemodynamically, dc shock may be necessary. For digitalis-induced PVT, intravenous Dilantin or potassium are the drugs utilized. Propranolol may be useful for treating catecholamine-induced ventricular tachycardia. Procainamide and quinidine may be used successfully in place of lidocaine or Dilantin in some patients. In those with refractory or recurrent PVT, amiodarone, a class III antiarrhythmic agent, or some of the newer class I agents [such as tocainide (see Appendix A)] may be used. In some patients with refractory ventricular tachycardia, overdrive suppression of the ectopic pacemaker is accomplished through the use of an artificial cardiac pacemaker. As with most other arrhythmias, treatment or elimination of the direct or underlying cause is always important.

Torsades de Pointes   An atypical form of ventricular tachycardia was described for the first time in 1966 by Dessertenne.[8] The term *torsades de pointes,* which translated means "twisting of the points," was used to describe a ventricular tachyrhythm in which there was a phasic variation in the polarity and amplitude of the QRS seemingly around an isoelectric line (Fig. 11-43). The rhythm is usually initiated by a late diastolic VPC occurring on a prolonged T-U wave. It may terminate spontaneously or degenerate into ventricular fibrillation. The ventricular rate is generally between 150 and 250 beats per minute and the R-R cycles are irregular. Most electrocardiographers believe this rhythm must always be associated with a prolonged QT interval. If the QT interval is not prolonged but all other characteristics of the rhythm disturbance exist, the rhythm is identified as *polymorphous ventricular tachycardia.*

The exact arrhythmogenic mechanism of torsades de pointes is not clearly understood. Some believe the reentry phenomenon is responsible for the rhythm; however, Dessertenne believed the arrhythmia was due to competing sites of enhanced automaticity. Research studies for the purpose of identifying the genesis of this rhythm disorder continue to be implemented.

As noted previously, torsades de pointes is associated with prolonged QT intervals. Consequently the rhythm disturbance should be anticipated in patients who are predisposed to long QT intervals. Quinidine therapy and electrolyte imbalance are the most common causes of the arrhythmia.

Differentiation between torsades de pointes and polymorphous ventricular tachycardia is important in order that appropriate therapeutic measures may be instituted. Agents which prolong repolarization and, therefore, lengthen the QT interval [such as class IA antiarrhythmics (see Appendix A)] should be avoided in a true torsades de pointes ventricular tachycardia. Treatment measures for this rhythm may include isoproterenol, defibrillation, or atrial or ventricular overdrive pacing. In contrast, polymorphous ventricular tachycardia, with its normal QT intervals, seems to respond to class IA antiarrhythmic therapy.

Ventricular Fibrillation   *Ventricular fibrillation* (VF) is characterized on the ECG as rapid, irregular,

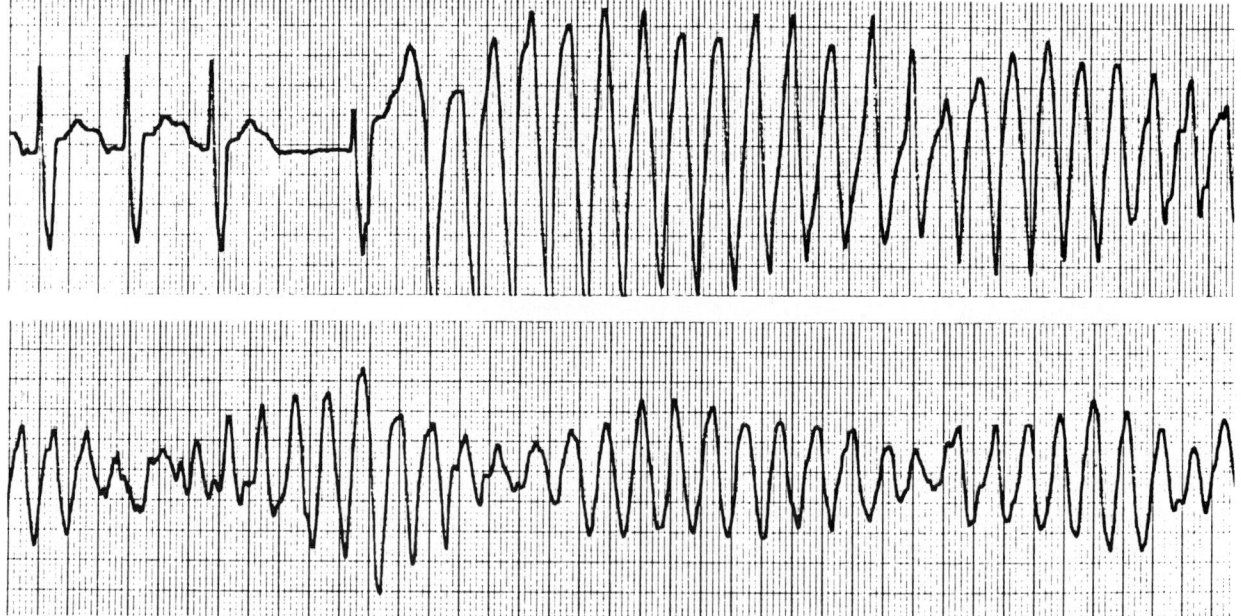

Figure 11-43 Torsades de pointes (continuous strip). Note the prolonged Q-T interval and the undulating-spindle look to the pattern. *Courtesy Dr. Alan Lindsay, Salt Lake City, Utah. From (M. B. Conover, electrocardiography, Mosby, St. Louis, 1984, p. 155. Copyright 1984 by The C. V. Mosby Company. Reprinted by permission.)*

and very bizarre waves (Fig. 11-44). When the waveforms are somewhat more regular and fairly uniform but without an isoelectric interval, the rhythm is identified as *ventricular flutter* (Fig. 11-45). In either case, definite P waves, QRS complexes, and T waves cannot be distinguished. The amplitude of the waves progressively diminishes as the cardiac function deteriorates, resulting in a very fine fibrillation immediately before cardiac death. The rate of the ventricular undulations varies from 150 to 500 per minute in VF and 180 to 250 per minute in ventricular flutter.

Various theories exist to explain the mechanism of ventricular flutter and fibrillation. Four specific theories, those of circus movement, multiple reentry, unifocal impulse formation, and multifocal impulse formation, are considered to best explain the rhythm disorder.

Ventricular fibrillation, as well as ventricular flutter, usually leads to sudden death unless the rhythm is immediately converted to a more normal rhythm. This rhythm disturbance may occur in a number of disease processes, both cardiac and noncardiac. The most commonly associated cardiac

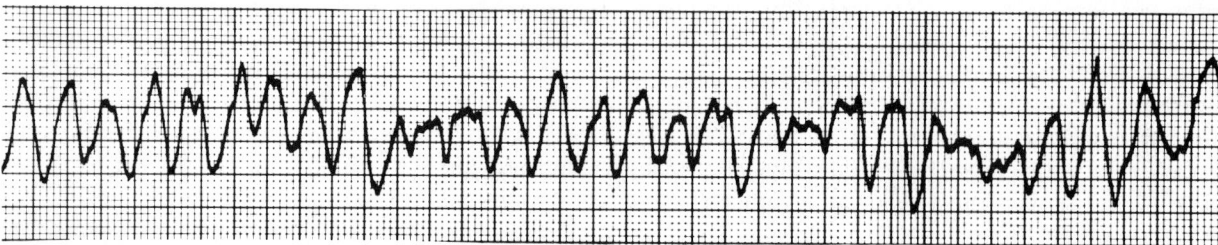

Figure 11-44 Ventricular fibrillation.

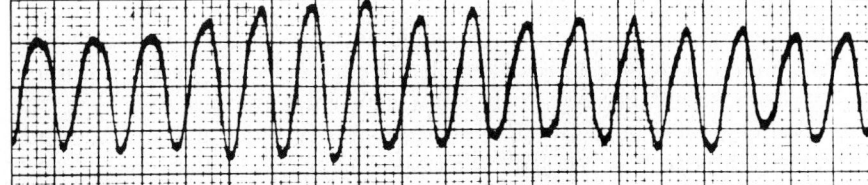

Figure 11-45   Ventricular flutter. There is a zigzag pattern without differentiation between the QRS complexes, S-T segments, and T waves. *(From H. H. Friedman, Diagnostic electrocardiography and vectorcardiography, McGraw-Hill, New York, 1985, p. 519. Copyright 1985 by McGraw-Hill Book Company. Reprinted by permission.)*

disease is coronary artery disease, particularly acute myocardial infarction. Digitalis intoxication may be the second most common cause. Marked electrolyte abnormalities also may lead to ventricular fibrillation if not treated quickly and effectively.

The treatment of choice for ventricular fibrillation and ventricular flutter is dc shock. Cardiopulmonary resuscitation techniques must be implemented until the defibrillator is available and readied for use. It is important to institute defibrillation measures as quickly as possible to ensure the greatest success of the resuscitative efforts.

Aberrant Ventricular Conduction versus Ventricular Ectopy

Aberrant ventricular conduction is defined as the temporary, abnormal intraventricular conduction of supraventricular impulses. Differentiation of supraventricular impulses with aberrant ventricular conduction from ventricular ectopic impulses is often difficult. Mistaken identification of the two in the clinical setting, though, can lead to inappropriate and ineffective therapy. Consequently, it is useful to review the causes of aberrant ventricular conduction and the clues which assist us in correctly identifying supraventricular impulses with aberrant ventricular conduction and ventricular ectopic impulses.

Aberrant ventricular conduction is usually caused by a change in ventricular cycle length. A direct relationship exists between the cycle length and the refractoriness of the His-Purkinje system; that is, the greater the preceding R-R interval, the longer the refractory period and the shorter the R-R interval, the shorter the refractory period.

Therefore, if a long R-R cycle is followed by a short R-R cycle, such as that created by a premature impulse, the impulse causing the shorter cycle is likely to arrive in the ventricles when portions of the ventricular conduction system are still refractory and aberrant ventricular conduction is favored.

Four conditions determine whether the supraventricular impulse will conduct normally or aberrantly. The first condition is the length of the R-R interval preceding the ectopic beat. Aberrant ventricular conduction is more likely to occur when the preceding cycle length is long, due to the relationship of cycle length and refractoriness. The second condition is the degree of the prematurity of the impulse. When the impulse is very premature, resulting in a short coupling interval, the premature impulse is more likely to encounter refractory conductive cells. The outcome will be aberrant conduction. The speed of AV conduction is the third determining condition. Rapid AV conduction increases the likelihood of aberrancy because it allows the impulse to arrive in the ventricles while the conduction system is still refractory. Conversely, if the AV conduction is slow, the impulse may arrive late enough that the cells are no longer refractory and the impulse conducts normally. The fourth condition determining aberrant ventricular conduction is the state of recovery of the excitability in the specialized ventricular conduction system. If there is unequal refractoriness of the bundle branches, conduction of the premature supraventricular impulse is likely to be abnormal.

The degree of aberrant conduction is dependent on the degree of the refractory period in the ventricles at the time of arrival of the supraventricular impulse. The aberrant conduction often resembles the conduction pattern identified with a right bundle branch block (see "Ventricular Conduction Abnormalities" in this chapter) because the right bundle has a longer action potential and refractory period than does the left and is, therefore, more susceptible to conduction failure (see Fig. 11-27). Less often, a left bundle branch block pattern may characterize the aberrant complex. The QRS interval may occasionally exceed 0.12 s in those with the right bundle branch block pattern and 0.14 s in those with left bundle branch block pattern.

Clues for the identification of aberrant ventricular conduction and for ventricular ectopic impulses are listed in Table 11-3.[6] However, even with these helpful hints, differentiation is sometimes difficult. Occasionally, intracardiac electrograms are needed to diagnose the problem.

AV Conduction Abnormalities

When conduction through the AV node is prolonged or prevented due to a prolonged refractory period in the AV junctional tissue, His bundle, or the His-Purkinje network, AV block is said to exist. The prolonged AV conduction is pathologic rather than functional or physiologic. AV blocks are classified as *incomplete* and *complete,* and the conduction disturbance may be described by degrees. Incomplete AV block includes first-degree, second-degree, and advanced or high-degree AV block. Complete AV block is also known as third-degree AV block. Any of these forms of AV block may be transient, intermittent, or persistent. Also, the degree of block may periodically change from one to another in the same individual.

First-Degree AV Block Prolongation of the P-R interval beyond 0.20 s characterizes *first-degree AV block* (Fig. 11-46). It should be noted that in this form of incomplete AV block each atrial impulse is conducted to the ventricles. The P-R interval is constant unless there is a change in the heart rate, in which case the P-R interval changes according to the length of the preceding refractory period (that is, the P-R interval lengthens when the heart rate slows and shortens when the heart rate is faster). The usual range for the prolonged P-R interval is 0.21 to 0.40 s but intervals as long as 0.80 s may appear.

Prolongation of the refractory period of the AV junction is thought to be the cause of first-degree AV block. Impaired conduction through the His bundle may also be the cause of the P-R prolongation. This prolongation of the AV refractory

Table 11-3 ECG Criteria Favoring Aberrant Ventricular Conduction and Ventricular Ectopy[6]

Aberrant Ventricular Conduction	Ventricular Ectopy
rsR′ pattern in V_1	Rsr′ or qR pattern in V_1
Initial vector of anomalous complex is usually identical to that of normally conducted beats	Initial vector of anomalous complex is dissimilar to that of the conducted beats
qRs pattern in V_6	QS or rS pattern in V_6
Definite relationship between preceding atrial activity and the anomalous beat	No relationship between preceding atrial activity and the anomalous beat
Abnormal complexes resemble conducted beats in same lead	LBBB[a] pattern in the precordial leads with a wide R wave in V_1
QRS morphology is similar to previous known aberrancy	QRS morphology is identical to previously known ventricular ectopic beats
Variable coupling	Fixed coupling usually
Long-short cycle sequences	Long-short cycle sequence but with fixed coupling
	Abnormally wide QRS complexes (> 0.12 s in left ventricular beats and 0.14 s in right ventricular beats)

[a] LBBB = left bundle branch block (see "Ventricular Conduction Abnormalities" in this chapter).

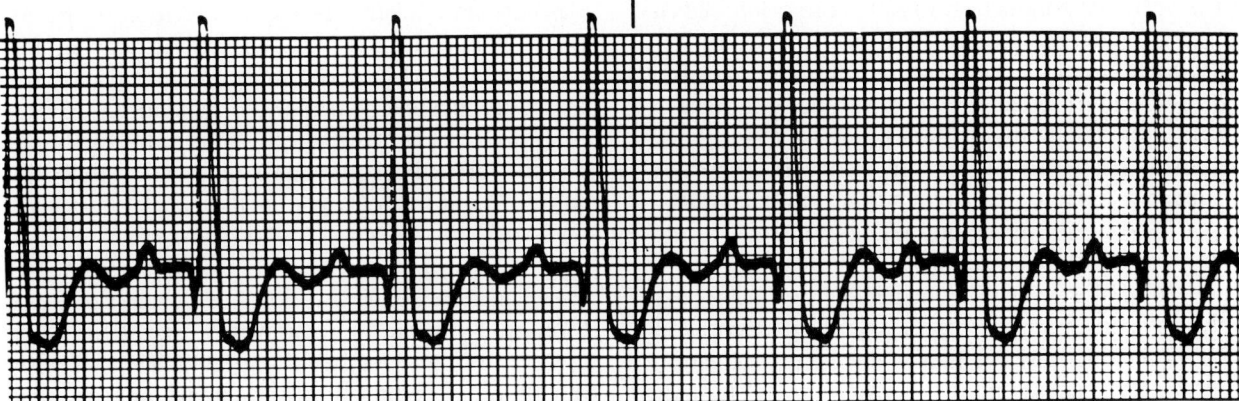

Figure 11-46   First-degree AV block. The P-R interval is approximately 0.24 s.

period or His bundle conduction time may occur in healthy individuals but is much more common in individuals with heart disease. When first-degree AV block appears abruptly, the related cause is likely to be digitalis intoxication, acute inferior myocardial infarction, or acute myocarditis. Less commonly it may be related to hyperkalemia or propranolol, quinidine, or procainamide therapy. First-degree AV block may occur in elderly people without established heart disease, in which case the cause may be chronic degeneration of the AV conduction system.

Therapy for first-degree AV block is generally not necessary but the cause should be investigated and corrected when possible. Individuals with first-degree AV block of recent onset should be closely monitored for the possible development of a higher degree of AV block.

Second-Degree AV Block—Mobitz Type I (Wenckebach AV Block)   *Second-degree AV block* can be divided into two types which are identified as Mobitz type I and Mobitz type II AV block. The former is more common than the latter. Second-degree AV block, Mobitz type I, is also known as *Wenckebach AV block*. This type of second-degree AV block will be discussed first.

Mobitz type I AV block (Fig. 11-47) is characterized on the ECG by the progressive prolongation of the P-R intervals until a single P wave is not followed by a QRS. The P-R interval after the blocked P will be the shortest and may be within the normal range or greater than 0.20 s. The R-R intervals become progressively shorter until the P wave is blocked, thus producing the longest R-R interval. This long R-R interval is shorter than two P-P intervals.

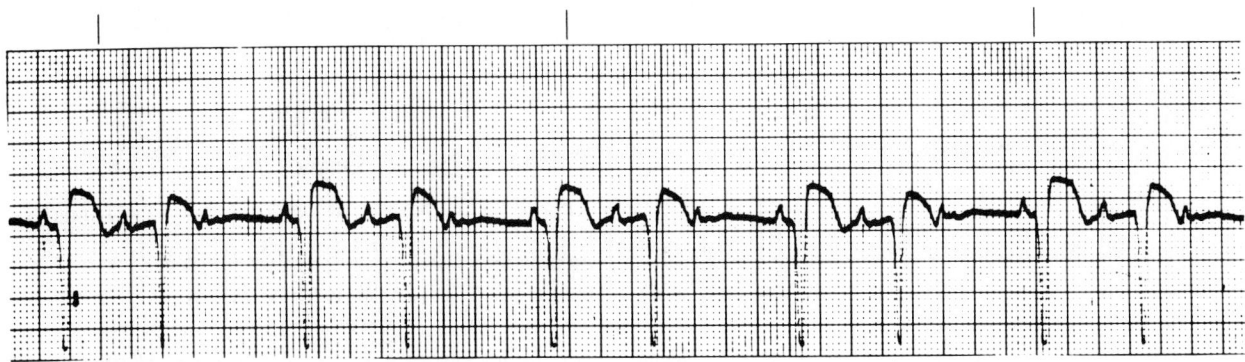

Figure 11-47   Second-degree AV block—Mobitz type I (Wenckebach AV block). The AV conduction ratio is 3:2.

The AV conduction ratio is commonly 3:2 or 4:3 but may be greater (5:4 or 6:5). If the AV conduction ratio is constant, the ventricular rhythm is regularly irregular. However, the AV conduction ratio may change from time to time, that is, change from a 3:2 to a 4:3 ratio or vice versa, thereby causing the ventricular rhythm to be quite irregular.

The period from one blocked P wave to the next is the *Wenckebach period*. It is important to note that the typical Wenckebach period is not always seen in Mobitz type I AV block (such as in 2:1 AV conduction). Frequently the P-R prolongation and the R-R shortening is not progressive. This may be due to an underlying sinus arrhythmia or to a varying vagal tone. If the Wenckebach period is quite long, several successive P-R intervals may show no measurable change.[5,6]

If the QRS complex is narrow in the presence of Mobitz type I AV block, the location of the block is usually in the AV node, or intranodal. This is true in 75 percent of cases. In the other 25 percent, the location of the block is the His bundle and, therefore, is infranodal. Noting the response of the rhythm to atropine or carotid sinus massage may offer a clue to the location. If the AV conduction ratio improves with carotid sinus massage and worsens after atropine administration, the block is infranodal. The opposite responses occur when the block is intranodal.[5] Occasionally a second-degree AV block, Mobitz type I, is associated with an existing bundle branch block, in which case the QRS interval is prolonged.[7]

The arrhythmogenic mechanism of type I AV block is thought to be prolongation of both the absolute and relative refractory periods of the AV node. This type of AV block is often transient and may be caused by mild digitalis intoxication, acute infection, uremia, electrolyte imbalance, or propranolol toxicity. In these instances the treatment for the arrhythmia is directed at alleviating the cause. Mobitz type I AV block is often associated with acute inferior myocardial infarction. The block is generally transient due to ischemia of the AV node and consequently does not usually require therapy. Only rarely does Mobitz type I AV block appear in otherwise healthy individuals. Generally the block is of little clinical significance in these cases and is thought to be related to hyperactive vagal tone.

Second-Degree AV Block—Mobitz Type II When P waves are periodically blocked from conducting to the ventricles without a progressive prolongation of the P-R interval or a progressive shortening of the R-R interval, the conduction defect is identified as *second-degree AV block* or *Mobitz type II AV block* (Fig. 11-48). The AV conduction ratio is commonly 3:2 or 4:3 and may be fixed or may vary. In this conduction disturbance the P-R interval of all conducted beats is constant. The QRS complex almost always exhibits a hemiblock, right or left bundle branch block, or bifascicular block pattern (see "Ventricular Conduction Abnormalities" in this chapter). The R-R interval including the blocked P wave is a multiple of the normal P-P interval.

A variation of Mobitz type II AV block is the 2:1 AV conduction ratio (Fig. 11-49). With this variation it is often difficult, if not impossible, to

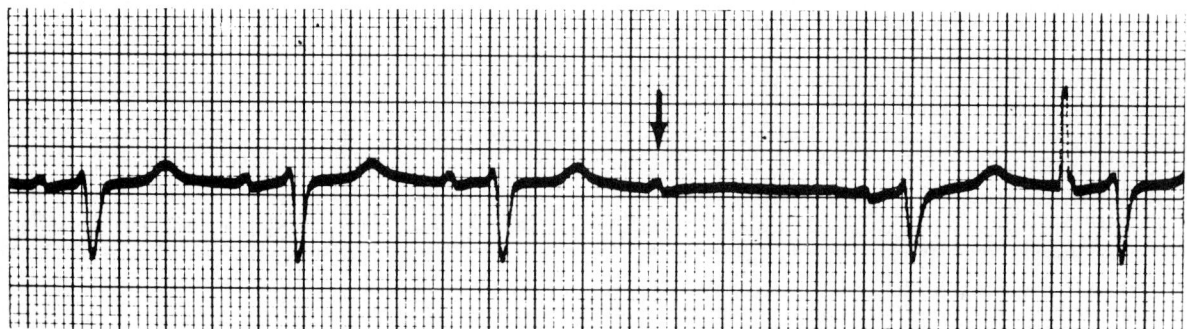

Figure 11-48 Second-degree AV block—Mobitz type II. The fourth P wave does not conduct a QRS. The P-R intervals for the conducted beats are slightly prolonged but constant. *(From A. E. Lindsay and A. Budkin, The cardiac arrhythmias, second edition, Year Book, Chicago, 1975, p. 78. Copyright 1975 by Year Book Medical Publishers, Inc. Reprinted by permission.)*

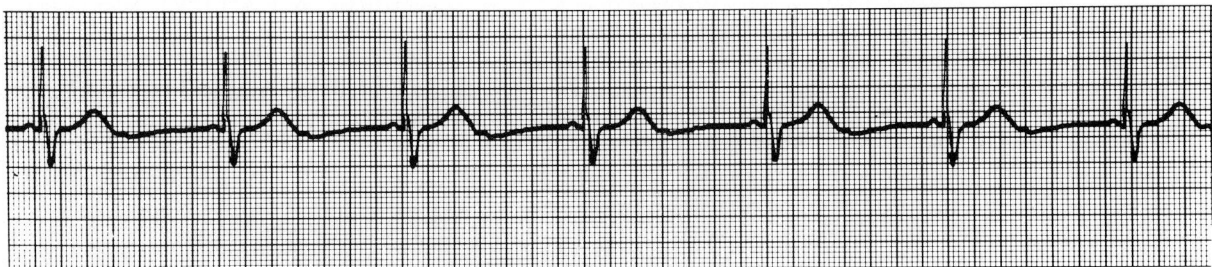

Figure 11-49   Second-degree AV block—Mobitz type II. The 2:1 AV conduction ratio is a variation of the Mobitz type II AV block. In this strip the low voltage nonconducted P waves appear immediately after the T wave. The QRS complexes are abnormally wide (0.12 s) which is usual for this AV conduction abnormality.

determine whether the conduction abnormality is a type I or type II second-degree AV block. A long, continuous recording of the rhythm may show an episode of changing conduction ratios and the behavior of the P-R interval and thus assist in the determination of the type of block. If the AV block decreases when the atrial rate is increased due to exercise or atropine administration, the block is likely to be a type I second-degree block. The AV block increases with an increased atrial rate secondary to these maneuvers when the block is a Mobitz type II.[5]

The location of the conduction abnormality in second-degree, type II AV block is almost always in the His-Purkinje system or infranodal. The exact location may be either within the His bundle itself (intra-His) or in the bundle branches. This explains why the QRS complex in Mobitz type II block has the appearance of a ventricular conduction abnormality. The block is in actuality a form of incomplete bilateral bundle branch block in the majority of cases.

Chronic Mobitz type II AV block is probably due to a degenerative sclerotic change in the His-Purkinje system. Acute Mobitz type II AV block is almost always caused by an acute anteroseptal myocardial infarction. Symptoms may include those associated with CHF and those of lightheadedness, dizziness, fatigue and syncope, and Adams-Stokes attacks. Because second-degree AV block, Mobitz type II, is usually a precursor of complete AV block secondary to complete bilateral bundle branch block, and because the type II AV block is almost always irreversible, a permanent artificial pacemaker may be indicated in all cases, irrespective of the presence or absence of symptoms.

Advanced AV Block   *Advanced* or *high-degree AV block* is recognized on the ECG when the AV conduction ratio is equal to or greater than 3:1 (Fig. 11-50). Usually the conduction ratios are even-numbered (such as 4:1, 6:1, or 8:1), with odd-numbered ratios being relatively uncommon. It is common to observe AV junctional escape complexes (less commonly ventricular escape complexes) when the conduction ratio is 4:1 or greater. When conduction ratios are very high the conducted beats, or ventricular capture beats, are relatively rare. Consequently, under these circumstances the rhythm resembles complete AV block except for the occasional conducted beat, and there is incomplete AV dissociation. Occasionally the underlying rhythm is atrial (that is, atrial tachycardia, flutter, or fibrillation) rather than sinus. In these situations the AV conduction ratio cannot be determined.

The P-R intervals of the conducted beats may be normal or prolonged. They are generally constant; however, they may be variable if Wenckebach phenomenon or concealed conduction occurs. The P-P intervals are usually regular but may be irregular if there is an abnormality in sinus impulse formation or conduction. The R-R intervals are almost always irregular. The QRS configuration is dependent on the site of the AV block and the origin of the QRS complex. The QRS complex of conducted beats is usually normal but may have a right or left bundle branch block configuration if there is an associated ventricular conduction abnormality. If the escape mechanism arises from the AV junction, those QRS complexes are normal in configuration unless there is a coexisting bundle branch block. The QRS configuration of ventricular escape beats is wide

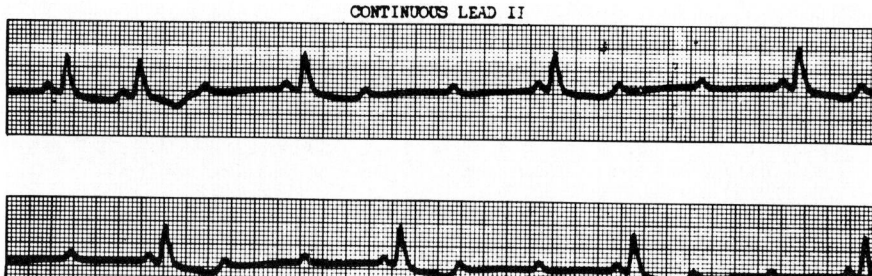

Figure 11-50   Advanced AV block. The first and second P waves are conducted at a constant P-R interval of 0.18 s. The third P wave is blocked, and the fourth is conducted. Then the AV conduction ratio becomes 3:1. The P-R interval of all the conducted beats is constant. *(From H. H. Friedman, Diagnostic electrocardiography and vectocardiography, McGraw-Hill, New York, 1985, p. 571. Copyright 1985 by McGraw-Hill Book Company. Reprinted by permission.)*

and bizarre. Ventricular fusion beats have varying QRS configurations.

Advanced AV block may be due to various mechanisms including those responsible for both Mobitz type I and Mobitz type II second-degree AV block. The site of the conduction abnormality may be intranodal, in which case AV junctional escape beats can control the ventricles; or infranodal, with the escape pacemaker being from within the ventricles. As with other forms of incomplete AV block, high-degree block may be caused by drug intoxication (such as digitalis, propranolol, and guanethidine), electrolyte imbalances, acute infections, acute inferior myocardial infarction, and acute anterior myocardial infarction. The clinical significance depends on the site of the block, the ventricular rate, the presence or absence of hemodynamic instability, and the underlying etiology, but is in general very similar to that of third-degree AV block. A temporary artificial cardiac pacemaker may be necessary initially and if the AV block is found to be infranodal and permanent, a permanent artificial pacemaker is indicated.

Third-Degree AV Block   As noted earlier, third-degree AV block is also known as *complete AV block*. This conduction abnormality is characterized on the ECG by separate and independent atrial and ventricular activity (Fig. 11-51). The atria are controlled by either sinus or ectopic atrial pacemakers which almost always generate impulses at a rate faster than the pacemaker which controls the ventricles. The ventricles are controlled by a pacemaker which is distal to the AV block. If the site of the block is intranodal, the AV junction usually serves as pacemaker with a rate of 40 to 60 beats per

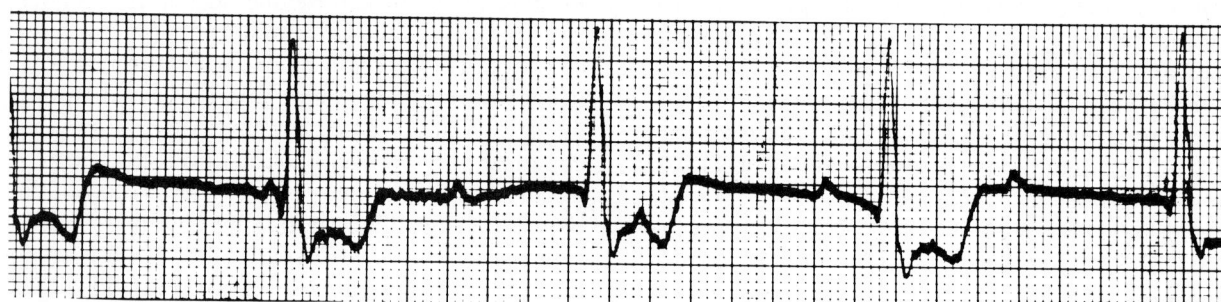

Figure 11-51   Third-degree AV block. Note the lack of association between the atria and the ventricles as indicated by the totally variable P-R intervals and nonconducted P waves, some of which are in the S-T segments and T waves.

minute; however, if the block is in the His bundle or the bundle branches the pacemaker site is below that site in either the His bundle or the His-Purkinje system and at a rate of 20 to 40 beats per minute.

The P-P interval is often regular when the sinus node acts as the atrial pacemaker but may be irregular if there is a sinus arrhythmia or intermittent SA block. The R-R intervals produced by the junctional or ventricular escape complexes are also usually regular; however, they too may be irregular if there are multiple pacemaker sites, irregular discharges of the pacemaker, or exit blocks of varying degrees.[7] The P-R interval is totally and completely irregular because of the complete dissociation of the atria and ventricles. The configuration of the QRS is dependent on the site of the subsidiary pacemaker. Normal QRS complexes result when the AV junction paces the ventricles. However, if the pacemaker site is below the bifurcation of the His bundle, the QRS is wide and bizarre.

Third-degree AV block may be caused by digitalis intoxication, acute inferior myocardial infarction, or acute myocarditis. In these instances the block is usually transient and due to a block in the AV node. When an acute anterior myocardial infarction causes the complete AV block, the block is usually infranodal and permanent. Complete AV block may also be caused by congenital malformation of the AV node and by chronic degenerative changes of the His-Purkinje network in the elderly. Both these conditions also produce permanent blocks. Occasionally AV block is caused by cardiac surgery or trauma.

A variety of signs and symptoms may be associated with third-degree AV block. If there is underlying heart disease or congestive heart failure, signs and symptoms secondary to those problems may be observed. Complete AV block secondary to congenital malformation may produce no symptoms. Symptoms associated with acquired complete AV block are dependent on the severity of the underlying heart disease and the rate of the ventricular pacemaker. With slow ventricular rates, severe symptoms are likely to be due to the resulting reduction in cardiac output.

Treatment for acute complete AV block almost always involves the use of a temporary artificial cardiac pacemaker, particularly when the site of the block is infranodal, the ventricular rate is very slow, and the individual is severely symptomatic. Emergency measures such as administration of epinephrine or isoproterenol may be tried and cardiopulmonary resuscitation may be necessary until a pacemaker can be placed. If the block proves to be permanent, a permanent artificial pacemaker will be necessary. Individuals with congenital complete AV block may go for years without symptoms or need of therapy; however, most will eventually require implantation of a permanent artificial cardiac pacemaker when they reach middle age and begin to develop symptoms.[7]

AV Dissociation

Mention of AV dissociation has been made on several occasions when describing various rhythm disturbances (such as nonparoxysmal AV junctional rhythm, accelerated ventricular rhythm, Mobitz type II AV block, and third-degree AV block). It is important to note that AV dissociation is never a primary rhythm disturbance but is always secondary to some other cardiac rhythm disturbance. By definition, AV dissociation implies that the atria and ventricles beat independently. Consequently, the P waves, atrial flutter waves, or atrial fibrillation waves bear no relationship to the QRS complex.

Three primary rhythm disturbances produce AV dissociation. The first is slowed or impaired sinus impulse formation or SA conduction. Specific arrhythmias of this type include sinus bradycardia, sinus arrest, and SA block. The P wave, if there is one, will originate in the sinus node and the QRS will be generated by a faster AV junctional or ventricular escape pacemaker. The second major rhythm disturbance producing AV dissociation is acceleration of the impulse formation in an AV junctional or ventricular pacemaker. The atrial pacemaker under these circumstances may be the sinus node or an ectopic atrial pacemaker. The ventricles are controlled by an accelerated or tachycardic AV junctional or ventricular pacemaker which discharges faster than the pacemaker controlling the atria. The last cause of AV dissociation is AV conduction disturbance. Rhythm disorders of this variety are advanced AV block and complete AV block. In addition, AV dissociation results when the ventricles are paced by an artificial cardiac pacemaker independent of the atrial mechanism.

AV dissociation may be incomplete or complete. Incomplete AV dissociation occurs when there is an intermittent or occasional relationship between the atria and ventricles. When no capture beats exist and the atria and ventricles consistently beat independently, complete AV dissociation is said to be present.

The clinical significance of AV dissociation rests with the underlying causative rhythm disorder and the presence or absence of organic heart disease. The dissociation itself is not treated directly; rather, therapeutic measures are directed toward the basic rhythm disturbance and the underlying heart disease or drug toxicity.

Ventricular Conduction Abnormalities

The ventricular conduction system is comprised of the distal portion of the His bundle, the bundle branch system, and the Purkinje network (Fig. 11-52). The bundle of His is a thin conductive pathway connecting the AV node with the bundle branches. At its distal end the His bundle bifurcates into the left and right bundles. The left bundle branch arises almost perpendicularly from the common bundle, whereas the right bundle is a more direct extension of the His bundle. The right bundle branch extends along the right side of the inter-

ventricular septum until its subdivisions merge with the Purkinje network.

There is lack of agreement regarding the anatomic structure of the left bundle branch. Many believe that it almost immediately subdivides into the left posterior and the left anterior fascicles. The posterior fascicle extends inferiorly and the anterior fascicle spreads superiorly beneath the left ventricular endocardium. Many individuals may also have a third subdivision which has been identified as the septal fascicle of the left bundle branch (see Fig. 11-52).[6] For the purposes of this discussion it is assumed that there are fascicular divisions of the left bundles even though some investigators dispute this concept.

The subdivisions of the bundle branch system blend into the Purkinje network. This network is widely distributed throughout both ventricles, making it possible for impulses to conduct rapidly to all sections of the ventricular muscle.

Figure 11-9 illustrates the sequence of normal ventricular activation which was described earlier in this chapter. When this activation sequence is disturbed due to conduction abnormalities within the ventricles, distortions in the QRS complex result. Ventricular conduction abnormalities may arise from either of the bundle branches, the divisions

Figure 11-52 Schematic representation of the conduction system of the heart. Note especially the ventricular conduction system. *(From H. H. Friedman, Diagnostic electrocardiography and vectorcardiography, McGraw-Hill, New York, 1985, p. 22. Copyright 1985 by McGraw-Hill Book Company. Reprinted by permission.)*

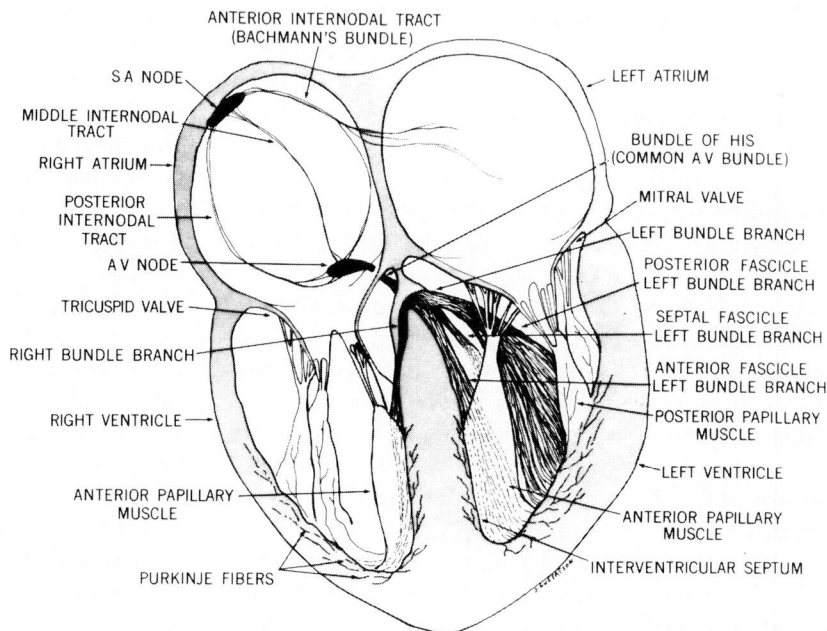

of the left bundle, or a combination of sites. The most common forms of intraventricular conduction abnormalities are *right bundle branch block (RBBB)* and *left bundle branch block (LBBB),* with the incidence of the two being about equal. When these conduction disturbances occur the bundle which is not blocked conducts normally, depolarizing its respective ventricle. The bundle which is blocked is unable to conduct the impulse to the ventricular fibers, so the associated ventricle will be depolarized abnormally and late. Under normal conditions both ventricles are activated simultaneously.

Bundle branch blocks are generally associated with QRS intervals of 0.12 s or greater in the frontal plane leads. Left bundle branch block frequently prolongs the QRS more than does RBBB. If the QRS duration is between 0.10 and 0.12 s the bundle branch block is considered to be incomplete. It is described as a complete block only when the QRS interval is equal to or greater than 0.12 s.

Right and left bundle branch blocks are frequently caused by the same diseases which are responsible for producing AV blocks. However, bundle branch blocks are more often associated with coronary artery disease, aortic valve disease, and hypertension. These blocks are rarely idiopathic in origin. They are generally chronic and permanent but may appear intermittently.

Fascicular blocks, or *hemiblocks,* alter the activation sequence of the left ventricle and in so doing, alter the vector of the QRS complexes. Consequently, left anterior and posterior hemiblocks result in left and right axis deviation respectively. They do not, however, significantly alter the QRS interval.

Hemiblocks may occur alone or in association with blocks at other sites. A RBBB may coexist with either a left anterior hemiblock (LAH) or a left posterior hemiblock (LPH), creating what is sometimes described as a *bifascicular block.* Blockage of the right bundle and both fascicles results in a *trifascicular block* which is an expression of a *bilateral bundle branch block.*

In this chapter the ventricular conduction abnormalities of right bundle branch block, left bundle branch block, left anterior hemiblock, and left posterior hemiblock will be discussed and their ECG findings described. Discussion of the more complex ventricular conduction abnormalities of bifascicular and trifascicular block are reserved for electrocardiographic textbooks.

Right Bundle Branch Block   When conduction through the right bundle is blocked the right ventricle is depolarized later than the left ventricle. The QRS duration is prolonged to account for the additional time required for the right ventricle to be activated. A characteristic change in the QRS results from the abnormal ventricular activation sequence. Figure 11-53 illustrates the pattern of activation when RBBB is present. Note that the septum depolarizes in its normal left-to-right direction, producing a small r wave in V_1 and a small q wave in V_6. The left ventricle is the next area to be depolarized and results in the inscription of an S wave in V_1 and an R wave in V_6. The last area to be depolarized is the right ventricle. An R' wave in V_1 and a deep and slurred S wave in V_6 represent this electrical activity.

When the ventricles depolarize abnormally, they also repolarize abnormally, resulting in a T wave change. This T wave alteration is said to be *secondary* to the QRS alteration. In the case of RBBB the secondary T wave change results in a T axis that is approximately 180° from the QRS axis. For example, in leads V_{1-3} the QRS complex of RBBB is predominantly upright; the T wave is inverted and asymmetrical with the downward slope being more gradual and the upward stroke being more rapid. When combined with the S-T segment it takes on the appearance of a backward check mark.

The ECG criteria for RBBB can be summarized as:

1. A QRS interval ≥ 0.12 s
2. An rSR', or M-shaped QRS in the right precordial leads (V_{1-3})
3. Deep and slurred S waves in the left leads (I, aVL, V_{4-6})
4. Secondary S-T, T wave changes in the right precordial leads (V_{1-3})

Figure 11-54 is an ECG from a patient with RBBB. Note the presence of each of the four diagnostic criteria.

Other clinical conditions may produce an rSR' in V_1 and should be differentiated from RBBB. A key factor in the differential diagnosis is the QRS

Figure 11-53 Schematic representation of ventricular depolarization in right bundle branch block. See text for description. *(From H. H. Friedman, Diagnostic electrocardiography and vectorcardiography, McGraw-Hill, New York, 1985, p. 181. Copyright 1985 by McGraw-Hill Book Company. Reprinted by permission.)*

VENTRICULAR DEPOLARIZATION IN RIGHT BUNDLE BRANCH BLOCK

SEQUENCE OF VENTRICULAR ACTIVATION

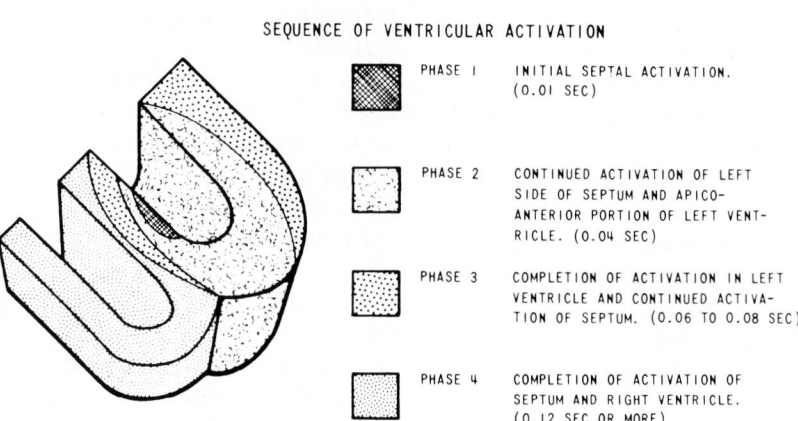

PHASE 1 INITIAL SEPTAL ACTIVATION. (0.01 SEC)

PHASE 2 CONTINUED ACTIVATION OF LEFT SIDE OF SEPTUM AND APICO-ANTERIOR PORTION OF LEFT VENTRICLE. (0.04 SEC)

PHASE 3 COMPLETION OF ACTIVATION IN LEFT VENTRICLE AND CONTINUED ACTIVATION OF SEPTUM. (0.06 TO 0.08 SEC)

PHASE 4 COMPLETION OF ACTIVATION OF SEPTUM AND RIGHT VENTRICLE. (0.12 SEC OR MORE)

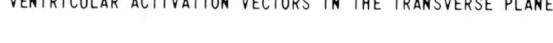

VENTRICULAR ACTIVATION VECTORS IN THE TRANSVERSE PLANE

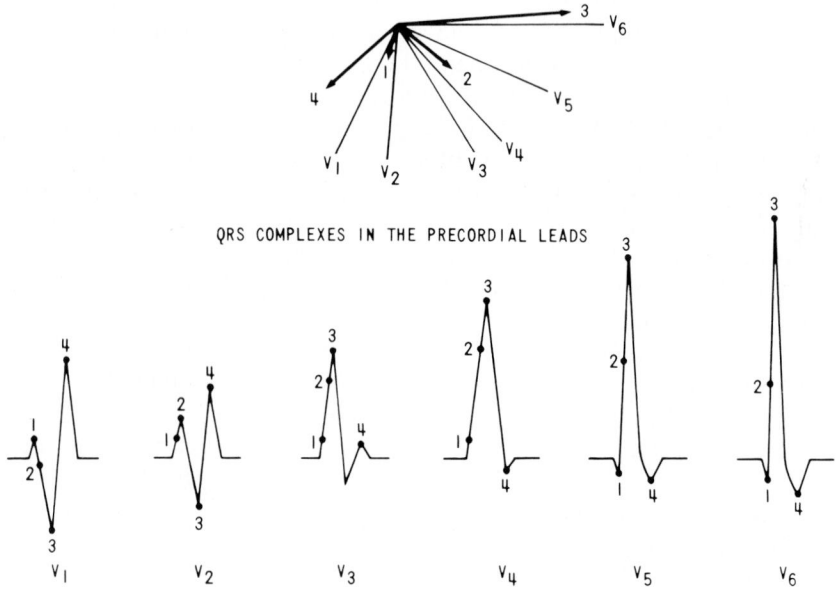

QRS COMPLEXES IN THE PRECORDIAL LEADS

interval which is less than 0.12 s except when RBBB is present. Normal variants, right ventricular enlargement (especially diastolic overload), straight back syndrome, true posterior myocardial infarction, and Wolff-Parkinson-White syndrome (type A) may mimic the ECG changes of a true RBBB.

Right bundle branch block may appear in apparently healthy individuals and those with organic heart disease. It may be identified in people with coronary artery disease, systemic hypertension, cardiac tumors, cardiomyopathy, rheumatic heart disease, and congenital heart disease. Atrial septal defects are often associated with RBBB patterns. Acute pulmonary embolism or infarction should be suspected when RBBB of sudden onset appears. Acute CHF, acute myocardial infarction, and acute pericarditis may produce intermittent RBBB.

Left Bundle Branch Block   Blockage of the left bundle results in an alteration of the normal activation of the ventricles beginning with septal depolarization (Fig. 11-55). Rather than the usual left-

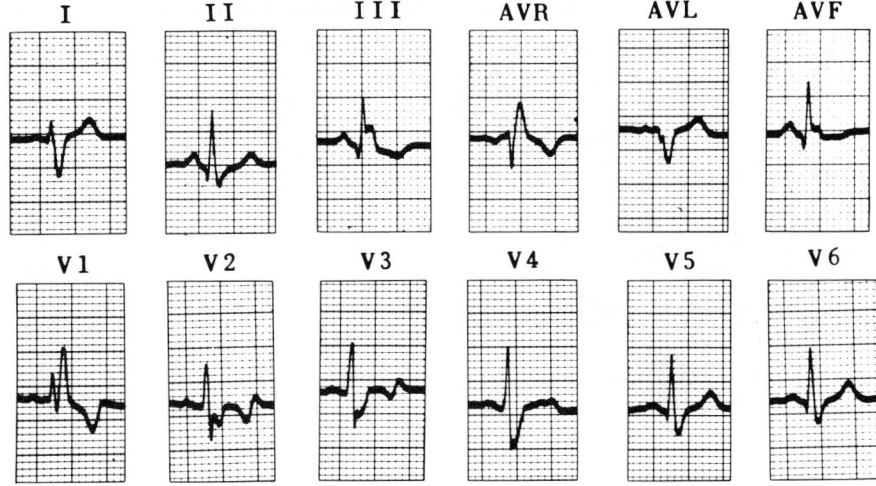

I II III AVR AVL AVF

V1 V2 V3 V4 V5 V6

Figure 11-54 Right bundle branch block. The QRS interval measures 0.12 s. There are wide S waves in leads I, V_5, and V_6. An rSR' complex with a delayed intrinsicoid deflection is present in V_1. The T wave changes are secondary to the block. *(From H. H. Friedman, Diagnostic electrocardiography and vectorcardiography, McGraw-Hill, New York, 1985, p. 182. Copyright 1985 by McGraw-Hill Book Company. Reprinted by permission.)*

to-right depolarization, the septum must depolarize in a right-to-left direction. This change in the initial vector of the QRS produces the loss of the initial r wave in V_1 and the septal q wave in V_6. Occasionally, though, the septal vector is overpowered by the right ventricular electrical activity, in which case there may be a small r wave inscribed in V_1. Following septal and right ventricular depolarization is left ventricular depolarization. Because conduction is abnormal and outside the Purkinje network, the activation time for the left ventricle is prolonged. This results in a prolonged QRS interval and the development of a broad, slurred S wave in V_1 and an R' wave in V_6. The QRS axis may be normal but more often is deviated to the left. Secondary S-T, T wave changes will be present in the left leads. It should be noted that if primary T wave changes (see "Myocardial Infarction" in this chapter) replace the secondary S-T, T wave changes in the presence of a bundle branch block, myocardial ischemia should be suspected.

The diagnostic ECG criteria for LBBB are summarized as:

1. A QRS interval $\geq$ 0.12 s
2. Absence of septal q waves in the left leads (I, aVL, V_{4-6})
3. rsR', M-shaped QRS, or broad R waves in the left leads (I, aVL, V_{4-6})
4. Broad QS or rS waves in the right precordial leads (V_{1-3})

5. Secondary S-T, T wave changes in the left leads (I, aVL, V_{4-6})

These criteria are apparent in Fig. 11-56.

Left bundle branch block must be electrocardiographically differentiated from Wolff-Parkinson-White syndrome (type B), anteroseptal myocardial infarction with nonspecific intraventricular conduction defect, idioventricular conduction defect, idioventricular rhythm, and an artificial cardiac pacemaker-induced ventricular rhythm.[7] The QRS interval and clinical history may provide clues to the correct diagnosis.

The most common cause of LBBB is considered to be hypertensive heart disease. Less often it may be associated with aortic stenosis, cardiomyopathy, and congenital heart disease. It is very rare for LBBB to exist in an individual with an apparently healthy heart. The elderly are much more likely to have LBBB than RBBB. If an individual develops LBBB in the presence of an anteroseptal myocardial infarction or vice versa, the patient's prognosis is considered to be serious.

Left Anterior Hemiblock Usually impulses conduct through the left anterior and left posterior fascicles simultaneously (Fig. 11-57A). The left anterior fascicle normally conducts impulses to the Purkinje fibers of the anterior and lateral walls of the left ventricle. However, when conduction through the anterior fascicle is blocked, the anterior and

Figure 11-55 Schematic representation of ventricular depolarization in left bundle branch block. See text for description. *(From H. H. Friedman, Diagnostic electrocardiography and vectorcardiography, McGraw-Hill, New York, 1985, p. 192. Copyright 1985 by McGraw-Hill Book Company. Reprinted by permission.)*

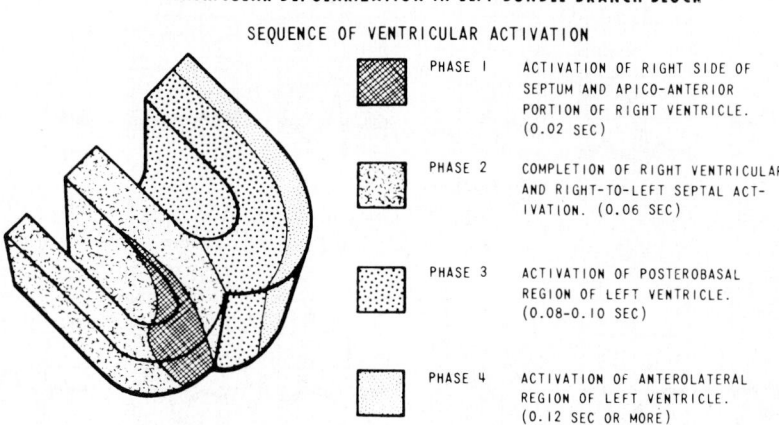

VENTRICULAR DEPOLARIZATION IN LEFT BUNDLE BRANCH BLOCK

SEQUENCE OF VENTRICULAR ACTIVATION

PHASE 1 — ACTIVATION OF RIGHT SIDE OF SEPTUM AND APICO-ANTERIOR PORTION OF RIGHT VENTRICLE. (0.02 SEC)

PHASE 2 — COMPLETION OF RIGHT VENTRICULAR AND RIGHT-TO-LEFT SEPTAL ACTIVATION. (0.06 SEC)

PHASE 3 — ACTIVATION OF POSTEROBASAL REGION OF LEFT VENTRICLE. (0.08-0.10 SEC)

PHASE 4 — ACTIVATION OF ANTEROLATERAL REGION OF LEFT VENTRICLE. (0.12 SEC OR MORE)

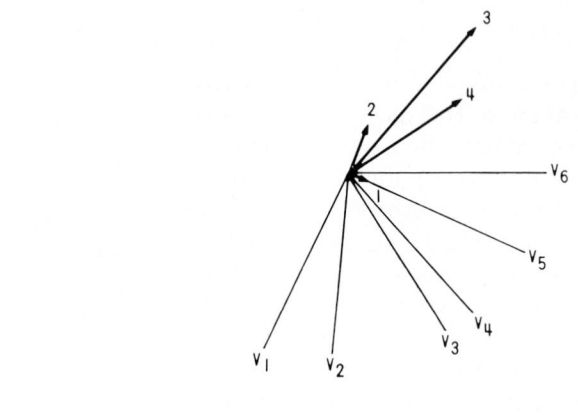

VENTRICULAR ACTIVATION VECTORS IN THE TRANSVERSE PLANE

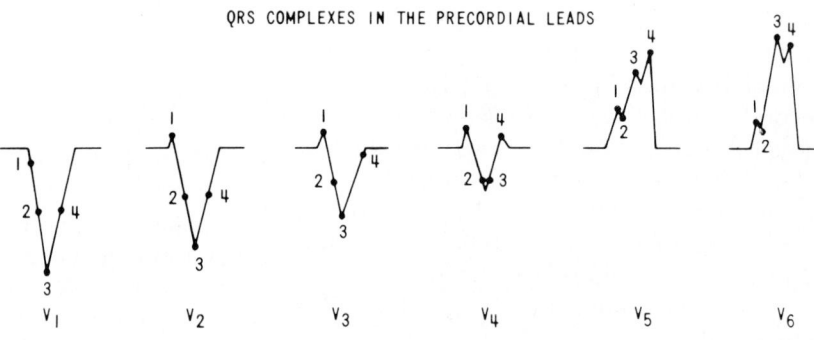

QRS COMPLEXES IN THE PRECORDIAL LEADS

lateral walls must be activated by retrograde conduction from the posterior fascicle. The retrograde activation, which is directed left and superior (Fig. 11-57*B*), occurs late and is essentially unopposed by other electrical activity. Consequently, the left and superior forces cause the mean vector of the QRS to shift leftward and superiorly creating left axis deviation on the ECG (Fig. 11-58). Initial forces are directed rightward and inferiorly, thus producing an initial q wave in leads I and aVL and an initial r wave in the inferior leads (II, III, and aVF).

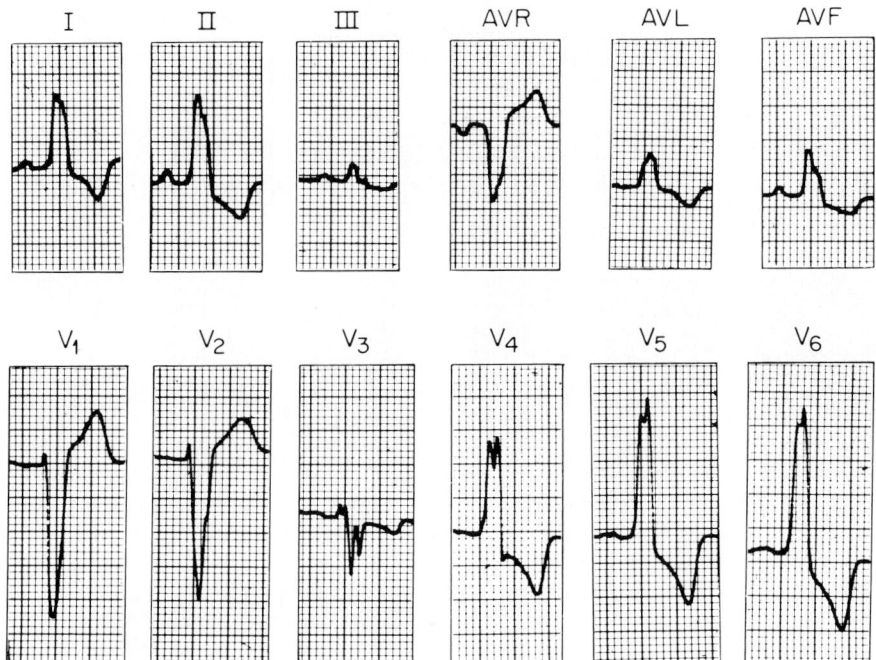

Figure 11-56 Left bundle branch block. The QRS complex measures 0.14 s. A broad, biphasic R wave with a delayed intrinsicoid deflection is present in leads V_5 and V_6, and also in lead I. Significant, too, is the absence of Q waves in leads I and aVL and the left precordial leads. Note, also, the absence of an S wave in lead I. *(From H. H. Friedman, Diagnostic electrocardiography and vectorcardiography, McGraw-Hill, New York, 1985, p. 194. Copyright 1985 by McGraw-Hill Book Company. Reprinted by permission.)*

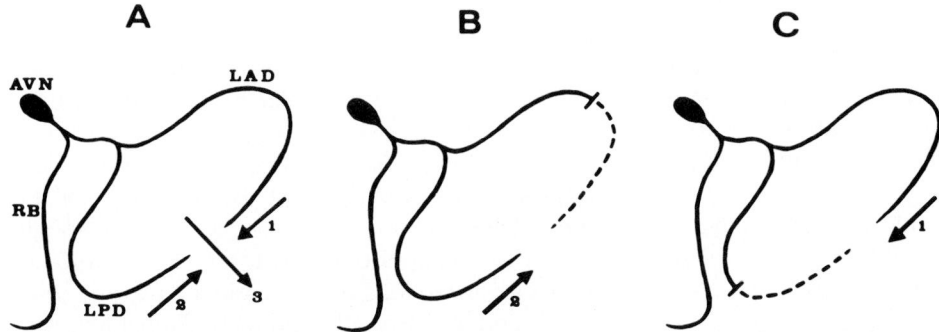

Figure 11-57 Hemiblocks. When both the anterior and posterior divisions of the left bundle branch system are intact (A), the left ventricle is activated through both divisions (vectors 1 and 2) so that the resultant forces of vectors 1 and 2 will produce vector 3. However, when one of the two divisions of the left bundle branch system is blocked, the impulses must travel through the intact division only. That is, in anterior hemiblock (B) vector 1 is no longer present and as a result the left ventricle is activated through the intact posterior division (vector 2). In this case the electrical axis shifts to the left and superiorly (marked left axis deviation). For the same reason, posterior hemiblock (C) produces right axis deviation because the left ventricle is activated through the intact anterior division (vector 1). RB: right bundle branch; AVN: AV node; LAD: left anterior division; LPD: left posterior division. *(From E. K. Chung, Electrocardiography. Practical application with vectorial principles, Appleton-Century-Crofts, Norwalk, CT, 1985, p. 89. Copyright 1985 by Appleton-Century-Crofts. Reprinted by permission.)*

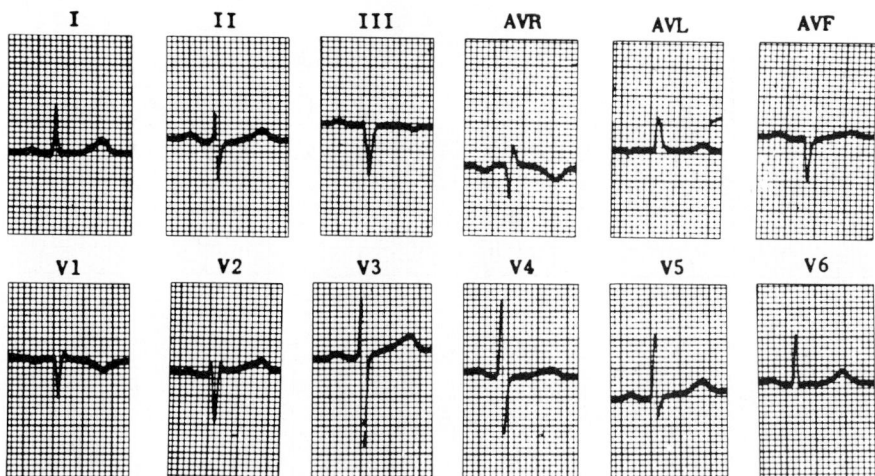

Figure 11-58 Abnormal left axis deviation ($-45°$) due to left anterior hemiblock in a patient with chronic coronary artery disease. The electrocardiogram is otherwise normal. There is an R' wave in leads V_1 and V_2, which indicates the terminal QRS vector, in addition to being directed leftward and superiorly, also points anteriorly. *(From H. H. Friedman, Diagnostic electrocardiography and vectorcardiography, McGraw-Hill, New York, 1985, p. 201. Copyright 1985 by McGraw-Hill Book Company. Reprinted by permission.)*

The major ECG criterion for left anterior hemiblock is marked left axis deviation. There are conflicting opinions in the literature regarding what constitutes marked LAD. Two authors[2,5] consider axis deviation of $-30°$ to $-90°$ as suitable criteria for marked LAD and others[6,7] state that $-45°$ to $-90°$ are the suitable limits. This author uses $-45°$ as the lower limit for marked LAD and the criterion measure for LAH.

The electrocardiographic criteria for the diagnosis of left anterior hemiblock may be summarized as:

1. Marked left axis deviation ($-45°$ to $-90°$)
2. qR complex in leads I and aVL; rS complex in leads II, III, and aVF
3. A QRS interval < 0.12 s

It is important to note, however, that other clinical conditions (such as emphysema, ventricular preexcitation, hyperkalemia, acute pulmonary embolism, and inferior myocardial infarction) may cause marked LAD and mimic in other ways the ECG findings of left anterior hemiblock. The presence of these conditions must be ruled out before true left anterior hemiblock can be diagnosed.

Left Posterior Hemiblock The left posterior fascicle conducts impulses to the inferior and posterior walls of the left ventricle. When this fascicle is blocked, impulses must be conducted to these areas via the anterior fascicle. The activation of the inferior and posterior left ventricular walls is late and the impulses are directed inferiorly and rightward (Figure 11-57C). These late forces are essentially unopposed and produce right axis deviation of the mean QRS vector. The initial QRS forces, though, are directed superiorly and to the left causing an initial r wave in lead I and an initial q wave in leads II, III, and aVF. Even though the terminal forces of the QRS occur late, the QRS interval is usually less than 0.12 s.

Figure 11-59 depicts the ECG changes associated with a left posterior hemiblock. These changes can be summarized as follows:

1. Marked right axis deviation ($+105°$ to $+180°$)
2. A small r wave (rS complex) in lead I and a small q wave (qR complex) in lead III
3. A QRS interval < 0.12 s

As with left anterior hemiblock, left posterior hemiblock can only be diagnosed with certainty when

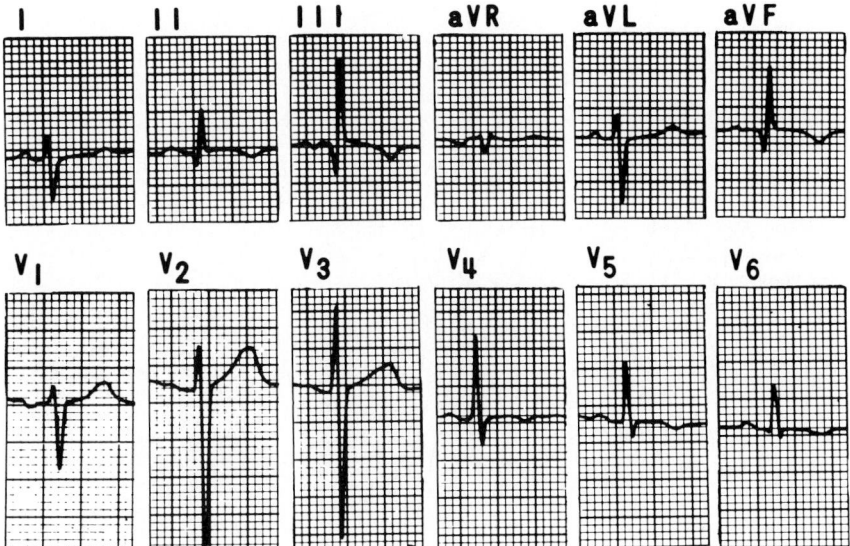

Figure 11-59   Left posterior hemiblock in a patient with recent inferior myocardial infarction. There is abnormal right axis deviation (about +120°) with an
rS pattern in leads I and aVL, and qR patterns with relatively tall R waves in
leads II, III, and aVF. The abnormal Q waves and inverted T waves in the
inferior leads indicate a recent inferior myocardial infarction. The patient had
diffuse, severe, occlusive disease of all major coronary vessels demonstrable on
arteriography. *(From H. H. Friedman, Diagnostic electrocardiography and vectorcardiography, McGraw-Hill, New York, 1985, p. 205. Copyright 1985 by
McGraw-Hill Book Company. Reprinted by permission.*

all other factors which might cause RAD are ruled
out. These factors include a vertical heart, chronic
obstructive lung disease, right ventricular enlargement, and lateral wall myocardial infarction.

Left posterior hemiblock rarely occurs as an
isolated lesion. More often it coexists with RBBB
(bifascicular block), inferior wall myocardial infarction, or both. This block may also be found,
though less commonly, in individuals with cardiomyopathy, calcific aortic stenosis, and hyperkalemia.[7]

Wolff-Parkinson-White Syndrome

Wolff-Parkinson-White (WPW) syndrome is a form
of ventricular preexcitation which was first described in 1930. The syndrome, characterized by a
short P-R interval and an abnormal configuration
of the QRS complex, is sometimes known as the
bundle of Kent syndrome or the anomalous atrioventricular excitation syndrome. The rhythm disturbance occurs when an anomalous atrioventric-

ular conductive pathway, usually the bundle of
Kent, allows the atrial impulse to bypass the AV
node and excite the ventricles sooner than would
be normally expected. The Kent bundle may be
located between the free walls of the atria and
ventricles or between the atrial and ventricular
septa (Fig. 11-60).

When the atrial impulse is able to bypass the
normal AV conductive pathway in the AV node and
His bundle, the normal AV conduction delay is not
exhibited on the ECG. Consequently, the P-R interval
is less than normal and usually between 0.08 and
0.12 s (Fig. 11-61). If, however, there is a preexisting
AV conduction defect, the P-R interval may be
prolonged and appear normal in the presence of
WPW syndrome. The P wave is normal unless there
is a coexisting cardiac disease.

The QRS complex in WPW syndrome is almost
always prolonged (0.10 s or more). Occasionally it
may be less than 0.10 s with the range being 0.08
to 0.16 s. The duration of the QRS interval is

Figure 11-60 Diagram-matic representation of the bundles of Kent. See text for discussion.

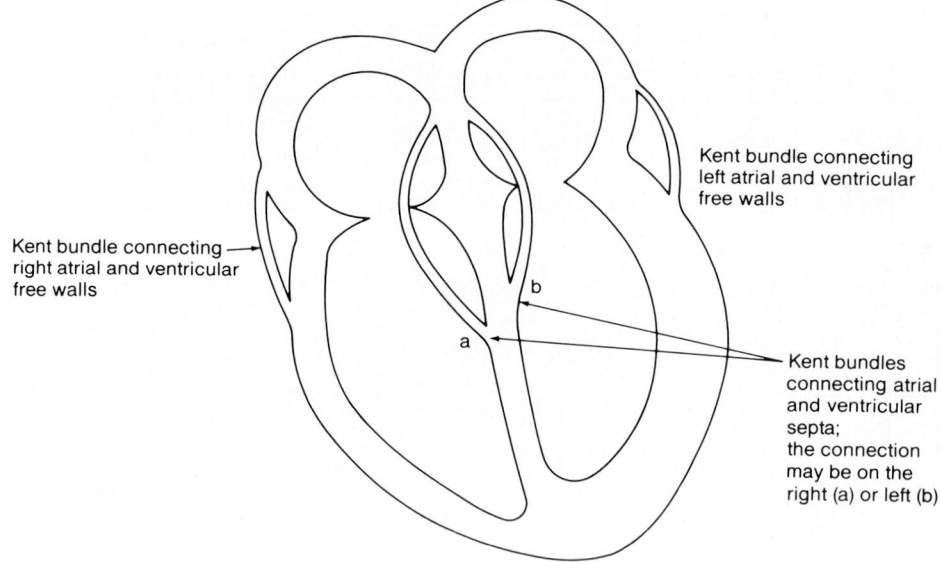

Kent bundle connecting left atrial and ventricular free walls

Kent bundle connecting right atrial and ventricular free walls

Kent bundles connecting atrial and ventricular septa; the connection may be on the right (a) or left (b)

frequently inversely proportional to the P-R interval (Fig. 11-61) and is dependent on the degree of preexcitation. The sum of the P-R interval and the QRS interval (P-S interval) (Fig. 11-61) usually is within the normal range.

The most important finding in WPW syndrome is the presence of the *delta wave*. The delta wave is the initial slurring of the QRS complex (Fig. 11-61). This slurred initial component of the QRS complex should be present in all leads but may be

Figure 11-61 The uninterrupted line indicates anomalous conduction in WPW syndrome, whereas the broken line indicates normal conduction. Note the short P-R interval, the delta wave, and the secondary T wave change. The P-S interval is within the normal range. See text for further discussion.

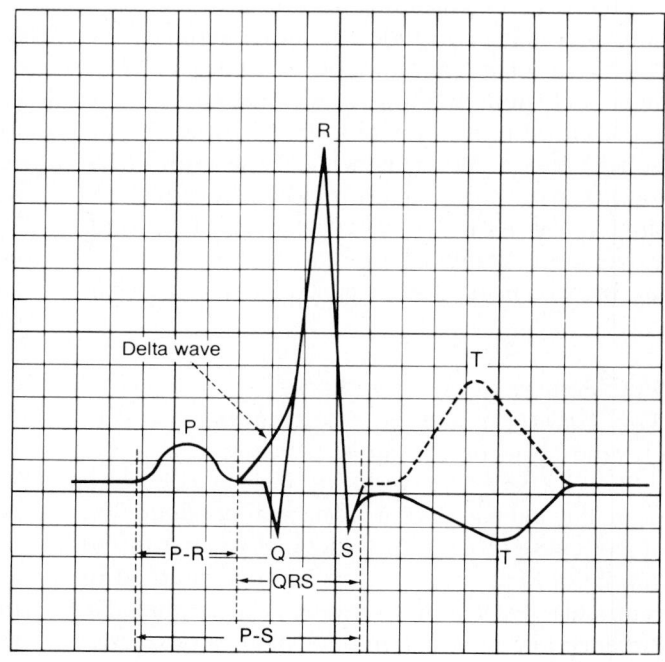

more visible in some leads than in others (Fig. 11-62).

Associated with the abnormal sequence of ventricular activation is abnormal repolarization; consequently, secondary S-T and T wave changes are present (Fig. 11-61). Usually the displacement of the S-T segment and the polarity of the T wave are opposite to the direction of the delta wave and the major QRS deflection.

Wolff-Parkinson-White syndrome has been traditionally classified into two types, A and B. The basis of the classification is the morphology of the QRS complex in the precordial leads. Type A WPW is characterized by an upright delta wave and QRS in all the precordial leads (Fig. 11-62). Lead V_1 shows a dominant R wave with R, RS, Rs, RSr', or Rsr' patterns and lead V_6 exhibits Rs or R deflections.[6] At first glance type A WPW may resemble a right bundle branch block. In type B WPW (Fig. 11-63) the delta wave and the remainder of the QRS complex are predominantly negative in V_{1-2} but upright in the left precordial leads. Conse-

quently, V_{1-2} show an rS, QS, or qrS pattern and the left chest leads show tall R waves. Type B resembles the ECG characteristic of left bundle branch block and is more common than type A. Other rare forms of WPW which cannot be classified into one of the existing types have been identified. Wolff-Parkinson-White type C is one such rare form which may be identified by positive delta waves in leads V_{1-4} and negative delta waves in leads V_{5-6}.

In general, preexcitation in type A WPW occurs in the posterobasal region of the left ventricle. In type B cases the posterobasal region of the right ventricle is preexcited. In both types depolarization proceeds from epicardium to endocardium from the point of preexcitation. However, current methods of electrocardiographic testing demonstrate a poor correlation between the location of the bypass tract and the electrocardiographic pattern of the QRS. Therefore, the traditional classification system of type A and B is being used less frequently.

The most important clinical manifestations of WPW syndrome are paroxysmal tachyarrhythmias.

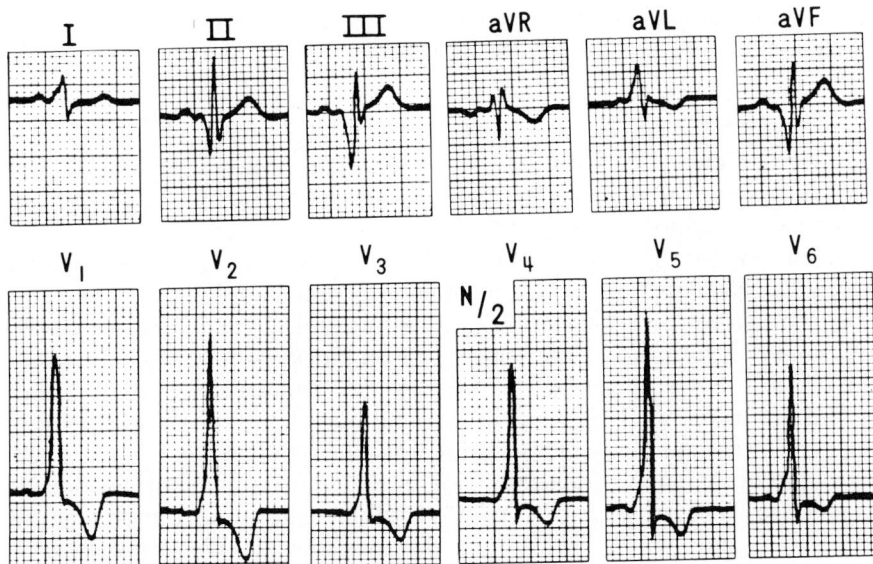

Figure 11-62   Wolff-Parkinson-White, type A. The P waves are normal, the P-R interval is short, the QRS complex is broad, and delta waves are present. The prominent Q waves in leads II, III, and aVF may lead to the erroneous diagnosis of an inferior myocardial infarction. The upright QRS complexes in both right and left precordial leads are characteristic of type A WPW. *(From H. H. Friedman, Diagnostic electrocardiography and vectorcardiography, McGraw-Hill, New York, 1985, p. 229. Copyright 1985 by McGraw-Hill Book Company. Reprinted by permission.)*

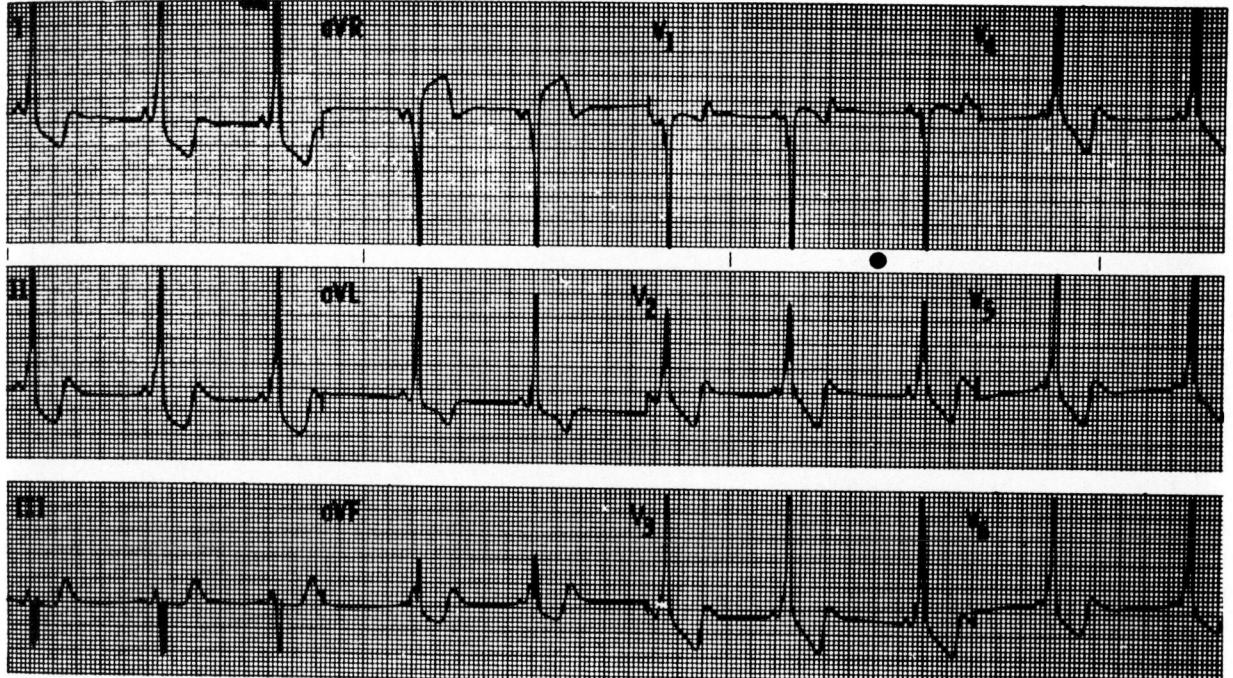

Figure 11-63 Wolff-Parkinson-White, type B. The rhythm is sinus arrhythmia with sinus bradycardia (rate 53 to 60 beats per minute). Left ventricular enlargement and left bundle branch block resemble this ECG and may be erroneously diagnosed. Note the short P-R interval, the delta wave, and the secondary S-T, T wave changes. *(From E. K. Chung, Electrocardiography. Practical applications with vectorial principles, Appleton-Century-Crofts, Norwalk, CT, 1985, p. 311. Copyright 1985 by Appleton-Century-Crofts. Reprinted by permission.)*

They have been reported in 13 to 80 percent of the cases with the incidence being closely related to the population sampled; 13 percent in routine ECGs from clinically healthy individuals and 40 to 80 percent in hospitalized or cardiac clinic patients known to have the syndrome.[5,6] Paroxysmal supraventricular tachycardia is the most common form of tachyarrhythmia seen in patients with the syndrome. The tachycardia is a reciprocating or reentrant tachyrhythm which is often initiated by a single premature atrial or ventricular extrasystole. When the impulse of excitation proceeds antegrade through the AV conduction system and returns to the atrium via the bypass tract in a retrograde fashion, the delta wave is not observed, the QRS interval is normal, and the rate ranges between 140 and 250 beats per minute. Atrial flutter and fibrillation are less common than PSVT in WPW syndrome, but when they are present, the atrial impulses are conducted to the ventricles via the accessory path-

way and result in wide, bizarre QRS complexes. The ventricular rate may range from 220 to 360 beats per minute.

Wolff-Parkinson-White syndrome, both type A and B, must be differentiated from a number of other ECG abnormalities. Type A may resemble right bundle branch block, right ventricular hypertrophy, true posterior myocardial infarction, and inferior myocardial infarction. Type B may resemble anterior myocardial infarction and inferior myocardial infarction in addition to left bundle branch block. WPW syndrome and atrial flutter may be mistaken for paroxysmal ventricular tachycardia or ventricular flutter.

Therapy for WPW is not warranted if no tachyarrhythmias are associated with the syndrome. Prevention of and treatment for tachyrhythms secondary to WPW syndrome, however, is often necessary. Vagal maneuvers may be useful in treating paroxysmal reentrant tachyrhythms, although many patients require antiarrhythmic drug therapy, either acutely or for long-term maintenance. In crisis situations of extremely rapid ventricular response to atrial fibrillation or flutter, direct current shock may be needed. When the tachyrhythms are refractory to conventional therapy, artificial pacemaker or surgical therapy may be implemented.

The choice of the most appropriate drug for treating WPW-associated tachyrhythms is dependent on the specific electrophysiologic properties of the drug and on the site of the reentry mechanism (that is, the AV nodal conductive pathway or the accessory pathway). The goal of drug therapy is to change the conduction times in the pathways so that reentry is impossible. Table 11-4 lists the effect of various antiarrhythmic drugs on the refractory period of the normal and anomalous pathways. Propranolol is frequently the drug of choice for normal QRS tachyrhythms associated with WPW syndrome, whereas quinidine and procainamide are used for long-term treatment of reentrant tachyrhythms which are transmitted via antegrade conduction through the accessory pathway. Digitalis may be useful in treating tachyrhythms conducted antegrade through the AV node conduction system and retrograde through the bypass tract. However, this drug may enhance the antegrade conduction through the accessory pathway and should be used with caution in conjunction with other antiarrhythmic agents in

patients with WPW syndrome and atrial fibrillation or atrial flutter. Amiodarone and verapamil have been found to be useful in treating various tachyrhythms in WPW syndrome.

Nursing Management of Patients with Cardiac Dysrhythmias

The relationship between the electrical and mechanical cardiac events as well as their combined effects on cardiac output have been described earlier. It is this relationship that causes patients who are known to have or who are susceptible to developing rhythm disturbances to require close monitoring by the critical-care nurse. The nurse must recognize those patients who are at risk for cardiac arrhythmias, the potentially lethal arrhythmias, the hemodynamic consequences of rhythm disorders, and the usual or probable therapeutic interventions for the various dysrhythmias.

From the previous presentation regarding specific rhythm disorders it is clear that organic heart disease places patients in jeopardy for developing cardiac dysrhythmias. However, critically ill individuals suffering from a variety of other body system disorders or trauma are also prone to cardiac rhythm disturbances. Neurologic trauma may result in abnormalities in the cardiac centers of the brain. Abnormal pulmonary function may cause hypoxia which affects the heart's ability to extract the amount

11-4 Effect of Drugs on the Refractory Periods of the Normal AV and Anomalous Pathways

	Effective Refractory Period	
Drugs	A-V Node	Accessory Pathway
Propranolol	Lengthened	No change
Digitalis	Lengthened	Shortened
Lidocaine	No change	Lengthened
Quinidine	Shortened	Lengthened
Procainamide	No change	Lengthened
Phenytoin	Shortened	Variable
Amiodarone	Lengthened	Lengthened
Verapamil	Lengthened	Variable

Adapted from E. K. Chung, Electrocardiography, practical applications with vectorial principles, Appleton-Century-Crofts, Norwalk, CT, 1985, p. 331. (Copyright 1985 by Appleton-Century-Crofts. Adapted by permission.)

of oxygen necessary for cellular metabolism. Altered renal function may cause electrolyte imbalances which create an abnormal ionic environment for cardiac cells. Consequently, continuous monitoring of the cardiac rhythm is recommended for all critically ill patients, and telemetry monitoring is frequently necessary for certain patients in the acute care setting.

Given the right circumstances, any dysrhythmia may have potentially lethal consequences. However, certain rhythm disorders are known to produce almost immediate life-threatening hemodynamic alterations. In general, any rhythm disturbance that produces a very slow or a very rapid ventricular rate is suspect. In addition, those arrhythmias which are known to initiate lethal tachyrhythms should be closely monitored, as should those which warn of impending serious rhythm disturbances. Vigilance on the part of the nurse is critical if the life-threatening consequences of cardiac rhythm disturbances are to be prevented and/or treated.

Prevention of and treatment for cardiac dysrhythmias is becoming increasingly complex. New antiarrhythmic agents are being tested and marketed with increasing frequency. Advanced technology is enhancing the ability to produce more complex and physiologically comparable cardiac pacemakers and internal cardiac defibrillators. These advances in science and technology require that the critical-care nurse be more knowledgeable regarding the vast array of possible therapeutic interventions. Often it is the nurse who is expected to initiate antiarrhythmic therapy in the emergency situation. Additionally, the nurse is expected to anticipate appropriate antiarrhythmic interventions to ensure ready availability in the critical-care environment.

In addition to recognizing and treating cardiac dysrhythmias, the critical-care nurse must be able to recognize the ECG criteria for other cardiac and noncardiac abnormalities which include chamber enlargement, myocardial infarction, and electrolyte imbalance. Also, the critical-care nurse must be familiar with the effects of drug therapy on the ECG. A discussion of these topics follows.

Chamber Enlargement

Characteristics of cardiac *hypertrophy,* the increase in the size of the cardiac muscle fibers secondary to increased pressure loads, and cardiac *dilatation,* the increase in a chamber's diameter secondary to increased volume loads, are virtually indistinguishable on the ECG. Consequently, the term *chamber enlargement* has been adopted by many to refer to either hypertrophy or dilatation of a cardiac muscle mass or chamber. Diagnostic ECG criteria for atrial and ventricular enlargement will be presented in this section.

Atrial Abnormality, Enlargement, or Hypertrophy

The normal configuration for the P wave has previously been described (see "Waves, Complexes, and Intervals" in this chapter). When the voltage, duration, morphology, and direction of the P wave are abnormal, it usually indicates either the enlargement of one or both of the atrial chambers or an intra- or interatrial conduction defect. The specific diagnosis for the P wave alteration cannot be made with certainty by electrocardiography; therefore, the term *atrial abnormality* more correctly describes alterations in P wave morphology and is being used more frequently for this purpose. However, *atrial enlargement* is the term which is used in this chapter only because it is the term which is commonly used in clinical practice.

Left Atrial Enlargement   Depolarization of the left atrium is represented on the ECG by the mid- and late portions of the P wave. Therefore, if activation of the left atrium is abnormal, the ECG reflects the abnormality via changes in the mid- and terminal components of the P wave. Diagnostic criteria for left atrial enlargement (LAE) are:

1. P-terminal force in leads V_{1-2} equal to or greater than 1 mm in both width and depth (Fig. 11-64)
2. P wave duration prolonged at 0.12 s or more
3. Notched and slurred P wave with a peak-to-peak interval of 0.04 s in leads I, II, and aVL (Fig. 11-64)
4. Ratio of the duration of the P wave to the P-R segment greater than 1.60[5]
5. P axis between 0 and $+45°$ in the frontal plane

Figure 11-65 is an ECG from a patient with mitral stenosis. Note the ECG characteristics of LAE.

Left atrial enlargement is commonly the result of mitral valve disease, particularly mitral stenosis. For this reason, the term *P mitrale* is often used

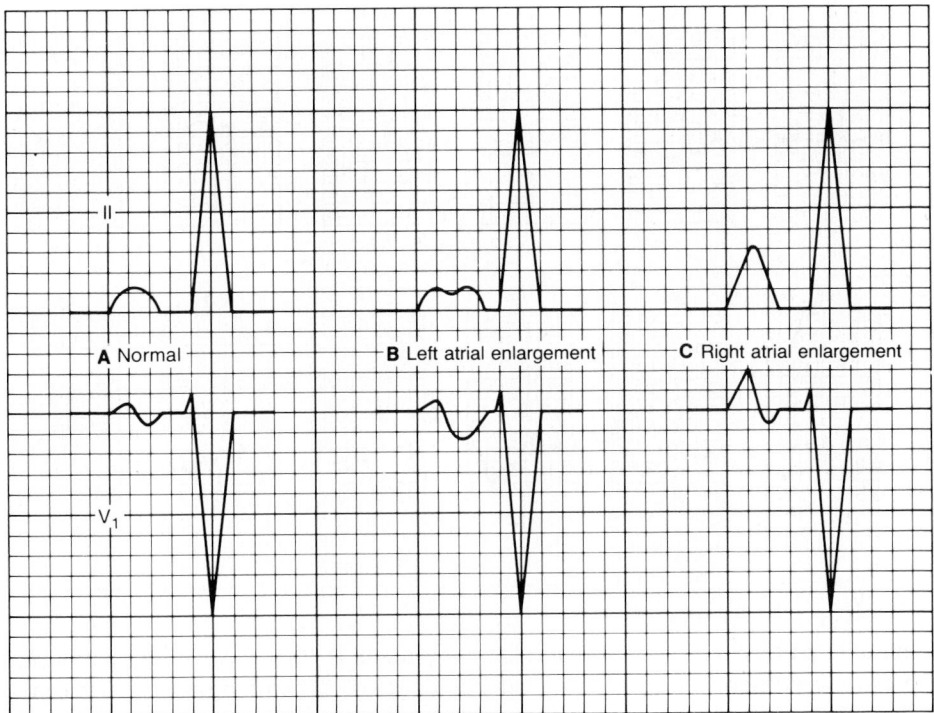

Figure 11-64   P waves reflective of left atrial enlargement (B) and right atrial enlarge-
ment (C) in comparison with normal atrial P waves (A) in leads II and V_1. *(From E. K.
Chung, Electrocardiography. Practical applications with vectorial principles, Appleton-
Century-Crofts, Norwalk, CT, 1985, p. 44. Copyright 1985 by Appleton-Century-Crofts.
Adapted by permission.)*

when referring to the P wave of LAE. A useful clue
for remembering the ECG criteria of LAE is to
associate this term with the "M-shaped" (for mitral)
or wide, notched P wave characteristic of *left* atrial
enlargement.

Other conditions in which the ECG characteristics of left atrial enlargement may be found
include aortic valve disease, coronary artery disease,
acute myocardial infarction, acute pulmonary edema,
constrictive pericarditis, idiopathic hypertrophic
subaortic stenosis (IHSS), dilated cardiomyopathy,
coarctation of the aorta, endocardial cushion defects, and other conditions causing diastolic overloading of the left ventricle. Patients with systemic
hypertension also frequently demonstrate characteristics of LAE on their ECGs.

Right Atrial Enlargement   The initial component
of the normal P wave reflects depolarization of the
right atrium. Hence, when there is enlargement of

the right atrium the initial component of the P wave
is altered. Diagnostic criteria for right atrial enlargement (RAE) are:

1. Tall, peaked (or tent-shaped) P waves with a
   height of 2.5 mm[5,6] or more in leads II, III, and
   aVF (Fig. 11-64)
2. Normal P wave duration
3. P axis of 75° or greater in the frontal plane
4. A positive deflection of the P wave in leads V_{1-2}
   with a height of 1.5 mm[5,6] or more (Fig. 11-64)

Figure 11-66 illustrates the ECG changes found
in a patient with RAE. The patient in this example
had cor pulmonale, which is a common cause of
RAE. The term *P pulmonale* is used to describe the
tall, thin, peaked P wave of RAE secondary to chronic
lung disease, coronary artery disease, acute left
ventricular failure, and hypoxemia.[6] It should be
noted, however, that actual right atrial enlargement
is only demonstrable in about one-half of the

Figure 11-65   Left atrial and right ventricular enlargement and right ventricular strain in a patient with mitral stenosis. The P waves are broad and notched. There is a qR pattern with an inverted T wave in lead V_1. The S-T segments are depressed and the T waves inverted in the precordial leads. *(From H. H. Friedman, Diagnostic electrocardiography and vectorcardiography, McGraw-Hill, New York, 1985, p. 132. Copyright 1985 by McGraw-Hill Book Company. Reprinted by permission.)*

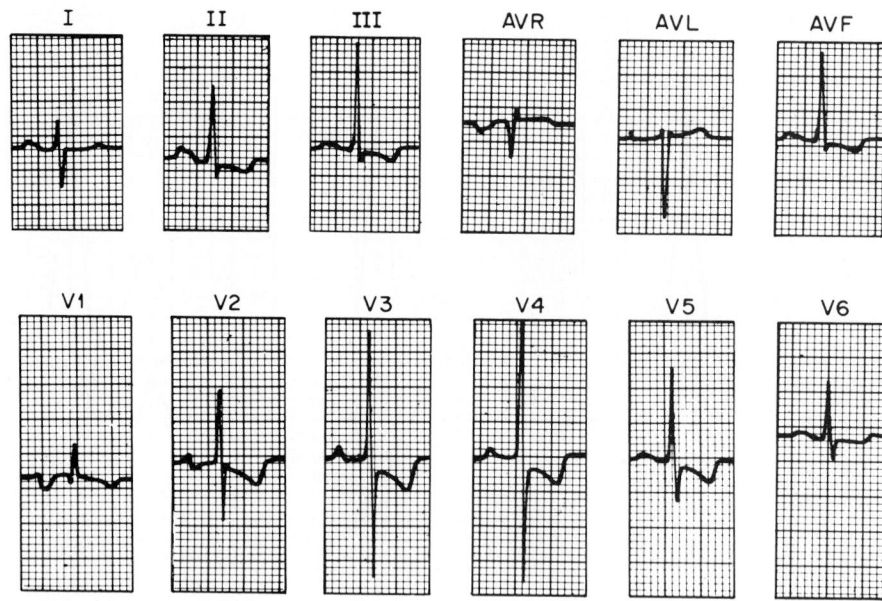

patients displaying the P pulmonale pattern. Occasionally, the P pulmonale pattern represents left atrial enlargement or another condition. P pulmonale in association with the finding of an abnormal P terminal force in lead V_1 and in the presence of left ventricular enlargement (LVE) favors LAE as the cause of the P pulmonale pattern. The converse of this, P pulmonale without the P terminal force in lead V_1 and LVE, but with ECG changes consistent with right ventricular enlargement (RVE) or pulmonary disease, favors RAE.

Biatrial Enlargement   When both atrial chambers are enlarged the characteristics of both right and left atrial enlargement coexist on the ECG. The diagnostic criteria for biatrial enlargement are:

1. Tall (2.5 mm or more) and wide (3 mm or more) P waves in the limb leads
2. Large diphasic P waves in the right precordial leads (V_{1-2}) with the initial component greater than 1.5 mm and the terminal component deeper and wider than 1 mm
3. Tall, peaked P waves (greater than 1.5 mm) in V_{1-2} and wide, notched P waves in the limb leads or left precordial leads (V_{5-6})[5,7]

It is important to note that the electrocardiographic findings for biatrial enlargement are largely dependent on the degree of atrial abnormality.

Biatrial enlargement is found clinically in people with various congenital heart diseases, cardiomyopathy, and rheumatic heart disease.

Ventricular Hypertrophy or Enlargement

Prior to considering the electrocardiographic findings associated with ventricular enlargement it is useful to review the characteristics of the normal ECG (Table 11-2), paying particular attention to the amplitude, R wave progression, intrinsicoid deflection, and axis of the QRS; the configuration of the S-T segment; and the direction and shape of the T wave. This review is important because ventricular enlargement alters these elements of the ECG.

It is unfortunate that the actual diagnostic criteria for left, right, and biventricular enlargement are not as sensitive as one would like. For this reason numerous electrocardiographic indicators for the diagnosis of ventricular enlargement have been published. Only the more commonly used criteria are presented here.

Left Ventricular Enlargement   Left ventricular enlargement (LVE) may be secondary to either systolic overload or diastolic overload. Systolic overload of the left ventricle occurs when there is resistance to left ventricular ejection. Common causes of LVE secondary to systolic overload are systemic hypertension, aortic stenosis, and coarc-

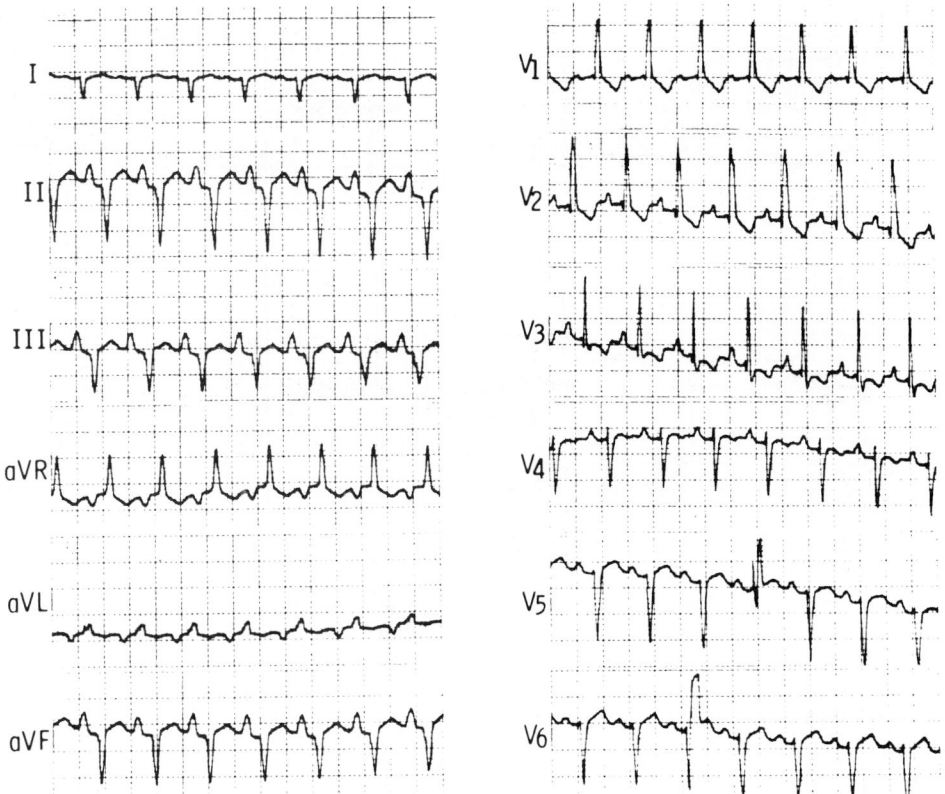

Figure 11-66   Right atrial and ventricular enlargement and right ventricular strain in a patient with advanced chronic cor pulmonale. The P waves are tall and peaked. The QRS axis is +250°. There are tall R waves in leads V₁ through V₃ with secondary T wave changes. *(From E. K. Chung and D. K. Chung, ECG diagnosis. Self assessment, Harper & Row, New York, 1972, p. 9. Copyright Harper & Row, Publishers, Inc. Reprinted by permission.)*

tation of the aorta. Diastolic overload of the left ventricle occurs when there is increased diastolic volume and pressure. The common causes of this type of overload include aortic insufficiency, mitral insufficiency, patent ductus arteriosus, and ventricular septal defect.

The most notable electrocardiographic change in LVE secondary to either systolic or diastolic overload is increased voltage of the QRS (Fig. 11-67). Frequently the duration of the QRS is prolonged slightly, but it is not greater than 0.12 s. The QRS axis may be deviated to the left. Occasionally the onset of the intrinisicoid deflection is delayed. The direction of the S-T and T vectors in the left limb and precordial leads is altered so that they point in a direction opposite to that of the

QRS. This S-T, T wave change is known as the *left ventricular strain pattern* and resembles a backward check mark (⌄). The S-T segment slopes gradually downward into the initial component of the T wave and the terminal component of the T wave slopes upward more rapidly. The strain pattern is generally associated with LVE secondary to systolic overload and is found more often in long-standing LVE. The pattern is intensified when dilatation and failure set in. It is important to note that the typical strain pattern found in systolic overload of the left ventricle is absent in diastolic overload of the chamber (Fig. 11-68). Rather, the T waves are tall and upright in the left precordial leads of patients with diastolic overload of the left ventricle. In addition, the depth of the Q wave and the height

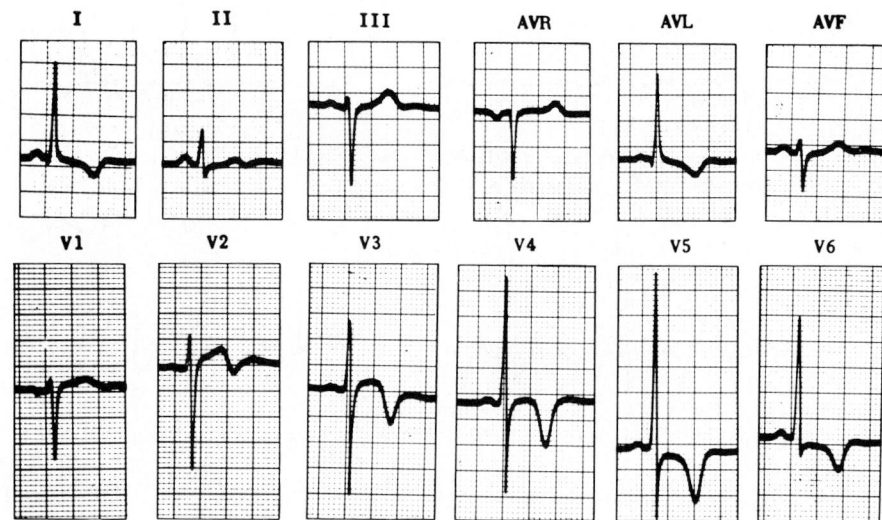

Figure 11-67   Left ventricular enlargement and strain. There is high voltage in leads aVL and V_5. The R in V_5 exceeds 30 mm. The QRS axis is $+15°$. The S-T segments and T waves show changes characteristic of the strain pattern. This is an example of systolic overloading of the left ventricle in a patient with hypertensive heart disease. *(From H. H. Friedman, Diagnostic electrocardiography and vectorcardiography, McGraw-Hill, New York, 1985, p. 142. Copyright 1985 by McGraw-Hill Book Company. Reprinted by permission.*

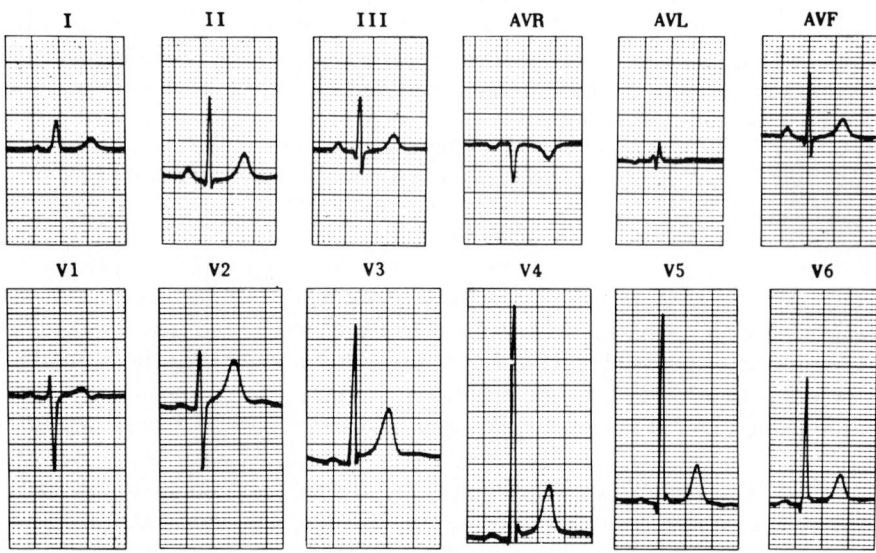

Figure 11-68   Left ventricular enlargement in an adult with aortic insufficiency. There is no deviation of the electrical axis. There is high voltage of the R waves in lead V_4 and V_5. The sum of the maximum R wave (lead V_4) and the maximum S wave (lead V_1) in the precordial leads exceeds 45 mm. The S-T segments and the T waves are normal. This is an example of diastolic overloading of the left ventricle. *(From H. H. Friedman, Diagnostic electrocardiography and vectorcardiography, McGraw-Hill, New York, 1985, p. 142. Copyright 1985 by McGraw-Hill Book Company. Reprinted by permission.)*

of the R wave in leads V_{5-6} is greater in diastolic than in systolic overload LVE.

Romhilt and Estes[9] developed a point score system for the diagnosis of LVE. This is considered to be one of the better methods for diagnosing LVE and is reproduced in Table 11-5. Other criteria also may be used to diagnose LVE (Table 11-6).[2,5–7] The electrocardiographic diagnosis of LVE is made when one or more of these criteria are identified and the QRS is less than 0.12 s.

It must be pointed out that diagnosis of LVE based only on voltage criteria may result in a false positive diagnosis. This is because there are some normal individuals whose ECGs show increased voltage in the absence of LVE. These individuals may be particularly thin, elderly, and emaciated or may be adolescents or young adults. False positive diagnoses may also be made when LVE is diagnosed in the presence of complete or incomplete LBBB. Accurate diagnosis of LVE may only be made when the LBBB is intermittent.[7] False negative interpretations may be made in some individuals whose ECGs fail to record voltages exceeding maximum normal values.[6] Consequently, when making an electrocardiographic diagnosis of LVE it is wise to

Table 11-5 Romhilt and Estes Point-Score System for the ECG Diagnosis of Left Ventricular Hypertrophy[9]

Characteristics		Points
1. QRS amplitude:		3
(R or S in limb lead	20 mm or more, or	
S in V_1 or V_2	30 mm or more, or	
R in V_5 or V_6	30 mm or more)	
2. S-T segment (S-T segment deviation in a direction opposite to that of the main deflection of the QRS):		
Without digitalis		3
(With digitalis)		(1)
3. Left atrial involvement (P terminal forces in V_1 is $\geq$ 1 mm in depth and $\geq$ 0.04 s in duration)		3
4. Left axis deviation $\geq -30°$		2
5. QRS duration $\geq$ 0.09 s		1
6. Intrinsicoid deflection in V_5 or $V_6 \geq$ 0.05.		1
	Maximum total	13

Five points are read as LVH.

Four points are read as probable LVH.

Table 11-6 Diagnostic Criteria for Left Ventricular Enlargement[2,5–7]

Voltage of the QRS[a]

Limb leads:	
R in I + S in III	More than 25 mm, or
R in I	More than 13 mm, or
S in aVR	More than 14 mm, or
R in aVL	More than 11 mm, or
R in aVF	More than 20 mm
Chest leads:	
S in V_1 or V_2 + R in V_5 or V_6	
In adults > 30 years old	More than 35 mm
In adults 20–30 years old	More than 40 mm
In adults 16–20 years old	More than 60 mm, or
R in V_5	More than 26 mm, or
R in V_6	More than 20 mm, or
R + S in any V lead	More than 45 mm

Intrinsicoid Deflection (optional for diagnosis)[a]

V_1 and V_2	Normal
V_5 and V_6	$\geq$ 0.045s

S-T Segment and T wave changes[a]
Left ventricular strain pattern in V_4 to V_6; in I, II, and aVL when mean QRS axis is horizontal; and in II, III, and aVF when the mean QRS axis is vertical.

[a] These criteria are applicable only if the duration of the QRS is < 0.12 s.

carefully evaluate other factors such as body build, thickness of chest wall, and the underlying disease process.

Right Ventricular Enlargement   Like LVE, right ventricular enlargement (RVE) may be secondary to either systolic or diastolic overload. Pulmonary stenosis, pulmonary hypertension, tetralogy of Fallot, mitral stenosis, and chronic cor pulmonale are potential causes of systolic overload of the right ventricle. Diastolic overload may be caused by atrial septal defect or tricuspid insufficiency. If the resultant hypertrophy of either type of overload is mild, the ECG may not be sensitive enough to detect changes. Consequently, only marked RVE can be electrocardiographically diagnosed with certainty (Fig. 11-65).

Early ECG changes consistent with RVE are right axis deviation of the QRS and alteration of the R:S ratio in lead V_1. These changes result from the electrocardiographic dominance of the right ventricular muscle mass. The diagnostic criteria for

RVE are summarized in Table 11-7. Note that these criteria do not include a prolongation of the QRS interval. This is because activation of even a markedly enlarged right ventricle requires no more time than does the activation of the normal left ventricle.

The electrocardiographic findings associated with RVE may resemble those of other cardiac abnormalities. Specifically, RVE must be differentiated from a normal vertical heart, RBBB, posterior wall myocardial infarction, WPW-type A, left posterior hemiblock, and pseudo-right axis deviation because of a high lateral wall myocardial infarction. The QRS duration may serve as a clue when distinguishing between RVE and RBBB. The presence of a delta wave will assist with the differentiation of RVE and WPW. Distinguishing between primary and secondary S-T, T wave changes will aid in the correct diagnosis of RVE versus myocardial infarction.

Biventricular Enlargement Electrocardiographic diagnosis of biventricular enlargement is extremely difficult, especially in adults. The electrical potential generated from the increased muscle mass of both ventricles may cancel each other so that no ECG changes indicative of ventricular enlargement are present. If one ventricle is more hypertrophied than the other, evidence of enlargement of the dominant ventricle appears. Only rarely are the signs of both left and right ventricular enlargement present on the ECG.

The diagnostic criteria of biventricular enlargement are summarized in Table 11-8.[7] These findings may be present in ECGs from individuals with various congenital lesions, cardiomyopathy, and multivalvular lesions.

Myocardial Infarction

An extended loss of blood supply to the myocardium which results in tissue death or necrosis is

Table 11-7 Diagnostic Criteria for Right Ventricular Enlargement[5 – 7]

1. Right axis deviation
2. R:S ratio in $V_1 > 1.0$ and in $V_{5-6} \leq 1.0$
3. Tall (or relatively tall) R wave in V_1
4. RR' pattern in V_1
5. Deep S waves in I, aVL, and V_{4-6}

Table 11-8 Diagnostic Criteria for Biventricular Enlargement[7]

1. Left ventricular enlargement pattern in the precordial leads and right axis deviation
2. Right ventricular enlargement pattern in the precordial leads and left axis deviation
3. Tall (or relatively tall) R waves in all precordial leads
4. Equiphasic QRS (RS pattern) complexes in the midleft precordial leads (Katz-Wachtel phenomenon)

termed *myocardial infarction (MI).* During an acute infarct, the necrotic tissue is surrounded by an area of injured myocardium and an area of ischemic myocardium (Fig. 11-69). Each of these areas of abnormality, infarction, injury, and ischemia, produces characteristic changes in the ECG which make it possible to diagnose the specific tissue abnormality.

Characteristic ECG Changes

Necrotic myocardial tissue does not have the ability to depolarize or repolarize. Leads in which the positive electrode faces the infarcted tissue, described as *indicative,* or *direct leads,* "look through" the infarcted tissue and record the electrical activity from the opposite side of the heart (Fig. 11-69). The indicative leads "see" the electrical potential move from the endocardial to the epicardial surface on the opposite myocardial wall. Because the wave of depolarization is moving away from the positive electrode, a negative deflection or Q wave is recorded on the ECG. *Reciprocal leads,* those in which the positive electrode faces the portion of the heart opposite to the infarction, record the normal endocardial to epicardial depolarization of the unaffected tissue. Because this wave of electrical potential is directed toward a positive electrode, a positive deflection or R wave is produced (Fig. 11-69). The R wave is frequently larger than normal due to the lack of opposing forces at the site of the infarct.

As noted earlier, Q waves produced by septal depolarization are normal in certain leads (Table 11-2). Q waves caused by myocardial infarction may be distinguished from normal Q waves because they are larger and last longer. Pathologic Q waves, those which are the result of myocardial infarction, are equal to or greater than 0.04 s in duration and/or are equal to or larger than 25 percent of the following R wave.

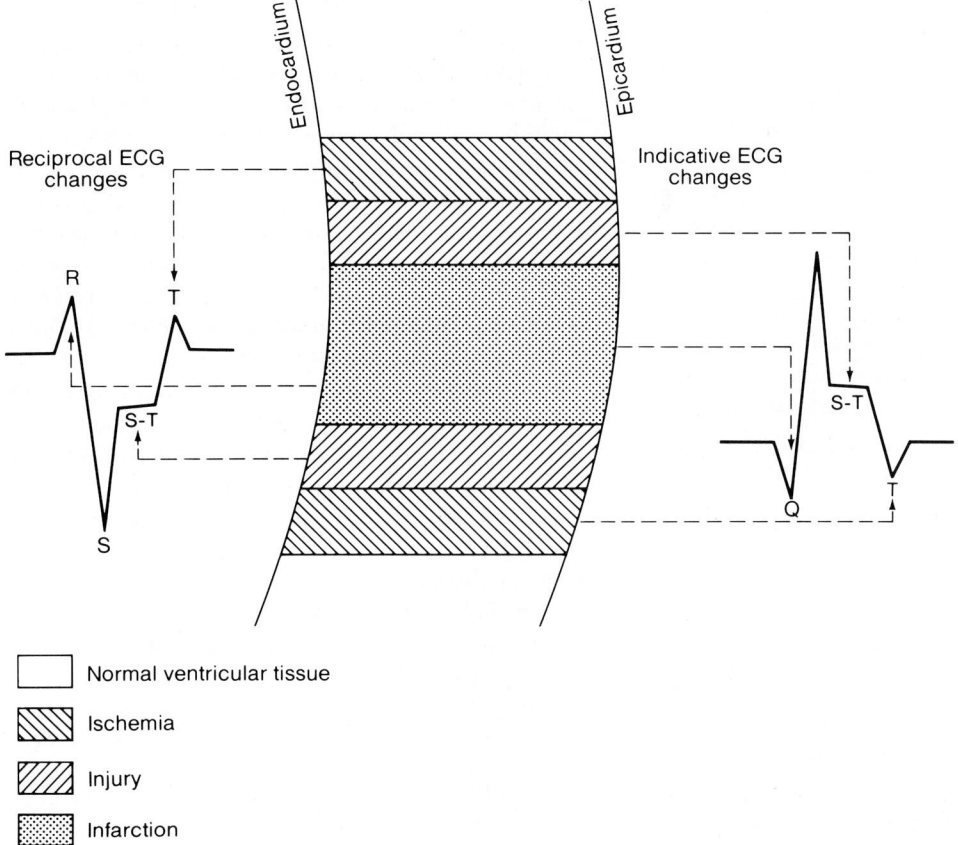

Reciprocal ECG changes

Indicative ECG changes

Figure 11-69   Transmural myocardial ischemia, injury, and infarction. During the acute myocardial infarction, the electrocardiogram discloses all three states. Indicative lead changes are shown on the right. Reciprocal lead changes are on the left.

☐ Normal ventricular tissue

▨ Ischemia

▨ Injury

▨ Infarction

The injured tissue surrounding the necrotic myocardium depolarizes incompletely and, therefore, remains electrically more positive than uninjured tissue at the end of depolarization. The relative positive electrical potential produces S-T segment elevation in the indicative leads and S-T segment depression in the reciprocal leads (Fig. 11-69). The elevated S-T segment is typically convex upward and terminates into an inverted T wave. The inverted T wave may or may not be evident, depending on the age of the infarct.

Myocardial ischemia associated with an MI manifests itself on the ECG as primary inversion of the T wave in the indicative leads. These T waves are symmetrically inverted as opposed to the asymmetrically inverted T waves associated with ventricular strain and bundle branch block. Primary in-

version of the T wave is thought to be due to the delay in the repolarization process which causes the ischemic zone to be electrically more negative than the unaffected area. The positive electrode facing the ischemic zone records an inverted T wave because it "sees" this increased negativity. Reciprocal leads record tall peaked T waves (Fig. 11-69).

The ECG changes associated with myocardial infarction can be summarized as follows:

Indicative lead changes:

1. Q waves equal to or greater than 0.04 s in duration and/or equal to or larger than 25 percent of the associated R wave
2. S-T segment elevation
3. T wave inversion

Reciprocal lead changes:

1. Tall or relatively tall R waves with the initial vector greater than 0.04 s in duration
2. S-T segment depression
3. Tall, peaked T waves

In order to diagnose a myocardial infarction with certainty, changes in the QRS complex, S-T segment, and T wave must be present.

Transmural versus Subendocardial Infarction

As discussed in Chap. 21, myocardial infarctions may be classified into two types: *transmural* and *nontransmural*. The previously described ECG changes generally apply to transmural infarcts. Subepicardial and intramural infarcts result in ECG changes very similar to those of transmural infarcts. Subendocardial infarcts, though, produce somewhat different changes and are more difficult to diagnose with certainty.

Subendocardial infarction generally refers to infarction involving less than the inner half of the total thickness of the ventricular wall. The most consistent ECG findings associated with acute subendocardial infarction are S-T segment depression and elevation of the terminal component of the upright T waves in the leads facing the epicardial surface overlying the infarcted subendocardium. QRS changes are more variable. Typically, there is no appreciable change in the QRS complex, but some patients with subendocardial infarcts do demonstrate abnormal Q waves. Because of the variability of the ECG changes associated with subendocardial infarction, it is probably best that the diagnosis of this infarct type not be made from the ECG alone.

Localization of Infarcts to Anatomic Site

The anatomic site of infarcts can be located by identifying the leads in which diagnostic characteristics of myocardial infarction appear. Generally, only the leads which exhibit QRS changes are used for this purpose. Leads in which only S-T segment and T wave changes are recorded are not usually helpful in localizing the infarct, but they may provide information regarding the extension of the injured and ischemic zones.

There are generally considered to be four major infarct sites, the anterior, lateral, inferior, and posterior walls of the left ventricle (Fig. 11-70). Anterior wall infarcts are frequently more specifically described as anteroseptal, anteroapical, anterolateral, and extensive anterior wall infarcts. Lateral infarcts are occasionally described as high lateral or superior lateral infarcts. Inferior wall infarcts are sometimes identified as diaphragmatic wall infarcts. Historically, the term *posterior* was used to describe what we now know to be inferior infarcts, so it is not uncommon to find posterior infarcts referred to as "true" posterior infarcts in order to distinguish between the old and new terms.

Infarcts localized in the anterior, lateral, and inferior walls produce indicative ECG changes on the ECG. This occurs because positive electrodes for specific leads face these infarcted sites. Posterior wall infarcts, however, are diagnosed when reciprocal ECG changes occur in the anterior leads. This is due to the fact that there are no positive electrodes facing the infarcted posterior wall; consequently, the reciprocal leads must be relied upon for diagnostic information. Following is a list of the myocardial infarction sites and the associated ECG criteria.

Anteroseptal MI—Q or QS waves in leads V_{1-3} and sometimes V_4 (Fig. 11-71)

Anteroapical (midanterior or localized anterior) MI—Q or QS waves in leads V_{2-4} with normal rS waves in lead V_1 and Q waves in leads I, aVL, and V_6 or decreased amplitude of the initial R waves in V_{1-4} (Fig. 11-72)

Anterolateral MI—Q or QS waves in leads I, aVL, and V_{4-6} (Fig. 11-73)

Extensive anterior MI—Q or QS waves in leads I, aVL, and V_{1-6} (Fig. 11-74)

Lateral (superior or high lateral) MI—Q or QS waves in leads I and aVL (Fig. 11-75)

Inferior (diaphragmatic) MI—Q or QS waves in leads II, III, and aVF (Fig. 11-76)

Posterior ("true" posterior) MI—Tall or relatively tall R waves in leads V_{1-3} with the initial R wave duration equal to or greater than 0.04 s and the R/S ratio equal to or greater than 1 (Fig. 11-77)

Myocardial infarctions of more than one area may occur simultaneously or they may occur at

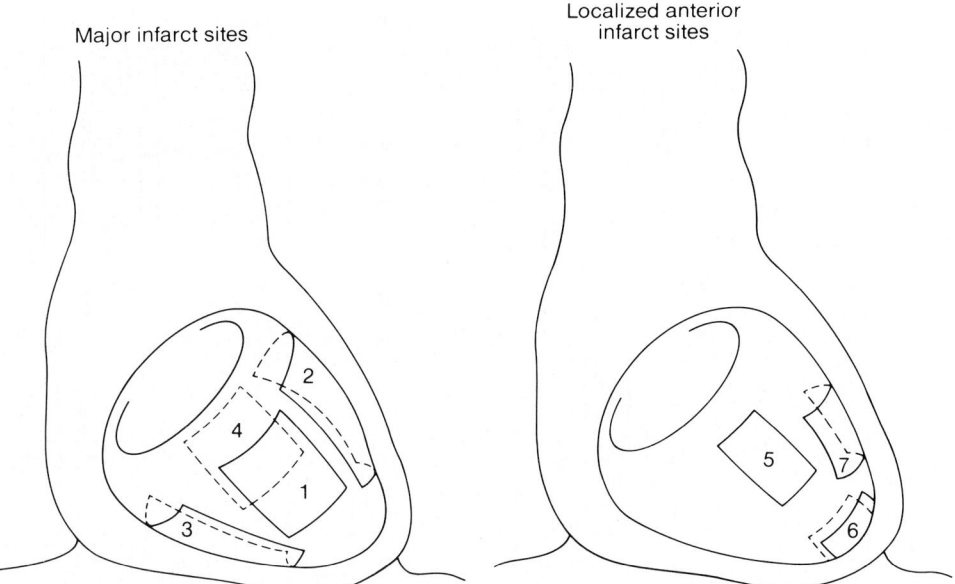

Major infarct sites

Localized anterior
infarct sites

Figure 11-70   Major sites of myocardial infarction in the left ventricle. (1) anterior wall, (2) lateral wall, (3) inferior wall, and (4) posterior wall. Anterior infarcts can be further localized to the (5) anteroseptal, (6) anteroapical, (7) anterolateral, and extensive anterior walls. *(From H. H. Friedman, Diagnostic electrocardiography and vectorcardiography, McGraw-Hill, New York, 1985, p. 247. Copyright 1985 by McGraw-Hill Book Company. Adapted by permission.)*

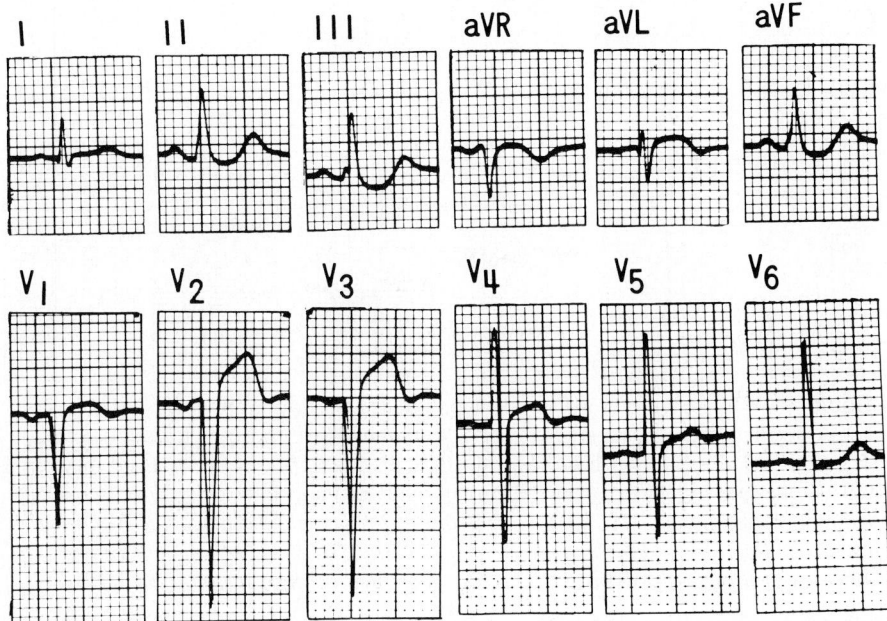

Figure 11-71   Acute strictly anterior or anteroseptal myocardial infarction. There are QS complexes in leads V_1 through V_3, with absence of Q waves in V_4 to V_6. The S-T segments are elevated in V_1 through V_5 and leads I and aVL, which indicates anterior subepicardial injury. Reciprocal S-T segment depression is present in leads II, III, and aVF. *(From H. H. Friedman, Diagnostic electrocardiography and vectorcardiography, McGraw-Hill, New York, 1985, p. 249. Copyright 1985 by McGraw-Hill Book Company. Reprinted by permission.)*

Figure 11-72 Acute localized anterior or apical myocardial infarction. A QS complex is present in lead V_3, and a qrS deflection is seen lead V_4. The R waves are preserved in leads V_5 and V_6. The S-T segment elevation in leads V_1 to V_4 indicates that the infarct is acute. Residuals of an old inferior myocardial infarction are seen in the inferior extremity leads. *(From H. H. Friedman, Diagnostic electrocardiography and vectorcardiography, McGraw-Hill, New York, 1985, p. 250. Copyright 1985 by McGraw-Hill Book Company. Reprinted by permission.)*

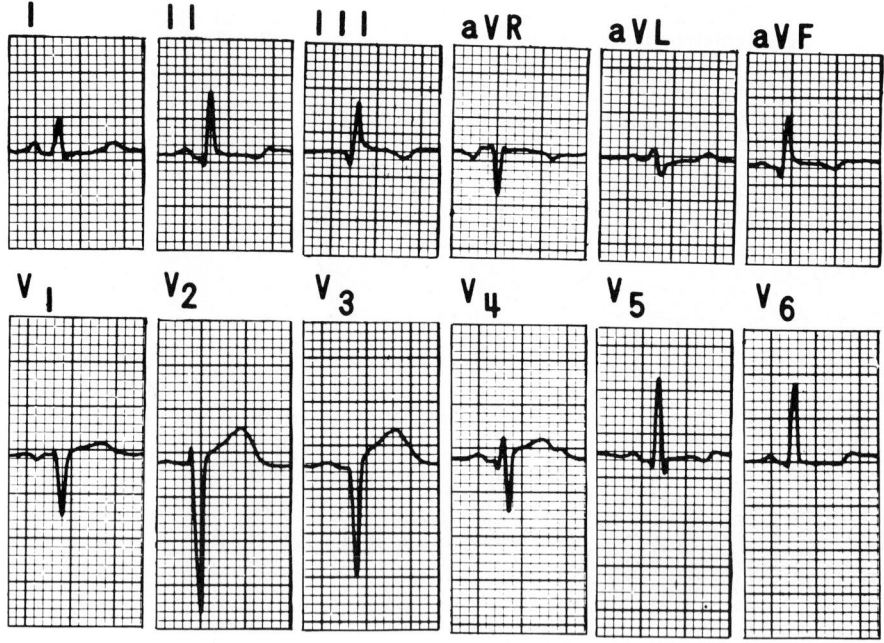

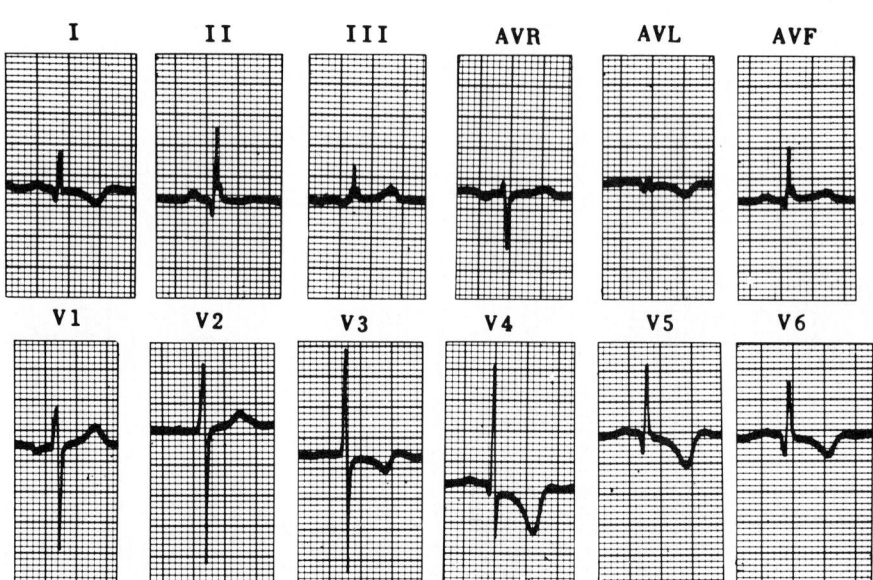

Figure 11-73 Recent anterolateral myocardial infarction. Abnormal Q waves are present in leads I, aVL, V_5, and V_6. The S-T segments are more or less isoelectric. The T waves are symmetrically inverted in leads I, aVL, and V_3 to V_6. Both the initial 0.04-s QRS and the T vectors are directed rightward and inferiorly, away from the location of the infarct. *(From H. H. Friedman, Diagnostic electrocardiography and vectorcardiography, McGraw-Hill, New York, 1985, p. 251. Copyright 1985 by McGraw-Hill Book Publishing Company. Reprinted by permission.)*

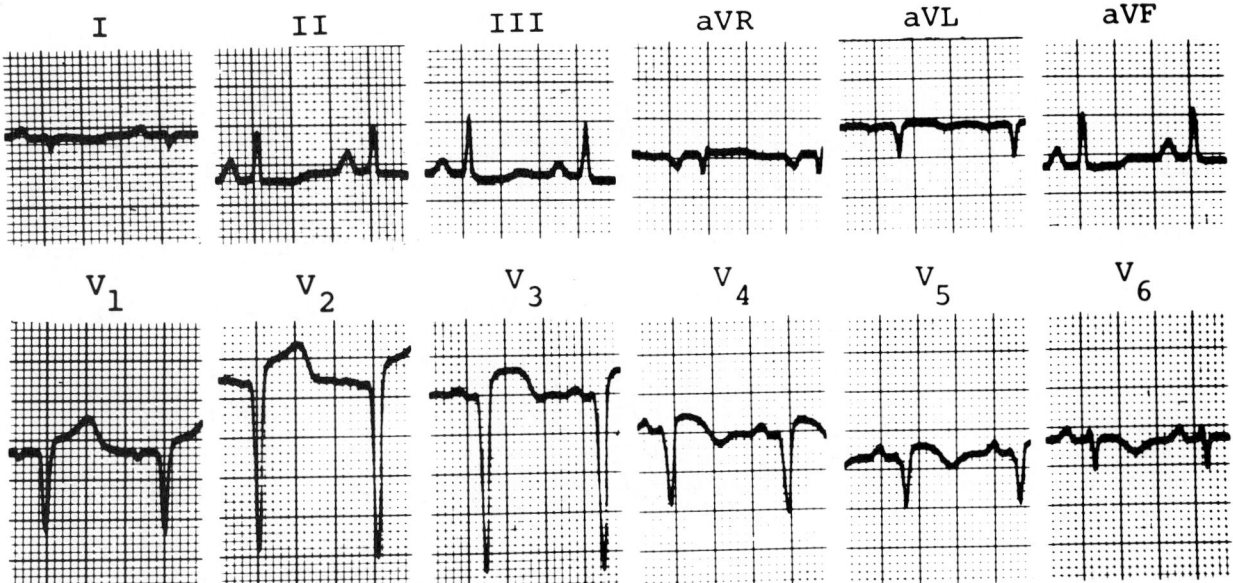

Figure 11-74   Acute extensive anterior myocardial infarction proven by autopsy. The ECG shows the loss of anterior QRS forces throughout all precordial leads with S-T segment elevation and T wave inversion. QS deflections are also present in leads I and aVL. This tracing was recorded 1 week after the onset of chest pain. The patient died of cardiogenic shock. At autopsy it was estimated that about 50 percent of the left ventricle was infarcted. *(From T. Chou, Electrocardiography in clinical practice, Grune & Stratton, Orlando, FL, 1986, p. 151. Copyright 1986 by Grune & Stratton, Inc. Reprinted by permission.)*

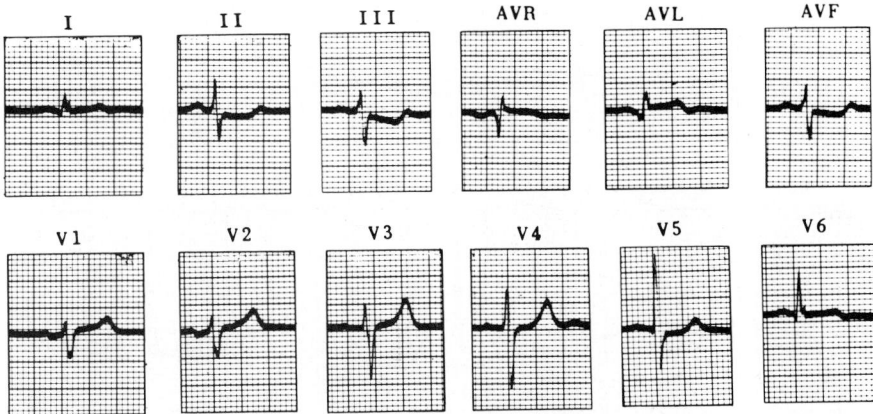

Figure 11-75   Acute superior or high lateral myocardial infarction. There are wide Q waves in leads I and aVL and broad R waves in leads III and aVF. The S-T segments are elevated in leads I and aVL, with reciprocal depression in leads II, III, and aVF. The initial QRS vector points inferiorly and rightward; the S-T vector superiorly. *(From H. H. Friedman, Diagnostic electrocardiography and vectorcardiography, McGraw-Hill, New York, 1985, p. 252. Copyright 1985 by McGraw-Hill Book Company. Reprinted by permission.)*

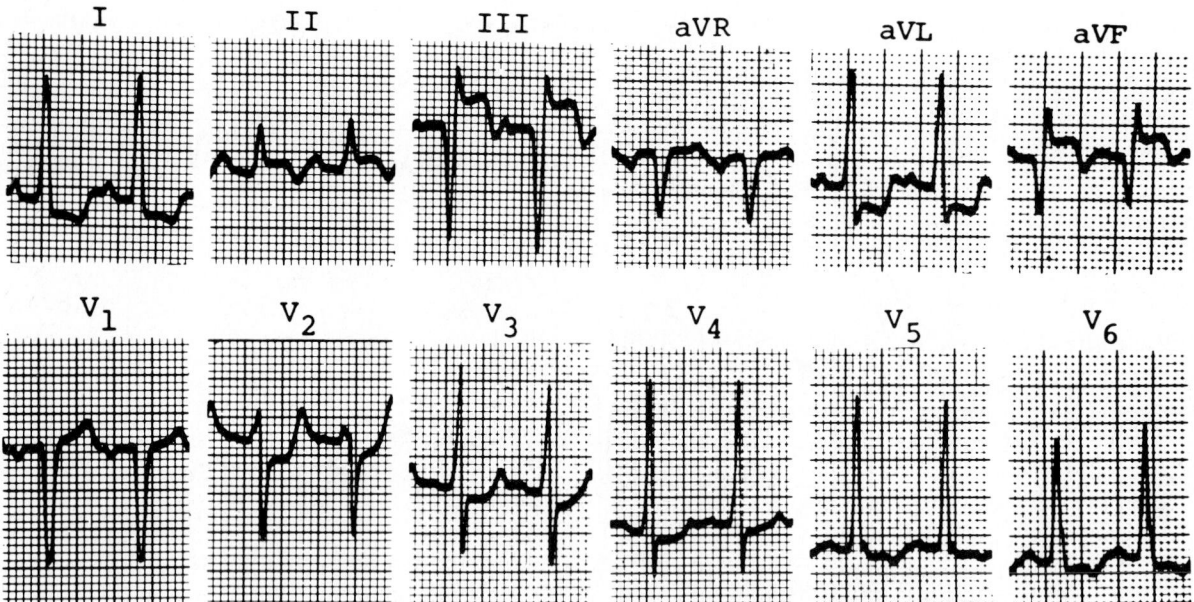

Figure 11-76 Acute inferior myocardial infarction proven by autopsy. In the ECG the P wave in lead V_1 suggests left atrial enlargement. The abnormal Q waves in leads III and aVF with S-T segment elevation and T wave inversion in leads II, III, and aVF are consistent with acute inferior myocardial infarction. There is reciprocal S-T segment depression in leads I and aVL and the precordial leads, especially leads V_2 to V_4. The high voltage of the R wave in lead aVL strongly suggests left ventricular enlargement. *(From T. Chou, Electrocardiography in clinical practice, Grune & Stratton, Orlando, FL, 1986, p. 153. Copyright 1986 by Grune & Stratton, Inc. Reprinted by permission.)*

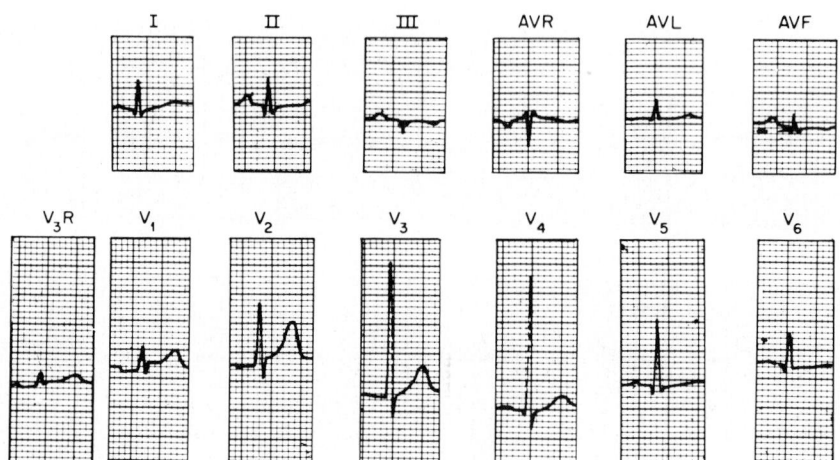

Figure 11-77 True posterior myocardial infarction. There are tall, broad R waves and tall symmetrical T waves in V_{3R}, V_1, and V_2. The patient had a typical clinical picture of myocardial infarction at the time the ECG was taken. *(From H. H. Friedman, Diagnostic electrocardiography and vectorcardiography, McGraw-Hill, New York, 1985, p. 253. Copyright 1985 by McGraw-Hill Book Company. Reprinted by permission.)*

separate times. Common infarct combinations are inferior and lateral and inferior, posterior, and lateral. Less common are simultaneous anterior and inferior infarctions. On occasion the right ventricle is the site of the infarct. This infarct can be recognized when the findings of an inferior MI are associated with S-T segment elevation in leads V_1, V_{3R} and/or V_{4R} (Fig. 11-78).

Evolutionary Changes of Acute Transmural Myocardial Infarction

Myocardial infarctions are often electrocardiographically described in stages using terms such as hyperacute, acute, recent, and old. The *hyperacute* stage is the initial stage occurring within minutes to hours after the onset of pain. Because it is a very transient stage it is often missed or observed only in the ECG obtained in the emergency department. The ECG findings are rising S-T segments with tall, peaked T waves and generally normal QRS complexes.

An *acute* infarct produces the usual S-T segment elevation and Q wave development in the direct leads and S-T segment depression and R waves in the reciprocal leads. This stage occurs within 7 to 12 h after the onset of pain and continues for several days. As the S-T segment moves toward the baseline, the inverted T wave begins to appear and the Q wave reaches its full size. The S-T segment should return to normal within the first 2 weeks after the initiation of symptoms. If S-T segment elevation persists for longer than this, one should consider the development of a ventricular aneurysm.

Recent infarcts are recognized electrocardiographically by the typical Q and T wave changes in the indicative leads. This stage occurs within weeks after the onset of pain and lasts for a few months. The T wave may remain inverted for several months or even years. *Old* infarcts are those in which the T wave has returned to normal and only the typical QRS abnormalities remain on the ECG. Occasionally the Q waves of an old infarct will disappear after several years. Because of the variability in the length of the recent stage, it may be useful to define an infarct as "old" when it is known to have existed for at least 2 months.[5]

It should be noted that none of the above stages can be precisely described or dated. It is, therefore, desirable to obtain serial ECGs and to rely on the clinical history and pertinent laboratory data of the patient so that a more accurate description can be supplied.

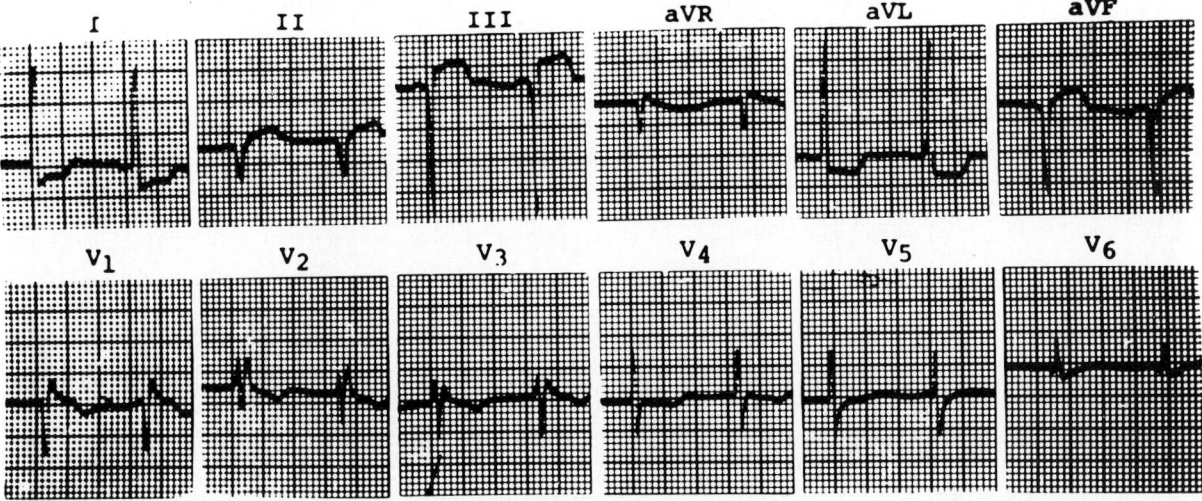

Figure 11-78   Acute right ventricular infarction associated with acute inferior left ventricular infarction proven at autopsy. The tracing shows acute inferior myocardial infarction, left ventricular enlargement, and incomplete right bundle branch block. There is also S-T segment elevation in lead V_1 to suggest right ventricular infarction. *(From T. Chou, Electrocardiography in clinical practice, Grune & Stratton, Orlando, FL, 1986, p. 156. Copyright 1986 by Grune & Stratton, Inc. Reprinted by permission.)*

Differential Diagnosis of Infarct Patterns

The ECG changes characteristic of myocardial infarction may resemble changes associated with other cardiac and noncardiac abnormalities. Therefore, a false diagnosis of myocardial infarction may be made. Following is a list of various abnormalities and the infarct pattern(s) which they may mimic.[7]

Left ventricular hypertrophy and left bundle branch block—anteroseptal, anteroapical, or inferior MIs

Chronic obstructive pulmonary disease and right ventricular hypertrophy—inferior, posterior, anteroseptal, or anteroapical MIs

Left anterior hemiblock and left axis deviation—inferior or anteroapical MIs

Cardiomyopathy—any MI pattern

Idiopathic hypertrophic subaortic stenosis (IHSS)—inferior, posterior, or inferoposterolateral MIs

Wolff-Parkinson-White syndrome—inferior, anteroseptal, or posterior MIs

Chest deformity—inferior, anteroseptal, anteroapical, or anterolateral MIs

Ventricular aneurysms, pericarditis, cerebrovascular disease, pulmonary embolism, and hyperkalemia also may create ECG changes that mimic infarcts.

Careful observation of the ECG and its recorded findings as well as close attention to the clinical history and physical examination help to prevent incorrect electrocardiographic diagnoses.

Effects of Electrolyte Imbalance

Recalling how the movement of electrically charged ions causes the action potential to occur, it is easy to understand how abnormalities in electrolyte concentrations can have an effect on the ECG. Two electrolytes in particular, calcium and potassium, can seriously alter the electrical functioning of the heart. Consequently, it is important for the critical-care nurse to recognize the effects of hypocalcemia, hypercalcemia, hypokalemia, and hyperkalemia on the ECG.

Hypocalcemia

Calcium enters the cell during phase 2 of the action potential. This phase is associated with the Q-T interval on the surface ECG (Fig. 11-4). If the concentration of calcium is low the movement of calcium into the cell will be prolonged. Consequently, a prolonged Q-T$_c$ interval is recorded on the ECG (Fig. 11-79). The degree of prolongation is inversely proportional to the calcium concentration. The Q-T$_c$ prolongation is due to S-T segment prolongation rather than to an increase in the

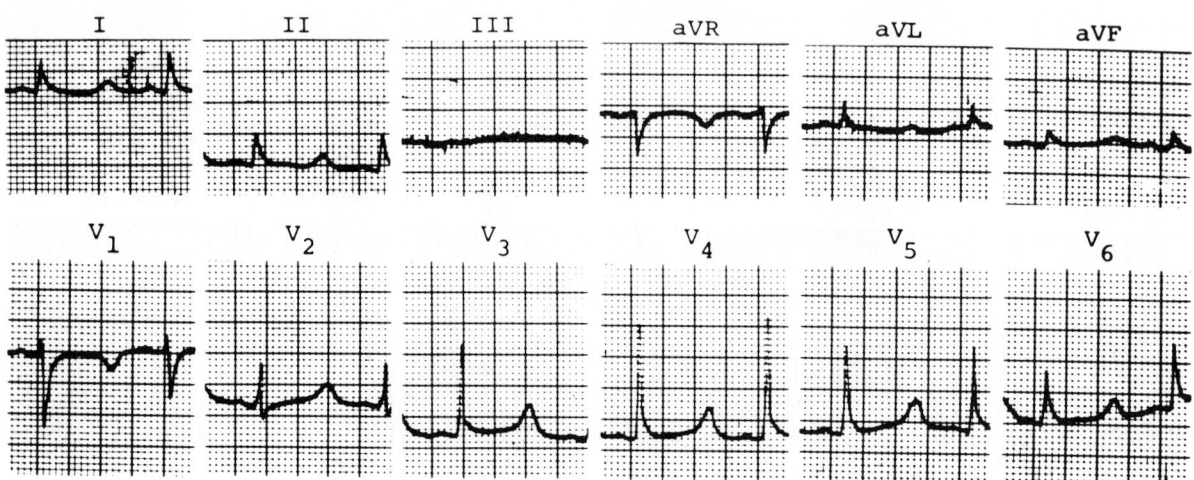

Figure 11-79 Hypocalcemia. The patient is a 69-year-old patient with uremia. The serum calcium level was 5.6 mg/100 mL. In the ECG, there is a prolongation of the Q-T interval, mainly because of lengthening of the S-T segment. *(From T. Chou, Electrocardiography in clinical practice, Grune & Stratton, Orlando, FL, 1986, p. 574. Copyright 1986 by Grune & Stratton, Inc. Reprinted by permission.)*

duration of the T wave. Morphologic changes of the T wave are common, however, and are manifested as either peaked, flattened, or sharply inverted T waves. The T wave changes may be most pronounced in the right precordial leads. Changes in the P, P-R, QRS, and U are not generally seen.

Hypercalcemia

Elevated concentrations of calcium produce shortened S-T segments on the ECG and therefore cause a decrease in the Q-T$_c$ duration (Fig. 11-80). Occasionally, the S-T segment is so short it cannot be identified on the ECG. As the calcium concentration reaches and exceeds 16 mg/100 mL, the duration of the T wave may increase, causing the Q-T$_c$ to appear normal. The morphology of the T wave generally does not change, however. The P wave and the QRS complex are generally not affected by hypercalcemia, but the U wave may increase in amplitude.

Hypokalemia

The electrocardiographic changes resulting from hypokalemia are due to an alteration of the ventricular action potential, particularly phase 3. Probably the first hint of a low potassium concentration appears when a prominent U wave is identified (Fig. 11-81). The U wave is considered to be prominent when its amplitude is greater than 1

mm or is taller than the T wave in a given lead. The cause of the change in the U wave is not well understood. Associated with the prominent U wave are S-T segment depression and decreased T wave amplitude. The changes become apparent when the serum potassium falls below 3.0 meq/L. Very low concentrations of serum potassium may cause prolongation of the QRS complex and an increase in the amplitude and duration of the P wave; however, both of these changes are uncommon. All the ECG changes of hypokalemia are usually best seen in the mid-precordial leads.

It is important to note that hypokalemia generally does not prolong the Q-T$_c$. When the Q-T$_c$ appears to be prolonged it is usually the result of an inaccurate Q-T measurement. This occurs because the U wave is superimposed on the end of the T wave or the U is mistaken for the T wave. Great care must be taken so that a Q-U interval is not recorded as a Q-T interval.

Hypokalemia is known to cause a variety of cardiac dysrhythmias. Patients are more susceptible to developing these arrhythmias when they are receiving digitalis and are hypokalemic. The incidence of arrhythmias secondary to hypokalemia alone is quite low. Supraventricular arrhythmias which may occur due to hypokalemia include paroxysmal atrial tachycardia with block, first-degree AV block, and second-degree AV block, Mobitz

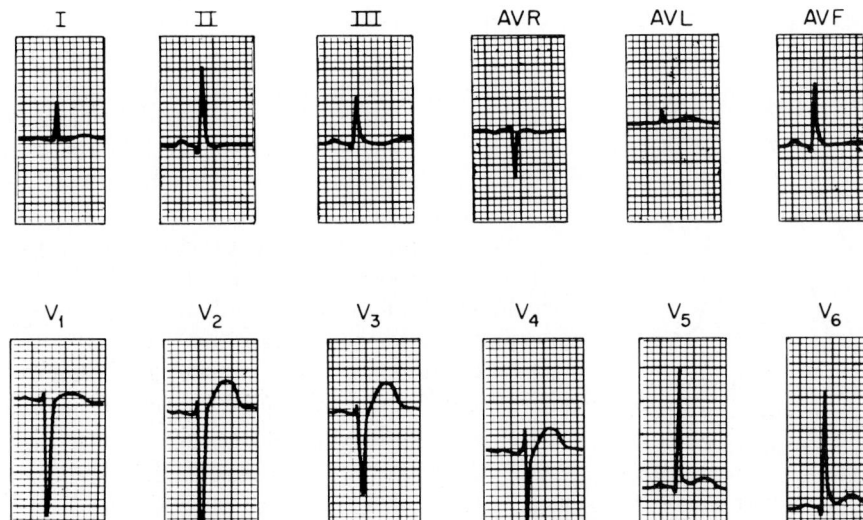

Figure 11-80 Hypercalcemia. There is a shortening of the Q-T$_c$ interval and virtual absence of the segment from the beginning of the Q to the onset of the T wave (Q-$_o$T). The serum calcium was 18.7 mg/100 mL. *(From H. H.. Friedman, Diagnostic electrocardiography and vectorcardiography, McGraw-Hill, New York, 1985, p. 346. Copyright 1985 by McGraw-Hill Book Company. Reprinted by permission.)*

Figure 11-81 Hypokalemia. The U waves are large and the T waves flattened. The T/U ratio is less than 1.0 in leads II and V_3. The U wave in V_3 exceeds 2 mm. The S-T segments have a shallow, troughlike appearance in the limb leads. The serum potassium was 2.2 mg/L. *(From H. H. Friedman, Diagnostic electrocardiography and vectorcardiography, McGraw-Hill, New York, 1985, p. 343. Copyright 1985 by McGraw-Hill Book Company. Reprinted by permission.)*

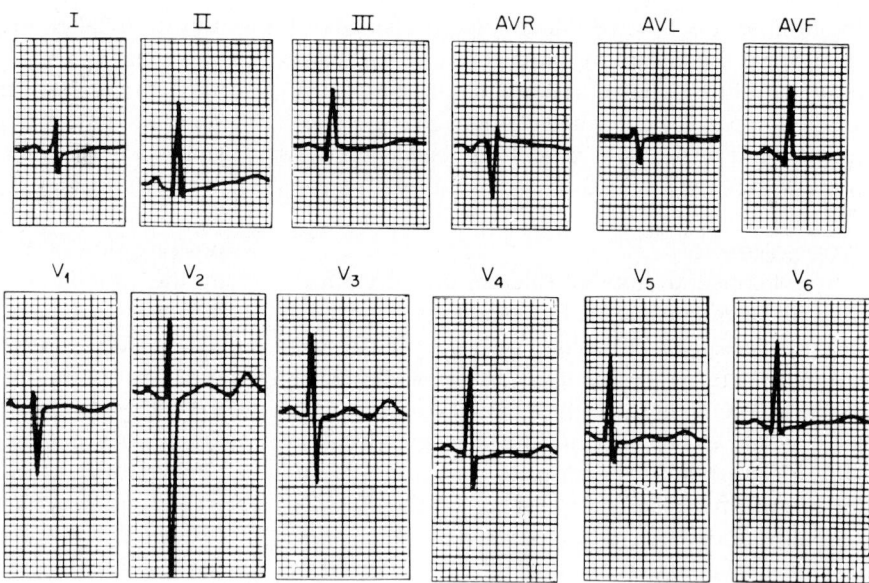

type I. Ventricular arrhythmias include premature ventricular complexes, ventricular tachycardia, and ventricular fibrillation.

Hyperkalemia

High serum potassium levels are manifested on the ECG in a variety of ways. Figure 11-82 shows the progressive changes produced by hyperkalemia. The first and probably most common ECG change

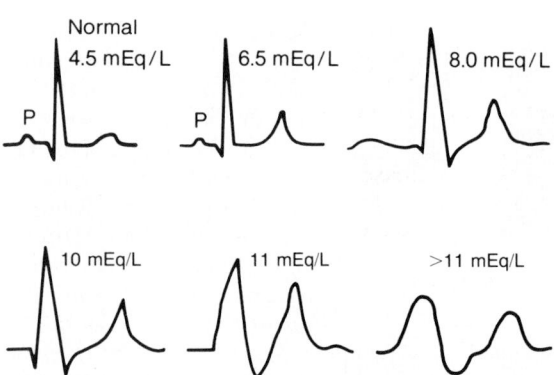

Figure 11-82 Effects of hyperkalemia on the ECG. The initial change with hyperkalemia is peaking of the T wave. With progressive elevations in serum potassium, there is loss of P waves, alteration of the S-T segment, lengthening of the QRS duration, and finally ventricular fibrillation. These changes do not necessarily occur with a specific serum potassium level. See text for further discussion.

is that of narrow, tall, peaked, tent-shaped T waves. This change, which may be seen in all leads, occurs when the serum potassium level is from 5.5 to 6.5 meq/L (Fig. 11-83). As the levels rise from 6.5 to 7.5 meq/L, the morphology of the P, S-T, and QRS begins to change; the P wave amplitude decreases, the S-T segment is either depressed or elevated, and the QRS widens slightly. At advanced levels of hyperkalemia, 7.5 to 8.5 meq/L, the P wave flattens and becomes broader, the QRS widens markedly, and various forms of AV nodal and bundle branch blocks appear. When the serum potassium exceeds 8.5 meq/L, the P wave disappears; the QRS continues to broaden, resulting in various forms of intraventricular conduction blocks; and ventricular arrhythmias, namely ventricular tachycardia, flutter, and fibrillation, and idioventricular rhythm followed by ventricular standstill may appear.

As is evident from the previous discussion, electrolyte imbalances can seriously affect the electrical function of the heart and, if not diagnosed and treated effectively, can lead to death. The critical-care nurse should be constantly alert for electrolyte imbalances and should monitor the ECG for any associated changes.

Effects of Drug Therapy

The administration of various cardiac and noncardiac drugs can result in direct changes in the cardiac

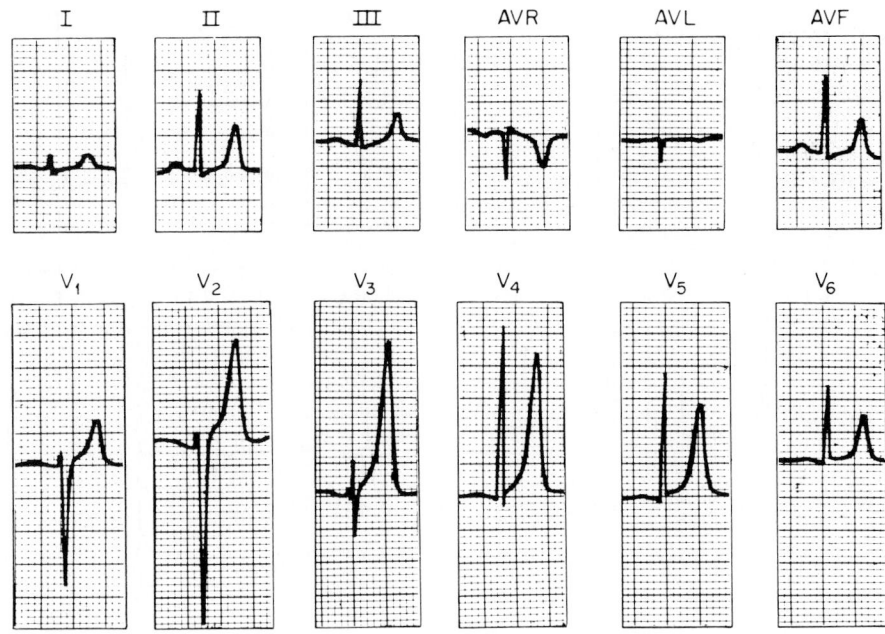

Figure 11-83 Hyperkalemia. The T waves are typically narrow, symmetrical, tall, and peaked. The serum potassium was 6.2 meq/L. *(From H. H. Friedman, Diagnostic electrocardiography and vectorcardiography, McGraw-Hill, New York, 1985, p. 339. Copyright 1985 by McGraw-Hill Book Company. Reprinted by permission.)*

action potential and, consequently, in the ECG. Many of the ECG drug effects are positive or therapeutic. Unfortunately, though, some effects can mimic pathologic changes from cardiac disease processes, thus leading to incorrect diagnoses, or can cause serious impulse formation and/or conduction abnormalities which if not recognized and treated can lead to the death of the patient. The critical-care nurse should be aware of the drugs most likely to alter the ECG and should monitor the patient for the associated changes.

Digitalis

Digitalis, through either direct or indirect effects on the heart, can alter in varying degrees the automaticity, excitability, and conductivity of cardiac cells. These effects are the result of the drug's ability to inhibit the active transport of sodium and potassium across the cell membrane (direct effect), increase vagal tone (indirect effect), or both.[5] Some of these effects occur with therapeutic doses and others occur with toxic doses.

Therapeutic doses of digitalis decrease automaticity of pacemaker cells in the SA node and the atria and increase automaticity in the AV junction and the His-Purkinje system. Digitalis-induced junctional and ventricular tachyarrhythmias are the result of the latter action. The drug in usual dosages

decreases excitability in atrial and His-Purkinje cells but increases ventricular excitability. Conductivity of atrial and AV junctional cells is depressed by therapeutic doses of the drug. Digitalis speeds the repolarization in the ventricular myocardium, resulting in S-T segment depression and flattened T waves in epicardial leads with upright QRS complexes. Therapeutic digitalis effects on the normal ECG (Fig. 11-84) can be summarized as:

1. Depression of the S-T segment
2. Depressed T wave amplitude, which may result in diphasic or negative T waves
3. Shortening of the Q-T_c interval
4. Slightly increased U wave amplitude

The ECG changes produced by digitalis are usually best observed in leads II, III, aVF, and the left precordial leads.

In abnormal ECGs, digitalis may produce prolongation of the PR interval as well as the other changes noted for normal ECGs. Digitalis may slow the ventricular rate in atrial fibrillation or terminate the arrhythmia. However, it is important to note that the drug produces varying effects in the ECG when other atrial tachyrhythms are present. The arrhythmias may be stopped, continued, or accelerated. In other words, atrial tachycardia may change to flutter, to fibrillation, and then to sinus rhythm.

Figure 11-84   Digitalis effect. The S-T segments are depressed and concave upward. The T waves are of decreased amplitude. The Q-T interval is shortened. *(From H. H. Friedman, Diagnostic electrocardiography and vectorcardiography, McGraw-Hill, New York, 1985, p. 329. Copyright 1985 by McGraw-Hill Book Company. Reprinted by permission.)*

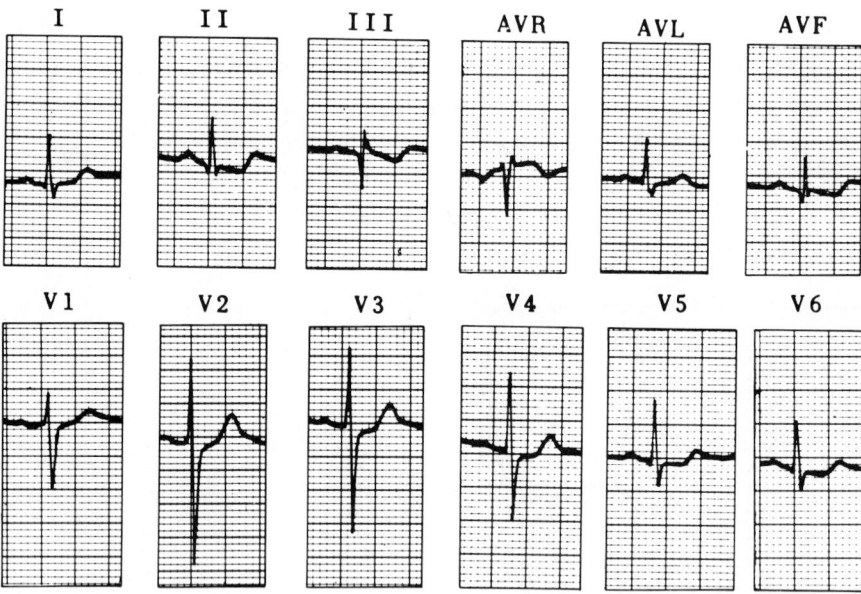

Toxic levels of digitalis can cause increased automaticity in the SA node and atrial pacemaker cells. Sinoatrial conductibility is impaired by high drug levels and the ventricular refractory period is often shortened. Toxic effects of the drug may produce a great number and variety of arrhythmias, including NJT, VPCs, sinus bradycardia, Mobitz type I AV block, AT with varying block, APCs, JPCs, SA block, SA arrest, MAT, atrial flutter or fibrillation, PVT, VF or flutter, and VS. Therapeutic measures for these arrhythmias are discussed in the section of this chapter which pertains to the specific rhythm disorders.

Quinidine

Quinidine is a Class I antiarrhythmic agent which has a depressant effect on the heart. Its primary electrophysiologic effects are: (1) little or no change in automaticity of the SA node; (2) depressed atrial automaticity, excitability, and conductivity and prolonged atrial refractoriness; (3) little or no effect on AV conduction; (4) depressed automaticity, slowed conduction velocity, and prolonged refractoriness of the His-Purkinje system; and (5) depressed ventricular conductivity and excitability. Its therapeutic effects on the ECG (Fig. 11-85) can be summarized as:

1. Notched, flat, or inverted T waves, usually asso-

ciated with prolonged T wave duration and increased U wave amplitude
2. Prolonged Q-T_c intervals
3. Absent S-T segment elevation or depression
4. Slightly widened and notched P waves
5. Slightly prolonged P-R intervals

Quinidine can also produce toxic effects which may or may not be related to dosage. Ventricular arrhythmias secondary to quinidine, for example, are not dose-dependent and are probably caused by reentry. Other ECG disturbances produced by the toxic effects of quinidine are: varying degrees of AV block, intraatrial block and/or atrial standstill, marked Q-T prolongation, widening of the QRS complex, and ventricular tachyarrhythmias, particularly torsades de pointes.

Other Drugs

Other antiarrhythmic agents and drugs which act on the autonomic nervous system can produce changes in the ECG. Appendix A describes the various antiarrhythmic drugs and their effects on the electrophysiologic properties of the heart. Sympathomimetic drugs enhance automaticity, excitability, and conductivity, whereas sympathetic blocking agents have the opposite effect.

Phenothiazines and antidepressant drugs such as amitriptyline and imipramine depress intracar-

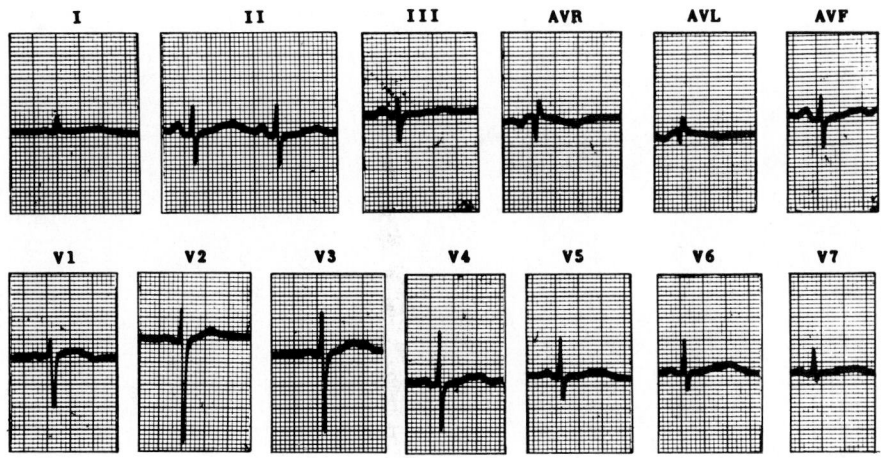

Figure 11-85 Quinidine effect. The Q-T interval is prolonged, the T waves are flattened, and the U waves are prominent. *(From H. H. Friedman, Diagnostic electrocardiography and vectorcardiography, McGraw-Hill, New York, 1985, p. 332. Copyright 1985 by McGraw-Hill Book Company. Reprinted by permission.)*

diac conduction. With high doses, the S-T segment may become depressed and the T wave flattens or is inverted. Q-T$_c$ prolongation, increased U wave amplitude, AV and ventricular conduction defects, and cardiac arrhythmias may also be produced.

Conclusion

As the previous discussion illustrates, a number of pathologic and physiologic alterations can have an effect on cardiac electrical activity. It is the responsibility of the critical-care nurse to monitor for and recognize these effects and to initiate appropriate therapy when necessary. This chapter has provided information to prepare the nurse for these actions.

References

1. Guyton, A. C. (1981). *Textbook of medical physiology.* Philadelphia: Saunders.

2. Marriott, H. J. L. (1983). *Practical electrocardiography.* Baltimore: Williams & Wilkins.

3. Wells, J. L., MacLean, W. A. H., James, T. N., & Waldo, A. L. (1979). Characterization of atrial flutter. Studies in man after open heart surgery using fixed atrial electrodes. *Circulation, 60,* 665–673.

4. Wells, J. L., Karp, R. B., Kouchoukos, N. T., Maclean, W. A. H., James, T. N., & Waldo, A. L. (1978). Characterization of atrial fibrillation in man: Studies following open heart surgery. *PACE, 1,* 422–437.

5. Chou, T. C. (1986). *Electrocardiography in clinical practice.* Orlando, FL: Grune & Stratton.

6. Friedman, H. H. (1985). *Diagnostic electrocardiography and vectorcardiography.* New York: McGraw-Hill.

7. Chung, E. K. (1985). *Electrocardiography. Practical applications with vectorial principles.* Norwalk, CT: Appleton-Century-Crofts.

8. Dessertenne, F. (1966). La tachycardie ventriculaire a deux foyers opposes variable. *Archives Mal Coeur, 59,* 263–272.

9. Romhilt, D. W., & Estes, E. H. (1968). A point score system for the ECG diagnosis of left ventricular hypertrophy. *American Heart Journal, 75,* 752–758.

12 Nutrition

Sheila M.
 Campbell

In 1974, Butterworth described the effects of malnutrition on hospitalized patients.[1] Following this historic article, several studies were published which documented the extent of malnutrition that existed at that time in medical and surgical patient populations. The dire consequences of malnutrition in critically ill patients, including pneumonia, wound dehiscence, increased rate of sepsis, failure to wean from respirators, and, ultimately, increased mortality, have been chronicled in the medical literature.

During the last 15 years, nutritional support has become an accepted part of medical care because of development of special techniques for delivery of nutrients. Recognition of malnutrition as a co-morbidity factor under the newly established Prospective Payment System for Medicare beneficiaries has also heightened awareness of the necessity to provide nutritional support to patients. This enlightened view is reflected by the increasing number of hospitals which have established interdisciplinary nutrition support teams. Nutritional care of patients can be accomplished in the absence of a formal nutritional support team by integrating principles of nutrition support into daily care of patients.

The purpose of this chapter is to provide information regarding normal nutritional requirements and the ways in which these are altered by disease and critical illness. Nutritional status assessment techniques and risk factors are defined. Specialized modalities for supplying nutrients are described. This knowledge should enhance the ability of the nurse to address nutritional needs of the critically ill patient.

Special acknowledgment is given to T. G. Campbell, L.P.N.; Margaret Campbell; Ella Schwartz, R.N.; and Marcia Nahikian-Nelms, M.Ed., R.D., for their assistance in preparation of this manuscript.

Normal Nutritional Requirements

The intricate biochemistry of nutrition approaches the metaphysical. However, there are some constants which facilitate understanding and are useful in daily practice.

Energy

Every organism has an obligate, minimum need for energy. This energy requirement is the amount necessary to carry on minimal, necessary body processes. *Basal energy expenditure (BEE)* is defined as the energy required to maintain life-sustaining mechanical, transport, and synthetic processes while the body is completely at rest, at standard room temperature, and in a postabsorptive state. Basal energy expenditure can be measured by indirect calorimetry. Metabolic measurement carts which indicate a patient's oxygen consumption and expression of carbon dioxide are a means of quantifying BEE by indirect calorimetry. Use of metabolic carts to measure BEE is increasing in research and intensive care units, but in most clinical settings, BEE is still usually estimated through the use of the Harris-Benedict formula (Fig. 12-1).[2] This formula provides an estimate of BEE which takes into account the effects of age, sex, and body size. Basal energy expenditure is the basis on which total energy requirements are estimated. In the clinical setting, *resting energy expenditure (REE)* is calculated; this takes into account energy requirements for minimal activity and metabolism of nutrients. Resting energy expenditure is expressed as BEE + 10–15 percent.

Basal energy expenditure is elevated by disease and critical illness (Table 12-1). Energy needs of the critically ill patient are primary and, in the face of deficit calorie input, will be met by catab-

BEE for males = 66 + (13.7 x W) + (5 x H) — 6.8 x A)
BEE for females = 665 + (9.6 x W) + (1.7 x H) — 4.7 x A)
W = body weight in kg
H = body height in cm
A = age in years

Figure 12-1   The Harris Benedict formula for calculating basal energy expenditure.

olism of organ and muscle protein and adipose tissue. Use of lean body mass as an energy source represents a potentially fatal cost to the critically ill patient, since every body protein has a function. As body protein is catabolized to meet energy requirements, body function is lost.

Protein

Protein has many functions in the body. It is a vital structural component of muscle and organ tissue, erythrocytes, white blood cells, hormones, and antibodies. Proteins play a role in metabolism, as enzymes and coenzymes. Serum proteins regulate fluid and acid-base balance by maintaining osmotic pressure and serving in buffer systems.

The most important function of dietary protein is to provide amino acid precursors for synthesis of these vital body proteins. There are 20 to 25 naturally occurring amino acids. Eight of these amino acids are termed *essential* since they are necessary to prevent deficiency disease symptoms. Essential amino acids cannot be made by the body, but must be consumed from the diet. Nonessential amino acids are as necessary for synthesis of new body proteins as are essential amino acids. How-

ever, nonessential amino acids can be made in the body from ingested substrates.

In order for the body to create new proteins, substrate amino acids must be present in appropriate amounts and in specific ratios. The *all or none rule* states that the body cannot synthesize protein molecules required for growth, repair, or maintenance if all precursor amino acids are not present in favorable ratios. The all or none rule accentuates the importance of providing adequate nonprotein calories along with dietary protein so that protein can be used to create new body proteins rather than be used as an energy source.

The recommended daily allowance (RDA) for protein intake in adults is 0.8 g protein per kilogram of body weight. Protein requirements for the critically ill patient are usually greater than the RDA requirement levels (Table 12-2). There are a number of factors which contribute to the elevated protein needs in critically ill patients, including depletion of body protein through tissue losses from injury, surgery, and/or starvation; and drainage of serous protein through fistulas, open wounds, and/or abscesses. Catabolism of body protein is enhanced during illness or trauma due to the accompanying increase of BEE, and presence of stress-related catabolic hormones. Certain therapeutic modalities including steroid and chemo-

Table 12-1   Energy Requirement during Various Critical Illnesses

Condition	Energy Requirements
Major surgery or trauma	35–40 kcal/kg IBW*
Head injury	35–50 kcal/kg IBW*
Acute or chronic renal failure	35–45 kcal kg dry body weight
Cancer	35 kcal/kg IBW*
Chronic obstructive pulmonary disease	25–35 kcal/kg IBW*

* IBW = ideal body weight.

Table 12-2   Protein Requirements during Various Critical Illnesses

Condition	Protein Requirements
Burns	1–4 g/kg IBW*
Cardiac cachexia	1.5–2 g/kg IBW*
Major surgery or trauma	1.5–3.5 g/kg IBW* (acute)
	1.5 g/kg IBW* (stable)
	14–22% of total kcal needs
Head injury	
Renal failure	
Peritoneal dialysis	1 g/kg dry body weight
Chronic ambulatory peritoneal dialysis	1.2–1.5 g/kg dry body weight
Hemodialysis	1.5 g/kg dry body weight
Cancer	1–1.5 g/kg IBW*
Chronic obstructive pulmonary disease	1.5 g/kg IBW*

* IBW = ideal body weight.

therapy, other drug therapies, and radiation also enhance loss of body proteins.

Often, patients who suffer protein losses are not provided sufficient amounts of nonprotein calories, which increase protein requirements because in this case protein is used as an energy source as well as for synthesis of new body protein.

Carbohydrate

The major function of dietary carbohydrate is as a protein-sparing energy source. Dietary carbohydrate provides 4 kcal per gram. Carbohydrate in the form of glucose is the only energy source which can be used by the central nervous system, red and white blood cells, neutrophils, and fibroblasts. These cells are termed *obligate glycolyzers.* This has special significance for the critically ill patient since obligate glycolyzer cells are found at the frontiers of wounds and in granulating tissue. If insufficient carbohydrate is available to meet glucose demands of glycolyzer cells, protein will be catabolized (via gluconeogenesis) to supply glucose.

No RDA for carbohydrate has been established. However, it has been recommended that a minimum of 50 to 100 g of digestible carbohydrate be consumed daily to prevent ketosis. Because glucose is the fuel of choice for many cells which are important for recovery of the critically ill patient, these patients may require much more than the minimal amount of carbohydrate.

Fat

Dietary fat is a concentrated source of energy. Fats provide 9 kcal per gram. Fats are also important as sources of fat-soluble vitamins and the essential fatty acids, linolenic and linoleic acids. Linolenic and linoleic acids must be provided from the diet or other exogenous sources, because they cannot be manufactured by the body. Although it is unusual for adults to develop symptoms of essential fatty acid deficiency, patients maintained on fat-free parenteral nutritional solutions or tube feeding formulas having very low fat content are at risk of developing symptoms of essential fatty acid deficiency.

There is no specific dietary recommendation for fat. However, adequate amounts must be con-

sumed so that requirements for essential fatty acids are met. These requirements can be met if 1 to 2 percent of total dietary calories are provided by fat. Although fat provides more than twice the energy per gram of carbohydrate, fat is not a source of glucose. This has special significance for the critically ill patient who requires glucose to fuel glycolyzer cells. Additionally, the ability of the critically ill patient to metabolize and use large amounts of fat may be impaired due to altered circulating levels of certain hormones and enzymes.

Vitamins

Vitamins do not supply energy or nitrogen to the body but are important in metabolic reactions and are required for growth and maintenance of tissue. Vitamins are classified as *fat-soluble* (vitamins A, D, E, and K), or *water-soluble* (vitamins C, B-12, niacin, riboflavin, thiamine, B-6, and folacin). Most vitamins cannot be synthesized by the body and must be provided by the diet or other exogenous sources. Exceptions to this are vitamins K, thiamine, folacin, and B-12, which can be synthesized in varying amounts by microorganisms present in the human gut; and niacin and vitamin A, which can be formed in the body if their precursors are present. Vitamins are essential to prevention of a variety of vitamin deficiency diseases. These diseases are not common among the general American population, but symptoms may occur in hospitalized patients who have greater than normal needs for vitamins or who are supported by nutritional solutions which do not meet requirements.

The RDAs for vitamins are expected to reflect average requirements for most healthy adults. Specific requirements for each vitamin required by critically ill patients are unknown. It *is* known that requirements for intravenously administered vitamins are different from the RDA for orally administered vitamins, and standards for IV dosages of vitamins have been established.[3] This has special significance for critically ill patients, since often their nutritional requirements are met by parenteral feeding.

Minerals and Trace Elements

Twenty-one minerals are known to be essential to human nutriture. Minerals which are required in very small amounts are referred to as *trace elements*. Minerals function in the body as constituents of enzymes and hormones, and as structural components. They have important roles in regulating metabolism, acid-base, and fluid balance. Minerals cannot be synthesized by the body and must be provided by the diet. Recommended daily allowances are established for calcium, phosphorus, magnesium, iron, zinc, and iodine but because there is less information regarding requirements for other minerals, no RDAs have been established for them.

Because minerals play an integral role in regulating body processes, it is probable that the critically ill patient may require amounts which vary from the RDAs or suggested dietary intakes. It is wise to closely monitor a patient's serum levels of minerals and supplement as necessary.

Nutritional Risk Factors

Frequently patients enter the hospital in a marginal nutritional status. In addition, disease, injury, and surgery cause metabolic stress that elevates protein and calorie needs of patients. Studies show that up to 50 percent of patients develop malnutrition during their hospital stay.[4-6] Malnutrition has catastrophic effects on the ability of the critically ill patient to tolerate and recover from illness or injury. This is because the body cannibalizes its own tissues to provide energy needed to meet elevated demands for REE. When autocannibalism occurs, new body proteins are not synthesized; plasma proteins are depleted, impairing immunocompetence, so the patient is at risk for infection; and structural proteins are not produced, so wounds do not heal.

The most common types of malnutrition occurring in the critically ill population are *marasmus* and *kwashiorkor*. Marasmus, or severe cachexia, is a chronic condition characterized by wasting of body fat and muscle tissue, and results from deficient intake of both calories and protein. Marasmus is easily diagnosed by clinical examination. The marasmic patient does require nutritional repletion, but is likely to withstand short periods of metabolic stress because immunocompetence and wound healing ability are relatively intact. If nutritional insults are prolonged, the marasmic patient is at a particular disadvantage because he or she does not have significant reserves of endogenous nutritional substrates on which to draw.

Kwashiorkor is the result of acute protein deficiency and can develop in as short a period as 2 weeks. Typically, patients who develop kwashiorkor are those undergoing acute metabolic stress and being supported on protein-free intravenous dextrose solutions. Development of kwashiorkor is a grim prognostic indicator for the critically ill patient because of associated incompetence of the immune system. Impairment of the immune system is reflected by depressed values for total lymphocytes, and lack of reactivity to skin test antigens. Immunoincompetence creates the potential for development of postoperative sepsis. Kwashiorkor is more lethal to the critically ill patient than marasmus, and is more difficult to diagnose. The patient appears well-nourished because muscle and fat stores remain intact. Diagnosis depends on evaluation of laboratory data. Kwashiorkor can be diagnosed when total lymphocyte count is less than 1500/mm³, and serum albumin is less than 2.8 g/100 mL. The levels of circulating plasma proteins (such as lymphocytes, albumin, and transferrin) are rapidly depleted because of their short half-life. Because exogenous protein is not available for synthesis of replacement proteins, circulating levels rapidly fall. Nutritional support of the patient with kwashiorkor is vital to recovery. Without adequate nutritional input, the patient is at increased risk of sepsis, development of complications, and, ultimately, death.

Because the presence of malnutrition may increase the incidence of morbidity and mortality for patients experiencing metabolic stress, especially when imposed on poor nutritional status, it behooves health care professionals to identify patients who are at risk of developing nutritional deficiency in order to prevent malnutrition-related complications. Many risk factors can be identified during nursing assessment. Inquiries regarding the ability of the patient to ingest an adequate oral diet; history of and/or impending drug treatments, radiation, and/or surgery; presence of conditions of nutrient loss or increased nutrient need; and over- or underweight or unexplained changes in weight (Table 12-3) can be useful in identifying patients who may develop complications after surgery, ill-

Table 12-3 Nutritional Risk Factors

Presence of the following conditions or observations indicates the potential for malnutrition in a patient.

General

Are conditions which cause nutrient loss (e.g., malabsorption syndromes, draining abscesses or wounds, protracted diarrhea, etc.) present?

Are conditions in which there is an increased need for nutrients (such as fever, thermal injury, trauma, surgery, sepsis, chemo- or radiation therapy, etc.) present?

Has the patient been NPO for 10 days or more?

Does the patient describe food allergies, lactose intolerance, or limited food preferences? Is the patient more than 120 or less than 80 percent of ideal body weight, or had recent unexplained weight change?

Is the patient on a modified diet such as clear or full liquid, or one restricted in sodium, calories, protein, and/or carbohydrate?

Is the patient receiving tube feeding or parenteral nutritional solutions?

Gastrointestinal (GI)

Does the patient complain of nausea, indigestion, vomiting, diarrhea, or constipation?

Does the patient have glossitis, stomatitis, or esophagitis?

Does the patient have mechanical difficulties with chewing or swallowing?

Does the patient have any fistulas?

Does the patient have a partial or total GI obstruction?

What is the patient's dental status (edentulous? state of repair?)

Cardiovascular

Does the patient have ascites or edema?

Is the patient able to perform activities of daily living?

Genitourinary

Does input approximately equal output?

Does the patient have an ostomy?

Is the patient on hemo- or peritoneal dialysis?

Respiratory

Is the patient receiving mechanical ventilatory support?

Is the patient receiving oxygen via nasal prongs?

Integument

Does the patient have pressure areas on sacrum, hips, ankles, etc.?

Does the patient have rashes or dermatitis?

Are mucous membranes dry or pale?

Extremities

Does the patient have pedal edema?

Is the patient cachexic (evidenced by decreased skin turgor, reduced buccal fat pads, or general marasmic appearance)?

ness, or injury which are secondary to malnutrition. Patients who exhibit a number of nutritional risk factors are candidates for more extensive assessment of nutritional status.

Nutritional Assessment

Nutritional assessment is the thorough evaluation of major body compartments to assess protein and energy status. This evaluation is accomplished through the use of anthropometric measurements, laboratory data, and clinical examination (Fig. 12-2).

Lean Body Mass

Height, weight, midarm circumference, and calculation of midarm muscle circumference are anthropometric measurements used to evaluate lean body mass. It is accepted practice to compare the patient's values to standard values. However, these standards do not allow for individual differences and may be

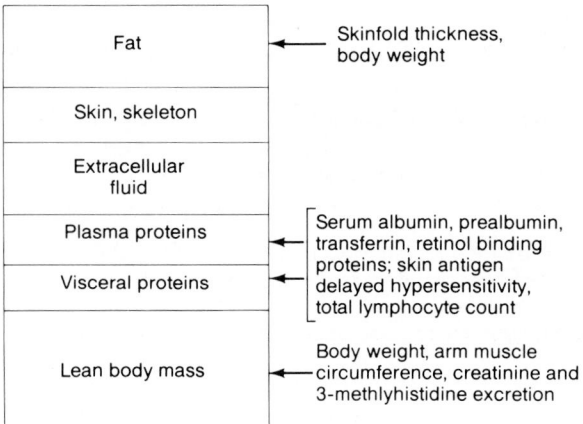

Figure 12-2 Parameters important in assessment of nutritional status.

a source of error. It is more valuable to use the usual status of the patient as the reference for initial and serial anthropometric measurements.

A 24-h urine collection for analysis of creatinine and 3-methylhistidine, metabolites of muscle catabolism excreted in the urine, provides biochemical data useful in assessing muscle protein turnover. A predictable amount of these metabolites is excreted daily. Total urinary excretion falls, in relation to declining lean body mass, which occurs during malnutrition. Creatinine-to-height ratio (*creatinine height index*) is calculated by dividing the amount of creatinine actually excreted during a 24-h period by the predicted value. A creatinine height index of less than 80 percent indicates depletion of lean body mass.

The nurse must assure that a complete 24-h urine collection is made. If the collection is incomplete, a false high turnover rate for muscle protein may be assumed. Since excretion of creatinine and 3-methylhistidine depends on renal function, a potential for error exists in cases of impaired renal function.

Energy Stores

Estimation of adequacy of fat or energy stores is accomplished by evaluation of body weight and skinfold measurements. Body weight should be expressed as a percentage of usual weight so that a potential error is avoided which may arise from

comparing a patient's weight values to standard weight values. Rapidity of weight loss is particularly important to assess, since nutritional status of the critically ill patient is extremely labile. It is important, whenever possible, to weigh the patient on admission and at routine intervals, at the same time of day and using the same scales, so that changes in weight are recognized and monitored. Measurement of skinfold thickness is another index of body energy stores. Skinfold measurements are taken using calipers. Consistent and meticulous technique is required for reliable measurements. The patient's values for skinfold thickness should be interpreted in relation to other anthropometric measurements.

Visceral Protein

Visceral protein status is assessed by evaluating serum concentrations of certain transport proteins. Serum albumin, transferrin, prealbumin, and retinol-binding protein have been used to assess visceral protein status because of their short half-life. These plasma proteins reflect protein malnutrition because their serum concentrations fall rapidly in the face of protein deficiency. Serum albumin and transferrin levels are most commonly used in the clinical setting because they are more easily obtained and their half-life is sufficient to reflect protein depletion while being less affected by medications, therapies, and the general clinical condition of the patient. Serum albumin and transferrin concentrations of less than 3.0 g/100 mL and 200 mg/100 mL, respectively, indicate visceral protein depletion. However, these values must be interpreted with caution because dehydration or administration of blood products may falsely produce a high concentration of albumin and transferrin. Liver disease can cause a decrease in circulating levels of all transport proteins which is not related to nutritional status.

Nitrogen Balance

Nitrogen (N) balance is usually evaluated during nutritional assessment. It is not a measure of somatic or visceral protein status, but is used to estimate adequacy of protein input. A 24-h urine collection is made and assayed for total urinary urea nitrogen (UUN) content. Nitrogen content is reported in milligrams per 100 mL. This value is used to calculate N balance using the formula:

$$\text{N balance} = \left(\frac{\text{24-h protein intake}}{6.25}\right) - (\text{UUN} + 4\,\text{g N})$$

Positive nitrogen balance, or nitrogen homeostasis, is desired. Negative nitrogen balance indicates a catabolic state and requires an increase in protein input.

Immunocompetence

Protein malnutrition negatively affects immunocompetence by depressing neutrophil chemotaxis, total lymphocyte count (TLC), and skin reactivity to common antigens. Immunosuppression renders the critically ill, malnourished patient particularly vulnerable to infection. The immune system is assessed by determining the TLC and delayed cutaneous hypersensitivity to antigens. The total lymphocyte count is derived from a complete blood cell count with differential count. The total lymphocyte count is calculated by multiplying the percentage of lymphocytes by the white blood cell count (WBC):

$$\text{TLC} = \frac{\%\ lymphocytes \times WBC}{100}$$

A TLC of less than 1500 mm³ is indicative of an impaired immune system.

Skin testing with common antigens (such as mumps, streptokinase-streptodornase, *Candida albicans, Tricophytin,* tuberculin) for delayed hypersensitivity assesses immune function at the cellular level. A *positive skin test* is defined as an induration of 5 mm or more at the site of antigen injection within 24 to 72 h. *Anergy* is defined as no response to the antigen. Anergy to skin testing indicates immunosuppression which may be related to malnutrition. The immune system can also be depressed by steroids, radiation, and chemotherapy. Therefore, evidence of immunosuppression in patients receiving these therapies does not necessarily indicate poor nutritional status.

Nutritional assessment consists of data collected by a variety of methods. Evaluation of nutritional status should be dynamic, and not based on data from a single source. The currently available parameters which provide nonspecific data regarding nutritional status must be reviewed as a whole to accurately evaluate and monitor the nutritional state of a patient. In addition, a thorough knowledge of the health history and biopsychological status of the patient is necessary for accurate interpretation of nutritional status assessment data, because factors other than nutritionally relevant ones can influence test results. The most important use of nutritional status assessment in the care of the critically ill is identifying patients who have the potential for developing malnutrition, preventing its occurrence, monitoring nutritional therapy, and treating existing cases of malnutrition.

Methods for Providing Nutritional Support

Enteral feeding by tube has been used for centuries while parenteral nutrition has been commonly used only since the early 1970s. Both are important techniques for providing nutritional support to the patient who cannot meet nutritional needs through an oral diet. Due to continuing improvements in techniques, equipment, and formulas, use of tube feeding and parenteral nutrition is increasing for in- and outpatients.

Enteral Feeding by Tube

Nonvolitional enteral feeding was first used in 1598 when a stiff, hollow tube was used to deliver nutritional solutions into the esophagus. The practice of enteral feeding continued to develop, and by the late 1800s, stomach pumps were in common use in insane asylums for forced feeding of recalcitrant residents. In spite of advancements, enteral nutrition by tube was not well tolerated; the assistance of four strong men was required to restrain the patient during administration of mixtures of beef broth, sugar, egg, and milk. In 1910, use of a rubber tube having a small lumen and a distal metal weight was advocated because it enhanced patient comfort and tolerance to nasoenteric feeding. By the 1970s, small-diameter, weighted feeding tubes made from biocompatible materials were commercially available. At that time, tube feeding formulas were handmade in the hospital kitchen from baby foods or blenderized house diets. Commercial availability of prepared formulas was spurred by development of special liquid diets which were consumed by astronauts during early space flights. In the ensuing years, a plethora of commercial formulas has been introduced.

Indications

There are two major criteria which qualify patients for oral supplementation or enteral feeding by tube. Enteral nutritional support is indicated for patients who have a totally or partially functioning gastrointestinal (GI) tract and are unable or unwilling to ingest enough nutrients via an oral diet. Candidates include patients who are hypermetabolic due to disease, sepsis, or trauma; those who are unable to eat due to mechanical dysfunction such as esophageal or pharyngeal stricture or obstruction, maxillofacial surgery, swallowing impairment due to cerebrovascular accident or other neurological disorder, and those who are unwilling to eat because of nausea, vomiting, or anorexia.

Patients who are able to eat an oral diet but unable to ingest enough to meet their nutritional requirements may benefit from supplementation of the diet with flavored tube feeding formulas. Oral supplements may be consumed directly from the container, or may be incorporated into foods to increase nutritional value of the meal.

Formulas

Formulas for tube feeding or oral supplementation are available which are especially suited to the disease state, GI function, nutritional needs, and absorptive capacity of the patient. However, the choice is difficult when one attempts to identify an appropriate formula from the bewildering array of the more than 70 that are commercially available. Formula selection can be simplified when formulas are grouped into generic categories. Type and quantity of nutrients in formulas are important criteria in assuring patient absorption and tolerance of tube feeding. Enteral formulas can be categorized as *polymeric* or *monomeric,* to indicate the form in which the nutrients are provided in a given formula.

Nutrients in polymeric formulas are in complex form and require digestion. Polymeric formulas range from those made from blenderized foods to those compounded from protein isolates, vegetable oils, and carbohydrates. Lactose has been eliminated as a carbohydrate source from most compounded formulas because patients with primary lactase deficiency do not tolerate it. Since secondary lactase deficiency may result from critical illness, the critically ill patient is also unlikely to tolerate lactose.

The caloric density of most of these formulas is 1 cal per milliliter, although some provide 1.5 or 2 cal per milliliter. The higher-calorie formulas are useful in meeting elevated energy requirements of the critically ill patient.

Most commercially prepared enteral formulas provide 14 to 17 percent of calories as protein. Patients whose protein needs are elevated due to trauma, sepsis, or thermal injuries may require formulas which have higher protein concentrations.

Polymeric formulas are intermediate in osmolality and are tolerable, at full strength, to the nonstressed patient. More care must be given in administering a polymeric formula to the critically ill patient. The critically ill patient may require slow initiation of an isotonic formula to enhance tolerance. Nurses should observe the patient for tolerance of the formula as evidenced by absence of abdominal distention, nausea, vomiting, or diarrhea. Polymeric formulas are useful as tube feedings for patients who have digestive and absorptive capacity. Many of these formulas are flavored or have a tolerable, bland taste, making them useful as oral dietary supplements.

Monomeric formulas provide nutrients in simple or "predigested" form, and very little digestion is required before nutrients can be absorbed. Monomeric formulas are compounded from nutrient sources ranging from simple crystalline amino acids and glucose molecules, to slightly more complex sources such as di- and tripeptides and modified corn starch or glucose oligosaccharides. These formulas are very low in fat. Most monomeric formulas are powdered and require reconstitution. Caloric density depends upon final dilution, but at full strength they provide 1 cal per milliliter.

Monomeric formulas are particularly hypertonic (550 mOsm per kilogram of water or more) because their short-chain nutrient sources contribute many osmotically active particles to the solution. Tube feeding using hypertonic formulas is often initiated with a dilute concentration to allow for gut adaptation to the osmolar load. Monomeric formulas are extremely unpalatable due to the short-chain nutrient sources. They should not be used for oral supplementation.

A number of specialty formulas are available which are intended for use in cases of trauma, renal failure, ventilator dependence, or hepatic encephalopathy. These formulas are often used for nutritional support of the critically ill patient. The actual benefit derived from use of specialty formulas in reducing morbidity or mortality in the clinical setting remains to be proven. Moreover, the high cost of these formulas precludes routine use.

Modular nutritional components are sources of single nutrients. Carbohydrate, fat, and protein modules are commercially available and are used to supplement individual nutrients of prepared formulas, to produce formulas specifically designed to meet nutritional requirements of individual patients. Single-nutrient modules are especially useful in enteral nutritional support of the critically ill patient because the modules provide the flexibility often needed to meet special nutritional requirements.

Equipment and Supplies

Tubes specifically designed for enteral feeding are available in sizes ranging from a no. 5 French (1.7 mm) to a no. 16 French (4.3 mm); the size most frequently used is a no. 8 French (2.6 mm). The small lumen of feeding tubes greatly enhances a patient's comfort, and reduces risk of aspiration.

Nasoenteric feeding tubes are constructed of silicone, polyurethane, or polyvinylchloride. Silicone and polyurethane are biocompatible materials that do not react with gastric juices. Tubes made from polyvinylchloride or other plastics, such as NG suction tubes, react with gastric juices and must be replaced more frequently than silicone or polyurethane tubes, and, therefore, are not ideal for use as feeding tubes.

Because silicone and polyurethane tubes are softer than plastic tubes, they are more comfortable, but require an aid for insertion. Feeding tubes which use rigid outer guide tubes as insertion aids are available; however, the large diameter of the guide tube is a source of discomfort to the patient during intubation. Stylets are more frequently used

to facilitate insertion of feeding tubes. Most tubes have been redesigned so that the outlet ports are at the distal tip of the tube which eliminates the possibility of mucosal damage because the stylet cannot exit through an outlet port.

Tubes tend to "sleeve up" over the stylet during removal. Some manufacturers have alleviated this problem by applying a lubricious coating to the interior of the tube. When the tube is in place, the stylet can be easily removed after the lubricant is activated by injection of about 10 mL of water into the tube. There have been some reports that, because tubes tend to collapse under negative pressure, it is difficult to check gastric residue by aspiration from feeding tubes. This is thought to be due to the softness and small lumen size of feeding tubes. Silicone tubes collapse more easily than those made from polyurethane because silicone tubes do not have very great tensile strength. Silicone tubes also have a greater tendency to rupture and stretch. Polyurethane is a superior material for feeding tubes because it has greater tensile strength.

Feeding tubes are available with and without weighted boluses. Weights are thought to help maintain tube placement, although there is some question regarding their efficacy. Most weights are made of tungsten or stainless steel to eliminate problems relating to disposal of mercury which was used initially.

Enterostomies are frequently used for long-term tube feeding. Gastrostomies and jejunostomies are most common but esophagotomies are also used. Large-bore Levin-type tubes, Foley catheters, or rubber tubing are commonly used as surgically placed feeding tubes. These tubes are uncomfortable, and esthetically unappealing and are relatively easy to dislodge or displace. Since they are not made from biocompatible materials, they require frequent replacement. Moreover, overinflation of the balloon on Foley catheters may cause intestinal obstruction or rupture.

A number of enterostomy tubes specifically designed to alleviate or prevent these problems have recently become available. Needle catheter jejunostomy tubes are very small caliber, polyethylene tubes which can be introduced into the jejunum via a large-bore needle or trocar. These tubes are placed in the jejunum during abdominal surgery, and feeding can begin shortly after surgery. Their major disadvantage is that the very small lumen will not permit delivery of viscous formulas, necessitating exclusive use of monomeric formulas.

The majority of gastrostomy tubes require surgical placement. Percutaneous endoscopic gastrostomy (PEG) tubes can be placed via a gastroscope under local anesthesia, obviating the need for a surgical procedure.

Prior to the early 1970s enteral feeding pumps were not widely used in hospitals. Tube feeding was delivered by bolus administration or continuous gravity drip. As use of hyperosmolar feeding solutions increased, it was found that patients tolerated them better if feedings were delivered by slow, continuous infusion. Use of small-caliber feeding tubes also stimulated use of infusion pumps to assure controlled delivery of more viscous formulas, because such formulas would not flow freely by gravity drip through small feeding tubes. Pump-assisted enteral feeding assures accurate and reliable delivery of large volumes of formula. Use of a pump assures that the patient receives formula by a slow, continuous drip, which reduces gastric pooling, thereby decreasing the potential for aspiration.

Intravenous (IV) infusion pumps have been used to deliver enteral feedings. However, in most hospitals, use of IV pumps to deliver enteral feeding is limited because pump-assisted infusion of IV solutions is of higher priority than delivery of pump-controlled enteral feeding. Use of IV pumps may not be ideal for delivery of enteral formulas because most of these pumps are designed to sense clear fluids, and may not deliver accurate volumes when pumping opaque tube feeding formulas. The most recent generation of enteral feeding infusion pumps employs microprocessors which assure accuracy rates of ± 5 percent. The newest pump models provide flexibility in range of flow rate settings because the rate can be advanced in 1-mL increments; older models offer a variety of rate settings ranging from increments of 5 mL to 50 mL. Most enteral pumps operate on both direct current and battery power. The option for battery-powered operation is an important consideration as more patients are discharged to continue tube feeding as outpatients. Feeding pumps are generally lightweight and easy to operate, making their use even more feasible in the outpatient setting. Enteral feeding pumps feature audible and visual alarms which indicate malfunction, battery status, and inadvertent change of flow rate.

The tubing and other disposable supplies used with a specific pump are not compatible between various makes of pumps. This feature may increase cost of supplies, but assures accuracy and safety, because tubing is specifically calibrated to the pump for which it is made, and decreases the potential for accidental connection of enteral feeding solutions to IV lines.

Administration

Formula is delivered via the tube either into the stomach or the small intestine. Choice of a feeding site depends on the condition of the patient. Feeding into the stomach is the method of choice for the alert patient who has an intact gag reflex and an adequate rate of gastric emptying. Feeding into the stomach is advantageous because, unlike the small intestine, the stomach can tolerate high osmotic loads with less incidence of GI side effects. Most formulas are well tolerated by patients receiving gastric feeding. Bolus feedings are tolerable for the patient who has a gastric feeding tube. The relatively large volume of the stomach allows it to tolerate boluses of 200 to 250 mL.

Critically ill patients often have a depressed level of consciousness, artificial airways, depressed gag reflex, extreme debilitation, or decreased intestinal motility. Patients having these conditions are not candidates for nasogastric tube feeding because they are at a higher risk for aspiration of gastric contents. Although insertion of nasoduodenal or nasojejunal tubes is more difficult than passage of nasogastric tubes, transpyloric tube placement decreases the risk of regurgitation and aspiration of gastric contents. In addition, use of the small bowel makes early postoperative feedings possible because the small intestine is unaffected by gastric ileus.

Procedures used for insertion of nasoenteric feeding tubes have been well described elsewhere. Placement of the tube into the stomach is accomplished by gently advancing the feeding tube through the most patent nostril until an appropriate, premeasured length is inserted. If small bowel placement is desired, an additional 50 cm is inserted.

The tube should pass into the duodenum by normal peristaltic action within 24 to 48 h, which can be enhanced by having the patient lie on his or her right side. An oral or intravenous dose of metaclopramide to stimulate gastric emptying may also facilitate passage of the tube into the duodenum.

In spite of the presence of weighted boluses, it is possible for feeding tubes to migrate or become dislodged, and it is necessary to secure the tube to the patient. Paper tape does not adhere well to silicone or polyurethane feeding tubes. Adherence of tape to feeding tubes may be improved by first wiping the portion of the tube to be taped with alcohol, then with benzoin, and finally, placing the tape on the feeding tube. Use of a transparent, moisture-vapor permeable dressing is an alternative to using paper tape (Fig. 12-3).

Formula may be administered by a variety of methods. Bolus, or intermittent, feeding is best tolerated by the patient who has a gastric feeding tube. Bolus feeding is advocated by some because it is similar to normal meal patterns and gastric distention resulting from boluses of formula may stimulate digestion. This method is more time-consuming than pump-assisted feeding because to avoid GI complications, formula should not be administered faster than 30 mL per minute. More-over, because of decreased absorptive function of the GI tract and delayed gastric emptying time, rapid delivery of boluses may lead to gastric pooling. This can increase the potential for reflux and pulmonary aspiration of gastric contents.

The critically ill patient, and those receiving feeding into the small intestine, benefit from continuous delivery of formula. Continuous drip feeding may be accomplished by gravity or by the use of a pump. When feeding a hypertonic solution, continuous drip administration is preferred because it is associated with fewer GI complications than bolus administration because pump-assisted tube feeding assures accurate, constant delivery of formulas. Gravity flow is less easy to regulate.

Regardless of the method of delivery, feeding should be initiated in small volumes and advanced slowly. It is still common practice to begin tube feeding with diluted formula, advancing to full strength over the course of 2 to 3 days. This practice is usually unnecessary for patients who have adequate GI function. Such "starter regimens" have been found to reduce nutrient intake while not significantly improving tolerance to feeding.[7] Generally, tolerance is assured if full-strength isotonic formulas are begun at flow rates of 30 to 50 mL per hour, advancing in increments of 30 to 50 mL per day, until the desired volume is reached. Feeding can be advanced from isotonic to hypertonic formulas after gut adaptation has occurred.

Enteral feeding by tube is associated with some of the same complications which occur with parenteral feeding. Careful nursing care and monitoring of the patient's progress can help avoid the development of these problems. Use of routine procedures (Table 12-4) can assist in providing comprehensive care of the patient receiving tube feeding.

Complications

Side effects which may occur during tube feeding can be classified as GI, mechanical, or metabolic. Most can be alleviated through proper monitoring and management.

Gastrointestinal complications, including nausea, vomiting, diarrhea, gastric retention, and malabsorption are often considered unavoidable consequences of tube feeding. However, most complications can be relieved or prevented.

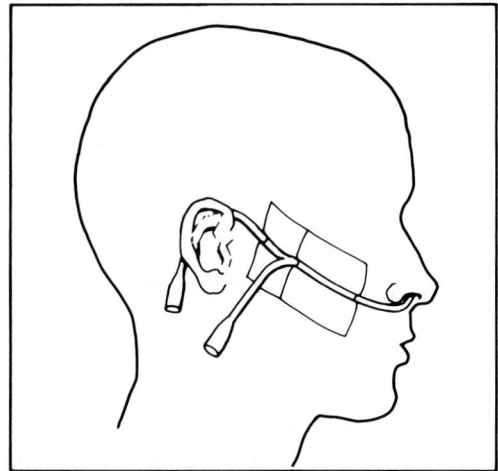

Figure 12-3 Use of a transparent moistureproof dressing to anchor feeding tubes. [*Reprinted with permission from D. Patricia Gray and Paul D. Smith, Nutritional Support Services, 4(7):37–38, 1984.*]

Table 12-4 Routine Procedures for Care of the Tube-fed Patient

Procedure	Frequency	Rationale
Confirm tube placement and patency.	Prior to bolus feeding or every 4–6 h	To prevent aspiration and avoid delivery of formula to sites other than GI tract
Check gastric residuals (use a 30-mL syringe or larger).	Prior to bolus feeding or every 4–6 h	To assess tolerance and prevent aspiration
Hold feedings and notify physician if residual is > 150 mL or patient exhibits signs of intolerance.	As necessary	To prevent aspiration and alleviate symptoms
Elevate head of bed 45° for patients who have depressed gag reflex (this may be unnecessary for alert patients).	During feeding and 30 min following feeding	To prevent aspiration
Hang feeding for 8 h or less.		To decrease chance of patient intolerance due to bacterial overgrowth
Monitor gravity drip flow rates.	Every hour	To enhance tolerance by maintaining even flow rate of formulas
Irrigate feeding tube with 30–50 mL water.	After each bolus or every 4–6 h and following medications	To maintain patency of feeding tube and supplement fluid intake
Provide oral and nasal hygiene.	Daily and as necessary	To enhance comfort
Clean or replace feeding container.	Every 8 h	To maintain sanitation of system and decrease chances of patient intolerance due to bacterial contamination
Replace pump or gravity drip tubing.	Every 24 h	To maintain sanitation of system and decrease chances of patient intolerance due to bacterial contamination
Evaluate and document:		To monitor patient tolerance and progress and avoid complications
Urine glucose and acetone	Every 4–6 h initially, 3 times/day when stable	
Intake and output	Daily	
Stool frequency and consistency	Daily	
Body weight	Daily initially, 1 time/week when stable	
Plasma electrolytes	2–3 times/week initially, 1 time/week when stable	
Blood glucose	2–3 times/week initially, 1 time/week when stable	
Blood urea nitrogen and creatinine	2–3 times/week initially, 1 time/week when stable	
Clinical observations	Daily	

Diarrhea is the most commonly reported GI side effect of tube feeding. There may be numerous etiological factors that simultaneously contribute to diarrhea, each of which may require therapy before diarrhea can be resolved. Stool frequency may be due to rapid infusion of hyperosmolar enteral solutions, although it may occur because of bacterial contamination of formula or malabsorption of specific components of formulas. Protein-calorie malnutrition, resulting in hypoalbuminemia and atrophy of intestinal absorptive surfaces, may cause diarrhea by decreasing absorption of nutrients from the GI tract. Frequent stools induced by antibiotic therapy may be mistakenly attributed to tube feeding. Bolus feeding is often associated with diarrhea and other GI symptoms because there is a propensity to overwhelm the absorptive capacity of the gut.

Most GI symptoms can be relieved or prevented by beginning feeding with an isotonic formula and slowly advancing the infusion rate. Use of a feeding pump to control the rate of infusion is also helpful in decreasing the incidence of GI side effects. It may be necessary in the case of malabsorption to change formulas to eliminate the offending component. The critically ill patient is frequently intolerant of lactose, due to lactase deficiency. Almost all commercial formulas are lactose-free; however, lactose intolerance may still be an etiologic factor in development of GI complications if milk products are added to formulas. This may have greater significance as more patients are discharged from the hospital to continue tube feeding at home using homemade formulas which include lactose-containing foods.

Fat is frequently malabsorbed by patients receiving commercial formulas. This problem may be addressed by changing to a formula with a different fat source or one with a lower overall fat content.

Tube feeding formulas are rich media for bacterial growth. Administration of bacterially contaminated formulas has been associated with diarrhea; therefore scrupulous care must be taken to avoid contaminating the formula and administration system. Moreover, formula should not hang longer than 8 h. Some authors have suggested that the best way to minimize risk of bacterial contamination is by the use of sterile formula packaged in a closed administration system.[8]

Mechanical complications may be decreased through choice of an appropriate feeding tube, proper monitoring of tube placement, and adequate care of the tube. Mechanical side effects frequently arise from use of large-bore tubes which are extremely uncomfortable for the patient, and are associated with pulmonary aspiration of gastric contents. Meticulous attention to monitoring tube placement and gastric residue is also important to decreasing potential for aspiration by assuring that feeding is only administered to the GI tract, and that gastric pooling does not occur. Taping the tube in place is useful in maintaining tube position. Care must be taken in taping nasoenteric tubes to avoid pressure on the nostril. Ostomy sites must be carefully dressed to avoid tissue irritation.

Feeding tubes must be carefully and frequently irrigated to maintain patency, which is particularly important if these tubes are used to deliver medications. Feeding tubes should be flushed before and after administering medications. Whenever possible, liquid medications should be ordered. When this is not possible, medications should be thoroughly crushed or dissolved in water before administering. It is advisable to check with a pharmacist when medications must be delivered via a feeding tube. Crushing or dissolving drugs may alter their absorption or action. There may also be potential for drug–nutrient interactions.

In the event of occlusion, a stylet should not be used to clear the tube because of the possibility of rupturing the tube and damaging intestinal mucosa. Before removing an occluded tube, an attempt can be made to clear the tube by instilling a solution of ¼ tsp meat tenderizer in 60 mL of water, followed with clear water 10 min later. If this maneuver is unsuccessful, tube replacement is necessary.

Metabolic complications of tube feeding occur relatively frequently but can be prevented if patients are properly managed. Hypertonic dehydration is commonly labeled *tube feeding syndrome*. Tube feeding syndrome can occur when hypertonic, high-protein formulas are delivered without sufficient free water. Patients who are unable to communicate their feelings of thirst are particularly susceptible. It is necessary to supplement fluid intake of tube-fed patients, even though most isotonic formulas contain approximately 75 to 80 percent moisture. Usually, 1 mL of water is required for each calorie provided by tube feeding formula. Overhydration, or *refeeding edema,* can occur when feeding is reintroduced to severely malnourished patients. Patients with cardiac, renal, or hepatic insufficiency are also candidates for development of edema. Refeeding edema is treated by decreasing the rate of feeding, then gradually advancing the rate when the fluid status of the patient normalizes. Use of a 1.5- or 2-cal-per-milliliter formula assists in providing adequate nutrition while restricting fluid volume. Hyperglycemia occurs frequently in tube-fed patients. It is treated by decreasing infusion rate and administering insulin to maintain the blood sugar at 200 mg/100 mL.

Electrolyte abnormalities occurring as a consequence of tube feeding are relatively uncommon.

Such abnormalities usually arise from the underlying disease state rather than from enteral nutritional support. Hypophosphatemia may occur with rapid refeeding or secondary to insulin therapy. It can be avoided by slowly initiating feeding, and monitoring the patient's serum phosphorus levels.

Parenteral Nutrition

Patients received the benefit of intravenous glucose solutions as early as 1896. In 1952, a method for central venous access by percutaneous infraclavicular catheterization was developed by Aubaniac, which Dudrick in the late 1960s adapted to deliver hypertonic, IV nutritional solutions. The demonstration in 1967 that this technique could support weight gain and growth of human beings heralded the beginning of the modern history of parenteral nutritional support.

Indications

Parenteral nutrition (PN) has been used in cases of anorexia nervosa, prolonged ileus, inflammatory bowel disease, pancreatitis, neoplastic disease, and other conditions. Metabolic support by the parenteral route was conceived as an "artificial gut." Because of expense and the potential for life-threatening complications, it should ideally be used only in situations in which the GI tract cannot or should not work, or when the patient can tolerate some enteral alimentation, but not enough to meet metabolic requirements. Parenteral nutrition is often used in the critical-care setting because disease or trauma frequently renders the GI tract partially or totally nonfunctional. Critical illness may increase nutritional requirements such that it is not possible for the gut to tolerate the volume or caloric density of formulas which may be required to meet the nutritional needs imposed by some hypermetabolic states.

Routes of Access

Percutaneous placement of a polyethylene catheter into the superior vena cava via the subclavian vein is the most frequently used method for delivery of parenteral nutritional solutions. The catheter can be inserted at the bedside under local anesthesia but there is a potential for technical complications including arterial puncture, pneumothorax, or hemothorax, since the catheter is inserted blindly without benefit of fluoroscopy. Another problem is that polyethylene catheters are suitable only for short-term PN because the material of the catheter may cause thrombophlebitis, and the catheter can serve as a site for infection. Because of the potential for infection, the catheter should only be used for infusion of PN solutions.

It is common for the critically ill patient to require multiple central lines. This need can be met by inserting bilateral subclavian catheters, but this is not ideal because it doubles the chances of catheter-related complications and increases the care required to maintain critical IV lines. A multilumen, polyethylene central venous infusion catheter has been developed to meet the need for multiple lines. This catheter contains three separate lumens and can be placed through a single insertion site. The multiple lumens can be used to administer blood products, medications, chemotherapy, PN, and to withdraw blood samples. Each distinct line exits from the catheter at a different interval, obviating concern regarding potential incompatibilities between fluids.

If a lumen is used to deliver PN, no other fluids should be infused through it in order to maintain its integrity. The catheter is suitable only for short-term use because the plastic material is reactive with bacteria and can cause phlebitis. To avoid technical problems, an experienced physician should insert this catheter because it, like the single-lumen central venous line, is inserted blindly.

Right atrial Silastic catheters, commonly called *Hickman catheters* (Fig. 12-4), are used when long-term central venous access is required. Hickman catheters have a number of desirable features which make them feasible for long-term use. The silicone material of the catheter is nonthrombogenic and less reactive with bacteria than is polyethylene. The proximal Dacron cuff is a physical barrier to entry of bacteria to the systemic circulation. The cuff also facilitates engraftment of tissue to it, which helps to anchor the catheter. The catheter is inserted through a 4-in subcutaneous tunnel before it enters systemic circulation. Because there is less potential for infection with use of this catheter, it is possible to sequentially administer multiple infusions, and withdraw blood samples through Hickman catheters.

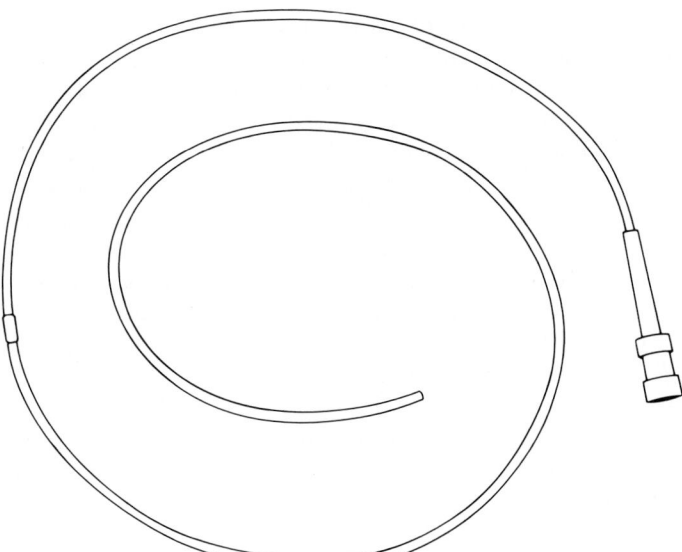

Figure 12-4   Hickman catheter.

It is not possible, however, to infuse incompatible solutions simultaneously through a single-lumen Hickman catheter. A double-lumen Hickman catheter was developed to provide an additional lumen for central venous access. The first lumen is used exclusively for delivery of PN solutions, and the second lumen is used to administer other IV solutions, blood products, and to withdraw blood samples.

Double- and single-lumen Hickman catheters are inserted in the operating room under continuous fluoroscopy, which reduces the incidence of technical complications that can occur from blind insertion of central venous lines. Use of the operating room and the need for a surgeons's expertise to place these catheters increases the cost of using them, and may discourage some physicians from using Hickman catheters solely for the purpose of PN.

Peripherally inserted silicone central venous catheters provide some of the same benefits as Hickman catheters, and they can be inserted at the patient's bedside. These *long-arm catheters* are placed in the right atrium, via a percutaneous route, with the aid of an introducing device.

The development of IV lipid emulsions as a calorie source has made peripheral delivery of PN a possibility. Before IV lipids were available, peripheral parenteral nutritional support was limited to *protein-sparing* therapy. This is because small-diameter peripheral veins cannot tolerate the hypertonic glucose solutions required to accomplish weight gain and nitrogen retention. The goal of protein-sparing therapy was to provide enough amino acids and calories in a tolerable concentration and volume to reduce catabolism of body protein by gluconeogenesis. It is obvious that this therapy cannot provide adequate calories for anabolism because 1 L of 10 percent dextrose in water provides approximately 400 calories.

Lipid emulsions provide 1.1 to 2 cal per milliliter, and one 500-mL bottle provides up to 1000 cal. Lipid emulsions are isotonic, and can be administered via a peripheral vein. Provision of a nutritionally complete PN solution is possible using a two-bottle system in which a lipid emulsion and an amino acid–dextrose solution are infused simultaneously through a Y connector into a peripheral IV catheter. For peripheral PN to be successful, there must be adequate venous access because, as with any peripheral IV line, sites must be changed frequently to avoid phlebitis. In addition, some patients, especially the critically ill, may not tolerate large doses of IV lipid emulsions.

Solutions

Parenteral nutritional support is often called *total parenteral nutrition,* or *TPN,* because it is possible to provide all three major substrates—protein, carbohydrate, and fat—along with vitamins, minerals, and trace elements, parenterally. Protein is provided in the form of crystalline amino acids that are commercially available in concentrations of 7, 8, 8.5, and 10 percent. The calories provided by protein usually are not included when calculating the amount of energy provided by PN solutions. This is because the ideal end point of amino acids is incorporation into somatic and plasma proteins. For this to occur, it is necessary to provide adequate amounts of nonprotein calories so that protein is not used as an energy source. The glucose concentrations most frequently used to supply nonprotein calories are 20, 50, or 70 percent glucose in sterile water. Intravenously administered carbohydrate provides 3.4 cal per gram, as compared to the 4 cal per gram provided by enterally administered carbohydrate.

Total reliance on glucose for energy is not ideal since its metabolism increases the cardiac output, respiratory quotient, and serum levels of catecholamines and insulin. Although glucose calories support nitrogen retention, associated weight gain may be due to increases in fat tissue and body water rather than muscle mass. Development of fatty deposits in the liver may occur when glucose is the only source of nonprotein calories. The critically ill patient is frequently insulin-resistant and significant hyperglycemia may result when glucose is the sole energy source. Moreover, because glucose is not a source of essential fatty acids, the patient is at risk of developing essential fatty acid deficiency if a source is not provided. However, at least 100 g of glucose are required to meet the need for glucose by obligate glycolyzer cells and to prevent gluconeogenesis. Provision of 20 percent of total calories as glucose will meet these minimum requirements.

Intravenous lipid emulsions are another source of calories and are ideally used with glucose to provide calories in PN solutions. Intravenous lipid emulsions are useful in preventing essential fatty acid deficiency and side effects associated with the sole use of glucose to provide nonprotein calories. It is usual to infuse a 500-mL dose of IV lipid twice a week to preclude essential fatty acid deficiency. Dosages for adults in excess of 2.5 g per kilogram of body weight per day should be avoided to prevent fat overload, because critically ill patients are unable to eliminate excessive amounts of lipid from the bloodstream.

Requirements for parenterally administered vitamins, trace elements, and electrolytes vary from enteral requirements because the gut is bypassed. However, it is necessary to supply adequate amounts of trace elements to the patient receiving PN. Maintenance levels of IV trace elements are least 2 mg zinc, 0.5 mg copper, 10 g chromium, and 0.15 mg manganese, but the critically ill patient, especially one with intestinal losses, requires more than these maintenance amounts.

A number of commercial PN solutions are available which contain maintenance levels of electrolytes. When PN solutions are mixed in the hospital pharmacy, 60 to 100 meq of sodium, 60 to 100 meq of potassium, 400 to 600 mg of phosphorus, 10 to 25 meq of magnesium, and 180 to 400 mg of calcium should be added to assure that minimum needs are met.

The critically ill patient may require electrolytes in amounts that vary from these maintenance amounts. Patients receiving antibiotics such as carbenicillin, ticarcillin, and tobramycin may require increased amounts of potassium, since these antibiotics can cause significant urinary losses of potassium. Diuretics and amphotericin also may precipitate hypokalemia through renal losses. Potassium can also be lost through the GI tract via diarrhea and small bowel drainage. Significant losses of bicarbonate may occur in the patient who has large gastric output.

Many IV fluids, and certain antibiotics, such as carbenicillin and ticarcillin, contain considerable amounts of sodium. It may be necessary to delete sodium from PN solutions for patients receiving sodium-containing antibiotics and fluids in order to decrease sodium intake.

Phosphorus requirements may be elevated for patients receiving phosphate-binding antacids. Steroid therapy can cause renal losses of phosphate. Phosphate requirements may be increased by parenteral feeding itself because phosphate is required to metabolize glucose.

Patients receiving PN often develop hypomagnesemia simply because magnesium is overlooked when writing orders for PN solutions. Patients receiving cisplatin, amphotericin, steroids, or diuretics may require increased amounts of magnesium.

Complications

Complications associated with PN can be categorized as technical, septic, or metabolic. Technical complications are those which occur during or related to catheter insertion. The most common technical complications are pneumothorax, air embolism, catheter embolism, arterial puncture, and subclavian vein thrombosis. These complications are more frequently associated with blind percutaneous placement of subclavian catheters. The frequency with which technical complications occur is inversely related to the experience of the physician inserting the catheter. Technical complications occur less frequently when catheters are inserted under continuous fluoroscopy. There is great potential for catheter-related sepsis; therefore the nurse should adhere to strict aseptic technique when hanging PN solutions and caring for the catheter and tubing.

The most common metabolic complication of PN is glucose intolerance. Most patients tolerate glucose infusions of 400 to 500 g delivered over a 24-h period. Patients who are stressed, diabetic, severely malnourished or debilitated, or undergoing steroid therapy, may, however, exhibit hyperglycemia and glucosuria. Blood glucose levels in excess of 200 mg/100 mL accompanied by urinary spillage of 2 g glucose per 100 mL urine may lead to development of hyperglycemic, hyperosmolar, nonketotic coma.

Conversely, hypoglycemia may occur with sudden cessation of hypertonic glucose solutions. When discontinuing PN solutions, the infusion rate should be tapered to 50 mL/h for two hours before turning off the infusion.

Electrolyte abnormalities may occur rapidly with PN, especially in the critically ill patient. Aberrations in serum levels of potassium, phosphorus, and magnesium are common.

When lipid emulsions are used, the nurse should report abnormalities in a patient's values for liver function tests, serum cholesterol, triglycerides, and free fatty acids.

Administration

During initiation of PN, 1 to 2 L of the solution are infused during the first 24-h period. The severely stressed or critically ill patient may require significant amounts of insulin to maintain acceptable blood glucose levels during the initial period. After 24 h, the infusion rate can be increased in increments of 500 to 1000 mL per day, until the volume necessary to meet nutritional requirements is attained.

Occasionally, PN solutions are "cycled" to provide a period of time each day during which no nutritional solutions are administered. Cycling PN solutions is thought to induce a "postabsorptive state" similar to that following ingestion of an oral meal. Cycling is claimed to prevent or resolve fatty liver deposits which can occur with continuous PN. Cycled PN is also useful when the number of IV lines is limited and Hickman catheters are used to deliver medications, chemotherapy, blood products, and other IV fluids, as well as PN.

Parenteral nutrition is cycled by beginning the infusion at one-third the final desired rate for 1 h. During the second hour, the infusion rate is increased to two-thirds the desired final rate. The full infusion rate is reached during the third hour, and the infusion continues at that rate for the next 8 to 10 h. When the cycle is complete, the infusion rate is tapered off by one-third in the following 2 h. It is not necessary to hang 10 percent glucose following cycles of PN administration because the infusion is tapered slowly to prevent rebound hypoglycemia.

The use of lipid emulsions in cyclic PN makes it possible to provide adequate calories in a volume that can be administered over a 12-to-14-h period. Fat emulsions may be delivered by gravity drip or with the use of a pump. They may be delivered through a separate IV line or simultaneously with amino acid–glucose solutions through a Y connector into the central line. Lipids should be connected to the extension tubing as closely as possible to the hub of the catheter. The lipid container should be hung lower than the PN container. These actions are necessary to prevent backflow of the lipid emulsion. Lipid emulsions should not be mixed with amino acid–glucose solutions, vitamins, or electrolytes, except in the pharmacy, because of possible incompatibilities.

When the patient is able to resume an oral diet, he or she should be weaned from PN, especially if the patient has been without oral intake for a long time, because the gut may atrophy during periods of disuse. The patient may experience symptoms of malabsorption due to decreased absorptive surface of the gut and reduced production of the digestive enzymes maltase, sucrase, and lactase. Concentrated sugars, milk products, and fats should be reintroduced slowly to the diet because these foods are frequently malabsorbed by the patient who has been NPO. Transition to an oral diet should be individualized according to the tolerance of the patient. Generally, following the traditional dietary progression from clear liquid to full liquid to low residue, and finally to a regular diet will assure patient tolerance.

The patient should continue to receive PN until he or she is able to ingest approximately 75 percent of the nutritional requirements via an oral diet. Commercial nutritional supplements can be used to reach this goal, but care must be taken that they do not contribute to malabsorption. Several widely used nutritional supplements provide more than 50 percent of calories as carbohydrate, the majority of which is sucrose. The high fat content of most nutritional supplements also may be a factor that contributes to intolerance in patients who are being weaned from PN.

Nursing Responsibilities

Nursing interventions are aimed at preventing complications and enhancing a patient's tolerance and progress with PN. These responsibilities can be met by preparing the patient for and assisting the physician with insertion of the central venous catheter, preventing sepsis by proper maintenance of tubing and insertion site, and evaluating therapy. Most institutions have comprehensive policies and procedures for accomplishing these goals.

Technical complications which may occur during insertion of the central venous catheter can be reduced if the patient understands the procedure. Discussion of the need for the patient's cooperation in performing the Valsalva maneuver are helpful in reducing anxiety and increasing compliance during insertion.

When the PN catheter is inserted at the bedside, the patient is placed in the Trendelenburg position, with his or her head turned away from the insertion site and a rolled towel placed beneath the scapulae. The skin is prepared by shaving and defatting, followed by a povidone-iodine scrub. The patient is asked to perform the Valsalva maneuver at the time of catheter insertion, and is monitored during the procedure for evidence of complications such as pneumo- or hydrothorax, or cardiac irritability.

Since PN is administered directly into the systemic circulation, meticulous care must be given to the solution, line, and insertion site to prevent infection. The extension tubing should be changed every 24 h. Care should be taken to avoid contaminating the tubing spike when inserting it into the PN container. The patient performs the Valsalva maneuver while the tubing is quickly placed into the catheter hub. Maintenance of a sterile, occlusive dressing over the site is vital for prevention of infection. Gauze dressings should be changed three times a week, and transparent moisture-vapor permeable dressings should be changed once a week.

Procedures used with subclavian catheters must be varied when the patient has a Hickman catheter. Since the catheter can be "heparin locked" and clamped when not in use, patency must be restored before beginning an infusion. After the infusion is complete, the catheter must be flushed with 3 mL of a heparin-saline solution to prevent occlusion.

It is important to use padded clamps and to change the location of clamp sites to prevent wear on the catheter. This reduces risk of tearing or puncturing the catheter.

Other nursing responsibilities include monitoring the patient's progress and tolerance to PN. Progress should be evaluated by daily measurement of body weight to evaluate weight gain. The nurse is responsible for assuring that a complete 24-h collection of urine, which is used for estimation of nitrogen balance, is collected. Other nursing interventions include accurate measurement and recording of the patient's temperature, fluid input and output, and checking urine for presence of sugar and acetone. Abnormal serum electrolyte values should be indicated to the physician as soon as possible. The catheter insertion site should be inspected for redness or irritation during each dressing change and signs of infection should be reported to the physician.

Case Study

Mr. W was admitted with a diagnosis of acute myelogenous leukemia. His weight was 70 kg and his serum albumin was 2.8 g per deciliter. His initial daily nutritional requirements were calculated to be approximately 1700 cal and 56 g of protein. A single-lumen Hickman catheter was inserted and chemotherapy was begun.

Mr. W lost 5 kg due to nausea, vomiting, and anorexia secondary to induction therapy. His nutritional status was compromised further when he developed an opportunistic *Candida* infection throughout his GI tract that further impaired his ability to ingest and absorb an adequate oral diet.

Mr. W received sequential infusions of blood products, amphotericin, other medications, and other IV fluids through the Hickman catheter, so continuous infusion of PN was not possible. Cyclic PN was administered between 6:00 P.M. and 8:00 A.M. each day. Other necessary IV solutions were delivered through the catheter during the intervals when no PN solutions were infused.

Nutritional requirements were provided by two different solutions. During each cycle, 1500 mL of a solution consisting of 4.25 percent amino acids and 25 percent glucose provided 1175 cal and approximately 64 g of protein. An additional 500 cal were provided by 500 mL of 10 percent lipid emulsion infused concurrently with the amino acid–glucose solution.

Ten U of insulin were added to the amino acid-glucose solution during each cycle to prevent hyperglycemia. An in-line filter was not used since it was feared that insulin might adsorb to it, thus causing erratic delivery of insulin to the patient.

Serum electrolytes were evaluated each morning. Daily PN orders were written by the physician, based on the patient's electrolyte values. Electrolyte replacement was accomplished as much as possible by the nutritional solutions to obviate the need for peripheral IV lines for electrolyte replacement.

One week after cyclic PN began, evaluation of nitrogen balance showed that Mr. W had a negative nitrogen balance of 10 g of protein. The amount of protein in the PN solution was increased by changing the 4.25 percent amino acid concentration to 5 percent. The reformulated PN solutions provided 1675 nonprotein calories and 75 g of protein.

Mr. W received cyclic PN for 3 weeks. During that period, he evidenced elevated liver function tests. Although elevations in liver function tests can occur due to hepatitis (which may develop in patients receiving multiple blood infusions), PN was discontinued because it was possible that this was the reason for the elevated values. By this time, Mr. W had begun to ingest an oral diet. His complaints of nausea and vomiting had decreased although he was still anorexic. He was encouraged to increase his daily intake by sipping, over the period of several hours, one can (250 mL) of a 2-cal-per-milliliter, commercially prepared formula. This augmented his dietary intake by 500 cal per day.

At the end of 4 weeks, Mr. W was discharged, having achieved remission of his leukemia during a fairly uneventful hospital course. He had regained 4 kg of body weight and his serum albumin was 3.0 g/100 mL. He was encouraged to continue supplementing his diet with the commercial supplement and was given recipes which incorporated the formula in dishes he had enjoyed before his hospitalization.

Special Conditions

Burns

Thermal injury is tremendously devastating since it causes impressive pain, metabolic aberrations, and nutritional costs. Recovery requires long hospitalization and comprehensive nursing care. Involvement of the entire health care team is required because input from all disciplines is necessary to facilitate healing and discharge of the patient.

Effects on Metabolism
There are two distinct metabolic phases following thermal injury. The *ebb phase* is the period immediately following injury. Shock, hypovolemia, and decreased metabolic rate and oxygen consumption are the major metabolic events of this period.

The second, or *flow phase,* begins 2 to 3 days after an injury. This period is marked by hypermetabolism, hyperventilation, elevated skin temperature, and increased evaporative water loss. Hormonal response during this period includes increased secretion of glucocorticoids and mineralocorticoids. These hormones are responsible for mounting the "survival response" which includes mobilization of necessary energy substrates. Amino acids are transferred from skeletal muscle for conversion to glucose, via gluconeogenesis by the liver. Urinary loss of nitrogen occurs as lean body mass is catabolized to produce energy. Negative nitrogen balance is enhanced by elevated serum levels of glucagon and catecholamines. These hormones are antagonistic to insulin; therefore presence of increased serum levels of glucagon and catecholamines contribute to hyperglycemia, and continued release of amino acids from the periphery.

The etiology of hypermetabolism following thermal injury is multifactorial, and not completely understood. It is thought to be a result of readjustment of preburn metabolic activity to a higher level. Catecholamines are implicated as the primary mediators in this "reset" of metabolic rate. Elevated skin temperature and evaporative water loss contribute to hypermetabolism. These are also the result of adrenergic activity, which is directly proportional to the extent of the open wound, and continues to influence metabolic rate until wounds are healed or grafted.

The critically ill patient undergoing disease, surgery, or injury experiences metabolic stress similar to the burned patient; therefore, the pattern of metabolic response activated by thermal injury can serve as a model of the response of the body to any major stress.

Nutritional Requirements

Basal energy expenditure of the burned patient is increased tremendously. A recent study[9] indicates that nutritional needs are related to the extent of the open wound and not necessarily to burn size. Age and physical condition of the patient, prior nutritional status, and presence of chronic diseases are factors which also affect nutritional requirements.

Body weight and percentage of total body surface area burned (TBSAB) are necessary data for estimation of fluid and calorie requirements. The *rule of nines* is a rapid method for assessing burn size (see Chap. 55). This method is limited because it can be inaccurate, and it underestimates the body surface area of infants and children. Moreover, the rule of nines assesses burn size, not open wound size.

Because calorie and protein needs decrease as wound size diminishes through grafting and healing, nutritional requirements decline throughout convalescence. Therefore, the patient's nutritional needs should be routinely reevaluated to assure appropriate nutritional input.

Adequate provision of micronutrients is necessary for anabolism to occur. Although exact requirements are unknown, it is usual to supplement the diet of the burned patient with multivitamins, vitamin C, and zinc.

Nutritional Care

At one time malnutrition was considered an inevitable consequence of thermal injury. Malnutrition of the burned patient is associated with increased susceptibility to sepsis and increased morbidity and mortality in general. Loss of more than 20 percent of pre-burn body weight is common in patients with a large TBSAB. Weight loss of about 10 percent may be tolerated by the patient, but loss of 40 to 50 percent of the pre-burn weight is usually fatal, because this reflects corresponding loss of body function. The extreme weight loss which was once characteristic of large burns can be alleviated by use of xenografts, early wound closure, and use of nutritional support techniques.

During the ebb phase, wound care, fluid resuscitation, and major organ support are priorities. Nutritional support can begin when the patient is stable and has entered the flow phase, usually 48 to 72 h following injury.

Consumption of an oral intake may not be possible during the first 5 to 10 days following a burn injury because of nausea, vomiting, anorexia, gastric ileus, and decreased peristalsis. Following this period, the burned patient may experience loss of appetite due to pain and, ironically, because analgesic medications may depress appetite or cause nausea. Depression, pain, and physical inability to self-feed due to scarring of the hands and mouth are powerful deterrents to attaining adequate oral intake. Frequent wound debridement and dressing changes, physical therapy, and surgical procedures are necessary but timing of procedures may cause pain and a decrease in appetite which reduce intake further. Moreover, it is unlikely that the patient who has large burns or chronic disease, complications from injuries, or is in poor nutritional or physical condition prior to the injury, will be able to consume amounts of food necessary to meet nutritional requirements so vastly elevated because of the injury.

Frequently the burned patient needs *hyperalimentation.* Hyperalimentation is a misnomer often applied to special modalities of nutrition support. This term is misleading since it implies that provision of more nutrients than calculated requirements is desirable. Overnutrition may, in fact, be deleterious since there is a potential for toxic effects. Input of excessive amounts of parenteral carbohydrate has been implicated in development of fatty deposits in the liver and in liver dysfunction. Moreover, excess carbohydrate may impair pulmonary function. Although these effects may be tempered when nutrients are delivered enterally, input of superfluous amounts of any nutrient may elevate BEE.

Parenteral nutrition is the route of choice when paralytic ileus persists, or GI function is impaired following a burn. Often PN is used, even though the GI tract is functioning, simply because the patient cannot tolerate the necessary volume of enterally supplied nutrients.

When the gut is functioning, but the patient is unable to ingest an adequate oral diet, tube feeding should be employed. Continuous drip administration into the small bowel is the desired method for enteral support of burned patients.

Tube feeding formulas which provide 1.5 or 2 cal per milliliter are especially useful since they supply the amount of calories required in a tolerable volume. To meet specific requirements of individual patients, it may be necessary to alter the nutritional composition of a prepared formula by adding one or more modular nutritional components.

The nutritional needs of the burned patient with less than 20 percent TBSAB can usually be met through consumption of a high-calorie, high-protein diet supplemented with multivitamins. To avoid overwhelming the patient with the sheer volume of food, intake should be divided into several meals and nutritionally dense snacks. Commercial formulas may be used as between-meal nourishments, but it is difficult for the patient to consume large volumes. Patients complain that prepared formulas

used for oral supplementation rapidly become unpalatable because the consistency may be unpleasant, and the flavor may become tiresome. In addition, the satiety value of formulas may depress the patient's appetite for meals. Nutritional modules are useful for enhancing nutrient levels of the oral diet without altering the flavor of food. Carbohydrate, fat, and protein components can be added to food items (Table 12-5) to increase nutritional content.

When calorie requirements exceed 3500 per day, it may be necessary to use both enteral and parenteral routes to deliver nutrients. An oral diet, or enteral support by tube feeding, can be augmented by peripheral or central PN. At times, an oral diet, tube feeding, and PN may be used simultaneously to attain adequate nutritional input.

Regardless of the modality of nutrition support that is used, it is imperative to monitor the patient's nutritional care and status, to assure tolerance and progress toward an obtainable goal. Nutritional assessment should be dynamic so that changes in metabolic status and tolerance to nutritional therapy are noted and acted upon (see specific variables for monitoring in "Methods for Providing Nutritional Support" in this chapter). Care must be taken to consider the effects that burns and their treatment have on indices of nutritional status. Fluid shifts, dehydration, and transfusional therapy may affect serum concentrations of albumin, transferrin, and

Table 12-5 Examples of Use of Modular Nutritional Components to Enhance Nutrient Density of Common Food Items

Food Item	Calories	Protein (Grams)
6 oz coffee	0	0.0
6 oz coffee + 10 g Polycose*	38	0.0
4 oz chocolate pudding	160	5.0
4 oz chocolate pudding + 10 g Propac†	200	12.6
6 oz cream of tomato soup	160	5.0
6 oz cream of tomato soup + 10 mL Microlipid‡	205	5.0

* Carbohydrate module: Ross Laboratories, Columbus, OH.
† Protein module: Chesebrough-Ponds, Inc., Greenwich, CT.
‡ Fat module: Chesebrough-Ponds, Inc., Greenwich, CT.

prealbumin. Measurements of body weight and anthropometrics are difficult to obtain, and may be skewed by the presence of edema and dressings. Immunocompetence may be difficult to assess since total lymphocyte count is affected by tissue necrosis, infection, stress, and medications. Skin testing does have some utility for evaluating the immune system of burned patients; however, clinicians may not be willing to jeopardize potential skin donor sites.

In spite of these limitations, nutritional assessment remains the most effective method of appraising nutritional therapy. Use of clinical judgment in evaluating results further increases effectiveness of nutritional assessment in guiding metabolic support.

Cardiac Disorders

Heart disease in America is of epidemic proportions. In coronary and intensive-care units one sees the results of cardiac disease which was years in the making. Diet is a major etiological factor in the development of cardiac disease, and one of the few over which the patient is able to have direct influence. Nutritional therapy is an integral part of overall treatment of the patient with heart disease and it should become part of the total plan of care of the patient.

Nutritional Goals for Prevention of Cardiac Disease

Health, and the opportunity for prevention of disease through dietary manipulation has assumed increasing importance to the American population in recent years. This interest was reflected in the development of dietary goals by the U.S. Senate Select Committee on Nutrition and Human Needs in 1977. These goals were the subject of significant controversy, and have been revised. A summary of the 1985 *Dietary Guidelines for Americans* includes the following:

1. Maintain or attain ideal body weight through a balance of energy expenditure and intake.
2. Increase consumption of complex carbohydrates (starches), and naturally occurring sugars while reducing consumption of refined and processed sugars.

3. Decrease total dietary fat, especially saturated fat and cholesterol.
4. Reduce sodium consumption.
5. Moderate consumption of alcohol.

Coronary atherosclerotic heart disease is the most common underlying cause of morbidity and mortality from heart disease. Research has implicated almost every blood lipid fraction in the genesis of atherosclerotic heart disease. It is believed that dietary factors influence blood lipid concentrations. Thus the "Prudent Diet," espoused by the American Heart Association, was developed to aid Americans in reducing their risk of heart disease through dietary modification. The "Prudent Diet" provides specific recommendations which aid Americans in incorporating the U.S. Senate Dietary Guidelines into their daily dietary patterns.

In recent years the food industry has responded to the increasing interest in preventive nutrition on the part of the American public. Information regarding sodium, cholesterol, and fat content appears on food labels. A greater variety of palatable "dietetic" foods, including low-sodium, low-fat, and sugar-free items, is available. These developments are encouraging because these items are useful in enhancing adherence to restricted diets. Compliance with dietary restriction can be facilitated by assuring that the patient thoroughly understands principles of the diet before discharge from the hospital. A consultation from a registered dietitian is invaluable in teaching the patient to translate these modifications into a diet that can be maintained for life.

Coronary Atherosclerotic Heart Disease

Coronary artery disease (CAD) is the most common manifestation of cardiovascular dysfunction. Because elevation of low-density plasma lipoproteins is considered to potentiate development of atherosclerosis, some clinicians believe dietary modification aimed toward lowering circulating levels of the offending lipoprotein(s) is helpful. An exhaustive description of the dietary regimen for each type of hyperlipidemia is beyond the scope of this chapter but a summary of each diet is given in Table 12-6.

Another school of thought supports the use of the principles of the "Prudent Diet" for patients

Chapter 12 Nutrition **357**

Table 12-6 Summary of Dietary Modifications for Hyperlipoproteinemia

Dietary Modifications	Type I	Type IIa	Type IIb	Type III	Type IV	Type V
Limit calories (cal)	No	No	Yes*	Yes*	Yes*	Yes*
Limit protein	No	No	20% total cal	20% total cal	15–25% total cal	15–25% total cal
Limit carbohydrates	No	No	40% total cal	40% total cal	45% total cal	50% total cal
			←———— (Restrict concentrated carbohydrates) ————→			
Limit fat	12–20% total cal	No	40% total cal	40% total cal	20–35% total cal	12–30% total cal
Emphasize PUFA†	No	Yes	Yes	Yes	Yes	Yes
Limit cholesterol	No	100–300 mg/day	100–300 mg/day	100–300 mg/day	300–500 mg/day	300–500 mg/day
Limit alcohol	Yes	Yes	0–2 oz./day	0–2 oz./day	0–2 oz./day‡	Yes

* Restrict calories to the level necessary to obtain or maintain ideal body weight.
† PUFA = polyunsaturated fatty acids (found in vegetable sources).
‡ Moderate consumption of alcohol may be beneficial in some types of hyperlipidemia as it has been found to elevate serum levels of HDL.

who have atherosclerosis, or the potential for developing it, or for patients following coronary artery bypass surgery.

Coronary Artery Bypass Surgery

The patient recovering from coronary artery bypass surgery (CABS) has elevated protein and energy needs as a consequence of major surgery. Meeting the increased nutritional requirements of patients following surgical revascularization of the myocardium is complicated by the need to severely restrict sodium during the postoperative period. Prophylactic sodium restriction is helpful in reducing the potential for thrombosis of the graft which is associated with fluid retention. When dietary sodium is restricted to 1 g or less per day, intake of milk, bread, cereals, and some vegetables is limited. All salted, cured, and commercially prepared foods must be eliminated from the diet. Because fruit, fruit juices, and carbonated beverages contain only trace amounts of naturally occurring sodium, these foods may be consumed as the patient desires. Unfortunately, foods containing very low amounts of sodium are poor sources of protein. Low-sodium diets must be carefully planned by dietitians to be nutritionally adequate for the patient after CABS. But patients may be unable to consume an adequate diet following cardiac surgery because of unpalatability of the low-sodium diet, general weakness and fatigue, or medication-induced anorexia and gastric irritation. The nurse should encourage the patient to achieve adequate oral intake, in spite of the lack of salted foods, by teaching the patient that nutrients are vital for healing. If the patient continues to consume suboptimal amounts for more than 48 h, the physician should be apprised, and the dietitian consulted. It may be necessary to allow a familiar dish which may be relatively high in sodium content in lieu of other foods, to pique the patient's appetite. Lemon juice, vinegar, and sodium-free spices and seasonings can be used to add flavor to the otherwise bland diet.

If these measures are not successful, it may be necessary to add commercially prepared supplements to the diet. Low-sodium protein modules are useful to increase protein content of menu items. When nutritional supplements are used, communication between the nurse, dietitian, and patient is vital so that attainable dietary goals can be planned which are compatible with the dietary prescription.

The patient's instruction regarding a diet reduced in calories (if the patient is above ideal body weight), fat, and sodium should be initiated as soon as possible. The nurse can enhance willingness of the patient to learn by teaching the relationship of diet to the disease process, and the potential benefits to be derived from dietary modification. Consistent, individualized instruction from a dietitian, coupled with group diet classes are effective in teaching patients the principles of the modified diet. The patient's compliance can be facilitated if the nurse reinforces the formal diet instruction. Mealtimes can be ideal times for the nurse to review dietary principles such as sodium restriction and decreased fat intake, using the patient's menu and meal tray as visual aids. A number of patient-oriented publications, such as those prepared by the American Heart Association, are available which contain recipes and guidelines for practical application of the diet in everyday life.

An important factor that the nurse can contribute to the diet instruction process is a positive attitude. By emphasizing the salubrious effects of the diet, the nurse can enhance the willingness of the patient to comply with necessary dietary modifications which are vital to health.

Myocardial Ischemia and Infarction

Nutritional therapy for myocardial ischemia is aimed at reducing symptoms and preventing further damage to weakened myocardial tissue. Calorie restriction may be necessary to attain ideal body weight for height. Another goal of dietary therapy is to modify fat intake in order to alter blood lipid levels. A diet low in saturated fat, cholesterol, total fat, and concentrated carbohydrates is useful in lowering calorie density of the diet and may be useful in reducing serum lipid concentrations. Since consumption of large meals may cause pain due to displacement of the diaphragm, the patient should be counseled to eat small, frequent meals. Those patients who continue to experience pain following eating usually are instructed by their physician to take nitroglycerin before meals.

If myocardial infarction occurs, the patient usually receives the traditional dietary progression from nothing by mouth during the acute phase, progressing to liquids, and finally to a soft diet. Usually, some additional modifications are imposed on this traditional dietary regimen, to protect the weakened heart from further stress. Calories may be limited to preclude elevation of cardiac output. However, it must be remembered that depending upon the amount of tissue damage caused by the infarction, an adrenergic response may be evoked. This event is accompanied by an elevation in calorie and protein requirements. The clinical status of the patient must be monitored carefully so that caloric restriction which is imposed to decrease stress to the heart does not lead to nutritional depletion. Stimulants such as caffeine and extremes in food temperatures should be avoided. A moderate sodium restriction may be indicated, based on the clinical condition of the patient. Cholesterol and fat content of the diet should be limited. When the patient is able to resume consumption of solid foods, calorie level of the diet can be increased to the amount necessary to reach or sustain ideal body weight. Dietary instruction should begin during hospitalization so that the patient understands and is able to make the necessary modifications in the diet prior to discharge.

Congestive Heart Failure

Malnutrition, and *cardiac cachexia* associated with congestive heart failure (CHF), has been recognized for centuries. Classical cardiac cachexia develops over a period of time in the patient who has chronic CHF. Several factors are responsible for the development of cardiac cachexia in patients with CHF. One theory purports that diminished oral intake is a voluntary compensatory mechanism which prevents stress on the failing heart by reducing cardiac output. Anorexia may occur simply because the patient is too weak to ingest adequate amounts of food. Often medications such as digitalis, opiates, and diuretics are responsible for depressed appetite. The patient with CHF frequently describes vague GI discomfort and early satiety due to the presence of pulmonary edema, which further decrease oral intake.

Conditions of nutrient loss are common due to malabsorption and failure to transport nutrients as a result of splenic, hepatic, and pancreatic hypoxia. Excessive urinary nitrogen losses occur via a nephrotic-like syndrome that is secondary to poor cardiac perfusion.

The patient with CHF is hypermetabolic due to elevated temperature and thyroid activity, and increased energy requirements of specific tissues. Energy needs are elevated because of the effects of cellular hypoxia. Poor oxygen perfusion at the cellular level necessitates energy production via less efficient anaerobic processes.

Malnutrition has serious consequences for the patient with CHF. Malnutrition can cause reduced cardiac output, decreased left ventricular mass, and low radiographic total heart volume. Successful treatment of CHF should include treatment of underlying malnutrition. Nutritional therapy must be undertaken with care to avoid overloading the impaired cardiovascular system. Provision of superfluous nutrients is not desirable since this can overtax the heart by increasing metabolic rate, cardiac output, and oxygen consumption. It is important for the nurse to accurately measure and record fluid intake and output to facilitate accurate calculation of water requirements. Fluid intake is usually limited to 1000 to 1500 mL per day.

Sodium replacement is titrated to maintain serum sodium at approximately 140 meq/100 mL. It is usual for sodium input to be restricted to 0.5 to 2.0 g (22 to 65 meq) per day. The nurse should monitor serum sodium levels and report abnormal values to the physician.

Parenteral nutrition is used when GI symptoms preclude enteral feeding. Use of IV lipid emulsions in combination with parenteral amino acids and glucose is advantageous because lipids are calorically dense, and contribute only 500 mL to total daily fluid allowance.

Tube feeding with a 1.5-to-2-cal-per-milliliter enteral formula is a means of providing concentrated nutrients in a limited volume via the enteral route. The nurse should assess the patient's hydration status to assure that he or she does not become dehydrated while receiving a high-calorie tube feeding formula.

When the patient can tolerate an oral diet, frequent, small, soft, low-sodium feedings are appropriate. Modular nutritional components and prepared formulas are vital in supplementing an oral diet because the patient with CHF is quickly fatigued by the exertion of eating. Commercial nutritional products may be added to liquids and food items to enhance nutritional value.

Nutritional support of the patient with CHF must be undertaken with caution because both over- and underfeeding have negative consequences. Strict attention to serum electrolytes, input and output records, and nursing assessment of edema and heart and lung sounds are vital to avoid worsening heart failure as a consequence of nutritional therapy.

Hypertension

An association between sodium intake and the incidence of essential hypertension has been shown by epidemiological studies.[10] Other studies have revealed that individuals who have a propensity for developing hypertension are sensitive to dietary sodium at levels of 125 to 200 meq per day.[11] The "average" sodium content of the American diet is high, between 100 to 200 meq per day.

The action of medications used to manage hypertension is enhanced by decreasing the amount of sodium in the diet. Generally a 2-to-4-g sodium diet is prescribed. This level of restriction can be met if the patient is counseled to avoid canned, processed, and cured meats, and convenience foods, unless these items are labeled as low-sodium. Use of fresh or frozen vegetables in lieu of the canned variety further decreases dietary sodium. The patient should be specifically enjoined against consumption of salted snack foods since these are a significant source of sodium and low-nutrient calories.

If the patient is obese, weight reduction may be effective in lowering blood pressure. However, it is important not to impose too many dietary modifications at one time, because one runs the risk of overwhelming the patient with lifestyle changes.

Antihypertensive medications are also associated with loss of potassium. Simply encouraging the patient to increase consumption of potassium-containing foods is not sufficient to replace potassium losses. In cases when antihypertensive medications are used, the nurse should remind the physician that oral or IV potassium replacement is necessary.

Cardiomyopathy

Unfortunately, the amount of literature regarding nutritional support of the patient with cardiomyopathy is insufficient. It may be assumed that the patient is at nutritional risk for the same reasons as the patient with CHF. The poorly functioning heart muscle is less efficient, requiring more energy to accomplish less work than the normal heart. Oxygen starvation of tissues interferes with absorption, transport, and metabolism of nutritional substrates. The patient may be unable to consume adequate nutrients because of weakness and fatigue, early satiety, or anorexia due to medications. The patient with severe cardiomopathy may suffer from cardiac cachexia because of these conditions.

Nutritional therapy should be directed toward maintaining or improving the nutritional status and avoiding additional strain to the heart. The same guidelines which govern nutritional support of the patient with CHF may be applied to care of the patient with cardiomyopathy.

Valvular Disease

The most common causes of valvular disease in adults are rheumatic fever and calcification of the valve structures noted in older patients. During acute episodes of rheumatic fever, the goal of nutritional therapy is to support elevated requirements for energy and protein due to the hypermetabolism which results from fever and infection. Following recovery, prophylactic dietary modifications may include adherence to a mild sodium restriction (2 to 4 g per day), and a calorie level appropriate to obtain or maintain ideal body weight, because obesity adds to the strain on the heart.

Surgery and Trauma

The metabolic events following major surgery or multiple trauma are dictated by the changing hormonal milieu following injury. The body responds to significant trauma and surgery in the ebb and flow reactions described previously (see "Burns" in this section). Lesser injuries or elective surgeries do not significantly alter metabolism of body fuels or protein, although they do stimulate conservation of water and salt.

During the early flow phase, the healing wound has priority over other tissues for nutrients. The wound is in positive nitrogen balance because other tissues provide nutritional substrates through adrenergically stimulated autocannibalism. In the case of relatively minor surgery or trauma, input of large amounts of exogenous substrates is unnecessary, because metabolic requirements are not greatly increased and the patient is soon able to consume an adequate oral diet. If there is significant hypermetabolism, if nutritional input is absent or inadequate, or if sepsis and other complications occur, wound healing may suffer unless nutritional needs are met.

Frequently, surgical candidates are in poor nutritional status as a result of disease. Cancer, regional enteritis, and colitis are examples of conditions which often cause significant weight loss and impose nutritional costs in addition to those resulting from major surgery. Because patients with these conditions are already at nutritional risk, they may benefit from a period of nutritional repletion prior to surgery.

The goals for metabolic support following injury or trauma are prioritized as follows:

1. Provide fluid resuscitation and support organ function. Restoration of cardiovascular homeostasis in itself is useful in reducing catecholamine levels, thus decreasing the period of hypermetabolism which follows major tissue damage.
2. Repair wounds and damaged tissue. The degree of adrenergic response is related to the extent of the open wound. The hypermetabolic response evoked by catecholamines is abated when wounds are closed, fractures immobilized, and septic and contaminated areas drained.
3. Provide nutritional substrates when the patient is stable and capable of using them for anabolism. This period usually does not begin until 24 to 48 h following injury.

Nutritional Requirements

Nutritional requirements vary according to the degree of injury and resulting hypermetabolism. The patient undergoing minor elective procedures experiences limited, short-term alterations in nutritional requirements. Major surgery and trauma, on the other hand, elevate the patient's protein requirements because of the increased rates of protein synthesis and catabolism associated with these events. The elevation in protein synthetic rate accounts for some of the increase in energy expenditure experienced by patients recovering from surgery or trauma.

Because the response to injury includes obligate catabolism of amino acids, protein requirments during the acute stage may be high, but level off as the patient recovers. Protein input should be monitored closely by nitrogen balance studies because these patients may quickly become intolerant of nitrogen secondary to acute renal or hepatic insufficiency. During acute stress, protein appears to be most efficiently used when approximately 15 nonprotein calories are provided with every gram of protein. As the acute phase resolves, the optimal protein-to-nonprotein calorie ratio increases to 1:25. Vitamin and mineral supplementation is often given although there is little agreement regarding data on dosages of vitamins and minerals required by trauma and surgery patients.

Nutritional Care

Choice of the feeding route depends on GI functional capability, degree of stress and hypermetabolism present, the extent of preexisting malnutrition, and the risk of complications. Feeding by tube is the optimal route when there is adequate GI function, and the patient can tolerate the volume necessary to meet nutritional requirements. Use of the GI tract precludes development of mucosal atrophy which can occur when the patient is sustained on PN over a long period of time. Moreover, enteral feeding is associated with fewer complications, especially less hemorrhage of the upper GI tract, than is intravenous nutritional support. In spite of this, parenteral nutritional support is extensively used, particularly in cases of abdominal surgery, because it is thought that postoperative paralytic ileus precludes early use of the GI tract. Abdominal surgery or postoperative ileus does not necessarily contraindicate enteral feeding. While gastric and colonic ileus may persist for 24 to 48 h after surgery, motility of the small intestine recovers within hours. Therefore, it is possible to begin feeding into the small intestine via jejunostomy shortly after surgery. Traditionally, monomeric enteral formulas have been exclusively used for jejunostomy feeding. A recent study[7] has demonstrated that polymeric formulas administered jejunally are well tolerated and, unlike monomeric formulas,

can be initiated in full strength because polymeric formulas are relatively isotonic.

Protein-sparing IV solutions can be used in cases in which a relatively well-nourished patient may begin eating within 5 to 7 days of surgery. Patients who have large nutritional requirements and are not candidates for enteral feeding may require PN.

The patient undergoing metabolic stress may have a limited capacity to metabolize nutritional substrates. Intravenous infusions of about 2 to 3 mg of dextrose per kilogram per minute are generally tolerated. The energy needs of extremely hypermetabolic patients may be best met by a combination of glucose and lipid calories. Input of lipid emulsions should be limited to approximately 35 percent of total calorie requirements to assure the patient's tolerance of IV fat emulsions.

Nutritional care should be continually assessed and evaluated by the health care team. Because the metabolic consequences of surgery and trauma influence several major nutritional assessment parameters, identification of these effects is essential for accurate diagnosis of nutritional status. The fluid resuscitation which occurs following surgery or trauma affects several body compartments and may produce erroneous values when these body compartments are evaluated to assess the nutritional status of the patient. Fluid input may cause false elevation in body weight and other anthropometric measurements. Fluid retention may cause a false low value in serum protein concentrations because of dilution and extravasation from intravascular to interstitial spaces. Surgery and trauma are events which may affect common indices of a patient's nutritional status. Anergy may result from circulating immunosuppressive factor and increased supressor T cell activity, which is associated with surgery and trauma rather than nutritional factors.

While all of these changes are a result of metabolic stress, they are usually short-lived, and are not true indicators of a nutritional deficit. Even though indicators of nutritional status may not be useful in the initial period following injury, they do provide a guide for monitoring nutritional progress. Serial assessments are necessary to follow the dynamic metabolic course following surgery and injury.

Special Considerations

The adrenergic response to neurosurgery is similar to that mounted as a result of major injury. However, there are additional factors which must be considered when providing nutritional support to patients following neurosurgery or head injury. Increased energy requirements resulting from hyperventilation, increased cardiac output, fever, posturing, seizures, and general restlessness are superimposed on those energy requirements resulting from the effects of stress-related catecholamines. Steroid therapy further increases catabolic activity and nitrogen losses. On the other hand, paralysis, ventilatory support, and barbiturate coma decrease energy expenditure.

Factors which further complicate nutritional care of the neurosurgery patient include prevention of further brain damage which can occur secondary to cerebral swelling. This necessitates fluid restriction and diuresis with mannitol and Lasix. Fluid and electrolyte status can fluctuate dramatically as a result, and must be followed closely when providing nutritional support.

The obtunded patient is at risk of aspiration due to an inability to protect the airway, although the presence of an endotracheal tube or tracheostomy provides some protection. In addition, these patients are prone to vomiting because of nausea, nasogastric secretions, and changes in intracranial pressure. The presence of nausea, secretions, and changes in intracranial pressure do not preclude enteral feeding if appropriate precautions are taken (see "Enteral Feeding by Tube" in this chapter). Commercial formulas which provide 1.5 to 2 cal per milliliter are especially useful because it is possible to provide adequate protein and calories in a tolerable volume. Modular nutritional components can be used to further augment nutrient density of enteral formulas. Parenteral nutrition may be necessary if the patient is unable to tolerate the volume of enteral formula necessary to meet nutritional requirements, or if the risk of aspiration is too great.

Special nutritional care is required following surgery of the GI tract. Surgical intervention for complications of peptic ulcer disease includes drainage, vagotomy, pyloroplasty, and partial or total removal of the stomach and/or part of the small intestine. The postgastrectomy patient is prone

to develop the *dumping syndrome*. Dumping occurs when the hyperosmolar food mass rapidly enters the small intestine without first undergoing normal digestion and mixing in the stomach. Symptoms arise from 5 to 15 min after consuming a meal. Symptoms include bloating, pain, nausea, diarrhea, pallor, weakness, palpitations, sweating, and increased pulse rate. One method of dietary treatment for dumping includes providing foods in numerous small meals rather than three large ones. The diet should be relatively high in protein and fat without concentrated carbohydrates. The carbohydrates used should be complex, since these are less osmotically active than simple sugars. Fluid with meals should be restricted to 4 oz, because liquid enhances formation of osmolar solutes which can precipitate the dumping reaction. These dietary modifications are not necessary, however, in all patients following gastrectomy. Those patients who do suffer from dumping usually experience cessation of symptoms over time.

Following surgery of the small intestine, digestive and absorptive capability remains intact if the distal ileum, ileocecal valve, and the dueodenum are not excised. If more than 50 to 75 percent of the small intestine is resected, malabsorption and accompanying malnutrition may occur.

Short bowel syndrome occurs after a large amount of the bowel is removed. Malabsorption problems vary depending on the extent of excision of the small intestine, the part of small intestine resected, and the degree to which diseased tissue is excised. Nutritional therapy must be tailored to the individual needs of the patient. Fat and lactose are the nutrients most frequently malabsorbed. The consistency of the diet may require modification in order to omit roughage, depending on the patient's tolerance. In cases of extreme malabsorption, the patient may require tube feeding with a monomeric, low-fat formula. If very little absorptive surface of the GI tract remains, PN must be instituted.

Gastrointestinal Disorders

Diseases affecting the GI tract have the greatest potential for influencing the nutritional status of the patient because the GI tract is the site of ingestion, digestion, and absorption of nutrients. The category of GI disease includes a variety of malabsorption syndromes, inflammatory disorders, and other entities which may cause significant malabsorption and depleted nutritional status. Each condition requires specific treatment and nutritional care is individualized according to the patient's needs and tolerance.

Nutritional Requirements

Energy needs of the patient with GI disease are based on the current clinical status, presence of preexisting malnutrition, and function of the gut. The patient with chronic disease is frequently protein-depleted due to poor intake, dyspepsia, malabsorption, and increased losses. Special attention should be given to vitamin, mineral, and trace element nutriture. The GI patient is at risk for vitamin deficiency and mineral and trace element depletion because of increased losses and failure to absorb these micronutrients.

Nutritional Care

Peptic ulcer is the lesion of the GI tract most frequently seen. Peptic ulcers may occur in the lower end of the esophagus or in the stomach or duodenum. Acute cases are treated with antacids and by eliminating stimulants from the diet. Caffeine, alcohol, and spices are eliminated from the diet to decrease the production of acid. Small meals should be provided at regular intervals. Late-night snacking should be avoided since this is implicated in nocturnal production of acid. The traditional *Sippy diet,* which espouses very small, frequent feedings of milk and cream, has been proven to be noneffective, and is rarely part of modern treatment plans. The buffering capacity of milk is quite weak, and its protein content can actually increase acid production. Furthermore, the high cholesterol and saturated fat content of whole milk precludes its use in patients who have or are prone to develop atherosclerosis.[12] The patient who suffers recurrent or intractable ulcers generally requires surgical intervention to prevent erosion into adjacent structures or development of obstructions.

Malabsorption syndromes arise from three etiological factors: (1) dyspepsia due to lack of bile salts, digestive enzymes, or normal peristalsis; (2) inadequate absorption of nutrients because of a deficiency of enzymes or dysfunction of the intestinal mucosa; or (3) failure in assimilation of nu-trients secondary to obstruction of the lymphatic system, portal veins, or lack of transport mechanisms. Common malabsorption syndromes include celiac disease and inflammatory bowel disease. The patient with malabsorption syndrome is at nutritional risk because of ongoing failure to digest, absorb, and/or assimilate nutrients. Moreover, a diagnostic workup for malabsorption syndromes requires that the patient be NPO for several days prior to and during tests. Frequently this additional nutritional deprivation is superimposed on preexisting malnutrition.

Inflammatory bowel disease includes two distinct entities. *Crohn's disease* is a progressive inflammatory process which usually affects the large bowel, although it may affect any part of the GI tract. Healthy bowel tissue is interposed with diseased areas and, therefore, some normal absorption may occur. Acute and chronic inflammation of the GI tract may lead to significant weight loss. Lesions of the GI tract include all layers of the mucosa and submucosa, and development of fistulas is common, which represents an additional nutritional cost because nutrients may be diverted outside the GI tract via fistulas.

Ulcerative colitis affects mainly the large bowel, and sometimes the terminal ileum, and causes a diffuse inflammation of the mucosa, but does not affect the submucosa. Eventually the absorptive surface of the GI tract is destroyed as scar tissue fills the ulcerated areas. The patient experiences significant nutritional losses due to diarrhea which occurs secondary to malabsorption of nutrients. Water and electrolytes normally reabsorbed by the large bowel are also lost.

Treatment of acute ulcerative colitis includes a period of bowel rest. Although the well-nourished patient can tolerate 3 to 5 days of being NPO, generally the patient with GI disease does not have nutritional reserves on which to call so parenteral nutrition is an important adjunct therapy to prevent further nutritional decline in these patients. Following the acute stage of ulcerative colitis, the patient may be advanced to an oral diet which restricts lactose and fat. The degree of dietary restriction should vary according to the patient's tolerance of foods containing fat and lactose.

Bowel rest is required by the patient with Crohn's disease when it is in the active phase.

Parenteral nutrition is used frequently but tube feeding using a monomeric formula is possible when the patient is not critically ill, and when the GI tract is free of fistulas or obstructions. When the patient achieves remission, the diet can be progressed slowly, restricting fat and lactose.

Management of fistulas that have a variety of etiologies includes keeping the patient NPO which controls complications from fistula leakage. Several interesting studies have demonstrated that with adequate PN, fistulas may close spontaneously, obviating the need for surgical intervention.[13,14]

The patient suffering from acute pancreatitis also benefits from gut rest (to decrease output of pancreatic secretions), nasogastric suction, and supportive care. Resolution of pancreatitis usually occurs within 5 to 7 days. The patient who develops complications including prolonged ileus or pseudocyst requires nutritional intervention, preferably with PN. Administration of IV amino acids has been shown to stimulate some pancreatic activity, but much less than an oral diet or tube feeding using a polymeric formula.

Following a patient's nutritional progress by serial assessments of nutritional status is especially beneficial to the GI patient. While hydration status and effects of some medications must be taken into consideration when evaluating nutritional assessment parameters, interpretation of most measurements is fairly straightforward.

Renal Failure

Nutritional Requirements

A major goal of nutritional therapy for the patient with renal failure is to minimize uremic symptoms which occur when metabolites of protein cannot be excreted by the kidneys. Protein metabolites are generated from dietary protein and from catabolism of body proteins. Therefore, a tenet of nutritional therapy is to provide tolerable amounts of protein, accompanied by adequate amounts of nonprotein calories to prevent breakdown of muscle mass.

Input of protein which has *high biologic value (HBV)* is emphasized when planning nutritional care of patients in acute renal failure (ARF) and chronic renal failure (CRF). High biologic value protein sources (eggs, milk, meat, and fish) are those which contain a full complement of essential amino acids. Input of nonessential amino acids is limited so that endogenous urea is used by the body to synthesize nonessential amino acids. Provision of 70 percent of dietary protein as HBV protein facilitates reduction of serum urea levels because urea may be "recycled" to produce nonessential amino acids.

The type of dialysis used is a factor to consider when estimating protein needs. Continuous peritoneal dialysis (CAPD) solutions contain as much as 4.25 percent glucose per liter and are significant calorie sources. However, CAPD is associated with the greatest loss of protein, while lesser amounts are lost with intermittent peritoneal dialysis and hemodialysis.

Prior to initiation of dialysis, the amount of protein which can be tolerated by the patient with CRF is estimated based on the glomerular filtration rate (GFR). As the GFR declines, the amount of protein input must be also be reduced (Table 12-7).

Protein requirements for patients with ARF are more difficult to estimate. Acute renal failure is frequently accompanied by conditions which may evoke overwhelming catabolism and protein losses. However, enthusiasm for providing protein must be tempered by the knowledge of the inability of the kidneys to excrete the resulting metabolites.

The failure of the malfunctioning kidney to perform its normal regulatory and endocrine functions necessitates other nutritional modifications, including attention to electrolyte, vitamin, mineral, and fluid input. Water-soluble vitamins are usually supplemented since dialysis causes loss of these nutrients. Vitamin A is generally not supplemented because serum levels are frequently elevated in patients with renal failure. Vitamin D and calcium may be supplemented but require close monitoring.

Table 12-7 Recommended Protein Intake in Undialyzed Chronic Renal Failure Patients

Glomerular Filtration Rate	Recommended Protein Intake
20–25 mL/min	Up to 90 g/day
15–20 mL/min	Up to 70 g/day
10–15 mL/min	Up to 50 g/day

Trace elements, zinc, and iron are usually supplemented.

Sodium and fluid input must be titrated to the tolerance of the individual patient. Hyperkalemia, hyperphosphatemia, and hypermagnesemia are common in renal failure because of the inability of the kidney to excrete potassium, phosphorus, and magnesium. The potassium content of the diet is restricted to about 40 meq per day. Serum levels of phosphorus are controlled through use of phosphate binders. Intake of magnesium-containing compounds is restricted and serum magnesium levels should be monitored frequently.

Nutritional Care

The patient with renal failure frequently becomes malnourished as renal failure progresses. Uremia is associated with anorexia, nausea, and vomiting. Drugs used in CRF may cause GI upset, constipation, diarrhea, and anorexia. Moreover, the sheer volume of medications the patient is required to consume daily may contribute to the inability to consume adequate amounts of food. Poor oral intake is exacerbated by a necessarily limited diet. Every opportunity should be taken to increase the calorie content of the diet while remaining within the dietary prescription for protein, sodium, potassium, and fluid. This may be accomplished through the addition of fat, oil, and sugar during food preparation. Consumption of protein-free food items, such as hard candies, jam and jelly, syrups, and breads and cookies prepared from low-protein flour, can be encouraged. Addition of commercial fat or carbohydrate modules to menu items is useful because the modules are fairly neutral in taste, provide a fair number of calories, and contribute only small amounts of volume. If nutritional intake is not adequate or continues to decline, commercial nutritional supplements may be added to the oral diet.

Frequently the critically ill patient with renal failure requires aggressive nutritional support. It is important to prevent the breakdown of tissues that results from inadequate intake, because metabolites of catabolism of body protein contribute to uremia. There are at least two commercial tube feeding formulas available which are specially formulated for use with renal failure patients. These special formulas are relatively low in protein and electrolytes and high in calories. Protein is provided as essential amino acids. These formulas are not suitable for long-term use because they are nutritionally incomplete. Moreover, they are hyperosmolar and, therefore, a period of gut adaptation is required before they are tolerated at full strength. They are extremely unpalatable because of the presence of free amino acids, and, therefore, should not be used for supplementation of the oral diet. Due to these limitations, specialty formulas should be used only in cases of short-term protein restriction, when dialysis is not an option. It is possible to use a standard polymeric formula for enteral support of the patient with renal failure. Formulas which provide 1.5 to 2 cal per milliliter are useful for tube feeding patients with renal failure in whom volume restriction is necessary.

Another alternative for successful enteral support of patients with renal failure is use of modular components. Modular nutrient components can be added to standard formulas to provide for modifications of major nutrients and electrolytes required by individual patients.

Parenteral nutritional support may be necessary if the gut is nonfunctioning. Essential amino acid solutions are commercially available but there is controversy regarding whether their use is more efficacious than use of lower concentrations of solutions containing mixed amino acids.

Patients with renal failure have alterations in glucose metabolism, so that use of hypertonic glucose concentrations must be carefully monitored to prevent complications. Intravenous lipid emulsions are especially useful for the patient who is intolerant of large glucose loads. Moreover, IV lipids are beneficial when calorie requirements are high and fluid input must be limited. When lipid emulsions are used, serum triglyceride levels should be closely followed to assure patient tolerance to IV lipid emulsions.

Nutritional assessment is useful in order to follow the progress of patients with renal failure. Anthropometric measurements are useful in evaluating somatic protein and energy stores in the patient with CRF. These measurements are less useful in the patient with ARF since fluid status is extremely dynamic. Dramatic shifts in fluid balance can also affect the reliability of circulating proteins as markers of nutritional status in the patient with ARF. Visceral protein levels are more useful in CRF, especially when used in conjunction with parameters of somatic proteins.

Skin testing provides unreliable data regarding immune function in these patients. Estimation of nitrogen balance and creatinine height index is unreliable, if not impossible, in conditions of impaired renal excretion of nitrogenous waste products. Urea kinetics is a method which determines the rate of protein catabolism from the rate of urea generation. It is a tool which holds promise as a means of estimating nitrogen balance in the patient with renal failure.[15]

Cancer

Cachexia is the most widely recognized manifestation of cancer. The etiology of weight loss in the cancer patient is poorly understood, but a number of factors contribute to the development of malnutrition which frequently accompanies oncologic disease. Development of cancer cachexia occurs in three stages. Anorexia is the primary manifestation in the first phase, but its development is not well understood. One theory is that the tumor itself secretes "anorexigenic peptides," but isolation of these substances has yet to be accomplished. Nonetheless, early stages of cancer are typified by increasing anorexia accompanied by weight loss.

Energy requirements of cancer patients may be increased by the existence of "futile metabolic cycles," which use more energy than they produce. It has been shown that there is an increase in Cori cycle activity in some cancer patients. This Cori cycle activity produces energy via less efficient anaerobic processes.

Other factors which may contribute to cancer cachexia in the first stage are possible alterations in taste perception (although one recent study has discounted this as a major contributing factor),[16] development of food aversions, early satiety resulting from secretion of anorexigenic substances or mechanical effects of the tumor burden, or inability to digest or assimilate nutrients.

The second stage is characterized by initiation of antineoplastic therapies and imposition of mechanical effects of the tumor (such as obstruction of the GI tract). Resection of neoplastic masses has acute and long-term effects. Any major surgical procedure evokes the typical adrenergic response which initiates a hypermetabolic reaction (see "Surgery" in this chapter). Long-term effects vary according to the area and the extent of resection. Excision of tumors in the GI tract may produce difficulties in chewing, swallowing, digesting, and absorbing nutrients. Resection of the lip and tongue may interfere with the ability of the patient to retain food and saliva, to chew, and to manipulate food to the back of the mouth for swallowing. A partial laryngectomy makes swallowing difficult and a total laryngectomy renders the patient dysphagic for a period of time following surgery. In addition, the protective mechanism of the epiglottis is lost, placing the patient at risk for aspiration until the skill of swallowing is relearned. Surgical treatment of cancer involving the esophagus may be accompanied by early satiety, diarrhea, and steatorrhea. Weight loss is frequently a consequence of partial gastrectomy and always occurs with total gastrectomy. Gastrectomy may be accompanied by the dumping syndrome. Dyspepsia may occur as a consequence of resection of the pancreas, biliary system, or small intestine. Resection of the large intestine may be associated with temporary alterations in the ability to conserve water and electrolytes. However, these aberrations are short-lived because adaptation occurs fairly rapidly.

The effects of radiation therapy are dependent on dose, site, volume of tissue treated, and time over which the dose is given. The major nutritional effects of radiation occur when the GI tract is radiated. Acute effects include mucositis, stomatitis, esophagitis, nausea, vomiting, diarrhea, and loss of taste sensation, also known as *mouth blindness*. Later effects include malabsorption, dental caries, and radiation enteritis.

Chemotherapy is designed to destroy rapidly growing and dividing cancer cells, but normal cells which also experience rapid turnover are affected by chemotherapeutic agents. Because cells of the GI tract are rapidly growing, chemotherapy damages the GI tract, causing nausea, vomiting, diarrhea, malabsorption, and painful lesions. Moreover, nutritional status may be compromised because of possible hepatic, renal, and pancreatic toxicity of antineoplastic agents.

Patients in the third phase of cancer cachexia are extremely marasmic. The third phase of cancer cachexia is characterized by catabolism of somatic muscle and energy stores, depletion of circulating proteins, anergy, and asthenia.

The issue of nutritional support of the cancer patient is a controversial one. Opponents cite the failure of nutritional support to positively affect prognosis. Animal studies which show acceleration of tumor growth when provided with nutritional substrate may also deter clinicians from instituting metabolic support.

It is estimated that 45 percent of hospitalized cancer patients lose 10 percent of their body weight, and an additional 25 percent of patients lose 20 percent of their body weight. Weight loss is correlated with longer length of hospital stay, a significantly higher incidence of complications, and increased mortality. Depleted serum albumin levels are also associated with higher rates of postoperative infection. It is recognized that nutritional therapy is not primary or curative cancer treatment, but nutritional therapy does have the potential for decreasing the incidence of malnutrition-associated side effects. Proponents argue that nutritional support is important adjunct therapy for the cancer patient because there are few associated complications; the possibility for prevention or alleviation of weight loss and malnutrition exists, and provision of nutritional needs contributes to a general feeling of well-being on the part of the patient. Moreover, there is no evidence of inappropriate increases in tumor growth as a consequence of nutrition support. Discrepancies between tumor growth rate in animals versus humans can be explained by the fact that tumors implanted in animals grow rapidly and quickly achieve weights equal to 30 percent of the total weight of the animal. This is in contrast to tumors in human beings, which are slow-growing and reach no more than 5 percent of total body weight.

Nutritional Requirements

Increased energy requirements as a result of the primary disease is not universal among cancer patients. However, it should be noted that the cancer patient does not respond to long-term inadequate nutritional intake by decreasing basal energy requirements as do normal individuals. Antineoplastic therapies may elevate energy requirements. Negative nitrogen balance and low levels of circulating proteins may persist in spite of adequate protein input, until the tumor burden is reduced and/or antineoplastic therapy is completed. Negative nitrogen balance is thought to be related to an increased rate of protein catabolism accompanied by a decreased synthesis of body proteins.

Vitamin and mineral supplementation should be provided so that the RDA for these nutrients is met and to replete diminished stores. To date, data are inconclusive regarding optimal levels of supplementation of vitamins and minerals. Particular attention should be paid to maintaining serum levels of potassium, phosphorus, and magnesium, since these electrolytes are vital for anabolism and retention of nitrogen. Potassium may be lost by the cancer patient as a result of treatments including gastric suctioning, and potassium-losing diuretic and antibiotic therapies. Copious diarrhea and small bowel drainage may also represent significant losses of potassium. Hypophosphatemia may occur during refeeding when an adequate amount of phosphorus is not supplied. Use of steroids and phosphate-binding antacids is also associated with low serum phosphorus levels. Hypomagnesemia may arise from malabsorption, diarrhea, and small bowel drainage.

Nutritional Care

Dietary manipulations to deal with the sequelae of antineoplastic therapy have received wide attention in the literature. A summary is provided in Table 12-8. Dietary modifications must be individualized according to the patient's preferences, tolerance, and condition. Education regarding the importance of adequate nutritional intake and provision of encouragement and support of the cancer patient during mealtimes is most effective in encouraging intake. Flexibility in mealtimes is useful in enabling the patient to eat whenever and whatever he or she can. If it is impossible to individualize meal service times, intake may be maximized by keeping high-protein, high-calorie food items at the bedside or in the unit refrigerator so that the patient can take advantage of times when he or she feels able to eat. Appropriate and timely delivery of antiemetic medications is invaluable in assisting the cancer patient to overcome nausea in order to eat when

Table 12-8 Symptom-Specific Dietary Modifications

Symptom	Dietary Modification(s)
Anorexia	Small, frequent feedings.
	Emphasize high-calorie protein foods.
	Offer support and encouragement at mealtimes.
	Keep snacks available so patient can eat when appetite allows.
Dysgeusia	Serve foods at room temperature.
	Offer cold plates.
	Avoid specific foods patient cannot tolerate such as coffee or hot entrees.
Mouth dryness	Add sauces, gravies, au jus, margarine.
	Suggest pureed or liquid foods.
	Offer "slushes," popsicles, and juicy fruits.
Esophagitis	Offer soft or pureed foods.
	Avoid irritating seasonings, spices, and acidic foods such as citrus or tomatoes.
	Avoid extremes in temperature.
Stomatitis, mucositis	Avoid salty, acidic, highly seasoned foods, and carbonated beverages.
	Avoid extremes in temperature.
Early satiety	See dietary modifications for anorexia.
	Limit liquids with or just preceding meals.
Nausea, vomiting	Assure appropriate delivery of antiemetics.
	Avoid excessively sweet, strongly flavored or greasy foods.
	Delay eating until acute nausea subsides.
	Individualize diet to patient tolerance.
	Use carbonated beverages or salty foods to relieve nausea.

meals are delivered. If the patient is acutely nauseated and vomiting at mealtimes, he or she should not be encouraged to eat solid foods, but should be given antiemetic medication and encouraged to sip cool liquids until the nausea subsides.

Tube feeding may be required if the patient is unable to ingest adequate nutrients by mouth because of anorexia, nausea, or mechanical obstruction. Because antineoplastic therapy or preexisting malnutrition may cause immunosuppression in the cancer patient, care must be given to maintain the sanitary condition of the tube feeding formula and system (see "Enteral Feeding by Tube" in this chapter). Dilution of the formula may be unwise because increased handling is required and may result in contamination of the feeding. Use of an isotonic, polymeric feeding, initiated at a slow rate, is the best way to assure tolerance and prevent infection. A monomeric, low-fat formula may be necessary, however, if the patient exhibits symptoms of malabsorption.

Parenteral nutritional support may be necessary if the patient suffers from significant malabsorption, intractable nausea and vomiting, or if the GI tract is nonfunctioning. Meticulous attention must be given to care of the catheter insertion site and delivery of PN solutions to avoid septic complications (see "Parenteral Nutrition" in this chapter). Right atrial Silastic catheters are frequently inserted prior to the beginning of chemotherapy to provide central venous access, to deliver chemotherapy, blood products, other medications, and PN solutions. It is possible to cycle PN solutions during hours in which the catheter is not being used for other infusions. While it is necessary to plan delivery of all IV solutions so that none are omitted, cyclic delivery of PN formulas is helpful to assure that adequate nutritional input is attained.

The validity of traditional nutritional assessment techniques in the cancer patient has been widely debated. Most parameters of nutritional status are significantly affected by the effects of cancer itself and by antineoplastic therapies. Oncology patients frequently experience alterations in fluid status. Alterations in hydration status may affect the reliability of any biochemical data which are expressed as concentration per volume (such as serum albumin, transferrin, and total lymphocyte count), as well as measurements of body weight and other anthropometrics. Steroids and chemotherapy cause immunosuppression which is not necessarily related to malnutrition. These therapies invalidate evaluation of the immune system in the effort to evaluate nutritional status. Moreover, some chemotherapeutic agents may cause hepatic and renal dysfunction. Liver or kidney insufficiency may cause alteration in serum levels of circulating proteins and in outcome of urine tests for creatinine excretion and nitrogen balance. Traditional nutritional assessment indices are useful in evaluating the nutritional status of the newly diagnosed cancer patient prior to institution of therapy. Serial assessments must be used in combination with sound clinical judgment to assure that nutritional status is being evaluated, and not simply the effects of therapy.

Pulmonary Disorders

The role that maintenance of adequate nutrition status plays in management of the patient with pulmonary disease has not been emphasized until recently. It has been reported that as many as 40 percent of patients suffering from chronic obstructive pulmonary disease (COPD) lose approximately 10 percent or more of body weight. Weight loss in COPD patients is associated with cor pulmonale, declining pulmonary function, and death. There are a number of contributing factors in the etiology of chronic weight loss in the COPD patient. Intake is often curtailed because the patient experiences fatigue and shortness of breath caused by the exertion of eating, and lack of appetite may develop as a result of chronic sputum production. Medications frequently prescribed for the patient with pulmonary disease include bronchodilators and steroids, known gastric irritants which may cause anorexia. Additional weight loss may be related to the increased energy required for the work of breathing. Malnutrition manifested by the COPD patient is generally of the marasmic type. Marasmus is recognizable on physical examination by general cachexia. The COPD patient usually has compensated for this chronically undernourished state as evidenced by relatively normal levels of circulating proteins. However, this patient is at significant nutritional risk should acute illness, infection, or trauma develop, because there are no nutritional reserves on which he or she can rely during periods of hypermetabolism.

The acutely ill patient on ventilator support is also at risk of developing malnutrition. Kwashiorkor-type malnutrition can develop rapidly if nutritional support is absent or inadequate because associated hypermetabolism causes rapid catabolism of somatic and visceral protein and energy stores, accompanied by a corresponding loss of body function.

Malnutrition has several deleterious effects which have particular significance for the patient with pulmonary disease. Lean body protein, including respiratory muscles, is catabolized during periods of hypermetabolism accompanied by inadequate nutritional input. Autocannibalism results in loss of respiratory function. Ventilatory drive is reduced as respiratory muscle mass is reduced and endurance of the remaining muscle tissue is impaired. Malnutrition is also associated with incompetence of the immune system and, thus the pulmonary patient who is unable to clear secretions has an increased risk of developing infection. Protein-calorie malnutrition causes depletion of serum albumin level which decreases oncotic pressure, and may result in pulmonary edema. All these malnutrition-related factors contribute to decreased inspiratory force, decreased vital capacity and functioning residual capacity of the lungs, impaired oxygenation, and increased minute ventilation. Presence of these effects impairs weaning from ventilator-assisted respiration.

Nutritional Requirements

Provision of overabundant amounts of nutrients to the pulmonary patient is as undesirable as is undernutrition. Input of excess calories, especially in the form of carbohydrate, is associated with an increased respiratory quotient (RQ). The RQ is the ratio of carbon dioxide produced to the oxygen consumed and it varies with the type of nutritional substrate being oxidized. Oxidation of fat results in an RQ of 0.7. When enough glucose is provided to meet basal requirements, RQ increases to 1.0. When more calories than necessary are provided, RQ rises above 1.0. An RQ above 1.0 is undesirable because this reflects production of carbon dioxide in excess of oxygen consumed, and it is associated with increased ventilatory workload. This is especially detrimental to the patient who is being weaned from ventilator support and the patient with chronic obstructive pulmonary disease. Therefore, it is beneficial for the patient who is being weaned from ventilator support and the patient with COPD to avoid provision of excess calories and to provide about 50 percent of energy requirements in the form of fat.

Provision of protein in excess of requirements should be avoided in patients with pulmonary disease. Oxidation of amino acids increases minute ventilation which may result in dyspnea.

Adequate vitamin and mineral nurriture is important for nutritional support of the pulmonary patient. Maintenance of normal serum phosphate levels is particularly important because hypophosphatemia has been related to respiratory failure. Hypophosphatemia may occur because of increased requirements for phosphate during hypermetabolism, movement of phosphate into the cells during metabolism of glucose, or infusion of phosphate-free PN solutions. Maintenance levels of vitamins, minerals, and trace elements should be provided and serum levels monitored to provide for increased requirements.

Nutritional Care

It is vital to provide nutritional care to pulmonary patients as early as possible to forestall the development of chronic malnutrition. A high-protein, high-calorie diet accompanied by oral vitamin and mineral supplementation is the nutritional therapy of choice for the patient with chronic pulmonary disease. Since distention of the stomach can interfere with movement of the diaphragm, the patient should be encouraged to "graze," consuming numerous small snacks throughout the day, rather than concentrating nutrients into three meals. Ingestion of liquids and semisolid foods seems to provoke less shortness of breath than consumption of solids. These foods should not provide empty calories, but should be nutritionally dense so that the patient benefits from the greatest nutritional input in the smallest volume possible. Addition of fats and carbohydrates to menu items is helpful to add calories. Imaginative use of eggs, milk, and cheese can boost protein content as well. Nutritional modular components and commercial supplements can increase nutrient density of the diet as well, although patients may object to their flavor and consistency.

If a patient is consuming an oral diet but is not able to meet total nutritional needs, tube feeding is necessary. It may be beneficial to cycle tube feeding. The tube feeding may be held during daytime hours so that the patient is able to eat small meals, and can be delivered by continuous drip at night. Continuous drip delivery of formula is especially beneficial to the patient on a ventilator, because this decreases the risk of aspiration. Pres-

ence of the airway cuff, particularly a soft cuff, should not be construed as total protection against aspiration, because it does not provide a total seal. Routine procedures designed to minimize the risk of aspiration, including proper patient position, determination of the presence of residual, adequate tube placement, and determination of tolerance of the tube feeding should be followed.

Tube feeding formulas which derive most of their energy content from carbohydrate are unsatisfactory for use in pulmonary patients. At least 20 to 50 percent of calories should be provided by fat. Most commercial formulas meet this requirement. The ratio of fat-to-carbohydrate calorie content of formulas can be enhanced through the addition of commercial fat modules. Recently, a high-fat formula specifically designed for use with patients with respiratory disease has become available. Its clinical efficacy has not yet been widely tested.

Parenteral nutritional support may be necessary in the extremely malnourished patient whose gut has atrophied to the extent that enterally supplied nutrients are malabsorbed, or if the gut is not functioning. A mixed parenteral diet which provides approximately 50 percent of calories as carbohydrate and 50 percent as fat is ideal. The septic and severely catabolic patient is the exception to this rule. Such a patient may not be able to metabolize significant amounts of lipid calories.

The critically ill, ventilator-dependent patient should be monitored closely to ascertain the effects of nutritional support on respiratory status. Such monitoring should include measurement of minute ventilation, breathing frequency, oxygen consumption, carbon dioxide production, and arterial blood gases.

Serial nutritional assessments should be performed to facilitate evaluation of nutritional therapy, but data should be interpreted with caution. Hydration status is variable in the patient with pulmonary edema or in one receiving steroid therapy. The presence of fluid overload may cause false low values in serum albumin and other serum proteins and contribute to falsely high measurements of body weight.

Summary

Recognition of the importance of nutritional support as part of health team management of critically ill patients is increasing. The continuing development of techniques, equipment, and formulas especially designed for nutritional support requires that the critical-care nurse remain abreast of the daily advances in nutritional support of critically ill patients.

Appropriate nutritional care of the critically ill patient must be initiated, monitored, and assessed by ongoing evaluation of nutritional status. This is accomplished through evaluation of anthropometric measurements, biochemical data, and clinical examination, in conjunction with clinical judgment.

Choice of the route of feeding depends on the patient's tolerance and presence of a functioning GI tract. Parenteral nutritional support is frequently the first choice for the critically ill patient. However, significant mechanical, septic, and metabolic complications can arise from its use. Enteral support by tube feeding should be considered for the patient having an intact GI tract. The advent of modern feeding tubes, formulas, and equipment makes tube feeding a viable method of nutritional support which is less costly and more physiologic than PN. Tube feeding requires the same degree of monitoring as does PN, but it is associated with fewer complications.

Nutritional requirements vary greatly according to the disease and clinical condition of the patient. It is important to carefully estimate nutritional needs of the patient before initiating nutritional support. By doing this, it is possible to choose a realistic goal for treatment, and to avoid complications arising from inadequate or overzealous provision of nutrients.

The nurse has the greatest contact with the patient, and has the knowledge of the patient's progress with nutritional therapy. Therefore, it is the nurse's responsibility to actively participate with the health care team in planning nutritional support of the critically ill patient.

References

1. Butterworth, C. E. (1974). The skeleton in the hospital closet. *Nutrition Today, 9,* 4–8.
2. Campbell, S. M. (Ed.) (1984). *Practical guide to nutritional care for dietitians and other health care professionals.* Birmingham: University of Alabama in Birmingham.
3. American Medical Association, Department of Foods and Nutrition. (1979). Multivitamin preparations for parenteral use. A statement by the Nutrition Advisory Group. *Journal of Parenteral and Enteral Nutrition, 3,* 258–262.
4. Bistrian, B. R., Blackburn, G. L., Vitale, J., Cochran, D., & Naylor, J. (1976). Prevalence of malnutrition in general medical patients. *Journal of the American Medical Association, 235,* 1567–1570.
5. Mullen, J. L., Gertner, M. H., Buzby, G. P., Goodhart, G. L., & Rosato, E. F. (1979). Implications of malnutrition in the surgical patient. *Archives of Surgery, 114,* 121–124.
6. Young, G. A., Chem, C., & Hill, G. L. (1978). Assessment of protein-calorie malnutrition in surgical patients from plasma proteins and anthropometric measurements. *American Journal of Clinical Nutrition, 31,* 429–434.
7. Keohane, P. P., Attrill, H., Love, M., Frost, P., & Silk, D. B. A. (1984). Relation between osmolality of diet and gastrointestinal side effects in enteral nutrition. *British Medical Journal, 288,* 378–380.
8. Anderson, K. A., Norris, D. J., Godfrey, L. B., Avent, C. K., & Butterworth, C. E. (1984). Bacterial contamination of tube-feeding formulas. *Journal of Parenteral and Enteral Nutrition, 8,* 673–678.
9. Kagan, R. J., Matsuda, T., Hanumadass, M., Castillo, B., & Jonasson, O. (1982). The effect of burn size on ureagenesis and nitrogen balance. *Annals of Surgery, 195,* 70–74.
10. McCauley, K., & Weaver, T. E. (1983). Cardiac and pulmonary diseases: Nutritional implications. *Nursing Clinics of North America, 18,* 81–96.
11. Tobian, L. V. (1979). Dietary salt (sodium) and hypertension. *American Journal of Clinical Nutrition, 31,* 2659–2662.
12. Taylor, K. B. Gastroenterology. In Schneider, H. A., Anderson, C. E., & Coursin, D. B. (Eds.). (1977). *Nutritional support of medical practice.* New York: Harper & Row, pp. 332–340.
13. Roback, S. A., & Nicoloff, D. M. (1972). High output enterocutaneous fistulas of the small bowel. *American Journal of Surgery, 123,* 317–322.
14. Soeters, P. B., Ebeid, A. M., & Fischer, J. E. (1979). Review of 404 patients with gastrointestinal fistulas. *Annals of Surgery, 190,* 189–202.
15. Bennett, N. (1984). Urea kinetics in the nutritional management of patients with renal failure. *Nutritional Support Services, 4,* 21–25.
16. Tant, A. S., Serin, J., & Douglass, H. O. (1982). Is taste related to anorexia in cancer patients? *American Journal of Clinical Nutrition, 36,* 45–48.

13 Pain

Susan B. Christoph

Notoriously, pain is cited as the one symptom which most frequently stimulates a person to seek assistance from a health care provider.[1] Pain is most often considered a protective mechanism and may indeed provide important clues to diagnosis and treatment. However, once pain has served its purpose it becomes deleterious. Critical-care nurses are all too familiar with the decreased lung volumes, increased oxygen consumption, and depletion of energy that occur when a patient must cope with pain. Perhaps nowhere can nursing efforts have a greater impact than in assisting the patient with pain management and control.

The subject of pain is a difficult one to approach because it is, at the same time, both well and poorly understood. Except for the rare individual born without pain sensation, everyone knows about pain from direct experience. It is part of all our lives; yet when we begin to study it scientifically, we realize how poorly we understand the phenomena involved. It seems that pain is one of those terms which engenders in everyone who hears it a general concept of what is meant, but which has been impossible to universally define.

The following chapter will outline the neurophysiology of pain, review theories of pain, and describe human responses to pain. Methods for the assessment of pain and current medical, surgical, and nursing interventions for the management and control of pain will be presented.

The Neurophysiology of Pain

Pain is a complex physical and psychological phenomenon. Physiologically it may be described as consisting of a sensory component (perception) and a reactive component (behavior) which occur in response to actual or impending tissue damage.[2]

Two factors make presentation of the neurophysiology of pain extremely difficult. First, the pain experience involves the entire body. Even for heuristic purposes, it is difficult to separate out either structures or functions specifically related only to pain. Pain is a subjective experience which depends not only upon the integrity of anatomic structures and physiologic functioning but also upon the integration of psychological factors.

Second, a veritable explosion of information has been gleaned from research over the past two decades. While "pieces of the puzzle" have been delineated, an overall picture has not fully evolved. Many research findings are contradictory and much of our information about pain is the result of educated speculation. Although much is known, there is little agreement about what causes a noxious stimulus to be perceived as pain. The translation and transmission of stimuli for interpretation by the brain as pain and the consequent reactions involve an extremely complex interplay of biochemical, physiologic, and psychological mechanisms.

The following section presents a brief overview of the nervous and endocrine systems as they relate to the pain experience. For an excellent detailed description of the nervous system the reader is referred to Rudy,[3] or Chap. 33.

The Nervous System

The basic anatomic and functional unit of the nervous system is the neuron (Fig. 13-1). Each

The opinions or assertions contained herein are the private views of the author and are not to be construed as official or as reflecting the views of the Department of the Army or the Department of Defense.

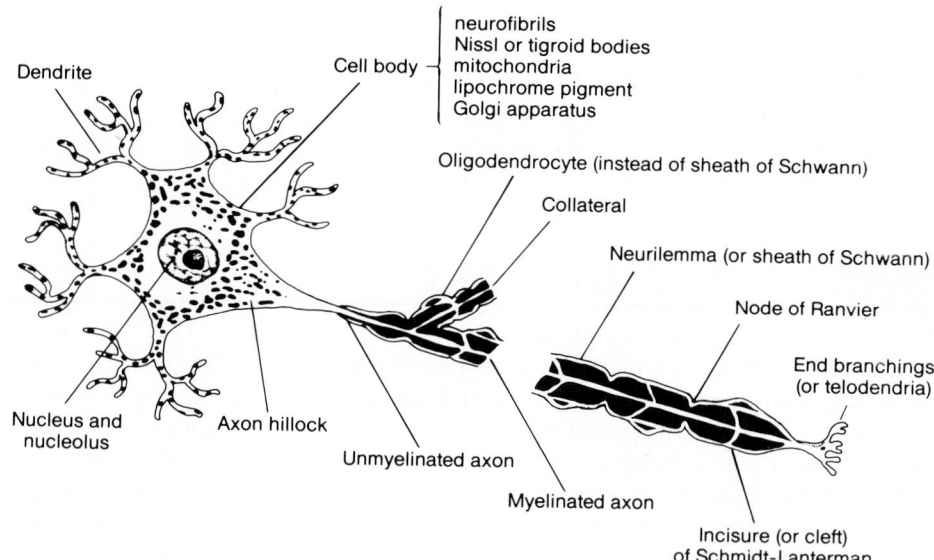

Figure 13-1   The neuron. *(From J. Bossey, Atlas of Neuroanatomy and Special Sense Organs, Saunders, Philadelphia, 1970, p. 5, with permission of the publisher.)*

neuron is composed of a cell body, the *soma,* receptor fibers or *dendrites* which transmit impulses toward the cell body, and a nerve terminal or *axon* which transmits impulses away from the cell body. The dendrites of the sensory neurons branch to form a tight-laced network throughout the body.

Somata, or cell bodies, are named according to location. Nerve cell bodies located outside the central nervous system are called *ganglia.* Nerve cell bodies located within the central nervous system are called *nuclei.*

Three types of neurons exist. *Afferent* neurons, or sensory neurons, are receptors and receive stimuli and transmit the resulting impulse to either *internuncial* neurons (the connector neurons) or to *efferent* neurons, which transmit the impulse to the effectors, such as muscles or glands.

In order for neurons to transmit information within the nervous system, all stimuli must be converted to nerve impulses. Nerve impulses are sometimes called *electrical impulses, chemical impulses,* or *neurochemical impulses.* As these names imply, the initiation of an impulse and its transmission result from action potentials which are created by changing concentrations of sodium, potassium, and chloride within the cell and the extracellular environment.

The special junction across which impulses are transmitted from the axon of a neuron to another cell (another neuron, muscle, or gland) is called a *synapse* (Fig. 13-2). At the terminal end of the axon are hundreds of swellings called *synaptic knobs.* Vesicles in these synaptic knobs contain inhibitory and excitatory transmitters which are released into the synaptic cleft when an impulse reaches the

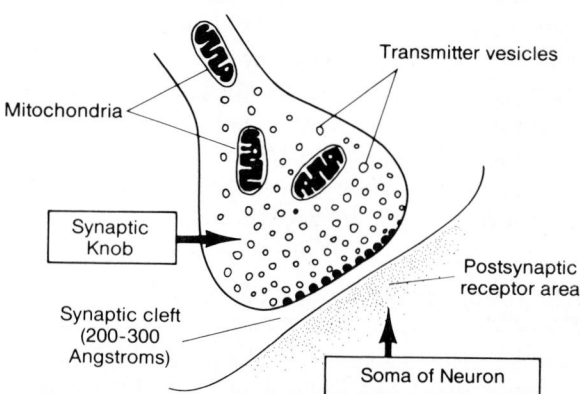

Figure 13-2   The synapse. *(From A. C. Guyton, Textbook of Medical Physiology, 7th ed., Saunders, Philadelphia, 1986, figure 46-5, p. 550, with permission of the publisher.)*

synaptic knob. Transmitters change cell membrane permeability at the postsynaptic receptor site.

The known excitatory transmitters include epinephrine and dopamine. Aminobutyric acid (GABA) and glycine are inhibitory transmitters. A number of identified transmitters, including histamine, acetylcholine, serotonin, norepinephrine, and the prostaglandins may act as either excitatory or inhibitory depending upon the transmitter-receptor interaction. A great deal of pain research is aimed at this cellular area, yielding exciting results which will be of great interest to the critical-care nurse.

The translation of the stimulus to electrical impulse and its transmission within the nervous system are influenced by at least eight interrelated physiologic variables of the receptor neuron: (1) threshold to mechanical distortion, (2) threshold to negative and positive temperature change, (3) peak sensitivity to temperature change, (4) threshold to chemical change, (5) stimulus strength-response curve, (6) rate of adaptation to stimulation, (7) size of receptive field, and (8) duration of after-discharge.[4] A full discussion of these variables is beyond the scope of this text. These concepts may be reviewed in any textbook of medical physiology. Suffice it to say that even at the basic level of translation of stimulus to nerve impulse, there is room for great variation.

Transmission of the nerve impulse is also influenced by the arrangement of groups of interconnected neurons (*neuronal pools*) and convergence and divergence. *Convergence* refers to the concept that a single neuron may be controlled by input from more than one nerve fiber from a single additional neuron or from a number of other neurons (Fig. 13-3). *Divergence* refers to the concept of a single nerve stimulating a number of output nerves (Fig. 13-4).

The nervous system is functionally divided (somewhat arbitrarily) into the peripheral nervous system and the central nervous system

The Peripheral Nervous System

The peripheral nervous system consists of all elements outside the central nervous system: the peripheral nerves, cranial nerves, spinal nerves, and the autonomic nervous system.

Sensory Receptors   Sensory information is transmitted to the central nervous system via the sensory

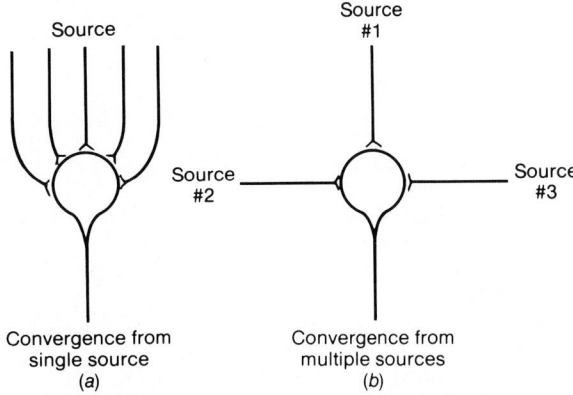

Figure 13-3   Convergence of multiple input fibers on a single neuron. (*a*), Input fibers from a single source. (*b*), Input fibers from multiple sources. (*From A. C. Guyton, Textbook of Medical Physiology, 7th ed., Saunders, Philadelphia, 1986, figure 47-6, p. 565, with permission of the publisher.*)

or afferent elements of the peripheral nervous system. The sensory or afferent neurons are traditionally classified into five types based on sensitivity. These five types of sensory receptors are listed in Table 13-1. Each of these receptors may contribute information to the pain experience. Large myelinated fibers which terminate as free nerve endings

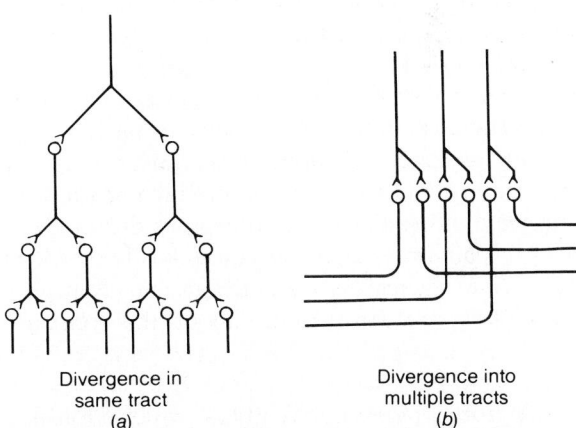

Figure 13-4   Divergence in neuronal pathways. (*a*), Divergence within a pathway to cause "amplification" of the signal. (*b*), Divergence into multiple tracts to transmit the signal to separate areas. (*From A. C. Guyton, Textbook of Medical Physiology, 7th ed., Saunders, Philadelphia, 1986, figure 47-5, p. 564, with permission of the publisher.*)

Table 13-1 Classification of Sensory Receptors

Mechanoreceptors
  Free nerve endings
  Merkel's disks
  Ruffini's endings
  Meissner's corpuscles
  Krause's corpuscles
  Pacinian corpuscles
  Golgi tendon receptors
Thermoreceptors
  Warmth/heat
  Cold
Nociceptors
  Free nerve endings
Electromagnetic Receptors
  Vision—rods and cones
Chemoreceptors
  Taste bud receptors
  Olfactory (smell) receptors
  Oxygen-sensitive (aortic and carotid bodies)
  Carbon dioxide-sensitive (aortic and carotid bodies)

are receptive to mechanical and thermal stimulation of low intensity and manifest adaptation.

Nociceptors (pain receptors) are the terminals of small A delta and C afferent fibers which have a relatively small receptor field and do not demonstrate adaptation. In fact, when a stimulus of sufficient strength initiates the impulse, discharges persist. Nociceptors are activated by strong thermal (less than 15°C or more than 50°C) or mechanical stimuli which may be destructive. Some nociceptors, the C-polymodal nociceptors, are activated by chemical stimuli.

Nociceptor excitability is enhanced by endogenous chemical substances. Tissue damage liberates certain substances including histamine, serotonin, bradykinins, and prostaglandins, which apparently lower the threshold of pain receptors. Substance P (PPS or pain-producing substance) has been identified as an excitatory substance and an excitatory transmitter but information about this remains vague.

Conductors The nerve fibers which transmit impulses from the nerve endings have been classified into groups based upon the character of sensation transmitted and the type of fiber.

The functions of proprioception, touch, pressure, and reflex activity are supported by mechanoreceptors and large, myelinated, rapidly conduct-

ing A alpha and beta fibers. The skin, subcutaneous tissue, viscera, muscles, and other deep structures are innervated by A delta fibers which are small, thinly myelinated, relatively rapidly conducting fibers. A delta nociceptors respond only to mechanical and thermal stimuli intense enough to produce tissue damage.

Unmyelinated, slowly conducting C fibers are also involved in pain perception. Approximately 50 percent of the C fibers supply receptors which respond to innocuous mechanical or thermal stimuli. Approximately 20 percent supply mechanical nociceptors, and 30 percent, thermal nociceptors.[5]

Pain sensation results from involvement of both the A delta and C fibers. A delta fibers are responsible for the transmission of well-localized, rapidly subsiding, pricking or sharp sensations; C fibers transmit poorly localized, long-lasting burning sensations.

The cell bodies of the sensory nerves are located in the dorsal root ganglia. Their axons enter the spinal cord and synapse with other cells in the dorsal horn (Fig. 13-5).

In addition to a sensory element, each spinal nerve has a motor element which transmits motor impulses via somatic fibers to specific voluntary muscle groups and via autonomic fibers to glands,

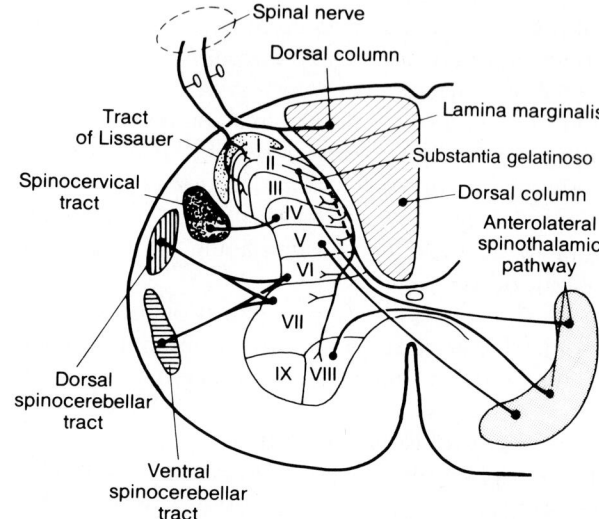

Figure 13-5 Cross-section of the spinal cord. *(From A. C. Guyton, Textbook of Medical Physiology, 7th ed., Saunders, Philadelphia, 1986, figure 50-4, p. 595, with permission of the publisher.)*

cardiac muscle, and smooth muscle. These elements leave the spinal cord via the ventral root.

Somewhat discrete, but definitely overlapping segments of the body are innervated by each spinal or cranial nerve. These body regions are called *dermatomes* (Fig. 13-6). Dermatome innervation corresponds to the segment of the body from which the viscera developed embryonically.

Autonomic Nervous System The autonomic nervous system regulates the viscera and circulation. It consists of two divisions: the *sympathetic system*

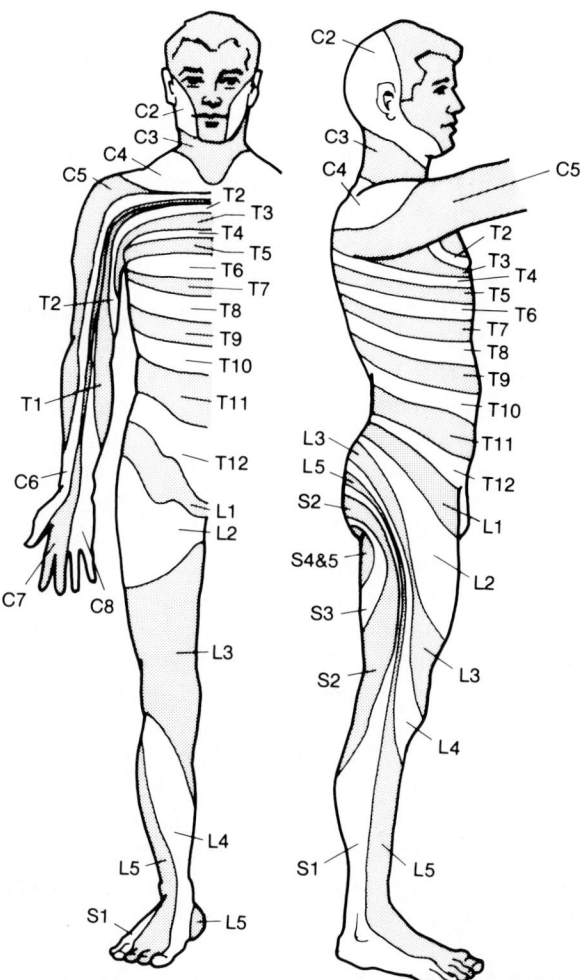

Figure 13-6 The dermatomes. *(From A. C. Guyton, Textbook of Medical Physiology, 7th ed., Saunders, Philadelphia, 1986, figure 49-12, p. 591, with permission of the publisher.)*

Table 13-2 Autonomic Nervous System Responses

Sympathetic
  Pupils dilate
  Sweat glands activated
  Increased heart rate
  Increased cardiac contractility
  Blood vessels constrict
  Bronchi dilate
  Decreased peristalsis of the stomach
  Liver releases glucose
  Gallbladder relaxes
  Decreased renal output
  Basal metabolism increases
Parasympathetic
  Pupils constrict
  Heart rate slows
  Contractility of heart decreases
  Bronchi constrict
  Increased peristalsis of the stomach
  Liver conserves or synthesizes glucose
  Gallbladder contracts
  Basal metabolic rate remains stable

and the *parasympathetic system*. The sympathetic portion is often called the *fight or flight system* because, in general, it activates functions necessary to respond to stress. The parasympathetic portion is sometimes called the *vegetative system* because stimulation results in bodily activities which conserve resources (Table 13-2).

Although these two divisions tend to balance each other, neither is purely excitatory or inhibitory. The autonomic nervous system comes under the influence of the central nervous system and is therefore susceptible to the emotions. How this occurs is largely unknown.

The Central Nervous System

The central nervous system consists of the spinal cord, the brainstem, and the brain.

Spinal Cord The spinal cord consists of gray matter and white matter. The gray matter is composed of unmyelinated fibers and cell bodies. It is divided into three zones: the anterior horn, which contains motor cells; the intermediate zone and lateral horn, which house autonomic cell bodies; and the posterior or dorsal horn, which contains axons from the peripheral sensory neurons. It is here that fibers carrying nociceptive impulses cross over to white matter and ascend to the brain via fibers.

The white matter is composed of both myelinated and unmyelinated fibers but contains no cell bodies. These fibers are grouped into tracts. Tracts may be ascending, that is, carrying impulses to the brain; or descending, that is, carrying impulses from the brain to the spinal nerves.

The *tract of Lissauer* extends from the periphery of the dorsal horn to the cord surface. Input consists primarily of fine fibers from cells in the dorsal root gelatinosa. These fibers run longitudinally and ascend or descend in the tract for one to six segments before entering the dorsal horn of the spinal cord.

The *dorsal horn* of the spinal cord is an intricate arrangement of neurons and synapses which allows modulation of impulses through excitation and inhibition. Excitation and inhibition are influenced by input from the periphery, adjacent neurons, the brain, and other parts of the central nervous system. The dorsal horn has been divided into six laminae based on the anatomic and functional characteristics of its cells.

Cells from all the lamina have connections with cells in lamina II and III. Some axons of lamina II and III cells project directly to the brain. This is the area known as the *substantia gelatinosa,* once thought to be the gate control mechanism central to gate control theory. Although not the only regulator of sensory input, a great deal of impulse modulation takes place in this area.

Of particular note is that cells in lamina V that receive pain impulses from visceral fibers also receive input from somatic fibers which may partially account for the mechanism of referred pain.

Axons from the cells of the dorsal horn project to various areas of the spinal cord and group together as *ascending tracts*. Three primary pathways are involved with carrying information from the spinal cord to the brain: the spinothalamic system, the dorsal column system (lemniscal system), and the propriospinal system.

The ascending tract most commonly referred to as the pain tract is the *spinothalamic tract.* This is due to its function of transmitting impulses from the spine to the thalamus, a sensory center in the brain, at which point one may first become conscious of pain. The spinothalamic tract is divided into the ventral spinothalamic tract and the lateral spinothalamic tract.

The ventral spinothalamic tract is composed of long fibers which connect to the thalamus and synapse with fibers that relay impulses to the somatic sensory cortex. This system processes discriminative information about location and intensity of peripheral stimulation, including touch and pressure.

The lateral spinothalamic tract is composed of long fibers which connect with the reticular formation, lateral pons, midbrain, and finally the intralaminar thalamic nuclei. This system transmits signals for intolerable aching and burning pain and thermal sensations. It is also involved with the reflex responses of ventilation, circulation, and endocrine function.

The dorsal column system consists of large myelinated fibers and is responsible for transmission and probably modulation of impulses related to touch, pressure, and proprioception.

The propriospinal system has two components: the reticular core and the spinoreticular tract. The reticular core consists of very short axon neurons which extend from the spinal cord to the thalamus. The spinoreticular tract is composed primarily of small C fibers which originate in the dorsal horn and terminate in the reticular formation where they synapse with neurons which transmit impulses to the intralaminar nuclei of the thalamus.

Historically it has been thought that descending tracts carried only motor information to effectors. It is now known that information about pain is carried from the brain to lower structures via descending fibers. Descending fibers of the corticospinal (pyramidal) and extrapyramidal tracts influence transmission in the dorsal horn and other parts of the spinal cord. The corticospinal tract transmits impulses to the skeletal muscles. The fibers of the extrapyramidal tracts, many of which act in collaboration with fibers of the corticospinal tract, mediate the more specialized functions with muscle tone, posture, and equilibrium.

Brainstem and Brain   As the spinal cord enters the skull it begins to enlarge to form the brainstem. The brainstem includes the medulla, the pons, and the midbrain. Through successive synapses impulses are transmitted to the thalamus which monitors and relays sensory input. The reticular formation, an area of small, densely packed cells and fibers, and anterior nuclei of the thalamus comprise the *reticular activating system (RAS)*. The RAS integrates information and influences transmission of the impulses back down the spinal cord and either directly or indirectly transmits impulses to all areas of the cerebral cortex. The role of the reticular formation is aversion to noxious stimuli and the development of concomitant behaviors.

The thalamus, hypothalamus, hippocampus, amygdala, septum, and cingulum comprise together the *limbic system,* which plays a major role in the modulation of the pain experience. Finally, surrounding these structures is the cerebral cortex, which integrates all information and influences behavior based on its cognitive-evaluative activities.

It is this very complex interplay of interpretation at the cortical/thalamic levels which leads to perception, that is, the awareness of noxious sensation, an interpretation and appreciation of it, and an attribution of meaning to it. It is this area of interpretation that gives pain its very individual and personal nature. This is what drives the behaviors we can observe, and this is the area we least understand.

It was previously thought that emotional or psychological factors affected only the emotional overtones or the reactive components of the pain experience. New data indicate that emotions can actually diminish or increase the sensory portion of the pain experience. How this occurs is largely unknown, but partial explanations may be found when the interactions of the endocrine system with the autonomic nervous system and the rest of the nervous system are more fully defined.

The Endocrine System

The endocrine system regulates functions of the body by secreting chemical substances (hormones) into the body fluids. As indicated earlier, the endocrine system is interrelated with the nervous system.

Adrenal Medullae

Of primary concern in a discussion of the neurophysiology of pain are the medullae of the adrenal gland which secrete their hormones only in response to appropriate nervous activity. The hormones epinephrine and norepinephrine are excreted in response to stimulation of the sympathetic portion of the autonomic nervous system and exert the same effects as direct stimulation of sympathetic nerves. This is of great interest to the clinician because it accounts in part for the role of fear and anxiety in pain perception.

The Endogenous Opiate System

The endogenous opiate system is a fairly recent discovery that has greatly influenced thinking about pain mechanisms. The isolation of stereospecific opiate receptors in the brain led to speculation that the body must produce its own analgesics. A number of opiate-like substances have been identified. These have been grouped into two categories: the *endorphins* and the *enkephalins*. Much less is known about a third group of endogenous opioids, the *dynorphins.*

The endorphins (a combination word from *endogenous* and *morphine*) are amino acid fragments of beta-lipoprotein, a peptide found primarily in the pituitary gland and parts of the hypothalamus. These fragments have a pharmacologic action similar to morphine. Endorphins identified so far include beta-endorphin, thought to be the most potent; gamma-endorphin; and alpha-endorphin.

Enkephalins, peptides found in both the brain and spinal cord, are localized to nerve fibers and their endings. Two enkephalins have been isolated: *met*-enkephalin and *leu*-enkephalin, so named to reflect their terminal amino acids methionine and leucine, respectively.

While volumes of information have been published on the endogenous opiate system, most findings are tentative. It is thought that both physiologic and psychological processes stimulate the release of endorphins and enkephalins. The beta-endorphins are apparently released in response to exercise and mood changes. The influence of psychological processes on the release of endogenous opiates may explain what is known as the placebo effect. The endogenous opiates are known to increase in concentration during and after the stress of surgery and decrease once narcotic analgesia (morphine) is administered.

The endogenous opiates may act as neuromodulators by increasing or decreasing the efficacy of the neurotransmitters or act directly themselves by stimulating parts of the brain's analgesic system. In general, the endorphins appear to be more potent analgesics and longer acting than the enkephalins.

New knowledge about the endogenous opiates may well assist in unraveling the mysteries of mind–body interaction.

Theories of Pain Perception

Though much is known about the neurophysiology of pain perception, significant gaps in knowledge exist. Three basic pain theories have evolved: the *specificity theory,* the *pattern theory,* and the *gate control theory.* Although none is fully explanatory, each has contributed to the understanding of the phenomena involved with pain perception and remnants of each are retained in present-day conceptions of pain.

The Specificity Theory of Pain Perception

Historically, pain was viewed entirely philosophically and described as a negative passion in opposition to the more desirable feeling of pleasure. Many negative connotations associated with pain persist in our religious and cultural beliefs. Starting in the nineteenth century researchers gathered a great deal of anatomic and physiologic data from which the competing specificity theory and pattern theory were generated.

In specificity theory, pain was considered a primary sense. This theory was a fairly simple one based on a straightforward path of impulse transmission from stimulus to brain. The specificity theory postulated that specific pain receptors were present in the tissues that responded to painful stimuli. When specific pain receptors could not be identified, it was suggested that the pain receptors were all of the free nerve endings. Although it is generally accepted that free nerve endings are the pain receptors, they are not specific to pain but rather are sensitive to a variety of stimuli, including painful ones.

Included in the specificity theory was the notion of a specific pain pathway (the spinothalamic tract) and a central pain center (the thalamus). The spinothalamic tract is still recognized as a major pain pathway but many other pathways have been identified and it is clear that, in addition to the thalamus, many parts of the brain are involved with the perception of pain. The specificity theory offered no explanation for the lack of a direct relationship between stimulus intensity and perceived pain or the diversity of perceived pain among subjects exposed to the same stimulus.

The concept of simple, straightforward neural receptor and conductor mechanisms led to the belief that the threshold for pain is the same for all individuals, i.e., that the stimulus that will invoke perception of pain is the same for all patients and that it is only the reaction to pain, an indication of tolerance, that differs from one individual to another. This view is still widely held.

In spite of refuting information, specificity theory continues to influence practice when pain is treated as a purely physiologic response or when it is inferred that the pain expected or perceived will be directly proportional to tissue damage.

The *chemical specificity theory* enjoyed popularity for a time and contributed significantly to the development of present-day concepts of pain. There is little question that tissue damage stimulates pain impulses. The question has been whether the stimulus from tissue damage is mechanical or chemical. The excitation of nociceptors by chemical substances has been frequently postulated. Lindahl[6] proposed that it was not the receptors that were specific to pain but rather the stimulus. The biochemical theory postulated that the pain-producing stimulus was an elevation of hydrogen ion concentration at the nerve ending. Isolation of many of the pain-producing substances gave support to this concept. This theory has been refined and incorporated into the more general theories while biochemical mechanisms underlying the transmission of pain generate continued research interest.

The Pattern Theory of Pain Perception

The various pattern theories of pain disposed of the notion of specific receptors and postulated that the brain recognized certain patterns of impulses as pain. The pattern theory, also known as the *intensive theory,* was based on the premise that it was the intensity of a stimulus and central summation that determined whether or not a sensation was perceived as pain.

Central summation referred to the concept that all information about the sensory stimulus was carried by small nerve fibers to the dorsal horn of the spinal cord where it was "summed up" and transmitted to the brain as a pattern which was recognized as pain. During the summation, because of the complexity of the arrangement of nerves within the spinal cord, reverberating circuits of noxious impulses could be set in motion. Normally, a control system prevented summation of normal stimuli to an intensity that could produce the "pain pattern." If this control system were not working, abnormal pain states would develop.

The Gate Control Theory of Pain Perception

Melzack and Wall[7] proposed a relatively new and divergent pain theory. The gate control theory, which has undergone considerable refinement within the last two decades, takes a holistic approach to pain and more than any other theory emphasizes that pain is not just a physiologic phenomenon. It offers an explanation for how psychological and sociocultural variables interact to influence the perception of pain intensity and quality. It retains the idea of pain receptors and also, to an extent, central summation, although these concepts have been somewhat revised based on expanded physiologic evidence.

According to gate control theory, the entire nervous system is involved in the modulation of both physiologic and psychological responses of the body, including the perception of and response to noxious stimuli. Peripheral nerves conduct excitatory signals to the spinal cord, to the transmission cells in the dorsal horn, and from there to the thalamus and cerebral cortex.

The major emphasis of gate control theory is that pain is modifiable. It was originally thought that this was accomplished by a gate mechanism located in the substantia gelatinosa of the dorsal horn (lamina II and III). The mechanism was dependent upon elaborate feedback loops. Opening and closing the gate to certain signals either enhanced or inhibited pain perception. The gate was opened when small fibers were activated and closed by stimulation of large-diameter nerves. The

resulting balance determined whether or not stimuli reached the central transmission cells in the dorsal horn. This area continues to be recognized as important for modulation of impulses; however, refinements of the theory have incorporated explanations for the influence of other factors on the pain phenomenon.

It is thought that noxious impulses may be modified at any point. The notion of opening and closing gates is probably too simple an analogy but remains a basic concept.

It is postulated that the whole brain acts as the pain center for recognition and interpretation and also as a modulator of sensory input. Impulses from the cerebral cortex and thalamus which are influenced by fear, anxiety, memory of past experience, etc., may be inhibitory (closing the gate by reducing anxiety) or facilitory (opening the gate when fear or anxiety is experienced). This part of the gate control theory presents a partial explanation for the influence of psychological and sociocultural factors on pain perception.

The perception of and response to pain is also modulated by the action system which is activated when the output of the transmission cells exceeds a critical level. The theory postulates that interpretation plus cognitive information influence the response to pain, and this explains the diverse, complex behavior observed in individuals reacting to noxious stimuli. Melzack and Wall[4] now think that these central mechanisms play a greater part in controlling the gate(s) than any of the peripheral mechanisms.

Responses to Pain Perception

It is clear that pain is more than just a physiologic experience; it is a psychological experience as well. The phenomenon of pain is a subjective experience which occurs in a total, integrated human being who has had a variety of physical, emotional, and intellectual experiences affected by sociocultural factors. As stated previously, both the sensory component and the reactive component of the pain experience are modified by all these variables. It is the reactive component of pain that can be directly observed and hence the aspect of this complex phenomenon that has been most studied.

Although many studies exist which attempt to delineate how various additional factors, including personality, mood, culture, and emotional state apparently mediate the perception of pain and reaction to it, relatively little is known. It would appear that differences in reactions to pain could be attributed primarily to tolerance rather than threshold. But evidence of the powerful influences of central mechanisms involving the brain, including memory and thought processes, on pain threshold at least partially negates this notion. One thing is clear: There is no "correct" way to react to pain.

Sociocultural Influences on Response to Pain

Sociocultural factors which apparently modify the pain experience include race, age, sex, marital status, educational level, and religious affiliation. While marital status, educational level, and religious affiliation clearly contribute to the sociocultural component of pain, it is difficult to discern whether race, age, and sex are solely sociocultural influences or actually physiologic influences. It may be that race, age, and sex are more related physiologically to the pain experience than is presently recognized. It is probable that these factors influence both the physiologic and the sociocultural components of the pain experience. They are included in this section merely as a convenience.

Although race has been shown to influence pain, the actual differences between the reaction (culturally influenced) or the tolerance and the threshold component (physiologically influenced) have been difficult to discern. Consequently, conflicts within the literature abound as to how race may affect pain.

Age is another variable which influences the perception of pain in a confusing manner. Some studies report increased threshold and tolerance with increased age, others report a decrease in pain tolerance with increasing age, and still others report no difference. It is known that cutaneous sensitivity decreases in the elderly, so superficial pain may not be as readily perceived. It should also be kept in mind that developmental stage and vocabulary will influence how the child will respond to pain.

Lower pain thresholds for females than for males have been described; however, the infor-mation regarding the influence of gender on pain is generally conflicting.

Sex, age, and race are also variables which take on a social orientation as to norms of expected behavior, which further clouds interpretation of results of studies which have attempted to determine how these variables influence pain.

Emotional and Psychological Influences

Emotional and psychological factors not only modify pain, they may even cause pain.

Anxiety

Anxiety has been commonly recognized as a component of the pain experience as well as a modifier of pain perception. Anxiety not only influences pain perception, but pain perception or the fear of pain stimulates anxiety (Fig. 13-7). Anxiety is a pattern of emotion, the major component of which is fear. It consists of a diffuse, unpleasant, often vague feeling of apprehension accompanied by one or more recurring bodily sensations. Anxiety is the consequence of threat perception. The exact relationship between anxiety and pain perception remains elusive due to the multiplicity of uncontrollable intervening variables. It is, however, generally accepted that a positive relationship exists.

Pain is an aversive event, one to be avoided. Patients relate that pain or fear of pain is the most distressing component of illness or injury. This fear of pain is the greatest influence on the patient's state of anxiety.

Situational Factors

The patient's response to pain will to a large extent be determined by the meaning and value attributed to pain. What does the pain mean to the individual in terms of a potential or actual threat? Pain may represent a threat of tissue damage. The patient may know that pain will herald a return trip to the operating room. Pain may offer a threat to body

⬆ ANXIETY ⬅——➡ ⬇ PAIN TOLERANCE
(⬇ PAIN THRESHOLD)

Figure 13-7 Direct relationship between anxiety and pain.

image, represent a serious illness, or define a threat to life itself. For the critically ill patient it may represent all these things and very realistically all may be present.

Prediction and Control

The components of a theory of personal control and its influence on pain perception and on anxiety have been difficult to delineate. It is known that prediction, timing, and reinforcement of perception of control are important.

In general, humans prefer predictable aversive events (pain) to unpredictable ones and suffer emotional, somatic, and cognitive disturbances when they are denied predictability. The lack of control over a threat (anticipated pain or actual pain) intensifies feelings of helplessness and stimulates anxiety.

Illness, injury, hospitalization, and prescribed treatments tend to be externalizing events which conflict with predictability and personal control. Illness and injury are certainly never planned. Although surgery may be planned, most patients are not well versed in handling pain and know little about pain management. Patients are subject to the restraints of the hospital organization and prescribed regimens which are directed by the staff. The threat of pain may be enhanced by both a perceived and a real lack of control since, traditionally, control over pain rests with the staff, i.e., the physician's prescriptions and the nurse's keys to the medication cabinet. The constraints of the unit's organization often hamper the patient's usual coping mechanisms. For the critically ill or injured patient this is particularly true. The reduction of uncertainty, which includes providing both predictability of the aversive event and a sense of control over it, seems to be the most powerful element in increasing pain tolerance.

Assessment of Pain

Pain is generally differentiated as *acute* or *chronic*. *Acute pain* refers to pain of sudden onset resulting from actual or impending tissue damage from injury or disease. It is limited in duration and either resolves due to healing or removal of the cause, or

it progresses to chronic pain. *Chronic pain,* on the other hand, refers to pain that has existed for 6 months or more. The pathology of chronic pain may or may not exist or be known. In most settings, it is important to differentiate chronic from acute pain so that appropriate care can be planned. The critical-care nurse will deal primarily with acute pain symptoms; therefore, this section will address the assessment of acute pain symptoms. The critical-care nurse should be aware, however, of the patient's history and recognize that the patient may suffer from chronic pain overlaid by acute pain.

The very nature of pain makes it a most difficult symptom to assess. Because pain is a subjective experience, it is generally agreed that the patient is the only real expert on what he or she is feeling. In truth, there are *no* reliable unvarying signs or symptoms of pain. The physiologic and psychological reactions to pain are as individualistic as the person who suffers it. Pain draws attention to itself and can influence all physiologic and psychological responses. The assessment of pain, therefore, involves the evaluation of a *constellation of pain indicators*. It is the grouping of associated symptoms that will be most helpful in delineating pain and developing strategies for its control.

Verbalizations

As simplistic as it may seem, the most reliable indicators of pain are the patient's own verbalizations. In fact, the most common operational definition of pain in practice today comes from McCaffery,[8] who states that "Pain is whatever the experiencing person says it is, existing whenever he [or she] says it does" (p. 11). The principal problem then becomes one of communication between the patient and the nurse to determine the nature of pain and what can be done to alleviate the noxious sensation.

The patient's description of pain can greatly assist the nurse with assessment of pain and the development of a plan for management. The nurse may have to aid the patient with directive questioning to get descriptions of the most important characteristics of the pain: location, intensity, quality, onset, duration, and variations. Listening carefully to the words chosen by the patient to describe these characteristics will provide important clues to the nature of the pain being experienced.

Location of Pain

Where is the pain being felt? It may not always be easy for the patient to localize the pain. It may be felt in more than one place or may cover an extensive area. The patient may be asked to point to the location of the pain on his or her own body, or on a drawing or doll. Complaints of pain or discomfort by the postoperative patient, for instance, may not be the result of incisional pain as assumed, but rather headache or sore throat as a result of anesthesia technique, discomfort at the site of intravenous infusion, or irritation from other associated apparatus such as nasogastric tubes. All would require very different intervention.

Superficial Pain Superficial pain refers to pain in the skin and mucous membranes. This is usually easy for the patient to pinpoint. Descriptive words of cutaneous superficial pain include *sharp, pricking,* or *burning. Sharp* and *pricking* are the words most commonly chosen to describe incisional pain.

Deep Pain Deep pain, pain of the structures within the body, is categorized as *visceral* or *somatic.* Deep pain is more difficult to localize than superficial pain due to the limited nociceptors in most viscera and multisegmental and overlapping innervation at the spinal level. Due to their location,

the deep structures have not developed a sensitivity to chemical, thermal, mechanical, or electrical stimuli. In addition, the patient may have more difficulty describing deep pain sensation due to lack of knowledge about internal body parts.[9]

Referred pain is pain in an area of the body distant from the tissue damage caused by injury or disease. Most often pain from the viscera is referred to an area on the surface of the body, but pain may be referred from one viscus to another or from one body surface to another. Understanding dermatome innervation (see Fig. 13-6) is important in assessing deep pain because the area of referred pain is usually supplied by the same spinal segment as the generating site.

Several typical patterns of referred pain can be described (Table 13-3). This has given rise to the notion that certain diseases may elicit unique descriptors. Again, it must be emphasized that while these patterns may yield clues, variations of these patterns will occur.

Intensity of Pain

The intensity of pain may range from mild discomfort or irritation to severe, completely debilitating pain. There is no direct correlation between stimulus and pain perception. The patient's report of intensity will be influenced by the patient's threshold and tolerance for pain. *Threshold* refers to the point at which pain is first perceived and has been thought to be fairly constant from person to person. Evidence now indicates that threshold varies from

Table 13-3 Patterns of Referred Pain

Involved Viscera	Sites of Pain
Heart	Pain radiates. Left side of body. Shoulder, axilla, inside of arm, neck, and jaw
Lungs and diaphragm	Scapular regions, shoulders
Esophagus	Lower neck, arm, sternum, substernal area
Stomach	Surface of body between xiphoid process of sternum and umbilicus
Gallbladder and biliary system	Midepigastric area to tip of right scapula
Pancreas	Midback and low epigastric regions
Large bowel	Hypogastric or lower abdominal region and periumbilical area
Kidneys and ureters	Flanks and groin area. Border of rectus abdominis muscle below the umbilicus
Bladder and testicles	Suprapubic area
Urethra	Penis or perineum
Uterus	Lower abdomen and low back

Source: After Rudy, E. B., *Advanced Neurological and Neurosurgical Nursing,* Mosby, St. Louis, 1983, with permission.

individual to individual and may vary within the individual from situation to situation. This has been difficult to discern because of vast differences in tolerance. *Tolerance* refers to the point at which an individual reports that he or she cannot or will not withstand the noxious stimulus. Because threshold and tolerance vary so greatly from individual to individual and within the same individual from one time to another, intensity may be extremely difficult for the nurse to judge.

Several tools have been developed to assist with the assessment of pain intensity. Most of these depend upon anchors at either end of a scale upon which the patient rates pain. The anchors are arbitrary.

The verbal rating scales ask the patient to rate pain based on 3 to 5 numerically ranked word descriptors. The pain score is the number of the chosen word and can be recorded for comparison with later complaints of pain or to evaluate the effectiveness of relief measures. The *visual analog scale* (VAS) is a 10-cm line with anchors of "no pain" at the left end, and "severe pain" or "pain as bad as it can be" at the right end. The distance in centimeters from the left end of the line to the point intersect marked by the patient on the line constitutes the measurement (Fig. 13-8). With the VAS there are an infinite number of points between the extremes which allows sensitivity for many grades of pain as experienced by the patient without forcing the patient to translate a feeling into words.

Quality of Pain

The quality of pain may be the most difficult characteristic for the patient to describe. The language of pain is varied and many patients lack the vocabulary to relate what they are feeling. As indicated previously, some indicators of superficial pain may include the descriptors *pricking* or *burning.* Deep pain is more likely to be described as *aching, throbbing,* or *radiating.* Intensity may be described as *gnawing* or *tiring.*

Please make a mark on the line (_____) that best describes the pain you are experiencing right now.

NO PAIN ——————————————— SEVERE PAIN

Figure 13-8   Visual analog scale.

The McGill-Melzack Pain Questionnaire (MPQ) (Fig. 13-9) is a measurement tool which can be administered either by an examiner or self-administered by the patient. It consists of four major classes of word descriptors, *sensory, affective, evaluative,* and *miscellaneous,* which are used by the patient to describe the pain experience. It provides quantitative information that is sufficiently sensitive to detect differences among different methods to relieve pain, and provides information about the relative effects of a given manipulation on the sensory, affective, evaluative, and miscellaneous dimensions of pain.

The MPQ yields three types of data which can be useful to the clinician: (1) a pain rating index (PRI), based on the sum of rank values for all words chosen in a given category; (2) the number of words chosen (NWC); and (3) the present pain intensity (PPI), based on the number-word combination chosen as the indicator of overall pain intensity.[9] The MPQ takes only 10 to 15 min to complete, can be read to the patient or self-administered, and yields valuable information about the pain experience. It can be particularly useful in the critical-care unit when the patient cannot or will not verbalize the pain experience or when it is difficult to evaluate the effectiveness of pain relief measures. For descriptions of administration and scoring methods see Melzack.[10]

Variations in Pain

In addition to the location, intensity, and quality of pain, it is important to determine whether or not it is associated with any other discernible factors such as movement, swallowing, changes in posture, etc. Time associations may be particularly diagnostic. Unfortunately, the patient often cannot or will not admit that pain is present. This is particularly true for the critically ill or injured patient. The nurse must therefore be aware of additional indicators that the patient is experiencing pain.

Physiologic Indicators

The physiologic indicators of pain result primarily from autonomic stimulation. Pain contributes to fear and anxiety, which elicit a sympathetic response. In addition, dual sensory input is provided by both visceral and somatic afferents.

McGILL-MELZACK PAIN QUESTIONNAIRE (MPQ)

Patient's name_____ Age_____ ID No._____

Diagnosis _____

Part 1. Where is your pain? Please mark on the drawings the areas where you feel your pain. Put "E" if external or "I" if internal.

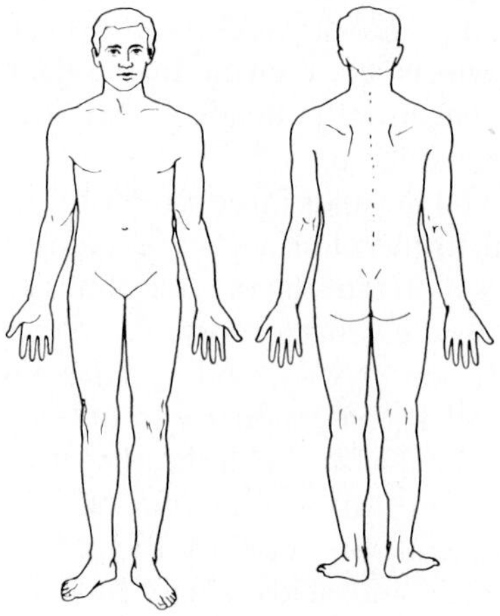

11	12	13	14	15
1 Tiring	1 Sickening	1 Fearful	1 Punishing	1 Wretched
2 Exhausting	2 Suffocating	2 Frightful	2 Gruelling	2 Blinding
		3 Terrifying	3 Cruel	
			4 Vicious	
			5 Killing	PRI-A———

16

1 Annoying
2 Troublesome
3 Miserable
4 Intense
5 Unbearable

PRI-E———

17	18	19	20
1 Spreading	1 Tight	1 Cool	1 Nagging
2 Radiating	2 Numb	2 Cold	2 Nauseating
3 Penetrating	3 Drawing	3 Freezing	3 Agonizing
4 Piercing	4 Squeezing		4 Dreadful
	5 Tearing		5 Torturing PRI-M———

TOTAL PRI ———

NWC ———

Part 2. What does your pain feel like?

Some of the words below describe your present pain. Circle ONLY those words that best describe it. Leave out any word group that is not suitable. Use only a single word in each appropriate group—the one that applies the best.

1	2	3	4
1 Flickering	1 Jumping	1 Pricking	1 Sharp
2 Quivering	2 Flashing	2 Boring	2 Cutting
3 Pulsing	3 Shooting	3 Drilling	3 Lacerating
4 Throbbing		4 Stabbing	

5	6	7	8
1 Pinching	1 Tugging	1 Hot	1 Tingling
2 Pressing	2 Pulling	2 Burning	2 Itchy
3 Gnawing	3 Wrenching	3 Scalding	3 Smarting
4 Cramping		4 Searing	4 Stinging

9	10
1 Dull	1 Tender
2 Sore	2 Taut
3 Hurting	3 Rasping
4 Aching	4 Splitting
5 Heavy	PRI–S———

Part 3. How does your pain change with time?

1. Which word or words would you use to describe the pattern of your pain?

1	2	3
Continuous	Rhythmic	Brief
Steady	Periodic	Momentary
Constant	Intermittent	Transient

2. What kind of things relieve your pain? _____
_____

3. What kind of things increase your pain? _____
_____

Part 4. How strong is your pain?

The following words represent pain of increasing intensity. Choose the number of the word which best describes your pain right now.

1	2	3	4	5
Mild	Discomforting	Distressing	Horrible	Excruciating

Figure 13-9 The McGill-Melzack Pain Questionnaire (MPQ). *(From R. Melzack, Pain, 1, 1975, 357–373. With permission of author and publisher.)*

Sympathetic Responses

Most sensory information is conducted via the visceral sympathetic pathways, the cardiac, and splanchnic nerves to their respective spinal segments. Therefore, acute pain elicits primarily sympathetic symptoms including pallor, increased respirations, increased heart rate, increased blood pressure, dilated pupils, and increased muscle tension. The systems that control cardiovascular function and modulate the perception of pain are closely coupled and directly influence each other. Of particular note to the critical-care nurse are the cyclical adverse effects that pain may have on the cardiovascular and respiratory systems. The sympathetic response to pain may result in inhibition of gastrointestinal and genitourinary function, resulting in ileus, distention, and decreased urinary function. It becomes obvious that untreated pain may significantly alter a patient's physiologic status and contribute to complications.

Parasympathetic Responses

The colon, rectum, and bladder are innervated through the sacral parasympathetic nerves and, therefore, deep pain involving these viscera may elicit parasympathetic responses including pallor, nausea and vomiting, decreased heart rate, and decreased blood pressure. The resulting hypotension may be so profound that fainting and loss of consciousness occur. Pain that evokes these parasympathetic responses results from ischemia or other pain-producing chemical stimulation, and overdistention or spasm of these viscera.

Obviously, these physiologic indicators may not be diagnostic in and of themselves and in fact may be the result of problems other than pain. They must be assessed in context with the patient's verbalizations and additional behavioral clues.

Behavioral Clues

Some observable behaviors are associated with the pain experience. These are variable and their existence depends in great part upon the patient's notion of what acceptable pain behavior is.

Moaning, groaning, crying, or screaming certainly indicate that something is wrong. On the other hand, the patient in pain may become withdrawn and fearful. Any change in affect, including excitement, irritability, anger, hostility, depression, unusual quietness, or withdrawal, may indicate that the patient is experiencing pain. Children are particularly prone to withdrawal as a means of coping with pain. Fear of how the pain will be treated (particularly fear of injections) often interferes with the patient's communication of the pain experience.

The patient in pain may hold the body or the painful part rigid and immobile in an attempt to limit pain. On the other hand, activity may increase. The patient may rock, or rub a painful body part. Clenched jaws or fists may be evidence that pain is present. Restlessness or seemingly purposeless activity may indicate pain and must be carefully assessed to differentiate from other causes such as hypoxia.

Inability to sleep or rest is also an indication that pain may be a problem. However, a patient may become so worn out from pain that he or she sleeps. It should never be assumed that because a patient is asleep, pain is not experienced. Unless treated, pain leads to fatigue and robs the patient of energy needed to cope with the stresses of hospitalization and illness.

Pain Management

The complexity of the phenomenon of pain calls for multidimensional, combination approaches to prevent pain and as interventions for its relief. The notion of a combination of approaches incorporated into a treatment package is sometimes called a *stress-inoculation package.* Such combinations have been shown to be far more powerful than singular interventions.

The nurse is in a unique position to direct the assessment of pain in the critical-care patient and coordinate the plan for pain management, for it is the nurse who spends the most time with the patient and who brings the holistic perspective to care. The development of the pain management plan must involve all personnel who contribute to the care of the patient but, most importantly, must also include the patient as an active participant. Participation of the patient must, as a minimum, involve him or her in the ongoing assessment of pain and evaluation of pain relief modalities. To the extent possible, the patient should be involved with deciding what combinations of pain relief modalities will be used.

The implementation of pain management based upon a multidimensional scheme requires a knowledgeable professional nurse with a broad background in the known neurophysiology of pain, the applicable theories of pain and pain modulation, and assessment and pain management skills.

Pain Prevention

The first goal of any pain management plan is to prevent pain and promote comfort. Much of this requires a back-to-basics kind of approach, but may be far more difficult than it sounds, for often the diagnosis and treatment of injury or illness involve the infliction of pain. Protection of the patient from painful stimuli and the provision of comfort measures are fully within the purview of the nurse. The goals of the pain management plan are to decrease the sensation of pain, relieve suffering, decrease the intensity of pain, increase pain tolerance, and promote comfort.

Physical Factors

Pain is so common an experience for certain illnesses or injuries that it is an anticipated consequence. Surgery, which includes incision, tissue manipulation, retraction, and excision is a vivid example of tissue damage that may well be expected to stimulate the pain experience. Diagnostic tests and treatment—debridement of a burn wound, for instance—may induce pain sensations.

No one would purposefully hurt a patient. However, in the bustle of a busy critical-care environment, it may be difficult to keep pain prevention "rules" in mind. Injured tissue must be handled carefully and further trauma avoided whenever possible. If the patient can move the injured part, he or she may be the best judge of how to avoid stimulating pain. Postoperative patients should have been taught preoperatively how to externally splint abdominal and thoracic incisions to minimize pain stimuli when deep breathing, coughing, and ambulating. These patients should be reminded how to do this and in some instances should be assisted.

The critical-care patient often has a myriad of equipment or apparatus attached to his or her person, which may be irritating. Attention to phys-

ical comfort details will reduce accumulation of sensory stimuli which may overburden the patient, thus reducing tolerance to pain. Relieving a dry mouth with ice chips or moistened gauze and applying petrolatum ointment to cracked lips relieve the critical-care patient of uncomfortable stimuli with which to contend. Not to be neglected is a clean, dry bed with sheets that are straightened and free of irritating wrinkles.

All drainage tubes should be checked frequently for patency to avoid distention of the drainage site. All apparatus attached to the patient should be checked frequently to ensure that it is secure and will not cause irritation of the tissues from movement and to avoid tension from pulling. Nasogastric tubes are especially prone to irritate the nares and pharynx and stimulate complaints of pain. Attention to anchoring the tube and protecting the skin with petrolatum jelly are important.

Good body alignment and frequent changes of position will help prevent muscle contractures and spasms. Support of injured parts will prevent muscular strain and muscular fatigue which may stimulate pain.

It almost goes without saying that control of the environment within the critical-care unit is difficult, if not impossible. The sensory overload that may occur with lights, noise, and activity may consume the patient's energy as well as decrease tolerance to pain. Insofar as possible, the nurse should promote a quiet environment with non-glaring lights and attempt to coordinate the whole treatment plan to provide periods of rest for the patient.

Although comfort and freedom from pain are not one and the same, it is known that attention to comfort measures may increase pain tolerance and decrease the sense of suffering a person in pain may experience. General comfort measures include attention to the patient and to the environment.

Psychological Pain Prevention Measures

Pain prevention measures may be directed toward the goal of increasing predictability and control of painful stimuli, thus decreasing anxiety. A number of strategies with demonstrated effectiveness have been devised.

The advantage of incorporating this component into the pain management plan is development and use of the patient's own resources to control pain. The patient's own resources can be transferred from one situation to another, assist in coping with future painful experiences, and preclude experiences which could lead to the development of increased susceptibility to pain (Fig. 13-10).

Informational control, letting the patient know what to expect and when, reduces fear of the unknown and thus anxiety. Providing preparatory information that includes sensory as well as procedural descriptions is most effective. The nurse should allow the patient as much decisional control as is realistic. The preferred site for an intravenous route, the timing of treatments, and the adjunctive pain relief modalities to be used are decisions into which the critical-care patient can have input.

The use of both avoidant and nonavoidant cognitive strategies for relief of pain, including distraction/diversion, imagery, music therapy, and humor can contribute to the patient's sense of control over the threat of pain. Behavioral pain relief techniques including biofeedback and relaxation can be very powerful components of a pain

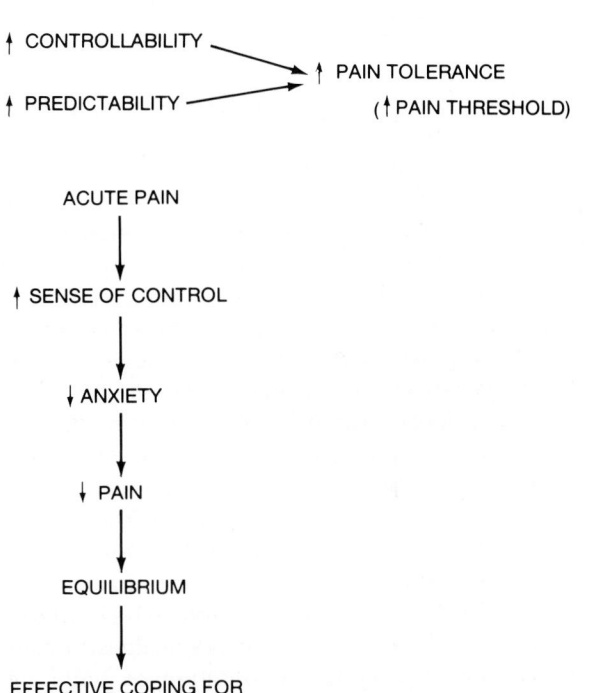

Figure 13-10 Wire diagram of explanation for how increasing control decreases pain perception.

management plan and should be incorporated whenever possible. These techniques are detailed further under specific intervention headings later in this chapter. It is the concept of increasing control that is important to this portion of the pain management plan.

Pain Relief

Several modalities are available for the management of pain. Pain relief modalities may be categorized as *invasive* or *noninvasive. Invasive modalities* are those that breach the body's barriers, such as the administration of a medication or alteration of the body surgically. Most, if not all, must be prescribed by a physician but may be suggested and/or implemented by the nurse. *Noninvasive modalities* may have internal effects but originate externally and do not breach the body's barriers. Most of these can be implemented independently by the nurse, although hospital policy may be influential in making this determination.[8]

Invasive Interventions

Pharmacologic Agents   Many pharmacologic agents have been incorporated into the armamentarium for pain relief. These drugs may be classified as *analgesics,* which are directed specifically toward relieving pain by altering sensation; or *analgesic adjuncts,* which alter a component of the pain.

Analgesics   The more commonly used analgesics are listed in Table 13-4. Just as there are no objective indicators for pain, there are no reliable indicators of analgesic requirement. Drugs are often prescribed based on weight, but weight does not seem to be a reliable predictor of analgesic need.

The analgesics are categorized as *non-narcotic* and *narcotic.* The non-narcotic analgesics are generally administered orally and are fairly weak. They have few side effects and may be very useful in conjunction with other modalities to provide relief of mild to moderate pain states.

Every drug has limitations in the form of dangerous or unpleasant side effects, or both. The undesirable effects of narcotic analgesics include respiratory depression, circulatory depression, nausea, vomiting, and the possible development of dependence. The narcotics cloud the sensorium

Table 13-4 Common Analgesics

Generic Name	Brand Name	Route of Administration	Length of Action (Hours)
Non-narcotics			
Aspirin	Hundreds	Oral	3–4
		Suppository	
Acetaminophen	Tylenol, Tempra	Oral	3–4
	Datril, Panadol	Suppository	
Ibuprofen	Motrin, Nuprin	Oral	3–4
Fenoprofen	Nalfon	Oral	3–4
	Many others		
Phenacetin		Oral	3–4
Narcotic			
Codeine	Codeine	Oral, IM, IV	2–4
Oxycodone	Percocet (combined with acetaminophen)	Oral	3–4
	Percodan (combined with A.P.C.)	Oral	3–4
Pentazocine	Talwin	Oral, IM, IV	2–3
Meperidine, Pethidine	Demerol	Oral (not efficacious) IM, IV	2–4
Morphine	Morphine	Oral, IM, IV	4–5
Hydropmorphone	Dilaudid	Oral, IM, IV	4–5
Methadone	Dolophine	Oral, IM, IV	4–5
Levorphanol	Levo-Dromoran Levorphan	Oral, IM, IV	4–5
Fentanyl	Sublimaze	IM, IV	4–5

and promote drowsiness, which may preclude the patient's ability to use other means of coping with pain (Fig. 13-11). In addition, analgesic effect is difficult to predict and often unsatisfactory. Even when analgesics are administered as requested, patients often suffer.

Concern for the side effects of narcotic analgesia has drastically limited treatment with narcotics which could be effective if used properly. While it is true that narcotics eventually cause addiction, this has never been a significant problem when they are used to treat acute pain. Respiratory depression occurs with the use of narcotics and the patient should be monitored carefully for adequacy of ventilation. This should be standard practice within the controlled environment of the critical-care unit and the possibility of respiratory depression should not preclude the use of narcotic analgesia when it is needed. In fact, narcotics can be titrated to produce appropriate analgesia by observing for normalcy of respiratory pattern with expiratory pause versus the shortened or absent

expiratory pause present in the respirations of a patient in acute pain.[11]

The patient should be evaluated for previous narcotic use for this will influence the doses of narcotics necessary to control pain. Patients who are physically dependent on narcotics, including those who have been in drug rehabilitation programs and are on a methadone maintenance schedule, will require larger doses of narcotics to prevent withdrawal symptoms during this vulnerable time.

The elderly patient is often undermedicated for severe acute pain because it is assumed that the elderly have a higher pain threshold or tolerate pain better. This is not necessarily so. The elderly patient should be assessed for concomitant physical problems, such as decreased circulation or decreased kidney and liver function, which would affect both uptake and clearance of analgesic drugs and therefore prolong the duration of action of these drugs. This does not change the amount of drug per administration needed to control pain for these patients. The nurse should also be alert for

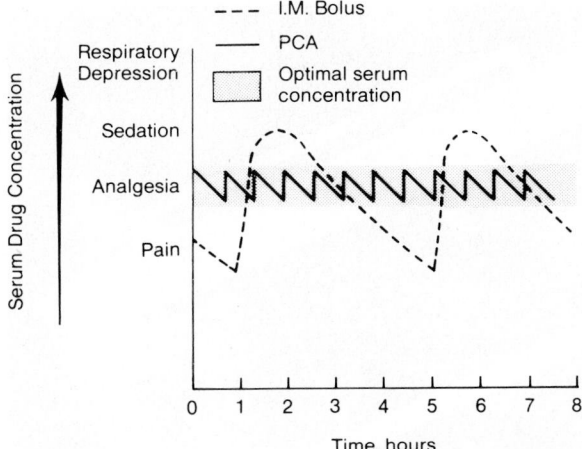

Figure 13-11   Narcotic analgesics exhibit a "hierarchy of response" to increasing serum drug concentrations. Typically there exists an optimal concentration where the patient is both analgesic and unsedated. Intermittent intramuscular injections of narcotics produce much wider swings in serum drug concentrations than do smaller, more frequently administered intravenous boluses. *(From R. L. Bennett and W. O. Griffen, Patient Controlled Analgesia, Contemporary Surgery, 23, 1983. With permission.)*

an increased likelihood of drug interactions if other medications are being administered for associated disease processes.

Austin relates that the plethora of new analgesics in the drug cabinet is not an indication that good analgesics have not been found, but rather that we are still not using appropriate methods of drug delivery.[12] For the critically ill or injured patient the intramuscular route of administration is clearly inferior. The peak levels of serum drug concentration are variable, partially due to the variable absorption rates from muscle. Small amounts of a narcotic administered frequently via the intravenous route to maintain serum drug concentrations control pain more effectively.

The *patient-controlled analgesic device (PCA)* (Fig. 13-12) is an electronically controlled infusion device which includes a timer and a mechanism for presetting doses of analgesics. This device allows the patient to self-administer analgesia as necessary. A lockout mechanism can be set to preclude inadvertent overdoses but initial evidence indicates that patients do a much better job of assessing the

dosage of analgesics needed to relieve pain without deleterious side effects than do either nurses or physicians. Blood serum concentrations are maintained at a more stable level, preventing the development of severe pain, which is more difficult to ablate without the development of drowsiness (Fig. 13-13). The beneficial aspects of this device are obvious; it combines individualized analgesic therapy based on each patient's subjective appreciation of pain with the reassurance and sense of control that patients derive from knowing that pain relief is readily at hand.

An interesting sidelight on trials of this device is that data indicate that patients need far more analgesia to relieve pain in the immediate postoperative period than was previously supposed, but that patients taper off their narcotic usage more quickly when they regulate administration themselves.

Pharmacologic analgesic adjuncts include drugs developed to alter a component of disease or injury that may contribute to the pain phenomenon, or to relieve associated symptoms of pain. Drugs may be used to relieve anxiety and apprehension, promote sleep, relax muscles, or reduce inflammatory processes. Table 13-5 presents some of the more commonly used analgesic adjuncts.

The pharmacologic approach essentially ignores the psychological and sociocultural factors known to influence pain perception, and interviews with patients indicate that few are satisfied with the way their pain was managed. Clearly, then, the use of analgesic drugs should not serve as the sole remedy for pain relief.

Nerve Blocks   Nerve blocks—the injection of local anesthetics or morphine close to nerves to block impulse conduction—are particularly useful for the relief of severe acute pain. These may be accomplished via singular puncture, as with the paravertebral (cervical plexus) block or the intercostal block, or as a continuous infusion, as used with continuous segmental peridural block.

The intercostal block, which provides complete relief of pain in the thoracic and abdominal regions, is particularly useful to treat unrelieved pain following thoracic and abdominal surgery, for patients with chest tubes, and for multiple trauma patients with rib fractures and flail chest. The

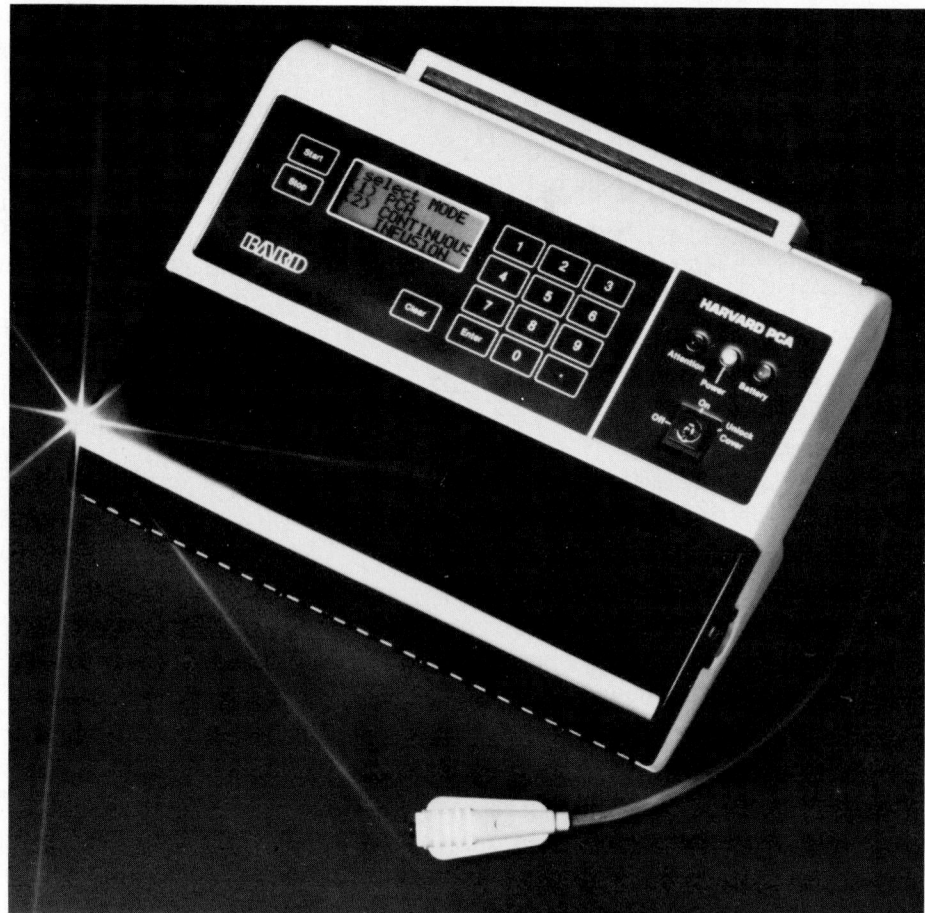

Figure 13-12   The patient-controlled analgesia device (PCA). *(With permission from Bard Electro Medical Systems, Inc., Englewood, Colorado.)*

advantage of a continuous infusion is that multiple painful punctures may be avoided if a block is necessary.

The major advantage of these central blocks is complete pain relief without central depression and, most importantly, no respiratory depression or interference with the patient's cough reflex. Therefore, ventilatory patterns can be improved and the patient can deep breathe and cough to cleanse the tracheobronchial tree.

The patient who has undergone nerve block should be observed closely for signs and symptoms of hypotension (particularly orthostatic), hypertension, toxic or allergic reactions to the anesthetic used, and respiratory dysfunction and paralysis. A block to relieve pain in the lower abdominal regions may induce urinary retention, so output should be monitored. If a continuous block is used, a catheter will remain in place. It should be handled using aseptic techniques and all precautions employed to avoid the hazards of infection.

Surgical Intervention   Surgical procedures for pain relief are generally regarded as the last resort after all other measures have failed. They may be employed to relieve pain associated with malignancy when life expectancy is limited.

Surgical procedures achieve pain relief through interruption of sensory pathways. Unfortunately, surgical procedures are short-term solutions and may result in neurologic damage. Central pain syndromes may result, and further neurologic dysfunction is almost a given. The critical-care nurse may be called upon to care for a patient who has

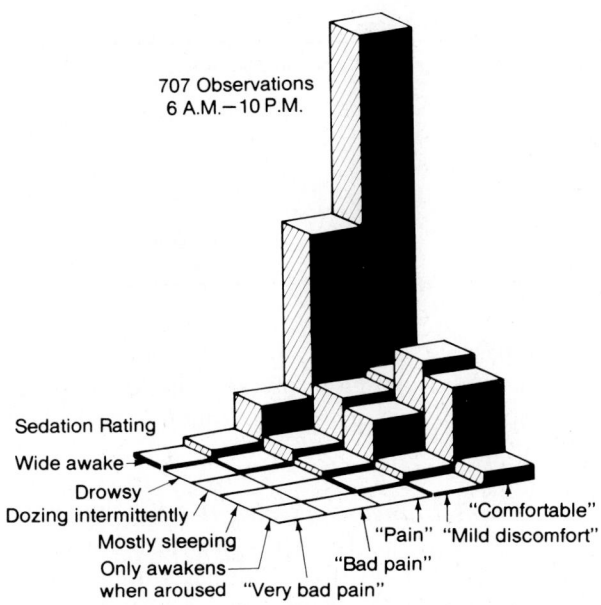

707 Observations
6 A.M.–10 P.M.

Sedation Rating
Wide awake
Drowsy
Dozing intermittently
Mostly sleeping
Only awakens
when aroused

"Comfortable"
"Mild discomfort"
"Pain"
"Bad pain"
"Very bad pain"

Analgesia Rating

Figure 13-13   Concurrent analgesia and sedation ratings made during normal waking hours (6 A.M.–10 P.M.) in a group of 50 patients using PCA following elective laparotomy. The majority of observations indicate a state of analgesia with minimal sedation. Optimal drug titration is effectively accomplished with PCA. *(From R. L. Bennett and W. O. Griffen, Patient Controlled Analgesia. Contemporary Surgery, 23, 1983. With permission.)*

undergone one of these operative procedures and should be familiar with them. Interruption of nerve pathways may be accomplished with the injection of neurolytic chemicals, cryodestruction, radiofre-

quency coagulation, or actual incision and resection. The more common procedures are listed in Table 13-6.

After such a procedure, all sensory innervation of the affected area is gone, including receptivity of pressure and temperature stimuli, so care must be directed toward preventing inadvertent injury. Postoperative care associated with spinal and cranial surgery is applicable to this patient. Due to possible disruption of neural pathways involved with the regulation of respiration, particular attention should be paid to respiratory patterns and neurologic function. Narcotic analgesia is generally not used for pain relief postoperatively because it masks the danger signals of increasing intracranial pressure and respiratory dysfunction. However, if pain is severe, narcotics may be necessary. In this case the surgeon should be consulted, prescriptions verified, and the patient monitored very carefully.

Noninvasive Interventions

Stimulation   Stimulation is a time-honored pain relief modality which may be employed independently by the nurse but probably is not used as often as it should be. Stimulation techniques may include the application of heat or cold, pressure, massage, and vibration. Transcutaneous electrical stimulation requires a prescription from a physician and specific knowledge for its use. It will be dealt with in the next section.

How the stimulation modalities work is not completely known and patients' responses tend to be very individualistic. Since many of these techniques are used in the home, the nurse can explore

Table 13-5 Pharmacologic Analgesic Adjuncts

Generic Group	Generic Name	Brand Name	Contributory Actions
Phenothiazines			Antiemetic
	Prochlorperazine	Compazine	Mild sedative
	Chlorpromazine	Thorazine	Narcotic potentiation
	Promazine	Sparine	Anxiety reduction
Butyrophenone			
	Droperidol	Inapsine	Narcotic potentiation
			Sedative
			Antiemetic
Synthetics			
	Chlordiazepoxide	Librium	Anxiety reduction
	Diazepam	Valium	Muscle relaxation
	Hydroxyzine hydrochloride	Atarax/Vistaril	Antiemetic

Table 13-6 Neurosurgical Procedures for Relief of Pain

Procedure	Pathway	Associated Surgery
Neurectomy	Cranial or peripheral nerves	Craniotomy
Rhizotomy	Anterior or posterior nerve root of spinal cord	Laminectomy
Chordotomy	Various pathways in cord	Laminectomy
Tractotomy	Anterolateral pathway in brainstem	Craniotomy
Intracranial stereotaxic procedures	Lesions created vary	Introduction of special instrumentation

with the patient what kinds of things feel good, relieve pain, and promote comfort. Many of them are interreactive.

Warmth or heat may be applied to a painful area and relief obtained through improved circulation and muscle relaxation. The application of heat is particularly useful to relieve the discomfort from intravenous solutions that have infiltrated.

Cold applications may also relieve pain. Cold packs or light ice packs may be soothing to a sore throat after surgery or relieve headache. Cold applications are also useful to relieve pain after orthopedic procedures and to relieve incisional pain. With both heat and cold applications, care must be taken to prevent injury to the skin.

Massage, especially back rubs, may be used to promote relaxation of the muscles. Massage coupled with heat or cold application is particularly effective.

Transcutaneous Electrical Nerve Stimulation (TENS) Transcutaneous electrical nerve stimulation (TENS) involves external stimulation of nerves through electrodes placed over the skin. The stimulation is produced by electric current activated by a battery-powered device (Fig. 13-14). The electric current produces a mild tingling or vibrating sensation over the area of application.

Controlled studies have demonstrated TENS to be particularly effective for the alleviation of

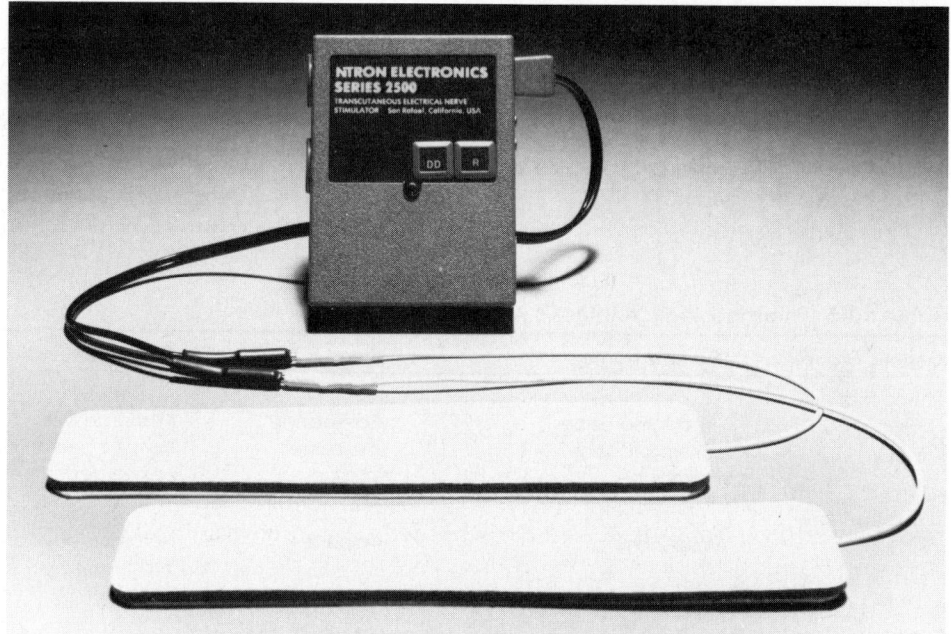

Figure 13-14 The transcutaneous electrical nerve stimulation device (TENS). *(With permission of NTRON International Sales Co., San Rafael, California.)*

chronic pain but TENS has also demonstrated potential effectiveness for relief of acute pain. It is not satisfactory as the sole modality. It seems to work better when the patient is drug-naive. Patients report that it potentiates relief from analgesics and gives them a sense of control over pain.

A number of different units are on the market. Most are simple to use. Generally, electrodes similar to those used for cardiac monitoring are applied to the area to be stimulated and the current flow adjusted until the patient reports discomfort. The current flow is then reduced until stimulation is felt but at a comfortable level. Each patient must decide this level for himself or herself. In the event a patient does not identify the stimulation as uncomfortable but a muscle response becomes apparent, the current flow should be reduced until it is obliterated. On many models, pulse rate and pulse width may be adjusted in a similar manner.

Since there are no deleterious side effects with TENS, it is an excellent adjunct for pain relief in the critical-care unit. It has been particularly effective for relieving the incisional pain associated with large thoracic and abdominal incisions. It may also be effective for relieving pain associated with chest tubes and sternal pain following open-heart surgery.

Initially, the use of TENS for patients scheduled for cardiac surgery or who have either internal or external pacemakers was contraindicated. Recent evidence indicates that it is safe for these patients to use TENS, although it should be used with caution and the patient observed closely for any adverse effects. TENS may interfere with electrical monitoring equipment and this should be observed. Caution should also be exercised when using TENS for patients who are taking anticoagulant medications, who are pregnant, or who have a diagnosis of myasthenia gravis.

Behavioral Techniques   Behavioral techniques for pain control can be very powerful and are particularly useful in the critical-care unit since they are safe and have few, if any, demonstrated side effects. Behavioral control involves the belief that one has a behavioral response available that can affect the aversiveness of an event.

Most of these techniques require concentrated and active thought processes. It should be noted that intense pain will adversely affect concentration and preclude success of these measures. If severe pain can be relieved through administration of narcotics, these techniques can substantially alter pain perception, increase tolerance, and reduce the need for narcotic analgesia.

Behavioral techniques include biofeedback, hypnosis, distraction, diversion, imagery, and relaxation. A patient's preference for one technique over another will have a substantial influence on its effectiveness. In addition, the nurse should be alert to behavioral techniques the patient may have previously developed, and augment these when possible.

Biofeedback, the use of instrumentation to provide information to the patient on the level of relaxation or tension, should be incorporated into the pain management plan if the patient has previously used this technique. It is not likely to be successful if original training must be started in the critical-care unit because it requires intense concentration. A disadvantage, of course, is that special equipment is needed. Likewise, hypnosis, which requires intense concentration, is usually not useful for severe acute pain; its use requires both a patient previously trained in the technique and a specifically trained practitioner.

The two most useful behavioral pain relief techniques for the critical-care patient are distraction and relaxation. Distraction involves focusing attention on stimuli other than the pain sensation and may take many forms, including guided imagery, music therapy, humor, and work. One of the most successful strategies that can be enhanced through nursing intervention is the distraction of visitors. Visiting hours in the critical-care unit are often unnecessarily restricted. Modifications should be made when visitors can contribute positively to care of the patient, particularly for something as important as pain control. The distraction and reassurance fostered through social support is extremely important. Burn patients tell us repeatedly that their greatest source of assistance in coping with pain is their families and other burn patients on the unit.

The development of distraction strategies is limited only by the imagination of the patient and nurse. The advantage of distraction is that it can be used at any age, but the nurse must plan the distraction with the patient to match age, developmental stage, and personal preference. Distraction techniques tend to be more successful when several sensory modalities (i.e., hearing, vision, touch, movement, smell, or taste) are included.

The disadvantage of distraction is that it can be quite fatiguing in the face of severe pain and the nurse must plan accordingly. For instance, the postoperative thoracic patient may tolerate pain well while being visited due to the distraction but once the visitors are gone feel worn out and be much less tolerant of pain and need narcotic analgesia to regain pain control.

Relaxation has been studied repeatedly as a pain relief adjunct with demonstrated effectiveness for increasing tolerance to pain and reducing narcotic analgesia necessary to control pain. Teaching the techniques and practice take time, which is seen by some as a disadvantage. However, there are major advantages in that relaxation is fairly simple to learn, noninvasive, has no known deleterious effects, and the patient can easily transfer the technique from one situation to another. The effective use of cognitive relaxation techniques appears to be dependent upon coaching but this may be another means by which the patient's family can contribute to care.

Relaxation is usually not effective when used as the sole pain relief modality but can be very useful to augment analgesics and increase tolerance by providing a sense of control over pain, which reduces anxiety.

Not to be negated are alternative methods for inducing relaxation, including back rubs or massage, light stroking, application of heat, and the reassurance of personal attention.

Evaluation of the Plan

Assessment of pain and the implementation of a pain management plan do not assure success in the relief of pain. Assessment must be continuous, the plan evaluated, and revisions made as necessary.

When evaluating the pain management plan the nurse should maintain a holistic approach, for pain is a holistic experience. Pain may affect any or all of the patient's physiologic or psychological responses. The nurse should stay open-minded about what may relieve pain and reduce suffering for very little is actually known about what does or doesn't work and why.

It should be kept in mind that it is usually easier to prevent severe pain than to relieve it and drastic measures may be needed to "get on top of the pain" once severe pain has taken hold. In addition, adjunctive measures may not immediately relieve pain but should be given a reasonable trial period. A case study may best illustrate these principles.

Case Study

Jamie D. is a 23-year-old white male construction worker admitted to the burn unit with partial and full thickness burns over 15 percent of his body, including abdomen and left arm. Jamie had been on a weekend camping trip. His burns were sustained from having his shirt catch fire when a kerosene lantern exploded as he was lighting it.

Initial surgical debridement of his burn wounds had been accomplished. Three days after his burn, Jamie was awaiting grafting. Continued treatment included removal of burn cream and reapplication twice a day. Morphine, 10 mg IV every 4 to 6 hours as needed, had been prescribed for pain but Jamie rarely complained and this drug had been administered sporadically.

On the fourth day after his burn, it was noted that Jamie was not eating well, a cause for concern due to the metabolic requirements of burn patients. In addition, it was noted that Jamie was becoming more and more withdrawn, an unusual response according to his wife. Upon directed questioning, Jamie admitted that he was suffering from "the worst pain I've ever had," but that he felt it was only appropriate since the accident had been "my own dumb fault."

During a care conference the burn team developed a pain management plan and initiated a pain management flow sheet (Fig. 13-15). A flow sheet can yield important clues to the effectiveness of a pain management plan as well as assist in the identification of associated integral problems.

Jamie's initial score on the visual analog scale was 9.5. It was decided that narcotic analgesia (the morphine prescribed) on a set schedule to maintain serum concentrations was needed to bring his pain under control. Administrations were planned to

PAIN MANAGEMENT FLOW SHEET

Patient's Name _____ ID No. _____

Diagnosis _____ Age _____

Pain rating scale used _____

Pain Management Plan _____

_____

_____

Date Time	Pain Score	Intervention	Vital Signs	Assoc S & SX	Comments include evidence of pain relief/Changes in plan

Figure 13-15 Sample pain management flow sheet.

provide peak concentrations prior to treatments so as to minimize further stimulation of pain, and treatments were planned so that he could have a period of rest before mealtime.

Meanwhile, Jamie was taught a relaxation exercise that included concentration on his breathing patterns. It was hoped that relaxation would augment the narcotic analgesia during treatments. Jamie tried this behavioral technique but did not feel that it enhanced pain control. Therefore, his love of hard rock music was incorporated into the overall plan by allowing him to use his portable radio with earphones as a distraction. He reported that this did not relieve the pain; however, he thought about the pain less and listening to music made treatments more "bearable."

Complete pain relief is usually not a realistically achievable goal for the burn patient. However,

the patient should not suffer severe, unrelenting pain. In this case, severe pain was reduced to a tolerable level with the use of narcotic analgesia and tolerance for the pain of continued necessary treatments was increased through the use of a behavioral technique geared to the patient's preference.

Jamie became more open to his environment and gained social support from other patients with whom he could work through the nature of his burn accident and explore what this pain meant. He gained valuable social support from his visitors, who also helped distract him from his pain. It took 36 h to bring Jamie's pain under reasonable control, after which distraction could be effectively used. The pain was then manageable, the narcotic dosages were tapered, and his appetite improved.

Pain is a challenge to both the patient who suffers it and the clinicians who attempt to alleviate it. A great deal of information about pain has been acquired and new findings are published every day. It is essential that critical-care nurses appreciate the complex nature of pain, develop holistic approaches to its management, and remain open to new pain relief techniques applicable to the critical-care patient that may be incorporated into practice.

References

1. Zborowski, M. (1969). *People in pain.* San Francisco: Jossey-Bass.
2. Weisenberg, M. (1977). Pain and pain control. *Psychological Bulletin, 84*(5), 1008–1044.
3. Rudy, E. B. (1984). *Advanced neurological and neurosurgical nursing.* St. Louis: Mosby.
4. Melzack, R., & Wall, P. (1983). *The challenge of pain.* New York: Basic Books.
5. Bonica, J. J. (1977). Neurophysiologic and pathologic aspects of acute and chronic pain. *Archives of Surgery, 112,* 750–761.
6. Lindahl, O. (1974). Pain—a general chemical explanation. In J. J. Bonica (Ed.), *Advances in neurology: International symposium on pain* (Vol. 4). New York: Raven Press.
7. Melzack, R., & Wall, P. (1965). Pain mechanisms: A new theory. *Science, 150,* 971–979.
8. McCaffery, M. (1979). *Nursing management of the patient with pain* (2d ed.). Philadelphia: Lippincott.

9. Meinhart, N. T., & McCaffery, M. (1983). *Pain: A nursing approach to assessment and analysis.* Norwalk, Connecticut: Appleton-Century-Crofts.

10. Melzack, R. (1975). The McGill pain questionnaire: Major properties and scoring methods. *Pain, 1,* 177–299.

11. Van Poznak, A. (1984). Role of respiratory patterns in the treatment of pain and anxiety. In M. E. Luczun (Au.), *Post anesthesia nursing.* Rockville, Maryland: Aspen Systems Corp.

12. Austin, K. L., Stapleton, J. V., & Mather, L. E. (1980). Multiple intramuscular injections—a major source of variability in analgesic response to meperidine. *Pain, 8,* 47–62.

Bibliography

Beecher, H. K. (1956). The Subject response and reaction to sensation. *American Journal of Medicine, 20,* 107–113.

Beyer, J. E., DeGood, D. E., Ashley, L. C., & Russell, G. A. (1983). Patterns of postoperative analgesic use with adults and children following cardiac surgery. *Pain, 17*(1), 71–81.

Christoph, S. B. (1985). A comparison of patient-controlled transcutaneous electrical stimulation with traditional analgesics for postoperative pain relief. Doctoral dissertation, The Catholic University of America. Ann Arbor, Michigan: University Microfilms.

Johnson, J. E., & Rice, V. H. (1974). Sensory and distress components of pain: Implications for the study of clinical pain. *Nursing Research, 23*(3), 203–209.

Kaiko, R. F., Wallenstein, S., Rogers, A., Grabinski, P., & Houde, R. (1982). Narcotics in the elderly. *Medical Clinics of North America, 66,* 1079–1089.

Scott, L. E., Clum, G. A., & Peoples, J. B. (1983). Preoperative predictors of postoperative pain. *Pain, 15,* 283–293.

Shade, S. K. (1985). Use of transcutaneous electrical stimulation for a patient with a cardiac pacemaker. *Physical Therapy, 65*(2), 206–208.

Siang-Yang Tan. (1982). Cognitive and cognitive-behavioral methods for pain control: A selective review. *Pain, 12,* 201–228.

Thompson, S. C. (1981). Will it hurt less if I can control it? A complex answer to a simple question. *Psychological Bulletin, 90*(1), 89–101.

Wells, N. (1982). The effect of relaxation on postoperative muscle tension and pain. *Nursing Research, 31*(4), 236–238.

White, P. F. (1985). Use of parenteral narcotics in the postoperative period: The concept of "on-demand" analgesia. *Current Reviews for Recovery Room Nurses, 15*(7), 118–123.

Zaloga, G. P., Hostinsky, C., & Chernow, B. (1984). Endogenous opioid peptides: Critical care implications. *Heart and Lung, 13*(4), 421–430.

14

Sleep and the Critically Ill Patient

Sarah J. Sanford

Introduction

Sleep is one of the most basic and natural processes in which all humans, in fact, all mammals engage. As an activity, it occupies roughly one-third of our lives, yet it is often taken for granted. Most commonly, the vital role sleep plays in the maintenance of high-level wellness is only appreciated when sleep has been lost or disrupted. Fortunately, otherwise healthy individuals usually need only adjust their activities or environment, and sleep normally to completely reverse the impact of previous sleep compromise, a process typically accomplished within several days.

In contrast, individuals admitted to critical-care units experience actual or potential life-threatening physiologic vulnerability. Continuous monitoring, intensive treatment, and aggressive interventions are the rule. As a result, critically ill patients are subjected to further compromise in the form of both qualitative and quantitative sleep disruptions. Compounding the problem is the patient's inability to adjust the environment to allow normal sleep. Thus, sleep disruption tends to have both potentially significant and cumulative effects.

The discussion that follows includes information regarding the nature and physiologic correlates of normal sleep as well as the nature and impact of disruptive influences inherent in the critical-care setting. A discussion of applying the nursing process to minimize sleep disruption follows.

Normal Sleep

Scientific research involving simultaneous monitoring of the EEG (electroencephalogram), EOG (electrooculogram), and EMG (electromyogram) has shown that sleep is composed of two very distinct types of activity: *REM,* or *rapid eye movement,* and *non-REM (NREM) sleep.* Far from the traditional view of sleep as a quiescent state, REM sleep involves intense physiologic activation, and for that reason is often referred to as *active* or *paradoxic sleep.* Non-REM sleep, on the other hand, is associated with progressive relaxation. It is divided into four stages (NREM 1 to 4) with NREM stages 3 and 4 often referred to as *quiet sleep.*[1]

REM Sleep

REM sleep was named for the characteristic, sporadic bursts of extremely rapid and conjugate eye movements seen on the EOG. These movements are frequently visible through the closed eyelid to an observer. The EMG during REM sleep is essentially flat and reflects hyperpolarization of neurons in the brainstem and spinal cord. This hyperpolarization prevents distal impulse transmission and results in immobility and functional paralysis of large postural and skeletal muscles. In contrast, cerebral cortical metabolic activity greatly increases during REM sleep, and, not surprisingly, the EEG closely resembles that of the waking state.[1]

Physiologically, REM sleep is associated with autonomic (sympathetic nervous system) activation. Overall oxygen consumption increases despite large muscle immobility, due to the intense cerebral metabolic activity. Clinically, cardiac output, blood pressure, and heart rate may become erratic and, at times, surpass waking values. In the presence of underlying cardiac disease, both nocturnal angina and ventricular arrhythmias have been documented. Respiratory rates during REM sleep are highly irregular, frequently very fast or very slow, and central apneic periods have been noted.[7]

REM sleep is frequently referred to as *dreaming sleep* because REM sleep periods are associated with dramatic, episodic dreams. Described as full color, vivid, and often bizarre experiences, REM sleep dreams may include auditory components and intensely emotional overtones. Not infrequently, REM sleep dreams are associated with paralysis and a perceived inability to move or escape. Some hypothesize that dreams in REM sleep provide the psyche with opportunities to deal with profound anxieties and psychologic concerns.

NREM Sleep

Of the four stages of NREM sleep, stage 1 is subjectively the lightest. The EEG is similar to that seen in waking, and it may most appropriately be viewed as a transition state. The EEG of stage 2 NREM sleep displays a pattern similar to that of stage 1, differing primarily in that the background wave frequency is slower, and characteristic waveforms called *sleep spindles* and *K complexes* are superimposed. Stages 3 and 4 NREM sleep are associated with very large, slow-frequency waves called *deltas* in the EEG. Thus, these two stages are commonly referred to as *delta* or *slow-wave sleep* (*SWS*). The primary criterion used to differentiate NREM stage 3 from stage 4 is the percentage of these slow delta waves on the EEG. Throughout NREM sleep, the EOG reflects gradual slowing or cessation of eye movements, and the EMG progressively declines in association with the profound muscle relaxation characteristic of NREM sleep. However, although low, the EMG during NREM sleep never is as low as that seen during REM sleep.[1]

Dominance of the parasympathetic nervous system characterizes NREM sleep; thus physiologic activation is low. Progression through NREM sleep is associated with declines in cardiac and respiratory rates, blood pressure, metabolic rate, and body temperature to basal levels. Premature ventricular escape beats have been documented during NREM stage 4 and, to a lesser extent, NREM stage 3, in patients with chronic cardiac disease and previous myocardial infarction.[2] Presumably, periods of marked bradycardia facilitate initiation of ectopic beats by irritable myocardial foci.

Cyclic Aspects of Sleep

Sleep is a cyclic phenomenon. The majority of time spent sleeping most commonly occurs rhythmically in a continuous bulk period once a day; within that period, sleep activity is composed of repeating cycles of sleep stages.

Sleep Cycle

Within the normal sleep period, NREM and REM sleep occur in a specific repeating pattern or *sleep cycle*. With the onset of sleep, there occurs a progression through NREM sleep, first from stage 1 through 4 and then back again to stage 2. From stage 2, a REM sleep period is entered. Following completion of REM sleep, stage 2 is again entered and the cycle is reinitiated (see Fig. 14-1). The average length of each sleep cycle is approximately 90 min (70 to 100 min) and is dictated by an intrinsic basic rest–activity cycle (BRAC) of the central nervous system.[1] Thus, a REM or active sleep period occurs about every 90 min.

The length of time within the 90-min cycles occupied by each sleep stage is determined by the cycle's temporal relationship to the total sleep period. Early in the sleep period, NREM stages dominate the cycle and REM sleep periods are very brief. As the sleep period progresses, the proportions reverse somewhat, and cycles near the end of the sleep period tend to be dominated by REM periods of longer duration. Thus, most NREM sleep occurs during the early sleep period, while the majority of REM sleep is obtained during the final hours.[1]

Daytime naps taken in the late afternoon are characterized by cycles relatively dominated by NREM sleep, as if the total sleep period had begun

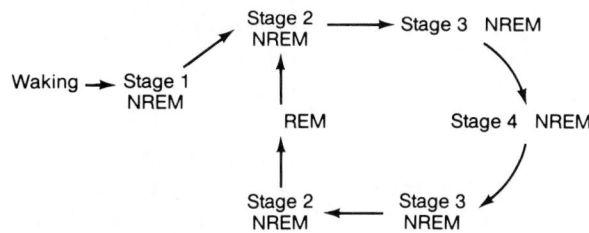

Figure 14-1   The sleep cycle. The average time between two REM sleep periods equals approximately 90 min.

early. Afternoon naps, therefore, can reduce NREM stages 3 and 4 sleep during the subsequent total sleep period. Morning naps, on the other hand, are characterized by cycles relatively dominated by REM, as if reflecting continuation of the preceding total sleep period.[1]

Circadian Rhythm

Intrinsic to humans is a self-sustaining internal biologic clock known as the *circadian rhythm*. Operating roughly every 24 h, the circadian rhythm pattern is comprised of consistent rhythms of peaks and troughs of hormone secretion rates, body temperature, humoral and metabolic parameters, and mental and emotional functioning.[3,4] Internal acclimatization to the sleep schedule is present when sleep activity occupies the trough or low phase of the circadian rhythm, in which case *circadian synchronization* is said to exist. Wakefulness and activity, on the other hand, occur during the higher phase or peak of the circadian cycle.

Ideally, internal acclimatization of the sleep schedule is maintained. Most commonly, the vast majority of total sleep time (TST) within a 24-h period occurs in one uninterrupted sleep period, the actual clock hours of which are determined by each individual's balancing of external factors such as employment schedule, social and family commitments, and societal influences such as availability of goods and services.

Sleep obtained during hours customarily spent awake and active, or trying to be awake and active during hours customarily spent in sleep activity, constitutes a *phase shift* and thus *circadian desynchronization*.[5] Desynchronized sleep is subjectively and consistently given a poor quality rating. It is associated with a decrease in arousal threshold and spontaneous awakenings are more likely. Anxiety, depression, restlessness, irritability, and decreased accuracy in task performance (judgment, reaction time) are characteristic findings.[5]

When the sleep–activity schedule changes, internal acclimatization must be reestablished. That is, *resynchronization* must occur. Individual resynchronization efficiency is variable. The minimum time required is thought to be 3 days, and during that time constancy of environment and schedule must be maintained. More commonly, the process of reacclimatization involves 5 to 12 days. Characteristically, resynchronization is associated with chronic fatigue, malaise, and a decreased ability to perform all life tasks.[5]

Theories of Sleep Functions

Sleep is vital to the maintenance of optimal physiologic and psychologic function. Beyond prevention of the syndrome associated with sleep deprivation, however, only theories about the precise functions of sleep exist.

Restorative Theory of Function

During slow-wave sleep, growth hormone (GH) is consistently secreted by the anterior pituitary.[1] Stimuli associated with growth hormone secretion include a reduced availability of energy substrate or increased energy demand. By virtue of the anabolic effects of growth hormone, effects which include action to prevent breakdown and promote synthesis of protein, elevated secretion of growth hormone during sleep is consistent with a physiologically recuperative function, particularly for tissues characteristically high in protein content such as cartilage and muscle. The finding that physical exercise during the day often produces increased proportions of stages 3 and 4 NREM sleep during the subsequent night has provided further evidence that NREM sleep is associated with physiologic recuperation. Presumably, depletion of energy substrates during exercise increases the need for anabolic restoration, which in turn results in increased NREM 3 and 4 sleep.[1]

Animal studies have implied that levels of cerebral neurochemical substances are replenished during sleep. Compared with animals allowed to sleep normally, sleep-deprived animals have been found to have depleted levels of cerebral glucose, adenosine triphosphate (ATP), and other high-energy phosphate compounds. Incorporation of phosphorus into both phosphoproteins and phosphopeptides is known to increase during sleep. The drowsiness characteristically associated with the postictal state is thought to represent a period of high-energy phosphate level restoration after the exaggerated cerebral and physiologic metabolic expenditure during seizure activity.[1]

Psychologic Theory of Function

Experts believe that information is reviewed and categorized during sleep. Contextual and conceptual input from the most recent day is thought to be sorted, selectively stored in memory, or cleared to make room for the upcoming day's input. Evidence for this theory is based largely upon the finding of inappropriate interpretation of reality and personality changes following sleep deprivation.

Precise mechanisms have not been defined; however, REM sleep is thought to be vitally involved in the maintenance of optimum mental and emotional function. Selective deprivation of REM sleep has been found to lead to disrupted interpretation of the environment; described manifestations range from disorientation and delusions to frank hallucinations. Personality changes found to be associated with REM sleep deprivation include withdrawal, increased suspiciousness, and paranoia.[1] Most researchers believe that information processing and storage activities occur during REM sleep.

Sleep Requirements

The precise length of the daily continuous bulk sleep period is highly variable between individuals. The same is true for the frequency, timing, and length of naps customarily engaged in across the population. Thus, other than the fact that no one has been documented as being able to survive without sleep, there are no universally accepted parameters for too much or too little. In general, the most useful standard is that amount of sleep that results in the subjective feeling of being rested and refreshed.[1]

Characteristic quantitative guidelines and patterns do exist, however, and reflect both age and gender. Typically, as age increases, total sleep time decreases, primarily as a function of decreasing percentages of NREM stages 3 and 4.[21] The percentage of sleep activity comprised of REM sleep is highest in the first week of life and gradually declines until young adulthood at which time the REM sleep percent-of-total stabilizes at between 20 to 25 percent, a percent that diminishes only slightly, if at all, with continued advance in age.[6] Increases in stages 1 and 2 NREM sleep also accompany advancing age, as do the number of spontaneous awakenings during the sleep period.[6] Thus, as age increases there appears to be a decreasing need for slow-wave sleep and in addition an overall decrease in the stability of sleep activity.

Gender also appears to play a role in determining individual sleep characteristics. Females typically demonstrate bulk sleep periods of longer duration than males. In addition, at all ages women characteristically display a slightly greater percentage of NREM stage 4 sleep than do men.[6]

Sleep Apneas

Two types of apneic events occur during sleep: central apneas with diaphragmatic arrest occurring characteristically during REM sleep, and obstructive apneas due to upper airway collapse, most commonly during REM but possible during NREM sleep as well. Both types of apneic events are known to be accompanied by arterial desaturation and hypoxemia; the degree of severity, however, is greatest during the obstructive type.[7]

Relaxation of the muscles that normally maintain the patency of the upper respiratory tract occurs during both REM and NREM sleep, but the degree of sleep-related hypotonia is generally most pronounced during REM sleep.[2] Clinically manifested as snoring, this sleep-induced oropharyngeal hypotonia promotes and perpetuates abnormal inspiratory subatmospheric intrathoracic pressures; negative values ranging from 50 to 150 cmH$_2$O have been documented in heavy snorers.[8] When applied to an already hypotonic oropharyngeal tract, such pressures result in a self-perpetuating tendency for narrowing, lengthening, and eventual collapse of the airway. The resultant airway obstruction, with attempted airflow against a closed glottis, results in both hemodynamic and electrocardiographic changes.

Systemic and pulmonary hypertension accompany obstructive apneic events; the degree of pressure elevation directly and positively correlates with the frequency of obstructive events. If apneic events are repetitive, that is, they occur throughout the sleep period during both REM and NREM sleep, pressure elevations can be severe. Systemic pressures as high as 200/120 (with awake supine control of 130/80), and 280/170 (with awake supine control of 160/94), and pulmonary artery pressures of 80/54 (control 30/20), and 68/40 (control 34/20), have been recorded after repetitive apneic events over a 5-h sleep period.[7] While hypoxemia-induced pulmonary vasoconstriction and sympathetic nervous system discharge, and increased systemic vascular resistance are undoubtedly involved, the marked intrathoracic pressure changes associated with attempted inspiration against a closed glottis may also contribute to the development of the hemodynamic findings characteristic of obstructive apneic events. Comparison of pressure changes associated with central versus obstructive apneas clearly demonstrates greater increases with the latter; hypoxemia and arterial desaturation are also more pronounced during obstructive apneic events.[7]

Arrhythmias, including bradycardias, sinus arrests, and, occasionally, second-degree heart blocks, have been documented during obstructive sleep apneas. Increased vagal tone is thought to be involved. Following resumption of airflow and removal of vagal stimulation, tachycardias are common. Overall, the electrocardiographic accompaniment of obstructive apneic events is thus a *brady-tachy syndrome*.[7]

Sleep apneas of 10 s or more duration are thought to affect at least 1 percent of the adult male population.[9] Individuals who experience either prolonged or repetitive episodes can suffer significant sleep loss. With arterial desaturation and hypoxemia, brainstem respiratory centers are activated and arousal is stimulated. With transition from sleeping to waking, airflow resumes as the sleep-induced hypotonia and/or diaphragmatic arrest are reversed. Such apnea-induced arousals have been documented at frequencies of five per hour; severe cases have been documented which involved as many as 300 to 500 apnea-induced arousals over the course of one night's sleep period.[9,10] Remarkably, other than reporting excessive daytime sleepiness or labored and disruptive snoring, individuals are often unaware that they experience sleep apneas.[10]

Daytime sleepiness and a history of snoring are commonly reported in individuals requiring treatment for chronic systemic hypertension. In light of the hemodynamic pressure changes asso-

ciated with repeated and/or prolonged apneic events, such a finding should not be surprising.[7]

Recovery of Lost Sleep: Rebounds

Loss of REM, NREM stage 4, and probably NREM stage 3 sleep, lead to development of debt-like phenomena. As is true of all others, sleep debts must be repaid. Following selective deprivation of these stages, *rebounds,* or consistent quantitative increases in the "debted" types of sleep occur in subsequent bulk sleep periods. Specifically, the stage for which the debt has been developed is entered both more often and from stages which normally do not precede the deficient stage.

Presumably, rebounds are compensatory. Growth hormone secretion increases during stage 4 NREM sleep rebounds and is thought to reflect anabolic restoration following depletion of energy stores as a result of increased time awake. Whether or not the reason is the need for physiologic restoration, stage 4 NREM sleep rebounds appear to assume a high priority. In the presence of coexisting NREM stage 4 and REM sleep debts, NREM stage 4 is consistently and preferentially rebounded.[6] REM sleep debts are thus more likely sustained, and accumulated, and REM sleep rebounds, when they occur, are likely to be intense and prolonged.

Sleep Pattern Disturbance in the Critical-Care Setting

Normal sleep in the critical-care setting is for all practical purposes impossible. Both environmental and situational factors result in sleep disruption.

Environmental Disruptions of Sleep

Critical-care settings are characterized by virtually continuous activity. Treatments and interventions are required and delivered 24 h a day. The environment thus directly impairs the ability of patients to experience effective sleep.

Loss of Day-Night Orientation
Many critical-care units either lack windows or are designed in such a way as to limit a patient's exposure to natural light. In addition, the need for

frequent interventions often results in the majority of unit lights being on continuously during most, if not all, hours of the day. Under such conditions patients are often unable to distinguish day from night.

Besides contributing to disorientation, loss of the usual day-night natural light cues alters pineal secretion of melatonin, a hormone thought to have natural sedative and hypnotic properties.[11,12] It has long been recognized that even small variations in natural light alter melatonin secretion in most mammals and similar relationships have recently been found in humans. In the absence of natural light, that is, when it is dark, melatonin secretion is increased. In contrast, the presence of natural light results in suppression of melatonin secretion. However, light of very high intensity is required to inhibit human melatonin secretion. Characteristically, intensity of a magnitude great enough to reduce melatonin secretion is achieved only by natural outdoor light and not by most artificial indoor light.

Patients receiving care in critical-care units, where natural light exposure is limited, not only lack the inhibition of melatonin which naturally occurs with outdoor light, but in addition are continuously exposed to artificial light. The result is a patient who experiences the effects of melatonin and thus is subjectively drowsy and sleepy but for whom time blurs and day blends into night.

Noise Level

Noise is constant in the critical-care setting. Contributors include mechanical equipment, activated alarms, ringing phones, computer printers, care-related sounds associated with suctioning and coughing, and, as well, the moans and cries of patients. Talking, laughing, and cajoling between and among nursing, medical, ancillary personnel, and patients further aggravate the situation.

Sound recordings in critical-care units have revealed noise levels between 45 to 85 dB.[13] Heavy traffic and busy restaurants have been recorded at roughly 80 dB. To allow sleep, sound levels not exceeding 40 dB are generally thought to be required; 35 dB or less are recommended.[14]

Compounding the problem is the unfamiliar, strange, and often frightening nature of many of the sounds. While individual reactions to specific noises vary, illness is known to lower the threshold of tolerable sound.[15] That excessive noise is a frequent complaint of patients admitted to critical-care units should not be surprising.

Situational Disruptions of Sleep

In addition to disruptive influences that occur as a result of the critical-care environment, a number of circumstantial factors either create discomfort or further inhibit the ability of patients to obtain effective sleep. Personal and social isolation, with complete dependence upon totally unfamiliar people; pain; loss of privacy; and loss of control all contribute to already existing anxiety and fear regarding the outcome of admission to the critical-care setting.[16] In addition, sedative and analgesic medications, administered to reverse the impact of these influences, often functionally contribute to inability to obtain effective sleep by altering sleep stage activity. The effects of medications are discussed in a later section.

Personal and Social Isolation

Patients admitted to critical-care units are completely removed from everything familiar to them. Family and significant others are allowed to visit only infrequently, and when they are permitted access, time is limited. In addition, usually only one or two visitors are allowed at a time. Communication is strained at best and often far from effective in reversing personal and social isolation.

Discomfort and Pain

Patients admitted to critical-care units often experience intense pain as a result of specific pathologies, physiologic insults, and therapeutic interventions. Nasogastric and pulmonary suctioning, and insertion and manipulation of invasive lines produce far from pleasant sensations. Compounding the impact are well-documented perceptions of forced and total immobilization, that is, the "tied down" syndrome.[16] Even if the patient is physically capable of adjusting or changing position, restrictions to movement in the form of respiratory assistance devices, traction, tubes and lines, and restraints applied to assure secure placement of all the above often prevent movement. Under such conditions, even seemingly minor sources of discomfort such as wrinkles, "being exposed," and/or being too cold or too warm assume exaggerated proportions and are often described as a major source of discomfort.

Anxiety and Fear

Anxiety and fear are not only standard emotional responses to any critical-care environment but in fact are considered essential. Lack of such responses may indicate severe depression, psychotic withdrawal, or denial.[15] At the heart of each patient's emotional response is recognition that the danger of death is real. Even though the thought of dying may not be at the level of immediate and conscious awareness, it is often manifested by hesitance, if not complete refusal, to ask about prognosis. Excessive verbalization expressing complete confidence in and trust of care givers, in other words, a "do what you have to do" approach, is not uncommon and may reflect severe anxiety.

Pharmacologic Agents

Care providers order and administer analgesic, sedative, and hypnotic agents in recognition of the prevalence of pain, anxiety, and fear in the critical-care patient population. Many of the commonly utilized agents are known to disrupt sleep.

Morphine sulfate increases drowsiness but simultaneously results in less intense, more disrupted sleep. Spontaneous arousals increase and proportions of total sleep time comprised by REM and NREM stages 3 and 4 decrease following its administration. Functionally, morphine sulfate results in relative increases in the lighter, that is, NREM 1 and 2, stages of sleep.[17]

Benzodiazepines are a class of sedative, hypnotic agents often administered to aid sleep. Commonly utilized are the long-acting agents *diazepam* (*Valium*) and *flurazepam* (*Dalmane*), the intermediate-range agent *temazeam* (*Restoril*), and the shorter-range, more rapidly acting agent *triazolam* (*Halcion*).

Diazepam (Valium) increases stage 1 NREM sleep and reduces both REM and slow-wave sleep. The degree of REM sleep suppression is dose-dependent—the larger the dose, the greater the REM sleep reduction. Slow-wave sleep suppression, on the other hand, occurs to the same extent at all doses within the therapeutic range. Thus, the overall effect of diazepam is to reduce deep sleep while simultaneously increasing light sleep.[18]

Flurazepam (Dalmane), if administered in doses less than 60 mg a day, may be an effective hypnotic agent. Conflicting reports do, however, exist. Both increases and decreases in stage 4 NREM and REM sleep have been reported.[17,19] The active metabolite of flurazepam (to which effects are attributed) demonstrates a half-life ranging from 24 to 100 h; thus, daytime sleepiness as well as other side effects, including decreased dexterity and cognitive performance, can occur even after cessation of this agent.[20]

Both temazeam (Restoril) and triazolam (Halcion) have a shorter half-life and more rapid onset of action than their longer-acting benzodiazepine counterparts. Sleep latency, that is, the time spent in bed before falling asleep, is decreased by both agents, and next-day side effects are far less commonly reported. However, these shorter-acting agents suppress to some extent both slow-wave and REM sleep.[17]

Barbiturates also disrupt sleep. *Amobarbital* (*Seconal*), *secobarbital* (*Tuinal*), and *pentobarbital* (*Nembutal*) markedly reduce REM sleep while simultaneously increasing stage 2 NREM sleep. *Phenobarbital* (*Luminal*) facilitates stage 4 NREM sleep but in doses greater than 200 mg also suppresses REM sleep.[19] Thus, utilization of agents from this sedative category, with the possible exception of low-dose phenobarbital, introduces the risk of promoting qualitatively altered sleep activity.

Nature and Impact of Sleep Disruptions in Critical Care

Three general types of sleep disruptions are commonly experienced by individuals admitted to critical-care units: *circadian desynchronization, sleep fragmentation,* and *sleep deprivation.*

Circadian Desynchronization

For patients admitted to critical-care units, *circadian desynchronization* is essentially unavoidable. Because of 24-h care requirements, patients are frequently awake at times during which they customarily sleep. Similarly, they sleep during times customarily spent awake. As a result, much of the sleep obtained is desynchronized and less than optimally effective. Such sleep is also more unstable because desynchronization is associated with a decreased arousal threshold, and an increased tendency for spontaneous awakenings.

Compounding the impact is the unlikelihood and difficulty of reacclimatization of sleep and activity schedules. Resynchronization requires adherence to a consistent sleep schedule in a constant environment. Because patient care activities in critical-care units are rarely consistent for 1, let alone 3 days, chronic desynchronization is likely. Sleep received is associated with a poor-quality rating, and with restlessness, anxiety, and decreased accuracy in task performance.

Sleep Fragmentation

In contrast to the normal practice of obtaining essentially all the 24-h quota of sleep in one uninterrupted period of repeating sleep stage cycles, patients in critical-care units are likely to experience frequently interrupted and sporadically occurring cycles. Whether due to treatment requirements or awakenings as a result of a decreased arousal threshold, repeated interruptions result in sleep fragmentation and with it an increased frequency of transitions between sleep stages.[21]

Phasic alterations in autonomic stimulation accompany sleep-stage transitions. If rapid, alterations in autonomic stimulation can increase myocardial irritability. Ventricular tachycardia has occurred in individuals forced to make sudden transitions between sleep stages, especially in and out of REM sleep.[2]

Sleep fragmentation may also jeopardize pulmonary function. Impaired arousal responses to elevations in the Pa_{CO_2}, decreases in the Pa_{O_2}, and the presence of a foreign substance, water, in the respiratory tract have been documented.[21]

Sleep Deprivation

Patients in critical-care units invariably experience deprivation of REM and probably NREM stages 3 and 4 sleep as well. Even if uninterrupted periods of sleep occur, it is highly unlikely that the length

of any one of those periods equals that of the customary sleep period. Because the majority of REM sleep is normally obtained during the later portion of the sleep period, REM quantity is decreased when the sleep period is shortened. Further, the use of a variety of sedative, hypnotic, and analgesic medications, as previously discussed, contribute to REM sleep loss as well as loss of NREM stages 3 and 4.

Sleep fragmentation further compromises REM and NREM stages 3 and 4 sleep. When sleep resumes after an interruption, the cycle essentially begins anew rather than returning to the stage from which arousal occurred. Repeated failure to complete full 90-min cycles therefore leads to relative dominance of NREM stages 1 and 2 sleep and loss of NREM 3 and 4 and REM sleep.[1]

In heavy snorers sleep deprivation, even of short duration (e.g., loss of one customary sleep period), has been found to increase both the frequency and duration of sleep-induced obstructive apneic events. Especially pronounced was the increase in length of REM-associated apneic events.[7]

Further physiologic vulnerability occurs as a function of selective loss of REM and NREM stage 4 sleep (and probably NREM stage 3 sleep). As previously discussed, deprivation of these sleep stages results in rebounds or consistent quantitative increases during bulk sleep periods that follow such loss.[1] As also noted, NREM sleep tends to be selectively rebounded in the presence of both NREM and REM sleep deprivation. While NREM sleep rebounds are physiologically benign, the same cannot be said of REM sleep rebounds. Because sympathetic nervous system discharge is pronounced during REM sleep, rebounds of this type of sleep can involve excessive myocardial stimulation and thus predispose patients with preexisting compromise to ischemia, infarction, and/or failure. Similarly, in the presence of preexisting neurologic insult, intense periods of REM sleep can result in significant elevations in intracranial pressure.[17]

REM sleep debts also predispose to significant disturbance in mental and emotional function. Perceptual disruptions can become severe and be manifested by disorientation, delusions, and even paranoia. Fear accompanying such disruptions can impair ability to relax, thus adding to already-existing difficulty falling asleep. When sleep does occur, it is likely desynchronized and characterized by a low arousal threshold. Staying asleep is thus also difficult. Finally, restlessness and anxiety associated with desynchronized sleep are likely to prompt the use of pharmacologic agents that further disrupt sleep. Unfortunately, perpetuation of both disturbed sleep and psychologic disruption is likely.

Using the Nursing Process to Limit Sleep Disruption

Normal sleep in the critical-care setting is essentially impossible. Environmental and situational disruptions to customary sleep patterns are inherent, rampant, and likely self-perpetuating without aggressive nursing therapy. Perhaps one of the biggest challenges to critical-care nurses is to integrate interventions designed to limit sleep disruption into the complex, ever-changing plan of care required for critically ill patients.

Assessment

Data regarding pattern and effectiveness of customary sleep activity need to be incorporated into the admission nursing assessment of all critically ill patients. Whether gathered from the patient or family, assessment data should include hours usually spent sleeping, both during the customary bulk sleep period and in naps, as well as usual timeframes for each activity. The customary sleep environment should also be described, including numbers of blankets and pillows utilized, use of night lights or other direct or indirect lighting, and the presence and type of noise customarily present, such as ticking clocks or other background noise (Table 14-1). Usual presleep routines and activities felt to enhance ability to sleep should also be described. Lastly, the presence of a history of snoring needs to be noted.

Once such data are known, information gathered subsequently during the patient's stay can be compared against this baseline to determine the presence and degree of any potential and developing sleep disruption. Ongoing assessments must reflect awareness of the need to monitor the effects the many disruptive factors in the critical-care environment have on a patient's sleep.

Table 14-1 The Sleep History

1. Customary sleep activity
   a. Bulk sleep period:
      Number of hours
      Usual clock time
      Environment
   b. Naps:
      Usual hours
      Length
      Environment
2. Sleep aids utilized
3. Presleep routines
4. History of snoring or chronic systemic hypertension

Potential Nursing Diagnosis: Sleep Pattern Disturbance

Sleep pattern disturbance refers to a situation in which an individual experiences, or is at risk for experiencing, altered quantity or quality of sleep compared to his or her own norm. Many pathophysiologic conditions are known to impair sleep. Impaired oxygen transport occurring in respiratory and circulatory disorders; impaired elimination (bowel or bladder) occurring with diarrhea, incontinence, constipation, or urinary retention; and impaired metabolism occurring in thyroid and hepatic disorders are just some examples.[22] Thorough discussion of the myriad of pathophysiologically induced influences upon sleep is beyond the scope of this chapter. Rather, the focus of the following discussion will be to minimize sleep pattern disturbances related to (1) circadian desynchronization, (2) sleep fragmentation, and (3) sleep deprivation.

Sleep Pattern Disturbance Related to Circadian Desynchronization

Guiding principles in planning and implementing nursing care to limit sleep pattern disturbance related to circadian desynchronization include providing periods of uninterrupted rest during hours customarily spent asleep and promoting structure in care activities to enhance resynchronization mechanisms.

The sleep history provides data regarding usual hours spent in bulk sleep periods and naps. While it is unlikely that specific times or prolonged periods can be completely or consistently protected, routine procedures should be scheduled to minimally disrupt these hours. When extensive nursing evaluations and other procedures that invariably waken the patient must be performed, maximum effort should be expended in coordinating and grouping interventions such that optimum use of the patient's time awake is achieved. Much information is available via sophisticated monitoring systems and patients should not be awakened for either singular or redundant data collection purposes.

The care provider who has the most extensive contact and knowledge of the patient, the responsibility for working with peers, other health team members, and representatives of other diagnostic and therapeutic departments to schedule activities around the patient's needs, clearly is the nurse. Daily laboratory tests, radiographic studies, patients' weights, and even baths are often routinely performed during hours when patients customarily engage in uninterrupted sleep. Such practices often evolve as a matter of routine distribution of work activities as opposed to consciously timed activities based upon each patient's unique situation.

A certain degree of desynchronization is unavoidable, thus nursing care should be planned and implemented to enhance reacclimatization between the sleep–activity and circadian cycles. Resynchronization can be enhanced in several ways. Exposure to natural light and maintenance of day–night orientation can be enhanced by assuring that unit blinds and drapes remain open. In this way, coordination between pineal melatonin secretion and the natural day–night sequence may be enhanced. Similarly, during hours of natural darkness, unit and other artificial lights should be dimmed. Easily visible, preferably self-illuminated, clocks should be made available, either on a nearby wall or on the bedstand. Frequent reminders of not only the hour of day but whether it is day or night may also help.

With the knowledge that resynchronization requires constancy in the sleep environment, effort should be made to maintain consistency and order in the patient's immediate environment. Continuity with direct care providers and simplicity and order in routine aspects of care may also be helpful, especially with longer-term patients. Specific positioning, with numbers of pillows and blankets

similar to those used at home, may be helpful in preparing the patient for sleep and rest periods. Finally, duplication of customary presleep routines or initiating a routine of, for example, a back rub or face wash may help prepare the patient for sleep.

Sleep Pattern Disturbance Related to Sleep Fragmentation

In planning and implementing care to minimize sleep pattern disturbance related to sleep fragmentation, it is important to remember that the sleep cycle averages 90 min in length. Unfortunately the frequency of vital sign recording and ongoing assessments of patients in critical care have typically evolved on an hourly schedule. Therefore, a starting point is careful assessment of the needed frequency of these activities and reorientation, if possible, to a schedule that allows 90-min uninterrupted intervals between. As previously noted, circadian desynchronization is likely in patients being provided care in critical-care units. As a result, the arousal threshold is likely to be decreased.

Illness is also known to lower the threshold of tolerable sound. Noise control must therefore be a pivotal component of the nursing care plan. Alarms should be purposefully activated and false alarms explained, as should the sounds associated with all care-related equipment in the patient's immediate environment. Names can be placed upon noise-producing objects to provide repeated orientation as to the nature and meaning of strange and unfamiliar sounds. Phones should be muted and computer printers covered. Liquid-containing humidifiers and chest drainage apparatus should be adjusted to "bubble" at the lowest possible intensity. Similarly, paging systems should be kept at the lowest possible volume.

Constant vigilance is required to limit noise between and among care providers. Long recognized as one of the largest single sources of noise in the critical-care setting, conversations and laughter must be continually monitored. Unit quiet periods and reminder signs may help.

Sleep fragmentation is known to be associated with increased frequency of transitions not only between sleep stages, but also between sleep stages and the awake stage. Such transitions are associated with phasic alterations in autonomic activation, especially with rapid movement from REM sleep to waking. As noted previously, rapid alterations in autonomic activation can produce myocardial irritability; ventricular arrhythmias have been documented in instances when arousal occurred as a result of auditory stimulation.[17] Therefore, when patients must be awakened, it is important to do so by gently touching the patient either shortly before or as the patient is spoken to. In this way the abruptness of the required transition may be decreased.

Sleep Pattern Disturbance Related to Sleep Deprivation

Frequent interruptions, a decreased arousal threshold, and an increased likelihood of spontaneous awakenings directly contribute to sleep loss. Such inability to complete sleep cycles, both within and in addition to the customary uninterrupted bulk sleep period, plus the direct effects of commonly used sedative, hypnotic, and analgesic medications, almost guarantee development of REM and NREM stages 4 and 3 sleep deficits.

NREM sleep debts are, for a number of reasons, less pronounced and somewhat easier to prevent and treat. Manifested primarily by fatigue, NREM sleep debts are, as previously noted, preferentially rebounded in sleep periods that occur following sleep loss. They therefore tend to be somewhat less cumulative than their REM sleep debt counterparts. Additionally, by scheduling planned family visits and other activity periods for the patient such as ambulation, physical therapy, and other out-of-unit treatments during the late afternoon hours, NREM sleep may be enhanced during the subsequent evening and night.

Limitation and treatment of REM sleep debts, on the other hand, present challenges both in terms of the symptomatology associated with such debts and the potential physiologic impact of REM sleep rebounds. Because REM sleep loss is associated with moderate to severe changes in mental and emotional function, disorientation, confusion, paranoia, withdrawal, and even hallucinations often complicate care requirements. Nursing interventions which reduce the need for abstract thought, reasoning, and memory should be utilized.

Specifically, reorientation efforts should focus upon the here and now, and present activities only.

Interventions should be explained step by step and include specific directions for the patient's role. Care givers should also identify who they are and why they are interacting even if only short periods of time have elapsed between contact with the patient. Care givers should not expect patients to be able to accurately interpret or recall very much about what is intrinsically a strange and unfamiliar environment. Finally, neither disorientation nor impairment of short-term memory should be treated as if the patient is also hard of hearing. Speaking loudly or directly into a patient's ear when hearing impairment is not a documented problem can add unnecessary distress to patients because of already-compromised sound tolerance and arousal threshold levels.

Because of the intense sympathetic activation associated with REM sleep, rebounds can pose potentially significant risks to patients. Decreasing the likelihood of intense and prolonged REM sleep rebounds should be an important nursing goal. High priority must be given to activities designed to limit the degree of REM sleep loss and therefore the accumulated REM sleep debt. Providing uninterrupted periods for rest and sleep facilitates normal cycling of stages. Repetitive complete cycles, preferably during hours customarily spent sleeping, may facilitate more normalized proportions of NREM and REM sleep within each cycle, unless significant sleep loss has already occurred and preferential NREM stages 3 and 4 sleep rebounds limit time spent in REM sleep. Naps should also be encouraged during the early morning hours, because sleep during these hours is characteristically high in REM.

The decision-making process regarding use of sedative, hypnotic, and analgesic medications should be deliberate. These agents can potentiate the sleep disruption associated with critical-care admission. Agents which block REM sleep contribute to and potentiate the preexisting REM sleep deficits occurring as a result of lacking or shortened bulk sleep periods and sleep fragmentation. NREM stages 3 and 4 sleep blockers can further compromise REM sleep by superimposing preferentially rebounded NREM sleep deficits.

Clearly, there are many instances when sedatives, hypnotics, and analgesics are completely indicated, but these agents should be part of a nursing plan that aggressively and comprehensively addresses agitation, anxiety, and restlessness. For instance, has communication with the patient included frequent, even repetitive, reassurances, explanations, and orientation to what is happening and why? Has the patient had optimal access to family or other key support people? Has the noise level in the unit been controlled and have extraneous, unfamiliar, or frightening sounds been explained? Is the patient appropriately restrained, that is, has reasonable self-movement been made possible within the context of needed therapeutic devices?

Relaxation and comfort should also be actively promoted. Has the patient's privacy been assured? Is the bed dry and wrinkle-free? Have back rubs, position changes, and adjustments in blankets or pillows been utilized to full advantage? Finally, when pain control is difficult, have analgesics been administered at regular levels to maintain blood levels, and have they been provided just before particularly painful procedures?

Ideally, through utilization of careful assessment and comprehensive interventions, sleep-disrupting pharmacologic agents should be administered at appropriate (neither too little nor too excessive) frequencies and quantities to minimize pharmacologically induced sleep debts. Equally important, however, is the assurance that, as such agents are no longer needed, dosages will be gradually reduced both during and after the critical-care stay. In this way the likelihood of intense and prolonged rebounds can be minimized. Also, communication of the plan to minimize sleep disruption must be part of the transfer process as the patient leaves the critical-care setting.

Evaluation

The effectiveness of interventions to minimize sleep disruption can be evaluated through ongoing, focused assessments in which actual experience is compared to reported sleep activity at home. The sleep history provides baseline data regarding the customary amount of time spent in bulk sleep periods and naps. Quantification of the potential overall sleep deficit can be estimated by both direct observation and review of the patient's record to ascertain the number and frequency of interventions and thus probable interruptions. If, for example, the patient's record indicates recording of vital signs and other interventions at hourly intervals

within a given 24-h period, it is likely that no complete sleep cycle was obtained. Administration of agents known to be REM or NREM sleep blockers would add further concern that the patient had received only the lightest type (stages 1 and 2 NREM sleep) of sleep during that period.

Additional data need to be gathered from the patient. How does sleep received compare to that at home? Are there specific deterrents to sleep that can be identified or are there interventions that might help the patient sleep? Answers to these questions can be utilized to adjust the care plan, establish specific objectives, and structure care activities to allow for undisturbed periods. Following sleep loss, the occurrence of rebounds is accompanied by increased efficiency in falling asleep. Thus, providing for even one or two uninterrupted 90-min blocks of time within a 24-h period may make a significant difference in the patient's report of sleep effectiveness.

Additionally, in the ongoing assessment of the patient's physiologic status, vigilance should be maintained for indications of significant sleep disruption. Unexplained deterioration of pulmonary status or persistent inability to control arrhythmias may reflect the effects of sleep fragmentation. Periods of pulmonary or systemic hypertension accompanied by a bradycardia-tachycardia electrocardiographic pattern could indicate undetected sleep-induced apneic periods made more frequent by sleep deprivation, especially if the patient has a history of heavy snoring or chronic systemic hypertension. Finally, inappropriate, confused behavior with disorientation may reflect desynchronization, while progression to anxiety, restlessness, withdrawal, suspiciousness, or delusions may reflect the presence of significant REM sleep debt.

Case Study: Disrupted Sleep Following Multiple Trauma

C. S., a 32-year-old woman, was admitted to an open-bay mixed medical-surgical intensive care unit following a motor vehicle accident in which she sustained multiple bilateral rib fractures, bilateral femur fractures, and a tibial fracture on the left. She presented with bilateral hemopneumothorax, cardiac and pulmonary contusion, and hypovolemic shock. Upon admission C. S. was intubated, chest tubes were inserted, and continuous ventilation with positive end-expiratory pressure (PEEP) instituted. She was also placed in extension traction.

Throughout her first 3 days in the ICU, C. S. was grossly unstable. Pulmonary deterioration was accompanied by cardiac arrhythmias and hypotension. Danger of compartmental syndrome in the left lower extremity prompted a fasciotomy. Throughout that period C. S. required almost two-to-one nursing care and was intermittently agitated, complaining of extensive chest and leg pain. She received intravenous diazepam and morphine sulfate on roughly an hourly basis.

By day six of her admission, C. S. began to stabilize but became increasingly agitated. In written communication to the nursing staff she requested that one particular respiratory therapist be "kept away" from her because "he [is] making me smoke." Later that day she tried to strike a nurse caring for her. In explanation she wrote "she [is] giving me LSD in my IV."

Extensive laboratory, radiographic, blood chemistry, and arterial blood gas determinations failed to provide an explanation for her mental state. Fat embolization was suspected but her vital signs and overall condition seemed to be improving. Her sedation was increased.

That night the chart was reviewed. It was discovered that from the time of admission C. S. had experienced three complete days during which she had received some intervention at a frequency of roughly every 30 min. During her fourth through sixth days, interventions had been performed on roughly an hourly basis.

Based upon these data, a sleep program was defined and initiated. C. S.'s care plan and status were reviewed. It was determined that she no longer needed hourly vital signs. Routine monitoring was placed on a 90-min schedule; activities that would awaken her, plus position changes, were scheduled for every 3 h. Between the hours of 3 A.M. and 6 A.M. and 10 A.M. and 11:30 A.M., every effort was made to provide C. S. with undisturbed periods. Curtains were drawn around her bed and signs were pinned to the curtains to remind care providers to maintain quiet. Routine radiographic and laboratory studies were coordinated to occur between 6 A.M. and 8 A.M. and results were obtained in time for usual physician rounds between 8 A.M.

and 10 A.M. Before each protected rest period, C. S. was positioned, given a back rub, and told that a rest period, during which time she should try to sleep, was going to occur. Visitors were asked to visit during the afternoon hours and allowed to stay until C. S. became fatigued. Restraints were removed when visitors were present and they were encouraged to talk to her about things with which she was familiar. All care providers were asked to introduce themselves and explain what they were doing during every contact with C. S. Finally, meperidine was substituted for morphine, and gradual weaning of diazepam began.

Within 24 h C. S. was noticeably less agitated and more oriented. She requested less pain medication and sedation. Her written communication ceased to contain bizarre statements and she became more cooperative. After 48 h C. S. was requesting infrequent analgesia and no sedation. She began to indicate that she knew sleep periods were coming when back rubs were offered. After 72 h C. S. seemed completely oriented and offered comments indicating she was looking forward to being able to go home.

Discussion

Prior to initiation of the sleep program, C. S. may have never received a complete sleep cycle. Contributing factors no doubt included the frequency of needed interventions, the open-bay unit and propensity for noise, anxiety related to the outcome of her extreme physiologic compromise and the strange environment, pain, and last but not least, administration of the agents diazepam and morphine. She was undoubtedly experiencing sleep fragmentation and deprivation. The sleep C. S. was able to obtain was more than likely desynchronized and limited to the lighter stages. At the point she displayed paranoia and confusion she was probably experiencing significant NREM and REM sleep debts.

The sleep program initiated addressed two fundamental needs. Undisturbed periods of rest were long enough to allow completion of a full sleep cycle. Similarly, specific sleep periods were also in 90-min increments, and, in addition, were scheduled to coincide with hours when REM sleep is likely. These actions no doubt facilitated a gradual beginning toward repayment of NREM and REM sleep debts.

Gradual reduction of the REM and NREM sleep-blocking agents, morphine sulfate and diazepam, also helped. Comfort measures, initiation of a brief presleep routine, and continual reorientation probably facilitated relaxation and ability to fall asleep.

C. S.'s fairly rapid improvement following initiation of a deliberate sleep program speaks not only to her resilience, but also to the increased efficiency in sleep following disruption. While she no doubt was still experiencing REM and probably NREM sleep debts 3 days after initiation of the sleep program, she was clearly much less symptomatic, easier to work with, and seemed far more tolerant of her situation.

References

1. Orem, J. (1980). Compendium of physiology of sleep. In J. Orem & C. D. Barnes (Eds.), *Physiology of sleep* (pp. 315–335). New York: Academic Press.
2. Miles, L. (1980). Sleep Pathologies. *Sleep, 3,* 171–185.
3. Moore-Ede, C., et al. (1983). Circadian timekeeping in health and disease, part 1. Basic properties of circadian pacemakers. *New England Journal of Medicine, 309,* 469–476.
4. Moore-Ede, C., et al. (1983). Circadian timekeeping in health and disease, part 2. Clinical implications of circadian rhythmicity. *New England Journal of Medicine, 309,* 530–536.
5. Czeisler, C., et al. (1983). Resetting circadian clocks in man: Applications to sleep disorder medicine and occupational health. In C. Guilleminault & E. Gugaresci. (Eds.). *Sleep/wake disorders: Natural history, epidemiology and long-term evolution.* New York: Raven Press.
6. Williams, R., et al. (1974). *EEG of human sleep-clinical applications.* New York: John Wiley & Sons.
7. Guilleminault, C. (1980). Sleep apnea syndromes: Impact of sleep and sleep states. *Sleep, 3,* 227–234.
8. Cirignotta, F. (1980). Some cineradiographic aspects of snoring and obstructive apneas. *Sleep, 3,* 225–226.
9. Cherniack, N. (1981). Respiratory dysrhythmias during sleep. *New England Journal of Medicine, 305,* 325–333.
10. Lavie, P. (1983). Incidence of sleep apnea in a presumably healthy working population: A significant relationship with excessive daytime sleepiness. *Sleep, 6,* 312–318.
11. Lewy, A. (1983). Effects of light on human melatonin production and the human circadian system. *Prog. Neuro-Psychopharmacol. and Biol. Psychiat., 7,* 551–556.
12. Lieberman, H., et al. (1984). Effects of melatonin on human mood and performance. *Brain Research, 323,* 201–207.
13. Seidlitz, P. (1981). Excessive noise levels detrimental to patients and staff. *Hospital Progress, 62,* 54–64.
14. Baker, C. (1984). Sensory overload and noise in the ICU: Sources of environmental stress. *Critical Care Quarterly, 6,* 66–80.
15. Kleck, H. (1984). ICU syndrome: Onset, manifestations, treatment, stressors, and prevention. *Critical Care Quarterly, 6,* 21–28.
16. Ballard, K. (1981). Identification of environmental stressors for patients in a surgical Intensive Care Unit. *Issues in Mental Health Nursing, 3,* 89–108.
17. Gordon, W. (1985). Sleep. Stanford, CA: Institute for Cortex Research and Development Seminar.
18. Greenblatt, D., et al. (1983). Drug therapy part I and II. *New England Journal of Medicine, 309,* 354–358, 410–416.
19. Nicholson, A. (1983). *Insomnia: A guide for medical practitioners.* Boston: Klawer Academic, Hingham, MA (MTP Press Limited, England).
20. Harvey, S. (1980). Hypnotics and sedatives. In A. Gilman, et al. (Eds.), *The pharmacological basis for therapeutics* (6th ed.). New York: MacMillan.
21. Phillipson, E., et al. (1980). The influence of sleep fragmentation on arousal and ventilatory responses to respiratory stimuli. *Sleep, 3,* 281–288.
22. Carpenito, L. (1983). *Nursing diagnosis application to clinical practice.* Philadelphia: Lippincott.

15

Thermal Regulation

Sister Maurita
Soukup, R.S.M.

The scope of practice for critical-care nursing[1] includes the critically ill person, the critical-care nurse, and the environment in which critical-care nursing is delivered. Thermal regulation challenges the critical-care nurse to meaningfully monitor and enhance positive interfacing of the environment and the person's ability to maintain a normal body temperature despite the stresses of illness.

Regulation of Body Temperature

In human beings, presently recognized thermal zones are as follows:

1. Superficial zone [ranges between 35.5° to 36.6°C (96° to 98°F) approximately]
2. Intermediate zone (ranges between superficial and core zone temperatures)
3. Core zone [37.5°C (99.5°F) approximately]

The *superficial zone* refers to the temperature of the skin. This temperature may be altered by a person's regional blood flow or environmental temperature changes. The *intermediate zone* refers to skeletal muscle and subcutaneous tissue temperatures which serve an insulating function to maintain core temperature. The *core zone* refers to the temperature of the body's inner organs such as the heart, liver, or brain. Generally, core zone temperature is several degrees higher than superficial zone temperature. However, if the ambient or environmental temperature is cold, the superficial zone temperature may be several degrees lower than core zone temperature. Conversely, if the ambient or environmental temperature is hot, the superficial zone temperature may be several degrees higher than core zone temperature (Fig. 15-1).

Thermoregulation refers to internal control of body temperature. Because of *homoiothermic* mechanisms, the core temperature in a healthy person is maintained within a very narrow range, normally fluctuating only within 0.5 to 1°C, regardless of age, sex, or the environmental temperature. Although normal temperatures vary among adults as well as within individuals (related to diurnal variations during a 24-h period, menstruation, or pregnancy), the range of 36.0° to 37°C (96.8° to 98.6°F) orally is generally accepted as normothermic. Body temperature is regulated by maintaining a balance between heat production and heat loss, which is coordinated by the autonomic and

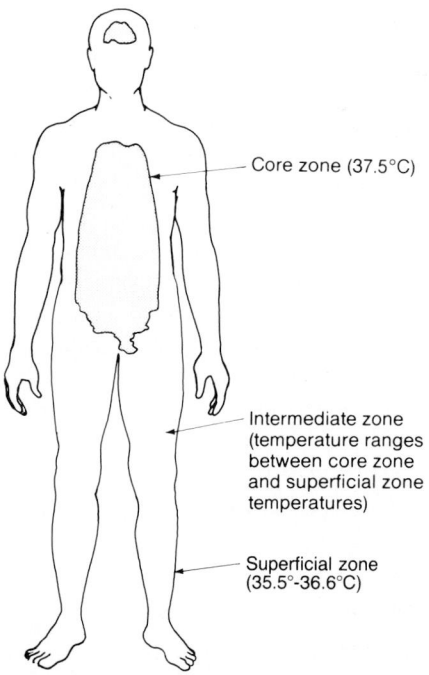

Core zone (37.5°C)

Intermediate zone (temperature ranges between core zone and superficial zone temperatures)

Superficial zone (35.5°-36.6°C)

Figure 15-1   Thermal zones.

neuroendocrine systems, with the hypothalamus acting as the thermostatic control center.

Heat Production

Through the process of cellular metabolism, heat is continually generated in the body. Food ingestion, carbohydrate, protein, and fat metabolism, basal metabolic rate, muscle activity, hormonal factors, and sympathetic nervous system stimulation contribute to heat production.

The sites of heat production vary. In a healthy adult during low energy expenditure (such as while resting), heat production occurs in the body's core areas—the trunk, the brain, and other vital organs. During high energy expenditure or increased muscle activity (such as exercising or shivering), the skeletal muscles are the primary site for heat production.

An increase in heat production occurs during an increased metabolic rate which can be related to moderate or heavy exercise, excessive food intake, thyroid hormonal secretion under normal temperature conditions, and release of epinephrine and norepinephrine through sympathetic nervous system activation. For the energy-compromised and hyperthermic person, minimal biopsychologic stress can increase heat production and even further increase temperature. In response to cold stimulation, skeletal muscle shivering can increase heat production more than two to five times. In contrast, chemical or *nonshivering thermogenesis* accounts for approximately a 10 to 15 percent increase in heat production among adults.

A decrease in heat production can result from normalizing body temperature or a reduction in metabolic rate related to hypopituitarism, myxedema, or malnutrition. Another cause could be muscular inactivity related to lack of mobility or loss of shivering response. Impairment of shivering can be found among persons with hypothalamic dysfunction, spinal cord lesions, or advanced age. Therapeutic control measures to minimize or inhibit shivering decrease heat production in thermoregulation.

Heat Loss Mechanisms

Normally, in a healthy adult heat loss is continuous through the skin and its ambient or environmental exposure. Heat loss mechanisms include *radiation, conduction, convection,* and *evaporation.*

Radiation refers to the transfer of heat between the body and the air in the form of rays. The direction of heat loss is from warm to cold until body and air temperatures are equal. The rate of heat loss is influenced by the difference between body and air temperature. For example, a hyperthermic person in a cool environment can experience heat loss at a faster rate than a normothermic person in the same environment. Loosely woven, lightweight clothing reduces heat loss by radiation.

Conduction refers to the flow of heat between two objects that are in contact, such as a normothermic person in contact with cold prepping solutions and lowered air temperatures in specialized procedure rooms. When temperatures between the two objects in contact equalize, conduction heat loss ceases.

Convection refers to heat transfer that is influenced by skin temperature, air temperature, and air velocity. An example would be the movement of cool air over a hyperthermic person. The sympathetic nervous system controls convective heat loss from the circulating blood to the skin. Exercise in a warm environment causes increased blood flow to the skin, increasing convective heat loss sometimes greater than nine times. However, in a cold environment, vasoconstriction inhibits convective heat loss to the skin.

Evaporation refers to the energy conversion of heat into vapor. Approximately 10 percent of body heat loss occurs during normal respiration. Evaporation heat loss in the form of perspiration is one of the primary methods for body cooling. When superficial or core zone temperatures rise, perspiration is initiated by hypothalamic activity. Perspiration is vaporized and body heat loss occurs. The faster the process of evaporation, the greater the body heat loss. Low humidity and air currents enhance evaporation and heat loss processes.

Mechanisms which increase body heat loss include enhancing vasodilation, especially to the superficial zone; sweat gland activity; respiratory rate; skin water vapor; exposure of body surface area to a cooler environment; air currents; and physical and subcutaneous fat insulation. Also, as core temperature rises 0.5° to 1°C, the body adapts by increasing heat loss.

Mechanisms which decrease body heat loss include vasoconstriction to the superficial zone, reducing exposure of body surface area to a cooler environment, sweat gland activity, adding insulation, alcohol abstinence, controlling against a hypothermic environment, and monitoring for piloerection ("goose bumps"). Piloerections are a warning sign of impending heat loss imbalance.

Hypothalamic Control

Internal regulation of physiologic responses related to heat production and heat loss mechanisms occurs in the hypothalamus, the thermoregulatory center of the brain. The hypothalamus receives superficial zone temperature information from the skin's thermoreceptors and core zone temperature information from the brain, heart, and other vital organs' thermoreceptors.

The hypothalamus sends information to the *cerebral cortex* for thought processing and voluntary behavioral activity for promoting normothermia; to *blood vessels* in the superficial zone, directing them to vasodilate or vasoconstrict; to *skeletal muscles* of the intermediate zone, causing shivering or increasing or decreasing muscle tone; and to the *anterior pituitary and adrenal medulla,* activating the neuroendocrine systems' response for balancing heat production and heat loss in body thermoregulation.

Temperature Regulation Disturbance

Inability to maintain an appropriate body temperature can be related to dysfunction in neuroendocrine thermoregulation, heat production, and/or heat loss mechanisms.

Altered neuroendocrine thermoregulation can include such causes as hypopituitarism, brain lesions, cerebrovascular accidents, tumors or insults, and spinal cord insult. Spinal cord trauma may impair regional vasoconstriction or vasodilation in peripheral blood flow, temporarily or permanently, such as in a person with quadriplegia. Hypothalamic function can be altered by surgical anesthesia, alcohol, pharmacologic interventions, and pyrogenic activities related to infection. In spinal anesthesia, hypothalamic control is inactivated; regional vasodilation and increased heat loss occur below

the level of the block. In general anesthesia, peripheral vasodilation and increased heat loss occur, with depression of the hypothalamic thermoregulatory activities. A genetic predisposition together with general anesthesia contribute to a disease known as malignant hyperthermia, which is lethal without medical emergency cooling interventions. Pyrogenic action, known as *pyrexia,* on the hypothalamus results in thermoregulatory control limits being reset above normal. In turn, hypothalamic activity initiates responses for increasing heat production and decreasing heat loss. Hypothalamic dysfunction occurs in critical hyperthermia [greater than 41°C (106°F) approximately] or in moderate hypothermia [less than 29°C (85°F) approximately]. When hypothalamic thermoregulatory control ceases and medical interventions are absent or unsuccessful, death is imminent.

Alterations in heat production resulting in thermoregulatory disturbance may result from diseases of neuroendocrine systems, excessive heat production and imbalance, paralysis, shivering impairment, inadequate nutrition, or hypoglycemia. Thyroid gland and adrenal medulla dysfunction alter hormonal production which, in turn, affects heat production by altering metabolic rate. Excessive heat production and imbalance, especially on humid, hot days, places at risk athletes and those persons engaged in vigorous or heavy energy expenditures. Regional paralysis, through reduction in muscle mass and tone, alters heat production. In malnutrition or hypoglycemia, oxygen is available but cellular metabolism is limited due to insufficient glycogen for chemical reactions.

Alterations in heat loss resulting in thermoregulatory disturbance can include dehydration related to sweating impairment, obesity related to excessive insulation, cardiovascular disease related to vasodilation impairment, and excessive heat loss imbalance. Heat loss imbalance may be localized to a group of muscles, as in *heat cramps,* or generalized throughout the body, as in *heat exhaustion,* which may progress into *heat stroke.*

Excessive heat production or heat loss places persons in either hyperthermic or hypothermic states which may range from mild to profound. The length of time spent in hyperthermia or hypothermia and the body's responses to interventions contribute to survival.

Hyperthermia

Hyperthermia refers to a body temperature above the normal physiologic level of 37.2°C (99°F) and the response of major support systems. Although controversial, hyperthermia can be described according to core temperature maintained:

1. Mild hyperthermia: 37.2° to 38.8°C (99°F to 102°F)
2. Moderate hyperthermia: 38.8° to 40°C (102°F to 104°F)
3. Critical hyperthermia: 40.5°C and above (105°F and above)
4. Malignant hyperthermia: 0.5°C per 15 min to 42.7°C (1°F per 15 min to 109°F)

Hyperthermia increases metabolic processes that can lead to organ distress or an irreversible state. Prolonged periods of moderate to critical levels of hyperthermia can cause increased metabolism, nerve dysfunction, breakdown of body protein, and coma and death. Causes of hyperthermia can include tissue injury related to infection or hormonal and pharmacologic agents. Within critical-care settings, persons frequently presenting in hyperthermia include those with medical diagnoses such as fever, heat stroke, or malignant hyperthermia.

Fever is the body's response to tissue injury, evidenced by excessive heat production. Temperatures may range from mild to critical hyperthermic levels, and present as intermittent or continuous, depending on cause. This can occur in one of two ways. First, the hyperthermic thermoregulatory control limits are reset at a higher level in response to temperature elevation, so that core temperature is regulated, but at a higher level. Second, the hypothalamic thermoregulatory center ceases to function, resulting in a rapidly rising temperature. This may be temporary (such as in heat stroke, malignant hyperthermia, or thyroid crisis, conditions which respond to medical interventions), or may be permanent, resulting in death.

A person experiencing hyperthermia related to fever progresses through three phases:

1. Chill phase
2. Hot phase
3. Defervescence phase

During the chill phase, as core temperature is rising there is an excess of heat production, with an imbalance or decrease in heat loss. Peripheral vasoconstriction, piloerection (goose pimples), increased muscle tone, and shivering occur. During the hot phase, core temperature reaches a new elevated level within the hypothalamic thermoregulatory center, and shivering ceases. In the defervescence phase, hypothalamic thermoregulatory limits are reset at a lower level and core temperature returns to a normothermic level.

Heat stroke is a medical emergency and refers to the end stage of heat exhaustion in which there has been prolonged exposure to high temperatures and humidity with dysfunction of the thermoregulatory center, resulting in a rapid rise in core temperature to a critical hyperthermic level. A high-risk complication during heat stroke is the potential for cardiovascular collapse related to myocardial thermal injury or increased pulmonary vascular resistance.

Malignant hyperthermia is a medical emergency and refers to a rapid rise in the core temperature of approximately 0.5°C every 15 min (1°F every 15 min), reaching critical levels for organ preservation and for life at 40.5° to 42.7°C (105° to 109°F). This is usually related to a genetic predisposition for and reaction to general anesthesia.

Critical-level hyperthermia refers to a core temperature above 40.5°C (105°F). Multiple body systems are affected. Hyperthermic cardiovascular effects include tachycardia, hypotension, altered electrodynamics, and the potential for cardiac arrest. Metabolic effects can include metabolic acidosis and electrolyte imbalance related to dehydration, while neurologic effects evidence an altered mentation ranging from confusion to coma. The risk for seizures is high. Hyperthermic pulmonary effects include hyperventilation, respiratory alkalosis, and the risk for cardiopulmonary arrest. Renal effects can result in acute renal failure, while gastrointestinal effects can include altered elimination patterns related to pharmacologic interventions, infection, immobility, and stress ulcers. Hyperthermic musculoskeletal effects are generally a depression of deep tendon reflexes, muscle discomfort, and twitching related to altered electrolytes, especially potassium in hypokalemia. Hematologic effects evidence an increased hematocrit resulting from excessive tissue damage. The risk for disseminated intravascular coagulation (DIC) is high. Psychoemotional effects depend upon the severity and reversibility of hyperthermia and the body's responses to complications, especially coma and acute renal failure (Fig. 15-2).

Hypothermia

Hypothermia refers to a body temperature below the normal physiologic level of 37°C (98.6°F) and the response of major support systems. Hypothermia can be classified according to the temperature maintained:

1. Mild hypothermia: 34° to 36.5°C (93.2° to 97°F)
2. Moderate hypothermia: 28° to 33.5°C (82° to 92.3°F)
3. Deep hypothermia: 17° to 27.5°C (62.6° to 81.5°F)
4. Profound hypothermia: 0° to 16.5°C (0° to 61.7°F)

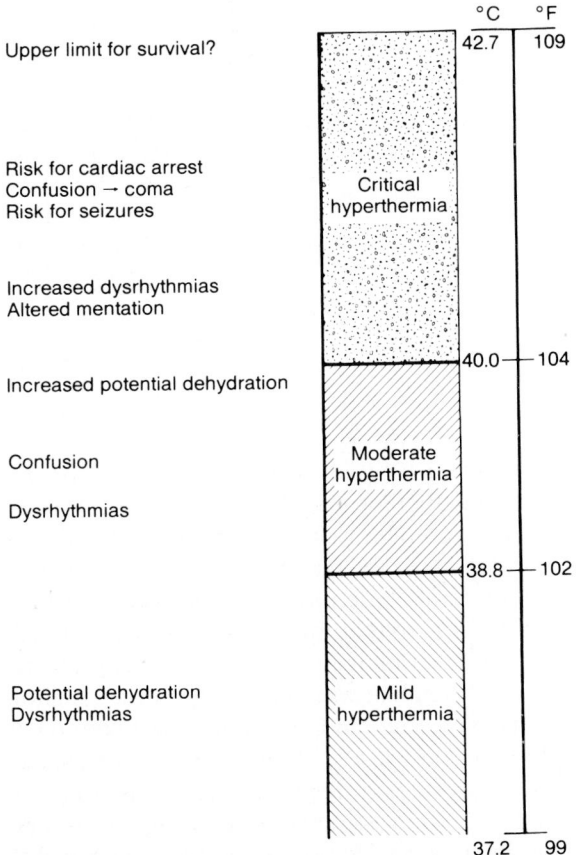

Figure 15-2 Hyperthermia levels with selected physiologic effects.

Hypothermia progressively depresses metabolic processes and nerve conduction, which may result in loss of thermoregulation, coma, and death.

Within a critical-care setting, persons may present with hypothermia due to varying causes. *Accidental hypothermia* often includes victims of drowning, those exposed to cold temperature insult, recipients of rapid infusions of refrigerated bank blood or intravenous solutions, and persons with increased heat loss, or thermoregulatory dysfunction, as well as decreased ability to produce heat. Disease states such as hypoglycemia, adrenal insufficiency, hypopituitarism, myxedema, and malnutrition decrease body heat production capabilities. Parkinson's disease and cerebrovascular accidents are examples of conditions that decrease muscle activity, including the ability to shiver. Conditions that increase heat loss include major surgery and pharmacologically induced hypothermia. Alcohol toxicity, antidepressants, antipyretics, sedatives, phenothiazines, barbiturates, and anesthetic gases are pharmacologic agents that can alter thermoregulation, resulting in hypothermia. *Elective hypothermia,* or cooling therapy, is used frequently in cardiovascular surgery and neurosurgery and is often prescribed for moderate to deep hyperthermic therapy, multiple trauma, acute cerebral ischemia, burn insults, thyroid crisis, and graft preservation.

Since distinct physiologic effects occur at various temperatures, understanding the significance of certain data can be critical to monitoring cooling or rewarming dynamics without major consequences. Fig. 15-3 illustrates selected physiologic effects of the various subsystems at specific hypothermic levels.

Hypothermic cardiovascular effects include an immediate response to hypothermia by peripheral vasoconstriction. Warm blood is shunted from the skin to the body core, increasing central blood volume. Temperature in the superficial thermal zone falls to prevent further heat loss. Hemodynamically, there is an initial increase in heart rate, cardiac output (CO), and mean arterial pressure (MAP) that is related to neural and hormonal responses. During this early phase of hypothermia, intermittent vasodilation to superficial zone tissues occurs through a compensatory mechanism, called the *Lewis phenomenon,* to prevent localized isch-

Figure 15-3 Hypothermia levels with selected physiologic effects.

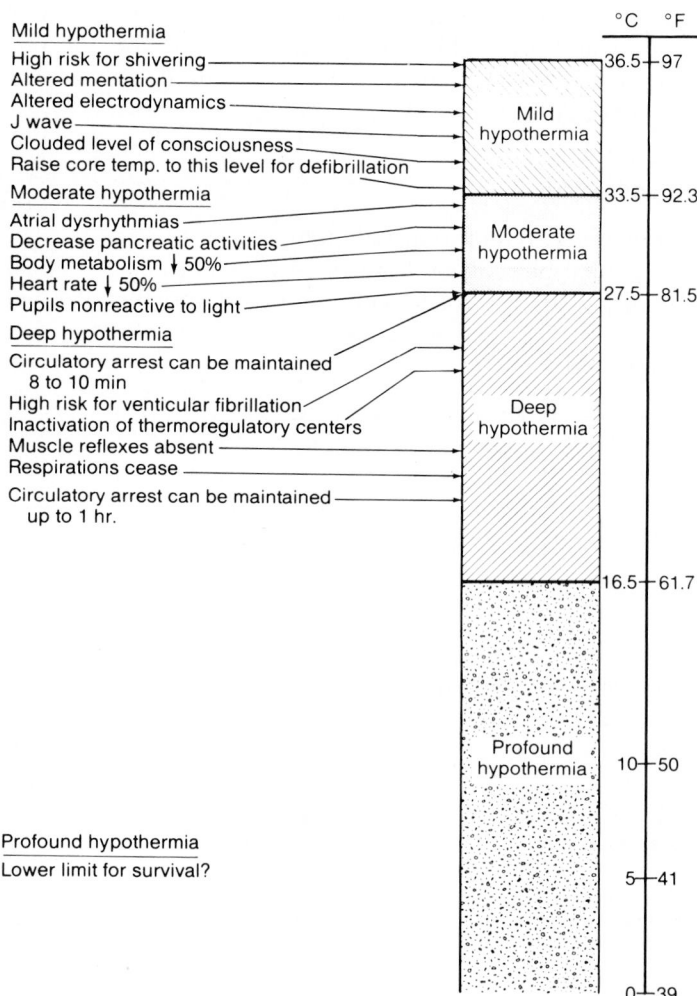

emia or frostbite. (This compensatory mechanism is inhibited as hypothermia progresses to lower levels.)

Following these immediate responses to hypothermia, there are further hemodynamic and electrodynamic alterations. The greatest reduction in heart rate usually occurs with the initial reduction in temperature without decreasing MAP. However, as core temperature falls, there is a decrease in heart rate, CO, and MAP. At 28° to 32°C, the heart rate may be reduced by 50 percent. Also, diastole is prolonged and contractility is increased. Dysrhythmias include bradycardia, atrial fibrillation, atrioventricular blocks, premature ventricular contractions, and ventricular tachycardia. Below 28°C

(82°F) there is critical prolongation of ventricular systole, lengthening of all ECG intervals, T wave inversion, and high risk for ventricular fibrillation.

Additional ECG manifestations associated with hypothermia include *muscle tremor artifact,* the *J wave,* and *delayed intrinsicoid deflection. Muscle tremor artifact* often precedes visible shivering. The *J wave,* a humplike wave occurring at the junction of the QRS complex and S-T segment and prominent in the left chest leads, is one of the most characteristic ECG signs in hypothermia and is useful in monitoring progression of hypothermia from mild to moderate levels. Its amplitude is proportional to the degree of hypothermia (Fig. 15-4). The *delayed intrinsicoid deflection* is also a sign of the degree

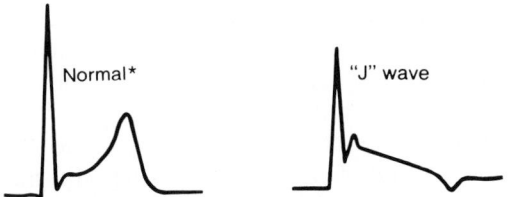

Figure 15-4 J wave: An acute elevation of the S-T segment during ECG monitoring, observed during moderate level hypothermia.

of hypothermia. A delay of over 24 percent is considered to be significant warning of impending ventricular fibrillation.

Generally, cardiovascular alterations during hypothermia therapy are evidenced by decrease in heart rate, CO, MAP, and diminished circulation to the hypothermic area. With a health history of altered hemodynamics related to a reduced cardiac output, hypothermia therapy can greatly enhance peripheral vasoconstriction and result in tissue hypoxia, anaerobic metabolism, and metabolic acidosis. Under electively controlled hypothermia, circulation to specific organs can be interrupted without risk of permanent damage.

Hypothermic metabolic effects are multifaceted. Initially, metabolic rate may increase up to six times the normal rate as a result of catecholamine stimulation and shivering. However, this is only temporary and as hypothermia progresses to a lower level, the metabolic rate also decreases. For each 1°C lowering of body temperature to 27.5°C (81.5°F), there is a 6.5 percent reduction in metabolic demands. At 30°C (86°F), total-body oxygen demand is reduced by 50 percent, and oxygen demand in the brain is reduced by 54 percent. During moderate hypothermia, there is maximal reduction in metabolic demands with minimal risk for complications. The critical physiologic level is 27.5°C; however, recognition must be given to a critical physiologic range for some individuals.

At 28 to 33.5°C, metabolic alterations include impairment of hypothalamic thermoregulation; increase in lactic acid, potassium, and calcium; reduction in hormonal response; suppression of thyroid activity; and reduction of normal adrenocortical activity. Depression of pancreatic activity inhibits insulin release, contributing to hyperglycemia. Since peripheral metabolic needs are decreased, hyperglycemia contributes to fluid shifting. Changes in hepatic function occur. Detoxification mechanisms are less active, bile becomes more dilute, and secretions slow. Below 28°C or during anesthesia, the hypothalamic thermoregulatory center is totally inactivated.

Hypothermic neurologic effects are directed first to depression of the higher centers of the brain to offer greater metabolic protection. For every 1°C lowering of core temperature, cerebral blood flow is decreased 6 to 7 percent. Shivering can increase core temperature but at the risk of increasing oxygen consumption 50 to 500 percent and with an already compromised cerebral blood flow status. During total-body hypothermia, there is a difference in the initial rate of brain and body core cooling, since the brain is normally 1°C colder at normothermia. During moderate hypothermia, however, the brain remains 1 to 2°C warmer than the core zone. During all phases of hypothermia, the systolic blood pressure is recognized as the most important factor in controlling cerebral blood flow.

At 35°C (95°F), mentation level becomes altered with experiences of amnesia and reduced coordination. Pain is still appreciated. At 30°C, orientation to person is reduced. At 30°C, there is a reduction in brain metabolism by 54 percent (provided that shivering is controlled), in cerebral blood flow by 30 percent, in cerebrospinal fluid pressure by 38 percent, and in brain volume by 20 percent. Pupils begin to dilate. Nerve conduction is depressed, resulting in paralysis. Electrical activity of the brain, inflammatory processes, and brain cell size and permeability are reduced. Below 25°C (77°F), there is absence of pupillary response to light and loss of reflex activity.

Hypothermic pulmonary effects initially produce an increase in respiratory rate; then the rate and tidal volume decrease in response to lowered metabolism. At 28 to 32°C (82 to 89.6°F), carbon dioxide production is diminished and the oxygen-hemoglobin dissociation curve is shifted to the left. Below 25°C, anatomic dead space is increased 50 percent and physiologic dead space is increased 28 percent, resulting in bronchial and alveolar edema, and respirations cease.

Early hypothermic renal effects include *cold-induced diuresis* with an increase in central blood volume as core temperature begins to fall 2 to 4°C. At 28 to 32°C, the rate of glomerular filtration is moderately reduced. At 32 to 35°C, there is stabilization of the specific gravity. Generally, renal function is not significantly altered until profound hypothermia is reached. Oliguria and azotemia are found among the hypothermic elderly, indicative of prolonged hypothermic exposure and dehydration.

Hypothermic gastrointestinal effects begin to offer risk at 28 to 32°C. Pepsin production continues while digestive activity is reduced. These effects, together with pharmacologic therapy, nasogastric suction, or stress of illness can contribute to such complications as gastric erosions, ileus, or altered elimination patterns.

Hypothermic musculoskeletal effects initially include vasodilation of muscle and visceral tissues which occur as a protective activity to threatened core zone cooling. During hypothermia, muscle tone diminishes. Below 25°C, muscle reflexes are absent.

Coarse muscular action of the body, or shivering, can be seen before actual changes in body temperature take place. The sequence of muscular action begins with facial muscles, progressing to pectoral muscles, and finally to muscles of the extremities. Shivering must be respected as a critical complication during all phases of hypothermia, elective hypothermia therapy, and rewarming. Metabolic demands can increase 100 to 500 times (equivalent to demands during heavy exercise) which, in turn, has serious implications if the core zone body organs are hypothermic.

Hypothermic immunologic effects continue to be researched. Depressed immunologic responses can be related to alterations in splenic and hepatic function during moderate to profound hypothermia levels.

Hypothermic hematologic effects include alterations in fluid balance and an increase in hemoglobin and hematocrit. Cold-induced diuresis, edema, decreased platelets, decreased white blood cell counts, and potential for DIC may occur. During hypothermia carbon dioxide concentration is lowered, and the oxygen-hemoglobin dissociation curve is shifted to the left, making it more difficult for red blood cells to release oxygen to the tissues. At 28 to 32°C, hemolysis is decreased. Below 28°C, metabolic acidosis can occur. To avoid intravascular aggregation, cooling rates should be less than 1°C per minute.

The psychoemotional effects related to hypothermia are individual. Generally, as hypothermia progresses, mentation is altered. Paradoxical undressing can occur in the moderate level of hypothermia. With dysfunction of hypothalamic thermoregulation and resulting vasodilation, clothing is removed in response to the temporary stress of warmth. This, of course, enhances hypothermic complications, especially among the pre-hospital, hypothermic elderly during winter. In spite of greater manipulation of life processes and multifarious stressors, psychiatric complications in hypothermia with anesthesia are reportedly lower at 28 to 37°C. Below 28°C, however, psychiatric complications increase.

Medical Therapies for Temperature Regulation Disturbances

Medical therapies for the critically ill person experiencing altered thermal regulation focus on holistic assessment, establishing priority medical diagnoses, implementing select clinical methods for therapeutic temperature control, and monitoring for and/or facilitating prompt early treatment for critical events and complications. In moderate to critical levels of hyperthermia and hypothermia, medical therapies include continuous monitoring of core temperatures, ECG, hemodynamic, and fluid balance monitoring. Arterial blood gases assist in determining the type of ventilatory assistance needed; however, generally a volume cycle ventilator is used in moderate to critical levels of altered thermoregulation. Laboratory profiles can include CBC, prothrombin time, partial prothrombin time, platelet count, serum glucose, amylase, creatine, electrolytes, and blood urea nitrogen (BUN); a drug screen and an alcohol level may be requested. Baseline ECG, chest x-ray, and CT scan can also be included in treatment plans. Clinical cooling or rewarming methods specific to hyperthermia or hypothermia states will be discussed separately.

Hyperthermia

Medical therapies for a person experiencing hyperthermia can include external surface cooling, pharmacologic therapy, and core cooling therapies until the core temperature reaches the normothermic range. Immediate initiation of therapy is critical for enhancing optimum reduction or control of core temperature, support of vital functions, prevention of complications, and survival. (Also, present research is recognized for electively induced hyperthermia combined with anticancer chemotherapy as a selected treatment modality; however, it will not be discussed since the clinical methods for induction are extracorporeal or whole-body microwave and these methods are not generally performed in the critical-care unit.)

External surface cooling is initiated immediately with ice bathing using vigorous skin massage to promote peripheral heat dissipation. This is promptly followed by cooling blanket therapy and ice bags over superficial major artery sites with the patient in an air conditioned or low-temperature environment. Core temperature monitoring is critical so that effects of therapy do not exceed 1°C reduction every 5 min.

Pharmacologic therapy includes antipyretics to reduce temperature, antibiotics to treat infection, and neuroleptic medications to control shivering and reduce mental confusion. If the client is intubated and on ventilatory-assist equipment, curare can be anticipated to control shivering and reduce the metabolic rate.

If these therapies are unsuccessful, other medical therapies such as gastric lavage, bladder irrigation, or rectal irrigation with iced isotonic solutions and peritoneal dialysis can be considered in reducing critical core temperatures to normothermia.

In malignant hyperthermia, anesthesia and surgery must be stopped immediately. All ventilatory and intravenous tubings are changed, followed by hyperventilation with 100% oxygen and IV administration of iced saline. External surface cooling and/or gastric, bladder, and rectal lavage are rapidly initiated. Sodium bicarbonate can be anticipated to correct metabolic acidosis. Dantrolene sodium, a direct-acting skeletal muscle relaxant, may be prescribed in a dosage of 1 mg/kg IV to a total dose of 10 mg/kg, to reverse effects of this critical event.

Hypothermia

Medical therapies may include prescribed elective hypothermic therapy or rewarming therapy for the person in hypothermia. Prescribed elective hypothermic therapy can utilize localized cooling, extracorporeal cooling, and external surface cooling clinical methods. Prescribed rewarming therapy can utilize active core rewarming, and external active or passive surface rewarming methods.

Localized cooling is usually an invasive therapy and is restricted to a specific body area or organ, such as in gastroesophageal hypothermia, inhalation, peritoneal dialysis, mediastinal irrigation, gastric lavage, colonic irrigation, cardioplegic hypothermic arrest, and cerebral hypothermia. *Extracorporeal cooling* is achieved through a direct approach of intravascular cooling during cardiopulmonary bypass or hemodialysis. *External surface cooling* is accomplished through noninvasive techniques of cold water immersion, air cooling, and use of ice packs and cooling blankets.

Surface cooling for achieving moderate hypothermia is a specific medical therapy frequently prescribed within the critical-care setting. Scientific advances in electrically controlled cooling blankets have enhanced quality and convenience in accomplishing this prescribed therapy. Surface cooling hypothermia focuses on three phases.

The *induction phase* of surface cooling requires assessment and control of environmental factors. To facilitate prompt induction, room temperature is reduced to 36°C (96.8°F), lighting is dimmed, and hypothermia blankets are precooled to between 5 and 10°C. A sheet blanket between hypothermia pads enhances induction without insulating against cooling. Ice packs or additional hypothermia pads, placed where major arteries lie close to the skin surface, can supplement cooling blankets. Temperature reduction is monitored closely with a rectal probe or other core temperature monitoring equipment. Hands and feet are protected with mitts. Below 32°C (89.6°F), 2 to 5 percent carbon dioxide is added to ventilations to enhance oxyhemoglobin dissociation by the Bohr effect and cerebral perfusion by vasodilation.

Early in the induction phase, there is a high risk for shivering, which demands close assessment and immediate treatment by IV medications or anesthesia. Initial manifestations are ECG muscle tremor artifact, visible facial muscle twitches, hyperventilation, and verbalized comfort level alterations.

Late in the induction phase, there is a high risk for drifting, or *afterfall*, which is continued body temperature reduction after the hypothermia blanket is turned off. Factors influencing this phenomenon include body size, muscle tone, age, vascular response, room temperature, and pharmacologic interventions. To prevent or reduce this complication, supplementary cooling supports and the top hypothermia blanket are removed and the lower hypothermia blanket control is reset to 2 to 5°C lower than the prescribed temperature.

Hypothermia induction should be prompt but always controlled. A maximal limit of 1°C lowering every 15 min should be respected. In 40 to 50 min, a 33 to 34°C hypothermic level can be achieved. Of significance during the induction phase is that the greater the area of body surface in contact with cooling, the faster the desired temperature is reached. The lower the temperature, the higher the risk for entry into the critical range. Finally, the more rapid the induction, the greater the afterfall.

The *maintenance phase* of surface cooling focuses on maintaining the prescribed hypothermic level while minimizing any adverse effects. Activities are individualized, requiring frequent evaluation and refinement. Generally, for every 1°C temperature reduction, vital signs are taken every 30 min, then every 2 h. The rectal thermistor probe is removed every 4 h, cleaned, and reinserted to ensure accurate readings; automatic controls are checked every 4 h. Eye care to protect corneal reflexes, thigh support stockings to prevent venous stasis, coughing and deep breathing, repositioning every 30 min, massaging pressure points, inspection of total body surface, and skin lubrication every 2 h are examples of necessary preventive health measures. A critical activity, also, during this phase is pharmacologic profile assessment because of possible cumulative drug effects and an additional

temperature reduction of 1 to 3°C from tranquilizers or opiates.

Rewarming is done purposefully to avoid increasing metabolic demands on a heart in hypothermia. Generally, rewarming should progress no faster than 2°C per hour. Vital core temperature and vital signs are monitored closely, usually at 15-min intervals. During this phase, assessment includes alertness for temperature overshoot, edema secondary to increased cell permeability, acidotic shock secondary to shivering, cumulative drug effects, altered ventilation, and fluid imbalance.

External passive rewarming therapy includes a warm, dry environment, removal from thermal stress, insulation to prevent heat loss, warm liquids, and application of blankets. *External active rewarming* therapy includes warming blankets and inhalation mask. External active rewarming should be used with critical assessment for rapid peripheral vasodilation and *afterdrop effect* of core temperature. The lowered core temperature can shift acidotic and hyperkalemic superficial zone circulation to the core zone, resulting in dysrhythmias, hypovolemia, and cardiogenic shock. *Active core rewarming* therapies include extracorporeal circulation; localized gastric, colon, peritoneal, or mediastinal irrigation; inhalation of warm gases; exchange transfusions; and warm IV fluid administration. Active core rewarming is used for treatment of profound hypothermia.

Medical therapies related to critical events are specialized. However, a person in profound to moderate hypothermia who experiences a cardiopulmonary arrest will need the core temperature raised to 32 to 33°C to optimize conditions for defibrillation. Pharmacologic interventions are to be used with caution due to decreased blood volume and ability to metabolize medications that are atropine-resistant. Dopamine, lidocaine, and Pronestyl are frequently used to improve altered hemodynamics and ventricular irritability.

Nursing Therapies

A critically ill person with altered thermoregulation related to hyperthermia, hypothermia, prescribed hypothermia, or prescribed rewarming therapy requires deliberative, holistic monitoring. Respect for physiologic parameters that reflect the status of thermoregulation dynamics, clinical competence in prescribed therapies, and responsibility for assessed client and family needs enhance meaningful participation and contributions in multidisciplinary health management.

Assessment of Temperature

Temperature assessment and monitoring, as with all monitoring, requires observation of alterations, rather than of absolute levels, and an assessment of the effects of these alterations on the person. A critically ill person experiencing altered thermoregulatory crisis needs continuous core temperature monitoring. Usually, the method preferred is the rectal thermistor probe; however, esophageal, thermodilution pulmonary artery catheter, tympanic membrane, or Foley catheter probes can also be used in select situations. If continuous monitoring of core temperature is not possible, the core zone temperature needs to be assessed no less than every 10 min during the crisis and/or electively prescribed cooling or rewarming therapies.

Thermal monitoring includes routine temperature monitoring even if rectal thermistor probe or safety alarms are used. Machine vibrations may cause deviations from prescribed settings; however, more frequently, inaccuracy of the electrical temperature display is related to a broken probe or a probe embedded in feces. Also, clinical thermometers or thermistor probes need to measure temperature within an approximate range of 20° to 42°C (64° to 108°F).

In temperature assessment of the critically ill person, influencing risk factors need to be considered. These can include the person's average core temperature, significant health history, medical therapies or surgical interventions affecting thermoregulation, medication profile compliance, environmental or ambient temperature, and usual response to temperature changes. Also, the person's usual response to heat production, such as the ability to perspire and drink fluids, as well as the person's response to heat loss, such as the ability to shiver, and alcohol or nicotine usage are important. Other factors to be considered in temperature assessment include sex, age, diurnal variations, and sites. Females tend to have more temperature fluctuations than males, which are related to hormonal factors. Infants and the elderly are at a greater risk for hyperthermia and hypothermia because of their altered responses to temperature changes. In considering diurnal variations, core temperature is highest between the hours of 4 P.M. to 6 P.M. and lowest between the hours of 1 A.M. to 4 A.M., with approximately 1 to 3 weeks for the cycle to reverse with workshift changes.

Average temperatures reported are influenced by sites. The axillary temperature reading is usually the least accurate and is approximately 1°F lower than the oral temperature. The rectal temperature reading is usually 1°F higher than the oral temperature reading. Finally, superficial zone thermal assessment contributes significant data to temperature assessment. Color, temperature, edema, diaphoresis, capillary refill, movement, and alterations in sensory perceptions, such as tingling and numbness, are contributing parameters.

Nursing Diagnoses

Nursing diagnoses for persons with thermoregulatory disturbances focus on biopsychologic, educative, and/or potential for complications, as shown below.

1. Alterations in thermal regulation related to:
    a. Hyperthermia (mild, moderate, malignant)
    b. Hypothermia (mild, moderate, profound)
    c. Inadequate control of temperature maintenance
    d. Temperature overshoot during rewarming
2. Altered comfort level related to:
    a. Hyperthermia
    b. Hypothermia
    c. Inadequate control of alterations in temperature maintenance
    d. Intolerance to decreased mobility
    e. Shivering
    f. Sleep deprivation
    g. Negative stressors such as noise stimuli, light intensity, or interruptions in sleep/rest cycle
3. Knowledge deficit related to:
    a. Supportive education specific to feelings, critical events, and hospitalization

b. Informational education specific to hyperthermia, hypothermia, body cooling or rewarming clinical methods, nutrition, elimination, stress control, medication profile, thermal risk factors, heat stroke, frostbite, and transfer continuity and discharge teaching

Complications may include one or more of the following diagnoses:

1. Potential for altered hemodynamics related to:
   a. Altered electrodynamics
   b. Fluid shifts
   c. Hypokalemia
   d. Rewarming therapy
   e. Diuresis related to hypothermia
2. Potential for altered electrodynamics related to:
   a. Myocardial oxygen deprivation
   b. Hypokalemia
   c. Altered hemodynamics
3. Potential for ineffective breathing patterns related to:
   a. Altered ventilations
   b. Acidotic shock
   c. Shivering
   d. Cumulative pharmacologic effects
4. Potential for critical event related to:
   a. Multiple dynamics present in thermal regulation
   b. Preentry cardiopulmonary arrest
   c. Health history of malignant hyperthermia episode
   d. Autonomic dysreflexia event
   e. Myocardial left ventricular dysfunction
5. Potential for altered skin integrity related to:
   a. Decreased blood flow
   b. Edema
   c. Pressure points
   d. Actual crystallization of tissue fluids in subcutaneous tissues
   e. Cutaneous vasodilation
6. Potential for altered tissue perfusion related to:
   a. Edema, alterations in blood flow
   b. Frostbite
   c. Sunburn
7. Potential for alterations in nutrition related to:
   a. Fluid and energy imbalance
   b. Anorexia
   c. Health history

8. Potential for alterations in bowel elimination related to:
   a. Pharmacologic effects
   b. Immobility
   c. Health history
   d. Ileus
9. Potential for infection related to:
   a. Vascular invasive catheters/techniques
   b. Foley catheters
   c. Tissue insult from prolonged and critical levels of hyperthermia or hypothermia
10. Potential for hyperthermia complications related to:
    a. Altered hemodynamics
    b. Pulmonary edema
    c. Hypotension during cooling therapies
    d. Fluid imbalance
    e. Cardiopulmonary arrest
    f. Hyperthermia
    g. Neurologic impairment
    h. Acidosis
    i. Renal failure
    j. DIC
    k. Rebound hyperthermia
11. Potential for hypothermia complications related to:
    a. Acute pancreatitis
    b. Stress ulcer
    c. Acute renal failure
    d. Hyperglycemia
    e. Coagulopathies
    f. Thromboembolism
    g. DIC
    h. Hepatic dysfunction
    i. Temperature overshoot during rewarming
12. Potential for rewarming complications related to:
    a. Hypovolemia
    b. Hyperkalemia
    c. Acidosis
    d. Dysrhythmias
    e. Cardiac arrest
13. Potential for hypersensitivity to cold (or heat) related to:
    a. Alterations in thermoregulation
    b. Health history of thermoregulatory dysfunction
    c. Allergies, autoantigen, or vasomotor disturbances

14. Potential for injury related to:
    a. Chemical drug reactions
    b. Instrumentation of prescribed hyperthermia or hypothermia therapies
    c. Microshock specific to temporary pacemaker therapy
    d. Thermal monitoring specific to broken probe, or probe embedded in feces
    e. Vascular invasive lines and monitoring
15. Potential for falls related to:
    a. Psychologic needs
    b. Alterations in thought processes
    c. Energy levels during progressive recovery phase

Goals

For the critical-care nurse caring for the person and family experiencing altered thermoregulation (moderate to critical levels), the following goals are offered:

1. Return client's body temperature to an appropriate normothermic level or electively induce prescribed hypothermia therapy safely and with minimal biopsychologic stressors.
2. Control comfort level.
3. Provide client and family with supportive and informational education.
4. Assess early and continuously for potential complications and facilitate therapeutic nursing interventions for prevention or treatment.

Interventions

Nursing interventions can include but are not limited to the following:

1. Implement an organized and systematic frequency of vital sign acquisition, especially core temperature. Holistic assessment of data should determine changes, client response to therapies, and trends in alterations. Communicate significant changes to multidisciplinary health team professionals.
2. Promptly facilitate prescribed rewarming or cooling methods (as discussed under "Medical Therapies for Temperature Regulation Disturbances"), utilizing thermal monitoring equip-

ment that is clinically appropriate and accurate. (Also, competent instrumentation of rewarming or cooling equipment is assumed.)

3. Control environmental factors to enhance heat production or heat loss, as appropriate.
4. Facilitate interventions for enhancing heat loss when appropriate, utilizing prescribed medications such as antipyretics, antibiotics, and steroids. Utilize cooling techniques such as cool baths, cooling blankets, ice bags to specific body areas where major arteries are located, and cold IV infusions. Assist the physician with invasive core temperature cooling methods.
5. Facilitate interventions for promoting heat production when appropriate, utilizing warm blankets, pharmacologic therapy, or blood warmers if blood is prescribed, or assist the physician with invasive core temperature rewarming methods.
6. Provide supplemental oxygen as prescribed.
7. Facilitate prescribed therapies for maintaining appropriate hydration and nutrition, including daily weights and fluid intake and output monitoring.
8. Assess skin integrity frequently, especially oral mucous membranes, regional sites, and burn, or frostbite sites.
9. Assess and maintain comfort level with prescribed medications.
10. Minimize and control stressors that would increase oxygen demands, such as mobility and excessive turning.
11. Anticipate potential for critical events and have ready crash cart, emergency medications, etc.
12. Assess readiness and utilize opportunities for supportive education and informational education with client and/or family during crisis, critical events, and progressive recovery phase. Document and plan for educational endeavors to continue after critical-care unit transfer, utilizing community resources if appropriate. Provide specific reinforcement teaching related to risk factors and prevention, including any new data for health profile, such as a health history of malignant hyperthermia.
13. Assess for early detection of potential complications and facilitate appropriate communication with physician. Implement appropriate therapies to prevent and/or treat these altera-

tions. (See "Nursing Diagnosis" for potential complications.)

Evaluation and Replanning

A person experiencing altered thermoregulation related to moderate or critical hyperthermia needs multidisciplinary health team coordination for rapid cooling, supplemental oxygen, fluid replacement therapy, and control of shivering. Cooling therapies can be terminated when core temperature is approximately 39°C (102°F) to minimize risk of temperature overshoot. As temperature is lowered, replanning becomes critical. Because of hemodynamic alterations, including plasma fluid volume shifting, the risk for pulmonary edema becomes high. Hypotension may be present, requiring an IV fluid challenge or pharmacologic interventions with agents such as dopamine or isoproterenol. Core temperature monitoring deserves priority in nursing assessment data as rebound hyperthermia can occur within 8 h after cooling and thermoregulatory instability can occur for weeks. Other progressive recovery phase interventions include ECG monitoring for detection and treatment of dysrhythmias, supplemental oxygen therapy for tissue hypoxia and increasing tissue oxygen demands, adequate fluids and nutrition, bed rest to minimize heat production and metabolic needs, pharmacologic interventions to correct acidosis and hypokalemia, and ongoing monitoring for complications. Complications of DIC, infection, renal failure, and neurologic deficits (e.g., coma present for a long period) are high risks in hyperthermia.

If critical level hyperthermia with coma persists, regardless of core zone cooling therapies, initial 24-h serum glutamic oxaloacetic transaminase (SGOT) level is extremely elevated, and renal failure is present, prognosis is poor. Family should be prepared for critical events, including death, and appropriate humanizing conditions for individualized needs facilitated.

A person experiencing altered thermoregulation related to moderate or profound hypothermia needs supplemental oxygen, IV fluid replacement, and therapeutic rewarming. As temperature is increased, active rewarming methods will be terminated when core temperature approaches 35.6°C (96°F) to control for potential complications of temperature overshoot. Frequent core temperature

monitoring is important for 48 h after rewarming therapy since some persons experience thermoregulatory instability. Replanning includes continued core temperature monitoring and ECG monitoring for altered electrodynamics, administration of supplemental oxygen, adequate fluids and nutrition, client tolerance to progressive activity to increase heat production and metabolic rate, pharmacologic interventions to control for comfort and metabolic alterations, care of frostbite areas (if present), and ongoing monitoring for complications. Potential for complications such as pneumonia, infection, thromboembolism, DIC, and renal failure need to be reassessed and included in planning needs during this phase.

Evaluation and replanning for client and family education are based on offering both supportive education and informational education. In both, continuity is important to enhance a multiprofessional therapeutic plan of care. Supportive education for the client and family focuses on attentive listening, crisis intervention during and following critical events, and/or grieving (loss of body part, critical health event, life-death issues) and minimizing negative stressors or emotional deterrents to learning. Following a knowledge-base assessment, informational education can include an overview of altered thermoregulation, pain control, a medical and nursing plan of care, critical-care unit, thermal risk factors, select clinical therapies, sequence of events, complications, adaptation to special requirements, transfer continuity, coping strategies, self-health responsibilities, community resources (if appropriate), and discharge teaching.

Case Studies

A person experiencing accidental or prescribed hyperthermia or hypothermia presents with individualized needs. These needs can change in importance and even in perspective within a given situation. It is anticipated that the following information will intensify responsibilities for planned individualized care rather than limit client and family needs to those selected.

Hyperthermia

Mrs. B. (33 years old, 5 ft 6 in, weighing 120 lb) was an emergency and direct transfer to the critical-care unit from an OR suite for continued emergency management of malignant hyperthermia which occurred during the induction phase of anesthesia; surgery was terminated. Except for this prescheduled L breast biopsy, Mrs. B.'s health status was documented as excellent, with no health history awareness for malignant hyperthermia.

Clinical assessment data: Rectal temperature, 105° (rapid onset); heart rate, 144; sinus tachycardia with PACs 6 to 10/min; blood pressure (cuff), 90/60; respirations, 44, tachypnea; skin, hot, flushed; profuse diaphoresis; voluntary muscle twitching; diminished deep tendon reflexes; and altered mentation level (related to anesthesia, pharmacologic preoperative medications, and hyperpyrexia).

Priority nursing diagnoses and interventions can be summarized as follows:

1. Altered thermoregulation related to malignant hyperthermia required prompt external surface cooling therapies utilizing alcohol ice baths, cooling blankets and ice packs; continuous core temperature, ECG, and hemodynamic (arterial pressure and CVP) monitoring; IV patency for fluid rehydration and medication administration; Foley catheter and hourly urines; arterial blood gases (ABGs) as requested; supplemental oxygen therapy; pharmacologic therapy to include Dantrium IV bolus (given orally after the crisis), antipyretics, and sodium bicarbonate to correct acidosis and hyperkalemia. Laboratory profile should include serial ABGs, electrolytes, CBC, serum enzymes, urinalysis, ECG, and chest x-ray.
2. Knowledge deficit related to malignant hyperthermia, critical event, and surgical follow-up planning required supportive and informational education.
3. Potential for complications related to critical event of malignant hyperthermia required ongoing assessment for altered electrodynamics, altered hemodynamics, signs and symptoms of renal failure, hematologic and neurologic alterations, and thermoregulatory instability.

Hypothermia

Mr. S. (92 years old, 5 ft 10 in, weighing 150 lb) was a direct admission to the critical-care unit from his apartment complex by ambulance, with his family physician awaiting his hospital arrival. Preentry information was limited. However, communi-

cation tapes evidenced that an ambulance was summoned and the family physician contacted following a friend's investigation after a Life-Line alert was received at the central base. Total time between Life-Line notification and hospital arrival was less than 40 min.

Clinical assessment data: Rectal temperature, 90°F; heart rate, 56, with sinus bradycardia (multifocal PVCs and J wave changes present); blood pressure, 80/50 (cuff); respirations, 8 per minute; skin cold with no evidence of frostbite; slow to respond to verbal and tactile stimuli, oriented only to name; fine tremors over body; pupils equal, dilated to 6 mm, nonreactive.

Priority nursing diagnoses and interventions can be summarized as follows:

1. Altered thermoregulation related to moderate-level accidental hypothermia, required continuous core temperature, ECG, and hemodynamic (arterial pressure and CVP) monitoring; passive external rewarming utilizing blankets and warm environment; IV access for pharmacologic interventions and warm IV fluid administration; nasogastric tube for warm fluid administration; Foley catheter; supplemental warm oxygen mist therapy. Laboratory profile should include serial ABGs, CBC, electrolytes, serum enzymes, urinalysis, ECG, and chest x-ray.
2. Altered comfort level related to rewarming therapy required pharmacologic interventions to control for shivering, controlling rest/sleep cycle interruptions, and gentle repositioning.
3. Knowledge deficit related to hypothermia, potential for critical event, risk factors and prevention required supportive education initially, informational education after the crisis, and reinforcement teaching (including affirmation of Life-Line compliance) prior to discharge.
4. Potential for complications related to hypothermia and rewarming required ongoing monitoring for altered electrodynamics, critical events, temperature overshoot, thermoregulatory instability, and renal, neurologic, or hematologic alterations.

In summary, the concept of thermal regulation is dynamic, with significant implications for the environment, critical-care nursing practice, and the person and family experiencing thermoregulatory disturbances. The future holds promise for knowledge advances in theory and clinical methods for optimizing health and quality of life.

References

1. American Association of Critical-Care Nurses. (1980) Scope of practice for critical-care nursing. Newport Beach, CA.

Bibliography

Atkins, E. (March 1984). Fever: The old and the new. *Journal of Infectious Diseases, 149,* 339–348.

Atkinson, L. & Murray, M. E. (1985). The need for temperature maintenance. In *Fundamentals of nursing—a nursing process approach.* New York: Macmillan, pp. 481–525.

Curley, F. J., & Irwin, R. S. (1986). Disorders of temperature control: Hyperthermia, Part I. *Journal of Intensive Care Medicine, 1,* 5–14.

Curley, F. J., & Irwin, R. S. (1986). Disorders of temperature control: Hyperthermia, Part II. *Journal of Intensive Care Medicine, 1,* 91–100.

Greany, D., & Brown, M. (April, 1986). Malignant hyperthermia, a concern for critical care nurses. *Focus on Critical Care, 13*(2), 52–57.

Delapp, T. (January 1983). Accidental hypothermia. *American Journal of Nursing, 83,* 62–67.

Elder, Paul T. (1984). Accidental hypothermia. In W. Shoemaker, et al. (Eds.), *Textbook of critical care.* Philadelphia: Saunders, pp. 85–93.

Kruse, D. H. (April 1983) Postoperative hypothermia. *Focus On Critical Care, 10,* 48–50.

Marty, J., & Sami Kamran. (1983). Hyperthermia. In J. Tinker, et al. (Eds.), *Care of the critically ill patient.* New York: Springer-Verlag, pp. 866–870.

Myers, R. (February 1984). Neurochemistry of thermoregulation. *Physiologist, 27,* 41–46.

Nadel, E. (March 1984). Temperature regulation and hyperthermia during exercise. *Clin. Chest Med. 5,* 13–20.

Regnier, B., & Harri, A. (1983). Accidental hypothermia. In J. Tinker, et al. (Eds.), *Care of the critically ill patient.* New York: Springer-Verlag, pp. 841–864.

16

Communication with the Critically Ill

Catherine Nuss
Kotecki

Introduction

"Sensitive and individualized verbal and non-verbal communication with the critically ill patient is a major method for bringing the art of healing into the highly scientific intensive care setting."[1] The art of communication in the critical-care unit is directed toward four goals, the first of which is to share information. The nurse needs accurate information about the patient's current health status, history of prior illness, current drug therapies, and emotional state. The patient and family need information about the patient's condition, prognosis, available treatments, and the cost of that treatment.[2] During the initial time of sharing information, a supportive relationship, based on trust and rapport, begins to be established.

A second goal is to prevent isolation and alienation of the patient and promote socialization to serve as a link from the premorbid state through intensive care to the patient's recovery and return to the community. The third goal is to acknowledge and accept the patient's feelings as they relate to the current illness, as well as future prognosis. "It often seems that a reluctance to join in a meaningful conversation with a critically ill patient is because of the fear that he will ask questions about the possibility of his own death."[3] As an outgrowth of the third goal, the nurse hopes to provide reassurance, instill hope, and assist the patient in future-oriented thinking and planning. This fourth goal is accomplished in a realistic manner or in a way that is appropriate to the patient's ability to understand and cope with the situation.

Communication is not just talking: It also includes listening to patients and responding to their cues, permitting them to lead the conversation, and directing them through areas of informational conversation so the nurse can formulate a plan of care. Effective communication in the critical-care unit assists the person in placing a potential life-changing event in perspective with respect to past behavior and future abilities. Effective communication also assists patients in making their needs known. In the face of physical disability, the nurse directs the patient to alternate channels of communication so that self-expression is not lost.

The communication process is important in critical care because it has been shown that nurses and patients have a physical reaction to each other, as well as a psychological reaction. Researchers from the University of Maryland have looked at patient–staff interactions with respect to a variety of physiologic responses. One study reviewed patients' cardiac responses to interviews in a coronary care unit.[4] They found that, while the patient had a varied reaction to being interviewed by the nurse, there was a change in heart rate in response to the interview. In 12 of the 19 patients, the heart rate increased significantly from preinterview levels. The postinterview heart rate was lower in 6 of the 19 patients. Further examination of the data revealed that the patient's heart rate decreased when the nurse spoke and increased when the patient spoke.

This study supported previous findings that the mere act of speaking influences a patient's heart rate and blood pressure. The author concluded, "In a series of studies, we have shown that a subject's verbal activity, the content of communication, status of the interviewer, and the content of the immediate social environment can all interact to produce rapid and highly significant shifts in blood pressure and heart rate in both normotensive and hypertensive subjects."[4]

Nurses and patients make an impression on each other. Communication is encouraged by positive nonverbal cues, by asking appropriate questions, encouraging patients to continue, mirroring what is said, and observing and following a patient's cues. In a study of nurse–patient interaction on a general nursing unit, nurses were found to block attempts at communication more than they encouraged it. This was done by asking closed or leading questions; missing or recognizing, but responding negatively to direct or indirect cues; use of cliché; maintaining superficiality; changing the subject; and avoidance.[5]

Value in Critical Care

The value of effective communication in the critical-care unit can be seen in three ways: (1) improved patient outcomes, (2) improved family–staff relationships, and (3) better staff-to-staff relationships. Effective communication has a direct and positive relationship with patient outcomes. Research that demonstrates this concerns nursing interventions to prevent delirium after cardiac surgery. Budd and Brown[6] found that an orientation program which focused on things that were meaningful to the patient, as well as keeping the patient oriented to time, person, place, and physical status, helped to decrease the incidence of postcardiotomy delirium.

Owens and Hutelmeyer[7] tested the hypothesis that patients who are educated preoperatively about the possibility of unusual sensory or cognitive experiences will either not have such experiences or will feel more comfortable, or more in control of the experiences, if they do occur. The hypothesis was supported and the authors concluded that, by supplying patients with information about what to expect and how to deal with it, they are better able to cope. The authors further stress that communication skills on the part of the nurse are needed to elicit responses from patients.

The reduction of anxiety when a patient is transferred out of the coronary care unit can also be linked to nursing interventions that have communication as a consideration. Schwartz and Brenner[8] examined the effectiveness of specific nursing interventions on reducing stress associated with coronary care unit transfer. They found that either communication with the nurse from the step-down unit, or the patient's family involvement in the transfer period, was a factor in reducing transfer stress. Overall, the experimental patients who received information about their transfer—either from the nurse or family members—scored lower in stress as reported by patient, family, and nurse, and had fewer cardiovascular complications after transfer.

Another way in which the value of communication in the critical-care unit is made apparent is by the ability of the nurse to influence a patient's care through family involvement. The family of the critically ill patient was initially identified as a source of stress for intensive care nurses.[9,10] Later, both positive and negative factors were identified regarding family involvement in the critical-care unit. One positive factor, a source of satisfaction for the critical-care nurse, was the development of a relationship between the nurse and the patient's family. Knowing more about the patient made it more rewarding to provide care.[10]

Other researchers[11] found that patients' interactions with family or friends were no more stressful than patients' interactions with the staff. Nursing staff members further discovered that they were able to direct the families' perception of the CCU experience to a more positive light through the use of intervention that alleviated anxiety and lack of information.[12,13,14]

Research efforts have also been directed toward determining the needs of families of critically ill patients. The thought is that, once the families' needs are met, they will be better able to help their loved ones cope with their illnesses.[15,16,17] Communicating with patients' families is now considered an important and positive part of the critical-care nurse's role.

Discord in interpersonal relationships among staff members and between nursing staff, physicians, and administration is frequently cited as the greatest source of critical-care job-related stress.[18,19] One study cited patient care as the most stressful factor, followed by the environment, the patient's family, administration, and interaction with other critical-care nurses.[20] Utilization of good interpersonal relationships and communication skills among the staff can ease some of the stress and tension that arises from working in a critical-care unit.

Basic Assumptions about Communication

Due to the special nature of the environment of the critical-care unit and the relationships among people in that environment, three assumptions about communications can be made:

1. Time pressure means that interactions between nurse and patient must occur in a compressed framework.
2. Critical illness as a result of physiologic compromise alters, interferes with, or destroys the patient's usual pathway of communication.
3. The nursing interview, the starting point of the nurse–patient relationship, is not a practical vehicle for communication in the critical-care setting.

Time is a governing factor in the critical-care nurse's day. The nurse has a tremendous responsibility for communicating with patients because extended and gradual time to develop the nurse–patient relationship is not possible. Very often, important information is gathered between tests or treatments. This may also be the only time available to talk with the patient and give comfort or support. A frequent nursing dilemma is how to conduct an interview with a patient who wants to discuss concerns, with time limiting what can be discussed.

Making the most of every patient interaction is critical. Sensitive care that realizes the patient's needs and yet incorporates the nurse's need for information makes the communication process challenging in critical-care nursing. Skilled communication techniques, eliciting the patient's feelings, assisting the acceptance of feelings and discussion of concerns, encompass and transcend the traditional nursing interview. The nurse who can compress these skills into the fast, demanding pace of the critical-care unit is justified in saying that the art of critical-care nursing is being practiced.

The physiologic status of critically ill patients frequently prohibits communication along usual pathways. Patients who are intubated or neurologically compromised are frequently unable to speak; this, coupled with time pressure, presents a challenge for communication in critical care. The nurse who has alternate methods of communication ready to use greatly assists the patient in making needs known. The many barriers that block the communication process are detailed later in this chapter. These barriers offer the critical-care nurse many opportunities to exercise skill and care.

The nursing interview is the traditional start of the communication process in nursing. Due to time constraints and physically compromised patients, the traditional interview is not practical in critical care. Most nursing texts on communication identify a beginning, middle, and end to the interview as well as more complex levels of interaction with the patient as the interview progresses.[21] Communication skills used in the nursing interview and at other times in the nurse–patient relationship are presented in Table 16-1.

In critical care, the important information that is usually gained in the nursing interview must be obtained in innovative ways. Instead of one nurse conducting the interview, many nurses over a period of time may gather information about the patient. Primary nursing in critical care facilitates the development of a nurse–patient relationship and the subsequent direction of care. A concise interview format developed for use in critical care is a helpful tool in gathering information, directing care, and identifying a patient's needs.

Each nurse–patient interaction in the critical-care unit must be maximized for the patient's benefit. Defensive or nontherapeutic behavior on the part of the nurse wastes valuable time and does nothing to further the nurse–patient relationship or help the patient (Table 16-2). An awareness on the nurse's part of communication skills, the pitfalls of defensive behavior, the influence of body language, innovative interviewing techniques, and maximum utilization of time will facilitate the communication process in critical care.

Theory and Model of Communication

Communication is the imparting or sharing of information, messages, feelings, and experience through signs, speech, gestures, or writing. Communication may be one way (e.g., giving of a command), or it may be two way (e.g., people carrying on a conversation). The process of communication, the sharing of ourselves with one another on levels ranging from the cursory to the intimate, is what makes us unique among the species of the earth. The process is as simple as the model in this section and, at the same time, as complex as all the variables that enter into it.

Table 16-1 Communication Skills and Their Purposes

Communication Skill	Purpose
Open-ended questions	To achieve information through clarification, elaboration, description, or comparison of a patient's thoughts and feelings
	To allow patients the freedom of response
	To establish an atmosphere of two-way communication
	To assess the type and level of a patient's vocabulary
Closed questions	To achieve specific information
	To allow a limited choice of response
Communicating support	To verbalize the feeling we see and hear being expressed
	To invite the patient to explore own feelings
Silence	To invite a response
	To observe nonverbal behavior
	To allow time for patient to collect thoughts
	To assess levels of anxiety (patient and nurse)
Tactics of Clarification	
Restatement (paraphrasing)	To clarify the meaning and accuracy of old information
	To demonstrate an understanding of what was heard
	To validate what has been said
Reflection of content	To explore new information
	To help patient develop and evaluate thoughts
Reflection of feeling	To put into words what we think or see being conveyed by a patient with respect to feelings and attitudes
	To clarify unspoken or incongruent impressions received from patients
Summarization	To review progress
	To pull together important ideas and facts at conclusion of interview
	To establish a basis for future interviews

Source: From E. C. Hein, *Communication in Nursing Practice*, 2d ed., Little, Brown, 1980. Reprinted with permission.

Table 16-2 Utilizing the Nursing Process in Defensive Behaviors

Defensive Behavior	Purpose or Need Served	Nursing Goal	Nursing Intervention	Effect
Nurse				
Self-focus	Maintain control Discharge anxiety	Reduce and channel anxiety	Self-intervention	Restores interview focus
Nonhelpful reassurance	Inadequacy in dealing with patient's problems	To restore patient's self-worth	Realistic, honest communication concerning patient's capabilities and worth	Effective humanistic interaction
Patient				
Personal questions; crying	To achieve mutuality during interview	Redirect interview	Refocus patient back to topic	Interview focus restored

Source: From E. C. Hein, *Communication in Nursing Practice*, 2d ed., Little, Brown, 1980. Reprinted with permission.

435

A model of communication is based on five components: (1) the stimulus, (2) the sender or encoder, (3) the message, (4) the channel, and (5) the receiver or decoder.[21,22] The short version of the communication process is called a *one-way* or *unilateral personal interaction*. In this type of communication, no response is elicited from the receiver of the message. The process occurs on a horizontal plane. In the long version of communication, called *two-way* or *reciprocal interaction,*[22] communication occurs in a circular manner. The sender's message is commented on by the receiver, causing further interaction by the original sender. Figures 16-1 and 16-2 show the two types of communication processes.

The *stimulus* is the event or occurrence that prompts the communication process to begin. It can originate from outside the sender, in the environment, as an event, object, or another person. For example, when sight of someone you haven't seen in a long time prompts you to say "hello," a stimulus occurs. The stimulus can also come from within the person, such as the need to tell someone of an idea or feeling. A frequent internal stimulus that prompts patients to begin the communication process is pain. Other physiologic mechanisms can also initiate the communication process.

In the critical-care environment, there are multiple external stimuli that can distract or take a person's attention away from the communication process that is going on. A new stimulus may override the patient's original request or an environmental stimulus may block out the request. For example, the patient feels pain and asks the nurse for medication, but at the same time the person in the next bed suffers a cardiac arrest. This new stimulus takes the nurse away from the original communication process, creating a new communication situation with a different person.

The *sender* of the message formulates the message and selects the channel in which to send it. This occurs in light of past knowledge and current experience with the person receiving the message. Cultural background is particularly important in the communication process in the critical-care unit. The nurse is part of a different culture—that of the hospital—than the patient, and, therefore, has different knowledge and experience than the patient. The sender's ability to communicate is reflected in the gesture, feeling tone, and intonation of the communication that he or she sends. Words, gesture, spatial distance, and facial expression are used to convey meaning.

The *message* is the concrete product of the sender's reaction to the original stimulus. A verbal message has two components, the *content* and the *code*. The sender not only selects what will be said, but how it is to be said. Message treatment is how the code and content are arranged to complement each other and convey meaning. The message must be logical, understandable, appropriate, and flexible for the situation. The meaning of a message can further be expressed by natural means or accessory means. *Natural means* are the person's mannerisms that make up voice language and body language. *Accessory means* are the resources that supplement the meaning of the message such as pictures, charts, the written word, or dramatics.[22] In the critical-care setting, the nurse must use both natural and accessory means of communication to ensure that the meaning of the message is understood by the patient. So many barriers to the communication process exist in the critical-care unit that the nurse must also assist the patient in message treatment. This ensures that the patient will be understood by others.

The *channel* that the message travels through to the receiver has two components: the *conveyor* and the *route*. The conveyor component appeals to the senses of the receiver and emanates from the senses of the sender. Thus, speech uses the conveyor or voice waves on the part of the sender and hearing on the part of the receiver. The conveyor can also be inanimate in forms such as the telephone, intercom, etc. The route that the message goes can be either direct or indirect. The direct route goes from the sender to the receiver; the indirect route uses an intermediary. The inter-

Stimulus → Sender → Reaction to stimulus → Message → Channel → Receiver → End

Figure 16-1 One-way communication model

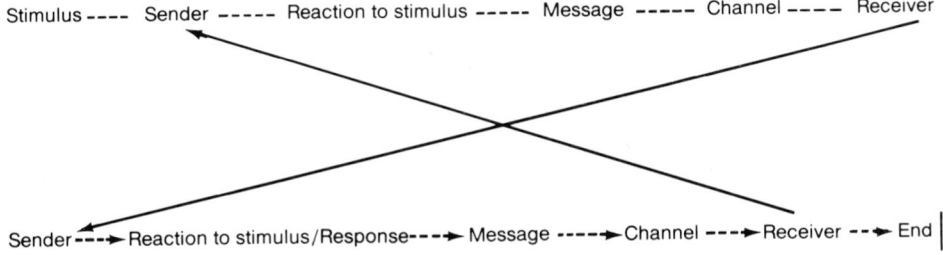

Figure 16-2   Two-way communication model

mediary can be either animate such as a patient's wife, or inanimate, such as a written message or tape recording.[22]

The message and the channel must complement each other for the message to be accurately received by the receiver. Mixed messages occur when the message and the channel do not complement each other, as when a person says "I love you" in an angry tone of voice. Careful, therapeutic communication avoids mixed messages by thoughtful consideration of the message treatment.

The *receiver* of the message is a unique individual, just as is the sender, and the sender's target. The receiver decodes the message which serves as a stimulus for a reply to the original sender. Thus, the cyclic manner of the communication process is begun, as the receiver becomes the sender.

The circular chain of communication is a theoretical model. In reality, many barriers to the communication process exist. The critical-care nurse must be aware of these barriers and understand when and where they are likely to occur, to help the patient select the correct channel of communication in light of apparent disabilities.

Barriers to Effective Communication in the Critical-Care Environment

Variables such as the environmental setting of the critical-care unit, the physical and psychological condition of the patient, and sociocultural differences between the health care system and the patient must be considered and addressed so that communication can take place. Barriers to effective communication are discussed in this section. Caus-

ative factors, etiology, and symptoms that interfere with the patient's ability to send, decode, and receive messages are discussed, as well as the social and cultural differences that exist between patients and nurses and which inhibit communication. The psychological barriers to communication, fear and anxiety, are considered in light of the patient's view of hospitalization. The environment of the critical-care unit, a subject of intense discussion since the inception of its forerunner, the open-heart recovery room of the 1950s, is considered first. Nursing strategies to overcome impaired communication as a result of these barriers are considered in a later section.

Environmental Barriers

Since its inception 25 years ago, the environment of the critical-care unit has been recognized as a contributor to a multiplicity of problems for patients, their families, and, more recently, for critical-care nurses themselves.[20,23,24] Sensory deprivation, alteration, overload, and sleep deprivation linked in the past to a preponderance of intensive care unit syndromes were closely associated with the setting and physical characteristics of the unit.[25,26] Early open-heart recovery units were large, crowded rooms with little attention paid to privacy or the provision of personal space for the patient. Curtains separated the patients' beds, although they were rarely used except in cases of emergency. Continual bright lights, noise, and a constant hum of activity offered little in the way of time orientation for the critically ill patient. The policy of keeping family, friends, and other people known to the patient out of the unit and on a controlled visiting schedule served to isolate the patient socially and culturally.

The patient in the early critical-care unit was faced with an incredible task in attempting to communicate with nurses without basis of social reference, time cues, or environmental cues, while at the same time suffering from a critical illness. As always, the key in this situation was the ability of the nurse in reaching out and assisting the patient make his or her needs known in an attempt to understand the environment.

Hackett, Cassem, and Wishnie[23] were the first to point out that the type of critical-care unit had an influence on the potential psychological hazards a patient might encounter. Coronary care units, out of deference to their population of cardiac patients, have made an effort to control the environment and maximize the healing process for patients while minimizing environmental stress. The private room, the hallmark of the coronary care unit, provides the necessary quiet, privacy, and environmental control that facilitates communication. By just being able to close the door and shut out all the outside noise and activity, the nurse and patient can concentrate on the sharing of information that will benefit the patient.

Over 50 percent of hospitals with critical-care units maintain combined medical–surgical coronary units which are more chaotic and, therefore, more stressful for patients.[23,27] Many advances in the design of critical-care units, particularly in coronary care units, have occurred in the last 10 years. More critical-care units are now built with the patient's comfort, as well as nursing efficiency, in mind. Units with private rooms, soundproofing, carpets, windowed doors, and sitting areas in patients' rooms for family members, are now seen across the country. Unfortunately, or perhaps inevitably, the traditional open-bed ward still exists.

What specific barriers do the nurse and the critically ill patient encounter in the critical-care units of today? Another look at the communication model may help provide answers. Considering the environmental context of the communication model, one could say that a stimulus that interferes with the channel or the message, inhibiting passage between sender and receiver, constitutes a barrier to effective communication. Three areas of interactions between the nurse, patient, and environment can provide such barriers. They are:

1. Lack of privacy.
2. Distractions that result in an incomplete message being sent or in the channel by which the message is to be sent being usurped by another message.
3. Lack of communication between the patient's previous environment and the present hospital environment.

Lack of Privacy

Hospitals are notorious for the lack of privacy they offer patients. Not only are patients' bodies subjected to intense scrutiny by a myriad of people largely unknown to them, but their very lives are placed under a microscope to be dissected by experts. That this occurs is an amazing testimony to the health profession's power and prestige. The critical-care environment is perhaps the worst offender of a patient's privacy with respect to the management of information. Few critical-care units have private conference rooms where the health care team can discuss the patient's prognosis, treatment regimens, and courses of disease with family members. Discussions are frequently held in lobbies, public waiting rooms, halls, and in the middle of the unit. Patients are likely to censor the message when they know that it will go out to a large number of people, or that there is no control over who has access to the information. Patients are very aware of other people, particularly other patients, in their environment. In the open-ward situation, they are able to compare their own health status with those around them. This may offer an erroneous picture of how the patient perceives his or her illness.

Lack of privacy is also a factor when extraneous sights, sounds, smells, people, and routines enter into the nurse–patient communication and override the message or channel in which the message is sent. An example of this is what occurs when chest tubes are bubbling so forcefully and the suction machine is hissing so loudly that the nurse cannot hear what the patient is saying. Noise levels in the CCU from machinery, as well as people, are usually high. This can be controlled by staff members lowering their voices, refraining from social talking and joking, and making certain that equipment surrounding the patient is working correctly, but at the lowest decibel level possible.[28]

Distractions

Distractions within the environment of the critical-care unit that compete for attention on the part of the nurse or patient are major barriers to communication. In the early days of the open-heart recovery room and critical-care unit, the ECG monitors, oscilloscopes, and equipment were distracting to patients because they were large, obvious, cumbersome, and noisy. Now, monitors and equipment are distracting to nurses and patients because they are such technologic wonders. Monitors have so many capabilities and functions that nurses may focus their attention on the monitors or equipment rather than on the patient. Increased public awareness of medical information fostered by the media also may cause the patient to focus attention on the equipment in an attempt to learn, recognize, or understand what is occurring.

Other distractions for the patient come from occurrences within the environment that the nurse may casually accept as part of the environment. Sound that is *noise* for the patient is particularly distracting when two people are trying to talk. Critical-care nurses may not be aware that sounds such as ventilators, suction apparatus, chest tubes, alarms on monitors, and infusion pump alarms are interfering with the communication process. To the nurse, they are part of the environment and are normal and acceptable. To the patient, they are unfamiliar sounds that need to be decoded and explained. At the very least, extraneous sounds in the environment cause a patient to wish for peace and quiet—at the very most, they provide a basis for misinterpretation of the environment.

Link to Other Environments

The final barrier exists when the attempt is made to confine the patient within the critical-care unit environment without recognizing that person as part of another environment. When the nonrecognition of a patient as an individual occurs, the nurse and hospital have set up another barrier.

Rules and regulations are needed in all institutions to standardize care and provide order. Certain policies and procedures can be bent in deference to patient and family preference to facilitate communication. When hospitals and nurses set up policies such as all baths between 5:00 and 6:00 A.M.; no valuables, jewelry, or personal clothing in the unit; and visiting 10 min an hour from 7:00 A.M. to 4:00 P.M.; the system sends a message that "individual preferences, personal items that identify you and your family, are not important to us." Many times, nurses expect that the illness at hand is uppermost in a person's mind when, in actuality, patients are more concerned with what's happening in the environment they left. The elderly lady worries about her dog, the businessman is concerned about his business, and the divorced mother of three wonders where her teenagers are. Without links to the outside, the patient may feel imprisoned within the system and may direct energies toward communication outside the system, rather than within.

Sociocultural Barriers

Culture is the reference point or orientation which shapes and guides our beliefs, actions, and reactions to others and the environment around us. "Communication is the medium by which our cultural heritage is maintained, conveyed, and translated as time passes. From this point of view, culture should invite, arouse, and excite the curious individual to seek out and discover the ways in which his own culture is expressed."[21] When two people from different cultures communicate, understanding that there is no "right" or "wrong" culture facilitates the communication process. Ethnocentric behavior or attitudes prevail when one believes the only "correct" culture is one's own. Ethnocentric health care professionals look down their noses at health care practices and ideas that are not in line with modern western medical thinking. When this message is conveyed to patients and their families, the communication barrier widens. Important information that the nurse needs to assist the person to optimum health may be withheld by the patient or family due to fear of ridicule or embarrassment when an ethnocentric attitude prevails.

Cultural relativism describes the attempt to understand each cultural trait in concert or with respect to the whole culture without being critical of the trait or culture. The nurse who practices cultural relativism doesn't pass judgments on cultural health care practices but attempts to create a bridge with the patient's cultural system and modern medicine to ensure optimal health for the patient.[29]

Elements within a culture having the greatest significance for nursing may include any one or all of the following components of society: (1) family organization; (2) care during birth, sickness, and death; (3) age- and sex-related values; (4) language; (5) time orientation; (6) sleep and hygiene habits; (7) modesty; (8) communication of satisfaction and dissatisfaction; (9) value of personal accomplishment; (10) food habits; and (11) religious orientation. In complex societies such as our own, people do not share a common culture, despite the fact that we may share a common language. The use of the term "cultural scene" may be more appropriate in determining cultural variations that exist within a large, complex society. Thus, certain of the previously mentioned cultural elements may characterize one cultural scene, while other elements may predominate in another.

Language

Language is a vital channel in which messages are received and sent. When language is unintelligible, whether due to a physiologic barrier such as aphasia, or to a cultural barrier such as language differences, communication does not occur, or occurs at a severely limited level. The cultural barrier of different languages between patient and nurse is one that may be frustrating and time-consuming at the least, and life-threatening at its greatest. Any attempt on the nurse's part to understand or speak the patient's language will be appreciated by the patient. If the nurse does not have a working knowledge of the patient's language and it is a common one in the area, the system should make it possible for the nurse to obtain an interpreter through which to communicate with the patient. Perhaps the single major factor that should be considered in caring for patients who speak a foreign language is that more time will be needed to provide nursing care.

Interpreters working in the critical-care area should be specifically trained to translate for patients and their families. Interpreters should know basic policy information about the unit, such as visiting hours, and the availability of other patient and family services. Translating is not just inter-

preting what a person has said. When translators are used, the nurse still directs the conversation along therapeutic lines. Factors that are important to consider when patient interpretation occurs are: the register at which the language is placed; the use of jargon, semantics, or polishing of phrases that may alter or change the patient's meaning; and the importance of anecdotal information in relation to the patient's health problem. A final factor to consider is that a person who speaks English as a second language may lose that ability in the face of stress from a critical illness.[30]

A patient's privacy and confidentiality are difficult to maintain when visitors, housekeeping, or dietary aides are pressed into service as translators. Family members are usually not trained in medical language or translating techniques and, although convenient, they may not be appropriate interpreters in certain situations. The nurse also must be sensitive to cultural variations regarding who is privileged to be spokesperson for the family. Although a younger daughter may have a good command of English, if the oldest brother is spokesperson, the nurse should make every attempt to communicate with him, or at least obtain his consent to talk with others of lesser stature in the family. This is particularly true in Asian cultures where age, or the oldest in the family, is accorded a high measure of respect.

Language barriers can be largely overcome through the use of skilled interpreters and an understanding of how language is translated. When translators are not available, or a patient speaks a little-known language, the nurse may press others into service to obtain information about the patient's language and culture. Sources of information about language include the hospital medical library, social services, and community-based organizations. Written material with basic information about the critical-care unit may assist some patients and families in determining what is occurring. Audiotapes in the person's language will also be helpful.[31] Without written or spoken language communication, gestures and facial expressions may be the only available means to communicate with the patient. Demonstration is helpful in teaching respiratory techniques. Small scale models of hospital equipment may help the patient relate hygiene needs to the nurse with minimal effort. Ingenuity and resourcefulness on the part of the nurse will facilitate communication and provide access to important patient information.

Nonverbal Communication

Nonverbal communications are those messages sent to others through the medium of our bodies. Eye contact, use of emotion, and territoriality are three areas that are included in nonverbal communication.

Two sayings, "the eye is the window of the soul," and "a clear eye reflects a clean heart" reveal a high value on face-to-face eye contact during communication. This concept is so ingrained in our western culture that expressions such as "he couldn't look me in the eye," or "she has shifty eyes," denote characteristics of a person who is devious, sly, or deceptive. That eye contact is closely associated with communication is further evident in expressions such as "We saw eye-to-eye on the matter." However, eye contact is a cultural variable. In some cultures, it is considered bad manners to look someone in the eye. In other cultures, downcast eyes are a sign of respect or submission to authority.

In the critical-care unit, eye contact is frequently not possible due to the position of the patient. Furthermore, when patients do attempt to make eye contact with the nurse, they may be admonished to "not move" or "stay still." Bright overhead lights shining directly in a recumbent patient's face discourage the person from even opening the eyes. The nurse is in a position to encourage or discourage eye contact through a patient's positioning and/or by controlling light intensity. To break down barriers to communication, the nurse needs to determine if eye contact is culturally desirable and then appropriately facilitate the communication process.

Expressions of emotion by the person's family to critical illness may be based on cultural variables such as ethnic origins, religious orientation, socioeconomic status, or geographic location. Past coping mechanisms during crisis situations or what the patient feels are expected emotions at a particular time are also aspects of how emotion is displayed in critical care. Stereotyping a patient's emotions based on ethnic origin is not accurate since a person's emotions are based on many variables.

The nurse who does not "expect" patients or families to emote in a certain way can do much to facilitate communication as each set of emotions is viewed in light of the circumstance or context in which it occurs. When inappropriate emotion is perceived, the nurse may well explore why the emotion is occurring, the feeling behind it, and the person's perception of the occurrence before "labeling" it as inappropriate.

Cultural biases become evident as territory and personal space are chosen and defined. Because of the status accorded to health care workers, nurses are offered frequent and easy access to a person's intimate space. *Intimate distance* of space occurs within 18 in of two people. Touch, the feel of one's breath, and body odors are exchanged within this distance. Personal space is the extension of ourselves to the point where we feel comfortable interacting with others. It may depend on how one feels about the person with whom one is communicating. A friendly look and smile signal a person to come closer, whereas a frown and crossed arms say "stay away."

Critical-care nurses working in a person's intimate space have the responsibility to provide the patient with sensory preparation on certain procedures. Draping and covering a patient to ensure modesty are essential. When asked by the patient to stop a certain procedure, the nurse should stop, even just for a moment, and reassess what is occurring. Would there be another way, or a different person or equipment that would ease the patient's discomfort? Respect, understanding, and compromise are needed in critical care to preserve a patient's autonomy.

Personal distance is between 1½ ft and 4 ft in distance. Nurses are more comfortable working in this range, as there is an increased flexibility in caring for the patient through touch and close contact but with the ability to move away from the patient. Conversation can range from serious talk to light banter. It is easier to change the subject in this distance, or avoid topics that may be disturbing to the patient or nurse. The foot of the bed is a comfortable, personal distance to assume for many health care professionals. Awareness of the patient's desires regarding distance and comfort zone when discussing topics of concern can help the communication process.

Social distance, 4 to 12 ft, is characterized by activity. The symbol of social distance is the nurses' station, where activity is directed. The nurses' station may be off limits to anyone but nurses and physicians, or it may allow more contact with families, technicians, and students. Within the social distance setting, a person can choose to join certain groups or persons, or ignore them by bustling through the unit and avoiding eye contact. Through the maintenance of social distance within the unit, the nurse may be able to step away from the patient for a moment or two and regain his or her thoughts, away from the demands that intimate personal distance contact places on an individual.[21]

Cultural Scene of a Critical-Care Unit

The phrase, *cultural scene,* describes an aspect of a large, complex culture that may be defined as "information shared by two or more people that defines some aspect of mutual experience."[32] The cultural scene of the critical-care unit varies from hospital to hospital, depending on local standards of care and custom. As a cultural scene, the critical-care unit of a hospital has its own written and spoken language. "Medicalese" attaches different meanings to commonly used phrases, has control over time-related events, and holds a scientifically based view of health and illness that may be very different from that of the people it cares for.

The scientific language that health care professionals use within the hospital setting constitutes a foreign language—complete with symbols and abbreviations. Many common or basic medical terms are misunderstood, misconstrued, or misinterpreted by the general public. In a study of lay understanding of medical terms, lack of understanding of the following terms was found to exist: virus, strep throat, herpes, tumor, Pap smear, and uterus.[33] Patients who were elderly, uneducated, or who lacked a medical background were identified as being less able to correctly define terms. Women had as much difficulty as men in their understanding of the terms "uterus" and "Pap smear." The educational level of the person proved to be the strongest indication of knowledge.

In another study, multiple misconceptions and interpretations of phrases commonly used in the hospital were found to exist. Interpretation of the phrase, "It'll only hurt a little," varied from a "quick pinch" to "will hurt a lot." These two studies point out that barriers do exist because of a difference between the health culture and the lay person, causing misunderstandings. A way to bridge misconceptions is to use the person's own language and terminology when possible, and repeat information in different ways.

The concept of time in the critical-care unit may be a source of misconception between patients and nurses in critical care. The usual time cues of day and night may be absent in the CCU. It is very unusual to find a critical-care policy that lets patients sleep through the night, although time for sleep and rest is recognized as important.[34] The normal time reference of day and night may be absent for the patient. The patient may perceive that many tests, tasks, or assessments could be omitted during the night to facilitate sleep. By contrast, the night nurse views the night as no less important a time in which to give comprehensive, complete nursing care.

Control of time in the critical-care unit is determined by the time schedule set up for the patient. There is a set time for hygiene, pulmonary toilet, assessments, vital signs, and laboratory work, despite what the patient feels or desires, or has done for most of his or her life. For many people, adjusting to a rigid time schedule of when things are done may be difficult and may place further stress on them. This is especially true if a patient is not a time-oriented person by culture and values.

Physiologic Barriers

The physiologic barriers that exist as a result of trauma and disease create the largest obstacles to nurse–patient communication. The patient's condition may change so rapidly that it is difficult to determine communicative abilities. One moment the patient may be speaking clearly and intelligently, then within an hour a drop in Pa_{O_2} may bring on confusion, apathy, and misperception about the environment. Physiologic conditions that exist as barriers to communication may be transitory or permanent. In addition, preexisting medical conditions may also impair communication. Finally, if the patient is elderly, special needs may exist as a result of the physiologic process of aging.

In viewing physiologic barriers in light of the communication model, it is apparent that the patient will be unable to encode messages to be sent out to the receiver, or decode the message of interpretation and response. Whatever the physiologic problem, communication breaks down with the patient's decreased physiologic responsiveness.

Cognitive Dysfunction

The cognitive processes of the human individual are at the basis of the communication process. Our thoughts are what we communicate. Memory aids us in bringing forth past learning and sharing our present interactions for future reference.

Comprehension, perception of surroundings, and feelings that make up awareness at a given time constitute a *thought*. *Memory* is the ability to recall a thought at least once, while *learning* is the storage of memories within the nervous system for future use. Each thought involves simultaneous action in portions of the cerebral cortex, thalamus, diencephalon, and reticular formation of the brain stem.

Any disturbance in the cerebral processes that generate memory, thoughts, perception, learning, or consciousness can be classified as *cognitive dysfunction*. Cognitive dysfunction can be transitory or permanent and can occur as a result of neurologic dysfunction (such as brain damage, an increase in intracranial pressure, or cerebral hemorrhage) or metabolic imbalances (resulting from metabolic acidosis, kidney failure, or hypoxia). Patients experiencing neurologic deficits may have alterations in all the processes of cognition and consciousness; patients with metabolic difficulty will experience altered levels of consciousness and changes in the sensorium.

The patient who suffers brain damage may experience alterations in general memory patterns because of lesions in the *Papez circuit,* which includes the hippocampus, mammilary bodies, mammillothalamic tract, and the anterior zones of the limbic regions. Loss of memory related to a particular experience may result when there are lesions in the area of the lateral temporal and parietal lobes.[35] Destruction of the temporal lobes in a person will cause loss of memory for recent events that have occurred within the previous 2 to 6 days. Long-term memory will not be affected. Knowledge of the area of neurologic damage that the patient has sustained is essential for the nurse to communicate with the patient and to have realistic expectations about what the patient will be able to communicate with the nurse.

Memory is classified as *instantaneous*—that which is recalled second by second, or minute by minute; or *fixed*—that which remains with a person for a few days up to a lifetime. Instantaneous memory is transitory and not stored for future use. The physiologic concept behind instantaneous memory is that an electrical stimulus in the cerebral cortex produces a reverberating circuit between the cerebral cortex and the thalamus. When the circuits become fatigued, the memory fades away. Fixed memory occurs when the memory becomes ingrained in the neuronal circuits. The minimal time at which memory can be fixed requires 15 to 20 min. Maximal fixation occurs at 1 h or more.

Certain areas of the brain can support memories for longer periods of time than others. Some areas of the brain, such as the temporal lobes, may be temporary storage areas. The corpus callosum serves as a link in memory storage between the two hemispheres. The exception to this is the cortices of the anterior portions of the temporal lobes, which all interconnect by fibers that pass through the anterior commissure. Therefore, there is a mechanism for storing memories between hemispheres with the quality of the memory remaining characteristic of the lobe.[35]

If recent memory is affected due to brain damage, the current situation may be interpreted in light of old memories. The patient may be appropriately oriented to place, i.e., the hospital, but may confuse it with a time 30 years ago. The hospital memory has been pulled to the forefront by other stimuli—smell, hearing, touch—but the patient "forgets" that it is the present, not the past. Interactions that are needed to impart new information are best repeated over and over so a new memory imprint can develop. Associating new experiences with old can be helpful in bridging memory gaps, thereby giving the patient a sense of security. The capacity to "forget" or lose new information in someone who has brain impairment cannot be overemphasized. Repetition that is presented in a consistent manner and assistance in bridging recent events to past memories can help a patient master a disability in communicating.

The level of consciousness that a patient presents is a traditional indicator of neurologic function. Changes in the level or stage of consciousness can serve as an indicator of the status of other physiologic conditions such as acid-base balance, hypoxia, and electrolyte balance. When these three areas of physiologic functioning are out of homeostatic balance, central nervous system deficiencies occur. The resulting symptoms may vary from lassitude and apathy to coma and will interfere with the communication process between nurse and patient.

Hypoxia is defined as the decreased availability of oxygen in the cells of the body. The effects of hypoxia on the nervous system may produce symptoms of lassitude, mental fatigue, and sometimes headache, nausea, and fatigue. In the critically ill patient, hypoxia may come on slowly or quickly as the patient's status changes. Good communication skills on the part of the nurse can reveal if the patient is experiencing a change in Pa_{O_2} levels, and alert the nurse.

The process of talking, assessing, and communicating with patients will not only bring to light emotional, cultural, and social concerns of the patient, but also can clue the nurse to subtle physiologic changes as well.

This point is further illustrated when an acid-base imbalance occurs, particularly in a uremic patient. When the blood pH falls below 7.0, central nervous system effects occur, beginning with a state of disorientation and ending with coma. The patient in a uremic crisis suffers from metabolic acidosis as well as electrolyte imbalance and azotemia. The patient's mental capacity for communication will be best several hours after renal dialysis, after body fluids have stabilized, and worst just prior to dialysis. What the renal patient can understand, assimilate, and remember about the care received, the disease, and hospitalization is very much dependent on the physiologic factors that influence the disease process. Timing conversations, teaching sessions, or the giving of important information at times when the physiologic barriers to communication are minimized will facilitate the communication process.

Electrolyte imbalance also contributes to cognitive dysfunctions. A person's electrolyte balance can change so frequently that many units have policies of drawing electrolytes every 2 to 4 h. Hypokalemia produces symptoms of malaise, irritability, confusion, mental depression, and speech changes. Hypercalcemia produces drowsiness, lethargy, depression, apathy, irritability, and confusion. Hyponatremia and hypernatremia both have an effect on the nervous system that is the opposite of each other. An electrolyte imbalance can interfere with a person's ability to think and act according to the surroundings. The nurse must assist the patient to communicate with regard for changing electrolyte status.

Finally, drug reactions and interactions must be included under cognitive dysfunction as causing potential barriers to communication. Lidocaine and corticosteroids, such as prednisone, are examples of two drugs which can produce side effects causing barriers to communication. Persons with either long-term or short-term corticosteroid use can experience alteration in mood and depression, making it difficult for them to communicate. Lidocaine's side effects can produce a decreased level of consciousness that makes talking and comprehension difficult.

Tracheostomy and Intubation

Critical-care nurses are experts in caring for the physical and mechanical needs of the patient who has a tracheostomy or who is intubated for purposes of mechanical ventilation. Meeting the patient's communication needs may be a different matter—frequently overlooked, but no less important.

When intubation occurs, either nasally or orally, the patient loses not only the ability to speak, but many facial expressions as well. Hands may be restrained to prevent pulling at the endotracheal tube, and gestures or the ability to signal may also be lost. The experience of tracheostomy may provoke fear and misunderstanding if the patient is not informed that speechlessness is temporary and can be reversed. In long-term critically ill patients, the use of the tracheal button to encourage speech (for brief times if permitted) can help the patient communicate his or her needs.

When the need for intubation is known in advance, perhaps for cardiac surgery, there is time to work out a system of communication between the patient and nurse. Frequently, the patient will be told that intubation will occur and what it means; the best way to communicate also should be added to this preparation. Writing messages, a method frequently relied upon by critically ill patients, is not always satisfactory. Arterial lines, blood lines, Swan-Ganz catheters in brachial arteries, or other intravenous lines, frequently prevent a person from writing. Even when a patient does write, it may be illegible because of the patient's position or inability to grip the writing materials. Sometimes patients try to write out entire sentences that are grammatically correct, a lengthy process causing fatigue on the part of the patient. In this situation, the patient should be asked to write pertinent nouns and verbs, saving time and energy.

Occasionally, patients will have an alternate method of communicating that is unknown to the nurse, causing the nurse as well as the patient to become frustrated. The author recalls three patients who, when they found they couldn't speak, utilized American sign language for the deaf, Morse code by blinking the eyes, and Native American sign language. Discussion regarding alternative ways of communicating can decrease frustration and anxiety.

If flash cards or message boards are used, it is helpful if the patient can be familiarized with them before intubation or tracheostomy. The critical-care nurse knows areas of concern that the person may encounter after being intubated. These may include difficulty in breathing, sore throat, pain, etc. A discussion of such areas and development of clues or cues for each will facilitate the communication process.

Frequently, intubation in the critical-care unit occurs on an emergency basis. The patient becomes hypoxic, loses orientation to his or her surroundings and, prior to respiratory arrest, is intubated. After intubation, when the airway is cleared, the patient is given a high concentration of oxygen, and once again becomes aware of the surroundings. The realization that he or she is unable to speak may produce feelings of fear or anxiety that result in reactions ranging from withdrawal to violence. Before the patient becomes alert, the nurse should begin to talk to the patient. After the patient has become noticeably oriented, reminders of what is occurring and why should be forthcoming. That the inability to vocalize is reversible is another important statement the nurse should make. As soon as possible, the nurse should try to interpret attempts at communication and discover what the patient feels is important. Giving information in a calm, slow voice, and touching a person gently and firmly can help the patient feel more in touch with the environment. Since the communication process

can take time and patience in a newly intubated patient, the ideal situation is one in which one nurse is present to calm the patient, provide reassurance and determine needs, while another nurse cares for the patient's physical needs.

New devices, such as fenestrated tracheostomy and endotracheal tubes, may prove helpful in assisting intubated patients to communicate. Speaking endotracheal tubes and voice amplifiers are other important technological developments.

A study of nurse–patient interaction of 20 intubated patients showed that communication was usually nurse-initiated.[36] Out of 217 observed interactions between patients and nurses, only 34 were patient-initiated. Of the 34, four were expressions of anger with the rest being positive interactions. One-third of the positively initiated actions by the patient were responded to in a negative way by the critical-care nurse. Examples of positive interactions on the part of the nurse were praise or encouragement, explanations, or directions. Positive patient responses were initiations of nonverbal communication that were not hostile. Negative nursing actions were silence during care or disapproval of actions. Hostility or physical anger on the part of the patient was viewed negatively.

This study found that the most common nursing action or reaction to patients was silence, with patients responding negatively to that silence. The researchers concluded that critical-care nurses in their study "may have been unable to recognize and/or deal with their patient's responses to illness and hospitalization, or they may have been unable to deal with their own reaction to the patient or situation."[36]

This study overwhelmingly points out that intubated patients may wait for the nurse to initiate communication and, when nothing is forthcoming, remain silent. When patients are unable to speak due to tracheostomy or intubation, the critical-care nurse has the responsibility to initiate communication verbally or nonverbally and to try to understand what the patient communicates back.

Another study that points out the need for verbal communication and touch for intubated patients concerns the perceptions of patients given pancuronium bromide.[37] In this study, five patients, all men, were asked their recollections and perceptions of the period they were paralyzed with pancuronium bromide. (Patients who receive pancuronium bromide are aware of their environment, but cannot respond to it; it has no effect on the central nervous system.) All subjects were able to recall some aspects of their intubated period: Four of five patients recalled being intubated. One subject was not told what was going to be done and he wondered what was happening to him. Verbal stimuli, when directed to the patient, or just occurring in the general area, was recalled by three patients. The author recommends planned auditory stimuli to provide communication with the patient and the use of touch as a method of reassurance.[37]

Aphasia

Aphasia is the loss of the ability to process, understand, or express words as thoughts, symbols, or ideas in a manner which communicates the intent of the sender to the receiver. Three main types of aphasia are generally identified: *receptive, expressive,* and *global.* The critical-care nurse may encounter aphasia as part of a patient's primary problem, such as a brain abscess, or as a secondary problem, as in the case of a patient who needs care for a duodenal ulcer and who has also had a cerebrovascular accident. Rehabilitation of the patient who experiences aphasia takes time and occurs over a period of months. Full rehabilitative potential is not usually reached until the patient has been discharged from the hospital.[38,39]

In light of this, the critical-care nurse works with the aphasic patient who is not ready for speech therapy, who may be physiologically unstable, and whose neurologic sequelae are still evolving, thereby presenting a changing pattern of communicative abilities. Time and patience are needed to help the patient become aware of how the disability affects his or her relationship to the environment and others. The anatomic approach to understanding aphasia correlates lesions in the cerebral cortex with causes of aphasia. It is the approach most frequently taken and will be utilized in this discussion. Table 16-3 lists characteristics of the different types of aphasia.

The left hemisphere is considered dominant for speech in most people, although connection and transmission of impulses occur in both hemispheres through the thalamus and mesencephalic areas. It is generally accepted that 90 percent of right-handed people have language dominance in

the left hemisphere and 50 to 60 percent of left-handed people have language dominance in the left hemisphere. Some people have a right hemisphere dominance for language or mixed language function divided between the two hemispheres. The tendency for hemisphere dominance is thought to be hereditary. Through learning and use, the hemisphere's dominance further develops. This is illustrated by the case of young children with lesions in their dominant hemisphere. Usually, speech function is not totally lost but is taken over by the noninjured hemisphere. The nondominant hemisphere's role in speech and language can be further developed if the dominant hemisphere's lesion is slow-growing.

In *sensory aphasia* the basic deficit occurs because of the destruction of the area of auditory comprehension, located at the superior part of the superior temporal convolution. The person is able to hear sounds and words, but is unable to comprehend them. This is also reflected in the patient's inability to "hear" oneself speak. Resulting speech is lacking in content, although it is correct in grammar, rhythm, and articulation.[39] *Literal paraphasia* is said to exist if incorrect sounds are substituted, as "bat" for "cat." In *verbal paraphasia,* one word is substituted for another, such as "fork" for "spoon." The communication barrier that exists in the patient with sensory aphasia makes it difficult to determine the patient's meaning in a sea of verbiage. Quite often, the patient is unaware that communication is ineffective, although in time the realization occurs that something is amiss. The patient is more likely to become angry with others at their lack of communicative ability.

Expressive aphasia results when there is a lesion in the area of the inferior frontal gyrus of the frontal lobe, anterior to the facial and lingual areas of the motor cortex.[40,41] The ability to formulate a sentence originates in Broca's area, and is transmitted to the motor cortex where transmission of impulses to motor speech areas produce speech. The motor cortex is responsible for control of movement of the lips, jaw, tongue, soft palate, and vocal cords. The frustration that the patient feels is a result of the inability to articulate the thought that has formed in his or her mind. Features of speech are presented in Table 16-4.

"Because Broca's area is so near the left motor area, disease often affects the ability to speak of

Table 16-3 Characteristics of Aphasia by Type

Type	Alternate Names	Anatomic Area of Involvement	Speech Characteristics	Language Comprehension
Expressive aphasia	Broca's aphasia, nonfluent aphasia, motor aphasia, anterior aphasia, apraxia of speech	Lateral Inferior portion of frontal lobe of dominant hemisphere	1. Slow, labored speech. 2. "Telescoping" the omission of small words or ends of nouns and verbs. 3. Poor naming ability. 4. Ability to repeat more than one word is poor. 5. Writing is similar to speech pattern. 6. Reading comprehension good. 7. May be fluent at swearing or humming.	Good
Receptive aphasia	Wernicke's aphasia, fluent aphasia, sensory aphasia	Superior temporal convolution of dominant hemisphere	1. Fluent speech, normal rate, rhythm, good grammar. 2. Content of speech is lacking. 3. Content of writing similar to speech. 4. Poor reading comprehension. 5. Repetition is poor. 6. Object naming poor.	Poor. Lacks auditory comprehension.
Anomic aphasia	General agnosia	Angular gyrus, near Wernicke's area	1. Speech fluent or rhythmic. 2. Difficulty in naming objects or places. 3. Circumlocutory speech.	Good
Conduction		Arcuate fasciculus, between frontal and temporal lobes sphere	1. Difficulty in repeating words, substitutes incorrect sounds (literal paraphasia). 2. Substitutes incorrect words (verbal paraphasia).	Good
Global		Several areas in dominant hemisphere	1. Combination of characteristics, depending on area of involvement.	Poor to good, depending on area of involvement.

Table 16-4 Features of Speech

Form

Articulation: The effort to produce speech.

Rate of speaking: Normal average of 100–125 words per minute.

Melody: Intonation of a sentence with patterns of stress and rising and falling of pitch.

Phrase length: The number of words uttered between pauses, with no reference to grammatic structure. (Estimate runs of uninterrupted words while listening to patient.)

Content

Word choice: Meaningful content words (nouns, principal verbs, adjectives, adverbs) that carry the information load of the sentence. Patient may use a few highly meaningful substantive words or be circumlocutory, using many words to talk around subject without precision.

Syntax: Grammatic structure, which may include filler words (articles, prepositions, pronouns, auxiliary verbs, verb and noun inflections, conjunctions).

Paraphasia: Substitution of one letter for another and/or one word for another.

Fluency

Fluent: Produced at a normal or hypernormal rate, with normal speech, rhythm, and melody; good articulation, and normal or hypernormal phrase length.

Nonfluent: Slow, laboriously produced, with abnormal speech, rhythm, and melody; poor articulation, shortened phrase length, preferential use of substantive words (nouns, main verbs) rather than grammatic words—often telegraphic or agrammatic.

Source: From G. V. Baykin, Strategies for Increasing Communication with the Dysphasic Patient, *Dimensions of Critical Care Nursing,* vol. 3, 1984, pp. 279–281. Copyright 1984, by J. B. Lippincott and Company. Reprinted with permission.

those with right-sided paralysis, whereas left-sided paralysis almost never results in speech disturbances."[42] The converse is also true, that melodic areas for singing and automatic speech located on the right side of the brain, enable those with expressive aphasia to hum, sing, or curse with fluency.

The person with expressive aphasia is very aware of the inability to communicate. Resulting feelings of anger, hostility, hopelessness, depression, and withdrawal may further widen the communication barrier. When conversing with the patient, the nurse should allow more time than usual and stick to one main topic per short conversation time. The nurse needs to be aware of his or her own verbal style in order not to present the expressive aphasic patient with an additional sea of verbiage.

Anomic and *conduction aphasia* refer to two types of lesions that occur in the association between Broca's and Wernicke's area. *Anomic aphasia* occurs when there is a lesion in the angular gyrus. The speech of the anomic individual is fluent and rhythmic, but there is difficulty naming objects or places. The patient engages in circumlocutory speech in an attempt to make meanings known.

Conduction aphasia exists when there is a lesion in the arcuate fasciculus that prevents trans-

mission of neuronal impulses from Wernicke's area to Broca's area. Comprehension is intact but the speech is characterized by literal paraphasias. The affected person will have trouble repeating words spoken by another.[41]

Global aphasia exists where there is damage to multiple areas in the left cerebral cortex and the person is left with few language skills. Poor comprehension and inability to name objects and repeat words, coupled with nonfluent speech, make communication difficult with this patient. Perhaps the best hope for communication lies in recognition of sign language, gestures, pantomime, or cues.

The importance of the thalamus as a link between the hemispheres and between the lower brain levels and the cortex is noteworthy. The cerebral cortex is an outgrowth of the thalamus and, as such, has corresponding areas. Thus, stimulation of certain thalamic areas of the brain also invokes a similar cerebral cortex response, and vice versa. Activation of areas of the mesencephalon transmits diffuse signals through the thalamus to the cerebral cortex to produce the state called wakefulness. Without these transmissions, sleep occurs.

The actual areas of the cerebral cortex related to receptive and expressive aphasia are small in relation to the total size of the cerebral area. The remaining areas are called *association areas*. A large association area extends out from the motor cortex. These association areas coordinate incoming sensory data and may influence motor function in the light of sensory data. The aphasic patient presents the critical-care nurse with a special challenge in the communication process. The nurse must alter existing patterns of communication to fit the physiologic deficits of the patient. In turn, the nurse helps the patient use alternate means of communicating when speech is incomprehensible.

Dysarthria

Dysarthria exists when a person has difficulty in articulating single sounds or phonemes of speech. "The dysarthric person experiences deficits in articulation, enunciation, resonance and rhythm caused by paralysis, muscular weakness, incoordination or abnormal enervation."[39] The cause can be classified as neurologic or functional in origin. Damage to the cranial nerves which control speech is just as damaging as trauma to the pharynx, larynx, or tongue. Dysarthria may be a sequela of intubation if the pharynx is damaged through repeated or traumatic intubation. *Dysphonia* is the term applied to guttural or inappropriate laryngeal speech. Table 16-5 lists cranial nerves that are important in the motor aspect of speech.

Aphasia and dysarthria are not synonymous nor do they always occur concomitantly, although at times they may. The dysarthric person may or may not have comprehension difficulties. Careful nursing assessment of the person's mental faculties are warranted when a person displays difficulty in speaking.

Age

As medicine and technology become more advanced, more and more elderly people are treated and released from critical-care units. Because the process of aging brings with it physical, mental, and social change, elderly patients present a different challenge in the critical-care unit than do younger or middle-aged patients. Mary Opal Wolanin,[43] noted gerontologist, identifies seven ways in which the elderly patient differs from younger patients. Loss of physiologic reserves, especially cardiac and immune defense reserves, places the elderly in a debilitated state quite easily. Even minor illnesses may take a long time for recovery. Critical illnesses may exhaust all body systems reserves, leaving the person with no resources.

Table 16-5 Cranial Nerve Involvement in Dysarthria

Cranial Nerve	Distribution	Symptoms
CN V	Motor fibers innervate masseter, temporal pterygoid and digastric muscles.	1. Inability to chew, move jaw. Keeps mouth closed due to a degeneration of motor nucleus of CN V. 2. Inability to open mouth due to spasm of masseter muscles as in lockjaw.
CN VII (facial nerve)	Motor fibers innervate temporal, facial muscles of cheek, eye; muscles around mouth and neck (platysma) muscle.	1. Lack of facial expression. 2. Facial expression that is not symmetrical between both sides of the face. 3. Inability to produce sounds made by the lips such as b, m, v.
CN IX (glossopharyngeal nerve)	Motor fibers that innervate pharynx and tongue. Motor fibers that innervate pharynx and larnyx.	1. Difficulty in swallowing 2. Difficulty in articulating guttural sounds 3. Dysphonia 4. Absence of speech
CN XII (hypoglossal nerve)	Motor fiber innervation of tongue, anterior portion.	1. Inability to articulate lingual sounds: l, t, d, n.

The sequelae of past disease may have an impact on present illness. Many elderly patients have fought major infections without the help of penicillin. The effects of past disease may further reduce physiologic reserves. Chronic disease is also a part of growing older. The elderly person's chronic disease may also develop into an acute phase as a result of current illness. This is particularly true of the cardiopulmonary system. Multisystem failure may also occur.

Sensory perceptual deficits occur concomitantly with a loss or decrease in the senses of vision, hearing, touch, or smell. Coupled with the psychological and social changes that the person experiences, the elderly may feel isolated from others and the environment. Finally, ethical issues about the person's care arise because of advanced age.

A confused state in an elderly person is the biggest barrier to communication in that age group. Since confusion can happen so quickly and easily, and since it happens so frequently, nursing efforts need to be directed to preventing confusion in the elderly to ensure open lines of communication.[44]

Two causes of confusion in the elderly critically ill patient, lack of cardiovascular reserve and altered environment, are considered in relation to the ability to communicate. The loss of cardiovascular reserve in the elderly patient is a result of several factors. A decrease in the force and strength of cardiac contractility leads to a decrease in stroke volume.[45] This, coupled with irregularities in the conduction system, leads to a decrease in cardiac output. Peripheral venous pooling, aggravated by poor smooth muscle tone and inactivity, contribute to the low cardiac output. The low cardiac output contributes to a decrease in cerebral perfusion. A decrease in pulmonary perfusion as a primary problem or as a secondary complication of low cardiac output can further exacerbate confusion in the elderly through the mechanisms of hypoxemia. The slightly hypoxic elderly patient can express extreme signs of confusion, due to a lack of cardiovascular reserves. Awareness that the lack of physiologic reserves in the patient can contribute to confusion and result in a communication barrier is needed on the part of the nurse.

When placed in a critical-care unit, the patient may become disoriented very quickly and be unable to communicate physical and emotional needs. This is because the older person's home environment offers so many cues. The patient may be unable to see the clock very well, but the way the sun hits the kitchen table tells one the time of day. When the elderly person enters the critical-care unit, these home cues are lost, and the person may have no clues to orientation in a new surrounding.

Further complicating the matter is the age barrier between the nurse and patient. The nurse moves efficiently and briskly, while and the patient may be slow. When the nurse takes interest in the patient's concerns, one bridge is built. Discussing what goes on at home builds another bridge and can provide valuable information about health practices. Discussing the past as related to the present, or as a means of retaining orientation, builds yet another bridge.

Psychological Barriers

Psychological sequelae of critical illness and responses to the critical-care unit are well documented in the critical-care literature. But the nature of the psychological trauma has changed, just as the critical-care experience has changed. A review of an early work by Kaplan[46] points out the impact that lifelong cardiac disease had on the patient's personality development. Patients who had rheumatic heart disease for most of their lives and then underwent mitral commissurotomy had a difficult time adjusting to their new "well" status. The premorbid illness personality was difficult to reconcile to the new physical health status because of the disruption of the old psychological coping patterns and establishment of new psychological adaptive mechanisms.

The "intensive care unit syndrome," "ICU psychosis," and "postcardiotomy delirium" are terms applied to the symptoms of hallucination, illusions, time disorientation, and general confusion that occur after cardiac surgery and confinement in the open-heart recovery room.[47,48] The course of psychological sequelae attributed to postcardiotomy delirium was short-lived and resolved before the patient left the hospital. This is in contrast to the difficulties the mitral commissurotomy patient continued to experience after discharge. ICU psychosis has become a general term and is now applied to a variety of situations which include both medical and surgical patients.

Specific symptoms of psychological sequelae of intensive care are identified differently by reviewers and researchers. Kimball[49] identified three categories of psychological response in the critical-care unit: delirium, catastrophic reaction (a severe passive response to anxiety), and euphoria. The euphoric response constitutes a type of denial to the situation and is characterized by a sense of well-being. Scalzi notes four behavioral reactions: anxiety, denial, depression, and aggressive sexual behavior following acute myocardial infarction.[50]

In an attempt to examine all factors that might affect the psychological experience of the patient in the critical-care unit, Maron listed depression, withdrawal, anxiety, regression, hallucinations, and delusions, and cautioned that labels such as "ICU psychosis" may provide recognition of a psychological problem but fail to differentiate the mechanisms that may be involved.[51]

In the classic study by Hackett and Cassem, attention given by nurses to patients' psychological, social, and educational needs, as well as physical needs, went a long way toward alleviating psychological distress that patients might have otherwise experienced.[23] In the study, over 80 percent of patients experienced anxiety, and 60 percent depression. Areas cited as being important in minimizing psychological stress and thereby preventing "ICU syndrome" were the familiarity of the patient with his or her nurse, the familiarity of the nurse with the monitor and other equipment, frequent assessments and checking of the patient, information provided with respect to oxygen and fluid therapy, and the prompt arrival of the nurse when needed. This study clearly demonstrates that the willingness of the nurse to serve as an interpreter or bridge between the critical-care unit environment and the patient was a factor in eliminating psychological distress.

Anxiety

Anxiety is a feeling that may be similar in quality to fear but is not referable to an object in the environment; it arises from a disruption in the adaptive resources within the individual. In contrast, fear is the feeling aroused by the perception that danger exists in the environment. It arises from a stimulus external to the person. Anxiety and fear are two common psychological reactions in the critical-care unit that can cause a communication barrier between nurse and patient. Fear, because of its concrete orientation, is easier to identify and dispel than anxiety. For example, the patient may be fearful of needles and other painful objects, and the nurse can focus efforts on making the patient comfortable and providing reassurance concerning painful procedures involving needles.

Anxiety is not as easy to define, since it is related to the patient's own experience. Anxiety may result from the possibility or the idea of one's death, loss of power, prestige, loss of financial independence, etc. Two extremes of anxiety, catastrophic reaction and euphoric reaction, create communication barriers for the critical-care nurse to address. The patient who is experiencing a catastrophic reaction is often mute and immobile. It is difficult to communicate comfort, information, or support that may be needed. In contrast, the euphoric patient cannot accept or work through the situation, and instead presents a picture that everything is going very well. This may include laughing and joking about grave concerns. Careful, directed, and probing conversation with these patients, based on the knowledge of concerns of the critically ill patient, can direct or assist the patient in working through the causes of the anxiety. Ancillary personnel can be referral sources for problems that concern post-hospital care, finances, transportation, and the like. A further awareness that there are times when the patient is likely to experience anxiety—on admission, on transfer out of the CCU, and on discharge from the hospital—can help the nurse plan meaningful communication with the patient.[50] The anxiety a patient is experiencing must be dispelled or reduced to a manageable level before home instructions or other important information can be successfully provided.

Assessment and Diagnosis of Communication Impairment

Many communication barriers may exist in critical care. Barriers arise because of the environment, or the physiologic or emotional complications of critical illness, and because of sociocultural differences between the nurse and the patient. Whether the nurse engages in a formal paper and pencil assessment or performs a mental checklist assessment of the patient is not of consequence. What is important is that the nurse is aware of these potential barriers to communication, can identify when and how they will exist, and assesses frequently for these occurrences. This section discusses the assessment of communication impairment in the critically ill person.

Each critical-care unit has its own defining characteristics and physical arrangement. The staff, physicians and nurses, the type of hospital, and type of patients determine the ambiance of the unit. When performing an assessment of the environment to determine if there are communication barriers the following questions should be asked:

Is there provision of privacy with respect to the environment, confidentiality of information about the patient, and awareness of the patient's personal space?

What elements are present in the environment (i.e., noise, equipment, lighting) that distract the patient's or nurse's attention?

What maintains or facilitates the link between the patient's previous environment and the present one?

These questions serve as a starting point for the assessment process. The characteristic most likely to affect privacy is the layout of the unit. Whether or not private rooms are available for the patient is not as important as the attention that the nurse gives to creating an *atmosphere* of privacy for the patient. Closed curtains, doors, screens, and proper draping of the patient provide for his or her individuality. Probably the best way to assess for this is to stand at some central point in the unit—the nurse's station, the entryway, the central supply cart—and look around the unit. What can be seen? Row upon row of undraped patients? Or closed doors, curtains, and appropriately covered patients? This observation is done with cognizance of the fact that what is in plain view of the nurse is in plain view of other ancillary personnel as well.

Another aspect of a patient's privacy is the way in which confidential information about the patient is kept or disseminated. Obviously, the patient and significant others should be informed of information in a timely manner with respect for the patient's privacy. Do discussions about a patient's care occur in the middle of the unit? When this occurs out of necessity, it is the manner and decibel level in which they are conducted that has the potential to impinge on the patient's privacy.

Each nurse who cares for a patient should ask the following questions: Do I request permission to enter the patient's personal space? Do I tell the patient what I am doing, why, and when to expect discomfort? Do I stop and let the patient rest when it is requested of me? If "yes" is answered to these questions, it is fairly likely that the nurse is respecting the patient's personal space. If "no" is answered, the nurse might reconsider ways of interacting with patients. Since the patient usually waits for the nurse to initiate the communication process, the nurse must make a conscious effort to communicate with even seemingly unresponsive patients.

An assessment of each individual critical-care unit will yield individual quirks in the unit with respect to the environment and patient population. A coronary care unit is generally quiet. A cardiothoracic unit may be filled with the sounds of bubbling chest tubes, chest physiotherapy, and the frequent coughing and deep breathing exercises of patients. Once again, each nurse must assess the unit for auditory and visual distractions and attempt to minimize them. Alarms should be low, with flashing pump and monitor lights outside the patient's visual field. Lighting should be soft and indirect, or not directed into the patient's eyes. The nurse might look along the patient's visual field to see what is in line: a tangle of IVs, monitors, and equipment, or a picture, clock, or window or doorway to the outside? Distractions in the patient's environment lead to an overload of meaningless information and inhibit the communication process by usurping the patient's energy and taking his or her attention away from the nurse.

Patients in the midst of critical illness experience disruptions in their lives, and they may bring other, more pressing problems to the critical-care unit. The nurse should evaluate the care rendered the patient to determine if the patient's emotional and spiritual needs are being taken into consideration. Are personal hygiene habits taken into account? Can special visiting times be arranged for small children or elderly parents? It is surprising to learn that many patients are more concerned with people or situations left in the home environment than with the current illness, but this does occur.

An obvious communication barrier exists with the person who cannot speak or who is having difficulty speaking. Two lines of assessment can be pursued to determine if a difficulty in speaking is due to a functional or organic problem, to determine the extent of a barrier. Table 16-6 provides a systematic way of assessing a person's ability to communicate through speech. The patient's reac-

Table 16-6 Assessment of Speech Skills

Speech Skill	Nursing Assessment
Communication Reaction and/or response to environment, spoken word	Note patient's response to greeting and self-introduction. Observe patient's reaction to environment (opens eyes, follows sound and/or noise with eyes, head, or both).
Speech Output Word choice Fluency Grammar	Obtain sample of speech output to communicate. Initiate conversational speech with topic relating to patient's current illness—how and when it happened. Or: Allow patient to introduce topic for conversational speech.
Comprehension Ability to understand questions Ability to repeat words and sentences Ability to carry out motor acts Ability to understand words and phrases	Note patient's ability to understand the meaning of words spoken. Determine patient's ability to follow simple commands with appropriate motor acts. Rephrase questions to improve comprehension if patient has difficulty recognizing words and/or objects that fall into categories or classes.
Nonverbal Behavior Facial expression Movement of hand, head, etc. Other emotional responses	Observations of all nonverbal behavior.
Verbal Behavior Word-finding difficulty	Describe output (fluent or nonfluent). Identify reduction in spontaneous speech and effort to produce speech. Note character of speech errors (grammar, verbal substitutions, etc.). Record ability to self-monitor speech errors. Observe if patient is self-critical. Monitor and record nonverbal expressions associated with effort to self-correct. Analyze speech sample to identify communication problem. Record assessment as baseline; monitor for changes from baseline.

(Continued)

Table 16-6 Assessment of Speech Skills (Continued)

Speech Skill	Nursing Assessment
Nonlinguistic Factors	
Orientation	Differentiate nonlinguistic findings which may alter communication—confusion, memory deficits, etc.
Mental state	
Attention span	
Paresis and/or plegia	Pay particular attention to disorders of eye movements and visual field defects as possible nonlinguistic cause for poor performance.
Visual deficits	
Response to verbal stimuli	Observe context-related nonverbal responses.
No verbal output (mute)	Monitor motor responses, gesture, and other behavior.
	Obtain information from family regarding words and behavior associated with daily body functions.
	Observe spontaneous use of pantomime.
	Record inability to associate word and concept.

Source: Adapted from G. V. Baykin, Strategies for Increasing Communication with the Dysphasic Patient, *Dimensions of Critical Care Nursing*, vol. 3, 1984, pp. 279–281. Copyright by J. B. Lippincott and Company. Reprinted with permission.

tion to others, speech output, comprehension, nonverbal behavior, and other factors can be evaluated. An assessment of the patient's mental status is valuable in determining if his or her inability to communicate is due to a decreased level of consciousness or to overt emotional or cognitive impairments. Table 16-7 presents guidelines for assessing mental status.

Just as the environmental attributes of a critical-care unit differ, so does the cultural milieu of patients. In the United States, different ethnic groups prevail in different areas of the country. Many border states have an influx of foreign nationals as patients. The cultural variations which exist among national groups make it essential that critical-care nurses be familiar with the ethnic groups frequenting a health care system. Assessment of cultural differences should proceed along the following line of questioning: What language barriers are evident in terms of language spoken, use of slang, or English as a second language? What cultural variations exist that need to be considered when caring for a patient? What aspects of territoriality and intimate space are appropriate to observe in a given situation? What health or religious beliefs might affect the way the patient assimilates the critical illness?

Nursing Diagnosis and Interventions for Impaired Communication

Nursing diagnosis has been widely developed and accepted in clinical and academic practice since the first national group for classification of nursing diagnosis met in 1973. Over 50 diagnostic categories have been currently generated by the North American Nursing Diagnosis Association. Each category of nursing diagnosis contains the following: the title, etiologic and contributing factors, and defining characteristics. There are two aspects to the term "nursing diagnosis" that should not be confused, for it is both a problem-solving process and a statement of a patient's problem that nursing is educationally prepared and licensed to treat. When completing nursing care plans, nursing diagnosis can be used along with identification of other patient problems to direct and evaluate nursing care. By itself, the nursing diagnosis is not complete without correlating it to factors that emphasize a cause and effect relationship. Thus, the phrase "related to" must link the two parts of the nursing diagnosis: the nursing diagnostic label. The descriptive terms that follow the phrase "related to" are derived from the list of etiologic and contributing factors listed under the category.

Table 16-7 Assessment of Mental Status

Parameter	Nursing Assessment
General Appearance	Note overall appearance of patient in bed: Does he or she look comfortable? What is body position in bed (fetal, erect, etc.)?
	Note facial expression of patient: Does he seem worried or anxious? Is he frowning, smiling?
	Validate facial expression or body position by asking patient how he feels.
Emotional Status	
Anxiety	Note signs of apprehension, restlessness tremors, inability to concentrate, hold a conversation, focus on a task, or respond to her situation. Is she hyperalert?
Denial	Note signs of avoidance of discussion of illness or treatments.
	Note inappropriate laughing, talking, or boasting.
	Note plans for the future that are not realistic.
Level of Consciousness	
Awareness	Assess the patient's response to the environment and those in it. Is it appropriate, correct, and based on fact?
	Record level of consciousness. Is the patient sleepy, difficult to arouse, etc.?
Orientation	Note and record patient's orientation to person, place, and time, utilizing new questions to each assessment period.
	Determine if the patient has limited or altered awareness or precise awareness.
	Note whether disorientation is a result of misinterpretation of environmental cues or from receiving incorrect information.
Cognitive Functioning	
Short-term memory	Determine patient's ability to remember by asking questions related to events prior to interview time, but within a 2-to-4-hour span.
Long-term memory	Determine patient's ability to remember past events by asking him to recite medical history, or events which occurred prior to hospitalization. Validate responses to recent and remote occurrences in patient's history.
Ability to learn	Document ongoing efforts of patient teaching and responses.
	Discuss with patient new information that has been given frequently and throughout the day and patient's response to it.
	Present new information in a variety of ways; i.e., through pictures, tapes, and written word.
	Validate and record what patient remembers.
	Discuss how new information will be applied in current lifestyle.

Impaired Verbal Communication

"Impaired verbal communication" is a nursing diagnosis that can be utilized in conjunction with the material discussed in this chapter. *Impaired verbal communication* is defined as: "The state in which the individual experiences, or would experience, a decreased ability to speak appropriately or understand the meaning of words."[62] Etiologic and contributing factors of this nursing diagnosis can be classified as pathophysiologic, situational, and developmental. Table 16-8 lists the factors under each of these areas. Table 16-9 lists defining characteristics which one should look for when placing a person in this nursing diagnosis. Many problems that occur as a result of the patient's

Table 16-8 Etiologic and Contributing Factors to the Nursing Diagnosis: Impaired Verbal Communication

General Area	Specific Factors
Pathophysiologic	Cerebral involvement:
	Aphasia
	CVA
	Brain damage
	CNS depression
	Increased ICP
	Tumor
	Hypoxia
	Infection
	Neurologic impairment:
	Vocal cord paralysis
	Trigeminal neuralgia
	Cranial nerve involvement of CN V, VII, IX, XII
	Respiratory impairment
	Laryngeal edema
Situational	Surgery:
	Intubation
	Tracheostomy
	Tracheotomy
	Laryngectomy
	Surgical procedure of head/ neck, face, and mouth
	Pain
	Oral deformities
	Speech pathology:
	Stuttering
	Lisping
	Lack of privacy
Developmental	Age:
	Physical limitation due to advanced age or youth
	Mental retardation
	Psychological barriers

Table 16-9 Characteristics of the Nursing Diagnosis: Impaired Verbal Communication

Defining Characteristics
Stuttering
Slurred speech
Difficulty in finding correct word
Substitution of words
Unusual use of profanity
Weak or absent voice
Shortness of breath
Decreased auditory comprehension
Inattention to auditory cues
Confusion
Inability to speak dominant language

inability to communicate have been discussed in this chapter. Nursing care plans utilizing the nursing diagnosis system are included as the conclusion to this chapter so the nurse can see how nursing diagnosis can be used in specific instances of communication impairment, as well as obtain further information about specific nursing interventions for patients' problems. These nursing care plans present strategies for the nursing diagnosis, "impaired verbal communication."

Goals

1. The patient will demonstrate improved ability to communicate with others as evidenced by:
   a. Decreased frustration (absence of uncontrolled anger, crying etc.)
   b. Initiating patient/nurse contacts
   c. Utilization of a mutually accepted form of communication
2. The patient will understand what is being communicated and will respond.
3. The patient will be able to make his or her needs known despite cultural and language differences and will relate feelings of acceptance rather than isolation.

Nursing Interventions

1. Anticipate and reduce frustration associated with inability to communicate.
   a. Anticipate patient's feelings of frustration, encourage demonstrations of controlled crying or anger in order to vent frustration and provide for positive communication.

b. Anticipate patient's needs.

c. Reassure the patient verbally by touch and frequent checks.

d. Maintain a positive attitude that reassures the patient you will work with him or her to assure initial understanding.

e. If a procedure is planned that will render the patient speechless (i.e., intubation or tracheostomy) develop prior signals and cues to facilitate communication.

f. Record signals or cues that patient responds to on nursing care plan.

2. Assist the patient initiating contact with the nurse.

a. Place call bell or dinner bell within patient's reach.

b. Discuss with the patient your desire to fulfill his or her general needs, many of which you know because of your experience, and individual needs which the patient will need to communicate to you.

c. Allow time to stand at bedside without tasks to be done so the patient can make needs known.

d. Wait for the patient's response to the nurse's questions.

3. Assist the patient in determining what format of communication will best meet the need.

a. Assess the patient's speech skills and mental status (see Tables 16-6 and 16-7).

b. Clearest understanding of what is being said comes when the patient uses pantomine in conjunction with words. Encourage the patient to gesture, and mouth words or write notes and mouth words or write and gesture.

c. Use aids that assist patients, discard aids that confuse patients.

d. In laryngectomy patients utilize amplifier; allow laryngectomy patient hospitalized for other medical problems to use amplifier.

e. If respiratory status of tracheostomy patient allows, show patient how to cover tube to speak. Remind patient that speech will be softer, more raspy than usual, will require effort, and may produce shortness of breath. Use speaking cuffed tracheostomy tube if available.

f. Assist patient in completion of sentences of difficult words.

4. General interventions for communicating with the aphasic patient include:

a. Respond to the patient as an adult.

b. Speak slowly, clearly, and enunciate clearly.

c. Remain on one topic of conversation.

d. Allow up to 10 to 30 s for the patient to respond to questions.

e. Reduce environmental stimuli such as TV or radio when talking with patient.

f. Make periods of communication short to avoid tiring patient.

g. Screen visitors to avoid tiring the patient.

h. Encourage and support the patient with statements that reflect her feelings when she is unable to articulate them.

5. Interventions for the patient with receptive aphasia are based on the understanding that the patient's comprehension of the written and spoken word is poor.

a. Direct patient to the proper word when circumlocutory speech is present.

b. During therapy sessions, introduce sentences for the patient to complete since object naming may be poor.

c. Encourage and support the patient and family through teaching and attendance at therapy sessions.

6. Interventions for the patient with expressive aphasia, who has generally good word understanding but poorly articulated, slow speech requiring great effort:

a. The patient may find singing or swearing easier than speaking. Singing familiar songs, or putting sentences to a tune may help the patient express himself. Small words may be omitted in sentences. Encourage the patient to use nouns and verbs.

b. Introduce one word or phrase for the patient to repeat. Therapy sessions should be short, less than 30 min. Exercises should be changed as the patient tires. The patient should not be worked to the point of fatigue.

c. Models of items utilized in activities of daily living, such as a toilet, chair, etc., can assist the patient to make his needs known.

d. Support and encouragement from the family can greatly help the patient. The family should receive teaching regarding the patient's therapy. Attendance at therapy sessions may be beneficial before discharge. The family should be taught that the rehabilitation process continues for 6 months to 1 year after the initial episode.

7. Determine which of the following interventions would be appropriate for the non-English-speaking patient:

   a. Utilize hospital policy for caring for a foreign-language-speaking patient.

   b. Use interpreters, language guides, tapes, picture books, or flash cards to help the patient feel comfortable and receive needed information.

   c. Identify alternative sources of information if preceding are not available, such as the hospital library, local community library, community groups, or social support services within the hospital.

   d. Allow more time to give information when scheduling teaching sessions.

   e. Use gesture, signs, models, or pictures when language is not possible. The tone of voice, maintaining eye contact, and touch will help reassure the patient.

   f. Utilize personnel trained as interpreters. Avoid using ancillary hospital personnel, taking them from their jobs, or using family members, who may not know hospital policy or medical terminology.

   g. Allow enough time, as the communication process is time-consuming.

   h. Direct interpreters to the most important areas first, to save the patient's energy.

8. Monitor use of medical terminology by patient's care givers:

   a. Offer explanations of medical terms used by others. Rephrase explanations, directions, or information so the patient can understand them.

   b. Utilize the patient as the point of reference, not the equipment: "You have a slow heartbeat," not "The monitor shows a bradycardia."

9. Identify nonverbal cues from the patient, and establish respect for patient's intimate space and emotions.

   a. Maintain eye contact when talking with patient.

   b. Provide for pleasant visual stimuli such as poster, window, etc.

   c. Remove disturbing scenes from patient's line of vision.

   d. Ask patient's permission to expose private body parts.

   e. Maintain patient's dignity through the use of drapes when performing procedures.

   f. Do not persist in performing a procedure if the patient is in pain, or asks for a rest period. Try another approach or get assistance.

   g. Inform the patient when procedures are to be done, how long they will take, and what they will entail.

   h. Ask patient his feelings regarding intimate distance, how he feels about his care givers, and if he would like things handled in a different manner.

10. Identify facial expressions and confirm patient's feelings.

11. Assist patient in expression of emotions, and provide the privacy needed for expression.

Additional Nursing Strategies for Impaired Communication

Facilitating Understanding through Alternate Means

Communication involves more than talking with and listening to patients. This chapter has presented several ways to overcome communication barriers. In addition, strategies such as therapeutic touch, speech therapy, use of assistive devices, and nursing care plans can assist the nurse in meeting a patient's communication needs. Some techniques reviewed in this section have a physiologic basis, others are based on principles of psychotherapy, while others have their origin in Eastern meditation rituals. Some of the following techniques involve specialized training, while others do not; some also may be labeled as unconventional. Each nurse is encouraged to examine his or her own abilities and determine which of the following techniques might be useful to each critically ill patient.

Empathy

The idea of the empathetic helper as a vital part of the healing or helping relationship was pioneered in the 1960s. According to this philosophy of a helping relationship, the helper is rated on a five-point scale from one to five: One represents hurtful or negative helping behavior and five represents the highest level of empathy, showing that the helper has understood the patient's message, sought clarification and further information, and assisted in the patient's exploration of the meaning of the message. Those in the helping professions should rate above three on the scale to be considered empathetic to their patients. Surprisingly, research has shown that without a training program, those in the helping professions generally rate below the three level. After a training program has been instituted, health professionals are generally found to improve their scores, and can be classified as empathetic to their patients.[52,53]

Empathy can be defined as the attempt to understand from another person's point of view what that person is experiencing. It is different from sympathy, in which one relates one's own experience to another person's experience. When the critical-care nurse practices empathy with patients, an attempt is made to determine what patients' comments mean and how the nurse can help patients help themselves. If the patient says "That pattern on my monitor sure looks funny," the nurse is not being empathetic if the response is "Oh, don't worry, it looks fine." An empathetic response would investigate the patient's line of thinking—Is there concern that the monitor is broken and the pattern is not accurate? Is there concern that the heart is "funny" or that something is wrong? Or is the patient seeking information about the monitor and how it displays an ECG? The simple response, that "it looks fine" is not the best, because it does not explore the real meaning underlying the patient's comment. Exploration of casual comments made by patients can lead to an exchange of information and feelings that goes beyond a superficial level and that benefits the patient.

The use of empathy in the critical-care unit can be a valuable tool with patients who are angry, acting "inappropriately," or who are uncommunicative. Verbal skills on the part of the patient need not be intact for this technique to be utilized. It may be of assistance to the verbally impaired patient who has intact hearing and understanding. This may be the case when the nurse is empathetic about the patient's inability to speak.

Transactional Analysis

Interpersonal relationships were analyzed and categorized by Berne[54] and later Harris[55] and popularized as *transactional analysis* (TA). Transactional analysis in the health care system has been used in management and in critical care.[56,57] There are several components of transactional analysis, including structural analysis, games, and scripts. The most basic component and the one most frequently utilized in the health care setting is structural analysis. Structural analysis views the human personality as being composed of three ego states, the *parent ego,* the *child ego,* and the *adult ego.* Interactions between people occur in one of these ego states. Ego states change continually and may be dependent on the situation, the message from the other person, the general health of the person, and past coping abilities.

The milieu of the critical-care unit has been likened in the past to a family situation, where the physician and head nurse are the parents, and the staff nurses and residents are the children. Perhaps the reason for the increase in the popularity of TA in the health care setting is the dependent, childlike state of the critically ill patient. The critical-care unit nurse may seem to be the parent figure to the patient. For TA to be helpful in the communication process in the critical-care unit, the nurse must use it as a way to analyze interactions between patients and staff and determine if they are helpful or harmful to the patient.

In general, adult-to-adult ego state responses would be considered the ideal of most interactions. Child-child would not be considered as helpful to the patient as the patient would not benefit from the interaction. The parent-to-child interaction may help the critically ill patient through the illness until enough ego strength is gathered for the patient to move back again to the adult state. Further study in the area of TA can assist the nurse in understanding patterns of interaction with other people and approaches to therapeutic interactions.

Nursing Care Plans

One very traditional way of facilitating understanding is the use of standardized nursing care plans (NCP) for a specific type of patient or family communication need. Breu and Dracup[58] developed a standard NCP for use with patients who had a grieving spouse. Regular nursing interventions based on needs identified through nursing research provided a continuum of care that facilitated communication.[59]

This format of utilizing the NCP to direct efforts at communication is one that is easily adapted to most critical-care units. The use of nursing diagnosis and assessment to identify communication problems sets the NCP process in motion. The NCP serves as a guide to all those who come in contact with the communication-impaired patient by identifying types of interactions best suited for sending and receiving messages to and from the individual patient.

Use of Touch

The use of therapeutic touch as a nursing intervention with the intent to heal was pioneered by Dolores Krieger.[60] Therapeutic touch can be distinguished from casual touch or reassuring touch because of the training it requires. Patients who are treated by a trained practitioner report a feeling of warmth when the practitioner lays hands on the patient. A sense of well-being, calmness, or relaxation may also be reported. When physiologic data are monitored there may be a rise in hemoglobin values.[60] Nurses trained in therapeutic touch are able to effect change in their patients' feelings of anxiety, as well as in physiologic data.[21,60]

Casual touch, when applied frequently and in a consistent manner, may be of great use in comforting, reassuring, and communicating with patients.[61] Casual touch, touch that occurs within the course of nursing treatments or examinations, differs from therapeutic touch in that it requires no special training and does not have healing as its intent.

Casual touch is essential for the patient with a communication impairment such as blindness, deafness, or stroke. The firm, reassuring touch of the critical-care nurse can overcome many communication barriers. Each individual nurse can utilize casual touch in everyday nursing practice in critical care.

Hand-holding is a variation of casual touch that may promote a patient's comfort and a sense of calmness or reassurance for the patient. The nurse sits or stands at the patient's bedside for a prescribed period of time each day and holds the patient's hand. This time of human contact, without any nursing or medical procedures, gives the patient the opportunity to talk with the nurse. If the patient is unable to communicate verbally with the nurse, this time of human contact may reassure the patient that the nurse cares for the patient as a person beyond the nursing responsibilities.

Devices

Technologic devices will surely become more cost effective and available in the next decade. Personal computers can be fitted with software that allows a person to enter a typed message, which activates an electronic voice message, thus allowing the person to "speak." As computers come closer to the bedside in critical-care nursing, it may be practical for patients to bring software used at home so that they can communicate in the hospital setting. Since electronic voice packages are fairly expensive, they are not practical for short-term use. Drawbacks to the use of electronic voice packages for computer systems are that the patient must be able to concentrate and also must be able to use a keyboard. Patients who are critically ill might have difficulty using computers in the critical-care setting. A more promising development is the speaking cuffed tracheostomy tube which allows the patient being mechanically ventilated to speak, while maintaining the airway. This device is a modification of a standard double cuffed tracheostomy tube. A separate air hose source is supplied by a thin tube attached between the inner and outer cannula. The air is directed through an air channel toward the vocal cords. Thus air passes across the vocal cords and vibration occurs, which results in laryngeal speech. These are just two technologic developments that can facilitate communication between the nurse and the critically ill patient.

References

1. Obier, K., & Haywood, L. J. (1973). Enhancing therapeutic communication with acutely ill patients. *Heart and Lung, 2,* 49–53.
2. Ritchie, J. A. (1981). Meeting the information needs of the critically ill. *Dimensions in Health Service, 58,* 15–17.
3. Baxter, S. (1975). Psychological problems of intensive care—1. *Nursing Times,* 922–923.

4. Thomas, S. A., et al. (1982). Patients' cardiac response to nursing interviews in a CCU. *Dimensions of Critical Care Nursing, 1,* 198–205.

5. Clark, J. M. (1981). Communication in nursing. *Nursing Times,* 12–18.

6. Budd, S., & Brown, W. (1974). Effect of a reorientation technique on postcardiotomy delirium. *Nursing Research, 23,* 341–348.

7. Owens, J. F., & Hutelmeyer, C. M. (1982). The effect of preoperative intervention on delirium in cardiac surgical patients. *Nursing Research, 31,* 60–62.

8. Schwartz, L. P., & Brenner, Z. R. (1979). Critical care unit transfer: Reducing patient stress through nursing interventions. *Heart and Lung, 8,* 540–546.

9. Eisendrath, S., & Dunkel, J. (1979). Psychological issues in intensive care unit staff. *Heart and Lung, 8,* 751–758.

10. Dunkel, J., & Eisendrath, S. (1983). Families in the intensive care unit: Their effect on staff. *Heart and Lung, 12,* 258–560.

11. Fuller, B. F., & Foster, G. M. (1982). The Effect of family/friend visits vs. staff interaction on stress arousal of surgical intensive care patients. *Heart and Lung, 11,* 457–463.

12. Gardner, D., & Stewart, N. (1978). Staff involvement with families of patients in critical care units. *Heart and Lung, 9,* 105–110.

13. Chatham, M. A. (1978). The effect of family involvement on patients' manifestations of postcardiotomy psychosis. *Heart and Lung, 7,* 995–999.

14. Doerr, B. C., & Jones, J. W. (1979). Effect of family preparation on the state anxiety level of the CCU patient. *Nursing Research, 28,* 315–316.

15. Molter, N. E. (1979). Needs of relatives of critically ill patients: A descriptive study. *Heart and Lung, 8,* 332–339.

16. Rasie, S. M. (1980). Meeting families' needs helps you meet ICU patients' needs. *Nursing '80, 10,* 32–35.

17. Rodgers, C. D. (1981). Needs of relatives of cardiac surgery patients during the critical care phase. *Focus on Critical Care, 10,* 50–55.

18. Friedman, E. H. (1982). Stress and intensive care nursing: A ten year reappraisal. *Heart and Lung, 11,* 26–28.

19. Gardner, D., Parzen, Z. D., & Stewart, N. (1980). The nurses' dilemma: Mediating stress in critical care units. *Heart and Lung, 9,* 103–106.

20. Oskins, S. L. (1979). Identification of situational stressors and coping methods by ICU nurses. *Heart and Lung, 8,* 953–960.

21. Hein, E. C. (1980). *Communication in nursing practice* (2d ed.). Boston: Little, Brown.

22. Wedenback, E., & Falls, C. E. (1978). *Communication: Key to effective nursing.* New York: Teresias Press.

23. Hackett, J. P., Cassem, N. H., & Wishnie, H. A. (1968). The coronary care unit; an appraisal of its psychological hazards. *The New England Journal of Medicine, 279,* 1365–1370.

24. Daley, L. (1984). The perceived immediate needs of families with relatives in the intensive care setting. *Heart and Lung, 13,* 231–237.

25. Ashworth, P. (1979). Sensory deprivation 2, the acutely ill. *Nursing Times,* 290–293.

26. Helton, M. C., Gordon, S. H., & Nunnery, S. L. (1980). The correlation between sleep deprivation and the intensive care unit syndrome. *Heart and Lung, 9,* 464–468.

27. Kinney, M. (1981). Survey of critical care nursing practice, Part II. Unit characteristics. *Heart and Lung, 10,* 1051–1054.

28. Hansell, H. N. (1984). The behavioral effects of noise on man: The patient with "intensive care unit psychosis." *Heart and Lung, 13,* 59–65.

29. Leininger, M. (1984). Transcultural nursing: An essential knowledge and practice field for today. *The Canadian Nurse, 80,* 41–45.

30. Diaz-Duque, O. F. (1982). Overcoming the language barrier: Advice from an interpreter. *American Journal of Nursing, 82,* 1380–1382.

31. Kubricht, D. W., & Clark, J. A. (1982). Foreign patients: A system for providing care. *Nursing Outlook, 30,* 55–57.

32. Spradley, J. P., & McCurdy, D. W. (1972). *The cultural experience, ethnography in complex society.* Kingsport, TN: Kingsport Press.

33. Spiro, D., & Heidrich, F. (1983). Lay understanding of medical terminology. *The Journal of Family Practice, 17,* 227–229.
    Heidt, P. (1981). Effect of therapeutic touch on anxiety level of hospitalized patients. *Nursing Research, 30,* 32–37.

34. Johnson, S. H. (Ed.). (1982). Emotional care in the ICU, St. Lukes Hospital, Milwaukee. *Dimensions in Critical Care Nursing, 1,* 166–171.

35. Mahoney, E. K. (1980). Alterations in cognitive functioning in the brain-damaged patient. *Nursing Clinics of North America, 15,* 283–292.

36. Salyer, J., & Stuart, B. J. (1985). Nurse-patient interaction in the intensive care unit. *Heart and Lung, 14,* 20–24.

37. Vitello-Cicciu, J. M. (1984). Recalled perception of patients administered pancuronium bromide. *Focus on Critical Care, 11,* 23–35.

38. Pickersgill, M. J., & Lincoln, N. B. (1983). Prognostic indicators and the pattern of recovery in aphasic

stroke patients. *Journal of Neurology, Neurosurgery and Psychiatry, 46,* 130–139.

39. Piotrowski, M. M. (1978). Aphasia: Providing better nursing care. *Nursing Clinics of North America, 13,* 543–554.

40. Marshall, R. C., & Phillips, D. S. (1983). Prognosis for improved verbal communication in aphasic stroke patients. *Archives of Physical Medicine and Rehabilitation, 64,* 597–600.

41. Louis, M. C., & Povse, S. M. (1980). Aphasia and endurance: Considerations in the assessment and care of the stroke patient. *Nursing Clinics of North America, 15,* 265–282.

42. Blanco, K. M. (1982). The aphasic patient. *Journal of Neurosurgical Nursing, 14,* 34–37.

43. Wolanin, M. O. (1984). Considering the elderly critical care patient. *Dimensions in Critical Care Nursing, 3,* 196–197.

44. Foreman, M. D. (1984). Acute confusional states in the elderly: An algorithm. *Dimensions in Critical Care Nursing, 3,* 207–215.

45. Hamner, M. L., & Lalor, L. J. (1983). The aged patient in the critical care setting, *Focus on Critical Care, 10,* 22–29.

46. Kaplan, S. M. (1956). Psychological aspects of cardiac disease: A study of patients experiencing mitral commissurotomy. *Psychosomatic Medicine, 18,* 221–233.

47. Blachy, P. H., & Starr, A. (1964). Postcardiotomy delirium. *American Journal of Psychiatry, 121,* 371–375.

48. Kornfeld, D. S., Zimberg, S., & Malm, J. R. (1965). Psychiatric complications of open heart surgery. *The New England Journal of Medicine, 273,* 287–290.

49. Kimball, C. P. (1969). Psychological responses to the experience of open heart surgery: 1. *American Journal of Psychiatry, 126,* 348–359.

50. Scalzi, C. C. (1973). Nursing management of behav-ioral responses following AMI. *Heart and Lung, 2,* 62–69.

51. Maron, J., et al. (1973). Toward a unified approach to psychological factors in the ICU. *Critical Care Medicine, 1,* 81–84.

52. La Monica, E. L., et al. (1976). Empathy training as the major thrust of a staff development program. *Nursing Research, 25,* 447–450.

53. Williamson-Kirkland, T. E., & Williamson-Kirkland, R. N. (1982). Rehabilitation medicine: Follow-up study on teaching communication skills. *Archives of Physical Medicine and Rehabilitation, 63,* 31–33.

54. Berne, E. (1961). *Transactional analysis in psychotherapy.* New York: Grove Press.

55. Harris, T. A. (1969). *I'm OK, you're OK: A practical guide to transactional analysis.* New York: Harper & Row.

56. Quinn, D. (1984). What makes us tick. *Nursing Mirror, 159,* 21–24.

57. Hill, R. L., & Simon, B. (1984). Transactional analysis: A better patient approach. *Focus on Critical Care 11,* 11–16.

58. Breu, C. S., & Dracup, K. A. (1978). Helping the spouse of critically ill patients. *American Journal of Nursing, 78,* 51–53.

59. Dracup, K. A., & Breu, C. (1978). Using nursing research findings to meet the needs of grieving spouses. *Nursing Research, 27,* 212–216.

60. Krieger, D. (1975). Therapeutic touch: The imprimatur of nursing. *American Journal of Nursing, 75,* 784–787.

61. Steffee, D. R., Sutu, K. A., & Delcalzo, P. V. (1985). More than a touch: Communicate with a blind and deaf patient. *Nursing '85, 15,* 36–39.

62. Carpenito, L. (1983). *Nursing diagnosis: application to clinical practice.* Philadelphia: J. B. Lippincott.

17

Teaching and Learning

Anne Elizabeth
Belcher

Introduction

At no previous time in the evolution of critical-care nursing has patient education assumed the position of importance which it now enjoys. The major reason for the increased emphasis on this essential nursing function is the impact of the prospective payment system on health care. By limiting hospitals' reimbursement for services rendered, the government, and eventually other third-party payors, make each day of patients' stay a critical one—not just for the provisions of care but also for comprehensive teaching and discharge planning.

For many patients, the intensive care unit may be the only patient care setting where they are hospitalized. In addition, increasing numbers of these patients are being discharged to go home in a stable but critically ill condition. As a result of these changes in the delivery of critical care, nurses should be addressing such patient education issues as:[1]

How can discharge planning be provided in light of staff reductions, increased patient acuity, and nurses' resumption of previously non-nursing functions?

How should patient teaching be modified for the critically ill patient?

What indicators of patients' readiness to learn should be used in critical-care settings?

How long must a patient be in the hospital in order to receive adequate discharge planning and patient education?

How should the special learning needs of the elderly be addressed when planning and implementing patient education?

Defining Patient Education

Patient education, viewed as a part of the nursing process, is a planned, organized activity in which are considered the patients' individual right and need to know about health maintenance and promotion, prevention of illness, treatment, and rehabilitation. It is not only a patient's right but also a nursing responsibility.

Narrow[2] defines patient teaching as "The process of helping a person to learn those things that will enable him to live a longer and/or fuller life and helping him learn how to reach his optimal level of physical and mental health." The emphasis on process is an important one; the American Hospital Association[3] described planned patient education as a process which includes the conduct of a needs assessment; the setting of objectives; the development of an action plan; and the implementation, documentation, and evaluation of that plan.

The target population for patient education is those individuals and their families who have entered the health care delivery system for diagnosis, treatment, and rehabilitation. The services developed in response to patient and family educational needs should include information regarding ways to use various health care services, preparation for medical and nursing procedures, assistance in managing disease during hospitalization and after discharge, and behavior modification for health promotion and disease prevention.

Current Status and Future Directions

The goals of patient education are (1) to inform individuals about health, illness, and disability, and the ways in which they can improve and protect their own health, including more efficient use of the health care delivery system; (2) to motivate people to want to change to more healthful practices; (3) to help persons learn the skills needed to adopt and maintain healthful practices and lifestyles; and (4) to advocate changes in the environment which facilitate healthful conditions and behavior.

Patient education has assumed what has been called "a degree of motherhood status"; everyone agrees that it is an essential service and every health profession wants to be involved in it. The issues on which critics now focus are those of:

1. Access—for whom should services be provided?
2. Patient privilege—what should be taught?
3. Professional privilege—who should teach it?
4. The nature of evaluation—process or outcome?

One of several reasons for the increased interest in patient education is its income-producing potential, its efficiency-enhancing effect on health services. Burke[4] notes that educated patients are more likely to comply with prescribed therapy; experience lessened stress and anxiety; and sustain shorter hospital stays, fewer emergency room admissions, and reduced mortality. Miller[5] also notes that patients who have had preoperative instruction spend less time in the hospital, have fewer postoperative complications, experience less pain, and resume normal activities sooner.

The self-care perspective on patient education[6] has as its goal the anticipation of risk, derived from patients' perceived needs and preferences. The patient-learner determines alone or in collaboration with the nurse the content, teaching and learning methods, and criteria for evaluation. This approach results in lessened patient dependency on the nurse and other health care providers.

The focus of self-care education is on increased awareness of the hazards of health care, the "how-tos" of reducing the risk of iatrogenic illness, and methods for changing the health care system to conform to patients' needs and preferences. This approach relies on the knowledge and skills which the patient already has, such as traditional family health practices or home remedies, or autonomous self-healing. The nurse's key strategy is to encourage circumstances wherein problem-

posing skills of the patient are acknowledged and supported.

Given the current climate of forced shorter hospitalization, increasing demands on available time, and the need to give acutely ill patients highly technical information as quickly as possible, nurses must learn to teach patients and families more effectively in less time. Harrell and Frauman[7] suggested the following cost-containment strategies for patient education: (1) teach patients in groups with printed or audiovisual materials; (2) train other, less costly personnel such as volunteers to do some aspects of patient education; and (3) focus on assessing individual patient needs and directing learning activities.

A philosophical issue which affects the process of patient education in a variety of ways is that of beliefs about learning. While most learning theorists define learning as an enduring change in behavior,[8] there are educational program planners who prefer to focus on learning as gaining new knowledge or skills. One's perspective on learning thus guides the selection of teaching strategies and, more importantly, the criteria used for learner evaluation. It is certainly less time- and resource-consuming to view learning as primarily the attainment of information and abilities, but the long-range goal of self-care cannot be assured unless there is a focus on resultant changes in patient and family behavior.

Factors Which Affect Teaching and Learning

Factors frequently identified by nurses as hindering patient teaching are low patient motivation; poor availability and quality of teaching aids; noise; lack of sufficient time; patients' impaired sensory perception, that is, poor eyesight or poor hearing; poor reading ability; and lack of family involvement. Other nurse-related factors include the *lack* of (1) patient teaching as a priority, (2) knowledge regarding the content, (3) teaching skills, (4) communication among members of the health care team, and (5) resultant *lack* of continuity of instruction and evaluation.

The enhancement of patient motivation, a complex challenge, will be discussed in a separate section, as will the availability and quality of teaching aids. Nurses can learn to control noise in a variety

of ways such as putting a sign on the patient/
classroom door, prearranging quiet time, using
settings distant from noise sources, and selecting
teaching times when there is decreased activity in
the area. Nurses can also more effectively manage
their time by using "routine" patient contacts for
teaching—for example, during the bath or meals—
by supplementing one-to-one or classroom instruction with self-instructional audiovisual materials,
and by sharing teaching activities with colleagues.
Patients' impaired sensory perception may require
assistive devices such as corrective lenses, a magnifying glass, a hearing aid, posters, and other
enlarged image or print media. Patients with poor
reading ability will also benefit from visual aids
such as photographs, diagrams, movies, and videotapes. In some instances it is necessary to involve
the family and/or significant others in patient teaching sessions so that they can assist the patient with
self-care. Teaching these persons may also heighten
their involvement in and commitment to the patient's self-sufficiency.

Dealing with nurse factors requires a variety
of strategies. Corkadel and McGlashan[9] described
a series of classes designed for staff nurses which
addressed the areas of role clarification and resource utilization, nurse–patient rapport, content
review, learning needs assessment, assessment of

readiness to learn, teaching strategies, and documentation. Hinthorne[10] developed a Patient Teaching Flow Sheet to help nurses perform and
document patient teaching (see Tables 17-1 and
17-2). Whitehouse[11] also designed a patient teaching
record which included general topics as well as
specific information presented, documentation of
time and teacher, comments shared by the nurse
and patient, and an evaluation section. Planned
conferences using real patient situations can serve
as both a learning experience for the staff and an
instructional planning session for the patient. Whatever methods are used to overcome nurses' real
or perceived barriers to patient teaching, nursing
administration should evidence its support through
the provision of time, money, and recognition to
the nursing staff.

Learning Needs Assessment

Assessment of the patient's learning needs has as
its purposes the anticipation and/or recognition of
learning needs, establishment of mutually identified
educational goals, the determination of the preexisting knowledge base, and the correction of misinformation. Assessment can be accomplished
through patient and family interviews, written ques-

Table 17-1 Hinthorne's Directions for the Use of the Patient
Teaching Flow Sheet

1. As the patient is admitted and you are interviewing him for the patient profile you
   have an excellent opportunity to assess the patient's learning needs. Enter these in
   the column "Teaching Needs" in terms of patient behavior. See Table 17-2.
2. At this time you can decide the teaching methods that would be most
   appropriate for this patient. Enter these in the column "Teaching Approach." See
   example.
3. As the staff initiates these approaches, the date is entered. This communicates to
   all members of the health team just exactly what the teaching plan is. Thus
   anyone on the staff can initiate an approach at the time most conducive for
   patient learning.
4. When the patient demonstrates that he has achieved the objective, note the date
   and sign it.
5. If the patient is unable to learn (confused, forgetful) please note this across the
   top of the Teaching Sheet.
6. If you are able to teach the family or significant others, please note this across top
   of sheet, ie. "Daughter Taught."
7. In these cases use the sheet as you would for the patient. Family should be
   included in all teaching situations when possible.

Source: R. Hinthorne, Teaching nurses how to teach patients. *Nursing Management,* 1983, *14*(9),
30–33.

Table 17-2 Problem Oriented Flow Sheet for General Patient Teaching

Medical Record	Problem Oriented Flow Sheet—General				
Problem Numbers and Titles (*Do Not Abbreviate*)					
Patient Teaching				Verbalizes and/or demon.	
Teaching Needs	**Teaching Approach**	**Date**		**know.**	**Signature**
Identify action	1. Write out for patient	5/1			
dosage, side effects	2. Explain as you give	5/1			
of Digoxin	medicine x 3 day				
Lasix	3. Question patient	5/4		5/4	D. Miller
Select proper food-2 GmNa	1. Dietition consult	5/2			
Hi K	2. Hand out list	5/2			
	3. Discuss			5/6	D. Miller
Explain A & P of heart	1. "Video" I am Joe's Heart	5/4			
	2. Discuss				
Recognize symptoms which	1. Hand out list	5/6			
require medical attention	2. Discuss				

Source: R. Hinthorne, Teaching nurses how to teach patients. *Nursing Management*, 1983, *14*(9), 30–33.

tionnaires, chart audit, review of the research literature, evaluation of relevant health care and illness statistics, and conferences with nurse colleagues and other members of the health care team. Much can be learned by listening with a third ear—that is, hearing what the patient does *not* say as well as what is said. Facilitative responding, listening carefully and reflecting back to the patient the feelings and content of statements, may help both patient and nurse to identify general and specific learning needs.

"Therapeutic seeding," described by Corkadel and McGlashan,[12] is a technique used to "plant ideas" via suggestion in the patient's mind. Given time to think about the idea, the patient can then identify personal learning needs. An example of this technique is "Many of our cardiac patients have questions about their postdischarge diet. Perhaps you have some, too."

Factors Affecting Learning Needs

Each patient's learning needs are affected by such factors as knowledge, past experience, values, priorities, and willingness to change. Determining the patient's preexisting knowledge, skills, and/or attitudes provides a point of reference for identifying learning needs. The patient may reveal incorrect or inaccurate knowledge or skills which need to be corrected as soon as possible in order to build on a sound base. The adult's past experience in life and as a learner can either help or hinder learning. Positive self-esteem regarding oneself as a person and as a learner can heighten the patient's desire to learn and willingess to change, whereas failures in life and in learning may cause fears and anxiety in the patient which prevent learning. In addition, past experiences which are in conflict with what the patient is asked to learn may result in resistance to change.

Adults value information and skills which help them to live their lives more happily and more productively, which help them both to avoid and solve problems, and to be self-directed and independent. The adult's priorities for learning relate to these goals and may seem, to the nurse, to be trivial or unimportant, such as living on a restricted diet, maintaining or regaining sexual function, or resuming the role as family wage earner. However, the nurse should encourage the patient to share these priorities so that mutually satisfying goal setting can be done.

Age can be a useful indicator of a patient's priorities, according to Taylor.[13] For example, teenaged to young adult patients consider appearance the highest priority. Learning about bowel, bladder, or sexual function is also a high priority; other teaching is secondary until these needs are addressed. Middle-aged patients also consider appearance an important priority; they want to understand problems with bowel, bladder, or sexual function but are uncomfortable discussing them and worry most about family acceptance of changes in body image. Elderly patients consider function a higher priority than appearance, are uncomfortable discussing bodily functions, and accept the inevitability of loss affecting body image, especially if it prolongs life or brings comfort.

Learning from Patients about Their Needs

Barrett and Schwartz,[14] interested in what and how much patients want or need to know, administered a questionnaire to 15 hospitalized patients. While the knowledge level varied with regard to causes, effects, and prognosis of the illness, treatments, and tests, most said they wanted to know (1) the name of the illness, (2) how the illness affected their body, (3) what to expect about recovery, (4) what to expect from medical tests, and (5) how the condition would affect their life.

While most patients want at least some information about their illness and treatment, some would rather "let the doctor decide" or have a family member receive the information. Periodic reassessment of this patient's "need not to know" should be done and questions answered as they are posed by the patient.

Patients also have much to teach nurses, which in turn makes patient teaching more individualized and effective. Taylor[15] offers several tips for learning from patients about their needs:

1. Discover what the patient already knows.
2. Ask the patient about his or her treatment; for example, "How have you been doing this procedure?" or, "Which way is best for you?"
3. Reinforce book learning with real-life examples.
4. Do not be defensive about a patient's criticism.
5. Learn from the things the patient doesn't say, including nonverbal behavior such as strained facial expression, nail biting, excessive eating, or smoking.

Need and Readiness to Learn: Potential Obstacles

Individualizing a patient's instruction requires an in-depth assessment of the patient's current knowledge, skills, and attitudes; previous health and educational experiences; preferred learning modes; and cultural, social, and economic factors. Stanton[16] (Fig. 17-1) developed a diagrammatic representation of the factors which she believes govern both patients' needs and their readiness to learn. These include intellectual capacity, developmental stage, personal characteristics, prior experiences, sociocultural group, religious group, prevalent life needs, and stage of illness. Any number of these factors may also be obstacles to a patient's learning. For example, Caron and Roth,[17] in studying the effectiveness of a peptic ulcer regimen teaching program, identified three specific sets of obstacles: the patient's lack of understanding of certain key concepts, such as acid neutralization; erroneous concepts previously learned, for example, the ineffectiveness of antacid therapy; and fears and concerns present at the time of illness, including fear of loss of job or spouse.

Murray and Zentner[18] described these and other prohibitors to teaching and learning which need to be acknowledged and considered in planning for a patient's learning:

1. Language or reading response—individuals decode instructional messages in relation to background situations, prejudices, and moods, which affect belief and comprehension.
2. Culture—new ideas and practices are judged in relation to existing customs and beliefs.
3. Myths and unconscious resistance.
4. Personal prejudices related to race, personality, status, sex, etc.

To overcome language as a prohibitor, a variety of audiovisual aids should be used as adjuncts to verbal explanations, such as motion pictures, videotapes, slides, and photographs. In response to culture as a prohibitor, there are a variety of useful strategies: (1) Consult important persons whose prestige can lend influence to the recommended change in behavior, and then refer to them in teaching sessions; (2) develop a feeling for the culture's beliefs, attitudes, knowledge, and behav-

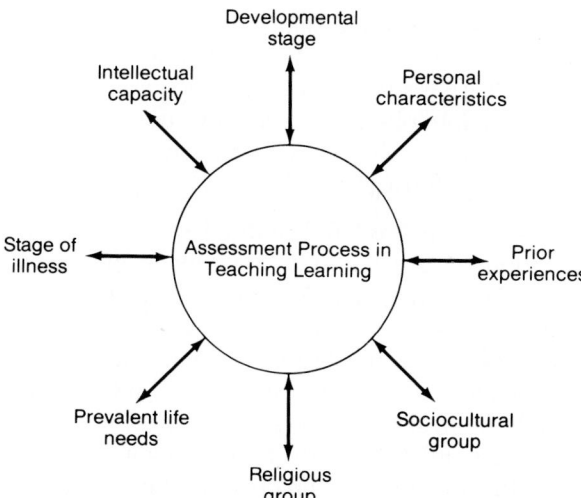

Developmental
stage

Intellectual
capacity

Personal
characteristics

Stage of
illness

Assessment Process in
Teaching Learning

Prior
experiences

Prevalent life
needs

Sociocultural
group

Religious
group

Figure 17-1 Stanton's diagrammatic representation of factors which govern need and readiness to learn.

ior; (3) be aware of subcultures' variations; (4) identify family and/or community decision makers; (5) appeal to the group's desire for health; and (6) help the individual and family to maintain a realistic perspective on effects of changed behavior.

Myths need to be identified and refuted with facts and figures whenever possible; they may be the basis for both conscious and unconscious resistance. Personal prejudices may inhibit the effectiveness of both nurse and patient. Recognition of these feelings as well as open discussion and negotiations regarding their resolution are essential if this barrier is to be overcome.

The stage of the patient's illness affects readiness to learn, which is described as a state of being both willing and able to make use of instruction. Lee[19] refers to these stages of illness as *impact, regression, acknowledgment,* and *reconstruction.* These are briefly described as follows:

1. *Impact*—the patient's initial emotional reaction to a trauma/illness. Feelings of anxiety, fear of dying, loss of control, despair, and discouragement are evident.
2. *Regression*—sets in with physiological stability; denial is the defense mechanism usually used by the patient in flight from reality. This stage gives the patient time to prepare for dealing with the crisis. Some patients express their fear of the loss of belonging and love through anger,

others joke about the illness, or make unrealistic plans for postdischarge activities.
3. *Acknowledgment*—also called the *mourning period,* when the patient's self-esteem and self-confidence are at an all-time low. The patient reviews precrisis events in order to identify and prevent the recurrence of its causes; the patient may also acknowledge his or her change in body image.
4. *Reconstruction*—brings hope for the future with the patient's renewed sense of self-worth and potential.

No teaching should begin in the impact stage, although the patient's and family's questions should be answered, and nursing actions explained. In the regression stage, teaching should be realistic, presented in a nonthreatening manner, and with reality given in small doses. Effective teaching can best begin in the acknowledgment stage, when the patient accepts and often asks for explanations and educational materials. Reconstruction may be enhanced by a focus on rehabilitation training, with instruction offered in a positive, nonblaming manner.

Other factors which have a strong influence on the patient's readiness to learn are comfort, energy motivation, and capability. Comfort is both physical and psychological and should be provided during each teaching session. Physical discomfort may be due to pain, nausea, fatigue, hunger, thirst, weakness, or dizziness. Emotional discomfort includes fear, anxiety, worry, depression, and anger. The patient's energy level is related to the physical status preillness as well as to the current stage of illness, psychological status, and stress level.

Motivation to Learn

Motivation is an important variable which must be considered, both in assessing learner readiness and in selecting teaching strategies. In its truest sense motivation is concerned with what gains individuals' attention, what directs their actions, and what keeps them learning (changing their behavior). While both intrinsic and extrinsic factors have been identified as contributing to one's motivation, the most frequently cited variables are:

1. A positive orientation toward learning, as evi-

denced by such behaviors as persistence, a high need for achievement, a high level of aspiration, a positive self-concept, and positive feelings about past learning experiences.
2. Curiosity about things, events, people, and relationships.
3. A need for social recognition.
4. Desire for conformity.
5. The desire to avoid failure.

According to many nurse-teachers, patients are motivated if they want to do the things the nurse thinks they should want to do, such as quit smoking, eat "right," exercise regularly, or stop worrying. In reality, patients are motivated to learn and do those things which help them to solve problems and avoid distress.

Some principles of motivation to use in working with patients are:

1. A sense of satisfaction has the most positive effect on future motivation.
2. Learners, in general, progress only as far as they need to in order to achieve their objectives or goals.
3. Genuine participation, not pretended sharing, enhances learner motivation at each step of the learning process.
4. To the extent possible, there must be freedom from discouragement or threats.
5. Feedback must be closely connected to learners' efforts when they are evaluating their own performance.
6. Both positive reinforcement, such as praise and attention, and negative reinforcement, including removal of discomfort and lessening of fears, should be used to increase the likelihood of a response recurring.
7. Always help the patient to see the applicability of the desired knowledge, skills, and attitudes to the solution of personally identified problems.

Capacity to Learn

The patient's capacity to learn is comprised of the following factors:

1. Aptitude—the amount of time required by the learner to actually learn the behavior or information. Aptitude is affected by the learner's individual differences and past experiences.

2. The ability to understand instructions.
3. The opportunity or time allowed for learning.
4. The learner's perseverance, which is affected by motivation, physical stamina or endurance, ability to cope with frustration, and number of external distractions.[20]

Often the patient's ability to understand instructions is a function of knowledge of hospital vocabulary. Byrne and Edeani,[21] in a follow-up to earlier studies, found a significant difference between nurses' perceptions of patients' knowledge and patients' actual understanding of medical terminology. While knowledge of medical terms had increased significantly over the last two decades, many black adults (44 percent), Hispanic adults (33 percent), and white adults were reported as functionally or marginally illiterate.[22] Apse and Stetler[23] found that the better educated the patient, the better the understanding of medical terms, and the older the patient, the fewer clinical terms known. It is suggested that not only should nurses make themselves and their colleagues more aware of this issue, but also that (1) fewer technical terms be used in patient education materials, (2) patients be oriented to hospital terminology, and (3) a handbook of commonly used medical terms be compiled and distributed to patients. The patient's and family's feedback should be elicited to determine if there is comprehension of the instruction given.

Instructions should also be specific and simple, such as "take the tablet three times a day with food," rather than "take the tablet after every meal." Repeat instructions both verbally and in printed materials whenever time and resources permit.

Cognitive Dissonance

It is important to be aware of the impact of cognitive dissonance on a patient's learning. The basic premise of this concept is that (1) one's knowledge, beliefs, and attitudes are generally consistent with one another; and (2) if given information which is not consistent, one experiences discomfort which may (3) motivate one to change, or (4) reinforce the "correctness" of present knowledge, beliefs, and attitudes.[24] For example, a male patient who smokes, when taught that smoking causes cancer, believes this to be true. He may subsequently (1) quit, (2) rationalize that he is not susceptible and continue to smoke, or (3) accept the risk and continue to smoke. If the nurse observes that the patient has done (2) or (3), he or she may discuss the inconsistency between knowledge and behavior with him. The patient may then do one of the following to modify the inconsistency:

1. Revise his initial decision to fit more closely the nurse's belief in the dangers of smoking.
2. Lessen the importance of the nurse's perceptions by such actions as questioning the available statistics.
3. Look for other aspects of the problem on which to agree, for example, some types of cigarettes are more dangerous than are others.
4. Change his perception of certain aspects of the situation by scheduling a chest film or implementing an exercise plan.

Other strategies which the patient might use to cope with the dissonance are denial, projection (criticize the nurse), or suppression, to name a few.

The nurse can help the patient resolve the dissonance in a manner which results in abstinence from smoking by focusing on the underlying issues such as stress, peer pressure, or weak self-image; by helping him to plan step-by-step alterations, for example, changing to a brand of cigarettes lower in nicotine, or smoking only a certain number of cigarettes each day; or by referring him to a credible smoking cessation program and support group.

Specification of Objectives

The formulation of objectives should be accomplished by the nurse in collaboration with the patient. As Stanton[25] points out, specifying learner behaviors is helpful for the following reasons:

1. It makes clear to teacher and learner what the expected outcome(s) is (are).
2. It guides the teacher in selecting appropriate content, learning activities, and/or media.
3. It directs the teacher toward valid methods of evaluating learner outcomes.

It is important to differentiate among the domains of learning—cognitive (thinking), psychomotor (doing), and affective (feeling)—in order to teach and evaluate in a valid and fair manner. Simple words and phrases should be used so that both

nurse and patient are clear regarding the expected outcomes. For example, objectives relating to dietary modification might be:

1. Cognitive—name five foods high in sodium.
2. Psychomotor—prepare a green, leafy vegetable using low-sodium seasoning.
3. Affective—report the daily substitution of fresh fruits for salt snacks within 1 week.

Teaching Techniques

Although some teaching techniques are more effective than are others with certain patients and in certain situations, there are no specific rules to apply in their selection. It is important that the technique correlate with the learning objectives, that it be familiar and nonthreatening to the patient, and that the teacher have previous experience with and/or comfort in its use. Murray and Zentner[26] organized teaching techniques according to desired patient behavioral outcomes:

1. Acquiring generalizations about experiences—lectures, symposiums, reading, audiovisual materials, and discussion based on printed materials.
2. Applying information to experience—problem-solving discussions, laboratory experiments, case studies, group activities such as role playing and simulation.
3. Skill development—role playing, coaching, demonstration, and return demonstration.
4. Creating new attitudes—reverse role playing, simulation games, and experience-sharing discussion.
5. Changing values—biographical or autobiographical reading, drama, experienced speakers, support groups, and values clarification activities.

Varied Teaching Strategies

As a patient educator, the nurse needs a varied repertoire of strategies from which to choose. Many of those to be described are traditional but still useful; others are relatively new and worthy of consideration.

Lecture is useful for providing information to large numbers of persons in an efficient manner.

The teacher retains control of the content, the time, and the amount and nature of interaction. Lecture is most appropriate when memory and logical organization of information are required.

Demonstration is appropriate for instruction in psychomotor skills. The teacher serves as a model of attainable skill and can provide immediate feedback to the learner when a return demonstration is requested. Anatomic models and equipment enable the learner to see and touch as well as listen, all of which enhance learning skills.

The use of *discussion* actively involves the patient as learner by encouraging his or her input and questions, with an opportunity for feedback and reinforcement. The peer group can provide another, perhaps more influenced, level of pressure for change to which the patient may be more responsive.

Adom and Wright[27] found in their study of hospitalized adults that two-thirds preferred *group teaching,* perhaps because they felt less alone in a group in which their fears and questions were voiced by others as well as themselves. In addition, the patients in this study gained reassurance from shared feelings in the group setting, perceived that sufficient time and attention had been given to them as individuals, and felt well prepared for surgery. Nurses, however, indicated a greater preference for individual teaching, perhaps because they were more familiar and comfortable with this method. Nevertheless, nurses perceived that group teaching was more time-effective and, therefore, of increasing value with shortened length of stay and decreased staff.

Simulation games and *role playing* are effective in actively involving patients in learning. They are particularly useful for providing a relatively safe environment in which to test new or modified attitudes, values, and beliefs.

Independent study is especially beneficial to patients who enjoy learning on their own, with the teacher serving as guide, facilitator, and evaluator. The variety of audiovisual and printed materials available provides the flexibility and individualization which many learners prefer.

Charts, graphs, diagrams, posters, and photographs can be used to supplement verbal or written descriptions and to provide added detail or relationships. These are particularly useful when the learner needs to see the object, activity, or concept being discussed.

Audiotapes are difficult for patients to use for learning because of the concentration required and the dependence on only the sense of hearing. If supplemented with printed materials or slides, they are more effective. Audiotapes are most appropriate when the patient needs to learn to differentiate between or among sounds such as heart sounds, dialysis machine, or volumetric infusion pump.

The 16-millimeter movies are useful for group instruction, especially if the objectives specify movement or interaction, both verbal and nonverbal. Elderly patients and the learning disadvantaged are particularly responsive to this medium. Slides, transparencies, and filmstrips can be integrated with other media (audiotapes) and methods (lecture) and can be presented at variable rates, which is particularly helpful to middle-aged and elderly patients, who may need more time to study the pictures or print.

Videotapes provide visualization and action, are a familiar medium to most, and can be stopped at intervals for a patient's questions if a teacher is present. Some patients cannot keep up with the fast-paced format; others dislike the "talking heads" with whom they cannot interact. Many hospitals and other health care institutions are developing centralized patient education channels on television. If this format is available to and utilized by patients, the nurse should be available to answer patients' questions and to evaluate their learning.

Relatively new to the catalogue of patient education media is the computer, which offers an active learning environment. Computer-assisted instruction offers patients the advantages of self-paced learning, frequent testing for comprehension with immediate feedback, individualized questions and information, and simulation of real-life situations.

Selecting and Evaluating Media

Many nurses and patients contract a condition known as "media-itis," which is caused by an overdose and/or prolonged exposure to inappropriate visual and auditory stimuli. This condition is a direct result of the belief that each instructional session should contain audiovisual materials and that everyone learns more effectively when they are utilized.

In making decisions regarding the appropriateness of using these materials for patient education, there are several factors to be considered:

1. The objective(s) to be attained by the learner.
2. The size of the group.
3. The availability of equipment.
4. The nurse's skill in using equipment.
5. The location of the program.

Having made the decision to utilize audiovisual materials for patient teaching, another series of questions needs to be answered:

1. Do the visuals (slides, photos, posters) portray scenes, people, and items familiar to the patient?
2. Do the visuals contain material which may be offensive to the patient's cultural background (clothing, lifestyle, or character)?
3. Are the verbal cues appropriate to the patient's level of literacy? Are terms defined? Is medical terminology kept to a minimum?
4. If the objective is to teach the patient a skill, is there an opportunity to practice?
5. If the objective is to modify the patient's attitudes, beliefs, or values, does the program ask for a commitment to action?
6. Are correct responses provided to the learner?
7. With regard to the medium's content, one should determine whether the information is accurate and up to date, presented at the appropriate developmental and literacy levels, and has been approved by recognized and respected health care associations.
8. Does each picture or sequence of pictures represent a single concept?
9. Is the graphic information legible?
10. Are the visuals properly lighted so that details are easily seen?
11. Are the voices clear? Music appropriate to mood?
12. Does the program have an identifiable introduction, body, and conclusion?
13. Does the introduction gain and maintain the patient's interest? Identify the objective of the presentation? State the reasons (if applicable) for the patient's participation? Relate health conditions to patient events? Show the need for change? Demonstrate workable action? Is there enough repetition?
14. Does the program appeal to and maintain learner interest?

Use of Printed Materials

In developing printed teaching materials, there are a number of principles which, if applied, should make these materials more effective and useful. These principles are as follows:

1. Use a title which describes clearly the purpose and contents of the material, such as "Sexual Function after Myocardial Infarction."
2. Use purpose statements—e.g., when the information should be used (as prescribed, as needed), and what materials are needed (quiet room, comfortable clothing).
3. Present information clearly and concisely (number items, organize from simple to complex, provide rationale for actions).
4. Highlight possible errors or precautions ("It is important to . . . ," "Caution . . . ," "Be sure to . . . ,").
5. Select visuals to meet the objectives and facilitate learning, then use them correctly (label figures, diagrams, charts), use clear photographs, eliminate distractions.
6. Use easy-to-read type and other visual devices such as different type styles and sizes, color, arrows, boxes.
7. Test the material for readability using such tools as the Smog Readability Formula. Do not assume that patients read at the level of their completed education. Glazer-Waldman, Hall, and Weiner[29] found in a sample of 81 literate patients that only 40 percent could read at the sixth-grade level.

Focus on Sensory Information

Preparing patients for diagnostic or therapeutic procedures has traditionally focused on specific information such as the equipment to be used, and the steps in the procedure. McHugh, Christman, and Johnson[30] found that sensory information was also helpful to patients in coping. These authors defined sensory information as "information about our environment that is acquired by way of our sensory modalities—sight, hearing, touch, taste, and smell." Their proposition was that giving patients information about typical experiences which they could anticipate during a procedure would help them form realistic mental images (schemata), which would lead them to expect certain things to occur. A series of studies indicated that (1) patients told about sensations created by pumping a blood pressure cuff on the arm to the level of 250 mmHg reported less distress than those not informed, (2) patients given sensory information coped more effectively with gastroendoscopic examinations, and (3) preparatory information decreased the length of the postoperative hospital stay for patients undergoing cholecystectomy. Patients in these studies were given sensory information describing both objectives and subjective features of the event, including length of the procedure, nature and location of objects in the environment, and physical sensation.

Guidelines for giving patients preparatory information were provided:

1. Describe but do not evaluate physical sensations ("It will ache or burn" but not "You'll really feel awful").
2. Tell patients the cause of the sensations.
3. Focus on commonly occurring aspects of the experience.

General indicators of the effect of a diagnostic or therapeutic procedure on a patient include the amount of sedation needed, verbal and facial expressions, degree of cooperation, and subsequent length of hospitalization.

Evaluation of Teaching and Learning

The process of evaluation usually receives the least attention in patient education, perhaps because it is viewed as too time-consuming and difficult to implement with patients. One way in which the process is facilitated is through the development of measurable learner objectives and outcomes which guide the selection of measurement procedures and the judgment of learner attainment.

The use of written tests may be useful with patients, although one must be concerned with validity (does the test measure what it is supposed to measure?), reliability (generalizability), readability, and practicality (ease of administration and grading), and resources needed (paper, pencil, desk).

Observation is another useful tool, particularly if a checklist or rating scale is developed which includes the desired outcomes in measurable terms. Psychomotor skills are best evaluated with a performance rating scale or checklist completed during a learner demonstration.

Antecdotal notes are useful for noting a patient's behaviors in all domains—cognitive, psychomotor, and affective. Both objective and subjective data can be included from which a judgment can be made.

Patient interviews serve a dual purpose. They can be used to (1) measure changes in knowledge and attitudes, and (2) elicit the patient's opinions about the teaching program and instruction. It is useful to record patients' compliments and complaints as a basis for improving the effectiveness of the teaching. Family members and significant others should also be asked to offer their opinions on the effectiveness of the teaching session or program.

Documentation of patient instruction and learner outcomes is essential. It serves as an indispensable form of communication among health care professionals to ensure continuity and as a legal record of a patient's attainment. The patient's record should also reflect the patient's and family's response to teaching, including doubts, fears, satisfaction, and confidence.

Communication should also occur via nursing care plans, planning conferences, and nursing rounds to name a few. All methods of communication provide an opportunity to evaluate the effectiveness of instructional programs.

Broader foci for evaluation in patient education have been suggested by Price and Cordell.[31] Their premise is that scientific methods must be applied to the patient teaching and learning process in order to validate the process. Some of the more frequent areas of investigation, which can serve as the basis for replication as well as new ideas, include:

1. Changes in patients as a result of educational experiences.

2. Amount and type of a patient's behavior as it relates to changes in attitudes toward wellness.
3. Surveys of techniques, materials, evaluation methods, etc.
4. Effects of "teaching style" on patient education outcomes.
5. Comparison of group and individual instruction.

Helpful Hints

Murray and Zentner[32] list suggestions for effective patient teaching which have a common-sense appeal, enhancing their value to the nurse teacher:

1. Be consistent in your approach to the patient and family.
2. Show enthusiasm for the content and its value to the patient.
3. Present yourself as a role model (neat, erect, alert, calm).
4. Know your content and present it in an organized manner so that the patient has confidence in what you are saying.
5. Continuously evaluate the effectiveness of your teaching, seeking input from peers and patients.
6. Use available teaching methods, resources, and referral systems as appropriate.
7. Communicate verbally and in writing with other nurse-teachers regarding the patient's level of understanding and attainment of objectives.
8. Respect the patient as an individual with wants and needs which may differ from those of the health care system.
9. Give the patient the rationale for any guidelines or prescriptions.
10. Do not equate ability to learn with educational level.
11. Distinguish between learning ability and misunderstandings caused by cultural, ethnic, religious, or developmental differences.
12. Learn about the patient in order to identify teachable moments.
13. Stimulate the patient's desire to learn rather than using such external motivators as threats or bribes.
14. Give frequent feedback and reinforcement.

Some of the most rewarding aspects of nursing are derived from patient education. As Woldum et al.[33] point out so clearly in their philosophical perspective on the nurse as patient teacher:

1. Believe in yourself as a teacher and in the value of this role in your practice.
2. See yourself as an extension of the patient.
3. Seek peer support for your teaching activities.
4. See yourself as an important advocate for the patient without encouraging dependence.
5. Risk questioning your beliefs about patient education in order to be open to new perspectives.
6. Let the patient teach you whenever possible.
7. View every communication with the patient as a form of instruction.
8. Be aware of, acknowledge, and collaborate with other health care providers in providing patient teaching.
9. Accept responsibility and accountability for documenting patient education.
10. Experiment with innovative and creative teaching and evaluation techniques.

In this era of prospective payment, high technology, and growing consumer awareness, the nurse faces the challenge of educating a more complex and knowledgeable patient population. Use of the teaching–learning process, which includes the assessment of learner needs, specification of objectives, selection of teaching techniques, and evaluation of teaching and learning enables the critical-care nurse to provide cost-effective patient education while maintaining quality patient care.

References

1. Alspach, J. (1985). Out with the old and in with the new: Discharge planning in critical care. *Critical Care Nurse, 5*(6), 1.
2. Narrow, B. (1979). *Patient teaching in nursing practice.* New York: John Wiley & Sons, Inc.
3. American Hospital Association. (1982). Policy and statement. The hospital's responsibility for patient education services. Chicago: Author.
4. Burke, C. (1985). Patient education and cost containment. *Computers in Healthcare, 6,* 38–42.
5. Miller, A. (1985). When is the time ripe for teaching? *American Journal of Nursing, 85*(7), 801–804.
6. Levin, L. (1978). Patient education and self-care: How do they differ? *Nursing Outlook, 26,* 170–175.

7. Harrell, J., & Frauman, A. (1985). Prospective payment calls for boosting productivity. *Nursing & Health Care, 6*(10), 535–537.

8. Bigge, M. (1976). *Learning theories for teachers.* New York: Harper & Row.

9. Corkadel, L., & McGlashan, R. (1983). A practical approach to patient teaching. *The Journal of Continuing Education in Nursing, 14,* 9–15.

10. Hinthorne, R. (1983). Teaching nurses how to teach patients. *Nursing Management, 14*(9), 30–33.

11. Whitehouse, R. (1979). Forms that facilitate patient teaching. *American Journal of Nursing, 79*(7), 1227–1229.

12. Corkadel, L., & McGlashan, R. (1983). A practical approach to patient teaching. *The Journal of Continuing Education in Nursing, 14,* 9–15.

13. Taylor, P. (1982). Patient teaching: Keys to more success more often. *Nursing Life, 2,* 25–32.

14. Barrett, N., & Schwartz, N. (1981). What patients really want to know. *American Journal of Nursing, 81*(9), 1642.

15. Taylor, J. (1984). Are you missing what your patients can teach you? *RN, 47,* 63–69.

16. Stanton, M. (1985). Teaching patients: Some basic lessons for nurse educators. *Nursing Management, 16,* 59–62.

17. Caron, H., & Roth, H. (1978). An evaluation of a program for teaching clinic patients the rationale of their peptic ulcer regimen. *Nursing Digest, 6,* 56–57.

18. Murray, R., & Zentner, J. (1976). Guidelines for more effective health teaching. *Nursing 76, 6,* 44–53.

19. Lee, J. (1970). Emotional reactions to trauma. *Nursing Clinics of North America, 5,* 577–587.

20. Wolf, V., & Quiring, J. (1971). Carroll's model applied to nursing education. *Nursing Outlook, 19*(3), 176–179.

21. Byrne, F., & Edeani, D. (1984). Knowledge of medical terminology among hospital patients. *Nursing Research, 33*(3), 178–181.

22. Kozol, J. (1985). *Illiterate America.* Garden City, NJ: Doubleday.

23. Apse, A., & Stetler, C. (1985). Avoiding terms of bewilderment. *Nursing 85, 15,* 42–43.

24. Miller, J. (1974). Cognitive dissonance in modifying families' perceptions. *American Journal of Nursing, 74*(8), 1468–1470.

25. Stanton, M. (1985). Teaching patients: Some basic lessons for nurse educators. *Nursing Management, 16,* 59–62.

26. Murray, R., & Zentner, J. (1976). Guidelines for more effective health teaching. *Nursing 76, 6,* 44–53.

27. Adom, D., & Wright, A. (1982). Dissonance in nurse and patient evaluations of the effectiveness of a patient-teaching program. *Nursing Outlook, 30,* 132–136.

28. U.S. Department of Health and Human Services, National Institutes of Health, National Cancer Institute. (1982). *Pretesting in health communications. Methods, examples and resources for improving health messages and materials.* Bethesda, MD: NIH.

29. Glazer-Waldman, H., Hall, K., & Weiner, M. (1985). Patient education in a public hospital. *Nursing Research, 34*(3), 184–185.

30. McHugh, N., Christman, N., & Johnson, J. (1982). Preparatory information: What helps and why. *American Journal of Nursing, 82*(5), 780–782.

31. Price, J., & Cordell, B. (1984). Patient education evaluation: Beyond intuition. *Nursing Forum, 21*(3), 117–122.

32. Murray, R., & Zentner, J. (1976). Guidelines for more effective health teaching. *Nursing 76, 6,* 44–53.

33. Woldum, K., Ryan-Morrell, V., Towson, M., Bower, K., & Zander, K. (1985). *Patient education. Foundation of practice.* Rockville, MD: Aspen Systems Corporation.

18 Coping

Doris S. Greiner

Introduction

Critically ill people behave in an endless variety of ways, yet patterns are detectable, enticing the clinician to think that there must be ways to classify behaviors such that interventions are dictated. Though this is not the case, there are keys to ordering observations that suggest interventions that will aid patients in living with and learning from their experience. The purposes of this chapter are to provide a structure for ordering observations about coping behavior and to describe individual differences with sufficient richness of detail so that the structure will not constrict observation. Interventions based on theory and research about individuals and families in particular contexts, over time, are suggested.

Helping individuals cope involves a decision-making process based on information about patient and family, context, and time. It can be a high-priority item in an assessment process or it can reasonably wait until higher priority needs of the patient are met. This is the first stage in the decision-making process.

Assumptions that underlie all that follows are that (1) individuals have developed competencies for coping with the complexities of their lives, (2) assessment of coping requires keen observation and openness to individual differences, and (3) intervention involves assisting individuals and families to mobilize their own energies, and draw on these existing competencies. When effective, intervention involves assisting individuals to move beyond coping to active problem solving.

Assessment of Previous Coping Behavior

Information about the previous coping behaviors of a critically ill patient is gathered throughout the patient's stay. The initial information, usually elicited from family members or friends, sets the direction of observation and cannot be underestimated in importance. Remaining aware of each person's point of view that may differ from that of the patient or others involved is a particular challenge of this period. It is for this reason that, at minimum, a two-column approach to records kept of the assessment is suggested, one for information received from the patient, the other for that received from others, specifying which others.

Psychosocial assessment, no matter what the form, easily lends itself to attempting to gather more data than will be used. This is a mistake. The reason for making the assessment is to plan intervention that will assist the patient to cope more effectively. Gathering extensive information because it might, or could theoretically, be useful is wasteful of patient and professional energy.

In a thorough discussion of assessment procedures using a mathematical decision theory model, Mariotto and Paul[1] discussed the four R's for judging the usefulness of assessment procedures. These can be practically applied to any assessment situation. The concepts are representativeness, replicability, relevance, and relative cost. *Representativeness* refers to the degree to which information obtained matches the needs of decisions to be made based upon it, and covers the categories of needed information. *Replicability* refers to interobserver agreement. The high degree of interdependence in nursing practice makes working toward such objectivity an even more crucial matter. *Relevance* equates with appropriateness. Ideally limited assessment information can contribute to many decisions. Any item of assessment information that contributes to many decisions is highly relevant. *Relative cost* of the assessment continues to be elusive. The amount of professional time needed is limited, especially when an ongoing or cumulative

478

approach is used, and at this time extensive and invasive technical procedures are not involved. The extent to which a patient's energies are conserved for active healing purposes by a representative, relevant, and replicable assessment that leads to coping and problem solving has yet to be established as cost-effective. All indications suggest that it is.

Usual Ways of Coping with Difficult Situations

The purpose of this information is to identify clues to patient behaviors in anticipation of helping the patient draw on those familiar patterns where possible. It also provides anticipatory information about possible difficulties ahead for the patient, family, and staff. As such it can be used as a base for creative problem solving. For example, a patient who is very goal-directed and who confronts problems directly can benefit from having small attainable goals suggested which can be carried out during and/or between procedures. As soon as feasible, this same person can be helped to identify personal goals. A person who is usually compliant and seeks direction from others responds much more favorably to on-the-spot direction. In this case,

Table 18-1 Coping Assessment

1. What are the patient's usual ways of coping with difficult situations?

Patient _____ Other sources (specify relationship) _____

2. Previous experience with critical care and/or serious illness.

Patient _____ Other sources _____

3. Who are important people to have close by, or people who help with coping?

Patient _____ Other sources _____

Designated family contact person: _____

4. Additional observations, e.g. developmental issues, usual role(s).

Patient _____ Other sources _____

small goals to work toward would be unnecessary at best and anxiety-evoking at worst.

Again, it is usual that initial information about coping comes from family. Always note the sources of information, remembering that relationship variables influence each person's point of view. Also note that each question applies equally well to the family member with whom one is speaking. A family member's usual way of coping may be of crucial significance in putting a patient's behavior into an understandable context. A detailed family assessment is not usually possible. Information about usual family patterns is found in a later section. The point initially is to note information from each source and about each source.

Anxiety is almost always high early in the critical-care experience. Asking questions about previous approaches to coping can be a useful focus of attention if the anxiety is not too high. If the patient or family member is unable to focus on the questions asked, redirect attention to specific, concrete aspects of the immediate situation, and return to this category at another time.

Previous Experience with Critical Care or Serious Illness

Critical-care specialty units have been available in hospitals long enough so that most people have had either direct experience or familiarity through the experiences of friends or acquaintances. Television is also a powerful resource for familiarizing people with otherwise mysterious environments and technologies. The combined effect of previous experience is easy to overlook. Asking about earlier critical-care experiences or serious illness can help identify both positive and negative expectations based on past experience. Once these events have been identified, the patient and family can be helped to draw on what was useful. Small things that the nursing staff can easily do or provide are often discovered in this context. When previous experience has been negative, help is needed to focus on the current experience and to identify ways in which this experience is different.

Important People to Have Close By

The subject of social support, like that of coping, has been the focus of extensive research. It is an area in which automatic assumptions are frequently made about the way things should be. These assumptions can often be traced to one's own experience, values, and/or desires for a more ideal world. For example, ideally people should talk calmly about problems, husbands and wives should be close, and adult children should care about aged parents in a gentle, understanding way. The nurse should question assumptions, and not make them automatically. Who are the people the patient needs nearby? Are these people private or talkative? Are people available to be supportive, especially to family, who might be being overlooked?

In addition to assumptions, a frequent deterrent to effective assessment in this area is a belief that the nurse must somehow meet patient and family needs for social support. Existing networks of support can stay active or be activated, often with minimal staff effort. This not only decreases the alienating effects of a critical illness, it provides a link from past to future, keeping this often relatively brief critical phase of illness firmly placed in the ongoing context of the family's life.

The question of whom the patient needs nearby is one to be repeated periodically. It is a question that directs thinking for anxious people toward potentially useful resources. Without this direction, the staff can easily become the focus of a patient's need to talk, which might be as usefully met by someone who does not also have the responsibility for all other aspects of care of the patient.

In the social network of some patients, many people are involved. Identifying one person who can serve as a liaison between staff, family, and friends can be very helpful for all concerned in keeping information exchange efficient and effective. Many families have a member who automatically functions in this role. Drawing on this skill explicitly can be useful.

Additional Observations

Developmental issues with which a family is coping is an example of information to be gathered in this category. For most people an experience with critical illness is a shocking, unexpected event. It always occurs within the context of the family's life, however. For example, an 18-year-old son, the youngest of three children, left the country for a planned year abroad the day that his father had emergency heart surgery. Some form of disruption is expected when a last child leaves home. This information was useful for staff in understanding particular concerns of this family. The critical illness added an additional burden to an already disrupted family system.

Knowing the roles each person assumes in the family or living situation can be important. Information about this aspect of the patient's life may not be particularly pertinent to the acute phase of illness. However, awareness that a person's usual roles can be temporarily filled by others may be a source of immense relief to some people. Others may feel useless when it becomes clear that someone else can take their place. For example, in families which adhere rigidly to traditional roles of husband as provider and wife as homemaker, for either to be sick and have that role capably assumed by the other can be very personally threatening to the patient. This becomes an added bit of evidence that as an ill person, life is without usefulness or meaning. Careful observation in this category is warranted.

Coping Behavior

Four definitions of coping from the voluminous literature on the subject have been chosen to give direction to the description of coping behavior. Though much of what follows is directed specifically to coping in serious or crisis situations, research findings and theoretic constructs related to normative coping are selectively included. The work of Pearlin and Schooler[2] falls in this second group. They refer to coping as the things "people do to avoid being harmed by life strains." These authors made the fundamental assumption that people are actively responsive to external forces, many of them social in origin. Action is clearly an element of this definition. The terms *strain* and *stress* are used interchangeably, and the authors were careful to clarify their idea of stress. *Stress* is defined as the experience of emotional upset as reported by subjects, and was clarified as different from other feelings of emotional distress by its specificity. First, stress was determined by particular threatening situations, and second, it had clearer boundaries than, for example, anxiety and depression, which

may develop from prolonged distress but are by nature more diffuse.

Lazarus and colleagues have worked for several decades in the area of coping and have elaborated a more detailed definition. *Coping* means "the constantly changing cognitive and behavioral efforts to manage specific external and/or internal demands that are appraised as taxing or exceeding the resources of the person" (p. 141).[3] This definition addresses what these researchers identify as limitations in other approaches to understanding coping. Coping is clearly a process rather than a single act. It is limited to those situations which evoke conscious appraisal, rather than being inclusive of automatic behavior, for example, psychological defenses. It includes the person's efforts, regardless of their effectiveness. By using the term *manage,* an attempt has been made to avoid confusing the terms *coping* and *mastery.* Certainly, coping may lead to mastery, but many coping behaviors described in the literature can be more adequately described as managing rather than eliminating or overcoming stress. In this definition psychological stress is implied. "Psychological stress is a particular relationship between the person and the environment that is appraised by the person as taxing or exceeding his or her resources and endangering his or her well-being" (p. 19).[3] Stress, defined as a relationship between demands of the environment and the person's appraisal of those demands, is different from a more usual conceptualization of stress as either stimulus or response.

Weisman says that coping is "what one does about a problem in order to bring about relief, reward, quiescence, and equilibrium."[4] This definition contains the three elements of a problem, what one does or does not do, and outcome. Weisman's work is both clinically and research-based, primarily in the area of coping with cancer.

White suggested observing the situations in which the term coping is used.

> We tend to speak of coping when we have in mind a fairly drastic change or problem that defies familiar ways of behaving, requires the production of new behavior, and very likely gives rise to uncomfortable affects like anxiety, despair, guilt, shame, or grief, the relief of which forms part of the needed adaptation. Coping refers to adaptation under relatively difficult conditions (pp. 48–49).[5]

Life is a series of adaptations. From the most simple problem solving or decision making about daily tasks to meeting the most complex environmental and internal demands imaginable, adaptation can be conceptualized as striving toward compromise. Coping behavior is called forth on the more complex end of this continuum. Critical illness and the critical-care environment demand coping for most people.

Operationally defined, coping is a process in which an individual experiences (1) internal and/or external events which evoke (2) an awareness of demands that exceed obvious resources, precipitating (3) behavior that in thought and/or observable action seeks relief from the felt threat of the demands, and (4) changes as awareness of the demands changes over time.

The structure for ordering observations of coping behavior thus involves direct observation of patients and families as well as elicited information from patients and families. Each individual's appraisal of the situation and personal resources dominate the experience and give direction to identifying assistance needed.

Personal characteristics have been demonstrated to positively influence coping. Hardiness—that is, a high degree of internal control—commitment, and responsiveness to challenge contribute to feeling positive about oneself.[6,7] Closeness and commitment in relationships are closely related and are strong positive variables in the work of Pearlin and Schooler.[2] The characteristic of flexibility is cited by numerous authors.[2,7,8,9] Self-consciousness and attention to internal clues act as precursors to active coping. Persons low in self-consciousness do not monitor critical clues resulting from stressful events; consequently, they do not access information that would permit coping.[10]

Figley[11] (p. 18) has identified 11 universal characteristics within a family context which differentiate functional and dysfunctional coping:

1. Ability to identify the stressor
2. Viewing the situation as a family problem, rather than as merely a problem of one or two of its members
3. Adopting a solution-oriented approach to the problem, rather than simply blaming
4. Showing tolerance for other family members

5. Clear expression of commitment to and affection for other family members
6. Open and clear communication among members
7. Evidence of high family cohesion
8. Evidence of considerable role flexibility
9. Appropriate utilization of resources inside and outside the family
10. Lack of overt or covert physical violence
11. Lack of substance abuse

Moving from universal considerations, Figley[11] summarizes factors that influence an individual's coping skills in emergency situations. Previous experience with very similar situations, personal hardiness, an ability to concentrate under pressure, and an internal locus of control are the factors named. A person with an internal locus of control believes that personal decisions and actions can make a difference. One is not totally vulnerable to external forces. A person with an external locus of control experiences very little possibility for personally influencing, or controlling, the course of life.

Another set of factors[11] that influences the amount of stress experienced pertains to the situation. The first is sociality, or the extent to which there is communication among fellow victims. Ignoring the degree to which the experience is humiliating or degrading is the second factor. The last is a sense of helplessness to influence or stop the situation. Thus, the nature of the emergency, individual coping ability, and situational factors interact to account for the intensity of the distress experienced.

Figley lists the following characteristics of catastrophic stressors which differ from normative stressors:

1. The amount of time one has to prepare
2. Previous experience with the stressor
3. Sources of guidance available to manage the stressor
4. The extent to which others have experienced the stressor
5. The amount of time spent in a "crisis" state
6. The degree to which there is a sense of loss of control or helplessness
7. Loss
8. Disruption and destruction

9. Danger experienced by people exposed to the stressor

10. The quantity and quality of the emotional impact of the stressor

11. Medical problems associated with exposure to the stressor (p. 14)[11]

The relevance of these characteristics to either patient or family is noteworthy.

The crisis of physical illness has been the focus of much study. From general crisis theory,[12] Moos and Schaefer[13] identify the three types of coping skills needed in coping with physical illness. These types are appraisal-, problem-, or emotion-focused. Examples of each are:

1. Appraisal-focused coping:
   a. Logical analysis and mental preparation
   b. Cognitive redefinition
   c. Cognitive avoidance or denial
2. Problem-focused coping:
   a. Seeking information and support
   b. Taking problem-solving action
   c. Identifying alternative rewards
3. Emotion-focused coping:
   a. Affective regulation
   b. Emotional discharge
   c. Resigned acceptance

These authors suggest that failure to cope in a realistic and timely manner in the first phase of a critical illness has enduring side effects. However, not all authors and researchers agree with this position.

In summary, coping is multidimensional. Changes occur in coping and its outcomes over time and across contexts. Many factors affect coping possibilities. These factors are only partially described by the available research to date. Coping as a concept is closely related to competence. The person and family attempting to cope with a threat may need assistance to draw on existing competencies. The potential exists for developing new competencies in every crisis or threatening situation.

Defense Mechanisms and Self-Concept

The relationship between coping and defense mechanisms is yet to be fully understood.[4] Defense mechanisms have a familiarity and thus an assumed truth about them for many professionals providing health care. They tend to be conceptualized as static or fixed, negative or unhealthy, and as phenomena about which little can be done with assurance. This belief does not dismiss an implication that something should be done.

In the original psychoanalytic development of the concepts known as defense mechanisms, they were related to neurotic defense against anxiety that had to do with past fears. White[5] has aptly pointed out that they have evolved with a concealed assumption of cowardice on the part of an individual who is unwilling to face reality. Carefully considered, they can be hypothesized as connecting links to an individual's past fears, many of which are presumably evoked in current threatening situations.

Defenses are evoked automatically, usually out of the conscious control of the individual. Defense mechanisms serve a life-preserving purpose in the face of overwhelming anxiety. This can, however, be a static solution because they close cognitive and emotional awareness of one's current situation. Problem solving cannot occur if individuals are unaware of a problem or threat. A close and elusive relationship exists between awareness and lack of awareness in individuals. Intervention can be especially effective in this in-between state, when it can be identified.

When the priority is to help people stay directed toward coping and increasing competence, awareness of clues to defenses on the part of the patient and family members can be very useful. A tendency on the part of staff to adopt an awareness of defended behavior as a static state is problematic. Observing for signs of defenses must be paired with observing for signals of readiness on the part of an individual to increase awareness. Anxiety inhibits that elusive space between awareness and unawareness. Intervening directly as an increase in anxiety is noted can make it possible for the patient to cope more effectively.

Anxiety is a state of tension within a person which arises when an interpersonal need for security and/or freedom from tension is not met. Anxiety is communicable, that is, it is experienced empathically with significant others.[14] It is without direction; that is, by its very nature it is a barrier to foresight or seeing beyond the anxiety to future states of being. The higher the level of anxiety, the less the person experiencing the anxiety can see beyond it. It is a basic human reaction resulting specifically in a felt need to change one's current state of being. Anxiety is an automatic response to a decrease in security which triggers automatic relief behaviors, ways of increasing comfort. Anxiety is not fear, though its observable manifestations may be identical. Fear, however, is directed. What one fears can be identified, named, and usually managed. What cannot be named evokes the anxious response. Asking patients or family members to name their fears can be exceedingly effective in reducing anxiety.

One defense mechanism that has been discussed extensively, especially in relation to coronary care, is denial. The findings of a reassessment of denial in coronary care patients[15] are enlightening. Nineteen patients were asked to talk about their experience and concerns. No conscious attempt was made to direct the interview away from anxiety-provoking content initiated by the patient. All patients expressed indicators of mutilation and death anxiety. Fourteen expressed indicators of denial. Significant heart rhythm changes did occur; however, further analysis revealed no relationship between heart rate and denial. The researchers concluded that patients in a CCU discussed their problems when given an opportunity and that they elaborated on their problems more frequently than they denied them. Patients are actively engaged in coping with their problems and it is important to provide them with an opportunity to share concerns. The researchers concluded that the questions asked and clinical expectations of the interviewer were different than those reported in earlier studies.[16,17,18] In this study the interviewer elicited patients' concerns but did not suggest things they might be concerned about. Also, it is proposed that the outcome might have been different if the interviewer had felt anxious about the potential for harmful effects from the interview. These are both crucial points to consider in planning intervention.

Horowitz[19] has developed a model for understanding psychological processes that occur in response to serious life events. Aspects of that model contribute to a fuller understanding of defense mechanisms, self-esteem, and stage of illness. The concept of control is used in the model,

instead of defense mechanisms, "in order to avoid imparting value judgments to the process, as adaptive or maladaptive, developmentally conservative or progressive, consciously or unconsciously operative ... Controls serve to maintain a state and determine transition from one state to another" (p. 252).[19] Thus, Horowitz is one researcher whose studies question the assertion that failure to cope in a realistic and timely manner has enduring side effects.

The Horowitz model suggests that the basic controls as ways of coping are *inhibition* and *facilitation*. To be more specific about what is inhibited and what is facilitated, three levels of increasing abstraction are described. At the first level, information of varying types and forms is selected or inhibited. At the second level, this information is connected with self-images and role models to form revised or new schemata that give patterns to the information as the person thinks about all that is happening.

Format selection is the term used for the third level of abstraction. The amount of time allowed to consider the threatening situation and the mode of thinking relate to format selection. Viewing threats over short or long periods of time, problem solving or fantasizing, use of words or images in thought, and allowing external or internal sources of information are all examples of modes of thinking. For example, some individuals ask continually for information from others and tend to ignore their own subjective experience. It is as though they feel pain only if they are told a procedure will be painful. At the other extreme are the individuals who are acutely sensitive to subjective experience, and less able to think about information that comes from external sources, for example, the nursing staff.

The fundamental assumptions of this model are that a serious stress-inducing life event necessitates action to alter the situation, or revision of inner models of organizing thinking to conform to a new reality. No one has just one self-image or role relationship model. Each person has several important models which are revised throughout life. The earlier models are not lost and can be reactivated in response to serious threats. Competent self-images may be replaced with one of incompetence which becomes dominant for periods of time. Frequent vacillation between them might also be common. This nonstability of self-concept is a very usual observation in critical-care settings and is a usual part of the process of moving forward with life, incorporating the current crisis into one's total experience of life.

Stages of Illness

The Horowitz[19] model is also useful in considering stages of illness. In the early stage of a critical illness, information is exceedingly hard to grasp. A coping effort that allows small bits of information is often observed. "Dosing" is the descriptive term. Denial, repression, suppression, avoidance, and use of drugs that block awareness are more exaggerated efforts at inhibition of information. Failure to control information at this early stage may be experienced as intrusion and emotional flooding. Attempts to think about information one has regarding the threatening situation may be observed in people who contemplate or often seem lost in thought. Rumination and inability to think clearly may be indicators of failure to control or inhibit information being received.

Changes in the need to control what one knows and what is happening over time are observable in the critical phase of illness. Cassell[20] discussed changes that often happen as loss of connectedness, loss of a sense of omnipotence, failure of reason, and loss of control. In the first stage, withdrawal from usual life-style and from relationships is postulated as a necessary step to garner energy, emotional and physical, to contend with the illness. The loss of omnipotence is usually noted as denial in those who are goal-directed and who are used to being in unquestionable control. At the other end of the control continuum, panic is experienced and indications of the intense emotion that accompany panic are observed. Failure of reason occurs as patients attempt to think about their illness but do not have the knowledge or strength to comprehend or sort out the complexities. During the experience of critical illness, loss of emotional control may be observed. Angry outbursts, demanding and aggressive behavior, and obsessive attention to one aspect of experience may be seen. Remembering that this stage is useful

and necessary for the patient to move toward regaining control may not make it easier to be the target of the angry outbursts.

Two aspects of the critical-care environment that influence the patient's experience over time and that are directly related to staff behavior are noise and sleep deprivation. Hansell[21] reviewed the relevant literature and stated that it has been well established that sensory overload and deprivation relate to behavioral aberrations. Both of these possibilities exist in critical care. Sensory overload and disruption with unwanted sensory stimulation make restorative sleep very difficult, a fact that contributes to the development of the related behavioral aberrations often referred to as "critical-care psychosis," or the "intensive care unit syndrome." Helton, Gordon, and Nunnery[22] measured disorientation, combativeness, hallucinations, paranoia, and delusions in critical-care patients. Cumulative scores of the incidence of these experiences were correlated with sleep-deprived and non-sleep-deprived states. Sleep-deprived patients had a significantly higher incidence of mental status alterations, according to the measures used in this study. The two intensive care units used for the study differed in the incidence of altered mental states. In one unit efforts were made to control lighting and disruption at night, but in the other unit there was constant lighting, open doors to patients' rooms, and frequent sounding of alarms. Six of the seven subjects who exhibited mental status alterations were from the second unit. Chapters 6 and 14 discuss these factors in more detail.

Using a repeated-measures design, King[23] identified coping strategies used by patients undergoing coronary artery bypass grafting. The 50 subjects, 42 men and 8 women, were interviewed before surgery, the day before discharge, and 3 weeks after discharge. Information-seeking was the most frequently used coping strategy at all stages. Turning to others, not family, for information was an early coping strategy. Usual sources of information were professionals and others who had experienced the procedure. Just before discharge and after the patient was at home, the family became the primary source of information. Direct action was a category that was used to a limited degree at first. Direct action increased over time, suggesting that when it is obvious that something can be done, it often is done. Imagery-rehearsal-vigilance was the lowest presurgery strategy but was used at time of discharge. Knowing about home and imagining oneself coping with being there was reported as useful. Not knowing the hospital environment made rehearsal difficult or impossible at an earlier stage. Attention deployment–avoidance was a strategy used frequently at first, but used less over time. This finding would fit with the concept of "dosing" previously discussed. Positive thinking was the one strategy that did not change in incidence of reported usefulness in this study. Though not all patients could or did use positive thinking, those who did, reported using it consistently. The findings in this study are based on the experience of patients who had some time to prepare for hospitalization, and offer useful comparison points for observations of coping strategies used by patients whose illness is completely unexpected.

Individual and Family Coping Patterns

Throughout the material presented, patients and families have been the focus. Coping always occurs in a context. While it is evident that the patient has particular stresses, different than those of family members, categories of coping responses are not that different. A loss is being experienced. Time is necessary to make the transition from the preillness state to one in which the illness is incorporated into the family's life experience. In order to take in the information that is needed to make this transition, most individuals exert some efforts at control of the amount and nature of information taken in. It is usual for patients to indicate *information overload* by their behavior. Family members are more often trying desperately to *access information,* at times with behavior that has an opposite effect. The tendency of staff is to avoid demanding family members, if possible. Withdrawn, quiet patients are not noticed.

Many studies of families in recent years have been subsumed into the larger category of social support. Like the concept of coping, the concept of social support has varied meanings and interpretations. A distinct advantage to the concept is that it can be used to connote the unique personal relationships that constitute an individual's support network, cutting across formal boundaries like the family, church, or self-help groups. A disadvantage to the concept is that it has tended to be used cross-sectionally in studies, inadequately accounting for the process involved in giving and receiving social support. Inadequate attention has been paid to the difference in normative support and crisis or emergency support. In addition, social support is often indicated as having a moderating effect on stress that enhances coping effectiveness. It is with great care that the studies of social support should be read. The general current assumptions can be made in the hope that future study will lead to more accurate detail. These assumptions are that each person in the patient's support network may be a source of support and/or may be needing support from the patient. The larger the active support network, the more complex these relationships become. The smaller the network, or family, the more intense the relationships often may be.

In observing emotional reactivity in families, Bowen[24] observed that when anxiety or tension increased between any two people, a third would be triangled to relieve the anxiety between the two. For example, rather than speaking directly to each other about personal concerns, two people might talk about a third person. Or, one person talks to another about the third rather than talking to the third directly. In both cases triangles are in motion. Bowen suggests that a dyad, that is, two individuals, is never stable, the smallest stable emotional unit being a triangle. When the anxiety between two cannot be contained by triangling a third, a fourth person may be triangled, starting the formation of a series of interlocking triangles. This concept extends the interpersonal definition of anxiety, suggesting patterns of relief behavior that to the informed observer become increasingly clear and provide a base on which to plan intervention. Nurses are frequent candidates for becoming part of anxious triangles with patients and family members.

Intervention

Four categories of nursing action toward intervention are set forth. They are *support, boundary marking, anxiety intervention,* and *information processing.*

Support

This category is chosen with some trepidation because it has been the catch-all category of nursing textbooks and care plans and can stay general enough to be useless. However, no word better describes the activity of the nurse in assisting with coping. The emotional tasks as outlined above are faced by the patient and family. Depending on the particular characteristics and skills of each, their approaches to the tasks are varied. The patient and family need support in order to do what they can do. Orem[25] used the phrase "helping others to do for themselves" or "doing with" and differentiates it from teaching others to do for themselves. When support is being considered as an intervention, it is crucial to have knowledge regarding the desired outcome of the person or family being supported. Knowledge of both the goals and identified limitations to meeting those goals is essential. Resources of the nurse are added to resources of the patient and family so that each person is able to act in his or her own behalf.

Support includes helping people make use of the information they already have. It also includes helping people gain and maintain adequate control so they can take in new information and solve their problems. Support requires knowledge of usual developmental issues that may be integrally related to the goals that the patient and family are trying to reach. Support always means taking clues from the patient and family about what must be done. This is very different from telling people what they must do.

Boundary Marking

Boettcher[26] has identified this core environmental variable. Nursing as a professional group has responsibility for regulation of the environment. Nursing can exercise a major influence in delineation of space, time structuring, and controlling supplies for patients and families. Interventions in this category recognize the adaptive value of privacy, sleep, specific communication, control over interruption, and noise. Consistent with the recommendations of Helton, Gordon, and Nunnery,[22] nurses can reduce the amount of noise and light, especially at night. Procedures can be planned where possible to provide maximum uninterrupted sleep time. Conscious efforts to reduce noise must always begin with monitoring one's own behavior. Noble's[27] finding, that critical-care patients found the most disturbing stimuli to be those which resulted from staff members' communication with each other, continues to be informative. Staff members can get into habits that are much noisier than each person realizes. Such habits form easily and die hard.

Anxiety Intervention

Intervening directly when anxiety is increasing involves helping the patient to name what is being experienced. People use many terms to describe such feelings. Find out what is meant by the terms the patient uses and, if possible, use the terms that have meaning to that person. This is followed by helping the patient think about specific concerns that may have triggered the anxious feelings. Patients can also be helped to identify ways they have used in the past to control increasing anxiety. In novel situations these past behaviors may not be immediately recalled, but with help to focus on remembering past experience, useful precedents may be found. This also serves to focus attention on ideas that are related to but not as directly threatening as the thoughts and feelings that had precipitated the anxious experience.

It is useful to remember that anxiety is communicable. At times, the nurse's first awareness of a patient's increasing anxiety is a feeling of personal distress. When one becomes aware of such clues while giving care, one is in an excellent situation for asking questions about what the patient is experiencing. This facilitates thinking about the experience which can be helpful in regaining emotional control.

Information Processing

The importance of seeking and providing information as an active intervention strategy cannot be overemphasized. Consideration of information is closely linked to the concept of communication. Like the concept of support, communication is often used loosely and serves to sidetrack serious consideration of the subject. Communication is an intricate process. In a recent rethinking of communication in the delivery of nursing care, Kasch[28] makes the observation that communication in health care has tended to be linked to therapeutic communication. Attempts to understand it theoretically have been closely linked to therapy and counseling paradigms. "Extending the counselling paradigm to the domain of nursing tends to ignore the constraints on communication in the health care context and the intense commitment to task activity that characterizes the delivery of nursing care" (p. 74).[28] Recognizing the intensity of demands to perform physical care tasks in the critical-care setting as an influence on communication and more specifically on information handling is imperative.

With these global considerations in mind, the specifics of information pertinent to the critical-care setting are outlined in Table 18-2. Several studies provide useful research-based data about patient and family needs for information. According to one, the foremost needs of family members during the first 72 h after admission to an intensive care unit were "to be informed of their relative's condition, to be kept informed as honestly as possible, to have a chance to speak with the doctor, and to know that the relative is receiving the best care possible. They care least of all about being alone, having friends or children visit, or having such personal needs as food or coffee available" (p. 234).[29] Stillwell[30] studied the importance of visiting to family members and found an increased need to see the relative frequently when the family perceived an increase in the severity of the patient's condition. She suggests that this might serve a coping function for some family members by validating the seriousness of the patient's condition and fostering crisis resolution in the family. Nurses have an active role in establishing and enforcing visiting policies. Frequency of visits can be tailored

to the needs of patient, family, and staff. Visiting is a way of exchanging information which is powerful beyond the use of words.

Conflict between physical care needs of the patient and intense emotional needs of both patients and families has been identified as a continuing issue for critical-care nurses. In a thoughtful discussion of both positive and negative aspects of increased family involvement with critical-care staff, Dunkel and Eisendarth[31] point out that mutual trust can be developed among family and staff members. Family members can provide positive feedback to staff in a way that the patient is too sick to do. They can bring word of their relative after transfer, helping to establish continuity and to decrease isolation of critical-care staff from the larger context of patients' lives. As nurses become grief counselors, their role is broadened and their failure to save life is eased. In this context, it is suggested that helping the family with grief also can bring personal closure for nurses.

However, involvement with family members ultimately may also increase the sense of loss that nurses experience, which may be perceived as a negative aspect of involvement with families. Other negative factors identified by Dunkel and Eisendarth[31] were fear of family interactions and judgments which interfered with patient care by setting unrealistic goals for practice. One cannot do everything. Peer pressure can be fostered when families connect positively with one nurse, and other nurses cannot live up to real or assumed family expectations.

Rasie[32] interviewed different patients and their family members to determine perceived needs. Recurring themes found were that the family members (1) had needs to relive the critical incident that led to the critical illness and hospitalization, (2) were fearful of criticizing staff and felt compelled to defend the quality of care, and (3) had a strong desire for medical information but uncertainty about obtaining it. Based on these and related findings one family intervention program has been developed[33] incorporating the following elements: an initial family assessment that identifies specific information and education needs, a telefamily program in which a daily call is made to an identified member of the family, a teaching pamphlet explaining equipment and procedures with space for

Table 18-2 Information as Intervention

The nurse *gives* information about:	The nurse *gets* information about:
The illness	Physical self
The procedures	Emotional self
The environment	Questions, concerns
The staff	What might help with
Usual patient reactions to a specific condition	coping

individualized information, and a volunteer program. Carefully screened and trained volunteers staff the family waiting room, providing information that may assist family members to meet personal needs and obtaining information regarding the patient when appropriate. They also provide an invaluable service in allowing family members to relive the critical incident and to discuss their observations repeatedly. As the Horowitz model described, this need to review one's experiences is usual. The review serves a powerful function in regaining control in the coping process.

Confronting Life and Death

Coping in critical care cannot adequately be discussed without considering the reality that death haunts the lives of staff and patients alike. The way a particular person or family contends with the knowledge of the tenuous hold we all have on life is as varied as the ways of coping. Many people do not think seriously about their own deaths until middle adulthood, at which point a life trajectory may be envisioned, usually extending into old age. Life-threatening illness challenges such a vision for patients, families, and for staff members, long before middle age.[34] Death rather than discharge from the critical-care unit is a reality for more than 50 percent of the patients admitted to some units. Not all patients want to, or will, talk about this reality. Staff members make choices consistently about how much of this reality they can stay aware of and still focus on life-supporting tasks. These are not always conscious choices, but when they are, staff members live with the memory of those choices. Coping with the emotional threat that the idea of death and/or the death of a particular patient evokes is both plight and privilege. The more emotional comfort any health professional can come to feel in this situation, the more available they can be to patients and families, and to each other.

All patients interviewed in the study of denial previously cited made statements indicative of death anxiety and concerns related to death, regardless of diagnosis or degree of illness.[15] These researchers concluded with recommendations for open-ended interviews which allow patients to discuss their concerns, including death-related concerns. As has

been suggested in other contexts, *being with* and *accepting* what patients say can be more important than *doing,* and more difficult.[35] Being available to hear patients' concerns is not always possible.

So many variables influence the lives of people associated with critical care, whether offering or receiving service. Awareness of life and death issues and the potential for emotional pain in confronting them is an ongoing challenge. Attempts to deny their existence can be costly. Exclusive focus on the death side of the equation restricts constructive work with life. Likewise, exclusive focus on maintaining life disallows the fundamental life experience of confronting death. Each person's beliefs, experience, stage of development, and felt connection with supportive others influence the degree to which a balance can be found between these two extremes and when lost, regained.

The discussion of death leads back to life and in this context, the life of the nurse. The way critical-care nurses cope with the stress of work, whether or not death is the issue in focus, is a continuing concern. The assumption that critical-care nursing is more stressful than other types of nursing has not been consistently supported by research,[36,37] but no one questions that it is stressful.

One review of literature regarding stress and coping in ICU nursing led two authors to conclude that excessive workloads and understaffing are stressful. Emotional reactions to loss, conflict between staff members, and insecurity in the face of great responsibility are also stressors. Coping involved talking things out, developing technical proficiency, sharing past experiences, and drawing on what had been learned.[38] At about the same time Stehle revisited studies of critical-care nursing stress.[39] Though most of the 19 studies reviewed substantiated work in the units as stressful, intervention strategies and their evaluation were absent. Most of the work neglected to examine personal coping responses specific or beneficial to the nurses themselves. While many suggestions are made to nurses regarding useful strategies, ranging from personal meditation and seeking spiritual guidance to team-building programs provided by the employer, definitive information from critical-care nurses is needed regarding their own approaches to coping. Each nurse's approach to coping with the distress of providing critical care is personally shaped. Whether private or interpersonally active methods are valued, consciously identifying one's own resources is encouraged, as is facing the distress that requires a coping response directly.

Summary

Coping behaviors take many forms. Assessing previous coping behaviors of patients and families is useful for drawing on existing family resources from the outset in an experience with critical illness. Coping is a process which can be facilitated by decreasing demands, increasing resources, and continually appraising the results of these efforts with patients and families.

The self-concept of patients and families is threatened in the process of accommodating to the demands of the current situation. Each person attempts to control the threats by actively inhibiting or facilitating conscious awareness of information and stimulation from the environment.

Stages of illness influence the kinds of coping behaviors that are likely to be observed, as well as usual individual and family coping patterns. These stages suggest intervention usually appropriate to them. The interventions discussed, boundary marking, support, anxiety intervention, and information processing, all apply at each stage. However, it is usual that in early stages of a critical illness, the nurse is in the position to establish definitive boundaries for patients and families. In later stages this can be a process in which people involved participate more actively. The nature of the support required for each patient and family will only become clear after assessment. Patients and families are supported in doing for themselves what they need to do. Anxiety intervention is activated whenever anxiety is observed to be increasing. When individuals are helped to think about what they are experiencing in anxious situations, they are more able to effectively use the available information for problem solving.

Information processing is an active intervention process that involves selective gathering of information from patients and families. It involves providing information to them in doses that are manageable. It also means reviewing information with them repeatedly, not expecting that anyone has information just because they have already been told.

Coping in critical care involves a constant confrontation with issues of life and death. Being with people who are experiencing enormous threats and losses can be both plight and privilege for the nurse. Knowing one's own approaches to coping and nurturing one's emotional resources continues to be a particular challenge to critical-care nurses.

References

1. Mariotto, M. J., & Paul, G. L. (1984). The utility of assessment for different purposes. In M. Mirabi (Ed.), *The chronically mentally ill: Research and services* (pp. 73–83). New York: SP Medical & Scientific Books.
2. Pearlin, L. I., & Schooler, C. (1978). The structure of coping. *Journal of Health and Social Behavior, 19,* 2–21.
3. Lazarus, R. S., & Folkman, S. (1984). *Stress, appraisal, and coping.* New York: Springer.
4. Weisman, A. D. (1979). *Coping with cancer* (p. 27). New York: McGraw-Hill.
5. White, R. W. (1974). Strategies of adaptation: An attempt at systematic description. In C. V. Coelho, D. A. Hamburg, & J. E. Adams (Eds.), *Coping and adaptation* (pp. 47–68). New York: Basic Books.
6. Kobosa, S. C., Maddi, S., & Kahn, S. (1982). Hardiness and health: A prospective study. *Journal of Personality and Social Psychology, 1,* 168–177.
7. Murphy, L. B. (1974). Coping, vulnerability and resilience in childhood. In G. V. Coelho, D. A. Hamburg, & J. E. Adams (Eds.), *Coping and adaptation,* (pp. 69–100). New York: Basic Books.
8. Dimsdale, J. E. (1978). Coping-every man's war. *American Journal of Psychotherapy, 32,* 402–413.
9. Fife, B. L. (1985). A model for predicting the adaptation of families to medical crisis: An analysis of role integration. *Image: the Journal of Nursing Scholarship, 17,* 108–112.
10. Suls, J., & Fletcher, B. (1985). Self-attention, life stress, and illness: A prospective study. *Psychosomatic Medicine, 47,* 469–481.
11. Figley, C. R. (1983). Catastrophes: An overview of family reactions. In C. R. Figley, & H. I. McCubbin (Eds.), *Stress and the family II: Coping with catastrophe* (pp. 3–20). New York: Brunner Mazel.
12. Caplan, G. (1964). *Principles of preventive psychiatry.* New York: Basic Books.
13. Moos, R. H., & Schaefer, J. A. (1984). The crisis of physical illness: An overview and conceptual ap-

proach. In R. H. Moos (Ed.), *Coping with physical illness. 2: New perspectives* (pp. 3–25). New York: Plenum Medical.

14. Sullivan, H. S. (1953). *The interpersonal theory of psychiatry.* New York: Norton.

15. Thomas, S. A., Sappington, E., Gross, H. S., Noctor, M., Friedmann, E., & Lynch, J. J. (1983). Denial in coronary care patients—an objective reassessment. *Heart and Lung, 12,* 74–80.

16. Browne, I. W., & Hackett, T. P. (1967). Emotional reactions to the threat of impending death. *Irish Journal of Medical Science, 496,* 177–187.

17. Hackett, T. P., Cassem, N. H., & Wishnie, H. (1968). Psychological hazards of coronary care unit. *New England Journal of Medicine, 279,* 1365–1370.

18. Hackett, T. P., & Cassem, N. H. (1974). Development of a quantitative rating scale to assess denial. *Journal of Psychosomatic Research, 18,* 93–100.

19. Horowitz, M. J. (1979). Psychological response to serious life events. In V. Hamilton, & D. M. Warburton (Eds.), *Human stress and cognition: An information processing approach* (pp. 235–263). New York: John Wiley & Sons.

20. Cassell, E. J. (1979). Reactions to physical illness and hospitalization. In G. Usdin, & J. M. Lewis (Eds.), *Psychiatry in medical practice* (pp. 103–131). New York: McGraw-Hill.

21. Hansell, H. N. (1984). The behavioral effects of noise on man: The patient with "intensive care unit psychosis." *Heart and Lung, 13,* 59–65.

22. Helton, M. C., Gordon, S. H., & Nunnery, S. L. (1980). The correlation between sleep deprivation and the intensive care unit syndrome. *Heart and Lung, 9,* 464–468.

23. King, K. B. (1985). Measurement of coping strategies, concerns, and emotional response in patients undergoing coronary artery bypass grafting. *Heart and Lung, 14,* 579–586.

24. Bowen, M. (1978). *Family therapy in clinical practice.* New York: Jason Aronson.

25. Orem, D. E. (1980). *Nursing concepts of practice* (2d ed.). New York: McGraw-Hill.

26. Boettcher, E. G. (1985). Boundary marking. *Journal of Psychosocial Nursing, 23*(8), 25–30.

27. Noble, M. A. (1979). Communication in the ICU: Therapeutic or disturbing? *Nursing Outlook, 3,* 195.

28. Kasch, C. R. (1983). Interpersonal competence and communication in the delivery of nursing care. *Advances in Nursing Science, 6,* 71–88.

29. Daley, L. (1984). The perceived immediate needs of families with relatives in the intensive care setting. *Heart and Lung, 13,* 231–237.

30. Stillwell, S. B. (1984). Importance of visiting needs as perceived by family members of patients in the intensive care unit. *Heart and Lung, 13,* 238–242.

31. Dunkel, J., & Eisendarth, S. (1983). Families in the intensive care unit: Their effect on staff. *Heart and Lung, 12,* 258–261.

32. Rasie, S. (1980). Meeting families' needs helps you meet ICU patients' needs. *Nursing, 10,* 32.

33. Hodovanic, B. H., Reardon, D., Reese, W., & Hedges, B. (1984). Family crisis intervention program in the medical intensive care unit. *Heart and Lung, 13,* 243–249.

34. Pattison, E. M. (1977). *The experience of dying.* Englewood Cliffs, NJ: Prentice-Hall.

35. Wright, L. K. (1985). Life threatening illness. *Journal of Psychosocial Nursing, 23*(9), 7–11.

36. Cronin-Stubbs, D., & Rooks, C. A. (1985). The stress, social support, and burnout of critical care nurses: The results of research. *Heart and Lung, 14,* 31–39.

37. Keane, A., Ducette, J., & Adler, D. C. (1985). Stress in ICU and non-ICU nurses. *Nursing Research, 34,* 231–236.

38. Caldwell, T., & Weiner, M. F. (1981). Stresses and coping in ICU nursing. I. A review. *General Hospital Psychiatry, 3,* 119–127.

39. Stehle, J. L. (1981). Critical care nursing stress: The findings revisited. *Nursing Research, 30,* 182–186.

4

Cardiovascular Patient-Care Problems

19

Anatomy and Physiology of the Cardiovascular System

Joan Vitello-Cicciu

Functional Anatomy

Introduction

When considering the anatomy and physiology of the cardiovascular system, it is helpful to begin with a sense of awe and admiration for the heart as a remarkably simplistic organ in which motion is continuous during a lifetime. The appreciation for the importance of the living heart perhaps was considered by William Harvey in the seventeenth century when he looked into the chest of an animal and noted "that there is a time when it moves, and a time when it is motionless."[1]

As knowledge expanded regarding this remarkable organ, it was noted that this organ had two fundamental tasks: (1) to pump blood without interruption in order to supply oxygen and nutrients to the billions of cells within the body, and (2) to be able to adjust its pumping action in order to supply more or less blood to the tissues upon demand.

It is believed that a thorough knowledge of cardiovascular anatomy and physiology provides the foundation on which treatment for cardiovascular disorders can be directed. John Morgan[2] further substantiates this perspective by commenting, "As every disease we labour under is a disorder of the vital animal or natural functions; a thorough acquaintance with these in their sound state is implied before we can pretend to understand their morbid affections, or how to remedy them." Thus, this chapter is intended to provide the foundation of this knowledge.

The authors gratefully acknowledge the contribution of Lin Weeks to the first edition.

External Appearance

Anterior View

The heart is a cone-shaped muscle situated in the middle of the mediastinum where it is overlapped by the two pleural sacs. It occupies most of the space between the posterior surface of the sternum and the anterior surface of the vertebrae. The heart is projected approximately two-thirds to the left of the midsternal line in what is known as the *levo-cardiac position*.

The normal heart size in the average adult is approximately 12 cm long and 9 cm wide. The weight varies in individuals depending on age, sex, and so forth. The upper part of the heart is called the base and is formed by the right and left atria. The great vessels are suspended from the base. The lower part of the heart is called the apex, which rests on the upper surface of the diaphragm.

The anterior surface of the heart consists mostly of the right ventricle (Fig. 19-1). The pulmonary trunk arises upwards from the right ventricle and bifurcates into the left and right pulmonary artery under the arch of the aorta. The right atrium is situated above the right ventricle. The groove known as the *atrioventricular (coronary) sulcus* separates these two chambers. The curved shape of the right atrium forms the right lateral border of the heart in the frontal plane. The superior vena cava forms the upper right margin. It can be visualized entering the right atrium from above through the pericardium.

The left lateral border or apex of the heart consists of the left ventricle (LV). The *anterior interventricular sulcus* is another groove which demarcates the right from the LV. The remaining portion of the left border of the heart is formed by the left atrial appendage and the pulmonary trunk.

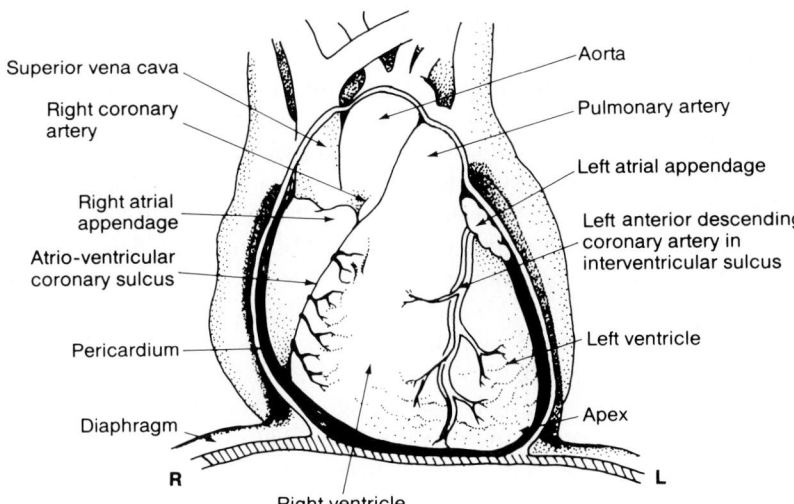

Figure 19-1   Schematic drawing showing the normal relations of the pericardium, great vessels, ventricles, and atria as viewed in the frontal position. R = right; L = left.

The aorta arises behind the pulmonary trunk from the LV. The space between the aortic arch and pulmonary trunk is called the *aortic window*. The ligamentum arteriosum and the left recurrent laryngeal nerve reside in this space.

Cardiac Tissue

Pericardium

The heart and roots of the great vessels are contained in a relatively fixed position by the pericardium, a fibroserous sac. This sac contains two surfaces known as the *fibrous* and *serous pericardium*. The fibrous pericardium is the outer surface which consists of white, glistening fibrous tissue giving the pericardium its shape and appearance. The serous pericardium consists of two linings known as the *visceral* and *parietal layers*.

The visceral pericardium or epicardium lines the surface of the heart. It also covers a small portion of the venae cavae, aorta, coronary blood vessels, and nerves. The parietal layer is continuous with the visceral layer and intimately adheres to the fibrous pericardium. This layer is also attached by ligaments to the manubrium, the xiphoid process, vertebral column, and diaphragm. The visceral and parietal layers are separated by the pleural cavity or space which contains about 10 to 20 mL of thin, clear pericardial fluid. This fluid acts as a lubricant between the contracting surfaces of the visceral and parietal layers.

The compliance of the pericardium is limited, and thus contains the heart in a stationary position, as previously mentioned. Since it resists stretching, it also functions to prevent acute cardiac overdistention. In addition, the pericardium serves as a barrier to infection and neoplastic invasion.

Myocardium

The myocardium is the cardiac muscle tissue that comprises the largest portion of the heart wall. It is composed of three major types: (1) the specialized conduction fibers, (2) the atrial muscle fibers, and (3) fibers of the ventricles. Each type will be discussed later in this chapter.

Endocardium

The endocardium is the innermost tissue layer of the cardiac wall. It contains connective tissue, elastic fibers, and endothelial cells which line the heart chambers and valves and is in continuation with the tunica intima layer of the great vessels. These endothelial cells form a smooth surface for blood contact to deter clot formation.

Cardiac Chambers

Atria

The right and left atria serve as volume reservoirs and conduits for blood that is being sent into the ventricles. The atria are divided by the interatrial septum which contains the fossa ovalis. The right atrium (RA) is a thin-walled structure approximately 2 mm in thickness. The inflow tracts, specifically the superior and inferior venae cavae, which deliver unoxygenated blood, enter through the posterior wall of the atrium, known as the *sinus venarum.* The opening to the coronary sinus which drains venous blood from the coronary circulation is located between the inferior vena cava and the tricuspid valve.

The left atrium (LA) is not usually seen in the anterior view. It lies posterior and to the right of the left ventricle. The wall thickness is approximately 3 mm, which is slightly thicker than the RA. Four pulmonary veins serve as inflow tracts bringing oxygenated blood from the lungs through the posterolateral wall of the LA. The posterior wall of the LA comprises most of the posterior surface of the heart and is anterior to the esophagus and thoracic aorta.

Ventricles

The right and left ventricles function as the pumping chambers of the heart (Fig. 19-2). The right ventricle (RV) is an anterior crescent-shaped structure which lies underneath the sternum. It contains trabeculations, or fibromuscular bands, from which the papillary muscles originate. These trabeculations serve as stabilizers for pacing catheters. The RV is approximately 3 to 5 mm in thickness and can be divided into an inflow and outflow tract. The inflow tract consists of the trabecular muscles and the tricuspid valve which directs incoming blood from the RA toward the smooth-walled infundibulum or outflow tract. The infundibulum forms the superior aspect of the chamber. It is divided from the inflow tract by a band of muscle, the *crista supraventricularis,* which joins other constrictor muscles from the outflow tract to direct blood superiorly and posteriorly out through the pulmonic valve. During ventricular systole, this chamber contracts like a bellows to eject venous blood through the pulmonary artery into the pulmonic circulation.

The LV is an egg-shaped structure. It is three to five times thicker than the RV with a wall thickness of 13 to 15 mm. This wall thickness reflects the degree of high-pressure work that is required by the LV. The LV free wall is the portion of the LV exclusive of the septum. A small portion of the LV and the interventricular septum form a blunt tip referred to as the *cardiac apex.* Because of the forward tilt of the heart, the movement of this apical portion during ventricular contraction is referred to as the *point of maximal impulse (PMI)* or *apical impulse,* which can be located on physical examination at the fourth to fifth intercostal space at the midclavicular line. The funnel-shaped inflow tract, consisting of the mitral annulus, both mitral leaflets, and their chordae tendineae, directs blood in from the LA. Blood flows in an anterior leftward motion and is ejected from the LV through the outflow tract in a superior rightward direction at a

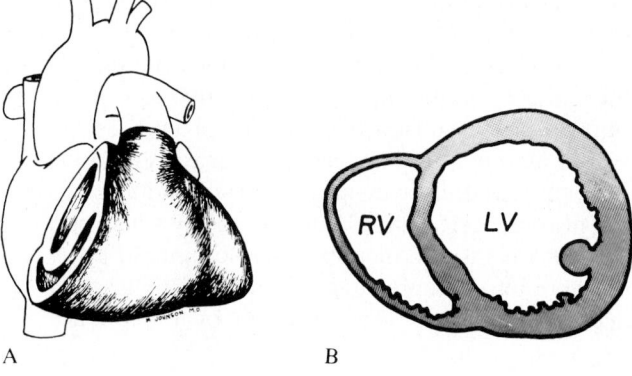

Figure 19-2   The striking structural difference between the left and right ventricular chambers. The interventricular septum protrudes into the right ventricle, causing a crescent shape which is in marked contrast to the circular left ventricle. (*From J. Willis Hurst (ed.), The Heart, Arteries, and Veins, 4th ed., McGraw-Hill, New York, 1974).*

A   B

90° angle to the inflow tract. The LV pumps like a corkscrew when ejecting blood out to the aorta.

Cardiac Valves

Three functional properties of the cardiac valves are (1) preventing regurgitation of blood from one chamber to another, (2) permitting rapid antegrade flow without imposing resistance on that flow, and (3) withstanding high-pressure loads. Valves open and close in response to pressure gradients; i.e., valves open when pressure in the preceding chamber is higher and close when the gradient reverses. Though medical science has been attempting for over three decades to prosthetically mimic these functions, the most sophisticated technology has resulted in a very poor second to the engineering marvels of the atrioventricular and semilunar valves.

The AV valves are structurally the more complex of the two sets of valves (Fig. 19-3). Situated between the atria and ventricles, the tricuspid valve on the right and mitral valve on the left are functionally very similar. Each has a fibrous supporting ring, the annulus, and has two large primary cusps (leaflets) which are opposite one another and connected via chordae tendineae, which descend as if from an inverted parachute to the papillary muscles. Note that the chordae tendineae arise from the large anterior and posterior cusps

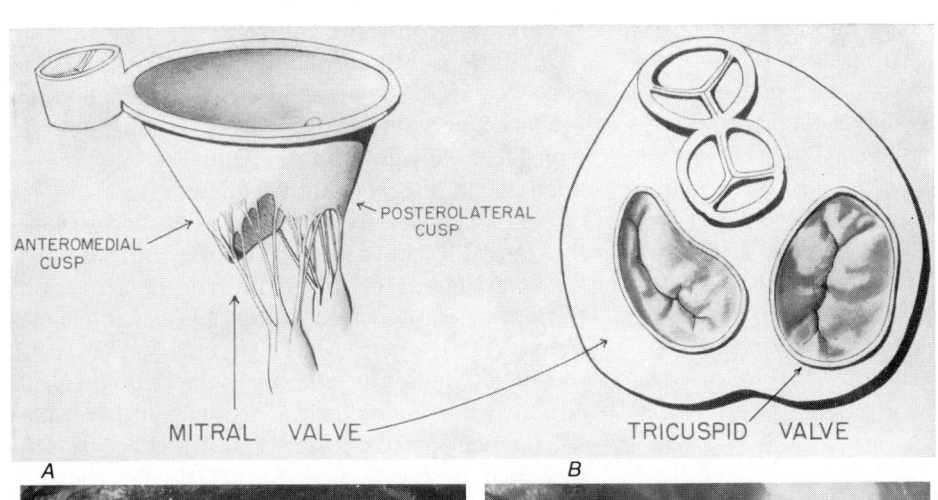

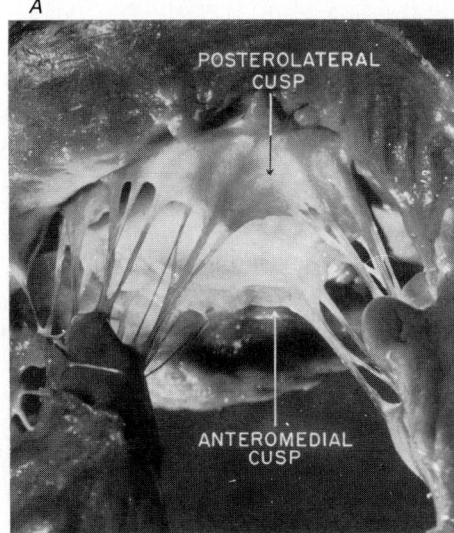

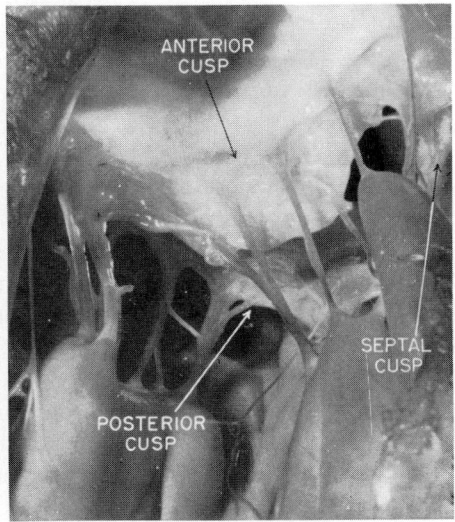

Figure 19-3 Anatomical structure of atrioventricular valves. (*A*) The funnel-shaped mitral valve is schematically demonstrated on the left, with the two cusps attaching via chordae tendineae to individual sets of papillary muscles. (*B*) Schematic representation of the closed mitral and tricuspid valves. Though very similar structurally, the tricuspid has a larger intermediate cusp which attaches to a third set of papillary muscles. (*After W. Spalteholz, Hand Atlas of Human Anatomy, Lippincott, Philadelphia, 1933.*) (*C*) Excision of a normal left ventricle to demonstrate the cusps of the mitral valve and attachment to papillary muscles. (*D*) View of the tricuspid valve from within the right ventricular chamber. (*From Robert Rushmer, Cardiovascular Dynamics, Saunders, Philadelphia, 1970. Used by permission of the publisher.*)

of the mitral valve and individually insert into two sets of papillary muscles. The tricuspid has a third intermediate cusp (septal) which inserts with the anterior and posterior cusps into a total of three sets of papillary muscles.

During ventricular filling, the valves serve as a conduit as they transfer blood from the atria to the ventricles (Fig. 19-3). With ventricular contraction, the papillary muscles exert tension on the chordae; this tension tends to allow the valve leaflets to balloon upward and draw together. Should the chordae tendineae rupture or the papillary muscle suffer acute ischemia, the result can be severe valvular regurgitation or insufficiency.

The semilunar valves each consist of three cuplike cusps which are symmetrical. Structurally, they are very dissimilar to the AV valves; since a much greater pressure load is imposed on these valves, their design is much simpler. Following termination of ventricular systole, the high pressure within the pulmonary artery and aorta drops, causing retrograde flow of blood toward the ventricles, thus filling the aortic and pulmonary cusps with blood and snapping them shut. The event can be seen on the normal arterial waveform and is known as the *dicrotic notch*.

The *sinuses of Valsalva* are two outpouchings immediately behind the semilunar cusps. In the aorta, they serve to prevent obstruction of the coronary ostia by the valve cusps.

Coronary Artery Anatomy

The right and left coronary arteries arise from the coronary ostia in the aortic root (Fig. 19-4). The left coronary artery almost always emerges from a single ostium in the coronary sinus of the aorta, while the right coronary sinus sometimes gives rise to two ostia, the smaller of which becomes the conus artery.

The left main coronary artery is of variable length but divides, usually within 2 to 10 cm, into the left anterior descending (LAD) and left circumflex arteries. The branches of the main vessel take a diagonal route over the left ventricular free wall and are frequently referred to as the *diagonal left ventricular branches*. They are generally situated

between the anterior descending and circumflex arteries. The LAD supplies the LV ventricular free wall, the septum, and portions of the right ventricle. In addition, it usually supplies the anterior as well as portions of the posterior and inferior apex. The circumflex usually emerges at a 90° angle from the main left coronary and courses toward the lateral left ventricle and apex. Branches from the circumflex supply the posterior and lateral walls of the left ventricle. In about 10 percent of persons, it gives rise to the AV nodal artery; in such cases the left coronary and its branches supply the entire left ventricle and septum.

The right coronary artery arises from the right aortic sinus and courses down the right atrioventricular sulcus. In 85 to 95 percent of hearts, it makes a 90° turn and crosses the crux of the heart and becomes the posterior descending artery.

If the conus artery does not originate directly from the aorta, it is the first branch off the right coronary artery (RCA). The sinus node artery emerges from the RCA in approximately 50 percent of persons; in the remainder it emerges from the circumflex. In the majority of cases the RCA supplies the RA and RV and gives rise to branches supplying the inferior surface of the LV. The determination of right or left coronary artery dominance is made by evaluating whether the right coronary artery or the left circumflex artery crosses the crux (the point at which the interventricular sulcus and coronary sulcus meet on the posterior wall) to become the posterior descending artery (PDA). The heart is said to have right coronary dominance if the right coronary artery becomes the PDA. The AV nodal artery arises from the right coronary in right-sided dominance and supplies the AV node and bundle of His.

Interarterial vessels connect or anastomose with each other. These foster collateral circulation and can be found through the full thickness of the myocardium. The greatest amount of collaterals is located near the endocardial surface. The number of these collaterals can increase in response to demand imposed by atherosclerotic heart disease, chronic anemia, or hypoxemia.

Coronary venous drainage is accomplished via the thebesian veins on the RA and RV, and the anterior cardiac veins, which course over the an-

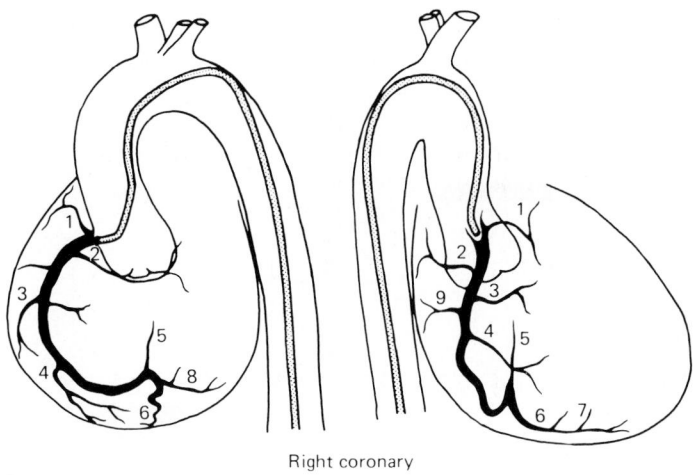

Right coronary

a

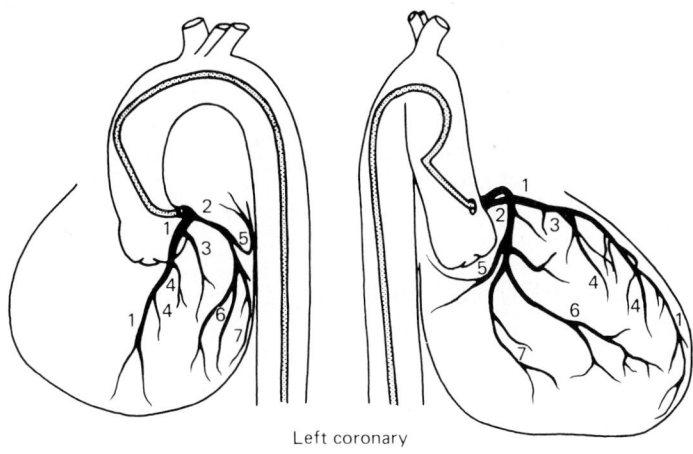

Left coronary

b

Figure 19-4 Normal coronary anatomy from right and left posterior oblique positions. (*a*) Right artery: (1) conus branch, (2) sinus node artery, (3) muscular branches to right ventricle, (4) artery of acute margins, (5) AV nodal artery, (6) posterior descending, (7) posterior septal, (8) posterolateral branches, (9) arterial branch. (*b*) Left coronary artery: (1) anterior descending, (2) circumflex, (3) diagonal branches, (4) septal branches, (5) atrial circumflex, (6) marginal artery, (7) posterolateral branches. (*Adapted from Stephen Ayres and V. Gianelli, Cardiology: A Clinicophysiologic Approach. Courtesy of Appleton Century Crofts, New York, 1971.*)

terior right ventricular wall. Left ventricular venous drainage occurs mainly through the coronary sinus and its branches.

Lymphatic System

The lymphatic vessels are the principal routes by which protein and other large particulate matter can be removed from the interstitium; it is fundamentally a drainage system. The distribution of the lymphatics parallels that of the venous system in that they both have extensive superficial and deep collecting systems. Only cartilage, epithelium, and tissues of the central nervous system lack lymph

supply. In addition to returning fluid and protein to the circulation, the lymphatic system removes debris such as bacteria, toxins, and degenerating tissues.

Cardiac Nerves

Innervation of the heart is accomplished by both cholinergic fibers from the vagus nerve and by adrenergic fibers from the upper thoracic spinal cord through the cardiac plexus via superior, middle, and inferior cervical ganglia.

Vagal fibers are predominantly found in the SA node, AV node, and atrial muscle fibers. The right vagus nerve fibers supply the SA node and function to control the heart rate and force of atrial contraction, whereas the left vagus nerve supplies chiefly the AV node.

Sympathetic nerve fibers extend to the atria and ventricles. Most of these fibers influence ventricular contraction. Vagal fibers also extend to both ventricles, but do not seem to affect ventricular contraction as do the sympathetic fibers.

Sensory fibers also transmit impulses through the cardiac nerves up to the central nervous system. These sensory fibers are located in the pericardium, ventricular walls, and coronary blood vessels.

Systemic and Pulmonic Circulation

The walls of the aorta and large arteries are extremely thick and tough. Functionally, they serve to transport blood under high pressure to the tissues through their role as a pressure reservoir. With left ventricular ejection, the walls within the aortic arch distend as the arterial pressure rises, resulting in transmission of a pressure pulse down the aorta and on into the arteries. When the ventricular contraction ceases, the arterial pressure gradually falls, but sufficient tension remains within the walls to drive blood through the capillaries to the tissues and overcome peripheral resistance. By so doing, the systemic arterial pressure of approximately 90 mmHg maintains forward flow, as demonstrated in Fig. 19-5. The elasticity of the aorta allows it to act as a compression chamber and reservoir during LV ejection which converts pulsatile to continuous flow in diastole. This process is called the *windkessel effect*.

Between the arteries and veins lie the capillaries, whose walls are composed only of endothelial cells. The thin capillary walls are essential in permitting rapid diffusion of substances between the blood and tissue. Because of their very small caliber they can support pressures of up to 100 mmHg in the lower extremities during standing. At heart level, the capillary pressure is normally between 20 and 30 mmHg.

The veins are very thin-walled and normally are under very low pressure. They accommodate large volumes of blood with very little fluctuation in pressure. Contrasted with the arterial circulation,

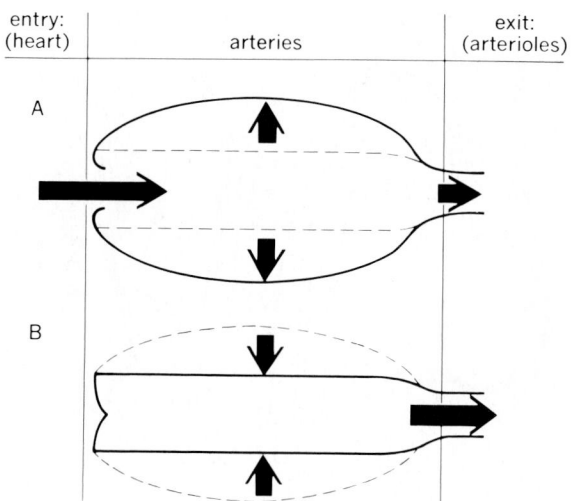

Figure 19-5 During systole much of the blood is stored in the elastic arteries, although some forward flow does occur. In diastole the stored tension within the walls, or elastic recoil, is instrumental in modifying pulsatile flow into constant flow throughout the cardiac cycle. (*From Robert M. Berne and Matthew N. Levy, Cardiovascular Physiology, 3d ed., Mosby, St. Louis, 1977. Used by permission of the publisher.*)

in which even small increases in volume can induce large pressure fluctuations, the principal function of the venous system as a low-pressure, variable-volume reservoir becomes apparent. In fact, almost three-quarters of the systemic circulation is stored within the venous circulation in the large capacitance veins (Fig. 19-6). Note the very small amount of blood within the capillaries, where the most important function of the cardiovascular system occurs.

Similarly, the pulmonary vasculature is thin-walled and distensible, with relatively short branches. Since the pulmonary branches have much larger internal diameters than do the systemic arteries, the distensible pulmonary vasculature accommodates the same stroke volume as the systemic arterial circuit.

The pulmonary artery extends approximately 4 cm beyond the right ventricle before dividing into the right and left arteries which carry venous blood from the right ventricle to the pulmonary capillaries. Two pulmonary veins from each lung carry oxygenated blood to the left atrium. The four pulmonary veins have similar compliance to the

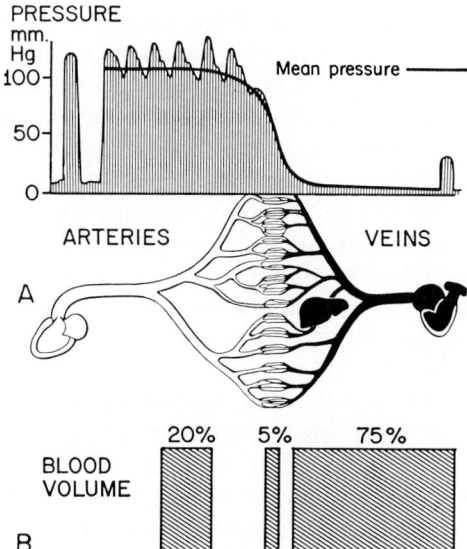

Figure 19-6   The volume of blood stored in the distensible venous circulation is between 60 to 75 percent and can change dramatically. Arterial volume, however, remains at about 20 percent of total blood volume and does not vary significantly. (*From Robert Rushmer, Cardiovascular Dynamics, Saunders, Philadelphia, 1970. Used by permission of the publisher.*)

veins of the systemic circuit. Oxygenation of the lungs themselves is performed by the bronchial vessels, which arise from the aorta and drain into the left atrium via the pulmonary veins to contribute a slight mixing of venous with arterial blood—approximately 1 to 2 percent of the cardiac output.

Anatomy of the Conduction System

The cells which are involved in conducting an electric current are known as the *pacemaker* or *automatic cells.* They are discussed in greater detail in Chap. 11. Located at the junction of the superior vena cava and the right atrium lies the normal pacemaker of the heart, the *sinoatrial node* (SA node). An electric impulse is initiated at this node and travels through the internodal pathways to the *atrioventricular node* (AV), located in the right atrium, directly above the tricuspid valve and anterior to the coronary sinus. Once the impulse travels through the AV node, it courses along the common *bundle of His,* which divides almost im-

mediately into the right and left bundle. The left bundle further divides to form two direct pathways to the anterior and posterior papillary muscle. The impulse then travels and permeates through the many small fibers of the *Purkinje network,* beginning at the endocardium, and finally terminates within the ventricular myocardium.

Structure of the Myocardium

The cells that comprise the cardiac muscle are the specialized electrical conduction cells known as pacemaker cells (previously discussed) and the *working myocardial cells.* These working myocardial cells consist of atrial and ventricular fibers which are involved in the contractile force of the heart. The pacemaker cells are somewhat smaller in size than the ventricular fibers.

The cardiac muscle as a whole is often compared to skeletal muscle because of its striated appearance and color as well as some of its functional characteristics. It should be noted, however, that myocardial muscle shares many similarities with certain types of visceral smooth muscle such as the ureter, uterus, and gastrointestinal tract. These muscles appear to have inherent rhythmicity and to be able to conduct a wave of excitation in a manner similar to that of the myocardium.

Microscopically, an individual myocardial cell is approximately 40 to 100 μm in length and 10 to 20 μm in diameter.[3] The long end of each cell is connected by a thickened portion of the sarcolemma known as an *intercalated disk.* These disks may vary in type, but they serve functionally as a barrier between cells. It should be noted that although these disks serve to separate cells, these cells as a whole still function as a syncytium or as a single cell because these disks offer little electrical resistance, allowing the electric current to spread simultaneously throughout the fibers.

Surrounding each cell is the surface membrane known as the sarcolemma. It is composed of the plasmalemma, which is a semipermeable membrane layer, and the glycocalyx. In the center of each cell is the nucleus. Lysosomes are located near the nucleus. These vesicles contain hydrolytic enzymes which have the potential of lysing cellular membranes and other cellular components.

Myofibrils are long rodlike structures which give the heart muscle its striated appearance. These structures run the length of a cell and are composed of repeating units called the *sarcomeres*. The sarcomere is the contractile unit within the myofibrils arranged in parallel rows along the long axis (Fig. 19-7). The average length of a sarcomere is 1.6 to 2.2 μm. Multiple sarcomeres are found in any given cell extending from one Z band to the next. Extending from each Z band toward the middle of the sarcomere can be seen the thin filament which is predominantly composed of the protein actin. The thick filaments of myosin are found in the middle of the sarcomere, the A band where they overlap with the thin actin filaments. The central light area or H zone is occupied only by the thicker filaments, while the I band contains only the actin filament.

It is postulated that cross bridges protrude from the myosin filaments at regular intervals, and it is these cross bridges which, during contraction, cause lateral movement of the actin and myosin filaments so that they slide past one another, bringing about the development of tension and shortening within the muscle. During contraction, it appears that the widths of the I band and H band shrink as the actin is drawn past the myosin and the Z bands draw closer together, while the A bands remain of one length, both during stretching and contraction of the fiber. The physiology of mechanical contraction will be discussed in further detail in the next section, "Excitation-Contraction Coupling."

In close proximity to the sarcomeres are the mitochondria, which are vitally important in cardiac metabolism. These bodies are the source of high-energy compounds such as ATP (adenosine triphosphate) needed for production of chemical energy for myocardial contraction as well as for synthesis of nutrients. The prodigious oxygen demands of the heart can be appreciated by noting that between 30 and 50 percent of the myocardium

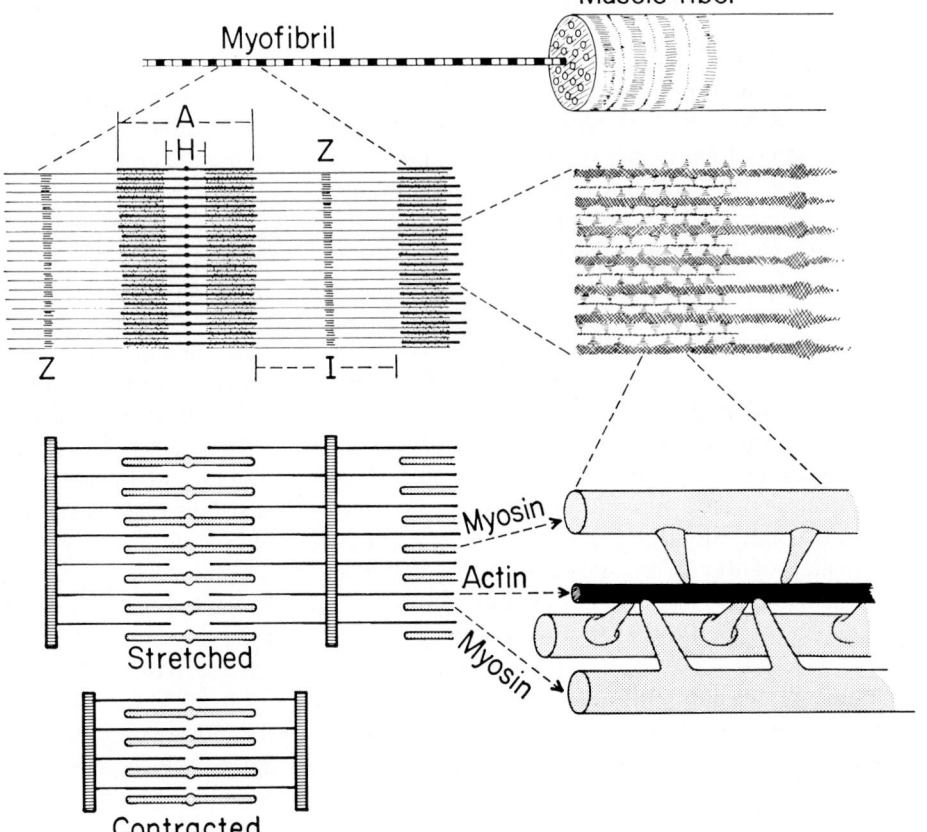

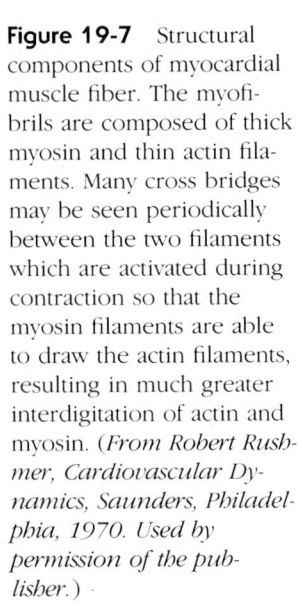

Figure 19-7 Structural components of myocardial muscle fiber. The myofibrils are composed of thick myosin and thin actin filaments. Many cross bridges may be seen periodically between the two filaments which are activated during contraction so that the myosin filaments are able to draw the actin filaments, resulting in much greater interdigitation of actin and myosin. (*From Robert Rushmer, Cardiovascular Dynamics, Saunders, Philadelphia, 1970. Used by permission of the publisher.*)

is occupied by mitochondria. When ischemia exists within the heart, the balance between energy supply and demand can become most precarious. There is some suggestion that a deficiency of ATP may be an important factor in the determinant of infarct size and in the development of cardiac failure.[3]

Additional intracellular components consist of the *transverse tubular system* and the *sarcoplasmic reticulum*. The transverse tubular system is considered to be the place at which the electrical action potential permeates through the cell to trigger muscle contraction and acts as an intracellular transport system for calcium. The sarcoplasmic reticulum is a tubular network surrounding each myofibril. This network stores calcium internally and is thought to release this intracellular calcium once an action potential has been generated. Once calcium is released, it migrates to the myofibrils where it is involved in binding of the actin and myosin molecule. A more in-depth discussion of the role of calcium in myocardial contraction is found in the next section, "Excitation-Contraction Coupling."

Excitation-Contraction Coupling

In order to comprehend cardiac physiology, it is essential that the electrical and mechanical events be understood. The electrical events have been discussed in Chap. 11. This section discusses the mechanical events which are preceded by electrical events. The method by which the electrical wave of depolarization at the cell membrane produces the mechanical contraction is known as *excitation-contraction coupling*. The major pathologic alterations in myocardial contractility have their basis in the degeneration of this very complex and intricate mechanism.

Calcium seems to have a dual role in cardiac contraction: as a trigger for initiation of contraction and as a regulating factor for the contractile process. The method for release of calcium from its storage place in the sarcoplasmic reticulum appears to result from the CA^+ ions which enter the cell during the plateau of the action potential. These CA^+ ions are theorized to release large quantities of CA^+ from the sarcoplasmic reticulum, allowing activation of the contractile process.[3] Thus, depolarization of the cell membrane initiates the release of the internal store of CA^+ into the cytoplasm. When the wave of depolarization stimulates the release of CA^+, the ion activates myosin to interdigitate with actin.

Interdigitation of the actin and myosin filaments depends upon two more proteins which are present within the thin filaments: *troponin* and *tropomyosin*. During relaxation these two proteins appear to inhibit activation of the myosin cross bridges. When calcium is released during excitation, however, the inhibition is reversed and calcium is bound to troponin so that the myosin cross bridge is activated to draw the thin filament toward itself. It appears that the amount of calcium available to bind with troponin has a direct bearing on the strength of the cardiac contraction.

During repolarization of the muscle, relaxation occurs as calcium is pumped back into the reticulum until its concentration is insufficient to utilize ATP and cross bridges can no longer be formed. Complete recovery of the cells coincides with the return of calcium to its storage sites.

Other potential influences on cardiac contractility are those caused by abnormal extracellular concentrations of electrolytes, specifically calcium and potassium. Increased concentrations of potassium can cause hyperpolarization of the resting membrane and result in cardiac arrest. Hypercalcemia can induce systolic arrest of the heart, while a decrease in serum calcium can have deleterious effects on contractility.

The Frank-Starling Phenomenon

Similar to that of the skeletal muscle fiber, the force of myocardial contraction is a function of the initial muscle length. The classic studies by Frank in 1895 demonstrated that the myocardial fiber responds with a more forceful contraction when it is stretched. Also referred to as the *length-tension relationship*, the results of Frank's work further demonstrated that there are physiologic limits to the relationship; excessive stretch of the muscle fiber results in development of less tension, resulting in a decrease in contractility.

Maximal force is developed at a length of 2.2 µm. It is at that length in which the actin and myosin filaments are able to provide the greatest number of cross bridges, or force-generating sites. When stretch exceeds a length of 2.4 µm, less interdigitation of thick and thin filaments occurs and fewer contractile sites are activated. Wiggers, and later Starling, continued Frank's work by studying the heart in an isolated heart-lung preparation and demonstrated that the length-tension relationship for the sarcomere can be applied graphically within the heart by substitution of ventricular filling pressure for tension and end-diastolic volume for fiber length.

The normal ventricle is very compliant. Initially the ventricle can accept large increases in volume without a significant increase in pressure. This concept can be illustrated in what is known as the Frank-Starling curve (Fig. 19-8). Physiologic limits operate here as well. However, should increases in ventricular end-diastolic volume cause

an elevated filling pressure within the ventricle, further increases in diastolic filling result in a decrease in ventricular performance, the so-called descending limb of the Starling curve (Fig. 19-8A). In the normal heart, optimal tension is achieved at a filling pressure of about 10 to 12 mmHg, which corresponds to a fiber length of 2.2 μm. Usually, end-diastolic pressure is approximately 0 to 7 mmHg and myocardial length about 2 μm, resulting in normal ventricular performance on the ascending limb of the curve.

The Cardiac Cycle

In order to comprehend cardiac physiology, it is essential that the sequential relationships between the electrical and mechanical events be understood. Figure 19-9 demonstrates the interrelation of those events along with the resulting pressure and volume changes within the cardiac chambers.

Correlation of Electrical and Mechanical Activity

With generation of an action potential within the sinus node and corresponding movement of calcium into the cells, atrial depolarization occurs and a P wave is recorded on the electrocardiogram. Atrial pressure rises immediately thereafter and atrial contraction occurs, adding an additional third to the volume of blood which becomes the ventricular diastolic filling volume. The resulting waveform causes the *a* wave demonstrated in Fig. 19-9 during pressure monitoring. Within 0.2 s following atrial depolarization, the wave of excitation activates the ventricles, resulting in the ventricular action potential and the inscription of the QRS complex, and generating ventricular contraction and the resulting rapid rise in ventricular pressure. The QRS complex, then, precedes ventricular systole very slightly. The contraction of the ventricles causes two additional waveforms within the atria: (1) The *c* wave occurs early and probably results from a combination of factors which include bulging of the AV valves retrograde into the atria; and (2) the *v* wave is seen later, following ventricular systole, and results from atrial filling and the reflection of the increase in atrial pressure on the closed AV valves.

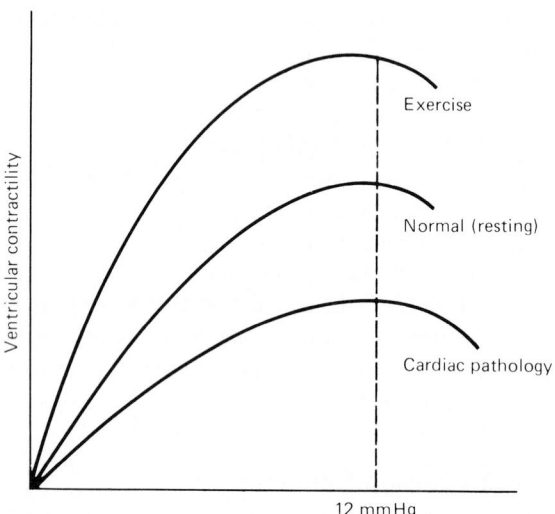

Left ventricular end-diastolic filling pressure (LVEDP)

Figure 19-8 Schematic drawing of the Frank-Starling law of the heart. (*A*) Stretching of the myocardial fiber will within physiologic limits produce an augmentation of ventricular contraction. Since myocardial fiber length cannot be measured, left ventricular end-diastolic filling pressure (LVEDP) is utilized to assess ventricular ejection. Peak ventricular ejection generally occurs at a ventricular filling pressure of 12 mmHg, represented by the dashed line. (*B*) Sympathetic effects can shift the curve to the left, resulting in more rapid increase of ventricular ejection. (*C*) Pathology can shift the curve to the right, causing greater filling pressures for the same or lesser ventricular ejection volume. Thus, filling pressures greater than 12 mmHg are generally required in the diseased heart for optimal performance.

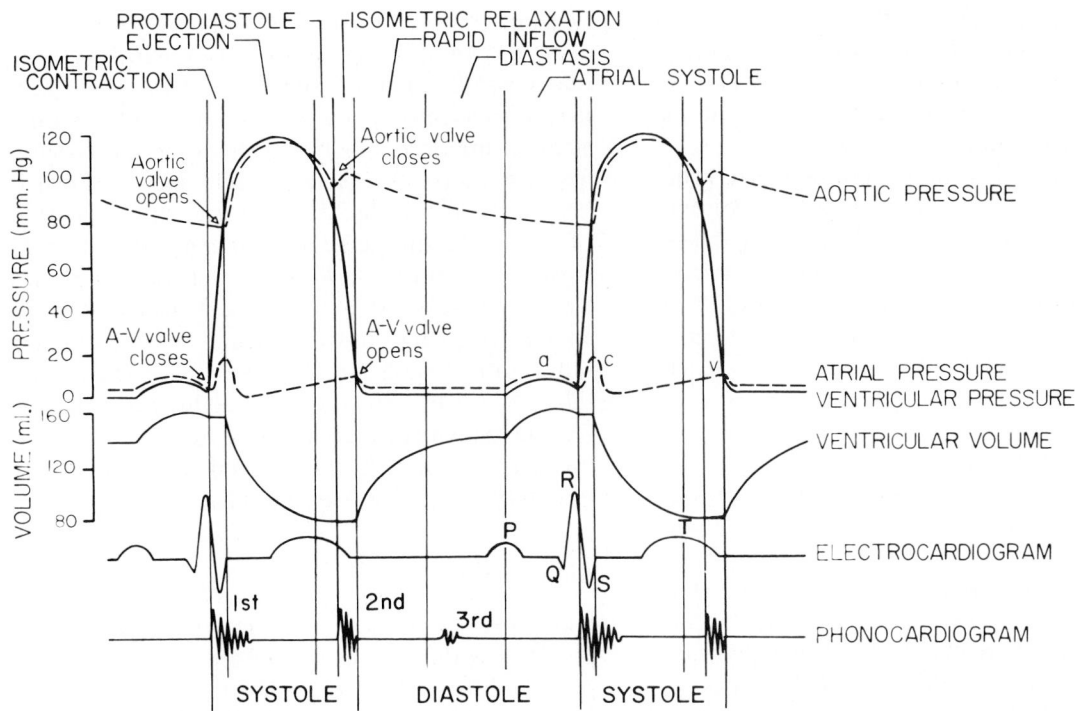

Figure 19-9   Interrelationship of the electrical and mechanical events in the cardiac cycle. Also depicted are the heart sounds (phonocardiogram) and intraventricular volume. (*From Arthur C. Guyton, Textbook of Medical Physiology, Saunders, Philadelphia, 1970. Used by permission of the publisher.*)

The T wave signals the beginning of ventricular repolarization. Atrial repolarization cannot be measured because it occurs simultaneously with ventricular systole and the resulting ventricular relaxation. Hence, ventricular diastole follows the T wave.

Ventricular Systole

The initial portion of ventricular contraction is directed at raising pressure within the chamber. As described previously, the sharp rise in pressure is caused by contraction of the papillary muscles which exerts pressure on the chordae tendineae so that the leaflets of the AV valves are drawn closer together. The resulting pressure increase closes them tightly. The early component of ventricular contraction is called *isovolumic* or *isovolumetric*. Since all four valves are closed, the contracting muscles elevate ventricular pressure without a change in volume. This period includes lengthening of some as well as shortening of other ventricular muscle fibers and is termed isovolumetric, meaning "maintenance of a constant volume."

At the point that intraventricular pressure exceeds the diastolic pressure within the outflow tract, approximately 80 mmHg in the aorta (Fig. 19-9) and 8 mmHg in the pulmonary artery, the semilunar valves are opened and ejection begins. In the initial portion of ventricular ejection, left ventricular pressure rises above that of the aorta, producing a very rapid flow. Later in ejection, ventricular pressure drops below aortic pressure, resulting in a diminished velocity of outflow. The amount of blood ejected from each ventricle under resting conditions, the *stroke volume,* is about 70 to 80 mL.

Right Ventricular Ejection
The geometric differences between the two ventricles were mentioned earlier (Fig. 19-2). Right ventricular ejection performance resembles that of a bellows, since the surface area of the two walls is large in relation to the area contained between

them, and very slight movement from the free wall toward the septum is quite effective in accomplishing systolic ejection. Shortening of the length of the right ventricular muscle occurs as well, but this is not as effective as the bellows action.

It is apparent that the right ventricular structure is suited for performance as a high-volume, low-resistance pump; severely deleterious effects can occur from an acute pressure load on the right ventricle, such as a massive pulmonary embolism. Currently under much investigation is the effect of right ventricular ischemia and infarct on cardiac performance.

Left Ventricular Ejection

Contraction within the LV receives most of its power and efficiency through the reduction of circumference. In contrast to the RV, the left chamber has a small surface area in relation to its volume. The law of Laplace ($P = T/R$) states that the muscle tension (T) necessary to maintain a level of pressure (P) is reduced as the radius (R) is decreased. A chronically dilated, hypertrophied ventricular chamber requires greater muscle tension, and, therefore, a greater energy supply, to sustain a given ventricular pressure. Because the LV with each ejection must overcome a pressure gradient of over 90 mmHg, it is structurally designed as a high-pressure pump. When subjected to excessive volume loads, however, the resulting ventricular dilatation can cause severe compromise of left ventricular efficiency.

With cessation of ventricular contraction and the resulting pressure drop within the arteries, closure of the semilunar valves occurs and systolic ejection ceases. Under resting conditions, the ejected stroke volume equals 50 to 60 percent of ventricular diastolic volume. The residual volume is influenced by many factors; among them are contractility, outflow resistance, and heart rate.

Similar to the early ejection period, the initial period of ventricular diastole is called the *isovolumic* or *isovolumetric relaxation,* in which a precipitous drop in ventricular pressure occurs without a change in volume. Because of increased accumulation of blood within the atrial chambers during ventricular systole, atrial pressures rise significantly. With reduction of diastolic pressures to levels less than those within the atria, the AV valves open and the rapid filling phase begins. Phenomena such as

diastolic recoil or diastolic suction significantly affect the rapid filling phase, during which ventricular volume apparently increases without a significant elevation of filling pressure. Rushmer emphasizes the importance of diastolic recoil in explanation for the more complete systolic ejection which occurs in tachycardia.[4] He postulates that a portion of the contractile tension occurring during systole is stored within the walls of the left ventricle; with sudden diastolic relaxation, the ventricular walls appear to spring outward during early ventricular filling. This diastolic recoil causes a drop in diastolic filling pressure, thus greatly augmenting filling. During tachycardia, when filling time is very brief, this phenomenon becomes even more important in contributing to a rise in cardiac output.

Atrial Systole

Following the period of early ventricular filling, blood flow diminishes and effectively ceases. This phase, which is the middle one-third of diastole, is known as the *period of diastasis* and occurs only if the ventricular diastolic period is sufficiently long. Since there is no blood flow and the AV valves are open, the pressures within the atria and ventricles are equal during the period of diastasis. With atrial excitation, atrial contraction occurs. The amount of blood entering the ventricle during atrial contraction is variable and is influenced by the following factors: (1) duration of the P-R interval, (2) heart rate, and (3) chamber filling pressures. Blood flow resulting from atrial contraction will follow the path of least resistance, forward into the LV or retrogradely into the great veins.

The atrial contraction is not essential for adequate cardiac performance in normal individuals. During exercise or any increase in metabolic demand resulting in tachycardia, however, the atrial contribution can be significant, particularly if the heart rate becomes so rapid that it affects the rapid filling phase.

Heart Sounds

The exact cause of the heart sounds remains controversial, but they occur, at least in part, as a result of the sudden acceleration and deceleration of blood within the ventricular chamber at the time of valvular closure and muscular contraction. Heart sounds reflect the mechanical events of the heart. The reader is referred to Chap. 20 for more detailed discussion of heart sounds.

Components of Arterial Pressure

Systolic Pressure

The normal LV ejects the majority of its stroke volume (SV) during the early period of ventricular systole, the rapid ejection phase. As was described earlier in this chapter, the left ventricular pressure momentarily exceeds aortic pressure (Fig. 19-9). Following the rapid ejection phase, the peak systolic pressure is reached, which is determined by the mass of ventricular volume, the rate of ejection, and the compliance of the arterial vessels. A relatively small stroke volume injected into a distensible aorta will produce a small increase in aortic pressure, while a very rapid ventricular ejection into a rigid arteriosclerotic vessel will produce significant elevations in arterial pressure.

Diastolic Pressure

During ventricular diastole, arterial pressure falls to a low level just prior to the next contraction. The rate of pressure drop is influenced by many factors; among them are the systolic pressure, the rate of flow through the periphery (peripheral runoff), and the length of diastole. End-diastolic pressure is determined mainly by total peripheral resistance and heart rate.

Mean Arterial Pressure

The average pressure throughout the phasic cardiac cycle is known as the *mean arterial pressure*. It can be measured by recording the area under the curve of an arterial pressure tracing and dividing the area by the concurrent time period. Normally, the mean is slightly less than the average of the systolic and diastolic pressures and it can be grossly approximated by adding one-third of the pulse pressure (difference between the systolic and diastolic pressures) to the diastolic pressure. The average adult with a systolic pressure of 120 mmHg and a diastolic pressure of 80 mmHg has a mean arterial pressure of 96 mmHg.

The mean pressure will vary directly with systolic and diastolic fluctuations. In the newborn it is normally about 70 mmHg but it is approximately 100 to 110 mmHg in the adult. With arteriosclerosis the arterial mean pressure can rise to 140 mmHg. Because the mean arterial pressure is the average pressure responsible for the arterial to venous pressure gradient, it has a very important influence on tissue flow.

Pulse Pressure

Pulse pressure is defined as the difference between the systolic and diastolic pressure. Thus, it can be affected by factors which determine systolic or diastolic pressure, particularly arterial capacitance or stroke volume.

The pulse pressure, according to Berne and Levy,[5] can be utilized to assess both arterial capacitance and stroke volume. Normally the pulse pressure is approximately 40 mmHg. If a reduction in arterial compliance occurs, for example, as in arteriosclerosis, a greater pulse pressure will result than if the arterial wall were normally distensible, thus causing increased left ventricular work and energy requirements. Increases in total peripheral resistance resulting from conditions such as hypertension will obviously increase arterial pressure if the same volume is to be maintained.

Heart rate, then, will change the pulse pressure according to the degree by which stroke volume and compliance of the arterial tree are changed. If a tachycardia and the resulting normal increase in arterial pressure are accompanied by a drop in arterial compliance, pulse pressure will be increased, assuming stroke volume is constant. Conversely, if the volume of blood ejected from the left ventricle is reduced without a change in arterial compliance, the pulse pressure will usually decrease. In summary, factors which tend to increase systolic pressure and/or cause a drop in diastolic pressure will tend to augment the pulse pressure.

Transmission of the Arterial Pulse Wave

Since the left ventricular stroke volume is ejected with such force and velocity, it tends to accumulate in the aortic root (the first portion of the aorta), causing stretching and increased tension within the aortic wall. The transmission of the stretching and development of tension into each adjacent section of the aorta and arterial vasculature results in a measurable pressure waveform and palpable pulse within the peripheral arterial circulation. The rate at which the pressure waveform is transmitted depends upon arterial compliance.

The shape of the arterial waveform changes as the pressure pulse reaches the more peripheral segments of the arterial tree; the systolic peak becomes significantly higher, as much as 20 to 40 mmHg higher within the brachial and femoral arteries than in the central aorta due to an increase in the pulse pressure; and the dicrotic notch (point of closure of the aortic valve) becomes increasingly more distorted and eventually disappears. In addition, a peak is often seen on the diastolic portion of the peripheral arterial waveform. The changes in morphology of the transmitted aortic waveform decrease with age, and in older individuals with severe arteriosclerosis there may be relatively little difference between central and peripheral waveforms.

Control of Cardiac Output

Cardiac output is defined as that amount of blood which is pumped from the left ventricle into the aorta per minute. Although the right ventricle ejects an equivalent amount of blood into the pulmonary artery, it is not included in measurement of total cardiac output. *Venous return* is considered as the amount of blood which is returned to the right atrium. Venous return may differ from the cardiac output for short periods of time because blood can be stored in some areas of the circulation; the cardiac output and venous return are eventually equivalent amounts and are inextricably related to one another.

The normal volume of cardiac output is about 5600 mL/min or 5.6 L in the average male. Because the cardiac output varies considerably in accordance with body size, the cardiac index is utilized to achieve an accurate estimate of blood flow in proportion to body surface area. The average 70-kg male has an estimated standard cardiac index of approximately 3 L/min.

Cardiac output is defined as the product of the heart rate and the amount of blood ejected from the left ventricle with each contraction, which is the stroke volume. The control of cardiac output resides in the ability of the heart to alter either its frequency of beating or the stroke volume. Alteration of heart rate is chiefly controlled through innervation of the autonomic nervous system, while alteration of the stroke volume involves a much more complex group of control mechanisms (Fig. 19-10). With sympathetic stimulation, the cardiac output can more than double by utilizing the systolic and diastolic reserve capacities. The normal resting cardiac output is achieved through the product of a resting stroke volume of 80 mL and a resting heart rate of 70 beats per minute. The heart rate can increase to an effective rate of 180 beats per minute while the ventricles respond to the inotropic sympathetic effects. If only the rate of the SA node is increased by electrical stimulation or specific localized sympathetic excitation upon the SA node, without generalized peripheral effects, cardiac output will probably not increase.

The *stroke volume* is defined as the difference between the diastolic volume within the left ventricle and the residual volume of blood within the ventricle following systole. The major factors which influence stroke volume are diastolic filling (preload), afterload, and contractility.

Diastolic filling (*preload*) is dependent upon total blood volume and peripheral circulatory regulation. Atrial contraction can augment diastolic filling by as much as 35 percent. Increase in stroke volume is effected by the length-tension relationship of the Frank-Starling mechanism within physiologic limits. The effects are augmented through the inotropic effects of the sympathetic nervous system.

Afterload or *wall tension* during left ventricular ejection is determined primarily by aortic end-diastolic pressure but is influenced by other factors influencing resistance as well: aortic distensibility, peripheral vascular resistance, and characteristics of the blood itself, namely, the mass of the column of blood in the aorta and the viscosity of the blood. The effect of afterload on the normal ventricle is possibly augmentation of contractility insofar as a smaller afterload will enable the heart to contract more rapidly. This relationship is often referred to

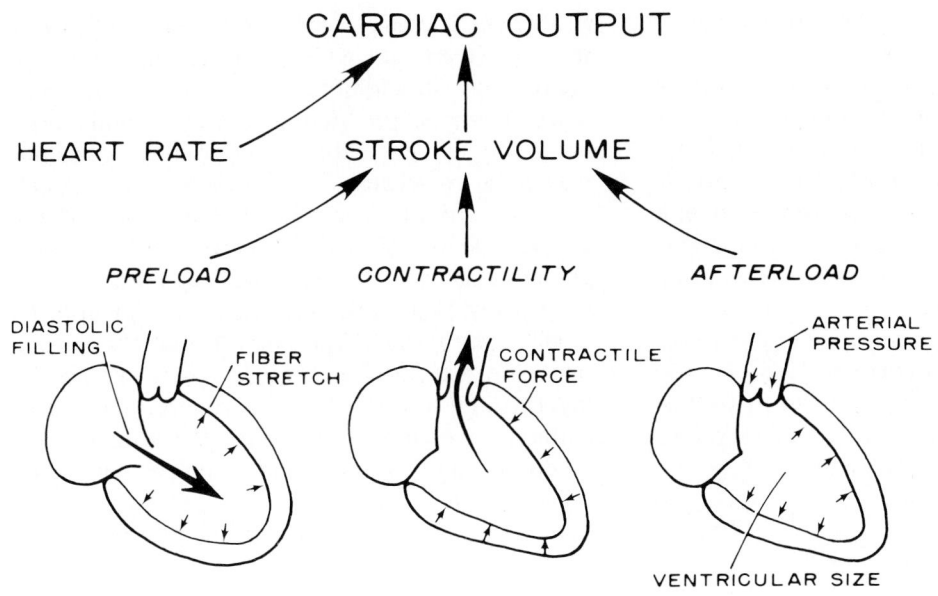

CARDIAC OUTPUT

HEART RATE   STROKE VOLUME

PRELOAD   CONTRACTILITY   AFTERLOAD

DIASTOLIC
FILLING   FIBER
STRETCH   CONTRACTILE
FORCE   ARTERIAL
PRESSURE

VENTRICULAR SIZE

Figure 19-10   Factors influencing cardiac output. Among the complex variables which affect cardiac output are changes in heart rate and four factors which influence stroke volume: (1) diastolic filling pressure, (2) ventricular distensibility, (3) arterial pressure, and (4) myocardial contractility. *(From S. Price and L. Wilson, Pathophysiology, McGraw-Hill, New York, 1978. Used by permission of the publisher.)*

as the *force-velocity relationship.* Within the diseased heart, however, severely deleterious effects may result from the resistance imposed by normal aortic impedance (afterload).

Ventricular contractility is determined by a very complex relationship between many factors involved in ventricular structure and dimensions. Cardiac dilation impedes effective contractility because of the Laplace relationship.

Cardiac output, then, is dependent on the interrelationships developed between (1) venous return or diastolic filling pressure, (2) heart rate, (3) stroke volume, (4) myocardial contractility, and (5) aortic end-diastolic pressure.

Venous Return

Cardiac output and venous return are, in the broad sense, inseparable. The heart can obviously pump no more blood than it receives from the peripheral circulation; therefore, venous return and cardiac output must eventually be equal, although temporary differences can exist.

Guyton describes the role of the heart as permissive in its regulation of cardiac output.[6] Up to a physiologic limit of 13 to 15 L/min, the heart will pump the amount of blood that returns to the right atrium. If venous return exceeds that amount, sympathetic stimulation is required. The normal resting venous return is approximately 5 L/min; therefore, the normal cardiac output is also 5 L/min.

Control of Heart Rate

The normal adult heart beats at a frequency of between 60 and 80 beats per minute. Although the principal regulators of cardiac rate are the nerves of the parasympathetic and sympathetic nervous systems, it is important to review the intrinsic control mechanism within the heart, namely, the property of automaticity (Chap. 11).

Specialized cardiac myofibrils can drive the denervated heart. There have even been reports of implantation of pacemaker cells which have been successful in controlling the heart. Usually the denervated heart beats at a rate somewhat slower than when under the influence of the nervous system. The heart rate does not increase in response to exercise or stress until influenced by the circulating catecholamines (norepinephrine and epinephrine, which are secreted from the adrenal medulla). Clinically, the heart may be denervated or mimic denervation in a variety of circumstances:

(1) cardiac transplantation, (2) vagolytic effects produced by atropine and beta-blocking effects of propranolol, (3) depletion of the normal stores of norepinephrine through antihypertensives such as reserpine, and (4) depletion of norepinephrine resulting from cardiac pathology such as chronic ventricular failure. The latter two conditions exhibit their effect through mitigation of the sympathetic effect resulting from a reduction in norepinephrine release from the sympathetic nerve endings.

The function of the extrinsic neural and humoral controls is generally integrative; they increase the functional effectiveness of the heart as well as acting as a higher control center, and one therefore capable of more specialized action.

Autonomic Control

The divisions of the automatic nervous system exhibit tonic influence on the heart rate. Increased parasympathetic stimulation along with reciprocal decrease in sympathetic activity results in a drop in rate. Acceleration of the heart rate is produced by the opposite action of the two divisions of the nervous system.

The parasympathetic cardiac fibers originate in the medulla and have their innervation primarily in nodal tissue and the atria. Animal experimentation has revealed that the right vagus nerve affects the sinoatrial node predominantly, and that the left vagus has its greatest effect on atrioventricular (AV) conduction tissue. Some ventricular innervation occurs at the base of the ventricles near the conduction tissue. However, ventricular muscle is relatively unresponsive to acetylcholine and thus the parasympathetic effect on the ventricles is presumed to be insignificant.

The effect of vagal stimuli is transient since the acetylcholine is rapidly dissipated by the enzyme cholinesterase, of which the SA and AV nodes have abundant stores.

The sympathetic nerve fibers arise from the thoracic spinal cord and penetrate the myocardium in a manner similar to the parasympathetic nerve fibers; that is, left and right fibers appear to be functionally specific. Under experimental conditions, the left sympathetic fibers appear to augment cardiac contractility more than they accelerate the heart rate. The right sympathetic fibers selectively increase heart rate with relatively little effect on contractility. In addition, fibers from the right primarily innervate the SA node and atria, while those from the left have their predominant influence within the ventricles.

In contrast to acetylcholine, norepinephrine remains active following release from the nerve endings; relatively little undergoes degradation within the tissues. Most of the remaining norepinephrine is taken up again by the nerve terminals. Norepinephrine acts on the beta receptors within the myocardium (most of the adrenergic receptors within the nodal regions and myocardium are beta receptors) and on the alpha receptors within the coronary arteries.

The antagonistic interaction between acetylcholine and the catecholamines is very complex and poorly understood. Normally, in the resting heart, the parasympathetic system predominates in controlling the SA node. In addition to these neurotransmitters, the heart rate is also controlled by the cardioregulatory center and baroreceptors.

Cardioregulatory Center

Impulses from the cerebral cortex can have a substantial effect on the heart rate; fear, excitement, and anger can all induce significant acceleration in rate. Areas within the hypothalamus can also effect changes in the heart rate. Experiments have demonstrated that sympathetic fibers descending from the medulla can be separated into accelerator and augmentor fibers and, further, that the augmentor sites are more prevalent on the left, the accelerator on the right. A cardioregulatory center is frequently assumed to exist and carry out upper nervous control of cardiac function.

Baroreceptor Reflex

An elevation in right atrial pressure sufficient to cause distention causes a reflex acceleration of heart rate. In 1915 Bainbridge hypothesized that tachycardia resulted from a vagal reflex. The effect of the Bainbridge reflex is somewhat controversial, but recent study has supported the existence of "accelerator" receptors located in both atria which excite the nervous system and elicit diuresis by reducing the secretion of antidiuretic hormone (ADH).[5]

Stretch receptors within the ventricles have been identified within the epicardium and deep within the myocardium. A potent stimulus can induce bradycardia, hypotension, and a drop in the respiratory rate.

The reciprocal relationship between arterial pressure and heart rate has been called *Marey's law of the heart*. The stretch receptors within the carotid sinus and aortic arch respond to an increase in arterial pressure with a reflex bradycardia. The pulmonary vasculature responds to distention with a reflex reduction in rate. The well-known carotid sinus reflex, similar to occipital pressure, can produce a bradycardia and can frequently convert a tachyarrhythmia to normal sinus rhythm.

The carotid sinus reflex is so sensitive in some individuals that tight collars or sudden movement of the head can cause syncope through induction of bradycardia and hypotension. Such syncopal reactions can be produced by many other types of stimuli. Called a *vasovagal response,* the reaction can be elicited by stimulation of the upper respiratory tract during endotracheal suctioning and during intubation of the trachea and the esophagus.

Since the gastrointestinal tract has afferent fibers leading to the medulla, nausea and vomiting in addition to rectal stimulation can be associated with a reflex bradycardia. Generally, stimulation of visceral pain fibers can cause a marked bradycardia. Pressure on the eyeball, in addition to painful stimulation of skeletal muscle, may elicit a significant reduction of heart rate. Conversely, somatic pain in the skin frequently produces tachycardia.

The phenomenon of phasic acceleration and deceleration in heart rate simultaneous with inspiration and expiration occurs frequently and is known as *sinus arrhythmia*. Since intrathoracic pressure drops during inspiration, resulting in an increase in venous return, sinus arrhythmia has been attributed to stimulation of the Bainbridge reflex, causing increased heart rate. With the corresponding increase in left ventricular output and resulting rise in arterial pressure, a decrease in heart rate occurs through excitation of the aortic baroreceptors. Pulmonary stretch receptors may be operative as well in the bradycardia associated with sinus arrhythmia.

Control of Stroke Volume

The fundamental control mechanism for the stroke volume is the Frank-Starling law of the heart. Though the experiments done by Starling were in isolated hearts on heart-lung machines and many complex variables exist within the intact animal and human heart, the basic qualitative relationships regarding ventricular performance can be extrapolated and applied to ventricular function.

When the Starling mechanism was mentioned earlier in this chapter, it was referred to as an intrinsic method for autoregulation of cardiac performance. Its most basic effect is to guarantee equal stroke volumes from the right and left ventricles, should there be a momentary increase in volume; thus the term *autoregulation*. The mechanism through which the heart can automatically respond is one it shares with all striated muscle: the length–tension relationship. Increasing the length of the ventricular fiber (preload) in practice, measured as filling pressure (Fig. 19-8*B*), shifts the curve to the left, augmenting ventricular contractility.

The normal left ventricle is extremely distensible and accepts increases in diastolic volume, or preload, without significant increase in ventricular filling pressure (end-diastolic pressure). Generally, peak contractility occurs at a fiber length of 2.2 μm or 12 mmHg. Further increases in filling pressure beyond the physiologic limits of the length–tension relationship will result in a reduction in effective ventricular performance. Once fiber length reaches 4 to 4.5 μm corresponding to a filling pressure of 14 or 15 mmHg, the rate of rise in ventricular end-diastolic pressure occurs very rapidly.

In the noncompliant, stiff ventricle, the situation is very different. A higher filling pressure results for the same fiber length, which results in a shift in the performance curve to the right, as shown in Fig. 19-8*C*. The end result, then, is a reduction in ventricular performance while simultaneously causing higher filling pressures.

There is evidence that other types of autoregulation can occur within the heart which are not related to an increase in preload or ventricular fiber length. Afterload, or increased peripheral resistance (aortic), may result in ventricular adaptation by augmenting ventricular contractility (Anrep effect). Other examples of the augmentation of ventricular contractility can be seen in tachycardia and with premature beats. Berne and Levy theorize that the increased contractility seen with elevation of heart rate is based on increases in intracellular calcium (treppe phenomenon).[5] Similarly, the phenomenon known as *postextrasystolic accentuation* may be the result of elevated intracellular calcium. It is well known that a premature beat generally produces a feeble contraction, which probably relates to low concentrations of calcium. The fact that the beat following the premature (extrasystolic) beat is usually much stronger relates not only to the increased time for diastolic filling during the long pause following the premature beat, but, according to Berne and Levy, may be potentiated by increased concentrations of intracellular calcium as well.[5]

Myocardial Contractility

Rushmer points out that the factors which cannot be ascribed to the length–tension relationship are usually combined to mean contractility, a fact which confuses the meaning of the word.[4] Rushmer groups the following variables under the concept of contractility: (1) the degree of systolic emptying, (2) rate of muscle shortening, (3) rate of tension development, (4) ejection velocity, (5) inotropic effects, (6) vigor of contraction, and (7) rate of myocardial shortening.[4] In addition, the ratio of pressure development and resulting myocardial tension (dP/dT) is frequently utilized as a determinant of contractility.

Neural Control of Myocardial Contractility

Sympathetic innervation has already been reviewed with respect to control of the heart rate. The atria are liberally supplied with both parasympathetic and sympathetic nerves, while the ventricles are mainly supplied by sympathetic nerves. Generally, the sympathetic nerves are effective in augmentation

of contractility; the parasympathetic nerves function to diminish the strength of ventricular contraction.

The amount of sympathetic activity can be estimated by comparing the quantity of norepinephrine within the atria, in the SA and AV nodes, and within the ventricles; ventricular concentration of norepinephrine is triple that in the atria and nodes.

Sympathetic Nervous System

Sympathetic stimulation within the heart is inotropic; within the atria, stimulation can cause a 20 to 30 percent increase in atrial contractility. The effect of sympathetic activity within the ventricle is, of course, more complicated and is dependent upon the relationship of the factors listed earlier which influence contractility in addition to affecting heart rate. The stroke volume may or may not increase; the primary benefit from the inotropic effect of sympathetic activity is thought by some investigators to be the increased rate and velocity of pressure change, ventricular outflow, and change in ventricular dimensions. The net result is ejection of the same or slightly higher stroke volume in a much shorter period of time, and more frequently per minute, thereby increasing cardiac output. The results of sympathetic effects on cardiac function are summarized in Fig. 19-11.

Parasympathetic Nervous System

The vagal inhibitory effect on the nodes and other conduction tissue within the atria and AV junction are very potent. Recently the existence of parasympathetic influence within the ventricle has been demonstrated. Its effect is the reverse of sympathetic: Left ventricular pressure falls, as does the maximum rate of pressure development.

Effect of Electrolyte Imbalance

Hyperkalemia can result in extreme cardiac dilation and bradycardia. If extreme hyperpolarization is caused by the increased extracellular potassium concentration, no action potential will be generated and asystole will ensue. An acute increase in serum potassium to 8 meq is sufficient to cause death through this mechanism.[6]

Hypercalcemia results in tetany, probably resulting from the excitatory effects of calcium on the

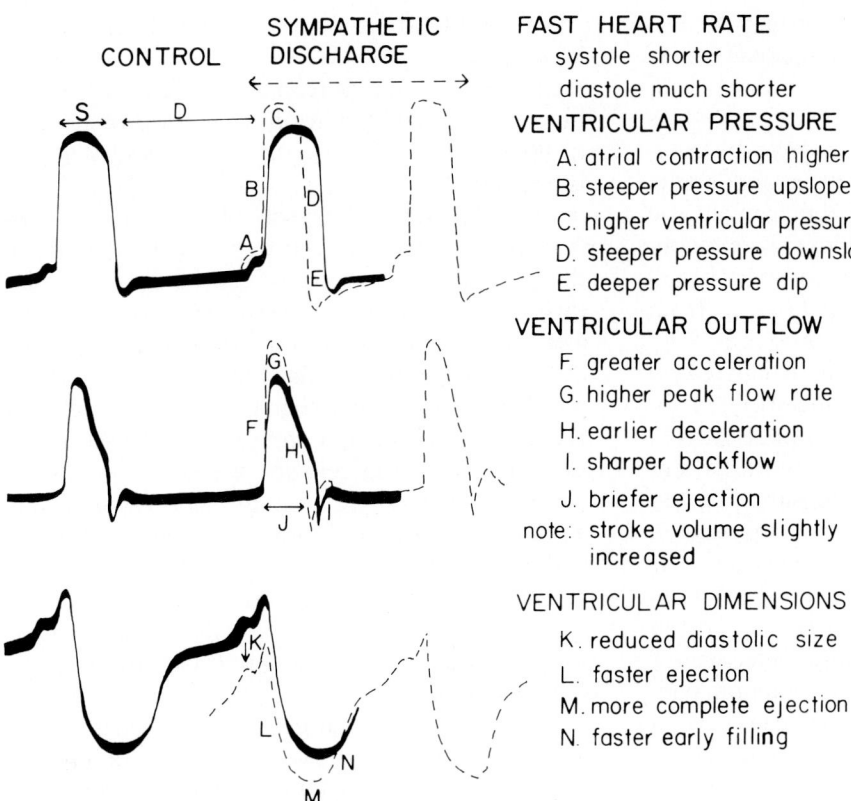

CONTROL | SYMPATHETIC DISCHARGE

FAST HEART RATE
systole shorter
diastole much shorter

VENTRICULAR PRESSURE
A. atrial contraction higher
B. steeper pressure upslope
C. higher ventricular pressure
D. steeper pressure downslope
E. deeper pressure dip

VENTRICULAR OUTFLOW
F. greater acceleration
G. higher peak flow rate
H. earlier deceleration
I. sharper backflow
J. briefer ejection
note: stroke volume slightly increased

VENTRICULAR DIMENSIONS
K. reduced diastolic size
L. faster ejection
M. more complete ejection
N. faster early filling

Figure 19-11 Summary of sympathetic effect on cardiac performance. The major results of sympathetic discharge are in increasing the following: (1) ventricular functioning, (2) heart rate, (3) pressure rise and fall within ventricles, (4) ejection velocity, (5) change in velocity (acceleration), (6) deceleration, and (7) change in ventricular dimensions. (*From Robert Rushmer, Cardiovascular Dynamics, Saunders, Philadelphia, 1970. Used by permission of the publisher.*)

contractile process. Clinically this is rarely seen, since tetany would more likely result in respiratory arrest prior to exhibition of significant effects from hypercalcemia.

Coronary Blood Flow

In the resting state, coronary flow is about 5 percent of the cardiac output (100 to 150 mL/min). As metabolic demands increase, blood flow can increase to more than four to five times the resting value. The myocardial oxygen extraction remains fixed at 65 to 70 percent of stroke volume, regardless of physiologic conditions, which provides arterial P_{O_2} of 18 to 20 mmHg and a venous oxygen saturation of about 30 percent. That is the lowest value for venous oxygen saturation in the body. The heart functions exclusively on aerobic metabolism and cannot sustain an oxygen debt as can skeletal muscle. The most basic regulator, then, of coronary flow is the degree of oxygen need. Since oxygen extraction is maximal, the sole mechanism for meeting increased oxygen demand is an increase in coronary flow.

Coronary blood flow is intermittent; it is dependent on phasic aortic pressure and faces significant resistance within the myocardium. External compression during systole causes severe reduction of flow within the left ventricle. Although the right ventricle is subjected to the same factors, the lower right ventricular pressures result in relatively mild changes in coronary flow. The left ventricular coronary flow, however, occurs almost exclusively during ventricular diastole. In addition, the thickness of the left ventricular wall results in some variance in flow from endocardium to epicardium. Normally, however, the endocardium is compensated during diastole for the increased systolic epicardial flow. With pathologic conditions such as severe atherosclerosis, severe reduction of flow can occur within the endocardium.

Since the major regulator of coronary flow is oxygen deficiency, it is believed that hypoxia causes coronary arteriolar dilation, but whether it is directly or from the release of neurotransmitters is unclear. The primary method appears to be automatic regulation of flow through arteriolar constriction and dilation. Influence of the sympathetic nervous system or of catecholamines (norepinephrine and epinephrine) is complex; coronary blood flow increases either through dilation or from increased heart rate and perfusion pressure.

Factors which can contribute to increased myocardial oxygen consumption include: (1) increased heart rate, (2) rise in arterial pressure, (3) increased contractility, and (4) increased fiber tension. The last of these, myocardial tension, plays an extremely important role in determining oxygen consumption, particularly in the event of ventricular decompensation. The Laplace relationship states that a dilated ventricle will utilize increased tension to maintain adequate stroke volume, even against a normal arterial pressure. That phenomenon, coupled with coronary atherosclerosis, can have a deleterious effect on cardiac efficiency in the failing heart.

Collateral circulation within the vasculature is apparently present from infancy in the form of arterial anastomoses and is particularly plentiful within the ventricular septum, apex, right ventricular anterior surface, and in the atria. Epicardial anastomoses exist between all three major coronary vessels of the left ventricle. The crucial determinant for success of the anastomoses is the rapidity with which occlusion occurs, because the anastomotic connections become functional only when there is a long-standing need for increased flow. Other determining factors in the development of adequate collateral circulation are the location of the anastomosis to the occluded artery and the amount of disease in adjacent vessels.

Special Features of the Vascular Circulation

Blood Flow Determinants

An important determinant of blood flow is viscosity. There are several factors which influence the vis-

cosity of blood; principal among them are the hematocrit and the internal diameter of the vessel. An increase in the percentage of cells within the blood, the hematocrit, from the normal of 40 to 70 or 80, can triple the viscosity and seriously impair blood flow.

Within the small vessels, blood flow decreases markedly. Because of the decrease in velocity of flow, blood viscosity can increase tenfold. Following division of an artery or vein, the cross-sectional area of the branches taken together exceeds that of the vessel of origin. Since the volumes of blood moving through each segment of the circulation are equal, changes in a cross-sectional area necessarily influence the velocity of blood flow. In the aorta, blood travels very rapidly, slows significantly within the capillaries (large cross-sectional area), and accelerates in the veins, where the cross-sectional area once again is smaller. The relatively slow capillary blood flow provides sufficient time for exchange of oxygen and nutrients through the capillary walls.

Blood flow is directly proportional to the pressure difference between two ends of a vessel and inversely proportional to the resistance imposed by characteristics within the vessel. The relationship is expressed in Fig. 19-12, for which any vessel within the circulation is depicted. Were there no pressure difference or gradient between P_1 and P_2, there could be no blood flow. The resistance, which includes any factor that serves to impede flow, can be calculated from measurements of blood flow and pressure gradients within the vessel.

In a resting individual, blood flow within the circulation occurs at a rate of approximately 100 mL/s. The normal arterial to venous pressure gra-

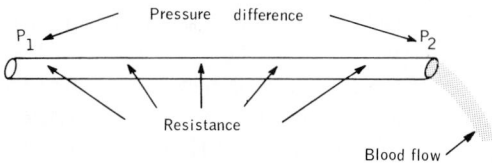

Figure 19-12 Factors influencing blood flow: pressure resistance and pressure gradient (P_1 and P_2). (*From Arthur C. Guyton, Textbook of Medical Physiology, Saunders, Philadelphia, 1970. Used by permission of the publisher.*)

dient within the total circulation is around 100 mmHg. The resistance within the circulation (total peripheral resistance), then, is 100 mL/s to 100 mmHg, or one peripheral resistance unit (PRU). Another method for measurement of total peripheral resistance is obtained by relating the cardiac output and arterial pressure. An individual with a cardiac output of 5000 mL/min and arterial pressure of 100 mmHg would have a calculated peripheral resistance of 0.02 PRU. The systemic resistance will vary considerably when vasoconstriction or vasodilatation occur, increasing with the former and dropping as vascular capacity is increased through vessel dilatation.

The effect of vessel diameter on blood flow is graphically demonstrated in Fig. 19-13. In Fig. 19-13A, increasing the vessel diameter by fourfold results in an increase in blood flow by 256-fold with no change in pressure gradient. The basis behind such marked changes in flow with relatively small changes in vessel diameter is explained in Fig. 19-13B. Blood flows within a vessel in layers; the layers closest to the vessel wall experience the greatest "drag" and move very slowly, while the layers farther away from the vessel wall move with increasing velocity. The phenomenon is known as *streamlining,* or *laminar flow.* The greater the

internal diameter of the vessel, the greater the number of layers that can form, thereby increasing flow.

The major factors influencing blood flow are often expressed through Poiseuille's law,[5] which states that the flow ($\dot{Q}$) of fluid through a tube is directly proportional to the pressure gradient ($P_1 - P_2$) across the tube, to the fourth power of the radius of the tube (r^4), and inversely proportional to the length of the tube (L) and the viscosity (n) of the fluid:

$$\dot{Q} = \pi(P_1 - P_2)r^4 \div 8Ln$$

with $\pi/8$ serving as a geometric proportional value. Resistance, then, increases in direct proportion to the viscosity and length of the vessel, but decreases in direct proportion to the vessel diameter (the fourth power of the radius of the vessel) and pressure gradient.

Although the relationships of Poiseuille's law are helpful in isolating the dynamics of blood flow, there are several factors which hinder a qualitative application. The formula is based on a system of rigid tubes which, unlike distensible blood vessels, cannot increase in both length and diameter; in addition, there are other factors unique to the fluid characteristics of blood which are not considered in the Poiseuille relationship.

The caliber of blood vessels is unquestionably significant in determining pressure gradients and flow through various segments of the circulation. Approximately 80 percent of the pressure drop occurs in the terminal arteries and arterioles (Fig. 19-14). The resistance imposed by the arteriolar circulation must, in addition, be related to the cross-sectional area. Since the different types of vessels lie in a series arrangement with one another and the various vascular beds are parallel, it is apparent that the total flow is a sum of the individual flows through each vascular bed (Fig. 19-14). Since resistance is increased both by an increase in cross-sectional area and by a reduction in vessel diameter, it follows that the resistance of each individual resistance bed exceeds the total systemic resistance. The resistance of the renal circulation, for instance, will exceed that of the total peripheral circulation, since far greater volumes of blood will flow through the total circulation than through the renal vasculature.

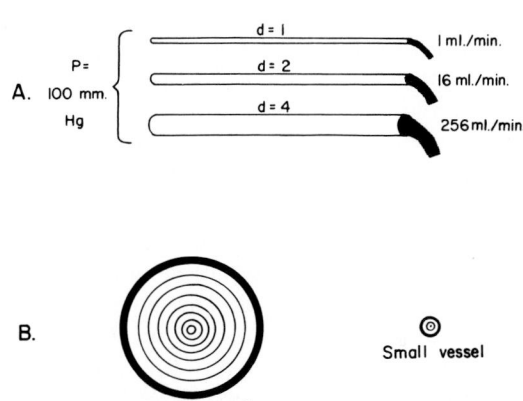

Figure 19-13   Effect of increasing vessel diameter on (*A*) blood flow increasing velocity of (*B*) concentric rings of blood flowing at varying velocity; the farther away from the vessel wall, the more rapid the flow. (*From Arthur C. Guyton, Textbook of Medical Physiology, Saunders, Philadelphia, 1970. Used by permission of the publisher.*)

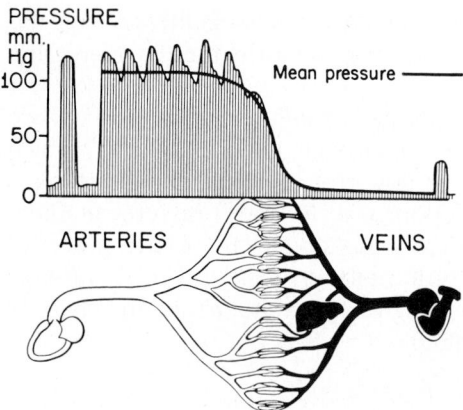

Figure 19-14 Resistance and resulting loss of pressure within the circulation. Arterial pressure diminishes very rapidly in the small resistance vessels of the circulation. In the venous vessels the pressure gradient is very low.

Law of Laplace

The law of Laplace, which was used earlier to explain the relationship between cardiac dilation and resulting increase in oxygen consumption, is operative as well within the vascular system. The relationship as applied to blood vessels states that the tension sustained by the wall of a cylinder is directly proportional to the product of the pressure within the cylinder and its radius. In other words, the smaller a blood vessel, the less the amount of tension required to maintain a given pressure. At normal aortic and capillary pressures, the tension necessary to support the pressure exerted on the wall of the aorta is over 10,000 times as great as that in the capillary.

Vascular Smooth Muscle

Vascular smooth muscle shares some characteristics of cardiac and skeletal muscle. The contractile process operates in a similar manner, since it is contingent on the action of the proteins actin, myosin, and troponin-tropomyosin. In addition, the ability of certain of the smooth muscles to exhibit automaticity has already been reviewed. Since it is very difficult to separate the structural components of smooth muscle, no consistent pattern of myofibril organization has been observed. The actual mech-

anism which causes vascular smooth muscle shortening is unknown, since the relationship of the actin and myosin filaments during contraction and the mechanism for calcium release can only be inferred. The relationship between stimulation and contraction seems to vary, although the contractile time of smooth muscle is generally much more prolonged than that of cardiac and skeletal muscle. Neural and hormonal stimuli (epinephrine, angiotensin) usually elicit a contractile response.

The sympathetic nervous system innervates a majority of the arterial and venous circulation. Arterioles apparently have a relatively greater concentration of neuromuscular connections, which is in keeping with their role as resistance vessels. It is this property of relative contraction or relaxation which determines the tone of vascular smooth muscle. Although sympathetic control is very important, it is crucial to understand that the routine control of the peripheral circulation is independent of extrinsic mechanisms.

Arterial Circulation

The essential feature of the arterial circulation is its function as a pressure reservoir in order to convert its intermittent ventricular ejection into relatively constant flow i.e., the windkessel effect. The intrinsic properties of normal arteries which permit such a function have been reviewed. The fact that the arteries are capable of storing a portion of energy received from the heart during systolic contraction within their elastic walls is critically important in maintaining flow to the tissues in a pulsatile circulation. The greater the distensibility or compliance of the arterial circulation, the more constant is blood flow during diastole and systole. In addition, the arterial circulation has an important influence on the workload imposed on the heart. Since the phasic pumping of the heart requires much more energy expenditure from the heart than would be demanded for steady flow, the capability for the normal arterial circulation to transmit pressure throughout the diastolic phase of the heart results in a decrease in cardiac workload. On the other hand, loss of the property of elastic recoil within the arterial circulation can profoundly increase cardiac work.

It is known that the major resistance within the peripheral circulation is exerted by the extremely muscular arterioles and their precapillary sphincters. The distention properties of the venae cavae and of the aorta are exemplified by a comparison of the relative diameter, wall thickness, and proportion of elastic tissue with those of the arteriole and sphincter (Fig. 19-15). It is through constriction and dilation of these resistance vessels, thereby changing internal diameters, that blood flow is distributed to the tissues. Note that the capillary walls contain only endothelial tissue, a structural composition which is highly appropriate for rapid diffusion. Although much of the arterial pressure head is dissipated prior to reaching the capillary bed, the capillaries must be able to withstand significant pressure in order to effect a sufficient pressure gradient for maintenance of blood flow.

Capillary Dynamics

Normally the regulation of blood through the vast capillary network is controlled very precisely. An exact amount of blood is provided to the tissue in accordance with its metabolic demands. Blood flows continuously through the arterioles and then into metarterioles through the precapillary sphincter and on into the capillary. Two types of capillaries can be seen in Fig. 19-16: thoroughfare channels (TC), which serve as direct channels from the arteriole to the venule, and the true capillaries (C). By reviewing Fig. 19-16, it will be recalled that the capillaries are not invested with muscle, while the thoroughfare channels are supplied with smooth muscle which is more pronounced at the arterial end.

Through dilation and constriction of the precapillary sphincters, thoroughfare channels, and the arterioles, blood flow is controlled according to the specific needs of a group of cells. Since the process involves rhythmic movement of the vessels, it is also called *vasomotion*. With dilation of these vessels, a steeper pressure gradient occurs and therefore an increase in blood flow. With constriction, the arterial pressure gradient is decreased, resulting in either reduction or cessation of blood flow.

The most important method for exchange of substances through the capillary wall is diffusion. Though there are many factors which affect the rate at which a substance diffuses across the capillary wall, the chief influence is derived from the concentration gradient between the two sides of the membrane. The greater the difference between the

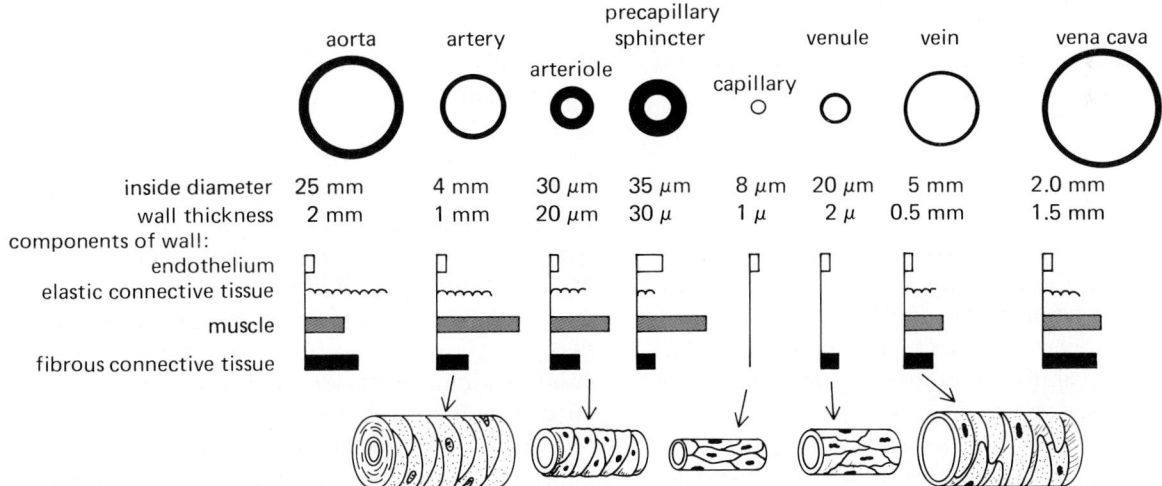

Figure 19-15 Schematic representation of anatomy of circulatory vasculature. Comparisons of internal diameters, musculature, wall thickness, and vascular components. (*From D. Luciano, A. J. Vander, and J. H. Sherman, Human Function and Structure, McGraw-Hill, New York, 1978. Adapted from A. C. Burton, Physiol. Rev. 34:619, 1954.*)

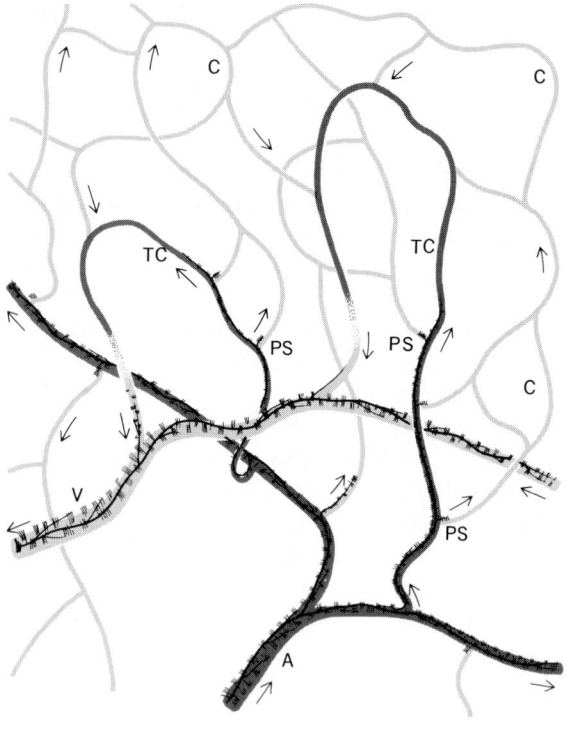

A = arteriole   C = capillaries
V = venule   PS = precapillary
TC = thoroughfare channel   sphincter

Figure 19-16 Schematic representation of the micro-circulation. The arrows indicate blood flow direction. Circular structures on arteriole and venule indicate smooth muscle fibers, and branching solid lines are indicative of sympathetic nervous innervation. (*From A. H. Vander, J. H. Sherman, and D. S. Luciano, Human Physiology, 2d ed., McGraw-Hill, New York, 1975. Adapted from B. W. Zweifach, Fed. Proc. 24:1074, 1965. Used by permission of the publisher.*)

concentrations of any substance, the more rapidly will it diffuse across the cell membrane. Tiny passageways connect the interior of the capillary with the exterior. Substances which are insoluble in the lipid capillary membrane can diffuse only through these capillary "pores."

Starling Equilibrium

Maintenance of fluid within the vascular system is the very basis of capillary dynamics. According to the Starling equilibrium, or law of the capillaries,

filtration or reabsorption of fluid across the capillary wall depends on the interrelation of four forces. Figure 19-17 depicts the four major factors involved in fluid transfer: (1) capillary pressure, which tends to filter fluid out of the capillary membrane to the tissues; (2) interstitial fluid pressure, which maintains a negative value, tending to draw fluid back into the interstitium; (3) plasma colloid osmotic pressure (oncotic pressure), which promotes absorption of fluid through osmotic attraction back into the capillary; and (4) interstitial fluid colloid osmotic pressure, which osmotically attracts fluid into the interstitium (tissue space).

The hydrostatic pressure (blood pressure) within the capillaries cannot be directly measured. It is not a constant value since it is dependent upon the arterial and venous pressures and the pre- and postcapillary resistance. The capillary pressure is assumed to be between 25 and 32 mmHg at the arterial end. Guyton[6] approximates the normal functional mean capillary pressure to be about 17 mmHg and the average pressure at the venous end to be about 10 mmHg.

The tissue pressure is also difficult to measure directly but is thought to be approximately -7 mmHg, a partial vacuum since it is less than atmospheric pressure. The tissue pressure should not be considered without relation to the lymphatic system, since the latter appears to maintain negativity of the interstitium.

Strategic factors in preventing fluid loss from the capillaries are the plasma proteins. The major determinant in the maintenance of the colloidal osmotic pressure is the protein, albumin. Since the protein molecule is so large, it cannot diffuse readily into the tissue space, but the few molecules that do diffuse into the interstitium are removed by the lymph system. In addition, a phenomenon known as *Gibbs-Donnan equilibrium* enhances the osmotic attraction of proteins. Since proteins are anions, they attract an equal number of cations, predominantly sodium, in order to achieve electrical balance. This increases the osmotic attraction of proteins by about 50 percent. In addition, the Donnan effect increases in proportion to increasing concentrations of proteins. In other words, additional grams of protein over the first few have much greater oncotic attraction than do the original few grams, a fact which makes hypoalbuminemia in-

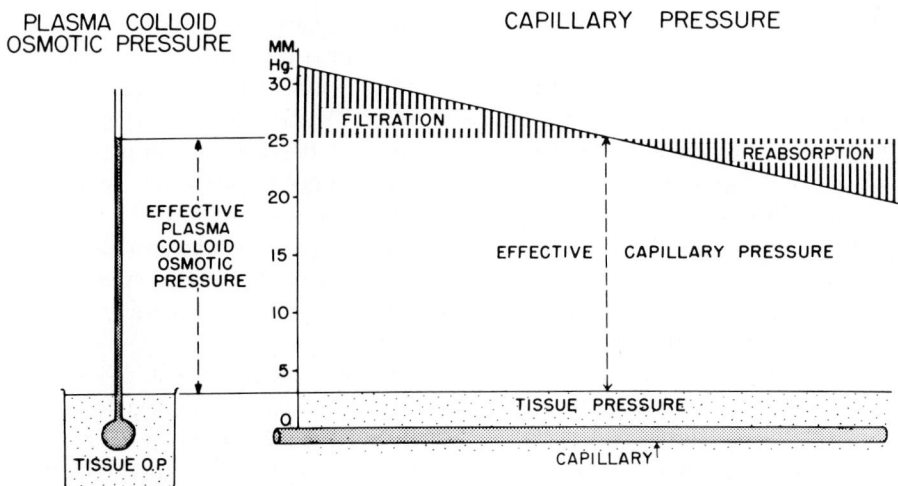

Figure 19-17   Capillary fluid exchange. Factors favoring filtration occur at the arterial end of the capillary and reabsorption at the venous end. The determination is the result of a balance between four pressures: (1) arterial and venous capillary mean pressures, (2) plasma colloidal pressure, (3) tissue colloidal osmotic pressure, and (4) interstitial fluid pressure. The lymphatic system is involved in maintenance of normal capillary dynamics. See text for further explanation. (*From Robert Rushmer, Cardiovascular Dynamics, Saunders, Philadelphia, 1970. Used by permission of the publisher.*)

creasingly significant. The oncotic pressure is estimated to be about 28 mmHg. Within the interstitium, the oncotic pressure is approximately 4.5 mmHg.

The pressures, when combined, favor filtration, or movement outward, at the arterial end of the capillary. The low hydrostatic pressure at the venous end of the capillary reverses the balance. There the oncotic pressure exceeds the filtration (outward) force, and reabsorption into the venule occurs. The Starling equilibrium states that in a steady state, the positive filtration forces favoring diffusion outward at the arterial end of the capillary are equal to the forces favoring reabsorption at the venous end. The total amount of fluid leaving the circulation is almost equal to the amount of fluid being reabsorbed in the venous end. The small amount of excess fluid and protein which accumulates within the interstitial space is removed by the lymphatic drainage system.

Edema Formation

It is immediately evident that a significant increase in capillary pressure, which causes an imbalance of filtration and reabsorptive forces, can result in an accumulation of fluid within the tissues. Similarly, edema can result from a reduction of oncotic pressure, or an increase in the permeability of the capillary such that excessive protein is lost from the plasma, causing reduction of oncotic pressure within the plasma, and from an increase in colloid osmotic pressure within the tissue spaces. There are two major protective mechanisms against the development of edema within the pulmonary vasculature: (1) The pulmonary capillary pressure is substantially lower, about 7 mmHg; and (2) the negative interstitial pressure is thought to be approximately −17 mmHg, both of which favor absorption from the alveolus into the interstitial fluid spaces.

Exchange across Capillary Membrane

The permeability of the capillaries is not consistent in all tissues. Lymph flow can be used to determine capillary permeability, and the lymph flow from the heart, lungs, intestines, and kidneys reveals a higher concentration of protein than does that from the skin and connective tissues. The liver capillary system is far more permeable than the others, which results in a protein concentration within the lymph flow almost equal to that of plasma.

Other factors affecting the rate of exchange of substances across the capillary are: (1) the area of capillary available for filtration, (2) thickness of the capillary wall, (3) viscosity of the filtrate, and (4) the sum of hydrostatic and osmotic pressures, as discussed earlier.

Although filtration and absorption are critically important in the maintenance of normal capillary dynamics, they play a relatively minor role in the normal exchange of substances. It is diffusion which provides the governing factor in the exchange of water, gases, waste products, and substrates across the capillary membranes. Since the principal limiting factors of diffusion are concentration gradient, molecular size, and lipid solubility, small molecules like water and glucose diffuse with little restriction.

The major factor which determines the rate of lymph flow is the interstitial fluid pressure. A rise in tissue pressure, which can result from a rise in capillary pressure, reduction in oncotic pressure, increase in capillary permeability, or increase in tissue oncotic pressure, will accelerate lymph flow.

As in the veins, lymphatic vessels are liberally supplied with one-way valves which prevent backflow and contribute to the lymphatic pump. Contraction of the muscles, passive movements of parts of the body such as respiration or abdominal movement, arterial pulsations, and external compression of the tissues all stimulate the lymphatic pump. In addition, there is evidence that certain lymphatics possess independent contractility which performs similarly to a type of peristalsis. About 120 mL of lymph per hour flows through the thoracic system of a resting adult. Although it is a very small volume in comparison to total capillary exchange, were protein not removed by the lymph vessels, it would significantly increase tissue oncotic pressure and cause severe edema.

Venous Circulation

The veins function not only as conduits for blood flow, but as a variable-volume reservoir, thereby helping to regulate cardiac output. Marked changes in venous capacity can occur without a significant effect on venous pressure. Thus the veins are a capacitance system. *Capacitance,* as defined by Berne and Levy, is the increment of volume accommodated per unit change of pressure.[5] Assuming normal arterial and venous pressures, a 1-mmHg increase in venous pressure would accommodate 20 times more blood within the venous system than within the arterial system for the same pressure change.

Since the pressure at the point of outflow from a series of tubes to a large extent determines the pressure gradient, an understanding of the right atrial pressure and its role as reflecting the central venous pressure (CVP) is important. Three factors contribute to the regulation of right atrial pressure or the CVP: (1) capacitance of the venous system (C), (2) total blood volume (V), and (3) the pumping ability of the heart (P). Normally the mean right atrial pressure, or CVP, is about equal to the atmospheric pressure around the body, which is zero. With hypervolemia or ventricular failure resulting from a reduction in contractility or pumping ability, the CVP may rise to very high levels. The effect within the peripheral veins is a backing up of blood, resulting in distention. Usually, many of the large veins which lie adjacent to the ribs and abdominal organs are almost totally collapsed, therefore offering considerable resistance to venous flow. Normally the pressure gradient between peripheral venous pressure and right atrial pressure is approximately 6 to 10 mmHg. As right atrial pressure climbs above its norm, blood begins to distend the large veins, correspondingly decreasing resistance; elevated peripheral venous pressure is therefore not seen until the later stages of failure, or until all the collapsed veins have opened, which is usually seen when right atrial pressure exceeds 4 to 6 mmHg.

Effects of Hydrostatic Pressure

The pressure resulting from the weight of water within a chamber is called *hydrostatic pressure*; at the surface of the fluid, the pressure equals atmospheric, but for each 13.6-mm distance under the surface, pressure increases 1 mmHg. In a standing, immobile person with a normal right atrial pressure (zero), venous pressure within the feet will be 90 mmHg. The same relationship exists within the arterial system.

Were the arterial pressure within the same individual equal to 100 mmHg, arterial pressure at the feet would approximate 190 mmHg. It is only at the phlebostatic axis, which is at the level of the tricuspid valve, that venous pressures are not significantly affected by hydrostatic influence. Regardless of the position of the body, the pressure will not vary more than about 1 mmHg.

The venous pump and the valves enable the standing individual to overcome hydrostatic pressure as long as muscle compression occurs. As in the lymphatic vessels, the veins are supplied with unidirectional valves so that muscle compression causes blood to flow back toward the heart. In the quietly standing individual, of course, the venous pump cannot function, and extravasation of fluid from the capillaries into the tissues can occur fairly rapidly, causing edema and possibly significant loss of volume from the vascular space.

Although the resistance imposed by the veins and venules does not approach that of the arterioles, it is important to note that constriction and dilation of the postcapillary venous vessels can cause marked changes in blood volume. Constriction of the venules will produce an increase in capillary pressure and result in enhanced filtration of fluid from the capillary. Dilation, along with precapillary constriction, can result in expansion of blood volume and dehydration of the tissues.

Control of Arterial Pressure

Everyday control of variations in arterial pressure is exercised mainly by the circulatory reflexes. Were it not for this vital integrative role, arterial pressure and thereby vital cerebral and cardiac perfusion could be dangerously compromised by changes in position, or by extreme localized demand for increased flow. When simply assuming the erect position from the supine, the tendency is for cerebral arterial pressure to drop precipitously; however, by excitation of the circulatory reflexes, increased sympathetic tone through vasoconstriction maintains cerebral flow.

Circulatory Reflexes

The most important of the cardiovascular reflexes are the baroreceptors, or stretch receptors. Although baroreceptors are situated within the walls of most large thoracic and neck arteries, the highest concentrations are within the carotid sinus, which is located in the internal carotid artery slightly above the bifurcation of the external and internal carotid arteries. With a rise in arterial pressure, the baroreceptors respond extremely rapidly through inhibition of the vasomotor center in the medulla and stimulation of the vagal center (Fig. 19-18). The vagal center functions primarily as a countercheck on the heart in that excitation produces bradycardia, while inhibition results in tachycardia. The overall effects of the baroreceptors are vasodilatation due to suppression of the vasomotor center, and reduction of heart rate and contractility, which results in a decrease in arterial pressure. Conversely,

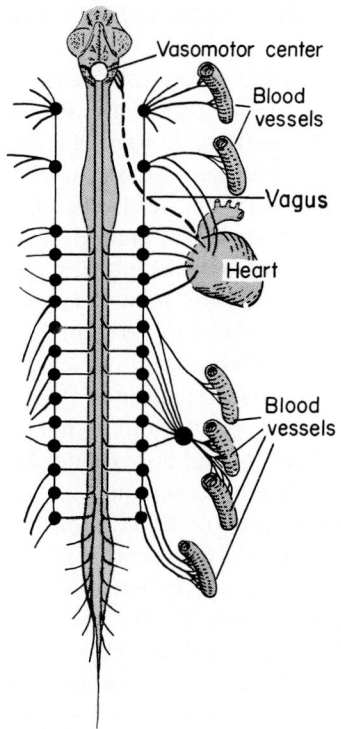

Figure 19-18 Neural control (vasomotor center) of the circulatory system through sympathetic and vagal nervous innervation. (*From A. C. Guyton, Textbook of Medical Physiology, Saunders, Philadelphia, 1970. Used by permission of the publisher.*)

arterial pressure is augmented through opposite effects of the baroreceptors—should there be a drop in arterial pressure. Because these neural receptors mitigate increases and decreases in arterial pressure, they are called *buffer nerves,* and the baroreceptors are a buffer system.

The baroreceptor response can be obviated if the hypertension or hypotension persists for a protracted length of time. The major effect of the circulatory reflexes exists in acute changes. However, over a longer time period, the baroreceptors simply adapt by decreasing their rate of excitation to normal, although the blood pressure remains very high or very low.

Other Types of Cardiovascular Reflexes

The chemoreceptors, which are located at the bifurcation of the internal and external carotid arteries and within the aortic arch, are sensitive to hypoxia and hypercapnia, which causes stimulation of the vasomotor center and results in elevation of arterial blood pressure.

The atrial baroreceptors, called low-pressure receptors, include two types of receptors. The A receptors are synchronous with the *a* wave of atrial contraction, while the B receptors are stimulated by the *v* wave occurring during atrial filling. Experimentally, these receptors, when stretched, have demonstrated a slight reflex vasodilatation of peripheral arterioles, which in turn may decrease arterial pressure.[6] These receptors are stretched in response to an increase in blood volume within the atria. It is thought that stimulation can also cause an increase in urinary flow, and either a decrease or increase in heart rate, and reduction of arterial pressure, at least experimentally.

Spinal cord receptors become evident following cervical spinal cord transection. Initially following the trauma, arterial pressure drops but can eventually return to near-normal levels, probably through local sympathetic vasoconstriction.

Other potential reflexes occur within the pulmonary vasculature. Distention of the pulmonary vessels can cause reduction in both heart rate and arterial pressure. Distention of the abdominal viscera may elicit a depressor response. Lastly, pain can cause either vasoconstriction or vasodilatation;

usually, however, pain elicits a sympathetic response.

The cardiac and respiratory reflexes are very closely related. It can be safely surmised that anything affecting the respiratory center will also stimulate the vasomotor center. Elevations of P_{CO_2} and reduction of pH produce vasoconstriction. Conversely, vasodilatation results from a drop in P_{CO_2} or rise in pH.

Intrinsic Control

Through variations in capillary pressure which are a direct result of changes in arterial pressure, changes in vascular volume via capillary-to-tissue fluid shifts can effectively participate in arterial pressure control. Although capillary fluid shift takes longer than the cardiovascular reflexes to become fully effective (about 1 h), this system can be twice as effective as the baroreceptors in restoring normal ranges of arterial pressure. The reader is referred to the previous discussion on capillary dynamics for a review of normal fluid balance.

Long-Term Regulation

The crucial role of the kidney in long-term regulation of arterial pressure cannot be overemphasized. It is estimated that an increase in arterial pressure from 100 mmHg to 200 mmHg can increase water and sodium excretion approximately sixfold. Hypotension, of course, has the opposite effect of increasing reabsorption of water and salt, thus augmenting blood volume and therefore pressure. The importance of aldosterone in selective water and salt reabsorption or excretion was reviewed earlier.

The kidneys can begin to respond to an acute situation within a few hours; for complete effect, though, several days are necessary.

Variables Affecting Circulation

The actual method by which each local tissue is able to regulate its blood flow is unknown, but several theories have been proposed. Since a decrease in the available oxygen supply or increase in the metabolic activity of tissue causes an immediate increase in blood flow, it is postulated that hypoxia is a stimulant for the phasic opening and closing of the precapillary sphincters. Another possibility is that an unknown vasodilator substance accumulates within the tissue as a result of increased metabolic activity. Vasodilators which have been proposed as possible vasodilator substances are carbon dioxide, adenosine, and hydrogen.

Autoregulation

A phenomenon which has received considerable attention is the ability of the vessels to maintain blood flow in the face of marked changes in arterial pressure. Changing arterial pressure from a low of 80 mmHg to 175 mmHg has remarkably little effect. The principles previously discussed are able to obviate the effects of acute changes in pressure.

Another example of a type of autoregulation is known as *reactive hyperemia*. Occlusion of arterial flow to a specific organ or vascular bed will result in a quadrupling of flow to the affected area following removal of the occlusion. This phenomenon may be observed in an extremity following occlusion via a tourniquet—for example, the arm may be seen to redden considerably, and dilation of blood vessels is observed, following occlusion.

If the change in arterial pressure persists for an indefinite period of time or if the metabolic demands of a tissue increase chronically, a system of long-term autoregulation develops over a period of days and weeks. An example of this type of chronic local autoregulation probably occurs with coarctation of the aorta. Coarctation is a congenital condition in which an area of partial occlusion occurs within the aorta and causes an extremely high pressure above the occlusion and a lower than normal pressure below it. Despite the enormous pressure gradient, blood flow to the upper and lower body appears to be equal within several weeks.

Earlier in this section, an almost linear correlation was made between the vascularity of the tissue and its metabolic demands: the higher the activity, the more vascular the tissue. It appears that this increase in vascularity may develop on demand. For an example, consider coarctation once more.

Should the arterial pressure below the coarctation drop to 80 mmHg, the number of vessels probably increases, so that blood flow is not compromised. In the upper extremities, however, where the arterial pressure may be 220 mmHg, the reverse situation occurs; the vessels decrease both in number and in size. The rate at which the tissue can adjust its vasculature undoubtedly relates to many factors, not the least of which is age.

Collateral circulation can be considered as a mechanism of chronic long-term autoregulation. In the discussion relating to the coronary circulation, the observation was made that the anastomotic connections were assumed to be present from early life but that their use as channels for blood flow only occurred following occlusion or insufficiency within a vessel. The same pattern for utilization of collateral vessels appears to exist in most vascular systems.

Fluid Balance

A review of the intrinsic control mechanisms within the circulation would be incomplete without at least brief attention to the integral role of the blood and extracellular fluid volumes on circulatory control, and of the key role of the kidney in maintaining fluid balance. Proper function of the intrinsic vascular mechanisms in maintenance of adequate tissue perfusion is dependent on sufficient blood volume and an adequate pressure gradient (arterial pressure) to move blood through the circulatory system.

Simplistically, extracellular fluid volume is maintained through daily ingestion of fluid and sodium. With increases in the extracellular fluid volume, proportionate amounts will remain in the plasma as increased blood volume until the point at which capillary balance is lost and fluid extravasates into the tissues, resulting in edema.

As blood volume increases, venous return to the heart is increased, causing a rise in both cardiac output and arterial pressure. With an increase in arterial pressure, the rate of urine production correspondingly increases in order to restore plasma and extracellular fluid volumes to their normal levels. For example, the rate of glomerular filtrate formed within the kidneys at a normal arterial pressure of 100 mmHg is approximately 1 mL/min. Elevating the arterial pressure to 150 mmHg will increase the rate of filtrate production to about 4 mL/min.

Neural Control of Circulation

Located within the medulla and a portion of the pons is the vasomotor center, depicted in Fig. 19-18. From the vasoconstrictor portion of the vasomotor center, sympathetic fibers descend to synapse in the thoracolumbar region of the spinal cord and to innervate all major blood vessels except the capillaries. Through this massive innervation of the entire vasculature, sympathetic stimulation results in alteration of arterial and venous resistance.

The vasomotor center is able to maintain sympathetic vasoconstrictor tone through continual transmission of impulses, the frequency of which is increased or decreased in relation to stimulation received from the cardiovascular reflexes and hormones. This continual activity of the vasomotor center causes release of the sympathetic hormone norepinephrine from the nerve endings, and elicits through its alpha-adrenergic effect on the blood vessels a partial state of contraction, or tone.

Within the vasomotor center, near the vasoconstrictor center, lies a depressor or inhibitory portion. Its function is, at intervals, to inhibit impulse transmission from the vasoconstrictor center, thus permitting vasodilation.

The major effect of neural control is demonstrated within the microcirculation. Though innervation exists in all major vessels, it is through constriction of the resistance vessels that localized reduction in blood flow is effected, and through constriction in the venous or capacitance vessels that circulating blood volume is increased. In response to any increase in metabolic demand, whether exercise or shock, circulating blood volume is increased and cardiac contractility enhanced through an elevation in venous return to the right side of the heart. Arterial pressure, in addition, is augmented by arterial and venous vasoconstriction.

Control of the vasomotor center can be exercised by other higher nervous centers. Areas within the diencephalon, mesencephalon, and pons can have either a stimulative or suppressive effect.

The hypothalamus as well can have a powerful influence on neural control of the vasculature. Many coordinative responses which involve the circulatory system are known to center within the hypothalamus: temperature control, osmotic regulation of circulating plasma through water balance, and cardiovascular responses to exercise. Experimental excitation of the hypothalamus is known to produce vast alterations in arterial pressure, heart rate, and cardiac contractility. Lastly, vasomotor control can be affected to some extent by the cerebral cortex, as investigation of areas such as biofeedback and relaxation therapy have demonstrated.

Sympathetic Nervous System

The sympathetic vasodilator fibers emerge from the motor cortex and hypothalamus. Upon excitation, these fibers release acetylcholine from their nerve endings, as evidenced by the name, *sympathetic cholinergic fibers*. Normally, this system probably plays a relatively insignificant role in circulatory control; however, if the normal vasoconstrictor response is blocked by a pharmacologic blocking agent or the customary stores of norepinephrine are reduced by reserpine, sympathetic stimulation can result in active vasodilatation.

The existence of beta-adrenergic receptors within the skeletal muscle has been confirmed using isoproterenol; stimulation of beta receptors produces vasodilatation.[5] In addition, epinephrine under certain circumstances can cause vasodilatation within skeletal and cardiac vasculature.[6] Since the two effects can be elicited, the terms *alpha* and *beta receptors* were proposed to name the binding sites within vascular smooth muscle controlling each. Neural control of the beta-receptor system is undetermined; however, it is doubtful that circulating catecholamines (epinephrine and norepinephrine) have a significant role in the everyday neural control of peripheral blood flow.

Parasympathetic Nervous System

Vascular innervation by the parasympathetic nervous system exists only in the head, viscera, bladder, and genitalia; within the skin and the majority of the muscles, there are no parasympathetic nervous connections. Thus the vasodilatation evoked by acetylcholine, the neurohumoral transmitter of the parasympathetic system, while potent, is limited to certain vascular beds. It is possible that the vasodilatation which accompanies eating and follows parasympathetic stimulation of the salivary glands may be caused partially by acetylcholine, by the production of the enzyme bradykinin (which produces vasodilatation), or by a combination of both.

Hormonal Influences on the Circulation

The most important of the humoral or hormonal substances is aldosterone. Secreted by the cortex of the adrenal gland, aldosterone is important in regulation of blood volume through its control over sodium and water concentrations within the extracellular fluid. Stimulated by a decrease in cardiac output, total body volume, or reduction in sodium concentration, aldosterone promotes increased renal tubular reabsorption of sodium and, indirectly, chloride and water. The end result is an increase in plasma and extracellular fluid volume.

Epinephrine, norepinephrine, and acetylcholine exert their major influence when released at sympathetic and parasympathetic nerve endings. Stimulation of sympathetic nerves also prompts the adrenal medulla to secret epinephrine and norepinephrine as circulating catecholamines. The major vascular effects of these neurohumors were reviewed earlier.

Vasodilator substances known as *kinins* can be identified within the blood following obstruction of flow or decrease in oxygen. Little is known about kinins other than their very potent vasodilator effect. *Bradykinin* and *kallikrein* are two kinins which can be activated with relative ease, and which function throughout the circulation.

Angiotensin is formed through the release of renin from the kidney. When renin acts on another substance to produce angiotensin 1, an activating enzyme converts angiotensin 1 to angiotensin II. The mechanism for renin release is uncertain, but it is believed to be governed by variations in arterial pressure because increased renin secretion follows hypotension. Renal vascular constriction and low serum sodium also influence the rate of renin production. Angiotensin has very powerful vasoconstrictive effects on the arterioles, but there is

apparently little or no significant influence on the venous system. The renin mechanism has, in addition, an important role in raising aldosterone secretion in response to hypotension and reducing it in response to elevations in arterial pressure.

Similar to angiotension, *vasopressin* is a potent vasoconstrictor which acts primarily on the arterioles. It is produced in the neurohypophysis and is secreted by the posterior pituitary gland. Its influence on the peripheral circulation appears to be relatively minor. The primary function of this hormone is in controlling the volume of water reabsorbed across the renal tubule.

Serotonin is concentrated predominantly in the intestinal and other abdominal tissue as well as within platelets. It can have very powerful vasodilator as well as vasoconstrictor effects. The role of serotonin in controlling the peripheral circulation is obscure.

Histamine is probably not involved in normal circulatory control. Almost every tissue within the body releases histamine in response to injury. The result is local vasoconstriction, surrounding vasodilatation, and edema. Histamine causes intense dilation of the arterioles and constriction within the venous system, a combination which produces edema. The hormone is involved with allergic responses and tissue injury such as burns in addition to trauma.

Pulmonary Circulation

Although the systemic and pulmonary circulations together form the cardiovascular circuit, there are very important differences between the two circuits (Fig. 19-19). The pulmonary circulation is a low-pressure, low-resistance system which has a limited perfusion area. The high-pressure, high-resistance systemic circulation, on the other hand, must supply the variable requirements within the entire body, thus requiring many controls and adaptation to a great variety of vascular conditions that have been previously discussed.

Functional Anatomy

There is no corollary to the arteriole within the pulmonary circuit. That fact, in addition to the

Figure 19-19 Functional differences between pulmonary and systemic circuits. (*From Robert Rushmer, Cardiovascular Dynamics, Saunders, Philadelphia, 1970. Used by permission of the publisher.*)

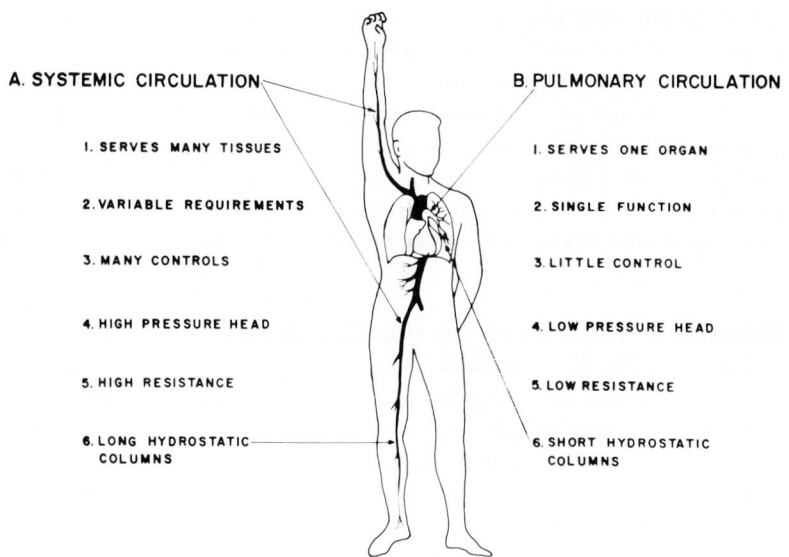

A. SYSTEMIC CIRCULATION

1. SERVES MANY TISSUES
2. VARIABLE REQUIREMENTS
3. MANY CONTROLS
4. HIGH PRESSURE HEAD
5. HIGH RESISTANCE
6. LONG HYDROSTATIC COLUMNS

B. PULMONARY CIRCULATION

1. SERVES ONE ORGAN
2. SINGLE FUNCTION
3. LITTLE CONTROL
4. LOW PRESSURE HEAD
5. LOW RESISTANCE
6. SHORT HYDROSTATIC COLUMNS

factors previously mentioned which contribute to the compliance of the pulmonary vessels (large internal diameter of the vessels and the enormous cross-sectional area of the pulmonary vasculature), results in a resistance imposed on the right ventricle which is about one-eighth that imposed on the left ventricle.

Atrial contraction occurs just prior to right ventricular contraction and contributes a small amount of blood as well as a slight rise in diastolic pressure within the right ventricle. Immediately following atrial contraction, the pressure within the right ventricle continues to rise, closing the tricuspid valve, until the pressure is equal to pulmonary pressure (22 mmHg) and can open the pulmonic valve. With the opening of the valve, right ventricular and pulmonary pressures are essentially the same, and blood flows into the pulmonary artery. During right ventricular relaxation, the right ventricular pressure falls, the pulmonary valve shuts, and the normal diastolic pressure of around zero resumes within the ventricle. Following systole, pressure within the pulmonary artery drops to about 8 mmHg.

The pulmonary veins, like the peripheral veins, are collapsed at low pressures; with distention, they open, thereby offering negligible resistance to flow. It is for this reason that as much as a 7-mmHg change in pressure within the left atrium,

the point of outflow for the pulmonary veins, will have little effect on pulmonary arterial pressure. If the left atrial pressure exceeds about 7 mmHg, however, the pulmonary system begins to assume the characteristics of a system of almost rigid tubes, thereby causing retrograde transmission of pressure to the pulmonary artery and right ventricle. Normally the right ventricle can sustain an increase in systolic pressure of 10 to 20 mmHg. Above a systolic pressure of 40 mmHg, however, the increased resistance causes an increase in right atrial pressure and resulting signs and symptoms of right ventricular failure.

Functions of the Pulmonary Circuit

In addition to its major function in diffusion of oxygen and carbon dioxide, the pulmonary circuit can function as a variable-volume reservoir. Normally about 12 percent (600 mL) of the circulation is contained within the pulmonary vasculature at any one time. When the supine position is assumed, a considerable amount of blood can be displaced into the pulmonary vasculature. There is a volume of blood which can be contained within the lungs and can be displaced as necessary without significantly increasing pulmonary pressure.

The cardiac output can increase to three or four times normal before causing an elevation in pulmonary pressures. The sole purpose, of course, of circulation through the lungs is oxygenation, but it is important that the blood circulate without elevating the energy demands on the heart. An increase in pulmonary pressure imposes just such an increase in metabolic demand.

Lastly, the lungs are well adapted for filtration of emboli, foreign bodies, air bubbles, and other particles because of their extensive dual blood supply, which is a result of the bronchial arterial supply running parallel to the pulmonary vessels.

References

1. Harvey, W. (1941). An anatomical disquisition on the motion of the heart and blood in animals. In F. A. Willius, & T. E. Keys (Eds.), *Cardiac classics*. St. Louis: Mosby.

2. Morgan, J. (1968). A discourse upon the institution of medical schools in America. In M. B. Strauss (Ed.), *Familiar medical quotations*. Boston: Little, Brown.

3. Braunwald, E., Sonnenblick, E. H., and Ross, J. (1984). Contraction of the normal heart. In E. Braunwald (Ed.), *Heart disease*. Philadelphia: Saunders.

4. Rushmer, R. F. (1981). *Cardiovascular dynamics*. Philadelphia: Saunders.

5. Berne, R. M., & Levy, M. N. (1981). *Cardiovascular physiology*. St. Louis: Mosby.

6. Guyton, A. C. (1981). *Textbook of medical physiology*, 6th Ed. Philadelphia: Saunders.

20 Data Acquisition from the Cardiovascular System

Joan Vitello-Cicciu
Janet S. Eagan

Nursing History

The clinical evaluation of any cardiovascular (CV) patient admitted to a critical-care unit consists of a nursing history, physical assessment, and data from diagnostic procedures. When a seriously ill patient is admitted to a unit, he or she may be incapable of providing a history. In this instance, any available data should be obtained from significant others, ambulance drivers, helicopter personnel, or previous records. When no history can be gathered, the critical-care nurse must rely on subsequent data obtained from the physical assessment and diagnostic procedures.

Ideally, the nursing history should be obtained from the patient on arrival in a unit, but life-threatening medical problems that need immediate assessment and intervention must take precedence. One of several frameworks for obtaining a nursing history has been proposed by Gordon.[1] Before discussing this framework, an understanding of Gordon's views of the scope of nursing is a prerequisite.

Gordon[2] divides the scope of nursing into two focuses. The first deals with the patient's medical problems. These are viewed as "collaborative problems" between medicine and nursing and are most frequently encountered in the critical-care setting. The other focus deals with purely "nursing problems," referred to as "nursing diagnosis." Gordon[1] defines these diagnoses as "actual or potential problems which nurses by virtue of their education and experience are capable and licensed to treat."

Nursing diagnoses are formulated based on the data obtained from the nursing history. To facilitate the collection of admission history information, Gordon[2] has suggested 11 assessment categories. These categories are referred to as *func-tional health patterns*. Utilization of this model encompasses a biopsychosocial perspective of the patient. This holistic view is important in understanding that a problem in one pattern area may affect function in other areas.

A detailed explanation concerning each pattern is beyond the scope of this chapter. However, a list and description of each 11 functional health patterns can be found in Table 20-1. In addition, specific questions related to each pattern that can facilitate the collection of information is also found in Table 20-1.

Once the nursing history is completed and the nursing diagnoses have been identified, a plan of care should be formulated that is aimed at resolving the patient's problems. This plan of care is based on the steps of the nursing process. Thus, goals, interventions, and evaluation will be the elements contained in a nursing care plan developed to treat these problems. In addition, to facilitate psychological as well as physiologic recovery, the plan of care should include the patient's significant others.

Physical Assessment

The next step in the clinical evaluation of a cardiovascular patient is performance of a physical assessment. Included in this process are inspection, palpation, percussion, and auscultation. The cardinal areas for inspection, palpation, percussion, and auscultation are illustrated in Fig. 20-1.

Inspection

The observations noted on inspection should include level of consciousness, posture, facial expressions, and mobility. In regard to the skin, the critical-

Table 20-1 Gordon's 11 Functional Health Patterns

Functional Health Patterns	Description	Questions Relating to Patterns
1. Health perception and health management pattern	Describes client's perceived pattern of health and well-being and how health is managed	What brought you here to the hospital? How has your health been before this incident? Are you taking any medications or following any special regimens to maintain your health? What do you feel has caused this illness?
2. Nutritional and metabolic pattern	Describes pattern of food and fluid consumption relative to metabolic need and pattern indicators of local nutrient supply	Any recent weight loss or gain? Could you describe your daily food intake? Do you follow any dietary restrictions? Any problems with healing, dentures, or digestion?
3. Elimination pattern	Describes patterns of excretory function (bowel, bladder, skin)	Any problem moving your bowels? How often? Any problem urinating? How frequently do you have to urinate? Do you wake up at night to urinate?
4. Activity and exercise pattern	Describes pattern of exercise, activity, leisure, and recreation	Describe the type, amount, and frequency of exercise you do on a regular basis. Does your occupation require exercise? Do you have sufficient energy for all your activities?
5. Cognitive and perceptual pattern	Describes sensory, perceptual, and cognitive pattern	Describe your vision and hearing. Any changes? Any trouble feeling hot or cold? Describe your memory. Any changes? What's the easiest way for you to learn something?
6. Sleep and rest pattern	Describes patterns of sleep, rest, and relaxation	How many hours do you sleep each night? Do you have trouble falling asleep or with early awakening? Do you take anything or follow a nightly ritual to induce sleep?
7. Self-perception and self-concept pattern	Describes self-concept pattern, perceptions of self (e.g., body comfort, body image, feeling state)	How would you describe yourself to another? What are your strengths and weaknesses? What do you feel about your life? Future goals?
8. Role and relationship pattern	Describes pattern of role engagements and relationships	What are your primary responsibilities? Who makes decisions? Any major changes recently? Who are the most significant persons available to you?
9. Sexuality and reproductive pattern	Describes client's pattern of satisfaction and dissatisfaction with sexuality pattern; describes reproductive patterns	Any changes or problems with your sexual relations? For female question, self-breast exam. For males, testicular exam.
10. Coping, stress, and tolerance pattern	Describes general coping pattern and effectiveness of the pattern in terms of stress tolerance	What are the major stressors in your life? How do you feel you handle stress? How have you handled a past crisis? Any significant losses or changes in your life?
11. Value and belief pattern	Describes pattern of values, beliefs (including spiritual), or goals that guide decisions or choices.	Is religion important to you? List three things you value most in life. Would you like to see a member of the clergy?

Adapted from M. Gordon, *Manual of Nursing Diagnosis.* New York: McGraw-Hill, 1982.

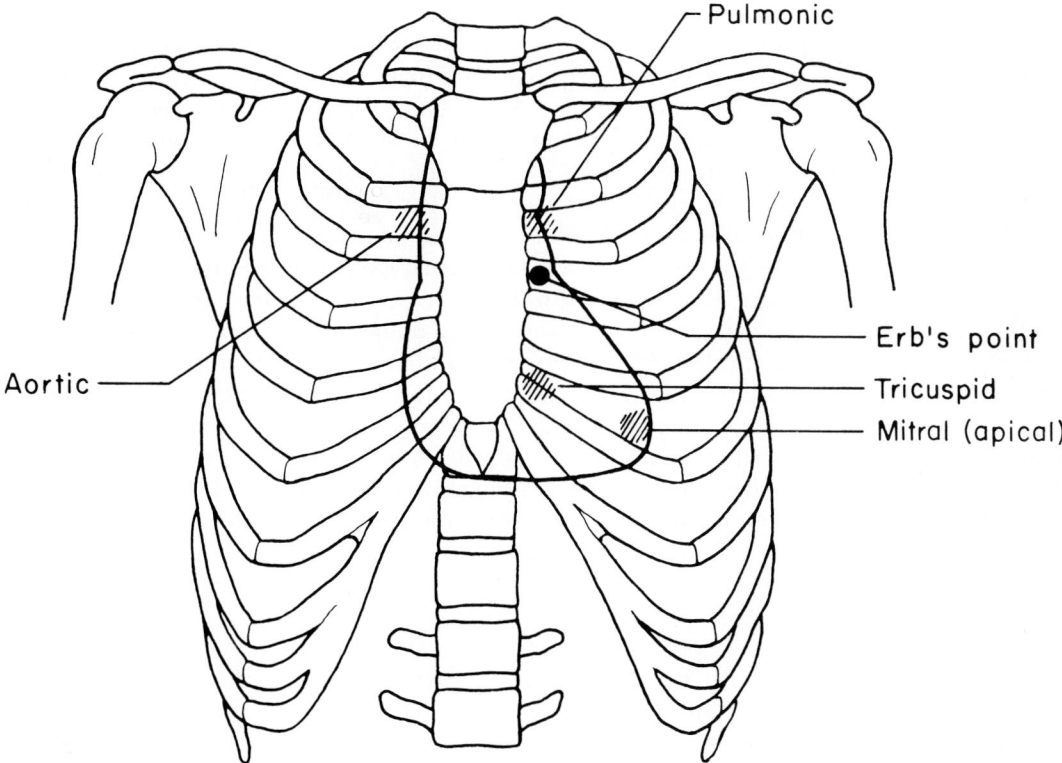

Figure 20-1   Cardinal areas for inspection, palpation, and auscultation. (*From E. Hochstein and A. L. Rubin, Physical Diagnosis, McGraw-Hill, New York, 1964. Used by permission of the publisher.*)

care nurse should look for cyanosis, pallor (anemia), ruddiness (polycythemia), glossy or shiny skin surface (Raynaud's disease), the presence of ulcers (vascular insufficiency), loss of hair, petechiae, jaundice (liver congestion due to right-sided heart failure), and peripheral edema. Inspection should also reveal the presence of bounding pulses occurring in the upper extremities. Corrigan's pulse is an example of a bounding arterial pulsation which can be present in severe aortic regurgitation.

The eyes can reveal underlying cardiovascular disorders. Exophthalmus, or protrusion of the eyeball, can occur in advanced congestive heart failure in the presence of severe pulmonary hypertension and significant weight loss.[3] The presence of corneal arcus, a circumferential light ring around the iris, is frequently associated with hypercholesterolemia and premature atherosclerosis. Roth's spots, which are white spots in the center of hemorrhages, can

occur in infective endocarditis. Yellow plaques called xanthelasmas may be found in patients with atherosclerosis.[4]

The ear lobes may reveal diagonal creases, called McCathy's sign. These creases may be an indicator of coronary artery disease (CAD). They have also been noted in patients who present with acute myocardial infarction.[5]

The nails may evidence clubbing in the setting of hypoxemia or infective endocarditis. There may also be splinter hemorrhages in the nail beds and Osler's nodes, which are painful, tender red nodules associated with emboli in infective endocarditis.

The chest may reveal pectus excavatum, a depressed sternum often associated with aortic aneurysms. The abdomen may be enlarged and tender from venous congestion as a sequela of right ventricular failure. The lower extremities should be inspected for edema, clubbing, petechiae, and absence of hair.

Venous Pulsations

The internal and external jugular veins should be inspected for abnormal pulsations and elevated pressure. The normal venous pulse includes two outward pulsations known as the *a* and *v* waves. A third positive, the *c* wave, which is graphically recorded using instrumentation, can rarely be detected clinically and thus has no significance in the assessment of the venous pulse.[6] The *a* wave corresponds to right atrial contraction, and is seen just prior to the first heart sound. It occurs after the *p* wave on an ECG. The *v* wave is produced during diastole as a result of atrial filling and corresponds in time to ventricular contraction. It follows the second heart sound and can be seen after the QRS complex. In order to visualize these pulsations, the head of the bed should be elevated 15 to 45° with a pillow placed directly under the patient's head and shoulders so as not to cause neck flexion. In inspecting the venous pulse, the nurse should observe a "double flicker," with both *a* and *v* waves being of equal prominence.[6] Giant *a* waves, for example, are seen in any condition which impedes emptying from the right atrium into the right ventricle. Thus, large *a* waves can be seen in tricuspid stenosis and with such arrhythmias as junctional rhythms, complete heart block, premature ventricular contractions, and ventricular tachycardia. Conversely, the *a* wave is absent in atrial fibrillation.

The *v* wave is affected when any condition increases or decreases the right atrial (RA) pressure during diastole. For example, tricuspid insufficiency can produce amplified *v* waves because of the retrograde flow of blood into the right atrium.

Ideally, the internal jugular vein should be used when measuring jugular venous pressure (JVP). This vein courses under the sternocleidomastoid muscle, in parallel with the carotid artery. When the internal jugular cannot be visualized, the external jugular vein may be used. The angle of Louis is used as a zero reference point. Also known as the sternal angle, it is a bony protrusion on the sternum found at the second intercostal space, and is located 5 to 7 cm above the right atrium (Fig. 20-2).

Measurement of the JVP is begun by drawing an imaginary horizontal line from the sternal angle away from the body. The patient should be positioned in bed at 30 to 45° of truncal elevation to locate the highest point of jugular pulsations. Another horizontal imaginary line is drawn from this point. The vertical distance from this horizontal line at the height of the column of blood to the other horizontal line at the sternal angle is the measurement made in centimeters. Documentation of this pressure may be written as follows: The internal jugular pulse is 3 to 5 cm above the sternal angle at 45° of truncal elevation.

Another method used to calculate the jugular pressure is to add the vertical distance in centimeters to the 5 to 7-cm distance known to exist from the sternal angle to the right atrium. As an example, if the vertical distance is 5 cm, the central

Figure 20-2 Measurement of JVP: Calculated by measuring the distance between angle of Louis and height of column of blood visible in the internal jugular vein.

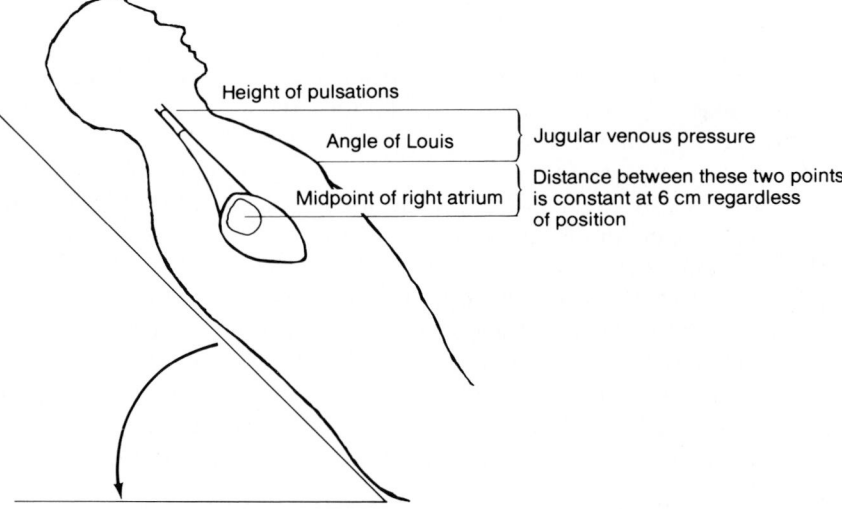

Height of pulsations

Angle of Louis

Midpoint of right atrium

Jugular venous pressure

Distance between these two points is constant at 6 cm regardless of position venous pressure can be estimated to be 10 to 12 cm. Elevation of the JVP can occur with congestive heart failure, right ventricular infarcts, tricuspid valvular defects, and constrictive pericarditis.[7]

Carotid Arterial Pulsations

The critical-care nurse should inspect the carotid artery for bounding or weak pulsations. Abnormal large bounding pulses may be associated with hypertension, complete heart block, hypoxia, anemia, or anxiety states. A weak pulse may be related to left ventricular failure, aortic stenosis, or any other condition which causes diminished stroke volume.

Anterior Chest Pulsations

Pulsations should also be observed on the anterior chest. Table 20-2 lists the abnormalities of the heart detected by inspection and palpation. Possible etiologies are also listed.

Respiratory Movement

In concluding the inspection procedure, the nurse should observe for the adequacy of chest expansion, the use of accessory muscles to breathe (may be an indication of respiratory distress), and the quality and quantity of the respiratory rate.

Palpation

Precordial palpation is done to confirm and qualify visible findings and detect the presence of other normal and abnormal pulsations or vibrations. The nurse should be positioned on the right side of the patient. Palpation begins by placing the palmar surface of the fingers and hand over visible areas of pulsation and then moving over the entire precordium, palpating in a systematic manner. When areas of pulsation or vibration are felt, the fingertips are used to denote the rate, rhythm, and intensity of the pulsation.

Beginning at the base of the heart, the nurse then palpates for pulsations, thrills, and heaves or vibrations in the aortic area at the second or third intercostal space (ICS) to the right of the sternum. A thrill in this area may signify aortic stenosis and abnormal pulsations may be suggestive of an aortic aneurysm. Palpation of this area is enhanced when the patient is sitting up or leaning forward.

Table 20-2 Abnormalities of the Heart Detected by Inspection and Palpation

Precordium	Abnormality	Examples of Possible Cause

Aortic area
  2d and 3d interspaces to right
    of sternum
	Forceful pulsation
	
	Thrill
		Rheumatic heart disease
		Systemic hypertension
		Ascending thoracic aortic aneurysm
		Aortic stenosis

Pulmonary area
  2d and 3d interspaces to left
    of sternum
	Forceful pulsation
	
	Thrill
		Essential pulmonary hypertension
		Left-to-right intracardiac shunt
		Mitral stenosis, pulmonary embolism, diffuse
		    pneumonia
		Obstruction of right ventricular outflow tract

Right ventricular area
  Lower sternal border to the
    immediate right and left of
    sternum
	Thrill
	Lift or heave
		Ventricular septal defect
		Obstructions of right ventricular outflow tract
		Mitral stenosis
		Left-to-right intracardiac shunts
		Skeletal deformities

Left ventricular area
  4th to 6th interspaces
  Left midclavicular line or
    beyond
	Strong apical impulse or ab-
	    normally large PMI
	
	Dyskinetic apical impulse
	Thrill
	Gallop
		Left ventricular hypertrophy
		Aortic valve diseases
		Left ventricular aneurysm
		Mitral valve disease
		Myocardial dysfunction, mitral or aortic valve
		    disease, HCVD

Epigastric area	Strong pulsation of abdomi- nal aorta Pulsation of liver	Abdominal aortic aneurysm Congestive heart failure

In the pulmonic area (second or third ICS to the left of the sternum), a slow, sustained, forceful pulsation may be associated with pulmonary hypertension or mitral stenosis. Erb's point, located in the third intercostal space on the left sternal border (LSB) should be palpated, since murmurs of aortic and pulmonic origin may be referred to this area. Gradually, palpation is continued over the parasternal area until the right ventricular area is reached. An abnormal pulsation of the right ventricular area may be indicative of right ventricular (RV) enlargement. A substantial heave may suggest pulmonic stenosis, mitral stenosis, or left ventricular (LV) failure. Palpation of the epigastric region is then done to detect the presence of pulsations. The apical area is palpated next to determine the strength of the point of maximal apical impulse (PMI). The PMI, which is the palpable apical impulse, is about the size of a quarter, and is normally felt in about half the population. The apical area is most easily palpated with the patient either in the left lateral decubitus position or seated and leaning forward. Thrills in this area may be associated with mitral stenosis or regurgitation. A displaced PMI occurs with LV hypertrophy. In addition, a systolic bulge suggestive of an LV aneurysm may be present in the apical area. Location of areas of palpation and abnormalities that may be detected by such inspection may be found in Table 20-2.

Abnormal arterial pulsations may occur as a manifestation of diminished left ventricular function, increased cardiac output (CO), or may be secondary to arrhythmias. Configurations of normal and abnormal arterial pulse waves are illustrated in Fig. 20-3.

Percussion

Percussion is no longer routinely used in the cardiovascular assessment because of imaging capabilities. When percussion is used, it is performed to outline the left and right borders of cardiac dullness, although the findings may not be as reliable as palpation. This technique may often be omitted from a routine physical assessment.

Auscultation

Auscultation of the heart includes listening to the rate and rhythm of the heartbeat, evaluating normal heart sounds, and determining the presence or absence of extra heart sounds, murmurs, and pericardial friction rubs.

Figure 20-3 Arterial pulse waves.

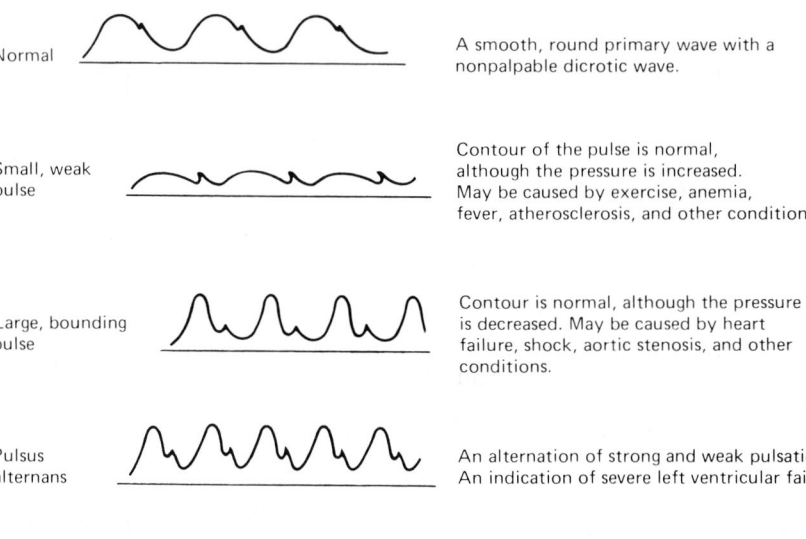

Normal — A smooth, round primary wave with a nonpalpable dicrotic wave.

Small, weak pulse — Contour of the pulse is normal, although the pressure is increased. May be caused by exercise, anemia, fever, atherosclerosis, and other conditions.

Large, bounding pulse — Contour is normal, although the pressure is decreased. May be caused by heart failure, shock, aortic stenosis, and other conditions.

Pulsus alternans — An alternation of strong and weak pulsations. An indication of severe left ventricular failure.

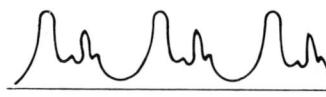

Bigeminal pulse — A coupling rhythm that reflects a normal beat quickly followed by a premature ventricular contraction. May resemble a pulsus alternans.

Examining the heart by auscultation ideally begins with a warm, well-lighted, and particularly quiet space. The patient is placed in the same positions for auscultation as palpation: lying, left lateral, sitting, and leaning forward. Both the diaphragm and the bell of the stethoscope are used.

The entire precordium, including areas of radiation (axilla and carotid arteries), is auscultated; however, particular attention should be paid to the areas in which valve closure sounds are best heard. These areas include the aortic area at the second right intercostal space adjacent to the sternal border, the pulmonic area in the second left intercostal space, the tricuspid area situated at the fifth left intercostal space near the sternal edge, and the mitral or apical area located at the fifth left intercostal space medial to the midclavicular line.

The examiner may begin with the diaphragm of the stethoscope at the aortic area, at which the second heart sound (S_2) is loudest, move to the pulmonic area, and inch the stethoscope down the left sternal border to the mitral or apical area. Another approach is to begin at the apical area at which the first sound (S_1) is loudest and move upward to the left sternal border and across the sternum to the aortic area. Beginning at the aortic or the apical area first, the examiner listens to and assesses the rate and rhythm of the heart to establish a baseline for comparison in each area examined. The course of auscultation is then reversed using the bell of the stethoscope.

In each area auscultated, the following components of the cardiac cycle are assessed:

1. The characteristics of S_1 (intensity, splitting, effects of respiration)
2. The characteristics of S_2 (intensity, splitting, effects of respiration)
3. The presence or absence of extra sounds in systole and diastole
4. The presence or absence of murmurs in systole and diastole
5. The presence or absence of pericardial friction rubs

Heart Rate and Rhythm

The normal rate and rhythm of the heart are determined by the conduction system. In the normal heart, the small bundle of fibers comprising the sinoatrial (SA) node initiates the cardiac impulse. Known as the *cardiac pacemaker,* the SA node is located in the wall of the right atrium at the entrance of the venae cavae. The SA node automatically discharges an electrical impulse which is then conducted throughout the atria to the atrioventricular (AV) node, another small bundle of cardiac fibers located in the posterior lower right atrium near the septum. After a slight delay, allowing for completion of atrial systole, the impulse is conducted through a bundle of electrically specialized conducting tissue, the *His bundle.* The bundle divides into right and left branches, each passing down the corresponding side of the interventricular septum, and then spreads into a fine network of Purkinje fibers. These fibers infiltrate into all portions of the ventricular myocardium. The impulse reaches the ventricles almost simultaneously and excites the muscles, causing ventricular contraction.

Variations in the rate and rhythm of the heart are classified as dysrhythmias and are caused by (1) variation in the rate of discharge of the SA node, (2) ectopic impulses which compete with the SA node, or (3) abnormal conduction of impulses from the SA node through the heart. (See Chap. 11 for further discussion of cardiac electrical activity.)

Normal Heart Sounds

Normal heart sounds are vibrations produced, at least in part, by the closure of valves and by the flow of blood through the heart. The first heart sound (S_1) is a high-pitched sound but is slightly lower in frequency and longer in duration than the second heart sound (S_2).

An S_1 is louder than an S_2 at the apex. If any difficulty arises in differentiating between S_1 and S_2, the timing of S_1 correlates with that of the carotid pulse and it is usually heard as one sound. The S_1 sound occurs as a result of closure of the atrioventricular [mitral (M_1) and tricuspid (T_1)] valves and can be heard over the entire precordium but is heard best at the apex.

Since the pressure gradients are greater on the left side of the heart than on the right side, sometimes there will be a minimal difference in closure of the mitral and tricuspid valve. This interval between M_1 and T_1 is referred to as a split of the first heart sound which produces an audible separation between these two components of S_1.

The second heart sound is high-pitched and slightly shorter in duration than S_1. The S_2 sound occurs upon closure of the semilunar (aortic and pulmonic) valves and may be heard most audibly at the base of the heart. It may vary in character when related to loudness as does S_1; however, particular attention should be given to the "splitting" phenomenon of S_2 which explains why two sounds are heard when listening. Other variations of S_2 will be presented following this discussion.

Splitting of S_2 may be physiologic or pathologic. Physiologic splitting is audible on inspiration at the pulmonic or aortic area when the aortic valve (A_2) closes before the pulmonic valve (P_2) as in the normal heart. This accentuated asynchronous closure of A_2 and P_2 on inspiration is due to an increased venous return to the right ventricle during inspiration. The prolongation of right ventricular systole delays closure of the pulmonic valve, increasing the time interval between closure of A_2 and P_2.

Pathologic splitting of S_2 indicates the presence of disease. When the split does not vary with inspiration or expiration, it is referred to as *fixed splitting,* and occurs in such conditions as pulmonic stenosis and atrial septal defect. *Wide splitting* refers to an increase in the normal splitting time of S_2 on inspiration along with an S_1 split. This occurs in right bundle branch block in which prolonged electrical conduction delays right ventricular contraction and pulmonic valve closure. *Paradoxical splitting* refers to a reverse phenomenon in which splitting of S_2 occurs on expiration rather than inspiration. In left bundle branch block, a delay in left ventricular contraction may cause the aortic valve to close after the pulmonic valve, producing a single sound on inspiration and a split sound on expiration.

In further assessing S_2, attention should be given to the intensity of the aortic and pulmonic components of S_2. An accentuated aortic component of S_2, as heard in arterial hypertension and aortic regurgitation, results from an increase in arterial pressure which forces the aortic valve to close. A diminished aortic component of S_2 occurs when the arterial pressure is low, as in shock, and aortic valve closure is soft. Aortic stenosis also produces a diminished second sound because the valve leaflets are relatively immobile.

An accentuated pulmonic component of S_2 occurs when back pressure in the pulmonary artery increases and forces the pulmonary valve to close, as in pulmonary hypertension. Other conditions in which an accentuated P_2 is heard are mitral stenosis, left ventricular failure, and atrial septal defect. A diminished pulmonic component of the second heart sound is also heard in pulmonic stenosis when the pressure against the pulmonic valve is less than normal.

Extra Heart Sounds

Extra heart sounds can basically be classified in relation to location in the cardiac cycle and are named and described accordingly. The sounds are heard either in systole or diastole, except for pericardial friction rubs, which are heard in both systole and diastole.

Ejection clicks may be heard in the early, middle, or late phase of cardiac systole. These clicks are thought to be related to prolapse of either the mitral or tricuspid valve. Early systolic ejection clicks are either aortic or pulmonic in origin and occur immediately after S_1. Aortic ejection clicks are heard at the base and apex of the heart and occur in diseases of the aortic valve and in aortic aneurysms. The click does not change with respiration.

Pulmonic ejection clicks are heard in the pulmonic area, diminish with inspiration, and occur in pulmonic stenosis. Middle and late systolic clicks are not as well defined as early systolic clicks, but are frequently associated with systolic murmurs of mitral regurgitation.

The opening snap (OS) of mitral stenosis is a high-pitched, short, snappy sound heard in the early phase of diastole. An OS is best heard along the LSB medial to the apex; however, it does radiate widely and can be differentiated from a third heart sound (S_3) because it occurs earlier in the cardiac cycle.

The third heart sound (S_3) can be physiologic or pathologic. It is a common and usually normal finding in children and young adults. In the middle-aged and older person, however, it is considered abnormal and usually indicative of LV failure. In fact, the presence of an S_3 sound should be searched for in any patient with a cardiac condition. It is a low-pitched sound which occurs early in diastole during rapid ventricular filling, resulting in vibrations in the left ventricle. An S_3 sound can be heard best at the apex with the bell of the stethoscope.

The fourth heart sound (S_4) may also be physiologic or pathologic. It may be occasionally heard normally in young children, but not as often as is an S_3. It is usually an abnormal sound which is believed to be a late ventricular filling sound resulting from the accelerated flow of blood into the ventricles produced by atrial contraction. It is a low-pitched sound which occurs late in diastole just before the first heart sound. It is heard best at the apex with the bell of the stethoscope. A pathologic S_4 is usually associated with hypertensive cardiovascular (CV) disease, coronary artery disease, or aortic stenosis. It may be the first evidence of CV disease and can be an important contribution to the data regarding the CV system of a patient.

A pericardial friction rub is usually described as a transient scratching, grating, or squeaking high-pitched sound indicative of pericarditis. It is heard best with the diaphragm of the stethoscope in the region between the apex and left sternal border. The timing of the pericardial friction rub is associated with cardiac movement and consists of three short components: atrial systole, ventricular systole, and ventricular diastole. Often, two components are heard; however, all three components are diagnostic and help to differentiate a pericardial rub from a pleural friction rub, which has two components.

Gallop Rhythm

Gallop rhythm is a term used to describe the rhythm of the heart when an S_3, S_4, or both sounds are perceived by auscultation and possibly palpation. The presence of an S_3 sound is referred to as a *protodiastolic gallop*. The term *summation gallop* is used when presystolic (S_4) and protodiastolic (S_3) gallops combine to form a single, loud, evenly spaced sound in diastole. Gallop rhythms are heard best with the bell of the stethoscope.

Murmurs

Murmurs are audible vibrations which originate within the heart and great vessels. These sounds represent turbulence of blood flow caused by (1) an increased rate of blood flow through normal structures (such as is caused by exercise), (2) the forward flow of blood across a partially obstructed or narrowed valve (such as in valvular stenosis), (3) blood flow into a dilated chamber, or (4) the backward flow of blood across an incompetent valve or defect (such as in valvular insufficiency).

Murmurs are usually classified as *systolic, diastolic,* or *continuous* because of the location in the cardiac cycle. To determine the significance of a murmur, certain factors must be identified and described in the process of cardiac assessment. These factors include:

1. The timing of the murmur within the cardiac cycle which may be in early, or late systole, or in diastole, or it may be considered holosystolic
2. Characteristics
   a. Intensity (graded on a scale from 1 to 6)
      (1) Difficult to hear; barely audible, very faint
      (2) Very soft, but can be heard without straining
      (3) Moderately loud
      (4) Loud
      (5) Very loud, but requires stethoscope chestpiece to be placed on chest
      (6) Extremely loud; heard with chestpiece off chest
   b. Pattern (crescendo, decrescendo, or diamond-shaped)
   c. Pitch (high, medium, low)
   d. Quality (harsh, musical, blowing, or rumbling)
3. Location on the precordium (location of greatest intensity, that is, the apex, tricuspid, aortic, or pulmonic area)
4. Radiation (areas in which the murmur is less audible, but still perceptible)
5. Posture and exercise (the body position or activity under which murmur is heard)
6. Stethoscope chestpiece used to hear the murmur (bell or diaphragm)

Systolic Murmurs

Systolic murmurs may be physiologic or pathologic and occur between S_1 and S_2 sounds. They may be further described as *early systolic* or *midsystolic* because of their relationship or proximity to S_1 and S_2 sounds.

There are basically two types of systolic murmurs: *ejection* and *regurgitant*. Systolic ejection murmurs occur when ventricular contraction forces blood, under high pressure, forward through the aortic valve, pulmonic valve, or septal defect into normal or dilated vessels which are at lower pressures.

Systolic ejection murmurs occur with such conditions as aortic and pulmonic stenoses. Aortic and pulmonic stenoses produce midsystolic murmurs that are diamond-shaped, medium-pitched, and harsh, and heard with either the bell or diaphragm chestpiece.

Regurgitant murmurs occur in systole when the mitral or tricuspid valves do not close sufficiently to prevent the backflow of blood into the atria during ventricular contraction as seen in mitral and tricuspid insufficiency or mitral valve prolapse. These murmurs are holosystolic and heard over their respective valvular areas. They are both high-pitched and blowing, with the intensity remaining relatively the same. Mitral and tricuspid regurgitant murmurs differ characteristically in the effect of respiration and manner of radiation. The intensity of the murmur of tricuspid regurgitation increases with inspiration and may radiate only to the left midclavicular line. The murmur of mitral regurgitation does not change with inspiration and radiates into the left axilla. They are best heard with the diaphragm chestpiece.

Diastolic Murmurs

Diastolic murmurs occur after S_2 and before S_1 and are also further classified as early, mid-, late, or holosystolic. Diastolic murmurs are usually pathologic and may be *ejection, filling,* or *regurgitant* in nature.

The ejection or filling murmur of mitral stenosis may range from a very faint to a loud rumble with a crescendo or descrescendo pattern. It is low-pitched, heard best with the bell chestpiece, and usually localized at the apex in a very small area.

Regurgitant murmurs as in aortic insufficiency occur when blood flows back into the ventricle at the beginning of diastole, continuing throughout the diastolic phase in a decrescendo pattern. The intensity varies from very faint to loud, depending on the degree of valvular insufficiency. It is a very

high-pitched, blowing murmur which is heard best with the diaphragm chestpiece at the aortic area. (See Chap. 24 for further discussion of valvular murmurs.)

Continuous murmurs are less common and represent the presence of both systolic and diastolic murmurs. These are evident in conditions in which arteriovenous communication exists, such as patent ductus arteriosus.

Data from Diagnostic Procedures

The third and final component in the clinical evaluation of a patient involves the interpretation of data obtained from diagnostic procedures. This section will focus on those procedures which enable the critical-care team to assess a cardiovascular patient.

Atrial Electrograms

The recording of atrial electrograms (AEGs) can significantly facilitate the bedside diagnosis of complex rhythm and conduction disturbances. The surface ECG will generally permit an accurate identification of the QRS complexes and an assessment of the ventricular activation sequence. The recognition of the low-amplitude P wave, however, can be unreliable, especially in patients with ECG baseline artifacts, tachyarrhythmias, and conduction disturbances. The atrial electrogram overcomes this problem by recording the atrial activity as a large amplitude A wave that can be readily identified. Atrial electrograms can be recorded as either unipolar or bipolar signals (Fig. 20-4). The unipolar atrial electrogram is a recording of the electrical difference between the atrial electrode and the skin electrode and has the appearance of a conventional ECG with amplification of the P wave. A standard electrocardiographic amplifier can be used to record a unipolar atrial electrogram by connecting the left arm lead to an atrial electrode and the right arm lead to a skin electrode with the lead selector in the I position. Most electrocardiographic amplifiers also require an additional skin electrode as an indifferent reference lead (generally the right leg). Recording the atrial electrogram as a unipolar signal has the advantages of requiring only a single

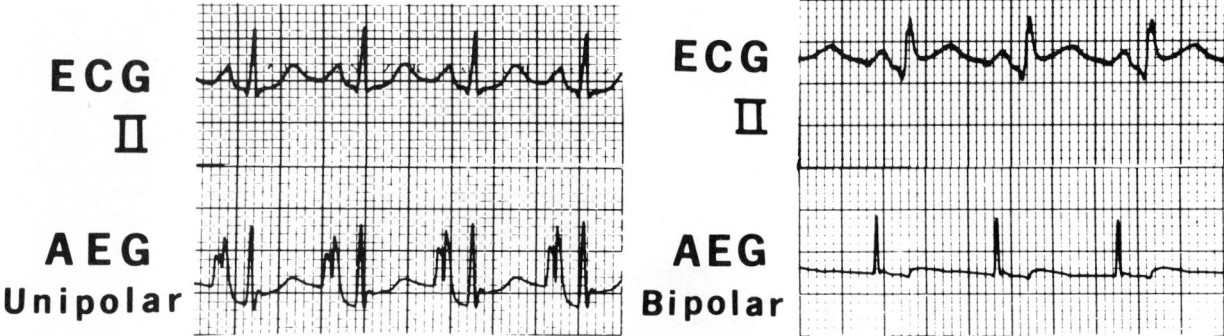

Figure 20-4   Simultaneous recording of lead II electrocardiogram and unipolar atrial electrogram (AEG) or bipolar atrial electrogram. See text for definition and recording techniques.

atrial electrode and of providing information about both the atrial and ventricular rhythm on a single data channel. The disadvantages include baseline noise introduced via the skin electrode and superimposition of the atrial and ventricular signals. The bipolar atrial electrogram is a recording of the atrial electric impulses recorded from two atrial electrodes and consists of isolated A waves.

A standard electrocardiographic amplifier can be used to record a bipolar electrogram by connecting one atrial electrode to each arm lead and recording with the lead selector in the I position. With computerized ECG machines, it is possible to obtain both a bipolar and unipolar tracing by attaching with alligator clamps both arm leads to two atrial wires and attaching the conventional limb leads to each leg. By changing the format and using the manual mode, one can obtain a simultaneous lead I, II, and III. Lead I is the bipolar lead and leads II and III are the unipolar leads. Since the bipolar atrial electrogram records only information about the atrial rhythm, a simultaneous ECG is required to evaluate the relationship between the atrial and ventricular rhythms. The advantages of recording the atrial electrogram as a bipolar signal include a high signal/noise ratio and isolated atrial signal without interference from ventricular activity. The disadvantages are the requirement for two atrial electrodes and the need for a second data channel to display the simultaneous ECG. The polarity of the atrial electrogram can be reversed by interchanging the lead connections.

Atrial electrograms can be recorded from epicardial electrode wires, electrode catheters, per-

manent pacemakers, and esophageal electrodes. Patients undergoing cardiac surgery can have electrode wires sutured to the atrial epicardium and brought out through the chest wall for temporary postoperative atrial electrogram recording and pacing. The routine placement of two epicardial atrial wires and one ventricular wire has proved to be extremely valuable in the management of these patients. Prior to discharge, the wires are pulled free and removed.

Transvenous electrode catheters can be used to record atrial electrograms to pace the atrium in patients who do not have indwelling epicardial wires. By having a pair of electrodes on the shaft of a specially designed pulmonary arterial catheter, atrial electrogram recording and atrial pacing can be combined with hemodynamic monitoring via a single right heart catheter (Fig. 20-5). With the electrodes positioned high in the right atrium near the junction with the superior vena cava, stable high-quality atrial electrograms can be recorded and the atrium can be paced for several days as indicated. In addition to direct fluoroscopic visualization, the electrode position can be determined by monitoring the appearance of the bipolar atrial electrogram (Fig. 20-6). At the tricuspid valve, the electrogram consists of an A wave corresponding to the P wave on the ECG and a V wave corresponding to the QRS complex on the ECG. When the electrode pair is withdrawn into the lower right atrium, the electrogram changes to a predominant large negative A wave and a very low amplitude V wave, whereas in the high right atrium the atrial electrogram changes to a biphasic and then to a

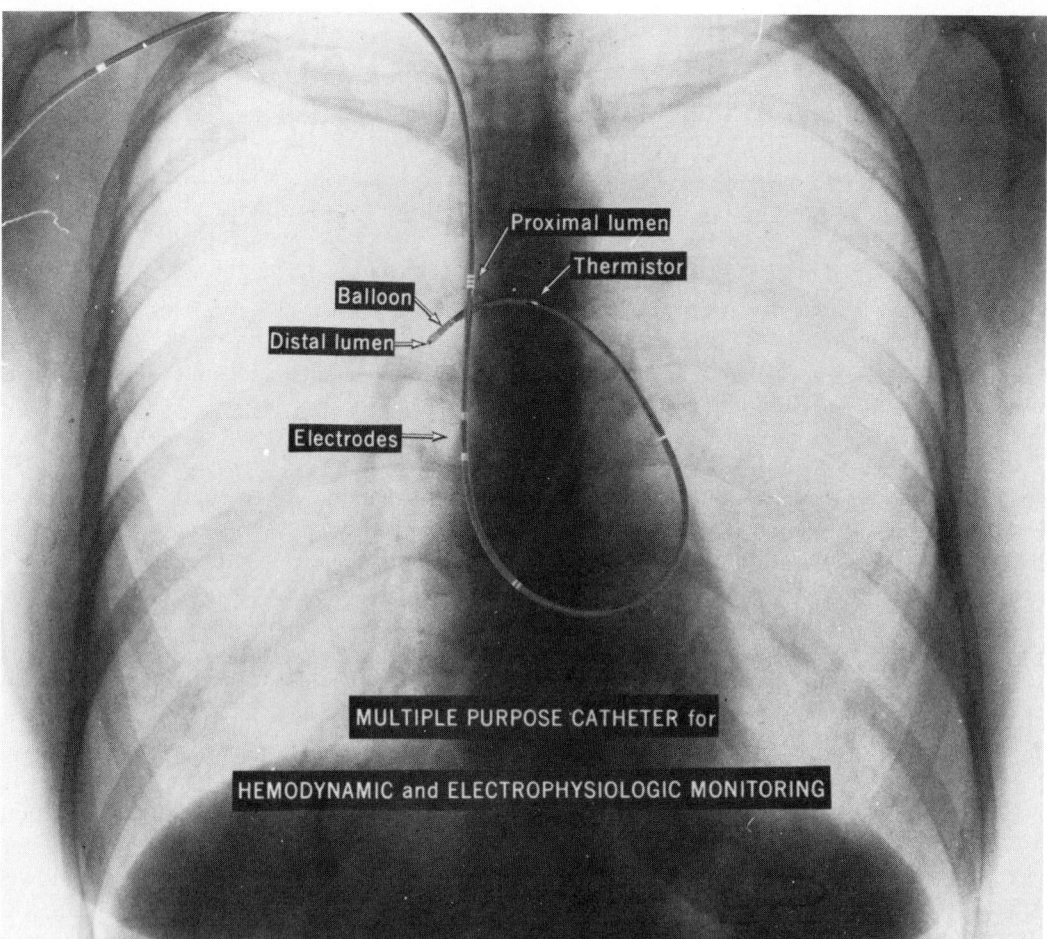

Figure 20-5   The multiple-purpose pulmonary triple lumen catheter with atrial electrodes is shown superimposed on a chest x-ray. (*From J. A. Mantle et al.: A multipurpose catheter for electrophysiologic and hemodynamic monitoring plus atrial pacing, Chest 72:285–290, 1977. Reproduced by permission.*)

positive A wave. When the electrode pair is withdrawn completely from the right atrium into the superior vena cava, an atrial electrogram can no longer be recorded.

Atrial electrograms can also be recorded by passing an electrode catheter down the esophagus and positioning the electrodes at the level of the atrium. This approach has the advantage of being noninvasive but cannot be used for atrial pacing. An esophageal "pill electrode" with fine connecting wires can be more easily swallowed and left comfortably indwelling for many hours for electrogram monitoring even while eating. Since the pill electrode is well tolerated by patients and can provide

a high-quality atrial electrogram, this noninvasive technique makes the use of atrial electrograms practical for a much larger patient population with complex arrhythmias.

Independent of the technique used for recording the atrial electrogram, great care must be exercised to protect the patient from microshock. All recording equipment must be electrically isolated from current leakage of less than 10 μA. Precautions must be used to avoid additional sources of current leakage from electric beds, televisions, radios, razors, or hair dryers. To prevent accidental contact with potential sources of current, the electrode terminal connectors should never be left uncovered. Frequent periodic checks of the recording equipment for ground faults and current leakage are mandatory.

Atrial electrograms are useful in the evaluation of patients with tachyarrhythmias, atrioventricular dissociation, heart block, and premature beats. Specific examples in which an atrial electrogram may be necessary to establish correct diagnoses include the differentiation of ventricular tachycardia versus supraventricular tachycardia with bundle branch block, atrial tachycardia (or flutter) with 2 to 1 conduction versus sinus tachycardia, and premature ventricular contractions (PVCs) versus aberrantly conducted premature atrial contractions (PACs). The ability to accurately identify both the atrial and ventricular complexes simplifies these electrocardiographic dilemmas into a straightforward rhythm analysis and diagnosis.

Blood Tests

To determine whether a patient has sustained a myocardial infarction (MI), a clinician evaluates the patient's pain history, associated electrocardiographic changes, and elevations of serum enzyme levels. The enzymes frequently assessed are creatine phosphokinase (CK) and lactate dehydrogenase (LDH). Previously a third enzyme, serum glutamic oxaloacetic transaminase (SGOT), was also assessed when making this diagnosis. However, due to its lack of specificity, clinicians today primarily utilize the CK and LDH total enzymes and isoenzymes when diagnosing an MI. These enzymes are released from myocardial cells that have undergone necrosis. Roberts[8] estimates that 30 to 60 min of prolonged ischemia can result in cellular membrane damage and resultant enzyme leak.

LDH can be isolated in serum within 8 to 12 h after infarction, peaks in 3 days, and returns to baseline within 10 to 14 days. An elevated LDH value is not specific for myocardial infarction because this enzyme is also found in liver, kidney, and red blood cells. Therefore, an elevation of LDH may be recorded in liver and kidney abnormalities as well as in hemolyzed blood samples.

In order to increase the specificity of utilizing LDH to confirm the diagnosis of MI, one needs to examine the five isoenzymes of LDH, which are LDH_1, LDH_2, LDH_3, LDH_4, and LDH_5. Cardiac muscle contains a predominance of the LDH_1 isoenzyme.

Under normal circumstances, the serum level of LDH_1 is less than LDH_2. After infarction, the heart

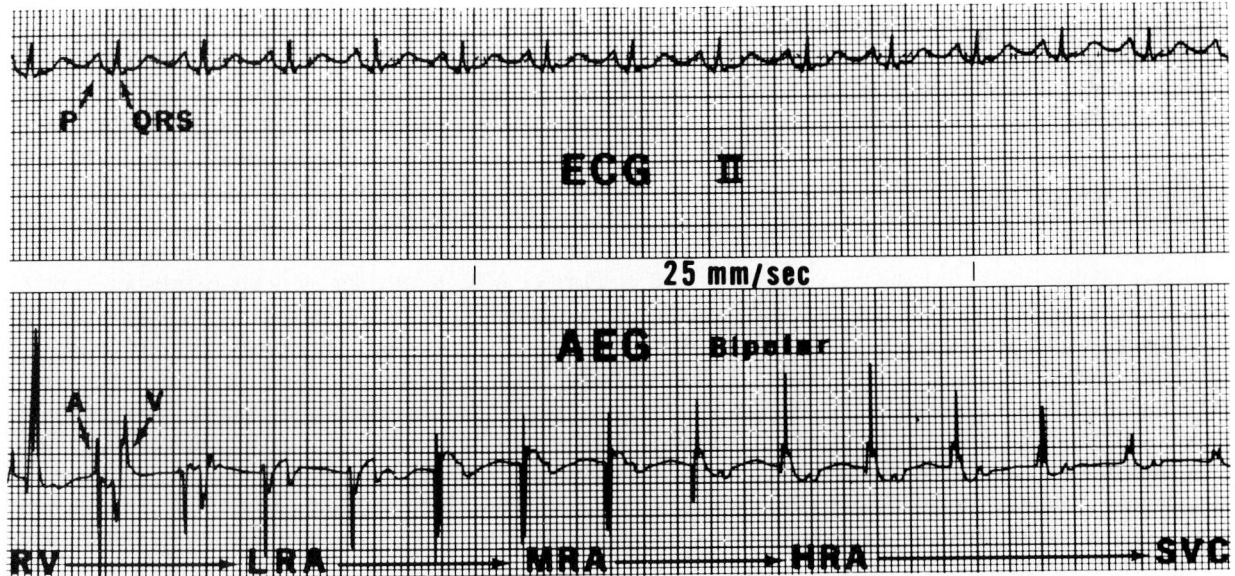

Figure 20-6   Simultaneous recording of a lead II electrocardiogram and an atrial electrocardiogram. (*From ACCN's Clinical Reference, 1st edition.*)

releases LDH which includes LDH_1. This results in an elevated total LDH level as well as a level of LDH_1 greater than LDH_2. Galen[9] reports that this "flipped" pattern in LDH isoenzymes is present within 48 h in 80 percent of acute infarctions.

The cardiac enzyme creatine phosphokinase (CK) is more sensitive in diagnosing MI than LDH or SGOT. CK is mainly contained in heart and skeletal tissue and to a lesser extent in the gastrointestinal tract and brain. CK can be detected in the serum approximately 4 h after an MI, peaks in 12 to 24 h, and returns to baseline in 72 to 96 h.

Although the most sensitive of the three enzymes, total CK may be elevated in conditions other than MI. Elevated CK levels are seen with repeated intramuscular injections or postoperatively. Evaluation of the isoenzymes of CK, especially the MB isoenzyme, is necessary to increase the specificity of the test.

The CK-MB isoenzyme is found predominantly in cardiac muscle tissue. It is released into the serum after infarction and necrosis of cardiac tissue occurs. At present, it is the most specific laboratory enzymatic test indicative of an MI.

Serial samples of cardiac enzymes are required after a suspected MI in order to monitor their pattern of release, indirectly quantify the extent of the infarction, and document stabilization of the myocardium. The literature cites many sampling intervals ranging from 4- to 6-h intervals to 12-h intervals.[9-12] Trends in enzyme release should be closely monitored regardless of the sampling interval employed.

Cardiac Catheterization

From an historical perspective, cardiac catheterization has evolved over the last 55 years since the first attempt by Werner Forssman in 1929 to pass a catheter into his own right heart. The 1930s saw the perfection of right heart catheterization by such investigators as Klein, Padillo, Cournand, and Richards.[13] The technique of left heart catheterization was first introduced by Zimmerman and Lason in the 1950s. Seldinger created the percutaneous technique, which is the currently accepted procedure for both left and right heart catheterization, in 1953. In 1959, Sones developed selective coronary arteriography, which has become the "gold standard"

in the cadre of diagnostic procedures for coronary artery disease.

Cardiac catheterization is defined by Grossman[13] as an invasive hemodynamic and angiographic procedure performed for various diagnostic purposes. As a hemodynamic procedure, the data which can be obtained include chamber and vessel pressures, volumes, waveforms, and calculations of cardiac outputs.

Angiography, which is the injection of contrast material into the ventricle (ventriculography) or coronary artery (arteriography) is employed when visualization of the chamber or artery is necessary. Filming methods such as cineangiography or angiocardiography provide visualization of ventricular motion. This is especially helpful in looking for wall motion abnormalities, ventricular function, valvular defects, septal defects, and aneurysms.

Right Heart Catheterization

With right heart catheterization, a catheter is inserted through either the basilic vein or femoral vein. It is sequentially introduced through the right heart chambers into the pulmonary artery. Through this catheter, pressures, volumes, and tracings of the right atrium, right ventricle, pulmonary artery, and pulmonary artery wedge position may be obtained for evaluation.

Right-Sided Valvular Function   Tricuspid and pulmonic valvular function can be assessed for the purpose of determining the presence and/or severity of stenosis or regurgitation. In evaluating stenosis, for example, the physician can determine the presence of a pressure gradient (normally, there should be none) and calculation of the valve orifice size. If valvular stenosis is present, ventriculography can be employed to indicate mobility and calcification of the valve leaflets. Tricuspid regurgitation is evaluated on the basis of waveform tracings and the degree of regurgitation seen angiographically. The grading of regurgitation ranges from 1+ to 4+, whereby 4+ is the most severe gradation. The evaluation of pulmonic regurgitation is accomplished by looking for a widened pulmonary arterial pressure, an increase in right ventricular end-diastolic pressure, and demonstration of regurgitation via ventriculography.[13]

Shunts In addition to valvular assessment, left-to-right shunts can be detected during the angiography procedure. This is accomplished by drawing blood samples sequentially from the pulmonary artery, right ventricle, right atrium, superior vena cava (SVC), and inferior vena cava (IVC). A significant finding for the presence of a shunt is a "step up" in blood oxygen saturation found during this retrograde sampling. The visualization and localization of a shunt are further elucidated via angiography.

Cardiac Outputs Cardiac outputs (CO) can be obtained in the catheterization laboratory via four different methods: quantitative angiography, the Fick method, the indicator dilution method, and the thermodilution method. The latter method, thermodilution technique, will be discussed in the section, "Hemodynamic Monitoring."

Quantitative angiography involves obtaining ventricular end-systolic (ESV) and end-diastolic volumes (EDV) from the ventriculogram. Once these volumes have been obtained, stroke volume (SV) can be determined by subtracting the end-systolic volume from the end-diastolic volume (SV = ESV − EDV). Total CO is then calculated. It should be noted that this cardiac output differs from that obtained by the Fick method. The Fick cardiac output is the forward cardiac output. From a clinical standpoint, this would have significance in valvular regurgitation in which some of the total cardiac output flows in a retrograde pattern. Thus, the regurgitant volume could be easily obtained by simply subtracting the forward CO from the total CO (regurgitant volume = total CO − forward CO).

The Fick method is based on the principle proposed by Fick in 1870. This principle states "that in a steady state, the flow of blood through an organ (such as the lungs) is equal to the amount of a substance (oxygen) absorbed by the blood flowing through the organ (consumption), divided by the difference in oxygen concentration between the blood entering and leaving the organ (arteriovenous O_2 difference)."[16] This formula can then be computed as follows:

Cardiac output

$$= \frac{\text{Oxygen consumption (mL/min)}}{\text{Arteriovenous } O_2 \text{ difference (mL/100 mL blood)}}$$

Normal oxygen consumption is approximately 250 mL/min. The arteriovenous O_2 difference is about 50 mL. Thus, the cardiac output is normally about 5 L/min. If this cardiac output is adjusted to the body surface area, the value is referred to as the cardiac index.

The indicator-dilution method for determining CO involves the injection of green dye (indocyanine green) into the right atrium; the concentration of the indicator is sampled at a peripheral site downstream, after the indicator has adequately mixed with the blood. A blood sample is continually withdrawn through a photoelectric instrument called a *densitometer*. A curve is recorded from the densitometer whereby the CO is calculated through computers from the known amount of the indicator that was injected and the area of the time concentration curve.

Left Heart Catheterization

Left heart catheterization is performed either through a retrograde approach from the femoral artery to the aorta and then through the aortic valve, or through a transseptal approach across the right atrium through the foramen ovale into the left atrium. Hemodynamically, left-sided pressures and volumes are assessed. Elevations of left-sided pressure can result from such CV disorders as myocardial infarction, cardiomyopathy, hypertension, cardiogenic shock, and valvular disease.

Left-Sided Valvular Function Pressure gradients across the valve orifice are determined in order to assess for either mitral or aortic stenosis. The valve orifice is visualized during angiography for mobility and calcification. The aortic valve is evaluated at this time for the presence of bicuspid or unicuspid defects.

Heightened v waves on the left atrial tracing are diagnostic of mitral regurgitation. Severe regurgitation is determined when the v waves are greater than twice the mean left atrial pressure.[13] In advanced mitral regurgitation, it is also common for the patient to have a reduced cardiac output. During the catheterization procedure, the regurgitant fraction will also be calculated. The formula is as follows:

Regurgitant stroke volume = total left ventricular stroke volume − forward stroke volume

Elevated *a* waves and a significant systolic pressure difference between the LV and aorta are the findings on catheterization which indicate aortic stenosis. Angiographically, the stenotic orifice can be visualized during systole along with the mobility of the cusps. Aortic regurgitation is determined by a widened aortic pulse pressure and elevated end-systolic volume. The amount of blood regurgitated can be as great as 60 percent or more of the forward stroke volume and occurs mainly in early diastole.

Left Ventriculography   Left ventriculography is also useful in providing the following information: (1) anatomy and function of the ventricle, (2) presence and location of ventricular aneurysms, (3) abnormalities in wall motion, (4) presence of ventricular septal defects, (5) calculation of LV wall thickness and mass, and (6) LV ejection fraction.

Abnormalities of wall motion are commonly seen in patients with prior myocardial infarcts. It has been suggested that 65 percent of patients referred for coronary artery disease workup demonstrate abnormal ventricular contraction patterns at rest. The critical-care nurse should become familiar with such abnormalities. These abnormalities will be further discussed in Chap. 21 regarding myocardial infarction.

Coronary Arteriography

Coronary arteriography, developed by Sones in 1959, is usually performed to assess the coronary arterial circulation. This procedure defines the presence and extent of coronary arterial lesions. It also assists physicians to quantify the degree of stenosis as well as to assess collateral circulation. These findings are then used to determine the feasibility of performing percutaneous transluminal coronary angioplasty (PTCA) or coronary artery bypass surgery (CABG). In addition, the presence of vasospasm can be determined by coronary arteriography. Another recent application of this procedure is to facilitate use of thrombolytic agents such as streptokinase during the evolution of an MI.

Conclusion

The mortality associated with cardiac catheterization is relatively low. Morbidity noted with left heart catheterization is significantly greater than that noted with a right-sided procedure. One of the more serious complications associated with left heart catheterization via the femoral approach is the formation of a thrombus which can occlude the femoral artery. Careful vascular checks need to be performed. Dissection of a coronary artery also may occur with arteriography. Hemorrhage at the insertion site is another complication that necessitates applied pressure at the site of insertion upon withdrawal of the catheter.

Chest X-Ray

The chest x-ray is a convenient, noninvasive method for assessing the cardiac silhouette, its chambers and great vessels, and the pulmonary system. Cardiac enlargement, valvular calcification, aortic dilatation, thoracic tumors, pulmonary infiltrate, pleural effusion, hemothorax, and pneumothorax are all the common abnormalities recognized with the standard posterior-anterior and lateral views. The radiographic findings of pulmonary edema, pulmonary hypertension, left-to-right cardiac shunts, and various types of congenital heart disease are also reasonably specific.

Portable chest films taken in the anterior-posterior (AP) view in the critical-care setting are different from those posteroanterior (PA) films taken in the x-ray department. These AP films are taken in such a way that the x-ray beam passes from front to back instead of posteriorly to anteriorly, which places the heart farther from the x-ray film than in the PA projection and thus casts a larger shadow on the x-ray film. The result is that the AP film provides poor visualization of the cardiac silhouette, which limits its diagnostic value. Moreover, heart size cannot be compared accurately between AP and PA projections but can be compared with similar sequential AP or PA projections.[14]

The assessment of left ventricular function and pulmonary venous pressures from a chest x-ray lacks both sensitivity and specificity. A cardiothoracic ratio of greater than 1:2 is a late sign of left ventricular failure and may also occur from right ventricular dilatation and pericardial effusions. The estimation of pulmonary vein engorgement is subjective in light of the fact that an x-ray pattern of pulmonary edema may be present when the pulmonary venous pressure is normal. Fluid that leaks into the alveolar space may be noted on x-ray for up to 24 h after pulmonary venous hypertension has been reversed, and noncardiac causes of pulmonary edema produce an x-ray picture of pulmonary edema with normal pulmonary venous pressure.[14]

Other extraneous findings which may be noted on chest x-ray include valvular prostheses, epicardial pacing wires, sternal closure wires after cardiac surgery, mediastinal or pleural chest tubes, endotracheal tubes, electrocardiogram leads, and pacemakers.

In the critical-care setting, the patient should be positioned in an erect position if possible. The portable chest x-ray should be taken during deep inspiration because this is a factor which affects the size and contour of the heart.

Echocardiography

Echocardiography is a noninvasive technique which utilizes high-frequency ultrasonic waves to yield information about cardiac structures and function. This technique employs a transducer capable of both sending and receiving sound waves. This transducer contains a piezoelectric substance which, when stimulated by an electric current, expands and contracts to produce mechanical energy which produces waves that are sent outward. Conversely, when a sound wave is reflected back toward the transducer, it converts this mechanical energy back into electric energy which can be recorded.

Feigenbaum[16] cites the advantages of utilizing ultrasonic waves as being that (1) they are reflected by very small objects, (2) they can be directed, and (3) they obey the laws of reflection and refraction. The disadvantages are that they are poorly transmitted in a gaseous medium; therefore, good transducer-to-skin contact is imperative.

During an echocardiogram, the patient is placed in a supine position and the transducer is placed on the chest wall. An ultrasonic coupling gel is used to facilitate sound wave transmission. The technician directs ultrasonic sound waves toward the heart and records the echos of these waves as they reflect back from various cardiac structures. This procedure is usually quick and painless for the patient.

Types of Echocardiograms

Currently, there are three types or modes of echocardiograms: *unidimensional, two-dimensional,* and *Doppler.*

Unidimensional Echocardiograms   There are three modes of unidimensional echocardiograms available: A mode, B mode, and M mode. The A mode monitors the amplitude of returning signals or sound waves and converts them to spikes which can be visualized and recorded on an oscilloscope. The stronger the wave the taller the height of the spike. The B mode transforms the returning sound waves to dots which are displayed on the oscilloscope, in which the stronger waves evidence brighter dots. Lastly, the M mode, which is the most common, records both amplitude and motion. The M-mode echocardiogram has the advantage of enabling the physician to study cardiac structures in motion as they function at various points in the cardiac cycle.

The M-mode echocardiogram utilizes a single beam of ultrasonic waves and measures the distance of structures from the transducer in a vertical axis with time on a horizontal axis. Therefore, although called unidimensional, M-mode echocardiography actually is comprised of two dimensions, distance and time. The major disadvantage of this type of echocardiography is that it lacks spatial orientation. Figures 20-7 and 20-8 are examples of M-mode echocardiograms.

Two-Dimensional Echocardiograms (2-D)   The two-dimensional or 2-D echocardiogram records returning sound waves on a planar image, thus allowing a spatial orientation for viewing cardiac structures. This is accomplished with a more advanced transducer that emits a planar beam of sound waves, not a single beam. The disadvantage of a 2-D echocardiogram is that it cannot record a complete heart chamber or valve as a whole. Composite views must be examined in order to avoid missing important data.[9] An example of this type of echocardiogram is found in Fig. 20-9.

Doppler Echocardiograms   Unlike unidimensional and two-dimensional echocardiograms which record returning sound waves, Doppler echocardiograms record the velocity of moving objects by

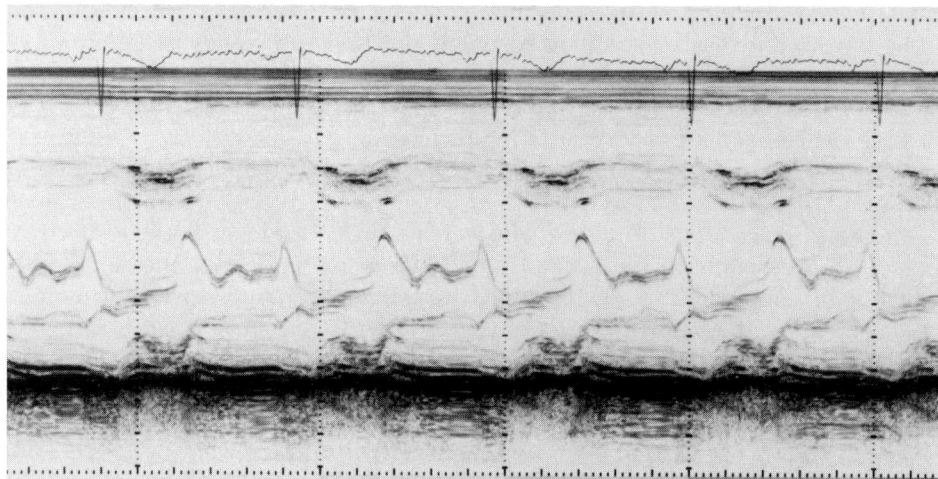

Figure 20-7 Normal mitral valve (M-mode echocardiogram).

measuring the frequency of change of emitted and reflected ultrasonic waves. The clinical applicability of this technique is in assessing the circulation in peripheral arteries and veins, examining blood flow in the heart and great vessels, and in assessing regurgitant valvular disorders. The disadvantages of this technique are the following: (1) it cannot record a high velocity, (2) it cannot record velocities that lie within structures greater than 13 cm from the transducer, (3) it cannot be recorded on a graphic display, and (4) much variability exists with the different angles at which the transducer is held.

A new development in this field has been the introduction of pulsed Doppler echocardiography.

When combined with the previously described continuous Doppler technique, pulsed Doppler echocardiography has the advantage of recording views of the heart while also examining Doppler signals. Since many of the disadvantages previously cited for continuous Doppler echocardiography remain with the pulsed technique, more research is needed to further refine this mode of echocardiography.

Clinical Applications

Echocardiography can be utilized to noninvasively study cardiac function, valvular disorders, complications resulting from a myocardial infarction, the

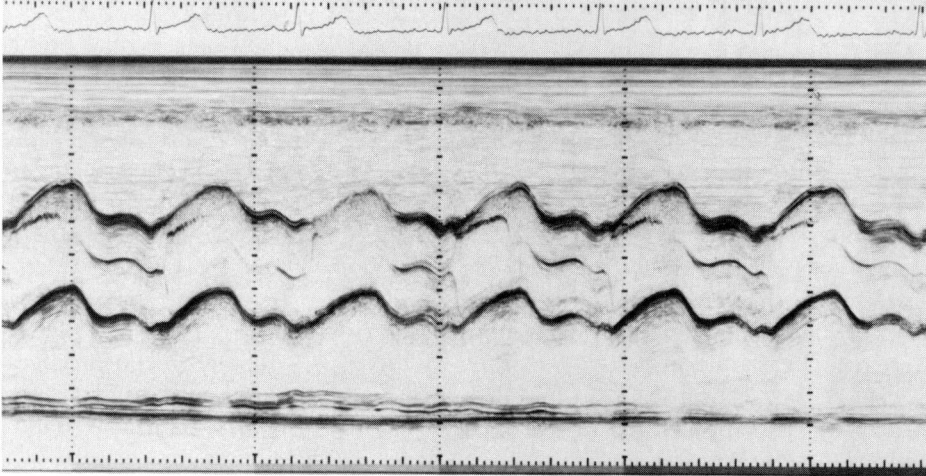

Figure 20-8 Normal aorta/aortic valve/left atrium (M-mode echo).

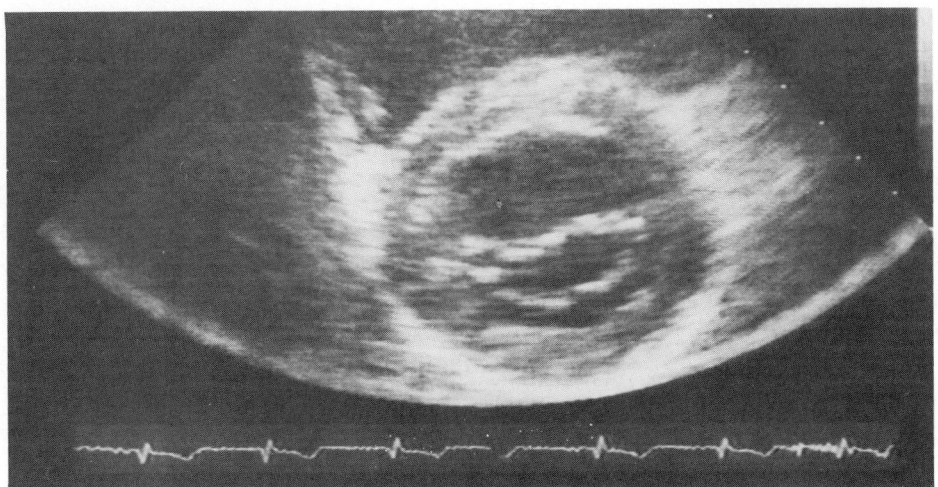

Figure 20-9A   Normal mitral valve parasternal short axis. (2-D echocardiogram).

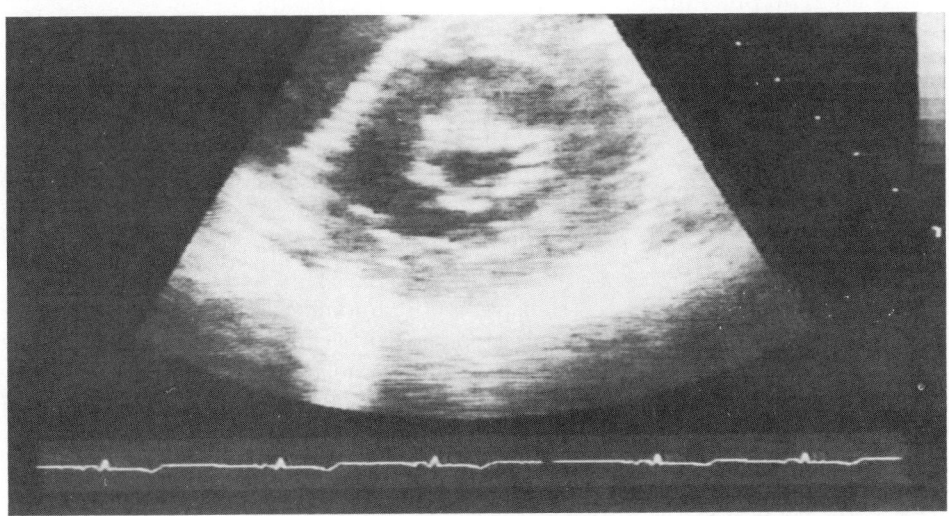

Figure 20-9B   Mitral stenosis. (2-D echocardiogram).

functional effects of ischemia, cardiomyopathy, pericardial effusions, endocarditis, and congenital heart defects.

Assessment of Cardiac Function   Information regarding left ventricular performance can be calculated with the aid of echocardiography. A shortening fraction which reflects performance, similar to an ejection fraction, can be estimated from measurements of the left ventricular end-systolic (DES) and end-diastolic dimensions (DED) gained from an echocardiogram.

Mitral Stenosis   Both the M-mode and 2-D echo are useful in evaluating mitral stenosis (MS). Evidence of fibrosis or calcification of the valve leaflets which commonly is found in MS exists when there is an increased number of reflected echos. Thickening of the leaflets, minimal leaflet separation during diastole, and abnormal valve motions are other M-mode findings of MS. Two-D echocardiography can also quantify the size of the valve orifice.

Other echocardiographic data to support the existence of MS are the effect of MS on other cardiac structures. Left atrial dilatation and occasional pulmonary hypertension as a result of the outflow obstruction caused by MS may be documented. Figure 20-9A and B illustrate normal and stenotic mitral valves.

Lastly, Feigenbaum[17] cites that the echocardiogram is useful to evaluate whether a mitral valve replacement (MVR) or a commissurotomy is required for MS. This is an important decision because the implications of an MVR are more serious than those of a commissurotomy. An in-depth discussion regarding this valvular defect is found in Chap. 24.

Mitral Regurgitation   Regurgitant lesions are better evaluated by Doppler echocardiography than by other modes of echocardiography because this method detects turbulent blood flow indicative of regurgitant lesions. Two-dimensional and unidimensional echocardiography is useful in providing data to support the diagnosis of mitral regurgitation (MR) by assessing left atrial dilatation. This occurs as the left atrium expands to compensate for the regurgitant volume. An increased left ventricular stroke volume is recorded as blood exits the left ventricle through two outflow tracts, normally via the aortic valve and abnormally through the incompetent mitral valve. Lastly, an increased left ventricular end-diastolic dimension is noted due to the increased volume in the left ventricle. The reader is referred to Chap. 24 for more information regarding MR.

Mitral Valve Prolapse   Due to changes in the mitral valve structure, the mitral valve balloons or protrudes backward into the left atrium during ventricular systole in mitral valve prolapse (MVP). Both 2-D and M-mode echocardiograms are helpful in documenting the abnormal backward motion of the mitral valve in MVP. More information on MVP is located in Chap. 24.

Aortic Stenosis   The diagnosis of aortic stenosis (AS) via echographic data is supported by the findings of thickened and/or calcified leaflets, decreased separation of the leaflets during systole, and doming of the valve on the 2-D echocardiogram. Absence of these characteristics does not completely exclude the diagnosis, however. Figure 20-10A and 20-10B contrast a normal and stenotic aortic valve.

The use of pulsed Doppler echocardiography may be helpful in the diagnosis of AS by documenting turbulent blood flow in the aorta. Lastly, the presence of left ventricular hypertrophy, secondary to this outflow tract obstruction, can often be calculated with echocardiography. More information on AS may be found in Chap. 24.

Aortic Insufficiency   As in mitral regurgitation, Doppler echocardiography is useful in assessing the turbulent blood flow that results in the regurgitant lesion of aortic insufficiency (AI). Direct evaluation of AI by echocardiography is not a useful technique; therefore, indirect assessments of the secondary effects of AI on the left ventricle and mitral valve serve as supportive data for this disorder. Dilatation of the left ventricle due to volume overload as well as heightened septal motion reflect AI. Lastly, fluttering of the mitral valve from the regurgitant diastolic flow through an incompetent aortic valve is diagnostic of AI.

There are data to support the usefulness of echocardiography in determining the optimum time for an aortic valve replacement, as documented by Feigenbaum[17] and Fernandez.[19] Aortic insufficiency is further discussed in Chap. 24.

Tricuspid and Pulmonic Valvular Disorders   Tricuspid stenosis exhibits motion abnormality on an echocardiogram similar to that of mitral stenosis. Evidence of tricuspid regurgitation can be found by calculating the degree of secondary right ventricular dilatation from volume overload and the degree of turbulent regurgitant blood flow by Doppler echocardiography. The pulsed Doppler echocardiogram also aids in the diagnosis of pulmonic valvular regurgitation.

Septal Defects   Wenger and Hellerstein[18] report that ventricular septal defects occur in about 1 percent of patients who sustain an acute transmural MI. Echocardiography is very useful in isolating the defect, estimating its severity as a result of secondary hemodynamic changes, and documenting the amount of shunted blood. Two-D echocardiography is useful in identifying both ventricular and atrial septal defects by direct visualization. The M-mode echocardiogram provides data to support this diagnosis by evaluating the hemodynamic consequences of

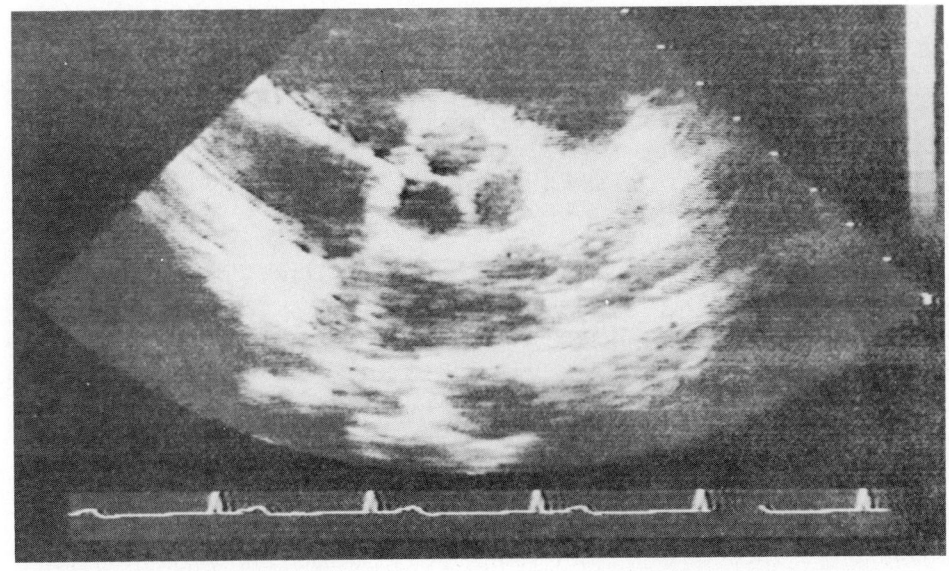

A

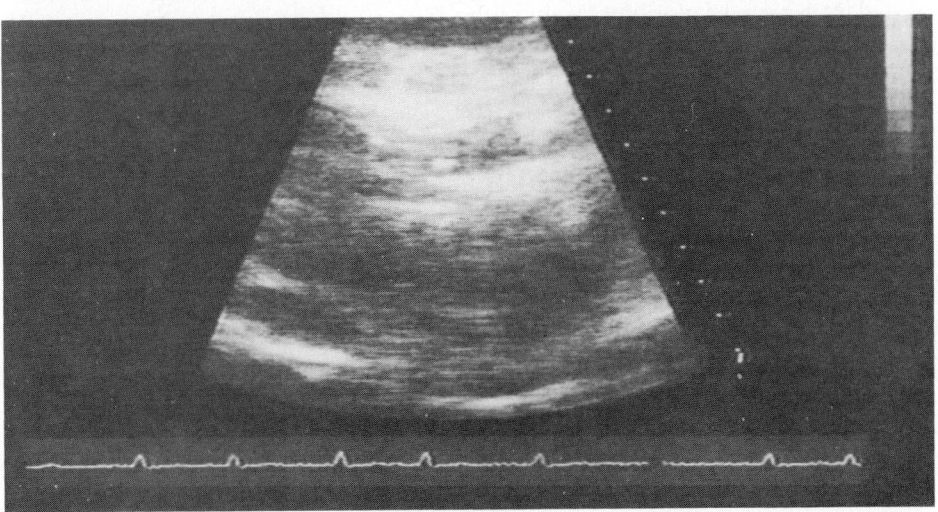

B

Figure 20-10A & B *A.* Normal aortic valve (2-D echo) contrasted with (Fig. 20-10*B*) aortic stenosis.

enlargement in chambers affected by the shunt. Doppler echocardiography is also useful in evaluating turbulent bloodflow which results from blood shunted through a septal defect.

Lastly, a technique called *contrast echocardiography* is helpful in evaluating shunts. In this technique, agitated normal saline solution is injected via a brachial vein. The path of the bubbled normal saline solution is followed on an echocar-

diogram. Shunts are detected if bubbles traverse the septum and do not follow the normal pathway.

Papillary Muscle Rupture Necrosis of the left ventricular papillary muscles is common with an acute MI and exceeds a 50 percent incidence in patients with a fatal MI, but papillary muscle rupture occurs in less than 1 percent of patients who sustain a fatal MI.[18] Echocardiographic evidence of papillary muscle rupture consists of prolapsing of a part of a mitral valve leaflet during systole.

Aneurysm   The incidence of a ventricular aneurysm secondary to a transmural MI is approximately 20 percent as supported by Wenger and Hellerstein.[18] Echocardiography is useful in estimating the size of an aneurysm as well as myocardial function. Feigenbaum[17] states that 2-D echocardiography is superior to M-mode echocardiography in detecting these abnormalities and in assessing residual ventricular function. An aneurysm is suspected if there is dilatation, thinning, and dyskinesis of a part of the ventricular wall. For more information regarding complications of an MI, refer to Chap. 21.

Evaluating Thrombi   Thrombi can be clearly visualized by use of echocardiography as their densities reflect echos. Because 15 to 20 percent of patients with an acute myocardial infarction develop thrombi,[19] the echocardiogram may be useful in documenting thrombi and thereby guide management.

Evaluating Ischemia   During systole, the left ventricular wall normally thickens. Ischemic tissue does not thicken during systole and can, therefore, be identified and quantified by echocardiography.

Cardiomyopathy   Two types of cardiomyopathies can be evaluated with the aid of echocardiography, *dilated* (congestive) and *hypertrophic*. In dilated cardiomyopathy, echocardiographic findings reveal a dilated and poorly functioning left ventricle with possible involvement of other cardiac chambers as well as the mitral valve. While 2-D and M-mode echocardiography evaluate chamber changes, pulsed Doppler echocardiography is useful in assessing coexisting mitral regurgitation.

Echocardiographic findings in patients with hypertrophic cardiomyopathy illustrate left ventricular hypertrophy. Unlike the findings noted in dilated cardiomyopathy, there is no cardiac enlargement, and there is a hypercontractile state.

The echocardiogram is the "gold standard" for diagnosing one form of hypertrophic cardiomyopathy, idiopathic hypertrophic subaortic stenosis (IHSS). Two classic features of IHSS are abnormal septal hypertrophy, causing an outflow obstruction of the left ventricle, and an abnormal systolic anterior motion (SAM) of the mitral valve secondary to this obstruction. Early midsystolic closure of the aortic valve may also be present secondary to the outflow obstruction. For additional information on cardiomyopathies, the reader is referred to Chap. 23.

Pericardial Effusions   Pericardial effusions can be visualized on both M-mode and 2-D echocardiograms. Two-D echocardiograms, however, allow for the most accurate quantification of pericardial effusions, especially if the fluid is loculated. Since fluid is less dense than tissue, a pericardial effusion appears on an echocardiogram as an echo-free space between the pericardium and the epicardium. Feigenbaum[17] states that the echo provides a sensitive indicator of cardiac tamponade from an effusion which is noted as compression of the right ventricle.

Endocarditis   Vegetations associated with valvular endocarditis can often be recorded by echocardiography. If present, the vegetations usually affect one valve leaflet to a greater degree than others and appear asymmetrical. When valvular function is impaired, secondary changes in cardiac chambers may be recorded on the echocardiogram. Absence of these findings, however, does not entirely rule out the possibility of endocarditis.

Electrocardiography

Electrocardiography depicts important information regarding the electrical forces produced by the heart during the cardiac cycle. The electrocardiogram (ECG) is a simple, noninvasive recording taken from the body surface in contrast to atrial electrograms or His bundle recordings, which are taken within the tissue. The reader is referred to Chap. 11 for a more in-depth discussion regarding electrocardiography.

The ECG is useful as a clinical tool in depicting abnormalities associated with certain cardiac pathology. For example, atrial enlargement and ventricular or biventricular hypertrophy can be detected on an ECG. These chamber enlargements may be related to a valvular defect, systemic or pulmonary hypertension, heart failure, or a cardiomyopathy. Specific ECG changes will be discussed in each chapter relating to coronary artery disease, valvular defects, hypertension, and cardiomyopathy.

In addition to being used as a diagnostic tool, the ECG is also affected by drugs and electrolytes. Drugs such as digoxin and quinidine alter the normal appearance of an ECG. Digoxin, for example, produces a scooping effect in the S-T segment and quinidine prolongs the QT interval. Electrolytes such as potassium and calcium also affect the ECG. Variations in potassium levels produce changes in the T wave morphology (hyperkalemia) or the appearance of U waves (hypokalemia). Calcium levels either shorten (hypercalcemia) or lengthen (hypocalcemia) the QT interval.

Caution needs to be exercised in relying on the ECG. Although the 12 leads provide 12 different views of the heart in assessing for abnormalities, the ECG alone should not be used solely to make a clinical diagnosis.

Electrophysiologic Studies

Cardiac electrophysiology is a new discipline in cardiology and cardiovascular nursing. Simply defined, it is "the direct study and manipulation of the electrical activity of the heart utilizing electrodes placed inside the cardiac chambers."[20] This technique provides information regarding sinus node function, atrioventricular conduction, and tachyarrhythmias. Cardiac electrophysiology guides medical therapy by yielding data regarding the effectiveness of various antiarrhythmic drugs on tachyarrhythmias and determines which type of pacemaker is most effective in terminating sustained tachyarrhythmias. Lastly, through the technique of cardiac mapping, cardiac electrophysiology assists in locating the origin of dangerous, repetitive arrhythmias and in directing surgical interventions.

A cardiac electrophysiologic study is performed in a controlled environment. It requires the use of catheters with multiple electrodes at their distal ends capable of stimulating the heart and of recording its response. Figure 20-11 illustrates common placement sites for these catheters. Although Michelson, Spielman, and Greenspan[21] point out that the catheter may be placed within the outflow tract of the right ventricle as well as the left ventricle, the more common sites are high

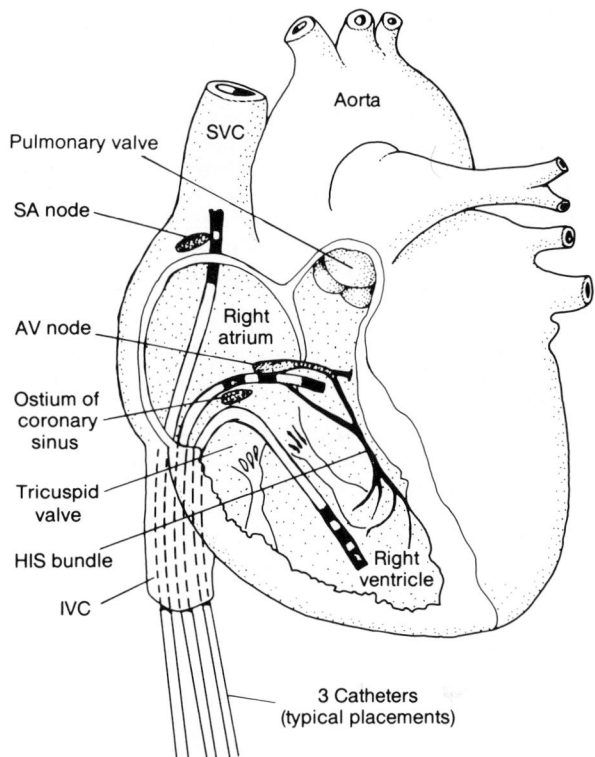

Figure 20-11 Common placement sites for catheters used in electrophysiologic studies. (*From J. Vacek, W. Smith, & J. Phillips, Cardiac Electrophysiology: An overview, Practical Cardiology, 10(13), 83–97, 1984.*)

in the right atrium, across the tricuspid valve, in the apex of the right ventricle, and in the coronary sinus.

The multiple catheter electrodes are then connected to a switchbox. The switchbox designates the electrode used for monitoring and stimulating. It is connected to a console that records and displays electrical activity on an oscilloscope.

Passive Applications of Cardiac Electrophysiology

Vacek, Smith, and Phillips[20] classified the uses of cardiac electrophysiology into three categories: *passive, active,* and *interventional* (refer to Table 20-3 for a complete list). The passive applications of cardiac electrophysiology are merely observational in nature. The catheter electrodes record the electrical activity in various cardiac structures. If an abnormal pathway exists such as in heart block or

Table 20-3 Assessment and Applications of Cardiac Electrophysiology

Passive

Intrinsic pacemaker site and activity
Sequence of atrial, conducting-system, and ventricular activation
Characteristics of AV node and His bundle
Observation of spontaneous phenomena
  Heart block
  Intraatrial or intraventricular conduction abnormalities
  Tachyarrhythmias
Overt bypass-tract presence and position

Active

SA-node function and conduction of impulses through peri-SA-node tissues (sinus-node recovery time, SA
  conduction time, response to carotid-sinus massage or drugs) (direct measurement of SA-node activity still
  experimental)
AV-node and His bundle properties in response to pacing or premature stimuli (or both) (internal changes
  and assessment of dual AV-node pathways)
Tachycardia initiation and termination
Concealed bypass-tract presence and position; response of both overt and concealed bypass tracts to pacing
  or premature stimuli (or both)
Mapping of endocardium for sites of tachycardia initiation and wavefront propagation characteristics

Interventional

Trials of the effects of drugs on induced tachyarrhythmias or on conduction properties of various portions of the
  cardiac electrical system
Consideration of efficacy and practicality of implantable pacemakers and defibrillators
Cold ablation (cryoablation) or electrical (direct-current shock) ablation of AV node or bypass tracts when part
  of a reentrant tachycardiac circuit is unresponsive to pharmacological manipulation

Reprinted with permission of J. Vacek, W. Smith, & J. Phillips, (1984). Cardiac electrophysiology: An overview. *Practical Cardiology,*
1984, *10*(13), 83–97.

conduction via an accessory pathway, it is recorded. Since such events may be transient, they often go undetected when only passive cardiac electrophysiology is utilized.

Active Applications of Cardiac Electrophysiology

During cardiac electrophysiologic testing, the heart can be stimulated and its response assessed, which is helpful in provoking transient arrhythmias. Sinus node disorders, atrioventricular conduction disturbances, supraventricular tachycardias (SVT), and ventricular tachycardias (VT) can be evaluated with this technique.

Ventricular Tachycardia   For patients with a history of malignant ventricular tachycardias, provoking the arrhythmia, studying its cause, and the location of origin yield valuable information to guide therapy. There are a number of protocols for programmed premature stimulation, all of which require a basic rhythm that is either sinus or paced. A ventricular or atrial premature beat is then stimulated to occur in late diastole. This beat is then programmed to occur earlier and closer to the T wave of the previous beat until the effective refractory beat is reached or the desired rhythm provoked. The effective refractory period is the longest distance between the patient's baseline rhythm and a programmed extra systole that does not produce a ventricular response. If one extra systole fails to produce a ventricular response, the procedure is repeated with a second or third programmed beat.

The desired end point when evaluating patients with a history of malignant ectopy is usually to elicit VT. Podrid and Lambert[22] cite that, if well tolerated, this rhythm can be terminated in 88 percent of patients with a programmed extra systole. To decrease the risk of provoking sustained VT, some authorities use nonsustained VT as an end point.

In addition to studying factors affecting VT, cardiac electrophysiology employs mapping to locate the origin of the VT reentrant arrhythmia. Two types of mapping techniques exist: *endocardial* and *epicardial*.

In endocardial mapping, multiple percutaneous electrodes are implanted on the heart, approximately 15 to 20 sites on the left ventricle, three on the right, and three sites over any aneurysm. Recordings are taken with the patient in sinus rhythm and again during VT. The location of the earliest activation time correlates to the location of the reentry circuit. During the mapping, which is a surgical procedure, the location is verified with a finger probe which measures the activation time in the endocardium

Epicardial mapping is also performed during surgery and involves applying electrodes directly to the epicardium. Again, the earliest activation time is sought. Since mapping is performed while the patient is on bypass, bypass time is lengthened. A prolonged bypass time exposes the patient to a number of potential complications. Podrid and Lambert[22] also report that in 10 to 15 percent of these patients, VT cannot be replicated; therefore, the origin cannot be identified.

Supraventricular Tachycardia   Cardiac electrophysiologic studies are utilized to define the mechanism of supraventricular tachycardia (SVT) and, therefore, are helpful in treating patients with symptomatic medical refractory SVT. AV nodal reentry (Chap. 11) is the most common cause of SVT as supported by Denes and Ezri,[23] and Kienzle, Doherty, Marcus, and Josephson.[24] This reentry circuit can be located in the AV node or accessory pathways between the atria and ventricles. These pathways are endowed with different properties of conduction. Once the mechanism responsible for the SVT is isolated, drug therapy aimed at the specific site of the problem can be instituted.

Drugs affecting the AV node are employed if the node is the site of reentry. Digoxin, verapamil, and beta-blocking medications prolong the conduction time and refractory period of the AV node and may be helpful. If the problem is the retrograde accessory pathways, drugs such as procainamide, quinidine, and disopramide, which alter the conduction properties of the retrograde pathway, may be used.[24]

Cardiac electrophysiologic studies are useful in guiding therapy in patients with a preexcitation syndrome. These patients experience arrhythmias secondary to accessory pathways. Ezri[25] states that the major benefit of studying this group of patients is to avoid using drugs that may exacerbate the arrhythmia.

Atrioventricular Conduction Disturbances   Cardiac electrophysiologic studies are useful to examine transient conduction disturbances, to locate the site of the disturbance, and to discern the need for permanent pacemaker implantation. This technique is helpful in evoking transient His-Purkinje disease for which a permanent pacemaker may be indicated. It is also useful in evaluating symptomatic patients with bifascular block to determine the need for permanent pacing. Lastly, this technique is beneficial in assessing asymptomatic patients with chronic heart block.

Sinus Node Disorders   The usefulness of cardiac electrophysiologic testing for sinus node dysfunction or sick sinus syndrome is controversial because this arrhythmia is often identified by less invasive techniques. Denes and Ezri[23] and Ezri[25] feel the decision regarding pacemaker use in these patients should be based on clinical symptomatology at the time of occurrence of bradyarrhythmias.

Cardiac electrophysiologic testing is useful in patients with undocumented cardiac syncope. It provides objective data regarding sinus node function.

Applications of Cardiac Electrophysiology

Assessing the Effectiveness of Antiarrhythmic Therapies   Cardiac electrophysiologic studies provide objective data regarding the effectiveness of various antiarrhythmic medications. Data from certain investigators have shown that antiarrhythmic therapy may potentiate arrhythmias.[26] Although work by Naccarelli et al.[27] alludes to the benefits of basing antiarrhythmic treatment on the data obtained from electrophysiologic study, the effectiveness of this approach remains controversial.[28]

Determining the Mode of Implantable Pacemakers/ Defibrillators   Pacemakers can terminate arrhythmias by a number of mechanisms: overdrive pacing, underdrive pacing, or direct countershock. Cardiac electrophysiologic testing helps determine which pacemaker mode is most effective in terminating a patient's arrhythmia, and thus guides therapy.

Cold or Electrical Ablation Electrophysiologic testing is used in extreme circumstances to isolate and destroy accessory pathways of the arrhythmogenic area by cryoablation or direct electric shock. Careful studies of the patient's coronary circulation need to be conducted prior to the procedure. This procedure is contraindicated if the area is located near a major artery due to the threat of a significant myocardial infarction.

Complications

At present, there is insufficient data regarding the risk of cardiac electrophysiologic testing. Kaufmann and Schwartz[29] report a 1 to 2 percent morbidity rate. Potential complications secondary to cardiac electrophysiologic testing are the following: excessive bleeding, hematoma formation at the catheter insertion site, catheter-induced vascular dissection, phlebitis, thrombophlebitis, pneumothorax, and pulmonary emboli. The risk of cardiac perforation and infection is small. The need for cardioversion from sustained VT or fibrillation is approximately 20 percent, as cited by Podrid and Lambert.[22]

Hemodynamic Monitoring

Invasive hemodynamic monitoring in the critical-care setting has become a safe, convenient bedside technique used to monitor pressures and waveforms in critically ill patients. Online continuous monitoring is invaluable when caring for the critically ill in whom hemodynamics may change rapidly. Through the use of various catheters, the critical-care team is provided with valuable information concerning pressures, waveforms, oxygen saturation, cardiac outputs, and venous or arterial blood gas parameters.

Therapy in the critically ill patient is often directed at maintaining an adequate cardiac output. Those variables which directly regulate cardiac output include preload, afterload, contractility, and heart rate (Chap. 19). Heart rate is controlled by both the parasympathetic and sympathetic nervous system. Changes in rate brought on by neural control will directly affect cardiac output by altering ventricular filling time. For example, in the setting of bradycardia (parasympathetic influence) the ventricular filling time is prolonged, while a tachycardia (sympathetic influence) reduces it. Alterations in ventricular filling time will in turn affect stroke volume and subsequently cardiac output. In the setting of diminished cardiac output, both direct and indirect, or derived, parameters are useful in assessing preload, afterload, and contractility which determine appropriate therapy.

Right ventricular preload is assessed in the critical-care setting using such parameters as central venous pressure (CVP) or right atrial pressure (RAP). Parameters used to assess left ventricular preload include pulmonary artery end-diastolic pressure (PAEDP), pulmonary artery wedge pressure (PAWP), and left atrial pressure (LAP). The parameters which are used to reflect right or left ventricular afterload, respectively, are pulmonary arterial pressure, pulmonary vascular resistance, aortic end-diastolic pressure, and systemic vascular resistance. Lastly, right and left ventricular stroke work indices are the derived parameters used to indirectly assess contractility in the critical-care setting.[30] Another derived parameter which can be obtained via hemodynamic monitoring is the rate-pressure product (RPP), which is used as an indirect determinant of myocardial O_2 consumption (Chap. 19).

Catheters

Arterial Line (A-Line) Catheter Use of an indwelling arterial catheter (A-line) is common in many critical-care units. These catheters permit constant monitoring of peripheral arterial pressures and frequent blood sampling. Indwelling arterial catheters can be placed in the radial, ulnar, brachial, femoral, or pedal artery, either percutaneously or via a surgical cutdown procedure. The radial artery is the site most frequently cannulated. Prior to radial insertion, assessment of circulation to the distal extremity should be performed via Allen's test.

In addition to these intraarterial catheters, the central aorta can be cannulated with an intraaortic balloon (IAB) catheter. This catheter has two lumens: one which transports gas to and from the balloon, and a second one which serves as a central aortic A-line.

The data which can be obtained from an A-line are systolic, diastolic, and mean pressures. These pressures will be discussed in more detail later in this section.

The most frequent complication of arterial line use results from accidental disconnection of the catheter from the transducer. This complication can be minimized if careful attention is paid to maintenance of intact connections. Other complications of A-line use are thrombus, local obstruction with resultant distal ischemia, embolization, and infection.

Right Atrial or Central Venous Pressure Catheters
Right atrial pressure (RAP) catheters or central venous pressure (CVP) catheters are used to measure the mean pressure of the right atrium. The RAP or CVP measurement is obtained by either a water manometer or a transducer. If a water manometer is used, the reading is recorded in cm H_2O. If, however, the transducer is employed, the reading will be recorded in mmHg. Due to the different molecular weights of substances (water or mercury) used to obtain the measurement, the readings are not interchangeable. Because mercury is 1.34 times heavier than water, conversion from a mercury reading to a water reading requires multiplying the pressure by 1.34.

Example: 7 mmHg $\times$ 1.34 = 9.38 cmH$_2$O

As with arterial catheters, RAP catheters can be inserted in a variety of sites. The subclavian vein is the optimum site for RAP catheter insertion, although cannulation of the internal jugular, cephalic, antecubital, basilic, saphenous, and femoral veins are alternatives. The approach taken can be either by percutaneous or surgical cutdown procedure. Once inserted, a confirmatory chest x-ray is required to verify the position of the catheter. Some complications associated with RAP catheter insertion and position include pneumothorax, hemothorax, pulmonary embolism, perforation of the right atrium or ventricle, air embolism, and cardiac tamponade.

Pulmonary Artery Catheter   A pulmonary artery (PA) catheter is a flow-directed, balloon-tipped catheter. This catheter measures the pressure in the right side of the heart and in the pulmonary vasculature. Newer generations of these catheters include (1) the thermodilution pulmonary arterial pacing catheter, which permits atrial, ventricular, or A-V sequential pacing; (2) a fiber-optic catheter which allows continuous monitoring of mixed venous oxygen saturation (SVO$_2$); and (3) a catheter with additional lumen ports for fluid resuscitation.

Prior to the insertion of any type of PA catheter, the patient must be assessed for underlying complete left bundle branch block (LBBB), because there is a small risk of developing a right bundle branch block (RBBB) during insertion, and complete heart block might result. Hurst[31] advocates the prophylactic insertion of a temporary pacemaker or a pacing thermodilution PA catheter in patients with a preexisting LBBB. A new alternative in patients with an LBBB is to have an external transthoracic pacemaker on standby during the insertion.

A pulmonary artery catheter may be inserted via a brachial, subclavian, or femoral vein and is advanced into the right atrium, through the tricuspid valve into the right ventricle, and finally out the pulmonic valve into the pulmonary artery. When the catheter is traversing the right ventricle, the small balloon at its distal end is inflated to allow the normal cardiac circulation to direct the catheter into the pulmonary artery, and to minimize the potential of catheter-induced ventricular irritability. Pressure readings from the RV are obtained only on insertion of the catheter.

Once the catheter is in the pulmonary artery, systolic, diastolic, mean, and wedge pressures can be obtained. The pulmonary artery wedge pressure (PAWP) can be obtained by inflating the balloon at the distal tip of the catheter with air, permitting the pulmonary artery catheter to advance until it occludes a pulmonary arterial branch. When the balloon is inflated, blood flow in this branch is impeded from the right side of the heart toward the lungs. The distal part of the catheter records the pressure that is reflected backward through the capillary bed from the left atrium. During diastole, the mitral valve opens, allowing the pressure in the left ventricle to be transmitted through the left atrium backward against the tip of the pulmonary artery catheter. This reflected left ventricular pressure is captured by the catheter when the balloon is inflated and is referred to as the pulmonary artery wedge pressure (PAWP). Once the catheter has been inserted, a confirmatory chest x-ray is necessary for validation of placement if fluoroscopy has not been used.

Special attention should be paid to the potential problems which may result from the use of these catheters, which include (1) catheter-induced ventricular irritability, which may warrant lidocaine to be kept at the bedside during insertion; (2) catheter whip artifact caused by acceleration forces induced by ventricular systole, which may require high-frequency filters; (3) balloon rupture, which requires careful attention to prevention of overinflation; and (4) catheter migration to other areas, which requires repositioning of catheters and documentation of proper placement by chest x-ray. Complications inherent in a PA catheter use include infection, pulmonary infarction, pulmonary artery rupture, pulmonary embolism, and air embolism.

Left Atrial Catheter   The left atrial (LA) catheter may be inserted in some patients following cardiac surgery. While the distal end of the LA catheter lies in the left atrial appendage, it exits through a small incision to the right of the mediastinal incision near the epigastric area and permits recording of left atrial pressures (LAP).

Because the LA line enters the left heart circulation, the presence of any foreign material such as air or debris poses the risk of embolization to the brain or coronary arteries and, therefore, frequent inspection of the LA line should be performed. Gentle aspiration of foreign material is imperative. In addition, the administration of any drugs through this catheter is usually not permitted. Complications associated with use of the LA catheter include emboli, infection, bleeding associated with withdrawal, and cardiac tamponade.

Special Considerations Regarding Monitoring Systems

In assembling the equipment for hemodynamic monitoring, sterile technique needs to be maintained. Prior to initiating hemodynamic monitoring, each transducer must be leveled, balanced, and calibrated. Leveling is performed so that the transducer will be positioned at the height of the right atrium. The most accurate method to accomplish this is to position the air–fluid interface of the transducer stopcock at the fourth intercostal space in the midaxillary line. This location is often referred to as the phlebostatic axis. Balancing refers to a zero reference (usually atmospheric pressure). This is attained by positioning the transducer stopcock so that the transducer is opened to air. Then the transducer is calibrated to a known pressure. The procedure varies with each monitor; moreover,

some newer monitors have internal calibration factors. It is recommended that specific guidelines by each manufacturer be followed.

Once these tasks have been accomplished, the system must be kept patent by a constant flow of heparinized solution via an intraflow device. This device allows for a constant 3 to 4 mL per hour flow. This flush solution also needs to be pressurized by some means to prevent backup of blood into the catheter.

Certain considerations need to be addressed to ensure accuracy of pressure readings. These include (1) catheter and tubing length, (2) type of tubing used, (3) catheter diameter, (4) secure connections, and (5) air bubbles and blood clots. The catheter and tubing length should be kept to a minimum. Tubing that is too long may result in an overshoot of the systolic pressures and lowering of diastolic pressures. Therefore, the recommended length of tubing is 3 to 4 ft. The tubing must also be stiff and noncompliant because soft, compliant tubing may cause distortion from the absorption of transmitted pressure by the compliant tubing. This in turn will create falsely low pressure readings. The diameter of the catheter is another consideration, but is probably of least importance. In the clinical setting, there is a trade-off between using a large-size catheter which ensures an adequate signal transmission, or a smaller catheter which reduces the risk of thrombosis. Catheter size is thus largely dependent on physician preference and the patient's size.

Air bubbles and blood clots pose an additional problem in that they are both compressible and produce a decrease in the amplitude of the wave. Thus, the critical-care nurse needs to eliminate each.

In addition to these considerations, the critical-care nurse needs to take special precautions regarding electrical hazards. There is an inherent risk for developing microshock in patients with catheters placed directly in the heart.

Hemodynamic Parameters

In the critical-care unit, it is important for nurses to be able to identify, monitor, and interpret hemodynamic parameters. This section focuses on only those parameters which assess cardiac output, stroke volume, preload, afterload, contractility, and myocardial oxygen consumption. A summary of these parameters is found in Table 20-4 along with normal values and formulas.

Cardiac Output   The cardiac output is obtained via the pulmonary artery catheter using the thermodilution method, which involves injecting a known temperature solution into the blood and measuring the resultant change downstream. Iced or room temperature solution is injected via the proximal port of the PA catheter, producing a temperature change in the blood that is detected by a thermistor located at the distal end of the

catheter. A computer records the thermodilution curve and calculates a digital value from the area under this curve.[32] It is recommended that the injectate be injected in less than 4 s to prevent distortion of the temperature concentration curve. It has been suggested that CO be measured during end-expiration. Riedinger and Shellock[33] dispute the necessity of taking CO at end-expiration because of the fact that most current CO computers have corrected for the potential problem of respiratory-associated baseline drift by electronically averaging the blood temperature over a shortened period of time prior to the injection of indicator solution.

Table 20-4 Summary of Hemodynamic Parameters

	Normal Values	Calculations	Definition
CO	4–8 L/min	$SV \times HR$	Blood ejected from the heart into systemic circulation per minute
CI	2.5–4.0 L/min	$\dfrac{CO}{BSA}$	Cardiac output adjusted for body size
SV	60–135 mL per beat	$\dfrac{CO \times 1000}{HR}$	Volume of blood ejected from the ventricle per beat
SVI	45–85 mL/m^2 per beat	$\dfrac{SV}{BSA}$	Stroke volume adjusted for body size
CVP	2–6 mmHg 2.7–12 cmH$_2$O	1 mmHg = 13.6 mmH$_2$O or 1.36 cmH$_2$O	Reflects filling pressure of RV and mean pressure of systemic veins (i.e., venous return)
PAEDP	8–10 mmHg		Reflects filling pressure to LV (usually 1–5 mmHg higher than PAWP)
PAWP	5–15 mmHg		Reflects filling pressure of LV if no obstruction exists between catheter balloon tip and LV (i.e., mitral stenosis)
PVR	155–255 dynes/s/cm^{-5}	$\dfrac{(PAM - PAWP) \times 80.0}{CO}$	Resistance to RV ejection offered by pulmonary pressure
SVR	950 to 1300 dynes/s/cm^{-5}	$\dfrac{(MAP - CVP) \times 80.0}{CO}$	Resistance to LV ejection offered by aortic pressure
RVSWI	8.5–12 g/m^1	$\dfrac{RVSW}{BSA}$	Work performed by RV to generate pressure per beat, adjusted for body size
LVSWI	35–85 g/m^1	$\dfrac{LVSW}{BSA}$	Work performed by LV to generate pressure per beat, adjusted for body size
RPP	<12,000	$SYS. BP \times HR$	Indirect determinant of $M\dot{V}_{O_2}$ consumption

This averaging offers a stable baseline during the period of cardiac output measurement eliminating the need for proper timing of the injection.

The thermodilution method provides a quick, accurate assessment (± 20 percent) of the CO. A major disadvantage, however, is the potential for inaccuracy when thermodilution is used in low output states, intracardiac shunts, or pulmonary/tricuspid regurgitation, arrhythmias, or mechanical ventilation.

Many conditions may result in a decreased CO. Tachycardia is one example that may precipitate a low CO because of a decrease in ventricular filling time and a reduction in stroke volume. Additional conditions which lower CO are factors which reduce preload such as massive vasodilatation, diuresis, dehydration, third space shifting of fluids, arrhythmias, and increased intrathoracic pressure. Factors such as ischemia, myocardial infarction, and negative inotropic drugs also yield a lower CO by decreasing contractility. Lastly, any factor that increases afterload or the vascular resistance such as hypothermia, increased sympathetic stimulation, or hypertension may limit CO. Conversely, variables which cause an increase in CO include exercise, anxiety, certain atrioventricular shunts, and sepsis in the early stage.

Cardiac Index The cardiac index (CI) is more precise than CO in reflecting LV output because it takes into account the individual patient's body size. The CI represents a patient's CO in relation to his or her body surface area. Any factors which decrease or increase CO will directly affect the cardiac index (Chap. 19).

Stroke Volume The SV is obtained by dividing the cardiac output by the heart rate. Factors which affect preload, afterload, and contractility directly affect SV.

Stroke Volume Index (SVI) The SVI is a sensitive measurement of stroke volume because it reflects the body surface area of an individual. The normal SVI value and formula are in Table 20-4.

Preload Parameters The CVP or RAP is a determinant of the right ventricular end-diastolic pressure or preload and is recorded as a mean pressure. This mean pressure corresponds to RV end-diastolic

pressure because during diastole when the tricuspid valve is open, there is communication between the right atrium and ventricle. In the past, these pressures were considered to be a reliable measure of left ventricular preload, but with the advent of pulmonary arterial catheters, these pressures were found not to accurately reflect LV preload.

The RAP and CVP reflect venous return to the right atrium; thus, any condition which reduces venous return results in a decrease in these pressures. Some of these conditions include hemorrhage, shock, third space shifting, burns, diuresis, vomiting, venous pooling, and increased intrathoracic pressure. Interventions used in some of these circumstances are aimed at augmenting venous return such as with the administration of crystalloid or colloid therapy. Conversely, interventions used to decrease these pressures include diuretics and venodilators. The positioning of patients is another variable which may alter venous return. For example, patients in the semierect position may experience a decrease in venous return and those who are recumbent may have an increase in venous return.

The waveform of a right atrial tracing characteristically has three positive pressures (*a, c, v*) and two negative descents (*x, y*) (Fig. 20-12). An explanation of each waveform and correlation to the ECG are found in Table 20-5.

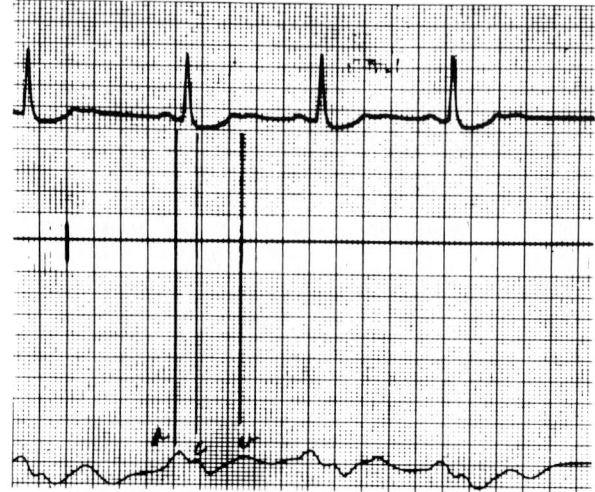

Figure 20-12 Normal right atrial pressure waveform showing *a, c, v* waves and *x* and *y* descents. (*Used with permission of Hewlett-Packard, Waltham Division.*)

Table 20-5 Summary of Right Atrial, Pulmonary Artery Wedge, and Left Atrial Waveforms

Waveforms	Normal Right Atrial	Correlation to ECG	Pulmonary Artery Wedge Pressure or Left Atrial	Correlation to ECG
a	Produced by atrial contraction; precedes arterial pulsation	Corresponds in time to PR interval of ECG	Produced by left atrial systole	Follows P wave of ECG
x	Negative descent caused by a reduction in pressure after atrial contraction		Decline in pressure related to a decrease in LA volume	
c	Depicts movement of the tricuspid valve toward the atrium	Corresponds to RS-T junction on ECG	Produced by closure of mitral valve—may not be seen	
v	Represents ventricular systole	Corresponds to T-P interval	Results from filling of LA and bulging back of mitral valve during ventricular contractions	Follows QRS complex on ECG
y	Reflects a decrease in RA volume during passive filling of RV		Reflects decrease in LA during passive filling of LV	

Adapted from E. Daily, & J. Schroeder, *Techniques of Bedside Hemodynamic Monitoring*, 3d ed. St. Louis: C. V. Mosby, 1985.

Left ventricular preload parameters such as the pulmonary artery end-diastolic pressure (PAEDP) are obtained via the PA catheter. The PAEDP is obtained during diastole. It will approximate the PAWP with the exception of such conditions as mechanical ventilation, elevated pulmonary vascular resistance, heart rates which exceed 130 beats per minute, chronic obstructive lung disease, and pulmonary embolism. The PAEDP is usually 1 to 4 mmHg higher than the PAWP.

The PAWP is a dampened, time-delayed version of a left atrial pressure tracing. It is a reflection of left ventricular filling pressure and is extremely useful in managing cardiac patients. Readings should be obtained at the end of expiration. Results from studies have indicated that both PA and PAW pressures can be accurately measured with the backrest of the bed elevated from 0 to 45°.[34] Conditions which do not enable the PAWP to be used as a reflection of left ventricular preload include mitral stenosis, mitral regurgitation, left atrial tumors, and pulmonary venous obstructions. Elevations in the PAWP occur in the setting of left ventricular failure.

The advantages of obtaining a PAWP in reflecting left ventricular performance are obvious. The disadvantages are (1) threat of balloon-induced pulmonary artery rupture and hemorrhage as a result of repeated balloon inflation and (2) migration of the catheter to a distal artery yielding a permanent wedge tracing and potential pulmonary infarct if not repositioned. The risk of pulmonary artery rupture or infarct can be minimized with careful adherence to the procedures for balloon inflation (1½ cc maximum). Frequent balloon inflations may not be necessary when the PAEDP approximates the PAWP.

The normal PA wedge tracing has a characteristic atrial pattern described in the CVP parameter section. A more detailed explanation of this waveform along with correlation to the ECG is found in Table 20-5 and Fig. 20-13.

An abnormal PA wedge tracing is found in mitral regurgitation. An elevated *v* wave tracing is considered to be the hallmark of this type of valvular defect. In mitral regurgitation the PAWP does not accurately reflect LVEDP and results in a higher than normal value.

The left atrial pressure (LAP) is the third parameter used to assess LV preload. The major limitation of LAP monitoring is that the catheter can be placed only during cardiac surgical procedures and thus is not a commonly obtained pressure in critical-care units. However, the LAP is the most

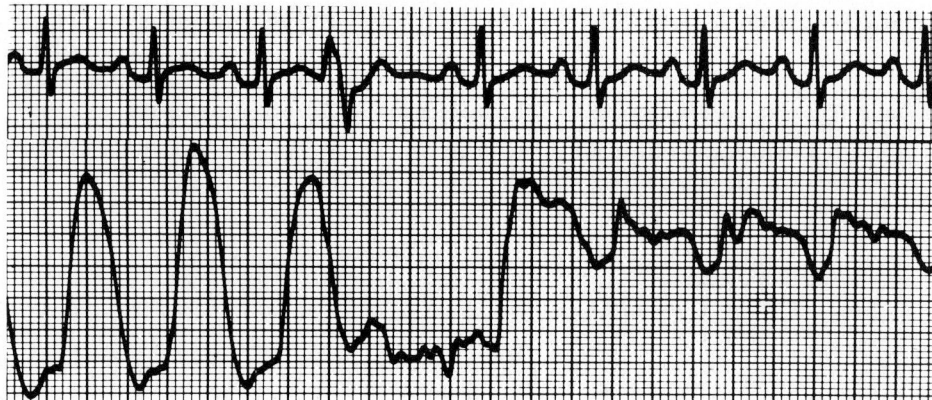

Figure 20-13   Normal PA and PAW pressure waveforms showing *a* and *v* waves and *x* and *y* descents the PAW tracing. (*Used with permission of Hewlett-Packard, Waltham Division.*)

accurate estimation of LVEDP in the absence of mitral valve disease. The waveform is the exact tracing as found in Fig. 20-14. The detailed description of the positive and negative descents of LAP will also be found in Table 20-5.

Afterload Parameters   Right ventricular afterload can be evaluated using the pulmonary vascular resistance whereby the systemic vascular resistance, and aortic end-diastolic pressure may be used as a reflection of left ventricular afterload. The formulas to calculate these derived parameters are found in Table 20-4.

Pulmonary vascular resistance (PVR) is a measure of impedance or resistance by the pulmonic arterial circulation to RV ejection. It can be calculated with a programmed calculator or by using the formula found in Table 20-4. Certain conditions elevate the PVR and may cause a subsequent reduction in cardiac output. These include hypoxia or hypercapnia, which induces vasoconstriction; acute respiratory distress syndrome; positive end-expiratory pressure; pulmonary embolism; pulmonary interstitial edema; chronic obstructive lung disease; inflammatory states; and mitral stenosis. The critical-care nurse needs to be aware of conditions that may increase the PVR and report them to the physician.

Systemic vascular resistance (SVR) is a measure of resistance by the systemic arterial circulation to LV ejection. Certain states or conditions will elevate the SVR and cause a reduction in CO such as vasoconstriction, inotropic agents, polycythemia vera, and hypovolemic/cardiogenic shock, all of which cause increased sympathetic stimulation. Afterload reducers such as nitroprusside or nitroglycerin are frequently employed in the above conditions. Decreases in SVR will occur with vasodilatation, moderate hypoxemia, vasodilator agents, and anemic states.

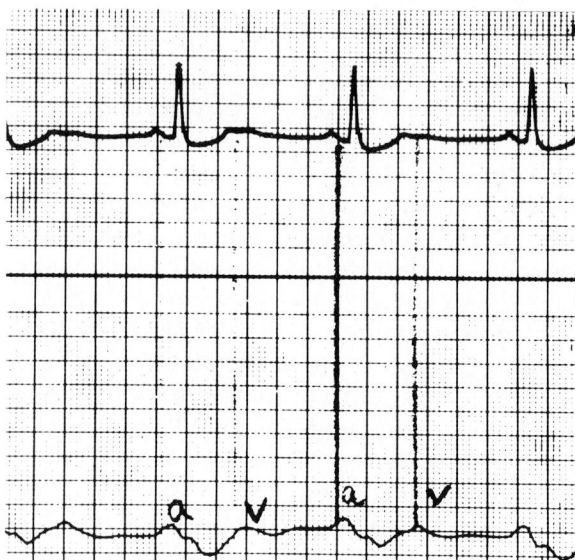

Figure 20-14   LA pressure waveform demonstrating similarity to PAW waveform. This pressure is normal. (*Used with permission of Hewlett-Packard, Waltham Division.*)

Another parameter which can be used as a reflection of afterload is the aortic end-diastolic pressure. This pressure correlates to the pressure that the left ventricle must overcome to open the aortic valve during the phase of isovolumetric contraction and can be easily obtained from an arterial catheter. Conditions which elevate or decrease the SVR produce similar changes in aortic end-diastolic pressure.

Contractility Parameters There are no direct methods of measuring contractility, but an indirect value may be obtained by calculating the amount of work that the right or left ventricle does during systolic ejection. These indirect measures of contractility are referred to as *right ventricular stroke work* (RVSW) and *left ventricular stroke work* (LVSW).

The RVSW parameter measures the amount of work the right ventricle generates per beat when ejecting blood and is based on the calculation for work: Work = pressure generated × volume of blood pumped. It is a product of the mean arterial blood pressure and stroke volume. The conversion factor of 0.0136 converts pressure to work. It can be calculated either by a programmed calculator or using the formula cited in Table 20-4. A decrease in RVSW is suggestive of a right ventricular infarct which can depress contractility. The right ventricular stroke work index (RVSWI) is a more precise determinant of RV stroke work in that it reflects the body surface area of a patient.

The LVSW is a measurement of the amount of work the left ventricle generates per beat during ventricular ejection. It is similar to RVSW in that it is based on the calculation of work. The LVSW is a product of the MAP and the SV. In the presence of depressed contractility and decreased LVSW, inotropic agents are needed to strengthen cardiac contraction. An increase in LVSW may be related to conditions in which there is an increase in MV_{O_2}. This increase in MV_{O_2} can be detrimental in patients with coronary artery disease, who by virtue of their disease have diminished blood supply and may develop further ischemia because they are unable to satisfy the demand for O_2. The LVSWI is also a more exact measurement of SW in that it is indexed to the patient's body surface area.

Rate-Pressure-Product The rate-pressure-product (RPP) is an indirect assessment of myocardial oxygen consumption and is calculated as the product of systolic blood pressure and heart rate. If the RPP is greater than 12,000 it indicates an increase in MV_{O_2}, which is an important consideration in patients who have ischemic heart disease and are vulnerable to further damage when demand exceeds supply.

Conclusion

Bedside hemodynamic monitoring permits an objective assessment and continuous monitoring of patients with acute cardiovascular problems. The major determinants of CO previously discussed can be assessed by the parameters mentioned in this section. In low CO states, it is important for the critical-care nurse to evaluate the contribution of individual variables to reduced ventricular ejection. Through this evaluation process, the nurse can gain an understanding of the therapeutic interventions necessary to optimize CO.

Magnetic Resonance Imaging (MRI)

Magnetic resonance imaging (MRI) is one of the newest, noninvasive diagnostic techniques available. Although used by chemists in the 1940s to study molecular structures, MRI is now being utilized as a diagnostic imaging technique and as a technique to provide in-vivo cellular metabolic information.

Nucleons, protons, and neutrons that comprise an atomic nucleus are the structures of interest in MRI. Atoms with an odd number of nucleons or atomic mass have both a charge and an inherent spin around their axes. Since any moving charge creates a magnetic force, these spinning atomic nuclei have their own magnetic fields or moments. Morganroth, Parisi, and Pohost[35] compared magnetic moments to microscopic bar magnets and found them similar. A substance is composed of many nuclei whose magnetic moments occur randomly. When subjected to an external magnetic field, random magnetic moments align themselves in either a parallel or antiparallel relation to the external field which creates a stronger net magnetic force parallel to the external field.

If these nucleons are further subjected to a second force or radiofrequency, they are pulled from their equilibrium with the first external magnetic field. If this radiofrequency force is discontinued, the nucleons return to their prior position of alignment with the external field and release a signal known as *free induction decay*. This signal is one type of data analyzed in MRI. A second type of data obtained by MRI is the relaxation time or the time it takes for a nucleon to return to its original position after exposure to a radiofrequency force.[35] The relaxation time of nucleons differs depending on the tissue type, presence of disease, and differences in tissue water content.

Magnetic Resonance Spectroscopy

MR spectroscopy transforms the free induction decay signal into a frequency spectrum and provides data revealing the chemical composition of nuclei. These data are useful in studying cellular metabolism and the effect of disease or interventions. Hydrogen 1, carbon 13, sodium 23, fluorine 19, and phosphorus 31 are nuclei that are sensitive to magnetic resonance scrutiny.

NMR spectroscopy with phosphorus 31 (^{31}P) provides insight into cellular metabolism. Phosphorus 31 is contained in adenosine triphosphate (ATP) and creatine phosphate, substances vital to cell viability. Ratner and Pohost[36] cite laboratory data derived from rat and rabbit hearts which reveal that monitoring ^{31}P levels yields helpful data regarding myocardial anoxia, ischemia, infarction, and intracellular pH.

Clinical applicability of this technique in monitoring cardiac metabolism is currently being studied. Fossel, Morgan, and Ingwall[37] utilized ^{31}P spectroscopy to document variations in high-energy phosphorus concentrations throughout the cardiac cycle. In addition, the peak of the ^{31}P has been shown to be related to cellular pH by Ingwall.[38]

The applicability of this information to clinical practice is discussed in the literature. ^{31}P spectroscopy has been utilized to examine the effectiveness of propranolol in reducing ischemic arrest-induced acidosis.[39] Others have utilized ^{31}P spectroscopy to document the effect of potassium cardioplegia and hypothermia on high-energy phosphates and cellular pH during ischemia.[40]

Magnetic Resonance Imaging Study

MR imaging utilizes the free induction decay signal and relaxation time to construct a three-dimensional image. The nucleon studied in MR imaging is the proton because of its abundance in humans and its sensitivity to MRI. Hydrogen is the proton of choice in MR imaging.

Imaging a moving object, such as the heart, poses a threat to image clarity. To minimize image distortion, gating or timing the delivery of the radiofrequency force to a consistent period in the cardiac cycle was accomplished. Ratner and Pohost[36] and Viamonte[41] state that gating to the electrocardiogram is the method of choice to minimize image distortion and has resulted in improved imaging.

One advantage of MR imaging over x-ray is its superiority in differentiating tissues because MRI detects changes in tissue chemistry that precede changes in structure. MR imaging can detect brain metastasis, infarcts, signs of demyelinating diseases, and some types of dementia earlier than CAT scanning; this is possible by documenting edema in the tissues surrounding a tumor. Viamonte[41] has highlighted its superiority in identifying early bone ischemia that may be undetected by CAT scan or x-ray. Since bone is not visible with MR imaging, Viamonte[41] states that it is the test of choice in evaluating the brain and spinal cord.

In some instances, MR imaging can differentiate malignant from benign tumors. It does not detect calcification and, therefore, fails to diagnose one-third of all calcified nonpalpable carcinomas. It also cannot distinguish inflammation from a neoplasm.

The applicability of MR imaging in evaluating the cardiovascular system is varied. MR imaging permits viewing the heart on a multitude of planes and yields visualization of the cardiac chambers, ventricular wall, aorta, pulmonary artery, and septum during systole as well as diastole. Early detection of lipid deposits on coronary artery intima is possible. Also, the existence of dissection and clot can be clearly documented by MR imaging. Figures 20-15 and 20-16 depict cross-sectional views of the heart taken with MRI.

Contraindications

MRI is contraindicated in patients with pacemakers or neurostimulater devices because, for example, the pacemaker may be reprogrammed or changed to an asynchronous mode. Patients with aneurysm clips undergo this technique because of the danger of dislodging the clips.

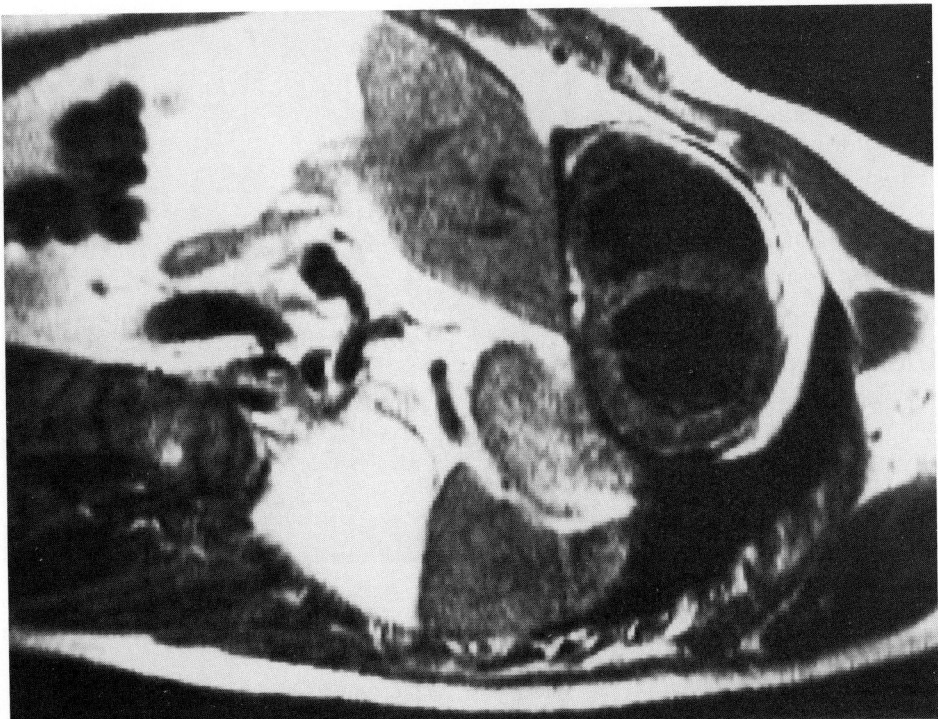

Figure 20-15 Cross-sectional view of heart taken by MRI.

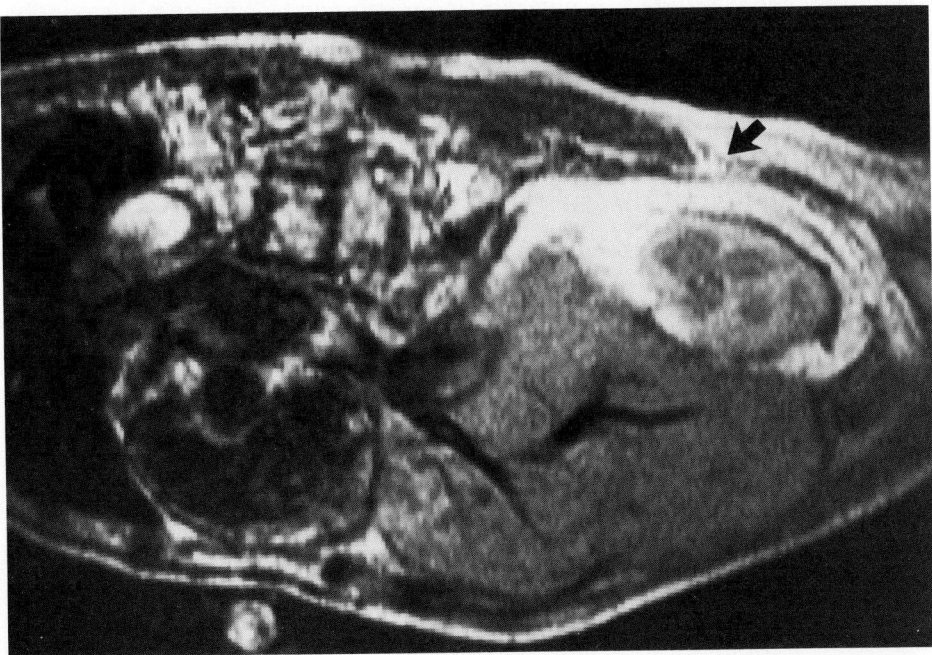

Figure 20-16 Cross-sectional view of heart taken by MRI.

Safety

To date, there is no report of ill effects associated with MRI. The only potential ill effect from the magnetic and radiofrequency fields is tissue heating, but Morganroth et al.[35] state that this has not been actualized even when higher magnetic fields were employed. Finally, unlike x-ray or radionuclide techniques, MRI does not utilize ionizing radiation.

Radionuclide Testing

Radionuclide tests or nuclear scans are techniques that utilize radionuclide substances to study cardiac function, perfusion, or injury. These substances emit energy as gamma rays when they convert from an unstable to a stable form. Gamma rays, the radioactive decay of the radionuclide substance, are monitored by a device known as a gamma scintillation camera.

Myocardial Infarct Imaging Techniques

Myocardial infarct imaging is a radionuclide technique that identifies the size and location of a myocardial infarction. For certain subsets of patients, this technique is necessary to confirm the diagnosis of an MI. In patients who experienced an MI days before admission, have muscle disease, and have electrocardiographic (ECG) findings of a left bundle branch block, previous MIs, paced rhythm, or subendocardial changes, enzymatic and ECG evidence of an MI may be inconclusive, and diagnosis may depend on a myocardial infarct imaging study.

Technetium pyrophosphate (^{99m}Tc), the radionuclide utilized in myocardial infarct imaging, was previously utilized for bone scanning. In myocardial scanning, ^{99m}Tc accumulates in infarcted tissue and is detected as an area of increased concentration or a "hot spot" by the gamma scintillation camera. (Fig. 20-17).

Although the exact mechanism by which the ^{99m}Tc is deposited in necrotic myocardium is disputed, some theories have been postulated. One such theory is the binding of the radionuclide with damaged mitochondria; a second theory alludes to the role of calcium crystals present in necrotic tissue as postulated by Wacker[42] and Anderson.[10]

Myocardial infarct imaging can identify an MI within 10 to 12 h of infarction. The imaging reaches

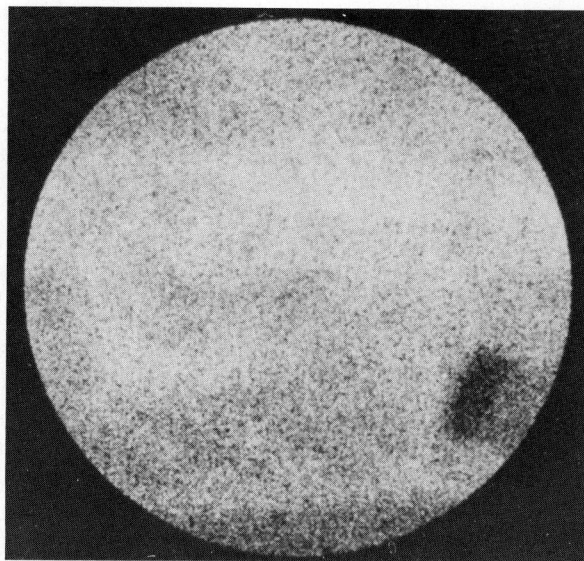

Figure 20-17 Pyrophosphate scan depicting area of increased uptake.

a diagnostic peak within 72 h and is negative after 4 to 5 days. Identification of an MI that has occurred 7 to 10 days earlier is not feasible.

Myocardial infarct imaging relies on myocardial blood flow, calcification, and size of infarction for uptake of ^{99m}Tc. Technetium pyrophosphate uptake is more concentrated in areas surrounding an infarction than in the center. In a large anterior MI, for instance, the damaged myocardium may appear as a doughnutlike area of increased uptake, corresponding to the zone of injury, surrounding a center area of decreased uptake which corresponds to the necrotic or infarcted tissue. Areas of calcification are also associated with increased uptake. Lastly, 3 g or more of infarcted myocardium must be present for imaging to be diagnostic. Gerson[43] and Willerson[44] have identified new three-dimensional techniques that permit the imaging of smaller infarcts.

Although very specific in identifying an MI, ^{99m}Tc scanning is a useful diagnostic tool for a variety of cardiac conditions. Viral myocarditis, trauma, left ventricular aneurysms, unstable angina, tumor, calcification of valves, and amyloidosis are examples. Willerson[44] identified other conditions, excluding MI, that result in positive findings such as decreased myocardial perfusion secondary to hypotension, delayed clearance secondary to renal insufficiency, or excessive injection of the radio-nuclide. It has been found that persistently abnormal results are associated with more severe disease, congestive heart failure, and persistent angina.[45]

Myocardial Perfusion Imaging Techniques

Myocardial perfusion imaging is a radionuclide technique which quantifies, as the name implies, myocardial tissue perfusion. Thallium, ^{201}Tl, is the most frequently utilized radionuclide in this procedure because its activity resembles that of potassium. Once injected, thallium accumulates within viable myocardium via the sodium-potassium–ATPase system. Uptake is therefore dependent on coronary circulation and viable myocardium. Areas of decreased uptake, or "cold spots," correlate with ischemic and infarcted tissue.

Thallium scans are useful to locate and quantify the size of an MI. The role of ^{201}Tl exercise scintigraphy in diagnosing coronary artery disease has been documented by many authorities.[46–48]

Thallium exercise scintigraphy is the only radionuclide technique that differentiates between myocardial infarction and ischemia. During this procedure, the patient is exercised in a stress laboratory and is injected with ^{201}Tl once the point of peak exercise is reached. Imaging obtained at this point visualizes areas of decreased tracer uptake in the presence of significant stenosis resulting from decreased coronary blood circulation to areas beyond the stenosis. Because thallium uptake is dependent on coronary circulation, a cold spot is visualized (Fig. 20-18).

To differentiate between infarction and ischemia, a repeat scan is performed approximately 4 h after the ^{201}Tl injection. Ischemia is identified if reperfusion occurs in the previously documented cold areas.

Differing from ischemia, zones of infarcted tissue do not illustrate reperfusion on the repeated scan. Freund, Lewis, and Reduto[49] identify two advantages of ^{201}Tl exercise scintigraphy when compared to conventional exercise testing. One advantage is an increase in sensitivity and specificity when diagnosing coronary artery disease. A second is that this test allows for the evaluation of ischemia in patients with ECG evidence of left bundle branch block, left ventricular hypertrophy, and S-T segment changes associated with digitalis.

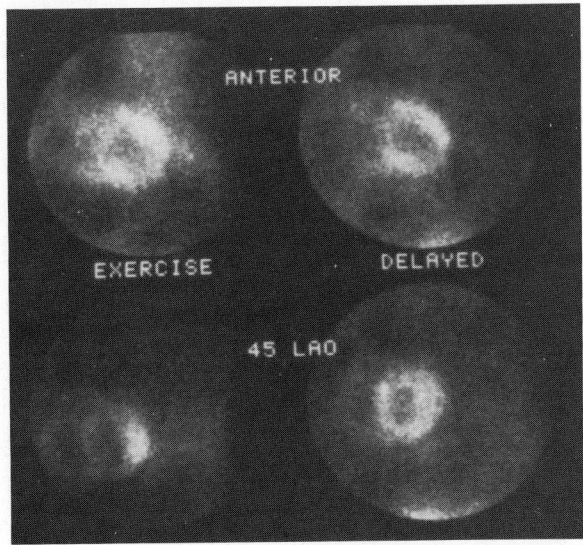

Figure 20-18   Exercise thallium scan with reperfusion indicating septal and inferoapical ischemia.

Although sensitive for coronary artery disease, Gerson[43] has cited other conditions that yield abnormal perfusion studies: sarcoidosis, aortic stenosis, cardiomyopathy, and metastatic carcinoma. These conditions must be excluded before a definitive diagnosis of coronary artery disease is made.

The prognostic implications from abnormal thallium scans are illustrated in the literature. Certain investigators have utilized results from thallium testing to identify high- and low-risk patients following an acute myocardial infarction.[50,51] The detection of multivessel disease by thallium scans has also been employed.[48]

Myocardial Function Imaging Techniques

Two radionuclide techniques allow for evaluation of ventricular function. Both require the injection of a radionuclide tracer.

One technique, the *first pass technique,* requires the injection of a bolus of a radionuclide tracer and follows it on the pathway through the heart. The major advantage of this technique is the ability to obtain data regarding ventricular size and function quickly.[52] The disadvantage is that incorrect patient positioning and variable injection techniques may alter the results.

Equilibrium scans are the second type of radionuclide scans that assess ventricular function.

Unlike the first pass technique in which scanning begins immediately after the bolus injection, in this technique there is a delay of several minutes after injection before scanning which allows the tracer to be mixed homogeneously within the blood. The scintigraphic camera is synchronized with the cardiac cycle and divides the R-to-R interval into multiple intervals or gates, the counts emitted by the radionuclide tracer in each gate are recorded, and a picture is made of the heart and its function throughout the cardiac cycle. The advantage of the equilibrium technique is in assessing regional wall motion and ventricular shape.[52]

These radionuclide tests may be combined with exercise stress testing to yield a variety of information. A higher sensitivity has been reported when combined exercise radionuclide angiocardiography was employed as opposed to conventional exercise testing.[53] The ability to assess the effectiveness of therapies as a second benefit of this procedure has also been noted.[47]

The effect of inadequate exercise levels on the sensitivity of the test must be considered when utilizing this technique and interpreting the results.[54] Lastly, it has been reported that the type of population undergoing exercise radionuclide ventriculography may also affect the sensitivity of the test.[55]

In conclusion, this section has provided an in-depth review of the current diagnostic tests used to evaluate the cardiovascular system. Although each test provides valuable information, the critical-care nurse needs to integrate information from the nursing history as well as the physical examination in order to direct patient care.

References

1. Gordon, M. (1976). Nursing diagnoses and the diagnostic process. *American Journal of Nursing, 76,* 1298–1300.

2. Gordon, M. (1982). *Manual of Nursing Diagnosis.* New York: McGraw-Hill.

3. Braunwald, E. (1984). The physical examination. In E. Braunwald (Ed.), *Heart disease.* Philadelphia: Saunders.

4. Silverman, M. E., & Hurst, J. W. (1986). Inspection of the patient. In J. W. Hurst, R. B. Logue, R. C. Schlant, & N. K. Wenger (Eds.). *The heart.* New York: McGraw-Hill.

5. Lichstein, E., Chadda, K., Naik, D., and Gupta, P. K. (1974). Diagonal ear lobe crease: Prevalence and implications as a coronary risk factor. *New England Journal of Medicine, 290,* 615–616.

6. Thompson, D. A. (1981). *Cardiovascular assessment.* St. Louis: Mosby.

7. Vaughan, P. (1984). Bedside assessment of the myocardial infarction patient. *Critical Care Nurse, 4* 60–77.

8. Roberts, R. (1981). Diagnostic assessment of myocardial infarction based on lactate dehydrogenase and creatine kinase isoenzyme. *Heart and Lung, 10,*(3), 486–504.

9. Galen, R. S. (1977). Myocardial infarction: A clinician's guide to the isoenzymes. *Resident and Staff Physician, 23,* 67–75.

10. Anderson, V. (1984). Cardiovascular laboratory testing procedures. In C. E. Guzzetta, & B. M. Dossey (Eds.). *Cardiovascular nursing.* St. Louis: Mosby, 219–251.

11. Fisher, M. L., Carlinger, N. H., Becker, L. C. Peters, R. W., and Plotnick, G. D. (1984). Serum creatine kinase in the diagnosis of acute myocardial infarctions. Optimal sampling frequency. *Journal of the American Medical Association, 249,* 393–394.

12. Woods, S. L., & Laurent-Bopp, D. (1982). Laboratory tests using blood and urine. In S. L. Underhill, S. L. Woods, E. S. Sivarajan, & C. T. Halpenny (Eds.). *Cardiac nursing.* Philadelphia: Lippincott.

13. Grossman, W. (1980). *Cardiac catheterization and angiography.* Philadelphia: Lea & Febiger.

14. Sanderson, R. G. (1983). Diagnostic techniques. In R. G. Sanderson, & C. L. Kurth (Eds.). *The cardiac patient.* Philadelphia: Saunders.

15. Sokolow, M., & McIlroy, M. (1981). *Clinical cardiology.* Los Altos, CA: Lange Medical Publications.

16. Feigenbaum, H. (1981). *Echocardiography* (3d ed.). Philadelphia: Lea & Febiger.

17. Feigenbaum, H. (1984). Echocardiography. In E. Braunwald (Ed.). *Heart disease.* Philadelphia: Saunders, 400–408.

18. Wenger, N., & Hellerstein, H. (1984). *Rehabilitation of the coronary patient.* New York: John Wiley & Sons.

19. Fernandez, G. (1983). Echocardiography for the general internist. *Comprehensive Medicine, 9*(10), 46–56.

20. Vacek, J., Smith, W., & Phillips, J. (1984). Cardiac electrophysiology: An overview. *Practical Cardiology, 10*(13) 83–97.

21. Michelson, E., Spielman, S. R., Greenspan, A. M., Farshidi, A., Horowitz, L. N., & Josephson, M. E. (1979). Electrophysiologic study of the left ventricle. Indications and safety. *Chest, 75,* 592–596.

22. Podrid, P., & Lambert, S. (1983). Electrophysiologic approach to ventricular arrhythmias: A review. *Cardiovascular Review & Reports, 2*(4), 231–237.

23. Denes, P., & Ezri, M. D. (1983). Clinical electrophysiology—a decade of progress. *Journal of the American College of Cardiology, 1,* 292–305.

24. Kienzle, M., Doherty, J., Marcus, N., & Josephson, M., (1984). When do electrophysiologic studies benefit arrhythmia patients? *Journal of Cardiovascular Medicine,* January 1984, 41–55.

25. Ezri, M. D. (1983). Electrophysiologic testing in the diagnosis and management of cardiac arrhythmias. *Chest, 84,* 481–491.

26. Velebit, V., Podrid, P., Lown, B., Cohen, B. H., & Grayboys, T. B. (1982). Aggravation and provocation of ventricular arrhythmias by antiarrhythmic drugs. *Circulation, 65,* 886–894.

27. Naccarelli, G. V., Prystowsky, E. N., Jackman, W. M., Heger, J. J., Rahilly, G. T., & Zipes, D. P. (1982). Role of electrophysiologic testing in managing patients who have ventricular tachycardia unrelated to coronary artery disease. *American Journal of Cardiology, 50,* 165–171.

28. Michelson, E. L., & Medina, R. P. (1985). Introduction to clinical electrophysiologic studies. *Cardiovascular Clinics, 16*(1), 1–36.

29. Kaufmann, L., & Schwartz, J. (1984). Diagnostic endocardial electrical recording and stimulation. *Annals of Internal Medicine,* 100(3), 452–454.

30. Palmer, P. N. (1982). Advanced hemodynamic assessment. *Dimensions of Critical Care Nursing, 1*(3), 139–144.

31. Hurst, J. M. (1984). Invasive hemodynamic monitoring: An overview. *Journal of Emergency Nursing, 10*(1), 11–22.

32. Sedlock, S. (1981). Cardiac output: Physiologic variables and therapeutic interventions. *Critical Care Nurse, 2*(1), 14–22.

33. Riedinger, M. S., & Shellock, F. G. (1984). Technical aspects of the thermodilution method for measuring cardiac output. *Heart and Lung,* 13(3), 215–222.

34. Chulay, M., & Miller, T. (1984). The effect of backrest elevation on pulmonary artery and pulmonary capillary wedge pressures in patients after cardiac surgery. *Heart and Lung, 13*(2), 138–140.

35. Morganroth, J., Parisi, A., & Pohost, G. (1983). *Noninvasive cardiac imaging.* Chicago: Yearbook Medical Publications.

36. Ratner, A. V., & Pohost, G. M. (1984). Nuclear magnetic resonance imaging of the heart. In E. Braunwald (Ed.), *Heart disease.* Philadelphia: Saunders, 400–407.

37. Fossel, E. T., Morgan, H. E., & Ingwall, J. S. (1980). Measurement of changes in high-energy phosphates in the cardiac cycle using gated 31P NMR. *Proceedings of the National Academy of Science, 77,* 3654–3658.

38. Ingwall, J. S. (1982). Phosphorus nuclear magnetic resonance spectroscopy of cardiac and skeletal muscles. *American Journal of Physiology, 242* 729–744.

39. Pieper, G. M., Todd, G. L., Wu, S. T., Salhany, J. M., Clayton, F. C., and Eliot, R. S. (1980). Attenuation of myocardial acidosis by propranolol during ischemic arrest and reperfusion. *Cardiovascular Research,* (14), 646–653.

40. Flaherty, J. T., Weisfeldt, M. L., Bulkley, B. H., Gardner, T. J., Golt, V. L., and Jacobs, W. E. (1982). Mechanism of ischemic myocardial cell damage assessed by phosphorus-31 nuclear magnetic resonance. *Circulation, 65,* 561–570.

41. Viamonte, M. (1985). New images of imaging. *Emergency Medicine, 17*(8), 52–67.

42. Wacker, F. J. (1980). Current status of radionuclide imaging in the management and evaluation of patients with cardiovascular disease. *Advances in Cardiology, 27,* 40–50.

43. Gerson, M. C. (1983). Myocardial imaging in myocardial infarction: Technetium vs. thallium. *Cardiovascular Clinics, 13*(3), 223–242.

44. Willerson, J. T. (1983). How reliable is myocardial imaging in the diagnosis of acute myocardial infarctions? *Cardiovascular Clinics, 13,* 33–50.

45. Olson, H. G., Lyons, K. P., Aronow, L. W. S., Brown, W. T., & Greenfield, R. S. (1977). Follow up technetium-99m stannous pyrophosphate myocardial scintigrams after acute myocardial infarctions. *Circulation, 56,* 181–187.

46. Berger, B. C., Watson, D. D., Taylor, G. J., Craddock, G. B., Martin, R. P., Teates, C. D., & Beller, G. A. (1981). Quantitative thallium-201 exercise scintigraphy for detection of coronary artery disease. *Journal of Nuclear Medicine, 22,* 585–593.

47. Bodenheimer, M. M., and Helfant, R. H. (1983). Exercise radionuclide angiography: Role in diagnosis and management of cardiovascular disease. *Cardiovascular Clinics, 13,* 243–251.

48. Gibson, R. S., Taylor, G. J., Watson, D. D., Stebbins, P. T., Martin, R. P., Crampton, R. S., & Beller, G. A. (1981). Predicting the extent and location of coronary artery disease during the early postinfarction period by quantitative thallium-201 scintigraphy. *American Journal of Cardiology, 47,* 1010–1019.

49. Freund, G., Lewis, B., & Reduto, L. (1983). Patient assessment: Laboratory studies. In K. Andreoli, V. Fawkes, D. Zipes, & A. Wallace (Eds.). *Comprehensive cardiac care.* St. Louis: Mosby.

50. Silverman, K. J., Becker, L. C., Bulkley, B. H., Burrow, R. D., Mellits, E. D., Kallman, C. H., & Weisfeldt, M.

L. (1980). Value of early thallium-201 scintigraphy for predicting mortality in patients with acute myocardial infarction. *Circulation, 61,* 996–1003.

51. Gibson, R. S., Watson, D. D., Craddock, G. B., Crampton, R. S., Kaiser, D. L., Denny, M. J., & Beller, G. A. (1983). Prediction of cardiac events after uncomplicated myocardial infarction: A prospective study comparing predischarge exercise thallium-201 scintigraphy and coronary angiography. *Circulation, 68,* 321–336.

52. Burrow, R. D., Strauss, H. W., Singleton, R., Pond, M., Rehn, T., Bailey, I. K., Griffith, L. C., Nickoloff, E., & Pitt, B. (1977). Analysis of left ventricular function from multiple gated acquisition cardiac blood pool imaging. Comparison to contrast angiography. *Circulation, 56,* 1024–1028.

53. Jones, R. H., McEwan, P., Newman, G. E., Port, S., Rerych, S. K., Scholz, P. M., Upton, M. T., Peter, C. A., Austin, E. H., Leong, K. H., Gibbons, R. J., Cobb, F. R., Coleman, R. E., and Sabiston, D. C. (1981). Accuracy of diagnosis of coronary artery disease by radionuclide measurements of left ventricular function during rest and exercise. *Circulation, 64,* 586–601.

54. Brady, T. J., Thrall, J. H., Lo, K., & Pitt, B. (1980). The importance of adequate exercise in the detection of coronary heart disease by radionuclide ventriculography. *Journal of Nuclear Medicine, 21,* 1125–1130.

55. Rozanski, A., Diamond, G. A., Berman, D., Forrester, J. S., Morris, D., and Swan, H. J. (1983). The declining specificity of exercise radionuclide ventriculography. *New England Journal of Medicine, 309,* 518–522.

21

Coronary Artery Disease

Joan Vitello-
Cicciu
Susan L. Stewart
Eileen Lovett
Griffin

Coronary heart disease is one of the most predominant health problems in our nation today. Each year over 600,000 people die of complications resulting from this disease process.[1] The major cause of coronary heart disease is coronary artery disease (CAD). This is a disease process characterized by progressive narrowing of the lumen of coronary arteries. This narrowing of the lumen is referred to as *atherosclerosis*.

According to Levy and Feinleib,[1] CAD is a disease process that affects all nationalities, all areas of the world, and all socioeconomic classes. The ramifications of coronary artery disease are not limited to its impact on morbidity or mortality alone. Additionally, complications of CAD such as angina pectoris, myocardial infarction (MI), congestive heart failure (CHF), and cardiogenic shock create physical, psychosocial, and economic hardships. Moreover, individuals who manifest these complications often require critical-care interventions which are costly and stress-provoking.

In the past 30 years, many advances have been made in the treatment of coronary artery disease and its complications. Medical and nursing research have provided many options to patients as well as to the members of the health care interdisciplinary team. Developments such as coronary artery bypass (CABG) surgery, intraaortic balloon counterpulsation, percutaneous transluminal coronary angioplasty, laser angioplasty, thrombolytic therapy, and cardiac rehabilitation programs have opened new doors for acutely ill cardiovascular patients and for the quality of life they may experience.

Newer drug therapies such as beta-adrenergic blocking agents, calcium channel antagonists, and longer-acting nitrates have also been developed. With all these advances, critical-care nurses need to expand their skill and knowledge base to maintain expertise in patient assessment and early intervention to prevent complications.

Atherosclerosis

Introduction

Atherosclerosis is a disease process which results in the development of thick, hard atherosclerotic plaques referred to as *atheromas* or *lesions* which obstruct the lumen in coronary arteries as well as in other medium-sized or large arteries. Plaque formation tends to develop in areas which have turbulent flow patterns such as in areas of bifurcation of vessels and where the diameter of vessels decreases.[2] In the coronary arteries, plaque formation predominates within the first 6 cm. Atherosclerosis manifests itself in varying forms, depending upon the organ it affects.

The clinical effects of these plaques are related to their space-occupying characteristics, which usually result in stenosis of the vessel, or to their propensity to develop a thrombus over a plaque, which may cause total occlusion of the vessel. For example, deposition of atherosclerotic plaques in the coronary arteries results in ischemic heart disease which can provoke angina or a myocardial infarction (MI). Lesions found in the coronary vessels may also be a source for emboli which can cause occlusions in distal vessels or in the collateral circulation. In the kidneys, these lesions may result in renal failure and/or renovascular hypertension. Atherosclerotic plaques in the cerebral arteries can induce organic brain syndrome and stroke. Atherosclerotic plaques may also account for the development of peripheral vascular disease in the lower extremities and aneurysms (because of weakening of the wall) in the lower abdominal aorta. It is hoped that through increased knowledge of the pathogenesis of atherosclerosis as well as the risk factors which contribute to its development that prevention, treatment, and regression of these clinically significant plaques may be accomplished.

Lesions of Atherosclerosis

The lesions of atherosclerosis include the fatty streak, the fibrous plaque, and the so-called advanced or complicated lesion. These lesions are located primarily within the intima (innermost layer which contains endothelial cells) of the coronary artery; however, with more advanced lesions involvement of the medial layer (contains smooth muscle cells) has also been noted.[3] Each intimal lesion is thought to contain three elements: (1) smooth muscle cells; (2) large amounts of connective tissue matrix consisting of collagen, elastic fibers, and proteoglycans; and (3) intracellular and extracellular lipid. In addition to these components, platelets and monocytes/macrophages are thought to contribute to the atherosclerotic process.[4] The facts regarding the genesis of the lesions remain controversial. However, there is consensus that these lesions progress over a period of years and that plaque formation is not only a preventable process, but a reversible one.

Fatty Streak

The fatty streak, found in infants and children, is considered by some to be the earliest lesion of atherosclerosis.[5] Although not considered to be clinically significant, these fatty streaks are thought to be the precursor of the more complex lesion, the fibrous plaque. Recent investigations support earlier hypotheses that fatty streaks in the young are often found at the same anatomic sites as the fibrous plaque at older ages, lending further credence to the precursor–product relation between these two types of lesions.[5] Additional investigations in the future should provide further support or refutation of this relationship.

The fatty streak is often described as a yellowish, grossly flat, lipid-rich lesion consisting of both monocytes and macrophages and some smooth muscle cells. The lipid found in these smooth muscle cells is chiefly composed of cholesterol and cholesterol esters. These lipid-rich cells are commonly referred to as *foam cells*. These lesions may balloon out and protrude slightly into the lumen of the artery but are usually not obstructive to blood flow. These fatty streaks have been found in the coronary arteries around age 15 and continue to accumulate in these vessels until the third decade of life.[3]

Fibrous Plaque

Fibrous plaques, or atheromas, are white, pearly elevations of the intima which may protrude into the lumen of the artery, causing occlusion of the vessel.[3] These lesions are thought to develop around the second decade of life. During the development of the fibrous plaque, the principal change that takes place within the intima of the artery is the proliferation of smooth muscle cells. Smooth muscle cells are not usually found in the intima. They are contained chiefly in the medial layer of the artery. It is thought that the proliferation of smooth muscle cells is derived from the cells in the medial layer, although the exact mechanism of this needs to be further elucidated.[4]

One hypothesis of this smooth muscle cell proliferation comes from the work of Ross and co-workers in the 1970s.[4] They observed that when the arterial intima was damaged platelets would stick or disintegrate on the damaged site, liberating a platelet factor known as the *platelet-derived growth factor (PDGF)*. This PDGF, in turn, promoted proliferation of smooth muscle cells.[4]

Recent investigations further support this concept and have found PDGF to promote smooth muscle migration from the media to the intima, and that the PDGF also binds to receptor sites on smooth muscle cells.[5] Once these smooth muscle cells proliferate in the intima, they form what is known as a fibrous cap, which protrudes into the lumen of the artery. This fibrous cap is the result of connective tissue formation by the smooth muscle cells and the accumulation of lipids.

The accumulation of lipids is chiefly cholesterol in the form of low-density lipoproteins (LDL) or β-lipoprotein. This specific fraction of cholesterol is metabolized from very-low-density lipoproteins known as VLDL, or pre-β-lipoprotein. The pre-β-lipoprotein transports mostly triglycerides, whereas

LDL carries about three-quarters of the total serum cholesterol.[6] These lipoproteins will be discussed in further detail in the section, "Risk Factors."

The deep central core of the fibrous plaque also contains lipid and cell debris which is thought to result from inadequate blood supply to the central core, resulting in cell necrosis.[3] This necrotic core appears on gross examination as having a soft, porridgelike consistency. Other constituents found in some fibrous plaques include fibrin, fibrinogen, albumen, and white blood cells.[7] The proportions of all the components of a fibrous plaque vary from plaque to plaque. These proportions also may differ during the evolution or regression of a certain plaque.

Advanced or Complicated Lesion

The advanced or complicated lesion is a degenerative fibrous plaque (Fig. 21-1). The lipid-rich necrotic central core as described previously is thought to increase in size and become calcified.[5] As this lesion degenerates, rupture of the fibrous cap may occur with hemorrhage into the plaque. This rupture may further lead to thrombus formation.[5] In the event of thrombus formation on the plaque, the clot increases the thickness of the plaque, resulting in a reduction of the size of the lumen of the vessel. This sequela may in turn precipitate a myocardial infarction or sudden death. Aneurysmal formation may also develop as a result of the medial layer undergoing atrophy as the intimal lesion progresses and the number of smooth muscle cells in the media are reduced.[5]

Pathogenesis of Atherosclerosis

The data from a number of investigations have indicated that the pathogenesis of atherosclerosis involves several cell types such as the arterial smooth muscle cells of the medial layer, endothelial intimal cells, and macrophages.[4] In addition, there are two major processes; namely, smooth muscle cell proliferation and lipid accumulation (previously discussed), which contribute to progressive atherosclerosis having clinical significance. Various theories have been proposed regarding the pathogenesis of atherosclerosis. These include the lipogenic or lipid insudation theory, the response to injury theory, the thrombogenic theory, and the monoclonal theory.

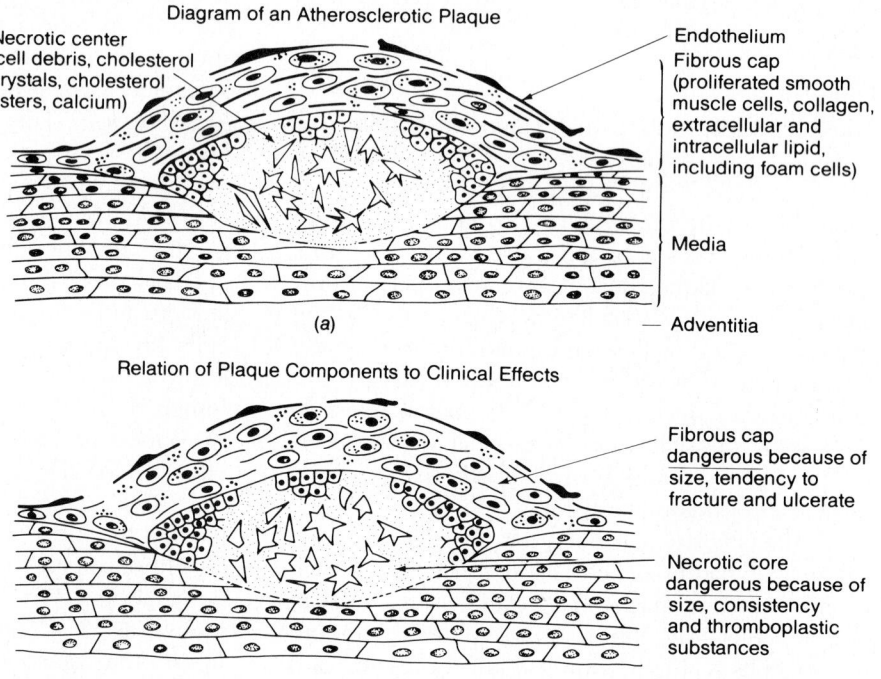

Figure 21-1 (*a*) Major components of the advanced or complicated (clinically important) atherosclerotic plaque. (*b*) Diagram depicting relationship of plaque components to clinical effects. (*Modified from R. W. Wissler, and D. Vesselinovitch. Animal models of regression. In G. Schettler, Y. Goto, Y. Hata, and G. Glose, eds., Atherosclerosis IV. Berlin: Springer-Verlag, 1977, p. 377*).

Diagram of an Atherosclerotic Plaque

Necrotic center (cell debris, cholesterol crystals, cholesterol esters, calcium)

Endothelium

Fibrous cap (proliferated smooth muscle cells, collagen, extracellular and intracellular lipid, including foam cells)

Media

Adventitia

(a)

Relation of Plaque Components to Clinical Effects

Fibrous cap dangerous because of size, tendency to fracture and ulcerate

Necrotic core dangerous because of size, consistency and thromboplastic substances

(b)

Lipogenic Hypothesis

According to the lipogenic hypothesis, markedly elevated levels of plasma low-density lipoprotein (LDL) in some individuals are associated with the development and progression of a fibrous plaque. The elevated levels of LDL may be a result of heredity, hypothyroidism, or ingestion of a high-fat or a high-cholesterol diet. According to Ross,[3] some studies in hyperlipidemic animals suggest that there are factors in LDL which promote proliferation of smooth muscle cells and the formation of a connective-tissue matrix by the smooth muscle cells. In addition, it is thought that with elevated levels of LDL, the high concentrations act as an irritant or chemical agent which weakens the endothelial barrier of the intima. Once injury has occurred to the vessel wall, LDL fractions seem to permeate into the intima and initiate proliferation of smooth muscle cells, although the exact mechanism is not known.[7] Further research in this area is warranted to extrapolate the exact mechanisms by which LDL is transported across the endothelial cells of the intima. This information regarding LDL transportation could then be used to develop some means to prevent this from occurring.

Response to Injury Hypothesis

According to the response to injury hypothesis, the endothelial cell which normally acts as a barrier that protects the intimal layer is injured by mechanical or chemical means.[8] This injury results in structural and/or functional changes to the endothelial cells, which include platelet adhesion, platelet aggregation, and proliferation of smooth muscle cells into the intima. The response to injury theory suggests that an abnormal response to injury may be precipitated by such risk factors as cigarette smoking, hypertension, and hyperlipidemia. In a revision of the response to injury theory, Ross[5] proposes that at least two pathways may lead to formation of intimal smooth muscle proliferative lesions (Fig. 21-2). One pathway suggests that, in experimentally induced hypercholesterolemia, injury to the endothelium may induce a growth factor secretion and also attachment of monocytes to the endothelium. The attached monocytes themselves may continue to secrete growth factors. Once the subendothelial migration of the monocytes occurs (referred to as *macrophages* once they are inside the cell), fatty streak formation appears to develop, along with the release of other growth factors such as PDGF. The fatty streaks are thought to become directly converted to fibrous plaques through release of these growth factors. Platelet adherence is promoted in certain cases when the macrophages lose their endothelial cover. The platelets also release PDGF which in turn can induce both smooth muscle migration and proliferation.[5]

Other investigators have found that the monocytes which adhere to the endothelium are transformed into macrophages once the monocytes migrate into the intima.[9] Additionally, these macrophages have been found to be scavengers of plasma lipoproteins and cholesterol, promoting lipid accumulation in the intima.

The second pathway suggests that the injured endothelium remains intact but results in a growth factor released by the injured cells. This release of a growth factor is thought to stimulate migration of smooth muscle cells from the media into the intima. As previously mentioned, the smooth muscle cell proliferation is then thought to incite fibrous plaque formation and further lesion progression. Ross[5] suggests that this second pathway may be the result of those previously stated risk factors such as hypertension and cigarette smoking, or diabetes causing injury to the endothelium.

Thrombogenic Theory

The thrombogenic theory or encrustation theory proposes that a thrombus is the first stage of a fibrous plaque and that the thrombus is transformed into a mass of dense connective tissue known as *fibroblasts.*[7] Smooth muscle cell proliferation occurs and migrates into the thrombus. Most researchers have incorporated this hypothesis into the response to injury theory such that with endothelial injury there is platelet stickiness, aggregation, and release of granules leading to thrombus formation.[7] It has been mentioned before that Ross[5] and coworkers demonstrated in animals that platelets release PDGF, which causes migration and proliferation of smooth muscle cells from the media into the intima. Prevention of intimal proliferative lesions induced by endothelial injury can be accomplished by preventing platelets from aggregating at sites of endothelial injury through pharmacologically preventing platelet interactions, which is the premise

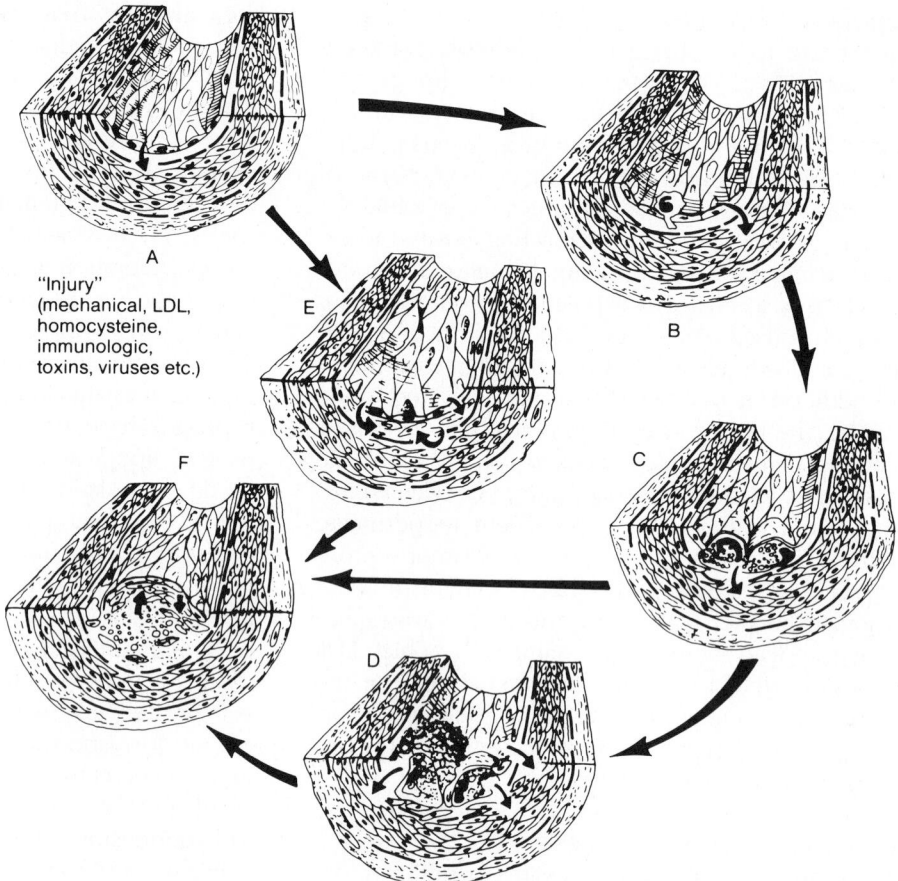

"Injury"
(mechanical, LDL,
homocysteine,
immunologic,
toxins, viruses etc.)

Figure 21-2 Advanced intimal proliferative lesions of atherosclerosis may occur by at least two pathways. The pathway demonstrated by the clockwise (long) arrows to the right has been observed in experimentally induced hypercholesterolemia. Injury to the endothelium (A) may induce growth secretion (short arrow). Monocytes attach to endothelium (B), which may continue to secrete growth factors (short arrow). Subendothelial migration of monocytes (C) may lead to fatty-streak formation and release of growth factors such as PDGF (short arrow). Fatty streaks may become directly converted to fibrous plaques (long arrow from C to F) through release of growth factors from macrophages or endothelial cells or both. Macrophages may also stimulate or injure the overlying endothelium. In some cases, macrophages may lose their endothelial cover and platelet attachment may occur (D), providing three possible sources of growth factors—platelets, macrophages, and endothelium (short arrows). Some of the smooth muscle cells in the proliferative lesion itself (F) may form and secrete growth factors such as PDGF (short arrows). An alternative pathway for development of advanced lesions of atherosclerosis is shown by the arrows from A to E to F. In this case, the endothelium may be injured but remain intact. Increased endothelial turnover may result in growth-factor formation by endothelial cells (A). This may stimulate migration of smooth muscle cells from the media into the intima, accompanied by endogenous production of PDGF by smooth muscle as well as growth factor secretion from the "injured" endothelial cells (E). These interactions could then lead to fibrous plaque formation and further lesion progression (F). (*From R. Ross. The pathogenesis of atherosclerosis—an update. New England Journal of Medicine, 314:488–500.*)

for giving antiplatelet drugs or thrombolytic agents.[5]

Monoclonal Theory

The monoclonal theory proposes that each atherosclerotic lesion is begun from a single smooth muscle cell and the remaining proliferative cells within the lesion are descendants or clones of that single cell. This hypothesis was first proposed by Benditt and Benditt.[3] These investigators relate the monotypic lesion to a benign neoplasm that may be a sequela of cell transformation by mutagenic agents such as toxins, viruses, or chemical agents. However, additional research seems to be required to support or refute this hypothesis, because additional research has provided conflicting data.[3]

It appears that a great deal of new information is emerging at the cellular and molecular level regarding the genesis of atherosclerosis. Most of the data have been based chiefly on animal research, so caution needs to be exercised in extrapolating results from animal studies to humans, primarily because the experimentally induced atherosclerotic plaque in animals has been found to develop differently from the human atherosclerotic lesion. Furthermore, successful attempts to cause regression of animal plaques should not be entirely applied to humans until carefully controlled randomized studies in humans is attempted. Thus, the concept that atherosclerosis in humans is a preventable or reversible process as has been demonstrated in animal research, will need further clarification through human investigation. Moreover, substantial inquiry into the role of certain risk factors into the pathogenesis of atherosclerosis will also be necessary.

Risk Factors

Recognition of risk factors associated with the development of CAD has been attained chiefly through epidemiologic studies. Several studies were undertaken in the 1940s and 1950s to identify the factors associated with the incidence of CAD.[1] As a result of these studies, it was observed that the rate of occurrence differed by such demographical factors as age, race, sex, and geography.[6] In addition, hyperlipidemia, hypertension, hyperglycemia, and obesity were found to be associated with an in-

creased incidence of the disease.[10] Other factors linked with an increased prevalence of CAD were cigarette smoking, lack of exercise, stress, oral contraceptives, and personality traits.[11] Data also indicate that there may be a familial or genetic predisposition to the development of CAD.[6,12]

In grouping all these risk factors, two categories emerge. The first includes those risk factors regarded as unavoidable or unmodifiable. Included in this group are age, sex, heredity, and geography. The second group consists of those risk factors considered avoidable or modifiable, including hypertension, hyperlipidemia, cigarette smoking, hyperglycemia, obesity, physical inactivity, personality traits, and oral contraceptives. Moreover, all these risk factors (unavoidable and avoidable) tend to have a multiplicative or synergistic effect on each other, such that multiple risk factors present in one individual tend to multiply the risk of developing CAD far more than one single risk factor alone.

Because CAD has been linked to life-style and habits, the following modifications of those avoidable risk factors have been recommended by the American Heart Association (AHA):[13]

1. Cessation of cigarette smoking
2. Control of hypertension by diet and/or medication and weight reduction
3. Decrease of serum cholesterol levels by reducing dietary saturated fat and cholesterol
4. Reduction of caloric intake to achieve ideal body weight
5. Engage in moderate exercise
6. Control of diabetes mellitus
7. Monitor use of oral contraceptives

Prevention of the risk factors described above involves *primary* and *secondary* measures. *Primary* prevention involves risk factor modification before clinical manifestations of coronary artery disease occur. *Secondary* prevention of risk factors refers to those measures begun to minimize the progression of CAD or prevent recurrences of catastrophic events such as MI in patients with documented CAD.

Unavoidable Risk Factors

Age, Sex, and Race

The mortality rates from CAD in the United States from 1950 to 1977 indicated that male mortality rates were much higher than those for females in both white and nonwhite populations.[1] For example, in comparing both white males and females between the ages of 35 and 44, male mortality was 5.2 times greater than that of females. By contrast, the same age group in nonwhite males and females revealed a male mortality rate that was 2.8 times greater than that of females in the group. It is interesting to note that during this same period of 1950 to 1977, the incidence of CAD in both white and nonwhite females increased dramatically after menopause.[1]

It is also noteworthy that in comparing white and nonwhite male mortality rates from 1950 to 1977 in the United States, that prior to 1968, nonwhite men had lower rates than white men; however, since 1968, nonwhite males have had higher rates up to the age of 65.[1] By contrast, in nonwhite and white females, the nonwhite females have had higher mortality rates than their white female counterparts throughout the period of 1950 to 1977.[1]

Certain ethnic groups in the United States, such as Japanese men residing in Hawaii or California, the Eskimo in Alaska, and men in Puerto Rico, have a much lower incidence of CAD than Caucasians.[1] Furthermore, Japanese men residing in Japan have a lower incidence of CAD than their male counterparts living in Hawaii or California. Therefore, when looking at Japanese men, for example, in various countries, one must consider how long they have lived in those locations and their life-style differences such as diet, working habits, and living conditions. Perhaps ethnic origin, which is unmodifiable, is related to life-style, which can be modified within a certain race.

Heredity

Although coronary artery disease is considered to be of uncertain genetic background, most researchers agree that it tends to be familial. Some families appear to have a predisposition to premature development of atherosclerosis, excluding those with known hyperlipidemias. Furthermore, it has been noted that both male and female relatives of men who died of coronary disease before 55 years of age had a fivefold and twofold higher risk of developing CAD, respectively.[14]

Geography

The incidence of CAD is variable throughout the United States and in other countries. A higher incidence of CAD has been reported along the southeastern Atlantic coast of the United States and in the industrialized states of the midwest and northeast, while a lower incidence has been noted in the Great Plains and some of the mountain states.[1] These rather clear regional differences in the incidence of CAD have not been adequately explained, although these differences have led to interest in the possibility that certain environmental conditions such as temperature, weather conditions, and altitude might have some influence.

The highest incidence of CAD in the world is found chiefly in industrialized nations, with the exception of Japan, which has one of the lowest incidences of CAD.[1] A plausible explanation for the increased incidence of CAD in industrialized nations is related to the difference in dietary habits, life-style, and affluence in those nations that have increased technology as compared to those poorer populations.

Avoidable Risk Factors

There are major risk factors which are considered avoidable. Among these avoidable risk factors are major and minor ones. The major risk factors include hypertension, hyperlipidemia, cigarette smoking, and hyperglycemia.

Hypertension

Hypertension is associated with an increased risk of developing CAD. It is often referred to as the "silent killer" because an individual may have the disease for up to 10 to 20 years or longer and may not be cognizant of its existence. By the time hypertension is discovered, damage to vital organs may be present. It is thought that the mechanism by which hypertension is related to CAD is that the chronic, persistent tension in the arterial walls that hypertension exerts, leads to injury and/or structural changes in the intimal layer of the coronary vessels.[3] These changes act to accelerate the development of atherosclerosis which may in turn lead to angina and myocardial infarction.

Systolic blood pressure elevation has been found to be a better predictor of the risk of developing CAD than diastolic blood pressure, especially in the elderly.[1,6,15] Until recently, most clinicians were concerned with elevations in the diastolic blood pressure rather than elevations in systolic blood pressure.

A sequela of hypertension, namely left ventricular hypertrophy (LVH), is also strongly associated with the risk of a coronary event. This finding comes from the Framingham study whereby it was documented that 44 percent of deaths related to CAD were heralded by electrographic evidence of LVH.[12] This ventricular enlargement is a compensatory mechanism to the increase in wall tension exerted to overcome high aortic pressure gradients. Thus, left ventricular hypertrophy develops when there is continued impedance to left ventricular ejection. Left ventricular hypertrophy as noted on an ECG is depicted by increased voltage of the QRS complexes and the typical "R wave plus S wave" voltage that is greater than 35 mm in certain precordial leads.

Identification and early treatment of hypertension is imperative in preventing the complications associated with prolonged, elevated blood pressure. The reader is referred to Chap. 22 for further discussion of hypertension.

Hyperlipidemia or Hyperlipoproteinemia

Wissler[4] states categorically that, among the numerous risk factors for the development of atherosclerosis, one of the best documented is the association between blood lipids and CAD. It is interesting to note that scientific data have indicated that no population with a severely reduced dietary intake of cholesterol has developed atherosclerotic heart disease.[4] In various studies it has been found that development of atherosclerosis does not occur until a certain threshold amount of cholesterol-rich lipoproteins has been reached in the body.[1] This threshold tends to be quite variable and is dependent on the individual as well as the presence of other risk factors. The etiology of sustained levels of serum cholesterol (hypercholesterolemia) in atherosclerotic heart disease may be genetically induced, secondary to a metabolic disorder, such as hypothyroidism, or caused by the elevated intake of a high-fat, high-cholesterol diet.

The term *hyperlipidemia* is used in reference to an elevation of one or both of the commonly known lipids referred to as cholesterol and triglycerides. These lipids are insoluble in plasma and are, therefore, transported in the serum in the form of lipoprotein complexes. According to Levy and Feinleib,[1] prospective studies have shown inconclusive results in implicating serum triglycerides as a coronary risk factor. In contrast, results from several prospective studies have unequivocally indicated that the risk of CAD in an otherwise healthy person is directly related to the concentration of plasma cholesterol.[16] Moreover, clinicians are now measuring the plasma cholesterol in terms of the lipoproteins rather than evaluating the total serum cholesterol.[16]

Lipoproteins are produced in the gut and liver and each has distinct functions in transporting exogenous and endogenous lipids.[17] An elevation of lipoproteins is referred to as *hyperlipoproteinemia*. Lipoproteins are broken down into the following subgroups or fractions, based on their density and chemical breakdown: chylomicrons, very-low-density lipoproteins (VLDL), intermediate-low-density lipoproteins (ILDL), low-density lipoproteins (LDL), and high-density lipoproteins (HDL).

Chylomicrons are derived from exogenous dietary fat. They are metabolized in the small intestine. Chylomicrons are composed mainly of triglycerides and small amounts of cholesterol. When released into the systemic circulation, they are hydrolyzed rapidly by the enzyme lipoprotein lipase. After chylomicrons undergo hydrolysis in the circulation, they are transported to the liver for the removal of cholesterol. After 12 to 14 h of fasting, chylomicrons are usually absent in plasma, and their presence in fasting plasma is considered to be an abnormal finding. Elevations of chylomicrons have not been linked with premature CAD.[1]

Another type of lipoprotein, very-low-density lipoproteins (VLDL), are also known as pre-*β*-lipoproteins. The main functions of VLDLs are to transport triglycerides from the liver to peripheral tissue and to serve as a precursor for LDL. Increases in triglyceride levels are associated with high dietary intake of carbohydrates. An excess of VLDL is associated with hypertriglyceridemia and premature atherosclerosis.[1]

Intermediate-low-density-lipoproteins (ILDL) are an intermediate form in the metabolism of VLDL to LDL. In certain types of hyperlipoproteinemia ILDL-like particles have been associated with premature coronary artery disease.[1]

Low-density lipoproteins (LDL) are obtained from the breakdown of VLDL. They serve primarily to transport large amounts (50 to 75 percent) of cholesterol from the liver to peripheral tissues. Another term for LDL is *ß*-lipoprotein. This lipoprotein has been most directly linked with CAD because patients with elevated levels of LDL tend to have CAD more often than those with normal levels of LDL. It has been found that patients with this type of hyperlipoproteinemia have concomitant hypercholesterolemia.[6]

High-density lipoproteins (HDL) are produced in the hepatocyte and secreted from the liver. These lipoproteins have been implicated in having a protective effect against atherosclerosis.[1] The cause and effect of this inverse relationship remain to be elucidated. It is also thought that the ratio of HDL to LDL may be a *better* predictor of coronary risk than either value alone, although some studies have indicated that HDL may remove LDL cholesterol from tissue.[16] High concentrations of HDL are noteworthy in such groups as children and premenopausal women, who tend as groups to have low coronary risk. It has also been found that exercise, reduction in obesity, cessation of cigarette smoking, and, lastly, consumption of al-

coholic beverages, may elevate HDL levels.[6] Recently, subfractions of both LDL and HDL have been identified through in vitro studies.[4,6] LDL_1 is thought to be the fraction involved in the atherosclerotic process in humans, whereas HDL_2 may be the protective fraction against atherosclerosis.[4]

A summary of the biochemical and clinical features of the lipoproteins previously discussed is found in Table 21-1. Additional information regarding the catabolism and clinical features is also provided in this table.

Hyperlipidemias are classified into five types based on evaluation of laboratory data. Table 21-2 lists these categories and illustrates the lipoprotein abnormality found in each type.

Cigarette Smoking

Cigarette smoking has been considered one of the major health hazards in this country. Cigarette smoking has been associated with even more deaths from CAD than from all the cancers it can cause. According to the Framingham study, cigarette smokers had a risk of CAD two to four times greater than the risk for nonsmokers.[18] The risk is also multiplicative or synergistic in that moderate cigarette smoking doubles or triples the susceptibility to CAD when associated with other risk factors.[6] Other factors associated with an increased risk of

Table 21-1 Biochemical and Clinical Features of Lipoproteins

Family	Origin	Function	Clinical Features of Elevated Level
Chylomicrons	Intestine, from dietary fat	Transport of dietary fat	Eruptive xanthoma, lipemia retinalis, organomegaly, pancreatitis
VLDL	Liver and small bowel, from carbohydrates, free fatty acids, medium-chain triglycerides	Transport of endogenous trigylcerides	Glucose intolerance; hyperuricemia
ILDL	VLDL	Unknown	Glucose intolerance; hyperuricemia; premature atherosclerosis; tuboeruptive, tendinous, and palmar planar xanthoma
LDL	VLDK; ILDL (? alternative source)	Unknown	Premature atherosclerosis, corneal arcus, tendinous and tuberous xanthoma, xanthelasma
HDL	? Intestine ? Liver	? Facilitates cholesterol ester and triglyceride metabolism	No associated abnormality

Adapted from R. I. Levy and M. Feinlieb, Risk Factors for Coronary Artery Disease and Their Management. In E. Braunwald (ed.), *Heart Disease*, Philadelphia: Saunders, 1984.

Table 21-2 Classification of Hyperlipidemias

Type	Lipoprotein Abnormality
I	Chylomicrons markedly increased VLDL, LDL normal or low
IIA	Increased LDL, VLDL normal
IIB	Increased LDL and VLDL
III	Increased ILDL; enriched VLDL present, in excess
IV	Increased VLDL, LDL normal
V	Chylomicrons markedly increased; increased VLDL, LDL normal or low

developing CAD include the age one started smoking, the number of years one smoked, the number of cigarettes smoked per day, and how deeply one inhales the smoke.[1,6] Furthermore, the risk of infarction has also been shown to correlate with the number of cigarettes smoked for both women and men.[1] In addition, women who take oral contraceptives and smoke have a significantly increased vulnerability to myocardial infarctions.

Some mechanisms by which cigarette smoking may induce coronary artery disease include the following:

1. The inhalation of cigarette smoke may result in exposure of arterial cells to mutagens that alter the smooth muscle cells and result in proliferation of these cells.[3]
2. Higher levels of LDL, cholesterol, and triglycerides as well as lower levels of HDL have been found in men and women who smoked more than 15 cigarettes daily as compared to nonsmokers.[6]
3. Cigarette smoking was found to increase the adhesiveness of platelets, perhaps leading to thrombus formation.[1]
4. Carboxyhemoglobin has been found to interfere with coronary oxygen supply.[1]
5. Increased myocardial demand for oxygen secondary to nicotine inhalation has been noted.[1]
6. Nicotine causes release of catecholamines, which increases heart rate and myocardial oxygen (MV_{O_2}) consumption.[1]

Further research is necessary, however, to identify the specific cellular mechanisms that are altered by cigarette smoking.

It has been suggested that cessation of cigarette smoking decreases the risk of atherosclerosis and may induce regression of lesions. The risk decreases about 50 percent within the first year following cessation and approaches the same risk as that of nonsmokers in about 2 to 10 years. Also, the level of HDL has been found to increase, while levels of LDL decrease once cigarette smoking has been discontinued.[1,6]

Hyperglycemia

The Framingham study clearly identified a relationship between CAD and hyperglycemia which was as strong for men as it was for women.[11] It has been found that the type of diabetes was also significant. For example, type II or adult-onset diabetes was associated with more deaths from CAD than type I or juvenile-onset diabetes, in which there were more deaths from renal disease.[11] Both male and female adult-onset diabetics (type II) have a 50 percent greater incidence of developing CAD than type I diabetics.[11]

Several complex mechanisms between hyperglycemia and CAD have been proposed. The first involves the effect of insulin and glucose on the arterial wall. High serum insulin levels may incite proliferation of smooth muscle cells and synthesis of cholesterol and triglyceride.[19] Secondly, hyperglycemia may cause increased adhesiveness of platelets as well as other abnormalities of coagulation, setting the stage for thrombus development.[19] Lastly, there are some data indicating that diabetics tend to have decreased levels of HDL, increasing their vulnerability to CAD.[1]

Control of hyperglycemia alone has not been shown to eliminate the risk of CAD. It appears that concomitant risk reduction of other factors such as obesity, hypertension, and hypercholesterolemia may be necessary to decrease the risk.[6]

Minor Risk Factors

Minor risk factors have been associated with an increased incidence of CAD; among these are obesity, physical inactivity, personality traits, and oral contraceptives. These will be highlighted in the ensuing discussion.

Obesity

Obesity is considered to contribute significantly to the severity of such major risk factors as hypertension, hyperglycemia, and hyperlipidemia. Patients who are obese also tend to have higher levels of LDL linked to premature atherosclerosis and lower levels of HDL. Furthermore, it has been suggested that obesity may alone be a risk factor in such populations as the young and the Japanese men in Hawaii, who otherwise have few risk factors predisposing them to CAD.[1]

Physical Inactivity

Until about a decade ago, very few people were aware of exercise as a factor associated with decreased coronary risk. Several studies have shown that HDLs are decreased below normal in sedentary people compared to elevated HDL levels noted in people following both short- and long-term exercise.[6] According to Wenger and Schlant,[6] the following favorable effects are achieved through exercise: (1) decreased weight, (2) increased cardiovascular functional capacity, (3) reduced myocardial oxygen demand, (4) decreased platelet adhesiveness and improved fibrinolysis, and (5) electrical stability of the myocardium. These effects suggest that regular exercise is a positive influence for decreasing the risk of CAD than is physical inactivity, although additional research is necessary to confirm exercise as a direct factor in the prevention of coronary artery disease.

Personality Traits

Personality and behavioral traits are the psychosocial factors that are the most consistently related to coronary artery disease. The Western Collaborative Study showed that men with type A personality traits developed coronary artery disease at two times the rate of individuals with a type B personality.[20] The Framingham study also supported this fact.[1]

Individuals with type A personality are characterized by a chronic struggle to obtain an unlimited number of items from the environment in the shortest period of time, despite environmental constraints. These individuals characteristically behave in a hostile, impatient, aggressive, and highly competitive manner. In contrast, the type B personality tends to be more patient, less aggressive, and is not as concerned with either deadlines or any habitual sense of time urgency.

To date, the exact mechanism whereby personality traits contribute to the pathogenesis of CAD is unknown. However, people with type A personalities tend to have increased circulating catecholamines. These endogenous amines may cause hypertension and abnormal platelet function, contributing indirectly to the development of atherosclerotic heart disease.[6,21]

Oral Contraceptives

The use of oral contraceptives seems to be related to an increased risk of CAD, especially in postmenopausal women. The risk of myocardial infarction is also associated with those premenopausal women who concomitantly suffer from hypertension and diabetes. Another significantly high risk group for the development of an MI are women who take oral contraceptives and who smoke cigarettes, as has been previously mentioned.[1]

Oral contraceptives have also been found to raise blood pressure and alter serum levels of lipoproteins. These contraceptives create disturbances in the clotting cascade and favor thrombus formation. It has also been noted that contraceptives which contain progestin tend to decrease levels of HDL cholesterol, whereas those contraceptives containing estrogen tend to increase the levels of cholesterol.[1]

Conclusion

Data from both epidemiologic and clinical studies indicate that coronary artery disease in humans may be due to multiple risk factors and not only to hypercholesterolemia as noted in basic research findings. Reduction of risk factors through primary prevention is thought to have the most beneficial effect if done before clinical findings of CAD become evident. Data indicating the ability to hinder or reverse CAD in humans by modification of risk factors is unequivocal. One study known as the Multiple Risk Factor Intervention Trial (MRFIT) attempted to modify three factors specifically, hypertension, cigarette smoking, and hyperglycemia, in 12,866 high-risk men aged 35 to 57 through a special intervention program. The results from this study did not document a mortality benefit over a 6-year period.[1,6] In contrast, the results from the Lipid Research Clinics Coronary Primary Prevention trial demonstrated for the first time a direct cause-and-effect relationship between plasma lipoproteins and cholesterol levels with morbidity and mortality from coronary artery disease.[22] This trial was a randomized double-blind study in which the efficacy of lowering cholesterol levels in reducing the risk of coronary artery disease was tested. The sample population consisted of 3806 middle-aged men with type II hyperlipoproteinemia (elevated LDL levels). The treatment group (1906 subjects) received the bile acid cholestyramine. The control group (1900 subjects) received a placebo for 7.4 years. Both groups were also placed on a moderate cholesterol-lowering diet. Low-density lipoprotein levels were elevated for each group along with the primary end point of coronary heart disease, death and/or definite nonfatal myocardial infarction. The data revealed that the treatment group had lower levels of low-density lipoproteins in comparison to the placebo group. The treatment group also had a significantly decreased incidence of CAD in comparison to the placebo group. This trial provided a strong cause-and-effect relationship between low-density lipoproteins in the pathogenesis of coronary heart disease.[22]

The importance of each risk factor may also be influenced by the genetic composition of each individual. Thus, each individual differs in susceptibility to each of the risk factors. Lastly, newer approaches to the prevention, treatment, or progression of CAD continue to be developed through additional research that discovers how each of these risk factors is related to the specific cellular structural and/or functional interactions that lead to atherosclerosis.

Angina Pectoris

In the majority of cases, angina pectoris is associated with an atherosclerotic lesion causing greater than 75 percent occlusion of the lumen of a specific coronary artery. Angina pectoris is a symptom of myocardial ischemia which literally means "choking of the chest," from the Greek word *anchein,* meaning "to choke." It is a manifestation of the disparity between myocardial oxygen demand and supply. The ability of the heart to increase blood flow when there is an increased oxygen demand is limited by the intraluminal obstruction of the atherosclerotic lesion. This fixed arterial obstruction in turn leads to an insufficient arterial oxygen supply in the coronary vasculature and results in ischemia and

chest pain, especially when the demand exceeds the supply. This type of angina is often referred to as *classic, effort,* or *exertional angina,* because the fixed coronary artery lesion impedes myocardial blood flow, leading to ischemia at a certain level of exertion.

A different type of angina presents itself typically at rest, suggesting that a discrepancy in supply suddenly exists as the demand remains relatively constant. This finding led investigators, notably Prinzmetal and coworkers in the 1950s, to probe for functional changes in the lumen of the coronary vessel.[23] They were able to document the presence of coronary vasoconstriction or coronary vasospasm in patients who experienced pain spontaneously at rest, and in whom ST segment elevation was depicted on the ECG during pain. Prinzmetal referred to this rest pain as *coronary spasm,* or *variant angina.* Variant angina can occur in two subsets of patients: those with atherosclerotic lesions and those with normal or near-normal coronary arteries.

There are two ends of a spectrum for patients who present with angina. The first is *effort* or *exertional angina,* in which ischemia is secondary to increases in myocardial oxygen demand, and the second is *coronary spasm* or *variant angina,* in which ischemia is secondary to reduction in supply induced by vasoconstriction of a coronary artery. The term *mixed angina* is referred to by some clinicians as a combination of pure exertional angina and coronary vasospasm.[24] Typically, these patients have a fixed obstruction with concomitant vasoconstriction (spasm) which precipitate ischemia, with or without increased oxygen demand.

There are other causes of angina. These include systemic hypertension, aortic stenosis or regurgitation, cardiac dysrhythmias, anemia, and hyperthyroidism.

Physical Assessment

The chest pain of classic angina pectoris is typically described as substernal chest discomfort or pain with a sensation of pressure or heaviness which occurs with activity and is relieved by rest. The pressure may be associated with a burning or itching in the chest. This chest discomfort gradually increases in intensity and is followed by a gradual fading away. Occasionally, some diabetic patients may not complain of chest pain, only dyspnea, because they may have developed peripheral neuropathy which prevents chest pain from being experienced.

The sensation of angina may appear in many locations but the most common is the middle or lower sternum, or over the left precordium, which in some patients may be confused with indigestion. Patients may complain of left shoulder pain or upper arm pain that may be mistaken for arthritis. When pain extends down the arm, usually the fourth and fifth fingers are involved. Patients may rarely complain of jaw pain. Occasionally, patients describe pain in the posterior thorax or intrascapular area. If a careful assessment is not made, the pain may be attributed to back ailments. When describing angina, patients commonly use their fist to describe the location of discomfort rather than pointing with their finger (Levine's sign).

Patients may also develop associated symptoms during an anginal attack. These symptoms include nausea, vomiting, diaphoresis, dyspnea, and exhaustion. They may appear pale or dusky with signs of labored breathing. Their skin may be clammy and cool. Certain cardiac dysrhythmias may occur with angina related to transient ischemia of a small area of heart tissue. In addition, patients may experience an increase in heart rate and blood pressure. Usually these signs and symptoms subside with resolution of the anginal attack.

Stimuli which may provoke an anginal episode include physical activity, cold or hot weather exposure, heavy eating, sexual intercourse, emotional stress factors, cigarette smoking, and rapid-eye-movement (REM) sleep. Physical activity commonly provokes an anginal attack because it increases myocardial oxygen demand. The discomfort usually occurs during the attack, rather than after the activity. The "second wind" phenomenon refers to a small group of patients who characteristically develop symptoms during the activity, but whose discomfort disappears while the activity is continued.

Exposure to hot or cold weather places an increased workload on the heart, thereby increasing myocardial oxygen demand. Heavy eating may precipitate an anginal attack because there is an increase in gastrointestinal oxygen demand which, in turn, increases cardiac output to the gut, thereby placing more demand on the heart. Sexual inter-

course also increases the workload on the heart and, therefore, causes an increased demand. Emotional stress factors such as anger, fear, and enthusiasm are known precursors of angina in that they increase circulating catecholamines which increase heart rate and contractility, thereby increasing myocardial oxygen demand. Angina is believed to be precipitated by cigarette smoking because the nicotine is thought to stimulate the release of Adrenalin which increases the work of the heart. Angina is also thought to occur during rapid-eye-movement (REM) sleep because of stimulation of the sympathetic nervous system which, in turn, increases myocardial oxygen demand by increasing heart rate, blood pressure, and contractility.[25]

The duration of angina pectoris precipitated by effort is usually 1 to 5 min, once the patient discontinues the activity. However, angina provoked by emotional stress factors typically lasts longer than effort angina because emotional factors are not as easy to control as physical activity.[26]

The chest pain of coronary vasospasm or variant angina is typically similar to classic or effort angina, but differs in that the chest pain occurs at rest. This rest pain often presents in a cyclic or predictive pattern in that the chest pain occurs around the same time every day in a particular patient. Notably, this rest pain tends to occur in the early morning hours. Kirshenbaum[27] suggests that the etiology of this occurrence may be related to increased levels of endogenous circulating catecholamines present in the body from 3 to 5 A.M. Associated symptoms include syncope, dyspnea, and palpitations.

Precipitating factors of variant angina have also been identified. For example, cigarette smoking, alcohol, and cocaine have been implicated in inciting variant angina.[27–29] This type of angina has also been reported in non-bypassed coronary arteries following myocardial revascularization.[30]

Categories of Angina

Stable Angina

Stable angina is also referred to as *classical angina,* and is usually triggered by physical exertion or emotional stress as previously discussed. This type of pain is noted to be unchanged over several months. The pain typically lasts 1 to 5 min and is relieved by rest. Thus, each attack of stable angina is similar to the previous episode and is relieved by the same mode of therapy.

Unstable Angina

Unstable angina, preinfarction angina, or *crescendo angina* are the terms used to describe the first episode of angina, rest angina, postinfarction angina, or stable angina when there has been a change in the timing, frequency, intensity, duration, and quality of stable angina. This type of angina is easily provoked with lower exercise workloads than stable angina. There is increased severity of pain with unstable angina, typically lasting longer (10 min), despite rest and the use of sublingual nitroglycerin. Moreover, this type of angina is harder to control with other pharmacologic therapy and may mimic the symptoms of a myocardial infarction. The patient with unstable angina may also be in jeopardy for myocardial infarction and sudden death.

Silent Ischemia

The term *silent ischemia* (asymptomatic myocardial ischemia) has received much attention lately in the medical literature. It has been defined as the presence of objective evidence of ischemia (as shown by electrocardiographic, exercise test, or radionuclide findings) in asymptomatic patients with or without documented coronary artery disease.[31,32] There are currently three subsets of patients who may evidence silent ischemia: (1) those who have no accompanying symptoms of angina but show ST segment shifts on exercise testing or ambulatory ECG monitoring, (2) those with asymptomatic postinfarction who demonstrate ST segment changes on exercise testing or ambulatory monitoring, and (3) those with angina pectoris who have multiple episodes of silent ischemia as documented by 24-h Holter monitoring.[31,32] According to Pratt,[31] it is postulated that patients with silent ischemic episodes may have higher pain thresholds than others. It is also theorized that this syndrome may be related to a reduction in myocardial oxygen supply secondary to vasospasm in contrast to an increase in myocardial oxygen demand as noted in classic angina.[32] Lastly, there have been no studies previously which have evaluated the efficacy of drug therapy on reducing the number of silent ischemia attacks and whether or not reducing the incidence of these attacks will have any effect on morbidity or mortality for these patients. Future research will hopefully resolve these many unanswered questions about this important syndrome.

Diagnostic Procedures

Electrocardiogram

The electrocardiogram (ECG) at rest is of limited importance in the diagnosis of angina pectoris related to atherosclerotic heart disease, except in diagnosing an old myocardial infarction. Normal resting ECGs have been noted in approximately 50 to 70 percent of patients with stable angina pectoris.[26] Transient ST depression of 1 mm or greater has been recorded in some patients during an episode of angina pectoris and has also been observed in patients experiencing silent ischemia but no pain.[26] This ST segment depression is characteristic of myocardial ischemia.

In variant angina, the ECG is probably one of the most diagnostic tools. Typically, during this type of angina the ECG will display transient ST segment elevations in the leads relative to the ischemic areas. Interestingly, there have also been reports of ST segment depression in such patients.[33] Evaluations of ST segments are considered by many as pathognomonic for coronary spasm, but in no way permit the diagnosis of the presence or absence of an atherosclerotic lesion at the site of the spasm.[27] Concomitant with this typical finding of variant angina may be a multitude of dysrhythmias. Ventricular dysrhythmias such as premature beats, ventricular tachycardia, or ventricular fibrillation may present in such patients. Atrioventricular block such as second- and third-degree heart block may also occur during chest pain indicative of spasm of the right coronary artery.[27]

Holter or ambulatory monitoring is useful in the evaluation of patients suspected of having atherosclerotic heart disease, silent ischemia, or coronary spasm. It enables clinicians to document ischemic changes such as ST segment depression during activities and over an extended period of time.

The exercise electrocardiogram is another worthwhile tool used to reveal ECG changes during and after exercise in contrast to the resting ECG in patients with stable angina pectoris. It is usually contraindicated in patients displaying unstable angina pectoris. Exercise stress testing can be accomplished using a bicycle ergometer, treadmill, or the master two-step test. The patient is exercised under controlled ECG monitoring conditions until certain findings are noted or until the patient reaches a predetermined heart rate. A positive stress test is indicated by the following: (1) onset of ST segment depression within the first 3 min of exercise, (2) persistent ST segment depression 8 min after exercise, (3) downward sloping or 2-mm ST depression for at least 0.8 s, or (4) hypotension.[26] These findings also suggest multivessel or left main disease involvement. It is important to note that both false positives and false negatives have been documented using the exercise stress test.[34,35] False-positive tests occur with greater frequency in the population with a less positive (less than 2-mm ST depression) exercise test and in premenopausal women.[35]

The exercise stress test is of limited value in patients with coronary vasospasm because spasm rarely occurs during exercise. However, a recent normal exercise test in a patient who then presents with a pain history similar to unstable angina should alert clinicians to the likelihood of coronary spasm.[27] The exercise stress test is also useful in diagnosing silent ischemia in asymptomatic patients after a positive stress test.

Radionuclide Imaging

Radionuclide imaging with thallium and radionuclide angiography with technetium are tools useful for evaluating patients with suspected CAD or to determine the extent and severity of the disease during exercise stress testing. Patients with stable angina are candidates for either test. The patient with unstable or variant angina usually is not a candidate for such testing.

In the thallium exercise stress test, thallium is injected once the patient becomes physically exhausted or develops angina. Following injection, myocardial scintigraphic images are obtained to reveal regions of underperfusion that develop with exercise. The amount of thallium present in each region is determined by two factors: (1) the amount of coronary blood flow to that region, and (2) the degree of viable myocardium. Ischemic or infarcted myocardial regions receiving little or no blood flow

accumulate minimal or no amounts of the injected thallium. Such regions are referred to as "cold spots" and are suggestive of the presence of coronary artery disease.[36]

Nuclear imaging with technetium bound to human serum albumin or red blood cells allows evaluation of global and segmental ventricular performance. This test is more useful in diagnosing myocardial infarction and is further described in that section.

Cardiac Catheterization and Coronary Arteriography

The data from cardiac catheterization and coronary arteriography are used to assess the hemodynamic status of the heart, left ventricular performance, and the presence, severity, and/or distribution of coronary artery disease. These invasive tools are also used to ascertain whether a particular patient may be a suitable candidate for either medical or surgical interventions.

Left heart catheterization is performed to obtain left ventricular (LV) and aortic pressures as well as volumes. There appears to be a correlation between abnormal elevations of left ventricular end-diastolic pressures or decreased cardiac output and the number of vessels with more than 75 percent occlusion of the lumen. The severity of vessel disease does not, however, solely have a reciprocal relationship with hemodynamic abnormalities.[37] The left ventricular end-diastolic pressure may also be elevated as a reflection of decreased left ventricular compliance or LV failure or both. Decreased compliance or failure may be a sequela of acute ischemia or scar formation from a previous MI.

Left ventricular angiography permits visualization of LV wall motion and determination of the ejection fraction. During diastole, the normal configuration of the outline of the LV cavity is that of an ellipsoid (Fig. 21-3). During systole, the ventricular walls are squeezed inward, especially the anterior and posterior walls. At the peak of systolic ejection, the normal appearance of the LV cavity is thought to resemble a pear core or an ice cream cone in the right anterior oblique (RAO) projection.[37] Abnormalities (asynergy) are noted whenever the LV outline either enlarges in one area or loses its normal characteristics (Fig. 21-3). In pa-

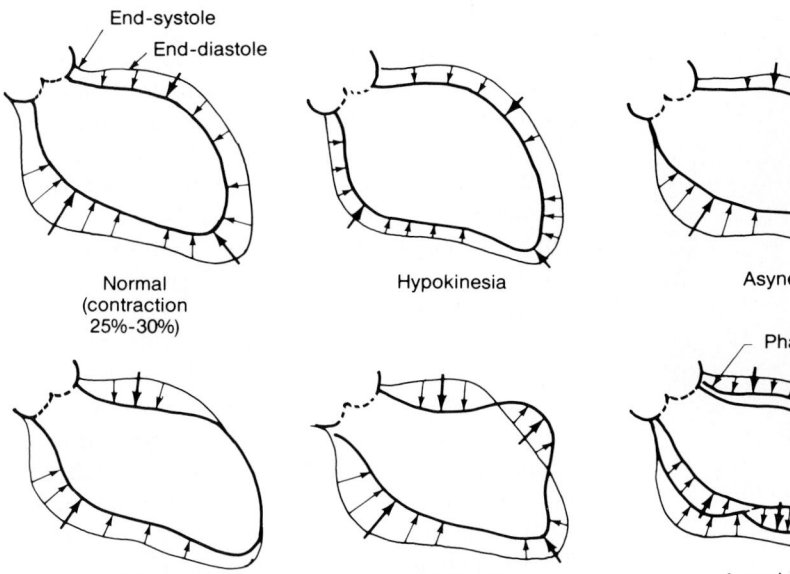

End-systole
End-diastole

Normal
(contraction
25%-30%)

Hypokinesia

Asyneresis

Akinesia

Dyskinesia
(paradoxical
systolic expansion)

Phase 1
Phase 2

Asynchrony

Figure 21-3 Figures which depict normal and abnormal cardiac contraction. Arrows represent motion from end-diastole to end-systole. (*From M. V. Herman and R. Gorlin. Implications of left ventricular asynergy. American Journal of Cardiology, 23:588, 1969.*)

tients with angina, asynergy has been noted during anginal attacks that cause ischemia but is reversible once the ischemic episode resolves.[37]

Ejection fractions are calculated from the ventriculogram and are a reflection of the systolic performance of the left ventricle. The normal ejection fraction is approximately 60 to 75 percent of the total left ventricular end-diastolic volume. A decrease in ejection fraction of less than 40 to 50 percent is indicative of impaired left ventricular function in patients with angina.

Coronary arteriography allows for assessment of the presence and grading of the severity of atherosclerotic lesions. An artery, except the left main, which has a reduction in the orifice of 75 percent or more is considered to have a clinically significant obstruction. A lesion in the left main coronary artery is considered significant when the obstruction is 50 percent or greater. Approximately 85 percent of patients with a clinical diagnosis of CAD have been found to have atherosclerotic lesions and 79 percent of these patients are found to have clinically significant obstructions.[38]

The indication for cardiac catheterization and coronary arteriography in patients with stable angina is not as urgent as in patients with unstable angina who require more immediate interventions. Those stable patients are often referred for an elective cardiac catheterization when symptoms are causing limitations in life-style and the need for surgery may become an issue. These patients may also require catheterization to confirm the presence of CAD. Unstable patients, on the other hand, are felt to be candidates for immediate catheterization.[26] When possible, these patients are medically stabilized prior to catheterization. Unstable angina patients are often found to have severe obstruction and multivessel disease.

Coronary arteriography also permits definitive diagnosis of the presence of coronary artery spasm (Fig. 21-4). This is often accomplished with the intravenous injection of ergonovine maleate, an agent found to induce uterine smooth muscle contraction in obstetric patients. The usual response to ergonovine in a patient with variant angina is near or total occlusion of an artery.[27] This test also helps to differentiate pure coronary artery vasospasm from spasm superimposed on a fixed lesion, previously referred to as a *mixed lesion*. Therapeutic interventions are directed differently once this distinction is made. The safety of the ergonovine test has, however, been questioned. It is recom-

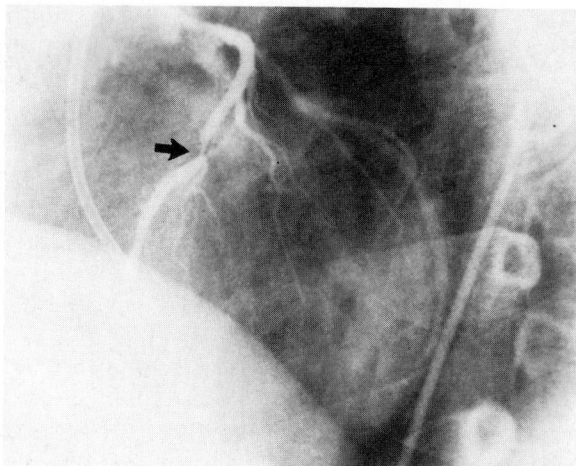

Figure 21-4 Arteriography of a patient who develops spasm (arrow) in the artery during the catheterization procedure.

mended that this test only be performed in settings whereby the immediate injection of intravenous nitroglycerin or calcium channel antagonists can be administered to prevent irreversible spasm which may lead to an MI.[37]

Therapeutic Interventions

Admission to a critical-care or coronary care unit is usually reserved for patients who present with the first episode of angina, or have suspected variant angina requiring confirmation, or for unstable angina. Patients are often admitted to rule out myocardial infarction. The goal of treatment for these patients is aimed at either increasing the coronary blood supply or decreasing the myocardial oxygen demand or both. This goal may be accomplished through medical or surgical interventions. Certain patients with CAD may also be offered other alternatives such as percutaneous transluminal coronary angioplasty (PTCA) or laser angioplasty.

Medical interventions for patients with CAD include pharmacologic therapy, dietary modifications, reduction of other risk factors, activity modification, and counterpulsation. Patients with pure vasospasm are treated medically with pharmacologic agents unless a mixed lesion is documented. Discussion will focus on all current treatment modalities for each subset of patients.

Pharmacologic Therapy

There are currently three classes of agents used for patients with CAD or spasm. They include nitrates, beta-adrenergic blocking agents, and calcium channel antagonists.

Nitrates are the first-line agents employed for both angina and coronary spasm. Nitrates act by dilating vascular and selected smooth muscle throughout the body, primarily causing venous dilatation and, to a lesser degree, arterial dilatation. The venous dilatation decreases venous return to the right side of the heart (preload). The reduced preload, in turn, reduces wall tension which decreases the oxygen requirements or demand. The minimal arterial dilatory effect causes a slight decrease in blood pressure. Nitrates are also thought to exert an effect on the coronary arteries specifically to increase coronary blood flow in some patients with coronary obstruction and to increase collateral blood flow to ischemic myocardium.[39] In contrast, patients with normal coronary arteries may exhibit a decrease in coronary blood flow with nitrates.[40] Nitrates are administered in sublingual, oral, intravenous, and topical forms.

Nitrates are classified into short-acting nitrates and longer-acting nitrates. Nitroglycerin, a shorter-acting nitrate, is often used sublingually to alleviate an acute anginal attack or episode of coronary spasm because of its rapid onset of action, or it can be used as prophylaxis prior to an activity which is known to precipitate an attack.

Intravenous or intracoronary nitroglycerin is often employed after provoking spasm with ergonovine maleate. Continuous intravenous infusion of nitroglycerin may be used to control angina. The longer-acting nitrates such as isosorbide dinitrate and isosorbide 5-mononitrate are used to increase exercise tolerance and prevent further anginal episodes or spasm attacks. Table 21-3 summarizes the effects of the commonly used nitrates.

Beta-adrenergic blocking agents are used solely or in combination with nitrates for treating stable and unstable angina. Recent investigations suggest that combined therapy may be more effective in treating stable angina than either nitrates or beta blockers alone.[41] The mechanism of action of the beta blockers is to inhibit the binding of catecholamines at receptor sites. These drugs compete at binding sites to block the effects of catecholamines.

Such blockade selectivity inhibits both inotropic and chronotropic actions produced by beta-adrenergic stimulation. The clinical effect of these drugs, therefore, is a reduction in the resting and exercising heart rate, a reduction in myocardial contractility, and a reduction in myocardial oxygen consumption. Most of the beta blockers have been found to increase exercise capacity in coronary artery disease and to increase diastolic filling time, permitting an increase in coronary perfusion time.

The use of beta blockers in coronary spasm is controversial. Some clinicians believe that beta blockers control the symptoms of variant angina by blocking the adrenergic effect which may induce coronary spasm.[42] Others believe that beta blockers may be detrimental because these agents have been found to decrease coronary blood flow and increase coronary vascular resistance, and are considered to be ineffective for spasm because of their failure to exert vasodilatory effects on coronary blood flow.[43] Labetolal, a new type of adrenergic blocker, has both alpha- and beta-blocking activity. A preliminary report suggests that it may be useful in blocking and reducing the frequency of vasospasm but it requires further study. Current recommendations are that beta blockers be avoided unless used concomitantly with a vasodilator.[42]

Propranolol (Inderal) is the most widely used beta blocker for control of angina as well as for dysrhythmias and hypertension in CAD. It is usually contraindicated in second- or third-degree heart block, bronchial asthma, cardiogenic shock, congestive heart failure, and with concurrent use of any adrenergic-stimulating psychotropic agent. Propranolol is also known to have a quinidinelike effect which depresses cardiac function and, therefore, the patient should be monitored for manifestations of congestive heart failure.

Metropolol (Lopressor) is a beta blocker which is more cardioselective in that it has more effect on the B_1 receptors of the heart than B_2 receptors. It is used for angina and hypertension and can be used judiciously with bronchospastic disease. Both propranolol and metropolol have short half-lives requiring frequent dosages. Nadolol (Corgard) and Atenolol have longer-half-lives, permitting less frequent dosages (one dose a day) for patients who have difficulty complying with drug regimens.

Calcium channel antagonists have been widely used in the last several years for angina. The primary mechanism of action of these agents is inhibition of the movement of calcium ions across myocardial and vascular smooth muscle, which produces (1) vasodilatation of the coronary arteries and collateral vessels; (2) a decrease in myocardial contractility, which leads to a decrease in myocardial oxygen demand; (3) vasodilatation of the peripheral arteries, resulting in a decrease in systemic blood pressure; and (4) a decrease in cardiac conduction.[44] Because of the coronary vasodilator effect, these drugs are useful in angina and spasm. Compared to the nitrates, the onset of action of calcium channel antagonists is somewhat slower, but they are much longer-acting.[45]

The three calcium channel antagonists that are most widely used are verapamil (Isoptin, Calan), diltiazem (Cardizem), and nifedipine (Procardia). All of these have been found to be effective in

Table 21-3 Summary of Commonly Used Nitrates

Drug	Route of Administration	Dosage	Onset of Effect	Duration of Effect
Nitroglycerin (Nitrostat; Susadrin)	Sublingual	0.3–0.6 mg	30 s	15–30 min
Nitroglycerin (Nitrostat SR; Nitro-Bid)	Oral	2.5–19.5 mg	1 h	2–4 h
Nitroglycerin (Nitro-Bid; Nitrodisc; Nitro-Dur; Nitrol ointment; Transderm)	Transdermal	1–2 in (ointment) 10–60 cm² (patches)	1 h	6–24 h
Nitroglycerin (Tridil)	Intravenous	10–200 µg/min	Immediate	—
Isosorbide dinitrate (Isordil; Sorbitrate; Dilatrate)	Sublingual	2.5–10 mg	5 min	1–2 h
Isosorbide dinitrate (Isordil; Sorbitrate; Dilatrate)	Oral	10–60 mg	30 min	4–6 h
Isosorbide 5-mononitrate (ISMO)	Oral	10–40 mg	30 min	8–21 h

Modified from J. Cohn, Drug Used to Control Vascular Resistance and Capacitance. In J. S. Hurst, et al., *The Heart*, New York: McGraw-Hill, 1986.

stable angina, reducing anginal attacks and improving exercise capacity. Each drug works differently on the heart to produce clinical effects.

Verapamil and diltiazem have been shown to decrease the heart rate by depressing the rate of sinus node discharge and attenuating the conduction velocity through the atrioventricular (AV) node. This negative chronotropic effect is useful in controlling tachyarrhythmias associated with CAD. Nifedipine is not useful in tachyarrhythmias because of the reflex tachycardia associated with its use. All three agents have been found to depress cardiac contractility; therefore, each has a negative inotropic effect. In addition, nifedipine exerts the greatest vasodilatory effects of these agents.[44]

Various clinical trials have supported the use of all three calcium channel antagonists for coronary spasm and rest pain associated with unstable angina.[42,44] These drugs have been able to block spontaneous and drug-induced spasm.

Patients with unstable angina in which medical management is difficult may require a combination of long-acting nitrates, a beta-adrenergic blocker, and calcium channel antagonists. In a randomized double-blind trial, combined therapy of nifedipine, nitrates, and propranolol reduced the number of unstable anginal attacks and reduced the number of patients requiring surgery for relief of chest pain.[46] The hemodynamic effects of each of these different types of drugs may be efficacious. However, adverse reactions such as heart block, severe bradycardia, and congestive heart failure mandate careful patient selection and surveillance.[44]

Antilipid agents are not useful for angina but may be reserved for some patients with familial hyperlipidemia who have been unsuccessful with dietary modifications.[47] The efficacy of their use in preventing CAD or preventing coronary events such as an MI in humans remains controversial, although recent data from the Lipid Research Clinics Program have demonstrated an effectiveness as previously discussed in the risk factor section.[22] The antilipid agents include cholestyramine, colestipal, nicotinic acid, clofibrate, probucol, and neomycin. Cholestyramine (Questran) and colestipal (Colested) are cholesterol-binding resins that have been found to decrease LDL and total cholesterol levels.[6,47-49] Nicotinic acid has been shown to lower LDL levels by decreasing the hepatic synthesis of VLDL.[6] It may

also increase HDL levels and is useful in hyperlipidemia types II, IV, and V. Clofibrate (Atromid S) reduces VLDL levels and plasma triglycerides.[6] Clofibrate has also been associated with serious side effects such as cardiac arrhythmias and sudden death. Probucol (Lorelco) lowers total cholesterol level but appears less effective in reducing LDL levels as compared with nicotinic acid.[6] It may also decrease HDL levels. Neomycin decreases LDL levels by promoting fecal excretion of bile salts, and decreasing cholesterol absorption, thereby decreasing total serum cholesterol. It has been shown to have ototoxic and nephrotoxic effects and may interfere with the absorption of digitalis.[6,47-49] In conclusion, these antilipid agents are not innocuous. Most of them have serious side effects and are potentially toxic. Their use should be reserved for high-risk patients with serious types of hyperlipidemia.

Activity Modifications

Patients with stable angina are encouraged to engage in activities which do not precipitate an anginal attack. Walking is often one of the recommended exercises. Those patients who wish to engage in more vigorous activity should participate in a supervised structural exercise program to gradually increase their exercise capacity, so as not to precipitate anginal attacks. Prior to engaging in any activity which may precipitate angina, the use of prophylactic nitroglycerin is encouraged.

The type of exercise is also an important variable in the patient with CAD. Isotonic exercise involving the large muscle groups is favored over isometric exercises, which may actually increase myocardial oxygen demand.[50] Patients should also be instructed not to engage in isotonic exercises immediately after a large meal because of the shunting of blood flow to the gastrointestinal tract.

Activity restrictions are frequently employed for the patient with unstable angina. Because of the seriousness of this type of angina, patients are often hospitalized, placed on bed rest, and administered combined pharmacologic agents. If their condition improves, gradual ambulation is encouraged. However, if despite medical therapy the condition worsens, these patients will require interventions such as counterpulsation, percutaneous transluminal coronary angioplasty, laser angioplasty, or coronary artery bypass surgery before progressive activity is undertaken.

Dietary Modifications

The study which provided evidence that dietary modifications and drug therapy (antilipids) was effective in lowering blood cholesterol and LDL levels was the Lipid Research Clinics Coronary Primary Prevention Trial.[22] This study has been previously discussed in the section, "Risk Factors." A consensus development conference was convened in 1984 by the National Institutes of Health[49] for the twofold purpose of reviewing the scientific evidence from this study and making specific recommendations on blood cholesterol reduction. The panel concluded that the scientific evidence "established beyond a reasonable doubt that lowering definitely elevated blood cholesterol (specifically blood levels of low density lipoprotein cholesterol) reduces the risk of heart attacks due to coronary heart disease."[51] This panel also made recommendations that men and women with certain blood cholesterol levels in specific age groups be considered for some intervention plan (see Table 21-4). It was recommended that the patient with a moderate risk of CAD be treated with dietary modification, whereas the patient at high risk should be treated intensively by dietary changes and, when ineffective, should then be treated with pharmacologic agents.[51] Therapeutic interventions are aimed at reducing plasma cholesterol levels to 180 mg/dL for adults under age 30 and to 200 mg/dL for those 30 years or older. In addition to reducing the plasma cholesterol level, special attention is paid to LDL levels and HDL levels obtained from a lipid analysis. Plasma LDL levels are often compared to HDL levels as a ratio such as LDL/HDL when the LDL level ranges between 100 to 200 mg/dL. Patients with an LDL/HDL ratio of 5:1 should be considered for drug therapy. However, if a patient has an LDL level which exceeds 200 mg/dL, aggressive drug therapy concomitant with diet restrictions is warranted regardless of the HDL level.[51]

Dietary modifications that lower cholesterol levels include restricting total fat, saturated fat, and cholesterol. In addition, weight reduction is another important component of a dietary plan. Foods such as poultry, fish, shellfish, lean red meats, and low-fat dairy products should be encouraged. Amounts of fruits, vegetables, breads, grains, and legumes also should be increased. Those foods which should be avoided include fried foods and foods that are high in saturated fat such as palm and coconut oil (found in nondairy creamers).

The consumption of fish has received much attention in the last several years primarily because of the eicosapentaenoic acid (EPA) contained in fish oil. Kromhout, Bosschieter, and Coulander[52] followed a group of men in the town of Zutphen, the Netherlands, for 20 years. In the 20-year follow-up, an inverse relationship was observed between fish consumption and death from coronary heart disease. Fish contains EPA, which has been shown in vitro to be the precursor of platelet thromboxane A_3 and of prostaglandin I_3. Thromboxane A_3, unlike thromboxane A_2, has demonstrated no platelet-aggregating power. In addition, prostaglandin I_3 has been shown to be an effective antiaggregating substance. The high levels of EPA are, therefore, theorized to lead to an antithrombotic state because of reduced platelet aggregation.

Platelet aggregation, which has been previously discussed in the section, "Pathogenesis of Atherosclerosis," may promote smooth muscle cell proliferation leading to atherosclerotic lesions. Thus, the effects of EPA may influence the pathogenesis

Table 21-4 Classification of Adults at Moderate and High Risk Requiring Treatment

Age	Moderate Risk	High Risk
20–29	Greater than 200 mg/dL	Greater than 200 mg/dL
30–39	Greater than 220 mg/dL	Greater than 240 mg/dL
40 and over	Greater than 240 mg/dL	Greater than 260 mg/dL

Source: Classification of adults at moderate and high risk requiring treatment (from National Institute of Health Consensus Development Conference Statement). *Lowering Blood Cholesterol to Prevent Heart Disease,* 5(7), 1985, Bethesda, Md.: DHHS.

of atherosclerosis by this mechanism as well as by other means.[53]

Lastly, Kromhout, Bosschieter, and Coulander concluded from their study that one or two fish dishes per week may have some preventive value against the development of atherosclerosis.[52] Additional studies are required to substantiate their conclusions and provide more insight into the correlation between consumption of fish and coronary heart disease.

Reduction of Risk Factors

Patients with CAD should be motivated to adopt healthier life-styles and to minimize their risk factors. As was previously mentioned, the number of risk factors can have an additive or synergistic effect on the development and progression of CAD and, therefore, these factors need to be controlled individually as well as collectively.

Patients with documented or suspected CAD should be encouraged to stop smoking cigarettes, filtered and nonfiltered. They should also be instructed to adhere to pharmacologic regimens to reduce high blood pressure when present.

Stress reduction is important for the patient who is under a great deal of stress. Critical-care nurses need to encourage the verbalization of feelings and explore ways of reducing stressful life events. Often, such patients and significant others require follow-up counseling.

Obesity is another risk factor requiring careful consideration. The overweight patient should be encouraged to change his or her eating habits to lose weight and maintain optimal body weight. Furthermore, results from the Framingham study suggest that weight reduction may decrease the risk of CAD and increase the functional exercise capacity in patients with CAD.[54]

Patients with systemic hypertension require careful management. Pharmacologic agents such as beta blockers and diuretics are recommended for the control of hypertension, especially for patients with systolic pressures over 160 mmHg or diastolic blood pressures over 95 mmHg. In certain patients with mild hypertension, the initial intervention may be to alter concomitant risk factors such as obesity, sedentary life-style, excessive alcohol intake, and use of oral contraceptives.[6]

It appears that management of hyperglycemia alone does not prevent atherosclerotic development but multifactorial risk reduction in association with control of hyperglycemia is important.[6] In patients with clinical manifestations of atherosclerosis, dietary restrictions as well as drug therapy may be employed.

Dietary restrictions include decreased saturated fats, complex carbohydrates, and sodium intake, especially for patients who are hypertensive or who have congestive heart failure. Drug therapy may include oral hypoglycemic agents or exogenous insulin preparations. The critical-care nurse should also be aware that diabetic patients on nonselective beta-blockade therapy may not manifest the sympathetic response during hypoglycemic reactions; thus careful consideration must be given to avoid hypoglycemia in patients receiving beta blockade therapy.

Intraaortic Balloon Pump

For unstable angina patients, intraaortic balloon pumping is considered as a means of reversing ischemia and protecting the myocardium if all conventional modes of therapy have failed, including bed rest, intravenous calcium channel antagonists, and nitrates. Ischemia must be documented according to clinical, hemodynamic, and electrocardiographic criteria. Persistent refractory ischemia is considered an indication for balloon pumping in certain institutions.

The intraaortic balloon pump has demonstrated efficacy in the reversal of myocardial ischemia for unstable angina patients.[55] During balloon pumping, a favorable balance between myocardial oxygen supply and demand can be restored by the simultaneous increase in coronary perfusion pressure and the reduction in cardiac work achieved with this intervention.

The intraaortic balloon pump (IABP), a counterpulsation device, was first introduced into the critical-care setting in 1969. Currently, it is the more widely used left ventricular assist device in comparison to the external pressure circulatory assist (EPCA) device. The IABP is an invasive unit while the EPCA is noninvasive. The following discussion will pertain only to the IABP as it is employed more frequently for unstable angina patients.

The intraaortic balloon catheter (available in several sizes and either with a single or double lumen) is introduced either percutaneously or by surgical cutdown into the femoral artery. The catheter is then advanced in a retrograde fashion to be positioned to lie in the descending thoracic aorta 1 to 2 cm distal to the orifice of the left subclavian artery. Once in position, the catheter is connected to a console and passage of either helium or carbon dioxide (manufacturer's preference) in and out of the balloon catheter is accomplished by the console.

The mechanism of the device is simply one of synchronized displacement of blood in the aorta by the actual inflation and deflation of the balloon. The inflation-deflation cycle is precisely set (timed) by the clinician. The balloon is inflated and deflated in synchrony with the mechanical events of the cardiac cycle. The timing of balloon inflation and deflation is opposite that of ventricular systole. Therefore, balloon activation is referred to as *counterpulsation*.

The timing of inflation is to occur at the beginning of diastole. To accurately adjust the timing of inflation, the arterial waveform is used. The dicrotic notch which depicts aortic valve closure (beginning of phase I in diastole) must be identified on the arterial trace. The balloon is then inflated at the dicrotic notch on the arterial waveform. Minor corrections are recommended to adjust the timing from a radial or femoral arterial line to account for slight delays in waveform transmission from the aorta to these distal recording sites. If a central aortic root line is used, then precise inflation at the dicrotic notch is suggested. The clinician is encouraged to refer to his or her specific manufacturer's recommendations regarding inflation delays for the device being used. This inflated balloon displaces a volume of blood equal to its own volume size, resulting in a pressure elevation in the aorta, referred to as the *diastolic augmented pressure*.

Deflation of the balloon is set to occur just prior to the next aortic valve opening, specifically during isovolumetric contraction of the left ventricle (phase I systole). As gas is removed from the balloon, the intraaortic volume is decreased and, therefore, aortic end-diastolic pressure is reduced. This reduction in aortic pressure lowers the pressure which the left ventricle must overcome to eject its stroke volume during the next systole. The balloon deflation, therefore, facilitates systolic unloading and emptying. The waveform achieved during balloon deflation should depict a 10-to-15-mm lowering of the balloon aortic end-diastolic pressure in contrast to the patient's unaugmented aortic end-diastolic pressure.[56]

The physiologic effects of balloon inflation and deflation are significant. During balloon inflation, elevation of the diastolic pressure (diastolic augmentation) has important effects in terms of coronary flow and tissue perfusion. Coronary flow is phasic because the branches of the coronary arteries are deeply embedded in the myocardium. During systole these intramyocardial branches are compressed, increasing the resistance to flow. During diastole, however, the coronary vascular resistance is minimal; therefore, coronary filling occurs primarily during diastole. The timing of pressure augmentation during balloon pumping is, therefore, optimal. Elevating diastolic pressure increases coronary perfusion pressure and potentially increases coronary blood flow and oxygen supply.

However, despite the fact that coronary perfusion pressure is elevated by balloon pumping, variable effects on total coronary blood flow have been documented.[55] In some instances, total coronary blood flow is elevated by diastolic augmentation; in others it is unchanged or even reduced. This variability results because the dominant mechanism controlling coronary blood flow is autoregulation within the coronary bed—not coronary perfusion pressure. Autoregulation is an intrinsic mechanism altering coronary blood flow in response to tissue need for oxygen. The process of autoregulation maintains a precise balance between myocardial oxygen supply and demand. Local tissue hypoxia or oxygen lack is the most potent stimulus for increasing coronary blood flow and oxygen supply through coronary vasodilatation. Conversely, a reduction in oxygen demand produces a corresponding reduction in coronary blood flow through vasoconstriction. Because counterpulsation reduces myocardial work and oxygen demand, overall coronary blood flow may be reduced during balloon pumping via autoregulated vasoconstriction, despite the elevation of aortic diastolic pressure.

Typically, absolute increases in total coronary blood flow are noted when the myocardium has been underperfused because of hypotension prior to initiation of balloon pumping.[55] In this instance, the myocardium is flow-deprived by the low-pressure state and is maximally dilated by the resultant tissue hypoxia. Consequently, elevation of pressure elevates flow. However, in the absence of hypotension, the balloon essentially supplements the autoregulatory process, offering a reserve in coronary perfusion pressure and oxygen supply.

In contrast to the variable effects on total coronary blood flow, favorable localized effects on flow do occur with diastolic augmentation.[55] Flow to myocardium threatened by significant obstructive lesions is pressure-dependent. The normal autoregulatory ability is impaired by disease. Therefore, flow to these potentially ischemic regions improves with elevation of diastolic pressure.[55] In addition, the balloon may increase coronary collateral development. In summary, diastolic augmentation increases the available myocardial oxygen supply, may improve the distribution of coronary blood flow to potentially ischemic regions of the myocardium, and improves peripheral tissue perfusion.

Balloon deflation has significant effects because it facilitates systolic emptying of the ventricle and, therefore, afterload reduction.[55] Afterload reduction produces a number of physiologic alterations. Because the resistance to ventricular ejection is reduced, the systolic pressure the left ventricle must generate to open the aortic valve and eject blood is correspondingly lower. As a result, the ventricle does not have to generate as much pressure during systole, and cardiac work is reduced. Finally, a reduction in cardiac work lowers myocardial oxygen demand and oxygen consumption. In essence, afterload reduction improves myocardial efficiency and reduces cardiac work and oxygen demand. Clinically, the effect of balloon deflation is, therefore, manifested by an increase in cardiac output and a reduction in left ventricular end-diastolic pressure, left atrial pressure, and pulmonary wedge pressure.

In summary, the physiologic effects of intraaortic balloon counterpulsation is an elevation of diastolic pressure and a lowering of systolic pressure so that cardiac work is reduced, while tissue perfusion is maintained. Myocardial oxygenation is improved with a reduction in oxygen demand and an increment in oxygen supply. All of these effects are desirable especially for unstable angina patients with persistent ischemia who are at high risk for infarction.[55]

The absolute contraindications to intraaortic balloon pumping are anatomic considerations. For the most part, the relative contraindications involve ethical issues that must be decided at the discretion of the patient, family, and physician.

Absolute contraindications to IABP therapy are the following: (1) aortic aneurysm, (2) aortic dissection, (3) aortic valve insufficiency, and (4) severe aortoiliac disease.[57] Aortic wall damage precludes insertion because of the hazard of progressive damage with potential aortic rupture secondary to the mechanical stress of pumping. Balloon inflation in the setting of aortic valve insufficiency increases the retrograde flow into the left ventricle during diastole, worsening the underlying dysfunction. Severe aortoiliac disease significantly increases the incidence of arterial trauma and peripheral embolization. Extensive atherosclerosis in the peripheral arterial vessels may prevent passage of the balloon catheter through the femoral artery. If balloon pumping is required urgently, consideration may be given to an alternative approach intraoperatively through the aortoiliac system or retrograde via the ascending aorta into the descending aorta.

Nursing care of the patient undergoing balloon pumping does not differ significantly from the care of any critically ill patient. Only those considerations unique to the care of patients on the balloon pump are considered in this section.[55,57] It is assumed that nurses caring for these patients possess a sound knowledge of hemodynamic monitoring, cardiac pacing, cardiac rhythm analysis, and patient assessment. Expertise in these areas is essential to provide safe and effective patient care during balloon pumping.

It is a nursing responsibility to create an environment that is safe and efficient for patient care and balloon insertion. A room plan should be developed with designated locations for essential equipment and supplies, including defibrillator, pacemaker, intubation equipment, emergency medications, monitor, IV poles with transducers, infusion pumps, bed, balloon console, operating room light, instrument tray, and waste receptacles. A minimum of two oxygen outlets and two vacuum outlets for endotracheal and operative field suction should be available for surgical insertion. An equipment cart containing all miscellaneous supplies required during insertion is an invaluable addition. As a rule, setting up the cubicle according to a predesignated plan can be accomplished within half an hour by one nurse.

An initial clinical assessment must be completed prior to insertion. The following information is critical to the anticipated insertion procedure. Status of peripheral pulses must be determined. Pulses must be checked and the quality recorded. Significant peripheral vascular disease may prevent the passage of the balloon catheter through the iliofemoral system and increase the risk of arterial trauma during insertion. Also, postinsertion assessment of pulses is meaningless without accurate baseline data for comparison. A history of bleeding tendencies or medication sensitivity must be noted. Anticoagulants and antibiotics are routinely administered during the insertion procedure. The patient's expectations and preparation for the procedure must be assessed to guide subsequent teaching and support efforts. Depending on time constraints and the presenting problem, additional information elicited should be tailored accordingly.

Once the admission procedure is completed, the first priority is to establish quality electrocardiographic and hemodynamic monitoring signals. The electrocardiogram is of primary importance during balloon pumping because it provides the triggering signal for balloon action. To effectively coordinate balloon and cardiac action, the balloon console must sense the R wave of the electrocardiogram. To ensure that the console senses only the R wave and not other ECG waves, a lead should be selected that demonstrates maximal R wave amplitude and minimal amplitude of all other ECG components, including pacing artifacts. This is most easily accomplished by recording a 12-lead ECG, reviewing all leads, and identifying the lead with the required ECG configuration. The electrodes can then be placed on the patient's chest to duplicate the desired lead. If none of the standard 12 leads is adequate, the electrodes can be systematically moved over the precordium until the ideal electrode placement is identified.

Insertion of the arterial line is the next priority when a double-lumen catheter is not inserted. An arterial line is necessary to accurately time balloon action. The arterial tracing represents the mechanical activity of the heart, whereas the ECG reflects the electrical activity. Because the intraaortic balloon is a mechanical assist device, accurate synchronization can only be obtained utilizing the arterial tracing. On certain consoles, the ECG trace is used as a guide for "initial" timing adjustments prior to initiation of pumping. This is possible because a rough relationship exists between the electrical and mechanical cycle. Ventricular contraction begins approximately at the R wave and continues through the peak of the T wave; consequently, a deflation marker can be placed in the P-R interval with the inflation marker superimposed on the peak of the T wave. Once pumping begins, precision timing is possible only by observing the arterial tracing for waveform alterations indicative of effective balloon pumping.

The arterial line is usually inserted in the radial artery. Although arterial tracings obtained directly from the aortic root would best reflect the balloon effect relative to aortic valve closure and opening, aortic root pressure monitoring cannot be obtained unless a double-lumen intraaortic balloon catheter is used. Radial arterial monitoring is a useful alternative because it has minimal waveform delay and distortion despite the peripheral location. Femoral arterial monitoring can also be used; however, the greater anatomic distance from central aortic events produces more wave transmission delay and waveform distortion. The left radial artery is usually selected rather than the right, because the balloon lies just below the left subclavian artery. If the balloon is displaced slightly upward in the aorta, the waveform obtained via the left radial artery will become damped, providing a valuable diagnostic index of balloon location, particularly useful during insertion.

Immediately prior to insertion, the insertion site is prepped and the patient is draped. The drape should be arranged so that the patient's head is uncovered and access to all lines and pacing wires is maintained. The most common oversight once this environment is created is to forget that the patient is not under general anesthesia. The patient must remain the pivotal figure during insertion, and continual attention must be given to his or her needs and perceptions. Mild sedation may be advisable during the procedure, if tolerated. However, the most important tranquilizer is ongoing support and interaction with the nurse. The nurse must interpret events and establish appropriate expectations for the patient, minimizing the opportunity for misperception.

The percutaneous route is the most commonly used method at present. In brief, the insertion procedure consists of the following events: The common femoral artery having the strongest pulse is selected and the incision site is infiltrated with local anesthesia, usually lidocaine 1% without epinephrine. The femoral artery is then cannulated with a flexible guide wire to permit passage into the lower abdominal aorta. Larger arterial dilators are progressively placed over the guide wire until a sheath can be introduced into the artery. The smoothly wrapped balloon catheter is then inserted through the sheath and passed over the guide wire into the thoracic aorta. Accurate placement is ascertained by measuring the catheter tip at the angle of Louis and marking with a ligature the location on the catheter indicating the point of exit through the femoral site.

Once the catheter is properly placed, the balloon is carefully unwrapped and sutured to the leg prior to connection to the pump console. Then counterpulsation may be initiated. Balloon location must be confirmed immediately after insertion either by fluoroscopy or a stat chest film.

Proper timing is adjusted from the arterial tracing. Timing should be set by trained personnel, because inappropriate timing can increase cardiac work and compromise myocardial function.

During the insertion, specific nursing interventions can be anticipated, based on events encountered during the procedure.[55] The patient's comfort is the foremost concern. Adequate local anesthesia should be administered to avoid any sensation of pain at the insertion site. Typically, the patient's greatest discomfort is secondary to the immobility required by the procedure. The patient should be instructed not to move, particularly not to flex the leg; and he or she must be assured that the nurse will provide comfort measures. Most patients are able to cooperate and do not require

restraint. During the procedure, transient leg numbness may be experienced. Patients must be aware that this is normal and will not last long. Any pain must be reported to the nurse to ensure appropriate intervention. Angina may be precipitated and must be controlled with medication during insertion. Back pain, if acute and sudden, may indicate dissection, warranting immediate notification of the physician.

To prevent infection, sterile conditions must be ensured during insertion. Room activity must be minimized. Everyone in the room should be gowned and masked. A broad-spectrum antibiotic may be administered one-half hour before insertion and every 6 h for at least 24 to 48 h.[55]

Anticoagulation may also be indicated because insertion of a foreign substance into the vasculature can initiate clotting along the blood–foreign substance interface of the balloon. Despite the fact that the balloon is antithrombogenic, many institutions implement anticoagulation during balloon pumping. If anticoagulation is desired, an initial dose of heparin is administered intravenously approximately 3 min prior to the insertion. Heparinization is subsequently maintained either via continuous infusion or divided bolus doses. Low-molecular-weight dextran or Rheomacrodex may be administered at 10 to 20 mL/h, either alone or in conjunction with heparin after the balloon is in place. Rheomacrodex reduces the platelet aggregation precipitated by the balloon.

Once the balloon is in place, peripheral pulses must be checked immediately to ensure that blood flow to the extremity distal to the balloon is not compromised. The balloon catheter in the iliofemoral system should not impede blood flow distally to the leg. Diminished peripheral pulsation can be secondary to transient arterial spasm, arterial occlusion by the catheter or a thrombus, or peripheral embolization. Inadequate perfusion of the leg may necessitate balloon removal to preserve limb viability. On occasion, the balloon can then be reinserted on the contralateral side to maintain balloon pumping.

During balloon pumping in the critical-care unit, selected nursing considerations are most easily summarized according to systems. As would be expected, the cardiovascular system warrants close attention. The hemodynamic and clinical response to balloon pumping should be evaluated every 15 to 60 min as the patient's condition dictates.

Patients requiring pumping for refractory myocardial ischemia usually experience either complete relief from pain or a reduction in the frequency of ischemic episodes. Recurrent angina on the balloon pump should immediately be brought to the attention of the responsible physician, since more aggressive therapy might be required to control the ischemia.

Evaluation of perfusion to the involved extremity should be performed hourly. Peripheral pulses and skin temperature and color should be checked relative to preinsertion status. It is essential that the quality of posterior tibial and dorsalis pedis pulses be assessed and recorded. The Doppler flow technique can be used to locate difficult-to-palpate pulses. When evaluating pulses, the opposite leg can be used for comparison, but it must be remembered that either leg can be the site of embolization from the aortoiliac tree. Peripheral pulses, when located initially, should be marked to facilitate subsequent localization. See Chap. 25 for further discussion.

Timing must be evaluated and adjusted as needed. Even if timing adjustments are not the responsibility of nursing, nurses must be able to distinguish between normal and abnormal arterial waveform configurations. Quality hemodynamic signals must be preserved to ensure the accuracy of timing adjustments and to permit valid interpretation of hemodynamic status. In addition, because balloon triggering depends upon the ECG signal, electrode security must be maintained.

Hematologic studies must be evaluated closely to detect abnormalities. Platelet counts may fall because of disruption of platelet integrity by the balloon surface and the mechanical trauma. Rheomacrodex infusion at 10 to 20 mL/h minimizes this fall in platelets. Rarely is the administration of platelets required unless active bleeding is noted in the presence of thrombocytopenia. Hematocrits may also fall secondary to the inevitable blood loss during insertion and subsequent blood sampling. Anticoagulation status should be monitored closely with anticoagulation precautions in effect.

Respiratory considerations during balloon pumping are straightforward. The balloon should not interfere with respiratory care or chest physical therapy. The only modifications in these are positional. The head of the bed should not be elevated over 45°, nor should the involved leg be flexed at the hip. Either one of these maneuvers could kink and crack the balloon catheter at the site of insertion in the groin, or could displace the catheter proximally into the aortic arch, potentially traumatizing the intima. The patient can be turned from side to side with only mild angulation of the affected extremity. The balloon leg should be restrained if the patient's cooperation cannot be achieved. During chest physical therapy, avoid inducing artifact in the electrocardiogram, because it is the ECG that provides the triggering stimulus to the balloon.

Renal parameters are significant because renal perfusion is a sensitive index of cardiac output. Persistent oliguria on the balloon can be secondary to an inadequate cardiac output. However, unexplained oliguria should prompt assessment of balloon-related causes. The position of the balloon should be reevaluated on x-ray. Poor perfusion of the kidneys could also indicate renal embolization during insertion.

Similarly, neurological or psychological signs and symptoms can have multiple origins. Disturbances of mentation can be secondary to low cardiac output, embolization, hypoxia, or psychosis. Careful evaluation and documentation is, therefore, required. Psychological stress needs to be addressed in these patients. Patacky and coworkers[58] found that patients who were placed on the IABP perceived more stress than patients who were not on the IABP. They also noted that patients reported other major stressors while on the IABP, which were: (1) admission to CCU, (2) being unable to move about freely in bed because of equipment, (3) frequent sleep interruptions, (4) the noise around them, and (5) the lack of knowledge and understanding of their illness and treatment. The implications for nursing based on this study indicate that stress can be minimized by clear explanations regarding the CCU environment, routines, and equipment components of patient care to patients and their families; providing emotional support by listening to patients and families; and establishing an atmosphere to promote communication. Efforts to reduce sensory overstimulation and sleep deprivation are essential.

The number of indwelling catheters and the high frequency of invasive procedures predisposes these patients to infection. If surgery is necessary, preoperative infection increases the likelihood of endocarditis and other septic complications postoperatively. Therefore, strict sterile technique must be maintained during line management and dressing changes. Antibiotic coverage must not be overlooked for 24 to 48 h after insertion. Signs and symptoms of infection must be monitored closely.

Ideally, the indication for weaning is evidence of potential hemodynamic independence. However, on occasion, the balloon must be removed because of ischemia to the involved extremity. The contribution of the balloon pump to circulatory support can be progressively reduced over a period of hours. The weaning process can be accomplished either by gradual reduction in the frequency of balloon support or in the volume of balloon inflation. The first method is preferred. Most units have a weaning control to reduce the ratio of patient-to-balloon cycles. Typically, patients are weaned from 1:1 to 1:8 over a period of hours. The duration of weaning depends on the patient's condition and the physician's preference. The primary nursing responsibility is to evaluate the patient's tolerance of the weaning process. Specific orders should be obtained prior to initiation of weaning to guide the weaning process. The criteria for resumption of balloon pumping at a higher frequency should be predetermined. Indications for substituting other pharmacologic means of support, such as vasopressors or volume, should be established. Weaning intolerance is evidenced by rising pulmonary wedge pressure, falling mean arterial pressure, falling cardiac output, oliguria, cardiac arrhythmias, or chest pain.

It must be remembered that despite the fact that the patient's stability is the usual indication for balloon removal, the procedure should be approached with the same care as balloon insertion. Careful planning is essential to avoid unnecessary complications. The environment must be organized to permit ready access to all equipment and supplies and to maintain sterile conditions in the critical-care unit. The patient must be prepared psychologically and physically for the procedure. Antibiotics

may be reinstituted one-half hour before removal begins. The patient is draped and the balloon is removed. Firm pressure must be applied over the insertion site for 30 min to 1 h. Pulses should be evaluated during removal and immediately thereafter. Balloon removal represents the final stage of the weaning process, and patients should be observed closely for tolerance.

Percutaneous Transluminal Coronary Angioplasty

Percutaneous transluminal coronary angioplasty (PTCA) is a procedure which is used to dilate occluded coronary arteries. In 1964 Dotter and Judkins first introduced this procedure in the treatment of peripheral vascular disease to improve vascular patency.[59] They used a catheter and guide wire to dilate arterial narrowings of the femoral and iliac arteries. It was not until 1977 when Dr. Andreas Gruentzig developed a double-lumen catheter small enough to be used in the coronary circulation that PTCA became an alternative treatment modality for CAD.

Little is understood of the mechanism by which the technique improves vascular patency. Originally, Dotter and Judkins postulated that the luminal diameter of the occluded vessel was increased by compression of the atheromatous intima.[59] Atheromatous lesions are solid and are incompressible unless empty spaces are present within the atheromas, something which has not been found histologically. According to Hall and Gruentzig,[60] several histological changes may be a consequence of the controlled injury which occurs when the balloon catheter exerts lateral force against the occluded vessel wall. These changes include compression, splitting, or redistribution of the plaque and stretching of the wall. The fibrous cap is disrupted and the exposed debris contained within the cap is removed by phagocytosis. During the healing process, endothelialization occurs concomitantly with plaque mobilization, which results in an increased diameter of the occluded segment and improved blood flow through the once stenotic area.[60]

The patient who may undergo PTCA must also be a suitable candidate for surgery in the event of complications. Thus, this patient must fulfill the criteria for surgery and indicate a willingness to have the PTCA procedure. This procedure is used for lesions in any of the three coronary vessels except the left main coronary artery, but the ideal candidate usually has one or two proximal or midvessel stenoses. Bentivoglio and Van Raden[61] reported that coronary angioplasty success was significantly higher for lesions in the proximal segment of the coronary artery (70 percent) than those in the mid- or distal segments of the artery (50 percent). The lesion or lesions should be noncalcified smooth plaque without sharp margins or irregular borders. Patients chosen for PTCA usually have stable angina which has caused lifestyle changes or unstable angina of short duration (less than 6 months) despite optimal medical therapy. The patient may also have multivessel disease and still be considered a candidate for PTCA.

Due to improvements in skill and technology, patients with multivessel disease are benefiting from PTCA. Usually, dilation of the more severe lesion is attempted first to ascertain the probability of successful angioplasty.[62] If the more severe lesion cannot be dilated, the patient will need surgery. Interestingly, the success rate in patients with multiple dilations is comparable with that seen in patients with single vessel disease; the rate of complication is also similar.[62]

It is generally agreed that left main coronary artery stenosis should not be dilated because of the danger of total vessel occlusion and the degree of myocardium at risk.[62] Lesions at the coronary ostia are typically resistant to dilation and are also associated with a high rate of restenosis. Patients with severely reduced ventricular function are also not considered suitable candidates for PTCA.

The procedure for PTCA is very similar to the procedure for cardiac catheterization. Informed consent is obtained prior to the procedure and the patient is kept NPO the day of the procedure in the event that surgery becomes necessary. A guiding catheter is inserted via a femoral or brachial artery and advanced retrograde into the ascending aorta. Some physicians may also insert a transvenous pacing lead into the pulmonary artery to permit emergency cardiac pacing as well as to serve as a marker for the location of the lesion during the procedure.[60] As the guiding catheter is introduced, angiography is performed to identify the lesion and to provide a view for passing the catheter. A

dilatation catheter with the balloon attached is advanced through the guiding catheter into the stenotic area of the artery. Pressure measurements are obtained to determine the pressure gradient across the stenosis which serve as a quantitative parameter to ascertain success of the procedure. When the catheter has been strategically placed over the area of occlusion, the balloon is inflated in a stepwise fashion until it reaches 4 to 10 atm of pressure. The balloon is inflated for approximately 15 to 30 s and then deflated. Balloon inflations can be repeated until the residual pressure gradient decreases approximately 20 percent or until the gradient is less than 16 mmHg. Angiography is also repeated to visualize the distal flow (Fig. 21-5). Once favorable results have been achieved, or if the patient should exhibit evidence of myocardial ischemia, the dilatation catheter and guiding catheter are removed. With a femoral approach, a sheath is left in place and the patient is then transferred to a nursing unit.

Patients may also be started on IV nitroglycerin prior to the procedure and remain on it during the procedure. In addition, some patients receive sublingual nifedipine and intracoronary nitroglycerin if coronary spasm is suspected or demonstrated. During the procedure, patients usually receive heparin to prevent thrombus formation, which is stopped when the procedure is finished. The femoral sheath is removed 4 to 6 h after the heparin is stopped to allow for metabolism of the heparin and prevent bleeding. Some patients need calcium channel antagonists after the procedure. After successful PTCA, patients receive antiplatelet drugs or Coumadin.

A registry of patients who have undergone PTCA has been maintained by the National Heart & Lung Blood Institute (NHLBI). This registry compiles data on the results of this procedure. According to the NHLBI, complications occurred in 289 patients or 9.4 percent of the 3079 PTCA patients on whom data were available.[63] Death occurred in 29 hospitalized patients with greater incidence of multivessel disease. Mortality was higher in females and in patients over 60 years of age. Nonfatal myocardial infarction was a complication in 154 or 5 percent of these patients and 202 patients or 6.6 percent required emergency coronary artery bypass grafting because of inability to bypass the occlusion or

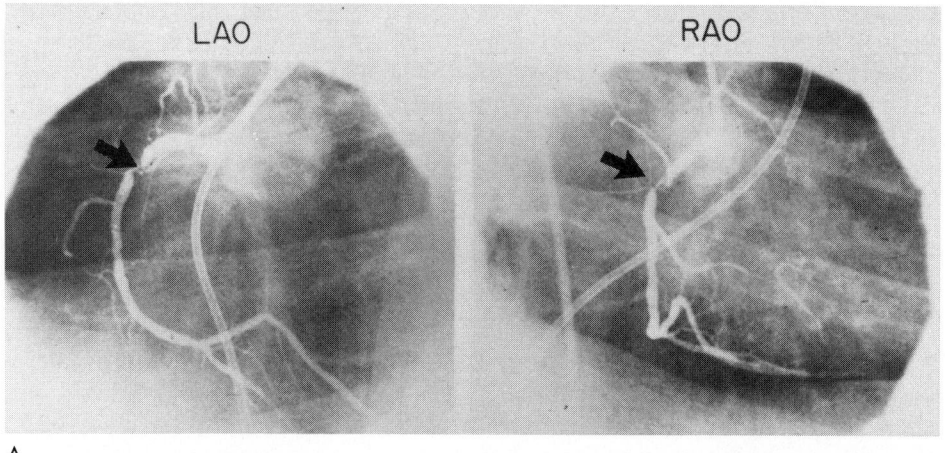

Figure 21-5 (*A*) Arteriography of a patient in the LAO and RAO projections, which depict a proximal RCA lesion (95 percent) stenosis amenable to angioplasty. (*B*) After PTCA, in the same patient, flow has been established through the vessel as depicted by the arrows.

damage to the coronary artery.[63] Restenosis remains the most difficult problem associated with PTCA.

Statistics from the NHLBI PTCA registry indicate that out of 1880 patients in whom an initial PTCA was deemed successful, 203 of those patients required a repeat PTCA on the same arterial segment that had restenosed. There was no associated mortality with the repeat PTCA procedure and the success rate was 85.2 percent.[64]

So far, according to the statistics from the NHLBI PTCA registry, restenosis does not present with a life-threatening problem (myocardial infarc-

tion or death). It is also interesting to note that repeat angioplasty yields a low complication rate. The majority of patients do not develop restenosis and report no further complaints of angina.[65]

Researchers are attempting to identify factors that may identify patients for whom restenosis is likely. In a study reported by Thornton et al.,[66] 248 patients were randomized to aspirin or warfarin (Coumadin) therapy following successful PTCA. All patients were restudied angiographically 3 to 6 months later, and the overall recurrence rate of restenosis was 32 percent. However, the recurrence rate among patients treated with aspirin was 27 percent compared to a 36 percent recurrence rate in patients treated with Coumadin. Although this finding was not statistically significant, it is of interest in regard to the use of aspirin which has fewer side effects than Coumadin.[66]

Presently, cardiologists choose a balloon catheter smaller than the calculated adjacent artery for use in a PTCA. Some authorities propose that successful results can be achieved with optimal selection of the balloon-artery ratio and balloon pressure application. Furthermore, it has been suggested that anatomic or procedural factors may be responsible for restenosis.[67] Future research is needed in relation to anatomic or procedural factors which could be responsible for restenosis. Further inquiry into the role of antiplatelet drugs and calcium channel blockers must also be addressed as to their effects on restenosis.

The patient's condition at the conclusion of the PTCA procedure dictates the intensity of care. Most patients are monitored for at least 4 to 6 h on a cardiac monitor for signs of myocardial ischemia. Isoenzymes are drawn on return from the catheterization laboratory. After the femoral sheath is removed, adequate assessment of the site for bleeding or hematoma formation is completed. The patient may ambulate several hours later.

If the patient should develop chest pain soon after the procedure, standard acute coronary care procedure is followed and includes a 12-lead ECG to document ischemia, vasodilator or drug therapy to relieve pain, and serial CK and isoenzymes (CK and LDH) to document the presence or absence of significant myocardial damage. If the pain persists, indicating an abrupt reduction in blood flow due to reocclusion of the dilated artery, the patient may be returned to the catheterization laboratory for repeat angiography and, perhaps, angioplasty.

Laser Angioplasty

Lasers have been used in medicine for over 15 years. They have been employed by a variety of disciplines such as dermatology, gastroenterology, gynecology, and otolarynology. "Laser" simply means *l*ight *a*mplification by *s*timulated *e*mission of *r*adiation. At present, there are three common laser types used in medicine: the CO_2 laser, the neodymium-Yag laser, and the argon laser.

The argon laser at present appears to be most applicable to coronary atheromas because the continuous wave operates in the blue-green range of the visible spectrum, and is easily absorbed by red tissue. This type of laser is also compatible to optical fiber coupling, is reliable, and easy to operate. The argon laser is being used to vaporize atheromatous lesions, open total occlusions, and decrease calcified as well as noncalcified plaque in animals. Tissue damage may still develop because of incorrect estimation of the plaque size and calcification. Absorption of the wavelength by ions, water, and blood may attenuate the delivery of laser energy. Charring along the atherosclerotic plaque, thermal injury, rupture of the artery, and thrombi formation have also been reported.[68,69]

Macruz and coworkers[70] described in 1980 the use of lasers as a treatment modality to revascularize obstructed coronary atheromas. Since then, both in-vitro and in-vivo animal studies, along with several human studies, have evaluated the use of lasers and their effect on plaque.[71-73]

Choy and coworkers[73] were the first to report the use of laser angioplasty in humans at the time of bypass surgery. Results from most of the animal and human studies indicate that one of the foremost complications of lasers is a high perforation rate, which will make human application problematic. The high perforation rate is thought to be attributed to the type of laser delivery system.

Recently, a new laser delivery system, the laser probe, has been perfected (Fig. 21-6)[74]. This laser probe converts argon laser energy to heat in a rounded metallic tip at the end of a fiber-optic fiber. The rounded tip permits laser thermal energy to be emitted circumferentially inside the vessel, instead of being distributed as a narrowly directed beam, as is the case in a bare fiber-optic fiber.[74] The laser probe has been used in animals with favorable results and has recently been employed in patients with severe peripheral vascular disease.[72] Catheter developments modified this laser probe system to make it applicable to human coronary arteries and it has recently been employed by Sanborn[74] in several patients requiring both laser and balloon angioplasty.

Much work remains to be done in the area of laser angioplasty. Some researchers feel lasers are too complex, requiring frequent adjustments

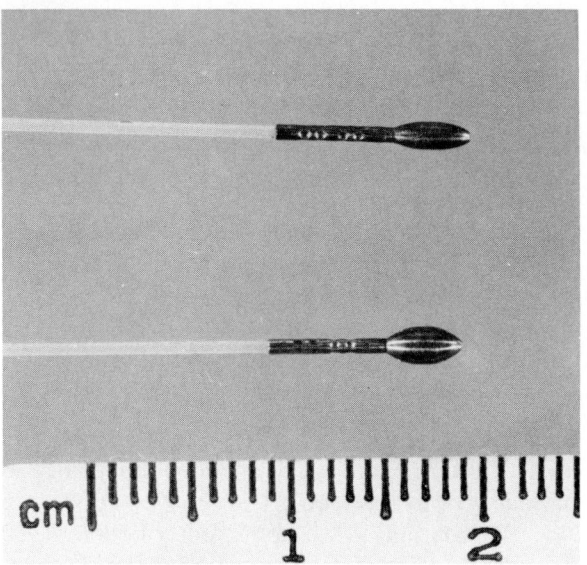

Figure 21-6 Illustration of the new laser probe delivery system. Used to vaporize atheromatous lesions.

and maintenance, and may prove to be too inconsistent for medical application. At present, laser therapy is unlikely to replace balloon angioplasty, but may be used as an adjunct to balloon angioplasty or CABG surgery.[68]

Surgery

Coronary artery bypass grafting (CABG) is the predominant surgical intervention for CAD. Some centers are also doing coronary endarterectomies for coronary artery disease. These interventions will be discussed in greater detail in a later section of this chapter.

Nursing Therapies

Patients admitted to a coronary care unit or a critical-care unit are usually those patients who manifest symptoms of unstable angina requiring further evaluation. Unstable angina patients may present at the time of admission with chest discomfort. Immediate attention must be given to providing relief of the discomfort; the drug of choice is usually nitroglycerin. The degree and intensity of the discomfort or pain determine the route of administration of nitroglycerin. Most often, if pain resolution cannot be obtained with oral or sublingual nitrates,

which is likely with unstable angina, intravenous therapy is required. A second priority on admission is the application of electrodes for continuous ECG monitoring to observe for ischemic changes. It is also necessary during an anginal attack to obtain a 12-lead ECG so as to document the presence of ischemic changes in leads viewing the area of ischemia. After these priorities have been addressed, the critical-care nurse should obtain a nursing history, including patient assessment, and identify the patient's problems based on the data obtained. Early interventions aimed at resolving these problems as well as minimizing or preventing potential problems are then implemented. In addition to the nursing history, the physical assessment and data from diagnostic procedures are incorporated in the data base.

Gordon's functional health patterns, as described in Chap. 20, provide a framework upon which a biopsychosocial nursing history may be obtained.[75] The reader is referred to that chapter for a more detailed explanation of these health patterns. As part of the nursing history, specific information regarding cardiac risk factors, family history of heart disease, and pain history, especially activities which precipitate discomfort or pain, is elicited. Previous medical history, medication history, occupation (may be a source of stress), and anticipated changes in life-style secondary to coronary artery disease should also be obtained.

The physical assessment of the unstable angina patient provides minimal information because the examination usually depicts normal data. Specific signs and symptoms during an anginal attack have been previously described. Auscultation of heart sounds during an anginal attack may reveal a paradoxical splitting of the second heart sound (S_2), pulsus alternans, or the presence of a transient S_3, or a fourth heart sound (S_4). In addition, there may also be a transient systolic murmur of mitral regurgitation secondary to papillary muscle ischemia. Most of these findings are considered nonspecific findings in unstable angina patients because they are often associated with stable angina or acute MI.[37]

Laboratory data may reveal elevated serum cholesterol levels and specific lipoproteins. Cardiac enzymes should not be elevated unless necrosis is present.

Once the data base is completed, both actual or potential problems may be identified. These problems are classified into collaborative diagnoses or nursing diagnoses. A nursing care plan aimed at alleviating or preventing either type of problem may be formulated from the data base. Patient outcomes, nursing interventions, and evaluation will be discussed for collaborative and actual diagnoses.

Collaborative Problem

Alteration in comfort: Pain (angina) related to decreased tissue perfusion.

Goal

The patient's frequency, intensity, duration, or quality of chest pain pattern will not deteriorate while in the critical-care setting.

Nursing Interventions

1. Instruct patient to immediately notify nursing staff of pain or chest discomfort.
2. Observe for nonverbal cues such as facial grimaces, restlessness, and posturing suggestive of pain or discomfort.
3. Monitor and document pain characteristics such as intensity, duration, localization, and radiation; and associated and alleviating factors so as to discern angina from other etiologies.
4. Administer medications such as nitrates, beta blockers, and calcium channel antagonists to relieve or prevent chest discomfort or pain.
5. Assess the patient's response to prescribed medications in order to determine the degree of relief obtained.
6. Explore with patient what factors precipitate or aggravate pain and then discuss possible changes in daily activities or life-style that may be necessary to prevent angina attacks.
7. Decrease physical activity during anginal attack.
8. Remove or reduce stress-provoking stimuli from a patient's environment, such as bright lights, loud, sudden noises, and frequent interruptions.
9. Provide for long, uninterrupted restful periods by organizing plan of care with other health care disciplines.
10. Obtain a 12-lead ECG during chest discomfort and report ischemic changes.
11. Employ energy conservation measures.

Evaluation

Patient will verbalize or demonstrate a decrease in frequency or intensity of pain as evidenced by (1) a decreased use of pharmacologic agents, (2) a decrease in nonverbal cues, (3) a decrease in incidence of pain, and (4) a decrease in duration and intensity of pain. Patient will also be able to verbalize factors that precipitate or aggravate pain and describe preventive actions.

Actual Nursing Diagnosis

Ineffective coping related to knowledge deficit of disease process.

Goal

Patient will demonstrate effective coping behaviors while in the critical-care setting.

Nursing Interventions

1. Assess impact of illness on patient and significant others.
2. Observe for signs of ineffective coping.
3. Encourage patient and family communication with nursing staff.
4. Inform patient and significant others of the disease process.
5. Discuss the disease process.
6. Discuss risk factors that contribute to the development of CAD and identify which of those risk factors are present and can be modified.
7. Instruct patient regarding signs and symptoms of angina that may occur as well as signs and symptoms of progression to an MI.
8. Assist with identification of appropriate resources available to the patient and/or family which may be utilized to help patient cope with the disease process.
9. Provide positive reinforcement with patient's use of effective coping mechanisms.
10. Begin instruction regarding medications—specifically their actions, side effects, and prophylactic use of antianginal drugs. Stress importance of adhering to prescribed medications.
11. Begin to explore necessary life-style changes as a result of disease process.
12. Consult with dietician to provide menus and substitutions compatible with patient's taste.

Evaluation

The patient is able to verbalize feelings and can identify his or her strengths in coping with illness. The patient will be able to recognize effective coping mechanisms and demonstrate use of them. Patient will be able to identify and utilize resources which may assist him or her to cope with illness.

The potential nursing diagnoses for the patient with unstable angina include:

1. Potential for decreased activity tolerance related to deconditioning
2. Potential for anxiety related to knowledge deficit regarding CAD
3. Potential for disturbance in self-concept related to patient/family responses to changes in lifestyle
4. Potential for injury related to failure to follow prescribed regimen

Along with these nursing interventions, critical-care nurses need to be aware of the physician's plan of therapy. Most patients with unstable angina stabilize or progress into such coronary events as MI or congestive heart failure. If progression occurs, the patient may also require counterpulsation or surgery. The critical-care nurse needs to prepare the patient and significant others for these interventions and also provide teaching regarding diagnostic procedures such as cardiac catheterization or gated blood pool scans.

The prognosis of unstable angina has improved over the last decade. This improvement can be attributed to advances in drug therapy, modification of risk factors, and more aggressive treatment modalities such as counterpulsation and PTCA. As additional information regarding the pathogenesis of atherosclerosis in CAD is elucidated, secondary prevention measures may improve this prognosis.

Myocardial Infarction

Introduction

As a serious complication of coronary artery disease, myocardial infarction (MI) remains the leading cause of death in the United States. The development of an MI is a manifestation of a serious interruption in blood supply to a segment of myocardium. As previously discussed, the supply is often fixed because of the formation of atherosclerotic plaques which partially occlude the lumen. It appears that an acute disruptive incident within an atherosclerotic coronary segment leads to sudden cessation of blood supply. This abrupt decrease in blood flow results in diminished or absence of oxygen supply to the heart resulting in ischemia, injury, and necrosis to the area of the myocardium supplied by that particular artery. The time course for damage to occur seems to be an interval ranging from minutes to several hours.[76,77]

Etiology of Myocardial Infarction

Myocardial infarction may be associated with any condition that produces prolonged, unrelieved ischemic episodes which cause irreversible damage and necrosis to myocardial cells. Unlike ischemic precordial chest pain (angina), which occurs as a result of an imbalance between myocardial blood supply and demand, an MI is caused by total obstruction in blood supply to a region of myocardium and is largely unrelated to myocardial demand.[77] According to Alpert and Braunwald,[78] the majority of MI patients have underlying atherosclerosis; however, these lesions are not thought to be responsible solely for occluding the coronary vessel.[76-79] Thrombosis has been implicated as the major precipitator of the abrupt interruption in blood supply. Coronary spasm and platelet aggregation have also been suggested as causative factors in the precipitation of an MI. These will be discussed in this section.

Thrombosis

It is evident from the literature that thrombus formation plays a major role in the etiology of an MI.[77-79] A thrombus which has been found to form over a previously narrowed atheroma (75 to 80 percent occluded) is usually the acute disruptive event which leads to total cessation of blood to the area of myocardium supplied by that atherosclerotic coronary artery. The precipitating events which incite thrombus formation appear to be plaque rupture, hemorrhage into the plaque, or erosion of the intima over the fibrous cap.[77] According to Factor and Kirk,[76] a number of studies have correlated coronary thrombosis with rupture or cracks of the thin fibrous cap and release of the plaque constituents into the coronary lumen. Plaque rupture may incite thrombus formation through one or a combination of mechanisms: (1) contact of platelets with denuded collagen, leading to thrombocyte adherence and the accumulation of a platelet plug; (2) release of tissue thromboplastin from the plaque contents, inciting the initiation of the clotting cascade; and (3) mechanical obstruction of the vascular lumen by the plaque components.

The incidence of thrombosis is thought to be 60 percent or greater as noted in postmortem investigations of subjects who had sudden cardiac death.[80] Because thrombus formation plays a major role in the evolution of an infarct, interventions have been aimed at dissolving clots. Such discoveries as thrombolytic agents have paved the way for unraveling the mysteries regarding the etiology of MI.

Coronary Artery Spasm

The concept of coronary artery spasm being a cause of myocardial infarction is fraught with controversy in the literature. The work of Prinzmetal, Kennamer, Merliss, Wada, and Bor brought to the forefront a reinvestigation of the mechanisms of rest angina.[23] In the 1970s, extensive clinical investigations documented the presence of spasm primarily in vessels with moderate or severe atherosclerotic lesions. Spasms were found not only involving the stenotic segment, but were also noted in proximal and distal segments.[81]

Maseri and coworkers indicated that spasm could be a possible cause for myocardial infarction.[82] Vincent, Anderson, and Marshall[83] reported a case study of a young woman who had a myocardial infarction in the presence of documented angiographically normal coronary arteries. It has been suggested that spasm predisposes to the formation of thrombi or to platelet aggregation, which may in turn lead to prolonged total obstruction and infarction. In contrast, Maseri and Chierchia[81] suggested that thrombi liberate potent coronary vasoconstrictors such as thromboxane A and serotonin, which may in turn precipitate sustained spasm over a long segment of a vessel preventing inflow from collaterals, and favoring the distal formation of thrombus. Another etiology for coronary vasospasm appears to be hypercontractility of the arterial wall associated with atherosclerosis.[84] Regardless of the controversy surrounding the underlying mechanism for coronary vasospasm, it is important for the critical-care nurse to appreciate the fact that spasm is implicated in the etiology of some MIs.

Platelet Aggregation

Blood flow turbulence at the site of a stenotic area creates a favorable milieu for platelet adhesion and aggregation.[81] Platelet aggregation results when injury to the myocardial tissue occurs because platelets migrate to the site of injury, and envelope the damaged surface. Moreover, these platelets are thought to release serotonin, adenosine diphosphate (ADP), catecholamines, and PDGF into the plasma. In turn, additional platelets adhere and aggregate at the site of vessel injury. The platelet aggregation can further impede blood flow at the area of stenosis, resulting in prolonged ischemic episodes and tissue necrosis.

Pathophysiology

Myocardial infarction usually develops distal to a totally occluded coronary artery. The amount of cells that become necrotic is determined by the amount of blood which is able to flow into the ischemic zone after the abrupt occlusion and by the duration of time it takes for flow to be resumed, if at all. Flow can be reestablished into the affected region, either retrograde via collateral vessels from distant coronary beds, or antegrade through clot lysis, or by retraction of a wall that has been in spasm.[77]

There is a sequential transmural pattern by which the jeopardized myocardium undergoes necrosis; it begins in the subendocardium and extends toward the epicardium. In the epicardial layers, tissue salvage is relative to the restoration of blood flow to this region or the presence of sufficient collaterals to this area to prevent tissue necrosis.[76]

It has been theorized that the time for prolonged, unrelieved ischemic episodes to cause cellular death can range from 25 min to several hours (3 to 6 h).[76-78] Cellular death is also dependent on the following factors: (1) the rate of development of the obstruction; (2) the coronary artery that is occluded; (3) the quantity of myocardium supplied by that artery; (4) the quantity of collateral flow available to the ischemic cells; and (5) the presence, site, and severity of any coronary artery spasm.[77,78]

Three types of irreversible cell injury can be identified histologically. These include coagulation necrosis, contraction band necrosis, and myocytolysis.[77] *Coagulation necrosis* is the type of necrosis that occurs when the blood supply to that region is permanently impeded. The tissue becomes pale or white in color. Within 6 to 12 h, the necrotic cells thin and stretch out. Over the course of several weeks, the necrotic cells are replaced by newly formed granulation tissue and within a year, the affected area becomes a dense collagen scar.

Contraction band necrosis is another type of necrosis which results from a period of prolonged ischemia followed by reperfusion of the area.[77] Thus, this necrosis occurs when myocardial blood flow is temporarily interrupted. The tissue typically appears as a red infarct which depicts the restoration of blood to the necrotic region. This reperfusion may cause some frank hemorrhage into the extracellular spaces. Patients in whom contraction band necrosis has been noted are those with spasm, those with nontransmural MIs, those who have died after cardiac surgery, or those who have had cardiopulmonary bypass which temporarily interrupted flow to the heart. This type of necrosis may also be noted on the margins of an acute infarct which is chiefly coagulation necrosis.

The third type of necrosis is *myocytolysis*, which is predominantly found on the border of infarcts or in the subendocardium.[77] Subcellular damage occurs with this type of ischemic cell injury along with a balloonlike degenerative appearance of these cells. Some of these cells have been found to survive for a time, although the ultimate fate of these damaged cells needs to be elucidated. When any of these cells die, they are replaced by scar tissue.

Intracellular Alterations

Myocardial cells normally utilize glucose (postprandial state and free fatty acids (unfed state) as an energy source to form adenosine triphosphate (ATP) during aerobic metabolism. With ischemia, there is a decrease in oxygenated blood supply to these cells and they revert to anaerobic metabolism. Glucose through the process of glycolysis (which

requires a supply of glycogen) becomes the main fuel source in anaerobic metabolism. The formation of ATP is severely reduced by anaerobic metabolism. Anaerobic metabolism supplies less than half the energy requirements of the cell.[85] In addition, lactic acid is produced by anaerobic metabolism, causing the intracellular pH to lower, resulting in acidosis. Acidosis, in turn, can inhibit the phosphorylation of glycogen to glucose, further reducing the production of ATP as well as depressing contractility.[85]

As a result of anaerobic metabolism, ischemic tissue is able to meet a significantly smaller proportion of its energy requirements. Therefore, when the demand exceeds the supply, the limited high-energy phosphate stores of ATP are depleted rapidly, resulting in the development of irreversible injury in the ischemic tissue. The injured cell membranes lose their functional integrity and leak their cytoplasmic contents into the circulation, releasing enzymes such as lactic dehydrogenase (LDH), creatine kinase (CK), and serum glutamic oxaloacetic transaminase (SGOT), which can be clinically measured.

Types of Infarcts

Infarcts may be divided into two major categories: *transmural* and *nontransmural*. A *transmural infarct* is described as myocardial necrosis which extends through the full thickness of the ventricular wall. The location of these infarcts can be anterior, lateral, inferior, or posterior, as depicted by the ECG. *Nontransmural infarcts* can be subdivided into (1) *subendocardial infarcts*, in which the necrosis is limited to the subendocardial surface; (2) *subepicardial infarcts*, in which necrosis is found on the epicardial layer; and (3) *intramural infarcts*, in which necrosis is seen in isolated sections of the myocardium without extending through the entire wall.

Most infarcts occur in the left ventricle and interventricular septum. However, in patients with inferior infarcts, approximately one-third sustain some damage to the right ventricle. Right ventricular infarcts are thought to occur in the setting of a transmural infarction of either the inferior-posterior wall or the posterior wall of the septum. Atrial infarcts have also been reported. These atrial infarcts tend to be manifested more on the right than on the left side, and in atrial appendages rather than in the lateral or posterior walls.[78] Patients with atrial infarcts frequently exhibit atrial dysrhythmias.

Location of Infarcts

The size and location of an infarct is dependent on several variables. These variables include (1) the site and degree of occlusion of the coronary artery, (2) the occurrence and intensity of coronary artery spasm near the occluded vessel, (3) the extent of the tissue supplied by that vessel, (4) development and extent of collateral blood vessels distal to the occluded vessel, and (5) O_2 requirements of the poorly perfused myocardium.[78]

In order to comprehend the locations of infarcts, the critical-care nurse must know which coronary artery supplies each area of the myocardium. As a review, the coronary arteries are classified as (1) the left main coronary artery, which extends about 5 cm from the left coronary ostium and subdivides into the left anterior descending (LAD) and left circumflex (LCX) artery; and (2) the right coronary artery (RCA). The coronary arteries and the area which each supplies are listed in Table 21-5.

The majority of anterior wall infarcts are caused by occlusion of the LAD. Other areas which may be affected by occlusions in the LAD are portions of the septum, anterolateral wall, papillary muscle, and inferioapical wall of the LV. Anterior infarcts tend to be larger than inferior infarcts and generally tend to have a greater degree of LV impairment in contrast to inferior infarcts. Anterior infarcts also tend to have a worse prognosis for patients than inferior infarcts, probably because of the greater extent of LV injury.[86]

Lateral or inferolateral wall infarcts of the LV can be attributed to occlusion in the left circumflex artery (LCX). Occlusions of the RCA can cause inferior, inferoposterior, as well as right ventricular (RV) infarcts.

True posterior infarcts usually result from occlusion in the LCX artery. These types of infarcts are somewhat more difficult to diagnose because there are no specific leads which directly face the injured area. Clinicians, therefore, look for reciprocal changes in leads V_1 and V_2 on the ECG. However, a recent investigation revealed that a Q

Table 21-5 Summary of the Coronary Arteries and the Major Areas and Structures Supplied

Coronary Artery	Major Areas and Structures Supplied
Right coronary	1. SA node (55%)
	2. AV node (90%)
	3. Bundle of His
	4. Right atrium and right ventricle
	5. Inferior/diaphragmatic surface of left ventricle
	6. Posterior one-third of septum
	7. Posterior/inferior division of left bundle
Left main	1. Massive LV area
Left anterior descending	1. Anterior wall of left ventricle
	2. Anterior two-thirds of septum
	3. Bundle of His
	4. Right bundle branch
	5. Anterior/superior division of the left bundle branch
	6. Posterior/inferior division of the left bundle branch
	7. Apex of LV
Left circumflex	1. SA node (45%)
	2. AV node (10%)
	3. Inferior/diaphragmatic surface of left ventricle
	4. Lateral wall of left ventricle
	5. Left atrium
	6. Posterior/inferior division of the left bundle branch

wave in V_6 is an excellent marker for posterior asynergy and is a useful criterion for the presence of a true posterior MI when there are concomitant Q waves noted in inferior leads on the ECG.[87]

Resolution of an Infarct

The resolution of an infarct begins at the periphery of the infarct and moves centrally. The formation of granulation tissue begins with subsequent phagocytosis of the dead myocardial cells by polymorphonuclear neutrophils and macrophages.[78] These necrotic cells eventually disappear and are replaced with scar tissue. These pathologic changes which occur in the postinfarction period are described in Table 21-6. The healing of an infarct under normal

Table 21-6 Summary of the Pathologic Changes Which Occur in the Postinfarction Period

Postinfarct Time	Pathologic Changes
0–6 h	No gross changes apparent.
6–18 h	Pale, bluish, and slightly swollen.
18–36 h	Tan or reddish purple with serofibrinous exudate on epicardium.
48 h	Gray and fine yellow lines appear at periphery and widen to extend through infarct.
8–10 days	Decreased thickness in wall in area of infarct due to removal of necrotic muscle by mononuclear cells. Cut surface of an infarct is yellow, surrounded by reddish-purple band of granulation tissue.
3–4 weeks	Extension of yellowish color through the necrotic tissue.
2–3 months	Infarcted area has gelatinous ground-glass or gray appearance which is then converted to a fibrous white scar.

Source: J. Alpert, and E. Braunwald, Acute Mycardial Infarction: Pathological, Pathophysiological, and Clinical Manifestations. In E. Braunwald (ed.), *Heart Disease,* Philadelphia, W. B. Saunders, 1984.

circumstances is resolved within 4 to 6 weeks, depending on the size of the infarcted area. Variables which could prolong the healing of an infarct are excessive LV dilatation, which predisposes to aneursym formation and extension of the infarct.[78]

Data Acquisition

History

The majority of patients (80 percent) admitted after an acute myocardial infarction present with chest pain.[26,78] The pain is typically more severe than angina, is prolonged (usually greater than 15 to 20 min), and most often, is unrelieved by nitroglycerin. When describing the pain, some patients report radiation or localization to the neck, jaw, back, shoulder, substernal region, left arm, or near the epigastric area, which may cause patients to think that they have indigestion and to treat themselves with antacids. Patients may be clutching their chest and sitting forward and may appear diaphoretic, pale, and restless, along with being nauseated, and

some may even vomit. Gastrointestinal symptoms such as nausea, vomiting, and hiccoughing are often associated with a vagal reflex.

Physical Examination

On physical examination, the overall cardiovascular status is evaluated. Patients generally look acutely ill, are in severe discomfort, and with facial grimaces indicative of pain. Their skin color may be either normal or a gray, ashen appearance, and the skin may be moist, warm, or cool.

Vital signs are affected by the autonomic nervous system. Excessive sympathetic stimulation as a compensatory mechanism can be seen in 40 percent of patients with an acute anterior infarction and in 25 percent of patients with an inferior infarction.[86,88] Under these circumstances, the blood pressure is elevated and the heart rate may be rapid and irregular due to premature ventricular contractions (PVCs). Sympathetic overactivity may be attributed to either pain or anxiety or to the stimulation of cardiac chemoreceptors by substances emitted from acutely ischemic or infarcted cells.[88]

Parasympathetic overactivity, the result of activation of the vagal reflex, has been reported in 30 percent of patients with anterior infarcts and in 65 percent of those experiencing an inferior infarct. This vagal reflex is often referred to as the Bezold-Javisch reflex.[88] The resultant bradycardia exhibited by these patients is often associated with concomitant hypotension. The hypotension is reversible when atropine and fluids are administered.

The respiratory rate is usually elevated immediately after an MI as a sequela of the pain and anxiety. The respiratory rate should return to normal once the pain and psychological stress are decreased, unless the patient develops ventricular failure.

An elevation in body temperature may occur 24 to 48 h postinfarction as a result of tissue necrosis. Acute pericarditis can also cause an elevation in body temperature 2 to 3 days following an MI.

Heart sounds are often muffled because of the reduced left ventricular contractility, but they are more distinctive as healing occurs. The presence of an S_4 sound is considered to be a common sign in patients with ischemic heart disease.[78] This sound is best heard at the apex. A fourth heart sound may be an indication of a decrease in LV compliance and reflect elevations in LVEDP. With RV infarcts, an S_4 is best heard at the left sternal border.

Patients with extensive infarctions may also have an S_3 sound, which reflects severe LV dysfunction, decreased LV compliance, and LV dilatation. An S_3 sound is a common finding with transmural anterior infarcts, in contrast with inferior or nontransmural infarcts. It is best heard at the apex with a patient in the left lateral decubitus position. It has been reported that the mortality of patients with a documented S_3 sound in the immediate postinfarct phase is higher than in those patients without this sound. In the presence of papillary muscle dysfunction, there may also be systolic murmurs resulting from acute mitral regurgitation. A pericardial friction rub may also be auscultated in the setting of an acute MI in approximately 20 percent of patients.[78]

Breath sounds need to be auscultated for baseline purposes as soon as possible after admission to a critical-care unit. Moist bibasilar crackles may be found in patients who subsequently develop left ventricular failure postinfarction.

In patients who exhibit RV infarcts, the jugular veins are distended. The jugular venous pressure is also elevated in cardiogenic shock and reduced in the presence of hypotension or hypoperfusion. Palpation of the carotid pulse indicates the status of the LV stroke volume. For example, a small, weak pulse is indicative of reduced stroke volume, while a sharp, brief upstroke is often felt in patients with mitral regurgitation, or a ruptured interventricular septum when there is a left-to-right shunt.[78]

Diagnostic Procedures

In addition to a history suggestive of MI, other data required to make the diagnosis include ECG abnormalities suggestive of ischemia, injury and necrosis, and serial enzymes. Discussion in this section will center on these data as well as information obtained from such procedures as echocardiography, radionuclide studies, and cardiac catheterization.

ECG   The pathologic changes which are seen in the majority of patients who sustain a transmural infarct include development of abnormal, persistent Q waves; elevation of the ST segment; and sym-

metrical inversion of the T wave. Ischemia produces ST segment depression as well as T wave inversion. Injury is depicted as ST segment elevation and T wave inversion. Infarction is noted with the appearance of pathologic Q waves which either exceed 0.04 s (1 mm) wide or are 25 percent (one-fourth), or one-third the height of the R wave in leads facing the infarcted area. These changes are often referred to as indicative changes.

The sequence of events of an MI as noted on the ECG begins with the hyperacute phase in which the ST segment and T waves are elevated in those leads facing the injured area. The T waves invert after several hours or days and pathologic Q waves eventually appear. As the infarct resolves, the ST segments revert to the baseline, and eventually the T waves return to normal. The pathologic Q waves persist for months to years, although some evidence refutes this commonly held belief.[26]

Reciprocal changes or mirror images of the ECG disturbances noted in the leads facing the injured area appear in those leads opposite to the site of injury. Notably, there are ST depressions. Many patients with inferior wall infarctions who demonstrate ST depression in V_1 to V_4 leads have been shown to have extensive global and regional wall dysfunction and are at high risk for further complications of ischemic heart disease.[86] Table 21-7 lists the sites of an MI and the leads associated with indicative and reciprocal changes.

Infarcts restricted to the subendocardial layers are treated aggressively because of recent data which suggest a mortality comparable to that of

Table 21-7 Sites of an MI and Leads Associated with Indicative and Reciprocal Changes

Type of Infarct	Leads with Indicative Changes	Leads with Reciprocal Changes
Inferior	2, 3, aVF	I, aVL and right and midprecordial chest leads V_1–V_4
Extensive anterior	I, aVL, V_1–V_6	2, 3, aVF, aVR
Anteroseptal	V_1–V_4	
Anterolateral	I, aVL, V_3–V_6	
High anterolateral	I, aVL	
Lateral	I, aVL, V_5–V_6	2, 3, aVF
True posterior	V_6 (Bar et al.[85])	V_1–V_2

transmural infarcts.[77] The ECG changes which occur with subendocardial injury may be localized or diffuse. The typical changes are ST segment depression concomitantly with T wave inversion. These changes are usually nonspecific in that they may also be a result of conditions such as acute pericarditis, ventricular hypertrophy, or electrolyte disturbances. Lead aVR is the only endocardial lead that may exhibit ST elevation in the setting of subendocardial infarcts.

Cardiac Enzymes   As was previously mentioned, enzymes are released from necrotic myocardial cells and enter the circulation. The most important of these enzymes are creatine kinase (CK) and lactic dehydrogenase (LDH), and are found to be elevated in an acute MI. Certain isoenzymes of CK and LDH are more specific for acute MI because these isoenzymes are located predominantly in myocardial tissue. The isoenzymes of CK specific for myocardial damage are the MB band of CK (CK-MB) which elevates 2 to 4 h after an MI. The isoenzymes for LDH are LDH_1 and LDH_2, which are changed to a characteristic "flipped pattern." Under normal circumstances, the value of LDH_2 exceeds that of LDH_1; however, in the setting of an MI, LDH_1 exceeds LDH_2.[89] More detailed explanation regarding these enzymes can be found in Chap. 20.

Echocardiography   Echocardiography is often employed as a method for estimating the extent of myocardial damage and for identifying regional wall motion abnormalities associated with an MI. It can also be used to detect intracardiac thrombi following an infarct. If thrombi are discovered, anticoagulant therapy may be warranted in this situation.

A study was conducted in which 43 consecutive patients with documented acute MIs had serial 2-D echocardiograms performed to predict the short-term clinical prognosis of the subject.[90] The researchers concluded that an echocardiogram obtained on the day of admission could be used to accurately define the extent and severity of the acute MI and could be used to predict whether the short-term clinical course would be complicated.

Two-dimensional echocardiograms may also prove useful in differentiating new from old infarcts.[91] In addition, other useful data can be ob-

tained by 2-D echocardiograms, such as the detection of small pericardial effusions in patients with postinfarction pericarditis, ventricular septal defects, and mitral regurgitation.[78]

Radionuclide Studies   Many advancements in nuclear cardiology have substantially improved diagnostic capabilities to detect an acute MI. Common radionuclide tests used in detection of an MI are the technetium (Tc) 99m pyrophosphate (PYP) scan, thallium 201 myocardial perfusion scintiography, and radionuclide ventriculography (RVG), also known as gated blood-pool scans. A newer diagnostic test is positron emission tomography, which will also be discussed in this section.

Thallium 201 and ^{99m}Tc PYP are both radioactive cell tracers which can be absorbed by either normal or abnormal myocardial cells. ^{99m}Tc PYP scans utilize hot spot imaging to detect myocardial infarction. In theory, technetium pyrophosphate binds to calcium in infarcted tissue; therefore, the accuracy of this test is dependent on the amount of calcium contained within necrotic tissue. It has been reported that the maximal sensitivity of this type of imaging is 24 to 72 h after an MI because the calcium in necrotic tissue is eventually reabsorbed.[89] It has been recommended that the use of pyrophosphate scans be limited to those patients in whom clinical and laboratory results are nondiagnostic.[36] Newer isotopes have been employed in humans and include ^{99m}Tc-labeled antimyosin antibody, which has been proposed to detect regions of myocardial necrosis, and indium III, which is an isotope used to image platelets at sites of cardiac thrombosis.[92]

Thallium 201 utilizes thallous chloride, which is chemically similar to potassium, as its isotope. This type of imaging is referred to as "cold spot imaging" in that infarcted tissue does not absorb this isotope and shows up as a blank or cold spot image. Thallium scans can be used in the evaluation of acute as well as old infarcts; however, there appear to be some doubts as to the accuracy of these scans. Newer techniques, such as thallium 201 tomography, and rubidium 82 positron-emitted tomography, may be useful for the localization of infarcts. In addition, magnetic resonance imaging (MRI) continues to be investigated and will probably play an important role in cardiovascular diagnosis in the future.[93] The reader is referred to Chap. 20 for a detailed description of these procedures.

Gated blood-pool scans, or RVGs, are used to assess cardiac function (ejection fraction), and to analyze wall motion abnormalities in infarcted areas by which aneurysms may be detected. It has been found that radionuclide ejection fractions tend to be lower in patients with anterior infarctions in contrast to inferior infarctions.[92] Gated blood-pool scans are not used to specifically localize infarcts.

Positron emission tomography (PET) is a recent advance in the diagnosis of the extent of an MI which assesses myocardial blood flow and cellular metabolism.[92] It is a noninvasive technique which allows measurements of local myocardial tissue concentrations of certain radioactive isotope tracers. Two tracers, F-2-fluoro-2-deoxyglucose (FDG) and N-13 ammonia, have been employed to identify and differentiate between myocardial ischemia and infarction in humans.[94] The FDG tracer is a glucose compound which measures glucose uptake in ischemic tissue. There is increased glucose utilization in ischemic cells because these cells are incapable of normally metabolizing free fatty acids (FFA) when becoming ischemic and revert to anaerobic glucose metabolism. The N-13 ammonia isotope tracer measures the degree of flow (perfusion) to myocardial tissue. Thus, areas which have necrotic tissue will not depict any uptake of the N-13 ammonia tracer.

When both tracers were used, the extent of the infarct as well as the degree of ischemic tissue could be noted.[94] It was found that neither FDG nor N-13 ammonia uptake occurred in necrotic tissue. This is regarded as a match or concordance between FDG and N-13 ammonia. On the other hand, it was found that in ischemic regions, there was an increase in the uptake of FDG but virtually no uptake of N-13 ammonia. This mismatch between the two tracers shows a discordant increase in FDG activity relative to N-13 ammonia which is found to be consistent with the increased extraction of glucose in ischemic myocardium.

Use of positron emission tomography is an exciting area of diagnostic advances, not only for detecting infarctions but ischemic regions as well. Further evaluation will be necessary to perfect this technique. Its application to other cardiovascular disorders such as cardiomyopathy may be enormous as well.

Cardiac Catheterization and Angiography   Data from cardiac catheterization following an acute LV infarction may reveal elevations in the LVEDP and LVEDV, as well as elevations in LVESP and LVESV. In addition, there is a reduction in the ejection fraction after an MI. Left ventriculography may reveal wall motion abnormalities, referred to as patterns of dysynergy or asynergy, as previously described. Figure 21-3 depicts these abnormalities in the right anterior oblique view. Under normal conditions, the LV cavity resembles an ellipsoid during diastole. During systole, the walls move inward such that at the peak of systolic ejection the LV outline resembles an ice-cream cone or a pear.[26] Hypokinesis is depicted as generalized reduction in wall motion, whereas akinesis is revealed as a segment in which there is no wall motion. Dyskinesis is the paradoxical bulging of a segment during systole. This paradoxical bulging occurs in patients soon after sustaining an MI (most often anterior infarcts) due to an initial increase in segmental LV compliance.[95] This wall motion abnormality leads to decreased stroke volume and a decrease in overall ejection fraction. Left ventricular compliance decreases in time as the infarct evolves, which, in turn, may lead to less dyskinesis and improvement in the ejection fraction. Correlations between the extent of the dyskinetic segment and clinical manifestations have also been noted.[95] These are found in Table 21-8.

Table 21-8 Correlation between the Extent of Dyskinetic Segment and Clinical Manifestations

Dyssynergy	Clinical Manifestations
1. Abnormal segment → 11% of the left ventricle	LVEDP rises above 12 mmHg
2. Abnormal segment → 14%	Decreased ejection fraction
3. Abnormal segment → 30%	Clinical evidence of LV failure
4. Abnormal segment → 40–50%	Clinical evidence of cardiogenic shock

Source: W. E. Donat and B. H. Weiner, Syndromes of Left Ventricular Failure. In J. M. Rippe, et al. (eds.), *Intensive Care Medicine*, Little, Brown, Boston, 1985.

Data from right and left heart catheterization in right ventricular infarctions may reveal an increase in right atrial (RA) pressure in contrast to pulmonary wedge pressures. The RA tracing may reveal elevated V waves in the presence of tricuspid insufficiency. In pure RV infarcts, left-sided diastolic pressures may be slightly decreased in comparison to right-sided pressures. The pulse pressures in the right ventricle and pulmonary artery may also be decreased.[96]

Therapeutic Interventions

Patients with acute myocardial infarctions are generally admitted into a coronary care unit for continuous ECG monitoring. Critical-care nurses in these units need sufficient training and expertise in the immediate recognition of life-threatening dysrhythmias. It has been clearly documented that most of the deaths which occur within the first 2 h after an MI are related to dysrhythmias and that the patient is at significant risk for dysrhythmias the first 24 h after an infarct. The appearance of PVCs is thought to be a precipitator of ventricular tachycardia; they need to be treated in the event that they increase in frequency or become coupled or multifocal. Prophylactic use of IV lidocaine in patients suspected of having an acute MI who are otherwise not sensitive to it has been advocated.[97]

Prompt attention is given to relieving chest pain in the patient with an MI, using small doses of morphine sulfate (4 to 8 mg) at 10-min intervals. Patients with a hypersensitivity to morphine can be treated with IV meperidine (25 to 50 mg) at 10-min intervals. Persistent or recurrent chest pain unrelieved by morphine sulfate can be treated with continuous IV nitroglycerin (NTG) which allows for a constant controlled blood level. Although there is no reported optimal dosage of NTG, it is recommended that the IV rate be titrated between 10 to 20 mg/min with an end point of pain relief, but short of causing symptomatic hypotension or severe headache.[98] Diazepam or phenobarbital is frequently used to provide sedation, especially in patients who exhibit anxiety.

In the past, bed rest was a controversial topic. It was not so long ago that patients were placed on bed rest after an MI for extended periods of time, until data revealed that bed rest was associated with numerous complications such as thrombophlebitis, pulmonary embolism, and pneumonia. There is evidence that orthostatic intolerance begins after as little as 6 h of bed rest. Winslow[99] recommends that nurses caution patients to change positions slowly and to assist and monitor the patient when he or she first gets out of bed. The amount of bed rest required for the acute MI is dependent on the complications present. In the uncomplicated MI, the patient is usually confined to bed for 24 h with bedside commode privileges.[26] During those 24 h, the patient should be instructed to perform lower extremity exercises such as ankle, plantar, and dorsiflexion while on bed rest. It is recommended that increased ambulation be attempted after 48 h. Wenger and Fletcher[100] suggest chair rest for periods of 30 min twice to three times daily after 24 h and increased ambulation such as walking to the bathroom and walking in corridors on days 4 and 5. Under supervised instruction, Wenger and Fletcher[100] recommend that exercise prescriptions involve 1 to 2 metabolic equivalents (METS) of activity with progression to 2 to 3 METS prior to discharge.

Recent investigations have indicated that a lack of scientific rationale exists for coronary precautions such as "no rectal temperatures," or "no vigorous backrubs."[101] The only restriction that appears to be well supported in research is the restriction of stimulant-type beverages. According to Kirchkoff,[101] the restriction of iced beverages may have some scientific basis only if the amount of fluid is about 600 to 800 mL, and if the patient is in the supine position, allowing the heart to be cooled. In support of these research findings, recommendations have been made to limit the intake of ice water to a glass or less at one time.

Oxygen therapy (100%) via nasal cannula or mask is routinely provided at 2 to 4 L per minute for the first 24 to 48 h unless the patient shows evidence of chronic obstructive lung disease or carbon dioxide retention. Clinicians vary in their opinion regarding whether oxygen therapy is beneficial for all uncomplicated MI patients, but concur that O_2 therapy is indicated for patients who are hypoxic.[26]

Patients are routinely given liquids on the day of admission to a critical-care unit and progressed to solid foods as tolerated. Some clinicians advise placing these patients on a low-sodium and low-fat diet.[26]

Prophylactic use of stool softeners is often recommended because constipation is a common sequela of bed rest and narcotics. This constipation may result in excessive straining at stool, which needs to be avoided.

Complications of Myocardial Infarction

Numerous complications are associated with acute myocardial infarction. Ventricular irritability is considered to be the most frequent complication in the first 48 h after an MI. Investigators have attempted to profile the patient at risk for developing ventricular dysrhythmias. According to Wessman,[102] studies have revealed the following:

1. Older patients who experienced episodes of ventricular irritability had greater frequency and severity of episodes than younger patients.
2. Gender was not significant.
3. There was a greater likelihood of ventricular dysrhythmias following an acute MI in patients with diseases such as Parkinson's disease, peptic ulcer, diabetes, or pulmonary disorders.
4. The presence of congestive heart failure, hypertension, angina, or palpitations was associated with a greater likelihood of developing ventricular dysrhythmias.
5. Patients with transmural as opposed to subendocardial infarcts had a higher incidence of ventricular irritability.
6. Patients with anterior infarcts had an increased risk for ventricular dysrhythmias.

It is important for the critical-care nurse to be able to identify MI patients at increased risk of life-threatening ventricular arrhythmias in order to institute preventative measures.

The prophylactic use of lidocaine in preventing primary ventricular fibrillation has been documented in the literature, but not universally implemented in practice.[103] The elderly patient on prophylactic lidocaine requires close monitoring for signs and symptoms of central nervous system disturbances due to decreased clearance of the drug.

Approximately one-third of patients with an MI develop sinus tachycardia (ST).[85] The etiology of ST varies from patient to patient, but factors associated with the development of ST include pain, anxiety, hypovolemia, vasoactive medications, LV failure, and RV infarcts. It must be noted that ST increases MV_{O_2} consumption, and also decreases diastolic filling time and coronary artery perfusion time. Thus, in the setting of an MI, ST should be treated directly or by removing the underlying cause.

Supraventricular dysrhythmias such as atrial flutter and fibrillation commonly occur in the post-MI patient. Atrial flutter occurs less frequently than atrial fibrillation in MIs. Atrial flutter is often associated with a 2:1 block and a rapid ventricular response. The critical-care nurse needs to be aware that the rapid ventricular rate may intensify hemodynamic compromise to MI patients and that excessive rates which exceed 100 beats per minute need to be reported quickly to institute early therapies.[85] Drug therapy may be unsuccessful in treating the rapid ventricular rate; therefore, early cardioversion or overdrive atrial pacing is recommended for patients with atrial flutter.[85,104] Atrial fibrillation may be more amenable to treatment with such drugs as digitalis, verapamil, or quinidine.[104]

Vagotonia following an acute MI may produce bradydysrhythmias. Sinus bradycardia is a frequent sequela of an inferior MI. This disturbance is usually not treated unless the patient manifests hemodynamic deterioration, in which case atropine may be administered as a vagolytic agent.

Ventricular conduction disturbances also may occur in the setting of an acute MI. It is often the critical-care nurse who must recognize these disturbances early in order to prevent deterioration to complete heart block. Insertion of a temporary pacing wire is generally indicated for patients following an MI for either prophylactic or therapeutic reasons. Those indications are found in Table 21-9. Prior to insertion of a pacing wire, these patients may require pharmacologic interventions such as atropine and Isuprel for significant hemodynamic compromise.

Prompt, continuous clinical assessment is necessary for the critical-care nurse to assist in the early recognition of congestive heart failure (CHF). The degree of LV failure is associated with the extent of the infarcted area as well as the degree

Table 21-9 Indications for Temporary Pacing Following Acute Myocardial Infarction

A. Prophylactic
   1. His-Purkinje block strongly indicated
      a. Usually anterior MI
      b. New RBBB and LAHB
      c. New RBBB and LPHB
      d. Alternating BBB
      e. Mobitz II 2° A-VB
      f. Complete heart block
   2. Possibly indicated
      a. 1° A-V block and old bilateral BBB
      b. 1° A-VB and new BBB
   3. A-V nodal block (pacemaker not indicated): usually inferior MI
B. Therapeutic
   1. Medically refractory bradycardia with symptoms (CHF, chest pain, syncope)
   2. Heart rate <50 beats/min
   3. Atrial or A-V sequential pacing for A-V dissociated rhythms and hemodynamic compromise

From J. C. Love, Conduction Disturbances following Acute MI. In J. W. Rippe, et al. (eds.), *Intensive Care Medicine*, Little, Brown, Boston, 1985.

of LV segmental contraction.[95] Clinical and hemodynamic criteria have been used to classify CHF[105] (Table 21-10). These criteria provide clinicians with a logical approach to therapy. For example, patients in subset II might require diuretic therapy, whereas patients in subset III should benefit from additional volume. Common signs and symptoms of CHF are dyspnea, tachypnea, crackles, and an S_3 gallop. The chest x-ray usually reveals pulmonary congestion. In addition, elevations of hemodynamic parameters such as LVEDP, LAP, and PAW are often noted along with a decrease in the cardiac index. Arterial blood gases may reveal hypoxemia depending on the severity of the heart failure.

Patients with anterior MIs tend to have more severe failure in contrast with inferior infarcts because the extent of damage is usually greater with anterior infarcts. In the acute setting, the goal of therapy for patients exhibiting LV failure is twofold: (1) to diminish blood volume and preload with the use of diuretics or nitroglycerin (NTG) and (2) to decrease afterload with intravenous vasodilators such as nitroprusside (Nipride). Oral vasodilators such as prazosin, captopril, and hydralazine, along with digitalis preparations, are used in the chronic phase of heart failure.

The most serious form of acute congestive heart failure is cardiogenic shock (subset IV), which is the leading cause of in-hospital mortality in MI patients. Cardiogenic shock usually occurs in massive MIs in which 40 percent or more of the LV is damaged.[95] Hemodynamically, these patients manifest marked hypotension (systolic BP <80 mmHg), low cardiac index less than 1.8 L min/m², decreased urinary output, elevated heart rates, and concomitant high filling pressures (pulmonary artery wedge pressure which exceeds 18 mmHg). They also have pulmonary congestion and arterial hypoxemia. A vicious cycle ensues in which there is continued myocardial ischemia related to decreased cardiac output and coronary blood flow which, in turn, leads to further ischemia. Therapeutic interventions

Table 21-10 Correlative Classification of Clinical and Hemodynamic Criteria after an Acute MI

Subset	Clinical Appearance	Hemodynamic Criteria	
I	No pulmonary congestion or peripheral hypotension	≤18 mgHg	>2.2 L/min/m²
II	Pulmonary congestion without peripheral hypotension	≥18 mmHg	>2.2 L/min/m²
III	Peripheral hypotension without pulmonary congestion	≤18 mmHg	<2.2 L/min/m²
IV	Pulmonary congestion and peripheral hypotension	≥18 mmHg	>2.2 L/min/m²

Adapted from J. S. Forrester, et al., Correlative Classification of Clinical and Hemodynamic Function after Acute MI. *American Journal of Cardiology*, 39:137–145, 1977.

include the use of inotropic agents such as dopamine and dobutamine to increase contractility and the use of vasodilators such as Nipride or NTG to reduce impedance to LV ejection (afterload) and, thereby, to increase forward flow.

Dopamine is also used in cardiogenic shock for its ability to increase renal blood flow. However, dopamine can be deleterious because it increases MV_{O_2} consumption and has a tendency to induce dysrhythmias. Nipride or nitroglycerin as vasodilators reduce afterload and allow the LV to eject a larger stroke volume, thereby decreasing the LV end-diastolic pressure. These drugs also decrease MV_{O_2} consumption; however, Nipride, because of its arterial vasodilatory properties, may decrease coronary artery perfusion. Thus, the critical-care nurse needs to be cognizant of these properties and possible complications that may result.

The intraaortic balloon pump, which was previously discussed, is also employed for MI patients. Sobel and Braunwald[85] identified three subsets of MI patients in whom the IABP is utilized: (1) those who are hemodynamically unstable and in whom support of the circulation is necessary for diagnostic studies to be performed for the purpose of assessing potential surgically correctable lesions; (2) in cardiogenic shock following an MI that is unresponsive to medical treatment; and (3) in the presence of persistent ischemic pain that is unresponsive to conventional treatment during the postinfarction state. The use of the IABP in the setting of cardiogenic shock does not improve overall mortality, and in fact many of these patients have become "balloon dependent," with a few being successfully weaned from the device. The overall mortality from cardiogenic shock due to extensive myocardial damage remains high, in the 80 to 90 percent range, despite aggressive interventions. However, there are certain circumstances whereby cardiogenic shock is exacerbated, including vagally induced hypotension, intravascular volume depletion, acute RV failure, and surgically treatable entities such as ventricular septal rupture, papillary muscle rupture, chordae tendineae rupture, and left ventricular aneurysms. When cardiogenic shock is induced by the aforementioned complications, it is usually reversible.

Right ventricular infarcts are a rare but important cause of cardiogenic shock. As previously mentioned, RV infarcts occur in the presence of inferior or inferioposterior infarcts of the LV. It has been estimated that RV infarcts occur in approximately 15 to 30 percent of all infarctions, but only 1 to 2 percent of these manifest shock.[96,106] Right ventricular infarcts can be diagnosed on the basis of the hemodynamic alterations which are noted in these patients. There is a disproportionate increase in the right atrial pressures in contrast with the pulmonary wedge pressures in the setting of normal pulmonary artery pressures. Radionuclide ventriculography may be helpful in detecting the RV infarct as evidenced by wall motion abnormalities and a decreased RV ejection fraction. Echocardiograms may also reveal RV dilatation. The ECG may be helpful in revealing posterior RV necrosis by the presence of a Q wave or ST segment elevation in lead V_4R.[107] The goal of therapy for these patients is to administer fluid therapy despite the apparent elevation in right atrial pressure. Inotropic agents (dopamine or dobutamine) may also be employed when volume alone is unable to correct hypotension.[94] Pacing such as atrioventricular sequential pacing is advocated for bradycardia or AV block.[95]

Acute mitral regurgitation is another complication which may occur after an MI and is caused by papillary muscle rupture (usually posterior medial papillary muscle) which usually occurs in inferior infarcts within the first several days after hospitalization.[78,108] Unfortunately, papillary muscles are subendocardial structures, which means that they are supplied by terminal end-branches of the coronary arterial system, rendering them highly vulnerable to ischemia. Infarction of a papillary muscle may also be limited to a subendocardial MI.

When a papillary muscle ruptures, there is incomplete closure of the mitral valve leading to acute regurgitation of blood from the left ventricle into the left atrium. The clinical manifestations of acute mitral regurgitation are pulmonary congestion, and a new, loud pansystolic murmur heard best at the apex with a thrill. If a pulmonary artery catheter is in place, the appearance of large v waves are noted. These patients require mitral valve replacement on an emergency basis. The IABP and/or vasodilators have been used as temporary measures in some cases prior to surgery in the hope of decreasing the regurgitation and encouraging forward flow which is accomplished by decreasing the resistance to LV ejection.

Another surgically correctable complication of an MI is rupture of the interventricular septum. Although a rare complication (1 to 2 percent), it requires surgical intervention because the mortality is high if left untreated. Characteristically, when there is a large septal rupture, a left-to-right shunt occurs with an abrupt and dramatic overloading of the right ventricle. These patients exhibit signs and symptoms of right-sided failure along with dyspnea and reduced LV forward output. Small ruptures may only manifest a new cardiac murmur.[106] Right and left heart catheterization and angiography confirm the diagnosis with a "step-up" in O_2 saturation in blood sampled from the pulmonary artery and right heart chambers as well as shunting of contrast material from left to right at the ventricular level. The use of IABP or vasodilators may be temporarily employed to reduce the resistance to LV ejection and, therefore, decrease the left-to-right shunt while the patient is awaiting surgery. Timing of surgery is controversial because some clinicians advocate medical management until scar tissue is formed to permit effective surgical repair.[26]

Left ventricular free wall rupture accounts for up to 10 percent of hospital deaths after MI.[76] Complete rupture of the free wall is thought to be caused by several factors, including thinning of the apical wall, marked intensity of necrosis at the terminal end-branches of the arterial blood supply, inadequate collateral flow, and the shearing effect of muscular contraction against a stiffened necrotic area. The profile of a patient at high risk for developing this dreaded complication includes a hypertensive, elderly female who has had a left anterior or lateral transmural infarct in the terminal area of the LAD. Ruptures commonly occur 3 to 5 days after infarction and some have been reported up to 4 weeks later.[78] A tear or a dissection hematoma in the necrotic area of the myocardium is the precipitating event leading to hemopericardium and sudden death from cardiac tamponade. Patients with LV free wall rupture can survive when the rupture is immediately recognized and surgically treated.

True ventricular aneurysms develop most often after an anterior transmural MI in approximately 12 to 15 percent of patients.[78] An aneurysm is a circumscribed, akinetic outpouching of the left ventricle which develops from increased wall tension that stretches the infarcted muscle. The aneurysm is a weak, thin-walled structure that bulges (dyskinesis) with each systolic contraction, occurring most often at the apex in the anterior wall of the left ventricle. Persistent ST segment elevations after 3 weeks following an MI is a characteristic yet not sensitive ECG finding of an LV aneurysm.[26] Two-dimensional echocardiography and radionuclide angiography are useful procedures in diagnosing an aneurysm. Mural thrombi may adhere to the aneurysmal wall, which puts patients at risk for systemic emboli. Other complications associated with ventricular aneurysms are CHF, angina pectoris, and ventricular dysrhythmias. Medical intervention includes treatment of CHF symptoms, prophylactic anticoagulation, and antiarrhythmic agents. When the patient with an aneurysm develops any of the above complications, an aneurysmectomy is recommended.

False (pseudo) aneurysms have been reported to occur in the post-MI phase and are usually due to an initial, incomplete rupture of the LV wall. The rupture is sealed with thrombus and a hematoma develops which prevents the sequela of hemopericardium. A false aneurysm is in direct contact with the LV cavity through a narrow opening. False aneurysms are problematic because of their tendency to rupture in contrast with true aneurysms that rarely rupture.[78]

Left ventricular thrombi are common findings in patients following an acute MI. They frequently occur with extensive infarcts and are located in the apex of the left ventricle.[78] These thrombi can be recognized on the echocardiogram. Prophylactic anticoagulation is used to prevent systemic emboli which may result from these thrombi.

Pericarditis can manifest in two forms. Early pericarditis is a direct inflammatory response to transmural damage in approximately 15 percent of patients between the second to fourth day after infarction. Late pericarditis is a delayed autoimmune response often referred to as *Dressler's syndrome*.[78,109]

Early pericarditis is clinically diagnosed by a pericardial friction rub which is transient in nature. Patients may also exhibit chest pain which may be confused with postinfarction angina or pain resulting from extension of an MI. This chest pain differs from angina in that it is positional and exacerbated with inspiration. The ECG may reveal diffuse ST segment elevation during the acute phase, which may also lead to confusion regarding extension of a preexisting infarct. However, it is imperative that the critical-care nurse be aware that these ST elevations are diffuse and exist in many leads (I, II AVL, AVF, V_3 to V_6) and that the patient will not develop pathologic Q waves. During the evolutionary phase of early pericarditis, the ST segment returns to normal and the T waves invert in most of the leads in which ST segment elevations existed. The T waves eventually return to the baseline configuration within days or weeks, although a few patients may be left with some degree of T wave inversion for an indefinite period.[109]

Treatment modalities in early pericarditis include antiinflammatory agents such as aspirin, indomethacin (Indocin), and nonsteroidal antiinflammatory drugs (ibuprofen) or steroids. The critical-care nurse should be aware of the possibility of cardiac tamponade when patients with early pericarditis receive systemic anticoagulants.[109]

Late pericarditis or Dressler's syndrome is not often seen in the critical-care unit because it usually occurs 2 to 4 weeks after the infarction.[78,108,109] The etiology of late pericarditis remains unknown; however, current investigations suggest that it is probably an autoimmune antibody response against certain pericardial or myocardial antigens that are produced by myocardial necrosis.[109] Clinical manifestations of Dressler's syndrome are persistent fever between 101 to 102°F, leukocytosis, malaise, and dull chest pain which is positional and intensified by deep inspiration. Patients often obtain pain relief by leaning forward. Pericardial friction rubs are also noted in this type of pericarditis. Antiinflammatory agents such as aspirin or ibuprofen are also employed in the treatment of this syndrome. Patients need to be told that this syndrome is self-limiting and usually requires no further medical intervention.

Limitation of Infarct Size

Numerous investigations have been undertaken to seek appropriate interventions aimed at limiting the size of a myocardial infarction by protecting the ischemic myocardium in the periphery of the infarcted area. Interventions either are sought to reduce myocardial oxygen demands or restore blood flow to the ischemic area. A brief review regarding the success and current recommendations of each will be discussed.

The venodilatory effects of nitrates have been found to decrease myocardial oxygen consumption and demand by decreasing preload. Intravenous nitroglycerin (NTG) has been investigated in some research centers to limit infarct size. The rationale for using IV NTG stems from clinical investigations which suggest that this drug dilates the large epicardial vessels and collateral channels and may, in patients with collateral vessels, increase flow into the ischemic area, subsequently reducing infarct size.[26] To date, no conclusive evidence has been found to warrant its routine use in post-MI patients, although some preliminary data suggest that IV NTG administered within a few hours after the onset of ischemic chest pain may decrease the probability of some patients developing CHF, extension of the infarct, and sudden death.[26] Thus, its clinical application may in time warrant routine use. However, additional research is necessary to validate its effectiveness for widespread usage.

According to Epstein and Palmeri, data supporting the efficacy of other vasodilators such as nitroprusside in reducing infarct size are inconclusive, and some data from clinical investigations suggest that nitroprusside may even increase ischemic injury or mortality when given early in the course of infarction.[79] If this is found to be accurate, the use of nitroprusside will be limited to the management of LV failure and systemic hypertension after an acute MI.

There is some limited evidence that suggests that verapamil, a calcium antagonist, may reduce infarct size.[79] Verapamil has been shown to be effective in alleviating coronary artery spasm refractory to nitroglycerin. Use of verapamil is restricted to the setting of recurrent, persistent chest pain after NTG administration becomes ineffective. Nifedipine, another calcium antagonist, failed to reduce infarct size in patients with acute MI in the Nifedipine Angina Myocardial Infarction Study.[110] Furthermore, calcium antagonists are contraindicated in patients who exhibit clinical evidence of CHF failure, heart block, or hypotension because of their negative inotropic effects.[79]

Use of beta-adrenergic blockade therapy to protect the ischemic myocardium from increased sympathetic discharge and limit infarct size, has been investigated. Data from some clinical trials are conflicting. Some data indicate a decrease in infarct size after IV use of Atenolol or Metoprolol, but frequent adverse side effects from this therapy have also been noted.[25] Epstein and Palmeri caution against using beta-blocking agents in the setting of spasm because these drugs may exacerbate the degree of ischemic injury by inhibiting β_2 receptors (vasodilators) located in the coronary circulation.[79]

Sobel and Braunwald[85] summarized the findings of all these studies and suggested that patients seen in the first 4 h after the onset of symptoms who are not candidates for thrombolytic therapy may benefit from the early use of beta blockers, and that "it is unlikely that beta blockade can reduce infarct size much later than six hours after the onset of the event, because by this time, the ultimate size of the infarct has been established in many patients" (p. 1321).[85]

The use of antiinflammatory agents such as corticosteroids in reducing infarct size remains controversial. There are conflicting reports in the literature, especially in regard to the frequency of administration. Sobel and Braunwald[85] indicated that a single large dose of methylprednisone was reported to decrease infarct size, yet Roberts, DeMello, and Sobel found an increase in enzymatically estimated infarct size in patients who received multiple doses of methylprednisone.[85,112] According to Sobel and Braunwald, based on recent experimental work, "it is possible that a single large dose of a corticosteroid may reduce infarct size without interfering with myocardial healing" (p. 1323).[85]

Sodi-Pollares et al. suggested that an infusion of glucose-insulin-potassium (GIK) may be beneficial in enhancing anaerobic glycolysis by the ischemic cell.[113] Mueller and Braunwald emphasized that a significant decrease in enzymatically measured infarct size has not been found to date with this infusion and that further investigation needs to be done.[111] The critical-care nurse needs to be aware that this treatment modality is contraindicated in patients with diabetes mellitus or renal failure.

Hyaluronidase was investigated in the Multicenter Investigation of the Limitation of Infarct Size (MILIS) trial. It is an enzyme obtained from a bovine testicular or microbial source that depolymerizes mucopolysaccharides and appears to lack adverse

hemodynamic and electrophysiologic effects. Animal studies have shown that this enzyme decreases myocardial ischemia and infarct size.[111,114] Data from the MILIS trial suggest that hyaluronidase may be effective in reducing infarct size, if given earlier than 9 h after onset of an MI.

According to Mueller and Braunwald, there is no evidence that anticoagulants or oxygen (hyperbaric) reduce infarct size in humans.[111] One study reported, however, that heparin reduced infarct size in dogs.[115] Additional investigation is needed before anticoagulants or oxygen can be accepted as therapy for limiting infarct size.

As previously mentioned, thrombosis is thought to be a frequent precipitator of acute infarcts. In fact, Alpert and Braunwald stated that "it is now clear that a transmural MI is usually (in more than 90 percent of the cases) caused by coronary thrombosis, as postulated by early investigators" (p. 1264).[78] As a result of this premise, thrombolytic agents have received a great deal of attention and intensive investigation since the first report in 1959 by Fletcher, et al.[116]

Thrombolytic therapy is aimed at dissolving thrombi or emboli by digestion of their supporting fibrin network. Thrombolytic drugs have been used in the treatment of deep vein thrombosis, arterial emboli, and pulmonary emboli, and have attained widespread application in the past 5 years for acute myocardial infarction. These agents can be classified into *non-clot-specific,* such as streptokinase and urokinase, or into *clot-specific,* such as the newer agent known as tissue plasminogen activator (rt-PA). Clot specificity refers to whether the drug activates circulating non-clot-bound plasminogen (non-clot-specific) or only activates plasminogen at the site of a clot (clot-specific).

Thrombolytic agents such as streptokinase, urokinase, and, more recently, rt-PA, can be administered by the intracoronary route which mandates its use only in institutions with cardiac catheterization facilities. These agents can also be administered intravenously, but higher dosages are usually required.

Studies have indicated that the success rate of streptokinase in thrombolysis varies depending on the duration of pain prior to administration of thrombolytic agents.[117–120] Because of the logistic limitations of administering intracoronary lytic agents in a timely fashion, the IV route may be advantageous. In a recent study, it was concluded that IV streptokinase was most effective when given within 1.5 h after the onset of pain.[117] Interestingly, subjects in this study were given IV streptokinase in a mobile care unit at home. It was also concluded that, in patients who received early prehospital intervention, LV function was preserved more than in patients who received IV streptokinase in the hospital.[117]

Braunwald[118] emphasized that thrombolytic therapy has not been considered to be unequivocally beneficial, although many clinical trials have suggested that this therapy does limit the evolving infarct.[117,119] However, there are inherent bleeding risks associated with streptokinase therapy[118] which necessitate that all patients at high risk for life-threatening bleeding complications be excluded from such therapy. The increased risk of bleeding associated with streptokinase prompted several investigators to evaluate the effects of rt-PA in humans, which revealed no apparent systemic activation of the fibrinolytic system.[121] This has spurred interest in rt-PA therapy. Other more recent agents include acylated-plasminogen-streptokinase activator complex (acyl-SK) and pro-urokinase and fibrin-specific monoclonal antibodies. These agents may be capable of inducing thrombolysis without causing severe bleeding. The efficacy of these drugs is still under investigation.

The National Heart, Lung and Blood Institute sponsored a large, ongoing, randomized, controlled multicenter trial, the Thrombolysis in Myocardial Infarction (TIMI) trial. Phase 1 of this trial is designed to evaluate the relative thrombolytic effectiveness and side effects of intravenous rt-PA and intravenous streptokinase. Data from the preliminary and later studies suggested that reperfusion was greater after administration of rt-PA than streptokinase. Similar complications were noted in both groups.[122–123]

Use of thrombolytic agents accomplishes lysis of the occluding thrombus with restoration of antegrade flow in the thrombosed vessel (Fig. 21-7). These agents do not, however, decrease the stenosis of the vessel. It has become quite clear that there is a high rate of reocclusion of the residual stenosis unless further intervention, such as coronary angioplasty or coronary artery bypass grafting, is performed.[120,124]

Several investigators have demonstrated the efficacy of concomitant streptokinase and coronary angioplasty in the MI patient. In one study, coronary angioplasty was performed in seven patients with acute myocardial infarction after receiving streptokinase and rapid reperfusion to all vessels was noted.[125] Gold performed coronary angioplasty in 28 patients with acute myocardial infarction following intracoronary administration of streptokinase.[126] In 16 of these patients, streptokinase failed to reopen the occluded coronary artery. In 11 of the 16 patients in whom streptokinase failed, coronary angioplasty recanalized the vessel. Thus, coronary angioplasty completely recanalized half of the vessels in which initial failure had occurred with streptokinase infusion. In the other 12 patients, coronary angioplasty was used to treat high-grade resistant stenoses after successful streptokinase infusion. Angioplasty was successful in 9 of the 12 patients. In this study, it was noted that the frequency of recurrent ischemic attacks was lower after successful coronary angioplasty than after streptokinase infusion alone. Restenosis or reocclusion occurred in 45 percent of the patients who had a successful coronary angioplasty following streptokinase administration for an acute myocardial infarction.[126]

O'Neill and coworkers randomly assigned 56 patients who presented within 12 h of their first symptoms of an MI to either PTCA or IC streptokinase therapy. They concluded that angioplasty was significantly more effective in reducing the underlying coronary stenoses in contrast to IC streptokinase.[127] Because it decreased the underlying stenoses, PTCA was also thought to be more effective in improving ventricular function. Sequential IV streptokinase therapy followed by PTCA was reported by Jung et al.[128] Ninety-five percent of patients had reperfusion.

Emergency PTCA has been used as a primary approach to limiting infarct size without the preceding use of a thrombolytic agent. The use of PTCA is limited to institutions with skilled technicians and fully equipped catheterization laboratory facilities, thereby reducing the general applicability of this procedure to all patients who present with an MI.

Counterpulsation using the intraaortic balloon pump has been shown to reduce infarct size in animals; however, no definitive evidence regarding

Figure 21-7 (A) Arteriogram of a patient which depicts abrupt cessation of flow (arrow) in the LAD of a patient who presented with an anterior MI. (B) The same patient received intracoronary streptokinase and had reestablished flow (arrow) to the affected myocardium.

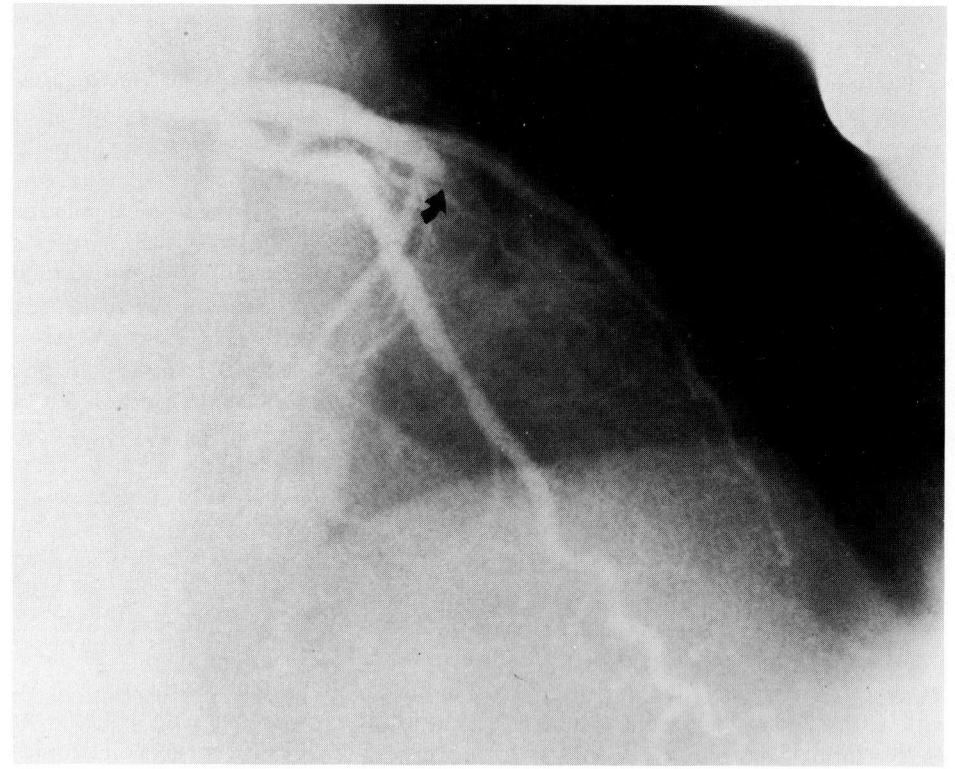

A

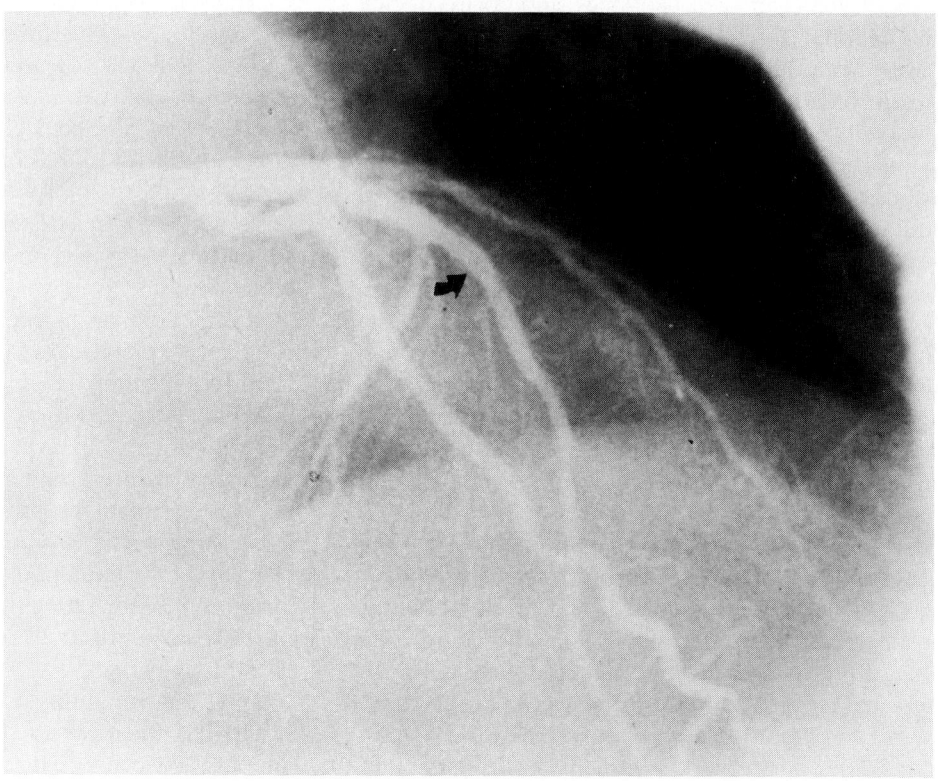

B

the limitation of infarct size in humans has been reported. Mueller and Braunwald reiterated that counterpulsation cannot be recommended for generalized use in an attempt to limit infarct size.[111]

Emergency CABG surgery has been employed in certain medical centers to limit infarct size. However, data suggest that this therapy can only be successful if revascularization takes place within the first 4 or 5 h after the onset of the acute event.[129,130] Logistically, this intervention is limited because of the difficulty in assembling personnel required to bring a patient to the hospital, then to the catheterization laboratory, and subsequently to the operating room. Because of the time involved in this process, emergency CABG surgery is restricted to in-hospital patients in whom an acute MI evolves. It is, therefore, unlikely for this therapy to be widely applied to all patients presenting with an acute MI because many patients are not in the hospital when they develop an MI.

Nursing Therapies

Those patients who manifest symptoms of an acute myocardial infarction are often placed in a coronary care unit. Patients evolving an MI may also present with chest discomfort. The drug choice is often morphine sulfate IV 2 to 4 mg q 1 h. In the first several hours of an acute MI, life-threatening arrhythmias may develop. Thus, continuous ECG monitoring is another priority upon admission to the unit. A third priority is the establishment of a patent venous access line for the administration of intravenous medications. The administration of O_2 therapy is regarded as another priority in some units. After these priorities have been addressed, the critical-care nurse needs to obtain a complete biopsychosocial assessment of the MI patient using Gordon's[73] functional health patterns as described in Chap. 20. This tool guides the nurse, along with the information obtained from the physical examination and diagnostic tests, in collecting data from which to deduce both collaborative problems, which have a medical etiology and in which a number of health care disciplines may participate in problem resolution, and solely nursing problems or diagnoses which may be treated within the scope of nursing.

Specific features to be noted on physical examination pertaining to the MI patient include height, weight, presence of edema, skin color and temperature, quality of respirations, presence and location of crackles, normal and abnormal heart sounds, cardiac murmurs, thrills, heaves or rubs, arrhythmias, blood pressure, jugular venous pressure, and mental status.

Laboratory data may reveal elevated serum enzymes such as LDH and CK with elevations in their respective isoenzymes. Data may also reveal an elevated sedimentation rate, elevated serum cholesterol, and specific lipoproteins.

Upon completion of the database, collaborative as well as nursing diagnoses may be identified. A nursing care plan aimed at alleviating or minimizing the patient's problems should be formulated and evaluated in order for problem resolution to be achieved. Patient outcomes, nursing interventions, and evaluation will be discussed for the collaborative and actual diagnoses.

The collaborative diagnosis for the MI patient is similar to that of the unstable angina patient in that chest pain is a major problem except that the MI pain is not due to a temporary reduction in tissue perfusion secondary to an imbalance in myocardial supply and demand, but to an abrupt cessation of blood supply which causes death of the myocardial tissue.

Collaborative Diagnosis

Alteration in comfort: pain (MI) related to decreased tissue perfusion to the myocardium, resulting in tissue necrosis.

Goal

Same as that stated in the unstable angina section.

Nursing Interventions

1–3. As stated in unstable angina section.
4. Administer analgesia such as morphine sulfate for pain as ordered to prevent increased intensity. Evaluate pain relief and effectiveness of interventions.
5. Check vital signs prior to admission of narcotics and after 30 min.
6. To promote psychological reassurance, assure patient that analgesia should relieve discomfort.
7. Assess the response to the analgesic agent by asking patient whether or not relief has been obtained using a scale of 1 to 10 (1 = low, 10 = high).

8. Instruct patient regarding the effects of analgesia.
9. Decrease physical activity during chest discomfort.
10. Avoid excessive sympathetic stimulation such as caffeine beverages, fever, volume depletion, and anxiety.
11. Obtain a 12-lead ECG during chest discomfort and report any changes.

Evaluation

Same as that stated in unstable angina section. The two nursing diagnoses identified for the patient with an MI include the one stated previously for the unstable angina patient, specifically, ineffective coping related to lack of knowledge regarding the disease process. The reader is referred to that section. The second diagnosis is noted below.

Actual Nursing Diagnosis

Activity intolerance related to: (1) decrease in myocardial workload capacity; (2) knowledge deficit regarding activity progression after infarction; (3) deconditioning effects of prolonged bed rest; and (4) potential sleep deficit secondary to care requirements.

Goal

Patient will have improved activity tolerance during hospitalization, as evidenced by: (1) the ability to demonstrate increased activity progression; (2) the ability to identify and minimize those factors which increase myocardial workload; (3) the ability to demonstrate a decrease in signs of cardiac decompensation such as excessive heart rate or a decrease in blood pressure or chest pain; (4) the ability to verbalize improvement of activity levels without experiencing chest pain.

Nursing Interventions

1. Assess prior activity level on admission to the critical-care unit.
2. Assist patient to complete those activities of daily living that do not lead to excessive increases in heart rate, blood pressure, respirations, or electrical disturbances such as dysrhythmias.
3. Plan and implement incremental increases in activity such as bed rest to chair to ambulation

so as not to abruptly increase myocardial workload.
4. Monitor blood pressure and heart rate prior to and immediately after activity and 3 min later.
5. Instruct patient regarding factors which increase myocardial workload, such as strenuous activity, stress, smoking, heavy meals, isometric exercises, and Valsalva maneuvers.
6. Instruct patient to stop an activity if the following signs of cardiac decompensation are present: increased heart rate, dyspnea, or chest pain.
7. Instruct patient to rest between activity periods.
8. Encourage passive and active ROM exercises while on bed rest.
9. Minimize the effects of postural hypotension by allowing bed to chair activity once the patient is hemodynamically stable, and by allowing patient to dangle feet at bedside.
10. Have patient plantar and dorsiflex feet while in bed to prevent stasis of blood.
11. Encourage frequent changes in body position while on bed rest.
12. Decrease environmental stimulation to promote sleep periods.
13. Assess quality and response to sleep by asking patient about his or her sleep periods.
14. Provide adequate rest periods for the patient between therapeutic care activities.

Evaluation

Patient demonstrates increased activity tolerance by demonstrating ability to progressively increase level of activity without developing chest pain. Patient verbalizes an increase in activity tolerance. Patient verbalizes decreased shortness of breath or fatigue with minimal activity. Patient demonstrates an appropriate heart rate, blood pressure, and respiratory rate with increased activity.

Potential nursing diagnosis have also been identified for the MI patient and include:

1. Potential for fear or anxiety related to diagnosis and prognosis of MI
2. Potential for disturbance in self-concept related to loss of healthy body image and role in family

The nursing management of a patient with an acute MI who becomes a patient in the critical-care setting is challenging. The patient often may develop serious potential complications as previously discussed in this section. Nursing personnel must constantly assess for these complications and institute preventive measures to minimize or prevent them. The critical-care nurse must also be aware of the various therapeutic modalities for the acute MI patient, to educate and prepare both the patient and significant others for such alternatives.

Coronary Revascularization

Introduction

Coronary artery disease was the last cardiovascular disease to which surgical therapy was successfully applied.[131] Numerous operative interventions, such as thoracic sympathectomy, epicardial abrasion, and placement of vascularized pedicles on the surface of the heart, were attempted from 1900 to 1960. None of these procedures was shown to provide sustained benefit and they were often associated with a high operative mortality.[37] The first successful surgery for coronary artery disease is usually credited to Rene Favalaro and his associates in 1967.[131] Favalaro's group utilized saphenous vein grafts to bypass obstructed coronary vessels and thus successfully revascularized ischemic myocardium. Since that time coronary artery bypass graft (CABG) surgery has become one of the most commonly performed operations in the United States. About 200,000 such procedures are performed in the United States each year.[26]

In concept, the procedure for coronary artery bypass surgery is a relatively straightforward technique. A conduit of the patient's tissue is connected to the aorta and anastomosed to the coronary artery distal to the site of blockage. Unlike medical therapy, which generally attempts to reduce myocardial oxygen demands, CABG surgery aims to increase MV_{O_2} by increasing blood flow to the myocardium, but it is not a cure for the underlying atherosclerotic disease process. The major goals of CABG surgery are to relieve symptoms, prolong survival, and improve the quality of life. However, much controversy exists concerning the degree to which surgical coronary revascularization actually achieves these goals. This is especially true with recent improvements in pharmacologic therapy and medical alternatives. Nonetheless, sophisticated surgical techniques, generally low operative mortality, and data

demonstrating improvement in patient symptoms and longevity have established surgical coronary revascularization as an acceptable, and in some cases, superior treatment for certain patients with coronary artery disease.[132]

Indications for Surgery

The criteria used to select patients for surgical myocardial revascularization are the subject of continued controversy and debate. Patients are generally carefully chosen on the basis of certain clinical, coronary arteriographic, and hemodynamic data. Improvement in longevity and relief of symptoms are the ultimate goals of surgical intervention.

Improvement in Longevity
For most patients the major issue concerning the treatment of coronary artery disease is longevity. Statistics regarding the effects of CABG surgery on survival are especially meaningful to patients without severe, chronic angina, but who fear a possible premature death.

In an attempt to identify objective criteria for coronary revascularization, several studies have described the long-term survival of patients with certain anatomic coronary lesions managed surgically or medically. In general, a stenosis of greater than 70 to 75 percent of the arterial lumen is considered significant,[37,133] and lesions in the more proximal portions of the coronary arteries are considered more lethal than distal blockages because they jeopardize larger areas of myocardium. Probably the most straightforward, undisputed indication for coronary artery bypass surgery is arteriographic documentation of left main coronary artery stenosis greater than 50 percent, regardless of symptomatology. Numerous investigations, including the VA Cooperative Study[134] and the large European Coronary Study Group,[135] have shown a significant increase in longevity when these patients are managed surgically rather than medically. These same studies, along with the more recent Coronary Artery Surgery Study (CASS),[133] documented that patients with triple-vessel coronary artery disease and decreased ejection fractions who undergo CABG surgery have significantly improved survival rates at five years as compared to patients treated medically. The indications for surgery in patients with triple-vessel disease and normal left ventricular function have been less clearly delineated. Although the European Study (1980) found an improved 5-year survival when these patients were managed surgically, the CASS Study (1983) found no difference in 5-year survival of patients in this group managed medically or surgically. The CASS Study (1983) demonstrated no difference in longevity in patients with double- or single-vessel disease managed with medicine or surgery. However, the European Study found a better survival curve in patients with double-vessel disease which involved the proximal left anterior descending coronary artery who were treated surgically rather than medically.

Relief of Symptoms

The most frequently cited indication for surgical intervention is disabling angina that is refractory to medical management.[131,136] Numerous studies have documented the superiority of surgical treatment over medical therapy in reducing symptoms.[137] Data have revealed that angina is abolished in 60 to 70 percent of patients; and 90 to 95 percent of patients have some symptomatic improvement following CABG surgery.[136,138] Although interruption of nerve fibers, intraoperative infarction of ischemic myocardium, and a placebo effect have all been postulated as contributing to the reduction in symptoms, the use of thallium perfusion scanning has demonstrated that a majority of patients with improvement in symptoms exhibit increased myocardial blood flow following CABG surgery.[139] Selection of patients based on symptoms is open to much variation, however. The amount of angina that is disabling is extremely subjective and dependent on the patient's life-style. Further, medical management may not be maximal because of patient noncompliance or differences in physician protocols. Despite these discrepancies, severity of symptoms is an important surgical consideration.

Unstable Angina

A related indication for coronary revascularization is unstable angina. Patients with angina of new onset that progresses rapidly in intensity and severity, patients with sudden acceleration of previous stable angina, or patients with pain at rest are considered to have unstable angina.[140,141] Patients who develop angina 1 week to 3 months following an acute myocardial infarction are also considered to be in this group.[136,141] Although hospitalization and aggressive medical management (including intraaortic balloon counterpulsation) are the initial treatments of choice for patients with unstable angina, urgent catheterization and surgery are indicated when angina or signs of ischemia persist.[136,140] Studies have documented low operative mortality and significant relief of symptoms when this group is treated with surgical intervention.[141]

Myocardial Infarction and Complications

Coronary revascularization in patients with evolving myocardial infarction has been attempted at some institutions in an effort to limit infarct size and preserve left ventricular function. The most beneficial results are achieved in patients with subendocardial rather than transmural infarcts, and occur when revascularization is accomplished within the first 6 h of symptoms.[129,130] However, because of the high operative mortality associated with this group of surgical candidates, and the increasing availability and success of thrombolysis, surgical intervention is not the usual treatment of choice in the uncomplicated MI patient.[136] Current data suggest that urgent operation is indicated for the postmyocardial infarction patient who develops significant congestive heart failure from acute rupture of the ventricular septum or papillary muscle,[142,143] and for patients who develop symptoms such as congestive heart failure, angina, or systemic emboli from a left ventricular aneurysm.[144,145]

Surgical Risks

Operative mortality of 1 percent or less has been reported in 90 percent of patients undergoing CABG surgery.[136,146] Certain factors, however, have been associated with significantly higher surgical mortalities and include left ventricular dysfunction, emergency operation, increasing age, female sex, the number of diseased vessels, and incomplete revascularization.

Before the development of hypothermic cardioplegia, severe left ventricular dysfunction was considered a contraindication to CABG surgery.[131] With recent improvements in myocardial preservation, studies have documented a significant reduction in operative mortality and improvement in symptoms in some patients with ejection fractions as low as 20 percent. In particular, patients with ventricular dysfunction whose primary symptom is angina may have ischemia with a viable myocardium. These patients have been shown to benefit significantly from surgical revascularization.[147] However, when low ejection fractions are associated with chronic congestive heart failure (in the absence of a ventricular aneurysm), CABG surgery does not appear to be beneficial.[136] In fact, data from a recent study indicated preoperative congestive heart failure as the factor associated with the greatest operative mortality in patients undergoing CABG surgery at Cleveland Clinic from 1980 to 1982.[148]

Cosgrove and his associates demonstrated that emergency operation, incomplete revascularization at the time of surgery, and an abnormal preoperative electrocardiogram were risk factors associated with high operative mortality. Further, women had a significantly higher operative risk than men (1.9 versus 0.7 percent) which is thought to be related to smaller vessel size in females.[148]

Surgical treatment of coronary artery disease in the elderly has been controversial. However, as this country's population has aged, the mean age of the CABG surgical patient has increased. Reports have indicated that patients in their seventh and eighth decade have undergone surgical coronary revascularization with relatively low operative mortality (2 percent).[136,148] Therefore, age per se does not appear to be a contraindication for surgery. However, investigators have documented a high incidence of neurologic complications following CABG surgery in patients over the age of 70.[148] Therefore, the presence of cerebrovascular disease or significant carotid artery stenosis may present especially great risk in the elderly CABG patient.

Patients with diffuse narrowing of the coronary vessels, poor distal runoff, and significant obstructions in intramyocardial vessels have been described as poor surgical candidates.[131] All these factors have been associated with reduced graft flow and possible subsequent graft closure. However, recent studies indicate that coronary revascularization is being successfully performed on patients with more diffuse coronary atherosclerosis.[146] The long-term result of surgical intervention in these patients is yet to be documented.

Obviously, the decision regarding surgical intervention in coronary artery disease must be individualized. Numerous factors concerning the patient's clinical, physiologic, and psychologic state must be considered. Potential benefits of surgery are carefully weighed against operative risk.

Choice of Conduits

Most commonly, coronary revascularization is accomplished with segments of the greater saphenous vein procured from the leg.[149] Advantages of utilizing this conduit include expendability, ease of procurement, usual proportionate size and adequate length, and relative durability under arterial pressures.[131] When previous vein stripping, varicosities, or disproportionate size make use of the greater saphenous vessel difficult, the lesser saphenous system (which is more difficult to harvest) or the cephalic or basilic veins of the arm (which are smaller and more fragile) have been successfully utilized.[131,149] With the vein graft in reverse position so that the venous valves do not obstruct blood flow, one end is sutured to a small opening made in the ascending aorta, and the other end is attached to an opening in the coronary artery distal to the atherosclerotic obstruction (see Fig. 21-8). In such a way a new conduit for blood flow is established between the aorta and the ischemic myocardium.

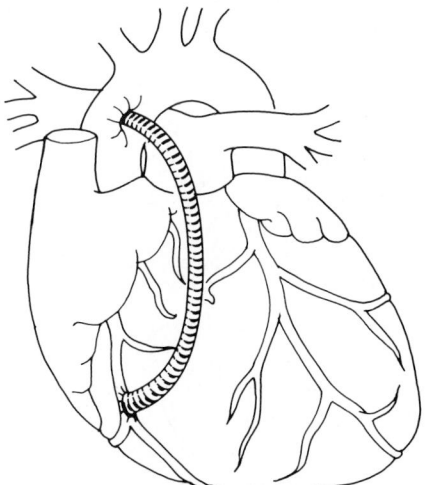

Figure 21-8 Aortocoronary artery saphenous vein bypass graft.

The "sequential" or "jump" graft is a variation of this "single bypass" procedure and has become increasingly popular since 1977.[150] This technique involves a single vein graft segment attached to more than one coronary artery (Fig. 21-9). The vein graft has one attachment to the aorta but bypasses more than one diseased vessel. The advantages to this procedure include increased distal runoff, fewer proximal anastomoses per bypass graft, and better utilization of available vein length.[151] So far, equivalent patency rates have been reported for single and sequential grafts, but theoretically, sequential grafts may increase long-term patency by establishing a higher rate of flow through the proximal portions of the graft.[146] However, possible kinking of this longer-type graft is a danger, and a proximal occlusion jeopardizes more than one coronary bypass location.[151]

The most frequently used alternative to the aortocoronary saphenous vein bypass is the internal mammary artery (IMA) graft. This procedure involves dissecting the internal mammary artery, ligating it from the chest wall, and anastomosing its end to the coronary artery. Blood flow to the ischemic myocardium is thus established via the normal internal mammary artery circulation (Fig. 21-10). This technique has gained renewed interest because of recent studies[152,153] demonstrating higher

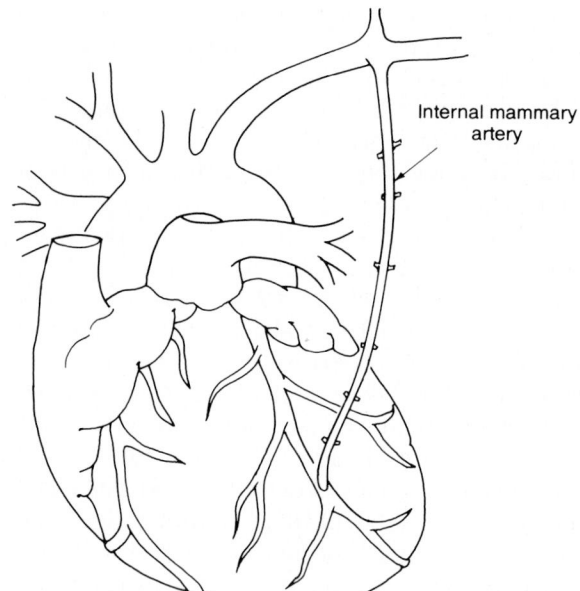

Figure 21-10   Internal mammary artery coronary artery bypass graft.

long-term patency of IMA grafts (88.5 percent at 1 year; 84.1 percent at 10 years) compared to saphenous vein grafts (76 percent patency at 1 year; 52 percent at 10 years). A recent study reported that 50 percent of all coronary revascularization procedures performed involved use of IMA grafts.[148] Other advantages cited by proponents of the IMA graft include the need for only one anastomosis, less size disparity between the graft and coronary artery, and the avoidance of a leg incision.[131] However, the internal mammary artery can only be used to vascularize vessels on the anterior surface of the heart, it requires extensive dissection, a longer operating time,[131] and has been associated with a slightly increased incidence of postoperative bleeding and pulmonary as well as wound complications.[154,155]

A troublesome problem during CABG surgery is the coronary artery with multiple obstructions, or a stenosis that is inaccessible on the surface of the heart. In an attempt to provide more complete myocardial revascularization, the use of intraoperative transluminal coronary angioplasty in the operating room is presently being attempted. Preliminary studies suggest that selective intraoperative angioplasty may be an important adjunct to effective

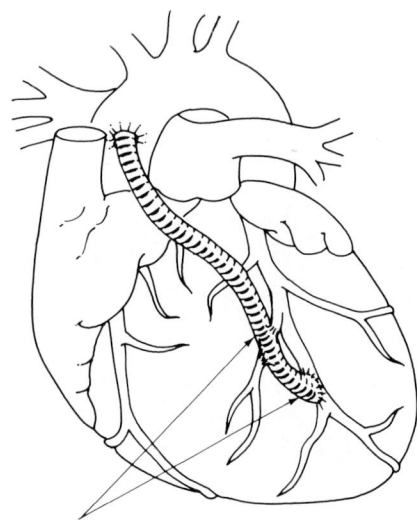

One saphenous vein, two anastamoses

Figure 21-9   Aortocoronary artery saphenous vein "sequential" bypass graft.

coronary revascularization.[156,157] Efforts are also under way to investigate the removal of focal coronary atherosclerotic obstructions by carbon dioxide and argon laser. Data from current studies show promise that laser therapy during cardiac surgery may ablate coronary artery lesions.[73,158,159] The future may hold exciting advancements in myocardial revascularization techniques.

Surgical Procedure

Coronary artery bypass surgery is most commonly performed via a median sternotomy incision. Cardiopulmonary bypass (CPBP) is used to provide an arrested heart during the most technically difficult part of the surgery, the anastomoses of the bypass grafts to the coronary arteries. Patients are routinely monitored throughout the procedure with an arterial line, pulmonary artery catheter, continuous electrocardiogram, and urinary catheter placed prior to surgery. After discontinuing CPBP, atrial, and frequently, ventricular epicardial pacing wires are placed on the anterior heart and tunneled through the chest wall where they are sutured to the skin. The wires are then accessible for use in cardiac pacing and electrocardiography. Prior to closure of the incision, mediastinal chest tubes are routinely placed within the pericardium and beneath the sternum (although the exact placement may vary). A pleural chest tube is usually needed after an internal mammary bypass graft. The chest tubes evacuate air and drainage, and most importantly, aid in monitoring mediastinal bleeding and preventing cardiac tamponade. Because of the length of anesthesia and the frequently associated respiratory dysfunction, CABG patients routinely remain intubated for 12 or more h following surgery.

Cardiopulmonary bypass is used almost exclusively in open cardiac operations and has a significant impact on patient outcome. Nursing care of the coronary artery bypass patient requires an understanding of the conduct of CPBP and its potential physiologic effects.

Cardiopulmonary Bypass

Cardiopulmonary bypass is a technique in which blood is diverted away from the heart and lungs into a machine (the heart-lung machine) that substitutes for the ventilatory and pumping functions of these organs. In 1953 Gibbon performed the first successful cardiac operation in which the patient was totally supported by CPBP.[160] Until this time, heart surgery was limited to closed, quickly performed procedures such as valve commissurotomy. The introduction of cardiopulmonary bypass, however, made it possible to repair intracardiac defects under direct vision.

CPBP has been used to sustain patients (especially newborn infants) with severe but potentially reversible respiratory distress, and in patients undergoing operations on the thoracic aorta. By far the most common utilization of CPBP, however, is to perform the function of the heart and lungs during cardiac surgery, and provide a motionless "empty" organ on which to carry out delicate surgical maneuvers.

The heart-lung machine drains blood from the heart, oxygenates it, and pumps it into the body. The perfusion apparatus consists of cannulas, reservoirs, pumps, filters, and an oxygenator.

Blood is diverted from entering the heart by a single catheter placed in the right atrium or by catheters placed separately in the inferior and superior vena cava.[160] An arterial cannula placed in the ascending aorta (or less commonly in the femoral artery) directs blood from the heart-lung machine to the patient. A small catheter is inserted into the aortic root in order to administer cardioplegia solution for myocardial preservation. In some cases a venting catheter may be passed into the left ventricle (directly or through the left atrium or pulmonary artery). The blood returning to the left heart during bypass via the thebesian veins and bronchial circulation can cause elevation of intraventricular pressure. Significant left ventricular distention is associated with a decrease in subendocardial blood flow and an increase in pulmonary vascular pressures, thus potentially contributing to postoperative cardiac and pulmonary dysfunction. Many surgeons do not routinely use the left ventricular venting catheter because of the danger of introducing air emboli with this device, and because of studies demonstrating the questionable necessity of this intervention.[132]

Components of Bypass System

Reservoirs   A reservoir is used to collect venous blood from the patient. The height of this reservoir below the level of the right atrium determines the blood flow from the patient by gravity. A smaller reservoir chamber is used to collect blood suctioned from the operative field (cardiotomy suction reservoir). This blood is then returned to the CPBP circuitry and the patient. Another reservoir contains cardioplegia solution.

Pumps   Two types of CPBP circuit pumps are the (1) nonocclusive roller and (2) impeller centrifugal rotating cone. The arterial pump is utilized to propel blood through the system. The flow pattern produced is a flat, nonpulsatile waveform. This pulseless flow pattern is clearly a major deviation from normal physiologic conditions. For many years extensive efforts focused on producing the normal physiologic pulse contour during CPBP because it was believed that this would improve the distribution of blood flow and thus reduce postoperative organ dysfunction. Present evidence suggests that pulsatile flow compared to nonpulsatile perfusion results in lower peripheral vascular resistance, increased oxygen uptake, and reduced lactate buildup.[161] Several studies have also demonstrated increased urinary output and creatinine clearance during pulsatile perfusion, as well as lower renin and vasopressin levels. Pulsatile pumps, however, are more complex than roller pumps and, therefore, more difficult to operate. Further, pulsation through the CPBP circuit may result in blood trauma from jet effects or may induce shearing of atherosclerotic plaques. At present, nonpulsatile flow is not associated with intolerable subsystem distortions during routine CPBP procedures. Currently, therefore, roller pumps and nonpulsatile flow are used in essentially all open-heart operations.[161]

Filters   Current methods of CPBP result in the production and release of numerous particulate, fat, and gaseous emboli. These can potentially adversely affect the performance of any organ subsystem. The use of blood filters within the CPBP circuit has resulted in major reductions in the quantity and size of emboli and reduced postoperative complications from this mechanism. It has been extensively documented that the greatest and most frequent source of emboli is generated from the cardiotomy suction system. Blood returning from this system, referred to as field aspirated

blood, has been shown to contain calcium fragments, suture, fat, fibrin, and other debris. Filtration of the cardiotomy return blood is, therefore, viewed as essential. Blood filters may also be used within the arterial line of the CPBP circuit to further reduce air and particulate matter returning to the patient.

Oxygenators   Oxygenation of venous blood diverted from the patient's right atrium occurs in the oxygenator of the CPBP circuit. Two types of oxygenators (Fig. 21-11) are presently utilized to perform the gas exchange function of the lungs. The *bubble oxygenator* accomplishes this oxygen interchange by bubbling oxygen through a vertical column of blood. Thus, a thin venous blood layer is in direct contact with finely dispersed gas bubbles. Concentration gradients result in oxygen diffusing out of the bubble into the blood and carbon dioxide diffusing from the blood to the bubble. In *membrane oxygenators,* blood and gas are not in direct contact, but are separated by a semipermeable membrane. Oxygen diffuses from the gas compartment through the membrane into the blood compartment, and carbon dioxide diffuses in the opposite direction. This design most closely simulates the human lung. Controversy exists concerning the superiority of one type of oxygenator over the other.[160,161] Bubble oxygenators are the most simple to use. However, the direct blood gas interface has been shown to cause more trauma to blood cells. Membrane oxygenators appear to cause less trauma to both formed and unformed blood elements but these devices are more difficult and time-consuming to use. Several studies have shown that when bypass time is less than 3 h the amount of trauma to blood elements is not significantly different between bubble and membrane oxygenators.[155,156]

Associated Factors

Despite improvements in equipment, the CPBP machine falls short of reproducing the normal functions of the heart and lungs. In order to circumvent this problem, several adjunct techniques are utilized to assure adequate total body perfusion and preservation of organ function during extracorporeal circulation. An explanation of these related factors is important in understanding the physiologic effects of CPBP.

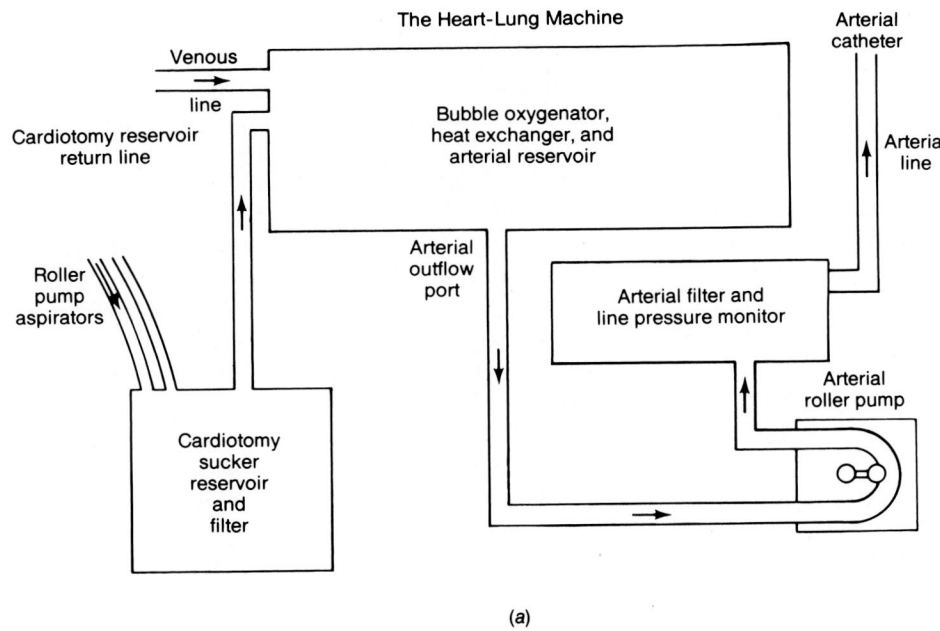

(a)

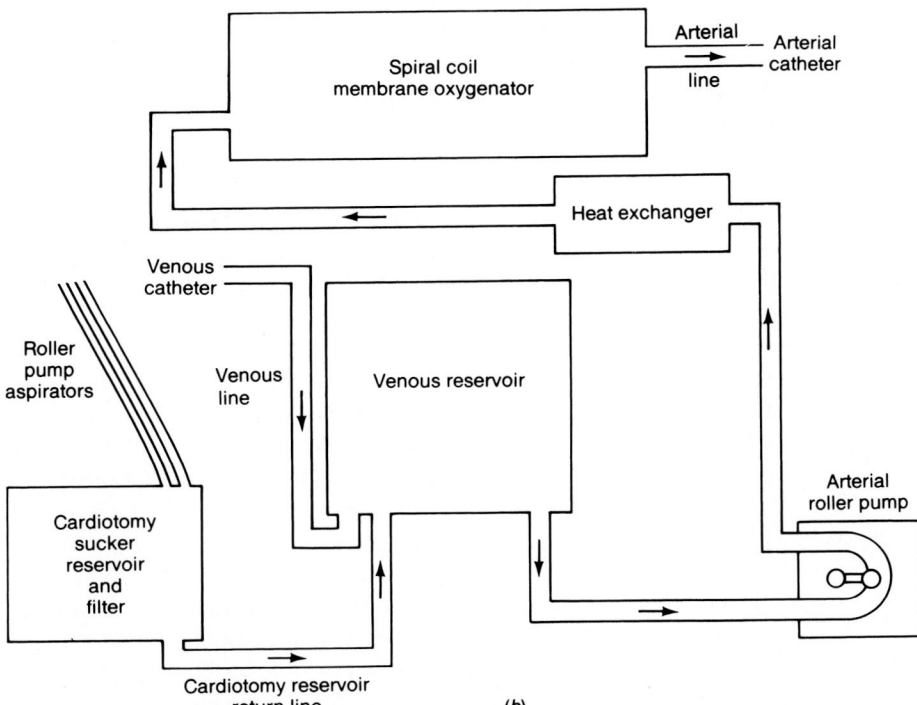

(b)

Figure 21-11 (*a*) Diagram of CPBP set up with a bubble oxygenator. (*b*) Diagram of a CPBP set up with a membrane oxygenator. (*Modified from L. Edmunds and L. Stephenson. Cardiopulmonary bypass for open heart surgery. In W. Glenn, ed., Thoracic and Cardiovascular Surgery. Appleton-Century-Crofts, Norwalk, CT, 1983.*)

Hypothermia   A commonly employed adjunct to CPBP is the use of systemic hypothermia. Metabolic processes are slowed as body temperature is lowered. Hypothermia provides for a margin of safety and helps reduce the occurrence of oxygen debts during extracorporeal circulation. It has been demonstrated that the metabolic rate is reduced approximately 7 percent for each 1°C lowering of body temperature. Generally, hypothermia is induced by cooling the bloodstream via a heat exchanger located in the venous, or more commonly on the arterial, inflow side of the heart-lung machine. This "core cooling" is more effective than surface cooling because the organs with the best perfusion and highest oxygen requirements are cooled most rapidly and completely.[162] The exact level of perfusion hypothermia employed varies with the specific requirements of the surgical procedure. Most commonly, temperatures of 28 to 32°C are utilized.[160,161] More profound hypothermia (as low as 18°C) has been utilized with total circulatory arrest in neonates and infants undergoing intracardiac repair of complex anomalies. Although hypothermia greatly reduces metabolic demands, it is not without untoward effects. Blood viscosity rises when the body temperature is lowered and may result in sluggish capillary and organ blood flow. Further, hypothermia causes oxygen to be more tightly bound to hemoglobin and, therefore, less available to the tissues. Rewarming of the patient is achieved by circulating warm water through the same heat exchanger. Although normal blood temperature is reestablished prior to the termination of CPBP, areas of the body which receive relatively low proportional blood flow may remain hypothermic. Body temperature may tend to drop in the first few hours after bypass as temperature throughout the body equilibrates.

Hemodilution   Prior to initiation of CPBP, the heart-lung machine must be filled with a priming solution in order to remove air from the circuit and provide adequate volume to fill the bypass apparatus and to augment the patient's vascular compartment. In the early days of cardiac surgery, large amounts of banked blood were used to prime the circuitry. Presently, virtually all cardiac surgery is performed with the use of a nonblood priming solution. The use of colloid and crystalloid nonblood priming solution results in a significant reduction of the patient's hematocrit (hemodilution). The optimal hematocrit during CPBP is controversial, but 25 percent is a commonly accepted hematocrit level.[160,161] While the patient's blood is maximally diluted at the onset of CPBP, the diluent tends to be lost from the perfusate, both in the interstitial space and the urine, as extracorporeal circulation continues.[161] Thus the hematocrit tends to rise progressively throughout perfusion but usually remains low (30 percent) in the immediate postoperative period unless transfusions are given. Although the lowered hematocrit reduces the oxygen-carrying capacity of the blood, decreases colloidal osmotic pressure, and may contribute to interstitial edema, the numerous advantages of hemodilution outweigh these factors. Most notably, hemodilution lowers blood viscosity and vascular resistance, thus counteracting the deleterious effects of hypothermia, and results in an improvement in capillary blood flow.[161] Hemodilution also decreases trauma to blood cells, thus reducing hemolysis and platelet denaturation. Postoperative renal and pulmonary dysfunction have been shown to be lower when hemodilution rather than blood priming solution is utilized. A decrease in postoperative bleeding has also been cited with hemodilution.[162] Finally, the decreased demand on limited blood bank supplies, as well as the decreased risk of transfusion reaction, hepatitis, and acquired immune deficiency syndrome give further support to the use of the hemodilution technique.

Heparin   Studies have shown indirect evidence that the Hageman factor (factor XII) is activated almost immediately after the start of CPBP by the massive contact of blood with nonbiological surfaces.[164] Heparin, therefore, is routinely administered immediately prior to and throughout the course of CPBP to inhibit factors V, IX, XI, XII, and thrombin. Because of the wide variation in individual responses to heparin, frequent measurement of the activated clotting time (ACT) during bypass is utilized to guide heparin administration. Heparin must be neutralized by protamine at the termination of CPBP, prior to closure of the chest, to assure adequate hemostasis.

Blood Flow   The goal of CPBP is to maintain near-normal cardiac output while the patient is being supported. Theoretically, perfusion rates should equal the basal conditions in adults, calculated as a cardiac index of 3 L/min/m² with an oxygen uptake of 125 mL/min/m². However, factors such as cannula size, intravascular volume changes, and altered venous return make the maintenance of these blood flow rates somewhat difficult throughout extracorporeal perfusion. Such high flows would also considerably increase blood trauma.[161] Data indicate that the basic flow rate of 2.4 L/min/m² ensures acceptable perfusion during CPBP.[160,162] Although oxygen-carrying capacity of blood is reduced (hemodilution), total body oxygen consumption is lowered (hypothermia); therefore, the body's metabolic demands can be met at these lowered perfusion rates.

With the start of CPBP, perfusion pressure tends to fall sharply, but after a brief period begins to rise. Perfusion pressures generally stabilize between 55 to 60 torr.[160,161] At flow rates of 2.4 L/min/m² and with the use of hypothermia and hemodilution as described, the mean arterial pressure level is usually well tolerated. Research data suggest that sustained mean perfusion pressures below 50 mmHg are associated with higher complication rates (especially cerebral complications).[160,161] Lower perfusion pressures may have especially untoward consequences in patients with high resistance atherosclerotic obstructions (common in the elderly). However, high pressures must also be avoided. Mean arterial pressures greater than 90 to 100 mmHg may increase the incidence of intracerebral bleeding in the heparinized patient. Mean arterial pressure during bypass is controlled between 60 to 80 mmHg with added volume or pharmacologic agents as indicated. Experience has demonstrated that CPBP can be conducted safely at flow rates of 2.4 L/min/m², and with a mean arterial pressure of 55 to 60 mmHg up to 4 to 6 h without major deleterious effects.[160]

Myocardial Preservation   Exclusion of the heart from circulation during CPBP provides a relatively bloodless field on which to perform delicate surgical procedures. However, extracorporeal circulation is also associated with interruption of normal myocardial blood flow. Preservation of myocardial function during CPBP is crucial to the patient's survival after open-heart surgery. Steps must be taken to preserve myocardial tissue and assure adequate cardiac function following the operative procedure. Specifically, interventions must be aimed at assuring a balance between myocardial oxygen demand and supply. Three techniques in particular have enjoyed widespread use: *coronary perfusion, global ischemic arrest with topical cooling,* and *hypothermic cardioplegia.*

One of the major advances in cardiac surgery was the development of hypothermic potassium cardioplegia in the 1970s. The best and most consistent myocardial preservation during CPBP has been achieved with this technique,[161,165] which is presently the preferred technique of cardiac surgeons.[164,166] The goals of chemical cardioplegia are to stop the heart safely and prevent significant myocardial damage. Although the exact composition of cardioplegic solutions varies, they all have some elements in common. Concentrations of potassium, magnesium, or procaine are used to cause immediate electromechanical asystole when infused through the coronary arteries into the myocardium.[167] This immediate arrest has been shown to eliminate the large energy expenditures associated with ventricular contraction, thus maintaining the integrity of the myocardial cell membrane.[161] Use of cold solutions (around 4°C) lowers myocardial temperature and significantly reduces metabolic requirements, thus protecting against ischemic damage during interruption of coronary blood flow. The addition of blood and/or glucose to the cardioplegia solution assures some energy supplies to the myocardium at this time. Buffers are often added to the solution to optimize pH, calcium and steroids may be used for myocardial membrane stabilization, and osmolarity is controlled to minimize myocardial edema.[132,167]

The conduct of CPBP with cardioplegic myocardial protection generally includes the following routines, although some variations are common.[136,151,168] A loading heparin dose is administered. The aorta and right atria are cannulated. Flow through the CPBP circuit is established with concomitant lowering of body temperature. Following adequate systemic cooling (28 to 32°C) the aorta is cross-clamped. The cardioplegic cannula is inserted into the ascending aorta. At this point the heart is arrested and cooled by infusing cold cardioplegic solution (4°C) into the aortic root via the cardioplegic cannula. If aortic regurgitation is present, selective cannulation of the coronary ostia is used to assure delivery of cardioplegia. The perfusion of the previously described cardioplegic solution into the coronary arteries results in immediate electromechanical asystole. One or more thermistors are usually inserted into the left ventricle and myocardial temperatures are lowered to 5 to 15°C.[136,161] Instillation of iced saline solution into the pericardial cavity is used to provide further myocardial cooling. At this point, with the heart arrested and a myocardial temperature of less than 15°C, the distal anastomoses of the coronary artery grafts are completed. Myocardial hypothermia is maintained throughout this part of surgery by intermittently infusing cardioplegia into the aortic root, and by injecting the solution into each new graft as the distal anastomoses are sutured.[161] When all distal anastomoses are completed, air is carefully evacuated from the heart and the aorta is unclamped. The heat exchanger is set to begin rewarming the patient, and any proximal vein graft anastomoses are completed. In the majority of patients cardiac activity returns promptly, but ventricular fibrillation can be easily converted with direct defibrillation. Once the patient is rewarmed, the CPBP cannulas are removed and protamine is given to reverse the effects of heparin. It is at this critical point that the heart resumes its normal workload and any ischemic damage is evident. Although use of hypothermic cardioplegia has been credited with significant reduction in operative mortality,[148] evidence suggests that a more subtle form of intraoperative myocardial damage may still occur.[167] Hopefully, further research will elucidate more effective methods of assuring myocardial preservation during CPBP.

Physiologic Effects of Cardiopulmonary Bypass

The patient's responses to extracorporeal perfusion are extremely complex, and potentially involve all body functions. In order to effectively care for the CABG patient, an understanding of the potential problems associated with cardiopulmonary bypass is imperative. A review of data from research reveals alterations in virtually all physiologic subsystems following CPBP. Table 21-11 presents research findings regarding the effects of CPBP and the potential postoperative problems often associated with those effects. It is evident that care of the patient who has undergone extracorporeal perfusion constitutes a major challenge in the acute care setting.

Postoperative Considerations

Because of the potential effects of CPBP on all body systems, the postoperative CABG surgery patient offers a major challenge in the critical-care setting. Potential problems commonly encountered in the postoperative phase have been elucidated based on knowledge of the operative procedure and the effects of CABP. This section will highlight the most predominant concerns.

Several studies have documented a significant decrease in left ventricular ejection fraction and cardiac index in as many as 90 percent of patients 2 h after CABG surgery.[169,170] Thus, transient left ventricular dysfunction may be common following coronary revascularization. The frequency of decreased cardiac output (CO) in the postoperative CABG patient makes it a problem of major importance. Many factors play dominant roles in adversely affecting the performance of the heart following cardiac surgery. Most importantly, these include the extent of preoperative cardiac dysfunction, the stress of the surgical intervention (anesthesia, CPBP, and surgical manipulation), and any uncorrected cardiovascular pathology.[161]

Heart rate and rhythm are important postoperative considerations in the management of CABG patients. It has been estimated that some cardiac rhythm disturbance occurs in up to 50 percent of all post-open-heart surgery patients, usually within the first 48 h following operation.[171] Supraventricular dysrhythmias, sinus bradycardia, sinus tachycardia, various degrees of heart block, junctional rhythms, AV dissociation, ventricular arrhythmias, and transient bundle branch blocks have all been reported in the postoperative patient.[172,173]

Epicardial pacing wires are a frequently used adjunct to the recognition and treatment of rhythm disturbances and to augment cardiac output in the postoperative cardiac surgery patient. Prior to closure of the sternum, pacing wires are commonly

Table 21-11 Effects of Cardiopulmonary Bypass in the Postoperative CABG Surgical Patient

Endocrine System

Effects of CPBP	Potential Problems
Catecholamine release	Elevated systemic vascular resistance as much as 44.6% in 75% of post-CPBP patients
Epinephrine 10 × baseline and norepinephrine 4 × baseline at 2–4 post-CPBP	Hypertension occurs in 33% of post-CAB patients
Elevated renin, angiotensin, and aldosterone levels	
Increase in antidiuretic hormone 30–40 × baseline during CPBP, returns to normal in 2–3 days	Excess sodium and water retention, and potassium excretion
Decreased ACTH levels and decreased cortisol response during CPBP	Danger of steroid inadequacy
Increased T_4 levels, decreased T_3 levels, and decreased TSH response	Danger of thyroid insufficiency
Elevated blood glucose levels and depressed insulin response	Ketoacidosis
	Hyperosmolar, hyperglycemic, nonketotic acidosis

Electrolytes

Effects of CPBP	Potential Problems
Dilution of serum potassium	Hypokalemia
Large potassium losses in the urine	Hypokalemia
Intracellular potassium shifts	Hypokalemia
Use of potassium cardioplegia	Hyperkalemia
Defective intracellular transport of glucose and potassium	Hyperkalemia
Dilution of serum sodium	Hyponatremia
Decreased urinary excretion of sodium, most marked on 2d postoperative day	Hypernatremia
Dilution of serum calcium and intracellular calcium shifts	Hypocalcemia
Dilution of serum magnesium and intracellular magnesium shifts	Hypomagnesemia
Magnesium losses in the urine	Hypomagnesemia

Imune System

Effects of CPBP	Potential Problems
Exposure to multiple sources of pathogens	
Decreased complement and immunoglobulin levels for up to 1 week	Lethal infections in general (pulmonary, mediastinal, urinary, blood) 1.1% of cardiac surgery patients die from postoperative infections
Suppression of the reticuloendothelial system	
Impaired phagocytosis and function of leukocytes	Mediastinitis occurs in 1.5% of cardiac surgical patients
Release of complement anaphylotoxins	A total body inflammatory reaction (?) "post-perfusion syndrome"

Coagulation System

Effects of CPBP	Potential Problems
Dilution, absorption, and destruction of coagulation factors in the CPBP circuit	Life-threatening hemorrhage occurs in 5–25% of post-CPBP patients
Heparin rebound after neutralization with protamine	
Platelet counts reduced by 30% and platelet function impaired for 3–5 days	

The Heart

Effects of CPBP	Potential Problems
Emboli, inadequate perfusion, inadequate myocardial cooling, and ventricular fibrillation may all contribute to myocardial ischemia and/or necrosis	Reported incidence of perioperative myocardial infarction varies from 5–20%

Continued

Table 21-11 Effects of Cardiopulmonary Bypass in the Postoperative CABG Surgical Patient (Continued)

The Heart	
Effects of CPBP	Potential Problems
Release of capillary damaging enzymes, lowered colloid osmotic pressure, high coronary perfusion pressures, and distention of the left ventricle contribute to myocardial edema Reperfusion injury (mechanism poorly understood)	Low postoperative cardiac output; up to 90% of patients show a decrease in ejection fraction 2 h post-CPBP

Renal System	
Effects of CPBP	Potential Problems
Decreased renal blood flow and decreased glomerular filtration rate Microemboli to renal vasculature Damage to RBCs with release of hemoglobin	Oliguric renal failure found to occur in 1.5% of post-CPBP patients

Fluids	
Effects of CPBP	Potential Problems
Increased total body water Increased extravascular fluid Decreased intravascular volume	Total body hypervolemia Interstitial edema and possible organ dysfunction Intravascular hypovolemia

Gastrointestinal System	
Effects of CPBP	Potential Problems

Catecholamine release and "stress response"
Coagulation defects
Emboli to pancreatic vasculature
Complement activation
Emboli to intestinal vasculature
Low perfusion state
	Gastrointestinal bleeding
	    Incidence of less than 1%
	Acute pancreatitis
	    Incidence estimated at 1.6% with a mortality of 86%
	Intestinal ischemia or infarction

Pulmonary System	
Effects of CPBP	Potential Problems
Complement activation, air and particulate emboli all contribute to alveolar–capillary membrane damage Hemodilution decreases colloid osmotic pressure and may contribute to interstitial pulmonary edema Minimal circulation to lung parenchyma during bypass may result in decreased surfactant production Alterations of ventilatory patterns during bypass (deflation, static inflation, or intermittent inflation) may contribute to atelectasis	Increased interstitial lung water Atelectasis Respiratory insufficiency

Central Nervous System	
Effects of CPBP	Potential Problems
Cerebral particulate emboli (especially fat emboli) and air emboli Alterations in cerebral blood flow (especially with perfusion pressures less than 50 torr) Systemic heparinization	Stroke (occurs in approximately 2% of post-CPBP patients) Transient motor deficits (occurs in approximately 0.3% of post-CPBP patients) Cerebral hemorrhage

Adapted from S. Stewart, *The Physiologic Effects and Nursing Implications of Cardiopulmonary Bypass.* Unpublished master's thesis, Boston University, Boston, 1985.

loosely sutured to the right atrial epicardium, and at times ventricular wires are also attached. These wires are then tunneled out through the anterior chest wall in the soft tissue below the sternum. In the event of a slow rhythm or heart block which compromises hemodynamics, the wires can be connected to a pacemaker generator for cardiac pacing. Pacing the heart at a rate slightly faster than the patient's spontaneous rate may also suppress atrial or ventricular ectopic beats and to augment cardiac output. Further, atrial tachyarrhythmias or recurrent ventricular tachyarrhythmias can frequently be terminated by overdrive pacing.

Atrial pacing wires are also a useful diagnostic tool in distinguishing supraventricular from ventricular arrhythmias. Tracings which reveal enhanced atrial activity can be obtained by an atrial electrogram (AEG). A unipolar atrial electrogram requires only one atrial pacing wire and records both atrial and ventricular activity. The bipolar AEG usually records only atrial activity and requires two atrial pacing wires. The utilization of AEGs provides a quick and safe method for dysrhythmia interpretation such as atrial fibrillation, atrial flutter (see Fig. 21-12), and premature atrial and ventricular contractions in the postoperative open-heart surgery patient. See Chap. 20 for further discussion.

In addition to heart rate and rhythm, stroke volume is another important determinant of cardiac output which must be considered postoperatively. Optimizing stroke volume requires management of its three determinants: *preload, afterload,* and *contractility.*

The postoperative CABG patient may experience alterations in preload for numerous reasons. The most obvious of these is fluid loss, which often occurs due to postoperative bleeding or urinary diuresis.

Studies indicate that post-CPBP urinary diuresis may be brisk, especially when dilute hyperosmolar priming solutions are used during the pump run.[174] Further, despite obvious postoperative interstitial edema, many cardiac surgery patients exhibit a decrease in intravascular volume for several days after the operation.

The profound vasoconstriction following CPBP and frequently documented low preoperative blood volumes in patients with coronary artery disease[175] may result in significant hypovolemia in these patients as they are warmed and vasodilate in the postoperative period. Some mediastinal bleeding following cardiac surgery is expected. However, chest tube drainage greater than 2 mL/kg/h, 2 or more h following surgery, is usually considered abnormal.[172] Coagulation abnormalities may occur from numerous effects of CPBP. These must be identified and treatment aimed at the specific defect.

Bleeding into the pericardial space may also result in cardiac tamponade. The increased volume and pressure within the pericardial space prevents adequate filling of the heart, reduces preload, and results in significant reductions in cardiac output.

Numerous factors predispose the post-CABG patient to significant elevations in systemic vascular resistance (SVR) and blood pressure, which are clinical determinants of afterload. These include the effects of CPBP, pain, agitation, shivering, hypoxia, hypercarbia, and withdrawal of antihypertensive medications.[176] Studies show that in the early postoperative period, hypertension occurs in 33 percent of patients following coronary artery bypass, and the majority of postoperative cardiac surgery patients exhibit a significant elevation in systemic vascular resistance. Such increases in afterload may critically intensify myocardial oxygen demands and significantly reduce cardiac output. As well as these effects on cardiac function, hypertension may cause disruption of fresh suture lines (especially aortotomy or coronary anastomoses), or result in cerebral bleeding in patients with widespread atherosclerotic changes.[177]

Despite optimization of heart rate, preload, and afterload, numerous factors can adversely affect the postoperative cardiac inotropic state. These include advanced preoperative myocardial disease, the effects of CPBP, operative trauma, and incomplete surgical repair. Postoperative hypoxemia, severe acid-base or electrolyte imbalances, or negative inotropic drugs may further reduce myocardial contractility in the postoperative CABG patient.[172] Finally, any impairment in myocardial contractility may be further exacerbated by an ischemic event. Despite present myocardial preservation techniques during CPBP, perioperative myocardial infarction has been reported in 4 to 6 percent of patients undergoing CABG surgery.[26]

Respiratory problems constitute the most frequent complication after all types of thoracic and

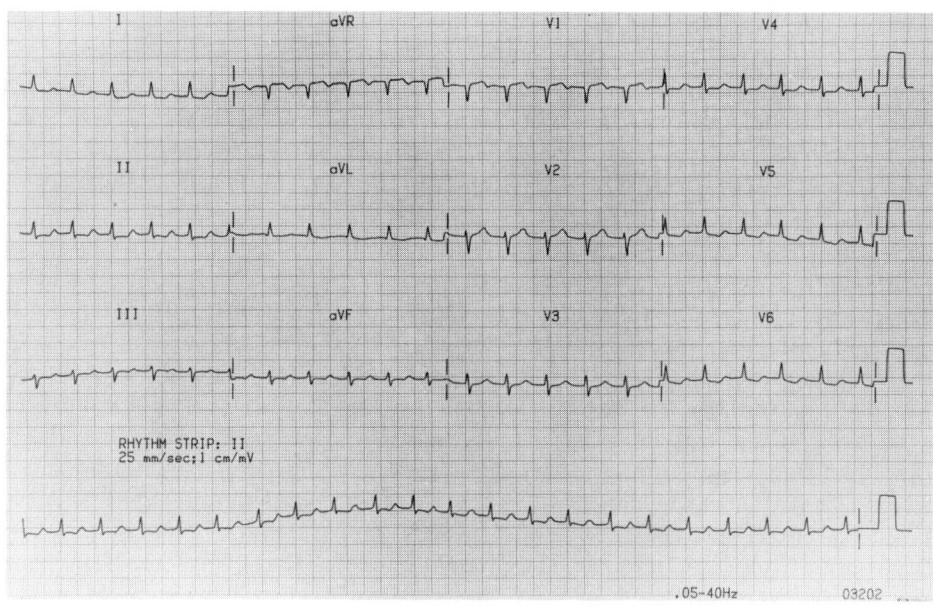

A

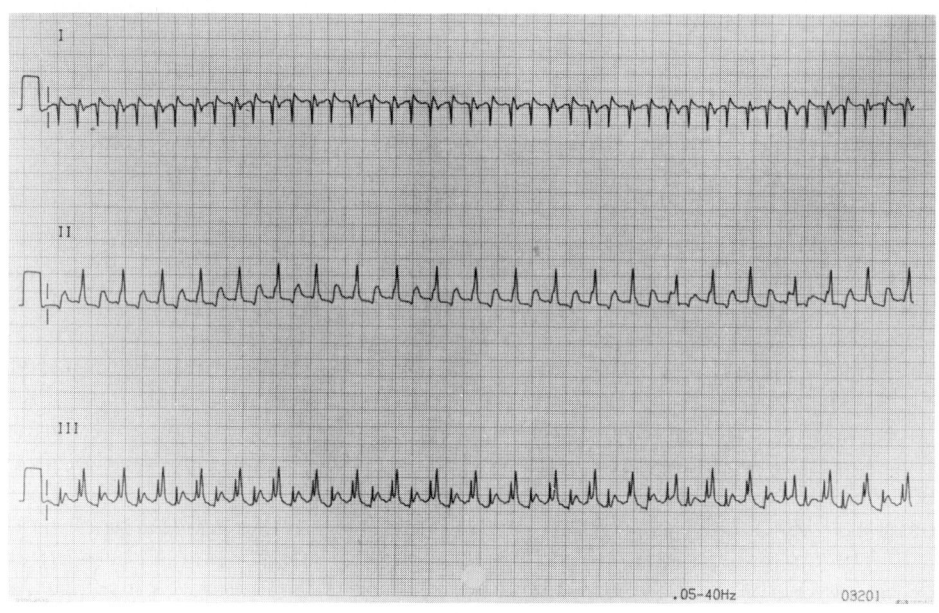

B

Figure 21-12   (A) Conventional surface 12-lead ECG in a 59-year-old man (CABGx3) who was 10 h postoperative. (B) Atrial electrogram obtained simultaneously with above surface ECG which revealed atrial flutter with 2:1 conduction in bipolar lead (lead I) and unipolar leads (leads II and III).

cardiac operations.[161] The overall incidence of pulmonary complications after open-heart surgery has been reported between 61 and 84 percent.[174] Gas exchange is frequently impaired in the postoperative cardiac surgical patient for several reasons. As outlined under "Cardiopulmonary Bypass," numerous effects of extracorporeal perfusion cause alveolar–capillary membrane injury, leading to increased interstitial lung water. In the presence of damaged alveolar capillary membranes, any elevations of left heart filling pressures (PAWP or LAP) may cause further extravasation of fluid and increased pulmonary interstitial fluid. These and other factors related to CPBP result in areas of atelectasis in the lung. In fact, the most common morphologic change in the post-CPBP lung is the presence of numerous scattered regions of atelectasis with nonventilated but perfused alveoli.[178] Low postoperative hemoglobin levels (hemodilution) may contribute to impaired gas exchange by lowering the oxygen-carrying capacity of red blood cells. Further, the effects of anesthesia, sedation, pain, and immobility may result in hypoventilation and further exacerbate atelectasis. All of these factors contribute to impairment in oxygen and carbon dioxide gas exchange in the postoperative CABG patient.

Another postoperative consideration is the incidence of stroke or transient motor deficits following CPBP, which has been reduced to 2 percent or less. A more frequently encountered problem has been behavioral changes following cardiac surgery which range from mild confusion to frank psychosis. Estimates of the incidence of such neurologic changes after CPBP range from 16 percent[179] to 70 percent.[180] Manifestations of postcardiotomy delirium (PCD) appear about 24 h after surgery and usually resolve within 24 to 48 h after transfer out of the intensive care unit. It is believed that numerous factors contribute to the syndrome of PCD. Some of these include advanced age, severe preoperative cardiac dysfunction, a history of psychiatric illness, sleep deprivation, and prolonged intensive care unit stay.[173,180]

Nursing Therapies: Preoperative Nursing Care

It is evident that cardiac surgery involves the potential for alterations in all body systems. The extensiveness of the procedure, and the implications of surgery on the heart, the seat of emotion, may result in tremendous psychological stress for the patient as well. Although each patient's plan of care must be individualized, certain interventions are necessary in the preoperative phase.

First, the nurse should perform and document a complete nursing history using Gordon's or another framework and physical examination on admission. This will enable the nurse to obtain a baseline profile, determine any present abnormalities and future changes, and formulate collaborative diagnoses as well as nursing diagnoses.

Second, the nurse should monitor for and document any clinical signs of compromised organ function preoperatively. In particular, this assessment should include the following data:

1. Neurologic: decreased LOC, neurologic deficits, weakness, impaired verbal response
2. Cardiovascular: Heart rate and rhythm disturbances, heart sounds, unequal blood pressure in both arms, decreased or absent peripheral pulses, edema, neck vein distention, and bruits levels
3. Respiratory: Breath sounds, tachypnea
4. Renal: Diminished urinary output
5. Gastrointestinal: Abdominal distention, absent bowel sounds
6. Immunological: Temperature, any localized infections

The nurse should also ensure that all diagnostic tests are completed and any abnormalities reported to the surgeon, including ECG, chest x-ray, arterial blood gases, CBC, electrolytes, coagulation profile, BUN and creatinine, cardiac enzymes, liver profile, and urinalysis.

In addition, the nurse will need to monitor the patient's response to medical interventions aimed at minimizing postoperative complications. These may include preoperative enema, pulmonary hygiene, electrolyte and other pharmacologic interventions. The nurse must instruct the patient in effective deep breathing and coughing exercises, and leg exercises to prevent postoperative pneumonia and venous stasis.

Some anxiety concerning the operative procedure and postoperative recovery is a universal response to open-heart surgery. This anxiety may range from mild to extremely high. Again, each plan of care must be individualized. One source of anxiety for the CABG patient is lack of knowledge concerning pre- and postoperative events. Much of nursing's role involves carefully executed patient and family teaching based on concepts of adult learning.

After all these aforementioned interventions have been accomplished, a plan of care should be formulated. Because most patients and their families exhibit some degree of fear concerning the operative procedure, one of the universal nursing diagnosis pertaining to preoperative cardiac surgical patients and families is fear related to perceptions of surgery and inadequate knowledge of events surrounding surgery and postoperative course. The following goals, interventions, and evaluation criteria will be discussed for this diagnosis.

Actual Nursing Diagnosis

Patient and family fear related to the perceptions of impending surgery and inadequate knowledge of events surrounding surgery and postoperative course.

Goal

The patient and family will demonstrate or verbalize a decrease in fear during the preoperative phase.

Nursing Interventions

1. Assess patient's and family's previous experiences with major surgery, stress levels, coping mechanisms, fears, and support systems.
2. Assist patient and family in recognizing and acknowledging specific fears.
3. Design an individualized teaching plan based on the patient's and family's knowledge of the operative procedure and events, and their readiness to learn.
4. Assist the patient and family in identifying signs that indicate increased fear, such as increased pulse, respirations and blood pressure, sweating, and changes in voice pitch or voice tremors.
5. Allow for continuity or consistency of nursing personnel in order to enhance trust and familiarity with nursing staff so as to minimize fears associated with unfamiliar environment.
6. Provide the patient and family with time to ask questions and follow through with accurate and realistic answers. Encourage the patient and

family to verbalize their fears with specific questions, such as, "What worries do you have?"
7. Offer realistic support and encouragement rather than vague comments such as "Everything will be okay."

Evaluation

The patient and family is able to verbalize specific fears regarding CABG surgery. The patient and family will be able to recognize fears and demonstrate appropriate problem-solving techniques to alleviate fears. Patient and family verbalize adequate knowledge of surgical and postoperative events.

Nursing Therapies: Postoperative Nursing Care

Although the complex care of CABG patients involves a concerted team effort, the safety with which the patient can be conducted through the immediate postoperative phase is "largely dependent on the minute-to-minute observations made by the critical care nurse" (p. 442).[165] The critical-care nurse acts as the first line of defense in detecting changes in the patient's condition and making effective interventions.

Postoperative nursing care focuses on identifying actual and potential problems and preventing complications. Nursing interventions are based on an accurate and ongoing patient assessment as well as comprehensive nursing history and preoperative data base.

In the immediate postoperative phase, left ventricular dysfunction often results in low cardiac output and inadequate tissue perfusion. The critical-care nurse should be concerned with preoperative myocardial function (especially pulmonary wedge pressure, ejection fraction, and cardiac index) as well as obtaining a detailed account of operative events in order to anticipate possible LV dysfunction. The major collaborative diagnosis in the immediate postoperative period is a decrease in tissue perfusion related to a decrease in cardiac output secondary to cardiac dysrhythmias, inappropriate preload status, and increased afterload and/or depressed myocardial contractility. The goals, interventions, and evaluation criteria will be discussed for this diagnosis.

Collaborative Diagnosis I

Decrease in tissue perfusion related to a decrease in cardiac output secondary to (1) cardiac dysrhythmias, (2) inappropriate preload status, (3) increased afterload, and/or (4) depressed myocardial contractility.

Goal

The patient will demonstrate an increase in or no further deterioration in tissue perfusion.

Nursing Interventions

1. Monitor the patient's ECG continuously with high and low alarms set and QRS volume on in order to detect any changes in heart rate or rhythm.
2. Document (with ECG) and report any changes in heart rate and/or rhythm and associated clinical response (BP, CI, peripheral pulses).
3. Monitor for and report any factors which may contribute to dysrhythmias in the post-CABG patient, such as acidosis, alkalosis, hypoxia, hypokalemia, or hyperkalemia.
4. Institute measures to warm the postoperative hypothermic patient because a low core body temperature may contribute to bradydysrhythmias.
5. Administer pain medication, offer the patient explanations and reassurance, and provide the patient with comfortable positioning in order to minimize sympathetic stimulation and catecholamine outpouring which may contribute to dysrhythmias.
6. Be prepared to immediately treat a hemodynamically compromising dysrhythmia by having cardioverter/defibrillator readily available (for treating ventricular fibrillation, ventricular tachycardia, or SVT) and pharmacologic agents on hand, especially atropine, for bradydysrhythmias.
7. Appropriately administer any ordered pharmacologic treatment, monitoring the patient's response and untoward side effects. In particular, this may include:
   a. Lidocaine: Intravenous (IV) bolus at 1 mg/kg for ventricular dysrhythmias, then administer a continuous infusion at 1 to 4 mg/min, followed by an additional 0.5 mg/kg IV bolus 5 to 10 min after the initial dose if ectopy still present. IV bolus should not exceed 3 mg/Kg.
   b. Verapamil: 0.075 to 0.15 mg/kg IV over 2 to 3 min for SVT (up to 10 mg).
   c. Atropine: 0.5 mg IV repeat at 5-min intervals. Total dose not to exceed 2.0 mg.[181]
8. Identify presence of atrial and/or ventricular temporary epicardial pacing wires and assure these are securely attached to external pulse generator with functioning batteries and with ordered settings.
9. Be prepared to initiate temporary pacing or change settings as directed by physician.
10. Document supraventricular arrhythmias by atrial electrocardiogram.
11. Prevent microshock and associated dysrhythmias by covering any exposed pacing wires with rubber gloves, using only grounded electrical equipment in room, and avoiding contact with any electrical equipment and the patient simultaneously.
12. Monitor all hemodynamic and clinical parameters for signs of hypovolemia, which include low PAWP, PAP, and CVP; increased HR; decreased BP and CI; weak peripheral pulses; cool, pale skin; and fluid output greater than intake.
13. While the hypothermic patient is being warmed, monitor all the above parameters every 5 min and be prepared to administer volume replacement as the patient's temperature rises and the vascular bed dilates, producing a relative hypovolemia.
14. Monitor all hemodynamic and clinical parameters for signs associated with bleeding and hemorrhage, which include chest tube drainage greater than 2 mL/kg/h, 2 or more h following surgery; bloody oozing from incisions or catheter sites; hematuria; bloody NG drainage; abnormal clotting studies; decreased hemoglobin and hematocrit values.
15. Be prepared to administer blood products, coagulation factors, or protamine sulfate appropriately as ordered.
16. Monitor all hemodynamic and clinical parameters for signs of hypervolemia, which may

include increased PAWP, PAP, and CVP; crackles; peripheral edema; jugular venous distention; and fluid volume intake in excess of output.

17. Report any of the above signs of hypervolemia and administer pharmacologic agents appropriately as ordered. These may include:
    a. Lasix or other diuretic agents given to increase urinary output and decrease intravascular fluid volume and preload.
    b. Nitroglycerin given by continuous intravenous infusion at rates up to 200 to 300 mg per minute to dilate the venous vascular bed and thus lower preload by decreasing venous return.

18. Position the hypervolemic patient in Fowler's position in order to aid in decreasing venous return.

19. Minimize fluid administration in the hypervolemic patient by concentrating intravenous medications in minimal fluid volume.

20. Monitor all hemodynamic and clinical parameters for signs of cardiac tamponade, which may include elevated and equalized CVP, PAD, LAP, and PAWP; decreased cardiac index; jugular venous distention; cool, clammy skin; diminished peripheral pulses; pulsus paradoxus; muffled heart sounds; sudden cessation of chest tube drainage.

21. Milk chest tubes every 15 to 30 min per physician order to maintain patency and prevent tamponade, but refrain from vigorous stripping of chest tubes, which may exacerbate bleeding problems because of high pressures produced by stripping.[182]

22. Monitor blood pressure continuously and immediately report a sustained systolic BP above 140 mmHg, or a mean arterial pressure above 90 mmHg.

23. Calculate systemic vascular resistance (SVR) q 1 h in the immediate postoperative period and report SVR greater than 1400 dyn/sec/cm⁵.

24. Monitor for clinical signs of peripheral vasoconstriction such as cool, pale, mottled extremities and sluggish capillary refill.

25. Administer pain medication and provide patient with comfortable positioning, reassurance, and emotional support in order to minimize catecholamine outpouring associated with discom-

fort and emotional stress which would further elevate SVR.

26. Institute measures to rewarm the hypothermic post-CABG patient with elevated SVR to decrease peripheral vasoconstriction. This may include warm blankets, blood warmers for transfusions, use of hypothermia blankets, or rewarming lights, and also increasing the temperature of the room.

27. Be prepared to administer afterload-reducing drugs appropriately. In particular, this may include sodium nitroprusside, a potent peripheral vasodilator administered via continuous intravenous infusion at a rate of 0.5 up to 8.0 μg/kg/min.[181]

28. Monitor for and maintain optimum preload and afterload as outlined above to enhance cardiac contractility and decrease myocardial oxygen demands.

29. Monitor hemodynamic and clinical parameters for signs of impaired myocardial contractility, which may include CI less than 2.5 L/min/m²; hypotension; tachycardia; crackles; cool, clammy skin; weak peripheral pulses; low urine output; and lethargy or restlessness.

30. Monitor for signs of myocardial ischemia, which may include ST segment elevation or depression on ECG, elevated CK-MB isoenzymes, and patient complaints of anginalike chest pain.

31. Institute measures to reduce myocardial oxygen demands wherever possible. These may include providing for a quiet, restful environment; treating pain expediently; offering comfort measures and emotional support to the patient; and timing procedures and interventions to allow for periods of rest between events.

32. Discontinue rewarming interventions when the patient's temperature is within 1 to 2 degrees of normal (98.6°F) to prevent temperature elevation which further increases myocardial oxygen demands.

33. Expediently report and treat shivering, hypertension, tachycardia, and fever, which all increase myocardial oxygen demands.

34. Provide for optimal myocardial oxygen supply by monitoring for and reporting hypoxemia by arterial blood gases or hematocrit values less than 30, and expediently reporting and treating

hypotension and hemodynamically compromising dysrhythmias.

35. Monitor for and report abnormalities that may further compromise myocardial contractility, such as acidosis or electrolyte imbalances.

36. Administer positive inotropic agents as ordered to enhance myocardial contractility and thus improve cardiac output. These may include:

   a. Dopamine: A chemical precursor of norepinephrine, given by continuous intravenous infusion. This drug acts on different receptors at varying infusion rates. 1 to 2 μg/kg/min exerts dopamanergic effects and increases renal and mesenteric blood flow. 2 to 10 μg/kg/min stimulates β_2 receptors, thus enhancing myocardial contractility and heart rate. Over 10 μg/kg/min causes more alpha stimulating effects resulting in vasoconstriction, rise in BP, and increased afterload.[181]

   b. Dobutamine: Direct beta-adrenergic receptor stimulator given by continuous infusion at rates of up to 10 μg/kg/min. Mainly enhances cardiac contractility with little vasoconstriction and less arrhythmogenesis than dopamine.[181]

37. Administer intravenous nitroglycerin as ordered to optimize myocardial oxygen supply. Nitroglycerine has been shown to dilate coronary arteries, increase coronary collateral blood flow, and relax areas of coronary artery spasm.[181] Thus, this drug may be effective in treating or preventing myocardial ischemia in the postCABG patient.[183]

Evaluation

The patient will demonstrate improved tissue perfusion as evidenced by (1) normal sinus rhythm without any hemodynamically compromising dysrhythmias; (2) cardiac index greater than 2.5 L/min/m², systolic BP greater than 90 mmHg, CVP and PAWP within patient's normal limits and absence of signs of hypovolemia, hemorrhage, hypervolemia, or cardiac tamponade; (3) systolic BP less than 140 but greater than 90, diastolic BP less than 90 but greater than 60, calculated SVR less than 1400 dyn/sec/cm⁵; (4) no clinical signs of hypotension, urinary output not less than 30 mL/h, no signs of

cool clammy skin, no diminished peripheral pulses, and warm, dry extremities with capillary refill less than 4 s.

Because respiratory problems are one of the most frequent complications after surgery, another collaborative diagnosis found in most CABG patients is impaired gas exchange related to atelectasis.

Collaborative Diagnosis II

Impaired gas exchange related to atelectasis.

Goal

The patient will maintain adequate gas exchange as evidenced by arterial blood gas values within normal limits, respiratory rate within normal limits, and absence of cyanosis.

Nursing Interventions

1. Monitor hemodynamic and clinical parameters for signs of hypoxia, which may include increased respiratory rate, use of accessory muscles of respiration, tachycardia, hypertension, confusion or restlessness, and low arterial P_{O_2}.

2. Institute measures to mobilize and remove secretions as well as open closed alveoli. These include turning and positioning the patient every 2 h, endotracheal suctioning as necessary followed by manual hyperinflation of the lungs, and head of bed elevated to promote diaphragmatic excursion.

3. Administer pain medication to decrease splinting and hypoventilation by the patient. Instruct the patient in use of a pillow or blanket to support the incisional area in order to increase comfort during deep breathing, coughing, and movement, and thus improve alveolar ventilation.

4. Monitor for signs of other complications which may further compromise gas exchange. These may include:

   a. Pulmonary edema: Crackles, elevated PAWP, elevated PAP, frothy pulmonary secretions

   b. Pneumothorax or hemothorax: Decreased or absent breath sounds, high peak inspiratory pressures, tracheal deviation

   c. Pulmonary embolus: Chest pain, hemoptysis, elevated PAP, cyanosis

   d. Gastric distention: Large, firm abdomen; absence of bowel sounds; diminished bilateral basilar breath sounds

5. Follow extubation with use of incentive spirometry and deep breathing exercises every 1 to 2 h.

6. Begin progressive patient ambulation as soon as possible postoperatively. This usually means getting the patient out of bed the day following surgery after removal of the endotracheal tube and pulmonary artery catheter.

Evaluation

The patient demonstrates an adequate gas exchange as evidenced by (1) the patient's arterial blood gases show P_{O_2} greater than 60 with an O_2 saturation above 85 percent, P_{CO_2} between 35 to 45, and pH of 7.35 to 7.45; (2) the patient's respiratory rate is less than 20 with no use of accessory muscles; (3) the patient's breath sounds are not decreased in lung fields with no crackles, rhonchi, or wheezes; (4) the patient exhibits no cyanosis; (5) sputum remains clear.

Anxiety is a common response to CABG surgery. In the postoperative period, the patient is faced with numerous potential sources of emotional stress. The median sternotomy and leg incisions, the presence of an endotracheal tube and chest tubes, and relative immobility because of equipment, are all obvious sources of discomfort for the post-CABG patient. It is well accepted that pain (discomfort) and anxiety can create a vicious cycle. Pain produces anxiety, which intensifies the pain, which results in greater anxiety.

During the period of endotracheal intubation, the patient's difficulty with communication may heighten feelings of helplessness and anxiety. Dependency on machines and medical staff may intensify the patient's fears of permanent disability and death, which, along with lack of knowledge regarding the progress of events, routines, equipment, and normal feelings, may also contribute to his or her emotional stress.[184]

Failure to alleviate or minimize anxiety may lead to adverse physiologic sequelae. The outpouring of catecholamines owing to the stress response can result in tachycardia, hypertension, and peripheral vasoconstriction, all of which increase myocardial oxygen demands and may have untoward hemodynamic consequences in the patient with coronary artery disease.

Therefore, the nursing diagnosis for a CABG patient is anxiety related to incisional pain, feelings of helplessness and/or lack of knowledge regarding the progress of events, routines, and/or equipment.

Nursing Diagnosis I

Patient anxiety related to pain, feelings of helplessness, or lack of knowledge regarding the progress of events, routines, and/or equipment.

Goal

The patient will not show extreme levels of anxiety as evidenced by his or her ability to rest quietly, to communicate concerns and needs, and to actively participate in all aspects of care.

Nursing Interventions

1. As the patient wakes up in the intensive care unit, the nurse should use a calm, controlled voice, offer frequent explanations, reorienting the patient to place, time, and events, including reminders that the operation is over.

2. Explain to patient why he or she is unable to talk (endotracheal tube in place). Take time to develop a mode for patient communication during intubation. This may include providing the patient with a writing pad and pen, or utilizing lip reading, or having the patient form letters with his or her fingers. Assure patient that a nurse is always within sight, and establish a method for patient to signal need for nurse's attention.

3. Encourage the patient to communicate sources of discomfort and assess the patient continuously for nonverbal cues of pain. In general, this may include facial grimacing, stiffness or reluctance in moving in bed, and splinting of body parts. Sympathetic nervous system responses are common when pain is of low or moderate intensity: pallor, tachycardia, increased BP, dilated pupils, increased respiratory rate, and skeletal muscle tension. When pain is more severe, parasympathetic responses may predominate: pallor, diminished heart rate, hypotension, nausea, vomiting, weakness, and prostration.[173]

4. Provide the patient with pain medication, anti-anxiety medications, comfortable positioning, and other comfort measures such as mouth care to promote patient comfort.
5. Encourage the patient to make some decisions in his or her care, even in the intensive care unit, to minimize feelings of loss of control and helplessness. This may be as simple as having the patient decide which side to turn to or how high to elevate the head of the bed.
6. Verbally communicate signs of progress to the patient and inform him or her of the next step in recovery.

Evaluation

The patient is able to verbalize effective ways of dealing with anxiety. The patient will verbalize or demonstrate a decrease in anxiety as evidenced by decreased respiratory and heart rate, tremors, shakiness, voice or pitch changes, and increased ability to deal with problems and to concentrate.

The CABG surgery patient is not an isolated individual, but the member of a family unit. The anxiety and stress of the surgical event is felt by the patient's significant others. The family is faced with the threat of loss of a loved one, feelings of helplessness in the intensive care environment, and lack of knowledge regarding the patient's condition and expected course of events. In recent years several studies have described the needs of relatives of the critically ill patient.[185–187] Rodgers' study looked specifically at needs of families of the cardiac surgery patient in the initial postoperative period.[186] Although the order of rank was slightly different, in all three studies, eight of the top ten ranked needs of families were identical. Table 21-12 is a compilation of the highest ranking needs.

Standards for Nursing Care of the Critically Ill emphasizes that the nursing care of CABG patients must include assessment and intervention in family needs.[188] Therefore, another nursing diagnosis identified is family anxiety related to feelings of helplessness and lack of knowledge regarding the patient's condition and expected course of events.

Nursing Diagnosis II

Family anxiety related to feelings of helplessness and lack of knowledge regarding the patient's condition and expected course of events.

Goal

Family members will show minimal or no anxiety as evidenced by their ability to express their questions and concerns and offer support to the patient.

Nursing Interventions

1. Take time to elicit questions and concerns from family members. Offer the family honest, simple explanations of events and equipment.
2. Encourage family members to address questions and concerns to physicians and reiterate the physician's explanations whenever necessary.
3. Offer the family members reassurance whenever possible. Make sure a phone number where the family can be reached is available at the patient's bedside.
4. Verbally communicate signs of the patient's progress to family members.

Table 21-12 The Highest Ranked Needs of Families of Critically Ill Patients

To feel there is hope
To feel that hospital personnel cared about the patient
To have my questions answered honestly
To know that I would be called at home for a change in the patient's condition
To have specific facts concerning the patient's progress
To know the patient's chances of recovery (prognosis)
To have explanations given that I could understand
To receive information about the patient's condition once a day

Compiled from Leske,[185] 1986; Rodgers,[187] 1983; Molter,[186] 1979.

5. Assist the family in communicating with the patient utilizing the methods established above.

Evaluation

The family will verbalize questions and concerns that contribute to the onset of anxiety.

The family will display a decrease in such behavioral symptoms as difficulty expressing oneself, selective inattention, indecisiveness, restlessness, and irritability. Family verbalizes relief of anxiety.

Other Nursing Considerations

Numerous other potential clinical problems may apply to the postcoronary artery bypass surgery patient. Nursing care must focus on monitoring for and identifying any abnormality in neurologic functioning after CABG surgery. Further, interventions directed at reorienting the patient to time, place, and person, providing for periods of uninterrupted sleep, allowing time for family-patient interaction, and providing the patient with familiar objects, sights, and sounds (radio, pictures from home) may help to decrease the incidence of psychological complications in the postoperative period.

The incidence of infection following CPBP is a concern in the postoperative period. Meticulous handling of all invasive lines and incisions, as well as monitoring for signs of infection, are vital nursing interventions in the postoperative CABG surgery patient.

The incidence of acute renal failure following CPBP is low. However, nursing care must include scrupulous monitoring of fluid intake and output, as well as monitoring of serum BUN and creatinine levels.

There are numerous sources of emboli during CPBP. The postoperative CABG surgery patient must be carefully assessed for any evidence of such a complication.

Identification of postoperative ileus, return of bowel sounds, and effective gastric decompression are important collaborative considerations in the post-CABG patient.

Results of Surgery

A significant problem following CABG surgery is bypass graft patency. Saphenous vein graft occlusion has been shown to occur at a rate of 10 to 15 percent within the first year after surgery.[189] Early graft closure has been attributed to disproportionate size of the vein, technical problems in anastomosis, trauma to the vein intima or coronary artery, poor distal runoff in the artery, graft kinking, and adhesions from postpericardiotomy syndrome. The annual graft closure rate a year or more after surgery decreases to approximately 2 percent per year.[26] Thus, grafts that remain patent the first year after surgery have a relatively slow failure rate. As previously discussed, IMA grafts have a higher long-term patency rate than saphenous vein grafts.

The progression of atherosclerosis in patients following CABG has been found in ungrafted coronary arteries as well as vein grafts, and is estimated to occur at a rate of approximately 10 percent per year.[136] Thus, modifying life-style and reducing risk factors in an attempt to slow the progression of coronary artery disease are important interventions in post-CABG patients.

The combination of vein graft closure and progression of atherosclerosis leads to the expected recurrence of angina in time. A review of research indicates that 5 years after surgery there is a return of angina in 20 to 30 percent of patients.[136,146] Although reoperation is becoming common, research reports indicate a second CABG procedure is associated with higher mortality and lower rates of angina relief than the initial CABG surgery.[190,191]

Despite less-than-ideal results in graft patency, the majority of patients report significant reduction in symptoms following CABG surgery, as previously mentioned. Associated with this reduction in symptoms has been documented improvement in postoperative exercise testing.[192] Data concerning improvement in ventricular function by CABG surgery has been conflicting. Most studies report no overall change in ventricular contractility after coronary revascularization. However, there is a subset of patients who exhibit ischemic ventricular dysfunction preoperatively but demonstrate improvement in left ventricular function with coronary revascularization.[146,189]

From data presently available, there is no evidence that CABG surgery decreases the long-term incidence of myocardial infarction in patients with coronary artery disease.[146,191] However, improvements in myocardial preservation have significantly lowered perioperative infarction rates over the past decade. Therefore the question of whether surgical revascularization can prevent myocardial infarction remains largely unanswered.

As previously reviewed, research has demonstrated that surgical intervention for coronary artery disease increases longevity in patients with significant stenosis of the left main coronary artery and in patients with triple-vessel disease and left ventricular dysfunction. Data from previous studies regarding improved survival in patients with single- or double-vessel disease or triple-vessel coronary artery involvement with normal ventricular function are controversial.

One of the most important roles and thus a measure of success of CABG surgery is gainful employment. In one study, Jenkins interviewed and tested 268 men and 50 women under the age of 70 years at 6 months after coronary surgical revascularization.[193] Jenkins found that 75 percent of the patients who were employed preoperatively returned to work after surgery. Twenty percent of the patients who were not employed prior to surgery reentered the work force. These results (similar to Hammermeister's study in 1978) are less than ideal since improvement in symptoms and functional capability after CABG surgery should allow individuals to be active in the work force.[194] The variables identified as influencing postoperative employment after CABG surgery include employment status prior to surgery, type of employment, educational level, financial status, age, reappearance of symptoms after CABG, and physicians' and employers' recommendations.[26] A significant correlation was found between patients not employed after surgery and the presence of left ventricular dysfunction. Some point to the data regarding return to work after CABG surgery as evidence of unsuccessful rehabilitation. Obviously, multiple complex personal and social factors are involved in this issue and continued research is necessary in this regard.

Despite the less-than-ideal statistics regarding return to work, Jenkins' study found numerous positive results. Angina was completely relieved in 69 to 85 percent of patients, disability days were reduced by more than 80 percent, anxiety, depression, fatigue, and sleep problems were reported to decline significantly, and vigor and well-being scores rose appreciably. Jenkins concluded that the ma-jority of patients are able to resume normal economic and social functioning within 6 months of CABG surgery.

Conclusion

Care of the patient undergoing coronary artery bypass surgery requires an understanding of the operative procedure, the indications for surgical intervention, and the outcomes of the choice of treatment. An understanding of the multiple physiologic effects of cardiopulmonary bypass is especially important. Armed with this knowledge base, nursing care can focus on assisting CABG patients to reach their "maximal health potential," both before and after surgery.

Cardiac Rehabilitation

Overview

Medical, surgical, and nursing care management of the patient with coronary artery disease is incomplete without discussion of rehabilitation. Despite successful treatment of the initial cardiac event, many patients become unnecessarily incapacitated, do not return to work, and report depression and a poor quality of life.

Cardiac rehabilitation is defined as "the process of actively assisting the known cardiac patient to achieve and maintain his optimal state of health."[195] The ultimate goal is to enable the cardiac patient, largely by his or her own endeavors, to regain pre-illness capabilities or make adjustments necessary for an active, productive life.[50] The key concept here is assisting the patient to function at the highest level compatible with his or her disease. In order to achieve this goal, rehabilitative efforts must be holistic in design, and involve a team approach which includes the patient himself or herself. The actual composition of the cardiac rehabilitation team varies widely from program to program, but an ideal list might include the following: cardiac patient and family, attending physician, primary nurse, cardiac rehabilitation clinical nurse specialist, cardiologist, physical therapist, occupational therapist, social worker, dietician, vocational rehabilitation counselor, chaplain, psychologist or psychiatric clinical nurse specialist, and pharmacist.

Although cardiac rehabilitation principles and techniques have largely developed from care of the postmyocardial infarction patient, the approach can be applied successfully to patients with other cardiac problems, including postcoronary artery bypass surgery, postcoronary angioplasty, valvular heart disease, and cardiac transplantation.

Cardiac rehabilitation programs are commonly divided into three phases. The two major components of these phases are progressive physical activity or exercise, and patient and family education and counseling. Each phase is characterized by slightly different objectives.[50,100,196]

Phase I	Hospitalization (7 to 10 days)
	"Early or in-hospital phase"
	Objectives: Minimize deleterious effects of bed rest and immobility, and provide education to adequately prepare patient for discharge.
Phase II	Convalescence (6 to 10 weeks)
	"Therapeutic or restorative phase"
	Objectives: Cardiac conditioning or training to pre-event levels (e.g., MI), reinforcement of patient education, and psychological support.
Phase III	Long-term (following completion of phase II)
	"Maintenance phase"
	Objectives: Retention of previous training, and stimulation for further progess.

Discussion of a total cardiac rehabilitation program is beyond the scope of this text. However, the critical-care nurse must have a basic understanding of concepts relating to phase I of rehabilitative care of the cardiac patient. In order to be most effective, rehabilitation efforts must begin at the time of admission. In particular, the critical-care nurse can be invaluable in minimizing the untoward effects of bed rest, preventing deconditioning, and decreasing the patient's anxiety to promote learning and adaptation.

Phase I: Activity

Despite intricate technological advances, bed rest still remains an initial important intervention in treatment of the patient with coronary artery disease in order to reduce myocardial oxygen demands. In fact, up until the 1960s, treatment of the acute myocardial infarction patient included a 6-week period of bed rest to allow for transformation of necrotic myocardium into firm scar tissue[197]). However, numerous studies have since documented the untoward effects of prolonged immobilization, which include a decrement of 20 percent or more in physical work capacity, hypovolemia, diminution in pulmonary ventilation, muscle degeneration, and venous stasis of blood.[50,197] As a result, early ambulation and activity is now recommended for the stable cardiac patient to reduce such problems. Early physical activity has not appeared to increase complications of myocardial infarction, and benefits from such intervention include prevention of deconditioning and lessened pulmonary atelectasis and thromboembolic complications.[100] In addition, early progressive ambulation permits more useful predischarge exercise testing, and shorter hospital stays. Finally, studies have documented that low-level exercise has numerous positive psychological effects in the postmyocardial infarction patient.[198] Physical activity and exercise appear to allay anxiety, prevent and limit depression, improve self-esteem, and decrease feelings of dependency.

The concept of METS (metabolic equivalents) is especially helpful to health care personnel, as well as patients and families in determining activity and exercise. One MET is defined as the energy expended per minute while sitting quietly in a chair. This correlates with an oxygen consumption of approximately 3.5 mL of O_2 per kilogram per minute. All activities can be quantified as multiples of this baseline. Charts of common activities and their respective MET levels are published in numerous texts. These charts provide nursing staff, patients, and families with useful guidelines.

A variety of structured programs for progressive patient activity is available. A frequently cited example of such a protocol is the "7-Step Myocardial Infarction Program" (Table 21-13) from Grady Memorial Hospital and the Emory University School of Medicine.[100] Such defined levels allow for progressive increase in the intensity, duration, frequency, and type of activity the patient performs. A structured protocol also enhances the documentation, communication, and evaluation of care.

Prior to initiation of progressive activity, the patient's physiologic condition must be stabilized.

Table 21-13 In-Patient Rehabilitation: Seven-Step Myocardial Infarction Program*

Step	Date	M.D. Initials	Nurse/PT Notes	Supervised Exercise	CCU/Ward Activity	Educational– Recreational Activity
				CCU		
1.				Active and passive ROM for all extremities, in bed. Teach patient ankle plantar and dorsiflexion—repeat hourly when awake	Partial self-care. Feed self. Dangle legs on side of bed. Use bedside commode. Sit in chair 15 min 1–2 times a day	Orientation to CCU. Personal emergencies, social service aid as needed
2.				Active ROM for all extremities, sitting on side of bed	Sit in chair 15–30 min 2–3 times a day. Complete self-care in bed	Orientation to rehabilitation team, program. Smoking cessation. Educational literature if requested. Planning transfer from CCU
				Ward		
3.				Warm-up exercises, 2 METs: stretching, calisthenics. Walk 50 ft and back at slow pace	Sit in chair ad lib. To ward class in wheelchair. Walk in room	Normal cardiac anatomy and function. Development of atherosclerosis. What happens with myocardial infarction. 1–2 METs craft activity
4.				ROM and calisthenics, 2.5 METs. Walk length of hall (75 ft) and back, average pace. Teach pulse counting	OOB as tolerated. Walk to bathroom. Walk to ward class, with supervision	Coronary risk factors and their control
5.				ROM and calisthenics, 3 METs. Check pulse counting. Practice walking few stairsteps. Walk 300 ft bid	Walk to waiting room or telephone. Walk in ward corridor prn	Diet. Energy conservation. Work simplification techniques (as needed). 2–3 METs craft activity
6.				Continue above activities. Walk down flight of steps (return by elevator). Walk 500 ft bid. Instruct on home exercise	Tepid shower or tub bath, with supervision. To OT, cardiac clinic teaching room, with supervision	Heart attack management: Medications. Exercise. Surgery. Response to symptoms. Family, community adjustments on return home. Craft activity prn

Continued

Table 21-13 In-Patient Rehabilitation: Seven-Step Myocardial Infarction Program* (Continued)

Step	Date	M.D. Initials	Nurse/PT Notes	Supervised Exercise	CCU/Ward Activity	Educational– Recreational Activity
				Ward		
7.				Continue above activities Walk up flight of steps Walk 500 ft bid Continue home exercise instruction; present information regarding outpatient exercise program	Continue all previous ward activities	Discharge planning: Medications, diet, activity Return appointments Scheduled tests Return to work Community resources Educational literature Medication cards Craft activity prn

* Grady Memorial Hospital and the Emory University School of Medicine. From N. K. Wenger and G. F. Fletcher, Rehabilitation of the Patient with Atherosclerotic Heart Disease. In J. W. Hurst, et al. (eds.), *The Heart*, McGraw-Hill, New York, 1986.

This means the patient must be free from any signs of cardiac arrhythmias, heart failure, hypotension, uncontrolled hypertension, and persistent or recurrent chest pain. Initially, patients with uncomplicated myocardial infarctions (representing about 40 percent of all MI patients) can perform partial self-care and feed themselves.[199] Patients who have undergone coronary artery bypass surgery are often progressed at a slightly faster rate. Studies have demonstrated that less energy is required to use the bedside commode than the bedpan,[200] and myocardial work is less in a sitting than in a recumbent position.[98] Therefore, MI patients are permitted bedside commode privileges from the time of admission, and are usually allowed up in a chair for 15 min once or twice a day within 24 h. Obviously, the amount and timing of activity must be individualized. Over 50 percent of the patients with acute myocardial infarction have transient complications during the initial phase of hospitalization, and therefore, progress more slowly through activity levels and convalescence.[199] In the acute phase of illness, the patient's activities should be limited to 1.5 to 2.0 METS. By the time the patient is transferred out of the intensive care unit, he or she is able to complete self-care in bed and sit in a chair 2 or 3 times a day.

The objective of activity prescription following transfer from intensive care is to increase cardiovascular function to a level that enables the patient to perform his or her usual self-care and home activities by the time of discharge. Exercise during this time is still of low intensity but of greater frequency and duration. An important nursing intervention during the time of progressive activity includes careful monitoring of the patient's physiologic responses. In particular, any of the following signs warrant immediate rest for the patient and reevaluation of the activity plan: extreme fatigue, weakness or dyspnea; chest pain; arrhythmia; ST segment displacement on ECG of 1 mm or more (up or down); an increase in heart rate by more than 20 beats per minute over resting heart rate; or a drop in systolic blood pressure of 20 mmHg.

Patients should be able to perform activities at an intensity of 3.5 to 4.0 METS at the time of discharge.[50,199] In order to further individualize exercise prescriptions, patients often undergo low-level stress testing. The highest heart rate attained without adverse effects is the heart rate patients are instructed to keep their exercise response below after discharge.

Phase I: Patient Education

Patient and family education is a major component of any cardiac rehabilitation program. Patients not only have a right to know what has happened to them and how they can help themselves, but achievement of the goal of "optimal health" requires the patient's active participation and understanding of his or her disease and treatment plan.

The process of educating the patient and family should begin at the time of admission and continue throughout the hospitalization. The teaching plan must be individualized and based on an assessment of each patient's baseline knowledge and readiness to learn.

Obviously, numerous barriers to learning for the cardiac patient may exist in the hospital setting. Nursing interventions are aimed at identifying and overcoming these barriers, which may include high anxiety, denial, depression, pain, sleep deprivation, effect of medications, lack of privacy, and numerous interruptions.

In the intensive care setting, anxiety levels may be too high to facilitate learning. During this time the focus of the patient's education must be on providing short, simple explanations and answers to questions, rather than in-depth knowledge. Education efforts for the remainder of the hospitalization should prepare the patient to function at his or her optimal level upon discharge and assure continued progression.

Formal group instruction is time-efficient and very effective in the hospital setting. However, to assure that all patient needs are met, this should be supplemented with individual patient education sessions. Methods of instruction include didactic presentation, films, tape recordings, and printed materials. Printed material supplemented with individual instruction has been shown to be more successful than either approach alone.[201] Further, patients must be carefully assessed for their ability to read and comprehend much of the printed cardiac teaching material available.[202] Despite barriers to learning, studies have demonstrated that cardiac patients who received instruction in the hospital showed an increase in knowledge at discharge.[203,204]

Although the exact content of the patient education component of cardiac rehabilitation may vary slightly from program to program, most authorities agree that information on the following topics should be included: hospital routines and tests, the disease process, cardiac risk factors, diet, medications, activity, psychological and emotional responses, and community resources. The patient and family need information regarding what is happening around them, the meaning of routine procedures, and some idea of what to expect in the near future. An understanding of basic cardiac anatomy and physiology is crucial for patients to comprehend what is happening to them. Included here should be information applicable to each patient's specific health problem, such as what is coronary artery disease, what is angina, what is a heart attack, the healing process after a heart attack, and what is coronary artery bypass surgery. Patients must also be informed of symptoms they might experience and how to deal with them, as well as guidelines for when to call the physician.

In order for patients to assume responsibility for their subsequent health care and life-style, they must be knowledgeable about the association of risk factors with coronary artery disease. Helping patients identify their own specific risk factors and planning modification of these are important outcomes of patient education.

Dietary restrictions should be individualized and dependent on the patient's weight, cholesterol levels, blood pressure, and left ventricular function. Patients and their spouses need individualized, specific guidelines and time to have their questions answered.

All patients should be able to state the name, dosage, schedule, and action of their prescribed drugs. In addition, it is imperative that they be instructed regarding the major potential side effects.

Besides individualized activity prescriptions, as previously discussed, the patient with cardiac disease needs special counseling regarding sexual activities. The patient and spouse may have numerous fears as well as guilt and lack of knowledge in this area. A detailed discussion of this topic is beyond the scope of this text, but the reader is referred to the excellent reference by Scalzi.[205]

Studies have documented common behavioral responses to the stress of cardiac events. These may include anxiety, denial, depression, anger, and sexual aggressiveness. Patients and spouses need reassurance that these responses are normal, and they need support throughout the period of adaptation.

Finally, any cardiac rehabilitation program must include information about community resources available to the patient and family. Knowledge of the nearest emergency room, the American

Heart Association, support groups, and who to call for help may be invaluable to the cardiac patient in coping at home.

Conclusion

As the cardiac patient's length of stay is shortened, there will be increasing demands placed on the cardiac rehabilitation team to assure optimal patient functioning after discharge. Continued research and evaluation of present cardiac rehabilitation programs are essential if patients' needs are to be met.

References

1. Levy, R. I., & Feinleib, M. (1984). Risk factors for coronary artery disease and their management. In E. Braunwald (Ed.), *Heart disease: A textbook of cardiovascular medicine.* Philadelphia: Saunders.

2. Guyton, A. (1981). *Textbook of medical physiology.* Philadelphia: Saunders.

3. Ross, R. (1986). Factors influencing atherogenesis. In J. W. Hurst, R. B. Logue, C. E. Rackley, R. C. Schlant, E. H. Sonnenblick, A. G. Wallace, & N. K. Wenger (Eds.), *The heart.* New York: McGraw-Hill.

4. Wissler, R. W. (1984). Principles of the pathogenesis of atherosclerosis. In E. Braunwald (Ed.), *Heart disease: A textbook of cardiovascular medicine.* Philadelphia: Saunders.

5. Ross, R. (1986). The pathogenesis of atherosclerosis—an update. *New England Journal of Medicine, 314,* 488–500.

6. Wenger, N. K., & Schlant, R. C. (1986). Prevention of coronary atherosclerosis. In J. W. Hurst, R. B. Logue, C. E. Rackley, R. C. Schlant, E. H. Sonnenblick, A. G. Wallace, N. K. Wenger (Eds.), *The heart.* New York: McGraw-Hill.

7. Cowan, M. J. (1982). Pathogenesis of atherosclerosis. In S. L. Underhill, S. L. Woods, E. S. Swarajan, & C. J. Halpenney (Eds.), *Cardiac nursing.* Philadelphia: Lippincott.

8. Cohn, P., & Vokonas, P. (1985). Pathophysiology of coronary artery disease in humans. In P. F. Cohn (Ed.), *Diagnosis and therapy of coronary artery disease.* Boston: Martinus Nijhoff.

9. Faggiotto, A., Ross, R., & Harker, L. (1984). Studies of hypercholesterolemia in the non-human primate. I. Changes that lead to fatty streak formation. *Atherosclerosis, 4,* 323–340.

10. American Heart Association. (1973). *Coronary risk handbook.* Dallas: American Heart Association.

11. Kannel, W. B. (1978). Recent findings of the Framingham study. *Resident and Staff Physician, 24,* 56–71.

12. Kannel, W. B. (1976). Some lesions in cardiovascular epidemiology from Framingham. *American Journal of Cardiology, 37,* 269–282.

13. American Heart Association. (1980). *Risk factors and coronary disease: A statement for physicians.* Dallas: American Heart Association.

14. Taylor, W. J. (1986). Genetics and the cardiovascular system. In J. W. Hurst, R. B. Logue, C. E. Rackley, R. C. Schlant, E. H. Sonnenblick, A. G. Wallace, & N. K. Wenger (Eds.), *The heart.* New York: McGraw-Hill.

15. Kaplan, N. (1984). Systemic hypertension: Mechanisms and diagnosis. In E. Braunwald (Ed.), *Heart disease: A textbook of cardiovascular medicine.* Philadelphia: Saunders.

16. National Institutes of Health Consensus Development Conference Statement. (1984). *Lowering blood cholesterol to prevent heart disease.* (Vol. 5, No. 7), Bethesda, MD: U.S. Department of Health and Human Services.

17. Illingworth, D., & Connor, W. E. (1985). Hyperlipidemia and coronary artery disease. In W. E. Connor, & J. D. Bristow (Eds.), *Coronary heart disease: Prevention, complications and treatment.* Philadelphia: Lippincott.

18. Kannel, W., & Stokes, J., III. (1985). The epidemiology of coronary artery disease. In P. Cohn (Ed.), *Diagnosis and therapy of coronary artery disease.* Boston: Martinus Nijhoff.

19. Boucek, R., Morales, A., Romanelli, R., & Judkins, M. (1984). Genetic considerations of coronary artery disease. In J. Sangston (Ed.), *Coronary artery disease: Pathologic and clinical assessment.* Baltimore: Williams & Wilkins.

20. Rosenman, R. H., Brand, R. J., Sholtz, R. I., & Friedman, M. (1976). Multivariate prediction of coronary heart disease during 8.5 year follow-up in the Western Collaborative Group Study. *American Journal of Cardiology, 37,* 903–910.

21. Williams, R. B., Friedman, M., Glass, D. C., Herd, J. A., & Schneiderman, N. (1977). Mechanisms linking behavioral and pathophysiological processes. In T. M. Dembroski, S. M. Weiss, J. L. Shields, S. G. Haynes, & M. Leinlieb (Eds.), *Coronary-prone behavior.* New York: Springer-Verlag.

22. Lipid Research Clinics Program. (1984). The Lipid Research Clinics coronary primary prevention trial results: 1. Reduction in incidence of coronary heart disease. *Journal of the American Medical Association, 251,* 351–374.

23. Prinzmetal, M., Kennamer, R., Merliss, R., Wada, T., & Bor, N. (1959). Angina pectoris. A variant form of angina pectoris. *American Journal of Medicine, 27*(88), 375–388.

24. Maseri, A., Chierchia, S., & Kaski, C. (1985). Mixed angina pectoris. *American Journal of Cardiology, 56,* 30E–33E.

25. Friedberg, C. K. (1972). *Angina pectoris.* (American Heart Association Monograph No. 37). New York: American Heart Association.

26. Hurst, J. W., King, III, S. B., Friesinger, G. C., Walter, P. F., & Morris, D. C. (1986). Atherosclerotic coronary heart disease: Recognition, prognosis, and treatment. In J. W. Hurst, R. B. Logue, C. E. Rackley, R. C. Schlant, E. H. Sonnenblick, A. G. Wallace, & N. K. Wenger (Eds.), *The heart.* New York: McGraw-Hill.

27. Kirshenbaum, H. D. (1986). Coronary spasm and variant angina. In J. M. Rippe, R. S. Irwin, J. S. Alpert, & J. E. Dalen (Eds.), *Intensive care medicine.* Boston: Little, Brown.

28. Sato, A., Taneichi, Y., Sekine, I., Okabe, F., Ueda, A., Takahashi, M., Ito, T., Su, K. M., Sada, T., Matsumoto, S., & Ito, Y. (1983). Prinzmetal's variant angina induced only by alcohol ingestion. *Clinical Cardiology, 4,* 193–195.

29. Schachne, J. S., Roberts, B. H., & Thompson, B. D. (1984). Coronary artery spasm and myocardial infarction associated with cocaine use. *New England Journal of Medicine, 310,* 1665–1666.

30. Buxton, A. E., Goldberg, S., Harken, A., Hirshfield, J., & Kastor, J. A. (1981). Coronary artery spasm immediately after myocardial revascularization. Recognition and management. *New England Journal of Medicine, 304,* 1249–1253.

31. Pra H. C. (1986). Silent ischemia. In R. Roberts (Ed.), *Current Perspectives in Coronary Care.* Selected Proceedings of Two Symposia in Bermuda and San Diego, August, 1986.

32. Glasser, S. (1986). Asymptomatic myocardial ischemia. In R. Roberts (Ed.), *Current Perspectives in Coronary Care.* Selected Proceedings of Two Symposia in Bermuda and San Diego, August 1986.

33. Shurbrooks, S. (1979). Variant angina: More variants of the variant. *American Journal of Cardiology, 43,* 1245–1247.

34. Hutter, A., & DeSanctis, R. (1980). The evaluation of patients with angina pectoris. In R. Johnson, E. Haber, & W. G. Austen (Eds.), *The practice of cardiology.* Boston: Little, Brown.

35. Berman, J. L., Wynee, J., & Cohn, P. F. (1978). A multi-variate approach for interpreting treadmill exercise tests in coronary artery disease. *Circulation, 58,* 505–512.

36. Holman, B. L. (1984). Nuclear cardiology. In E. Braunwald (Ed.), *Heart disease: A textbook of cardiovascular medicine.* Philadelphia: Saunders.

37. Cohn, P. F., & Braunwald, E. (1984). Chronic ischemic heart disease. In E. Braunwald (Ed.), *Heart disease: A textbook of cardiovascular medicine.* Philadelphia: Saunders.

38. Gensini, G. (1980). Coronary arteriography. In E. Braunwald (Ed.), *Heart disease: A textbook of cardiovascular medicine.* Philadelphia: Saunders.

39. Hopkins, D. G., & Harrison, D. C. (1986). Coronary artery spasm. In J. W. Hurst, R. B. Logue, C. E. Rackley, R. C. Schlant, E. H. Sonnenblick, A. G. Wallace, & N. K. Wenger (Eds.), *The heart.* New York: McGraw-Hill.

40. Cohn, J. N. (1986). Drugs used to control vascular resistance and capacitance. In J. W. Hurst, R. B. Logue, C. E. Rackley, R. C. Schlant, E. H. Sonnenblick, A. G. Wallace, & N. K. Wenger (Eds.), *The heart.* New York: McGraw-Hill.

41. Parmley, W. W. (1982). The combination of beta-adrenergic blocking agents and nitrates in the treatment of stable angina pectoris. *Cardiology Review Reports, 3,* 1425–1430.

42. Conti, C. R., Hill, J. A., Feldman, R. L., Mehta, J. L., & Pepine, C. J. (1986). Treatment of coronary artery spasm and variant angina. *Journal of Intensive Care Medicine, 1,* 66–74.

43. Frishman, W. H., & Sonnenblick, E. H. (1986). Beta-adrenergic blocking drugs. In J. W. Hurst, R. B. Logue, C. E. Rackley, R. C. Schlant, E. H. Sonnenblick, A. G. Wallace, & N. K. Wenger (Eds.), *The heart.* New York: McGraw-Hill.

44. Frishman, W. H., & Sonnenblick, E. H. (1986). Calcium channel blockers. In J. W. Hurst, R. B. Logue, C. E. Rackley, R. C. Schlant, E. H. Sonnenblick, A. G. Wallace, & N. K. Wenger (Eds.), *The heart.* New York: McGraw-Hill.

45. Kloster, F. E., & Bristow, J. D. (1985). Management of stable and unstable angina. In W. E. Connor, & J. D. Bristow (Eds.), *Coronary heart disease prevention, complications and treatment.* Philadelphia: Lippincott.

46. Gentenblith, G., Ouyang, P., Achuff, S. C., Bulkley, B. H., Becker, L. C., Mellits, E. D., Baughman, K. L., Weiss, J. L., Flaherty, J. T., Kallman, C. H., Llewellyn, M., & Weisfeldt, M. L. (1982). Nifedipine in unstable angina. A double blind randomized trial. *New England Journal of Medicine, 306,* 885–889.

47. Gotto, A. M., Jr., & Jones, P. (1983). How to lower the serum cholesterol. In J. W. Hurst (Ed.), *Clinical essays on the heart.* New York: McGraw-Hill.

48. AHA Special Report. (1984). Recommendations for

treatment of hyperlipidemia in adults. *Circulation, 69,* 1067A–1084A.

49. Gotto, A. M., Jr. (1984). Drug treatment of hyperlipidemia. *Modern Concepts of Cardiovascular Disease, 53,* 53–58.

50. Oberman, A. (1984). Rehabilitation of patients with coronary artery disease. In E. Braunwald (Ed.), *Heart disease.* Philadelphia: Saunders.

51. U.S. Department of Health and Human Services Public Health Service. (1985). *Cholesterol counts— steps for lowering your patient's blood cholesterol.* (NIH Publication No. 85-2699). Baltimore, MD: National Institute of Health.

52. Kromhout, D., Bosschieter, E., & Coulander, C. (1985). The inverse relation between fish consumption and 20 year mortality from coronary heart disease. *The New England Journal of Medicine, 312,* 1205–1210.

53. Glomset, J. A. (1985). Fish, fatty acids and health (Editorial). *New England Journal of Medicine, 312,* 1253–1254.

54. Ashley, F. W., & Kannel, W. B. (1974). Relation of weight changes to changes in atherogenic traits: The Framingham study. *Journal of Chronic Disease, 27,* 103–144.

55. Ford, P. J., & Buckley, M. J. (1981). Circulatory assistance. In M. R. Kinney, C. B. Dear, D. R. Packa, & D. M. Voorman (Eds.), *AACN's clinical reference for critical-care nursing.* New York: McGraw-Hill.

56. Craver, J. M., & Hatcher, C. R. (1986). Techniques of using the intraaortic balloon pump. In J. W. Hurst, R. B. Logue, C. E. Rackley, R. C. Schlant, E. H. Sonnenblick, A. G. Wallace, & W. K. Wenger (Eds.), *The heart.* New York: McGraw-Hill.

57. Quaal, S. J. (1984). *Comprehensive intra-aortic balloon pumping.* New York: Mosby.

58. Patacky, M. G., Garvin, B. J., Schwirian, P. M. (1985). Intra-aortic balloon pumping and stress in the coronary care unit. Patient's perceptions of psychological stress. *Heart & Lung, 14,* 142–148.

59. Dotter, C. T., & Judkins, M. P. (1964). Transluminal treatment of atherosclerotic obstruction. Description of a new technique and a preliminary report of its application. *Circulation, 30,* 654–670.

60. Hall, D. P., & Gruentzig, A. R. (1986). Technique of percutaneous transluminal angioplasty of the coronary, renal, mesenteric and peripheral arteries. In J. W. Hurst, R. B. Logue, C. E. Rackley, R. C. Schlant, E. H. Sonnenblick, A. G. Williams, & N. K. Wenger (Eds.), *The heart.* Philadelphia: Saunders.

61. Bentivoglio, L. G., Van Raden, M. J., Kelsey, S. F., & Detre, K. M. (1984). Percutaneous transluminal coronary angioplasty (PTCA) in patients with relative contraindications: Results of the National Heart, Lung and Blood Institute PTCA Registry. *American Journal of Cardiology, 53,* 82C–88C.

62. Cowley, M. J., Vetrover, G. W., DiSciascio, G., Lewis, S. A., Hirsh, P. D., & Wolfgang, T. C. (1985). Coronary angioplasty of multiple vessels: Short term and long term results. *Circulation, 72,* 1314–1320.

63. Dorros, G., Cowley, M. J., Janke, L., Kelsey, S. F., Mullin, S. M., & VanRaden, M. (1984). In-hospital mortality rate in the National Heart, Lung and Blood Institute percutaneous transluminal coronary angioplasty registry. *American Journal of Cardiology, 53,* 17C–21C.

64. Williams, D. O., Gruentzig, A. R., Kent, K. M., Detre, K. M., & Kelsey, S. F. (1984). Efficacy of repeat percutaneous transluminal coronary angioplasty for coronary restenosis. *American Journal of Cardiology, 53*(12), 32C–35C.

65. Kent, K. M., Bentivoglio, L. G., Block, P. C., Bourassa, M. G., Crowley, M. J., Dorros, G., Detre, K. M., Gosselin, A., Gruentzig, A. R., & Kelsey, S. F. (1984). Long term efficacy of percutaneous transluminal coronary angioplasty (PTCA). Report from the National Heart, Lung and Blood Institute PTCA Registry. *American Journal of Cardiology, 53,* 27C–31C.

66. Thornton, M. A., Gruentzig, A. R., Hollman, J., King, S. B., & Douglas, J. S. (1984). Coumadin and aspirin in prevention of recurrence after transluminal coronary angioplasty: A randomized study. *Circulation, 69,* 721–727.

67. Mata, L. A., Bosch, X., David, P. R., Rapold, H. J., Corcos, T., & Bourassa, M. L. (1985). Clinical and angiographic assessment six months after double vessel percutaneous coronary angioplasty. *The American College of Cardiology, 6,* 1239–1244.

68. Abela, G. S., & Conti, C. R. (1986). The use of laser in the treatment of coronary artery obstruction. In J. W. Hurst, R. B. Logue, C. E. Rackley, R. C. Schlant, E. H. Sonnenblick, A. G. Wallace, & N. K. Wenger (Eds.), *The heart.* Philadelphia: Saunders.

69. Crea, F., Abela, G. S., Fenech, A., Smith, W., Pepine, C. J., & Conti, R. (1986). Transluminal laser radiation of coronary arteries in live dogs: An angiographic and morphologic study of acute effects. *American Journal of Cardiology,* (1), 171–174.

70. Macruz, R., Martins, J. R. M., Lupinamba, A., Lopes, E. A., Varga, H., Penaaf, D. E., Caralaho, V. B., Armelin, E., & Decourt, L. V. (1980). Therapeutic possibilities of laser beams in atheromas. *Arq Bras Cardiology, 34,* 9–12.

71. Abela, G. S., Norman, S. T., Cohen, D. M., Franzine, D., Feldman, R. L., Orea, F., Fenech, A., Pepine, C. J., & Conti, R. C. (1985). Laser recanalization of

occluded atherosclerotic arteries in vivo and in vitro. *Circulation, 71,* 403–411.

72. Sanborn, T. A., Cumberland, D. C., Tayler, D. I., & Ryan, T. J. (1985). Human percutaneous laser thermal angioplasty. *Circulation, 72,* III–703.

73. Choy, D. S. J., Stertzer, S. H., Myler, R. K., Marco, J., & Fournial, G. (1984). Human coronary laser recanalization. *Clinical Cardiology, 7,* 377–381.

74. Sanborn, T. A., Faxon, D., Kallett, M., & Ryan, T. (1986). Percutaneous coronary laser thermal angioplasty. *Journal of the American College of Cardiology, 8,* 1437–1440.

75. Gordon, M. (1985). *Manual of nursing diagnosis.* New York: McGraw-Hill.

76. Factor, S. M., & Kirk, E. S. (1986). Pathophysiology of myocardial ischemia. In J. W. Hurst, R. B. Logue, C. E. Rackley, R. C. Schlant, E. H. Sonnenblick, A. G. Wallace, & N. K. Wenger (Eds.), *The heart.* New York: McGraw-Hill.

77. Bulkley, B. H. (1986). Pathology of coronary atherosclerotic heart disease. In J. W. Hurst, R. B. Logue, C. E. Rackley, R. C. Schlant, E. H. Sonnenblick, A. G. Wallace, & N. K. Wenger (Eds.), *The heart.* New York: McGraw-Hill.

78. Alpert, J. S., & Braunwald, E. (1984). Acute myocardial infarction: Pathological, pathophysiological, and clinical manifestations. In E. Braunwald (Ed.), *Heart disease.* Philadelphia: Saunders.

79. Epstein, S. E., & Palmeri, S. T. (1984). Mechanisms contributing to precipitation of unstable angina and acute myocardial infarction: Implications regarding therapy. *American Journal of Cardiology, 54,* 1245–1252.

80. Davies, M. J., & Thomas, A. (1984). Thrombosis and acute coronary artery lesions in sudden cardiac ischemic death. *New England Journal of Medicine, 310,* 1137–1140.

81. Maseri, A., & Chierchia, S. V. (1982). Coronary artery spasm: Demonstration, definition, diagnosis and consequences. *Progress in Cardiovascular Disease, 25*(3), 169–192.

82. Maseri, A., L'Abbate, A., Baroldi, G., Chierchia, S., Marzelli, M., Ballestra, A. M., Severi, S., Parodi, O., Biagnini, A., Distante, A., & Pesola, A. (1978). Coronary vasospasm as a possible cause of myocardial infarction: A conclusion derived from the study of "preinfarction" angina. *New England Journal of Medicine, 299,* 1271–1277.

83. Vincent, G. M., Anderson, J. L., & Marshall, H. W. (1983). Coronary spasm producing coronary thrombosis and myocardial infarction. *New England Journal of Medicine, 309*(4), 220–223.

84. Ganz, P., & Alexander, R. W. (1985). New insights into the cellular mechanisms of vasospasm. *American Journal of Cardiology, 56,* 11E–15E.

85. Sobel, B. E., & Braunwald, E. (1984). The management of acute myocardial infarction. In E. Braunwald (Ed.), *Heart disease.* Philadelphia: Saunders.

86. Alpert, J. S. (1985). A comparison of anterior and inferior myocardial infarction. In J. M. Rippe, R. S. Irwin, J. S. Alpert, & J. E. Dalen (Eds.), *Intensive care medicine.* Boston: Little, Brown.

87. Bar, F. W., Brugada, P., Wassen, W. R., Vander Werf, T., & Wellens, H. J. (1984). Prognostic value of Q waves, R/S ratio, loss of R wave voltage, ST-T segment abnormalities, electrical axis, low voltage and notching: Correlation of electrocardiogram and left ventriculogram. *Journal of American College of Cardiology, 4*(1), 17–27.

88. Hancock, E. W., (1982, June). Ischemic heart disease: Acute myocardial infarction. *Scientific American,* pp. 1–22.

89. Vinsant, M. O., & Spence, M. I. (1985). *Commonsense approach to coronary care.* St. Louis: Mosby.

90. Horowitz, R. S., Morganroth, J., Parrotto, C., Chem, C. C., & Meixell, L. (1981). Prognosis in acute myocardial infarction determined by serial 2-D echocardiography. *Circulation, 64*(Suppl. II), IV–94.

91. Chandrarantna, P. A. N., Ulene, R., Reid, C. L., Nimalasuriya, A., Kawanishi, D., Rosin, B., & Rahimtoola, S. H. (1983). Differentiation between new and old myocardial infarction by color encoding and time averaging two-dimensional echocardiograms. *Circulation, 68*(Suppl. III), III–3.

92. Zaret, B. L., & Berger, H. J. (1986). Techniques of nuclear cardiology. In J. W. Hurst, R. B. Logue, C. E. Rackley, R. C. Schlant, E. H. Sonnenblick, A. G. Wallace, & N. K. Wenger (Eds.), *The heart.* New York: McGraw-Hill.

93. Verani, M. S. (1983). Non-invasive diagnostic techniques in cardiology. *Comprehensive Therapy, 9*(10), 27–36.

94. Marshall, R. C., Tillisch, J. H., Phelps, M. E., Huang, S. C., Carson, R., Henze, E., & Schelbert, H. R. (1983). Identification and differentiation of resting myocardial ischemia and infarction in man with position computed tomography, 18F-labeled fluorodeoxyglucose and N-13 ammonia. *Circulation, 67,* 766–778.

95. Donat, W. E., & Weiner, B. H. (1985). Syndromes of left ventricular failure. In J. M. Rippe, R. S. Irwin, J. S. Alpert, & J. E. Dalen (Eds.), *Intensive care medicine.* Boston: Little, Brown.

96. Barnard, D., & Alpert, J. S. (1985). Right ventricular infarction. In J. M. Rippe, R. S. Irwin, J. S. Alpert, &

J. E. Dalen (Eds.), *Intensive care medicine*. Boston: Little, Brown.

97. Harrison, D. G. (1978). Should lidocaine be administered routinely to all patients after acute myocardial infarction? *Circulation, 58,* 581–584.

98. Valladares, B., & Lemberg, L. (1982). Intravenous nitroglycerine in acute infarction. *Heart and Lung, 11,* 383–385.

99. Winslow, E. H. (1985). Cardiovascular consequences of bed rest. *Heart and Lung, 14,* 236–246.

100. Wenger, N. K., & Fletcher, G. F. (1986). Rehabilitation of the patient with atherosclerotic coronary heart disease. In J. W. Hurst, R. B. Logue, C. E. Rackley, R. C. Schlant, E. H. Sonnenblick, A. G. Wallace, & N. K. Wenger (Eds.), *The heart*. New York: McGraw-Hill.

101. Kirchkoff, K. T. (1981). An examination of the physiologic basis for "coronary precautions." *Heart and Lung, 10,* 874–879.

102. Wessman, J. P. (1985). Preventing ventricular dysrhythmia following myocardial Infarction. *Dimensions of Critical Care Nursing, 4*(1), 24–32.

103. Barnaby, P. F., Barrett, P. A., & Lvoff, R. (1983). Routine prophylactic lidocaine in acute myocardial infarction. *Heart and Lung, 12,* 362–366.

104. Mills, R. M. (1985). Arrhythmias following myocardial infarction. In J. M. Rippe, R. S. Irwin, J. S. Alpert, & J. E. Dalen (Eds.), *Intensive care medicine*. Boston: Little, Brown.

105. Forrester, J. S., Diamond, G. A., & Swan, H. J. C. (1977). Correlative classification of clinical and hemodynamic function after acute myocardial infarction. *American Journal of Cardiology, 39,* 137–145.

106. Tommaso, C. L., Lesch, M., & Sonnenblick, E. H. (1984). Alterations in cardiac function in coronary artery disease, myocardial infarction and coronary bypass surgery. In N. K. Wenger, & H. K. Hellerstein (Eds.), *Rehabilitation of the coronary patient*. New York: John Wiley & Sons.

107. Sendon, J. L., Coma-Canella, I., Alcasena, S., Seoane, J., & Gamallo, C. (1985). Electrocardiographic findings in acute right ventricular infarction: Sensitivity and specificity of electrocardiographic alterations in right precordial leads, V_4R, V_3R, V_1, V_2 and V_3. *Journal of the American College of Cardiology, 6,* 1273–1279.

108. Waksmonski, C. A. (1985). Miscellaneous problems following acute myocardial infarction. In J. M. Rippe, R. S. Irwin, J. S. Alpert, & J. E. Dalen (Eds.), *Intensive care medicine*. Boston: Little, Brown.

109. Leon, M. B., & Cohen, L. S. (1984). Guidelines for patient management. In N. K. Wenger & H. K. Hellerstein (Eds.), *Rehabilitation of the coronary patient*. New York: John Wiley & Sons.

110. Pearle, D. L. (1984). Nifedipine in acute myocardial infarction. *American Journal of Cardiology, 54*(11), 21E–23E.

111. Mueller, J. E., & Braunwald, E. (1983). Can infarct size be limited in patients with acute myocardial infarction? In S. Rahimtoola (Ed.), Controversies in coronary artery disease. *Cardiovascular Clinics* (pp. 147–163). Boston: F. A. Davis Co.

112. Roberts, R., DeMello, V., & Sobel, B. E. (1976). Deleterious effects of methylprednisone in patients with myocardial infarction. *Circulation, (3)*(Suppl. I), 204–206.

113. Sodi-Pollares, D., Testelli, M. R., & Fishleder, B. L. (1962). Effects of an intravenous infusion of a potassium-glucose-insulin solution on the electrocardiographic signs of myocardial infarction. A preliminary clinical report. *American Journal of Cardiology, 9,* 166–181.

114. Milis Study Group. (1986). Hyaluronidase therapy for acute myocardial infarction: Results of a randomized, blinded, multicenter trial. *American Journal of Cardiology, 57,* 1236–1243.

115. Saliba, M. J., Covell, J. W., & Bloor, C. M. (1976). Effects of heparin in large doses on the extent of myocardial ischemia after acute coronary occlusion in the dog. *American Journal of Cardiology, 37,* 599–603.

116. Fletcher, A. P., Sherry, S., Alkjaersig, N., Smyrniots, S. E., & Jicks, S. (1959). The maintenance of a sustained thrombolytic state in man. II. Clinical observations on patients with myocardial infarction and other thromboembolic disorders. *Journal of Clinical Investigation, 38,* 1111–1119.

117. Koren, G., Weiss, A. T., Hasin, Y., Appelbaum, D., Welber, S., Rozenman, Y., Lotan, C., Mosseri, M., Sapoznikov, D., Luria, M. H., & Gotsman, M. S. (1985). Prevention of myocardial damage in acute myocardial ischemia by early treatment with intravenous streptokinase. *New England Journal of Medicine, 313,* 1384–1389.

118. Braunwald, E. (1985). The aggressive treatment of acute myocardial infarction. *Circulation, 71,* 1087–1092.

119. I.S.A.M. Study Group (1986). A prospective trial of intravenous streptokinase in acute myocardial infarction. *New England Journal of Medicine, 314,* 1465–1471.

120. Rentrop, K. P., Cohen, M., & Hosat, S. T. (1984). Thrombolytic therapy in acute myocardial infarction: Review of clinical trials. *American Journal of Cardiology, 54,* 29E–31E.

121. Van de Werf, F., Ludbrook, P. A., Bergmann, S. R., Tiefenbrum, A. J., Fox, K. A. A., de Geest, H., Verstraete, M., Collen, D., & Sobel, B. E. (1984). Coronary thrombolysis with tissue plasminogen activator in patients with evolving myocardial infarction. *New England Journal of Medicine, 310,* 609–613.

122. Williams, D., Borer, J., Braunwald, E., Chesebro, J., Cohen, L., Dalen, J., Dodge, H., Francis, C., Knatterud, G., Ludbrook, P., Markis, J., & Mueller, H. (1986). Intravenous recombinant tissue-type plasminogen activator in patients with acute myocardial infarction: A report from the NHLBI thrombolysis in myocardial infarction trial. *Circulation, 73,* 38–346.

123. TIMI Study Group. (1985). The thrombolysis in myocardial infarction (TIMI) trial: Phase 1 findings. *New England Journal of Medicine, 312,* 932–936.

124. Levin, D. C., Boxt, L. M., & Meyerovitz, M. F. (1985). Percutaneous transluminal coronary angioplasty. *Radiologic Clinics of North America, 23*(4), 597–611.

125. Pepine, C. J., Prida, X., Hill, J. A., Feldman, R. L., & Conti, C. R. (1984). Percutaneous transluminal coronary angioplasty in acute myocardial infarction. *American Heart Journal, 107,* 820–822.

126. Gold, H. K., Cowley, M. J., Palacios, I. F., Vetrovec, G. W., Akins, C. W., Block, P. C., & Leinbach, R. (1984). Combined intra-coronary streptokinase infusion and coronary angioplasty during acute myocardial infarction. *American Journal of Cardiology, 53,* 22C–125C.

127. O'Neill, W. D., Timmis, G. C., Baurdillon, P. D., Lai, P., Ganghadanhan, V., Walton, J., Ramos, R., Laufer, N., Gordon, S., Schork, M. H., & Pitt, B. (1986). A prospective randomized clinical trial of intra-coronary streptokinase versus coronary angioplasty for acute myocardial infarction. *New England Journal of Medicine, 314,* 812–816.

128. Jung, A., Lai, P., Juni, J., Bourdellon, P., Walton, J., Laufer, N., Buda, A., Pitt, & O'Neill, W. (1986). Prevention of subsequent exercise induced preinfarction ischemia by emergency coronary angioplasty in acute myocardial infarction: Comparison with intracoronary streptokinase. *Journal of the American College of Cardiology, 8,* 496–503.

129. Pluth, J. (1983). What is the status of coronary revascularization for the treatment of acute myocardial infarction? *Cardiovascular Clinics, 13*(1), 93–100.

130. Berg, R., Selinger, S., Leonard, J., Grunwald, R., & O'Grady, W. (1985). Surgical management of acute myocardial infarction. In K. McCauley, A. Brest, & D. McGoon (Eds.), *McGoon's cardiac surgery: An interprofessional approach to patient care* (pp. 61–74). Philadelphia: F. A. Davis Company.

131. Akins, C., & Austen, W. (1980). Aortocoronary bypass surgery in the management of coronary artery disease. In R. Johnson, E. Haber, & W. Austen (Eds.), *The practice of cardiology* (pp. 370–399). Boston: Little, Brown.

132. Roberts, A. (1983). *Coronary artery surgery: Application of new techniques.* Chicago: Year Book Medical Publishers, Inc.

133. CASS Principle Investigators and their Associates. (1983). Coronary Artery Surgery Study (CASS): A randomized trial of coronary artery bypass surgery. Survival Data. *Circulation, 68,* 939–950.

134. Takaro, T., Hullgren, H., & Lipton, M. (1976). The VA cooperative randomized study of surgery for coronary arterial occlusive disease II. Subgroup with significant left main lesions. *Circulation, 54*(Suppl. III) III–107.

135. European Coronary Surgery Study Group. (1980). Prospective randomized study of coronary artery bypass surgery in stable angina pectoris. Second interim report by the coronary surgery study group. *Lancet, 2,* 491–495.

136. Spencer, F. (1983). Bypass grafting for coronary artery disease. In D. Sabiston, & F. Spencer (Eds.), *Gibbon's surgery of the chest* (4th ed.). Philadelphia: Saunders.

137. Rahimtoola, S. (1981). Coronary artery bypass for chronic angina—1981: A perspective. *Circulation, 65,* 225–241.

138. Smith, H., Frye, R., & Piehler, J. (1983). Does coronary bypass surgery have a favorable influence on the quality of life? *Cardiovascular Clinics, 13,* 253–264.

139. Ritchie, J., Narahara, K., Trobaugh, G., Williams, D., & Hamilton, G. (1977). Thallium-201 myocardial imaging before and after coronary revascularization: Assessment of regional myocardial blood flow and graft patency. *Circulation, 56,* 830–936.

140. Akins, C. (1985). Indication and results of surgery in unstable angina and Prinzmetal's variant angina. In K. McCauley, A. Brest, & D. McGoon (Eds.), *McGoon's cardiac surgery: An interprofessional approach to patient care.* Philadelphia: F. A. Davis Company.

141. Rahimtoola, S., Nunley, D., Grunkemeier, G., Tepley, J., Lambert, L., & Starr, A. (1983). Ten year survival after coronary bypass surgery for unstable angina. *New England Journal of Medicine, 308,* 676–681.

142. Tepe, N., & Edmunds, L. (1985). Operation for acute postinfarction mitral insufficiency and cardiogenic shock. *Journal of Thoracic and Cardiovascular Surgery, 89,* 525–530.

143. Scanlon, P., Montoya, A., McKeever, L., Johnson, S., Sullivan, H., Bakhos, M., & Pifarre, R. (1984). Urgent surgery for ventricular septal rupture complicating acute myocardial infarction. *Circulation, 70*(Suppl. II), II–255.

144. Brawley, R., Magovern, G., Gott, V., Donahoo, J., Gardner, T., & Watkins, L. (1983). Left ventricular aneurysmectomy: Factors influencing post-operative results. *Journal of Thoracic and Cardiovascular Surgery, 85,* 712–717.

145. Najafi, H., Meng, R., Javid, H., Hunter, J., Golden, M., Manson, D., & Najafi, K. (1985). Post-myocardial ventricular aneurysm. In K. McCauley, A. Brest, & D. McGoon (Eds.), *McGoon's cardiac surgery: An interprofessional approach to patient care.* Philadelphia: F. A. Davis Company.

146. Lytle, B., & Loop, F. (1985). Elective coronary surgery. In K. McCauley, A. Brest, & D. McGoon (Eds.), *McGoon's cardiac surgery: An interprofessional approach to patient care.* Philadelphia: F. A. Davis Company.

147. Brockman, S., Cobanoglu, M., & Brest, A. (1985). The surgical management of coronary artery disease with myocardial dysfunction. In K. McCauley, A. Brest, & D. McGoon (Eds.), *McGoon's cardiac surgery: An interprofessional approach to patient care* (pp. 93–102). Philadelphia: F. A. Davis Company.

148. Cosgrove, D., Loop, F., Lytle, B., Baillot, R., Gill, C., Golding, L., Taylor, P., & Goormastic, M. (1984). Primary myocardial revascularization: Trends in surgical mortality. *Journal of Thoracic and Cardiovascular Surgery, 88,* 673–684.

149. Jones, E., & Hatcher, C. (1982). Techniques for the surgical treatment of atherosclerotic coronary artery disease. In J. Hurst (Ed.), *The heart.* New York: McGraw-Hill.

150. Miller, D., Ivey, T., Bailey, W., & Hessel, E. (1980). The practice of coronary bypass surgery in 1980. *Circulation, 62*(Suppl. III), III–95.

151. Reul, G. (1984). Revascularization of the ischemic myocardium. In D. Cooley (Ed.), *Techniques in cardiac surgery.* Philadelphia: Saunders.

152. Grondin, C., Campeau, L., Lesperance, J., Enjolbert, M., & Bourassa, M. (1984). Comparison of late changes in internal mammary artery and saphenous vein grafts in two consecutive series of patients 10 years after operation. *Circulation 70*(Suppl. I), I–208–I–212.

153. Lytle, B., Loop, F., Cosgrove, D., Ratliff, N., Easley, K., & Taylor, P. (1985). Long term (5 to 12 years) serial studies of internal mammary artery and saphenous vein coronary bypass grafts. *Journal of Thoracic and Cardiovascular Surgery, 89,* 248–258.

154. Culliford, A., Cunningham, J., Zeff, R., Isom, O., Teiko, P., & Spencer, F. (1976). Sternal and costochondral infections following open heart surgery. *Journal of Thoracic and Cardiovascular Surgery, 72,* 714–726.

155. Jansen, K. J., & McFadden, P. M. (1986). Post-operative nursing management in patients undergoing myocardial revascularization with internal mammary artery bypass. *Heart and Lung, 15,* 48–54.

156. Roberts, A., Faro, R., Feldman, R., Conti, C., Knauf, D., Alexander, J., & Pepine, C. (1983). Comparison of early and long term results with intraoperative transluminal balloon catheter dilatation and coronary artery bypass grafting. *Journal of Thoracic and Cardiovascular Surgery, 86,* 435–440.

157. Caralps, J. M., Crexells, C., Aris, A., Bonnin, O., & Oriol, A. (1984). Combined aortocoronary bypass and intra-operative transluminal angioplasty in left main coronary artery disease. *Annals of Thoracic Surgery, 37,* 291–294.

158. Gerrity, R., Loop, F., Golding, L., Ehrhart, L., & Argenyi, Z. (1983). Arterial response to laser operation for removal of atherosclerotic plaques. *Journal of Thoracic and Cardiovascular Surgery, 85,* 409–421.

159. Livessay, J. J., Leachman, D. R., Hogan, P. J., Cooper, J. R., Sweeney, M. S., Frazier, O. H., & Cooley, D. A. Preliminary report on laser coronary endarterectomy in patients. *Circulation, 72*–III, 302–1207.

160. Edmunds, L., & Stephenson, L. (1983). Cardiopulmonary bypass for open heart surgery. In W. Glenn (Ed.), *Thoracic and cardiovascular surgery.* Norwalk, CT: Appleton-Century-Crofts.

161. Litwak, R., & Giannelli, S. (1982). Open intracardiac operations employing extracorporeal circulation. In R. Litwak, & R. Jurado (Eds.), *Care of the cardiac surgical patient.* Norwalk, CT: Appleton-Century-Crofts.

162. Guyton, R., Williams, W., & Hatcher, C. (1986). Techniques of cardiopulmonary bypass. In J. Hurst, et al. (Eds.), *The Heart.* New York: McGraw-Hill.

163. Schwartz, A., & Geer, R. (1985). Cardiac anesthesia. In K. McCauley, A. Brest, & D. McGoon (Eds.), *McGoon's cardiac surgery: An interprofessional approach to patient care.* Philadelphia: F. A. Davis Company.

164. Davies, G., Sobel, M., & Salzman, E. (1980). Elevated plasma fibrinopetide A and thromboxane B_2 levels during cardiopulmonary bypass. *Circulation, 61,* 808–814.

165. Sanderson, R. (1983). The surgical cardiac patient. In R. Sanderson (Ed.), *The cardiac patient: A comprehensive approach* (pp. 409–458). Philadelphia: Saunders.

166. Buckberg, G. (1985). Progress in myocardial protection during cardiac operations. In K. McCauley, A. Brest, & D. McGoon (Eds.), *McGoon's cardiac surgery: An interprofessional approach to patient care.* (pp. 9–30). Philadelphia: F. A. Davis Company.

167. Cooley, D. (1984). Cannulation for temporary bypass. In D. Cooley (Ed.), *Techniques in cardiac surgery.* Philadelphia: Saunders.

168. Roberts, A., Spies, S., Sanders, J., Moran, J., Wilkinson, C., Lichtenthal, P., White, R., & Michaelis, L. (1981). Serial assessment of left ventricular performance following coronary artery bypass grafting. *Journal of Thoracic and Cardiovascular Surgery, 81,* 69–84.

169. Phillips, H., Carter, J., Okada, R., Levine, F., Boucher, C., Osbakken, M., Lappas, D., Buckley, M., & Pohost, G. (1983). Serial changes in left ventricular ejection fraction in the early hours after aortocoronary bypass grafting. *Chest, 83,* 28–34.

170. Angelini, P., Feldnam, M., Lufschanowski, R., & Leachman, R. (1974). Cardiac arrhythmias during and after heart surgery: Diagnosis and management. *Progress in Cardiovascular Disease, 16,* 469–495.

171. Litwak, R. (1982). Analysis, maintenance, and support of cardiac function after cardiac surgery. In R. Litwak, & R. Jurado (Eds.), *Care of the cardiac surgical patient.* Norwalk, CT: Appleton-Century-Crofts.

172. Markmann, P., & Wallace, P. (1985). Nursing care in the intensive care unit. In K. McCauley, A. Brest, & D. McGoon (Eds.), *McGoon's cardiac surgery: An interprofessional approach to patient care.* Philadelphia: F. A. Davis Company.

173. Jurado, R., & Osborn, J. (1982). Patient surveillance and general care. In R. Litwak, & R. Jurado (Eds.), *Care of the cardiac surgical patient.* Norwalk, CT: Appleton-Century-Crofts.

174. Utley, J., & Stephens, D. (1983). Fluid balance during cardiopulmonary bypass. In J. Utley (Ed.), *Pathophysiology and techniques of cardiopulmonary bypass.* Baltimore: Williams & Wilkins.

175. Estafanous, R., & Tarazi, R. (1980). Systemic arterial hypertension associated with cardiac surgery. *American Journal of Cardiology, 46,* 685–694.

176. Putnam, E., & Manners, J. (1983). Vascular resistance during cardiopulmonary bypass. *Anaesthesia, 38,* 635–643.

177. Turnbull, K., Miyagishima, R., & Gerein, A. (1974). Pulmonary complications and cardiopulmonary bypass: A clinical study in adults. *Canadian Anaesthesia Society Journal, 21,* 181–194.

178. Ellis, R. (1982). Cerebral dysfunction following cardiopulmonary bypass. In J. Utley (Ed.), *Pathophysiology and techniques of cardiopulmonary bypass.* Baltimore: William & Wilkins.

179. Sadler, P. (1979). Nursing assessment of postcardiotomy delirium. *Heart & Lung, 8,* 745–750.

180. McIntyre, K., & Lewis, A. (Eds.). (1983). *American Heart Association: Textbook of advanced cardiac life support.* Texas: American Heart Association.

181. Duncan, C., & Erickson, R. (1982). Pressures associated with chest tube stripping. *Heart & Lung, 11,* 166–171.

182. Conti, C., & Feldman, R. (1984). The use of nitrates in the treatment of ischemic heart disease. In J. Hurst (Ed.), *Clinical essays on the heart.* New York: McGraw-Hill.

183. Belitz, J. (1983). Minimizing the psychological complications of patients who require mechanical ventilation. *Critical Care Nurse,* May–June, 42–46.

184. Molter, N. (1979). Needs of relatives of critically ill patients: A descriptive study. *Heart & Lung, 8,* 332–339.

185. Rodgers, C. (1983). Needs of relatives of cardiac surgery patients during the critical care phase. *Focus, 10,* 50–55.

186. Leske, J. (1986). Needs of relatives of critically ill patients: A follow-up. *Heart & Lung, 15,* 189–193.

187. American Association of Critical-Care Nurses. (1981). *Standards for nursing care of the critically ill.* St. Louis: Reston Publishing Company.

188. Rahimtoola, S. (1984). Coronary bypass surgery for unstable angina. *Circulation, 69,* 842–848.

189. Lytle, B., & Loop, F. (1985). Elective coronary surgery. In K. McCauley, A. Brest, & D. McGoon (Eds.), *McGoon's cardiac surgery: An interprofessional approach to care.* Philadelphia: F. A. Davis Company.

190. Smith, H., Frye, R., & Piehler, J. (1983). Does coronary bypass surgery have a favorable influence on the quality of life? *Cardiovascular Clinics, 13,* 253–264.

191. Neill, W., Ritzmann, L., Okies, J., Anderson, R., & Selden, R. (1977). Medical versus surgical therapy for acute coronary insufficiency: A randomized study. In S. Rahimtoola (Ed.), *Coronary bypass surgery.* Philadelphia: F. A. Davis Company.

192. Jenkins, C., Stanton, B., Savageau, A., Denlinger, P., & Klein, M. (1983). Coronary artery bypass surgery: Physical, psychological, social & economic outcomes six months later. *Journal of the American Medical Association, 250,* 782–788.

193. Hammermeister, K., DeRouen, T., English, M., & Dodge, H. (1979). Effect of surgical versus medical therapy on return to work in patients with coronary artery disease. *American Journal of Cardiology, 44,* 105–111.

194. Comoss, P., Burke, E., & Swails, S. (1979). *Cardiac rehabilitation: A comprehensive nursing approach.* Philadelphia: Lippincott.

195. Lanoue, A. (1986). Cardiac rehabilitation. In B. Yee,

& S. Zorb (Eds.), *Cardiac critical care nursing*. Boston: Little, Brown.

196. Wenger, N. (1984). Early ambulation after myocardial infarction: Rationale, program components, and results. In N. Wenger (Ed.), *Rehabilitation of the coronary patient*. New York: John Wiley & Sons.

197. Stern, M., & Cleary, P. (1981). National exercise and heart disease project: Psychosocial changes observed during a low-level exercise program. *Archives of Internal Medicine, 141,* 1463–1469.

198. Sivarajan, E. (1981). Cardiac rehabilitation: Activity and exercise program. In S. Underhill, S. Woods, E. Sivarajan, & C. Halpenny (Eds.), *Cardiac nursing*. Philadelphia: Lippincott.

199. Wanka, J. (1970). Bedpan vs. commode in patients with myocardial infarction. *Cardiac Rehabilitation, 1,* 7–11.

200. Scalzi, C., & Burke, L. (1981). Education of the patient and family. In S. Underhill, S. Woods, E. Sivarajan, & C. Halpenny (Eds.), *Cardiac nursing*. Philadelphia: Lippincott.

201. Boyd, M., & Citro, K. (1983). Cardiac patient education literature: Can patients read what we give them? *Journal of Cardiac Rehabilitation, 3,* 513–516.

202. Budan, L. (1983). Cardiac patient learning in the hospital setting. *Focus, 10*(5), 16–22.

203. Murdaugh, C. (1982). Using research in practice—can cardiac patients be taught effectively in the critical care setting? *Focus, 9*(4), 11–14.

204. Scalzi, C. (1981). Sexual counseling. In S. Underhill, S. Woods, E. Sivarajan, & C. Halpenny (Eds.), *Cardiac nursing*. Philadelphia: Lippincott.

22 Hypertension

Mary-Michael
Brown
Judith Cook
Albright

Introduction

Hypertension is a major health problem in the United States today. It is the leading cause of cardiac-related death and disability and is one of the most significant risk factors for the development of heart attacks and strokes.

Critical-care nurses frequently care for patients with a primary diagnosis of hypertension, as seen in crises states, as well as for patients suffering from its secondary effects on target organs.

This chapter will present information concerning hypertension by (1) examining the normal mechanisms of arterial blood pressure, (2) describing classifications for high blood pressure, (3) considering the pathogenesis of hypertension, (4) reviewing available treatment options, and (5) discussing associated nursing care.

Normal Regulation of Arterial Blood Pressure

Arterial blood pressure is defined as the pressure exerted against the walls of the arteries. It is a product of flow and resistance, and is depicted in the formula:

Mean arterial pressure = cardiac output × total peripheral resistance, or MAP = CO × TPR

Cardiac output is considered the flow component, and total peripheral resistance is the resistance to blood flow within the vascular circuit. Anything that results in an elevation or reduction of either variable will influence blood pressure.

There are four mechanisms involved in the regulation of blood pressure: the cardiovascular, neural, hormonal, and renal components. The interplay of these four factors is necessary for proper blood pressure control.

The cardiovascular mechanism of blood pressure control is autoregulation, which is the innate ability of the cardiovascular system to adjust flow to coincide with variations in pressure. Blood vessels are intrinsically able to adjust their caliber to the needs of a specific region, a characteristic which is referred to as *inherent tone.* Additionally, the heart is able to adapt to changing volumes of venous return by altering stroke volume. Further, changes in vascular volume via capillary-to-tissue fluid shifts can effectively participate in arterial pressure control.

Everyday control of variations in arterial pressure is also influenced by neural reflexes. The reflexive regulation of blood pressure is mediated by baroreceptors and chemoreceptors. The baroreceptors are stretch receptors located primarily in the carotid sinus and aortic arch. Elevations in blood pressure cause these receptors to be stimulated. Once stretched by higher pressures, these receptors instigate an increase in urinary flow, either a decrease or increase in heart rate, and subsequently a reduction in blood pressure.

The chemoreceptors located in the carotid and aortic bodies are sensitive to chemical stimuli such as hypoxia and hypercapnea. In the presence of hypoxia or hypercapnea, stimulation of these chemoreceptors results in an elevation of blood pressure.

The hormonal mechanisms involved in blood pressure regulation are the renin-angiotensin system and aldosterone secretion. Under normal conditions, decreased blood pressure causes renin to be secreted into the circulation by the juxtaglomerular cells located in the afferent arterioles of the kidney. Renin, an enzyme, causes the plasma protein, renin substrate, to form the decapeptide angiotensin I. Angiotensin I is acted upon by angiotensin-converting enzyme in the lungs and is modified to the octapeptide angiotensin II. Angiotensin II is a powerful enzyme that causes an increase in blood pressure by three mechanisms: (1) rapid vasoconstriction of the arterioles, leading to an increase in total peripheral resistance; (2) decreased secretion of sodium and water by the kidneys, leading to a higher circulating blood volume and increased cardiac output; and (3) increased secretion of aldosterone, which causes additional sodium and water retention, once again enhancing blood fluid volume.[1]

Aldosterone, secreted by the adrenal cortex, exerts its effect on blood pressure through regulation of blood volume. The release of aldosterone is stimulated by a decrease in cardiac output, a decrease in total body blood volume, or a reduction in serum sodium concentration. Once stimulated, release of aldosterone promotes increases in renal tubular absorption of sodium directly, and water indirectly, the end result of which is an increase in plasma and extracellular blood volume, leading to increases in cardiac output and arterial blood pressure.

Definition of Hypertension

Hypertension is defined as a sustained elevation in mean arterial pressure. Because quantitative elevations of blood pressure vary with age, gender, and other factors, hypertension may be more specifically defined in adults as: (1) men under 45 years old: greater than 140/90 mmHg; (2) men over 45 years old: greater than 140/95 mmHg; and (3) women: greater than 150/95 mmHg.[2]

Classification of Hypertension

Hypertension may be classified by severity and cause in order to facilitate appropriate diagnostic testing and therapy. In terms of severity, hypertension is described as (1) "mild," if the patient's diastolic blood pressure is between 90 to 104 mmHg; (2) "moderate," with a diastolic blood pressure of 105 to 114 mmHg; and (3) "severe," if the diastolic blood pressure exceeds 115 mmHg.[2]

Categorizing hypertension by etiology provides three other divisions. These include (1) essential (primary, idiopathic), (2) secondary, and (3)

malignant. *Essential hypertension* has no known definitive etiology. *Secondary hypertension,* on the other hand, has an attributable, and ostensibly treatable, cause. *Malignant hypertension* represents those cases of hypertension that are emergent, life-threatening situations generally associated with diastolic pressures exceeding 140 mmHg.[2,3] It is of interest to note that both essential and secondary forms of hypertension may escalate to malignant episodes without effective treatment or by the influence of other precipitating events.

Consequences of Hypertension

While all organs are potentially affected by sustained elevations in blood pressure, four organ systems are the most frequent targets of hypertensive damage. These are the eyes, heart, brain, and kidneys. Dysfunction of these organs is primarily related to the vascular damage incurred as the result of chronically high blood pressure.

Vascular Changes

Sustained high blood pressure aggravates the development of specific vascular lesions. These include hyaline arteriosclerosis, hyperplastic arteriosclerosis, miliary aneurysms, atherosclerosis, and medial damage. Hyaline arteriosclerosis is a thickening of the intima and media which diminishes the lumen size. This type of damage most frequently affects the kidneys.[2]

Hyperplastic arteriosclerosis results from intimal injury from higher blood pressures. The intima is thickened by fibroblasts, the media is enlarged, and the adventitia becomes fibrotic.[2]

Miliary aneurysms form in small cerebral arterioles. They develop at points distal to areas of intimal thickening. Their rupture causes cerebral hemorrhages typically associated with hypertension.

Atherosclerosis includes the development of thrombus formation over plaques found in the arteries of the heart, brain, and kidneys. Medial damage may be noted in the aorta leading to aortic aneurysms and dissection. All of these lesions make the vessels less responsive to the body's autoregulatory system, and limit vessel lumen size, thereby promoting ischemia. (See Chap. 21 for further discussion of atherosclerosis.)

Target Organs

The eyes, through the fundoscopic examination, offer a direct visualization of the vascular status of the hypertensive patient. By assessing changes in the vascular system of the eyes (the only opportunity to view the vascular system noninvasively), the condition of the rest of the body's vascular system may be extrapolated. An increasing light reflex, narrowed vessel caliber, and arteriovenous crossing defects reflect vascular damage associated with the acceleration of arterio- and atherosclerosis by hypertension. As the high blood pressure becomes more severe, so do the vascular changes seen in the optic fundi. A classification system that categorizes these vascular changes is the Keith-Wagener Grade[4] (see Table 22-1). This system will be used more extensively in discussions concerning essential and malignant hypertension later in the text.

While the effects of hypertension may be seen in the eyes, the heart suffers most dramatically. The most common cause of death in hypertensive patients is cardiac in nature, most notably from coronary artery disease through myocardial infarction. This process usually evolves from the development of left ventricular hypertrophy, congestive failure, and ischemic damage as the heart attempts to pump against elevated systemic pressures.

Cerebral vascular changes are difficult to assess until the patient evidences encephalopathy from a stroke or hemorrhage from the high pressures exerted on damaged vessels. Renal dysfunction, on the other hand, is more easily detected with the development of nocturia, indicating the kidneys' inability to concentrate urine.

Table 22-1 Keith-Wagener Grade

KW1 = Minimal arteriolar narrowing and irregularity.

KW2 = More marked narrowing and arteriovenous nicking. Implies arteriosclerotic as well as hypertensive changes.

KW3 = Flame-shaped or circular hemorrhages and fluffy "cotton wool" exudates.

KW4 = Any of the above plus papilledema, i.e., elevation of the optic disk, obliteration of the physiologic cup, or blurring of the disk margins. By definition, malignant hypertension is always associated with papilledema.

Used with permission from M. Sokolow, Heart and Great Vessels. In M. Krup, M. Chalton, and D. Werdegan (eds.), *Current Medical Diagnosis and Treatment*, Lange Medical Publications, Los Altos, CA, 1985.

Familiarity with the types and consequences of hypertension assist in the initial evaluation of the patient with chronic elevations of blood pressure. The following section will review the sequence associated with the initial evaluation.

Initial Evaluation of Hypertension

In general, the diagnosis of hypertension is made after two or three blood pressure readings taken on different occasions are elevated above normal levels. The patient is then evaluated for causative factors (especially younger patients with moderate or severe hypertension) and the condition of target organs is assessed.

Initial History

The history includes ascertaining the duration of the patient's hypertension and if prior treatment has been received. Prior treatment modalities are reviewed to discover those that have been successful and those that have failed. Patients are assessed for ingestion of substances that may precipitate hypertension, such as excessive sodium intake, birth control pills, or other drugs. The patient is also screened for risk factors of hypertension including stress, being of the black race, obesity, a history of diabetes or gout, and a positive family history of hypertension.

Patients are assessed for cardiovascular disease and are questioned for symptoms of secondary causes of hypertension, which include anxiety, palpitations, flushing, weakness, and dizziness (associated with a pheochromocytoma); and personality changes, weight gain or loss (indicating endocrine disorders). Other symptoms, related to target organ damage, are (1) chest pain, associated with coronary insufficiency; (2) dyspnea, related to left ventricular hypertrophy; (3) visual changes, associated with retinopathy; (4) nocturia, associated with renal insufficiency; and (5) cerebellar changes, associated with cerebral vascular disease.

Initial Physical Examination

The physical examination of patients diagnosed with hypertension pays particular attention to serial blood pressure recordings, general physical presentation, and a specific systems assessment. This includes examining the neck for bruits and thyroid size; palpating the abdomen for masses or bruits; auscultating the lungs for crackles or wheezes; assessing the heart for sounds, rhythm, and size; and evaluating the extremities for pulses and edema.

Initial Diagnostic Tests

Preliminary diagnostic tests that are useful in newly diagnosed hypertension are a urinalysis, serum glucose, electrolytes, blood urea nitrogen or creatinine, hematocrit, and an electrocardiogram. The chest x-ray on initial workup has been found to provide useful diagnostic information in approximately 2 percent of patients in one study.[2] An intravenous pyelogram is limited to use in younger patients with recent development of hypertension and for patients noted to have abdominal bruits.[2] A fundoscopic examination is performed in order to assign a grade based on the Keith-Wagener classification (Table 22-1).

Plasma Renin Activity

Another laboratory test that is receiving considerable attention is serum determination of plasma renin activity (PRA). It is suggested that patients with low PRA have developed hypertension because of body fluid volume expansion. Conversely, patients with elevated PRA may evidence hypertension from the vasoconstrictive effects of angiotensin. PRA levels may benefit the clinician in the selection of appropriate drug therapy.[5] For example, diuretics may be prescribed for patients with low PRA while an angiotensin-converting enzyme inhibitor may be more beneficial in patients with high PRA.

Classification of Hypertension

Essential Hypertension

Essential hypertension, or a sustained elevation in mean arterial pressure without a discernable cause, takes its name from the German word *essentiale* meaning *idiopathic*.[2] Unfortunately, this description has mistakenly advanced the belief that high blood pressure was essential to pump blood through narrowed vessels. For this reason, Kaplan[2] prefers the term "primary hypertension" to "essential." However, the term "essential hypertension" seems to reflect the understanding of most groups of health care professionals and will be the preferred term in this text.

Essential hypertension accounts for approximately 90 percent of all reported cases of hypertension. It may be manifested in all levels of severity. While there is no consensus among researchers and clinicians regarding its cause, there are several working hypotheses. These hypotheses include (1) the autoregulatory hypothesis, (2) the renal salt retention model, and (3) the sodium transport hypothesis.

Autoregulatory Hypothesis

This hypothesis proposes that high cardiac output states are associated with hypertension. The increased cardiac output may be in excess of tissue needs for nutrition and waste removal. Therefore, by means of autoregulation, vessels constrict, resulting in diminished blood flow to tissues and causing an increase in total peripheral resistance. Thus, chronically increased blood pressure ensues to compensate for high-output states.

Renal Salt Retention Model

This model revolves around the concept of pressure natriuresis and renal function. Normally, as blood pressure increases, the kidneys secrete more sodium and water to reduce blood volume and hence lower blood pressure. This is known as *pressure natriuresis*.

Guyton[1] maintains that hypertensive individuals are unable to respond to higher arterial pressures by additional secretion of salt and water. This causes continued expansion of blood fluid volume, an increased cardiac output, and an elevated blood pressure. This cycle persists until a certain pressure is reached. Pressure natriuresis is eventually reactivated but with a chronically elevated blood pressure.[2]

Sodium Transport Hypothesis

Basically, this hypothesis proposes that hypertensive individuals have a genetic defect that prevents normal renal sodium excretion. It is postulated that this defect is overcome by the secretion of a natriuretic hormone. However, while enhancing sodium excretion, it is hypothesized that this natriuretic hormone ultimately increases intracellular calcium. Excess intracellular calcium leads to heightened vascular responsiveness (increased tone and reactivity). This ultimately causes increases in total peripheral resistance and, therefore, hypertension.[2]

It is possible that all three of these mechanisms contribute to the development of essential hypertension. Despite the lack of a specific etiology, the workup for essential hypertension continues to adequately plan for appropriate therapy.

Evaluation of Essential Hypertension

Essential hypertension may develop without accompanying symptoms. Because hypertensive individuals may experience few somatic complaints while target organ damage is perpetrated, essential hypertension has earned the name of the "silent killer." When symptoms are present, they may include a suboccipital morning headache, dizziness, fainting, epistaxis, tinnitus, and nocturia. Development of other symptoms is related to target organ involvement.

Damage to the heart may be manifested by left ventricular hypertrophy suggestive of congestive failure or cardiac muscle ischemia. Patients are evaluated for signs and symptoms of cardiac dysfunction by the history, physical, and laboratory findings.

Cerebral vascular damage associated with essential hypertension presents itself as cerebral artery infarction or hemorrhage. These vascular abnormalities may produce hemiparesis, sensory deficits, and dysarthria.[2] Extracranial vascular disease may be diagnosed by the presence of carotid bruits, transient ischemic attacks, and a unilateral headache.

As previously discussed, renal damage may be assessed by the findings of nocturia and proteinuria, reflecting the body's inability to concentrate and clear urine because of renal arteriolar sclerosis. This may ultimately result in renal failure.

Although essential hypertension predominates as the major type of high blood pressure, exploring and discovering secondary reasons may alter the treatment plan considerably.

Secondary Hypertension

Secondary hypertension, representing approximately 10 percent of diagnosed high blood pressure, is distinguished from essential hypertension by having an identifiable cause. Renovascular hypertension, hyperadrenocorticism (Cushing's syndrome and disease), primary hyperaldosteronism, a pheochromocytoma, and coarctation of the aorta are all causative agents in the development of secondary hypertension.

Renovascular Hypertension

In renovascular hypertension, renal artery stenosis (usually resulting from atherosclerosis or fibromuscular dysplasia) compromises blood flow to the affected kidney. Decreased renal blood flow stimulates renin secretion and, hence, enhances formation of angiotensin II. As previously discussed, the effects of angiotensin II ultimately cause an elevation in blood pressure.

Primary Hyperaldosteronism

Primary hyperaldosteronism results from excessive aldosterone secretion due to hyperplastic adrenal cortices or an adrenal adenoma. Increased levels of aldosterone enhance further sodium and water reabsorption. Sustained elevations in cardiac output ultimately cause sustained increases in mean arterial pressure.

Hyperadrenocorticism

Cushing's syndrome and Cushing's disease, respectively, result from hypersecretion of cortisol from hyperplastic adrenal cortices or a cortisol-secreting tumor usually located in the pituitary gland.[2] Excessive cortisol levels promote gluconeogenesis, reduce protein stored in body cells (except the liver), and mobilize and redistribute fatty acids. Development of hypertension related to elevated cortisol levels is not unlike the course associated with elevated aldosterone levels.

Pheochromocytoma

A pheochromocytoma is a tumor composed of chromaffin tissue. While usually located in the adrenal medulla, this tumor may localize wherever chromaffin cells exist, including the para-aortic sympathetic chain.[6] These tumors secrete catecholamines (predominantly norepinephrine) which exert an alpha-adrenergic effect on the peripheral vasculature (vasoconstriction) and a beta effect on the heart (increased force of contraction). Hypertension develops in response to a pheochromocytoma from the dual effects of increased catecholamines. These are (1) stimulation of body metabolism leading to an increased cardiac output, and (2) vasoconstriction leading to increased peripheral vascular resistance. Both increased cardiac output and increased total peripheral resistance lead to sustained elevations in the mean arterial pressure.

Coarctation of the Aorta

Coarctation of the aorta usually involves a diaphraghmatic constriction in the first 2 to 4 cm of the thoracic aorta beyond the left subclavian artery.[7] The aorta distal to the coarctation is usually dilated. Patients classically present with hypertension in the upper extremities and reduced blood pressure in the lower extremities. Degenerative vascular changes associated with hypertension become manifest in the proximal aorta. These changes may cause a decreased capacity and distensibility of the aorta which lead to the development of hypertension.[8]

Evaluation of Secondary Hypertension

The evaluation of secondary hypertension includes data collected from the studies mentioned in the evaluation of essential hypertensive patients. Data specific to the diagnosis and management of secondary hypertension follow.

Renovascular Hypertension   Patients with suspected renovascular hypertension may present with severe hypertension, complaints of flank pain, and the presence of an abdominal mass or bruit above the umbilicus, radiating laterally. Ultrasonography of the abdomen may determine kidney size, and arteriography of the abdominal aorta and renal arteries helps ascertain kidney size as well as the extent and location of stenosis. An intravenous pyelogram will usually reveal that one kidney is approximately 1.5 cm shorter, and there will be a delay in dye appearance on the ischemic side, and a delay in emptying due to the low flow of concentrated urine.

Plasma renin activity will usually be elevated. Renin may also be measured from the renal artery and both renal veins. The stenosed kidney will produce renin in amounts 1.5 to 2 times as great as the nonstenosed kidney, thereby identifying the dysfunctional kidney.

Hyperadrenocorticism   Patients with Cushing's disease and syndrome present with a typical cluster of physical characteristics. These include the appearance of a "moon-face," "buffalo-like torso," weight gain, and perhaps personality changes. Along with the routine hypertension workup, an overnight dexamethasone suppression test may indicate hyperadrenocorticism.

Primary Hyperaldosteronism   Patients with primary hyperaldosteronism may typically complain of muscle weakness or paresthesia, polyuria, and nocturia, which are often associated with hypokalemia, hypernatremia, and edema. Patients may have decreased plasma renin activity and increased serum and urinary aldosterone levels. A computerized tomography (CT) scan may assist in locating an adrenal tumor.

Pheochromocytoma   The patient with a pheochromocytoma may have symptoms that include tachycardia, palpitations, flushing, diaphoresis, glucosuria, and hypermetabolism. Laboratory tests required to diagnose these tumors are the vanillyl mandelic acid level in the urine and urinary catecholamine or metanephrine determination. A CT scan or a nuclear magnetic resonance scan may help to visualize tumors in the adrenal medulla. Segmental venous sampling, which measures plasma norepinephrine, may be required to localize the difficult-to-find tumor.

Coarctation of the Aorta   Patients with coarctation of the aorta may evidence blood pressure discrepancies between the upper and lower extremities. A chest x-ray may indicate rib notching and the electrocardiogram may show changes associated with left ventricular strain or hypertrophy. The arteriogram and/or cardiac catheterization may give most vivid proof of the coarctation.

Accelerated and Malignant Hypertension

Accelerated and malignant hypertension encompass the more extreme cases of hypertension. These acute elevations in blood pressure are characterized by a rapid rise in diastolic pressure frequently exceeding 120 to 140 mmHg which represents an emergent situation involving life-threatening cardiovascular changes in target organs.[3] Accelerated hypertension is defined by the presence of grade III fundi and a significantly elevated blood pressure (Table 22-1). Untreated, accelerated hypertension may rapidly progress to malignant hypertension.

Malignant hypertension is differentiated by the presence of grade IV fundoscopic changes that include papilledema (Table 22-1). Because of the continuum relationship between these two types of hypertension, and due to the similarity in pathologic and clinical features, the following discussion centers on malignant hypertension.

Malignant hypertension is typically accompanied by three types of pathologic changes. These are (1) arteriolar dilatation and contraction, (2) microangiopathic hemolytic anemia, and (3) arteriolar fibrinoid necrosis. Arterial dilatation and contraction result from increased amounts of circulating vasoactive agents (renin and angiotensin) associated with malignant hypertension. The turbulent blood flow created by the arteriolar activity causes microangiopathic hemolytic anemia and intravascular coagulation.[9] Fibrinoid necrosis is caused by failure of the autoregulatory mechanism which results in swelling and transudation of fluid into the walls of the arteries.[9] Necrotic areas that are found adjacent to these lesions are called *fibrinoid necrosis,* because the finely granular substance of which the lesions are composed have staining properties similar to fibrin.[3] Additionally, patients may present with hypertensive retinopathy, encephalopathy, acute renal changes, and cardiac decompensation.

Hypertensive Retinopathy

A classification of grade IV fundi must be present for a diagnosis of malignant hypertension, which includes severe arteriovenule (AV) narrowing, focal spasms, flame hemorrhages, cotton wool exudates, and papilledema (see Table 22-1). The AV narrowing is caused by the autoregulatory effort of vasoconstriction as the arterioles and veins try to respond to the sudden increased blood flow into the tissue. Frequently, autoregulation is insufficient, resulting in arteriolar dilatation, fluid transudation, exudates, and hemorrhages.

Hypertensive Encephalopathy

In addition to grade IV fundi, the individual with hypertensive encephalopathy presents with an al-tered level of consciousness, increased intracranial pressure, and possibly with seizures. The cause of these symptoms is due to cerebral ischemia. Lee[11] discusses two hypotheses regarding the causes of cerebral ischemia: (1) vasospasm, and (2) arterial dilatation. Vasospasm causes decreased blood flow, increased capillary permeability, and diffuse hemorrhages of cerebral capillaries resulting in cerebral edema and ischemia. Arteriolar dilatation caused by a failure of the autoregulatory mechanism of vasoconstriction results in increased permeability of the arterioles, which in turn leads to cerebral edema. The autoregulatory mechanism presumably fails when a threshold limit is exceeded and breakthrough dilatation occurs.

Acute Renal Changes

Vaziri[3] discusses three types of renal lesions associated with malignant hypertension: (1) proliferative endarteritis, (2) necrotizing arterialitis (arteriolar fibrinoid necrosis), and (3) necrotizing glomerulitis. Proliferative endarteritis is due to fibroblastic proliferation of connective tissue in the interlobular arterioles. This process causes narrowing of the lumen, resulting in parenchymal ischemia.

Necrotizing arteriolitis is the collection of a fibrinoid eosinophilic substance in the renal vessels. These changes are usually accompanied by cellular necrosis. Intratubular and parenchymal hemorrhaging are often present.

Necrotizing glomerulitis involves both fibrinoid necrosis and leukocyte infiltration of the glomeruli. Other cellular changes are present which can mimic chronic glomerulonephritis. Local scarring may occur, which results in decreased renal function at a later time.[3]

Cardiac Decompensation

Severely elevated arterial pressure greatly increases the workload of the myocardial muscle by increasing the demand for oxygen. The heart may not be able to adequately compensate and the individual may present with left ventricular failure, pulmonary edema, angina pectoris, or myocardial infarction. The acute stress of a rapidly and highly elevated mean arterial pressure (MAP), leading to an increased oxygen demand, may precipitate an acute cardiac event in patients with preexisting cardiac disease.

History

Initially, it is important to determine if the individual has a known history of essential hypertension. If not, the patient may be presenting in a crisis due to secondary causes, such as a pheochromocytoma. History of the present illness should include presence of visual or perceptual changes, chest pain, and urinary output status. Once a brief picture of the current situation is obtained, a physical examination will be performed.

Physical Assessment

The fundoscopic examination is essential in determining the current systemic vascular status. Individuals presenting with grade IV fundi will require immediate treatment with intravenous antihypertensive medications. Alternatively, an individual with grade III fundi may require a less aggressive, but nevertheless rapid treatment plan. A neurological examination will be performed to determine the presence of hypertensive encephalopathy. Signs and symptoms include altered level of consciousness, confusion, severe headache, nausea and vomiting, blurred vision, and seizures. Cardiac examination will include a 12-lead ECG to determine the presence of ischemic changes and axis deviation. Auscultation of the heart may reveal an S_3, S_4, or summation gallop. Crackles may be present on auscultation of the lung fields.

Data from Diagnostic Procedures

Microangiopathic hemolytic anemia is frequently present in malignant hypertension. Laboratory findings may include thrombocytopenia and increased fibrin degradation products as well as increased factor VIII. A significant fall in the hematocrit may also be present. Renal insufficiency will present with metabolic acidosis, azotemia, and hypocalcemia. Urinalysis frequently reveals the presence of blood and protein. Plasma renin activity may be markedly increased with an associated increase in aldosterone secretion and hypokalemia.[3]

Medical and Surgical Management

Essential Hypertension

The goal of treatment of essential hypertension is to reduce and maintain diastolic blood pressure

less than 90 mmHg.[2] This numerical figure was identified with landmark studies, such as the Veteran's Administration Cooperative Study,[12] and the Hypertension Detection Follow-Up Program,[13] which provided data indicating reductions in morbidity and mortality in aggressively treated hypertension.

Antihypertensive therapy is broadly divided into two modalities: nonpharmacologic and pharmacologic. Attainment of the goal of diastolic blood pressure of 85 to 90 mmHg may best be achieved by utilizing both forms of therapy.

Nonpharmacologic Therapy

Nonpharmacologic therapy is recommended in the treatment of mild hypertension in the absence of cardiovascular risk factors.[2,14] Nondrug therapy includes (1) dietary restriction of sodium and calories in the obese, (2) smoking cessation, (3) moderation of alcohol consumption, (4) dynamic exercise, and (5) stress reduction.[11,14] Nonpharmacologic therapy is sufficient if blood pressure control is achieved. It is also encouraged as an adjunctive measure in pharmacologically-based therapy for moderate or severe hypertension.[15]

Dietary Restrictions

The daily sodium requirement for the average American citizen (in order to accommodate daily water intake) is 3 g a day. The average citizen, however, ingests three to five times that amount. It is estimated that, by reducing sodium consumption to less than 5 g a day, mean arterial pressure may decrease by 10 mmHg.[14]

Increased body mass increases cardiac output but not the capacity of the aorta; therefore, obesity contributes to hypertension.[11] Chobanian[14] notes that a 25-lb weight loss may reduce mean arterial pressure by 10 mmHg. Comparatively speaking, therefore, weight control may be the least expensive antihypertensive therapy, as well as the one with the fewest side effects.[11] However, compliance with dietary restrictions must be considered as well.

Smoking Cessation

Introduction of nicotine into the body, associated with cigarette smoking, causes catecholamine discharge which increases heart rate and blood pressure. Smoking two cigarettes per day may cause a rise in mean arterial blood pressure by 12 mmHg.[11]

Cigarette smoking also reduces arterial oxygen content, which is problematic for those patients with coexisting coronary artery disease. Consequently, smoking cessation is strongly recommended for blood pressure reduction.

Alcohol Consumption

Consumption of 30 to 75 mL of 80 percent alcohol causes an increase in cardiac output and heart rate in normal adults without an accompanying change in peripheral vascular resistance. This is due to alcohol's vasodilatory effect and the compensatory effort by the visceral vasculature to vasoconstrict. These effects cause an increase in blood pressure.[11] Smaller amounts of alcohol daily (less than 30 mL) may not produce the aforementioned effects, and in fact, may reduce anxiety and offer protection from coronary heart disease.[2,11]

Exercise

Dynamic exercise (jogging, swimming, bicycling) may exert some favorable effects on blood pressure, especially if accompanied by weight loss.[14] On the other hand, isometric exercises (push-ups, chin-ups, weight lifting) may increase blood pressure and should be avoided.[2,14]

Stress Reduction

Stress reduction utilizing biofeedback, psychotherapy, transcendental meditation, and yoga may produce mild reductions in blood pressure.[14] Consequently, if these options are available and acceptable to a patient, they may prove to be beneficial.[2]

Pharmacologic Therapy

Pharmacologic therapy is advisable for all patients with a diastolic blood pressure greater than 100 to 105 mmHg, especially in the presence of target organ damage or cardiovascular risk factors.[2,11] While there are several ways to classify antihypertensive agents, there are generally seven categories of drugs used in the treatment of hypertension:

1. Diuretics
2. Beta-adrenergic blocking agents
3. Angiotensin-converting enzyme inhibitors
4. Arteriolar vasodilators
5. Alpha-adrenergic antagonists
6. Centrally acting drugs
7. Adrenergic neuron blocking agents

These drugs are administered using a stepped approach, which advocates initiating small doses of drugs from one class and sequentially adding drugs from another class until reduction in blood pressure occurs with minimal side effects[15] (see Fig. 22-1). Typically, diuretics or beta blockers are used initially. These are followed by sympatholytic agents, vasodilators, and antiangiotensin medications.[14,16] Table 22-2 represents those drugs that may be prescribed when treating essential hypertension via a stepped approach.

Another consideration when using the stepped approach is quantification of the patient's plasma renin level. For patients with a normal or elevated plasma renin level, some clinicians advocate beta blockers as first-line drugs. Conversely, they prescribe diuretics for patients with low plasma renin levels. However, Kaplan[2] challenges the utility of this practice based on the following argument: If all mildly hypertensive patients are started on a diuretic, those who respond well probably had a low renin level. Those patients who do not respond as favorably will logically have a second drug added in a stepped fashion, which may, in fact, lower the plasma renin level. Therefore, determination of plasma renin activity becomes largely an academic exercise when prescribing medication for essential hypertension.

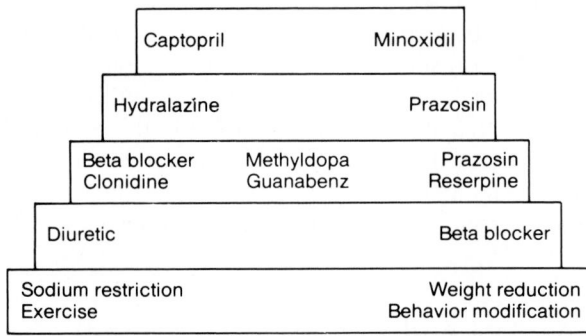

Figure 22-1 Stepped-care approach. *(Used with permission from A. Chobanian, Hypertension. In R. Wilkin and N. Levinsky, Eds., Medicine: Essentials of Clinical Practice (3d Ed.), Little, Brown, Boston, 1983.)*

Table 22-2 Commonly Used Oral Medications for the Treatment of Hypertension

Drug	Usual Daily Dose (mg/day)	Mechanism of Action	Major Side Effects
Diuretics			
Hydrochlorothiazide	25–100	Vasodilatation, ↓ plasma volume	↓ Serum K; ↑ serum uric acid, Ca,
Furosemide	40–80	Vasodilatation, ↓ plasma volume	lipids, glucose; digitalis toxicity
Metolazone	2.5–10	Vasodilatation, ↓ plasma volume	
Spironolactone	25–100	Aldosterone antagonist	Gynecomastia, menstrual irregularities, decreased libido, ↑ serum K
Triamterene	50–200	Inhibition of distal tubular Na-K exchange	↑ Serum K, ↓ renal function, nausea
Amiloride	5–10	Inhibition of distal tubular Na-K exchange	↑ K, nausea
Beta-adrenergic blockers			
Propranolol	80–320	↓ Renin, ↓ CO, central sympathetic effect, inhibition sympathetic transmission	Bronchoconstriction, CHF, peripheral vasoconstriction, bradyarrhythmias, hypoglycemia, masking of insulin reactions, impotence
Metoprolol	100–400	Same as propranolol but relative beta-1 selectivity	Similar to propranolol but less bronchoconstriction, hypoglycemia, or effects on insulin reactions
Nadolol	80–300	Same as propranolol but prolonged effect	Same as propranolol
Atenelol	50–100	Same as metoprolol, but longer effect	Same as metoprolol
Timolol	20–60	Same as propranolol	Same as propranolol
Pindolol	15–45	Same as propranolol but also intrinsic sympathomimetic activity	Same as propranolol but less bradycardia and less effect on cardiac output
Sympatholytic agents			
Methyldopa	500–1000	Central alpha-stimulation, ↓ renin	Somnolence, orthostatic hypotension, fever, focal hepatic necrosis, hemolytic anemia, impotence
Clonidine	0.2–0.8	Central alpha-stimulation, ↓ renin	Sedation, dry mouth, withdrawal rebound hypertension, impotence
Reserpine	0.1–0.25	Central catecholamine depletion	Mental depression, peptic ulcers, impotence, nasal congestion
Prazosin	2–10	Peripheral alpha-blockade, vasodilation	Orthostatic hypotension, syncope
Guanethidine	10–50	Catecholamine depletion, inhibition of norepinephrine reuptake by postganglionic nerves	Orthostatic hypotension, diarrhea, inhibition of ejaculation; action inhibited by tricyclic antidepressants
Guanabenz	8–16	Same as clonidine	Same as clonidine
Vasodilators			
Hydralazine	50–100	Direct vasodilator	Reflex increases in HR and CO, myocardial ischemia, systemic lupus erythematosus; headaches; diarrhea
Minoxidil	5–30	Direct vasodilator	Reflex increases in HR and CO, myocardial ischemia; Na retention, hypertrichosis, pericardial effusion
Angiotensin inhibitor			
Captopril	25–100	Converting enzyme inhibitor, ↓ aldosterone, ↑ bradykinin, ?sympathetic effect	Rash, proteinuria, leukopenia, taste loss

Used with permission from A. Chobanian, Hypertension. In R. Wildin and N. Levinsky (eds.), *Medicine: Essentials of Clinical Practice* (3d ed.), Little, Brown, Boston, 1983.

Secondary Hypertension

The treatment of secondary hypertension involves consideration of the patient's age, general health state, individual response to drug therapy, level of blood pressure, and presence of associated risk factors.[10,17] Therapeutic management of secondary hypertension may be comprised of less invasive medical modalities but usually includes surgical intervention.

Renovascular Hypertension

Medical management of renovascular hypertension consists of restrictions in dietary sodium and calories as well as administration of pharmacologic agents such as diuretics, beta blockers, alpha-adrenergic receptor stimulators, and vasodilators.[18] These measures are prescribed in an effort to offset the effects of a dysfunctional renin-angiotension negative feedback cycle. Doyle[18] comments that poor patient compliance, adverse side effects, and a sizable failure rate may favor surgical intervention. Medical management, too, may be associated with higher mortality rates than surgical management.[19]

The decision to treat renovascular hypertension with surgery depends on (1) the extent of disease in the renal arteries, (2) the degree of associated renal dysfunction, (3) the presence of severe refractory hypertension or poor patient compliance with antihypertensive medication, and (4) low predicted surgical risk.[18,20]

Among the operative procedures available for surgical management of renovascular hypertension are: (1) arterial replacement or bypass technique, (2) ex-vivo repair using microvascular techniques, (3) endarterectomy of the renal artery, (4) nephrectomy, and (5) percutaneous transluminal angioplasty. Arterial bypass surgery is preferred for patients whose renal artery evidences fibromuscular dysplasia.[20]

Ex-vivo repair of renal artery stenosis using microvascular surgical techniques may be used for (1) obstructive branches of the renal artery caused by fibromuscular dysplasia,[20] (2) aneurysms of the primary or secondary branches of the renal artery, and (3) renal artery dissection.

Endarterectomy of the renal artery is considered effective management for atherosclerotic lesions.[20] Transluminal renal angioplasty has been used most successfully for fibrodysplastic lesions, specifically medial fibroplasia.[14,18] Restenosis of the artery can occur and long-term patency rates are not yet available.[18] A nephrectomy may be considered if the arterial disease is unilateral and repair of the artery is impossible or hazardous.[20]

Hyperadrenocorticism

Medical intervention for secondary hypertension caused by hyperadrenocorticism (Cushing's syndrome and Cushing's disease) is used for symptomatic control in patients too sick to undergo surgery and for patients with inoperable cancer of the adrenal cortex with metastases.[21] Drug therapy and radiotherapy are available for these patients.

Three drugs commonly prescribed are metyrapone, $o,p' = $ DDD, and cyproheptadine.[21] Metyrapone inhibits steroid biosynthesis, resulting in a reduced plasma cortisol level.

A "relative" of the insecticide DDT, $o,p' = $ DDD (mitotane) produces direct cellular damage to the adrenal cortex. It is suggested primarily for the treatment of hyperadrenocorticism caused by adrenocortical carcinoma. Cyproheptadine, used in Cushing's disease, is an antiserotonin agent. It functions by inhibiting the hypothalamic serotoninergic mechanism that promotes ACTH release.[21]

Irradiation of the pituitary and/or adrenals may be indicated for those patients with adrenocortical hyperplasia who are not considered surgical candidates, or for those patients who are able to postpone surgery. [60]Cobalt is used for this radiotherapy and the effects are not evident for 6 to 12 months after irradiation.[21]

Target organs of surgical intervention include the pituitary and the adrenals. Excision of a pituitary adenoma is for the correction of Cushing's disease. Total bilateral adrenalectomy may be performed for adrenal hyperplasia associated with Cushing's syndrome.[22] Patients will require permanent steroid replacement therapy, but may find this preferable to experiencing Cushing's syndrome.[22]

Complications of surgical intervention are related to the debilitated physical condition of these patients preoperatively, and include infection, hemorrhage, pulmonary emboli, peptic ulcer, cardiovascular and renal failure, and corticosteroid withdrawal. These patients are highly susceptible to infection, especially fungal.[21] The patient's surgical incision may heal poorly, thus increasing the risk of a wound infection. Patients may develop respiratory infections, not only due to heightened susceptibility, but to preexisting obesity and muscle weakness (when present), which may prevent adequate pulmonary hygiene postoperatively.

Cardiovascular and renal failure may develop after surgery and is related to the patient's longstanding hypertension. Abrupt reduction in circulating corticosteroid levels may result in fever, depression, or frank psychosis.[21] Preoperatively, hypokalemia is corrected with replacement therapy and steroid replacement is postponed until the postoperative period.

The prognosis is good, if not curative, in patients who have adrenalectomies for hyperplasia. On the other hand, the prognosis is considered grave for patients with carcinoma of the adrenal cortex.[22]

Primary Hyperaldosteronism

Medical management of primary hyperaldosteronism is the preferred treatment when the etiology is bilateral nodular hyperplasia of the zona glomerulosa of the adrenal cortex.[21,22] Drug therapy includes spironolactone, amiloride, and triamterene. Spironolactone, an aldosterone antagonist, reduces sodium reabsorption while enhancing reabsorption of potassium. Doses exceeding 150 mg a day are avoided due to development of side effects such as impotence, gynecomastia, and orthostatic changes in the blood pressure.[22] Amiloride and triamterene, both potassium-sparing diuretics, may be useful as well.[21] Dietary restriction of sodium and supplementation of potassium may also reduce the effects of hyperaldosteronism.

Surgical treatment of primary hyperaldosteronism is indicated for patients with (1) adrenal hyperplasia on excessive spironolactone doses and chronically low potassium levels despite supplementation, (2) continuing damage to other organs from chronically elevated blood pressure, and (3) localized aldosterone-producing adenomas.[21,22] Preoperatively, patients are placed on a sodium-restricted, potassium-sparing diet. Spironolactone and amiloride are continued up to and until the day of surgery.

Operative procedures used in treatment of primary hyperaldosteronism include unilateral exploration with unilateral adrenalectomy, bilateral adrenalectomy, or a subtotal adrenalectomy. A unilateral adrenalectomy is the operation of choice for a well-localized tumor of one adrenal. This procedure precludes the additional administration of steroids postoperatively.

Bilateral total adrenalectomy is the preferred surgical procedure if hyperaldosteronism results from hyperplasia of the adrenal cortex. Subtotal adrenalectomy is considered controversial since steroid replacement becomes more complex due to residual adrenal tissue which continues to produce steroids.

Complications associated with adrenalectomies are hypoadrenocorticism and hyponatremia. Replacement with fludrocortisone and sodium is advocated until the remaining adrenal gland adjusts and once again secretes aldosterone.[21,22]

Pheochromocytoma

The goals of medical management of a pheochromocytoma and the related extra-adrenal tumors (ganglioneuromas) are twofold: (1) to gain immediate control of the blood pressure with medication, and (2) to restore blood volume depleted by sudden reversal of vasoconstriction by medication.[22] Medical therapy may be employed temporarily, such as preoperatively, or in episodic management of hypertension. It may also be utilized chronically for patients refusing surgery or with other deleterious medical conditions preventing surgery.[6]

Two modalities associated with medical management of a pheochromocytoma are medication administration and dietary restrictions. Alpha-blocking agents are used to obliterate the effects of norepinephrine in the peripheral receptors.[6] This action lowers blood pressure by diminishing vasoconstriction and ultimately facilitates restoration of normal blood volume.

Among the preferred medications to achieve alpha blockade are phenoxybenzamine (Dibenzaline), phentolamine (Regitine), and metatyrasine (Demser).[6,22,23] Other agents that may be enlisted to reduce blood pressure are vasodilators such as sodium nitroprusside (Nipride) and beta blockers such as propranolol (Inderal). Caution is practiced during introduction of beta blockers due to their ability to obscure the cardiovascular effects of reduced blood volume and vasodilatation.[6] Other drugs that may provide further relief of symptoms related to catecholamine release are prazosin (Minipress), verapamil (Isoptin), furosemide (Lasix) with digoxin (Lanoxin), and lidocaine (Xylocaine).

Dietary modifications mandate exclusion of caffeine, chocolate, and tyramine-containing foods, since these are capable of facilitating catecholamine release. Foods with a high tyramine content are pods of broad beans, aged cheeses, pickled foods, beer, red wine, yogurt, and liver yeast extract.[6] Additionally, drugs studiously avoided for the same reason are those containing histamine, tyramine, glucagon, and the monoamine oxidase inhibitors.

The usual and preferred treatment of a pheochromocytoma is surgical excision of the tumor.[6] This usually necessitates a bilateral adrenalectomy but is contingent on tumor location.[6,19,22]

The most common hazard postoperatively following tumor removal and/or bilateral adrenalectomy is hypotension; especially prone are patients who have not received alpha-blocking agents preoperatively. Hypotension may be intensified by the dramatic reversal of vasoconstriction after tumor removal as norepinephrine levels drop. A catecholamine infusion and blood volume expanders are indicated to maintain adequate tissue perfusion if hypotension occurs.[22]

Coarctation of the Aorta

The only treatment for coarctation of the aorta is surgery.[24] The lesion is excised, and an end-to-end anastomosis is done, or a synthetic graft may be used to repair the coarctation. Synthetic graft material is indicated in those patients with the aortic degenerative changes (calcification, fibrosis) associated with chronically elevated blood pressure.[7]

Two complications associated with surgical repair of coarctation of the aorta are paraplegia and paradoxical hypertension. Paraplegia is rare (less than 0.5 percent of patients), but it is considered catastrophic.[7,24] Paraplegia is thought to be related to lowering distal aortic pressures to less than 60 mmHg intraoperatively or prolonged duration of aortic clamp time in patients with inadequately developed collateral circulation.[7]

A paradoxical rise in blood pressure may be seen in the first 48 to 72 h after repair.[7] This is thought to be the result of sudden perfusion of visceral arteries that had been acclimated to lower perfusion pressures. This hypertensive state may lead to local damage causing mesenteric thrombosis, mesenteric arteritis, and intestinal necrosis. These states are usually associated with abdominal pain. Treatment is initially to relieve hypertension with medication.[24]

The prognosis following successful coarctation repair is considered good. Although residual hypertension may exist, it is controlled with medication.

Accelerated Hypertension

The therapeutic goal of treatment in hypertensive emergencies is to reduce arterial pressure rapidly in order to reverse and prevent serious target organ damage.[2,23,25] Kaplan[2] advocates lowering the diastolic blood pressure to 120 mmHg in the first 20 min of a diagnosed crisis while Vaziri[3] prefers reduction of diastolic blood pressure to 90 to 105 mmHg in the course of several hours. Finnerty[25] supports attempts to maintain diastolic pressure less than 100 mmHg with a urine output greater than 1 L a day. Regardless of the cause or suspected cause, immediate parenteral drug therapy is initiated to lower diastolic blood pressure (Table 22-3).

The drugs of choice to treat a hypertensive emergency are sodium nitroprusside (Nipride), diazoxide (Hyperstat), and trimethaphan camsylate (Arfonad).[26] Sodium nitroprusside is a potent vasodilator that relaxes both arteriolar and venous smooth muscle.[14,23,26] It is administered by a constant infusion starting with 0.5 μg/kg per minute and is titrated up to 5 to 10 μg/kg per minute according to the blood pressure. Its effect is dissipated in 2 to 3 min after cessation of the infusion. Because it reduces afterload and preload, it is especially beneficial in patients with myocardial damage.

Sodium nitroprusside is metabolized to cyanide then thiocyanate and is excreted by the kidneys. Patients may develop thiocyanate toxicity after infusions lasting longer than 48 to 72 h or in doses in excess of 200 μg per minute.[26] Serum thiocyanate levels greater than 10 mg/100 mL indicate toxicity and the patient may describe weakness, nausea, vomiting, tinnitus, muscle spasms, and disorientation.[14] Treatment of thiocyanate toxicity includes cessation of the infusion, peritoneal or hemodialysis

Table 22-3 Parenteral Drugs for Hypertensive Emergencies

Drug	Usual Dose	Route of Administration	Duration of Action	Major Side Effects
Immediate onset of action				
Diazoxide (Hyperstat)	5 mg/kg	Intravenous bolus	3–12 hr	Angina, sodium retention, hyperglycemia
Sodium nitroprusside (Nipride)	0.05–0.20 mg/min	Intravenous infusion	1–5 min	Nausea, muscular irritability, methemoglobinemia thiocyanate accumulation
Trimethaphan camsylate (Arfonad)	1–10 mg/min	Intravenous infusion	1–6 min	Renal impairment, ileus, urinary retention
Phentolamine (Regitine)	2–10 mg	Intravenous bolus	1–5 min	Tachycardia, hypotension
Onset of action within 15–60 min				
Methyldopa (Aldomet)	250–500 mg	Intravenous	2–8 hr	Somnolence, parkinsonism
Reserpine (Serpasil)	1.25–2.50 mg	Intramuscular	3–8 hr	Somnolence, gastrointestinal intolerance, parkinsonism
Hydralazine (Apresoline)	10–20 mg	Intravenous or intramuscular	1–6 hr	Angina, headache, tachycardia
Furosemide (Lasix)	40–80 mg	Intravenous	1–12 hr	Electrolyte imbalance

Used with permission from A. Chobanian, Hypertension. In R. Wilkin and N. Levinsky (eds.), *Medicine: Essentials of Clinical Practice* (3d ed.), Little Brown, 1983.

for patients with impaired renal function, correction of related metabolic disturbances (acidosis), and administration of hydroxycobalamin.[26]

Diazoxide is another potent vasodilator that exerts its effects primarily on arteriolar smooth muscle. It reduces peripheral vascular resistance and inhibits transcellular calcium flux. Because it also increases sympathetic activity, diazoxide may have limited use in patients with hypertensive crises related to myocardial ischemia, left ventricular failure, and aortic aneurysms.[23] Diazoxide may also produce hyperuricemia and hyperglycemia and consequently is used cautiously in patients with gout and diabetes.

Diazoxide may be delivered by intravenous bolus in less than 30 s since 90 percent will bind to plasma proteins and only the unbound drug exerts hypotensive effects. The initial doses of 75 to 100 mg by intravenous (IV) push may be repeated in 5 min if reduction in blood pressure is not achieved.[23] Maintenance doses of 100 to 300 mg by IV push are given every 3 to 4 h. Alternatively, Ginkus-O'Connor[26] proposes that administering 300 mg of diazoxide in 10 to 30 s by intravenous push,

followed by 150 mg over 5 s. Then one may either repeat the dose or give 25-mg doses by IV push every 10 min. This sequence may decrease the incidence of severe hypotensive episodes.

Side effects associated with diazoxide are sodium and water retention, palpitations, flushing, and inflammation or burning locally if the drug extravasates. Diuretics, such as furosemide, may be added to control salt and water retention. Normal saline or procaine may be injected intradermally to reduce pain associated with drug extravasation.[26]

Trimethaphan camsylate is a ganglionic blocking agent with effects similar to sodium nitroprusside. Delivered as a constant infusion, trimethaphan camsylate is titrated according to the blood pressure, usually administering 200 μg to 6 mg per minute. It starts working within minutes and stops immediately after cessation of the infusion. In doses exceeding 10 mg per minute, this drug mimics curare so the patient develops a higher risk for respiratory depression.[26] Other side effects of trimethaphan camsylate include reduction of renal blood flow and cardiac output, and its use is, therefore, limited in patients with renal dysfunction, but it may be beneficial in patients with aortic aneurysms. Other side effects include dry mucous membranes, gut hypomotility, and pupillary dilatation.

Other parenteral drugs used in treatment of hypertensive emergencies include hydralazine (Apresoline) and phentolamine (Regitine). Hydralazine lowers blood pressure by arteriolar vasodilatation and reduction of total peripheral resistance. Concomitantly, it increases heart rate and cardiac output, which limits its use in hypertensive crises associated with ischemic heart disease and aortic aneurysms. The usual dose is 10 to 50 mg every 6 h intravenously, but it may be administered intramuscularly to the patient without IV access.

Phentolamine, an alpha-adrenergic blocking agent, is specifically indicated in the treatment of a hypertensive crisis precipitated by a pheochromocytoma or ingestion of tyramine-containing products in addition to monoamine oxidase inhibitors. The usual dose of phentolamine is 2 to 5 mg by IV push. Side effects of phentolamine include tachyarrhythmias, angina, and dizziness.

Dialysis has been cited as a nonpharmacologic treatment for hypertensive crisis. In addition to its value in reversing the effects of uremia caused by malignant hypertension, dialysis is useful in removing excess fluid to facilitate blood pressure control.[3]

Nursing Management

Essential Hypertension

After the diagnosis of hypertension is established and medical or surgical management is prescribed, nurses typically initiate an individualized plan of patient care based on a holistic nursing assessment. This includes systematically collecting data, noting health practices, discerning responses to illness, and completing a physical examination (Chap. 1). The following portion of this text will describe the nursing process related to patients diagnosed with essential, secondary, and accelerated hypertension.

Nurses caring for patients with the medical diagnosis of essential hypertension are specifically interested in (1) presenting symptoms, (2) data from diagnostic tests, (3) findings on the physical examination, (4) presence of risk factors, and (5) the individual's response to essential hypertension. As previously noted, essential hypertension most frequently develops without a cadre of distinctive symptoms. However, for those patients that are symptomatic, a headache or a migraine is frequently described. The headache may be accompanied by dizziness, weakness, epistaxis, visual disturbances, diaphoresis, palpitations and numbness or tingling of extremities, angina, and dyspnea. Patients are assessed for changes in consciousness which may be related to cerebrovascular damage which includes emotional lability, memory deficits, and personality changes. Nurses note the onset and severity of symptoms and what patients use for relief of symptoms.

Patients are assessed for the presence of risk factors associated with high blood pressure. These include obesity, urban living, being black, smoking, excessive drug or alcohol intake, excessive sodium ingestion, use of birth control pills, or a history of diabetes. Further, patients at a higher risk are those who have family members with hypertension, atherosclerotic heart disease, and cerebrovascular disease. Nurses note findings of the diagnostic studies mentioned earlier which assist the physician in making the diagnosis of essential hypertension. Of particular interest are the results of the patient's electrocardiogram, chest x-ray, and laboratory work. On physical examination, nurses auscultate the patient's lung fields for evidence of crackles resulting from heart failure precipitated by long-standing high blood pressure. The cardiac assessment investigates the abnormal presence of S_3 or S_4 sounds. Nurses skilled in the fundoscopic examination note the presence of retinal changes such as flame hemorrhages, arteriovenous nicking, and cotton-wool patches.

While recording the patient's vital signs, nurses note the patient's blood pressure bilaterally and while the patient is supine, sitting, and standing, and at two or three different times during the day. Patients are also assessed for their individual responses to their medical diagnosis of hypertension. Potential nursing diagnoses may include alteration in comfort, alteration in health maintenance, knowledge deficit, ineffective coping, anxiety, alteration in nutrition, altered breathing patterns, and noncompliance.

This last diagnosis, noncompliance, has been a major focus by many health care providers due to its significant contribution to therapy failure. It is estimated that as many as 50 percent of patients do not comply with therapy.[2,27] It is especially significant for nurses who have been instrumental in describing this phenomenon as well as using data from nursing and other research to plan interventions to enhance patient compliance.[27-30]

The following plan may serve to typify the nursing assessment, diagnosis, planning, intervention, and evaluation related to the nursing diagnosis of potential noncompliance.

Potential Noncompliance

Potential noncompliance is defined as "the presence of risk factors for nonadherence to therapeutic recommendations following expressed intention to adhere or obtain therapeutic goals"[31] (p. 48). The goal is that the patient will express intention to follow therapeutic recommendations and exhibit behavior consistent with compliance to the therapeutic plan to decrease blood pressure upon hospital discharge.

Risk Factors

Patients receiving treatment for essential hypertension may be at risk for noncompliance due to lack of symptoms, chronicity of therapy, expense, and development of side effects.[11,14,32] Other factors that may influence a patient's compliance to therapy are misunderstanding, a poor relationship between the client and health care provider, and disbelief in the benefit of therapy. Other contributing factors are lack of family support, denial of illness, and perceived interruption of life-style.

Nursing Interventions

Nursing interventions to promote compliance are severalfold. First of all, nurses assess the patient for lack of knowledge, faith, or belief in therapy. The patient may be asked for his or her description of what hypertension is and why hypertension is problematic. The assessment may also include a description of the prescribed therapy and the consequences of failure to follow the prescribed recommendations. In addition, the patient can be asked what events might encourage compliance with the prescribed medications (e.g., experiencing debili-

tating symptoms). Second, nurses assess the patient's life-style for conflicting priorities. Patients may be asked to describe ways they will manage to reduce stress, take pills, and follow dietary restrictions in the home or workplace; what will make that difficult; and whether they foresee any barriers such as lack of family, or employer sanction and/or support. Third, nurses assess the patient's energy level to follow recommendations. Does the patient have enough energy to procure the prescribed drugs and does he or she have enough energy to take them? Further, nurses acknowledge a patient's problems with therapy and assist the patient to reduce side effects. Side effects may be minimized by advising the patient to take those drugs that cause nausea with food at mealtimes or to take diuretics at a time when their effect will not interfere with sleep or rest. Lastly, nurses simplify medical regimens and medication schedules, such as clustering daily medications at the same time, if possible.

Evaluation

Patients are evaluated for compliance to therapy by noting blood pressure on follow-up visits as well as number of hospital admissions for blood pressure control. Critical-care nurses may alert the nurses on general medical-surgical units to the number of hospitalizations the patient has experienced for acute management of hypertension and the patient's and family's perspective of contributing elements. If nonadherence becomes an issue, patients are assessed on a more in-depth level to discern reasons and possible measures that the patient and health care provider together may consider prior to hospital discharge.

Secondary Hypertension

The nursing care delivered to patients with secondary hypertension varies, depending on the specific cause of hypertension and its particular treatment. For example, the patient with a pheochromocytoma requires nursing interventions revolving around reduction of sympathetic activity, while the patient with coarctation of the aorta requires the nursing care associated with correction of this defect. In general, however, nurses in collaboration with the medical team strive to control hypertension by (1) drug therapy, (2) surgical intervention, and (3) nonpharmacologic, nonsurgical therapies.

Nursing interventions, in conjunction with these collaborative goals include:

1. Administering antihypertensive medications
2. Monitoring the patient's response to medications by noting blood pressure, heart rate, cardiac output, central venous pressure, pulmonary artery pressure, pulmonary artery wedge pressure, and urine output
3. Monitoring the patient for any untoward side effects and notifying the physician
4. Implementing dietary and activity restrictions
5. Assisting the patient's recovery from surgery

Evaluation generally includes noting the patient's response to these interventions by return of the blood pressure to normal levels.

Some nursing diagnoses that may be associated with secondary hypertension are (1) potential for infection, (2) potential for altered tissue perfusion, and (3) potential for alteration in fluid volume: excess.

Potential for infection or the "presence of risk factors for pathogenic microorganisms to produce injurious effects"[31] (p. 38) may be associated with patients recovering from an adrenalectomy for Cushing's syndrome. The nursing history includes assessment for the presence of risk factors for infection postoperatively such as: (1) chronically elevated corticosteroid levels preoperatively, (2) muscle weakness, (3) obesity, and (4) interruption of skin integrity (surgical incision).

Patients with muscle weakness and obesity and with chronically elevated corticosteroid levels require close scrutiny of their pulmonary status postoperatively. While all surgical patients are at risk for wound infections, these patients are at heightened risk due to suppression of their immune system.

Nursing interventions are designed to support the goal that patients will not develop any infection during hospitalization. These interventions include the following:

1. Note the presence of risk factors that predispose the patient to infection.
2. Auscultate the lungs every 8 h and 2° prn.

3. Assist the patient to turn, cough, and deep breathe every 2 h while awake and inspect sputum when produced.
4. Note the findings of the chest x-ray.
5. Assist the patient to get out of bed and ambulate as soon as possible.

Further, nurses:

1. Monitor the patient's temperature and are knowledgeable of the white blood cell count.
2. Inspect all opened skin areas every 8 h.
3. Clean wounds and cannulation sites per the ICU policy.
4. Render Foley catheter care per the hospital routine.
5. Send cultures of sputum, wound exudate, urine, and blood prn, noting the results.
6. Monitor vital signs at least every 4 h for increases in temperature and heart rate.

Patients are evaluated for the development of infection and appropriate referral and therapy are initiated for those patients who become infected.

Potential for alteration in tissue perfusion is a "deficit in blood supply to a part relative to metabolic needs"[31] (p. 126). This diagnosis represents an acute event in the patient recovering from surgical excision of a pheochromocytoma. These patients are at increased risk for alteration in tissue perfusion due to the sudden reversal of the alpha effects of catecholamines after the tumor is removed. Abrupt cessation of alpha stimulation may result in precipitous reductions in blood pressure, cardiac output, circulating blood volume, and an increased cardiac irritability. Hence, the patient is at high risk for an alteration in tissue perfusion.

The goal of nursing therapy is to prevent alterations in tissue perfusion by maintaining adequate blood volume, cardiac output, blood pressure, and cardiac rhythm in the immediate postoperative period. Nursing interventions designed for goal attainment include monitoring for (1) reductions in blood pressure, central venous pressure, pulmonary artery pressure, cardiac output, urine output, and increases in heart rate; (2) cardiac arrhythmias; (3) cyanotic color changes in the skin and mucous membranes; and (4) cold, clammy skin and fatigue. Nurses then alert the physician for any of the above findings while placing the patient in the Trendelenberg position, administering volume expanders, and initiating a catecholamine infusion and antidysrhythmic medication per the physician's request.

Patients are evaluated by maintenance of blood pressure, cardiac output, pulmonary artery pressure, central venous pressure, and urine output according to established parameters. Further, patients are evaluated for return of skin and mucous membrane color to normal.

Potential for alteration in fluid volume: excess is the presence of risk factors for increases in body fluid. This condition may be associated with the patient who is diagnosed with primary hyperaldosteronism. Nurses assess the patient for the presence of risk factors, including elevated aldosterone levels, high serum sodium levels, and hypokalemia. The goal of patient care is to prevent the development of fluid volume excess in patients by a series of interventions. These nursing interventions include the following:

1. Examine the patient for peripheral edema and distended neck veins.
2. Maintain an accurate account of fluid intake and output.
3. Note intake exceeding output.
4. Note changes in the specific gravity of the patient's urine.

Additionally, nurses:

1. Weigh the patient every day, at the same time of day and on the same scale.
2. Auscultate the patient's lungs every 8 h and prn for the presence of crackles.
3. Monitor the patient for shortness of breath.
4. Monitor the patient for changes in level of consciousness (LOC).
5. Note drops in the hematocrit indicating hemodilution.
6. Nurses also monitor the patient for increases in blood pressure, central venous pressure, pulmonary artery pressures, and cardiac output, as well as for electrolyte disturbances, particularly in sodium and potassium.

These preceding interventions help the nurse identify early trends indicating the development of fluid volume excess.

Nurses also administer potassium-sparing diuretics per the physician's request and note the effects. Patients may benefit from dietary restriction of sodium and provision of potassium supplements. Patients are also evaluated for the actual development of fluid volume excess. Nurses, together with the physician, then plan for changes in therapy.

Accelerated Hypertension

Patients diagnosed with a hypertensive crisis require the advanced and sophisticated care provided in critical-care settings. Routine monitoring of patients in a hypertensive crisis includes use of a continuous ECG, arterial line, CVP, and pulmonary artery catheter. Nurses, in conjunction with other health care team members, guide patient care to reflect three main goals: (1) prevention of the patient's death, (2) prevention of irreversible organ damage, and (3) reversal of existing organ damage.

Critical-care nurses, in collaboration with physicians, seek to accomplish these goals by (1) administering antihypertensive medications safely, (2) titrating antihypertensive medications to established parameters of the patient's blood pressure, (3) noting the resolution of the patient's symptoms of the crisis, (4) observing the patient closely for serious side effects of parenteral therapy, (5) reporting any trends or changes in the patient's condition, and (6) anticipating the use of certain drugs or equipment.

Nursing interventions are related to the following nursing diagnoses that may prove to be problematic for patients in a hypertensive crisis:

1. Potential for physical injury
2. Potential alteration in comfort
3. Potential for anxiety
4. Potential for alteration in fluid volume: deficit
5. Potential for alteration in fluid volume: excess

The potential for physical injury is the presence of risk factors for bodily injury.[31] Patients experiencing hypertensive crises are at high risk for physical injury due to changes in level of consciousness, uncompensated sensory loss, and increased bleeding tendencies. Changes in the patient's LOC are influenced by the presence of encephalopathy and associated seizures, agitation, stupor, or coma. Drug toxicity related to sodium nitroprusside infusions includes the symptoms of agitation and disorientation. Further, changes in the patient's LOC are related to the sequelae of antihypertensive drugs which may cause profound hypotension, including insufficient perfusion of the brain.

Uncompensated sensory losses place a patient at higher risk for physical injury. Visual disturbances may be present due to vascular changes in the fundi. Patients may have a hearing deficit due to tinnitus, a symptom of drug toxicity. Patients may be at increased risk for physical injuries related to their increased bleeding tendencies associated with a sodium nitroprusside infusion and the microhemolytic anemia related to malignant hypertensive vascular changes.

The goal of therapy is that the patient will not suffer a physical injury during the critical-care unit stay. Nursing interventions used to accomplish the goal include the following:

1. Note the LOC.
2. Implement seizure precautions per hospital policy.
3. Perform neurological checks every hour and prn, utilizing the Glasgow Coma Scale or other classification systems.
4. Report changes in the LOC promptly.
5. Implement routine protective care for patients in coma including skin and eye care.

Nurses also note therapeutic drug level reports as well as results of clotting studies and notify the physician of abnormalities; reorient patients prn; provide simple instructions, a clock, and a calendar; decrease sensory stimulation by lowering lights, limiting personnel, and clustering activity; restrain disoriented patients' prn as a last resort to protect them; and apply adequate pressure to puncture sites.

Patients are frequently evaluated for additional risk factors or resolution of other factors, as well as being evaluated for the development of a physical injury.

Potential for alteration in comfort: pain is described as the presence of risk factors indicating severe discomfort. Risk factors include: (1) invasive hemodynamic monitoring (arterial line, pulmonary artery catheter, central venous access, Foley catheter, possible endotracheal intubation), (2) head-

ache, dizziness, and (3) side effects of drugs (dry mouth, postural changes), and possible extravasation of antihypertensive drugs. The goal is for patients to experience limited discomfort during the critical-care unit stay.

Interventions include the following:

1. Assess the patient's pain level (being aware of facial grimacing, restlessness, and complaints of pain).
2. Dress and restrain cannulated areas to provide immobilization of catheters, yet maximizing patient movement.
3. Administer analgesics per patient request and established time parameters.
4. Provide hard candy, ice chips, and other mouth care to patients with dry oral mucous membranes.
5. Assist patients in gradual position changes (reducing the possibility of postural hypotensive episodes).
6. Assess for drug extravasation, elevating the affected extremity and applying cold to the extravasation site, or injecting normal saline or procaine intradermally per the physician's request.

Potential for anxiety is the presence of risk factors for an "increased level of arousal associated with expectation of a threat (unfocused) to the self or significant relationships"[31] (p. 156). Risk factors include: (1) an ICU setting (unfamiliar equipment, noise), (2) intense activity surrounding the patient, (3) lack of control (restrained extremities, impaired verbal communications with intubation), and (4) inarticulated fear of death. The goal of nursing care is that the patient will not experience acute anxiety during ICU stay.

Nursing interventions are as follows:

1. Orient the patient to personnel, surroundings, situations, and time.
2. Allow the patient to visit with family members if desired.
3. Establish eye contact when talking with the patient.
4. Briefly describe the therapeutic plan.
5. Calmly explain what the patient can do to help herself or himself.
6. Administer sedatives per established parameters.

7. Use the patient's preferred name.
8. Establish physical contact by touching the patient or holding the patient's hand.
9. Include the patient in conversations that are within their range of hearing.
10. Avoid staff conversation around the patient's bedside.
11. Return personal items as soon as possible (glasses, hearing aid).
12. Assure privacy.[33,34]

Potential for alteration in fluid volume: deficit is the "presence of risk factors for decrease in body fluid"[31] (p. 58). Risk factors include the introduction of rapidly acting vasodilators and administration of diuretics. The goal of therapy is to maintain adequate fluid volume levels as measured by established parameters for blood pressure, central venous pressure, pulmonary artery pressure, cardiac output, and urine output. Nursing interventions are as follows:

1. Continuously monitor the patient's blood pressure, central venous pressure, pulmonary artery pressures, cardiac output, and urine output.
2. Titrate medication per established parameters.
3. Administer intravenous fluid per the physician's request.
4. Report a decrease in the numerical values of hemodynamic monitoring.
5. Place the patient in the Trendelenberg position for emergent treatment of hypotension.
6. Maintain accurate intake and output records and note imbalances.
7. Monitor the patient for decreases in weight by weighing the patient every day at the same time on the same scale.
8. Analyze blood work for increases in the hematocrit, sodium, or blood urea nitrogen.
9. Note increases in the specific gravity.
10. Note the patient's skin turgor and mucous membranes for dryness.

Potential for alteration in fluid volume: excess is the state in which the individual is at risk of "experiencing vascular, cellular or extracellular fluid overload"[32] (p. 196). Risk factors are the administration of sodium- and water-retaining drugs, such as diazoxide, and the presence of impaired renal function. The goal of nursing therapy is to prevent fluid volume excess during the hypertensive crisis by maintaining established parameters for blood pressure, central venous pressure, pulmonary artery pressure, cardiac output, and urine output.

Interventions are as follows:

1. Continuously monitor the patient's blood pressure, central venous pressure, pulmonary artery pressures, and cardiac output.
2. Administer parenteral antihypertensives and diuretics.
3. Titrate medications per established parameters.
4. Report disturbances in laboratory tests (hemodilution, decreased sodium, decreased specific gravity) to the physician.
5. Note the physical findings of crackles, peripheral edema, distended neck veins, and an S_3 or S_4 heart sound.
6. Maintain intake and output records and note imbalances.
7. Weigh patient every day and note additional weight.

Patients are continuously evaluated for the addition or resolution of risk factors for these potential nursing diagnoses while experiencing a hypertensive crisis. Critical-care nurses, providing 24-hour-a-day care, monitor these patients and assist with their recovery.

Summary

This chapter has provided information about hypertension for the critical-care nurse. It is hoped that the review of the normal mechanisms of blood pressure, classification systems of hypertension, etiologic hypotheses, treatment modalities, and nursing care will assist the practitioner in the direct care of hypertensive patients.

References

1. Guyton, A. (1981). *Textbook of medical physiology* (6th Ed.). Philadelphia: Saunders.
2. Kaplan, N. (1982). *Clinical hypertension* (3d Ed.). Baltimore, Md.: Williams & Wilkins.
3. Vaziri, N. (1984). Malignant or accelerated hypertension. *Western Journal of Medicine, 140,* 575–582.

4. Sokolow, M. (1985). Heart and great vessels. In M. Krup, M. Chalton, & D. Werdegan (Eds.), *Current medical diagnosis treatment* (pp. 182–273). Los Altos, CA: Lange Medical Publications.

5. Buhler, R., Bolli, P., Kiowaski, W., Erne, P., Hulthen, U., & Block, L. (1984). Renin profiling to select antihypertensive baseline drugs. *The American Journal of Medicine, 77*(2A), 36–42.

6. Harris, R., & DelaRoca, R. (1984). Pheochromocytoma: A medical review. *Heart and Lung, 13*(1), 73–81.

7. Spencer, F. (1984). Congenital heart disease. In S. Schwartz, G. Shires, F. Spencer, & E. Storer (Eds.), *Principles of surgery* (4th Ed.) (pp. 733–806). New York: McGraw-Hill.

8. Nugent, E., Plauth, W., Edwards, J., Schlant, R., & Williams, W. (1986). Congenital heart disease. In J. Hurst, R. Logue, C. Rackley, R. Schlant, E. Sonnenblick, A. Wallace, & N. Wenger (Eds.), *The heart* (pp. 643–853). New York: McGraw-Hill.

9. Kincaid-Smith, P. (1977). Renal disease and hypertension. *Medical Clinics of North America, 61*(3), 611–22.

10. Dollery, C. (1985). Arterial hypertension. In J. Wyngarden & L. Smith (Eds.), *Textbook of medicine* (pp. 266–280). Philadelphia: Saunders.

11. Lee, K. (1982). High blood pressure. In S. Underhill, S. Woods, W. Sivarahzn, & C. Halpenny, *Cardiac nursing* (pp. 601–634). Philadelphia: Lippincott.

12. Veteran's Administration Cooperative Study Group on Antihypertensive Agents. (1967). Effects of treatment on morbidity in hypertension. *Journal of the American Medical Association, 202*(11), 116–122.

13. Hypertension Detection and Follow-Up Program Cooperative Group. (1979). Five year findings of the hypertension detection and follow-up program. *Journal of the American Medical Association, 242*(23), 2562–2571; 2572–2576.

14. Chobanian, A. (1983). Hypertension. In R. Wilkin & N. Levinsky (Eds.), *Medicine: Essentials of clinical practice* (3d Ed.) (pp. 217–233) Boston: Little, Brown.

15. Joint National Committee on Detection, Evaluation, and Treatment of High Blood Pressure. (1980). *The 1980 Report.* Bethesda, MD: NIH Publication No. 81–1088.

16. Hutchins, L. (1981). Drug treatment of high blood pressure. *Nursing Clinics of North America, 16*(2), 365–376.

17. Williams, G., & Braunwald, E. (1983). Hypertensive vascular disease. In R. Petersdorf, P. Adams, E. Braunwalk, K. Isselbacher, J. Martin, & J. Wilson (Eds.), *Harrison's principles of medicine* (10th Ed.) (pp. 1475–1488). New York: McGraw-Hill.

18. Doyle, J. (1985). Renovascular hypertension. *Critical Care Quarterly, 8*(2), 51–59.

19. Fry, W., & Fry, R. (1984). Surgically correctable hypertension. In S. Schwartz, G. Shires, F. Spencer, & E. Storer (Eds.), *Principles of surgery* (4th Ed.) (pp. 1003–1019). New York: McGraw-Hill.

20. Effeney, D., Wylie, E., Ehrenfeld, W., & W. Moore. (1983). Arteries. In L. Way (Ed.), *Current surgical diagnosis and treatment* (6th Ed.) (pp. 696–726). Los Altos, CA: Lange Medical Publications.

21. Bergland, R., & Harrison, T. (1984). The Pituitary and the adrenal. In S. Schwartz, G. Shires, F. Spencer, & E. Stover (Eds.), *Principles of surgery* (4th Ed.) (pp. 1475–1544). New York: McGraw-Hill.

22. Hunt, T., Biglien, E., Roizen, M., & Tyrrell, J. (1983). In L. Way (Ed.)., *Current surgical diagnosis and treatment* (6th Ed.) (pp. 683–695). Los Altos, CA: Lange Medical Publications.

23. Grossman, S., & Gunnells, J. (1981). Recognition and treatment of hypertensive emergencies. *Critical Care Cardiology, 11*(3), 97–116.

24. Ebert, P. (1983). The heart: Congenital diseases. In L. Way (Ed.), *Current surgical diagnosis and treatment* (6th Ed.) (pp. 363–384). Los Altos, CA: Lange Medical Publications.

25. Finnerty, F. (1981). Treatment of hypertensive emergencies. *Heart and Lung, 10*(2), 275–284.

26. Ginkus-O'Connor, N. (1981). Intravenous drugs used in treating hypertensive emergencies. *Heart and Lung, 10*(5), 848–855.

27. Foster, S., & Kousch, D. (1981). Adherence to therapy in hypertensive patients. *Nursing Clinics of North America, 16*(2), 331–341.

28. Edel, M. (1985). Non-compliance: An appropriate nursing diagnosis? *Nursing Outlook, 33*(4), 183–185.

29. Fink, J. (1981). The challenge of high blood pressure control. *Nursing Clinics of North America, 16*(2), 301–308.

30. McCombs, J., Fink, J., & Bandy, P. (1980). Critical patients' behavior in high blood pressure control. *Cardiovascular Nursing, 16*(4), 1–4.

31. Tanner, G., & Noury, D. (1981). The effect of instruction on control of blood pressure in individuals with essential hypertension. *Journal of Advanced Nursing, 6,* 99–106.

32. Gordon, M. (1982). *Manual of nursing diagnosis.* New York: McGraw-Hill.

33. Carpenito, J. (1983). *Nursing diagnosis: Application to clinical practice.* New York: Lippincott.

34. Duke University Hospital Nursing Services. (1983). *Guidelines for nursing care: Process and outcome.* Philadelphia: Lippincott.

23 Cardiomyopathy

Joan Vitello-Cicciu
Molly Johantgen

Introduction

Cardiomyopathy is a general term used to refer to a disease which affects the myocardial layer of the heart. Other general terms that are used synonymously with the the term cardiomyopathy are listed in Table 23-1.

More specifically, Goodwin, Roberts, and Wenger[1] classify cardiomyopathies into three types based on the pathophysiologic abnormalities of each: (1) *dilated,* or *congestive;* (2) *hypertrophic;* and (3) *restrictive,* or *obliterative.* In the dilated congestive type there is diffuse dilatation of all four heart chambers; thus, it is currently referred to as *dilated cardiomyopathy.* The hypertrophic form involves some degree of obstruction to the left ventricular outflow tract, while the restrictive type contains rigid walls caused by the fibrosis which has occurred. This rigidity restricts ventricular filling during diastole, causing the pathophysiologic alterations to those noted in constrictive pericarditis. These three types are illustrated in Fig. 23-1.

Aside from the pathophysiologic differences of the three types of cardiomyopathies, there are strong similarities: (1) by definition, the etiology is idiopathic, or unknown; (2) the myocardium is affected in all three types, and the pathologic changes may extend into the endocardial and pericardial layers; and (3) the sequelae of each form are often cardiomegaly and heart failure.

Wynne and Braunwald[2] further classify cardiomyopathies into *primary* and *secondary* forms. In the *primary form,* the heart is the only organ affected, and there is no involvement of valves or other cardiac structures. The cause of primary cardiomyopathy is not usually known (idiopathic). In *secondary cardiomyopathy,* the myocardial abnormality is related to another abnormality or condition and other organs are affected. Table 23-2 lists some of the secondary causes of the three types of cardiomyopathy.

Dilated Cardiomyopathy

The dilated type is the most common of the cardiomyopathies. The striking characteristics of this form are cardiomegaly and impairment of systolic pump function, which leads to congestive heart failure. Cardiomegaly is a result of the dilatation of all four chambers which gives the heart its globular-shaped appearance. The ventricles, however, are usually more dilated than the atria. Hypertrophy may or may not coexist with dilated cardiomyopathy, but the coronary arteries are most often free of disease.

According to Goodwin, et al.,[1] a variety of secondary disorders or conditions may precipitate this form of cardiomyopathy. They include alcohol, viruses (Coxsackie B virus, polio virus, influenza), hypertension, pregnancy (occurs in last trimester or 6 months postpartum), hyperthyroidism, and pheochromocytoma. The myocardial damage caused

Table 23-1 Synonyms for Cardiomyopathy

Diffuse myocardial disease
Idiopathic cardiomegaly
Idiopathic myocardial disease
Myocardiopathy
Myocardosis
Primary myocardial disease

The authors wish to acknowledge the assistance of Marianne Schreiber, R.N., and Karen Cuipylo, R.N., in reviewing this manuscript.

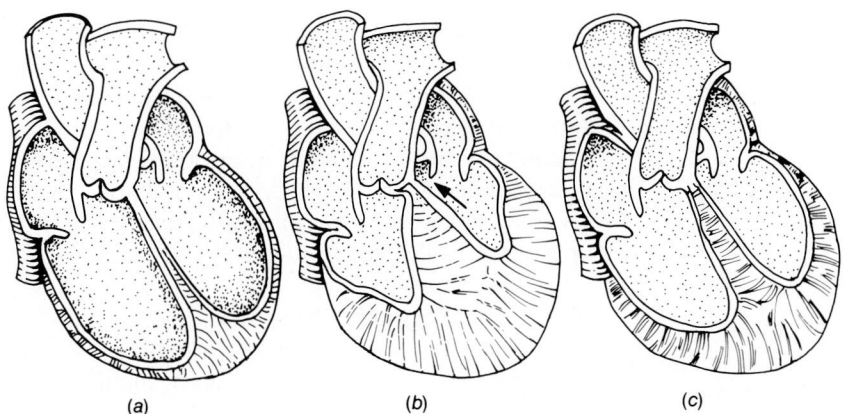

Figure 23-1 Types of cardiomyopathies: *A.* Dilated, congestive cardiomyopathy. *B.* Hypertrophic: Left ventricular outflow tract obstruction. *C.* Restrictive: Abnormal diastolic function; rigid, fibrotic ventricular walls which restrict ventricular filling.

by these secondary disorders may sometimes lead to extensive areas of fibrosis as revealed by histological examination.

Pathophysiology

The contractile function of the ventricles is impaired as the disease progresses. The inadequacy of the systolic pump leads to an elevated end-systolic volume (ESV). Poor contractility reduces the stroke volume as well as the ejection fraction.

Cardiac output may initially be augmented through compensatory increases in heart rate. Due to the lack of adequate cardiac reserve, however, cardiac output will decline in exercise or stress situations. Over time, both the atria and ventricles become dilated because of an increase in end-systolic volume; atrial dilation is due to restricted emptying of blood into the ventricle during diastole. This progressive chamber dilatation and resultant increase in fiber stretch cause eventual decreases in the rate and degree of myofibril shortening. According to the law of Laplace, dilation causes greater wall tension and increased workload. This increased workload is manifested as an increase in myocardial oxygen consumption (MV_{O_2}).

Retention of blood in the cardiac chambers due to increased end-systolic volume encourages thrombus formation. Postmortem examination has revealed the most common sites of intracavity thrombus formation, which are (in descending order of frequency): the left ventricle, the right ventricle, the right atrial appendage, and the left atrial appendage.[1]

Table 23-2 Secondary Causes

Dilated	Hypertrophic	Restrictive
Alcohol	Genetic (heredity)	Endomyocardial fibrosis
Hypertension	Systemic hypertension	Hemochromatosis
Pregnancy	Pheochromocytoma	Amyloidosis
Coxsackie B virus	Neurofibromatosis	Sarcoidosis
Arbovirus	Lentigenosis	Glycogen storage disease
Cobalt	Friedreich's ataxia	Lymphoma
Adriamycin	Norepinephrine	Neoplastic tumor
Daunorubicin		Scleroderma
Hyperthyroidism		Loeffler's endocarditis
Muscular dystrophy (Duchenne type)		
Limb girdle dystrophy		
Refsum's disease		
Emetine		

Adapted from J. Wynne and E. Braunwald,[2] and J. F. Goodwin, et al.[1]

In the end stage of this disease, cardiac output declines. Furthermore, the right side of the heart eventually fails as well, leading to biventricular failure accompanied by the clinical manifestations of systemic and pulmonic congestion.

Data Acquisition

History

Dilated cardiomyopathy occurs most commonly in middle age and affects men more frequently than women.[1] Symptoms of cardiomyopathy are insidious in nature. The initial insult is to the left ventricle; end-systolic volume begins to increase as does ventricular end-diastolic pressure. Progressive pulmonary symptoms are manifested as failure progresses, involving the left atrium and the pulmonary venous circulation. Dypsnea, initially on exertion, advances to orthopnea, then to paroxysmal nocturnal dypsnea (PND), and finally to dypsnea at rest. These prominant symptoms are frequently accompanied by complaints of fatigue and weakness.

Signs and symptoms of right-sided heart failure become evident in the end stage of the disease process, and include increased jugular venous distention (JVD), hepatomegaly, splenomegaly, ascites, and peripheral edema. Patients frequently complain of abdominal pain, reflecting congestion in the liver. There is danger of embolic phenomena should there be separation of mural thrombi with migration into the pulmonic or systemic circulation. The end stage of this progressive failure process is marked by a decline in cardiac output as left ventricular function is further impaired and compensatory mechanisms fail.

Physical Assessment

The patient with dilated cardiomyopathy will appear breathless on exertion, perhaps even at rest, depending on the stage of the disease. The skin may be cool, pale, and cyanosed. Peripheral edema, ascites, jugular venous distention, and pulsatile liver engorgement may be detected by palpation. Left, and occasionally right, precordial heaves may also be present but they will differ from those commonly felt in patients with pronounced ventricular hypertrophy, the latter being more sustained. The apex impulse is usually laterally displaced as a reflection of left ventricular dilation.

S_4 and S_3 heart sounds are often present on auscultation. These sounds may fuse together with rapid heart rates and form what is known as a summation gallop. Blood pressure auscultation frequently reveals a reduction in pulse pressure. This is related to an inadequate stroke volume. There also may be systolic murmurs, reflecting mitral and/or tricuspid valve regurgitation.

Data from Diagnostic Procedures

The chest x-ray often reveals enlargement of both ventricles and dilatation of the atria. Pleural effusions, sequelae of left ventricular failure, may also be present.

Sinus tachycardia may be exhibited on the electrocardiogram (ECG). This increase in heart rate is frequently seen in the presence of ventricular failure and is due to compensatory mechanisms aimed at augmenting cardiac output when stroke volume declines. Various atrioventricular conduction disturbances may also be evident, as well as left bundle branch block and supraventricular and ventricular tachyarrhythmias. Atrial fibrillation, a common supraventricular tachyarrhythmia, has been found in approximately 25 percent of patients with documented dilated cardiomyopathy.[1]

The appearance of pathologic Q waves may indicate the presence of extensive left ventricular fibrosis as opposed to necrosis. When Q waves are seen in these patients, however, coexisting myocardial infarction should be ruled out. The patient with cardiomyopathy may evidence abnormalities of the ST segment, T waves on the ECG, and chamber enlargement and axis deviation are often noted as well. Pulsus alternans, a morbid sign, indicates severe left ventricular failure.

The echocardiogram may reveal a ventricular cavity that is increased in size with poor left ventricular free wall movement. In addition, there may be concomitant dyssynergy of the septum. Two-dimensional echocardiography is useful in detecting thrombi in the cardiac chambers.

Left ventricular function is generally assessed using radionuclide techniques. Ventricular ejection fraction and end-systolic and end-diastolic volumes are useful in evaluating disease progression and the response to therapy.[3] Left ventricular function may also be assessed using echocardiography.

Cardiac status may be directly assessed using invasive methods commonly employed in the cardiac catheterization laboratory. Catheterization of the heart of patients in end-stage dilated cardiomyopathy reveals elevated volumes and pressures on both sides of the heart, reflecting biventricular failure. Both the left ventricular ejection fraction and cardiac output are decreased in dilated cardiomyopathy. Left ventriculography depicts enlargement of the chamber and abnormal wall motion. If thrombi are present in the ventricles, they may be visualized as a filling defect, and mitral regurgitation may also be observed.

Some investigators have employed the technique of transvenous myocardial biopsy to evaluate patients with dilated cardiomyopathy. Unlike its utility in evaluating cardiac transplant rejection, this procedure has not been shown to be of significant value in management of diseases of the myocardium.[4]

Plasma levels of carnitine, an important cofactor for the beta oxidation of fats, may prove useful in diagnosing cardiomyopathy. Tripp and Shug[5] reported data from 25 patients with diagnosed dilated or hypertrophic cardiomyopathy who were studied. Of these 25 subjects, 14 were found to have abnormally high levels of plasma carnitine. Additional investigation is needed to determine if plasma carnitine levels can be a useful marker for dilated cardiomyopathy.

Medical and Surgical Therapies

Medical treatment of dilated cardiomyopathy is palliative rather than curative in nature. Treatment is aimed at alleviating the symptoms of congestive heart failure and improving stroke volume. These end points become the collaborative problems that both medicine and nursing work collectively toward achieving.

Cardiac glycosides, such as digoxin, are used for their positive inotropic effects. Steroids are also used, but controversy remains regarding their value in management of this type of cardiomyopathy. While steroids have been found useful in treating patients with subacute myocarditis and dilated cardiomyopathy secondary to autoimmune disorders, reports in the literature reveal steroids to be of little or no value in treatment of established dilated cardiomyopathy.[6]

Diuretics are employed to decrease blood volume in patients in failure, and anticoagulation therapy is used to prevent systemic and pulmonary embolism. When tachyarrhythmias are poorly tolerated by the patient, antiarrhythmic agents are used. Lethal ventricular arrhythmias are also treated with these agents.

When the ECG reveals serious atrioventricular or intraventricular conduction defects, a pacemaker may be required. Patients exhibiting tachycardia at rest may benefit by the addition of beta-adrenergic blocking agents.[7,8] Prenalterol, a beta 1 agonist, has demonstrated promising results in management of refractory heart failure related to dilated cardiomyopathy.[9,10]

Another beta blocker, acebutolol (Sectral), has demonstrated the following effects: (1) reduction of myocardial energy requirements, (2) improvement of compliance, and (3) lowered arterial pressure.[11] However, the same study reports a significant increase of left ventricular end-systolic volume and end-diastolic volume and a reduction in contractility, as measured by the left ventricular stroke work index (SWI). These undesirable effects may lead to further patient deterioration, pointing to the fact that caution must be exercised when using this, or any beta-adrenergic blockade that significantly depresses myocardial contractility.[1]

Use of vasodilator therapy, to lessen symptoms of failure and increase exercise tolerance, is advocated by some authorities.[12] Vasodilators are classified according to action site. Arteriolar vasodilators, such as hydralazine and nifedipine, decrease arteriolar resistance and lessen impedance to ejection (afterload). With reduced impedance the left ventricle may empty its contents with less energy expenditure; thus MV_{O_2} consumption is reduced.

Venodilators decrease filling pressure (preload) by redistributing intravascular volume from the central to the peripheral vasculature. By redistributing venous volume the signs and symptoms of pulmonary congestion may be relieved. Nitrates are the more commonly used of the venodilators.

Balanced vasodilators, such as nitroprusside, prazosin, and captopril, have both arteriolar and venule effects. Their action is to reduce both afterload and preload. Vasodilator therapy is contraindicated when systolic blood pressure levels are below 100 mmHg, and in the presence of cardiogenic shock.[1]

Myocardial contractility may be enhanced through use of such positive inotropic agents as amrinone, dopamine, and dobutamine. Both metabolic and hemodynamic advantages, such as increases in cardiac output and coronary blood flow, have resulted from infusing dobutamine over a 3-day period into patients with dilated cardiomyopathy.[13]

The only surgical treatment for end-stage dilated cardiomyopathy is cardiac transplantation. Nearly half of the transplant procedures performed at Stanford University Medical Center are for patients with the diagnosis of dilated cardiomyopathy.[14] Mitral valve replacement may be used as a palliative measure for patients with concomitant mitral regurgitation, which may provide temporary relief of congestion.

Nursing Therapies

Patients with dilated cardiomyopathy typically experience multiple admissions to critical-care units during the course of the disease. According to Wold,[15] severe congestive heart failure, emboli, or arrhythmias are the reasons for most admissions; these require vigorous intervention by the health care team. In addition to implementing the various treatment modalities, the nurse is involved with guiding the patient and significant others in dealing with the human responses generated by this devastating disease.

Data from the patient's history, the nursing and medical physical examination, laboratory, and other diagnostic tests comprise a database upon which a personalized nursing care plan is formulated. Data acquisition using the functional health patterns assessment described in Chap. 20 is begun as soon as possible following admission of the patient to the critical-care unit.

Critical data which should be retrieved during the interview process include:

1. Description of dyspneic episodes and the measures that the patient has used to relieve the symptoms, as well as the situations that exacerbate them
2. The level of physical activity that the patient is capable of attaining
3. Dietary habits, including sodium and fluid intake
4. Past medical history, especially hypertension, arrhythmias, diabetes, and thyroid disease
5. Medications currently taken
6. Smoking habits
7. Alcohol consumption (alcohol could be the etiology of this form of cardiomyopathy)
8. Recent pregnancy, if applicable (another etiological factor of this disease)
9. Patterns of sleep
10. Recent weight gain or loss.

The data obtained from physical examination by the nurse should focus on the patient's overall cardiovascular status. Specific attention should be paid to inspection of general skin color, posture, pattern and depth of breathing, presence of ascites, peripheral edema, nail-bed changes, a tendency to use accessory muscles for breathing, the presence of jugular venous distention, muscle atrophy, and poor skin turgor.

Heart sounds, breath sounds, blood pressure, and bowel sounds should be auscultated. Palpation should include the location of the apex impulse, verification of heaves, abdominal distention, and peripheral pulses.

The complete database also includes nursing assessment of the level of factual awareness possessed by the patient and significant others regarding the disease. The plan of care should include periodic evaluation of the level of comprehension in order to avoid unnecessary anxiety and confusion by the patient. Moreover, the nurse must frequently evaluate the psychosocial impact of the disease on the patient and significant others.

Once the data from the nursing assessment, physical examination, and diagnostic tests are obtained, the nurse has a complete biopsychosocial database from which to identify both collaborative patient problems, which have a medical etiology and in which a number of disciplines may participate in the treatment protocol, and nursing diagnoses, which may be treated solely within the practice of nursing. The formulation of a plan of care aimed at alleviating these problems directs specific interventions and evaluation criteria for problem resolution to occur.

If the problem to be treated is a collaborative problem, the critical-care nurse's primary role is one of monitoring, assessing variables, and administering therapeutic interventions ordered by physicians. The nurse's role in regard to nursing diagnoses is to treat the problem through independent nursing interventions.

Nursing diagnoses for the patient with dilated cardiomyopathy are classified into actual, collaborative, and potential problems. Patient outcomes, nursing interventions, and evaluation of outcomes are discussed for the actual and collaborative problems listed below:

Actual: Activity intolerance related to fatigue secondary to limited cardiac reserve

Collaborative: Congestive heart failure related to ineffective systolic pump performance.

Nursing Diagnosis (I): Activity Intolerance Related to Fatigue Secondary to Limited Cardiac Reserve

Goal
The patient's present activity level will not deteriorate while in the critical-care setting.

Interventions

1. Initiate a schedule of activities which includes bed to chair for at least 20 min tid to prevent further deconditioning.
2. Help patient prioritize activities he or she values the most.
3. Develop progressive activity regimen with patient and physical therapy, occupational therapy, and significant others aimed at increasing patient's functional capacity.
4. Consult physical therapy (PT) for exercise training after discharge.
5. Consult occupational therapy (OT) for energy conservation activities.
6. Measure the patient's heart rate, blood pressure, respiratory rate, and emotional tolerance; and assess his or her ECG pattern before and following incremental increases in activity level.
7. Implement active and passive range-of-motion exercises.
8. Assess patient's readiness for instruction of energy conservation measures.
9. Plan adequate rest periods.

Evaluation: The patient demonstrates increased activity tolerance by reporting decreased fatigue

and heart rate; during activities respiratory rate and blood pressure will increase appropriately for the level of activity expended. The patient will verbalize factors that increase fatigue.

Collaborative Diagnosis (II): Congestive Heart Failure Related to Ineffective Systolic Pump Performance

Goal
The patient will show no further deterioration or will have improvement in congestive heart failure while in the critical-care setting.

Interventions

1. Monitor heart rate, blood pressure, pulmonary artery diastolic and/or wedge pressure, level of consciousness, urine output, arterial blood gases, and fluid balance, and report alterations.
2. Examine for tissue edema by palpation and note abnormalities.
3. Examine the jugular veins for distention and report increased distention.
4. Auscultate the lung fields for signs of pulmonary congestion and report increasing signs of congestion.
5. Assess hepatojugular reflux.
6. Auscultate the heart for S_3 sounds, which are indicative of failure.
7. Weigh the patient daily at the same time and on the same scale to assess fluid status.
8. Monitor the patient's response to prescribed diuretic therapy.
9. Consult with dietitian for specific food and beverage restrictions.
10. Restrict fluids as prescribed.
11. Administer vasodilator therapy as prescribed, and monitor effectiveness.
12. Assess the patient's and significant others' readiness for instruction regarding prescribed dietary and fluid restrictions.

Evaluation: The patient demonstrates no further deterioration or shows an improvement in congestive failure status as evidenced by (1) stable or improved ABGs with a decreased $F_{I_{O_2}}$ requirement, (2) a decrease or lack of crackles on auscultation, (3) absence of S_3 sounds, (4) stable weight, (5) decreased amount of tissue edema, (6) equal or negative fluid balance, and (7) optimal cardiac output.

Potential Nursing Diagnoses

Patients with a diagnosis of dilated cardiomyopathy face the following potential problems:

1. Disturbances in self-concept related to the patient's and significant others' response to chronic illness.
2. Fear and depression, related to the patient's and significant others' response to uncertain prognosis.
3. Disturbance of sleep patterns, related to excess fluid volume, fear and depression, and the critical-care environment.
4. Injury related to the use of numerous pharmacologic agents.
5. Ineffective individual and family coping, related to the patient's and significant others' response to the uncertainty of the chronic disease process.
6. Alteration in health maintenance related to knowledge deficit.

Management of the patient with dilated cardiomyopathy presents a particular challenge to the critical-care nurse. The patient leaves the critical-care unit following resolution of perhaps only one of a series of acute episodes. But the underlying disease persists. Thus, the patient and significant others are dependent on a continuity of both the physical and supportive care provided by critical-care practitioners. The patient's transition to an intermediate or general nursing unit can be made more smoothly when communication between the staff of both units is specific and comprehensive.

Hypertrophic Cardiomyopathy

Introduction

Hypertrophic cardiomyopathy (HC) has been described by many names, primarily in relation to its pathologic characteristics or clinical features. In the United States it has been known until recently as idiopathic hypertrophic subaortic stenosis (IHSS). It has also been known as hypertrophic obstructive cardiomyopathy (HOCM), asymmetrical septal hypertrophy (ASH), and muscular aortic stenosis.

The classic definition of HC is that of a disease of unknown etiology which characteristically has a hypertrophied, nondilated ventricle, in the absence of a cardiac or systemic disease which could produce left ventricular hypertrophy.[16]

Heredity appears to be an etiology of HC. An autosomal dominant trait has been linked to HC, with a varying extent of the disorder found in families. However, there have been reports of isolated cases not found in other family members.

Pathophysiology

The primary abnormalities which characterize HC are thickening of the ventricular septum greater than the left ventricular free wall, and disorganization of the myocardial fibers within the ventricular septum. Secondary abnormalities which are associated with HC include: (1) a fibrous plaque on the mural endocardium of the outflow portions of the septum, (2) a decrease in ventricular cavity size or lack of ventricular dilatation related to the hypertrophy of the septum and the left ventricular free wall's (LVFW) inability to distend outward, (3) anterior and posterior mitral valve thickening in response to the small ventricular cavity, and (4) left atrial dilatation in adults in response to the increased ventricular filling pressure.[1]

Varying patterns of hypertrophy occur within the ventricular septum which may include portions of the anterolateral LVFW. These patterns range from hypertrophy only in the anterior portion of the septum to hypertrophy which affects all regions of the left ventricle except the basal anterior ventricular septum (Fig. 23-2). The most common form of hypertrophy involves a substantial portion of ventricular septum and anterio-lateral LVFW. This form is most commonly associated with individuals who experience moderate to severe obstruction of the left ventricular outflow tract.

The etiology underlying the disorganization of the myocardial fibers of the ventricular septum is unclear. This disorganization and disarray has been noted in other diseases as well as in normal hearts, but the extent of cellular involvement is much greater in HC than in other cases. Two theories concerning the etiology of the myofibril disarray have been proposed. The first is that there is a congenital aberration of catecholamine function in the embryonic heart.[1] The second theory is that

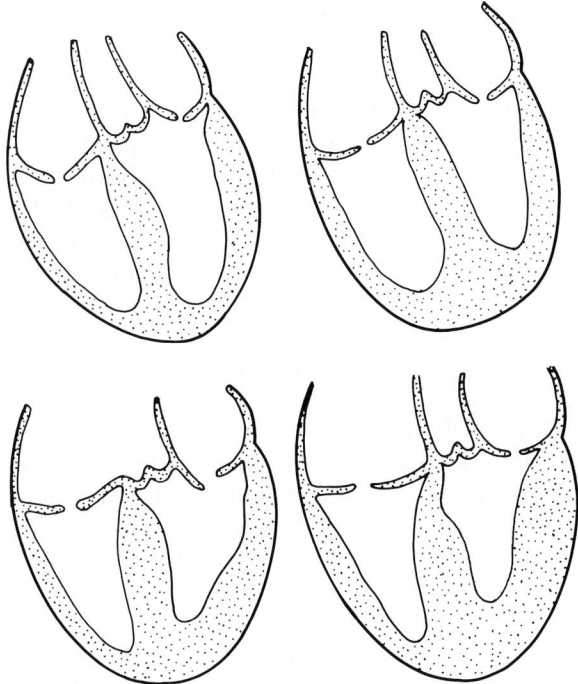

Figure 23-2   Types of hypertrophy: Type 1: Hypertrophy of anterior septum; type 2: Hypertrophy of entire septum; type 3: Hypertrophy of the septum and anterior-lateral LVFW; type 4: Hypertrophy of septum and LVFW except the basal anterior septum.

there is a primary abnormality of collagen which may lead to an abnormal and disorganized fibrous skeleton which in turn leads to the cellular disarray.[2]

Both the fibrous mural plaque and thickening of the mitral valve appear to be the result of trauma of the anterior mitral leaflet apposing the septum during systole. This defect is generally correlated with both a dynamic increase in the left ventricular outflow gradient in obstruction[17] and systolic anterior motion of the mitral valve.[18] Systolic anterior motion (SAM) is validated by echocardiogram and is depicted as the posterior leaflet coapting with a midportion of the anterior leaflet in the left ventricle during systole. Many individuals have some degree of mitral regurgitation related to SAM or to the abnormal bending and pulling of the papillary muscles from hypertrophy, especially when occurring in the anterio-lateral area.

The interaction of the asymmetric hypertrophy within the left ventricle and the chaotic architecture of the myofibrils produce several hemo-dynamic changes in the left ventricle. There is a decrease in ventricular compliance, a decrease in diastolic filling volume, and an elevated pressure gradient across the outflow tract when obstruction is present. The decreased ventricular compliance produces a prolonged diastolic filling time. The isovolumetric relaxation period is prolonged due to a delay in opening of the mitral valve because there is a prolongation in the rate of reduction of left ventricular pressure. There is a lengthening of the rapid filling period caused by the decreased end-systolic dimension. Finally, the initial systolic contraction is rapid and powerful, expelling the majority of the stroke volume in the first half of systole.[1]

Data Acquisition

Individuals with HC initially seek medical attention with a history of dyspnea, angina, palpitations, dizziness, or syncope. A small portion of people may remain asymptomatic but experience sudden death prior to diagnosis. The event which precedes the sudden death is unknown. Studies indicate that there is an increased prevalence of sudden death in individuals with HC and asymptomatic ventricular tachycardia (VT) as compared to those with HC but without VT as recorded by Holter monitoring.[19,20] Yet, a case study was published of a 52-year-old woman with HC who was monitored during a syncopal episode and found to have lost the left ventricular outflow tract murmur, and who had an unrecordable blood pressure, suggesting that a hemodynamic mechanism which reduced left ventricular volume may be the primary cause of death.[20]

Individuals with HC are often active, athletic people who are diagnosed during the second and third decade of life.[1] The presence of a pressure gradient is indicated on physical examination by three dominant signs. A systolic murmur of late onset is auscultated at the left sternal border and apex and radiates to the axilla. The murmur is increased by standing or performing a Valsalva maneuver. The systolic murmur reflects the late onset of a left ventricular outflow gradient and mitral regurgitation. The arterial pulse is abrupt and ill-sustained, and has a jerky quality due to the powerful initial contraction followed by a collapse in pressure from the obstruction. The apical systolic impulse has a triple characteristic (a bifid systolic impulse preceded by an atrial one), due to the initial contraction and obstruction, and a presystolic atrial contraction to fill the poorly compliant left ventricle.[1]

The electrocardiogram in HC reflects the hypertrophy and atrial abnormality. These abnormalities are depicted as an increase in QRS voltage and depressed T wave of left ventricular hypertrophy. In addition, other ECG abnormalities noted are Q waves in the inferior and left precordial leads, left anterior hemiblock, left atrial enlargement, a short PR interval, and asymptomatic ventricular arrhythmias.[19] Atrial fibrillation is present in approximately 20 percent of patients.

Echocardiography, which includes the standard M-mode and the wide-angle, two-dimensional mechanism, has been used to identify the extent and regions of hypertrophy noninvasively. Recently, magnetic resonance imaging has been used in concert with the echocardiogram to specify the areas of hypertrophy noninvasively.[21,22]

Cardiac catheterization is the definitive test used to diagnose HC and to evaluate the extent of obstruction when present. Endomyocardial biopsy of the left ventricular muscle via a catheter inserted during the cardiac catheterization procedure is a further adjunct in diagnosing HC.

A gated blood-pool imaging scan may be performed to determine the functional type of cardiomyopathy and myocardial perfusion. Furthermore, the use of Thallium 201 is helpful in identifying septal abnormalities and progression of the disease.

Medical and Surgical Therapies

Treatment protocols pertinent to the patient with HC are directed toward relief of symptoms and prevention of complications. The underlying pathophysiology of the disease provides the guideline for treatment. Interventions which increase or maintain left ventricular end-diastolic volume and reduce ventricular contractility are generally employed.

The primary pharmacologic therapy is beta-adrenergic blockade. The most commonly used agent is propanolol. Propranolol acts in the following manner: (1) it inhibits inotropic and chronotropic actions; (2) prolongs cardiac diastole, thereby decreasing contractility; (3) decreases myocardial

oxygen consumption; (4) improves the distensibility of the left ventricle; and (5) increases diastolic filling time.

The calcium-channel blocking agents, specifically verapamil, nifedipine, and diltiazem, are now being used as an alternative to beta-adrenergic blockade in the long-term management of HC. Verapamil is the more widely studied agent in HC and has produced significant increases in left ventricular stroke volume, a decreased heart rate, and increased exercise tolerance through increased diastolic filling.[23,24] Unfortunately, serious side effects can cause suppression of the SA node and inhibition of the AV node, vasodilatation, and a negative inotropic action. These properties may lead to hypotension and an increase in obstruction, pulmonary edema, and death.[25] Nifedipine has a greater vasodilatory effect and produces fewer conduction disturbances than verapamil. One study has shown that nifedipine prolongs left ventricular isovolumetric diastolic filling time and increases exercise tolerance.[26]

Diltiazem is the most recently studied calcium-channel blocker used in HC. Diltiazem has been shown to improve left ventricular relaxation and diastolic filling time without altering left ventricular systolic function.[27]

In those patients who exhibit frequent ventricular ectopy or ventricular tachycardia, amiodarone has been shown to decrease the frequency of atrial and ventricular tachyarrhythmias.[28] In addition, amiodarone has a weak beta-adrenergic blocking effect. Unfortunately, the drug's onset of action is five to ten days and cumulative effects may result.

Atrial fibrillation is regarded as a medical emergency in patients with HC. Loss of atrial kick and resultant tachycardia reduce left ventricular volume dramatically. Electrical defibrillation after heparin administration is indicated. The patient is maintained in sinus rhythm with the use of quinidine or digoxin when given in conjunction with propranolol.

In severe disease, the treatment of congestive heart failure is difficult. Generally, digoxin and diuretics are contraindicated but may be used in this clinical setting because there is little risk of provoking obstruction. When medical management is ineffective, septal mymotomy-mymectomy or mitral valve replacement may reduce the outflow obstruction.[1] In one study in which partial septal mymectomy patients were followed over a 10- to 20-year period, it was reported that in 26 of 36 surviving patients the surgery relieved the obstruction and mitral regurgitation, and concomitantly reduced symptoms.[29] Although mitral valve replacement has been advocated, the mymotomy-mymectomy alone has become the surgical procedure of choice.[2]

Finally, protection from infective endocarditis with antibiotic prophylaxis is indicated in patients with HC both prior to and following a surgical procedure. It has been reported that approximately 50 percent of individuals with HC without prophylactic antibiotic therapy develop infections involving the mitral and aortic valves.[30]

Nursing Therapies

The individual with HC who enters the critical-care area may fall within the following categories: (1) newly diagnosed, having recently incurred angina or a "sudden death" episode; (2) admitted to the hospital for other medical or surgical problems for which HC is a complicating factor; or (3) progressive disease in which congestive heart failure is being treated. Depending upon the category or stage of diagnosis, some of the nursing diagnoses may change.

Initially, a nursing history needs to be completed which focuses on: (1) the presenting symptoms, (2) time and duration of symptoms, (3) associated factors with onset of symptoms and relieving techniques of the symptoms, (4) background knowledge concerning the disease, (5) family history, (6) contributing diseases, (7) medications, (8) type of work or employment, (9) position in family, (10) hobbies, and (11) coping mechanisms. A physical examination including vital signs, pulse characteristics, ECG, and heart sounds indicates the clinical manifestations of HC.

The actual nursing diagnoses which are pertinent for HC are listed below. Patient outcomes, nursing interventions, and evaluation criteria are also discussed.

1. Alteration in health maintenance related to knowledge deficit regarding activity intolerance.
2. Ineffective coping related to fear of dying.

Nursing Diagnosis I: Alteration in Health Maintenance Related to Knowledge Deficit Regarding Activity Intolerance

Goal
The patient verbalizes health maintenance behaviors related to activity tolerance.

Interventions

1. Instruct patient on signs and symptoms of activity intolerance.
2. Instruct patient in methods of reducing LV outflow tract obstruction, such as avoiding dehydration, strenuous exercise, straining or Valsalva, very hot environments, and rapidly rising to a standing position.
3. Instruct patients regarding the potential side effects of prescribed medications.
4. Assess readiness for instruction in reducing exercise and physical work through energy conservation measures.

Evaluation: The patient reports lack of chest pain, syncope, and shortness of breath upon activity. The patient verbalizes methods to decrease obstruction. He or she can practice methods aimed at reducing obstruction.

Nursing Diagnosis II: Ineffective Coping Related to Fear of Chronic Fatal Disease

Goal

1. The patient and significant others are able to verbalize fears.
2. The patient and significant others evidence increased use of coping skills in reducing fear of dying.

Interventions

1. Keep lines of communication open among patient, significant others, and staff.
2. Identify patient's positive support system.
3. Explore patient's and significant others' stress-reducing coping methods which have been useful in the past.
4. Assess the patient's and significant others' readiness for instruction in methods of stress reduc-

ing activities. Assess ability to relate facts regarding disease process.

5. Provide support and reinforcement of adaptive behavior, such as problem solving, ability to make decisions.
6. Consult with significant others regarding desire for CPR training.
7. Consult and refer to appropriate professionals (e.g., chaplain, social service, psychologist, psychiatrist).

Evaluation: Patient verbalizes fears and positive coping methods for stress reduction. Patient identifies his or her support system.

Potential Nursing Diagnoses

Patients with a diagnosis of hypertrophic cardiomyopathy share many of the potential diagnoses previously discussed under "Dilated Cardiomyopathy." As well, there are two additional potential diagnoses that pertain to the fact that, as a group, these patients tend to be active, athletic people in their second or third decade of life, and the diagnosis of HC may necessitate a change in lifestyle. Therefore, the potential nursing diagnosis for such a cluster of patients includes:

1. Potential noncompliance with medical therapy related to a change in life-style.
2. Potential ineffective coping (significant others and/or patient) related to change in life-style and body image.

Restrictive Cardiomyopathy

Introduction

Restrictive cardiomyopathy is not commonly seen, yet resembles constrictive pericarditis in its clinical presentation. The distinguishing characteristic of the restrictive cardiomyopathy is that there is abnormal diastolic function resulting from abnormal cardiac stiffness.

Pathophysiology

Many specific pathologic processes may develop into restrictive cardiomyopathy, including myocardial fibrosis, hypertrophy, or infiltration, but the cause is often unknown (idiopathic). These proc-

esses increase rigidity of the ventricular walls and impede ventricular filling. Secondarily, restrictive cardiomyopathy may be caused by amyloidosis, hemochromatosis, glycogen deposition, endomyocardial fibrosis, fibroelastoses, neoplastic infiltration and pseudoxanthoma elasticum.[2]

The clinical and hemodynamic features of restrictive cardiomyopathy and constrictive pericarditis are similar but not the same. According to one authority, the left ventricular end-diastolic pressure in restrictive cardiomyopathy is greater than the right ventricular end-diastolic pressure, while in constrictive pericarditis both pressures are equal.[31] Restrictive cardiomyopathy does not demonstrate the extent of the deep and rapid early decline in ventricular pressure at the onset of diastole or the square root sign as in constrictive pericarditis. Finally, the left ventricular relaxation period is prolonged in restrictive cardiomyopathy but remains normal in constrictive pericarditis.[32] Table 23-3 summarizes the differentiating characteristics of restrictive cardiomyopathy from constrictive pericarditis.

Data Acquisition

Individuals with restrictive cardiomyopathy commonly present with chest pain, dyspnea on exertion, and fatigue. Exercise tolerance is limited because of the heart's inability to increase cardiac output. In advanced cases, an elevated central venous pressure and pulmonary artery pressure are present. Atrial pressure waveforms have a prominent y descent followed by a rapid rise and plateau, and the a wave is of equal amplitude to the v wave.[33] Jugular venous distention, peripheral edema, ascites, anasarca, and hepatomegaly may be noted. A concomitant S_3 or S_4 sound is commonly auscultated, with mitral valve and tricuspid valve regurgitation murmurs frequently noted.

The electrocardiogram frequently shows sinus tachycardia, which is a compensatory mechanism to maintain cardiac output. Atrial fibrillation occurs frequently with atrial dilatation. Biventricular hypertrophy with decreased voltage is also seen. High-degree A-V blocks occur with amyloid diseases.

The echocardiogram differentiates restrictive cardiomyopathy from other cardiomyopathies or constrictive pericarditis.[34] Embolic phenomenon and the degree of ventricular stiffness can be seen

Table 23-3 Characteristics Differentiating Restrictive Cardiomyopathy from Constrictive Pericarditis

	Restrictive Cardiomyopathy	Constrictive Pericarditis
Ventricular end-diastolic volume	Left > right	Equal
Square root sign	+ + + +	+ +
Left ventricular relaxation time	Prolonged	Normal
Left ventricular mass	Increased	Normal
Biatrial size	Increased	Normal
Left ventricular filling rate	+ +	+ + + +
Diastolic thinning of posterior wall	+ + + +	+ +
Interval between minimum cavity size and mitral valve opening	Prolonged	Normal

+ = increased.

as well. Radionuclide imaging techniques differentiate the systolic and diastolic function of the ventricles, including volumes and the ejection fraction. Cardiac catheterization defines the hemodynamic features and ventricular dynamics particular to restrictive cardiomyopathy.

Endomyocardial biopsy is sometimes used to further distinguish restrictive cardiomyopathy from constrictive pericarditis.[35]

Medical and Surgical Therapies

The medical treatment for restrictive cardiomyopathy is similar to that for congestive heart failure. Treatment is symptom-limiting and focuses on fluid restriction, diuretic therapy, anticoagulation, and digitalization if atrial fibrillation is present. Paracentesis may relieve pressure from ascites. When recurrent pericardial effusion occurs, pericardioperitoneal shunts have relieved tamponade.

Surgical treatment of restrictive cardiomyopathy is that of resection of thickened endocardial tissue. Mitral and tricuspid valve replacement is done when needed. Acute symptoms have been relieved with these surgical procedures, but long-term effectiveness is uncertain. Placement of a permanent pacemaker is done to relieve A-V blocks when they occur.

Nursing Therapies

As with the other cardiomyopathies, a careful and complete nursing history and physical examination guide the nurse in formulating nursing diagnoses, goals, and interventions. The primary nursing di-agnosis common for patients with restrictive cardiomyopathy is activity intolerance related to fatigue, but this type is secondary to restrictive diastolic filling. The collaborative diagnosis is congestive heart failure related to restrictive diastolic filling. The nursing interventions are the same as previously discussed in the dilated cardiomyopathy section.

Conclusion

In conclusion, the varying types of cardiomyopathy and related patient care have been discussed. It is imperative that the critical-care nurse differentiate these forms in order to understand the underlying pathology and anticipate potential problems. The exact prognosis of a patient with any type of cardiomyopathy is hard to accurately predict because the underlying pathologic progression varies. Treatment is aimed at alleviating the symptoms associated with the disease rather than the etiology because in most cases the cause is idiopathic. Specific causes of cardiomyopathy require additional therapeutic interventions.

These patients present a challenge to health care practitioners. The critical-care nurse will often see these patients during acute exacerbation of symptoms. Nursing care must be directed to minimizing some of these symptoms and providing the necessary education and support to cope with the fear and anxiety. The patient's and significant others' active involvement in a progressive plan of care in the critical-care setting may optimize the patient's quality of life.

References

1. Goodwin, J. F., Roberts, W. C., & Wenger, N. K. (1986). Cardiomyopathy and myocardial involvement in systemic disease. In J. W. Hurst, R. B. Logue, R. C. Schlant, & N. K. Wenger (Eds.), *The heart.* New York: McGraw-Hill.

2. Wynne, J., & Braunwald, E. (1984). The cardiomyopathies and myocarditides. In E. Braunwald (Ed.), *Heart disease: A textbook of cardiovascular medicine.* Philadelphia: Saunders.

3. Goldman, M. R., & Boucher, C. A. (1980). Value of radionuclide imaging techniques in assessing cardiomyopathy. *American Journal of Cardiology, 46,* 1232–1236.

4. Parrillo, J. E., Aretz, H. T., Palacios, I., Fallon, J. T., & Block, P. C. (1984). The results of transvenous endomyocardial biopsy can frequently be used to diagnose myocardial diseases in patients with idiopathic heart failure. *Circulation, 69*(11), 93–101.

5. Tripp, M. E., & Shug, A. L. (1984). Plasma carnitine concentrations in cardiomyopathy patients. *Biochemical Medicine, 32*(2), 199–206.

6. Mason, J. W., Billingham, M. E., & Ricci, D. R. (1980). Treatment of acute inflammatory myocarditis assisted by endomyocardial biopsy. *American Journal of Cardiology, 45,* 1037–1044.

7. Waagstein, F., Hjalmarson, A., Swedeberg, K. & Wallentin, I. (1983). Beta-blockers in dilated cardiomyopathies: They work. *European Heart Journal* (Suppl. A), 173–178.

8. Swedberg, K., Hjalmarson, A., Waagstein, F., & Wallentin, I. (1980). Beneficial effects of long-term beta blockade in patients with congestive cardiomyopathy. *British Health Journal, 44,* 117–133.

9. Guazzi, M. D., Qing, L. G., Olvari, M. T., Fiorentini, C., Loaldi, A, Bartorelli, A., Moruzzi, P., & Polese, A. (1982). Circulatory response to prenalterol in normal subjects and in patients with primary congestive cardiomyopathy. *Acta Medica Scandinavica, 659* (Suppl.), 233–250.

10. Kupper, W., Schutt, M., & Bleifeld, W. (1982). Effect of intravenous prenalterol on haemodynamics and myocardial lactate extraction in patients with left ventricular failure. *Acta Medica Scandinavica, 659* (Suppl.), 287–298.

11. Ikram, H., Chan, W, Bennett, S. I., & Bones, P. J. (1979). Hemodynamic effects of acute beta-adrenergic receptor blockade in congestive cardiomyopathy. *British Heart Journal, 42,* 311–315.

12. Camerini, F., Mestroni, L, Neri, R, & Humar, T. (1984). Vasodilators in left ventricular failure. *Italian Cardiology, 14,* 685–693.

13. Unverferth, D. V., Margorien, R. D., Altshuld, R., Kolibash, A. J., Lewis, R. P., & Leier, C. V. (1983). The hemodynamic and metabolic advantages gained by a three-day infusion of dobutamine in patients with congestive cardiomyopathy. *American Heart Journal, 106,* 29–34.

14. Hassell, L. A., Fowles, R. E., & Stinson, E. B. (1981). Patients with congestive cardiomyopathy as cardiac transplant recipients. *American Journal of Cardiology, 47,* 1205–1209.

15. Wold, B. (1983). Dilated cardiomyopathy: Considerations for the coronary care nurse. *Heart and Lung, 12,* 544–553.

16. Goodwin, J. F. (1974). Prospects and predictions for the cardiomyopathies. *Circulation, 50,* 210–219.

17. Shah, P. M., Taylor, R. D., & Wong, M. (1981). Abnormal mitral valve coaptation in hypertrophic obstructive cardiomyopathy: Proposed role in systolic anterior motion of the mitral valve. *American Journal of Cardiology, 48,* 258–262.

18. Pollick, C., Rakowski, H., & Wigle, E. D. (1984). Muscular subaortic stenosis: The quantitative relationship between systolic anterior motion and the pressure gradient. *Circulation, 69,* 43–49.

19. Maron, B. J., Savage, D. D., Wolfson, J. K., & Epstein, S. E. (1981). Prognostic significance of 24-hour ambulatory electrocardiographic monitoring in patients with hypertrophic cardiomyopathy: A prospective study. *American Journal of Cardiology, 48,* 252–257.

20. McKenna, W., Harris, L., & Deanfield, J. (1982). Syncope in hypertrophic cardiomyopathy. *British Heart Journal, 47,* 177–179.

21. Farmer, D., Higgins, C. B., Yee, E., Lipton, M. J., Wahr, D., & Ports, T. (1985). Tissue characterization by magnetic resonance imaging in hypertrophic cardiomyopathy. *American Journal of Cardiology, 55,* 230–232.

22. Higgins, C. B., Byrd, B. F., III, Stark, D., McNamara, M., Lanzer, P., Lipton, M. J., Schiller, N. B., Botvinick, E., & Chatterjee, K. (1985). Magnetic resonance imaging in hypertrophic cardiomyopathy. *American Journal of Cardiology, 55,* 1121–1126.

23. Bonow, R. O., Frederick, T. M., Bacharach, S. L., Green, M. V., Goose, P. W., Maron, B. J., & Rosing, D. R. (1983). Atrial systole and left ventricular filling in hypertrophic cardiomyopathy: Effect of verapamil. *American Journal of Cardiology, 51,* 1386–1391.

24. Hanrath, P., Schluter, M., Sonntag, F., Diemert, J., & Bleifeld, W. (1983). Influence of verapamil therapy on left ventricular performance at rest and during exercise in hypertrophic cardiomyopathy. *American Journal of Cardiology, 52,* 544–548.

25. Epstein, S. E., & Rosing, D. R. (1981). Verapamil: Its

potential for causing serious complications in patients with hypertrophic cardiomyopathy. *Circulation, 64,* 437–441.

26. Lorell, B. H., Paulus, W. J., Grossman, W., Wynne, J., & Cohn, P. F. (1982). Modification of abnormal left ventricular diastolic properties by nifedipine in patients with hypertrophic cardiomyopathy. *Circulation, 65,* 499–507.

27. Suwa, M., Hirota, Y., & Kawamura, K. (1984). Improvement in left ventricular diastolic function during intravenous and oral diltiazem treatment in patients with hypertrophic cardiomyopathy: An echocardiographic study. *American Journal of Cardiology, 54,* 1047–1053.

28. McKenna, W. J., Harris, L., Rowland, E., Kleinebenne, A., Krikler, D. M., Oakley, C. M., & Goodwin, J. F. (1984). Amiodarone for long-term management of patients with hypertrophic cardiomyopathy. *American Journal of Cardiology, 54,* 802–810.

29. Beahrs, M. M., Tajik, A. J., Seward, J. B., Giuliani, E. R., & McGoon, D. C. (1983). Hypertrophic obstructive cardiomyopathy: Ten to twenty-one year follow up after partial septal myectomy. *American Journal of Cardiology, 51,* 1160–1166.

30. Chagnac, A., Rudniki, C., Loebel, H., & Zahavi, I. (1982). Infectious endocarditis in idiopathic hypertrophic subaortic stenosis: Report of three cases and review of literature. *Chest, 81,* 346–349.

31. Hirota, Y., Kohriyama, T., Hayashi, T., Kaku, K., Nishimura, H., Saito, T., Nakayama, Y., Suwa, M., Kino, M., & Kawamura, K. (1983). Idiopathic restrictive cardiomyopathy: Differences of left ventricular relaxation and diastolic waveforms from constrictive pericarditis. *American Journal of Cardiology, 52,* 421–423.

32. Francis, V. R., Paulsen, W. H. J., Sagar, K. B., Engle, P., & Cowley, M. J. (1985). Improved echocardiographic differentiation of restrictive cardiomyopathy from constrictive pericarditis. *Circulation,* Suppl. III, 72(4), III–355.

33. Benotti, J. R., Grossman, W., & Cohn, P. F. (1980). Clinical profile of restrictive cardiomyopathy. *Circulation, 61,* 1206–1212.

34. Lekakis, J., Schick, E., Falk, R., & Plehn, J. (1985). Left ventricular diastolic function in differentiating constrictive pericarditis and restrictive cardiomyopathy. *Circulation,* Suppl. III, 72(4), III–355.

35. Schoenfeld, M. H., Supple, E. W., Dec, W. W., Fallon, J. T., & Palacios, I. F. (1985). Restrictive cardiomyopathy versus constrictive pericarditis: Role of endomyocardial biopsy in avoiding unnecessary thoracotomy. *Circulation,* Suppl. III, 72(4), III–355.

24 Valvular Heart Disease

Joan Vitello-Cicciu
Diane Panton
Lapsley

Acute Rheumatic Fever and Rheumatic Heart Disease

Acute rheumatic fever is a systemic connective tissue disease in which damage occurs to the collagen fibrils and to the ground substance of connective tissue. This disorder is characterized by inflammatory lesions which pervade connective and endothelial tissue. It has been linked to a group A beta-hemolytic streptococcal infection. Rheumatic fever is postulated to be an autoimmune response to the streptococcal organism. There is no definitive evidence as to the underlying mechanism by which damage occurs.[1] The incidence of rheumatic fever has declined according to recent statistics, probably as a result of prevention of hemolytic strep infections by use of penicillin. It develops in 1 to 3 percent of patients with a prior untreated streptococcal infection.[2] It is also documented that patients who have experienced previous attacks are increasingly susceptible to recurrent episodes and should be on continuous antibiotic therapy as prophylaxis against recurrences.[3]

Rheumatic heart disease (rheumatic carditis) is defined as a cardiac disorder which results as a sequel to a prior episode of acute rheumatic fever. It is the major acquired heart disease in children and the leading cause of death in the 5-to-24-year-old age group. There is a delayed diffuse inflammatory reaction as a result of acute rheumatic fever which can affect the pericardium, myocardium, and endocardium. The inflammatory reaction of acute rheumatic carditis will be discussed as it relates to the three layers. In the pericardium, the visceral and parietal layers become thickened and covered

with a fibrinous exudate. Serosanguineous fluid may accumulate, leading to pericardial effusion. During the healing process, the cells initiate the scarring process contributing to fibrosis and adhesions. These may result in adherence of the pericardium onto the epicardium; however, constrictive pericarditis usually does not occur.[4,5]

Rheumatic myocarditis is characterized by the presence of Aschoff bodies, which are areas of edema, destruction of tissue, and scarring. In addition to these Aschoff bodies, there is an extensive cellular infiltrate found in the interstitial tissue which is thought to cause ineffective contractility leading to cardiomegaly and heart failure.[4] The coronary arteries are usually not involved in this pathophysiology and remain free of disease.

Rheumatic endocarditis usually is limited to valvular involvement and does not infiltrate the mural endocardium. In descending frequency, the mitral, aortic, tricuspid, and rarely the pulmonic valves are affected. During the initial stages of valvulitis, there is inflammation and edema of the valve leaflets and formation of tiny beadlike vegetations referred to as *verrucae*. These verrucae grow along the lines of contact of the valve leaflets.

As the pathology progresses, blood, fibrin, and platelets are deposited along the coapting edges of the valves. They are also found in the commissures as well as in the chordae tendineae of the atrioventricular (AV) valves. According to McCarthy,[5] as sequelae of the above, the leaflets of the affected valves adhere to one another and fusion of the commissures develops. There is also shortening, fibrosis, and fusion of the chordae tendineae. In the later stages, granulation tissue develops and fibrotic changes occur leading to fibrosis and thickening with eventual calcification of the valve leaflets. These pathologic changes, which often take years

The authors wish to acknowledge the assistance of Karen Cuipylo, R.N., M.S.N., in reviewing the manuscript of this chapter.

697

to manifest, will produce either stenosis, or regurgitation, or combined stenosis and regurgitation of the involved valves. A more in-depth explanation of valvular stenosis and regurgitation will be forthcoming in this chapter.

Although not diagnostic, there are certain laboratory findings consistent with acute rheumatic fever. These consist of an elevated antistreptolysin O titer (ASOT) after the streptococcal infection, increased erythrocyte sedimentation rate (ESR) indicative of inflammation, and the appearance of a C-reactive protein (CRP).

The clinical features of acute rheumatic fever include: (1) systemic manifestations such as fatigue, malaise, and fever; (2) a migratory polyarthritis involving inflammatory movement from one large joint to another; (3) erythema marginatum, which is a painless, nonpruritic redness of the trunk and proximal extremities that is more pronounced with local heat; (4) Sydenham's chorea (rare occurrence), which is depicted as aimless, irregular movements and labile emotional state; (5) abdominal pain secondary to hepatic engorgement or inflammatory sinusitis; and (6) small, painless, subcutaneous nodules located over bony prominences which are often overlooked.

Treatment consists of bed rest, until the fever and acute manifestations abate. The streptococcal organism is treated with antibiotic (penicillin preferred) therapy. The acute phase of the disease usually resolves within 12 weeks.

Infective Endocarditis

Infective endocarditis is a disease which affects the lining of the heart whereby the valves are predominantly afflicted. It may be caused by an inflammatory lesion found in collagen vascular diseases or rheumatic fever, or by an infectious process that is caused by invading microorganisms.[5] The most common microbes involved are bacteria, fungi, yeasts, and rickettsiae. Of these, the gram-positive bacteria cause the highest incidence of reported cases. Rarer organisms implicated in this disease are viruses, parasites, mycobacteria, and chlamydia.

Infective endocarditis occurs most frequently in men over the age of 60. The left-sided valves of the heart are affected more often than the right side. Predisposing factors to infective endocarditis include parenteral drug abuse, insertion of indwelling catheters, dental procedures, urinary tract infections, skin and wound infections, congenital heart disease, rheumatic fever, cardiac surgery, and various instrumentation procedures. There is some discrepancy as to whether the overall incidence of this disease has declined because there has been an increased incidence of endocarditis in patients with prosthetic heart valves and in drug addicts, but a decreased incidence in nonaddict patients with native valves. Discussion in this section will be centered on native valves affected by endocarditis. Endocarditis in patients who have undergone valve replacement will be elaborated on in the section concerning valvular prostheses.

There seems to be a consensus in the literature regarding abolishing the previous classification of endocarditis into acute and subacute forms.[6,7,8] The reason for this is that many clinicians have discovered that acute cases of endocarditis could be converted to a subacute status with aggressive antibiotic therapy, and, conversely, subacute cases could suddenly develop life-threatening conditions.[9] However, it has been suggested that the clinical differentiation is important, because there remains a difference in clinical manifestations, duration of the course, nature of the complications, and final outcome between these two forms.[9,10]

In the acute form, the causative agents are of higher virulence. They include *Staphylococcus aureus*, *Streptococcus pneumoniae*, and *Neisseria menigitidis*. The onset of acute endocarditis is rapid as compared with a more insidious progression found in the subacute endocarditis. This type is associated with a fulminating course resulting in rapid destruction of the valves and a greater incidence of abscesses developing in the ring of the annulus.

The two most common invading organisms found in subacute endocarditis are *Streptococcus viridans* and *Staphylococcus epidermidis*. There is less valvular destruction, but they may cause large vegetations which may result in systemic emboli and occlusion of major arteries.[11]

Another feature that differentiates these two forms is the types of valves affected. Acute endocarditis usually affects normal valves, whereas subacute endocarditis is often found in previously damaged valves.

Regardless of the type, the pathologic process is essentially the same. One of the causative micro-organisms which is traveling in the bloodstream attaches itself to the endocardial lining of a normal valve, or a diseased, or prosthetic valve. Once attached, these organisms become enmeshed in deposits of fibrin, bacteria, platelets, and inflammatory cells which then are referred to as *vegetations*. These vegetations, which range in size and shape, settle on the valves and invade the leaflets. The color of the vegetations may vary initially from pink, red, yellow, or green, to gray when healed. Fungal infections are notorious for developing very large vegetations leading to emboli that can occlude large arteries.[9]

Vegetations interfere with normal alignment of the cusps and subsequently cause incomplete closure or regurgitation, which manifest as murmurs. The absence of a cardiac murmur has been reported in some patients (10 percent) with subacute endocarditis and in approximately one-third of patients stricken with acute endocarditis involving the left side.[9]

The clinical manifestations exhibited in patients with endocarditis are based on three underlying pathophysiologic mechanisms: generalized infection, valvular destruction, and embolism. Generalized infection accounts for such symptoms as weight loss, general malaise, anorexia, night sweats, and arthralgias. Fever is found in the majority of cases, but will vary depending on the type of infection. For example, the patient with acute endocarditis presents with a fever associated with shaking chills. With subacute endocarditis, the fever is usually an intermittent, low-grade type, and without shaking chills.

Regurgitant murmurs are associated with valvular destruction and correspond to the affected valve. For example, with mitral regurgitation, a systolic murmur results; with aortic insufficiency, the murmurs take the form of an early diastolic murmur. The regurgitation may become severe enough to produce hemodynamic alterations leading to congestive heart failure.

Embolism may result when fragments of the vegetations break off and travel downstream. Fragments on the right side of the heart may embolize to the lungs while fragments located on the left side may cause embolization to the cerebral and systemic circulation. Sepsis may occur at the site of embolic infarct in acute endocarditis, whereas secondary inflammatory reactions may result from emboli in subacute endocarditis. The spleen is reported to be the most common site of emboli in left-sided endocarditis along with the heart, brain, and kidneys. Thus, patients may manifest with splenomegaly, myocardial infarction, stroke, or renal infarction.

In addition, small emboli which migrate to the skin and mucous membranes result in certain classical findings such as Osler's nodes, Janeway's lesions, and Roth's spots. *Osler's nodes* are painful, tender, erythematous papules found in the pads of the fingers. *Janeway's lesions* are flat, tiny, irregular, non-tender red spots found on the palms of the hands and soles of the feet of some patients. *Roth's spots* are the result of retinal hemorrhages, appearing as white or yellow centers surrounded by red, irregular halos. In addition to these, patients may also exhibit splinter hemorrhages and clubbing.

The diagnosis of endocarditis is established by blood cultures. The offending organism is identified along with an assessment of the organism's sensitivity to antibiotics. In addition, anemia may also be present along with an elevation in the ESR. The white blood count (WBC) may be elevated in acute endocarditis, or it may be normal or subnormal in subacute endocarditis. In about 50 percent of cases, the urinalysis may reveal microscopic hematuria.[12]

Fluoroscopy and two-dimensional echocardiography have been found helpful in identifying vegetations and complications such as valvular ring abscesses. Figure 24-1 depicts a vegetation found on an aortic valve during echocardiography.

Medical treatment involves use of the appropriate bactericidal agent based on sensitivities. The dose of antibiotic is routinely based on bactericidal titer levels. Duration of antibiotic therapy is generally from 4 to 6 weeks. The critical-care nurse needs to be aware of the side effects of antibiotics and frequently assess the patient for signs and symptoms of toxicity.

The incidence of valvular replacement surgery is increasing in many centers. Current indications for surgery include patients who develop congestive

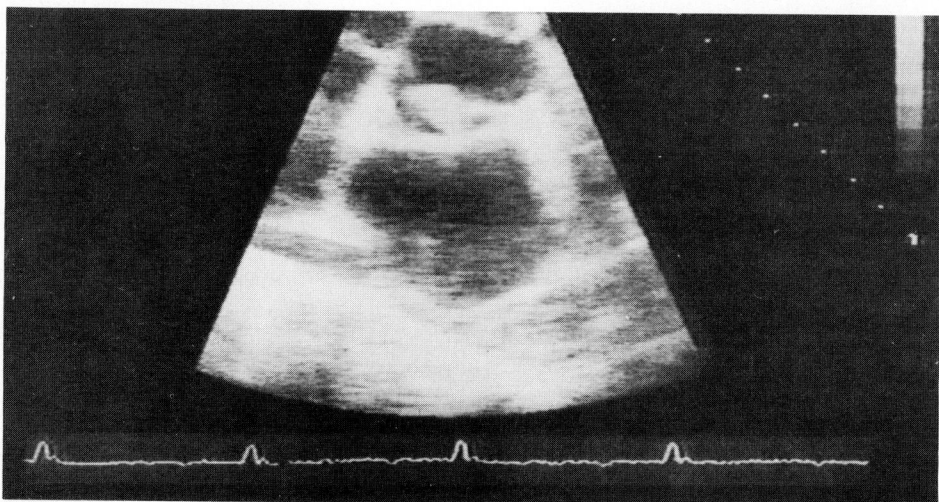

Figure 24-1 An example of a vegetation seen on an aortic valve.

heart failure from severe regurgitant valves, evidence of valvular ring abscesses, conduction disturbances, *Brucella* infection, prosthetic valve infection, and failure to control sepsis.[12] The goals of surgery are to remove infective tissue, and replace a diseased valve in order to restore valvular function.

In caring for patients with infective endocarditis, the critical-care nurse needs to employ strict aseptic technique as well as monitor for the previously mentioned complications. A widening of the pulse pressure, for instance, should alert the nurse to the possibility of worsening aortic regurgitation. Health teaching is important for both the patient and family, and should include antibiotic prophylaxis for instrumentation procedures, importance of maintaining proper oral hygiene, and discussion regarding the signs and symptoms of complications that should be immediately reported.

Valvular Dysfunction

Valvular dysfunction may result from either congenital or acquired causes. For many years, rheumatic heart disease accounted for nearly all of the acquired valvular heart disease.[13] The valves on the left side of the heart are more commonly affected due to the constant exposure to high pressures. Any abnormality of a valve, either congenital or acquired, exposes the valve to extraordinary hemodynamic stress and can thereby accelerate the

degenerative changes that cause dysfunction.[13] The degenerative changes causing a narrowing of the valve (mitral or aortic) orifice are classified as *stenosis*. Changes leading to valvular insufficiency due to improper closing of the mitral or aortic valves are classified as *regurgitation*.

Mitral Stenosis

Mitral stenosis, a narrowing of the mitral orifice, is usually caused by rheumatic fever.[14] Most patients who develop rheumatic heart disease from rheumatic fever are women. The latency period from the time of rheumatic fever to the onset of clinical symptoms of mitral stenosis is usually 19 years.[15]

Pathophysiology

The major long-term pathologic changes in the mitral valve caused by rheumatic fever are (1) fusion of the commissures; (2) fibrosis and thickening of the leaflets; (3) shortening, fibrosis, and fusion of the chordae and/or papillary muscles; and (4) calcification of the leaflets.[17] Thickening and shortening of the mitral valve structures result in a funnel-shaped valve with the valve orifice having a "fish mouth" or "buttonhole" shape.[14]

The normal mitral valve has a cross-sectional area of 4 to 6 cm². Normal flow across the valve is 150 to 200 mL per second of diastole.[16] There is usually no detectable pressure gradient across the normal mitral valve even when flow is increased with exercise.

As the valve area is reduced, the gradient across the valve increases. When the valve area is reduced to 3 cm², the gradient is approximately 2 mmHg; at 2 cm², the gradient increases to 4 to 6 mmHg, and at 1 cm², the gradient rises to 18 to 28 mmHg at rest.[15]

Critical mitral stenosis occurs when the mitral valve opening is reduced to 1 cm². This leads to elevations in left atrial pressure (LAP), which in turn leads to elevated pulmonary venous and pulmonary artery wedge pressure (PAWP). Dyspnea on exertion (especially after exercise, emotional stress, infection, or with atrial fibrillation) results from the increased rate of flow across the mitral orifice causing elevations in LAP. With a further rise to 25 to 30 mmHg, the LAP will exceed plasma oncotic pressure and episodes of orthopnea and/or paroxysmal nocturnal dyspnea (PND) develop. Right-sided heart failure may develop after chronic elevations in pulmonary capillary pressures produce pulmonary hypertension and exert increased and constant pressure against the right ventricle.

Years of elevated LAP lead to left atrial hypertrophy and may precipitate the development of atrial fibrillation. Systemic thromboembolic episodes occur in approximately 25 percent of patients with atrial fibrillation.[17]

Data Acquisition

History

The principal symptom of mitral stenosis is dyspnea. Dyspnea initially occurs with extreme exertion [New York Heart Association (NYHA) Class II], then with moderate exertion (NYHA Class III), and finally with minimal exertion with episodes of orthopnea, PND, or pulmonary edema (NYHA Class IV). Complaints of fatigue are also common with severe mitral stenosis. If atrial fibrillation has developed, patients may also complain of palpitations.

Other symptoms of mitral stenosis include hemoptysis, which may develop as frank pulmonary hemorrhage from a ruptured pulmonary vein; as frothy pink blood-tinged sputum from pulmonary edema; or as a result of pulmonary infarction.[2] Symptoms of "asthma" which develop after adolescence may also suggest mitral stenosis. Hoarseness

(Ortner's syndrome) may develop from compression of the left recurrent laryngeal nerve by a dilated left atrium, enlarged tracheobronchial lymph nodes, and a dilated pulmonary artery.[14] Systemic venous hypertension with increased jugular venous distention (JVD), hepatomegaly, ascites, splenomegaly, and peripheral edema develop when severe mitral stenosis leads to pulmonary vascular resistance and right-sided heart failure.

Thromboembolism may be the presenting symptom in some patients. The rhythm of most of these patients (80 percent) is atrial fibrillation. Thromboemboli accounted for one-fourth of all deaths in patients with mitral valve disease before the development of anticoagulation and surgical treatment. Patients who are over 35 years of age and have atrial fibrillation, a low cardiac output (CO), and dilation of the left atrial appendage are at the highest risk of emboli.[14]

Physical Assessment

Patients with severe mitral stenosis may appear with "mitral facies" (pinkish-purple patches on the cheeks). The degree of dyspnea will depend on the severity of the stenosis. Palpation reveals a point of maximum impulse (PMI) which is usually normal, and a right ventricular heave if pulmonary hypertension is present. An apical diastolic thrill may be elicited with the patient in a left lateral recumbent position.

Auscultation will usually reveal a loud S_1, normal S_2, and an opening snap heard with the diaphragm of the stethoscope. If these heart sounds are present, the classic diastolic rumble may be heard with the bell of the stethoscope near the apex with the patient in the left lateral recumbent position. The diastolic rumble and opening snap are often reduced with inspiration and augmented during expiration.[14] As the severity of mitral stenosis increases, and valve leaflets are markedly calcified or thickened, the S_1 sound will decrease in intensity while the diastolic rumble progresses from a mid-diastolic to presystolic to pandiastolic murmur.

Data from Diagnostic Procedures

The electrocardiogram (ECG) demonstrates a widened P wave in lead II that may be notched, bifid, or with a flat top (P mitrale) due to left atrial enlargement. Evidence of P mitrale is found in 90 percent of patients with significant mitral stenosis who are in normal sinus rhythm.[14] If the patient is in atrial fibrillation, the *f* waves are usually coarse (Fig. 24-2), although the voltage of the *f* wave is not an indication of left atrial size.[15] A right axis shift (mean QRS axis greater than +90°) usually occurs when the mitral valve orifice is less than 1.3 cm² and right ventricular hypertrophy has developed.

The chest x-ray may reveal a "double density" in the midportion of the cardiac silhouette, a "straight left heart border," or Kerley B lines.[17] Enlargement of the pulmonary artery, right ventri-

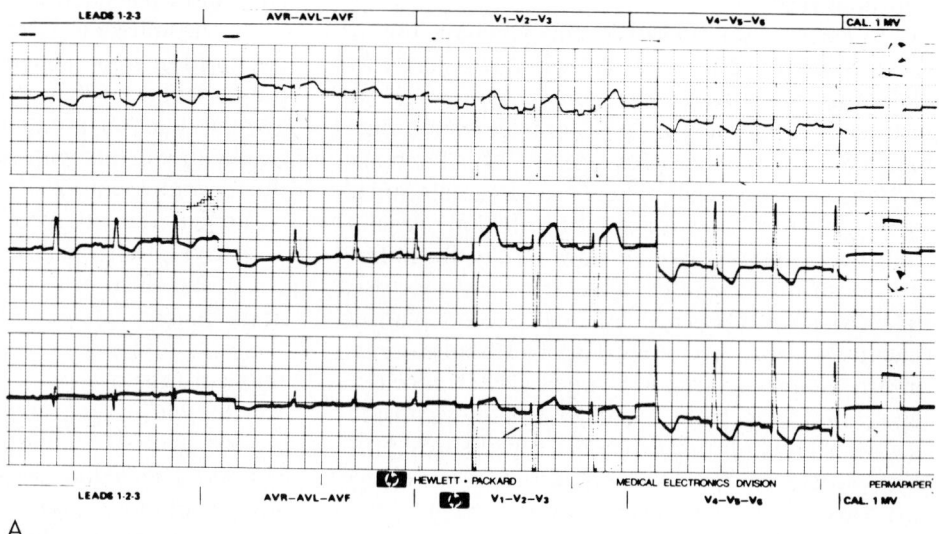

A

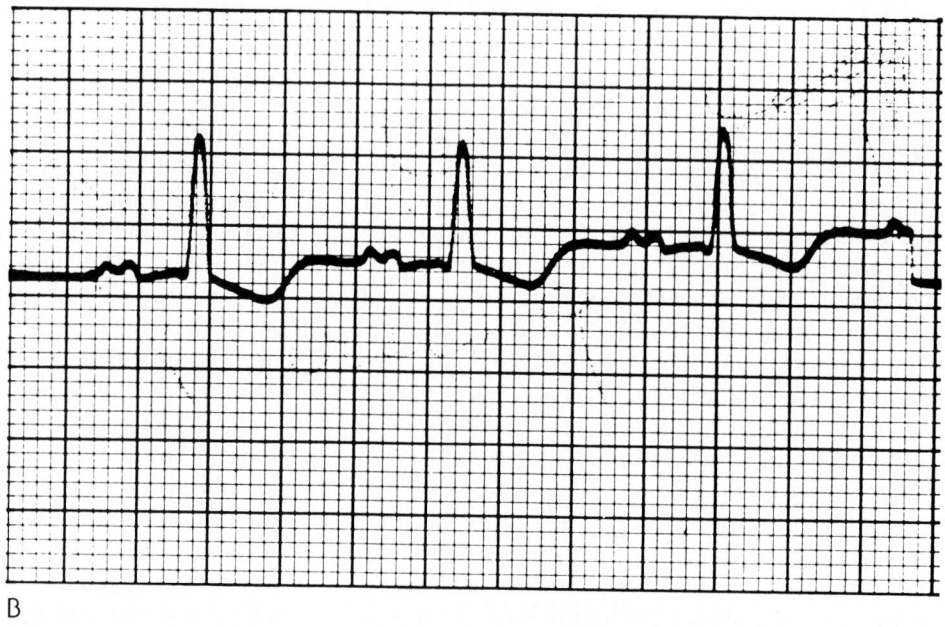

B

Figure 24-2 Electrocardiograms of a patient with mitral stenosis. *A.* 12-lead ECG of a patient with mitral stenosis. *B.* Lead II of same patient depicting mitral stenosis.

cle, and redistribution of fluid to the upper lobes become present when severe mitral stenosis leads to elevation of pulmonary artery pressures.

Echocardiographic evidence of anterior movement of the posterior mitral valve leaflet during diastole occurs in 90 percent of patients with mitral stenosis.[14] The degree of calcification of the mitral valve and measurement of left atrial size are also determined with the echocardiogram. (The reader is referred to Chap. 20 for a more in-depth discussion regarding echocardiography.)

Cardiac catheterization is useful to assess the severity of obstruction as well as adequacy of left ventricular contractility. It has been demonstrated that impaired left ventricular function is associated with poor surgical results.[17]

Medical and Surgical Interventions

Medical treatment of mitral stenosis is aimed at preventing complications such as systemic embolism or bacterial endocarditis, as well as treatment of atrial fibrillation. Prophylactic treatment for all patients with mitral stenosis includes penicillin prophylaxis for infections or surgical or any instrumentation procedures. Anemia or infections should be promptly treated. Occupations which demand strenuous physical exertion should be avoided.

Patients who become symptomatic are initially treated with oral diuretics and restriction of sodium intake. Patients with hemoptysis from elevated pulmonary vascular resistance are treated with sedation and aggressive diuresis. They should be instructed to sit in an upright position to facilitate breathing. A decrease in PAWP and congestion after sublingual nitroglycerin has been reported.[18] The relief of pulmonary congestion has been noted with combined dobutamine and isorbide dinitrate (Isordil) therapy.[19]

Arrhythmias, atrial fibrillation in particular, are treated with digitalis glycosides to slow the ventricular rate. For younger patients with mild mitral stenosis in whom atrial fibrillation has developed for the first time, cardioversion may help restore normal sinus rhythm. The patient must receive anticoagulation for 4 to 6 weeks prior to cardioversion if the duration of atrial fibrillation is known. Successful cardioversion should be followed by treatment with quinidine sulfate and digitalis glycosides to maintain normal sinus rhythm. Repeat cardioversion is not recommended if the patient reverts to atrial fibrillation while on adequate doses of quinidine sulfate or if the left atrium is significantly enlarged.[14] A group of investigators has demonstrated a low rate of successful cardioversion on patients who were symptomatic for over 3 years and with documented left atrial size of over 5.2 cm by echocardiogram.[20]

Braunwald[14] reported systemic embolism occurring in 1 to 2 percent of patients with mitral stenosis after electrical or chemical cardioversion. Risk of embolization increases in patients with paroxysmal atrial fibrillation and repeated conversions to normal sinus rhythm. Anticoagulant therapy is helpful in preventing venous thrombosis and pulmonary embolism, and reducing the frequency of systemic embolism in those patients who have experienced previous embolic episodes and who have had rheumatic heart disease and heart failure and/or atrial fibrillation.

It takes approximately 5 to 10 years after the onset of symptoms for most patients with mitral stenosis to progress from mild disability to total disability.[14] Mortality of medically treated patients at 10 years was 70 percent.[15] Surgery has been recommended for symptomatic patients, especially if thromboembolism has occurred. Patients in NYHA Class II and III are ideal surgical candidates with excellent results and low operative risk.[17] A major contraindication to surgery is active rheumatic endocarditis, which is rare.[14]

Patients who are in NYHA Class IV represent a slightly greater surgical risk. These patients should remain on bed rest with intensive medical therapy prior to surgery. If, despite intense diuresis, there continues to be a rise in blood urea nitrogen or creatinine, then surgery should not be delayed because medical therapy has reached its limit.[17]

The three surgical techniques for treatment of mitral stenosis are (1) closed mitral commissurotomy, (2) open mitral commissurotomy, and (3) mitral valve replacement. Closed mitral commissurotomy (CMC), which does not require cardiopulmonary bypass, is performed with the aid of a transventricular dilator and is an effective procedure for patients who do not also have mitral regurgitation, atrial thrombosis, or serious valve calcification with shortening or fusing of chordae. Postoperative improvement has been reported in 79 percent of patients, with 15 percent beginning to decline again after 5 years.[21] A high incidence of reoperation after the sixth and seventh (23.3 percent) and ninth and tenth (26.4 percent) years has been reported.[22] Others have reported that 86 percent of patients maintained excellent symptomatic improvement at the end of 15 years.[23] Low operative mortality for this type of surgery has been reported; 3 percent for the first CMC.[24]

Open mitral commissurotomy (OMC) has been termed the "precise" method of mitral commissurotomy. This technique, which requires cardiopulmonary bypass, allows for more precise visualization of the commissures as well as slitting of fused chordae or papillary muscles, and removal of left atrial thrombi.

Operative mortality of OMC has been reported to be between 0 to 4.4 percent and 10-year survivals have been reported to be between 81 to 95 percent.[25] Most patients who were NYHA Class III preoperatively improve to NYHA Class I or II postoperatively.

Mitral valve replacement is necessary for patients with an immobile, extremely calcified rheumatic mitral valve.[17] Hospital mortality for patients in NYHA Class IV has been reported to be 32 percent, while those in NYHA Class III were 3 percent.[26] Nine-year survival after mitral valve replacement was 72 percent.[26] Pulmonary hypertension was reported to decrease within 24 h of valve replacement for mitral stenosis.[27] The types of prosthetic heart valves which can be used to replace the native valve will be discussed at the end of this chapter.

Aortic Stenosis

Valvular aortic stenosis (AS) usually occurs from a congenital or degenerative origin rather than from a rheumatic cause.[14] Congenital malformations, which are more common in men, are usually unicuspid, bicuspid, or unequal valve leaflets. Any of these malformations may cause increased turbulent flow leading to fibrosis, calcification, and eventually to stenosis.[14]

Pathophysiology

The normal aortic valve orifice of 2.6 to 3.5 cm^2 is reduced in AS. This reduction causes obstruction to the flow of blood from the left ventricle into the aorta during ventricular systole. Left ventricular pressure increases, which results in an increase in systolic wall stress and leads to ventricular wall thickening (concentric hypertrophy). A systolic pressure gradient, known as an *aortic valve gradient,* develops between the left ventricle and aorta.[2]

The left ventricle hypertrophies as a compensatory mechanism to maintain an adequate cardiac output. A large pressure gradient across the aortic valve may be sustained for many years without a reduction in cardiac output, development of left ventricular dilation, or the development of symptoms.[14] Critical obstruction to left ventricular outflow occurs when the aortic orifice is less than approximately 0.4 cm^2 per square meter of body surface area, or when there is a peak systolic pressure gradient exceeding 50 mmHg in the presence of normal cardiac output.[14] Persistent pressure overload to the left ventricle may eventually lead to left ventricular dilatation, left atrial enlargement, and pulmonary and systemic vascular changes. Ultimately, the left ventricle may fail completely, leading to a critically low cardiac output.

Data Acquisition

History

Chest pain, syncope, and heart failure are the classic clinical manifestations of severe aortic stenosis. Exertional angina occurs in over 50 percent of patients with aortic stenosis and may be due to coronary atherosclerosis or to the markedly increased myocardial oxygen demand.[14] Dizziness or syncope, which occurs in 15 to 30 percent of patients, may result from (1) the abrupt decrease in cardiac output during effort without compensatory increase in systemic vascular resistance (SVR), (2) an abrupt fall in SVR in the presence of a fixed output, (3) or an arrhythmia.[28] Left ventricular failure eventually occurs with symptoms of fatigue, cough, progressive dyspnea on exertion, orthopnea, and paroxysmal nocturnal dyspnea.

Physical Assessment

Aortic stenosis will typically produce a harsh cres-cendo-decrescendo systolic ejection murmur which begins after the S_1 sound. This murmur is loudest at the second right sternal edge with radiation to the left lateral sternal edge and carotids and a thrill is often present. The murmur of aortic stenosis can be augmented by inhalation of amyl nitrite or by squatting or lying flat.[14] Delay in aortic valve closure often produces paradoxical splitting of the S_2 sound. Severe stenosis, however, does not produce an audible paradoxical split of S_2 since A_2 is inaudible in this case.

A widened pulse pressure with a normal diastolic pressure is common in compensated aortic stenosis. Narrowing of the pulse pressure may occur with decompensation. The prolonged ejection phase noted in aortic stenosis produces a slow rise of the arterial pulse which is best felt in the carotid artery. Left ventricular hypertrophy produces a sustained thrust or heave of the apical impulse. Displacement of the apical impulse downward and to the left occurs after left ventricular failure develops. The *a* wave on a jugular venous pulse becomes prominent once right ventricular compliance decreases sec-ondary to left ventricular failure.

Data from Diagnostic Procedures

The ECG demonstrates normal sinus rhythm with signs of left ventricular hypertrophy occurring from high-grade stenosis. Decompensated severe aortic stenosis may produce ECG evidence of left atrial hypertrophy. In one study only a small percentage (9 percent) of patients with aortic stenosis who died suddenly demonstrated normal ECGs.[28] Con-duction abnormalities such as first-degree atrioven-tricular block, bundle branch block, and intraven-tricular conduction disturbances are fairly common among patients with aortic stenosis.

Chest x-ray may demonstrate concentric hy-pertrophy of the left ventricle, poststenotic dilata-tion of the aorta, and calcification of the valve cusps. The heart shadow may depict a change in config-uration, but not in size. Cardiomegaly is visualized, however, with decompensated aortic stenosis.

The echocardiogram demonstrates a poststen-otic dilatation of the aorta, and left ventricular wall thickening. Dilatation of the left ventricle occurs with myocardial failure. Mobility of the aortic valve can also be assessed via the echocardiogram.

Cardiac catheterization is useful to determine the severity of obstruction and assess the functional status of the left ventricle as well as the coronary circulation. Chapter 20 provides a more in-depth discussion of the findings which may be obtained from cardiac catheterization.

Medical and Surgical Interventions

Medical therapy for the asymptomatic patient with aortic stenosis consists of antibiotic prophylaxis for the prevention of infective endocarditis. Those with high-grade lesions should be advised to avoid strenuous physical exertion. Digitalis glycosides are used when evidence of either an increased left ventricular volume or a decreased ejection fraction is noted. Diuretics should be used with caution since hypovolemia may decrease the elevated left ventricular end-diastolic pressure, decrease cardiac output, and produce orthostatic hypotension. The use of beta-blocking agents may depress myocardial function and may induce left ventricular failure.[14]

Atrial arrhythmias occur in less than 10 per-cent of patients with aortic stenosis.[14] The appear-ance of atrial fibrillation necessitates treatment with countershock, quinidine, or procainamide, because loss of atrial contraction may further impair left ventricular function.

Systemic emboli are rare in patients with aortic stenosis. Emboli which do occur are often due to calcific flecks coming from the aortic valve rather than from thrombi.

Patients with severe aortic stenosis with left ventricular dysfunction and myocardial ischemia have responded well to cautious administration of nitroprusside. Awan, DeMaria, Miller, Amsterdam, and Mason reported a decrease in left ventricular afterload, improved left ventricular function, and coronary flow after nitroprusside administration.[29]

Use of the intraaortic balloon pump (IABP) has also demonstrated marked clinical improve-ment in patients with decompensated aortic ste-nosis. One group of investigators reported that hemodynamic benefit from the IABP in these pa-tients was derived almost entirely from augmenta-tion of the diastolic coronary filling pressure because left ventricular systolic pressure was not decreased.[30]

Once patients with aortic stenosis become symptomatic with angina or syncope, the average survival time is 2 to 3 years. Patients with congestive heart failure demonstrate an average survival time of 1½ years.[14] Without surgery, mortality rates from onset of symptoms is approximately 25 percent at 1 year and 50 percent at 2 years, with more than half the deaths occurring suddenly.[14]

Surgical therapy primarily consists of aortic valve replacement with either mechanical or tissue valves. Surgical mortality ranges from 1 to 10 percent for patients without left ventricular failure and from 10 to 25 percent for those with left ventricular failure or a depressed ejection fraction.[14] Five-year survival has been reported to be less than 50 percent in medically treated patients while surgically treated patients' survival was 75 to 80 percent.[31] Even patients over the age of 60 at the time of surgery demonstrated improved left ventricular function and a 10-year survival of 57.5 percent using life-table analysis after surgical treatment.[32]

Innovative surgical techniques are being attempted on those patients in whom aortic valve replacement is not feasible. At one institution, a no. 21 Bjork Shiley valve was attached to the distal end of an 18-mm graft extending from the left ventricular apex to the descending aorta in a 82-year-old female with severe aortic stenosis (Fig. 24-3).

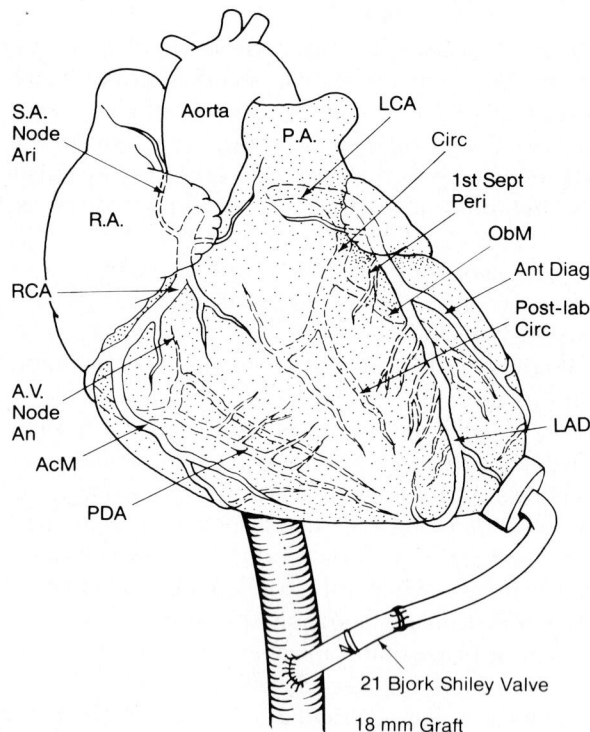

Figure 24-3 Drawing which depicts double outlet graft and insertion of a Bjork-Shiley prosthetic valve into an 82-year-old woman for aortic stenosis.

Mitral Regurgitation

Mitral regurgitation (insufficiency) occurs when the mitral valve fails to close completely, allowing blood to regurgitate back into the left atrium during ventricular systole. Pure mitral regurgitation occurs as a congenital condition which is present in neonates, infants, and young children, but is rare in adults.[33] In this condition, the mitral annulus is dilated without fusion of the commissures or obstruction to forward flow.

Chronic rheumatic heart disease remains the most common cause of mitral regurgitation. Other causes include isolated rupture of the chordae tendineae, mitral valve prolapse, ischemic papillary muscle dysfunction, and infective endocarditis. Mitral regurgitation results from a disruption of the functional components which may include the valve leaflets, papillary muscle, mitral valve annulus, chordae tendineae, or the left ventricle itself.

Pathophysiology

The degree of mitral regurgitation gradually increases over many years. The patient with chronic mitral regurgitation may remain asymptomatic for decades. The symptoms and outcome of chronic mitral regurgitation will depend on the rate of progression, onset of atrial fibrillation, development of pulmonary hypertension, and coexisting coronary artery disease.[16]

With chronic mitral regurgitation, the increased volume of blood ejected back into the left atrium will cause stretching and thinning of the atrial wall. The large, thin-walled atrium accommodates the large volume of blood ejected into it during systole. The left atrial pressure will decrease to near normal during ventricular diastole. The left ventricle dilates and becomes hypertrophied in response to the increased volume from the left atrium so that a sufficient cardiac output is maintained.[2] Pulmonary hypertension is not likely to develop in a patient with mitral regurgitation which has increased over time.

In contrast, patients with acute mitral regurgitation develop a rapid increase in left atrial pressure due to the sudden volume overload of a normal left atrium secondary to myocardial infarction, or chest trauma, which causes rupture of the papillary muscle or chordae. This sudden increase in left atrial pressure is reflected in the pulmonary vascular bed, producing interstitial edema which results in pulmonary edema.[33] Pulmonary hypertension may develop from compression of the pulmonary vascular bed. The left ventricle dilates rapidly without hypertrophy, producing a decrease in the ratio of left ventricular mass to left ventricular end-diastolic volume.[14]

The volume of mitral regurgitant flow in either chronic or acute mitral regurgitation depends on the size of the regurgitant orifice as well as on the pressure gradient between the left ventricle and left atrium. This volume of regurgitant flow is decreased by any agent which decreases left ventricular size (i.e., cardiac glycosides, diuretics, or vasodilators). Regurgitant flow is increased by any agent which increases LV size by increases in preload, afterload, or depression of myocardial function such as vasoconstrictors. A decrease in ejection fraction signifies severe impairment of contractility.

Data Acquisition

History

Patients with chronic mitral regurgitation initially complain of fatigue and, later, dyspnea on exertion. Palpitations may also occur. Symptoms of left ventricular failure frequently appear late in the course of chronic mitral regurgitation due to the gradual increase in volume overload. Hemoptysis is a rare finding in mitral regurgitation. A common complication of chronic mitral regurgitation is atrial fibrillation, which is related to the size of the left atrium and affects 75 percent of patients.[15] Other common complications include systemic emboli

(usually occurring in the presence of atrial fibrillation) and bacterial endocarditis.

Those who develop acute mitral regurgitation have been in relatively good health with an abrupt onset of symptoms. The intensity of symptoms and immediate prognosis depend on the cause and the amount of sudden volume overload to the left atrium. A patient with rupture of a few chordae from subacute bacterial endocarditis or trauma usually describes easy fatigue, dyspnea, pedal edema, and occasional intermittent chest pain, while a patient with rupture of a papillary muscle from acute myocardial infarction presents with severe hypotension and florid pulmonary edema.[34] In the latter instance, 75 percent of patients die within the first 24 h of rupture without surgical intervention and 95 percent die within the first 2 weeks.[34]

Physical Assessment

Chronic mitral regurgitation produces a carotid pulse which tends to collapse in quality from early closure of the aortic valve. This collapsing quality is less marked as the severity of mitral regurgitation increases and left ventricular failure increases. The hyperkinetic apical pulse will be displaced leftward and downward. A parasternal lift is usually present.

Auscultation of the patient with chronic mitral regurgitation reveals a widely split S_2 sound (A_2 early) accompanied by a short, mid-diastolic flow rumble. The hallmark of mitral regurgitation is a pansystolic, harsh, blowing murmur best heard at the apex and radiating to the axilla or back. This murmur can be increased or decreased with certain maneuvers. Maneuvers which decrease left ventricular volume by decreasing impedance to left ventricular outflow, decrease venous return, or increase myocardial contractility (such as sudden standing or inhalation of amyl nitrite) will result in a decreased murmur. Maneuvers which increase left ventricular volume by increase in venous return, decrease in myocardial contractility, bradycardia or increase in impedance to left ventricular emptying (such as squatting or administration of phenylephrine or methoxamine) will increase the murmur of mitral regurgitation.[14]

Patients with acute mitral regurgitation exhibit a rapid upstroke and fall-off of the carotid pulse. The jugular venous pressure may be elevated, indicating right ventricular failure. On palpation, the apical impulse may be prominent but is usually not displaced or sustained. A widely split S_2 sound (A_2 early) with increased P_2, as well as S_3 and S_4 sounds are present. An apical systolic murmur with a decrescendo character which may radiate throughout the chest is also present.

Data from Diagnostic Procedures

The ECG of a patient with chronic mitral regurgitation demonstrates normal sinus rhythm with left atrial hypertrophy in the early stage and then atrial fibrillation. As the degree of mitral regurgitation increases, evidence of left ventricular hypertrophy and associated ST-T wave changes secondary to strain may be present.

With acute mitral regurgitation, sinus tachycardia is the most obvious ECG sign. Volume overload of the left atrium may produce a large terminal negative force of the P wave in the precordial leads.

The chest x-ray of a patient with chronic mitral regurgitation initially demonstrates an increase in cardiac size due to left ventricular dilatation. As regurgitation increases, left atrial enlargement becomes evident. Pulmonary changes of upper lobe redistribution are seen when the left atrial pressure exceeds 12 to 18 mmHg. When left atrial pressure exceeds 18 to 20 mmHg, pulmonary edema is evident on the chest x-ray.

With acute mitral regurgitation, the chest x-ray shows little or no left ventricular or left atrial enlargement. Enlargement of the upper pulmonary vascular lobes as well as pulmonary edema are present on chest x-ray.

The echocardiogram is helpful in assessing the severity of regurgitation by measuring left ventricular end-diastolic dimension, septal and posterior ventricular wall motion, left atrial size, and ventricular contractility. Chronic mitral regurgitation usually produces a volume overload pattern and a large left atrium. Acute mitral regurgitation usually produces evidence of normal volume and some increase in left atrial size, a fluttering of the mitral valve leaflet, and a decrease (with ruptured papillary muscle) or hyperdynamic (with ruptured chordae) ventricular wall motion.

Radioisotope angiocardiography is useful for calculation of the ejection fraction and left ventricular cavity size to estimate the severity of chronic mitral regurgitation. Cardiac catheterization must be done prior to surgery but it is poorly tolerated by patients with acute mitral regurgitation. Cardiac catheterization is necessary to accurately quantify left ventricular size and contractility, the degree of regurgitation, and intracardiac pressures as well as other lesions or coronary artery disease. Dalen and Alpert[15] recommend that exercise hemodynamics be assessed in the catheterization laboratory for any patient with compensated chronic mitral regurgitation who demonstrates normal hemodynamics at rest. Catheterization data are useful in classifying the severity of mitral regurgitation as described by Dalen and Alpert:[15]

1. Minimal to mild mitral regurgitation (1 to 2+ on a scale of 4) = normal left ventricular end-diastolic pressure (LVEDP) and PAWP (less than 12 mmHg) at rest and exercise. Ejection fraction is greater than 55 percent.
2. Moderate chronic mitral regurgitation (3+) = marked dilatation of left atrium and ventricle. Normal or slightly increased LVEDP and PAWP at rest. Ejection fraction may be slightly decreased. Exercise may cause slight increase in ejection fraction and decrease in LVEDP due to vasodilatation, or cause an increase in LVEDP and PAWP secondary to pulmonary hypertension and an increase in mitral regurgitation.
3. Severe chronic mitral regurgitation (4+) = gross dilatation of left atrium and ventricle with increased LVEDP and PAWP at rest. Ejection fraction is less than 50 percent.

Data from cardiac catheterization are also used to determine a "regurgitant fraction," which is the ratio of blood volume regurgitated into the left atrium during systole divided by the total volume of blood ejected into both the left atrium and aorta by the left ventricle during systole. A correlation exists between the calculated regurgitant fraction and the degree of mitral regurgitation. A patient with severe chronic mitral regurgitation demonstrates a regurgitant fraction of 0.6 or greater.[15]

Cardiac catheterization for a patient with acute mitral regurgitation is necessary to determine the severity of regurgitation as well as the state of the left ventricle. A dilated, poorly contracting left ventricle may be a contraindication for surgery. Giant v waves on a PAWP tracing suggest an acute, severe regurgitation into a noncompliant left atrium.

Medical and Surgical Interventions

Medical treatment for all patients with chronic mitral regurgitation, even those who are asymptomatic, consists of antibiotic prophylaxis for any dental or surgical procedure. If atrial fibrillation develops, digitalis glycosides are given to control ventricular rate and anticoagulation is started to prevent systemic emboli. Patients with moderate mitral regurgitation (NYHA Class II) require the addition of a no-added-salt diet, but patients with moderately severe regurgitation (NYHA Class III) require addition of diuretics. If digitalis glycosides, a no-added-salt diet, and diuretics do not control left ventricular failure and the patient has severe regurgitation (NYHA Class IV), vasodilators are required.

For patients with acute mitral regurgitation, early stabilization is required to allow for identification of the responsible mechanical defect. Vasodilators are used to decrease preload and afterload because any increase in left ventricular volume may worsen mitral valve dysfunction. The PAWP should be maintained at 15 to 18 mmHg. Patients who are in shock or have severe coronary artery disease do poorly with vasodilators alone because the decrease in coronary perfusion pressure compromises left ventricular function. In this case, use of the intraaortic balloon pump should be considered to decrease afterload while maintaining perfusion pressure. Use of inotropic agents such as dopamine or dobutamine to increase arterial diastolic pressure must be monitored with caution because the increase in systemic vascular resistance may aggravate myocardial ischemia and mitral regurgitation.

For patients with chronic mitral regurgitation who are treated medically, 60 percent will survive 10 years after diagnosis. As previously mentioned, the occurrence of acute mitral regurgitation carries an extremely poor prognosis with medical treatment. Surgical mortality ranges from 2 to 7 percent in patients with pure or predominant chronic mitral regurgitation who are NYHA Class II or III.[14] Braunwald[14] recommends medical management for

4 to 6 weeks for those patients with acute mitral regurgitation prior to surgical therapy. The development of renal or pulmonary failure indicates a need for immediate surgical intervention. Five-year survival has been reported as 70 percent for patients with rheumatic mitral regurgitation and 30 percent for those with myocardial dysfunction secondary to ischemic heart disease.[14]

Surgical therapy is aimed at improving the patient's symptoms, relief of severe pulmonary hypertension, and decrease in LVEDV and mass. Patients with marked left ventricular dysfunction, however, may remain symptomatic even after surgical treatment. Patients may show a decrease in ejection fraction and an increase in end-systolic volume immediately after surgery because abolition of mitral regurgitation may increase afterload. These patients may require vasodilator treatment in the immediate postoperative period.

Surgical techniques used to treat mitral regurgitation are valve repair/reconstruction and valve replacement. Valve repair/reconstruction, in which the disrupted functional component is repaired, has shown stable functional results, a low surgical mortality, and an acceptable rate of reoperation.[35] It has been suggested that some of the left ventricular dysfunction observed after mitral valve replacement may be due to the excision of the native valve, whereas mitral valve repair retains the tethering effect of chordal attachments which may prevent postoperative dilatation.[36] David, Burns, Bacchus, and Druck[37] found a significant increase in exercise ejection fraction and stroke volume postoperatively in mitral valve replacement patients in whom the chordae and papillary muscles were preserved.

Mitral Valve Prolapse

Introduction

One of the most prevalent valvular abnormalities is mitral valve prolapse (MVP). It has been estimated that 5 to 10 percent of the population are afflicted with this condition. Typically, it is described as a displacement (prolapse) of the posterior cusp of the mitral valve in a posterior direction into the left atrium during systole. This syndrome has been given many synonyms—Barlow's syndrome, floppy mitral valve syndrome, and mitral leaflet prolapse—all of which are used interchangeably.

This syndrome has a propensity for women between the ages of 20 to 40 years, although it has been detected in males of all ages. It has also been suggested that there is a hereditary link because of a familiar tendency for MVP to occur in families. Moreover, transmission of this disorder is theorized to be an autosomal dominant trait.[14] In addition, MVP has a tendency to prevail concomitantly with such extracardiac defects as scoliosis, kyphosis, pectus excavatum, and carninatum. It has also been known to coexist with ischemic heart disease and mitral stenosis.

Pathophysiology

Mitral valve prolapse may result in mitral regurgitation. This occurs when the posterior leaflet bulges back into the left atrium during the maximal ejection phase of systole. This billowing back of the leaflet places stress on the chordae tendineae and papillary muscles, which decreases their ability to properly close the valve. As a result, blood is allowed to flow in a retrograde fashion into the left atrium during ventricular contraction instead of flowing forward through the aortic valve.

Data Acquisition

History

Most patients are asymptomatic with this syndrome. When symptoms do occur, patients usually report atypical chest discomfort, palpitations, minimal dyspnea, fatigue, and anxiety. The chest discomfort is atypical of anginal pain in that it is of longer duration, not precipitated by exertion, and manifested as brief attacks of severe, piercing pain localized at the apex. The critical-care nurse will need to differentiate this pain from angina, especially in an MVP patient who has coexisting coronary artery disease. Palpitations are usually the result of arrhythmias that may be a manifestation of the increased adrenergic tone found in patients with MVP. This outpouring of catecholamines could also be responsible for the dyspnea and anxiety which frequently accompany the palpitations.

Physical Assessment

Most cases of MVP are diagnosed on routine physical examination. The most specific sign of this syndrome is the presence of a nonejection click on auscultation. This click is depicted as a snapping extra heart sound which tends to occur in mid- to late systole. It is generally heard best at the lower left sternal border or at the apex. Positioning of the patient into the left lateral decubitus position or in an upright position enhances the click. The straining phase of a Valsalva maneuver or the inhalation of amyl nitrite will also produce a more audible click. The presence of an apical systolic murmur varies with the degree of mitral regurgitation. This systolic murmur is depicted as a late systolic crescendo-type which can be loud and musical. Murmurs which become holosystolic in nature are usually an indication of pronounced mitral valve prolapse resulting in a more severe form of mitral regurgitation.

Data from Diagnostic Procedures

The ECG may reveal some abnormalities in patients who are symptomatic with MVP. Typically, there can be inverted T waves and nonspecific ST segment changes in the inferior as well as left precordial leads. These changes can be a manifestation of the ischemia to the papillary muscles due to the strain placed on these muscles by the prolapsed valve leaflets.

A multitude of arrhythmias have been reported in some patients with this disorder, the most serious being ventricular tachycardia and ventricular fibrillation, which are found in patients who also manifest the aforementioned ECG changes.

Echocardiography, specifically two-dimensional, is regarded by some as the single best technique to define the disorder. Typically, what is seen on the echocardiogram is the posterior mitral valve leaflet bulging back into the left atrium during systole.[14]

Stress ECGs and thallium 201 exercise scans are employed when there is a need to differentiate MVP from coronary artery disease. This is especially important when patients with suspected MVP have chest discomfort.

Left ventricular angiography may be used when the degree of regurgitation needs to be evaluated. This invasive procedure is not, however, routinely done to confirm the diagnosis of MVP.

The angiographic procedure permits visualization of valve leaflet movement during systole. The integrity of the valve leaflets can also be seen during this procedure. It has been noted on angiography that some patients with MVP have decreased ventricular contraction, dilatation, and even calcification of the mitral annulus.[14] As an adjunct in evaluating the severity of the mitral regurgitation (MR), volumes and pressures are obtained to ascertain the hemodynamic consequences of the MR.

Medical and Surgical Interventions

Most patients with MVP are asymptomatic, as previously stated. In this subset of patients, no treatment is recommended unless ECG abnormalities are documented or signs of advanced MR are present. Asymptomatic patients need reassurance that their condition is benign and usually uncomplicated. They also need to be told that their prognosis for life is good.

Patients who are asymptomatic but who have a systolic murmur require sooner follow-up. The question of prophylaxis for bacterial endocarditis, which is a well-documented complication, remains controversial. Braunwald[14] recommends antibiotic prophylaxis in patients with a midsystolic click and/ or systolic murmur.

Beta blockers, especially propranolol, are employed for patients with documented arrhythmias and for the group of patients with increased adrenergic tone. Propranolol is also used to decrease the tension on the stretched chordae tendineae.

Digoxin has also been recommended for use in relieving chest pain in patients with MVP along with concomitant supraventricular arrhythmias. In a double-blind crossover study of 23 patients with MVP, digoxin reduced the incidence and severity of chest pain compared with control and placebo groups.[38] It also favorably affected the incidence of frequent supraventricular arrhythmias but was associated with a significant number of asymptomatic bradyarrhythmias. Thus, when digoxin is used, careful monitoring for bradyarrhythmias is warranted.

Surgical treatment of patients with MVP has been reported in the medical literature. Mitral annuloplasty is a surgical procedure useful in patients who present with such major symptoms as chest pain, arrhythmias, and dyspnea.[38] This procedure provides relief of one or more symptoms in 60 percent of patients as reported in a retrospective study.[41] Mitral valve replacement has also been performed in patients with refractory ventricular arrhythmias[40] and severe atypical chest pain.[39]

The majority of patients with MVP are never admitted to a critical-care unit. Only patients with severe MR or refractory ventricular arrhythmias are suitable candidates for admission to this setting. Nursing therapies for this subset of patients are the same as for patients with mitral regurgitation and are discussed under that section.

Aortic Regurgitation

Aortic regurgitation occurs when the aortic valve fails to close completely, allowing blood to regurgitate back into the left ventricle during ventricular diastole. This process may be either of a chronic or acute nature. Pathologic processes which affect the aortic valve, leading to chronic aortic regurgitation, are inflammation (due to rheumatic fever, syphilis, rheumatoid arthritis, etc.), structural (unicuspid, bicuspid, aneurysm), disruptive (trauma, infective endocarditis, dissection), congenital, or stress from hypertension.[42] Acute aortic regurgitation may occur from infective endocarditis, dissecting aortic aneurysm, chest compression injuries, spontaneous rupture of the valve cusps, or postoperative disruption of the valve leaflets during aortic valvuloplasty.[43]

Pathophysiology

Aortic regurgitation produces a volume overload to the left ventricle during diastole. The amount of regurgitant volume into the left ventricle determines if the volume overload is mild, moderate, or severe. Factors which determine the amount of regurgitant volume are (1) the area of the regurgitant valve orifice, (2) the amount of diastolic pressure gradient between the aorta and left ventricle, and (3) the duration of diastole.[42]

In chronic aortic regurgitation, the left ventricle compensates for the gradual increase in preload by dilatation and concentric hypertrophy. Patients with acute aortic regurgitation do not have time for this adaptation to occur. Therefore, patients with chronic aortic regurgitation develop an increased end-diastolic volume without increased end-diastolic pressure, while those with acute aortic regurgitation develop a dramatic increase in left ventricular end-diastolic pressure with only minor increases in end-diastolic volume.

Data Acquisition

History and Physical Assessment

Patients with chronic aortic regurgitation may be asymptomatic for decades. When symptoms do occur, the patient usually complains of chest discomfort and/or symptoms of congestive heart failure (especially dyspnea and fatigue). Patients with acute aortic regurgitation present with symptoms of severe left-sided failure (dyspnea at rest, orthopnea, paroxysmal nocturnal dyspnea, fatigue, exhaustion) which have occurred suddenly. Heart failure, in acute aortic regurgitation, is usually progressive and rapidly fatal unless surgical intervention is accomplished.[43] Symptoms of low forward cardiac output (fatigue and exhaustion) are overshadowed by symptoms of pulmonary congestion in patients with acute aortic regurgitation.

Hemodynamic findings of patients with acute, severe aortic regurgitation and chronic, severe, decompensated aortic regurgitation are similar except for the marked increase in left ventricular end-diastolic and end-systolic volume seen in the chronic patient. Arterial blood pressure usually demonstrates a low diastolic pressure (the Korotkoff sounds may even reach zero) in a patient with moderate or severe chronic aortic regurgitation. Because the systolic blood pressure is normal or increased, the patient with chronic aortic regurgitation usually demonstrates a widened pulse pressure, but patients with acute aortic regurgitation do not usually develop widened pulse pressures. The carotid arterial pulse will rise to a single, rapidly collapsing peak with acute aortic regurgitation. A pulsus alternans may be present in acute severe aortic regurgitation, but is unusual in patients with chronic aortic regurgitation.[44]

The apical pulse may be normal with acute aortic regurgitation. A parasternal lift indicative of right ventricular dilatation may be felt after pulmonary hypertension has developed. With chronic aortic regurgitation, the apical impulse is displaced to the left and downward. Left ventricular enlargement produces a large and forceful impulse. A water-hammer pulse may be present due to the forceful ejection of blood in early systole and regurgitation during early diastole.

On auscultation, the S_1 sound may be decreased or absent if premature closure of the mitral valve occurs, which makes it difficult to separate systole from diastole in acute aortic regurgitation. The S_2 quality varies, depending on the integrity of the aortic valve leaflet—if intact, the S_2 sound is well-preserved, but if destroyed, the S_2 is absent. An S_3 sound is a common finding in the patient with aortic regurgitation. The diastolic murmur of aortic regurgitation is best heard with the diaphragm of the stethoscope with the patient sitting up or leaning forward and expiring deeply.[42] The duration of the murmur is usually short, soft, and of medium pitch. With chronic aortic regurgitation of mild severity, the diastolic murmur occurs early with a decrescendo pattern. The Austin Flint murmur of antegrade flow across a decreasing mitral valve orifice is usually mid-diastolic with acute severe aortic regurgitation, and mid-diastolic and/ or presystolic with chronic severe aortic regurgitation.[43] A systolic ejection murmur is common in both acute and chronic aortic regurgitation.

Data from Diagnostic Procedures

The ECG will reflect left ventricular hypertrophy, especially in the precordial leads. Conduction disturbances may occur with aortic regurgitation secondary to inflammatory processes. The ECG is usually normal except for sinus tachycardia, without evidence of left ventricular hypertrophy with acute, severe aortic regurgitation.

As the severity of chronic aortic regurgitation increases, the left ventricular contour enlarges, producing a "boot-shaped" heart silhouette on chest x-ray. The aortic knob and ascending aorta become prominent in patients with moderate to severe chronic aortic regurgitation. Patients with acute aortic regurgitation do not demonstrate cardiac enlargement. These patients exhibit increased venous redistribution to the upper lobes because of pulmonary venous and capillary hypertension secondary to an increased left ventricular end-diastolic pressure and left atrial pressure.

Echocardiographic evidence of increased diastolic chamber dimension occurs with chronic aortic regurgitation but not with acute aortic regurgitation. The increased volume of the left ventricle during diastole may also cause fluttering of the anterior mitral valve leaflet.[42]

Cardiac catheterization is used to document the severity and extent of aortic regurgitation as well as left ventricular function. Aortic regurgitation is gauged on a 1-to-4+ scale according to severity (minimal to severe). No increase in left ventricular filling pressures occurs with compensated chronic aortic regurgitation. Left ventricular filling pressures increase as volume overload increases. Hemodynamic abnormalities occur at rest in 57 percent of patients in NYHA Class IV and 30 percent of patients in NYHA Class I, and with exercise in 100 percent of patients in NYHA Class IV and 47 percent of patients in NYHA Class I.

Medical and Surgical Interventions

Medical therapy for chronic aortic regurgitation consists of antibiotic prophylaxis for all patients. Once left ventricular failure develops, digitalis glycosides, diuretics, and vasodilators are necessary to improve left ventricular function as well as to reduce the aortic regurgitant fraction. The medical management in acute aortic regurgitation consists of minimizing congestive heart failure. Digitalis glycosides, diuretics, as well as nitroprusside (to maintain a PAWP between 16 to 20 mmHg), and inotropic agents (dopamine or dobutamine) to augment myocardial contractility may be necessary. Use of the intraaortic balloon pump (IABP) is contraindicated in patients with significant aortic regurgitation because the augmented diastolic pressure from the IABP is transmitted directly to the left ventricle, compounding the deleterious effects of valvular insufficiency.[45] One group of investigators has reported favorable hemodynamic effects using nifedipine and include a decrease in preload and afterload while maintaining left ventricular function.[46] These beneficial effects were demonstrated at rest as well as with exercise.[47] Patients with chronic aortic regurgitation have demonstrated long-term benefits of afterload reduction using hydralazine.[48]

The correct timing of surgery for patients with chronic aortic regurgitation is a debated issue.

Surgical mortality after aortic valve replacement was reported by Osamura and Tasaka[49] to be 12.9 percent compared with 35 percent mortality in medically treated patients. Patients with acute aortic regurgitation due to active endocarditis had an 80 percent mortality after surgery while those with chronic aortic regurgitation who had surgery within 3 years of symptoms of heart failure had a mortality rate of zero.[49] Braunwald[14] reported a mortality range of 5 to 10 percent in surgical patients. Early surgery for severe aortic regurgitation with left ventricular dysfunction has been recommended to prevent further left ventricular decompensation. After aortic valve replacement, patients who fail to show a decrease in heart size during the first 6 months have demonstrated a 57 percent mortality compared with 15 percent mortality for those who did show a decrease in heart size.[42] Evidence of severe left ventricular dysfunction preoperatively has been associated with poor postoperative prognosis.[50]

Nursing Interventions

A complete nursing assessment of the patient with valvular heart disease consists of a biopsychosocial assessment. Gordon's functional health pattern assessment is one type of assessment tool which provides such a holistic view of the patient (see Chap. 20).

This tool guides the nurse in gathering patient data regarding function within eleven areas called *functional pattern areas*. They include the following: health perception–health management pattern, nutritional and metabolic pattern, elimination pattern, activity and exercise pattern, cognitive and perceptual pattern, role-relationship pattern, sexuality and reproductive pattern, coping and stress tolerance pattern, and value-belief pattern.

When this information is combined with data obtained from the physical examination and diagnostic tests, the nurse has a complete biopsychosocial database from which to deduce both collaborative patient problems, which have a medical etiology and in which a number of disciplines may participate in the treatment, and nursing problems or diagnoses, which may be treatable within the scope of nursing. The nurse in planning care must identify and prioritize areas of patient problems. A plan of care aimed at alleviating the etiology of the patient's problem must be applied and evaluated for problem resolution to occur.

If the problem to be treated is a collaborative problem, the nurse then utilizes medical interventions prescribed by physician orders or parameters to optimally treat the disorder. Nursing enters into the treatment by individualizing those set orders for each patient to minimize the patient's discomfort and promote optimal treatment success by patient interaction, treatment planning, and continual assessment.

Nursing diagnoses for the patient with valvular dysfunction are classified into collaborative, actual, and potential problems. Patient outcomes, nursing interventions, and evaluation will be discussed for the collaborative and actual problem.

Collaborative Diagnosis I

Congestive heart failure secondary to (1) hemodynamic factors (preload, afterload, left ventricular dysfunction); (2) electrical factors (atrial fibrillation, sinus or atrial tachycardia, ventricular dysrhythmias, conduction disturbances); and (3) structural factors (papillary muscle dysfunction, ruptured chordae, calcification).

Goal
The patient will maintain optimum hemodynamic, electrical, and structural stability while in the critical-care unit.

Interventions

1. Monitor and assess the patient's blood pressure, pulse, respiratory status (dyspnea, orthopnea, pulmonary edema), heart sounds (S_1, S_2, systolic and diastolic murmurs), apical pulses, jugular venous distention, hepatic enlargement, and peripheral edema. Assessment should be done based on the patient's condition (every 10 to 15 min during unstable periods, every 4 h when stable).
2. Hemodynamic monitoring of arterial pressure, pulmonary artery pressure, pulmonary wedge pressure, and cardiac output to assess cardiac function. Measurements should be taken as prescribed by the physician based on the patient's condition.
3. Administer medications as prescribed: digitalis glycosides, diuretics, and vasodilators, and evaluate patient's response to therapy.
4. Monitor hemodynamic status of patient with intraaortic balloon pump (IABP) when applicable. Assess timing of IABP to assure maximum hemodynamic benefit to patient.
5. Assess degree of oxygenation by obtaining arterial blood gases and administer oxygen if necessary.
6. Assess the patient's fluid status (daily weight, intake and output, serum BUN, creatinine and electrolytes, urinary specific gravity).
7. Assess the patient for signs of cardiogenic shock (hypotension, tachycardia, urine output less than 30 mL/h, decreased peripheral perfusion, increased respiratory rate, mental status change).
8. Assess the patient's electrical conduction system by continuous ECG monitoring and 12-lead ECG recordings for evidence of electrical disturbances (such as sinus or atrial tachycardia, atrial fibrillation, ventricular dysrhythmias, or conduction disturbances).
9. Administer medications to control ventricular rate (digitalis glycosides, verapamil) and rhythm (quinidine sulfate, procainamide) as prescribed.
10. Assess for signs of acute mitral or aortic regurgitation (dyspnea at rest, fatigue, PND, pulmonary edema, hepatomegaly, hypotension, pedal edema). Collaborate with physician for therapeutic interventions (such as diuretics, fluid restriction, etc.).

Evaluation
Present stability is evidenced by electrical evidence of normal sinus rhythm, a controlled ventricular rhythm and rate.

Nursing Diagnosis I

Self-care deficit related to activity intolerance.

Goal
Patient's present activity level will not deteriorate while in the critical-care setting.

Interventions

1. Assess patient's classification of disease status according to NYHA classification system.
2. Assist patient to complete those activities of daily living that do not lead to excess increase in heart rate, blood pressure, respiratory rate, or electrical disturbances.
3. Provide adequate periods of rest for the patient between therapeutic care activities (such as completion of activities of daily living, therapeutic tests).
4. Plan and implement incremental increase in activity (such as passive or active range of motion while on bed rest, increase in active participation in activities of daily living).
5. Instruct the patient about signs of increased fatigue or exercise intolerance (such as increased heart rate, respiratory rate, shortness of breath).
6. Encourage patient to rest and/or decrease level of activity if the signs or symptoms of exercise intolerance are present.
7. Help patient prioritize activities most important for him or her to maintain.
8. Develop a plan to enable patient to achieve desired activities.
9. Assess the patient's readiness to learn energy conservation measures.

Evaluation

Patient demonstrates increased activity by reporting decreased shortness of breath. Patient verbalizes an increase in activity tolerance. Patient demonstrates an appropriate heart rate, blood pressure, and respiratory rate with increased activity.

Potential Nursing Diagnoses

Patients with a diagnosis of valvular dysfunction face the following potential nursing diagnoses:

1. Potential for injury related to infection on native or prosthetic valves or anticoagulation therapy
2. Potential ineffective coping secondary to knowledge deficit regarding illness, unmet expectations, unrealistic perceptions, or inadequate support systems
3. Potential sleep-pattern disturbances related to inactivity

The nursing management of a patient with valvular dysfunction who presents to the critical-care unit is challenging. The patient is in a state of hemodynamic instability whether it is related to acute valvular dysfunction secondary to another disease process (acute myocardial infarction) or to decompensation as a result of chronic valvular dysfunction. Intensive medical and nursing management is necessary to stabilize the patient and prepare for the possibility of valvular heart surgery.

Prosthetic Heart Valves

Introduction

The ideal prosthetic heart valve does not exist! Since the implantation of the first prosthetic valve in 1952 by Hufnagel, various types of prostheses (mechanical and biologic) have been introduced, but many of these have failed. Failure has often been attributed to poor hemodynamic performance, high incidence of thrombosis on the valve surface leading to obstruction and/or emboli, mechanical failure, cracking or fracture of valve components, excessive hemolysis, rapid degeneration, and wear of the device.[51,52] Characteristics that are considered desirable in the design of an ideal substitute valve include: (1) durability, (2) optimal hemodynamic performance, (3) absence of thrombogenicity, (4) minimal hemolysis, (5) resistance to infection, (6) quiet movement, (7) low cost, and (8) ease of insertion.[53,54]

Achieving optimal hemodynamic performance is considered one of the most important features of prosthetic heart valves. The aim in the design of an artificial valve is to permit laminar as opposed to turbulent flow. In order to achieve laminar flow, the direction of flow through the valve should ideally be central and smooth. If the construction of the valve is such that turbulent flow is created, then complications may develop, such as intimal proliferation, thrombosis formation leading to obstruction and/or embolization, and, finally, hemolysis. Furthermore, the transvalvular gradient which normally should be zero is increased with turbulent flow patterns.

In the discussion to follow, it will become obvious that although many significant advance-

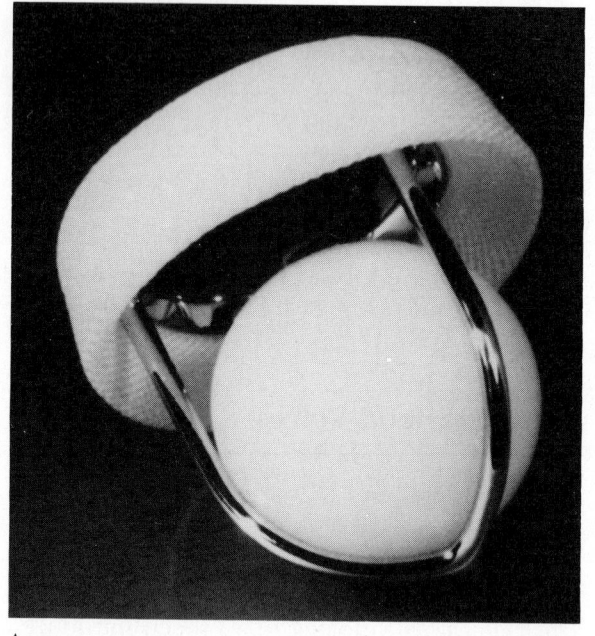

A

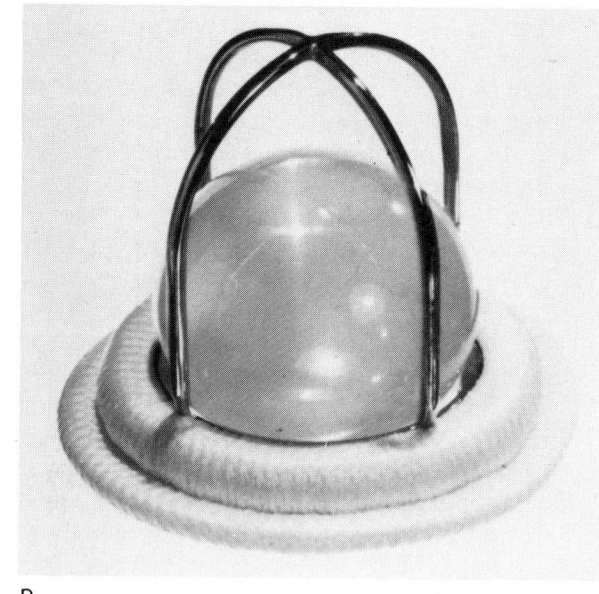

B

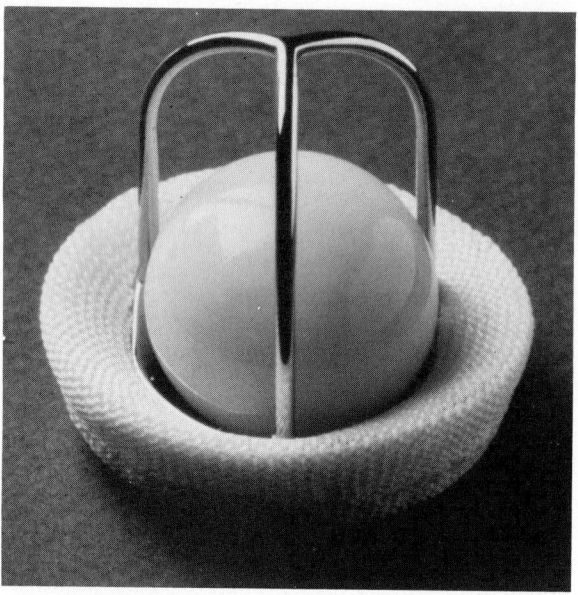

C

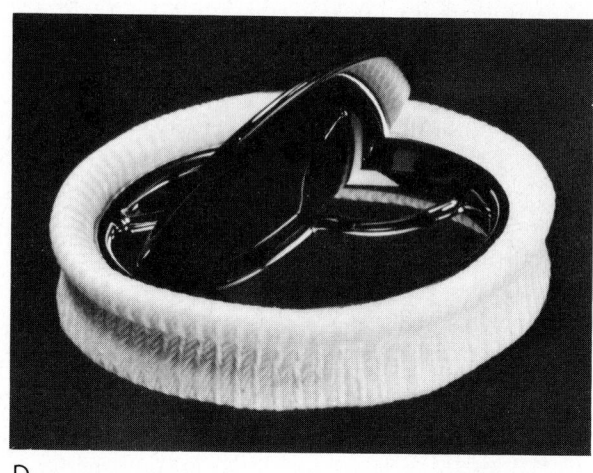

D

Figure 24-4 Prosthetic replacement valves: *A.* Starr-Edwards ball-cage valve, model 1200, aortic position. *B.* Starr-Edwards, model 6120. *C.* Starr-Edwards, model 1260. *D.* Bjork-Shiley, spherical disc valves, aortic position.

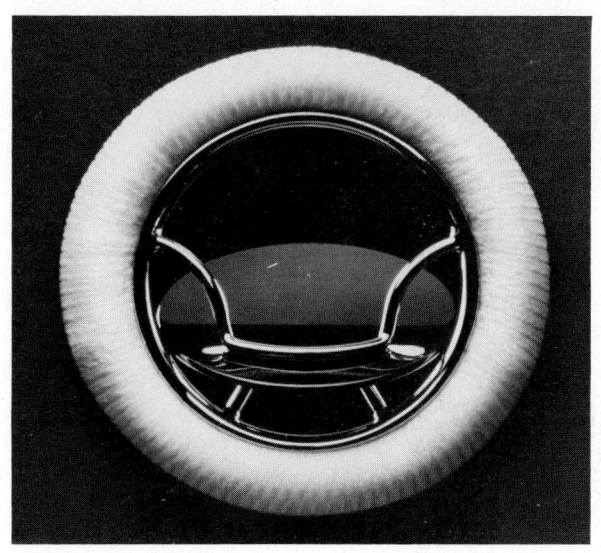

E

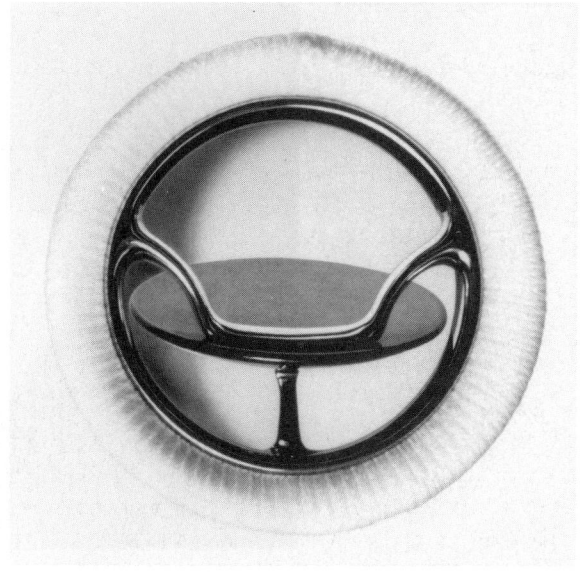

F

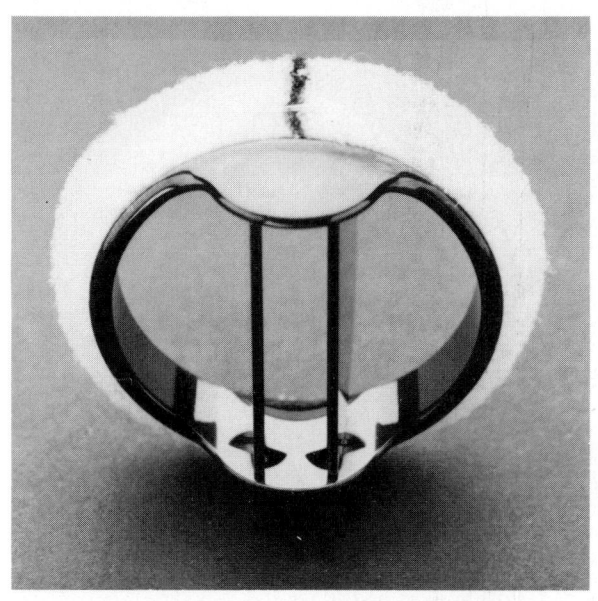

G

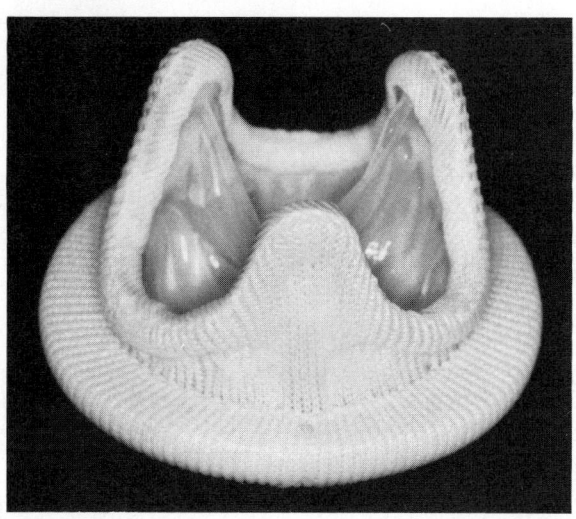

H

Figure 24-4 (Continued)   *E.* Bjork-Shiley, mitral position. *F.* Bjork-Shiley, monostrut valve. *G.* St. Jude medical heart valve, aortic position. *H.* Hancock porcine mitral valve.

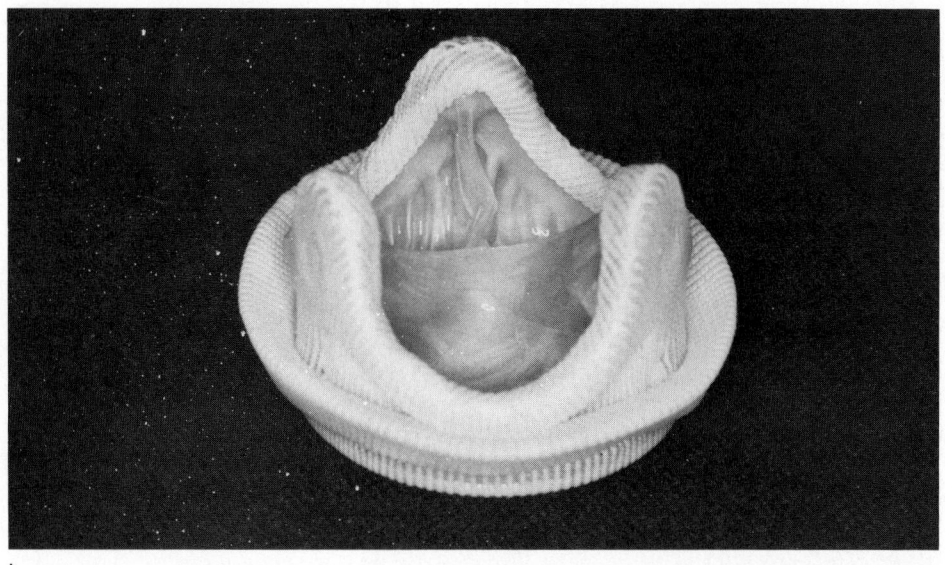

I

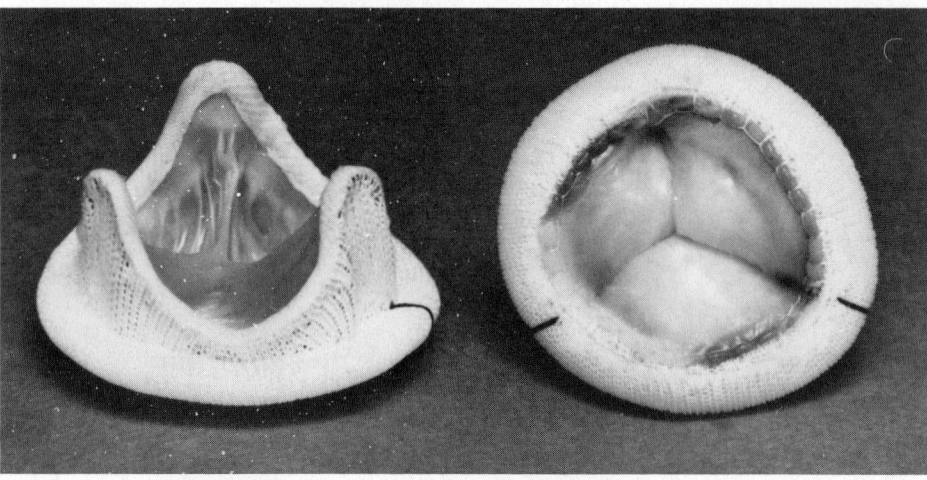

J

Figure 24-4 (Continued) *I.* Hancock porcine aortic valve. *J.* Carpentier-Edwards porcine valve, mitral position.

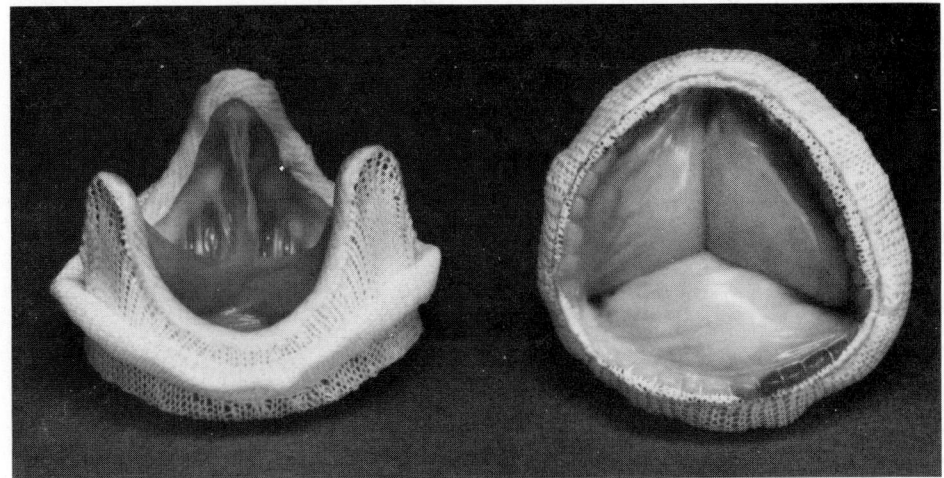

K

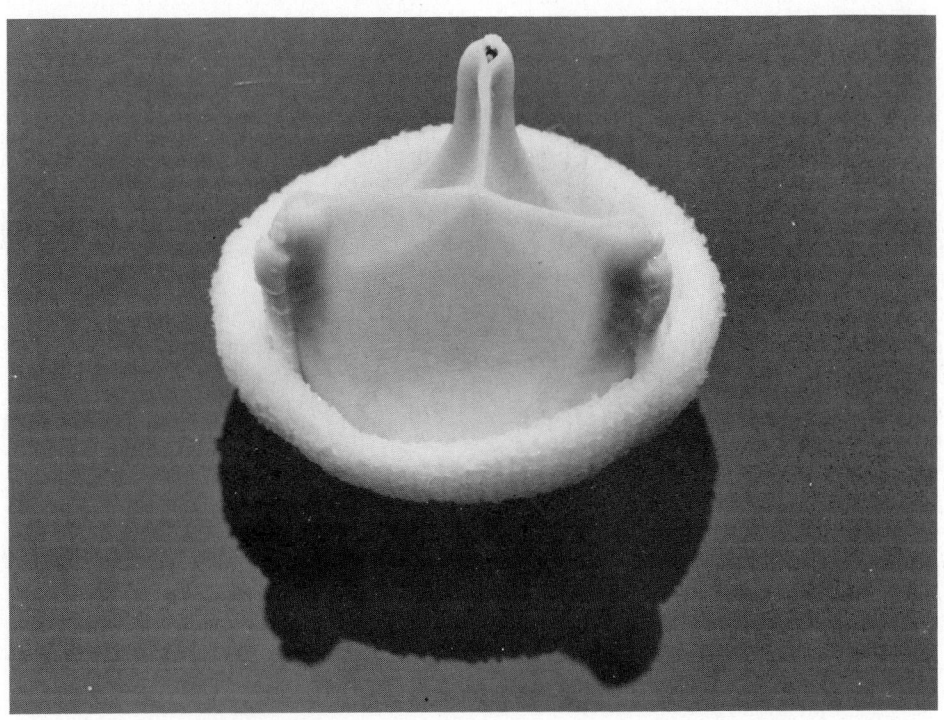

L

Figure 24-4 (Continued)   *K.* Carpentier-Edwards porcine valve, aortic position. *L.* Ionescu Shiley pericardial xenograft. *(A, B, C, J, and K courtesy of American Edwards Laboratories, Santa Ana, CA. D, E, F, and L courtesy of St. Jude Medical, Inc., One Lillehei Plaza, St. Paul, MN. H and I courtesy of Johnson & Johnson Cardiovascular, Anaheim, CA.)*

ments have been made in the development of artificial valves, no type of valve to date has successfully met all these ideal characteristics.

Mechanical versus Biologic (Tissue) Valves

Prosthetic heart valves are classified into two broad categories: (1) mechanical, and (2) biologic (tissue) prostheses. Mechanical valves include the two most commonly employed types, the caged-ball and tilting disk valves. Another type of mechanical valve that has virtually ceased to be implanted is the caged-disk valve. These valves were associated with a high degree of obstruction, thrombosis, and hemolysis.[54]

The caged-ball is the oldest type of valve. It has been used extensively since 1960. Models of this type include the Starr-Edwards, Harken, Smeloff-Cutter, DeBakey, Magovern, and Brownwell-Cutter. In the early years, some of these valves were associated with prosthetic disproportion in that these large, cumbersome valves were placed into small annuli which obstructed blood flow.[55] Since that time, use of the caged-ball prostheses has been recommended only in patients with aortic or mitral regurgitation in whom there is an enlarged left ventricle or ascending aorta.[54] These valves as a group also have a tendency to form thrombi, a problem which plagues all mechanical prostheses. Thus, patients with these devices require permanent anticoagulation therapy. Another undesirable problem is that these valves are audible.

Caged-ball prostheses also have less than desirable hemodynamic characteristics. Blood flow through these valves is not central, leading to all the complications mentioned with turbulent flow patterns. It is important to mention that hemolysis from a clinical standpoint is not problematic because the bone marrow under normal conditions is able to overcome the development of anemia and thrombocytopenia.[54] Another undesirable feature of these valves is that they are the most audible of all the prosthetic valves. This can be a nuisance to some patients.

The one important advantage of the caged-ball prostheses is durability. They are not as prone to rapid degeneration and wear and have an excellent record of being implanted for up to 20 years.[14]

The earlier models [Wada-Cutter, Lillehei-Kaster, and Bjork-Shiley (spherical disk model)] of tilting disk valves have been virtually discontinued since 1977. They have been replaced with a newer generation of valve models [Omniscience, Hall-Kaster, Bjork-Shiley (convexo-concave model), and St. Jude]. The overall major advantage in the design is the ability to permit semicentral or central blood flow in the case of the St. Jude model. Therefore, these valves have a minimal transvalvular gradient. They are not plagued as much with thrombi, although anticoagulation therapy is still recommended with all these models.

It was initially thought that the St. Jude valve might not require anticoagulants; however, case reports in the literature have indicated the formation of thrombi on this valve.[56] Failure to adequately anticoagulate patients may result in thromboemboli and fatal dysfunction (total obstruction of these devices). According to Braunwald,[14] the peak incidence of thromboemboli is in the first postoperative year. The uncertainty regarding the question of durability is attributed to the recent introduction of the St. Jude valve for valve replacements. Data collected in the next decade will assist in answering this question.

The first biologic tissue valve was implanted in 1962 by Heimbecker.[51] Since that time, a number of tissue types classified as isografts, allografts, and xenografts have been employed. Table 24-1 lists the various types of tissue valves and their source of origin.

In the 1960s, isografts were initially considered to be quite satisfactory. The use of the native pulmonic valve to replace the diseased aortic valve was first reported by Ross in 1967. He then replaced the native pulmonic valve with a homograft.[51] This technique has been virtually abandoned because of the prolonged operation time involved and the fact that durability could be attained with newer biologic valves. Fascia lata was fashioned to form a trileaflet aortic valve. Initially, the early results reported with this valve were excellent. After clinical investigation over several years, fascia lata valves were found to have a high incidence of endocarditis and rapid tissue degeneration.[51] Thus, long-term durability could not be achieved and they were discontinued in the early 1970s.

Table 24-1 Classification of Biologic Valves

Types	Source
Allograft (isograft)	Fascia lata, pulmonic valve
Homologous (allograft)	Cadaver aortic valve, dura mater
Heterologous (xenograft)	Bovine aortic valve, porcine aortic valve, bovine pericardium

Source: P. E. Oyer and E. B. Stinson, Biologic Valves. In W. W. L. Glenn, Ed., *Thoracic and Cardiovascular Surgery,* Norwalk, CT: Appleton-Century-Crafts Co., 1983.

Availability of allograft tissue limited its use. Procurement of sufficient numbers of donors has been unsuccessful in supplying the number of patients requiring valve replacement. However, allograft valves are still employed by some physicians in England and New Zealand.[55]

Currently, the most extensively used biologic valve is the xenograft. Xenograft valves which have been frequently implanted are the porcine (Hancock, Carpentier-Edwards) and the bovine pericardium (Ionescu-Shiley) molded from the pericardium of 16-to-18-month-old calves. The use of bovine aortic valves is restricted because of the inability to obtain a wide range of available sizes. The major advantage of the xenografts is their minimal thrombogenicity. Long-term anticoagulation therapy is generally not necessary. Isolated reports of thromboembolic events have occurred predominantly during the first 3 months with the xenograft implanted in the mitral position.[14] Therefore, anticoagulants may be ordered by some physicians for up to 6 months following mitral valve replacement. Circumstances that may require long-term anticoagulation with implanted xenograft valves are chronic atrial fibrillation, and patients with enlarged left atria or with documented thromboembolic events.[14]

The most serious disadvantage with the porcine xenograft is its clinical durability. Progressive deterioration and calcification on the valve surfaces of porcine tissue valves have occurred as early as 5 to 7 years postoperatively.[57] The question of durability for the bovine pericardial valve cannot be determined because it has only been clinically available since 1977.

Another disadvantage of the porcine xenografts relates to its structural design in small sizes. Small-sized porcine valves tend to have a small orifice size. This renders the valves stenotic and as a result they have higher transvalvular gradients than their mechanical counterparts in the same size. Moreover, when implanted into a small annulus they can be obstructive to flow. Furthermore, they are technically more difficult to insert. Thus, it is apparent that their use is prohibited in small annuli.

By contrast, the bovine pericardial valves do not seem to have this problem. The smaller sizes can be molded and fashioned in such a way as to have a wider orifice opening and better hemodynamic performance. Another advantage to the bovine pericardial valves is that they are easier to obtain in large quantities.

Selection of Prosthetic Valves

Considerations in choosing a prosthetic valve include: (1) age of the patient, (2) activities of daily living, (3) past medical history, (4) compliance and/or ability to follow an anticoagulation regimen, and (5) cardiac anatomy.[14,53,55] Critical-care nurses should be aware of these considerations in the physician's selection of an artificial valve. This knowledge enhances the teaching of patients and significant others regarding the advantages and disadvantages of each type of device.

Age can be an important criterion from the standpoint of durability. Braunwald[14] advocates the use of a mechanical valve prosthesis in patients under 65 who have no contraindications to anticoagulation. In patients over 65 the importance of durability is less of an issue, but the risk of hemorrhage from anticoagulants or noncompliance may be greater. Thus, the use of a tissue valve would seem warranted in this subset.

Tissue valves are preferred in patients whose activities of daily living increase the risk of bleeding. The question of which type of valve to implant in women of childbearing age remains controversial. Proponents of tissue valves believe that pregnancy in and of itself increases the risk of thromboembolism and that patients with mechanical valves who are anticoagulated have an increased risk of fetal hemorrhage during pregnancy.

Patients with a past medical history of bleeding usually receive a tissue valve as do patients in whom compliance and/or the ability to follow an anticoagulation regimen is doubtful. The elderly patient will often receive a tissue valve because of the potential problem with following an anticoagulation regimen.

Cardiac anatomy is another important consideration in choosing the prosthetic devices. Patients with small left ventricular cavities or tiny mitral annuli will probably benefit from the St. Jude valve or Ionescu-Shiley in comparison with the bulky caged-ball device or obstructive porcine xenografts.

Auscultation

In order to assess for possible malfunctioning of a prosthetic heart valve, an understanding of the normal auscultatory findings is appropriate. The opening and closing sounds associated with certain types of valves in either the mitral or aortic position will be discussed.

Caged-Ball Valves

Caged-ball valves are noted characteristically for their distinct, high-pitched, audible opening and closing sounds. There is a prominent opening click of these prostheses in both the aortic and mitral position which is notably louder than the mitral or aortic closure sound. The second or third right intercostal space (aortic) or the apex (mitral) are the preferred landmarks to auscultate these sounds. Caged-ball valves are associated with grade 2-3/6 early decrescendo or systolic ejection murmurs.[58] These murmurs are accentuated in conditions which augment the stroke volume. The presence of a diastolic murmur is not considered to be a normal finding.

Tilting-Disk Valves

The commonly used tilting disk valves, excluding the St. Jude model, generally are not associated with an audible opening sound in either mitral or aortic position but do produce distinct closing sounds.[58] Absence or diminution of a closing sound during sinus rhythm is considered to be an abnormal finding. Systolic murmurs are often noted in the mitral and aortic positions with tilting disk valves. A mitral prosthetic valve produces a 2/6 early to midsystolic ejection murmur, whereas an aortic prosthetic valve produces a basal early-to-midsystolic ejection murmur.

Tissue Valves

Porcine tissue valves have crisp, high-pitched opening and closing sounds which are typically less prominent than their mechanical counterparts. In the mitral position, approximately one-half of patients with implanted tissue valves have opening sounds which can be heard in the apical area. In addition, there may be apical diastolic rumbling or systolic murmurs. Prosthetic malfunction should be considered if a new diastolic murmur appears, or a change in the character or intensity of a murmur becomes apparent. Opening sounds are not generally heard in the aortic position; however, closing sounds are auscultated in many patients. A midsystolic murmur may be audible at the lower left sternal border. There should not be a diastolic murmur heard in the aortic position with tissue valves.

Complications

A detailed explanation of all possible complications associated with every type of valve is beyond the scope of this section. Discussion will focus on four major complications: inadequate valve seating, valvular obstruction related to thrombus formation or mechanical failure, thromboembolism, and prosthetic endocarditis.

Inadequate valve seating is usually related to suture displacement. There is a loss of adherence between the valve ring and the annulus. As a result, acute valvular regurgitation is manifested. These patients generally present with a poor postoperative convalescence, and develop congestive heart failure despite medical interventions. This complication should be suspected in patients who also develop a new regurgitant murmur. Treatment for this complication is to replace the valve.

Valvular obstruction related to thrombus formation or mechanical failure can be life-threatening or fatal if total obstruction occurs. Parameters by which to assess for this complication are a sudden or persistent decline in cardiac output, or a change in intensity or timing of a valve click. Echocardiograpy is useful in detecting this complication. Replacement of the prosthetic valve is usually necessary, especially if a mechanical failure is the precipitating factor.

Thromboembolism is usually a result of inadequate anticoagulation of patients. For this reason, nurses need to educate patients and significant others regarding the possibility of this complication. Prothrombin times are periodically necessary to ascertain proper blood levels. The most frequent organs to which arterial emboli migrate are the brain, heart, and kidneys. Therefore, careful assessment of the level of consciousness, cardiac function, and urinary output are necessary to clinically evaluate for the presence of emboli.

Prosthetic valve endocarditis (PVE) has similar clinical features to those discussed in the section related to infective endocarditis. Only the differences will be mentioned. Predisposing factors to this type of endocarditis are sternal wound infections or sternal osteomyelitis.[9] A decline in early PVE over the last two decades is probably related to prophylaxis antibiotic therapy and improved surgical technique.[59]

The most frequent causative microorganisms in both early (less than 2 months postoperatively) or late (more than 2 months postoperatively) PVE is *Staphylococcus epidermidis. Streptococcus,* when implicated, is seen in late PVE and carries a better prognosis than a staph infection.

The site of endocarditis varies with the type of tissue valve. For example, the majority of mechanical valves have the infection beneath the site of attachment and, as a result, ring abscess is manifested. The infection with tissue valves is usually limited to the cusps. Thus, if endocarditis should present it is better to have it on a tissue valve as compared to a mechanical valve.[52] When two prosthetic valves have been replaced, the infection for the most part involves the most downstream prosthesis.[52]

Clinical findings consist of a fever (95 percent of cases), leukocytosis (50 percent of cases), new regurgitant murmur (50 percent of cases) and (+) positive blood cultures (85 percent). Two-dimensional echocardiography has been found to be a useful diagnostic test for patients suspected of having PVE.[60]

Controversy remains regarding if and when valve replacement is necessary for PVE.[59] No consensus has been achieved about whether surgery, as an initial treatment performed very early after PVE is documented, will result in a lower fatality rate. The mortality rate in early PVE, defined as occurring within the first 60 days following valvular replacement, was found to be 71.4 percent versus late PVE (45.6 percent). According to Durack,[12] the decision to operate should also take into account the natural history of the type of PVE which has occurred. For example, streptococcal PVE usually responds medically, providing the patient does not develop failure, whereas a patient with fungal PVE should probably have valve replacement surgery.

In conclusion, cardiac valvular replacement is a routine cardiac surgical procedure performed for either valvular stenosis or regurgitation or both. Significant advancements have been made in the development of a suitable replacement for the native valve. Unfortunately, no one type of valve has proved to be a panacea.

Percutaneous Transluminal Valvuloplasty

For those patients with either mitral or aortic stenosis in whom surgical valve replacement is contraindicated or too high a risk (i.e., elderly, debilitated patients who have severe stenosis, patients with severe LV dysfunction, severe coronary artery disease, renal insufficiency, or chronic pulmonary disease), percutaneous transluminal valvuloplasty may offer some promise as an alternative to surgery. This procedure is performed with the use of a dilation balloon catheter which is inserted transvenously to inflate around the orifice of a stenotic valve. Initial studies have reported successful dilation of calcified mitral or aortic valves with such a catheter.[61, 62, 63, 64] Cribier, Savin, Berland, Rocha et al.[61] have postulated that the effects of aortic valvuloplasty could be the result of flattening or folding of the thickened calcified valvular leaflets, separation of fused commissines, or fracture of the calcified frame of the valvular cusps which reduce calcification to separate fragments and enable the valve to regain some suppleness. Although the exact mechanism of this procedure is still unknown, the premise for performing valvuloplasty is to create an increase in valve orifice area which will dramatically reduce the transvalvular gradient and improve flow.[14,61] Because of the newness of this procedure, long-term follow-up of these patients has not been accomplished. The next decade should provide valuable insight into the efficacy and long-term benefit of this alternative procedure.

References

1. Caplan, C. H. (1983). Diseases of the pericardium, myocardium and endocardium. In N. Levinsky (Ed.), *Medicine essentials of clinical practice.* Boston: Little, Brown.

2. Packa, D., & Vitello, J. M. (1984). Valvular heart disease. In B. Bullock & P. Rosendahl (Ed.), *Pathophysiology.* Boston: Little, Brown.

3. American Heart Association. (1977). Committee on rheumatic fever bacterial endocarditis: Prevention of rheumatic fever. *Circulation, 55,* 1–4.

4. Stollerman, G. H. (1984). Rheumatic and heritable connective tissue diseases of the cardiovascular system. In E. Braunwald (Ed.), *Heart disease.* Philadelphia: Saunders.

5. McCarthy, R. J. (1983). The medical cardiac patient. In R. G. Sanderson & C. L. Kurth (Eds.), *The cardiac patient.* Philadelphia: Saunders.

6. Lerner, P. I., & Weinstein, L. (1966). Infective endocarditis in the antibiotic era. *New England Journal of Medicine, 274,* 199–206.

7. Come, P. C. (1982). Infective endocarditis: Current perspectives. *Comprehensive Therapy, 8*(7), 57–70.

8. Arbulu, A., & Asfau, I. (1983). Infective endocarditis. In W. Glenn (Ed.), *Thoracic and cardiovascular surgery.* Norwalk, CT: Appleton-Century-Crofts.

9. Weinstein, L. (1984). Infective endocarditis. In E. Braunwald (Ed.), *Heart disease.* Philadelphia: Saunders.

10. Agarwal, A. K. (1985). Infective endocarditis. *Comprehensive Therapy, 11*(3), 17–25.

11. Caplan, C. H. (1983). Diseases of the pericardium, myocardium, and endocardium. In N. Levinsky (Ed.), *Medicine essentials of clinical practice.* Boston: Little, Brown.

12. Durack, D. T. (1986). Infective and non-infective endocarditis. In J. W. Hurst, R. B. Logue, C. E. Rackley, R. C. Schlant, E. H. Sonnenblick, A. G. Wallace, & N. K. Wenger (Eds.), *The heart.* New York: McGraw-Hill.

13. Pape, L. A. (1981). Pathogenesis and etiology of valvular heart disease. In J. E. Dalen, & J. S. Alpert (Eds.), *Valvular heart disease.* Boston: Little, Brown.

14. Braunwald, E. (1984). Valvular heart disease. In Braunwald, E. (Ed.), *Heart disease.* Philadelphia: Saunders.

15. Dalen, J. E., & Alpert, J. S. (Eds.) (1981). *Valvular heart disease.* Boston: Little, Brown.

16. Dalen, J. E. (1981). Mitral stenosis. In J. E. Dalen & J. S. Alpert (Eds.), *Valvular heart disease.* Boston: Little, Brown.

17. Isom, O. W., Shemin, R. J., & Whidden, L. L. (1983). Rheumatic mitral valve stenosis. In W. L. Glenn (Ed.), *Thoracic and cardiovascular surgery.* Norwalk, CT: Appleton-Century-Crofts.

18. Bornheimer, J. F., Kim, J. S., Sambasivan, V., & Biegler, T. L. (1982). Effects of nitroglycerin on supine and upright exercise in mitral stenosis. *American Heart Journal, 104*(6), 1288–1293.

19. Kawashita, K., Kambara, H., Kadota, K., Saimyoji, I. T., & Kawai, C. (1983). Radiocardiographic assessment of dobutamine and isosorbide dinitrite therapy in patients with mitral stenosis and pulmonary congestion. *Japan Circulation Journal, 47*(3), 283–288.

20. Flugelman, M. U., Hasin, Y., Katznelson, N., Kriwisky, M., Shefer, A., & Gotsman, M. S. (1984). Restoration and maintenance of sinus rhythm after mitral valve surgery for mitral stenosis. *American Journal of Cardiology, 54*(6), 617–619.

21. Dernevik, L., Brorsson, L., Wallentin, I., & William-Olsson, G. (1981). Improved results of closed commissurotomy for mitral stenosis using ultracardiography as selective ground. *Acta Medica Scandinavica, 210*(4), 283–286.

22. Sheares, J. H., Chia, F. K., Wu, D. C., Tan, K. T., & Tan, N. C. (1980). Surgery for mitral restenosis. *Annals of Academy of Medicine, Singapore, 9*(4), 468–473.

23. John, S., Bashi, V. V., Jairaj, P. S., Muralidharan, S., Ravikumar, E., Rajarajeswari, T., Krishnaswami, S., Sukumar, I. P., & Rao, P. S. (1983). Closed mitral valvotomy: Early results and long term follow ups of 3724 consecutive patients. *Circulation, 68*(5), 891–896.

24. Salerno, T. A., Neilson, I. R., Charrette, E. J., & Lynn, R. B. (1981). A 25 year experience with the closed method of treatment in 139 patients with mitral stenosis. *Annals of Thoracic Surgery, 31*(4), 300–304.

25. Breyer, R. H., Mills, S. A., Hudspeth, A. S., Johnston, S. R., Watts, L. E., Nomeir, A. M., & Cordell, A. R. (1985). Open mitral commissurotomy: Long term results with echocardiographic correlation. *Journal of Cardiovascular Surgery, 26*(1), 46–52.

26. Chaffin, J. S., & Daggett, W. M. (1979). Mitral valve

replacement: A nine year follow-up of risks and survivals. *Annals of Thoracic Surgery, 27*(4), 312–319.

27. Tryka, A. F., Godleski, J. J., Schoen, F. J., & Vandevanter, S. H. (1985). Pulmonary vascular disease and hypertension after valve surgery for mitral stenosis. *Human Pathology, 16*(1), 65–71.

28. Levinson, G. E. (1981). Aortic stenosis. In J. E. Dalen & J. S. Alpert (Eds.), *Valvular heart disease*. Boston: Little, Brown.

29. Awan, N. A., DeMaria, A. N., Miller, R. R., Amsterdam, E. A., & Mason, D. T. (1981). Beneficial effects of nitroprusside administration on left ventricular dysfunction and myocardial ischemia in severe aortic stenosis. *American Heart Journal, 101*(4), 386–394.

30. Folland, E. D., Kemper, A. J., Khuri, S. F., Josa, M., & Parisi, A. F. (1985). Intraaortic balloon counterpulsation as a temporary support measure in decompensated critical aortic stenosis. *Journal of the American College of Cardiology, 5*(3), 711–716.

31. McAnulty, J. H. (1984). Timing of surgical therapy for aortic valve stenosis, goals of therapy. *Herz, 9*(6), 341–345.

32. Murphy, E. S., Lawson, R. M., Starr, A., & Rahimtoola, S. H. (1981). Severe aortic stenosis in patients 60 years of age or older: Left ventricular function and 10 year survival after replacement. *Circulation, 64*, 184–188.

33. Kay, J. H., Carlish, R. A., & Dunne, E. F. (1983). Mitral insufficiency. In W. L. Glenn (Ed.), *Thoracic and cardiovascular surgery*. Norwalk, CT: Appleton-Century-Crofts.

34. Howe, J. P., & Alpert, J. S. (1981). Acute mitral regurgitation. In J. E. Dalen & J. S. Alpert (Eds.), *Valvular heart disease*. Boston: Little, Brown.

35. Nunley, D. L., & Starr, A. (1984). The evolution of reparative techniques for the mitral valve. *Annals of Thoracic Surgery, 37*(5), 393–397.

36. Bonchek, L. I., Olinger, G. N., Siegal, R., Tresch, D. D., & Keelan, M. H. (1984). Left ventricular performance after mitral reconstruction for mitral regurgitation. *Journal of Thoracic Cardiovascular Surgery, 88*(1), 122–127.

37. David, T. E., Burns, R. J., Bacchus, C. M., & Druck, M. N. (1984). Mitral valve replacement for mitral valve regurgitation with and without preservation of chordae tendineae. *Journal of Thoracic Cardiovascular Surgery, 88*, 718–725.

38. Saltissi, S., Crowther, A., Byrne, C., Clarke, S., Jenkins, B. S., & Webb-Peploe, M. M. (1983). The effects of oral digoxin therapy in primary mitral leaflet prolapse. *European Heart Journal, 4*, 828–837.

39. Malpartida, F., Arcas, R., Alegria, E., Monreal, F., &

Caro, D. M. (1980). Surgical treatment for chest pain in mitral valve prolapse. *Chest, 78*(1), 101–104.

40. Ross, A., DeWeese, J. A., & Yu, P. W. (1978). Refractory ventricular arrhythmias in a patient with mitral valve prolapse. Successful control with mitral valve replacement. *Journal of Electrocardiography, 11*, 289–295.

41. Reece, I. J., Cooley, D. A., Painvin, G. A., O'Kereke, O. U., Powers, P. L., Pechacek, L. W., & Frazier, O. H. (1985). Surgical treatment of mitral systolic click syndrome: Results in 37 patients. *Annals of Thoracic Surgery, 39*, 155–158.

42. Alpert, J. S. (1981). Chronic aortic regurgitation. In J. E. Dalen & J. S. Alpert (Eds.), *Valvular heart disease*. Boston: Little, Brown.

43. Benotti, J. R. (1981). Acute aortic insufficiency. In J. E. Dalen & J. S. Alpert (Eds.), *Valvular heart disease*. Boston: Little, Brown.

44. O'Rourke, R. A., & Walsh, R. A. (1986). Recognition and treatment of acute aortic regurgitation. *Journal of Intensive Care Medicine, 1*(1), 33–46.

45. Cutler, B. S. (1986). The intraaortic balloon and counterpulsation. In J. M. Rippe, R. S. Irwin, J. S. Alpert, & J. E. Dalen (Eds.), *Intensive care medicine*. Boston: Little, Brown.

46. Shen, W. F., Roubin, G. S., Hirasawa, K., Uren, R. F., Hutton, B. F., Harris, P. J., Fletcher, P. J., & Kelly, D. T. (1984). Noninvasive assessment of acute effects of nifedipine on rest and exercise hemodynamics and cardiac function in patients with aortic regurgitation. *Journal of the American College of Cardiology, 4*(5), 902–907.

47. Shen, W. F., Roubin, G. S., Hirasawa, K., Uren, R. F., Hutton, B. F., Harris, P. J., Fletcher, P. J., & Kelly, D. T. (1984). Abnormal left ventricular response to isometric exercise in pure, isolated aortic regurgitation: Beneficial effects of nifedipine. *American Journal of Cardiology, 54*(6), 605–609.

48. Greenberg, B. H., & Rahimtoola, S. H. (1980). Long term vasodilator therapy in aortic insufficiency. Evidence for regression of left ventricular dilatation and hypertrophy and improvement in systolic pump function. *Annals of Internal Medicine, 93*(3), 440–442.

49. Osamura, Y., & Tasaka, M. (1984). Observations on the timing of operative intervention for aortic regurgitation. *Japan Circulation Journal, 48*(10), 1162–1168.

50. Louagie, Y., Brohet, C., Lopez, E., Jaumin, P., Schoevaerdts, J. C., Ponlot, R., & Chalant, C. H. (1984). Early surgery for severe aortic regurgitation. *Journal of Cardiovascular Surgery* (Torino), *25*(4), 304–312.

51. Oyer, P. E., & Stinson, E. B. (1983). Biologic valves. In W. L. Glenn (Ed.), *Thoracic and cardiovascular surgery*. Norwalk, CT: Appleton-Century-Crofts.

52. Roberts, W. C. (1983). Complications of cardiac valve replacement. In W. L. Glenn (Ed.), *Thoracic and cardiovascular surgery.* Norwalk, CT: Appleton-Century-Crofts.

53. Weiland, A. P. (1983). A review of cardiac valve prostheses and their selection. *Heart & Lung, 12,* 498–504.

54. Geha, A. S. (1980). Mechanical valve prostheses. In W. L. Glenn (Ed.), *Thoracic and cardiovascular surgery.* Norwalk, CT: Appleton-Century-Crofts.

55. Bonchek, L. I. (1981). Current status of cardiac valve replacement: Selection of a prosthesis and indications for operation. *American Heart Journal, 101,* 96–106.

56. Nunez, L., Iglesias, A., & Sotillo, J. (1980). Entrapment of leaflet of St. Jude medical cardiac valve prosthesis by miniscule thrombus: Report of two cases. *Annals of Thoracic Surgery, 29*(6), 566–569.

57. Ferrans, V. J., Boyce, S. W., Billingham, M. E., Jones, M., Ishihara, T., & Roberts, W. C. (1980). Calcific deposits in porcine bioprostheses: Structure and pathogenesis. *American Journal of Cardiology, 46,* 721–734.

58. Smith, N. D., Raizada, V., & Abrams, J. (1981). Auscultation of the normally functioning prosthetic valve. *Annals of Internal Medicine, 95,* 594–598.

59. Mayer, K. H., & Schoenbaum, S. C. (1982). Evaluation and management of prosthetic valve endocarditis. *Progress in Cardiovascular Diseases, 25*(1), 43–54.

60. Cunha, C. L. P., Guiliani, E. R., Callahan, J. A., & Pluth, J. R. (1980). Echophonocardiographic findings in patients with prosthetic heart valve malfunction. *Mayo Clinic Proceedings, 55,* 231–242.

61. Cribier, A., Savin, T., Berland, J., Rocha, P., Mechmeche, R. Saoudi, N., Behar, P., & Letac, B. (1987). Percutaneous transluminal balloon valvuloplasty of adult aortic stenosis: Report of 92 cases. *Journal of the American College of Cardiology, 9*(2), 381–386.

62. McKay, R. G., Safian, R. D., Lock, J. E., Mandell, V. S., Thurer, R. L., Sehnitt, S. J., & Grossman, W. (1986). Balloon dilatation of calcific aortic stenosis in elderly patients: postmortem, intraoperative and percutaneous valvuloplasty studies. *Circulation, 74*(1), 119–125.

63. McKay R. G., Lock, J. E., Keane, J. F., Safian, R. D., Aroesty, J. M., & Grossman, W. Percutaneous mitral valvuloplasty in an adult patient with calcific rheumatic mitral stenosis. *Journal of the American College of Cardiology, 7*(6), 1410–1415.

64. Palacios, I. F., Lock, J. E., Keane, J. F., & Block, P. (1986). Percutaneous transvenous balloon valvotomy in a patient with severe calcific mitral stenosis. *Journal of the American College of Cardiology, 7*(6), 1416–1419.

25 Vascular Disease

Jeanne Doyle
Molly Johantgen
Joan Vitello-Cicciu

Aortic Disease

The arteries and veins are the roads and pathways by which the blood circulates through the body. The aorta is the largest of these conduits, delivering oxygenated blood directly from the heart. This chapter discusses abnormalities of the aorta and of the peripheral arteries and veins and the integral role that the critical-care nurse plays in the care of patients with such abnormalities.

Arterial Anatomy

The aorta is a large but thin and tough vessel which must absorb the pumping of approximately three billion heartbeats in an average lifetime. The aorta consists of the thin inner intima, thick media, and thin outer adventitia (Fig. 25-1). The aortic intima is a single endothelial layer which is easily traumatized. The media is composed of intertwining sheets of elastin arranged in a spiral design to increase strength. A small amount of smooth muscle and collagen lies between the elastic membranes, providing additional tensile strength and elasticity. The outer adventitia contains collagen and the vasa vasorum and lymphatics, which nourish the aortic wall.

The aorta is divided into (1) the ascending aorta, which arises from the base (aortic valve) of the heart and extends to the arch; (2) the arch of the aorta, from which the brachiocephalic and carotid vessels originate; (3) the descending thoracic aorta, which continues from the arch to the diaphragm; and (4) the abdominal aorta, which continues from the thoracic aorta to the aortic bifurcation.

The authors wish to acknowledge the assistance of Mary Michael Brown, R.N., in reviewing the nursing therapies sections of this chapter.

Pathophysiology

The most common underlying disease affecting the aorta is atherosclerosis. While atherosclerosis is initially an intimal process, hemorrhage into the plaques may invade the medial layer, causing weakening and generalized dilatation of the aorta. Atherosclerotic aneurysms characteristically affect the abdominal aorta below the renal arteries most severely and the ascending aorta least frequently. Advancing age has been linked with decreased elastin content within the aorta, which may contribute to weakness in the aortic wall.

Aortic Aneurysm

Risk factors associated with aortic aneurysmal disease parallel those involved in peripheral arterial occlusive disease. A study by Auerbach and Garfinkel demonstrated an increase in atherosclerotic plaque, ulceration, and calcification within the aorta in persons who smoked as compared to ex-smokers and nonsmokers.[1] Aneurysm formation was eight times greater in smokers than nonsmokers. Further, in a study by Norrgard, Angquist, and Johnson, 50 percent of patients with aneurysms had higher levels of triglycerides and low-density lipoproteins (LDL) and lower levels of high-density lipoproteins (HDL) than the control subjects.[2]

Hypertension increases injury to the endothelium and may accelerate medial degeneration because of increased hemodynamic stress in persons with underlying molecular defects of elastin and collagen. Medial degeneration, as previously noted, is part of the aging process. Further, acute hypertension has been shown experimentally to decrease blood flow to the vasa vasorum, thereby decreasing nutrient flow into the media and causing ischemia and weakening of that layer.

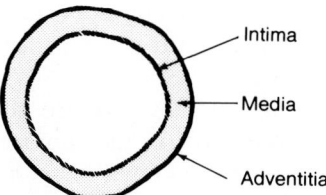

Figure 25-1   Cross-sectional representation of layers in arterial wall.

Aneurysms develop at areas of medial weakness. Once begun, aneurysm formation is promoted by the law of Laplace—a vicious cycle of increased tension on the aortic wall due to an enlarged wall diameter, which then increases the tension further, producing progressive dilatation of the aneurysm. The rate of expansion for a given aneurysm is unpredictable, and therefore there is no "safe" aneurysm.

Two types of aneurysm are seen in the aorta. *Fusiform* aneurysms result from a diffuse area of weakness producing a spindle-shaped deformity, whereas in *saccular* aneurysms a balloonlike dilatation is present. The lumen of an aneurysm usually contains layers of laminated clot, portions of which may break loose, embolizing to areas distal to the aneurysm[3] (Fig. 25-2).

The primary concerns with aneurysms are the risks of rupture of the aorta and aortic wall dissec-

tion. The incidence of aortic rupture is directly proportional to aneurysm size; there is a dramatic increase in the likelihood of rupture when the aneurysm is 6 cm in diameter or more. Aneurysms of smaller diameter are also at risk of rupture, but the incidence is far less. Aspects of aortic dissection are discussed later in this chapter.

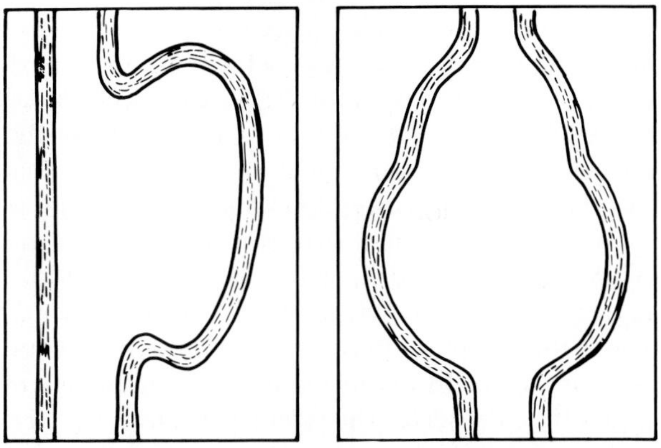

Marfan's syndrome is a nonatherosclerotic disorder of connective tissue, involving massive degeneration of elastic fibers in the aortic media, which can also result in aneurysm formation. Medial degeneration is most severe at the aortic root and ascending aorta; therefore, aneurysm of the proximal aorta is the most frequent manifestation noted in Marfan's syndrome. Marfan's syndrome is an inherited disorder which in its most complete presentation has four clinical characteristics, including a family history of the disorder, and skeletal abnormalities consisting of long extremities, particularly long hands and feet, a high arched palate, deformities of the thorax, and lax ligaments or sparse muscle mass. Ocular manifestations of subluxed or dislocated ocular lenses are attributed to lax supporting ligaments. In addition to aortic changes, myxomatous changes of the aortic and mitral valves may cause valvular incompetence.

Many persons with Marfan's syndrome present symptoms of aortic rupture or aortic regurgitation prior to age 40. Aortic dissection alone is less frequently noted in Marfan's syndrome than aortic rupture. Bacterial organisms which are blood-borne may enter the aortic wall from the lumen or the vasa vasorum and may damage the integrity of the wall, leading to aneurysm formation; secondary infection of an aneurysm at the site of damaged endothelial wall is commonly noted, because the damaged wall has lost its resistance to infection.

Syphilis, autoimmune disease, and trauma are also causes of aortic wall destruction which can result in aneurysm formation. Congenital anomalies such as coarctation of the thoracic or abdominal aorta are rare but may be associated with aneurysm formation (Table 25-1).

History and Physical Assessment

In general, patients who have an aneurysm are asymptomatic until the aneurysm reaches a size at which it impinges on other organs or begins to leak. Depending on the location of the aneurysm,

Most common kinds
of aneurysms

Saccular   Fusiform

Figure 25-2   Two most common types of aortic aneurysm.

Table 25-1 Underlying Causes of Aortic Disease

Hypertension
Atherosclerosis
Medial degeneration
   Age
   Marfan's syndrome
   Idiopathic cystic medial degeneration
Aortitis
   Bacterial aortitis
   Mycotic aneurysm
   Syphilitic aortitis
   Nonspecific aortitis
   Takayasu's disease
   Giant cell arteritis
   Ankylosing spondylitis
   Reiter's syndrome
Congenital anomalies
Trauma

Source: Adapted from Lindsay et al.[12] and Slater and DeSanctis.[5]

the physical examination may reflect pressure on or involvement of other organs.

Persons with ascending aortic aneurysms may be asymptomatic or may describe dyspnea and chest pain. Physical examination is significant for a widened pulse pressure, a bounding pulse, an aortic diastolic murmur, or an aortic valve regurgitation murmur.

An aortic arch aneurysm may impinge on the lungs, trachea, pulmonary artery, superior vena cava, innominate veins, or laryngeal nerve to produce symptoms of dyspnea, stridor, hoarseness, hemoptysis, cough, or chest pain. Physical findings may include distended jugular and arm veins, left vocal cord paralysis, abnormal pulsations of the upper anterior chest, signs of pleural fluid such as absent breath sounds or dullness on percussion, and signs of congestive heart failure such as crackles and an S_3.

The most common symptom of an aneurysm of the descending thoracic aorta is pain. The pain is often located in the posterior thorax, between the shoulders. However, some patients have pain in the lower back, abdomen, shoulders, arms, or neck. The pain is described as dull and intermittent or constant. Aneurysms of the descending thoracic aorta can rarely be detected by physical examination. A pulsatile mass at the base of the neck or left supraclavicular fossa may be noted if there is enlargement of the aneurysm, and hoarseness from

pressure on the laryngeal nerve sometimes occurs. Leaking of the aneurysm may cause a significant increase in pain and hemoptysis.

Abdominal aneurysms generally produce no symptoms until there is pressure on the lumbar nerves, inferior vena cava, or duodenum. Back pain that is dull and constant is caused by pressure on the lumbar nerves. Abdominal pain and bloating may indicate a stretching of the duodenum over an enlarging aneurysm.

Rupture of an aneurysm is the extravasation of blood beyond the walls of the aneurysm and must be recognized quickly. The clinical presentation depends upon location of the aneurysm and may include unremitting back or abdominal pain; severe tenderness of the mass in the abdominal aorta is suggestive of imminent rupture. The patient may present with a history of weakness, lightheadedness, faintness, nausea and vomiting, or unconsciousness consistent with rupture and hypovolemia. Rupture may initiate secondary disorders such as myocardial ischemia, pulmonary edema, or high-output failure.

Diagnostic Data

The diagnosis of an aortic aneurysm is frequently an incidental finding on a chest x-ray, abdominal film, or a routine physical examination. The aneurysm is further delineated by invasive and noninvasive methods including aortography, echocardiography, ultrasound, computerized tomography, and digital subtraction angiography.

In defining an aneurysm within the thorax, Doppler echocardiography of the aortic root and ultrasound studies of the descending thoracic aorta are noninvasive techniques which may be used. Computerized tomography (CT) may also be used to determine the size, location, and extent of the aneurysm and the amount of mural thrombus that may be present. Aortography and cardiac angiography define areas of obstruction and ischemia and outline the inner wall of the aneurysm. Unfortunately, aortography may fail to delineate the actual size of the aneurysm because of intraluminal thrombus formation. In instances when ascending aneurysms have caused aortic valvular insufficiency, the electrocardiogram may indicate left ventricular hypertrophy (increase in QRS voltage) and strain (ST depression and T wave inversion).[4]

Abdominal aortic aneurysms may be defined as to size, location, and extent through the use of ultrasound, abdominal x-rays, aortography, computerized tomography, or digital subtraction angiography. Digital subtraction angiography is a new technique which may yield information similar to aortography but eliminates the use of an intra-arterial injection.[5]

Medical and Surgical Interventions

Medical management of a patient with an aortic aneurysm involves frequent monitoring of aneurysmal size (as by ultrasound every 6 months) to indicate the need for surgical repair (at a diameter of 4 to 5 cm). Control of contributory risk factors such as hypertension, hypercholesteremia, hyperlipidemia, and smoking through modifications in diet, exercise, and medications and the cessation of smoking is also important. In the presence of a large aneurysm or rupture, operative repair is the only effective therapy.

For the patient facing elective surgical repair, medical therapy involves complete evaluation of the coronary arteries, carotid arteries, and peripheral vasculature through a comprehensive cardiovascular history and physical examination and may include an electrocardiogram, Doppler blood flow studies, and serum lipid profile, since atherosclerosis is the most frequent underlying cause of aneurysm formation. Significant coronary artery occlusions or carotid artery stenoses may precede repair of the aneurysm.

Leaking or rupture of an aneurysm is a surgical emergency. Treatment of hypovolemia, minimization of leakage with an external counterpulsation device, e.g., MAST trousers, and administration of intravenous fluids to maintain a systolic blood pressure of 80 to 100 mmHg are required with the onset of rupture.[6]

Surgical repair consists of replacing the section of the aorta which holds the aneurysm by a synthetic graft which is sewn into the normal aorta. Depending upon the area of aneurysm repair, the surgical procedures vary in the method of and the need for maintaining distal circulation. For aneurysms involving the ascending aorta and the aortic arch, cardiopulmonary bypass is needed, and aortic valve replacement may be required if aortic regurgitation is severe. In aneurysms below the left subclavian artery, the aorta is clamped proximally and distally while the surgical repair is done. The blood pressure is lowered and controlled by use of vasodilators, e.g., sodium nitroprusside.

Aortic Dissection

Acute dissection of the thoracic aorta occurs more frequently than rupture of an abdominal aortic aneurysm. If not treated, it has a 90 percent mortality rate.[7]

A longitudinal tearing of the aortic media by a dissecting hematoma is the primary feature of aortic dissection. The sudden laceration of the aortic intima opens the way for blood propelled by the force of arterial pressure into the media. The underlying pathogenesis of dissection may include (1) medial degeneration as noted in Marfan's syndrome, aging, and hypertension; (2) intimal damage as in atherosclerosis, syphilis, infection, or trauma; and (3) the shearing stress related to the beating of the heart, especially affecting the ascending aorta and related to the hemodynamic forces of the pulse wave.[8]

The types of dissection have been classified according to the areas most frequently affected within the aorta (Fig. 25-3). DeBakey types II and III arise from the ascending aorta: type II extends from the ascending aorta beyond the arch, while type III is confined to the ascending aorta. DeBakey type I begins in the descending thoracic aorta beyond the left subclavian artery and extends distally.

History and Physical Assessment

The prompt diagnosis and management of patients with acute aortic dissection has reduced mortality significantly.[7] Men are more frequently affected than women, and dissection most often occurs during the sixth or seventh decade of life. However, persons with Marfan's syndrome who experience acute dissection are usually in their early thirties. A history of long-standing hypertension is also common.

The most frequent presenting symptom of acute dissection is the onset of intense pain described as sharp, tearing, knifelike, or ripping in nature, occurring in the chest and spreading down into the back and to the abdomen. Pain may be

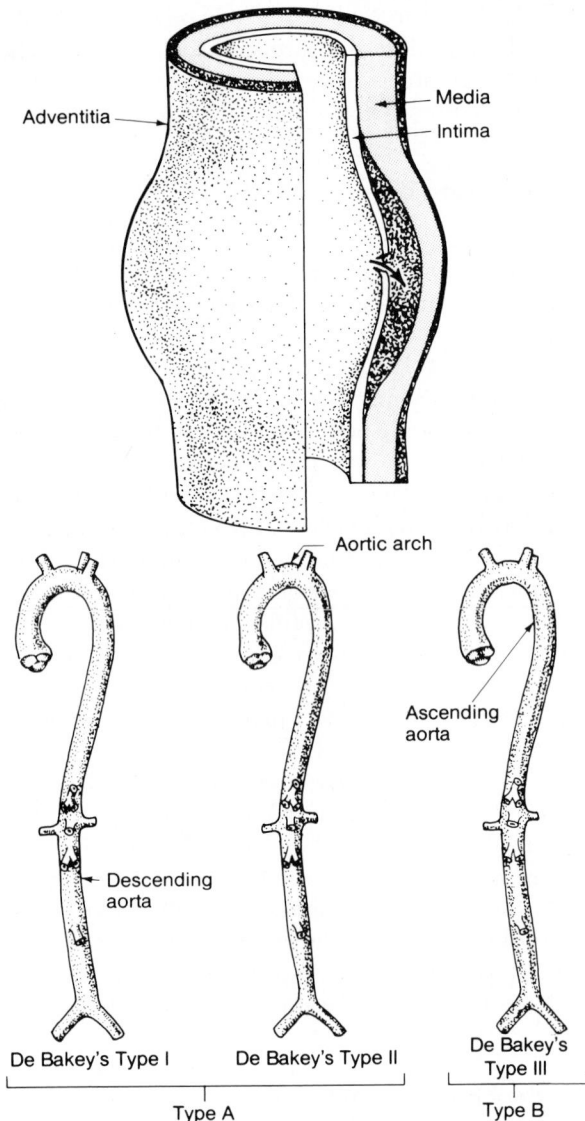

Figure 25-3 Aortic dissections classified according to DeBakey's typing. (*From Urk, F. & Oakes, A., Assessing the patient with acute aortic dissection. Focus Crit. Care, 10:16, 1983.*

confined only to the back or the abdomen. Determination of the location of the pain is useful in localizing the dissection.

The manifestations of aortic dissection are determined by the path taken by the dissecting hematoma: the circulation in major arteries originating from the aorta may be compromised, leading to myocardial infarction, cerebral insufficiency, cer-ebral vascular accident, paraplegia, necrosis of the bowel, or renal failure.

If the dissection has disrupted the aortic valve, precordial systolic murmurs are usually noted, and a diastolic murmur of aortic regurgitation with concomitant symptoms of pulmonary edema may be present. Strokelike symptoms of paralysis or hemiplegia may evolve from partial to complete occlusion of one or both carotid arteries. Nausea and vomiting with hematemesis or melanotic stools may indicate erosion of a thoracic dissection into the esophagus.[9] Blood pressure between the two arms may be significantly different, indicating compromise of blood flow into one or both subclavian arteries. Loss or decrease of femoral pulses with pain may indicate dissection into the aortic bifurcation, disrupting blood flow to the legs.

The patient with an acute dissection is in severe distress and presents with signs of shock (pallor, sweating, peripheral cyanosis, restlessness), yet the blood pressure is usually elevated. In some patients the systolic pressure may be greater than 200 mmHg.

Diagnostic Procedures

Initial blood studies of the patient admitted to the critical-care unit are usually within normal limits unless the patient is actively bleeding, in which case there is a decrease in red blood cell count, hemoglobin, and hematocrit valves. An admitting electrocardiogram assists in ruling out signs of myocardial ischemia or infarction. There may be signs of left ventricular hypertrophy as a sequela of hypertension.

The chest x-ray assists in confirming the diagnosis by detecting, e.g., a widening of the mediastinum with left pleural effusion, indicating possible rupture into the pleural cavity.[7] Further confirmation may be obtained by the use of computerized tomography and transesophageal echocardiography.[10] Aortography provides definitive diagnosis of aortic dissection, delineating the area of intimal tearing, false channels, compression of the true aortic lumen, and aortic valve competence.

Medical and Surgical Therapies

Once aortic dissection is suspected, immediate treatment is instituted to lower blood pressure and reduce the pulsatile force of left ventricular ejection. Reduction of both blood pressure and myocardial contractility to decrease the progression of the dissecting force through medication and rest is instituted in the critical-care unit until the patient is stabilized for further diagnostic procedures or surgery. Careful monitoring of blood pressure, cardiac rhythm, central venous pressure, pulmonary artery pressures, and urine output are required while antihypertensive drugs are administered, in order to detect complications such as hypotension, cardiac arrhythmias from the medication, and progression of dissection to cause ischemia or infarction of the renal, messenteric, or femoral arteries.

Sodium nitroprusside (Nipride) or trimethaphan camsylate (Arfonad, a ganglionic blocking agent), are frequently used in decreasing blood pressure. Sodium nitroprusside used alone can increase ejection force; thus simultaneous use of β-adrenergic blocking agents such as propranolol are essential to decreasing contractility. Propranolol is contraindicated if bradycardia, asthma, or congestive heart failure is present. Trimethaphan camsylate decreases blood pressure and myocardial contractility; however, tachyphylaxis, or rapid immunization to a toxic dose, is a common problem, so this drug is used less often than sodium nitroprusside. Reserpine given in doses of 1 to 2 mg every 4 to 6 h intramuscularly also decreases blood pressure and pulsatile force. However, the side effects of drowsiness, depression, and increased gastric acid formation, as well as difficulty in controlling the administration of the drug, reduce the frequency of use in medical management of aortic dissection.

Decrease of cardiac workload with diuretics such as furosemide or other loop diuretics contributes to limiting contractility and, therefore, progression of the dissection. Pain is managed primarily through reduction of blood pressure and limited amounts of morphine sulfate.

Patients with nonprogressive isolated dissection in an area of the aorta that does not affect major arteries may be treated medically. Persons of advanced age and those with severe associated disease or severe neurological injury caused by the dissection are not candidates for surgery. Other patients may choose between continued medical therapy or surgical intervention when their condition is stable (Table 25-2).

Table 25-2 Indications for Medical and Surgical Therapy in Acute Aortic Dissection

Medical
Initial stabilization of patient
Uncomplicated DeBakey type III dissection
Stable, isolated arch dissection
Chronic dissection—uncomplicated dissection presenting 2 or more weeks after onset
Inoperability because of advanced age, severe concomitant medical problems, or severe neurologic injuries

Surgical
Aortic valve regurgitation
Failure of drug therapy
Cardiac tamponade
Compromise of a major branch of the aorta
Types I and II dissection
Type III dissection complicated by compromise of vital organs, rupture, retrograde extension into the ascending aorta, or Marfan's syndrome

Source: Adapted from Finnerty,[11] Lindsay et al.,[12] and Slater and DeSanctis.[5]

Immediate surgical intervention is indicated when there is overwhelming aortic valve regurgitation, failure of drug therapy to control the progression of dissection, cardiac tamponade, or compromise of a major branch of the aorta.[11] Surgical therapy involves repair of the intimal tear and obliteration of the entry into the dissecting aortic wall. Dissections involving the ascending aorta (DeBakey types II and III) use cardiopulmonary bypass and cold cardioplegia. If there is aortic valve regurgitation due to dissection of the intima into the valve annulus, the valve is resuspended or replaced with a prosthetic valve. Splitting of the layer of the aortic wall in conjunction with underlying disease such as atherosclerosis may make the aorta very friable, difficult to suture, and susceptible to free bleeding. A tube graft is sutured in place, using Teflon strips to reinforce the suture line externally, within the true lumen and within the false lumen. The aneurysm wall is sutured around the graft for reinforcement and hemostasis (Fig. 25-4).

Repair of distal or DeBakey type I dissections consists in resection of the descending thoracic aorta above the origin of dissection, closure of the inner and outer layers of the false aneurysm by suturing, and replacement of the excised aorta with a graft.[12] Resuspension or restoration of major

Figure 25-4 Surgical repair of type III aortic dissection. (*a*) The clamps in place for a distal dissection. The distal clamp does not encompass the distal extent of the dissection. (*b*). The graft is in place and the adventitia is being closed. (*From Little, A. G. & Anagnostopoulos, C. E., Aortic dissections, in W. W. L. Glenn, Ed., Thoracic and Cardiovascular Surgery, 4th ed., Norwalk, Appleton-Century-Crofts, 1983, p. 1563.*)

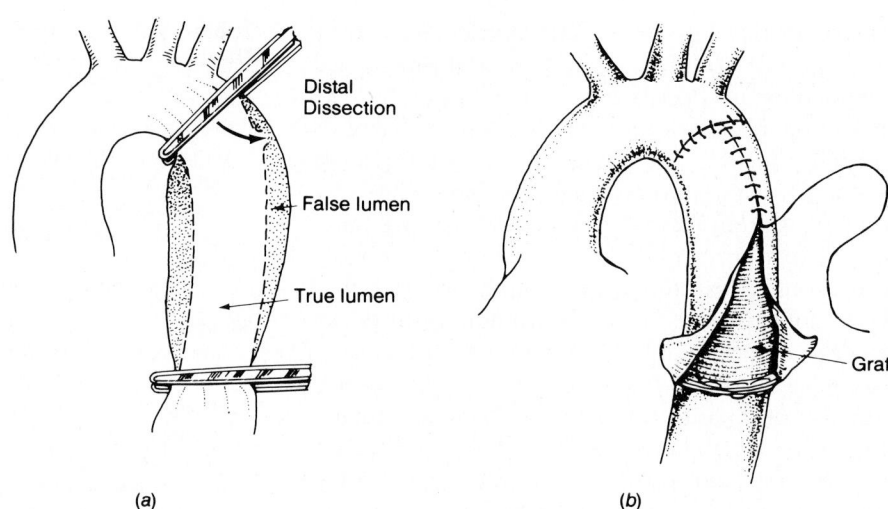

(a)   (b)

branches of the aorta may be necessary, depending upon the extent of the dissection.

Nursing Therapies

Nurses in the critical-care setting play key roles in the survival of patients with aortic aneurysms or acute aortic dissection. Discerning observation and assessment of the patient entering the critical-care environment assist in determining the diagnosis of rupture or dissection and expedite the provision of appropriate patient care.

Depending on the patient's level of consciousness and degree of discomfort, the following information can be ascertained from the patient or significant others as part of the initial nursing history:

1. A complete description of the pain, including its onset, duration, type, intensity, location, radiation, and any contributing factors which increase or decrease its severity
2. Past medical history of hypertension, carotid artery disease, coronary artery disease, peripheral vascular disease, Marfan's syndrome, syphilis, or severe infections
3. The presence and duration of symptoms such as hemoptysis, hematemesis, melena, hoarseness, dyspnea, changes in sensation or movement of extremities, or changes in vision.

The physical examination is a comprehensive physical assessment focusing on (1) blood pressure, both range and difference between extremities; (2) pulse pressure; (3) heart rate and rhythm; (4) pulse quality and bilateral changes in quality; (5) skin temperature and color; (6) heart tones; (7) presence of palpable heaves, thrills, or bruits in the anterior chest or abdomen; (8) breath sounds; (9) respiratory rate and depth and use of accessory muscles; (10) distention of jugular veins or upper extremity veins; (11) level of consciousness; (12) bowel sounds; (13) urine output; (14) presence of paresthesia or decreased motor function; (15) pain on palpation of the abdomen; and (16) decreased field of vision.

All too often the patient who presents acutely because of aneurysmal rupture or aortic dissection exhibits shock. The interventions by nurses are often aimed at minimizing or treating this shocklike state. In this case, shock is considered a collaborative problem as described by Gordon[13] (see Chap. 20). Most of these patients and their significant others are anxious, have a sense of impending doom, and exhibit ineffective coping because of the severity of the condition.

Nursing Diagnosis

Ineffective coping related to fear of dying secondary to acute hospitalization and severity of condition.

Goal

Use of appropriate coping skills by patient and significant others.

Interventions

1. Promote communication of patient and significant others with members of health care team.
2. Assess level of anxiety.
3. Provide a sense of empathic understanding through quiet presence and touch.
4. Inquire regarding patient's knowledge about the actual condition and prognosis.
5. Identify patient's positive support system.
6. Discuss with patient and significant others coping methods previously used.
7. Provide support and reinforcement of adaptive behavior such as problem solving.
8. Consult with appropriate resources (clergy, social service department, psychologist) to provide additional support.

Evaluation

Patient verbalizes fears and positive coping methods for stress reduction and identifies support system. Patient and significant others exhibit adaptive behaviors.

Other Diagnoses

Other potential nursing diagnoses that may be applicable for the patient with an aortic aneurysm or acute aortic dissection include:

1. Potential for alteration in comfort (pain) related to decreased tissue perfusion.
2. Potential for impaired physical mobility related to decreased tissue perfusion.
3. Potential for skin breakdown related to decreased tissue perfusion.

Peripheral Vascular Disease

Peripheral vascular disease (PVD) is defined as any pathophysiologic process which disrupts blood flow through arteries or veins of the extracranium, thorax, abdomen, and extremities, although the term is often used synonymously with lower extremity arterial insufficiency. Though rarely a cause of mortality in and of itself, PVD can result in profound morbidity in such forms as stroke, limb amputation, or chronic venous insufficiency. Additionally, symptomatic PVD often heralds the presence of "central" vascular disease, that is, coronary artery disease, with resultant risk of cardiac death and disability.

Because lower extremity arterial and venous diseases are the most commonly encountered clinical problems, they are the focus of this section.

Lower Extremity Arterial Disease

Pathophysiology

The leading cause of arterial insufficiency in the lower extremities is atherosclerotic occlusive disease. Other causes include acute thromboembolic problems, vasospastic disease (Raynaud's phenomenon), inflammatory processes (e.g., Buerger's disease, arteritis) and, less commonly, fibromuscular dysplasia, increased muscular compartment pressure, i.e., compartment syndrome, and congenital vascular diseases. Although a discussion of atherosclerosis forms the framework of this section, some of these other causes warrant brief mention.

Acute Arterial Occlusion   Acute disruption of arterial blood flow results from either thrombosis of a previously stenotic arterial lesion or embolism of blood clot or atherosclerotic debris into the arterial circuit. Abrupt arterial thrombosis usually results in more insidious symptoms, since preexisting arterial narrowing has often prompted the development of collateral arteries. Arterial embolism, on the other hand, causes very dramatic signs and symptoms of acute arterial insufficiency, namely, the six P's: pain, pallor, pulselessness, paresthesia, paralysis, and poikilothermia. Emboli most often originate from mural thrombi lining the myocardium in patients with chronic arrhythmias and/or ventricular dysfunction secondary to myocardial infarction. They can also originate from arterial aneurysms lined with thrombus (most often from the abdominal aorta or popliteal artery) or roughened intimal surfaces of stenotic arterial lesions. Depending on their size, arterial emboli can lodge anywhere from the aortic bifurcation, disrupting arterial flow to both legs, to tiny vessels in the toes.

When acute occlusion of arterial flow threatens the viability of the limb(s), immediate intervention in the form of arteriography, thrombolytic therapy, and/or surgery is indicated. These treatment options are discussed later in this section.

Vasospastic Disease   Vasospastic arterial disease is also known as *Raynaud's disease* or *phenomenon*. Raynaud's affects more women than men, and symptoms usually present from late adolescence to middle age. The hands are affected more commonly and severely than the feet.

Reported causes of Raynaud's disease include ineffective basal heat production, stress, and overstimulation of the sympathetic nervous system.

Raynaud's is triphasic in nature, the first phase being characterized by marked blanching of the skin, predominantly in the hands and feet, caused by severe vasoconstriction of the cutaneous blood vessels. During the blanching phase, patients complain of a cold, numb feeling in the affected digits. The second phase evidences cyanosis resulting from dilatation of cutaneous arterioles and venules. Because vasoconstriction is diminished in the final phase, reactive hyperemia characterized by reddish discoloration, burning, and throbbing pain are experienced.

Most mild cases of Raynaud's can be successfully managed with conservative measures such as avoiding extremes in temperature, particularly cold, and avoiding stress. Historically, drugs have proved to be of little value, although several recent reports describe the effectiveness of nifedipine in treating this syndrome.[14,15] With advanced Raynaud's, characterized by severe persistent vasoconstriction, full-thickness tissue necrosis may necessitate amputation of one or more digits.

Thromboangiitis Obliterans   Also known as *Buerger's disease,* thromboangiitis is an inflammatory occlusive disease involving small to medium-sized arteries and veins in the extremities. The existence of Buerger's disease as a distinct clinical entity is highly controversial among experts in peripheral vascular disease, although the current consensus is that the specific pathologic condition does exist, albeit with decreasing incidence in western cultures.[16] Unlike Raynaud's disease, Buerger's disease occurs more commonly in the lower extremities and predominantly in young male cigarette smokers. Histologically, the "lesion" of Buerger's disease is characterized by full-thickness inflammation of the vessel walls with associated thrombosis.

Signs and symptoms of Buerger's disease result from decreased arterial blood flow to tissues beyond the occlusive lesion and may parallel those of atherosclerotic arterial occlusive disease, discussed below. The diagnosis is usually determined from factors such as age of onset, associated risk factors, and the presence of venous as well as arterial involvement.

Atherosclerotic Occlusive Disease

Atherosclerosis is the leading cause of arterial occlusive disease in the extremities beyond age 30. Atherosclerosis is the most common form of arteriosclerosis obliterans and is histologically characterized by structural changes in the arterial wall as well as the development of intraluminal plaque, narrowing the route of blood flow through the artery.

Atherosclerosis is also characterized by accumulation of lipids and connective tissue in the arterial wall, increased intimal permeability and platelet aggregation secondary to injury, and proliferation of smooth muscle cells. The earliest precursor of atherosclerosis, the fatty streak, has been detected in autopsy specimens in the first decade of life. Although some fatty streaks are apparently reversible, others progress to fibromuscular lesions and on to complex nonreversible lesions containing lipids, platelets, fibrin, and cellular debris. Mature atherosclerotic lesions may be further complicated by intimal ulceration and intraplaque hemorrhage.

Risk Factors   The pathogenesis of atherosclerosis is exceedingly complex and undoubtedly multifactorial. Several modifiable risk factors have been linked with this process, most notably cigarette smoking, hypertension, and hyperlipidemia.

Smoking   Innumerable reports implicate cigarette smoking as the single independent risk factor most closely associated with atherogenesis, in both the coronary and the peripheral arteries.[17] Additionally, cigarette smoking adversely affects the course of existing arterial occlusive disease. Besides the marked vasoconstrictive effect of nicotine, inhalation of carbon monoxide in cigarette smoke increases circulating carboxyhemoglobin levels. Since carbon monoxide has a greater affinity for hemoglobin than oxygen, oxygen transport to ischemic tissues is impaired and hypoxic injury to the intimal lining of the artery results. Increased platelet aggregation and thrombus formation secondary to enhanced platelet adhesiveness have also been reported.

Hypertension It is well documented that persons with sustained hypertension are at increased risk of atherosclerotic development. The detrimental mechanism of hypertension is perhaps best explained by the constant trauma of elevated blood pressure, causing damage to and thus increasing the permeability of the intimal endothelium. This theory is further supported by the propensity for atherosclerotic plaque to develop at points of arterial branching or narrowing, where blood flow is turbulent and blood pressure increased.

Hyperlipidemia As previously mentioned, incorporation of lipoproteins into the arterial wall is the hallmark of atherosclerosis. Increased serum concentrations of cholesterol (190 mg per 100 mL blood) and/or fasting triglycerides (150 mg per 100 mL blood) as well as low-density lipoproteins and very-low-density lipoproteins are noted in relation to the incidence of atherosclerotic lesions in humans. Conversely, increased serum concentration of high-density lipoproteins has been shown to exert an antiatherogenic effect.

Other commonly implicated atherosclerotic risk factors include diabetes mellitus, advanced age, male sex, unfavorable family history, obesity, and psychophysiologic stress. The presence of more than one risk factor often exerts a multiplicative atherogenic risk.

Data Acquisition

A thorough history and physical assessment can provide the examiner with a nearly conclusive diagnosis of lower extremity arterial occlusive disease. In addition to a functional assessment of health patterns,[18] the nursing history should focus on (1) a detailed description of the patient's presenting complaint (emphasizing understanding), (2) a body systems review with specific questioning as to the presence of systemic atherosclerosis (e.g., history of stroke, transient ischemic attacks, angina, myocardial infarction, or renovascular hypertension), and (3) the presence of known atherosclerotic risk factors.

History Specific questioning about the presenting complaint (usually leg pain or discomfort), focusing on precipitating factors, character and location of pain, and relief methods, will often differentiate true ischemic pain from other potential causes of leg pain, such as neurogenic or musculoskeletal syndromes.

Arterial stenosis or complete occlusion in the presence of collateral vessels can precipitate symptoms of intermittent claudication distal to an occlusive lesion. Intermittent claudication is defined as muscular leg discomfort which is precipitated by exercise, is reproducible, and is relieved by a short period of rest. Depending on the location of the arterial obstruction, intermittent claudication may involve muscles of the calf, thigh, and/or buttocks. Cessation of exercise even for a minute or two relieves the discomfort. With risk factor modification and continuance of exercise, intermittent claudication is often self-limiting and may improve with time. The need for surgery is determined by the clinical course of the patient with intermittent claudication.

More extensive arterial occlusion often results in ischemic rest pain. As the name implies, blood flow in the limb is inadequate to meet even the basal metabolic tissue demands at rest. Pain is usually described as relentless, burning, and throbbing in the most distal portion of the limb, usually in a toe or toes and in the forefoot. Patients frequently describe the pain as being worse with leg elevation, necessitating sleeping upright in a chair so as to keep the ischemic limb dependent. Unlike intermittent claudication, ischemic rest pain is an ominous finding, heralding impending ulceration or tissue necrosis and threatening the viability of the limb unless adequate arterial circulation can be restored.

Physical Assessment In conjunction with a thorough history and systemic physical examination, assessment of the arterial circulation can confirm or exclude a diagnosis of arterial occlusive disease. Following Bates's framework of physical examination,[19] the examiner should employ the skills of inspection, palpation, and auscultation in order to thoroughly examine the arterial system. (Percussion is not applicable to examination of the arterial system.)

Inspection Inspection of a chronically ischemic lower limb often evidences several characteristic signs. Most obvious is the presence of atrophic skin and nail changes in the toes and foot. Typically, the nails are thickened, cornified, and misshapen. The skin of the foot is often thin, shiny, and scaly in appearance, due to atrophy of subcutaneous tissue. Since distal hair follicles are inadequately nourished, absence of hair growth is evident. Additionally, the ischemic limb is often cool or cold to touch.

Severe ischemia is often associated with position-related color changes in the foot. Elevation of an ischemic limb, even at a slight angle, results in the development of cadaveric pallor of the toes and foot. Blanching occurs because the capillary perfusion pressure is inadequate to pump blood "uphill" to the distal portion of the limb. In contrast, putting an ischemic limb in a dependent position (sitting) results in the development of dependent rubor and cyanosis. The toes and forefoot become red to deep blueish purple in color, secondary to pooling of blood in maximally dilated arterioles and venules. The time it takes to develop dependent rubor following leg elevation is directly proportional to the degree of ischemia.

Ischemic tissues are very susceptible to breakdown, and alterations in skin integrity are common. The ischemic limb should be carefully inspected for evidence of arterial ulceration or tissue necrosis (gangrene). Even minor trauma can result in skin disruption and the potential for infection. Also, patients with long-standing arterial insufficiency may suffer from ischemic neuropathy, increasing their risk of traumatic injury, which is exacerbated in diabetic patients with concomitant diabetic neuropathy.

Arterial ulcers are prone to develop on the toes, in the interdigital spaces, and over bony prominences, which are most susceptible to pressure and/or friction necrosis. Gangrene may develop following such simple trauma as stubbing a toe or wearing poorly fitting shoes.

Palpation Pulse assessment is the mainstay of a vascular examination. All peripheral pulses, including the carotid, brachial, radial, femoral, popliteal, dorsalis pedis, and posterior tibial, should be evaluated for quality and symmetry as well as presence or absence.

Weakness or absence of a pulse is indicative of stenosis or occlusion of an artery proximal to that anatomic location. For example, presence of a femoral pulse and absence of a popliteal pulse indicate obstruction of the superficial femoral artery.

Pulse assessment, like any skill, can be easily mastered with practice. If the examiner is uncertain as to whether a pulse is present, it is safest to document it as absent. Having a colleague count the patient's radial pulse aloud or checking the examiner's pulse may help differentiate the examiner's pulse projected through the fingertips from the patient's pulse. Keep in mind that one would not expect to palpate pulses in the foot of a markedly ischemic limb.

Auscultation Auscultation of the arteries may evidence a bruit over a stenotic lesion. In the presence of stenosis, bruits are most commonly audible in the carotid arteries, the abdominal aorta and its major branches, and the femoral arteries. A completely occluded artery will *not* project a bruit.

Noninvasive Diagnostic Procedures The Doppler ultrasound flowmeter can provide an adjunct to auscultation. This device amplifies the sound of blood flow through the vessel and often makes it possible to detect pulsatile flow through an artery in the absence of a palpable pulse.

Perhaps the most valuable noninvasive diagnostic test for lower extremity arterial disease, and certainly the most commonly employed, is segmental leg pressure measurement. Using the Doppler blood flow velocity detector and a technique identical to that of determining brachial blood pressure (Table 25-3), the examiner can compare the *systolic* blood pressure in the leg with that in the arm. Though determinations can be made at various levels in the leg, a quick test in routine clinical practice is to compare the higher of the dorsalis pedis or posterior tibial artery systolic pressure in each limb with the brachial systolic pressure. This comparison, known as the ankle/brachial index (ABI), is determined by dividing the "ankle" pressure by the arm pressure. The result

Table 25-3 Procedure for Use of Ultrasound Blood Flow Detector (Doppler) Flowmeter for Arterial Assessment of the Lower Extremity

1. Place a blood pressure cuff on the lower leg just above the ankle
2. Apply acoustic coupling gel to the Doppler probe or on the dorsum of the foot. This permits percutaneous transmission of high-frequency sound wave to underlying blood vessel. (Avoid using water-soluble lubricants or ECG transmission gel, as they are corrosive to the probe)
3. With the Doppler turned on, place the probe over the expected anatomic location of the dorsalis pedis (DP) artery. Manipulate the probe until *pulsatile** flow is audible
4. Holding the probe in place, inflate the blood pressure cuff until the pulse is obliterated. Slowly release the pressure in the cuff, recording the first audible return of pulse as the systolic artery pressure
5. Repeat procedure to determine systolic pressure in posterior tibial (PT) artery, behind medial malleolus
6. In the same manner, determine the brachial artery systolic pressure
7. Compare the ankle pressure (higher of DP or PT) to the arm pressure to calculate the ankle/brachial index (ABI)

Example:

$$\text{Ankle pressure} = 80 \text{ mmHg} = 0.66^{+}$$
$$\text{Brachial pressure} = 120 \text{ mmHg}$$

*Differentiate carefully between arterial pulsatile flow and consistent, windlike venous flow.
†May also be expressed as 66%, or 2/3 normal ABI of 1.00. The lower the index, the more severe the ischemia.

is most commonly expressed as a fraction, decimal, or percentage. With normal circulation, the ankle pressure should equal or exceed the brachial pressure (i.e., ABI ≥ 1.00). Patients with intermittent claudication often have an ABI in the symptomatic limb in the range of 0.4 to 0.8, and those with severe ischemic rest pain lie between 0.0 and 0.4.

Invasive Diagnostic Procedures   The "gold standard" against which all other diagnostic modalities is compared is arteriography, the roentgenography of the arteries after intraarterial injection of radiopaque contrast material which outlines the arterial circuit. A quality arteriogram will delineate the specific anatomic location of obstruction, clarify the underlying etiology (e.g., atherosclerosis vs. fibromuscular dysplasia), and depict the arteries proximal and distal to the obstructing lesion. Thus, it provides the vascular surgeon with a "road map" of the arterial circuit, clarifying the surgical treatment options. However, because a thorough health history and vascular assessment are nearly conclusively diagnostic, an arteriogram is indicated only when further intervention is planned, not solely to further strengthen the examiner's findings.

The nurse should be knowledgeable about the technique of arteriography in order to adequately prepare the patient for the procedure (see Chap. 20). The patient should be assured that throughout the procedure the heart function and vital signs will be closely monitored by the radiology staff.

Following the procedure, the patient requires careful nursing assessment. Arteriography carries with it the risks of intimal disruption at the site of catheter insertion, acute arterial occlusion, or arterial embolization, any of which may impair arterial inflow to the limb. These risks are most significant in patients with preexisting atherosclerotic disease. A significant change in circulatory status in the limb should be reported immediately to the physician.

The nurse should carefully monitor the patient's fluid balance for 72 h following arteriography or throughout the perioperative period. The rationale for this is twofold: (1) the contrast is hyperosmolar and precipitates an osmotic diuresis, and (2) the contrast is nephrotoxic and can precipitate acute tubular necrosis (acute renal failure), particularly in the diabetic patient with preexisting nephropathy.[20,21] Documentation of intake and output minimizes the risk of dehydration and provides a useful parameter by which to monitor renal function. Additionally, the postprocedure serum creatinine and BUN can be compared with the admission baseline results as another indicator of renal function.

Bed rest, with the punctured extremity immobile, is maintained for 8 to 12 h following the procedure to minimize the risk of disrupting the healing arteriotomy, with consequent hematoma or bleeding. Barring complications, the patient can resume sitting, ambulating, and routine daily activities following this period.

Medical Management of Arterial Occlusive Disease

The majority of patients with symptomatic lower extremity arterial occlusive disease—that is, those with intermittent claudication—are treated medically, the goal being control of modifiable risk factors such as cigarette smoking, hypertension, hyperlipidemia, diabetes mellitus, obesity, and stress, in the hope of preventing disease progression. Numerous reports studying the natural history of intermittent claudication conclude that with risk factor modification, particularly cessation of smoking, and routine exercise (walking is sufficient), only a small percentage of patients develop worsening symptoms or threatened limb viability within a 5-year follow-up period.[22,23]

Historically, vasodilating drugs have proved to be of little value in the treatment of peripheral arterial occlusive disease, because no known agent selectively dilates vessels in ischemic areas or in exercising skeletal muscle.[24] In fact, vasodilators may worsen symptoms, secondary to decreases in systemic blood pressure that further compromise flow to ischemic areas. Additionally, the efficacy of these drugs is limited by the fact that atherosclerosis has resulted in increased rigidity of the vessel walls, making them structurally incapable of dilating.

A recently published report of a multicenter trial, however, has evidenced an exception to the general rule that drugs are ineffective in treating intermittent claudication. Favorable objective results with the agent pentoxifylline (Trental) were reported to include increase of walking distance and minimization of limb paresthesias as compared with the placebo effects.[25] Pentoxifylline acts primarily by reducing blood viscosity and thus increasing blood flow in the microcirculation by increasing red blood cell flexibility and decreasing platelet aggregation and fibrinogen.[26] Future clinical trials are needed to substantiate these findings.

As mentioned previously, exercise in the form of walking to the point of discomfort, resting a short time, then continuing to walk is also an important component of treatment for patients with intermittent claudication. Although the cause of claudication—that is, inadequate oxygenation of working muscles—is similar to that of angina pectoris, an important distinction must be made. Persons with exertional angina must cease further exertion to preclude increases in myocardial oxygen demand and the risk of infarction, whereas stimulation of exercising leg muscles to the point of pain is thought to promote the development of collateral circulation. Although collateral vessels are normally insignificant in blood transport, they become important in bypassing a localized arterial obstruction, gradually increasing in size to carry more blood and thus stabilize or improve symptoms.[27]

Occasionally, patients with severe limb-threatening ischemia and rest pain are faced with a nonreconstructible situation (that is, diffuse disease with no bypassable lesion) or are prohibitive surgical risks because of coexisting medical problems. The goals of medical management of these patients are prevention of skin breakdown, ulceration, and infection, and treatment of gangrenous necrosis, if present. Gangrene is full-thickness tissue necrosis and is nonreversible even with an adequate blood flow. If the necrotic areas of the toes or foot are dry, they can be left open to air. The limb should be assessed daily for evidence of gangrenous progression. With purulent exudate, suggestive of infected necrotic tissue, wound cultures should be obtained and intravenous antibiotic therapy initiated. The draining area can be bandaged with a normal saline wet-to-dry dressing. A foot or lower leg x-ray can determine the presence of underlying osteomyelitis. If the infected necrotic limb precipitates systemic septicemia, local or limb amputation may be a lifesaving treatment.

Other nonsurgical treatment options include the use of percutaneous transluminal angioplasty and thrombolytic therapy, each being appropriate in certain clinical situations.

Percutaneous Transluminal Angioplasty In selected patients, percutaneous transluminal angioplasty (PTA) is a safe and effective treatment option. PTA involves mechanical dilation of a narrowed or occluded artery using a specially designed balloon-tipped catheter. The technique of PTA parallels that of arteriography, and preparation of the patient is identical. The balloon catheter is directed to the desired anatomic point using fluoroscopic control, and dilation is achieved by repeated inflations of the balloon tip to a predetermined size, minimizing the risk of overdistention and vessel rupture.

The atheromatous lesions that have proved to be most successfully managed with PTA are focal narrowings in the iliac or common femoral arteries. Refinements in technique and equipment are improving the results of PTA in arteries distal to the common femoral.

PTA actually causes a "cracking" of the intimal plaque, leaving behind a rough intimal surface which results in platelet aggregation and the potential for thrombus formation.[28] Therefore, following PTA, patients are often treated with anticoagulants or anti-platelet-aggregating agents, such as aspirin and/or dipyridamole (Persantine).

In the hands of a skilled vascular radiologist, and in patients who are at high risk for complica-

tions from surgical intervention, PTA can provide a safe, effective, and well tolerated treatment option.

Thrombolytic Therapy   The thrombolytic enzymes urokinase and streptokinase were approved for clinical use in 1979. In the peripheral arterial circuit, they can be used to treat acute thromboembolic events[29,30] as well as occlusion of arterial bypass grafts (Fig. 25-5). Additionally, in the venous circuit they are used to treat extensive deep vein thrombosis and massive pulmonary emboli.[31]

Streptokinase is obtained from bacterial culture (filtrates of group C beta-hemolytic streptococci), while urokinase is extracted from human urine or fetal kidney tissue culture. Both these thrombolytic agents work by converting plasminogen to plasmin, resulting in the degradation of fibrin clots, fibrinogen, and other plasma proteins.[32] They can be administered either intravenously

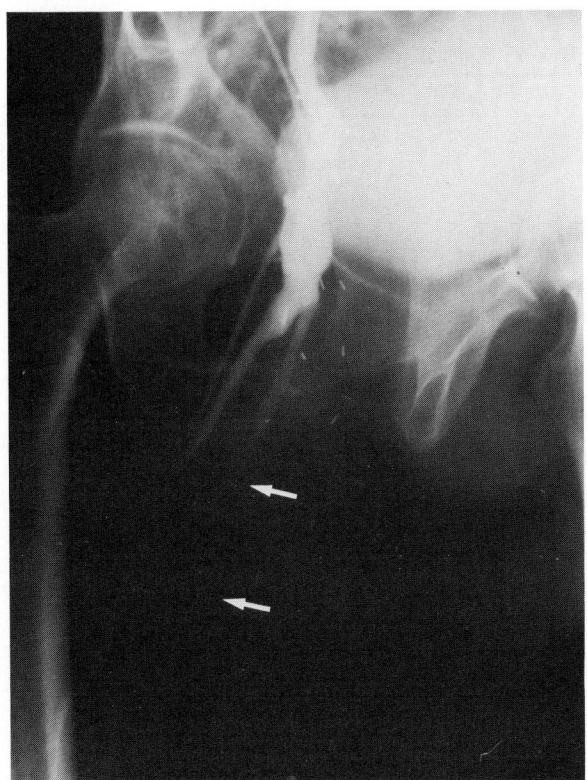

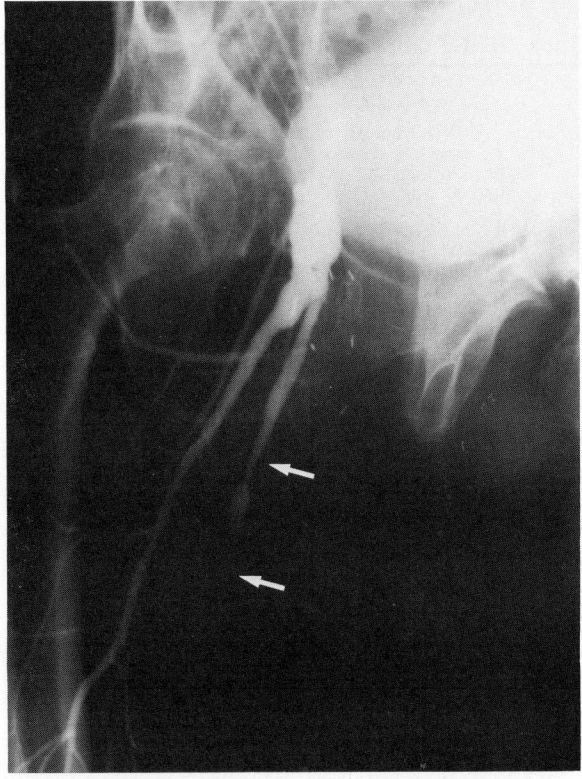

A   B

Figure 25-5   Arteriogram demonstrating (*A*) occlusion of right femoropopliteal bypass graft (arrows) and (*B*) partial patency of same graft following treatment with intraarterial urokinase.

(systemically) or directly into an arterial occlusion via a localizing catheter. Their action is immediate, and lysis is halted rapidly following discontinuation. Table 25-4 provides a comparison of dosage recommendations, methods of laboratory monitoring, adverse reactions, and cost of urokinase and streptokinase, the major difference being cost. Because of its source, urokinase is nearly ten times more expensive than its bacterial counterpart.

Activation of the fibrinolytic system is confirmed by prolongation of the thrombin time to two to five times the control value. The thrombin time should be checked 4 h after initiating treatment and every 8 to 12 h throughout therapy.[33]

Both agents are pyrogenic, though urokinase is less so. Fever is easily managed with antipyretics. Additionally, streptokinase has been associated with allergic reactions in 10 to 12 percent of patients, because preexisting antibodies to streptococci are common. Anaphylaxis can occur in 2 to 3 percent

of patients.[34] Symptoms of an allergic reaction are treated with antihistamines and/or steroids. These agents should be on hand before initiating treatment.

The major complication associated with the use of fibrinolytic agents is hemorrhage, which reportedly occurs in about 10 percent of patients but is only rarely life-threatening.[34] Nonetheless, patients treated with thrombolytic agents should not be concurrently treated with anticoagulants or antiplatelet agents.

Reports of successful results using thrombolytic therapy in peripheral vascular disease are increasingly frequent in current literature.[35,36]

Surgical Management of Arterial Occlusive Disease

Surgical intervention in management of arterial occlusive disease is indicated for patients with ischemic rest pain, with or without tissue necrosis.

Table 25-4 Comparison of Urokinase and Streptokinase as Thrombolytic Agents

	Urokinase	Streptokinase
Origin	Isolated from human urine or fetal kidney tissue	Filtrate of group C beta-hemolytic streptococci
Mechanism of action	Immediate-acting enzymatic protein which converts plasminogen to plasmin, resulting in breakdown of fibrin clot	Immediate-acting nonenzymatic protein which converts plasminogen to plasmin, resulting in breakdown of fibrin clot
Dosage/route of administration	IV: bolus of 4400 U over 10–20 min	IV: bolus of 250,000 IU over 20–30 min
	Maintenance dose 4400 U/h via controlled infusion pump	Maintenance dose 100,000 U/h via controlled infusion pump
	Intraarterial: up to 100,000 U/h*	Intraarterial: 5000–100,000 U/h*
	Available in powder form	Available in powder form
	Reconstitute with sterile saline	Reconstitute with sterile saline
Therapeutic monitoring	Thrombin time 2 to 5 times control (in seconds) assures lytic state	Thrombin time 2 to 5 times control (in seconds) assures lytic state
Adverse reactions	Pyrogenic	Pyrogenic
	Risk of hemorrhage	Risk of hemorrhage
		Allergic reaction, particularly in patients with recurrent streptococcal infection or retreatment with streptokinase
Cost	$2000 for 12 h treatment	$300 for 24 h treatment

*Wide variation in recommended dosage.

As mentioned previously, rest pain is premonitory of threatened limb viability without restoration of arterial inflow. In most cases, every attempt is made to preserve a limb, and amputation is limited to areas of full-thickness tissue necrosis (toe, forefoot). Unfortunately, limb amputation may be the only treatment option in cases of extremely diffuse atherosclerotic occlusion.

Arterial revascularization by means of bypass procedures is the most commonly employed surgical approach. Each patient must be considered individually when deciding on the best surgical option, taking into consideration factors such as the patient's general health, the location of the occlusive lesion along with the quality of the arteries proximally and distally, the availability of a suitable conduit with which to bypass the lesion, and the natural history of atherosclerosis.[37] Five-year survival rates are markedly lower in patients with clinically symptomatic systemic atherosclerosis than in age-matched asymptomatic patients, coronary artery disease carrying with it the most ominous prognosis.

The most commonly encountered arterial occlusive lesions are aortoiliac, superficial femoral, and tibial. Aortoiliac disease refers to arterial obstruction of blood flow into the lower extremities. It is often bilateral but may produce more severe symptoms in one leg. Symptoms range from exertional muscle pain and discomfort distal to the obstruction (as in the buttocks, thigh, and calf) to rest pain with or without tissue necrosis. Bypass approaches for aortoiliac occlusion include (1) aortobifemoral bypass (Fig. 25-6); (2) unilateral aortofemoral grafting, bypassing the more severely diseased iliac artery in the symptomatic extremity (Fig. 25-7); and (3) extraanatomic bypass, either axillobifemoral (Fig. 25-8) or femorofemoral (Fig. 25-9), restoring blood flow beyond an occlusive lesion. Extraanatomic bypass is safest in high-risk surgical patients. All these procedures are done with synthetic graft material, either Dacron velour or polytetrafluoroethylene (PTFE, Gore-tex).

Occlusive disease in the superficial femoral artery occurs most commonly in the mid to distal thigh, anatomically where the artery tapers and passes through the adductor canal posteriorly, above the knee (Fig. 25-10). The most common surgical approach in this situation is femoropopliteal bypass

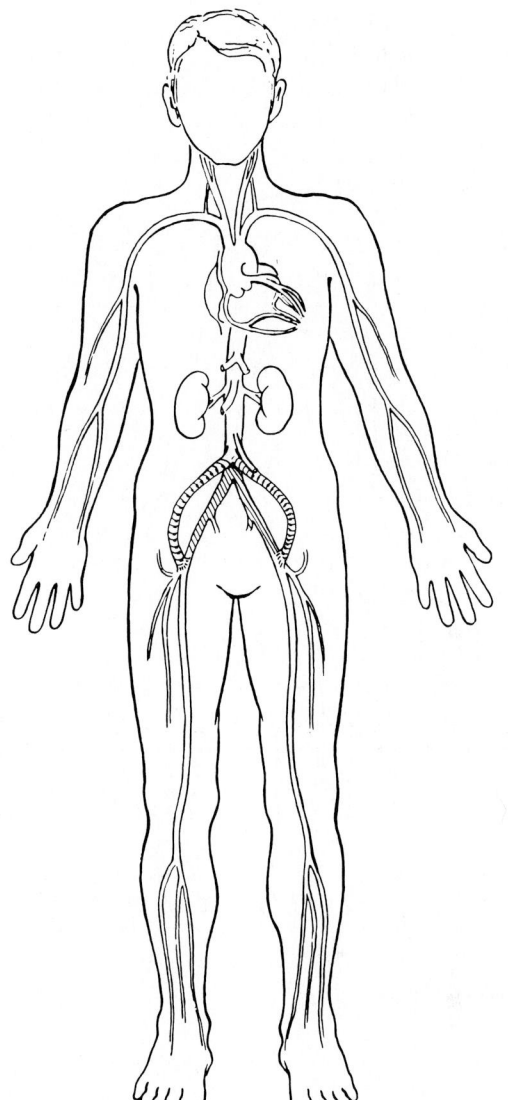

Figure 25-6   Artist's depiction of aortoiliac occlusion and revascularization—aortobifemoral prosthetic bypass graft.

anastomosed proximal and distal to the occlusion, with the conduit of choice being autogenous (usually saphenous) vein. The superiority of autogenous vein over synthetic materials in this location in terms of 5-year patency rates is cited frequently in the literature.[38,39]

Arterial obstruction of one or more tibial vessels is an especially common finding in the diabetic patient[40] and not unheard of in the non-

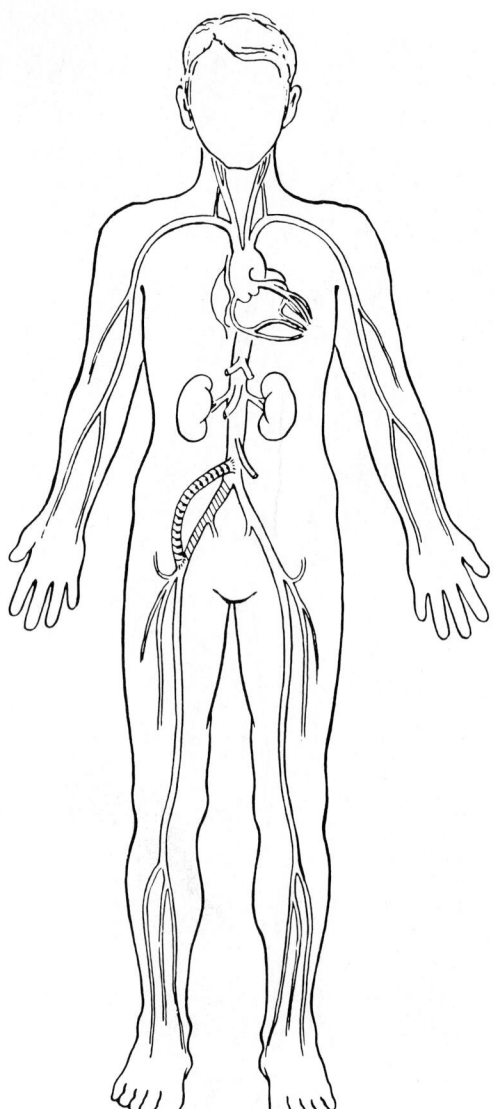

Figure 25-7 Right iliac artery occlusion and revascularization—unilateral aortofemoral prosthetic bypass graft.

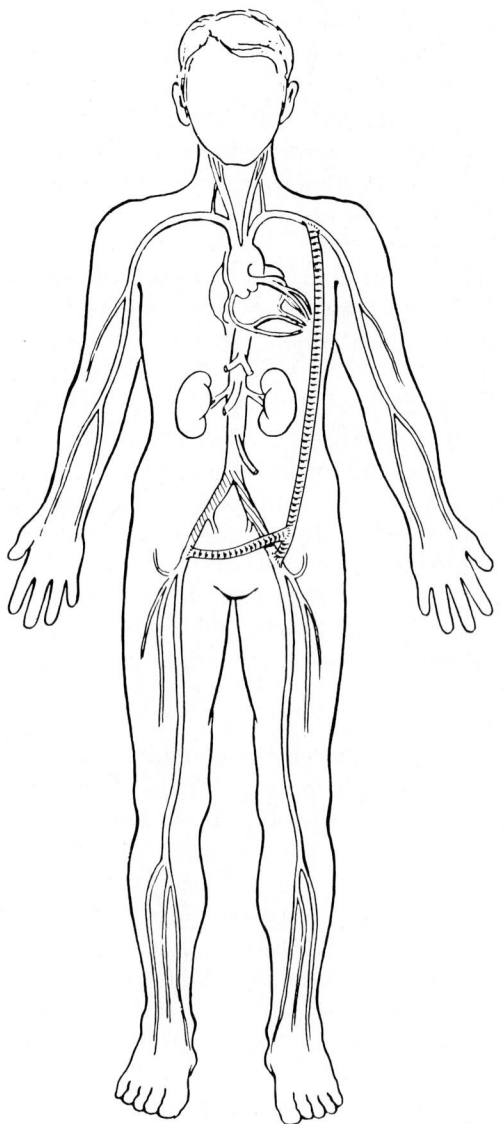

Figure 25-8 Aortoiliac occlusion and revascularization—left axillofemorofemoral prosthetic bypass graft.

diabetic smoker. As surgical techniques and instrumentation have improved, vascular surgeons have succeeded in improving patency rates to a distal tibial vessel. Depending on the quality of the vessels proximally, the bypass graft can originate at either the femoral or popliteal level. As with femoropopliteal bypass grafting, the conduit of choice is autogenous vein, which has superior long-term patency.

Until recent years, use of autogenous vein as an arterial bypass graft involved removing the vein, ligating its branches, and storing it in a preservative solution until the bypass was performed. Because of the presence of valves in the vein permitting unidirectional flow only, the vein had to be reversed before being anastomosed to the artery proximal and distal to the occlusion. Although the reversed vein technique continues to be commonly used, a

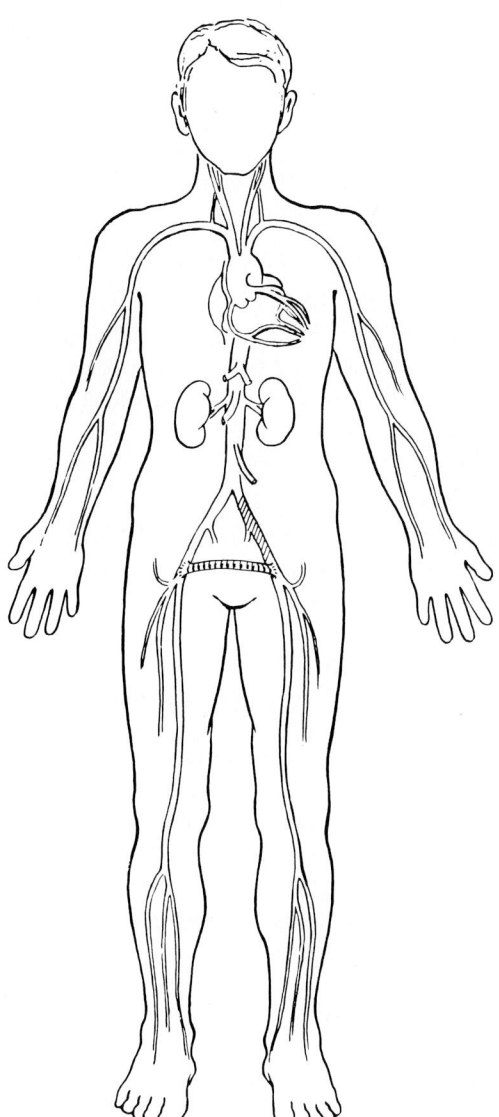

Figure 25-9 Left iliac artery occlusion and revascularization—right-to-left femorofemoral prosthetic bypass graft.

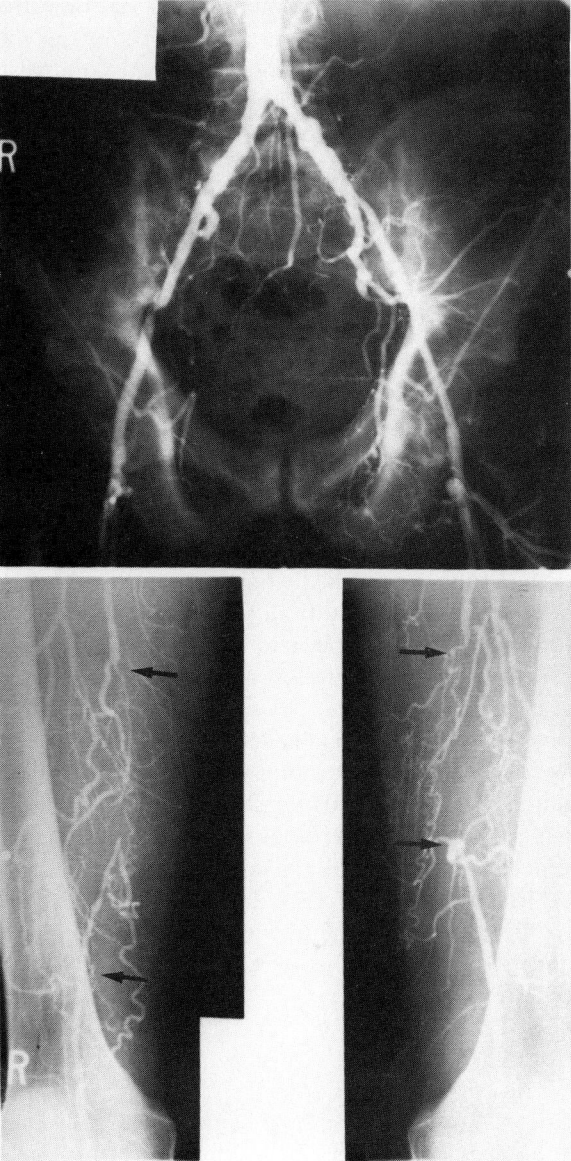

Figure 25-10 Arteriogram depicting diffuse iliac disease and complete occlusion of superficial femoral arteries, with reconstitution of popliteal arteries bilaterally (arrows).

more recently employed technique, known as *in situ vein grafting,* was introduced by Leather and Karmody in the early 1980s. With the in situ technique, the saphenous vein is left in place. After the vein is transected proximally and distally, a valvulotomy is used to cut the valve leaflets, permitting antegrade flow. The vein is sewn to the artery above and below the obstruction, and the proximal and distal veins are ligated. The literature

cites numerous reports of the success of this technique, although continued study is needed to determine its long-term efficacy.[41–43]

Apart from bypass procedures, surgical approaches to lower extremity arterial occlusive disease include endarterectomy, sympathectomy, and amputation. Endarterectomy involves opening the occluded portion of the artery and removing the obstructing plaque. Because this technique also necessitates excision of the artery's intimal lining, the denuded surface tends to be thrombogenic and prone to thrombotic occlusion. Thus endarterectomy is usually reserved for localized lesions in high blood flow areas, such as the carotid, aorta, and iliac arteries.

Though once commonly employed, surgical sympathectomy as a treatment option in atherosclerotic occlusive disease is of questionable value. The technique involves surgical transection of the lumbar sympathetic ganglia, resulting in permanent vasodilatation, albeit largely in skin vessels. The true usefulness of sympathectomy lies in the treatment of vasospastic disease, hyperhidrosis, and certain causalgias.[44]

Despite continually improving results with arterial revascularization, limb amputation may be the only treatment option to obliterate excruciating rest pain, gangrene, and/or infection. Consideration is given to preservation of as much of the limb as possible in order to facilitate rehabilitation. Below-knee versus above-knee amputation often means the difference between returning to ambulation with a prosthesis and total loss of independence, especially in the elderly patient. Limb loss is a devastating outcome. Providing emotional support to the patient and family, as well as recognizing and coordinating rehabilitation needs, are critical nursing roles.

Nursing Management of Lower Extremity Arterial Occlusive Disease

Nurses in the critical-care setting frequently encounter patients with severe lower extremity ischemia. They may be patients with severe cardiopulmonary dysfunction, or patients with brittle diabetes, or patients in end-stage renal failure with concomitant lower extremity atherosclerosis. The use of certain therapeutic modalities, such as intraaortic balloon counterpulsation or femoral artery catheters for dialysis access, may further impair already compromised arterial blood supply.

The nurse in this setting should carefully assess the adequacy of the patient's lower extremity circulation by means of a thorough history and physical examination as described previously. Nursing diagnoses and plans of care for patients with lower extremity ischemia and for surgical patients follow.

Nursing Diagnosis

Potential impairment of skin integrity of foot and leg related to alteration in tissue perfusion.

Goals

Patient (1) will not develop skin breakdown or necrosis of ischemic extremity; (2) will verbalize understanding of increased risk of skin breakdown; and (3) will take an active part in daily foot care.

Interventions

1. Prevent mechanical trauma:
   Minimize pressure of mattress and bedclothes by using heel protectors, footboard, and sheepskin pad at foot of bed.
   Use lambswool between toes to prevent interdigital friction necrosis.
   Moisturize ischemic foot and leg with alcohol-free lubricant lotion to prevent cracking of skin.
   Protect foot with shoe or slipper when patient is out of bed.
   Inspect ischemic limb every 4 h for evidence of pressure necrosis, especially at bony prominences such as phalanges, heel, and malleoli. Reposition ischemic limb every 2 h.
   Do not apply antiembolism stockings to ischemic limb.
2. Prevent thermal trauma:
   Avoid extremes in temperature. Do *not* use heating pads in attempt to enhance vasodilatation.
   Keep ischemic limb covered loosely with bedclothes. If socks are worn, remove frequently to inspect foot.
3. Prevent chemical trauma:
   Use only mild isotonic solutions on ischemic limb.
   Avoid use of enzymatic debriding agents or hypertonic bactericidal agents such as full-strength povidone-iodine solution.
   If foot soaks are prescribed, use mild soap solution and test water temperature before immersing ischemic limb.
4. Teach patient about necessity of meticulous foot care, reinforcing awareness of increased risk of

skin breakdown arising from compromised arterial circulation.

5. Encourage patient to participate actively in daily foot care.

Evaluation

Patient (1) did not develop mechanical, thermal, or chemical skin breakdown of ischemic limb; (2) verbalized understanding of increased risk of skin breakdown; and (3) took an active role in daily foot care.

Nursing Diagnosis

Alteration in comfort (ischemic resting pain) related to alteration in tissue perfusion.

Goals

Patient's resting pain will be minimized by nursing and medical or surgical intervention; after surgery, ischemic limb will be warm to the touch and ABI (ankle-brachial index) will be improved.

Interventions

1. Employ arterial positioning (if not contraindicated), using 6-in shock blocks at head of bed to achieve leg dependency.
2. Minimize tissue oxygen demands by limiting activity.
3. Avoid activities which promote vasoconstriction (e.g., cigarette smoking, exposure to cold).
4. Avoid restrictive clothing such as antiembolism stockings.
5. Administer analgesics per physician's prescription, and ascertain degree of relief by questioning patient.
6. Provide emotional support and utilize comfort measures such as touch, massage, music, and diversion.
7. Following surgical intervention, assess for objective evidence of improved arterial circulation (e.g., warmth, palpable pulses or improved ABI) and ascertain any changes in patient's symptoms.

Evaluation

Patient's rest pain improved with employment of nursing and medical/surgical therapies; after surgery, ischemic limb is warm to the touch and ABI is improved.

Nursing Diagnosis

Preoperative: Patient and/or family anxiety related to lack of knowledge about impending surgery.

Goal

Patient and/or family will not experience undue anxiety related to surgery.

Interventions

1. Encourage patient and family to explore concerns with nursing staff preoperatively (e.g., fear of death, limb loss, pain, potential complications).
2. Assess patient and family readiness to learn and reinforce preoperative teaching, reviewing perioperative routines and specific surgical plans (individualized for each patient).
3. Orient patient and family to critical-care setting and explain routine procedures.
4. If appropriate, teach patient leg and foot exercises to help promote venous return while at bed rest postoperatively and breathing exercises to minimize pulmonary compromise, allowing some control of recuperative process.

Evaluation

Patient and family asked questions to enhance their knowledge of impending surgery (to degree desired) and verbalized appropriate concerns, fears, etc.

Nursing Diagnosis

Potential altered tissue perfusion related to vascular surgical intervention.

Goal

Patient will maintain adequate tissue perfusion evidenced by palpable pulse(s), improved ABI, intact motion and sensation, and/or warm, pink limb.

Interventions

1. Assess pulses hourly for 24 h, then every 4 h, also Doppler pressure (may require physician order) in operated extremity.
2. Assess sensory and motor function of lower extremities.
3. Provide adequate hydration to assure normovolemia and avoid hypotension.

4. Monitor VS hourly for 24 h, then every shift unless directed otherwise.

5. Inspect operated limb for evidence of severe swelling, which may impede blood flow through the graft.

6. If marked edema develops, elevate foot of bed slightly and apply Ace bandage from foot to thigh (surgeon's order), *provided adequate arterial circulation has been restored).*

7. Record bilateral circumferential measurements of ankle, calf, and thigh daily.

8. Report any sudden change in tissue perfusion (e.g., loss of palpable pulse, acute nonincisional pain, change in color, motion, sensation) to physician immediately.

Evaluation
Patient maintained adequate tissue perfusion.

Nursing Diagnosis
Potential wound infection related to surgically induced skin disruption.

Goal
Patient will not develop wound infection.

Interventions

1. Assess surgical incision daily for evidence of erythema, induration, hematoma, warmth, drainage, etc.

2. Document appearance of wound and report any suspicion of infection to physician.

Evaluation
Patient did not develop incisional infection.

Other Nursing Diagnoses
Many patients undergoing lower extremity arterial bypass surgery also have concomitant cardiopulmonary dysfunction as well as pain and impaired mobility. Thus, other possible nursing diagnoses might include:

Potential decrease in cardiac output related to myocardial ischemia or infarction subsequent to surgical or anesthetic stress

Potential impairment of gas exchange related to altered tissue perfusion secondary to preexisting chronic obstructive pulmonary disease, general anesthesia, pain, and/or immobility.

Impaired mobility related to incisional pain

Alteration in comfort: pain related to surgical incision(s)

Astute nursing assessment and management of patients with lower extremity arterial occlusive disease affords the critical-care nurse the challenge of recognizing and preventing disastrous events which might indeed threaten the viability of an ischemic limb, as well as the opportunity to facilitate recuperation and minimize complications in the vascular surgical patient.

Lower Extremity Venous Disease

Normal Venous Anatomy and Physiology
Prior to the seventeenth century, blood was thought to be produced in the liver and to receive natural, vital, and animal spirits from other organs. William Harvey was the first to theorize that blood actually *circulates* through a system of blood vessels, the beginning and end point being the beating heart, with arteries functioning to carry oxygenated blood to all body cells and veins providing a return route for deoxygenated blood and waste products.

Histologically, the walls of veins are similar to those of arteries; they too have intimal, medial, and adventitial layers. The primary differences are that in veins there is less medial elastic tissue and the medial and adventitial layers are less clearly defined. Veins are capacitance vessels, capable of "storing" a tremendous volume of blood because of their relatively large diameter.

Major venous pathways parallel those of similarly named arteries (Fig. 25-11). Nearly all veins have valves permitting unidirectional flow toward the heart. The exceptions to this rule are those veins in the visceral venous system which drain blood to the liver for purification before it returns to the heart. In addition to returning blood to the heart, the venous system also functions to regulate vascular capacity and to maintain thermoregularity.

In the lower extremity there are three major systems of veins: superficial veins, communicating or perforating veins, and deep veins. The *superficial veins* course in the subcutaneous tissue layer and generally have fewer valves than deep veins. Examples of superficial veins in the leg include the greater and lesser saphenous vessels. The entire superficial system can be sacrificed, as in ligation

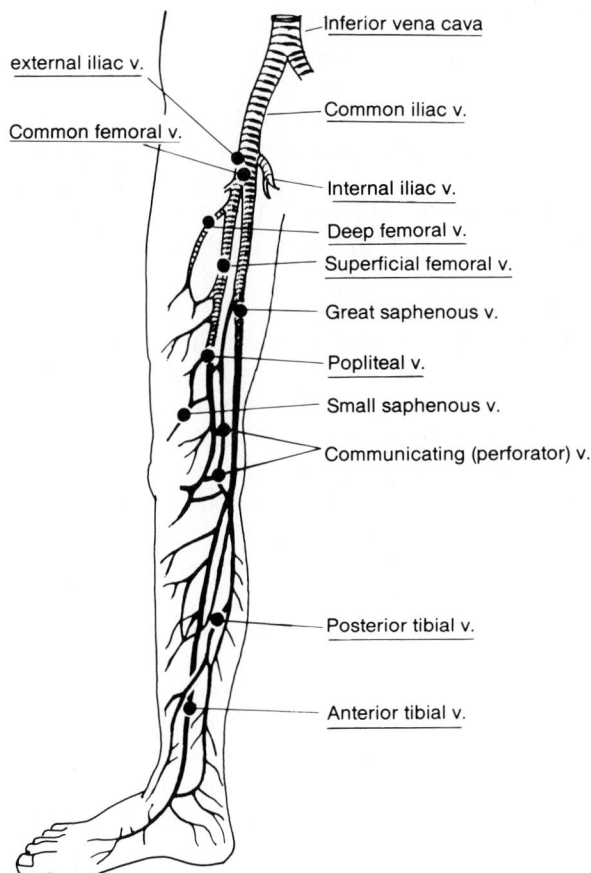

Inferior vena cava

external iliac v.

Common femoral v.

Common iliac v.

Internal iliac v.

Deep femoral v.

Superficial femoral v.

Great saphenous v.

Popliteal v.

Small saphenous v.

Communicating (perforator) v.

Posterior tibial v.

Anterior tibial v.

Figure 25-11 Major venous pathways of the lower extremity.

and stripping procedures, without leading to signs and symptoms of venous insufficiency. *Communicating or perforating veins* connect the superficial and deep systems. Valves in these vessels permit flow from the superficial to the deep system only. *Deep veins* course deeply within the leg musculature and are unquestionably the most functionally important vessels. They are normally responsible for at least 90 percent of venous outflow from the leg. Examples of deep veins in the leg are the femoral and popliteal veins.

Pathophysiology

The most common type of venous dysfunction is thrombosis, a narrowing or obstruction of venous outflow by intravascular clot formation. The terms *thrombosis* and *thrombophlebitis* are often used interchangeably, although thrombophlebitis in-

volves a noninfectious inflammatory component in addition to intraluminal clot formation.

A frequent site of intravenous thrombus formation is the valve cusps. Venous stasis in these cusps allows for accumulation and adherence of platelets and fibrin. Once initiated, the thrombus enlarges and eventually occludes the vessel lumen. If the thrombus only partially obstructs the lumen, it becomes covered by smooth endothelium (*recanalization*) and the process stops. It is also possible that the thrombus may dislodge and embolize distally in the venous circuit back to the heart and into the pulmonary arterial circulation (*pulmonary embolism*). If the thrombus does not become detached, it will become firmly adherent to the vein wall within 24 to 48 h and the body's intrinsic fibrinolytic system will gradually lyse the clot.

Thrombophlebitis can occur in either the superficial or the deep venous systems, but its consequences are more severe with deep vein involvement. Virchow, in 1846, identified three major elements promoting the development of venous thrombosis: hypercoagulability, venous stasis, and intimal damage, which have come to be known as *Virchow's triad*. Table 25-5 outlines common clinical causes of these elements. Table 25-6 lists risk factors associated with the development of deep venous thrombosis. Review of these factors quickly identifies the marked risk of deep vein thrombosis (DVT) in the critical-care patient population.

Table 25-5 Virchow's Triad

Hypercoagulability
  Blood dyscrasias (such as antithrombin III deficiency)
  Trauma
  Advanced malignant disease
  Estrogen therapy
  Systemic infection
  Cigarette smoking

Venous stasis
  Heart disease, especially congestive heart failure
  Dehydration
  Immobility
  Incompetent vein valves

Intimal damage
  Trauma
  Infection
  Venipuncture
  IV infusion of irritant solutions

Table 25-6 Risk Factors Associated with Development of Deep Vein Thrombosis

Prolonged bed rest
Cancer, especially pancreatic or prostatic
Advanced age
Obesity
Congestive heart failure
Previous venous disease
Pelvic surgery
Pregnancy, postpartum state
Lower extremity trauma

Superficial venous thrombosis is usually a self-limiting problem and is treated with conservative measures, which include elevation, application of moist heat, and administration of antiinflammatory agents such as acetylsalicylic acid. Antibiotics may also be prescribed if an infectious component is suspected.

Deep vein thrombosis may lead to two significant sequelae: pulmonary embolism and postphlebitic syndrome. *Pulmonary embolism* (PE) is the most acute consequence of DVT and is potentially lethal. Turpie and Hirsh report that PE occurs in over 500,000 patients annually and is fatal in more than 100,000.[45] Of these, 80,000 with massive PE die within 2 h of the onset of symptoms, often before the diagnosis is made.

The pathophysiologic effect of pulmonary embolism is dependent on the size of the obstructing clot and becomes significant when more than 25 percent of the pulmonary arterial circulation is occluded. With 25 to 30 percent occlusion, pulmonary artery pressure rises, indicating impending heart failure. Cardiac output remains normal until occlusion reaches or exceeds 50 percent. It is critical to keep in mind, however, that preexisting cardiac or respiratory insufficiency contributes significantly to premature cardiac failure. In addition to these hemodynamic effects, pulmonary emboli can also exert mechanical effects such as potential arrhythmias as the clot traverses the right side of the heart, bronchial artery dilatation, and decreased pulmonary blood flow.

The risk of PE is least when DVT is confined to the calf veins and increases proportionally with proximal propagation of clot. Iliofemoral DVT is associated with a significant incidence of PE.

Postphlebitic syndrome, also known as *venous insufficiency,* is a chronic consequence of DVT. It results from permanent valvular incompetence secondary to valve destruction by clot. The consequences of chronic venous insufficiency, most significantly venous ulceration, are infrequently encountered by the critical-care nurse and are, therefore, beyond the scope of this discussion.

Data Acquisition

History and Physical Assessment The clinical presentations of superficial and deep vein thrombophlebitis are markedly different. Superficial thrombophlebitis presents as a local inflammatory response, with erythema and tenderness in a localized area. The affected vein may be palpable as a subcutaneous cord. The most common sites of superficial thrombophlebitis are the upper extremity veins subsequent to intravenous infusions and the saphenous system of the lower extremities. Deep vein thrombophlebitis most commonly affects the major venous pathways in the lower extremity and is usually unidirectional. With DVT there are often systemic signs of inflammation such as low-grade fever. The most common clinical findings are generalized edema and resultant intense pain in the involved extremity.[46] Edema results from obstruction to venous outflow with venous engorgement and fluid transudation from the capillary bed into the extravascular tissue.

Additionally, the patient with DVT may exhibit a positive Homans' sign (sharp muscular calf pain on dorsiflexion), asymmetry in leg circumference, and/or a positive Pratt's sign (pain resulting from compression of the calf against the tibia). These findings are much less reliable, however.

The patient with PE may present clinically with an acute event leading to cardiac failure and death, but lesser degrees of PE may also present in patients who are asymptomatic or those with chest pain and dyspnea. In addition, tachypnea and tachycardia are common. Unexplained restlessness and apprehension, especially in a high-risk patient, should alert the examiner to the possibility of PE. Hemoptysis may or may not be present. Pleuritic chest pain may develop from pulmonary infarction. Recurrent small pulmonary emboli may lead to pulmonary hypertension and compromise of right ventricular heart function. With a massive PE, acute cor pulmonale, decreased cardiac output, hypoxemia, and shock develop.

Noninvasive Diagnostic Procedures   The noninvasive tests most commonly used to detect deep vein thrombophlebitis in current clinical practice are impedance plethysmography, phleborrheography, and Doppler venous evaluation. Each of these tests has inherent shortcomings, with different degrees of specificity and sensitivity according to the location of the thrombus and the experience of the examiner.

Thus, the ultimate diagnostic test for DVT remains contrast venography. Positive findings on venogram include filling defects, sharp termination of a column of contrast, and/or nonfilling of the deep vein system.

Several screening tests are commonly employed for patients with suspected pulmonary embolism. Laboratory evaluation includes analysis of arterial blood gases (ABGs), which usually evidence a decreased P_{O_2} (< 80 mmHg) and decreased P_{CO_2} secondary to hyperventilation. Serum enzymes may be analyzed to differentiate symptoms from those of a myocardial infarction (MI). Increased serum lactate dyhydrogenase (LDH) may be indicative of pulmonary infarction. An ECG is also routinely employed, again to differentiate between PE and acute MI. Chest x-rays, especially when used in conjunction with other studies, may help to rule out other possible causes of symptoms, such as pneumonia or pleural effusion.

Radionuclide lung scanning is a useful screening technique. The primary value of this test is that a normal perfusion scan virtually rules out a PE if done within 8 h of the onset of symptoms. The specificity of perfusion lung scanning is increased when combined with a ventilatory component. In addition to the injection of labeled albumin, the patient inspires xenon gas. A mismatch between the ventilation and perfusion scans (e.g., adequate ventilation with absence of gas exchange in the vasculature) is highly suggestive of PE. However, the ventilation component requires the cooperation of the patient and may be difficult or impossible to perform in some critically ill patients.

Invasive Diagnostic Procedures   Pulmonary arteriography remains the only conclusive diagnostic test for PE. This involves the injection of radiopaque contrast material into the pulmonary artery under fluoroscopy. It is considered diagnostic if an intraluminal filling defect can be identified or if there is sharp cutoff of lobar or segmental vessels.

Medical Management of Deep Venous Thrombophlebitis and Pulmonary Embolism

The goals of therapy for DVT and PE include prophylaxis, management during the acute phase, and long-term anticoagulation. The aim of prophylaxis is to reduce all elements of Virchow's triad: hypercoagulability, venous stasis, and intimal damage. This can be achieved by such measures as active or passive exercise for patients at bed rest, early ambulation whenever possible, leg elevation, use of graduated compression stockings, treatment with pneumatic compression boot devices, and administration of prophylactic minidose subcutaneous heparin in high-risk patients.[47]

Management during the acute phase of DVT and PE involves administration of anticoagulants, as well as symptomatic relief methods. Continuous intravenous heparin is the treatment of choice for both DVT and PE. The goal of therapy in DVT is to prevent propagation of the deep vein thrombus and to minimize the risk of embolization. The goal of therapy in PE is to treat the underlying cause and to prevent recurrent embolism. Heparin acts directly on both the intrinsic and extrinsic coagulation pathways, by inhibiting thrombin-mediated conversion of fibrinogen to fibrin. It also interferes with the action of several clotting factors and potentiates the actions of antithrombin III, an intrinsic anticoagulant. The goal of treatment is prolongation of the partial thromboplastin time (PTT) to $1\frac{1}{2}$ to $2\frac{1}{2}$ times control (in seconds). Heparin does not dissolve clot; however, the thrombus is lysed by the body's intrinsic fibrinolytic agents, which have more recently been employed to lyse extensive DVT or massive PE.[31,48]

Symptomatic relief methods for DVT include strict bed rest until acute symptoms subside, leg elevation, and application of warm, moist heat. With PE, strict bed rest with intensive care unit monitoring is preferable. Invasive hemodynamic monitoring via pulmonary artery catheter provides valuable information with respect to cardiac function. Cardiopulmonary support with digitalization to improve myocardial contractile function and administration of oxygen may be indicated. Additionally, use of antiembolization stockings assists in promoting venous outflow.

Long-term oral anticoagulation with warfarin sodium (Coumadin) is recommended for at least 6 months following acute DVT or PE, the goal of therapy being prevention of recurrence. Warfarin inhibits synthesis of vitamin K-dependent clotting factors by the liver by competitively interfering with vitamin K. Treatment with oral anticoagulants is initiated concurrently with heparin, and an overlap of 3 to 5 days is often necessary to ensure the therapeutic effectiveness of warfarin. The goal of treatment is prolongation of the prothrombin time (PT) to $1\frac{1}{2}$ to $2\frac{1}{2}$ times control (in seconds).

Surgical Management of Deep Venous Thrombophlebitis and Pulmonary Embolism

Only rarely is surgery indicated as a treatment for deep vein thrombosis—most often to protect a patient from initial or recurrent pulmonary embolism when conventional anticoagulation is contraindicated or has failed. Surgical options include pulmonary embolectomy and interruption of the inferior vena cava (IVC). Pulmonary embolectomy requires major thoracic surgery and is often undertaken as a "last resort" life-saving attempt, since the majority of patients suffering massive PE are hemodynamically unstable.

Extravascular interruption of the IVC involves abdominal surgery. A partitioning Teflon clip (Adams-DeWeese clip) can be applied to the cava which effectively partitions the lumen, preventing passage of large emboli. Caval clipping is sometimes done prophylactically during other abdominal surgical procedures (such as cholecystectomy or hysterectomy) in high-risk patients.

If patients are too ill to undergo abdominal surgery, an intravascular filter device can be inserted under local anesthesia in the radiology suite, using fluoroscopic control. The device, attached to a loading catheter, is threaded into the right internal jugular vein in the neck and positioned in the IVC just distal to the renal veins. The device is released from the catheter and lodged securely in place. It functions as a sieve, permitting filtration of emboli without obstruction of venous outflow. The two

most commonly used intracaval filter devices are the Mobin-Uddin "umbrella" and the Kimray-Greenfield filter (Fig. 25-12).

Nursing Therapies for Patients with Deep Venous Thrombophlebitis and Pulmonary Embolism

In nearly every patient cared for in an intensive care setting, be it medical or surgical, there are one or more factors which place the person at risk for the development of DVT and subsequent threat of PE. Prevention is the cornerstone of treatment. However, early recognition and reporting of the signs and symptoms of these pathophysiologic processes facilitate prompt intervention, which may avert life-threatening consequences.

Nurses in the critical-care setting routinely care for patients who are at high risk for the development of DVT and/or PE. They also provide care to those who are acutely symptomatic from PE. Therefore, a sound knowledge base regarding prophylaxis and treatment of these processes are essential nursing skills. The nursing diagnoses and plans of care outlined below are applicable to these problems.

Nursing Diagnosis

Potential circulatory impairment and obstruction of venous outflow in leg(s) and potential impairment of gas exchange due to alteration in pulmonary circulation subsequent to PE.

Goals

Patient will not develop DVT, as evidenced by absence of unilateral leg pain and/or edema; and will not develop PE, as evidenced by normal cardiopulmonary function.

Interventions

1. Minimize hypercoagulability:
Eliminate cigarette smoking.
Treat documented systemic infection with appropriate antibiotics per physician orders.
2. Minimize venous stasis:
Record fluid intake and output carefully to avert dehydration.
Apply antiembolism stockings or Ace bandages to lower extremities.

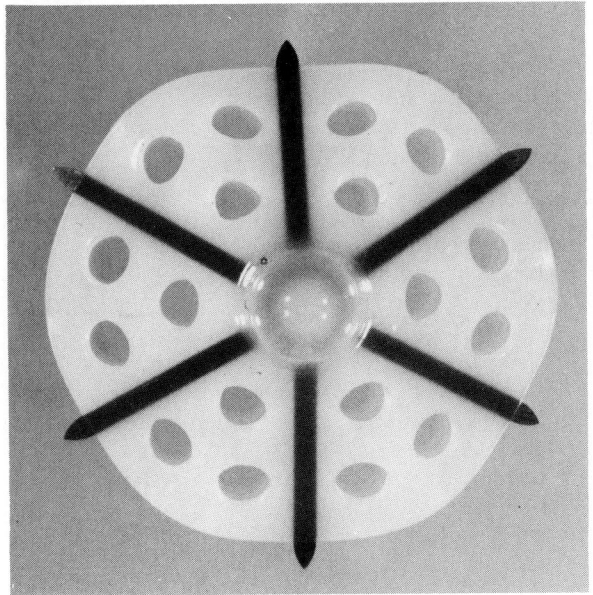 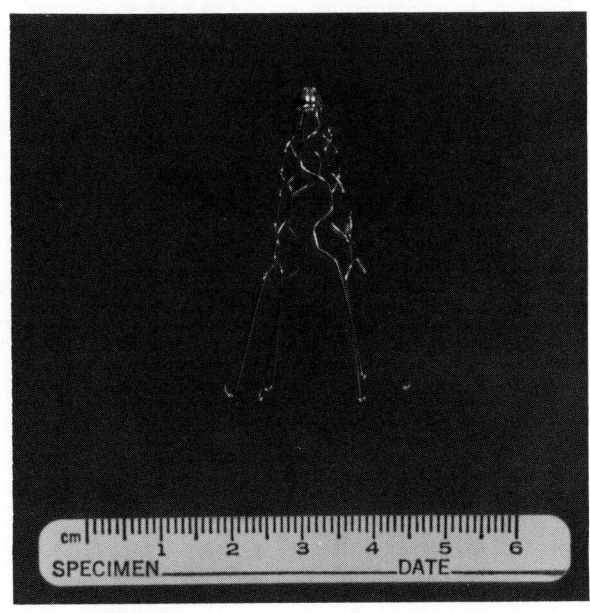

A   B

Figure 25-12   (*A*) Mobin-Uddin intracaval "umbrella" filter. (*B*) Kimray-Greenfield intracaval filter.

Elevate lower extremities above heart level to enhance venous drainage (if not otherwise contraindicated).

Perform active and passive range of motion exercises and frequent repositioning to promote venous return, especially in lower extremities.

Control signs of congestive heart failure with medications per physician's orders.

Evaluation
Patient did not develop DVT or PE.

Nursing Diagnosis
Potential impaired gas exchange and decreased cardiac output related to obstruction of pulmonary circulation by PE.

Goal
Patient will not develop impaired gas exchange or cardiac output.

Interventions

1. Administer anticoagulant medication per physician order—preferably IV bolus of heparin sodium followed by continuous infusion, utilizing regulatory infusion pump.
2. Monitor PTT as evidence of therapeutic effectiveness of heparin; regulate heparin dosage according to physician's order.
3. Monitor body secretions (e.g., urine, stool, nasogastric aspirate if any) for occult blood.
4. Monitor and document results of invasive hemodynamic tests, notifying physician of deteriorating arterial blood gas results, worsening pulmonary hypertension, persistent arrhythmias, or hypotension.
5. Give cardiopulmonary support (e.g., oxygen therapy or mechanical ventilation), digitalization, antiarrhythmic drugs, or fluid resuscitation per physician orders.
6. Monitor and document alteration in mental status which may reflect relative hypoxia.
7. Maintain bed rest in acute phase to minimize myocardial oxygen demand.

Evaluation
Patient did not develop impaired gas exchange or cardiac output.

Other Diagnoses

Other potential diagnoses include potential hemorrhage related to pharmacologic impairment of coagulation with heparin/coumadin therapy and anxiety (mild to severe) related to perceived life-threatening situation.

References

1. Auerbach, O., & Garfinkel, L. (1980). Atherosclerosis and aneurysm of the aorta in relation to smoking habits and age. *Chest, 78,* 805–809.

2. Norrgard, O., Angquist, K., & Johnson, O. (1985). Familiar aortic aneurysms: Serum concentrations of triglyceride, cholesterol, HDL-cholesterol and VLDL and LDL-cholesterol. *British Journal of Surgery, 72* (2), 113–116.

3. Donaldson, M. C., Rosenburg, J. M., & Buckham, C. A. (1985). Diagnosis of ruptured abdominal aortic aneurysm. *Connecticut Medicine, 49* (1), 3–6.

4. Kouchoukos, N. T., & Karp, R. B. Aneurysms of the ascending aorta. In W.W.L. Glenn (Ed.). (1983). *Thoracic and cardiovascular surgery* (4th ed.). Norwalk, CT: Appleton-Century-Crofts.

5. Slater, E. E., & DeSanctis, R. W. Diseases of the aorta. In E. Braunwald (Ed.). (1984). *Heart disease: A textbook of cardiovascular medicine.* Philadelphia: Saunders.

6. Baum, P. L. (1982). Abdominal aortic aneurysm? This patient takes AAA care. *Nursing, 12,* 34–41, 19.

7. Wheat, M. Acute dissection of the aorta. In K. McCauley, A. Brest, & D. McGoon (Eds.). (1985). *McGoon's cardiac surgery: An interprofessional approach to patient care.* Philadelphia: Davis.

8. Hammond, B. B. (1982). The patient with an acute aortic dissection: Assessment and management. *Critical Care Nurse, 2* (2), 46–52.

9. Axiotis, C. A. (1985). Dissecting thoracic aortic aneurysm perforating the esophagus and masquerading as peptic ulcer disease. *The Royal Society of Medicine, 78,* 160–161.

10. Borner, N., Erbel, R., Braun, B., Henkel, B., Meyer, J., & Rumpelt, J. (1984). Diagnosis of aortic dissection by transesophageal echocardiography. *American Journal of Cardiology, 54,* 1157–1158.

11. Finnerty, F. A., Jr. Treatment of hypertensive emergencies. *Heart Lung, 10,* 275–284.

12. Lindsay, J., Jr., DeBakey, M. E., & Beall, A. C., Jr. Diseases of the aorta. In J. W. Hurst, R. B. Logue, C. E. Rackley, R. C. Schlant, E. H. Sonnenblick, A. G. Wallace, & N. Wenger (Eds.). (1982). *The heart: Arteries and veins.* New York: McGraw-Hill.

13. Gordon, M. (1982). *Nursing diagnosis: Application to theory and practice.* New York: McGraw-Hill.

14. Porter, J. M., Taylor, L. M., Jr., & Baur, G. M. Drugs in vascular surgery. In W. S. Moore (Ed.). (1983). *Vascular surgery: A comprehensive review.* New York: Grune & Stratton.

15. Smith, C. D., & McKendry, R. J. (1982). Controlled trial of nifedipine in the treatment of Raynaud's phenomenon. *Lancet, 2* 1299–1301.

16. Porter, J. M., Taylor, L. M., Jr., & Baur, G. M. Nonatherosclerotic vascular disease. In W. S. Moore (Ed.). (1983). *Vascular surgery: A comprehensive review.* New York: Grune & Stratton.

17. Fielding, J. E. (1985). Smoking: Health effects and control. *New England Journal of Medicine, 313,* 491–498.

18. Gordon, M. (1985). *Manual of Nursing Diagnosis.* New York: McGraw-Hill.

19. Bates, B. (1979). *A Guide to Physical Examination* (2d ed.). Philadelphia: Lippincott.

20. Harkonen, S., & Kjellstrand, C. M. (1977). Exacerbation of diabetic renal failure following intravenous pyelography. *American Journal of Medicine, 63,* 939–946.

21. Eisenberg, R. L., Bank, W. O., & Hedgock, M. W. (1981). Renal failure after major angiography can be avoided with hydration. *American Journal of Radiology, 136,* 859–861.

22. Imparato, A. M., Kim, G. E., Davidson, T., & Crowley, J. G. (1975). Intermittent claudication: Its natural course. *Surgery, 78,* 795–799.

23. Coffman, J. D. Disease of the peripheral vessels. In P. B. Beeson, W. McDermott, & J. B. Wyngaarden (Eds.). (1979). *Cecil's Textbook of Medicine* (15th ed.). Philadelphia: Saunders.

24. Coffman, J. D. (1979). Drug therapy: Vasodilator drugs in peripheral vascular disease. *New England Journal of Medicine, 300,* 713–717.

25. Porter, J. M., Cutler, B. S., Lee, B. Y., Reich, T., Reichle, F. A., Scogin, J. T., & Strandnes, D. E. (1982). Pentoxifylline efficacy in the treatment of intermittent claudication: Multicenter controlled double-blind trial with objective assessment of chronic occlusive arterial disease patients. *American Heart Journal, 104* (1), 66–72.

26. Aviado, D. M., & Porter, J. M. (1984). Pentoxifylline: A new drug for the treatment of intermittent claudication. *Pharmacotherapy, 4,* 297–307.

27. Barker, W. F. (1975). *Peripheral arterial disease* (2d ed.). Philadelphia: Saunders.

28. Block, P. C., Myler, R. K., Stertzer, S., & Fallon, J. T. (1981). Morphology after transluminal angioplasty in human beings. *New England Journal of Medicine, 305,* 382–385.

29. Hess, H., Ingrisch, H., Mietaschk, A., & Rath, H. (1982). Local low-dose thrombolytic therapy of peripheral arterial occlusions. *New England Journal of Medicine, 307,* 1627–1630.

30. Berni, G. A., Bandyk, D. F., Zierler, R. E., Thiele, B. L., & Strandness, D. E. (1983). Streptokinase treatment of acute arterial occlusion. *Annals of Surgery, 198* (2), 185–191.

31. Rubin, R. N. (1981). The use of thrombolytic therapy in venous thromboembolic disease. *Connecticut Medicine, 45,* 551–554.

32. Wiener, M. G., & Pepper, G. A. (1985). *Clinical pharmacology and therapeutics in nursing.* New York: McGraw-Hill.

33. Bell, W. R., & Meek, A. G. (1979). Current concepts: Guidelines for the use of thrombolytic agents. *New England Journal of Medicine, 301,* 1266–1270.

34. Porter, J. M., & Taylor, L. M. (1985). Current status of thrombolytic therapy. *Journal of Vascular Surgery, 2,* 239–249.

35. Katzen, B. T., Edwards, K. C., Albert, A. S., & van Breda, A. (1984). Low-dose direct fibrinolysis in peripheral vascular disease. *Journal of Vascular Surgery, 1,* 718–722.

36. Sicard, G. A., Schier, J. J., Totty, W. G., Gilula, L. A., Walker, W. B., Etheredge, E. E., & Anderson, C. B. (1984). Thrombolytic therapy for acute arterial occlusion. *Journal of Vascular Surgery, 2,* 65–78.

37. Doyle, J. E. The person with lower extremity arterial occlusive disease. In C. E. Guzzetta & B. M. Dossey (Eds.). (1984). *Cardiovascular nursing: Bodymind tapestry.* St. Louis: Mosby.

38. Cranley, J. J., & Haffner, C. D. (1982). Revascularization of the femoropopliteal arteries using saphenous vein, polytetrafluoroethylene, and umbilical vein grafts: Five- and six-year results. *Archives of Surgery, 117,* 1543–1550.

39. Yeager, R. A., Hobson, R. W., Jamil, Z., Lynch, T. G., Lee, B. C., & Jain, K. (1982). Differential patency and limb salvage for polytetrafluoroethylene and autogenous saphenous vein in severe lower extremity ischemia. *Surgery, 91,* 99–103.

40. LoGerfo, F. W., & Coffman, J. D. (1984). Current concepts: Vascular and microvascular disease of the foot in diabetes. Implications for foot care. *New England Journal of Medicine, 311,* 1615–1619.

41. Hallin, R. W. (1983). In situ saphenous vein bypass grafting: Experience in 34 extremities over a 2 year period. *American Journal of Surgery, 145,* 626–629.

42. Connolly, J. E., & Kwaan, J. H. M. (1982). In situ saphenous vein bypass. *Archives of Surgery, 117,* 1551–1557.

43. Levine, A. W., Bandyk, D. F., Bonier, P. H., & Towne, J. B. (1985). Lessons learned in adapting the in situ saphenous vein bypass. *Journal of Vascular Surgery, 2,* 145–153.

44. Thompson, J. E., & Garrett, W. V. (1980). Peripheral arterial surgery. *New England Journal of Medicine, 302,* 491–503.

45. Turpie, A. G. G., & Hirsch, J. (1980). Venous thrombosis and pulmonary embolism: Guide to detection and prevention. *Hospital Medicine, 16,* 32–47.

46. Menzoian, J. O., Sequeira, J. C., Doyle, J. E., Cantelmo, N. L., Nowak, M., Tracey, K., Zimmerman, R., & Mozden, P. J. (1983). Therapeutic and clinical course of deep vein thrombosis. *American Journal of Surgery, 146,* 581–585.

47. Chamberlain, S. L. (1980). Low dose heparin therapy. *American Journal of Nursing, 80,* 1115–1117.

48. Bell, W. R. (1982). Thrombolytic therapy—a new realistic approach in treatment of thrombocclusive vascular disease. *Surgery, 92,* 913–914.

part 5

Pulmonary Patient-Care Problems

26 Pulmonary Data Acquisition

Vickie White Matus

Topography of the Chest

A basic understanding of the topography of the chest is essential in assessing lung function, since a working knowledge of the location of organs within the chest and structures of the thorax is important in distinguishing between normal and abnormal findings. It is important to remember that there are normal variations in structure among individuals.

The bony thorax consists of the sternum, ribs, and vertebral column. The sternum consists of the manubrium, body, and xiphoid process. The manubriosternal junction is called the *angle of Louis,* a reference point for locating the second costal cartilage and for measuring central venous pressure. There are 12 pairs of ribs. The first seven are individually connected to the sternum. The eighth, ninth, and tenth ribs are joined together by a common cartilage and attached to the sternum. The eleventh and twelfth ribs are not connected to the sternum and are called *floating ribs* (Fig. 26-1).

The lungs in midinspiration are located from the first rib anteriorly to approximately the seventh rib and from the first rib posteriorly to approximately the tenth vertebra or tenth intercostal space. This is demonstrated in Fig. 26-2 by the lung diagram area with the vertical lines. The lung in deep inspiration (represented in the same figure by the dotted inferior lung area) descends approximately 2.5 cm anteriorly, 5 cm posteriorly, and 7.5 cm laterally to fill the pleural cavity and part of the costophrenic sinus.

The lungs are relatively symmetrical. The right lung has three lobes: upper, middle, and lower. The left lung has two lobes: the upper and lower; however, the lingular segment of its upper lobe corresponds to the middle lobe of the right lung.

Each lobe is separated from the others by natural divisions of the lung called *lobar fissures.* The major or oblique fissure separates the upper and lower lobes bilaterally. The fissure is located posteriorly at approximately T3 or 4, extends to the fifth rib laterally at the midaxillary line, and around to the sixth intercostal space anteriorly. The minor or transverse fissure divides the middle and upper lobes of the right lung and is located at the fourth intercostal space anterior to the midaxillary line at the fifth rib (Fig. 26-2).

Each lung is further divided into segments. See Fig. 26-3 for the distribution of the lobar bronchi, their segmental branches, and the pulmonary segments. The *mediastinum* contains such structures as the heart, trachea, major bronchi, lymphatic structures, great vessels, thymus, and esophagus. Figure 26-4 shows the surface projection of the heart and large vessels. The right border of the heart is normally located 1 cm lateral to the right sternal border edge. It extends from the third rib superiorly down to the fifth intercostal space inferiorly. The left border begins superiorly at the third rib or third intercostal space approximately 1 cm lateral to the left sternal edge. It continues down diagonally to the sixth rib, approximately 5 cm from the left sternal border or 7 to 9 cm from the midsternal line.

Other areas of note anatomically are the diaphragm, liver, stomach, and spleen, as shown in Fig. 26-5. The diaphragm is a dome-shaped projection in the lower thoracic cage and is located (on midexpiration) at the fifth intercostal space on the right hemithorax and the sixth rib on the left hemithorax. The liver lies beneath the right diaphragm, with the superior border located at about the fifth rib, and extends downward to the eleventh rib.

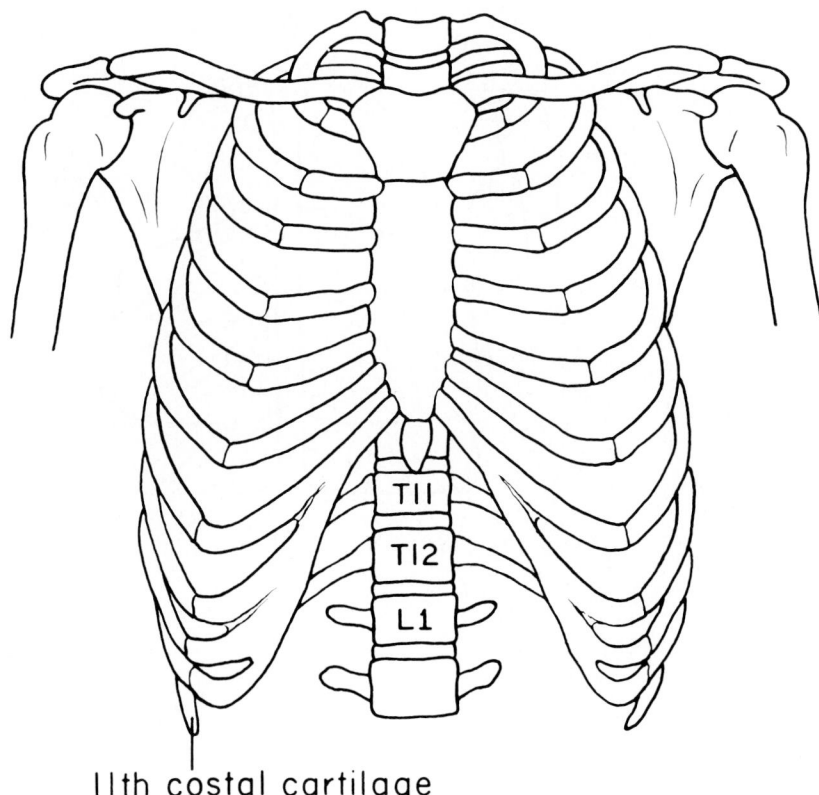

11th costal cartilage

Figure 26-1 Bony thorax. (*From E. Hochstein and A. L. Rubin, Physical Diagnosis, McGraw-Hill, New York, 1964.*)

The stomach normally contains an air bubble of variable size that yields a percussion sound of tympany in an area known as *Traube's semilunar space*. The tympanic sound is usually heard in the upper portion of the stomach under the left diaphragm and behind the sixth, seventh, or eighth intercostal space.

The spleen is located under the left lateral thoracic wall and extends down from the ninth to the eleventh rib.

Examination

The techniques utilized in assessing lung function are inspection, palpation, percussion, and auscultation. Adequate examination of the thorax and lungs can best be achieved with the patient in a sitting position and unclothed from the waist up, if possible. Adequate lighting is essential.

Inspection

The quality, rate, depth, and pattern of respiration should be observed visually. Men and children usually breathe diaphragmatically, while women often breathe thoracically or costally. Patients who appear to have labored respiration should be observed for use of accessory muscles of respiration (sternocleidomastoids, trapezii) and also for supraclavicular retraction.

There are many abnormal patterns of respiration (Fig. 26-6). The ratio of respiratory rate to heart rate is normally 1:4. Impedance to air inflow is frequently identified by the presence of laryngeal stridor or retraction of the intercostal spaces during inspiration. Prolonged expiratory times signify outflow impedance.

The thoracic cage is normally shaped like a truncated cone with the transverse diameter larger than the anteroposterior (AP) diameter. In addition,

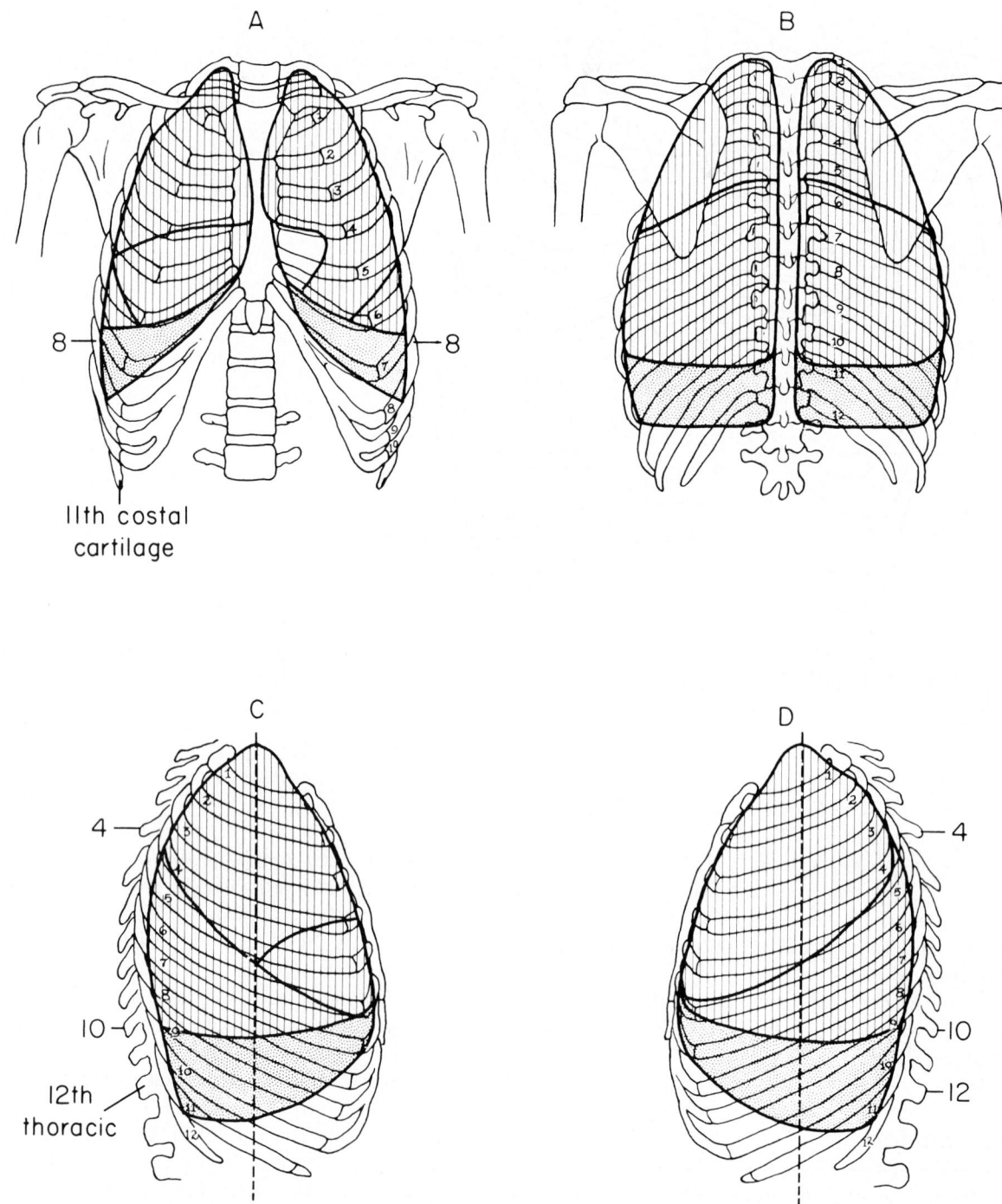

Figure 26-2 Surface projections of the fissures of the lung, borders of the lung, and pleura. (*From E. Hochstein and A. L. Rubin, Physical Diagnosis, McGraw-Hill, New York, 1964.*)

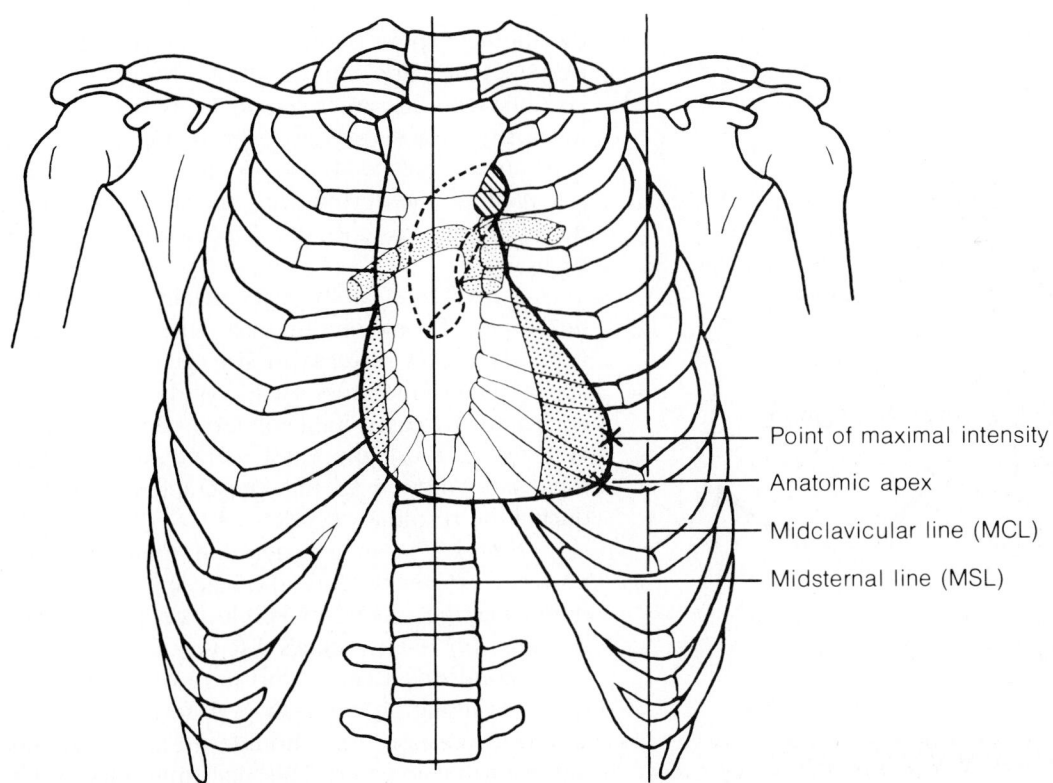

RIGHT LUNG AND BRONCHI

LEFT LUNG AND BRONCHI

Lateral   Medial

Lateral   Medial

SEGMENTS

1. Apical	6. Superior
2. Posterior	7. Medial Basal
3. Anterior	8. Anterior Basal
4. Lateral	9. Lateral Basal
5. Medial	10. Posterior Basal

A

SEGMENTS

1. Apical	6. Superior
2. Posterior	7. Not Present in Left Lung
3. Anterior	8. Anterior Medial Basal
4. Superior	9. Lateral Basal
5. Inferior	10. Posterior Basal

B

Figure 26-3 Lobar bronchi, their segmented branches, and the pulmonary segments. (*From S. Schwartz et al., eds., Principles of Surgery, 3d ed., McGraw-Hill, New York, 1978.*)

— Point of maximal intensity
— Anatomic apex
— Midclavicular line (MCL)
— Midsternal line (MSL)

Figure 26-4 Surface projection of the heart and large vessels. (*Modified from Hochstein and Rubin, Physical Diagnosis, McGraw-Hill, New York, 1964.*)

763

Figure 26-5 Surface projections of the diaphragm, liver, spleen, and stomach. (*From E. Hochstein and A. L. Rubin, Physical Diagnosis, McGraw-Hill, New York, 1964.*)

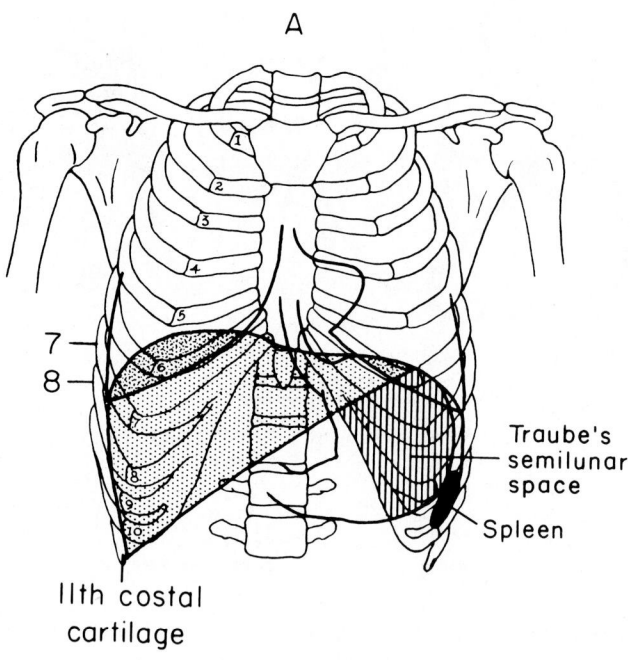

Traube's semilunar space

Spleen

11th costal cartilage

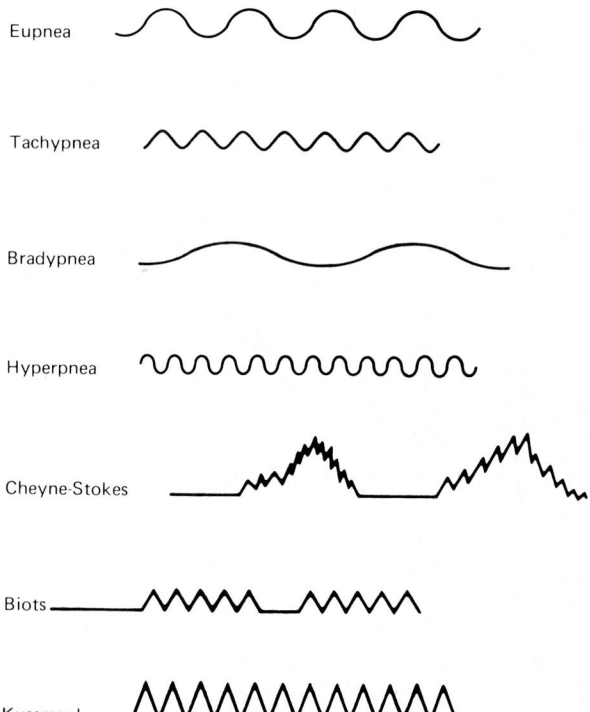

Figure 26-6 Abnormalities in rate and pattern of respiration.

the thoracic spine is slightly convex and makes a perpendicular line with the floor. Abnormalities of size and contour are referred to as barrel chest, kyphosis, scoliosis, kyphoscoliosis, pigeon breast, and funnel breast. These deformities have the potential of interfering with thoracic expansion; therefore, the existence of such deformities should be noted.

Barrel chest is characteristically seen in patients with chronic emphysema. The AP and transverse diameters increase in size, giving a circular appearance to the cross section of the thorax. The constantly increased lung volume in emphysema is believed to cause the chest to become barreled; thus, little motion of the chest appears evident during the respiratory cycle.

Kyphosis is an exaggeration of the normal posterior convexity of the thoracic spine. The condition may be caused by senile osteoporosis, ankylosing spondylitis, Paget's disease, or acromegaly.

Scoliosis is a lateral curvature of the thoracic spine resulting in an S-shaped formation. This abnormality causes one shoulder to be raised and the hip to be lowered. This deformity may result from polio, congenital deformities, thoracoplasty, spinal tumor, or muscular disorders.

Kyphoscoliosis is a deformity in which both kyphosis and scoliosis are present. The significance of this clinical entity is that the thoracic cavity may be so reduced that there is a decreased lung volume, which may severely compromise respiratory and cardiac function.

Pigeon breast, or pectus carinatum, is an abnormality of the thorax usually caused by rickets in childhood. During the active process of rickets, the upper ribs soften and bend inward. This forces the sternum forward, increasing the AP diameter and diminishing the transverse diameter.

Funnel breast, or pectus excavatum, is the opposite of pigeon breast. This abnormality is usually congenital and results when the softened ribs of the lower part of the sternum retract inward toward the spine and create a depressed area near the infrasternal notch. This decreases the AP diameter.

In addition to observing the size and contour of the chest, the examiner should keep in mind other abnormalities such as pulsations indicative of an aortic aneurysm, precordial lift due to cardiac enlargement, or nodules or masses of the thoracic cage, and should examine the axillary area for inflammation of hair follicles and enlarged lymph nodes.

Palpation

Palpation usually begins with assessing symmetrical expansion of the thoracic cage during respiration. The chest is palpated, using the palmar surface of the fingers, for sensitive or painful areas, subcutaneous crepitus (air bubbles under the skin), and tactile fremitus.

To assess *respiratory excursion,* have the patient sit upright. Stand facing the patient's back and grasp the patient's lateral rib cage, placing your thumbs at approximately the level of and parallel to the tenth ribs. Then draw both hands medially, pulling the underlying skin with them to position loose skin folds between the thumbs and spine. Ask the patient to inhale deeply. Observe the outward movement of your thumbs for range and symmetry of thoracic expansion. The technique can be modified for the bedfast patient by placing the hands over the anterior surface of the thorax at the level of the lower margin of the sternum and

performing the same maneuver but pulling the hands medially with the thumbs positioned together in the midline of the sternum and then instructing the patient to inhale deeply.

Tactile fremitus is the palpable vibration transmitted through the bronchopulmonary system to the chest wall when the patient makes a deep vocal sound. Using one hand over symmetrical areas or both hands over corresponding areas, place the palmar aspects of the fingers or the ulnar aspect of the hand on the chest and ask the patient to say in a deep voice, "Ninety-nine" or "one-two-three." A vibratory sensation should normally be felt over lung fields.

The sensation of tactile fremitus is usually uniform over most areas of the lung. When the right main stem bronchus is closer to the chest wall, however, fremitus is increased. Fremitus is also increased in conditions of lung consolidation such as pneumonia. Decreased fremitus occurs when the bronchus is obstructed or the pleural space is occupied by fluid, air, or solid tissue, as in pleural effusion, pneumothorax, or fibrosis.

Two other areas are important in palpation as related to lung function: determining the alignment of the trachea, since misalignment denotes a shifted mediastinum; and detecting palpable lymph nodes in the axillary and supraclavicular areas, which indicate localized or generalized inflammation or malignant disease.

To palpate for tracheal alignment, ask the patient to position the head in a relaxed neutral position. Locate the trachea in the suprasternal notch. Normally, it should be in the midline, with the spaces on each side of the trachea equidistant. Tracheal deviations usually result from masses in the neck or mediastinum or from pleural or pulmonary anomalies.

Percussion

Percussion of the chest provides further information regarding the status of lung function. The technique of manual percussion over the thorax is the same as that used for percussion over other body parts, as are the names given to characteristic percussion sounds. The noisy environment of a busy intensive care unit may make this technique of physical assessment less useful than others.

In the thoracic area, a practitioner may normally elicit a variety of sounds due to the presence of different structures making up the bony thorax and various organs located within the thoracic cage (Table 26-1). Normal lung tissue, however, produces only a resonant percussion sound.

The procedure for percussion may start with the apices and progress to the posterior and lateral thorax moving from top to bottom in a systematic manner. If percussion of the anterior chest seems warranted, keep in mind the location of the heart, mediastinum, and liver.

To percuss the apices, the patient should be in a sitting position facing you. Compare the supraclavicular areas on contralateral sides and note whether the areas are symmetrical.

For percussion of the posterior thorax, the patient is positioned with arms folded over the chest; the shoulders are bent forward in a sitting position if possible. A patient who cannot sit is placed in a left then right lateral decubitus position (remember that the lying position produces dullness in some areas because of the compression of the thorax against the mattress and the body weight itself).

The procedure, regardless of position, begins at the top of each shoulder, an area overlying each lung apex. Progress downward and percuss about a 5-cm area at a time, moving to symmetrical areas of each side of the thorax posteriorly and laterally. Avoid the scapular areas and spinal column. The lateral chest is percussed with the patient's arm positioned over the head.

To measure diaphragmatic excursion, ask the patient to inspire fully and hold the breath. Percuss along the midscapular line bilaterally from top to bottom until the percussion note changes from resonant to dull. Mark the point of transition bilaterally. Then have the patient exhale fully and hold the breath. Percuss upward from the transition line to a resonant percussion note and mark the point. Measure the excursion distance between the two lines. The normal diaphragm will move bilaterally from 3 to 5 cm. A 1-cm difference in bilateral movement may indicate an abnormality.

Auscultation

Auscultation of the lung is a means by which the practitioner can determine the effectiveness of airflow through the airways of the lungs. The origin of breath sounds is still being debated; however, it is generally believed that breath sounds are produced by air moving through the airways while the sound is transmitted out through the chest wall. Solid matter conducts sound waves better than air (a principle used by the American Indians when they placed an ear to the ground to listen for the hoofbeats of cavalry horsemen). Sounds transmitted through consolidated areas of the chest wall sound louder than normal, and, conversely, the chest sounds of an emphysematous patient will normally be very faint.

Auscultation of the lungs requires a quiet environment. The patient should be seated upright in a relaxed position; however, this is often difficult in a critical-care setting. Therefore, assistance may be needed to support the patient in a sitting position, or the patient may have to remain in a recumbent position and be turned to the left and right lateral

Table 26-1   Percussion Sounds

Note	Pitch	Intensity	Quality	Duration	Density	Examples of Location
Tympany	Very high	High	Musical	Long	More air than solid tissue	Gastric air bubble
Hyperresonance	Low	Moderately high	Slightly musical	Moderately long	More air than solid tissue	Emphysematous lung
Resonance	Moderately low	Moderate	Nonmusical	Moderate	Normal air to tissue ratio	Normal lung
Dull	Moderately high	Low	Nonmusical, muffled	Short	Fluid plus solid tissue	Liver, heart
Flat	High	Low	Soft thud	Short	Solid tissue	Bone, thigh

positions. Regardless of the position, the lungs are auscultated over each segment from top to bottom, anteriorly, posteriorly, and laterally. Instruct the patient to breathe with the mouth open. Breathing should be normal but deep enough to move secretions, if any are present. With the diaphragm of the stethoscope pressed snugly against the skin, listen over symmetrical areas of the chest. There are three types of sounds to listen for when auscultating the lungs: breath sounds, voice sounds, and adventitious or extra sounds. Patients who are receiving mechanical ventilation should be removed from the ventilator and given gentle bag ventilation by hand to decrease extraneous noise. Nasogastric suction and chest tube suction should be temporarily clamped, whenever possible, to decrease extraneous noise.

Breath Sounds

Three types of breath sounds are heard over the normal lung, depending on the area that is being auscultated: vesicular, bronchial or tubular, and bronchovesicular. Breath sounds can be described diagrammatically, as shown in Figs. 26-7 and 26-8. The upstroke denotes inspiration and the downstroke denotes expiration. The thickness of the line represents the intensity of the sound, and the height of the angle represents the pitch.

Vesicular breath sounds are soft, low-pitched sounds normally heard over most of the lung but

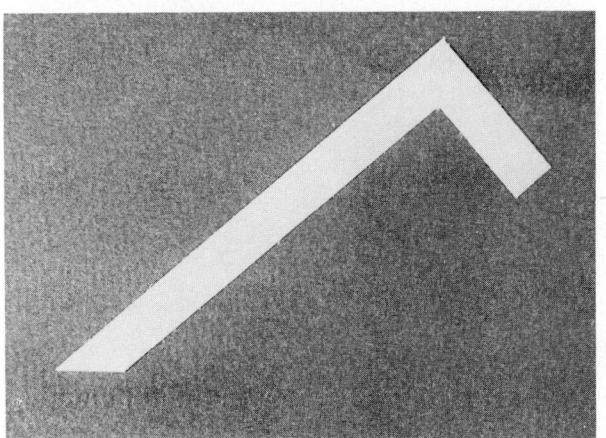

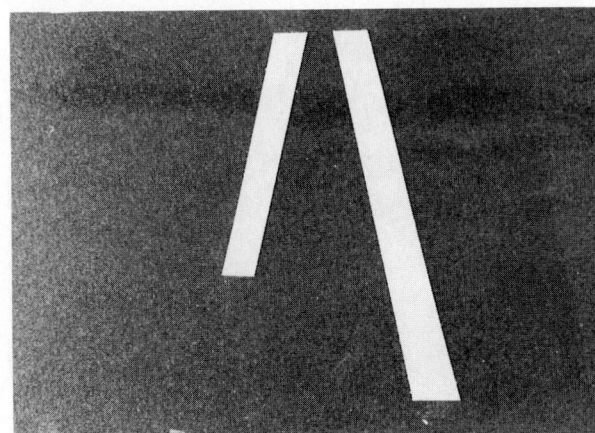

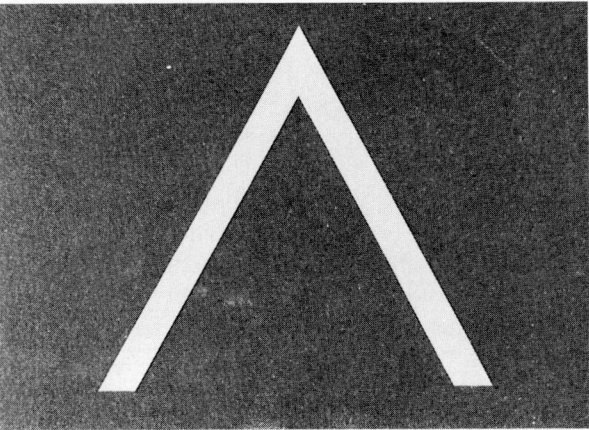

Figure 26-7   (*a*) Vesicular breath sounds. (*b*) Bronchial breath sounds. (*c*) Bronchovesicular breath sounds.

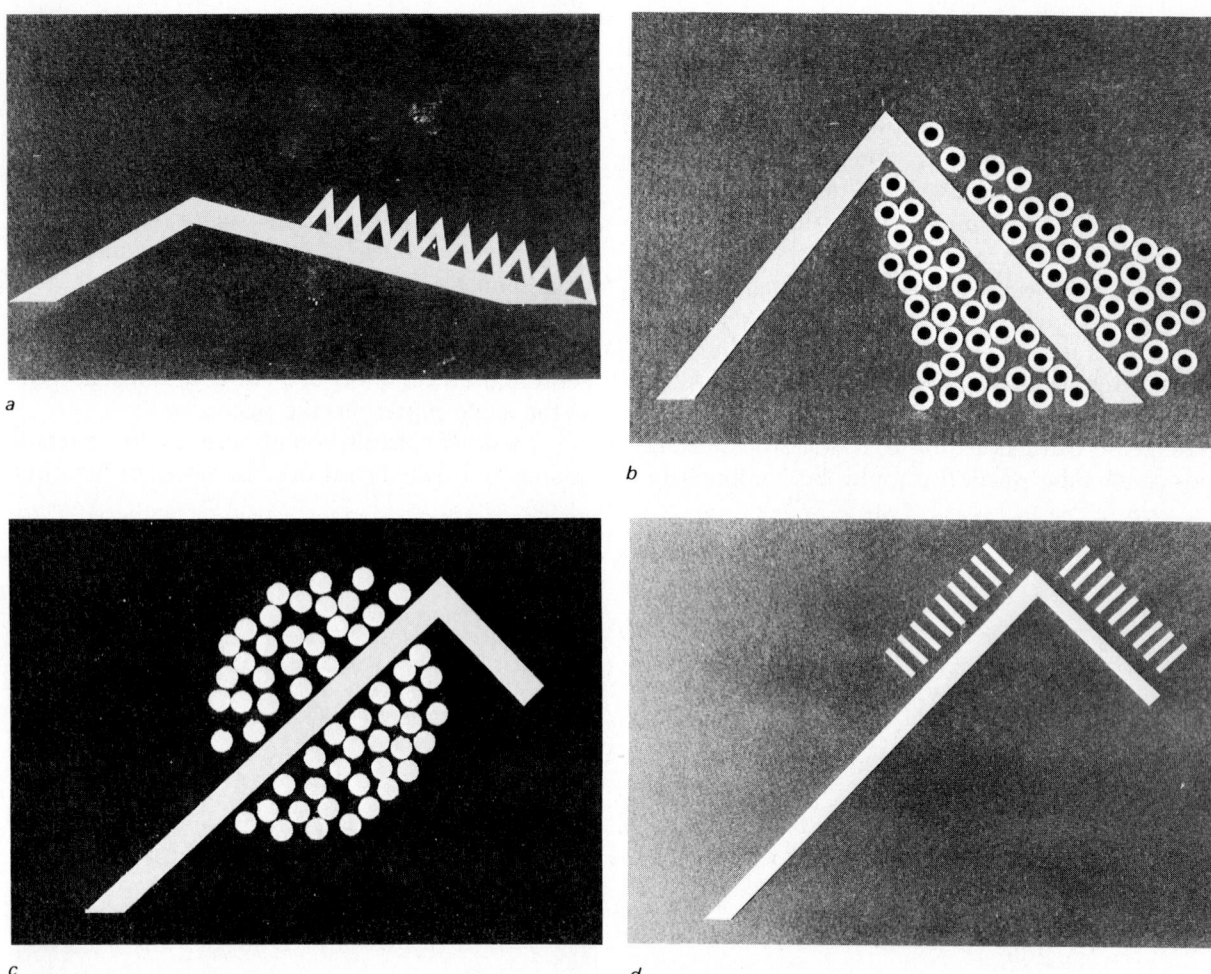

Figure 26-8   (*a*) Wheezes. (*b*) Rhonchi. (*c*) Rales. (*d*) Pleural friction rub.

heard best over the lower posterior and axillary region of the chest. The inspiratory phase is most easily heard because of the increased inspiratory flow rate. The expiratory phase is short (approximately one-third of the inspiratory phase) and faint because the expiratory flow is initially great, then diminishes through the expiratory cycle (Fig. 26-7).

Bronchial or *tubular* breath sounds are usually coarse, high-pitched sounds heard normally over the trachea. The expiratory phase is longer in duration than the inspiratory phase, and they are separated by a silent interval or gap. This type of sound heard elsewhere over lung tissue is indicative of extensive consolidative disease. The bronchioles

are patent and are surrounded by consolidated lung tissue.

Bronchovesicular breath sounds are a combination of bronchial and vesicular breath sounds. They are normally of moderate pitch and intensity. The inspiratory and expiratory phases are of equal duration and are normally heard near the major bronchi, below the clavicles, and between the scapulae, especially on the right. If bronchovesicular sounds are present elsewhere in the chest, early pulmonary disease should be suspected.

Voice Sounds

The types of voice sounds which are useful in diagnosing lung disease, primarily consolidation of lung tissue, are bronchophony, whispering pectoriloquy, and egophony.

Bronchophony is the transmission of louder and clearer voice sounds than one normally hears when auscultating the lungs. Listen with the stethoscope while the patient says "one, two, three" or "ninety-nine." The presence of bronchophony is indicative of consolidation.

Whispering pectoriloquy is tested for by having the patient whisper a combination of words such as "one, two, three." If there is consolidation, the whisper is clearly heard through a stethoscope. If there is no consolidation, the whisper is not heard.

Egophony is tested for by having the patient say aloud "eee." If the sound of the spoken *E* takes on a nasal quality and sounds like *A* (*E* to *A* change), consolidation is usually present.

Adventitious Sounds

Adventitious sounds are extra sounds heard in addition to breath sounds. There are basically four types of adventitious sounds: wheezes, rhonchi, rales, and pleural friction rubs (Fig. 26-8).

Wheezes are high-pitched, whistling sounds produced by airflow through narrowed tubes, resulting in severe turbulence. Wheezes occur primarily on expiration; however, with severe bronchial constriction they may be heard on inspiration.

Rhonchi are coarse, rumbling, low-pitched sounds produced by airflow over secretions in the larger airways. Rhonchi are heard on expiration and may be cleared by coughing or suctioning.

Rales are short, discrete, popping or crackling sounds produced by fluid in the small airways or alveoli. These sounds do not clear with suctioning or coughing.

Pleural friction rubs are creaking, leathery, loud, dry, coarse sounds indicative of pleural irritation. They are produced by the rubbing of the inflamed surfaces of two pleural layers against one another during respiration. Pleural friction rubs are heard at the end of inspiration and the beginning of expiration. They are heard best over the lower lateral aspects of the rib cage, since this area has the greatest amount of pleural movement during breathing.

Table 26-2 presents common respiratory problems of patients in critical-care units.

Diagnostic Tests

Chest X-ray

Serial chest x-rays (CXR) are used to monitor progression of disease and response to treatment. Portable views of the chest are usually obtained in critically ill patients because of the difficulties associated with transportation to the radiology suite. It is important to note that portable chest films vary

Table 26-2 Common Respiratory Problems of Critical-Care Patients

Disease	Tactile Fremitus	Percussion	Auscultation
Consolidation (e.g., pneumonia)	Increased	Dull	Bronchial breath sounds, rales, bronchophony, egophony, whispered pectoriloquy
Bronchitis	Normal	Resonant	Normal to decreased breath sounds, wheezes, and rhonchi
Emphysema	Decreased	Hyperresonant	Decreased intensity of breath sounds, usually with prolonged expiration
Asthma (severe attack)	Normal to decreased	Resonant to hyperresonant	Wheezes and rhonchi
Pulmonary edema	Normal	Resonant	Rales at lung bases, possibly wheezes
Pleural effusion	Absent	Dull to flat	Decreased to absent breath sounds, bronchial breath sounds and bronchophony, egophony, and whispering pectoriloquy above the effusion over the area of compressed lung
Pneumothorax	Decreased	Hyperresonant	Absent breath sounds
Atelectasis	Absent	Flat	Decreased to absent breath sounds

in their degree of sharpness and magnification and are never considered to be the highest quality film.

Immediately prior to obtaining a CXR the critical-care nurse should remove metallic objects which are in contact with the patient's thorax such as jewelry, ECG leads, safety pins, and snaps on the patient's gown and attempt to position ventilator tubing so that it does not obscure important views of the chest. The most common view obtained on the bed-rest patient is the posteroanterior, in which the x-ray beam is directed toward the patient, with the film plate behind the spine.

CXRs can detect common pulmonary disorders as well as anatomic abnormalities. They assist in determining the location and size of a lesion, assess pulmonary status, and verify proper placement of an endotracheal tube or central venous catheter. It is possible for serial CXRs to assist in the differentiation of pulmonary edema, parenchymal inflammation, and infection.

In the normal CXR the trachea has a tubelike appearance and is visible in the midline of the anterior mediastinal cavity. The heart is visible in the anterior left mediastinal cavity and should occupy approximately one-third of the thoracic cavity. The clavicle and ribs should be evaluated for fractures or misalignment if trauma is suspected. The bronchi are usually not clearly visible but have a tubelike appearance if surrounded by consolidated tissue. The parenchyma of the lungs is usually not visible throughout the lung fields, except for fine white lines radiating from the hilum which represent the pulmonary vascular tree. The height of the diaphragms should be compared (the right side is commonly 1 to 2 cm higher than the left). The costaphrenic angles should be well defined. Changes in the appearance of the CXR over time tend to be much more significant in monitoring the critically ill patient than any single film.

Pulmonary Function Tests

Pulmonary function tests (PFT) evaluate lung mechanics by measuring the volume of air a patient is able to move in and out during ventilation and estimating various lung capacities. It is essential that the patient be able to volitionally participate in a test in order to complete a full set of studies. This is frequently not possible in the critically ill patient, and selected subtests may have to suffice.

PFTs help determine whether an abnormality is functional or restrictive, assess the level of dysfunction, and assess the effectiveness of specific medications such as bronchodilators, as well as the side effects of other drugs such as beta blockers. They also help to assess the timeliness of weaning from mechanical ventilation. A full set of PFTs consists of spirometry, gas diffusion, and diffusing capacity (Table 26-3 and Fig. 26-9).

Ventilation/Perfusion Scanning

These two complementary tests involve the inhalation and the intravenous injection, respectively, of a radiopaque material. Both produce images of the agent's distribution throughout the lung, revealing abnormal patterns of ventilation or perfusion. While these tests are useful in a variety of disorders, they are most commonly used to diagnose pulmonary emboli in the critically ill patient. The results are expressed in terms of probability, and more invasive tests such as pulmonary angiography can validate the diagnosis (Fig. 26-10).

Pulmonary Angiography

This invasive test involves x-ray examination of the pulmonary circulation after injection of a radiopaque iodine contrast material through a catheter inserted into the pulmonary artery or one of its branches. It allows visualization of the pulmonary vascular bed and measurement of pressures at various sites during catheter insertion, as well as determination of cardiac output and pulmonary vascular resistance. Because of the attendant risks, this test is restricted to identifying defects in pulmonary vascular perfusion such as thrombi, aneurysms, and blood vessel displacement. It is used to confirm symptomatic pulmonary embolism (Fig. 26-11) when lung scans show no abnormalities, especially in the patient for whom anticoagulant therapy carries a particularly high risk. It also assists in the preoperative evaluation of pulmonary circulation in patients with congenital heart disease. Complications of pulmonary angiography include allergic reaction, arterial occlusion, ventricular arrhythmias, and myocardial perforation.

Table 26-3 Pulmonary Function Parameters Commonly Used in Intensive-Care Unit

Measurement of Pulmonary Function	Implications
Tidal volume (V_T): Amount of air inhaled or exhaled during normal tidal breathing	May indicate patient fatigue or onset of restrictive parenchymal process
Minute volume (MV): Total amount of gas breathed per minute	May indicate patient fatigue or onset of restrictive parenchymal process
Inspiratory capacity (IC): Amount of air that can be inhaled after a normal exhalation	Decreased IC indicates restrictive lung disease; one of the parameters used to determine patient's possibility of being weaned from mechanical ventilation
Functional residual capacity (FRC): Amount of air remaining in the lungs after a normal or tidal exhalation. This is the combined value of the expiratory reserve volume (ERV); amount of air that can be exhaled after a normal exhalation and residual volume (RV); amount of gas remaining in the lungs at all times	Decreased FRC is the hallmark of adult respiratory distress syndrome. Increased FRC reflects overdistention of the lungs, which may result from chronic obstructive pulmonary disease (COPD) or excessive use of positive end-expiratory pressure
Forced vital capacity (FVC): Dynamic measure of amount of gas exhaled after maximal inspiration	Decreased FVC indicates resistance to expiratory flow as in COPD
Forced expiratory volume (FEV): Amount of air exhaled in the first, second, and third second of FEV maneuver	May be prolonged in COPD. Improved FEV_1 following administration of beta blockers may indicate a degree of bronchospasm which prohibits further administration of the drugs

Direct Laryngoscopy

This technique allows direct visualization of the larynx through the use of a fiberoptic laryngoscope passed through the mouth or nose and pharynx. The larynx is observed at rest and during phonation. Laryngoscopy is performed to detect lesions, strictures, or foreign bodies of the larynx. It may also be used in conjunction with a biopsy to distinguish laryngeal edema from response to radiation or

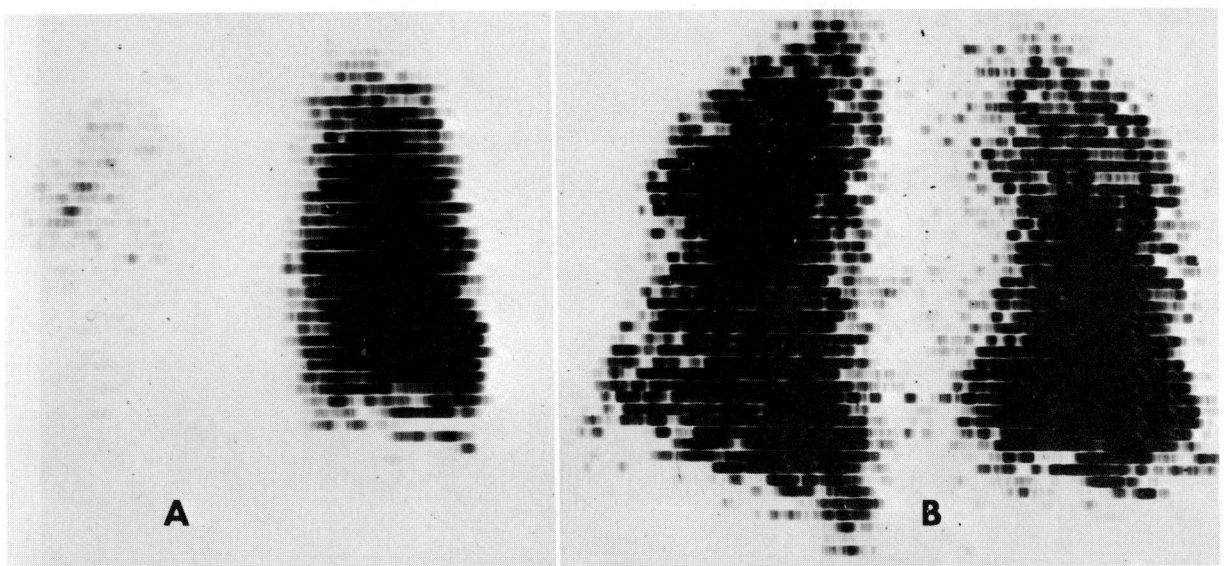

Figure 26-9 Pulmonary angiogram demonstrating absence of filling of left pulmonary arterial branches, indicative of large embolus obstructing left main pulmonary artery. (*From S. Schwartz et al., eds., Principles of Surgery, McGraw-Hill, 1979, p. 993.*)

Figure 26-10 Radioisotope scans following intravenous injection of macroaggregated albumin tagged with iodine 131. (*A*) Massive pulmonary embolus to right lung. (*B*) Small bilateral emboli evidenced by crescent-shaped objects. (*From S. Schwartz et al., eds, Principles of Surgery, McGraw-Hill, New York, 1979, p. 994.*)

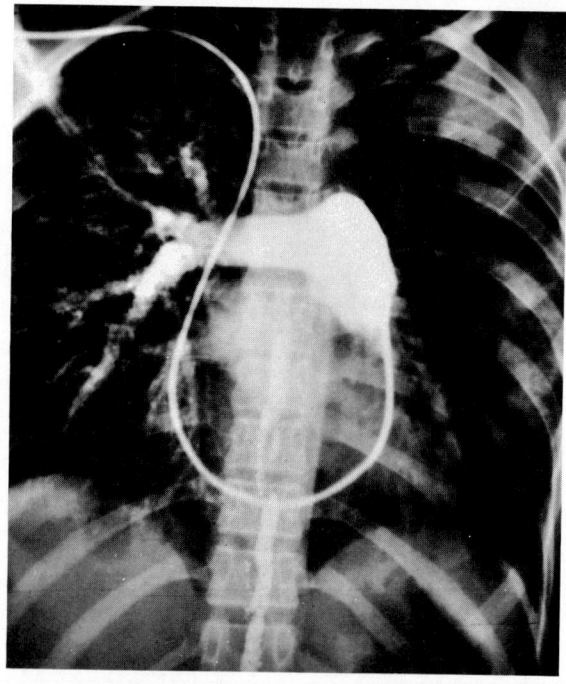

Figure 26-11 Division of total lung capacity into lung volumes and lung capacities. In the small diagrams surrounding the large central one, the shaded areas outline the *volumes* which constitute the various lung *capacities*. (*Adapted from J. H. Comroe, Jr., et al., The Lung: Clinical Physiology and Pulmonary Function Tests, 2d ed., Chicago, Year Book, 1962.*)

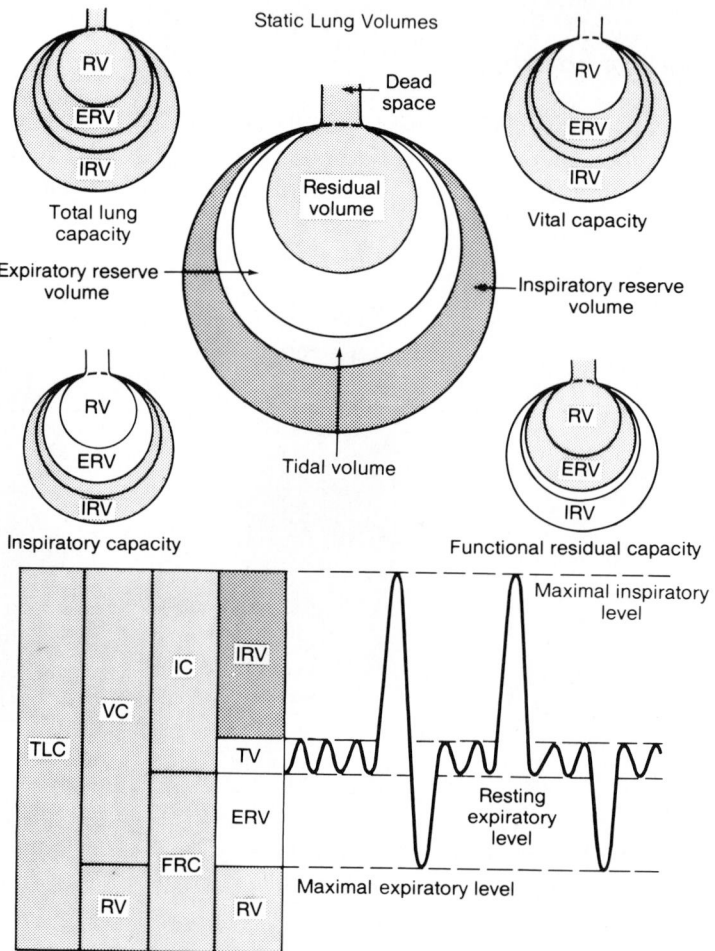

tumor and to examine the condition of the larynx following prolonged endotracheal intubation.

Bronchoscopy

The direct visualization of the trachea and tracheobronchial tree is now commonly performed by the fiberoptic bronchoscope. Its diagnostic value lies in the visual examination and identification of potential tumor, obstruction, or foreign body in the tracheobronchial tree, which aids in the diagnosis of carcinoma, interstitial pulmonary disease, and pulmonary infection by allowing procurement of a specimen for microbiologic and cytologic examination. It can also assist in locating a bleeding site or in determining the cause of a poorly functioning intubation.

Therapeutic benefits of a bronchoscopy include removal of a foreign body or mucous plug, treatment of atelectasis, drainage of an abscess, and improvement in bronchial clearance. Bronchoscopic findings are always correlated with radiographic, cytologic, and clinical data.

Transcutaneous O_2 Monitoring (TcP_{O_2})

TcP_{O_2} monitoring allows for continuous noninvasive assessment, through the use of an electrode placed on the skin, of the minute-to-minute changes that can occur in oxygen levels. The electrode has a heating unit to warm the skin, causing capillaries to dilate and thereby increasing blood flow. The monitor measures the amount of oxygen diffusing through the skin, which usually correlates with arterial oxygen levels. In neonates the correlation is high, making it possible to monitor the effect of treatment on oxygenation and avoid episodes of hypoxemia. The correlation in adults is less reliable, but the result is helpful in certain conditions.

Bibliography

Bates, B. *A guide to physical examination,* 3d ed., Philadelphia: Lippincott, 1983.

Burton, G., & J. E. Hodgkin. *Respiratory care,* 2d ed. Philadelphia: Lippincott, 1984.

Malasanos, L., V. Barkauskas, M. Moss, & K. Stoltenberg-Allen. *Health assessment,* 2d ed. St. Louis: Mosby, 1981.

27 Respiratory Disorders

Vickie White
Matus
Sheila A.
Glennon

Parenchymal Lung Disorders

Adult Respiratory Distress Syndrome (ARDS)

Catastrophic respiratory failure of sudden onset may occur in patients with previously normal or healthy lungs who sustain any one of a variety of pulmonary or systemic insults that cause diffuse injury to the lung. The initial insult may be any one of a diverse group of injuries, yet the histological response of the lung, regardless of the insult, is virtually identical. The fact that the lung has a characteristic clinical, physiological, and pathological response to acute injury, regardless of etiology, allows the critical-care practitioner to group a variety of illnesses which have one or more common phases under the singular heading of ARDS.

The lack of a single causative event and the absence of any specific diagnostic test for ARDS necessitates the use of a descriptive definition for this syndrome. The following constellation of pulmonary responses characterize ARDS:

1. Clinical: dyspnea, tachypnea
2. Radiologic: diffuse bilateral pulmonary infiltrates (an "alveolar pattern")
3. Physiological: decreased pulmonary compliance (i.e., increased "stiffness" of the lungs), impaired oxygen diffusion across alveolar capillary membrane (i.e., decreasing arterial oxygen tension nonresponsive to "standard" oxygen therapy)
4. Pathological: interstitial edema, intra-alveolar exudation, hemorrhage, microemboli, and hyaline membrane formation

The clinical hallmarks of this variety of respiratory failure include an initial insult, such as massive hemorrhage and hypovolemic shock, and a latent period during which pulmonary function appears normal, followed by respiratory decompensation. Initially the patient is tachypneic and dyspneic; the arterial oxygen tension decreases in spite of standard oxygen therapy. The arterial carbon dioxide tension is low initially (Pa_{CO_2} below 40 torr*) but rises rapidly in spite of the tachypnea as the respiratory insufficiency progresses.

The use of the term *ARDS* should not obscure the fact that the initial insult and mechanism of pulmonary injury vary widely. Therapy should be focused on two areas: supportive therapy to treat the secondary alterations in pulmonary function and maintain the patient, and treatment of the initiating or causal insult. Some of the causal factors seen in medical and surgical settings that are related to the development of ARDS are listed in Table 27-1.

Advances in emergency medical care during the Vietnam war period allowed for prolonged survival of trauma victims who previously would have died on the battleground. Two of the most notable advances were (1) rapid treatment and recovery from initial shock and trauma, and (2) rapid evacuation within 15 to 20 min to sophisticated treatment centers. Observations made during World War II were confirmed and extended to include development of respiratory failure after a posttraumatic latent period of 12 to 48 h. One reason for the apparently increasing incidence of ARDS over the years has been improvements in medical therapy and technology that facilitate the victim's survival of severe initial insults that lead to ARDS.

Pathology

Although there are a variety of causes of ARDS, the pathological changes are remarkably consistent. On

---

*A torr is a unit of pressure that is equivalent to 1 mmHg under standard conditions.

Table 27-1 Causal Factors Related to ARDS

Aspiration of gastric contents
Drug ingestion and overdose
Hydrocarbon ingestion
Trauma and hemorrhagic shock
Near drowning
Smoke and gas inhalation
Disseminated intravascular coagulation
Septic shock
Fat and air embolism
Severe pneumonitis (viral and other)
Oxygen toxicity
Postperfusion (cardiopulmonary bypass)
Anaphylaxis
Uremia
Hemorrhagic pancreatitis
Head injury
Homologous blood transfusion

gross examination at autopsy the lungs are heavy, congested, and hemorrhagic and have the appearance of liver. Such lungs sink when placed in water. Generally there is not a significant amount of secretions in the large airways, nor is there visible obstruction of the major vessels.

Frequently cited findings in ARDS include thickened alveolar walls, interstitial edema, intra-alveolar edema, and hemorrhage. Focal atelectasis is present. Congestion, plugging of small arterioles with fibrin and debris, and partial or even complete disruption of portions of the pulmonary vascular bed occur. Migration of the cellular material into the alveoli may be noted. There may be localized areas of alveolar wall necrosis and increased numbers of pulmonary macrophages.

Hyaline membranes are also noted on microscopic examination. They are probably formed from transudated plasma proteins and can increase the alveolar capillary membrane to 50 to 100 times its normal thickness. These membranes form a formidable barrier to gas diffusion.

Etiology

The support and management of all ARDS patients are similar yet vary somewhat according to the etiology. Mortality rates vary from 20 to 50 percent. A successful outcome depends upon recognition and treatment of all contributing factors. For example, the critically ill multisystem trauma patient

may have ARDS, fat embolism, sepsis, and posttraumatic pancreatitis as active problems. It is important to consider all possible contributing problems to facilitate proper management (Table 27-1).

The lung exhibits a limited number of responses to injury. ARDS is one type of response to a severe insult. Knowledge of the mechanisms of pulmonary injury is largely inferred rather than directly observed, with the exception of direct trauma and aspiration. It can also be assumed that some protective mechanisms exist, since not all patients having similar insults develop ARDS. The source of this protection is as yet poorly understood.

It is generally accepted that a period of pulmonary hypoperfusion is associated with the origin of most cases of ARDS. The precise mechanism by which this hypoperfusion develops into ARDS is not entirely clear, but it probably involves intravascular coagulation with subsequent thromboembolism within the pulmonary microvasculature (Fig. 27-1). It has now been proved that in ARDS of all causes the initial injury is to the capillary endothelium; however, there are many known mediators of lung injury which, if they do not initiate the syndrome, perpetuate it (Table 27-2).

Intravascular coagulation can develop from a variety of causes. Transfusion with mismatched blood, with resulting hemolysis, is a significant cause. Old blood itself is a source of microemboli, and the dead cells produce differing degrees of intravascular clotting. Other complications of shock states that lead to intravascular coagulation are tissue trauma mobilizing tissue thromboplastin, bacterial toxins through platelet aggregation with the release of thromboplastin, ischemia from endothelial cell damage, the release of tissue thromboplastin, and acidosis. Systemic microvascular obstruction with microemboli results in decreased tissue perfusion, progressive metabolic acidosis, and a secondary increase in coagulability.

Following resuscitation of the patient in a shock state, flow in the microcirculation is reestablished and the products of peripheral intravascular coagulation are flushed into the systemic circulation and carried to the vascular bed of the lungs. The filtering action of the pulmonary vascular bed removes gross and microscopic clots. Unstable circulating clots fragment until the microcirculation

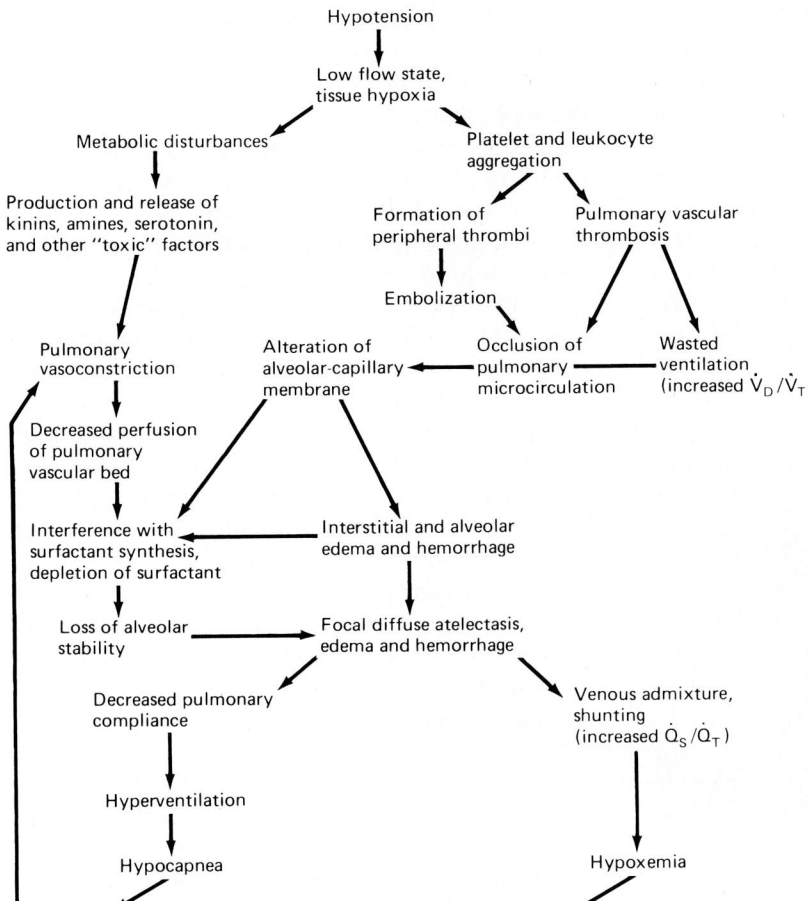

Figure 27-1 Pathogenesis and pathophysiology of ARDS. *(From K. Lake and J. Rumsfeld, The adult respiratory distress syndrome (shock lung), in G. G. Burton, G. N. Gee, and J. E. Hodgkins, Eds., Respiratory Care: A Guide to Clinical Practice, Lippincott, Philadelphia, 1977, p. 768.)*

of the lung is reached. Stasis here in the microcirculation invites further thrombosis because of endothelial cell damage distal to the emboli.

Thromboemboli cause pulmonary damage via at least two mechanisms: (1) release of potent bronchoconstrictors and venoconstrictors, and (2) mechanical obstruction of blood flow. Vasoactive

amines such as serotonin and histamine are released from platelet microemboli and produce microvascular constriction. Other agents, including bradykinin and catecholamines, are also released from white blood cell–platelet microaggregates and result in vasoconstriction, bronchoconstriction, and alterations in alveolar-capillary membrane permeability.

The primary target for all these forces is the alveolar-capillary membrane. There is hypoxia, lactic acidosis, and intravascular clotting. Hypoxemia and acidemia themselves increase pulmonary artery pressure and pulmonary vascular resistance. The capillary membranes are damaged by these insults and their permeability is increased, allowing extravasation of fluids into the interstitial space. Initially the fluid is a transudate, but as the leak increases,

Table 27-2 Mediators Implicated in ARDS

Coagulation products
Complement products
Platelets and platelet activating factor
Prostaglandins
Histamine
Bradykinin
Seratonin
Polymorphonuclear leukocytes

larger molecules such as proteins and formed blood elements leak out. Lymph channels which would normally remove this material are compressed by the extravasated fluid, further favoring interstitial fluid collection and retention (Fig. 27-2).

Perivascular edema and decreased capillary perfusion damage the alveolar type II pneumocyte, resulting in decreased surfactant production. The alveoli become increasingly unstable and tend to collapse unless filled with fluid from the interstitium. These alveoli, in either case, cannot participate in effective gas exchange, and this area becomes a

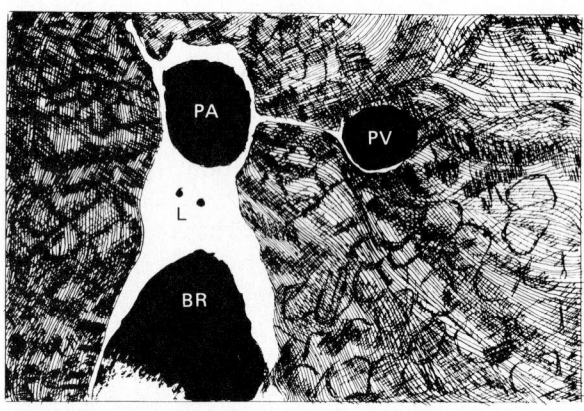

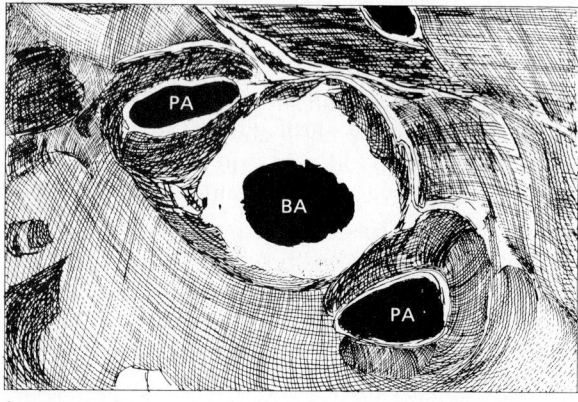

Figure 27-2 (*a*) Normal lung showing bronchus (BR), pulmonary artery (PA), and pulmonary venule (PV). The only visible interstitial space (L) is between the airway and the artery in which lymph vessels are located. (*b*) Massive fluid expansion of loose interstitial perivascular and peribronchial space. Note "halo" effect surrounding the pulmonary artery (PA) and the bronchial artery (BA). *(Courtesy of E. F. Lenihan.)*

mass of interstitial and alveolar edema with hemorrhage and atelectasis.

Pathophysiology

Pulmonary function abnormalities in patients with ARDS have been well described in several review articles. A reduction in functional residual capacity is a hallmark of this syndrome. Localization of edema fluid in the peribronchovascular interstitial space increases the normally subatmospheric pressure of the interstitial space. This reduces the transmural pressure gradient that helps to maintain patent airways. If these small airways close and remain closed, distal atelectasis and loss of lung volume occur. Lung volume also decreases as accumulating edema fluid begins to flood alveoli or as the alveoli become smaller in size because of the increasing surface forces.

Decreasing pulmonary compliance is another characteristic finding in ARDS. This means that greater than normal inspiratory pressure is needed to deliver the same tidal volume. This loss of compliance is directly due to increasing tissue elasticity or recoil caused by pulmonary congestion and the increasing alveolar surface forces resulting from loss or inactivation of surfactant. The decreasing compliance is indirectly a result of the overall decreasing lung volume. As compliance decreases, there is a progressive reduction in the volume of gas present in the involved lung units at functional residual capacity (FRC). If the process is severe, the volume of gas may be so small and the surface forces so great that the alveoli and/or terminal bronchioles collapse completely on deflation. When this occurs, the unit cannot reopen until a "critical opening pressure" has been exceeded during inspiration.

Hypoxia is an invariable feature of ARDS. A large number of gas exchange units do not contribute fully to the uptake of oxygen and elimination of carbon dioxide because of the processes described above. Alveoli that receive blood flow but no ventilation are sites of intrapulmonary shunting ($\dot{Q}s/\dot{Q}T$). In other areas where there is vasoconstriction and microembolization, "wasted" ventilation ($\dot{V}D/\dot{V}T$) exists. The net result over the entire pulmonary bed is $\dot{V}/\dot{Q}$ mismatching and hypoxemia.

A reflex increase in cardiac output and alveolar minute ventilation occurs in an attempt to compensate for the hypoxia and resultant acidosis. However, the lowered Pa_{CO_2} from hyperventilation increases both airway resistance and oxygen consumption and decreases dynamic compliance. All these effects contribute to additional pulmonary dysfunction. Increased inspiratory effort is needed to open previously closed alveoli. The increased inspiratory effort increases venous return to the right side of the heart, yet the total volume of the pulmonary circulatory bed is decreased because of coagulopathy and increased resistance. This causes further extravasation of fluid and formed elements into the interstitial space. As osmotically active particles leak through the damaged endothelial membrane and into the interstitial space, more water is drawn to them and the lungs become stiffer. The increased oxygen consumption required by the increased work of breathing is far too costly in the face of progressive hypoxemia.

The role of the central nervous system in ARDS has been suggested by many neurosurgeons. A model has been described in which cerebral hypoxia initiates the sequence by interfering with hypothalamic cellular metabolism. Descending sympathetic fibers are activated which pass through the cervical spinal cord and on to the vessels of the lung. The importance of these neurogenic factors is still unclear. Some head-injured patients without pulmonary or other major extracranial injuries show ventilation/perfusion disorders.

Diagnostic Findings

Recognition of ARDS in the late stages is relatively easy, yet diagnosis in the early, subtle stages is difficult unless members of the health care team are alert to its development in susceptible patients. Early diagnosis helps to avoid compounding the problem by mishandling oxygen, mechanical ventilation, and other therapeutic tools.

During the initial shock phase, therapeutic interventions are directed toward converting the low-flow state to a high-flow state by administration of the appropriate fluids and/or blood products to reverse the hypotension.

There may be few or no pulmonary symptoms at this time and for the next 12 to 48 h. Early symptoms include dyspnea, restlessness, and/or cough. Dyspnea, however, may not appear early in the young, healthy patient who can double or triple minute ventilation with ease. The initial finding in ventilated patients may be an increase in the peak inspiratory pressure necessary to deliver a given tidal volume (evidence of decreasing pulmonary compliance).

Abnormal findings on physical examination indicate that the disease process has already progressed beyond the early stages. Evidence of increased work of breathing such as hyperpnea, noisy respirations at a rapid rate, and intercostal and supracostal retraction may be noted. Cyanosis will be present if there is adequate capillary perfusion and more than 5 g of reduced hemoglobin. Pallor will be seen if perfusion is poor. Tachycardia, diaphoresis, and decreased mentation are seen frequently once the syndrome has progressed. Initially chest auscultation is normal, but rales, rhonchi, and bronchial breath sounds may be heard as the syndrome progresses to the later stages. Physical findings related to the underlying etiology, such as skin, conjunctival, and retinal changes in fat embolism and singed nasal hairs in pulmonary burns, should be sought.

Tests of gas exchange and pulmonary mechanics are useful in evaluating and managing ARDS. The hallmark of this syndrome remains a lowered arterial oxygen tension which is poorly responsive to increased concentrations of inspired oxygen. A more exact method of evaluating this is by calculating the alveolar-arterial oxygen gradient, $D(A\text{-}a)O_2$. This measure reflects the difficulty with which oxygen crosses the alveolar-capillary membrane (see Chap. 8). Normally the $D(A\text{-}a)O_2$ should be less than 15 to 20 torr on room air, but in patients with severe ARDS, values of 200 to 500 have been recorded. This test gives more information about the transfer of oxygen than the Pa_{O_2} alone, especially when followed serially. It is important to remember, however, that the A-a difference does not take into account changes in inspired oxygen concentration, cardiac output, or metabolic rate. Thus, when following the alveolar-arterial oxygen difference clinically, these variables must be continually assessed.

It is also useful to measure shunt fraction ($\dot{Q}s/\dot{Q}T$) in these patients (see Chap. 8). Normal persons spontaneously breathing have shunt fractions of less than 6 percent, and shunt fractions of less than 10 percent on a mechanical ventilator reflect a normal cardiopulmonary system. Until recently an $F_{I_{O_2}}$ of 100 percent was used to calculate "true shunt." Recent evidence in critically ill patients has shown that "physiological shunt" (which includes areas of low $\dot{V}/\dot{Q}$) is more clinically meaningful when calculated at an $F_{I_{O_2}}$ of 50 to 60 percent. In either case, the following guidelines are useful for evaluation of shunt fractions on ventilator patients:

1. A calculated shunt greater than 30 percent is generally considered incompatible with prolonged spontaneous ventilation.
2. Calculated shunts between 20 and 30 percent are considered compatible with spontaneous ventilation as long as the cardiovascular reserves are adequate and the status of the central nervous system and hepatorenal system are acceptable.
3. Calculated shunts less than 20 percent are considered completely compatible with prolonged spontaneous ventilation.[1]

Alveolar ventilation remains high until late in the course of ARDS. A Pa_{CO_2} of 35 to 45 torr in a very dyspneic, hypoxemic patient is not "normal," and when it does occur, it suggests that the seriously compromised lungs are no longer able to increase alveolar ventilation in response to hypoxemia and other stimuli.

The pH normally rises as Pa_{CO_2} falls (respiratory alkalemia). Failure to rise indicates that a metabolic acidemia is present. In the presence of shock and hypoxemia, this is most commonly the result of lactic acidosis. This can be confirmed by directly measuring serum lactate levels.

Tests of pulmonary mechanics show decreasing static and dynamic compliance. There is also a decrease in lung volumes, particularly FRC.

There is a real need for a sensitive test that can detect ARDS in an early phase when fluid is beginning to collect in the lung. Tests that measure lung water directly would obviously be desirable and might be a means for early diagnosis. A number of techniques have been used, but at this time none have proved their applicability to the clinical diagnosis of ARDS.

The radiologic picture of this syndrome is the result of movement of fluid out of the injured alveolar capillary into the interstitium and later into the alveolus. There must be a large increase in lung water before the chest roentgenogram becomes abnormal. The lungs frequently appear normal in the early stages of ARDS, although a considerable degree of microatelectasis may be present. Subtle findings such as thickened or blurred margins of bronchi or vessels may be seen first. Except for the absence of a large left ventricle, the roentgenogram of ARDS may be difficult to distinguish from that of cardiogenic pulmonary edema. Proper resolution demands films of good quality with sufficient contrast and good detail.

The first changes of fine reticulation progress to give the lung a ground glass appearance. A typical air-space alveolar pattern may be seen as fluid leaks into the alveoli. Terminally, when consolidation is seen, there may be few recognizable air spaces; at this point the term *white lung* is applicable.

There are no sensitive practical means for early detection of ARDS. Detectable changes are probably the result of significant water accumulation in the lung. Therefore, relatively minor alteration in tests of pulmonary function of patients who are at risk of ARDS should receive special attention. Early endotracheal intubation and mechanical ventilation should be considered as soon as abnormalities occur.

Figure 27-3 shows by means of x-rays the progress of a 35-year-old-man who was admitted with a gunshot wound through the right lobe of the liver. The bullet tract involved the base of the right lung. After admission to the hospital, the patient appeared well and breathed room air spontaneously. Pa_{O_2} was 67 and Pa_{CO_2}, 34; pH was 7.42.

Three days later, after developing severe respiratory failure, the patient was transferred to another institution. He had been given massive doses of diuretics and concentrated albumin solution and was receiving controlled mechanical ventilation (CMV) with 10 cmH$_2$O positive end-expiratory pressure (PEEP). Dopamine was needed to maintain blood pressure, and pancuronium was given because ventilation could not be synchronized with CMV. Pa_{O_2} was 48 and Pa_{CO_2}, 42; pH was 7.12 on $F_{I_{O_2}}$ of 1.0. Lactate level was 5.6 mmol/L, and the patient was oliguric.

The final x-ray was made 8 h after the patient was admitted to the second institution. He had received 2 U of whole blood and 4 L of crystalloid and was now receiving 26 cmH$_2$O PEEP; intermittent

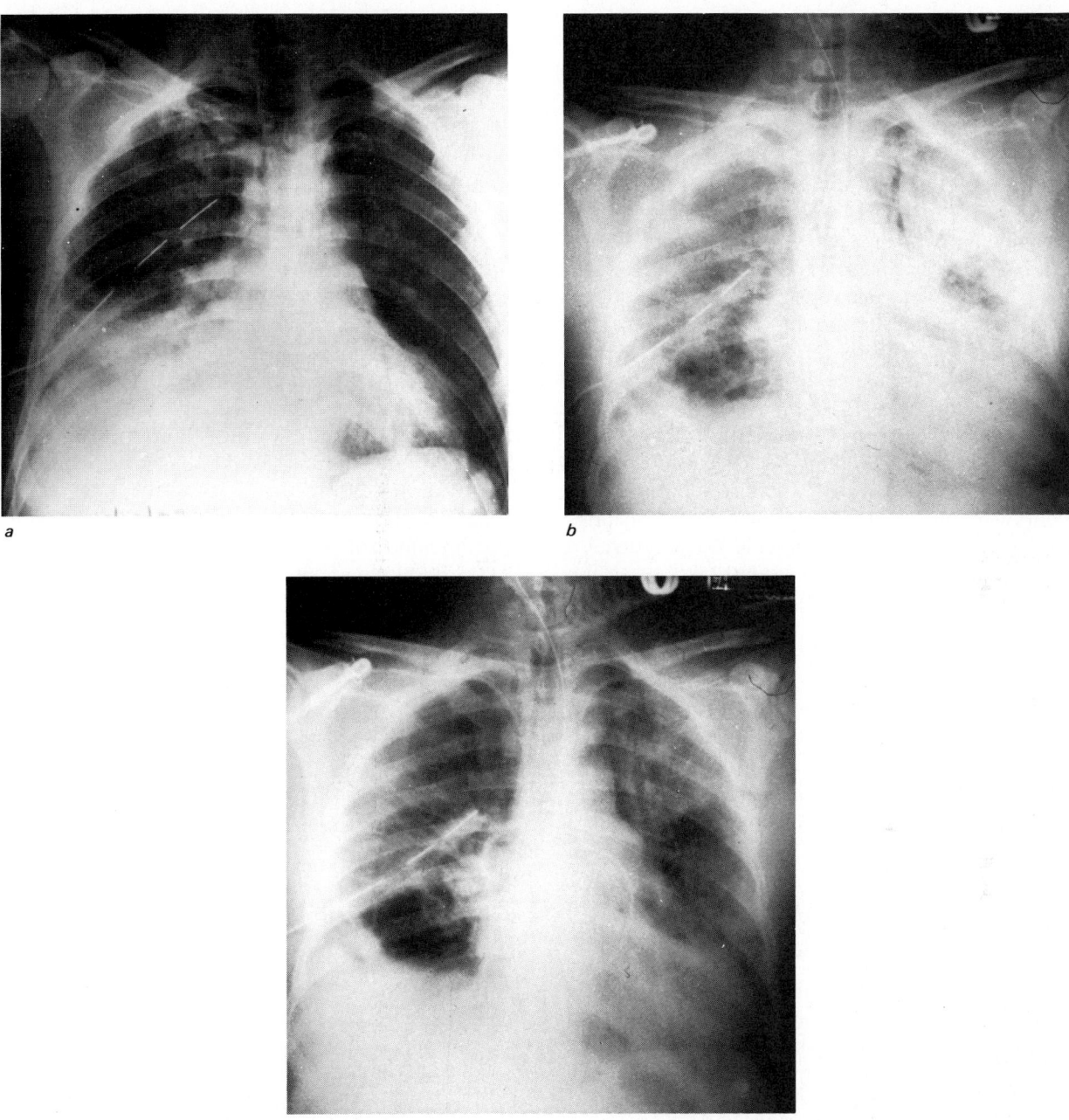

Figure 27-3   Chest x-rays of 35-year-old man with a gunshot wound through the right lobe of the liver. The bullet tract involved the base of the right lung. (*a*) After admission to the hospital, patient was breathing room air spontaneously and appeared well. (*b*) Three days later, after developing severe respiratory failure, the patient was transferred to another institution. (*c*) Patient 8 h after admission, having received 2 U of whole blood and 4 L of crystalloid. PEEP and IMV had begun.

mandatory ventilation (IMV) rate was six breaths per minute; Fi_{O_2} was 0.5. Pa_{O_2} was 92 and Pa_{CO_2}, 43; the pH was 7.37; the lactate level was 2 mmol/L. The patient was producing copious pink frothy sputum from the endotracheal tube and was nursed face down so that pulmonary edema fluid could be allowed to drain. He was not given suction during the first 36 h after admission, because secretions were being washed out by the pulmonary edema fluid. Circulatory integrity returned in 36 h, when the patient had normal renal function. He required some ventilatory support for another 5 days. By then he had returned to his admission weight, having voided the extra fluid given during resuscitation.

Patients with fully developed ARDS invariably require mechanical ventilation. The decision as to when to intervene with ventilatory support in patients with minor pulmonary function abnormalities suggesting ARDS may be difficult. Early intubation and ventilation are recommended because of the previously described cycle of edema, decreasing lung volume, and the appearance of hypoxia, leading to more edema and more volume loss, contributing to further hypoxia.

Endotracheal intubation should be performed initially. The widespread use of high-volume, low-pressure cuffs on endotracheal tubes has sufficiently decreased the rate of tracheal complications from these tubes so that today tracheostomy is not normally required unless prolonged mechanical ventilation is anticipated.

When mechanical ventilation is initiated in ARDS, tidal volumes of 10 to 15 mL per kilogram of body weight should be used. Volumes in this range are more effective in reducing or preventing atelectasis. When large tidal volumes are used with continuous positive pressure ventilation (CPPV), alveolar hyperventilation may be seen. Since a low Pa_{CO_2} has been shown to decrease cardiac output and increase oxygen consumption as well as airway resistance, it is important to keep the Pa_{CO_2} in the range of 35 to 45 torr. Additional mechanical dead space may be added to the ventilator circuit to achieve this, or the respiratory rate may be decreased, provided the patient can be assisted to breathe synchronously with the machine. One would not want to decrease tidal volume in order to

relieve the hyperventilation in these patients because of the atelectatic nature of the syndrome.

Many patients with ARDS are restless and tachypneic, which causes them to be overventilated when receiving CPPV and breathe out of phase with the ventilator. Sedation should be used to avoid these problems; usually intermittent small intravenous doses of morphine (3 to 5 mg given every hour) are sufficient. When larger doses of morphine are required to achieve adequate sedation, adverse effects from peripheral vasodilatation may become a problem. A neuromuscular blocking agent such as curare or pancuronium (Pavulon) is helpful to completely paralyze and control a restless patient. Patients who are receiving such agents are paralyzed but fully awake and aware of their surroundings. Small doses of opiates should be given in conjunction with these drugs.

The use of CPPV with PEEP has a well-documented role in the treatment of patients with ARDS. PEEP augments the reduced lung volumes seen in ARDS by producing a constantly positive distending pressure in the airways and alveoli. Intrapulmonary shunt is reduced because alveoli remain open and gases are available for diffusion throughout the respiratory cycle. The improved ventilation to gas exchange units that were previous sites of shunting or marked $\dot{V}/\dot{Q}$ abnormalities increases arterial P_{O_2} and reduces the aveolar-arterial difference. PEEP also physically expands alveoli and exerts gas pressure against the transudating fluid in the alveoli so that the volume of fluid that previously filled the lumen forms a layer on the alveolar surface wall through which gas diffusion can occur.

The use of PEEP with CPPV has certain limitations because of hazards associated with combining these two therapies. PEEP adds more pressure to the already high mean intrathoracic pressures needed to mechanically inflate stiff lungs with positive pressure. This high pressure is transmitted, in part, to the pleural space and great veins of the chest. Added pressure can compress these vessels and reduce venous return to the right side of the heart, thereby reducing cardiac output. This can lead to poor tissue perfusion and lactic acidosis. Pulmonary vascular resistance is also increased, which increases the work of the right ventricle in pumping blood into the normally low-resistance pulmonary bed. PEEP in excess of 15 cmH$_2$O has seldom been successful with CPPV.

The cardiac effects of PEEP are modified by its use in conjunction with spontaneous ventilation (continuous positive airway pressure, or CPAP) or with IMV. The combination of PEEP therapy with CPAP or IMV enhances the therapeutic potential of PEEP in ARDS (increased transpulmonary pressures) while reducing detrimental cardiovascular effects (control of intrapleural/mean intrathoracic pressure).

Patients requiring PEEP therapy for severe ARDS have an increased incidence of barotrauma when compared with a mixed population of intensive care unit (ICU) patients receiving mechanical ventilation without PEEP. This increase in barotrauma, however, is due to the severity of the parenchymal disease rather than to the level of PEEP therapy. It is now accepted that there are no absolute contraindications to the use of PEEP in ARDS.

The development of a flow-directed thermodilution catheter and cardiac output computer has allowed direct measurement of mixed venous and systemic arterial blood gases, central venous pressure, and pulmonary artery wedge pressure for monitoring cardiovascular compromise. This information is necessary to determine the relations between PEEP, intrapulmonary shunt, and cardiac output.

The availability of inexpensive programmable calculators allows long and tedious mathematical calculations to be done accurately, rapidly, and inexpensively. Cardiac function can be evaluated by preload, the degree to which the myocardium is stretched before contraction; contractility; and afterload, the resistance against which the blood is expelled. Preload is reflected by the pulmonary artery wedge pressure and central venous pressure. Contractility is evaluated in terms of the measured cardiac output and heart rate as well as the calculated left ventricular stroke work index and stroke volume. Afterload is obtained from calculations of pulmonary and systemic vascular resistance. The effects of ventilatory support can be evaluated along with their effects on the cardiovascular circuit and appropriate interventions instituted to support the cardiovascular system during ventilatory therapy.

The goal of PEEP therapy in ARDS is to reduce the physiological shunt enough so that adequate arterial oxygen content (adequate hemoglobin content plus adequate arterial P_{O_2}) is achieved without significant compromise of cardiac output while potentially detrimental alveolar oxygen concentrations are avoided.

Intensivists at some major centers use the techniques previously described to treat the patient to achieve a calculated intrapulmonary shunt of 20 percent or less. Other groups treat to achieve a P_{O_2} greater than 60 to 70 torr at an $F_{I_{O_2}}$ of less than 0.50. Regardless of blood gas values, should the patient exhibit signs of labored breathing, anxiety, or unexplained restlessness, inadequacy in the amount of mechanical ventilatory support being supplied should be considered.

Invasive cardiovascular monitoring is initiated whenever potential cardiovascular compromise is anticipated or when levels of PEEP greater than 15 cm of water are applied. Pulmonary wedge pressure which reflects left ventricular filling pressure can be optimized to a range of 13 to 17 torr in patients with documented cardiovascular dysfunction.[2] This is achieved by giving red cells or fluids as bolus IV infusions in an amount sufficient to maintain a reasonable cardiac output for the particular patient. Support of the cardiovascular function with fluid infusions or pharmacological agents is necessary only if the ventilatory support needed to achieve adequate pulmonary function decreases the usual pumping ability of the heart.

Medical Management

Fluid replacement in ARDS is an extremely controversial topic. The question focuses on the choice of colloids or crystalloids for fluid volume replacement. It has been proposed that intravascular volume should be replaced with colloids, since the major intravascular force keeping fluid within the capillaries is the protein osmotic pressure. Administration of colloids, then, would keep the protein osmotic pressure within the vascular space from diminishing. However, there is undoubtedly rapid equilibration of protein concentrations between vascular and interstitial spaces in the presence of a leaky capillary endothelium. There would be a loss of the oncotic pressure gradient across the capillary wall. The administration of colloids and the rapid exudation of protein into the interstitium may actually make the situation worse, since protein-rich fluid is cleared slowly from the interstitium and alveoli. Some physicians fear that resuscitation with colloids might increase lung water more than resuscitation with crystalloids. There is no clear-cut experimental evidence favoring either crystalloids or colloids for fluid replacement.

Crystalloid solutions have several real advantages in terms of present practicality. They are effective, readily available, and inexpensive. Colloids, on the other hand, are expensive and limited in supply. It would seem that in the absence of documented therapeutic benefits crystalloid solutions are preferable, since they can adequately replenish intravascular volume and restore functional extracellular fluid volumes. It seems reasonable to consider crystalloids early in the course of ARDS when the increase in permeability is greatest. Later, if the serum protein concentration is low, colloid solutions may be used. However, appropriate fluids must be used to maintain optimal cardiac output while instituting the treatment of choice—PEEP.

Successful employment of any regimen utilizing mechanical ventilation is dependent upon a knowledgeable and highly skilled nursing staff. The staff must understand the principles of mechanical ventilation and the interpretation of arterial blood gases and must have a high level of expertise in physical assessment, techniques of pulmonary toilet, and proper maintenance of cuffed endotracheal tubes. The nurse must also know how to assist in emergency procedures when indicated (e.g., development of bradycardia, emergency insertion of chest tube). If monitoring of the patient with a flow-directed thermodilution catheter is employed, the nurse must be familiar with care of the catheter and insertion site, must have visual recognition of the various pressure waveforms, and must be cognizant of the basic interpretation of numerical values associated with pulmonary artery and wedge pressures.

When perfusion of one lung is a major concern in addition to ventilation, the Rotorest bed, originally designed for orthopedic and neurosurgical patients, can be used with IMV and PEEP (Fig. 27-4 and Table 27-3). When the electrically driven motor is running, this bed rocks slowly from side to side. However, the bed can be stopped in any position, and a patient with unilateral pulmonary disease can be positioned so that the diseased lung is elevated and the unaffected lung is in the dependent position. Both ventilation and perfusion will be preferentially delivered to the unaffected lung, resulting in less perfusion of nonventilated areas in the diseased lung and producing a decreased intrapulmonary shunt and decreased microvascular pressure in that lung, all of which favor the egress of fluid.

Several indexes are available for the determination of adequate tissue oxygenation, although

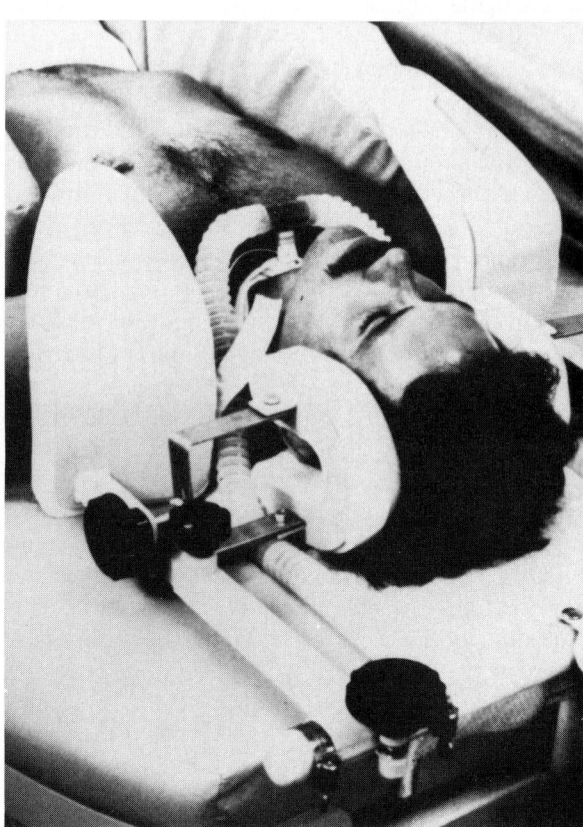

Figure 27-4 The Rotorest bed enables the critical-care practitioner to care for the patient who requires sophisticated mechanical ventilation with greater ease and patient comfort and offers a number of clinical advantages over conventional beds.

Table 27-3 Pulmonary Benefits of Rotorest Bed

Mobilizes secretions
Provides for continuous postural drainage
Decreases shunt by preferential positioning
Facilitates selective suctioning
Makes possible x-ray through table surfaces
Stabilizes ventilator tubing
Facilitates maintenance of chest tubes
Gives comfortable positioning for percussion and postural
  drainage
Eliminates disadvantages of prone positioning
Provides access for CPR or airway maintenance

no single value is useful unless taken in conjunction with others. Arterial P_{O_2} is accessible but provides little useful information, since it reflects oxygenation of blood that has not yet reached the peripheral tissues. A more precise estimate of tissue oxygenation is the correlation of arterial P_{O_2} with the mixed venous P_{O_2}. Most tissues compensate for inadequate oxygen delivery by increasing their extraction of the gas from arterial blood, thus widening the difference in oxygen content between arterial and venous blood and decreasing mixed venous P_{O_2} (drawn slowly from the distal lumen of the thermodilation catheter) below the normal 40 torr. Serum lactate levels (also measurable in the laboratory) will also rise as a result of the metabolic acidosis produced by poor oxygenation.

Indications for use and the beneficial effects of corticosteroids in ARDS are extremely controversial. Several theoretically beneficial effects of steroids may reduce the amount of edema resulting from injury. They may stabilize lysosomal membranes, preventing pulmonary damage from enzymes liberated from white blood cells, and they may reduce the amount of fibrosis following the acute phase of illness. There is, unfortunately, no clear experimental evidence to substantiate or refute these potential benefits.

Infection may produce or complicate the picture of ARDS. When infection is suspected, aggressive efforts should be made to identify the specific etiologic agent. This can usually be accomplished by Gram's stain and culture with sensitivity determinations of aspirated tracheal secretions. If more vigorous effort is needed, fiber-optic bronchoscopy can fairly easily be performed in patients receiving mechanical ventilation. Using the fiber-optic bronchoscope makes possible the use of a brush biopsy and bronchial lavage of localized areas. Needle aspiration and, rarely, open-lung biopsy may be required. Once an organism has been identified, appropriate therapy can be initiated utilizing the usual principles of antibiotic therapy. Cultures should be obtained if there is a change in the Gram smear, or they may be obtained on a routine basis (e.g., twice weekly) on severely ill patients at higher risk for development of infection.

Viral Pneumonia

Early descriptions of viral pneumonia were often confused by the presence of secondary bacterial pneumonias. Since bacterial pneumonias can be controlled with antibiotic therapy, the pathological changes of viral pneumonia within the lung are now being identified. In fulminating cases the alveoli are filled with fibrin, fluid, red blood cells, and macrophages. These patients have profound hypoxemias, often relatively unimproved by oxygen administration, and should be treated like ARDS patients. Prognosis is grave, and fortunately, these cases are rare. Far more common are cases of patchy areas of viral pneumonitis, occurring during an influenzal infection and not extensive enough to cause severe arterial desaturation. In fact, presenting signs and symptoms are less severe than the roentgenogram would suggest.

Although a viral pneumonia may be suspected clinically, the diagnosis is usually made retrospectively using serological studies. Pneumonia complicating viral influenza is commonly bacterial, although in the 1957 pandemic, fatal cases were recorded as resulting from purely viral pneumonia.

Pneumonia due to varicella virus may complicate severe chickenpox in adults and among adults constitutes 38 percent of the varicella cases[3]. Predisposing factors include chronic illness, steroid treatment, and treatment with antimetabolic drugs. The mortality from varicella pneumonia may be as high as 20 percent[4]. Pulmonary symptoms begin 2 to 5 days after vesicle eruption. Severe respiratory distress, cough, chest pain, and frequently hypoxemia and hemoptysis are typical, although milder cases also occur. Pleural friction rub, pleural effusion, and radiologic shadows have been described on the ipsilateral side in patients with intercostal herpes zoster, also thought to be caused by the varicella virus.

In addition to influenza and varicella viruses, measles and cytomegalovirus are the most commonly involved organisms in viral pneumonia. Whenever the viral pneumonia is severe, it rapidly progresses to a clinical picture of ARDS and should be treated as previously described.

Aspiration Pneumonia

Aspiration of acid gastric contents often results in a widespread, severe chemical pneumonitis with diffuse alveolar filling. Aspiration pneumonia actually occurs in three different forms: acute aspiration pneumonia (septic pneumonitis, or Mendelson's syndrome), chronic aspiration pneumonia, and lipoid pneumonia.

Acute aspiration pneumonia results from the aspiration of gastric contents, primarily hydrochloric acid. It is extremely severe and can be fatal. Predisposing conditions include trauma, burns, general anesthesia, comatose states, and the presence of nasogastric or endotracheal tubes. There is characteristically a latent period between aspiration and the onset of respiratory distress. Diagnostic findings are similar to those described previously with ARDS. The chest roentgenogram initially shows bilateral patchy pulmonary edema. Treatment is the same as previously described for ARDS. The use of steroids in acute aspiration pneumonia, as in ARDS, is controversial.

Chronic aspiration pneumonia is a localized consolidation of dependent portions of the lungs or of the bilateral midzones due to repeated aspiration of small quantities of infected pharyngeal secretions. It is particularly common in chronic alcoholic patients and drug abusers and in patients who are obtunded. Nasogastric and endotracheal tubes as well as swallowing defects and hiatus hernias are common predisposing factors. Infecting organisms are usually anaerobes or gram-negative bacilli; necrosis and abscess formation are common.

Lipoid pneumonia (oil granuloma) results from aspiration of milk, mineral oil, oily nose drops, etc. It presents radiologically as a chronic consolidation resembling carcinoma.

Radiation Pneumonitis

Radiation therapy to or near the lungs may result in acute radiation pneumonitis and/or radiation fibrosis. The reaction is limited to the area which has been irradiated, and therefore the condition is usually severe only when the irradiation is bilateral. The effect varies with the size of the radiation dose, the amount of lung that has been irradiated, and the rate of administration. It is more likely to occur in thin persons. It usually develops within a month or two after the initiation of therapy and appears on the roentgenogram as a soft, fluffy alveolar infiltrate. There is an associated loss of lung volume and the characteristic picture of an air bronchogram. Radiation fibrosis is a chronic restrictive abnormality that usually follows but may develop independently of radiation pneumonitis. The affected area of lung becomes small and firm, and the mediastinum may be shifted to the involved side with elevation of the hemidiaphragm. Cor pulmonale occurs if the process is sufficiently extensive.

Cardiogenic Pulmonary Edema

It is beyond the scope of this discussion to consider cardiogenic pulmonary edema in any depth. Like ARDS (noncardiac pulmonary edema), it is the result of excessive accumulation of lung water. In this case the cause is a failing left ventricle or excessive administration of intravenous fluids. Increased left atrial pressure increases hydrostatic pressure in the pulmonary capillary bed. The lung's lymphatics, which can normally handle moderately increased fluid loads with minimal increases in interstitial fluid accumulation, are overwhelmed. The increased intravascular hydrostatic pressure causes an increase in net filtration pressure. The capillary endothelium remains intact, but fluid transudates from the capillary into the interstitium and eventually into the alveolus. One major difference between ARDS and cardiogenic pulmonary edema is the loss of capillary endothelial integrity in ARDS. If the capillary endothelium remains intact in cardiogenic pulmonary edema, one would expect the fluid migrating into the alveoli to remain a transudate without the proteinaceous material seen in ARDS. In fact, when pulmonary edema fluid is due to high filtration pressures, the protein concentration of tracheal fluid is usually less than one-half that in plasma. In noncardiac pulmonary edema the alveolar fluid protein composition is much higher and similar to that of circulating plasma.

Severe cardiogenic pulmonary edema may be treated as previously described for ARDS, but with particular attention to cardiovascular functioning. Treatment includes optimizing preload, contractility, and afterload. The reader is encouraged to refer to Chap. 21 for detailed reading.

Oxygen Toxicity

The advent of outer space and underwater exploration has necessitated the development of new perspectives on oxygen exposure. As long as humans were restricted to life at or near sea level, the term $F_{I_{O_2}}$ was adequate to quantify oxygen exposure. This term reflects the fraction of total inspired gas that is pure oxygen. However, when humans are exposed to oxygen under hyperbaric conditions (increased barometric pressures), they develop oxygen toxicity at a lower $F_{I_{O_2}}$. Alternatively, under hypobaric conditions (lowered barometric pressures), oxygen toxicity does not develop even at a very high $F_{I_{O_2}}$. The term $P_{I_{O_2}}$ was developed to give a better index of exposure. It represents the partial pressure of inspired oxygen and is calculated by a formula that takes atmospheric pressure into consideration:

$$P_{I_{O_2}} = (P_a - 47) \times F_{I_{O_2}}$$

P_B is barometric pressure, and 47 represents the partial pressure of water vapor at body temperature. The $P_{I_{O_2}}$ is used to determine oxygen toxicity.

The term *atmosphere of oxygen* allows $P_{I_{O_2}}$ to be expressed in terms of atmospheric pressure. This term is calculated as

$$\text{Atmosphere of oxygen} = \frac{P_{I_{O_2}}}{760}$$

where 760 represents atmospheric pressure at sea level.

Oxygen is a drug, and like any other drug, its toxicity is determined by host tolerance, effective dose, and duration of exposure. Host tolerance is difficult to assess. There is tremendous species variation in response to oxygen. There is a great deal of variation between individual humans and, at times, in the same individual. Steroids, hypercarbia, and hyperthermia may facilitate the development of oxygen toxicity, and this may have some clinical significance, since most critical-care patients experience at least one if not all of these conditions in the critical-care unit. This information seems to contraindicate the use of steroids to treat the proliferative phase of oxygen toxicity, a common practice in some areas, and is a serious consideration against the use of steroids in ARDS.

Intermittent exposure seems to be the strongest minimizing factor in oxygen toxicity. This is an excellent area for future research. However, at present, critical-care practitioners are already using PEEP and CPAP to keep oxygen exposure as low as possible while maintaining adequate tissue oxygenation. It would be a gross error in judgment to jeopardize tissue oxygenation intermittently for the purpose of minimizing oxygen toxicity.

Clinical symptoms of early oxygen toxicity include tracheobronchitis beginning in the area of the carina, cough, and inspiratory pain. In the late stages of this phase, dyspnea may develop.

The late phase of oxygen toxicity affects the alveolar unit. It has been reported to develop after 4 days of exposure to 91% O_2 at 1 atm.[5] During this phase, noncardiogenic interstitial and later alveolar pulmonary edema develop. The clinical picture is the same as previously described for ARDS.

The end stage of oxygen toxicity is one of progressive consolidation and fibrosis of the lung. If the patient's total exposure to oxygen is within the toxic range and a compatible clinical picture is present, the diagnosis of oxygen toxicity can be made. Detection of this condition is valuable because, while it is potentially lethal, the chance for complete recovery exists once O_2 levels are reduced below toxicity level.

The pathological picture of oxygen toxicity is the same as that previously described for ARDS. The earliest changes are an exudative phase including capillary endothelial cell damage and loss of membrane integrity, interstitial edema, alveolar hemorrhage, and destruction of type I pneumocytes. Following the death of the type I alveolar cells, the basement membrane is exposed and covered with fibrin and cellular debris, leading to the formation of a hyaline membrane.

The proliferative phase which follows includes hyperplasia of type II pneumocytes. The alveoli become lined with these abnormal cells, and fibroblasts proliferate in the interstitium. Once this stage occurs, recovery is unlikely and permanent fibrosis of the interstitium is probable.

Hypoxemia is a frequent occurrence in critically ill patients; its damage is usually rapid, often irreversible, and sometimes fatal. Pulmonary oxygen toxicity is uncommon, variable in onset, and slow in developing. As previously stated, a patient should never be subjected to tissue hypoxia for the purpose of preventing oxygen toxicity. The best approach seems to be the judicious use of oxygen therapy to treat hypoxemia and tissue hypoxia without overtreating and needlessly exposing the patient to excessive amounts of the drug. PEEP and CPAP should be utilized to the extent possible to avoid subjecting the patient to an $F_{I_{O_2}}$ greater than 0.40 to 0.50.

Near Drowning

Submersion injuries are classified as drowning or near drowning. The drowning victim is one who dies within 24 h, while near-drowning victims survive for more than 24 h. Both injuries can be further classified as *wet,* when aspiration has occurred, or *dry,* when damage has been caused by asphyxiation without aspiration. In the dry group, intact laryngeal reflexes probably cause laryngospasm, thus preventing aspiration. The wet group are more likely to have been obtunded and to have experienced aspiration.

The type of injury seen in near-drowning victims depends on the toxicity of the fluid aspirated, the temperature, the nature of contaminants in the water (e.g., bacteria, protozoa, algae, sand) which may have been aspirated, and the duration of hypoxia. In animal studies, major differences were found between aspiration of seawater (3.5% NaCl) and hypotonic fresh water. In humans, however, the clinical picture is similar for both. Every near drowning is a response to a unique set of contaminants and environmental circumstances. Many submersion injuries are preceded or accompanied by

other primary events such as myocardial infarction, seizures, and spinal cord or head injuries due to a dive into shallow water. Near-drowning victims brought in for resuscitation should be carefully studied for other primary pathological conditions.

Hypothermia also has a dramatic impact in the near-drowning victim. Body temperature falls rapidly following submersion, since the thermal conduction properties of water are 32 times greater than those of air. Death before drowning may occur in healthy persons swimming in cold water. Cold water immersion causes hyperventilation, which may result in hypocapnia, disorientation, and possible loss of consciousness, leading to drowning.

Hypothermia also increases blood viscosity, slowing flow through the coronary arteries and other vessels. Shifting of the oxyhemoglobin dissociation curve to the left results in an increased affinity of hemoglobin for oxygen and decreased oxygen unloading.

The hypoxemia after human submersion is caused by a combination of interstitial and alveolar pulmonary edema similar to that previously described for ARDS. There is damage to pulmonary capillaries, decreased surfactant, and a hyaline membrane type of formation by proteinaceous material. There is a decrease in pulmonary compliance, increased dead space, and increased intrapulmonary shunt. Ventilation and perfusion are mismatched, and there is an increased alveolar-arterial oxygen difference.

When first seen, victims of submersion injury may show a variety of symptoms ranging from rales, rhonchi, and wheezes to cardiac arrest. A few may be relatively asymptomatic but proceed to develop ARDS within the next 24 h. All patients with a history of significant submersion should have medical observation for at least 24 h.

Therapeutic efforts for the pulmonary manifestations of near drowning are the same as those previously described in ARDS. The objectives of increasing lung volumes and matching ventilation with perfusion can be accomplished by the use of mechanical support with IMV ventilation, PEEP, and circulatory support when needed. Mask CPAP may prove beneficial in patients who are hypoxemic but can maintain a normal Pa_{CO_2}. Mask CPAP should not be used in patients who are obtunded or unconscious, because of the hazard of vomiting and aspiration.

There are reports of survival after prolonged submersion and cardiac arrest in very cold water. One report describes a submersion and cardiac arrest lasting approximately 40 min that was followed by survival without significant residual neurological deficits.[6] In such cases the decrease in metabolic rate, cellular metabolism, and oxygen consumption in the central nervous system and heart may have prevented damage from hypoxia. Resuscitation should be attempted in the hypothermic drowning victim even though prolonged submersion may have occurred.

Families and friends of near-drowning victims require a great deal of psychological support from critical-care unit personnel. Near drowning represents the extremely sudden onset of critical illness for which family members are totally unprepared. They have not had time to develop any coping mechanisms and certainly will be in the very earliest stages of the grieving process. ICU personnel should also be sensitive to the possibility that extreme guilt may plague the family members of these patients. If the victim is a small child, the parents may carry unrealistic amounts of guilt regarding supervision of the child. Regardless of the known circumstances surrounding the submersion incident, if family members or friends of the patient exhibit behavior indicating that they are having difficulty coping with the situation, an appropriate referral to a chaplain, psychiatric social worker, or psychologist should be initiated.

Acquired Immune Deficiency Syndrome (AIDS)

AIDS is characterized by the development of multiple severe opportunistic infections and rare neoplasms in previously healthy persons. The population at significant risk to date includes homosexual males, bisexuals, Haitians, intravenous drug abusers, recipients of large amounts of blood replacement products, and oncological and transplant patients receiving immunosuppressive therapy. Characteristic defects seen in the AIDS patient include depressed blastogenesis, lymphopenia with a selective decrease in T cells, and a marked depletion of helper T cells as compared with suppressor T cells.

A study of 15 AIDS victims including autopsy data reported in 1984 revealed that 100 percent of them had one or more episodes of serious respiratory illness which required hospitalization.[7] All patients exhibited signs of opportunistic infections, and the initial manifestation of the disease was pulmonary in 50 percent. The most common pulmonary pathogen was *Pneumocystis carinii,* alone or in combination with cytomegalovirus. Bouts of *Pneumocystis carinii* pneumonia had been successfully treated in two-thirds of the patients by trimethoprim-sulfamethoxazole (Bactrim, Septra) or pentamidine isethionate. This was the only pulmonary disease in which successful treatment was documented. Respiratory disease (ARDS) was the most common cause of death, and in 100 percent of the patients additional unsuspected pulmonary disease was diagnosed on autopsy—most commonly cytomegalovirus pneumonitis (14 of 15 patients).

Patients with pulmonary manifestations of AIDS complain most frequently of dyspnea and fever and exhibit bilateral diffuse pulmonary infiltrates on chest x-ray. Often tachypnea, fever, and dyspnea are more impressive than the radiographic findings. Bronchoscopic findings indicate a positive diagnosis in 70 to 80 percent of cases.

At present, only a minority of the infectious complications of AIDS can be successfully treated. The necessity for endotracheal intubation and mechanical ventilation is a grave prognostic sign; few patients with it survive to leave the hospital. Only a high index of suspicion, prompt diagnosis, and early treatment offer a prolonged, high-quality period of continued life for the AIDS victim.

Drug Overdose and Head Injury

Drug overdose and head injury produce, on rare occasions, a most devastating form of acute hemorrhagic pneumonitis. The effect of some agents, e.g., barbiturates, is to depress other system functions. Indirect effects on the lung may give rise to management problems in the recovery period.

Pathophysiology

Cerebral hypoxia has been indicated as a possible major cause for acute respiratory failure. This would account for the condition arising in head injury and the apnea or hypoventilation of drug overdose. The hypoxia and hypocapnia noted as early as the time of admission of patients with severe head injury may reflect increased intrapulmonary shunting and may progress to ARDS. Although pulmonary edema is an uncommon clinical problem in these patients, studies have suggested that extravascular lung water may be increased.

Acute hypoxia at the time of injury or with the intravenous injection of an excessive dose of heroin (*mainlining*) has been suggested as a possible cause of pulmonary failure by Severinghaus.[8] If a patient has a respiratory arrest, the resulting hypoxia gives rise to a massive sympathetic discharge, with a marked augmentation of cardiac output. At the same time, the pulmonary vascular resistance is much increased by hypoxia and possible acidemia. Consequently, there is an extremely high pulmonary artery pressure. This hypertension can be demonstrated to damage the pulmonary arterioles enough to allow considerable extravasation of blood. When the airway and ventilation are restored the circulation returns to normal, but the lungs have been severely damaged. By the time the patient is being cared for and life-saving maneuvers have been started, the noxious effects of hypoxia have seemingly vanished and the subsequent respiratory distress is labeled as an idiosyncratic reaction to heroin or pulmonary edema due to head injury.

Aspiration pneumonitis is another possible cause of failure in comatose patients who are not properly positioned and whose airways are not secured. Frequently it goes unrecognized because gastric juice with low pH often is clear, watery, and free from bile.

Medical Management

Head injury provides a special set of difficulties. The balance of adequate hydration of the body to maintain the circulation without causing cerebral edema makes the combination with acute respiratory failure particularly dangerous. High pressures from mechanical support of the lung can increase intracranial pressure. There does not appear to be a universally acceptable answer. Mild hyperventilation, which reduces cerebral edema, in combination with sufficient mechanical support of the lungs to maintain an arterial oxygen tension above

70 torr, with an inspired oxygen fraction of 40 to 45 percent, would seem a reasonable compromise. The use of IMV to minimize intrathoracic pressure that might be transmitted as venous pressure would also seem desirable. Monitoring cardiovascular and intracranial pressures may be helpful in determining the balance of therapy to reduce cerebral edema.

Drug overdose provides a lesser problem, in that volume loading and standard therapy for acute respiratory failure can be more easily managed without damaging the patient. Hydration should be just sufficient to maintain cardiac and renal function. If a low-output low-pressure state develops, inotropic support is permissible but is associated with a higher mortality.

In general, the basic principles of mechanical support of the lungs in both head injury and overdose patients are not rendered invalid by the patient's primary condition.

Atelectasis

One of the most common respiratory disorders in the critically ill patient is atelectasis. It may also be one of the most preventable complications of any hospitalized patient. By definition, *atelectasis* is collapse of alveoli or diminution of volume of lung units. Although it is a frequent complication of upper abdominal surgery, atelectasis may be caused by compression of lung tissue, as by tumors, effusions, pneumothorax, hemothorax, and empyema, as well as by any condition which decreases the inspiratory effort of the patient. This collapse may be lobar or segmental but is most often randomly spread throughout the lung (patchy atelectasis).

Pathophysiology

Three factors have been implicated in the collapse of alveoli: airway obstruction (*resorptive atelectasis*), ineffective ventilation, and decreased surfactant levels. Resorptive atelectasis results when gas is unable to reach alveoli because of obstruction. Mucous plug, foreign body, aspirated matter, and tumor material can all be causes of decreased ventilation to the alveoli. Once obstruction occurs, the gas distal to it is absorbed into the circulation. The absorption occurs because oxygen tension in the pulmonary arteries is lower than that in the alveoli. Thus, oxygen diffuses from the area of greater concentration. The higher the concentration of oxygen in the alveoli, the faster the absorption rate; thus the higher the FI_{O_2} of inspired gas at the time of the obstruction, the faster the alveolar collapse.

Obstruction of the larger lobar and segmental branches most certainly leads to collapse of lung tissue distal to it. However, atelectasis beyond this level is probably not caused by obstruction. Collateral ventilation usually permits passage of gas into the obstructed alveoli. Thus, resorptive atelectasis does not occur even with complete obstruction of peripheral airways unless underlying disease has prevented collateral ventilation.

Compression by space-occupying lesions of the chest decreases the number of ventilated alveoli. Ineffective ventilation is probably the main factor in postoperative atelectasis. Studies have shown that constant tidal volumes result in decreased lung volume, decreased compliance, and increased shunting. This collapse of alveoli is reversible by hyperinflation of the lung. Upper abdominal surgery may cause "splinting" during breathing, thereby lowering tidal volumes. Stasis of secretions due to ineffective cough further reduces the amount of gas available for gas exchange.

Surfactant, which has the property of lowering surface tension to prevent collapse, may be a significant factor in atelectasis. Decreased surfactant levels are thought to be a factor in promoting collapse of lung units. It has yet to be established whether these low levels are the cause or the result of atelectasis. It seems highly probable, however, that decreased blood flow decreases surfactant level.

Diagnostic Findings

Frequently, mild atelectasis is asymptomatic, but with inadequate treatment, the atelectatic areas may increase and lead to symptoms of hypoxemia. Acute onset of obstruction is marked with dyspnea, restlessness, and tachycardia. With extensive involvement, cyanosis may be evident. Structures in the mediastinum may shift toward the affected side when a collapse of a major portion of the lung occurs.

Generally, rales are heard on auscultation unless major collapse causes diminished or absent sounds. Characteristically, the blood gases show a decreased Pa_{O_2} and normal or decreased Pa_{CO_2}; the levels are dependent on the extent of shunting and the respiratory rate. Patchy atelectasis may be exhibited on chest x-ray as radiopaque areas bilaterally. Massive involvement may be demonstrated roentgenographically by increased density at the hilus and extending peripherally. The hemidiaphragm may be elevated on the affected side.

With persistent atelectasis, signs of pneumonia may be seen. Increased temperature, dyspnea, tachycardia, and cyanosis are generally evident. The accumulated secretions are a good medium for growth of bacteria, and this type of pneumonia is a frequent occurrence if therapeutic measures are not taken to open atelectatic areas to drain secretions.

Medical Management

Compression atelectasis is usually relieved once the precipitating cause is removed (e.g., drainage of effusion, removal of tumor), while hyperinflation of the lung will aid in opening atelectases of other causation. It has been suggested that deep breathing may stimulate surfactant mobilization.

Once atelectasis is present, secretions should be removed by coughing, endotracheal suctioning, or therapeutic bronchoscopy, if necessary. The best treatment is prevention. This task rests with the nurse or respiratory therapist and should never be overlooked. Preoperative teaching of coughing and deep breathing is essential to maintain efficient postoperative performance.

Frequent position changes, early ambulation, and vigorous chest physiotherapy are mandatory with any patient prone to atelectasis. Humidification and adequate hydration will keep secretions loose and enhance expectoration. Good nutrition is a vital part of therapy to prevent muscle atrophy, which can reduce inspiratory effort. The more chronic the atelectasis, the more vigorous these measures should be.

In the intubated patient, the use of high tidal volumes and/or PEEP can help to maintain open alveoli. Instillation of saline for irrigation during suctioning may loosen secretions and enhance removal. The use of bronchodilators and mucolytic agents may also prove useful.

Prophylactic measures should be instituted in all critically ill patients to prevent atelectasis. Position changes and chest physiotherapy are required for any patient for whom bed rest is prescribed.

Coughing and deep breathing are to be encouraged at routine intervals, since they are considered the first line of defense in prevention and treatment of atelectasis.

Bacterial Pneumonia

Bacterial pneumonia is a consolidative inflammation resulting from pathogenic microorganisms. It is a major source of additional morbidity and mortality in the critically ill patient.

The radiographic picture of bacterial pneumonia shows an alveolar filling pattern that is soft, fluffy, and poorly demarcated. If an entire lobe is involved, an air bronchogram may be the most outstanding marker. Lobular bacterial pneumonias are usually primary processes and not complications of preexisting disease. They present with an acute onset of fever, cough, dyspnea, chest pain, and hypoxemia.

Some bacterial pneumonias present radiographically as bronchopneumonia, with multiple poorly defined areas of alveolar consolidation involving one or both lungs. Organisms presenting in this fashion include *Streptococcus, Hemophilus influenzae, Pseudomonas, Serratia, Proteus, Escherichia coli,* and the anaerobes. *Staphylococcus* may produce a pattern of bronchopneumonia, particularly if the route of infection is hematogenous. Bronchopneumonias are often secondary to other predisposing conditions such as immunosuppressive therapy. Nosocomial pulmonary infections are commonly bronchopneumonias. The clinical criteria for pneumonia include leukocytosis, fever, purulent tracheobronchial secretions, and previously undetected infiltrates observed on chest x-ray. Pulmonary infection is commonly acquired through inhalation. Nosocomial bacterial pneumonia is most often associated with *Klebsiella, Staphylococcus aureus, Pseudomonas aeruginosa,* and *Escherichia coli.* It is usually distributed throughout the lung in a lobar or segmental pattern. A single lobe or segment is usually affected, although multiple areas of disease may appear simultaneously, especially with *Staphylococcus.*

Up to 60 percent of ICU patients may develop pneumonia, depending on the severity of their underlying disease. Specific etiologic diagnosis is commonly lacking because of contamination of specimens by oropharyngeal secretions. Significant predisposing factors in the development of nosocomial pneumonias include (1) concurrent antibiotic treatment, which predisposes the patient to colonization with resistant gram-negative bacilli of the oropharynx; (2) aspiration of oropharyngeal or gastric secretions; (3) bypassing of normal respiratory clearance mechanisms and subsequent implantation of bacteria onto alveolar surfaces; and (4) hematogenous spread to the lungs from distant foci.

Initial therapy of bacterial pneumonia is determined by Gram's stain of the sputum and later by culture. Antibiotic coverage may be started on the basis of the stain and modified later when culture results with antibiotic sensitivities are obtained. Dosage should be calculated as indicated on the package insert for *serious* infection and should be adjusted according to pre- and postadministration serum levels.

Prevention, not treatment, should be the primary approach to nosocomial bacterial pneumonias in the critical-care unit. Scrupulously sterile technique when using respiratory therapy equipment and during suctioning of patients is necessary. A program of infection control surveillance is essential in the modern critical-care unit.

Case Study: Parenchymal Disorders

The patient is a 34-year-old male, shot with a single steel-jacketed 9-mm bullet. The missile entered in the right axilla, shattered the C6 vertebra and posterior elements, and exited through the left side of the neck. After emergency treatment, he had a 12-h plane trip and was admitted to a teaching medical center. On admission he was noted to have quadriplegia with movement of only the right deltoid muscle, irregular spontaneous respirations using the diaphragm and sternocleidomastoid muscles, and a necrotizing exit wound in the left side of the neck. ABGs on $F_{I_{O_2}}$ 0.40 by face mask showed P_{O_2} 60, P_{CO_2} 48, pH 7.25. Mechanical ventilation was prescribed. Radiologic studies revealed a right clavicular fracture and intramuscular blood pushing the right apical pleura downward. No additional thoracic trauma was noted. Arterial angiography showed a right carotid jugular fistula, which was repaired in the OR via midline sternotomy by ligation of the right common carotid and subclavian arteries. The internal jugular vein was repaired. The neurosurgeon concluded that the spinal cord severance at C6 left no potential for neurological recovery, and a tracheotomy was performed in the OR. The exit wound, as well as obviously necrotized muscle, was debrided and the patient was admitted to the ICU on an MA 2 on F_{IO_2} of 0.40, TV 800, IMV 10. ABGs showed P_{O_2} 58, P_{CO_2} 40, pH 7.35. Dopamine was required to maintain blood pressure. The CXR at this time is depicted in Fig. 27-5. The patient had received 6 U of blood and Ringer's lactate solution and remained quadriplegic with the exception of right deltoid movement and spontaneous respiratory rate of 24. The intravenous antibiotic regimen was changed on the basis of cultures obtained previously and smears obtained in the OR. A total of 15 cm H_2O PEEP was added in increments to the ventilator circuit. Intravenous boluses of Ringer's lactate were administered to achieve a pulmonary artery wedge pressure of 14. The next set of ABGs were P_{O_2} 80, P_{CO_2} 40, pH 7.38.

Nursing Diagnosis

Impaired gas exchange related to inflammation of lung parenchyma, atelectasis, and intrapulmonary shunting.

Goal

Patient will demonstrate ABGs within acceptable levels.

Interventions

1. Provide mechanical ventilation and augment oxygenation as prescribed.
2. Assess ABGs prn and change ventilator parameters accordingly.
3. Assess respiratory status q 2 h.
4. Observe for signs and symptoms of pneumothorax secondary to PEEP.
5. Provide frequent rest periods between treatments to decrease oxygen demand.
6. Observe color, odor, and amount of secretions (indicating progression of disease or infection).
7. Turn patient q 2 h to minimize $\dot{V}/\dot{Q}$ shunting effects, or use Rotorest bed.

8. Use chest physiotherapy to facilitate open airways.

Nursing Diagnosis

Ineffective airway clearance related to tracheostomy, loss of muscles of ventilation, and increased viscosity of secretions.

Goal

Patient will maintain patent airway with no retained secretions, as evidenced by improvement on CXR and decreased rhonchi, loose clear secretions, and normal body temperature.

Interventions

1. Apply suction prn.
2. Perform tracheal lavage with nonpreserved saline prn.
3. Provide adequate humidification.
4. Turn patient laterally semiprone q 1–2 h or use Rotorest bed.
5. Give chest physiotherapy q 4 h.
6. Administer bronchodilators (if prescribed) prior to suctioning.

Nursing Diagnosis

Ineffective breathing pattern related to neurological compromise of muscles of ventilation, mechanical trauma, and decreased pulmonary compliance.

Goal

Patient will be weaned from mechanical ventilation.

Interventions

1. Establish baseline pulmonary function values and ABGs and obtain prescriptions to maintain these.
2. Consult with physician to establish acceptable ABG parameters for weaning.
3. Attempt to reduce IMV rate and then F_{IO_2} on the basis of previously determined respiratory parameters.

Nursing Diagnosis

Alteration in nutritional status related to mechanical trauma of neck and increased metabolic demands (trauma).

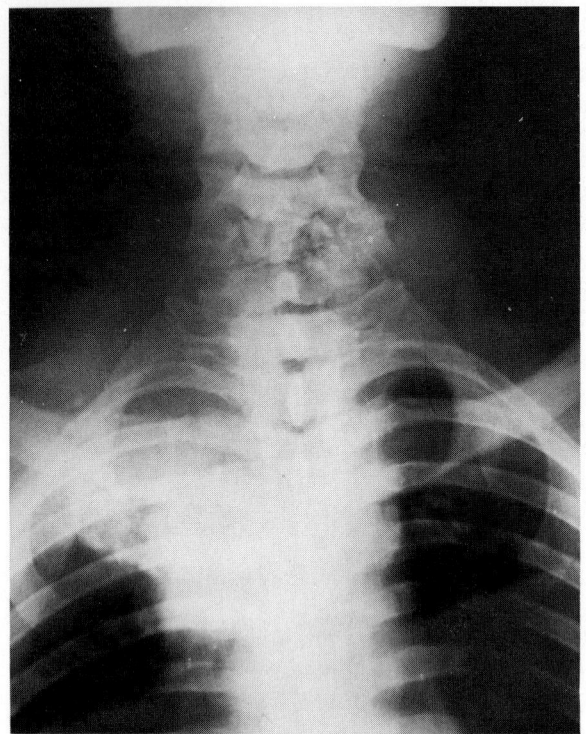

A

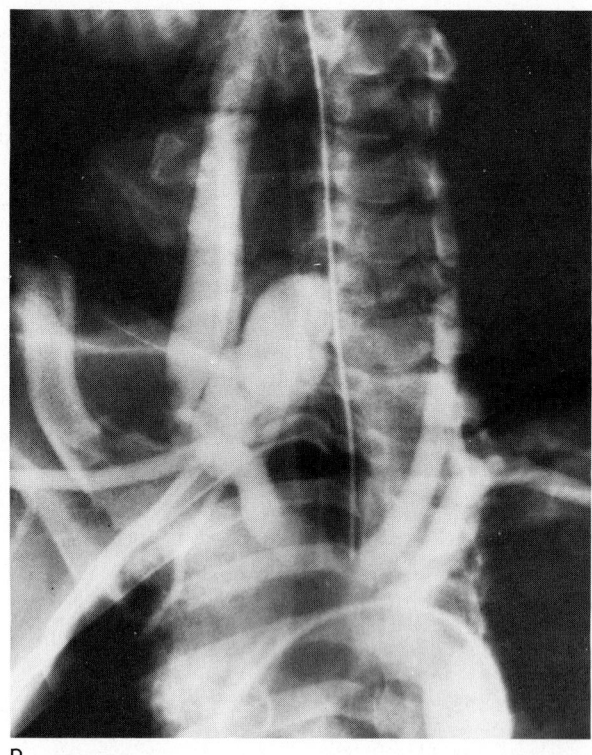

B

Figure 27-5 (*A*) X-ray taken 12 h after injury (see Case Study: Parenchymal Disorders) demonstrates crushed C6 vertebra, blood in muscles of right side of chest pushing right lung pleura downward, and exit wound of bullet in left side of neck. (*B*) Aortic flush angiogram performed 24 h after injury demonstrates right carotid-jugular fistula. Flow-directed catheter can be seen in position in the right side of the cardiovascular tree. (*C*) Postoperative x-ray demonstrates ARDS. Carotid-jugular fistula has been repaired via midline sternotomy.

Goal

Patient will maintain acceptable levels of serum albumin and protein and maintain present body weight.

Interventions

1. Provide caloric intake determined by physician via enteral or parenteral route.
2. Provide high-protein high-calorie nutrition.
3. Weigh patient daily.
4. Consult with dietician and keep daily calorie count.
5. Monitor fluid and electrolyte values.

Nursing Diagnosis

Potential for infection related to mechanical foreign bodies, retained secretions, and decreased ventilation.

Goal

Infection will be minimized by early detection. Patient will be protected from nosocomial infection.

Interventions

1. Vital signs q 2 h and prn.
2. Maintain IV lines per unit standards.
3. Use sterile suctioning technique and maintain tracheostomy per unit standards.
4. Follow Foley catheter care per unit standards.
5. Obtain culture and sensitivity of bodily fluids as requested.
6. Observe wound site and maintain sterility in dressing technique.

Nursing Diagnosis

Anxiety related to fear of dying, loss of verbal communication, and intermittent dyspnea.

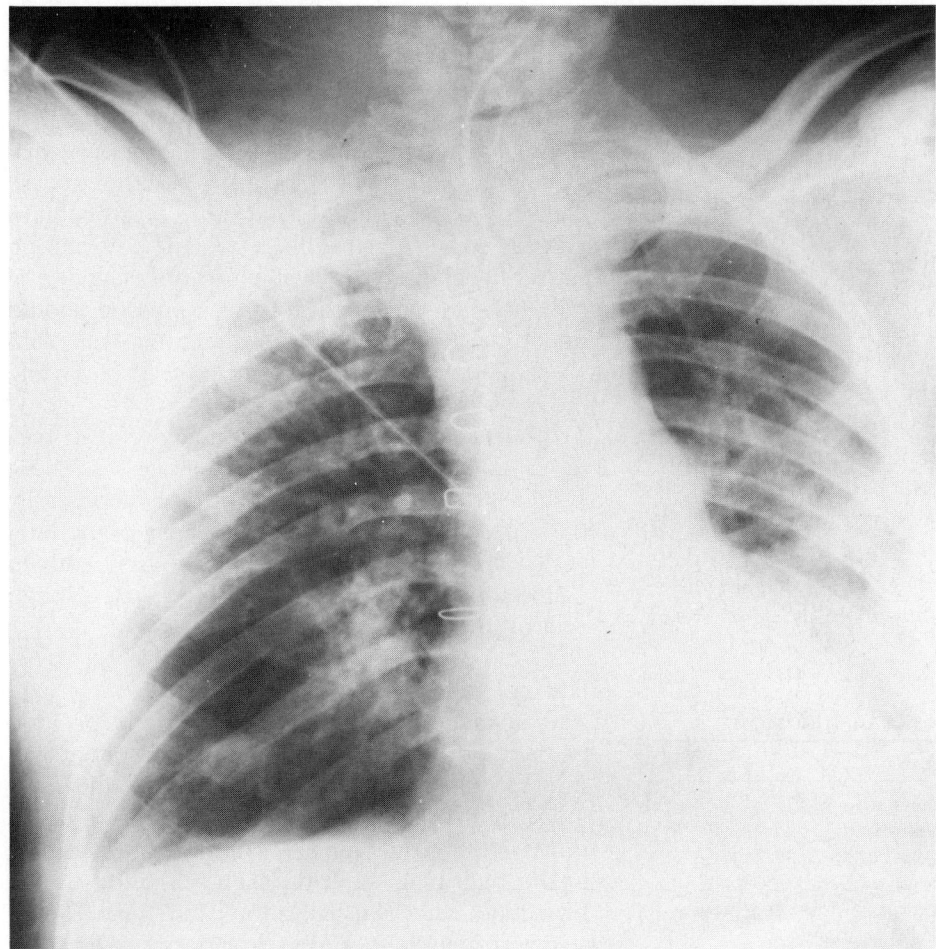

C

Goal

Patient will nonverbally communicate acceptance of present limitations.

Interventions

1. Establish a method of communication using patient's present level of function (e.g., eye closure or mouth movements).
2. Provide choices in timing or method of treatments among acceptable alternatives.
3. Provide for liberal schedule of family visitation.
4. Initiate consultation with psychiatric social worker or religious person and attempt to facilitate patient's communication with them.

Nursing Diagnosis

Family anxiety related to patient's poor prognosis.

Goal

Family will verbalize appropriate fears and demonstrate appropriate coping mechanisms.

Interventions

1. Reinforce physician's explanation of prognosis.
2. Encourage family to communicate their questions and fears to nursing staff.
3. Assist family in understanding the patient's status and physiological changes while avoiding focus on symptoms and false hopes.
4. Allow family to assist in daily care if they express an interest.
5. Contact psychiatric social worker or religious person as needed.

Restrictive Lung Disorders

Lung Abscess

Lung abscess is a pyogenic lesion of the lung parenchyma giving rise to a cavity. Most often it is attributed to the aspiration of foreign material into the respiratory tract. It may also arise systemically by hematogenous spread or may follow a lung infarct. Obstruction of the bronchioles and stasis of secretions contribute to the infection.

An aspiration abscess may be seen in any condition leading to a suppression of the cough reflex, including anesthesia, head injury, diabetic coma, drug overdose, epileptic or alcoholic coma, and near drowning. A detailed history should be sought from patients in whom lung abscess is suspected, since any one of these conditions can be found in up to 70 percent of the cases, alcoholic coma being the most common (Table 27-4). Oral

Table 27-4 Common Causes of Lung Abscess

Type of abscess	Cause
Aspiration abscess	Alcoholism
	Anesthesia
	Oversedation
	Coma (diabetic, epileptic, drug overdose, cerebrovascular accident)
	Oral infection
	Food or foreign body
	Laryngeal palsy
	Carcinoma of esophagus ("spillover" aspiration)
Malignant abscess	Necrotic bronchial carcinoma
	Bronchial obstruction and stasis of secretions
	Head and neck malignant tumor
Pulmonary embolus	Pulmonary infarct infection
	Septic emboli
	Fragments from bacterial endarteritis
Infection	Pneumonia
	Pyogenic bacteria (notably *Staphylococcus aureus*)
	Defective ciliary action
	Inefficient expectoration
	Infected cyst
	Necrotic lesion
	Subdiaphragmatic infection (usually liver)
	Open chest wound

infections such as pyorrhea or infected tonsils may be unrecognized causes of abscess formation if the debris is aspirated.

Tumors that cause abscess formation are usually malignant, the most common being bronchial carcinoma (squamous cell type). These tumors are likely to become infected and cause obstruction of lung segments by acting like a foreign body, causing stasis of secretions. Any patient with a diagnosis of lung abscess and no history of aspiration should undergo diagnostic testing for carcinoma. Very often chest therapy and antibiotics clear the abscess while the tumor remains undetected.

Necrosis of consolidated areas seen in bacterial pneumonia predisposes to abscesses. These cystlike sacs distend with inspired air and can easily burst into the pleura, causing collapse of the lung tissue. This mechanism is seen more frequently in children than adults because of the thin, less tough wall of the pleura in children.

Pathophysiology

The site of the abscess is determined by the position of the body during aspiration. The aspirate will travel to the most dependent region of the lung. Thus, in a supine patient the foreign material will move into the right lung (recall the anatomic angle of the right main stem bronchus). From the right bronchus, material usually moves into the posterior segment of the upper lobe or superior segment of the lower lobe.

Fibrous granulation tissue usually forms around most of the abscess while it becomes embedded in the parenchyma. The abscess may extend toward the pleural cavity but rarely ruptures into it. Pleuritic pain and pleural effusion due to irritation of the pleural space by the granulation tissue may occur. The abscess fills with pus, and the now granulated portion often erodes into a bronchus, resulting in the drainage of foul-smelling pus into the trachea. When the pleuritic pain is not significant, often the aspiration of pus is the first sign of abscess formation. The expectoration of the pus may lead to partial healing and cavity formation. However, inadequate drainage and chest therapy can lead to multiple small abscesses within the lung.

Diagnostic Findings

The onset of symptoms may be insidious or acute. Typically, general malaise and fever with or without pleuritic pain is seen. Over a number of days, fever with temperature spikes persists, pleuritic pain is evident, and there may be dyspnea, depending on the size of the abscess and its effect on lung tissue. The presence of foul-smelling pus in tracheal aspirate or expectoration clarifies the diagnosis. There may be blood-tinged purulent drainage due to bronchial erosion. Unfortunately, the symptoms are like those of pneumonia, and often the initial diagnosis is incorrect. For this reason the history is most important.

Physical examination shows a dullness to percussion and decreased or absent breath sounds with intermittent pleural friction rub, depending on the extent of abscess formation and its proximity to the pleural space. Rales may be present. Chest x-ray shows areas of consolidation which may indicate other disease entities. It is not until a fluid level is evident, usually indicating communication with the bronchus, that the diagnosis can be narrowed down to either empyema with bronchopleural fistula or a lung abscess.

Medical Management

The initial evaluation of the patient must determine the presence of anaerobic or aerobic pyogenic organisms. Early bronchoscopy may be desirable, followed by appropriate anaerobic and aerobic antibiotic therapy. Although the culture report should be followed closely to determine sensitivity, flora is usually mixed. In general, however, the antibiotic therapy should be changed according to clinical findings, not bacterial culture changes, when deterioration of the patient is noted.

The use of therapeutic bronchoscopy for drainage is somewhat controversial. Diagnostically, bronchoscopy can be used to rule out carcinoma or foreign body. It can also be useful in locating the site of the draining bronchus, thereby aiding positioning to facilitate drainage. Some clinicians believe that bronchoscopy should be reserved for those patients who do not respond to other treatment. It can be used to aspirate the abscess and to obtain specimens for diagnostic purposes. The fear of spreading infection to other parts of the lung, however, often deters clinicians from performing bronchoscopy.

The need for surgical treatment is rare but has been reported. The indications for surgery are (1) failure of the abscess to diminish in size, (2) continued toxicosis and sepsis, (3) suspicion of cancer, and (4) recurrent infection. Once the visceral and parietal pleura have become inflamed and pleural symphysis has occurred, surgery can be performed. Open drainage is the most common form of surgical intervention. The use of a double-lumen endotracheal tube is advocated to prevent spillage of the drainage to uninfected areas of the lung. Successful percutaneous drainage (*pneumonotomy*) has been reported. A cleansing bronchoscopy should be performed on both lungs after surgery is completed.

Pleural Effusion

The potential space between the visceral and parietal pleura is lined with a thin layer of fluid which constantly changes with the motion of the lungs. There are two types of fluid passage, classified according to the presence or absence of protein. Protein usually enters the pleural space by leaking from the pleural capillaries and is drained by the lymphatic system. Protein-free fluid flows from the parietal pleura via systemic capillaries into the pleural space and is absorbed into the visceral pleura by the pulmonary capillaries. This mechanism is dependent upon hydrostatic and colloid osmotic pressures across the space.

Systemic capillary hydrostatic pressure (parietal pleura) is higher than the pulmonary capillary pressure (visceral pleura), with colloid osmotic pressure the same in both systems. The pleural space has an osmotic pressure below that of the two capillary systems it separates. Thus the hydrostatic pressure in the systemic capillaries, coupled with negative pleural pressure, forces the movement of fluid from the parietal pleura into the pleural space. Conversely, the higher colloid osmotic pressure in the pulmonary capillaries results in a shift of fluid into the visceral pleura from the pleural space (Fig. 27-6). Since this movement of fluid is dependent on the various pressures, any hemodynamic changes in the cardiopulmonary system will be reflected in the formation and absorption of fluid in the pleural space.

Pathophysiology

A pleural effusion is excess fluid in the pleural space. It is usually thought of as a sign of disease, not a disease entity in itself. Effusions are classified

Figure 27-6   Process of pleural fluid formation and absorption in the pleural space. Fluid follows the direction of the black arrows because of pressure gradients. *(Adapted from R. W. Light, Pleural effusions, Med. Clin. North Am., 1977, 61:134.)*

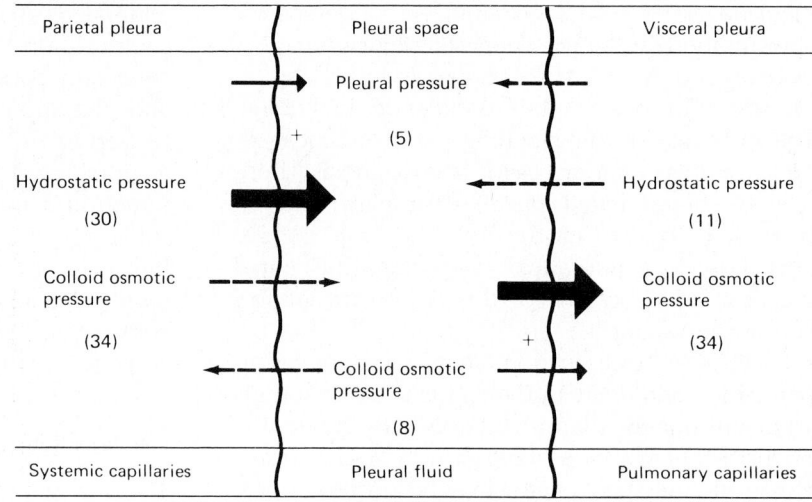

as transudate or exudate, with the distinction between them based on protein content.

Transudates are usually produced when there is a disturbance in the flow of protein-free fluid in the pleural space. Thus the protein content in transudates remains normal or less than 3 g per 100 mL. Pleural transudate is usually clear or pale yellow with a specific gravity of less than 1.015 and is usually bilateral. It is often termed *hydrothorax.*

Exudates usually result from disease of the pleural surface, due to either increased permeability of capillaries with resultant leak of proteins or an obstruction in the lymphatic system inhibiting drainage of proteins. Therefore, the protein content in exudates is high, usually more than 3 g per 100 mL. The specific gravity is increased (more than 1.016) because of the increased protein. The exudate is often dark yellow or amber in color and is usually unilateral.

Table 27-5 gives a partial list of the causes of pleural effusion categorized as exudate or transudate. It is necessary to differentiate the type of effusion in order to determine the cause. Transudates, since they are not caused by pleural disease, do not usually require the extensive diagnostic follow-up that is often needed for exudates.

A number of tests for pleural fluid are available to differentiate exudates from transudates and to diagnose the cause of exudates. Besides determination of the color, the amount of protein, and the specific gravity, other tests include the differentia-

tion of serum and pleural lactic acid dehydrogenase and protein levels, red cell count, white cell count with differential, pleural fluid cytologic study (for malignant cells), glucose and amylase levels, pH, and culture with bacteriologic stains.

Diagnostic Findings

Pleural effusions usually show a restriction of chest wall expansion on the affected side if the effusion is large. Dullness to percussion and absent or decreased breath sounds over the area are noted. If the effusion is infected or purulent, temperature elevation may be present. Dyspnea is common in

Table 27-5 Causes of Pleural Effusions

Transudates	Exudates
Congestive heart failure	Metastatic disease
Hypoproteinemia	Tuberculosis
Cirrhosis	Viral infection
Myxedema	Bacterial infection
Sarcoidosis	Pulmonary infarction
Meigs's syndrome	Systemic lupus
Constrictive pericarditis	erythematosus
Nephrotic syndrome	Pancreatitis
Peritoneal dialysis	Subphrenic abscess
	Trauma
	Whipple's disease
	Hepatic abscess
	Acute rheumatic fever
	Uremia
	Postmyocardial infarction
	syndrome

a rapidly accumulating effusion, while chronic or slow accumulation may cause no respiratory distress.

Chest x-ray abnormalities may be undetectable if the effusion is small (less than 100 mL). Larger effusions are seen as dense opacities. A level of fluid may be observed in a gravity-dependent position; thus, if the patient lies on the affected side prior to x-ray, fluid may be seen in the lateral chest wall.

Medical Management

Any pleural effusion should be subjected to a diagnostic tap (thoracentesis). Chemical, cytologic, and bacteriologic analyses may yield valuable information to determine cause.

The position of the patient during the procedure is important to prevent the occurrence of pneumothorax or hemothorax. A good position for a lateral or posterior tap is for the patient to sit on the edge of the bed and lean forward onto an over-bed table. The skin is cleaned with iodophor or iodine solution and anesthetized with local anesthetic. A tap requires insertion of the needle into the intercostal space along the upper surface of the lower rib. The presence of fluid confirms entrance into the pleural space. Usually no more than 1000 mL of fluid should be drained rapidly, and even less if the patient exhibits signs of respiratory distress. A pleural biopsy is also recommended at this time.

Recurrent pleural effusions present a management problem. Effusions from bronchial carcinoma and from metastatic tumors of extrathoracic origin fall into this category. Often a malignant effusion reaccumulates shortly after it is aspirated. Attempts are made to eliminate or reduce the number of recurrent effusions. The use of nitrogen mustard instilled in the pleural space has been reported to slow down the rate of effusion. Pleurodesis using iodized talc in an aerosol produces similar results.

The nurse must be aware of the conditions which precipitate effusions. Since malignant disease carries a high incidence of fluid accumulation, those patients being diagnostically worked up for lung cancer should have frequent chest auscultation. Any decreased or absent sounds, as well as signs of dyspnea, should be reported at once.

Kyphoscoliosis

Kyphoscoliosis is an orthopedic problem which may severely impair respiratory and cardiovascular function. Scoliosis is curvature of the spine laterally (twisted); kyphosis is curvature forward. This spinal deformity usually starts in adolescence as scoliosis and later becomes kyphotic. The condition may rarely be due to Pott's disease (tuberculosis of the spine), in which the kyphosis is more pronounced, or it may be due to poliomyelitis or rickets, or to osteoporosis in the aged. Unfortunately, the majority of cases are designated idiopathic.

Pathophysiology

The impairment of respiratory function results from distortions in the shape of the lung and the rib cage which prevent normal expansion. If there is a cone-shaped distortion, compression of the lung by the chest wall is usually more severe at the bases, with atelectasis and bronchopneumonia common findings. Overexpansion of the upper lobes may be evident. Rigidity of the chest wall is common with advancing age.

This rigidity of the chest wall and compression of the lung decrease the vital capacity, tidal volume, and alveolar ventilation and increase the work of breathing. The atelectasis alters the ventilation/perfusion ratio ($\dot{V}/\dot{Q}$) to increase shunting. The resultant hypoxemia and hypercapnia are pronounced in severe cases.

Constriction of the pulmonary vessels, primarily due to the compression of the chest cavity, may lead to pulmonary hypertension. The vascular resistance may be elevated from the effects of hypoxia, and the right ventricle may fail from continually forcing blood through the compromised pulmonary vasculature. The resultant right-sided heart failure and the ventilatory compromise are the usual cause of death.

Diagnostic Findings

The main clinical signs in a patient with severe kyphoscoliosis are similar to those in cor pulmonale. Severe dyspnea and rhonchi are often present in the late stages of the disease. Lung volumes reveal decreased tidal volume, minute volume, vital capacity, functional residual capacity, and expiratory reserve volume. Arterial blood gas analysis reveals decreased Pa_{O_2}, increased Pa_{CO_2}, and decreased pH due to effects of progressive respiratory failure.

Pitting edema of the extremities is noted if the patient is in heart failure. Chest x-ray interpretation is often difficult because of poor positioning. Radiologic findings consistent with pneumonia and atelectasis are present.

Medical Management

Initial management of the deformed chest wall in children is by correction of the chest wall by body casts. Some increase in vital capacity has been achieved. Operative procedures may be effective.

Ventilatory support is necessary for patients with acute respiratory failure from infection. High peak-inspiratory pressure may be useful in improving the compliance of the chest wall, thereby improving lung compliance. The relation between lung compliance and the amount of peak-inspiratory pressure is under investigation.

Treatment of kyphoscoliosis is purely symptomatic. Management of congestive heart failure and respiratory failure are described elsewhere in this book. Chronic therapy is similar to that of bronchitis. Recurrent infections, a common complication, are treated with antibiotics.

Case Study: Restrictive Disorders

A 58-year-old woman with a history of alcoholism and kyphoscoliosis is admitted to the emergency room with shortness of breath, pain on inspiration, and productive cough with purulent, foul-smelling sputum. ABGs and physical assessment lead to a diagnosis of lung abscess.

Nursing Diagnosis

Ineffective airway clearance related to copious pus drainage.

Goal

Abscess will clear.

Interventions

1. Give chest physiotherapy q 4 h.
2. Provide for postural drainage with proper positioning based on site of abscess.
3. Encourage patient to sleep in postural drainage position if possible.

4. Give coughing and deep breathing exercises q 2 h.

Nursing Diagnosis

Alteration in comfort (mouth) related to foul-smelling and bad-tasting purulent drainage.

Goal

Patient will maintain clean mouth.

Intervention

Give mouth care q 3 h using mixture of half 3% hydrogen peroxide and half water, sweetened with mouthwash.

Nursing Diagnosis

Alteration in comfort related to pleuritic irritation.

Goal

The patient will be free of pain.

Interventions

1. Medicate for pain half-hour prior to coughing, deep breathing exercises, and activities of daily living.
2. Use pillow to splint area during activities.

Nursing Diagnosis

Ineffective airway clearance related to retained secretions from nonproductive cough and inability to expand chest wall (kyphoscoliosis).

Goal

Patient will have no signs of infection and will have loose clear secretions.

Interventions

1. Teach effective coughing techniques.
2. Give nasotracheal suction prn.
3. Encourage adequate fluid intake.
4. Provide adequate humidification.
5. Turn patient laterally semiprone q 1–2 h or use Rotorest bed.
6. Give chest physiotherapy q 4 h.
7. Administer bronchodilators (if prescribed) prior to suctioning.
8. Observe for signs of infection (color, odor and thickness of secretions, temperature).

9. Provide frequent rest periods to decrease oxygen demand.

Obstructive Lung Disorders

Asthma

The term *asthma* is used to describe a recurrent, reversible airway obstruction with prolonged expiratory length, air trapping during attacks, ventilation perfusion mismatching, increased intrapulmonary shunt, cough, and tenacious sputum. The obstruction may be so mild that the patient experiences dyspnea only on exertion or so severe and prolonged that it results in respiratory failure or even death by asphyxiation. Symptoms may be intermittent with normal pulmonary function between attacks or may cause chronic debilitation from compromised pulmonary function.

The acute obstruction of asthma is a reversible process involving spasm of the smooth muscle in the bronchial walls. As the episode progresses, mucus from the lumina of the bronchi, together with edematous inflammation of the mucosa, further narrows the airways. The resultant ventilation/perfusion mismatch produces arterial hypoxemia.

Preventive care has decreased the morbidity associated with asthma in recent years, while more appropriate use of medications and respiratory therapy has improved the mortality associated with severe attacks.

Pathophysiology

Asthma reflects a hyperactive state of the bronchial airways to a variety of factors including extrinsic allergens. It is manifested by widespread airway narrowing that changes in severity either spontaneously or with treatment.[9] It has long been known that immediate hypersensitivity, mediated by immune globulin E (IgE), plays an important role in this syndrome.

Some clinicians identify a subgroup known as intrinsic asthma, or asthmatic bronchitis. This type of asthma is not mediated by IgE. Emotions and their impact on the sympathetic and parasympathetic nervous systems play a role in this process. Also, most persons with chronic obstructive pulmonary disease (COPD) have some bronchospastic component to their disease which can be considered intrinsic asthma.

A theory called *beta blockade* suggests that an imbalance exists in the normal sympathetic and parasympathetic nervous innervation of the airways. Beta-adrenergic receptors in the airways are responsible for bronchial smooth muscle relaxation when stimulated by cyclic adenosine monophosphate (cAMP). When there is no β_2 stimulation, cAMP is lower and bronchoconstriction occurs.

Cardiopulmonary blood vessels are also supplied with β_1 receptors. Stimulation of these receptors produces vasoconstriction and undesirable side effects, including tachycardia, possibly arrhythmias, and blood pressure alteration. Without beta stimulation, bronchoconstriction occurs in response to a variety of stimuli including hyperventilation, extreme temperature and humidity changes, emotional disturbances, infection, and the classic "allergic" response to extrinsic allergens.

In some persons, upper airway irritation may cause bronchoconstriction by stimulation of the vagus nerve. This parasympathetic stimulation may also enhance mucus secretion and be responsible for the cough and hyperventilation that accompany bronchospasm. Parasympathetic blockade using atropine may initially appear to be advantageous because of the drying of bronchial secretions that it produces, but it is contraindicated because of the increased risk of bronchial plugging. Parasympathetic and sympathetic forces create two opposing systems, then, with parasympathetic stimulation encouraging bronchospasm while sympathetic stimulation of both alpha and beta receptors favors bronchial relaxation.

Chemical mediator substances also influence the degree of bronchoconstriction. These mediators are released by mast cells in the pulmonary submucosa. Mast cell stimulation causes a release of these mediators, producing bronchoconstriction and/or vasodilatation. These include histamine, slow-reacting substance of anaphylaxis, prostaglandins, serotonin, and bradykinin. These mediators are inhibited by cAMP. Another effect that β_2 stimulation produces, in addition to its direct effect on smooth muscle, is bronchial relaxation, since such stimulation increases cAMP. Fig. 27-7 shows the effects of alterations in sympathetic and parasympathetic influence on the development of bronchospasm,

Figure 27-7 Sympathetic and parasympathetic influences on the development of bronchospasm.

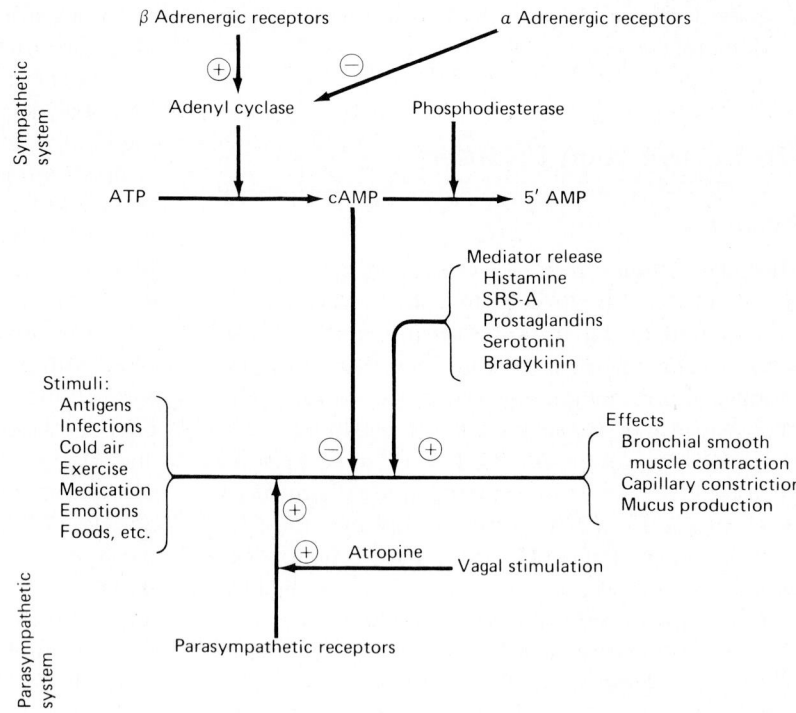

as well as the effects of mast cell mediator substances.

It is important to remember that severe bronchospasm involves more than just bronchoconstriction. Bronchial wall edema and mucus hypersecretion are also important contributors to pathophysiological changes during asthmatic crisis.

Once bronchospasm has developed, a variety of events follow, as shown in Fig. 27-8. Marked pulmonary hyperinflation may result. Total lung capacity may increase by up to 30 percent, and residual volume is markedly increased. An overinflated lung is stiff and compliance is low, and this increases the work of breathing. The patient then begins to perceive dyspnea, a hallmark of asthma attack. This process is aggravated by anxiety and a reflex hyperventilation.

As a result of hyperventilation, Pa_{CO_2} is usually low during an attack. If severe bronchospasm persists, however, the patient tires and cannot maintain hyperventilation. Pa_{CO_2} rises to normal and finally becomes elevated. Excessive sedation or narcotic administration decreases ventilatory drive and can hasten decompensation during an asthma attack.

Decreasing overall ventilation combined with ventilation/perfusion mismatching leads to hypercapnia, and mechanical ventilation is needed to maintain the patient.

Accumulation of secretions in airways leads to cough, which may stimulate more bronchospasm. Bronchial hygiene and maintenance of adequate hydration are important in controlling the problems associated with accumulation of secretions.

Hypercapnia is a late sign noted only in severe and prolonged asthma attacks. Hypoxemia is the common blood gas abnormality, resulting from the shunt created by uneven ventilation and perfusion. Oxygen therapy is needed to treat the hypoxemia, but assisted ventilation is necessary if the Pa_{CO_2} starts to rise.

In status asthmaticus the patient is severely distressed from the dyspnea and exhaustion. The patient is often unable to maintain adequate oxygenation and becomes cyanotic. Severely elevated intrathoracic pressures may interfere with venous return to the right ventricle; cardiac output falls, and vascular collapse may ensue. Dehydration due to fluid loss from hyperventilation may also contribute to impaired venous return. Cor pulmonale occurs late, when the situation is desperate. Tachycardia indicates the stress placed on the cardiovascular system. A pulse rate greater than 120 in a patient who has not taken alpha-adrenergic stimulating drugs (e.g., epinephrine) signifies the need for urgent measures.

Diagnostic Findings

The signs and symptoms of asthma reflect the distal airway obstruction and interference with gas exchange. The primary symptom is dyspnea, or breathlessness. The patient has difficulty forcing air out of the lungs and frequently wheezes in the attempt. Prolongation of expiration is audible on auscultation.

Cough is another symptom of bronchospasm in asthma. As the attack progresses, the cough becomes productive, dyspnea and wheezing increase, and the patient may speak only in short phrases. Preferential body position is seated, with forward tilt of the upper torso, arms braced, shoulders held high, and chest distended with little movement. There is retraction of the suprasternal notch and intercostal spaces.

In a very severe attack there may be so little air movement in the chest that a wheeze is not audible. Coughing is virtually impossible. The chest is hyperresonant and breath sounds are diminished. Heart tones are distant.

The pulse is rapid and thready. In severe episodes the pulse may be paradoxical, with diminished volume on inspiration. This is from decreased filling of the right atrium due to decreased lung compliance, itself a result of pulmonary overdistention and high intra-alveolar pressures. The patient becomes hypoxemic, cyanotic, and lethargic or unresponsive. Asphyxia is imminent unless the symptoms are reversed. The term *status asthmaticus* denotes the point in the course of asthma at which the bronchospasm can no longer be relieved by bronchodilators.

The duration of an asthma attack is variable. It may last 30 min to 1 h and be terminated by the use of medication or it may last for days or weeks. The frequency of attacks is even more variable.

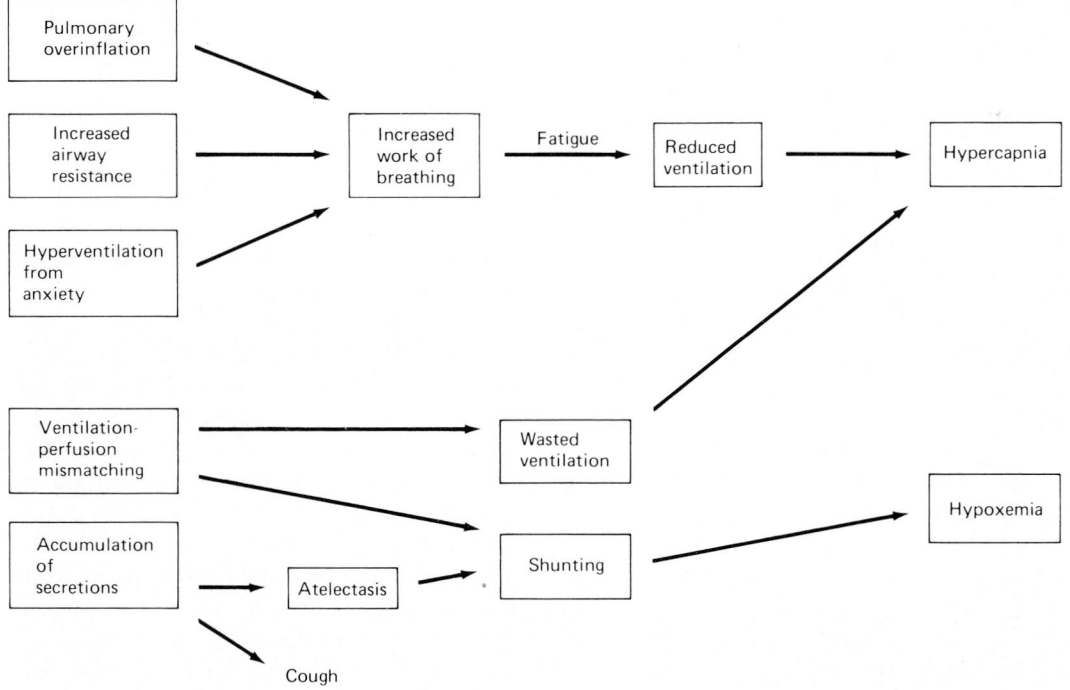

Figure 27-8 Consequences of bronchospasm.

Some patients have a single attack once or twice a year, while others are in chronic respiratory distress with frequent acute exacerbations.

The exact point at which patients in acute asthmatic attack will tire, become severely hypoxemic, and lose consciousness is unpredictable. Some patients are in status asthmaticus almost as soon as symptoms begin, but more commonly this condition occurs when there is a delay between the onset of symptoms and administration of medication. Patients receiving continuous high-dose therapy are more likely to present in status asthmaticus in the emergency room than those receiving seasonal or no medications.

The main abnormality in asthma is airway obstruction. Pulmonary function tests show decreased expiratory gas flow, including forced expiratory volume in 1, 2, and 3 s (FEV_{1-3}) and forced vital capacity (FVC). Functional residual capacity (FRC) is increased because of air trapping behind the bronchioles that have contracted in spasm during expiration. Pulmonary function usually improves after inhalation of a bronchodilator, indicating reversibility of the obstruction. During a symptom-free period the pulmonary function studies may be completely normal.

Radiology is not extremely valuable in asthma. During an asthma attack the chest film may show hyperinflation, identified by a low diaphragm. The heart may be long and narrow and the peripheral vessels poorly visualized. The film is more beneficial if taken during expiration, since the lowered diaphragm is more obvious. The main object in chest radiographs is to exclude the presence of other conditions or complications, especially pneumothorax. Secondary infections may sometimes be detected, and impacted mucus may be suspected from segmental collapse.

Medical Management

Precipitating factors in asthma attacks are identifiable by careful history taking, and many are readily avoidable. Asthmatic persons should avoid known bronchial irritants, promptly treat respiratory infections, and avoid drugs capable of inducing bronchospastic reactions, such as propranolol.

When a few specific allergens cause a large fraction of asthmatic episodes, hyposensitization injections may be helpful. This therapy induces the formation of IgG antibodies, which block antigen binding with IgE, although this is probably not the sole mechanism. In an unknown manner, hyposensitization also reduces IgE levels, at least in some cases. Unfortunately, hyposensitization is prolonged, expensive, and only partially effective.

Cromolyn sodium is an effective preventive agent in about 50 percent of asthmatic patients. This drug is not a bronchodilator but apparently blocks the release of chemical mediators of bronchospasm from the bronchial mucosa (Fig. 27-9). It is administered as a propelled powder from a hand-held inhaler and occasionally causes bronchial irritation on contact. Cromolyn sodium should not be given once bronchospasm has begun.

Vigorous bronchial hygiene is essential during periods of asthmatic exacerbation to keep airways clear and minimize ventilation/perfusion mismatching. Adequate fluid intake is necessary to prevent dehydration from hyperventilation and to liquefy secretions.

Inhaled bronchodilators should be used but not abused. Isoetharine combined with phenylephrine is useful as a metered preparation (Bronkosol) as well as by nebulization. It is a relatively selective β_2 agent and is particularly useful in bronchospastic patients who are hypoxemic and who have tachycardia or underlying coronary artery disease. Metaproterenol (Alupent, Metaprel) is claimed to have fewer cardiac stimulatory side effects than drugs like isoproterenol, but this requires further investigation. β_1 side effects of metaproterenol are probably as common as those of isoproterenol. Terbutaline (Brethine) has a higher β_2/β_1 ratio than either isoproterenol or metaproterenol and has negligible alpha activity. Oral administration of this drug has a marked tendency to produce muscular tremor and nervousness. Subcutaneous injections of terbutaline in doses of 0.125 to 0.25 mg, which may be repeated 30 min later, have proved useful in the critical-care setting. No more than 0.5 mg should be given in a 4-h period. Beclomethasone (Vanceril) is a metered inhaled steroid preparation which delivers 50 μg per puff. Investigations suggest that use of up to 2 mg per day is without significant steroid effect. Most asthmatic patients do well on smaller doses, and many

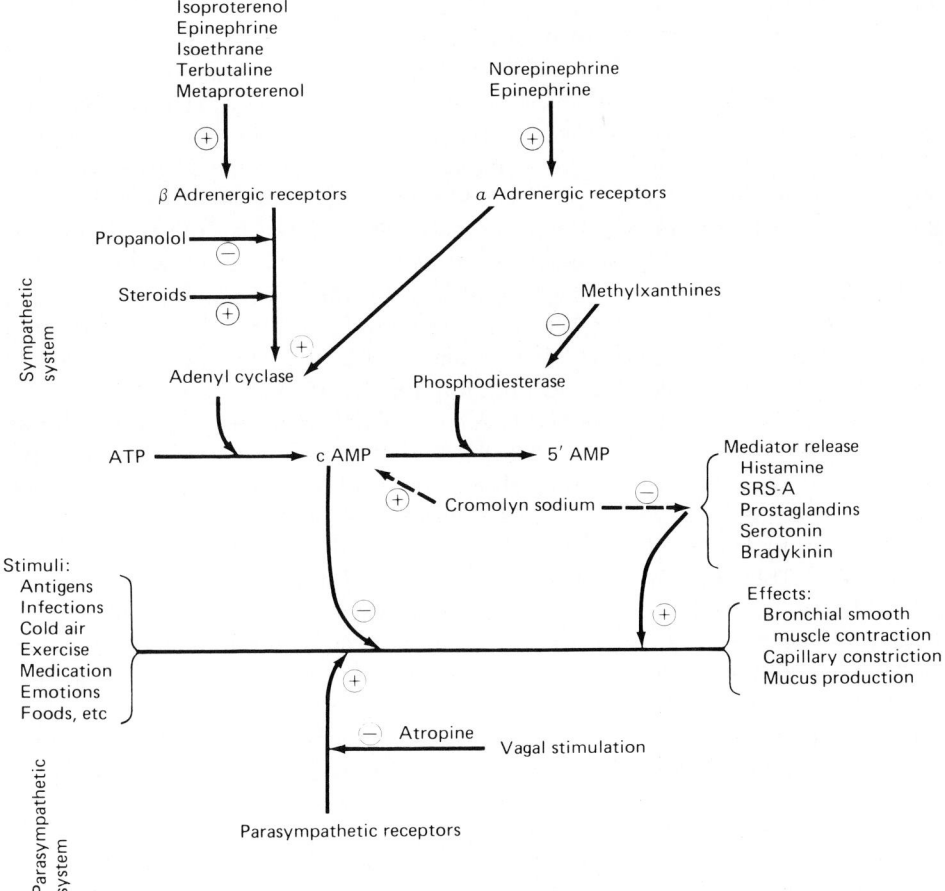

Figure 27-9   Interaction of pharmacologic agents with mechanisms of asthmatic bronchospasm.

steroid-dependent patients have been transferred from oral preparations, which cause Cushing's syndrome, to safer aerosol therapy.

The beneficial actions of steroids in asthma are not fully understood, but the following actions are believed to be of significant benefit: (1) prevention of antibody-antigen reaction by inhibition of antibody formation; (2) inhibition of formation or storage of mediators such as histamine; and (3) inhibition of nonspecific inflammatory processes. Steroids potentiate sympathomimetic drugs, probably by acting on β_2 receptors to produce smooth muscle relaxation and increase circulating levels of cAMP. The anti-inflammatory steroids (glucocorticoids) are beneficial in status asthmaticus of any cause.

Prednisone and prednisolone are oral steroid agents suitable for maintenance use. They are similar to hydrocortisone but more potent. During acute exacerbations they may be given in large doses of 40 to 70 mg per day for 5 to 7 days, titrated down to a maintenance dose of 5 to 20 mg per day. Cushing's syndrome can develop with prolonged use. Many asthmatic patients do well on alternate-day dosage schedules, which decrease the incidence of unwanted side effects. In cases of status asthmaticus in the critical-care unit, intravenous hydrocortisone (Solu-Cortef) can be given as 250 to 500 mg initially, followed by 100 to 250 mg every 3 h.

Patients with bronchospasm benefit greatly from any drug with bronchodilator capability. Epinephrine, 0.2 to 0.5 mL of 1:1000 solution by subcutaneous injection, was formerly used extensively, though now its use has been largely supplanted by methylxanthines (aminophylline) and inhaled drugs. Epinephrine has α, β_1, and β_2 effects, and thus, in addition to being a potent bronchodilator, has unwanted cardiovascular and nervous system side effects. It is dangerous to use in patients with underlying cardiac disease, especially the elderly.

Isoproterenol was once the most popular bronchodilator and is one of the most potent β_2 stimulators. It also has strong β_1 actions and carries a risk of dangerous inotropic and chronotropic cardiac stimulation. The β_1 cardiostimulatory effects of isoproterenol and its short duration of action are notable disadvantages compared with newer, more selective β_2 agents.

Methylxanthines are the most popular drugs used to treat bronchospasm today. They inhibit phosphodiesterase activity, thereby preventing breakdown of cAMP and favoring bronchial relaxation. Theophylline has many additional beneficial effects, including an increase in cardiac output, decrease in venous pressure, dilatation of pulmonary vascular bed, and improved renal circulation and cerebral stimulation.

The most serious common side effect of theophylline and its derivatives is increased gastric secretion, peptic irritation, and gastric bleeding. This is more common in oral preparations but is also a function of the blood level of the drug. Optimal therapeutic blood levels are close to toxic levels, and intermittent dosage may result in serum peak levels in the toxic range. Hepatic metabolism and renal excretion of the drug are often impaired, and for all these reasons, periodic serum drug levels should be monitored (preferably daily) in the critical-care unit. Gastric pH should be monitored whenever possible, and the use of antacids is recommended to minimize gastric complications.

Aminophylline is a synthetic theophylline derivative which is 20 times more soluble in water and can therefore be administered intravenously, whereas theophylline cannot. A loading dose of 375 to 500 mg in an average adult who has not recently taken aminophylline is recommended. This is followed by 50 mg/h via slow intravenous drip.

Treatment priorities for the patient in status asthmaticus with hypoxemia and increasing Pa_{CO_2} are as follows: (1) oxygen inhalation via mask with patient breathing spontaneously or with manually or mechanically assisted ventilation; (2) normalization of pH when necessary (pH less than 7.35) with IV bicarbonate, preferably in an intravenous drip titrated to maintain a desired arterial pH; (3) pharmacologic management of bronchospasm as described above; (4) supportive measures such as bronchial hygiene and fluid therapy; and (5) tracheal intubation, curarization, and sedation, used with controlled ventilation. If mechanical ventilation becomes unavoidable, the patient must be sedated and probably paralyzed to avoid fighting the ventilator because of the high risk of pneumothorax and cardiac arrest. A pleural chest drainage apparatus should be readily available on standby. The use of PEEP can be dangerous if large areas of the lung are already atelectatic because of overdistention of already open lung units. The use of expiratory retard achieves the effect of optimizing gas distribution but allows intrapulmonary pressures to reach atmospheric pressure at the end of expiration. Expiratory retard can also be added to a ball-valve mask apparatus for bag ventilation if mechanical ventilation can be avoided. The decision regarding the time at which to intubate may be a difficult one. The combination of respiratory distress and rising P_{CO_2} in the asthmatic patient indicates patient fatigue, and mechanical ventilation is necessary to prevent the development of severe respiratory failure.

Chronic Bronchitis

Chronic bronchitis is a syndrome arbitrarily defined as cough with sputum production during at least 3 consecutive months in at least 2 consecutive years.

Pathophysiology

The primary abnormality in this process is mucosal swelling, inflammation, and hypertrophy with excess production of thick, tenacious secretions in the airways. There is an increase in the size and number of mucus-secreting glands, which are overflowing with mucus. In the smaller bronchi and bronchioles, excessive numbers of mucus-producing goblet cells are found in the epithelial lining layer. Along the epithelial surface there is denuding of cilia in random fashion. Several inhalants have been implicated as causative agents in the development of chronic bronchitis, the most common of which is cigarette smoke. Other pollutants, such as oxides of nitrogen and sulfur dioxide, have been shown to diminish ciliary activity and stimulate hypersecretion of mucus. Patients with chronic bronchitis should be encouraged to stop their cigarette habit and examine their work environment for possible pollutants. Chronic bronchitis is primarily a reversible disease, since unlike emphysema, it does not cause permanent structural damage until late in the course of the disease.

Diagnostic Findings

Expiratory prolongation is notable on physical examination, as in the emphysematous patient. During acute exacerbations, inspiration may also be prolonged because of occlusion of airway lumina by secretions. Percussion is usually normal, and auscultation will reveal rales, rhonchi, and wheezes. The sounds are usually loud and are caused by secretions in the airways. Peripheral edema, hepatomegaly, and cyanosis are present in the patient with severe bronchitis and pulmonary hypertension (cor pulmonale).

On pulmonary function testing, flow rates during both expiration and inspiration may be reduced, although this is more pronounced on expiration. Patients with this condition have normal elastic recoil (in contrast to emphysema patients) and relatively normal diffusing capacities. Air trapping is consistent and depends on the severity of airway obstruction (Table 27-6).

Patients with chronic bronchitis are sometimes called "blue bloaters" because they are cyanotic, hypercapneic, and have right ventricular failure with peripheral edema. They are cyanotic and edematous because of the secondary cor pulmonale. All these changes are related to the severity of the disease process and the amount of ventilation/perfusion mismatch (primarily intrapulmonary shunt).

Medical Management

Treatment for chronic bronchitis is aimed at airway clearance. Bronchodilator therapy to control any bronchospasm present (previously described) and adequate hydration are essential. Expectorants such as glyceryl guaiacolate (Robitussin TG) may be helpful but are irritating to the stomach. Supersaturated solution of potassium iodine (SSKI) is frequently used but requires caution because of the side effects of parotid swelling, skin rash, hypothyroidism, and gastric irritation. When sputum becomes infected, appropriate antibiotic therapy should be used. Patients often have renewable prescriptions at local pharmacies and begin themselves on ampicillin or tetracycline whenever they note a change in sputum color or tenacity. There is controversy over whether the use of continuous antibiotic therapy for prophylaxis is of any value. Steroids and hyposensitization therapy are of no value. Chest physiotherapy is helpful for airway clearance.

Emphysema

Pulmonary emphysema involves the enlargement of the distal terminal bronchioles with alveolar fragmentation and destruction of the alveolar septa. Lung elasticity (elastic recoil) is progressively lost. Airway support is lost in emphysema because of the loss of parenchymal tissue, which normally gives structural support to the bronchioles and alveolar ducts. The terminal airways collapse during expiration. Patients with emphysema also tend to retain secretions and develop repeated infections easily.

Table 27-6 Pulmonary Function Profiles of Obstructive Pulmonary Diseases

Disease	Elastic Recoil	Static Compliance	Airway Resistance	Residual Volume/ Total Lung Capacity	Bronchodilator Response
Bronchitis	Normal	Normal	↑	Normal to ↑	+
Asthma	Normal (↓ in acute attack)	Normal (↑ in acute attack	↑		+ +
Emphysema	Decreased	Normal	Normal	↑	0

Approximately 80 percent of patients with chronic obstructive pulmonary disease have centrilobular emphysema in addition to chronic bronchitis. The major areas of destruction are the respiratory bronchioles. Another form of emphysema, *panlobular* or *panacinar,* is primarily caused by alveolar fragmentation. The most common cause of this emphysema is cigarette smoking. Also implicated are certain atmospheric pollutants such as oxidants, certain dusts, and cadmium vapors. One form of panlobular emphysema results from a genetic deficiency of the enzyme α_1 antitrypsin. This enzyme inactivates proteases from white blood cells which, when not inactivated, destroy lung parenchyma.

Pathophysiology

Ventilation, diffusion, and perfusion are all altered in emphysema. Ventilation is regionally decreased because of loss of elastic recoil, poor support of terminal airways, gas trapping, and poor alveolar gas mixing in the involved areas.

Pulmonary diffusion is reduced because of a loss of alveolar surface area and pulmonary vasoconstriction. Hypoxemia and pressure from adjacent distended alveoli may decrease perfusion to normal alveoli, further reducing capillary blood volume and decreasing diffusing capacity.

The perfusion abnormality is one in which hypoxemia causes generalized pulmonary artery constriction, shunting blood away from even relatively normal areas of lung.

Cor pulmonale usually occurs during exacerbations of the disease, late in its course, probably due to pulmonary hypertension produced by hypoxia, against which the right ventricle must pump. The ventricle, which normally pumps against low resistance, dilates.

Diagnostic Findings

A barrel chest deformity is characteristic of advanced emphysema. There is kyphosis, increased anteroposterior diameter, horizontal ribs, wide subcostal angles, and flat, immobile diaphragms. Hyperresonance to percussion, decreased breath sounds, and restricted chest wall movement are present. If crepitant rales are present, they will be heard bilaterally at the bases, particularly in those with cyanosis. Cor pulmonale, hepatomegaly, and peripheral edema may be present in severe cases. Prolongation of expiration is pronounced, and accessory muscles of respiration are used. The patient elects to sit upright with arms braced in the "emphysematous habitus." Heart sounds may be difficult to hear.

The chest roentgenogram shows typically low-lying diaphragms, overexpansion, and a long, narrow heart. The lung fields are hyperlucent, with pronounced vessels and diminished peripheral vascular markings. The lateral view may show flattened diaphragms and an increased retrosternal air space. Sometimes bullae can be identified by fine, hairlike margins and lack of vascular supply.

Pulmonary function testing shows increased residual volume (RV). The increased ratio of RV to total lung capacity (TLC) reflects expiratory airway collapse and airway trapping. Expiratory flow rates (FEV_{1-3}) are decreased because of loss of elastic recoil.

Arterial blood gas analysis usually shows hypoxemia. CO_2 retention may or may not be present. Patients who maintain good ventilation/perfusion matching (the "pink puffers") can maintain blood gases fairly well until late in the disease.

Medical Management

Emphysema is an irreversible disease for which care is only supportive. Improved activity performance and decreased morbidity have been demonstrated in patients who participate in pulmonary rehabilitation programs. Pursed-lip breathing adds a form of expiratory retard to the patient's spontaneous respiration and may improve gas distribution. Most patients find that it eases their dyspnea.

Home oxygen is useful for patients who cannot maintain a Pa_{CO_2} greater than 55 torr when breathing room air. Low-flow (1 to 2 L/min) oxygen at night is currently used to relieve pulmonary hypertension from hypoxemia and prevent secondary polycythemia.

Chronic obstructive pulmonary disease (COPD) is a combination of emphysema and chronic bronchitis with a varied component of bronchospasm. Emphysema, like chronic bronchitis, can usually be managed with controlled oxygen therapy, chest physiotherapy to clear airways, bronchial hygiene, antibiotics to treat infection, and cardiovascular support. Low-flow oxygen by nasal cannula is usually used to treat the patients. When Pa_{CO_2} is chronically elevated, breathing drive is regulated by hypoxemia. Oxygen should be carefully monitored to avoid excessive exposure of the patient, which might result in respiratory depression. Flow rates of 2 to 4 L/min are usually appropriate. Intrapulmonary FI_{O_2} varies since it is determined by the tidal volume of room air the patient also inhales. Oxygen by Venturi-principle face mask allows more precise administration of oxygen when necessary. Endotracheal intubation and mechanical ventilation are avoided if at all possible because of the high risk of complications and additional morbidity.

Criteria for endotracheal intubation and mechanical ventilation vary, but most agree that if Pa_{CO_2} increases above normal levels for that patient, and if acidemia and hypoxemia with mental obtundation are present, there is a need for more aggressive pulmonary support.

Continuous mechanical ventilation may impede venous return to the right side of the heart and therefore cardiac output. This occurs more commonly in patients with COPD, since their highly compliant lung tissue conducts the increased mean intrapulmonary pressure to the heart and great vessels with ease. Intermittent mandatory ventilation (IMV) can be successfully used in these patients. IMV offers the advantages of less influence on venous return as well as avoidance of the alkalemia, hypokalemia, and cardiac arrhythmias seen upon rapid reduction of Pa_{CO_2} on continuous mandatory ventilation.

Weaning presents little difficulty with IMV, since it essentially begins with the onset of mechanical ventilation. The patient does not need to "relearn" breathing and retrain respiratory muscles, because they have been continually used. It eliminates the fear and anxiety experienced by many patients with abrupt removal of the ventilator during conventional weaning. This is particularly significant for this group of patients, since anxiety increases their dyspnea and may increase bronchospasm, making weaning more difficult and very traumatic.

Psychosocial Aspects of COPD

The relation between the psychological and physical is closer, perhaps, in COPD than in most other chronic diseases. Many patients deal with their disease in one of two ways, and both are maladaptive. Some patients, when experiencing excitement, anxiety, or emotions like anger, become more active and hyperventilate. This adds more strain to their already maximally functioning cardiopulmonary systems and they become dyspneic. This dyspnea creates more anxiety, and a vicious circle ensues.

A second group of patients, possibly those who have observed the relation between their emotions and dyspnea, begin to fear emotion. They use mental defense mechanisms of isolation, denial, and depression to accomplish this. Nurses need to actively assess patients looking for these mechanisms and adjust the plan of care accordingly.

The patient's family also needs special support. With this disease complex the best they can hope for is extension of life and maximization of present level of function. They live from stage to stage of the disease with no hope for cure. They frequently have feelings of helplessness, fear, guilt, and anger. They usually feel so guilty about their feelings of anger that they frequently overprotect the patient. This definitely deters the patient from maximizing the level of functioning. The family of the COPD patient needs and deserves support from the medical and nursing staff. Referral to the psychiatric social worker or staff psychologist may be indicated.

Case Study: Obstructive Disorders

A 60-year-old male cigarette smoker with known COPD manifested primarily as chronic bronchitis with bronchospasm and mild emphysema is admitted to the ICU via the emergency room with a history of recent fever, purulent sputum, and thick, tenacious, foul-smelling green sputum.

Nursing Diagnosis
Ineffective airway clearance related to retained secretions, increased viscosity of secretions, and bronchospasm.

Goal
Patient will be able to expel clear, loose tracheobronchial secretions.

Interventions

1. Encourage oral fluid intake.
2. Teach and encourage effective cough techniques.

3. Provide adequate humidification.
4. Administer chest physiotherapy q 2–4 h.
5. Administer bronchodilators (if prescribed) prior to chest physiotherapy.
6. Give nasotracheal suction prn.

Nursing Diagnosis

Alteration in nutritional status related to increased metabolic demands and loss of appetite associated with dyspnea and fatigue.

Goal

Patient will maintain body weight.

Interventions

1. Provide high-calorie, high-protein diet in small, frequent feedings.
2. Allow frequent rest periods, especially prior to meals, to minimize dyspnea.
3. Get patient up in chair for meals to allow abdominal contents to fall, freeing thoracic motion and minimizing dyspnea while eating.
4. Weigh patient daily.
5. Encourage family to bring favorite foods from home.
6. Provide O_2 via nasal prongs during meals (if O_2 is prescribed) to prevent dyspnea associated with removal of mask for eating.
7. Consult with dietitian if indicated.

Nursing Diagnosis

Anxiety related to maladaptive smoking behavior with progressive pulmonary disease.

Goal

Patient will stop smoking cigarettes.

Interventions

1. Inform patient about relation of cigarette smoking to progression of disease.
2. Provide information about hospital and community resources for stopping smoking, e.g., self-help groups.
3. Assess smoking behavior of family members and intervene as indicated.

Nursing Diagnosis

Potential for recurrent pulmonary infections related to chronic pulmonary disease.

Goal

Patient will recognize early signs and symptoms of infection and seek medical attention early.

Interventions

1. Teach patient to recognize early signs of infection, such as change in color or consistency of sputum.
2. Reinforce patient's knowledge of good health habits such as good nutrition, avoiding crowded public places during seasonal outbreaks of viral infections, and asking physician about influenza vaccination.

Perfusion Lung Disorders

Pulmonary Thromboembolism

Pulmonary thromboembolism (PTE) is a common condition that complicates hospitalization today. The term is used to describe a blockage of a portion of the pulmonary arterial system by a blood clot arising from the systemic veins. Two factors concerning PTE should be considered. First, its incidence can be reduced if awareness of the high-risk factors predisposing to PTE leads to prophylactic treatment; and second, misdiagnosis is frequent because of the nonspecific signs and symptoms.

The incidence of PTE is estimated to be 650,000 annually, with a 30 percent mortality. The most common type of embolus is that arising in a peripheral vein. It is usually a result of deep vein thrombosis (DVT) in the lower part of the body, notably the calf and the plantar, common femoral, and superficial femoral veins.

Virchow, in 1846, described three contributing factors which predispose to thrombus formation: stasis, or reduction of blood flow, intercurrent illness, and vessel wall damage. Venostasis still remains a leading cause of DVT. Prolonged bed rest, immobility due to old age or muscular weakness, and obesity may decrease blood flow. Long intraoperative procedures in which cardiac output is reduced, such as neurosurgery, decrease limb perfusion. Myocardial infarction, atrial fibrillation, and congestive heart failure also decrease cardiac output. A history of any of these factors should alert those managing critically ill patients to the increased possibility of PTE.

Changes in coagulation factors as a cause of thrombus formation have been under investigation. Studies have shown that there is an increased incidence of venous thrombosis and PTE during pregnancy and in women taking oral contraceptives. Estrogens are known to promote coagulation and increase platelet aggregation. It is also believed that coagulation changes may precipitate thrombus formation in the postoperative period and after abrupt discontinuation of anticoagulation therapy. Damage to the endothelial wall of a vessel may be precipitated by venostasis, trauma, sepsis, or major body burns. Thrombus formation is enhanced by platelet adhesiveness and the release of serotonin. Both hypercoagulability and vessel wall injury are factors in thrombus formation, although they are usually seen in conjunction with venostasis. It is still uncertain whether they may cause thrombosis without accompanying stasis.

Pathophysiology

The formed thrombus can dislodge and travel through the circulation of the heart to rest in the pulmonary artery. Although the thrombus may dislodge spontaneously, the more common mechanism is the jarring of the clot from the vessel wall by mechanical forces. These forces include sudden standing, usually during initial ambulation, or changes in the rate of blood flow due to a Valsalva maneuver.

Smaller emboli tend to lodge in the distal branches of the pulmonary artery at the periphery of the lung. The severity of emboli is greater when a large number of small emboli travel to the lungs simultaneously or one large embolus blocks a larger vessel. The subsequent obstruction of blood flow in the pulmonary circuit has both respiratory and hemodynamic consequences.

Initially the number of perfused alveoli decreases, thereby increasing dead space or "wasted ventilation." Recall that ventilatory dead space results from lack of perfusion of ventilated alveoli. This yields a ventilation/perfusion ($\dot{V}/\dot{Q}$) mismatch. Because no gas exchange can take place, bronchoalveolar hypocarbia results (decreased alveolar CO_2). Hypocarbia contracts the bronchial smooth muscle, causing bronchoconstriction and alveolar shrinking. This constriction leads to maldistribution of ventilation and increased airway resistance and thus increases the work of breathing. The constrictive response may be viewed as a protective mea-

sure, since the amount of wasted ventilation is reduced. The inspired air is propelled into functioning alveolar units, rather than into the alveoli in which diffusion cannot take place. This mechanism is not enough, however, to normalize the $\dot{V}/\dot{Q}$ ratio.

Another mechanism that leads to alveolar collapse is the reduction of surfactant. Cessation of blood flow probably leads to reduced surfactant levels. This reduction may be due to the anoxic effects on the mitochondria of the alveolar type II cells which produce it. Atelectasis as an end result of bronchoalveolar constriction and decreased surfactant levels usually occurs 24 to 48 h after obstruction to blood flow.

Hemodynamic consequences seem to depend on the extent of pulmonary blood flow obstruction and the cardiopulmonary status prior to the episode. The primary consequence of obstruction is an increase in pulmonary vascular resistance. The right ventricle must maintain enough pressure to propel blood through this resistance; thus an increase in pulmonary artery pressure (PAP) is seen. If this pulmonary hypertension is severe enough, the right ventricle will fail. Tachycardia and decreased cardiac output are frequently seen at this stage. Frequently PTE is not totally obstructive and the cardiopulmonary responses may only be slight.

There is evidence that humoral responses (e.g., release of serotonin from platelets surrounding the PTE) may be involved in the constrictive response of the bronchioles and terminal lung units. This does not necessarily involve the areas affected by the embolus and often involves functioning alveoli. Thus one sees perfusion with little or no ventilation because of the constriction of the alveoli. This may lead to areas of atelectasis and shunting, possibly explaining the arterial hypoxemia frequently seen in PTE. Another factor contributing to increased shunting is pulmonary hypertension. The main response is the decrease in diffusion of gases in the lung. Thus, three main factors lead to ventilation/perfusion mismatching in PTE. One is the dead space effect of alveoli ventilated but not perfused because of the obstruction of blood flow from the thrombus. Another is the shunting of blood past nonventilated alveoli that have collapsed from atelectasis. A third response is no ventilation and no perfusion seen in silent units. The reader is referred to Chap. 8 for a more detailed description of ventilation/perfusion mismatch.

Pulmonary infarction as an end result of PTE is relatively uncommon. In most instances in which infarct develops, there is underlying pulmonary disease which has already impaired pulmonary circulation or increased pulmonary congestion, as seen in cardiac failure. It is characterized by marked consolidation, usually from hemorrhage, and is frequently associated with pleuritic pain from pleurisy or effusion. The infarct may necrotize and become infected, forming a lung abscess. Healing of involved lung usually results in some degree of pulmonary fibrosis.

Diagnostic Findings

One of the factors contributing to the misdiagnosis of PTE is the vagueness of the signs and symptoms. In general, sudden onset of dyspnea is the most common complaint. Unless the embolus is severe, this may be the only symptom. Massive PTE may produce chest pain, the origin of which is unclear. Tachycardia and increased intensity of the pulmonary S_2 heart sound can be found when there is pulmonary hypertension. Other less frequent findings include nonspecific rales, mild temperature elevation, gallop rhythm, and possibly signs of phlebitis. Hypotension with peripheral vasoconstriction and accompanying cyanosis may be evident.

When pulmonary infarct has occurred, the symptoms are usually more specific. Cough, hemoptysis (usually seen as blood-tinged sputum), and pleuritic pain are relatively common. There may be signs of consolidation, pleural effusion, and infection of the infarct. Bronchial breathing, pleural friction rub, and high fever are classic signs. It must be remembered that pulmonary infarct is *not* a common complication of PTE; therefore, the presence of these signs is rare.

Laboratory tests are usually not specific for PTE but are useful adjuncts to rule out other pulmonary disease. Leukocytosis is rare except in cases of infarction but may differentiate a diagnosis of pneumonia. Analysis of arterial blood gases is frequently useful, particularly in cases of massive PTE. Hypoxemia, hypocarbia, and respiratory alkalosis are common changes. Alveolar-arterial P_{CO_2} difference is widened because of increased dead

space. However, the presence of underlying pulmonary disease may make the blood gas readings hard to interpret. The main point to keep in mind is that arterial blood gas changes may help to confirm the diagnosis of PTE; however, normal arterial blood gases do not rule it out.

Chest x-ray and ECG findings are also vague. A normal chest x-ray, frequently seen, does not exclude the diagnosis of PTE. The changes, if any, are subtle but may include the following:

1. Differences in the diameter of normally equal size vessels, due to the fact that if one vessel is blocked the other may have to accommodate pulmonary blood flow
2. Abrupt cessation of a vessel due to obstruction
3. Shadow from a clot with no blood flow distally
4. Abnormal radiolucency due to absent or decreased blood flow (Westermark's sign)
5. Diaphragmatic elevation

ECG changes usually do not occur unless there is extensive embolization. A tall peak T wave, ST changes from right ventricular strain, and tachycardia may be present.

The use of perfusion and lung scanning can assist with the diagnosis. Once there is a suspicion of an embolus, based on a history of risk factors and any of the laboratory tests, a lung perfusion scan is usually done. Perfusion scan is performed by the injection of aggregates of serum albumin which are labeled with a radioactively tagged substance. The indicator is mixed in the heart and distributed with blood flow to the lungs. Thus scanning of the anterior, posterior, and lateral views of the lung can show the overall distribution of blood. A normal perfusion scan can rule out PTE. However, abnormal scans are seen in a multitude of pulmonary and cardiac diseases and do not establish the presence of PTE with absolute certainty. An abnormal perfusion scan which conforms to a lobe or segment increases the probability of embolism.

Ventilation lung scan determines the distribution of gas in the alveoli by detection of a radiolabeled gas. A defect in the ventilation lung scan that matches the perfusion scan is usually not seen in PTE unless infarction has occurred, and this can be demonstrated on chest x-ray. If there is no ventilation defect in the nonperfused area, the likelihood of PTE increases. However, if doubt persists, a pulmonary angiogram should be obtained if operative intervention is contemplated.

Pulmonary angiography is considered the standard definitive test for diagnosis of PTE. The technique involves the injection of radiopaque dye into the pulmonary artery. The presence of a filling defect or "cutoff" of an artery confirms the diagnosis. It should be noted that small peripheral emboli may not be seen by angiography, but these rarely cause symptoms of breathlessness or the usual consequences of embolism.

From this discussion it is easily concluded that the diagnosis of PTE is not a simple task. Anyone presenting with breathlessness warrants a detailed history specifically designed to ferret out risk factors. Prolonged bed rest, obesity, and cardiac failure are all significant findings. A history of recent hip fracture, malignant disease, pregnancy, use of oral contraceptives, burns, trauma, respiratory failure, or surgery should raise the question of possible pulmonary embolism. Although some of the reasons why these conditions precipitate PTE are still unknown, they merit consideration.

Medical Management

Treatment should include two main objectives: anticoagulation to prevent further thrombosis and cardiopulmonary supportive therapy. Continuous intravenous heparin remains the drug of choice for anticoagulant therapy. A coagulation profile should be drawn before heparin is administered.

An initial loading dose of 2000 to 3000 U of heparin may be given. Usually 800 to 1200 U/h is adequate to maintain proper anticoagulation. Periodic determinations of anticoagulant levels are necessary, twice per day initially and then once per day. Lee-White clotting time should remain at 25 to 35 min (about 2 to 2½ times normal). Partial thromboplastin time (PTT) should also be elevated to 2 to 2½ times normal (i.e., 50–80 S to 29–35 S).

Heparin therapy should be continued for approximately 7 to 10 days. However, this depends on a number of factors. When ambulation can be started, the extent of the venostasis and the preexisting condition of the patient should be considered before the therapy is discontinued. As long as the patient remains on prolonged bed rest, a significant risk factor, heparin therapy should be continued.

For example, the patient with acute respiratory failure and sepsis may require bed rest for longer periods, which predisposes to more thrombus formations. The transition from heparin to oral anticoagulants may be made as soon as the patient is up and about. Prothrombin time (PT) is used to determine the dosage of warfarin needed to maintain anticoagulation. The length of time anticoagulants are needed is dependent upon the existence of factors which predispose the patient to thrombosis.

Supportive therapy is required to maintain cardiopulmonary function. Oxygen administered by nasal cannula or endotracheal tube may be needed to maintain adequate oxygenation. The use of inotropics and pressors to maintain cardiac output has proved effective. Volume loading with dextran 40 may be used to increase pulmonary blood flow to previously unperfused segments. The increased and more evenly distributed flow has implications for increased arterial saturation. Dextran may also be helpful for its anticoagulation properties.

The use of streptokinase and urokinase for massive PTE with severe hemodynamic consequences has been advocated for their thrombolytic properties. Definitive studies have shown streptokinase and urokinase to produce earlier reduction of obstruction and more rapid restoration of hemodynamic properties than heparin alone. There is, however, no documented evidence of reduction of mortality or morbidity from PTE in either mode of therapy. Streptokinase is a secretory protein of hemolytic streptococci which is thought to activate plasminogen, a fibrinolytic enzyme precursor. Its effect should be noticed after 24 h of administration. Adverse reactions are bleeding and a low-grade fever. Urokinase, also an activator of plasminogen, is an enzyme found in human urine. Its maximum effect should be seen in 12 to 24 h.

Streptokinase and urokinase therapy should be followed by heparin/warfarin therapy to prevent further thrombosis and embolization. It appears that these substances can be used in massive PTE for those patients in whom surgical therapy is contraindicated.

Although the need for surgical intervention has decreased because of better pharmacologic agents, surgery may be necessary for those patients with massive pulmonary embolus (usually 50 percent obstruction). Patients who do not respond to conventional therapy and who exhibit life-threatening complications or those in whom anticoagulant therapy is contraindicated may require surgical intervention. Pulmonary embolectomy for these patients requires documentation by pulmonary angiography and the use of a cardiopulmonary bypass apparatus.

Vena caval ligation studies have shown an increasing number of patients who redevelop an embolism. Because of the dangers of increasing venostasis below the ligation, partial obstruction is being sought whenever possible. The intracaval "umbrella" causes progressive obstruction of the vena cava, allowing the body to adjust to the subsequent venostasis. The umbrella may be placed under local anesthesia and is associated with a reduced mortality rate. More recently the Greenfield filter (Fig. 27-10) has been used. It has proved to be safe, economical, and effective and is rapidly

becoming the method of choice because of its relatively low rate of complete caval occlusion.

Many clinicians believe that the main emphasis in the treatment of PTE should be prevention of deep vein thrombosis. Low-dose heparin therapy appears to be the most promising prophylactic measure. Doses of 5000 U subcutaneously every 12 h have been shown to reduce the incidence of thrombosis. Studies have also been conducted using warfarin, aspirin, and dextran 70. Minidose heparin therapy has resulted in few bleeding problems and no significant rise in clotting times or PTT.

Nonpharmacologic methods used to prevent thrombus formation are early ambulation, use of elastic stockings, leg elevation, and use of various exercise machines. It has not been proved that these methods result in any significant reduction in deep vein thrombosis, particularly in the high-risk patient. Intraoperative passive range of motion and the use of intermittent compression of the leg seem to retard venostasis and show promising results.

Clearly, clinical suspicion and the identification of high-risk factors in PTE are necessary for prevention. Once the predisposing factors are identified, prophylactic therapy may be instituted. The nurse must be aware of the subtle changes in patient status that might indicate PTE or deep vein thrombosis. Any slight change in heart rate and breathing pattern in a high-risk patient should initiate an investigation for PTE. Preoperative teaching of range of motion exercises and their rationale should be instituted with patients. Postoperative exercises and early ambulation should be carried out routinely. The dangers of prolonged sitting and crossed legs should be explained, particularly to the patient prone to thrombosis. The key to management of PTE patients is prevention and early detection.

Air Embolus

Entrance of air into the circulatory system under appropriate conditions can result in the same pathological changes as are found with solid particle emboli. Pathological conditions leading to symptomatic air embolus include intravenous infusion, tubal insufflation, pneumoperitoneum, uterine douches, surgical treatment of the neck, neuro-

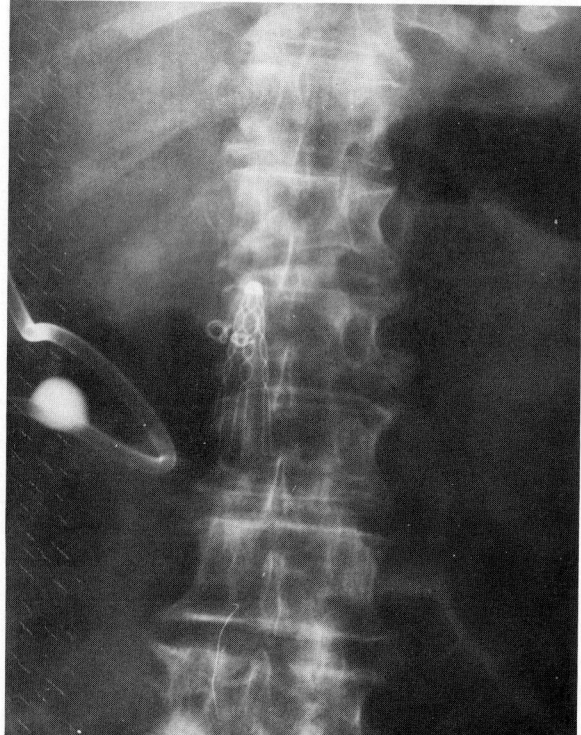

Figure 27-10 Greenfield filter can be seen positioned in the inferior vena cava. Foreign body seen in the right flank is a nephrostomy tube.

surgical procedures, open-heart surgery, retroperitoneal air injection, irrigation of nasal sinuses, chest trauma, and rapid decompression. It has been estimated that 100 mL of air can be lethal and lesser amounts can lead to frothing in the circulatory system. The symptoms are as much a function of rate of air entry into the circulation as of the absolute amount of air.

Air entering the bloodstream enters mainly through the venous system, because of the fact that venous pressure can reach levels below atmospheric pressure. Under such circumstances, if the venous system is open to the atmosphere, air enters the circulation. This accounts for the occurrence of air embolus during neurosurgical procedures done with the patient in the sitting position, surgery of the neck, and venous catheterization. Any portion of the venous system positioned above the level of the heart reaches a subatmospheric pressure and poses a threat of air embolus if the venous system is opened.

Use of the sitting position in neurosurgery risks the entrance of air into the patient's venous system when a vein is perforated. An added risk is encountered during surgery near the major venous sinuses of the brain, because their rigid walls fail to collapse when opened and large amounts of air can rush in.

Postcardiac surgery air embolus may develop if air has been trapped in the right or left side of the heart during surgery. The air in the left side poses a more serious problem, not only of myocardial ischemia but of the possibility of air passage through the aorta to the cerebral circulation. Air should be vented from the heart before cardiopulmonary bypass is discontinued.

When air embolism follows a central venous pressure (CVP) line insertion, air has been found to have entered via an opening in the catheter system, most commonly through a disconnected or broken CVP line. The catheter tip placed in the superior vena cava or right atrium is in a venous system that is subatmospheric during inspiration. Therefore, any part of the catheter system open to the atmosphere presents an opening for an inrush of air during inspiration. Catheters placed in veins of the neck may also give rise to air embolus because of negative venous pressure when the head is in the upright position.

The preceding paragraphs emphasize the role of subatmospheric venous pressure in causing air embolism; however, instances of increased air pressure as a cause have been reported. Chest trauma, tubal insufflation, and pneumoperitoneum may result in entrance of air into the venous system because of the increase in air pressure relative to venous pressure. In chest trauma, lung damage may result when communication is established between the venous system and bronchi. Forced expiration or mechanical ventilation can force air into the open venous system, resulting in air embolus. Tension pneumothorax can produce similar results.

Similar to air embolus is gas embolus, known as *caisson disease,* which occurs frequently in underwater divers and persons exposed to increased atmospheric pressure. Under high atmospheric pressure, increased amounts of hydrogen, oxygen, and nitrogen are dissolved in the bloodstream. If the ascent to lesser atmospheric pressure is too rapid, the three gases come out of solution. The hydrogen and oxygen are reabsorbed, but the nitrogen remains out of solution and portions coalesce, possibly resulting in large nitrogen bubbles that may obstruct the vascular tree. Clotting of small blood vessels may occur because of activation of a clotting cascade downstream of the bubbles and loss of plasma volume with hemoconcentration, due to transcapillary leakage of plasma water. The hyperbaric chamber reverses this process.

Diagnostic Findings

Air may enter the venous system at a slow infusion rate or as a large bolus. A small, slow infusion during normal respiration has been shown to initiate a gasp reflex, causing a large amount of air to be sucked into the veins. Signs and symptoms usually vary with the amount of air pulled into the venous system. It is believed that slow infusion of air results in decreased peripheral resistance and that the physiological changes seen are due to pulmonary vasculature changes.

ECG changes include a peaking of P waves and, later on, ST depression. When cardiovascular deterioration has been established, a churning noise ("mill wheel murmur") may be heard on auscultation. Central venous pressure gradually rises during slow infusion of air, while pulmonary artery pressure (PAP) increases early. At low infusion rates, blood pressure decreases and pulse increases. Signs of shock may be seen as peripheral resistance decreases.

With a bolus of air, cardiovascular collapse occurs because of an air lock in the heart. The rise in PAP is not seen, probably because the circulatory collapse can occur within seconds and the air is not pumped into the pulmonary artery. Heart failure in dogs has been shown to be precipitated by supraventricular tachycardia with 100 mL of air and ventricular tachycardia with 200 mL of air.

Medical Management

Since the effect of air embolus can be fatal within minutes, complete resuscitative methods should be initiated immediately. The patient should be placed on the left side in a head-down position (Durant's maneuver). This allows the air bubbles to float to the right atrium and away from the pulmonary artery. This may not prove effective alone or in cases of large air embolism, since inflow to the right side of the heart would also be obstructed. Intracardiac aspiration of air may be achieved through a subclavian or central line positioned in the right atrium. Success, however, depends on early detection and rapid aspiration. It has been demonstrated that large amounts of air can remain in the right side of the heart once clotting of blood has begun.

Air can also be removed from the right side of the heart by external cardiac massage. This is probably effective because the air is forced out of the heart into the pulmonary circulation, fragmenting into smaller air bubbles.

Whenever there is a possibility of air embolus, measures should be taken to prevent or detect its occurrence. During insertion of a central venous catheter, the patient should be placed in the head-down position, to increase venous pressure and prevent the sucking in of air. This technique also applies when treating patients with penetrating lung wounds. Positioning the patient with the laceration below the level of the right atrium may decrease the likelihood of air entering the system.

The use of an ultrasonic Doppler apparatus during neurosurgical procedures has been advocated to detect the presence of air embolus. With a clear, patent system and the transducer at the level of the right atrium, even minute bubbles of air can be detected. The Gardner antigravity suit (a circumferential pneumatic pressure suit) has been used to decrease postural hypotension, thereby increasing venous pressure and preventing air embolus. Its use, however, remains controversial.

Clinicans should be aware of the potentially lethal effects of air embolus whenever penetration of the venous system is contemplated. Proper positioning and the use of detection devices may aid in reducing overall mortality.

Fat Embolus

A complex and highly debated entity is fat embolization. This is a condition characterized by microembolization (usually 10 to 40 μm) of fat, resulting in obstruction of blood flow and inflammatory reactions around the vessels affected. Long bone fractures and major soft tissue trauma are the leading causes of fat embolus syndrome—thus the high incidence of the syndrome in the young and vigorous and the elderly. Occasionally, embolization follows osteomyelitis, cardiopulmonary bypass, burns, poisoning, pancreatitis, and renal transplantation. Characteristically, larger emboli lodge in the pulmonary vasculature, while the smaller globules travel through the circulation to other parts of the body.

The incidence of pathological fat emboli is far greater than their clinical manifestation. Embolization is often not heralded by clinical symptoms but is rather an incidental pathological finding in trauma patients who die of other causes. Some studies have demonstrated a 60 percent incidence of fat emboli, the majority being subclinical.

Fat emboli arise from the marrow of the injured bone and subcutaneous tissue where fat globules enter the venous circulation through ruptured veins, being drawn into the veins because of the difference in pressure in the damaged marrow and the venous system. The fat globules are in the form of neutral fat (saturated) and fatty acids (unsaturated). After the initial injury, the release of fat globules may continue intermittently, depending on the amount of patient manipulation. This theory is supported by the high incidence of fat emboli following long bone fracture and the fact that fat found in the lungs has been found to resemble marrow fat.

A chemical theory suggests that emboli are also formed from fat emulsions in the plasma. It is theorized that plasma lipids, in a hypercoagulable state, form with platelets and embolize. This process is probably triggered by the leakage of a small amount of fat from the marrow. The fact that other causes of fat emboli besides fractures have been described tends to support this theory.

Pathophysiology

The majority of emboli rest in the pulmonary vasculature. However, a small portion pass through the lungs and enter the circulation. The mechanism for the passage is still controversial. One theory suggests that a large number of emboli reach the lungs simultaneously and the lung is unable to filter all of them. Another cites local alveolar capillary dilatation or the effects of shunting, which allow emboli to pass through into the circulation. These emboli can travel to the brain, heart, kidney, skin, posterior pituitary, and eye.

The obstruction of pulmonary blood flow accounts for the number of alveoli ventilated but not perfused (alveolar dead space). However, the effects on the pulmonary vasculature and alveoli are probably similar to those described in ARDS. Intra-alveolar hemorrhagic edema may be associated with rupture of the capillaries. Parenchymal damage is frequently seen and is probably a result of local lipolysis and decreased surfactant production, which are in turn a result of edema and cessation of blood flow. The hypoxemia frequently seen in fat emboli is primarily due to shunting. This may be a result of three factors: considerable atelectasis from the intra-alveolar hemorrhage or inflammatory edema; precapillary shunting; and alveolar capillary dilatation, which allows an accelerated blood flow, inhibiting oxygenation of hemoglobin molecules.

Systemic fat emboli are usually liquid-deformable and most likely result in partial or temporary obstruction of vessels. As emboli penetrate the capillaries they break into smaller globules; this probably explains why systemic emboli are smaller than those found in the lung. Frequent passage through the circulation and the lungs make the emboli small enough to be eventually removed by phagocytosis. As the fat is broken down by lipases in plasma and macrophages, fatty acids are released which cause an inflammatory reaction.

Although there may be petechial eruption in the white matter of the brain, the main effects are from obstruction of smaller arteries in the gray matter, causing infarcts which may or may not be hemorrhagic. In the heart there may be areas of fatty degeneration, although symptoms are mild, if they exist at all, and the condition is reversible. Petechiae can also appear in the kidneys but have not been proved to cause tubular necrosis or renal failure. Fat emboli can cause blind spots in the eyes which resolve with no ill effects. Microemboli may be visualized in the retinal vessels. Skin rash, usually seen on the anterior chest and shoulders and in the axilla, is probably the result of embolization of the capillaries in the dermis. It has been suggested that thrombocytopenia may induce this petechial eruption, but this has not been definitely proved. Petechiae often appear in the conjunctiva of the eyelids.

Diagnostic Findings

Although severe fat emboli may develop rapidly and progress to coma and death, most clinical cases are asymptomatic and remain undiagnosed. Emboli reach the lung within minutes, and early signs of hypoxemia may be evident. Most patients have a Pa_{O_2} of 60 to 70 torr on admission following a long bone fracture. However, a more fulminant respiratory picture may develop, with Pa_{O_2} levels below 60 torr, along with the clinical signs of systemic emboli.

Classic symptoms can develop hours to 4 days after injury. Besides mild hypoxemia, subtle mental changes may appear in the first 24 h. Changes in patient behavior, slight disorientation, and increases in pulse and temperature may be early warning signs. If the embolization is partial, any of the cerebral, pulmonary, or skin rash effects may be absent. These symptoms usually disappear in about a week with adequate treatment.

More severely affected patients exhibit severe respiratory compromise similar to ARDS. Petechial rash usually appears within 24 h. Cerebral effects culminate in coma and death, most likely due to brainstem infarction.

Other findings include fat in the sputum due to leakage into the alveoli, lipuria, decreased hematocrit readings related to trapping of red cells, thrombocytopenia, and ECG changes. Elevated serum lipase levels appear about the third day after injury and may be a guide to prognosis.

Medical Management

Prevention of fat emboli following trauma and long bone fracture should be of prime concern when handling fracture patients initially. Care should be taken to splint the fracture as soon as possible and to avoid overmanipulation. Pneumatic tourniquets used during elective surgery on long bones has been advocated to minimize the possibility of fat reaching the lungs. The tourniquet should not be removed until the limb is immobilized in a splint.

The use of oxygen is clearly beneficial. It is thought that oxygen administration, besides correcting the hypoxemia, may inhibit passage of emboli through the lungs. Mechanical ventilation and the use of PEEP are required with severe respiratory compromise.

Heparin, aprotinin (Trasylsol), dextran, and steroids have all been advocated. However, the number of conflicting reports concerning the efficacy of these therapies indicates the need for further study. The possibility of dissolving larger fat globules into smaller ones and thus increasing the incidence of passage through the lungs into the circulation is a major deterrent to various lipolytic drugs. Lipolysis may also be harmful because of the local inflammatory reaction. The use of glucose and insulin to slow down this response has been suggested.

Nursing care of any patient following long bone fracture or trauma involves recognition of the subtle changes seen with fat emboli. The baseline admission data should include a good neurological assessment and evaluation of arterial blood gases. Any slight change in these parameters may indicate the beginning of a fat embolus syndrome.

Case Study: Perfusion Disorders

A 37-year-old female with a history of low back pain was admitted for treatment. After 2 weeks of bed rest and relief of back pain, the patient started ambulation and physical therapy. The first night following therapy the patient experienced shortness of breath and pain on inspiration. Arterial blood gas studies revealed a Pa_{O_2} of 50 torr. A diagnosis of PTE was made, and the patient was started on oxygen 5 l/min, given a bolus of 5000 U heparin, and started on a continuous infusion of 800 U heparin per hour.

Nursing Diagnosis

Ineffective breathing pattern related to pain on inspiration.

Goal

Patient will be able to cough effectively.

Interventions

1. Medicate patient half-hour prior to treatments and to coughing and deep breathing exercises.
2. Provide comfortable position for adequate aeration.
3. Teach breathing techniques using splinting with pillow.

Nursing Diagnosis

Impaired gas exchange related to $\dot{V}/\dot{Q}$ mismatching and atelectasis.

Goal

Patient will demonstrate ABGs within acceptable levels.

Interventions

1. Augment oxygenation as prescribed.
2. Assess ABGs prn.
3. Assess respiratory status q 2 h.
4. Assess cardiovascular status for increased pulmonary obstruction due to more pulmonary thromboembolism.
5. Provide frequent rest between treatments to decrease oxygenation demand.
6. Turn patient q 2 h to minimize $\dot{V}/\dot{Q}$ shunting effects.

Nursing Diagnosis

Potential for bleeding related to anticoagulant therapy.

Goal

Patient will not bleed, or, if bleeding occurs, it will be detected early.

Interventions

1. Give no intramuscular injections.
2. If venipuncture is necessary, hold the puncture site for 10 min.

3. Screen stools routinely for occult blood.
4. Screen urine routinely for red cells.
5. Test nasogastric fluid q 4 h for blood.
6. Administer antacid as prescribed.
7. If patient is at high risk for stress ulcer, measure abdominal girth every shift.
8. Prevent vigorous brushing of teeth and gums.

Chest Trauma

Pulmonary Contusion

Pulmonary contusion is usually characterized by damage to the lung parenchyma that results in localized edema and hemorrhage. It is often associated with more acute trauma (e.g., pneumothorax or hemothorax) and may go unnoticed until the hypoxic effects cause severe respiratory distress. Pulmonary contusion was widely recognized during World War II as "blast injury," caused by underwater detonation of high explosives or other forms of shock wave compression of the chest wall.

High-speed automobile accidents are presently a leading cause of lung contusion resulting from deceleration of the chest wall as it strikes the steering wheel. The contusion may be the result of direct force (the anterior portion of the lung striking the steering wheel), or a contrecoup effect of the posterior lung bouncing back against the rib cage. Blunt chest trauma and shotgun and high-velocity missiles often give rise to the same parenchymal damage. Because of the large number of automobile accidents and the increased incidence of bomb explosions related to terrorism, clinicians should be alert to the possibility of pulmonary contusion.

Pathophysiology

Rapid compression and decompression by a high-pressure wave results in parenchymal damage, hemorrhage, and edema. It is thought that the initial injury compresses the thoracic cavity and diminishes its size. The increase in intrathoracic pressure then compresses the lung, resulting in parenchymal damage. When decompression occurs, the lung springs back, causing rupture of the capillaries and the subsequent hemorrhage.

The degree of pathological change varies with the severity of the contusion. Less severe trauma usually produces focal areas of hemorrhage, while more severe injury can cause a firm purple lesion. The initial blow produces capillary damage and hemorrhage. The results of this hemorrhage and the vicious cycle effects are summarized in Fig. 27-11. The vascular damage from cellular debris is similar to the mechanism described in the section dealing with ARDS. In pulmonary contusion, the cellular debris from cell damage also contributes to the collapse of the alveoli. If the patient has multiple trauma, fat embolism is a likely additional cause of pulmonary failure. The reader is advised to review the section on ARDS for a more complete description of the pathophysiological changes.

Diagnostic Findings

There are problems with the recognition of pulmonary contusion. Often contusion is sustained without penetrating trauma to the chest. It has been observed that the more severe contusions are found in cases with no associated rib fractures. The belief is that there is a temporary deformity of the rib cage which compresses the lung or that the acceleration-deceleration effect causes the lung to strike the rib cage.

On the other hand, contusions associated with fractured ribs and flail chest often go unnoticed. It is probable that the hypoxic effects seen in flailing are primarily due not to the free-floating ribs but rather to the underlying contusion. This is discussed further in the section dealing with flail chest.

Another problem with the diagnosis of pulmonary contusion is the poor correlation of the initial signs and symptoms and the initial chest x-ray with the extent of the injury. A number of reports have shown that contusion may not appear clinically for 2 to 24 h after chest injury, with a lag of 4 to 6 h frequently found between the time of injury and an abnormal chest x-ray. The appearance of an abnormal roentgenographic pattern also does not correlate well with the extent of the injury. The less severe contusion may reveal patchy areas of ill-defined infiltrates which can progress to well-defined opacities. In its severest form the classic *white lung* may be seen.

Pulmonary contusion can be classified as mild, moderate, or severe. Physical symptoms vary accordingly. Patients with mild contusions usually present with tachypnea, tachycardia, and blood-

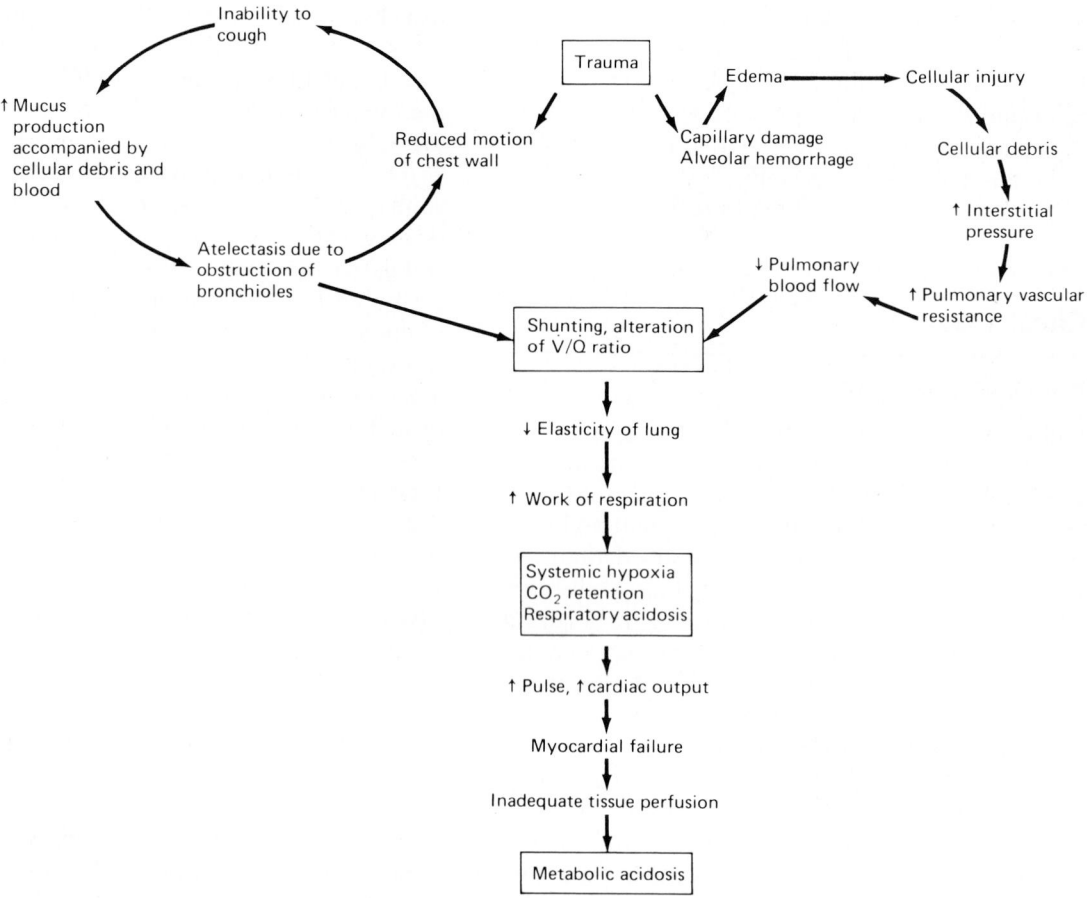

Figure 27-11   Pathophysiology of pulmonary contusion.

tinged secretions. There is an inability to cough effectively, probably because of the chest pain associated with the initial trauma. Rales may be heard on chest examination. Arterial blood gas measurements may reveal a slightly decreased Pa_{O_2} on room air and a decreased Pa_{CO_2} due to tachypnea.

If the contusion is more severe, the tachypnea, tachycardia, and rales persist. Secretions become more copious, and frank blood may become evident. The patient is unable to clear the secretions. Severe hypoxemia and CO_2 retention with a progressively widening alveolar-arterial gradient, $D(_{A-a})O_2$, indicate severe respiratory failure. Chest x-rays usually exhibit some abnormal findings at this stage, but they often do not correlate with the extensive damage. The white lung can appear hours later.

Medical Management

The primary goals in treatment of pulmonary contusion are early diagnosis, maintenance of a patent airway, and adequate oxygenation by maintenance of lung function. Because of the frequent lack of symptoms and confirmation of the extent of injury, the suspicion of contusion should be entertained in any chest trauma. Close observation of the patient for 24 to 48 h is highly desirable to detect signs of increased respiratory insufficiency. Once flailing, pneumothorax, and/or hemothorax are corrected, the Pa_{O_2} and $D(_{A-a})O_2$ should improve. Any subsequent signs of hypoxemia most likely indicate the presence of a contusion.

Mild contusion may be treated without ventilatory support. Oxygen by mask with good humidification may be all that is needed until signs of adequate oxygenation are seen. Vigorous chest physiotherapy and nasotracheal suctioning may be beneficial in helping to clear secretions. If these methods are not sufficient, therapeutic bronchoscopy may be used. Adequate relief of pain is needed to facilitate coughing and deep breathing.

Bacterial culture and sensitivity tests of sputum should be obtained periodically, since the damaged lung may be susceptible to infection. Broad spectrum antibiotics have not proved useful prophylatically, so coverage should be adjusted according to culture reports.

The patient with a mild contusion may be expected to have rapid resolution of the damage (3 to 4 days). However, there is a danger in diagnosing a mild contusion and treating without ventilatory support. Misdiagnosis of mild contusion is a distinct possibility when diagnosis is based on initial chest x-ray findings and presenting symptoms. The patient must be closely observed for signs of increasing hypoxemia as the extent of the disease becomes more apparent.

The more severe contusions require ventilatory support. Since many clinicians consider lung contusions in their severest form a disorder similar to ARDS, the ventilatory management is based on similar principles. Controlled mandatory ventilation or intermittent mandatory ventilation is necessary. The use of positive end-expiratory pressure is adjusted according to the criteria previously described for ARDS. The reader is advised to review the section on ARDS for nursing and medical management of pulmonary contusion in its most severe form.

Flail Chest

Paradoxical movement of the chest wall during respiration is known as *flail chest*. It is observed when the ribs are broken in two or more places, leaving them free-floating in the chest cavity. Flailing is frequently seen following blunt chest trauma or may occur iatrogenically during overzealous cardiopulmonary resuscitation. In the latter case the anterior rib fracture is often associated with costochondral separation.

Pathophysiology
The multiple rib fractures incurred during crushing injuries cause the chest wall to lose its continuity. During inspiration, atmospheric pressure exceeds intrathoracic pressure on the affected side, causing the chest wall to move inward. Conversely, on expiration, intrathoracic pressure exceeds atmospheric pressure, causing the outward motion of the chest wall until the thorax contracts, resulting in reduced pulmonary ventilation. The patient experiences pain and an inability to cough effectively. The increased work of breathing associated with noncompliant lungs, along with the lack of ventilated alveoli beneath the affected ribs, leads to atelectasis and hypoxemia. It should be noted that since flail chest from crushing injury is often associated with other pulmonary complications, including pulmonary contusion, pneumothorax, and hemothorax, the diagnosis of flailing should include a search for these other disorders.

Diagnostic Findings
The most apparent sign of flail chest is the paradoxical movement of part of the chest wall, although tissue swelling, chest wall hematoma, or poor inspiratory effort by the patient may mask this sign. Pain may be severe and increase with movement. The patient is usually short of breath, tachypneic, or tachycardic. If the flailing is related to other pulmonary injury or myocardial contusion, hypotension and cyanosis may be evident. Chest x-ray is useful in diagnosing rib fractures and the presence of underlying pulmonary trauma but *not* the presence or absence of flailing.

Medical Management
The main emphasis in treatment of flail chest is stabilization of the chest wall. Formerly this was accomplished by sandbagging the flail segment, chest wall traction with towel clips, or manual pressure during exhalation. The increase in atelectasis due to pressure on the chest wall has led many clinicians away from this type of management. Generally, if adequate oxygenation can be maintained with a manual inflation bag until ventilatory support can be established, mechanical stabilization is not necessary.

The concept of using controlled mechanical ventilation for treatment of flailing was introduced by Avery in 1956.[10] Other modes of support have included intermittent positive pressure breathing, control ventilation with PEEP, and more recently, intermittent mandatory ventilation (IMV) with PEEP. These techniques maintain chest wall expansion and prevent the rib cage from becoming permanently smaller when the fractures set, reducing the risk of permanent restriction of ventilatory function.

Allowing the patient to breathe spontaneously with some ventilator support (IMV) and positive pressure has some advantages. The patient receiving controlled ventilation may build up subatmospheric intrathoracic pressure trying to breathe spontaneously, thus increasing pain and the potential for dislodging ribs. With the use of IMV and PEEP, the patient does not "fight" the ventilator and the pressure needed to generate a breath is minimized. It has also been demonstrated that the use of IMV can reduce the time needed for mechanical ventilation.

The shorter ventilation period needed with IMV supports a theory that the effects of flail chest may be due not to the orthopedic problem but rather to the tissue damage. It was originally thought that PEEP improved oxygenation by reducing flailing. However, a number of clinicians believe that the hypoxemia is due to underlying pulmonary contusion, atelectasis, and the increased work of breathing. The fractured ribs and flailing may initiate the problem, but the contusion is probably responsible for the continued hypoxic effects.

Pain medication should be administered according to patient need. Controlled ventilation usually requires large amounts of sedation to keep the patient in phase with the ventilator. The use of IMV should not rule out pain medication but can reduce the amount needed. Pain, tachypnea, and tachycardia may increase oxygen consumption and defeat the purpose of ventilation. Morphine sulfate, 1 to 2 mg IV every hour, is enough to control pain without depressing respiration.

Pneumothorax

The entry of air into the pleural space with partial or complete collapse of the lung is defined as *pneumothorax*. Pneumothorax can be classified as closed or noncommunicating (simple); tension; and open or communicating (sucking wound). Since the severity, pathophysiology, and management of these conditions are different, they are discussed here separately. Normally the pleural space is potential rather than actual, occupied by only a thin film of fluid. Any disruption in this "traction" on the lung can cause serious effects on ventilation.

Simple or Closed Pneumothorax

The incidence of pneumothorax in patients sustaining blunt chest trauma has been reported to be as high as 50 percent. Automobile accidents, high falls, blows to the chest, and blast injuries are leading causes. Frequently the pneumothorax is a result of lung lacerations from fractured ribs. When there are no associated fractures, it may be a result of compression at the height of inspiration when alveolar pressure is high. A blow to the chest increases the pressure, causing rupture of the alveoli, escape of air, and collapse of lung tissue.

Spontaneous pneumothorax can be due to the rupture of an emphysematous bleb, cystic lung disease, pulmonary carcinoma, or tuberculosis. Iatrogenic causes include subclavian venous catheter insertion, intracardiac injection, thoracentesis, or positive pressure ventilation. Simple, or closed, pneumothorax has been so classified because of its self-sealing effect. Once the air has entered the pleural space, the lung seals and prevents further leak. Pneumothorax may be small (<15 percent), moderate (15 to 60 percent), or large (>60 percent).

Although pneumothorax usually produces symptoms, some patients are totally asymptomatic. In general, the larger the collapse, the more pronounced the symptoms. The presence of underlying pulmonary disease, however, may produce severe symptoms with even a small pneumothorax. Chest x-ray is helpful in establishing the presence of a small collapse or the extent of a larger one.

Shortness of breath and restlessness are classic signs. Chest pain radiating to the back, face, abdomen, and shoulders may be caused by stretching of the parietal pleura. The larger the collapse, the more likely are signs of increasing hypoxemia and inability to maintain adequate ventilation.

Inspection reveals decreased or absent motion of the chest wall and a tracheal shift toward the unaffected side. Subcutaneous emphysema is often present, particularly in the larger pneumothorax. Absent or decreased breath sounds and hyperresonance to percussion are common.

The treatment of closed pneumothorax is dependent upon the severity of the lung collapse and respiratory compromise. A small collapse may be followed by daily chest x-rays. One can expect the lung to reexpand at a rate of approximately 1.25 percent of the area per day. If the size continues to increase, insertion of a chest tube is the treatment of choice.

Symptomatic pneumothorax mandates the release of air. A chest tube is inserted into the second or third intercostal space at the midclavicular line. If at all possible, the patient should be in the upright or semiupright position. This helps to ensure that the underlying lung falls away from the chest wall. The skin should be cleansed with iodine or betadine, and sterile gloves should be used. After a 1- to 2-cm skin incision, the chest tube is inserted using a trocar or hemostat. When the chest tube is connected to underwater seal drainage, the presence of bubbling confirms the escape of air. The tube should be sutured into place and all tubing connections tightened or taped to prevent disconnection. A chest x-ray is taken after the procedure and repeated daily to monitor the reexpansion of the lung.

In caring for the patient with chest tubes connected to underwater seal drainage, one golden rule should be observed: chest tubes should *never* be clamped. The effects of tension pneumothorax from pressure build-up are far more damaging than the effects of an open pneumothorax from disconnection of the underwater seal. In the event of a bottle break or crack, the chest tube may be submerged in a bottle of sterile water until new equipment is available.

Pneumothorax is often associated with underlying pulmonary disease. Chest physiotherapy may still be done with the patient in a modified postural drainage position (flat) as long as the underwater seal remains intact and the water seal is below the level of the heart. Pain may inhibit vigorous physiotherapy, and therefore this patient should be premedicated and percussed for shorter periods more frequently. Once the chest tube is inserted, the patient may be turned from side to side. Care must be taken to prevent kinking of the tubing when turning the patient toward the affected side.

Recurrent or chronic pneumothorax may require additional therapy. Thoracotomy with decortication is reserved for those who have had multiple attempts at reexpansion of the lung. The procedure involves stripping of the parietal pleura from the apex of the lung to allow the visceral pleura to adhere to the chest wall. The mediastinal and diaphragmatic pleura are left intact. The leak in the lung may be repaired or resected during the procedure. Recurrence is relatively rare.

Tension Pneumothorax

Blunt chest trauma may also precipitate a tension pneumothorax. Although controlled mechanical ventilation, when used with positive end-expiratory pressure, has been associated with tension pneumothorax, the use of intermittent mandatory ventilation has reduced this occurrence. It is possible that the incidence of tension pneumothorax in severe pulmonary disease is related to the frequency of high peak pressures during lung inflation.

As air increases in the pleural space, tension increases. If the tear does not seal, a one-way valve effect is produced, allowing air to enter during inspiration but not to escape during exhalation. The intrapleural pressure, if not relieved, compresses the vena cava, causing decreased diastolic filling of the right ventricle, with a fall in cardiac output. The cardiovascular collapse is coupled with the compression of the unaffected lung because of intrathoracic pressure. The combination of decreased cardiac output and decreased ventilation is soon fatal unless immediate action is taken.

The patient with a tension pneumothorax is usually in marked respiratory distress. Tachypnea, cyanosis, tachycardia, and hypotension accompanied by restlessness and agitation are immediate danger signs. Subcutaneous emphysema is almost always present. If the patient is intubated, there is usually difficulty in ventilating manually because of high intrathoracic pressure. The shift of the trachea and mediastinum to the opposite side is acute, and breath sounds are absent. Often the affected side of the chest wall expands because of intrathoracic pressure.

Tension pneumothorax is an emergency situation, and treatment must not be delayed for any reason. Cardiopulmonary resuscitation is often ineffective for cardiovascular collapse until the tension inside the chest cavity is relieved. Insertion of a chest tube is the treatment of choice. If equipment for thoracotomy is not immediately available, a large-bore needle and syringe may be inserted into the second intercostal space to temporarily relieve the pressure. Because of the incidence of lung perforation from needle aspiration, this method should be used carefully. The use of a spring-loaded needle has been advocated. This needle has a sharp edge for insertion which springs back, leaving a blunt-end needle for escaping air. The use of this device has produced no evidence of lung perforation. These techniques, however, are only temporary measures; chest tubes should be inserted as soon as available.

Routine management is the same as that for simple pneumothorax. A functioning chest tube does not preclude the use of PEEP. If positive pressure ventilation is required for respiratory failure, it should be maintained once the chest tube is inserted and functioning, even if the lung collapse was caused by the PEEP. The persistent air leak will be relieved by the chest tube until the mechanical ventilation is no longer needed.

Open or Communicating Pneumothorax

Penetrating trauma to the chest wall causes the atmospheric air to have direct access to the pleural cavity, causing an open, sucking wound. Common causes are gunshot and stab wounds, although any defect of the chest wall can cause the open communication. Surgical intervention in the chest may also precipitate an open pneumothorax.

This injury involves the bulging inward of the affected lung during inspiration and an outward movement during exhalation. The affected lung's air is soon depleted, and it is unable to expand because of free air movement from outside into the pleural space. The unaffected lung receives air from the trachea *and* from the affected lung during inspiration. During expiration, air is exhaled into the trachea and into the unaffected lung. Thus this lung is moving deoxygenated air in and out, increasing functional dead space and causing carbon dioxide retention.

The most obvious sign of an open pneumothorax is the chest wall defect. The patient is usually in respiratory distress, tachycardic, and dyspneic. Subcutaneous emphysema is often present and expanding. Immediate action is needed to close the defect. Sterile gauze can be used until petroleum gauze can be secured with adhesive over the wound. Chest tube insertion is necessary to expand the

affected lung once the open air port has been sealed. When the patient is stabilized, surgical intervention may be necessary to explore and debride the wound. Irrigations with saline and broad spectrum antibiotics have been recommended.

Patients with open pneumothorax require close observation both pre- and postoperatively. Besides the pneumothorax, a hemothorax from a penetrating wound is possible. Infection from the instrument used to inflict the wound may precipitate empyema or pyopneumothorax (collapse of the lung from pus). Both of these complications may develop 24 to 48 h after trauma.

Hemothorax

Hemothorax is collapse of the lung from the accumulation of blood in the pleural space (Fig. 27-12). Blunt and penetrating chest trauma, as well as the iatrogenic causes previously indicated, may give rise to bleeding. The heart, lungs, great vessels, or any of the chest wall vessels are common sources of rupture. Usually this bleeding is self-limiting because of low pulmonary arterial pressure, throm-

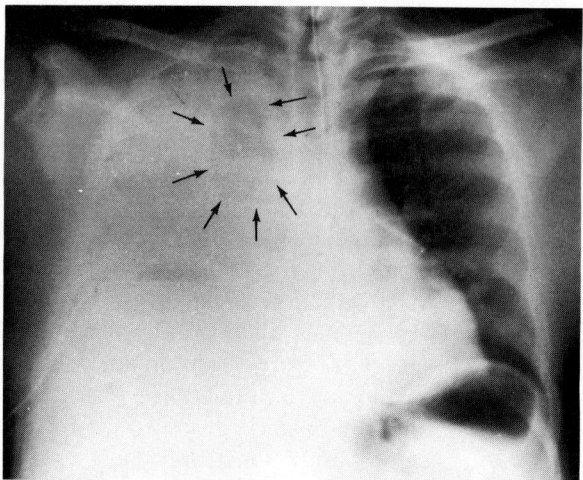

Figure 27-12   Chest x-ray of 32-year-old male following attempted right subclavian catheterization. Opacification of the right side of the chest is seen, with some mediastinal shift to the left. Arrows indicate collapsed right lung. At thoracotomy to control hemorrhage, 3 L of clotted blood was removed from the right pleural cavity and no bleeding point was found. The patient made a full recovery.

boplastin in the lungs, and compression of the site of bleeding by the pool of blood already accumulated.

Hemothorax has two main debilitating effects. First, the pool of blood causes the collapse of alveoli; second, the amount of blood loss can lead to hypovolemia. Severity of the condition depends upon the amount of lung tissue displacement and the amount and rate of blood loss.

Less than 400 mL of blood may cause little or no change in the patient's condition. Chest x-ray may show a loss of the acute costophrenic angle and a hazy appearance over the lower chest. Larger losses usually exhibit the classic signs of shock: pallor, tachycardia, hypotension, and restlessness, together with dyspnea and a tightness in the chest. Breath sounds range from diminished to absent, and there is dullness on percussion. Chest x-ray is useful in diagnosing the extent of fluid loss but may often be eliminated because of the severity of the shock.

The treatment of choice for self-limiting hemothorax is chest tube insertion. The patient should be in the upright or semiupright position when the chest tube is inserted in the fifth or sixth intercostal space at the midaxillary line. This helps to alleviate the risk of puncturing a high-lying diaphragm, spleen, liver, or colon. The tube is connected to underwater seal drainage with 20 to 30 cmH$_2$O suction. The chest tubes should be "milked" every hour to avoid obstruction by clots.

Massive hemothorax necessitates fluid administration for resuscitation. If the bleeding is not self-limiting, thoracotomy for repair of the site is necessary.

Case Study: Chest Trauma

A 27-year-old man is admitted to the emergency room after a car accident in which he struck the steering wheel. Physical examination and chest x-ray reveal a right pneumothorax, flail chest, no internal bleeding, and some patchy atelectasis. A chest tube is inserted to relieve the pneumothorax, and mechanical ventilation with a PEEP of 5 is prescribed.

Nursing Diagnosis
Impaired gas exchange related to atelectasis.

Goal
Patient will demonstrate ABGs within acceptable levels.

Interventions

1. Provide mechanical ventilation as prescribed.
2. Assess ABGs prn and change ventilator parameters accordingly.
3. Assess respiratory status q 2 h.
4. Provide frequent rest between treatments to decrease oxygen demand.
5. Observe color, odor, and amount of secretions (indicating progression of disease or infection).
6. Turn patient q 2 h to minimize $\dot{V}/\dot{Q}$ shunting effects or use Rotorest bed.
7. Give chest physiotherapy to facilitate open airways.

Nursing Diagnosis
Ineffective airway clearance related to endotracheal tube, flail chest, and increased viscosity of secretions.

Goal
Patient will maintain patent airway with no retained secretions.

Interventions

1. Give suction prn.
2. Perform tracheal lavage with nonpreserved saline prn.
3. Provide adequate humidification.
4. Turn laterally semiprone q 1–2 h or use Rotorest bed.
5. Give chest physiotherapy q 4 h.
6. Administer bronchodilators if prescribed prior to suctioning.

Nursing Diagnosis
Alteration in comfort (pain) related to broken ribs.

Goal
The patient will be free of pain.

Interventions

1. Medicate for pain half-hour prior to turning, chest physiotherapy, or ambulation.
2. Use pillow to splint area during activities.

References

1. Shapiro, B. A., et. al. (1982). Clinical application of glood gases. Chicago: Year Book.
2. Crexells, C., et. al. (1973). Optimal filling pressure in the left side of the heart in acute myocardial infarction. *New England Journal of Medicine, 289,* 1263.
3. Pek, S., & Gekas, P. W. (1965). Pneumonia due to herpes zoster. Report of a case and review of the literature. *Annals of Internal Medicine, 62,* 350.
4. Harper, J. R., et. al. (1969). Intermittent positive pressure ventilation in chickenpox pneumonia. *British Medical Journal, 3,* 637.
5. Hyde, R. W., & Rawson, A. J. (1969). Unintentional iatorgenic oxygen pneumonitis: Response to therapy. *Annals of Internal Medicine, 71,* 517.
6. Siebke, H., et al. (1975). Survival after 40 minutes submersion without cerebral sequelae. *Lancet, 1,* 1275.
7. Pass, H. I., et. al. (1984). Thoracic manifestations of acquired immune deficiency syndrome. *Journal of Cardiac Surgery, 88,* 654.
8. Severinghaus, J. W. (1977). Pulmonary vascular function. *Am Rev Resp Dis 115* (Part 2), 149–158.
9. American Thoracic Society (1965). Chronic bronchitis, asthma, and pulmonary emphysema: A statement by a committee on diagnostic standards for nontuberculous respiratory disease. *Am Rev Resp Dis 85,* 762.
10. Avery, A. E., Morch, E. T., & Benson, D. W. (1956). Critically crushed chests: A new method of treatment with continuous hyperventilation to produce alkalotic apnea and internal pneumatic stabilization. *Journal of Thoracic Surgery, 32,* 291–311.

Bibliography

Bone, R. C. (1984). The adult respiratory distress syndrome. *Respir. Care, 29:*3.

Cooper, K. R., & Marrow, C. F. (1984). Pulmonary complications associated with head injury. *Respir. Care, 29:*3.

Hechtman, H. (Ed). (1983). Symposium on critical illness. *Surg. Clinics of North America, 63:*2.

Hiller, F. C., Wilson, F. J., & Bone, R. C. (1983). *Pulmonary diseases: Focus on clinical diagnosis.* New York: Medical Examination Publishing Co.

Moss, C. (1974). The role of the central nervous system in shock: The centroneurogenic etiology of the respiratory distress syndrome. *Crit. Care Med. 2:*181.

Pass, H. I., et al. (1984). Thoracic manifestations of acquired immune deficiency syndrome. *Jour. Cardio. Surg., 88:*654.

Pepe, P. E., et al. (1982). Clinical predictors of the adult respiratory distress syndrome. *Amer. Jour. Surg., 144:*124.

Rodman, G. H. (1983). Posttraumatic respiratory failure: Role of fluid therapy. *Contemp. Anesth. Pract., 6:*119.

Shapiro, B. A., Cane, R. D., & Harrison, R. A. (1983). PEEP in acute lung injury. *Chest, 83:*3.

Shubin, H. & Weil, M. H. (1971). Shock associated with barbiturate intoxication. *JAMA, 215:*263–268.

Snow, R. L., et al. (1982). Pulmonary vascular remodeling in ARDS. *Amer. Rev. Resp. Dis., 126:*5.

Suffredini, A. F., et al. (1985). Acute respiratory failure due to pneumocyctis carinii pneumonia: Clinical, radiographic, and pathologic course. *Crit. Care Med., 13:*4.

Tafuro, P., Digamon-Beltian, M. & Cunha, B. (1984). Approach to hospital-acquired pneumonias. *Heart & Lung, 13:*5.

Tobin, M., & Grenvik, A. (1984). Nosocomial lung infection and its diagnosis. *Crit. Care Med., 12:*3.

Restrictive Lung Disorders

Snow, N., et al. (1985). Utility of pneumonotomy in the treatment of cavitary lung disease. *Chest, 187:*731–734.

Obstructive Lung Disorders

Dawson, A. & Simon, R. A. (Eds.) (1984). *The practical management of asthma.* New York: Grune & Stratton.

Montenegro H. D. (Ed.) (1984) *Chronic obstructive pulmonary disease.* New York: Churchill Livingston.

Perfusion Disorders

Bell, W. R., & Simon, T. L. (1982). Current status of pulmonary thromboembolic disease: Pathophysiology, diagnosis, prevention, and treatment. *Amer. Heart Jour., 103:*239–262.

Ellis, D. A. (1983). Subacute massive pulmonary embolism treated with plasminogen and streptokinase. *Thorax, 138:*903–907.

Greenfield L. J., et al. (1981). Greenfield vena caval filter experience. Late results in 156 patients. *Arch. Surg., 16:*1451–1454.

Kashuk, J. L., et al. (Sept. 1984). Air embolism after central venous catherization. *Surg. Gynecol, Obstet., 159:*249–252.

Loo, J. C. W., et al. (1983). Controlled multicenter pilot study of urokinase/heparin & streptokinase in deep vein thrombosis. *Thromb. Haemos.,* 3:50 pp. 660–663.

Negus, D., Cox, S. T., Reiedgood, A., et al. (1980) Ultra low dose intravenous heparin in the prevention of postoperative deep vein thrombosis. *Lancet, 1*:891–894.

Peltier, L. F. (July–Aug. 1984). Fat embolism. An appraisal of the problem. *Clin. Orthoped., 187,* pp. 3–17.

Stein, P. D., Willis, P. W. (1983). Diagnosis, prophylaxis, and treatment of acute pulmonary embolism. *Arch. Intern. Med., 143*:991–994.

Stevenson, R. C. K. (June 1985). Take no chances with fat embolism. *Nursing 85, 15*:6, pp. 58–63.

Theiss, W.; (Oct. 1983). Systemic fibrinolytic activity and inhibitor levels during treatment of deep vein thrombosis with urokinase and streptokinase. *Thromb. Haemos., 3*:50, pp. 664–667.

Urokinase Pulmonary Embolism Trial Study Group (1974). Urokinase—streptokinase embolism trial phase 3 results, a cooperative study. *JAMA, 229*:1601–1613.

Chest Trauma

Berte, J. (1977). *Pulmonary emergencies.* Philadelphia: Lippincott, p. 122.

Crofton, J., & Douglas A. (1981). *Respiratory Diseases,* 3d ed. London: Blackwell, p. 544.

Cullen, P., et al. (1975). Treatment of flail chest: Use of intermittent mandatory ventilation, and positive end-expiratory pressure, *Arch. Surg. 110*:1099–1103.

Keen, G. (1984). *Chest injuries: A guide for the accident department,* 2d ed. Bristol: John Wright and Sons.

Zuckerman, S. (1940). Experimental study of blast injuries of the lungs. *Lancet, 2*:219–224.

28 Mechanical Support of Ventilation

Sheila A. Glennon

Classification of Mechanical Ventilators

In recent years a vast number and variety of mechanical ventilators have become available. Because many different capabilities are represented by the various machines, an absolute classification is difficult. For the sake of simplicity, ventilators will be classified according to the mechanism most often employed to terminate the inspiratory phase.

Volume-Cycled Ventilators

The volume-cycled (or volume-preset) ventilators, such as the Emerson, Ohio 560, and Bennett MA-1, terminate inspiration after delivering a preset volume of gas. These ventilators will deliver the desired volume regardless of the pressure required to do so. The volume remains the same unless excessively high peak airway pressures are reached. To prevent potential lung damage due to high peak-inspiratory pressures, all volume-preset ventilators have a built-in safety release valve. The safety release pressure is set manually at about 10 cmH$_2$O above the peak-inspiratory pressure.

The inspiratory time is determined by adjusting the flow rate of the gas to be delivered. The more rapid the flow of gas, the shorter the inspiratory time. Conversely, the slower the flow rate, the longer the inspiratory time. Expiratory time is determined by setting a respiratory rate. Thus, if inspiratory time is adjusted and a certain number of breaths are to be given per minute, the remaining time is available for expiration. For example, if the tidal volume is preset for 1000 cm^3 and the respiratory rate is 10 per minute, this allows 6 s for each respiratory cycle. If the flow rate is adjusted so that inspiration of the desired tidal volume occurs in 2 s, then 4 s remains for expiration.

Many models of volume-cycled ventilators have a built-in oxygen selector and can be adjusted to deliver any concentration of oxygen from 21 to 100%. However, because of variable accuracy, the concentration should be frequently checked by a reliable oxygen analyzer.

Generally, the volume-cycled ventilators are more powerful and certainly more useful when ventilating patients with "stiff" lungs, such as victims of adult respiratory distress syndrome; the ventilator will continue to deliver a constant tidal volume regardless of the changes in airway resistance or in compliance of the lungs and thorax. Time-cycled ventilators, such as the Siemens Servo, achieve volume ventilation by a timing mechanism.

Pressure-Cycled Ventilators

The pressure-cycled (or pressure-preset) ventilators, such as the Bennett PR-2 and Bird Mark VII, terminate inspiration upon achieving a preset pressure. Gas flows to the patient until the preset pressure is reached throughout the system—ventilator, tubing, and patient's airways. When this pressure is reached, the gas flow is terminated and the patient passively exhales. Many pressure-cycled ventilators have some means of adjusting the gas flow rate, the sensitivity of the ventilator's response to the patient's own inspiratory effort and the respiratory frequency initiated by the machine.

One of the greatest disadvantages of pressure-cycled ventilators is that varying resistance interferes with gas flow, since flow is a function of pressure and resistance. This resistance causes a change in tidal volume, since volume is a product of flow and time. Thus, the delivered volume varies as resistance varies. If resistance does not vary appreciably, as in a young drug-overdosed patient, this ventilator may be used. However, it is inappropriate for patients with changing pulmonary resistance, as in acute bronchospasm and in postoperative states. These patients would receive varying volumes with each breath.

The relatively low pressure capability (top effective peak pressure is 30 to 40 cm from a 50-lb/in^2 source) is another disadvantage of pressure-cycled ventilators. A patient with very stiff lungs may need a pressure of 80 cm to deliver an adequate tidal volume.

External Body Ventilators

The external body ventilators assist the patient's spontaneous ventilatory effort by applying intermittent subatmospheric ("negative") pressures to the trunk of the body. For example, the body tank ventilator, or iron lung, may be of great value for the patient whose vital capacity is reduced to a value just below that needed for spontaneous ventilation. However, it is large, noisy, and restrictive.

Another example of this class of ventilator is the cuirass, which functions similarly to the iron lung. This is a rigid shell that covers only the thorax and abdomen. A disadvantage is the difficulty in attaining and maintaining a tight seal.

Modes of Ventilation

Various modes of mechanical ventilation are employed in the care of the critically ill today. They include controlled mandatory ventilation, assist-controlled ventilation, intermittent mandatory ventilation, and a more recent innovation, high-frequency jet ventilation. A variety of terms may be used to describe these basic modes of ventilation.

Controlled Mandatory Ventilation (CMV)

CMV totally regulates the patient's breathing. A set rate, tidal volume, or minute volume is dialed into the ventilator, which cycles automatically regardless of the patient's ability to breathe. This type of ventilation guarantees a set minute ventilation for the patient who cannot breathe spontaneously. It is ideal for totally paralyzed and/or apneic patients (such as those with neuromuscular dysfunction, severe brain damage, spinal cord injuries, drug overdose, or status asthmaticus).

For the patient who is able to initiate a breath, this type of ventilation becomes difficult to manage. Many patients "fight" the ventilator and require paralysis and sedation in order to maintain adequate ventilation without additional work of breathing or risk of cardiovascular compromise or barotrauma.

The respiratory rate and tidal volume should be regulated by the Pa_{CO_2}. Alkalemia due to a falling Pa_{CO_2} is a frequent problem and often requires the addition of "dead space" tubing.

The cardiovascular effects of CMV include decreased venous return and cardiac output. These can be related to both mechanical factors and alkalemia.

Assist-Controlled Ventilation (ACV)

ACV allows the patient to trigger a breath from the ventilator. The ventilator can be set to detect the patient's inspiratory effort and initiate inspiration. Once the patient triggers the ventilator, gas flow will be delivered to the patient until a preset tidal volume, pressure, or time limit has been reached. Should the patient stop triggering the ventilator, the control mode will take over at a preset rate. This method allows patients to initiate ventilation at their own rate but maintains a desired rate should the patient become apneic.

The advantage of ACV over CMV is that the patient sets the rate, rather than the clinician. The arguments to support this type of ventilation are based on the fact that patients use their own muscles to initiate the breath. Theoretically, there is a period when intrathoracic pressure decreases transiently before the ventilator delivers the tidal volume, thereby enhancing venous return and cardiac output. However, many clinicians dispute this theory, arguing that when the patient triggers, the ventilator will respond instantly, thereby mimicking CMV with its resultant cardiovascular effects.

As in CMV, the Pa_{CO_2} is used to determine the tidal volume and respiratory rate. Patients may require sedation, particularly if they are breathing too rapidly for the ventilator to complete a cycle.

Intermittent Mandatory Ventilation (IMV)

IMV allows the patient to breathe spontaneously from a gas reservoir while still receiving periodic mechanical hyperinflations. In this manner the patient's own spontaneous minute ventilation is augmented to a desired level by machine-delivered breaths. The sum of mechanical and spontaneous ventilation provides adequate alveolar minute ventilation. IMV is widely advocated for weaning, although many clinicians employ it from the start of mechanical ventilation.

There are numerous advantages to this approach to therapy. As mechanical ventilation is terminated the weaning process is facilitated. The patient has been spontaneously breathing during the entire course of therapy and gradually assumes the total responsibility for ventilation. It is not necessary to relearn breathing, and the patient's anxiety level is lower. IMV avoids the necessity for paralysis, and sedation, although it can be used with IMV, is needed significantly less often than with CMV.

The alkalemia seen in patients on CMV is diminished in patients on IMV, since these patients breathe spontaneously most of the time and mechanical ventilation is supplied only as needed. The patient is spared the increased oxygen consumption and difficulty of unloading oxygen from hemoglobin to the tissues which accompanies alkalemia.

Mechanically supplied breaths under positive pressure increase dead space (V_D/V_T), worsening the ventilation/perfusion ratio in patients whose primary disease process is characterized by $\dot{V}/\dot{Q}$ mismatching. The use of fewer machine-delivered breaths by employing IMV minimizes this effect.

The introduction of IMV has also helped to lower the incidence of pulmonary barotrauma from the use of positive end-expiratory pressure. The mean intrathoracic pressures are lower, since the high-pressure mechanically delivered breaths come less frequently and intrathoracic pressure is lower during spontaneous breathing.

A slight variation on IMV is synchronized intermittent mandatory ventilation. In this mode the ventilator delivers its mandated breath in synchronization with the patient's own inspiration.

IMV rate is determined by patient need on the basis of three criteria: the pH should be maintained within normal limits; the spontaneous respiratory rate should be 30 or less; and the Pa_{CO_2} should be maintained at the patient's normal level. This is particularly useful in patients with chronic obstructive pulmonary disease, who usually maintain a high Pa_{CO_2} while metabolically compensating to maintain a normal pH.

High-Frequency Jet Ventilation (HFJV)

HFJV is a relatively new type of ventilator therapy. This type of ventilation abandons the theory that alveolar ventilation can occur only when tidal volume exceeds anatomic dead space, the premise of all other types of ventilation.

The method employed is relatively simple, much like "panting" ventilation in the dog. The jet ventilator delivers low tidal volumes (100 to 300 mL) at rapid rates (60 to 100 breaths per minute). Gas delivery is from a pressurized source through a valve into a narrow cannula placed in the endotracheal tube (Fig. 28-1). The patient is also connected to a volume ventilator usually set for continuous positive airway pressure. As the jet stream is propelled into the tube, surrounding gases are entrained and propelled down the trachea. Exhalation is passive, and the inspiratory time (or ON time) is 33 percent, yielding a 1:2 inspiration/expiration ratio. Humidification is accomplished in two ways: the entrained gases are humidified via the cascade on a volume ventilator (used in con-

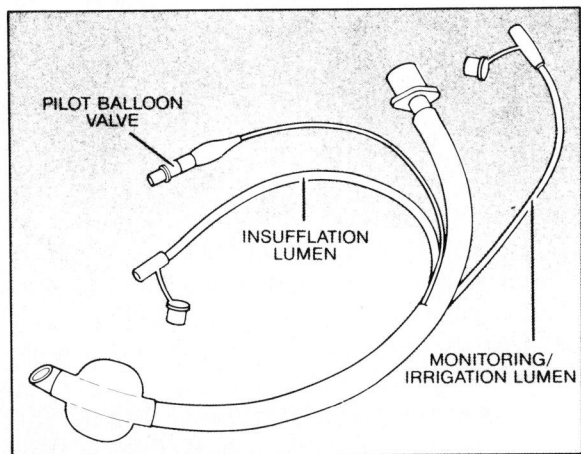

Figure 28-1   ET tube with jet cannula.

junction with the jet), and an infusion of normal saline into a port of the endotracheal tube (which exits just above and in front of the injector catheter tip) humidifies the jet gases.

Studies have suggested that HFJV provides low mean and peak airway pressures, lowers the incidence of barotrauma when high peak pressures are needed on conventional ventilation, decreases cardiovascular compromise, and facilitates weaning. At this time there are still many conflicting reports as to the validity of these claims. Research is continuing in the areas of its usefulness in cardiovascular surgery and neurosurgery, in augmenting pulmonary toilet and mucus clearance, and in ventilatory support during cardiopulmonary resuscitation. This type of ventilation has shown great promise in tracheoesophageal fistulas, bronchopleural fistulas, and oropharyngeal, laryngeal, and tracheal surgery.

Adjuncts to Mechanical Ventilation

Positive End-Expiratory Pressure (PEEP)

PEEP is positive resistive pressure applied to exhalation. This distending pressure in the airways and alveoli keeps small airways open throughout the entire ventilatory cycle. It increases functional residual capacity (or the volume of gas left in the alveoli at the end of exhalation) and removes the need to achieve a critical pressure during inspiration to reopen closed alveoli (commonly called *alveolar recruitment*). For these reasons, PEEP has been deemed essential in improving gas exchange and pulmonary function.

The clinical goal of PEEP is to achieve a Pa_{O_2} greater than 60 to 70 torr* and an FI_{O_2} of 0.5 or below with no significant decrease in cardiac output. It is commonly accepted that any patient receiving mechanical ventilation should receive low-level PEEP (5 cmH$_2$O). The use of PEEP to achieve the clinical goal in patients at risk for adult respiratory distress syndrome is well documented. PEEP should be increased or decreased in 3- to 5-cmH$_2$O increments.

Complications with the use of PEEP include cardiovascular compromise and pulmonary baro-

trauma. The cardiovascular compromise is easily corrected by administration of intravenous fluid or, in rare cases, inotropic or pressor agents. Levels below 10 cmH$_2$O rarely require inotropic or pressor therapy. The use of a flow-directed balloon catheter is warranted when high levels of PEEP are used to monitor fluid administration and inotropic support. Pulmonary barotrauma has been significantly reduced by the use of PEEP in conjunction with IMV rather than with CMV or ACV. The incidence of pneumothorax is increased with PEEP levels above 20 cmH$_2$O; this condition may be corrected by insertion of a chest tube.

Continuous Positive Airway Pressure (CPAP)

CPAP is PEEP applied to a spontaneously breathing patient and has the same physiologic effect of increasing functional residual capacity. It is useful in patients who require a positive distending pressure to maintain oxygenation but do not require mechanical ventilation. The term *expiratory positive airway pressure* has also been used to describe this adjunct, since the spontaneous inspiration of the patient results in negative pressure and the expiration results in positive pressure. The physiologic effects are the same.

Medical Management

Mechanical ventilation must be initiated whenever the patient's ventilatory function fails to maintain an adequate pulmonary blood gas exchange. It is emphasized that the clinical observation or measurement of pulmonary function (ventilation) does not reflect the adequacy of gas exchange (respiration). Arterial blood gas (ABG) determinations are essential to confirm a suspicion of impending acute ventilatory failure.

The clinical goals of mechanical ventilation are (1) to provide the pulmonary system with the mechanical power to maintain physiologic ventilation; (2) to manipulate the ventilatory pattern and airway pressures for the purpose of improving the efficiency of ventilation and/or oxygenation; and (3) to decrease myocardial work by diminishing the work of breathing and improving ventilatory efficiency.

---

*A unit of pressure equal to 1 mmHg.

Ventilators are generally set to provide a fairly high tidal volume of approximately 10 to 15 mL per kilogram of body weight at a relatively low respiratory rate of 10 to 14 breaths per minute and an FI_{O_2} of 0.4 to 0.5. Final adjustments of the mechanical ventilatory pattern ultimately depend on blood gas analysis. The physician should prescribe ventilator settings, ABG levels, sedation, and weaning parameters as guidelines for the nurse or therapist providing patient care on a routine basis.

The effectiveness of any life support system depends upon the patency of the airway. Endotracheal tubes, including nasotracheal, orotracheal, and tracheostomy tubes, are used to eliminate any soft tissue or laryngeal obstruction. A nasal tube is generally preferred for long-term intubation because (1) it is easier to stabilize; (2) it is easier to suction (longer catheters may be necessary); and (3) it is better tolerated by the alert patient. One disadvantage of nasotracheal intubation is that the tube diameter is limited by the nostrils and turbinates and meticulous care must be given to prevent pressure necrosis. Also, significant septal deviation may cause encroachment on the lumen of the tube, which does not affect ventilation but prevents the suction catheter from passing readily. Feeding by the oral route is generally poorly tolerated, although the patient can swallow water reasonably well.

Many respiratory problems, particularly those due to retained secretions, can be resolved during the 48 to 72 h of the more conservative endotracheal intubation if vigorous treatment is given. However, if prolonged ventilatory support is anticipated, tracheostomy may be performed at any convenient time following initial intubation. There are no specific criteria for the appropriateness of endotracheal versus tracheostomy airway management. Endotracheal tubes have been safely left in place for 5 to 14 days (and even longer); however, each clinical encounter must be decided on an individual basis. The primary concern is to prevent laryngeal trauma and granuloma.

Nursing Management

Coordination of care rendered to the critically ill patient is the responsibility of the nurse. Respiratory care given to the patient on a ventilator can be performed by a nurse or a respiratory therapist or a combination of the two. Who is responsible for respiratory care and ventilator maintenance in a particular institution is less important than who is coordinating that care. The nurse and the therapist must be aware of all treatments given to the patient and the response to those treatments. It is the nurse's responsibility to ensure that the patient is receiving the care necessary for a successful outcome. Teamwork and cooperation are essential.

Working nursing diagnoses are described with individual disease entities; but the two diagnoses discussed below are appropriate for any patient on a ventilator regardless of the disorder.

Nursing Diagnosis
Ineffective airway clearance related to placement of endotracheal tube.

Goal
Secretions will remain loose and not be retained.

Interventions

1. Provide humidification.
2. Suction prn.
3. Turn side to side and semiprone q 1 to 2 h.
4. Chest physiotherapy q 4 h.
5. Medicate prn to prevent "fighting" the ventilator.
6. Assess ABG levels prn.

It is imperative that the gas delivered through an artificial airway be 100 percent humidified at body temperature. Effective airway humidification may be accomplished by incorporating a heated humidifier into the ventilator so that the air reaching the patient's airway (37°C) is 100 percent saturated with water vapor. The humidifier must be heated, because an air mixture passing through water at room temperature is only 20 to 30 percent saturated when it is heated to body temperature in the tracheobronchial tree.

Humidifying devices and connecting tubing must be inspected at regular intervals. Condensed water within the tubing may either obstruct airflow or empty into the trachea. Condensed water should never be returned retrogradely to the sterile humidifier.

The intubated patient has an ineffective cough reflex and cannot exert a large intrathoracic pressure against a closed glottis; therefore, secretions must be suctioned from the airway. Tracheal suctioning should never be performed on a routine schedule; "every half-hour" may be too often for one patient and not often enough for another. Needless suctioning produces unnecessary tracheal irritation and should be avoided. Since secretions can be suctioned only from the main stem of the bronchi, it is essential that they be mobilized from the more distal regions by a regular schedule of patient repositioning.

The patient should be informed of the suctioning procedure, and the ventilator tubing should be disconnected after the inspiratory phase of respiration. When disconnected, the ventilator end of the tubing should be placed so that it does not become contaminated.

High concentrations of oxygen should always be administered for several inspirations prior to and immediately following tracheal aspiration so that myocardial hypoxia and cardiac arrhythmias may be prevented. This can be accomplished by turning the oxygen concentration dial on the ventilator to 100% (not forgetting to return it later to its preaspiration concentration) or by "bagging" the patient. A PEEP valve should be used on the bag when appropriate.

Strict adherence to sterile suctioning techniques is mandatory. These patients are generally debilitated and therefore more susceptible to infection. In addition, the mere placement of a tube in the airway greatly reduces the normal protective and defense mechanisms of the lungs. The catheter, about one-half the inner diameter of the tube, should be gently guided, not pushed or shoved, into the trachea. Suction is not applied while the catheter is being inserted. Lung collapse is possible if an excessive vacuum exists. For this reason, suctioning should not be done for longer than 8 to 12 s and the negative pressure should not be greater than 150 cmH$_2$O (for adults). Since each aspiration period lowers the P_{O_2} about 35 mmHg (the level being proportional to the amount and duration of negative pressure applied), it is unwise to make a second attempt at suctioning without first reoxygenating the patient. It is well known that oxygen tensions below 50 mmHg potentiate arrhythmias, and reported cases of cardiac arrest during or following tracheal suctioning are well

substantiated in the literature. All ventilator patients must have continuous electrocardiographic monitoring, and the monitor must be observed during the suctioning procedure.

The patient's position in bed determines which portions of the lungs are ventilated and perfused. Stasis of secretions in the bases and periphery of the lungs is enhanced by the all too frequently observed supine semi-Fowler's position. In this position it is difficult, if not impossible (particularly with positive pressure ventilation), for secretions to ascend from the bases of the lungs to the main stem of the bronchi where they can be reached by the aspirating catheter. Right and left lateral positioning, with the head of the bed gradually lowered, is tolerated by most patients connected to a ventilator (Fig. 28-2).

An optimum time to suction is just prior to position change. The patient's head should be turned at the same time as the rest of the body and kept in alignment. Extreme care must be taken to avoid twisting, hyperextending, or hyperflexing the neck, since these maneuvers traumatize the trachea. Arm and leg exercises are essential to maintain muscle tonus and joint range of motion. A program of breathing retraining and strengthening exercises should begin as soon as possible for patients with chronic airway obstruction. Deconditioning may be prevented and exercise tolerance increased by various arm and leg exercises, which should be synchronized with the breathing pattern while the patient is being assisted by the ventilator. Thus "weaning" is easier to accomplish.

As soon as medically stable, the patient should sit in a chair, even if only for brief periods of time, since this produces both physiologic and psychologic improvement. Continuous ventilatory assistance should not interfere with the patient's freedom out of bed (Fig. 28-3). For chronic ventilator patients, a walker can be equipped with a small ventilator to allow early ambulation.

A patient who is "fighting" the ventilator is restricting the respiratory cycle by actively "pushing out" while the machine is "pushing in." This dramatically decreases alveolar ventilation and increases intrathoracic pressure, consequently decreasing venous return and cardiac output. Patients who "fight" the ventilator are usually hypoxemic, underventilated, or uncomfortable because of an

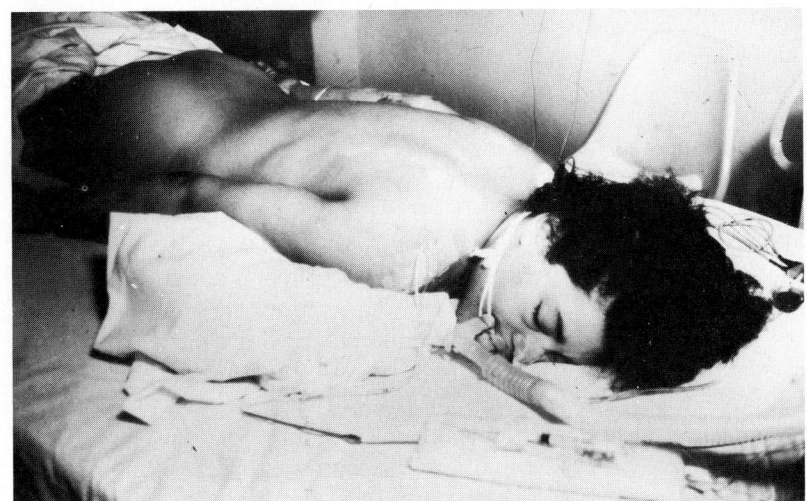

Figure 28-2 The semiprone position is one of the best to facilitate drainage of secretions with chest physiotherapy. Even though this patient has a Swan-Ganz catheter, arterial line, and hyperalimentation line, the position can be maintained with a towel under the shoulder to keep the anterior chest wall off the bed. Frequent position changes should include right and left semiprone, right and left 45° angle, and out of bed, if possible.

inappropriate filling waveform or are suffering pain and/or anxiety.

The individual clinical situation determines the frequency and timing of ABG studies. It generally takes about 15 to 20 min for a blood gas steady state to be reached after a ventilator adjustment, and the stability of the clinical situation should be assured before performing the arterial puncture.

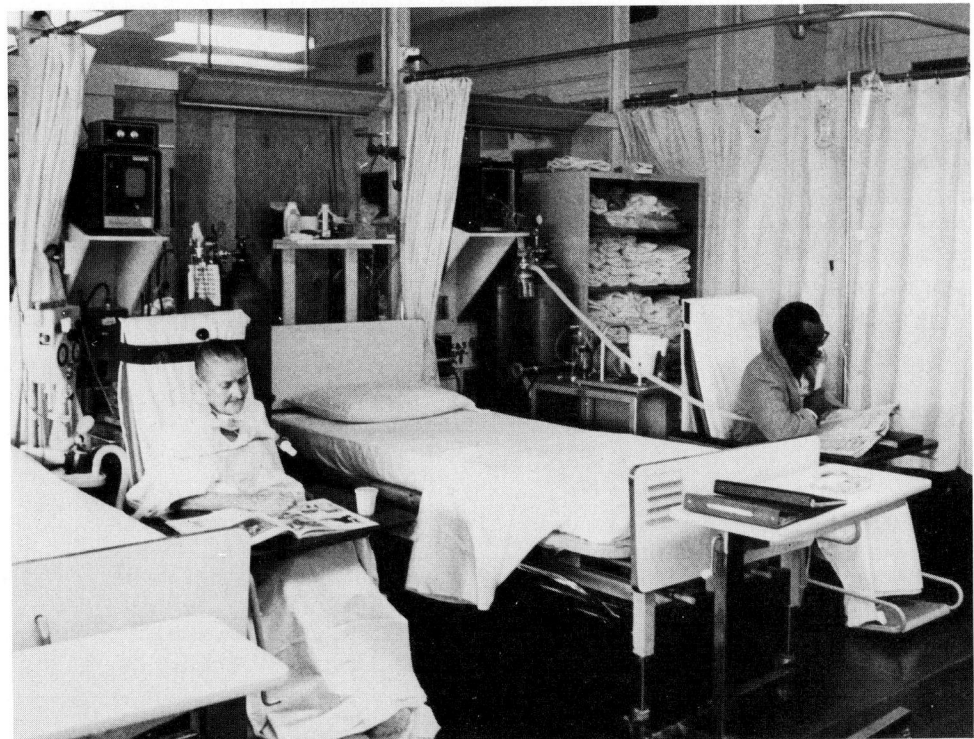

Figure 28-3 Patients should be out of bed as much as possible, and reading may occupy leisure time.

In this era of cost containment, the abuse of ABG testing has received considerable attention. It is to be expected that in the initial phases of respiratory decompensation multiple ABG measurements should be necessary to achieve an optimal ventilatory state. Once the patient is stabilized, however, routine ABG measurements should be eliminated. Indications for evaluating ABGs depend on the patient's clinical presentation. Certainly the patient whose vital signs are stable, who is alert and oriented and appears comfortable, does not require frequent ABG measurement. Even the patient who is being weaned may not require evaluation of ABG for every ventilatory change, if there is no indication of problems. ABG evaluation q 4 h or every shift is unnecessary when the ventilatory status is stable. Properly used ear oximetry or use of the oximetric catheter to measure oxygen saturation has been advocated to minimize the number of ABG measurements.

A Wright respirometer may be used to monitor the tidal volume and minute ventilation, thereby ascertaining the stability of the mechanical ventilation (Fig. 28-4). Frequent checking of the ventilator alarms and oxygen delivery are essential.

Nursing Diagnosis

Anxiety related to inability to communicate (endotracheal tube placement) and sensory overload and/or deprivation.

Goal

The patient will be able to communicate.

Interventions

As the treatment of conditions which once were rapidly fatal has become more successful, the patient requiring ventilatory assistance is exposed to much longer periods of uncertainty, general emotional distress, sensory deprivation, and monotony. The ventilators and monitors with their buzzers and flashing lights surround the patient like sentinels. Flow sheets chronicling the numerous physiochemical variables dangle from the bed and from every available hook. But the tears, pain, loneliness, fear, helplessness, and despair cannot be measured or computed. How easy it is to neglect the patient's emotional well-being because of the pressing demands to take care of the more tangible and task-oriented duties!

One of the most frustrating problems the patient experiences is communication. At a time when the patient's ability to breathe has reached a crisis point, a tube is passed between the vocal cords, thereby preventing speech. The need of the patient to communicate is intensified; the ability to do so is severely compromised. A Magic Slate or pencil and paper may be used. The intravenous apparatus should be placed, if possible, in the nonwriting arm.

Figure 28-4   A Wright respirometer is used to measure expired volume in patient on ventilator.

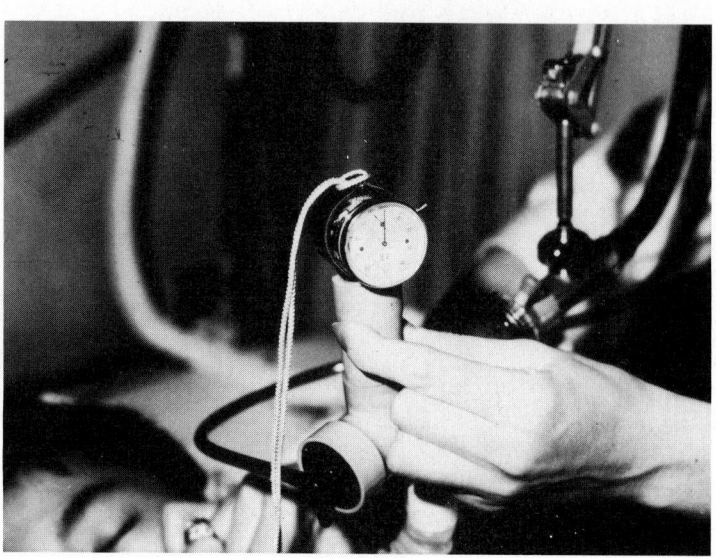

It is ironic that a patient suffering sensory overload may at the same time be deprived of the sensory perceptions needed for orientation. Artificial elimination of the day and night sequence, sleep deprivation, and almost constant bombardment by strange and obtrusive auditory and visual stimuli can produce severe behavior disturbances. Every effort should be made to organize care in such a way as to permit the patient to have disturbance-free rest periods during the day and quiet nights, interrupted only when absolutely necessary for clinical evaluation or treatment.

Orientation may be enhanced by windows, a visible clock, and a large wall calendar (with each day marked off as it passes). The family should be encouraged to talk about their activities, the news, and weather to help the patient keep in touch with reality. Many patients, of course, will not be able to respond, but they *can* hear and use the information to prevent confusion and disorientation. Family members should be encouraged to visit the patient, touch or hold the patient's hand, and participate in routine care whenever or however possible. The sight of a familiar object may relieve some of the anxiety produced by unfamiliar and frightening surroundings (Fig. 28-5). Background music interrupts the rhythmic monotony of ventilators cycling and monitors beeping and helps to relieve tension in both patients and staff.

Sitting in a chair frequently bolsters a patient's morale, and orientation is enhanced if eyeglasses, dentures, and hearing aids are returned to the patient as soon as practical. Combing the hair should not be overlooked. Long-term ventilator patients require activities and frequent stimulation. The family, volunteers, recreational therapists, and physical therapists should all be involved.

Weaning from Mechanical Ventilation

Modern respiratory care has demonstrated that the majority of patients appropriately committed to and maintained on mechanical ventilation readily tolerate its discontinuance when their disease process has been reversed. The criteria for weaning from mechanical ventilation are approximately the reciprocals of the indications for which ventilatory support was initiated. Since ventilatory support is primarily used for patients with profound gas transport abnormalities, its use may be discontinued only after therapy has been directed to correcting the pathophysiologic alteration. The ventilator does not cure; it is simply a temporary support system which "buys time" for correction of the underlying situation that precipitated its use in the first place. It is essential that other physiologic problems be minimized before the weaning process begins. Acid-base abnormalities, electrolyte imbalances, fever,

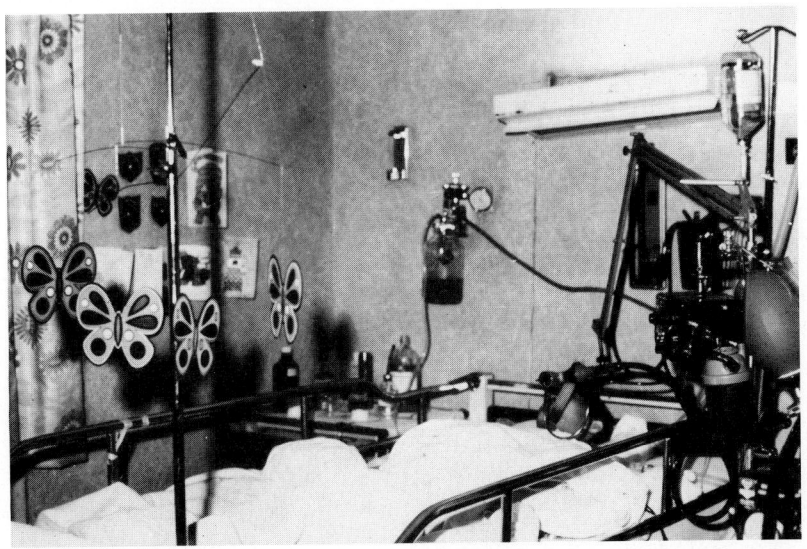

Figure 28-5 A familiar object brought from home, such as this child's butterfly mobile, will partially reduce the anxiety resulting from sudden exposure to strange surroundings.

anemia, infection, hypotension, arrhythmias, and nutritional problems should be corrected and stabilized prior to weaning. As in the discharge or transfer process, preparation for weaning should be implicit in the start of intubation and mechanical ventilation. Monitoring and correcting other problems during the course of therapy greatly facilitates the weaning process. Once it has been established that the patient is physiologically capable of independence from the ventilator, the weaning process should be directed toward the psychologic aspects of ventilator weaning.

Several physiologic tests have been established to serve as guidelines for determining the patient's readiness for ventilator discontinuance. These tests measure mechanical capabilities and effective oxygenation (Table 28-1).

With the patient who has been on mechanical ventilation for a short period of time (less than 36 h.), abrupt cessation of the ventilator may be successful. However, for the majority of patients requiring mechanical ventilation, the traditional T-piece method of weaning may be anxiety-producing and may actually prolong weaning. With the increased use of IMV, weaning time has been decreased with minimal psychologic and physiologic side effects. The purpose of IMV is to allow the patient's own breathing pattern to be maintained, but with positive-pressure breaths intermittently delivered by the ventilator; the positive-pressure breath is completely independent of the patient's own breathing pattern.

Prolonged ventilatory assistance leads to respiratory muscle weakness and markedly interferes with the patient's ability to breathe alone when disconnected from the ventilator. The incorporation of IMV as soon as it is clinically feasible (not when ventilator discontinuance is considered) is certain to decrease the time of ventilator support and the weaning process; and IMV allows a far more gradual transition from completely controlled ventilation to completely spontaneous ventilation.

One of the main advantages of IMV, particularly for patients with chronic airway obstruction, is that patients can adjust their own arterial carbon dioxide tension. Stabilization generally occurs at a higher tension than would have been provided with controlled ventilation.

Premature and unsuccessful attempts at weaning have adverse psychologic effects on the patient; therefore it is of utmost importance that the patient be both physically and psychologically prepared for ventilator discontinuation. When the ventilator is discontinued, the patient should be in a sitting position and humidified 40% oxygen should be readily available by mask.

When it is clinically advisable to remove the airway, the oropharynx and trachea should be suctioned and "bagged" with oxygen between suctioning attempts to prevent hypoxia. As the tracheal cuff is slowly deflated, the patient is given one big breath via the bag. As the tube is gently removed, the patient's automatic response is to either exhale forcibly or cough up any remaining secretions lodged in the vicinity of the cuff.

Following both ventilator discontinuation and airway removal, the patient should be observed for signs of respiratory insufficiency (increased respiratory rate, increased pulse, diaphoresis). Deep breathing and coughing exercises should be started immediately.

Complications of Mechanical Ventilation

Tracheal Tube Complications

Prolonged intubation may promote laryngeal trauma and massive gastric distention. Right main-stem intubation will produce alveolar hyperventilation,

Table 28-1 Weaning Parameters

Mechanical Tests	
Vital capacity	$\geq$10–15 mL per kilogram of body weight
Maximum inspiratory force	> -20 cmH$_2$O
FEV 1 s	>10 mL per kilogram of body weight
Minute ventilation (resting)	> 10 L/min
Tests of Oxygenation	
Pa$_{O_2}$	>60 torr on $\leq$0.4 Fl$_{O_2}$
Shunt	<15 percent
D(A-a)O$_2$ on 100% O$_2$	<300–350 torr
V$_D$/V$_T$	<0.6

atelectasis, and/or pneumothorax. Herniation of the cuff over the distal end of the tube causes airflow obstruction. Tracheal ischemia and necrosis are not as common today with the use of high-volume, low-pressure "floppy" cuffs. The intermittent deflation of these cuffs has no proven advantage in preventing mucosal necrosis. Any routine of inflation and deflation generally leads to careless reinflation and possibly higher cuff pressures. It is generally agreed that it would be optimal to have a high-volume cuff that could maintain an adequate seal at a resting tracheal mucosal pressure of 15 mmHg. The low-volume, high-pressure cuffs should *not* be used. The intraarterial pressure in blood vessels within the adult tracheal wall is approximately 30 mmHg, and the high-pressure cuffs are capable of exceeding pressures of 300 mmHg.

Ventilator Malfunctions

Some of the potentially serious ventilator malfunctions include mechanical breakdown, overheating of the inspired air, inadequate nebulization, and alarm failure. An extremely common error in the suctioning procedure is neglecting to turn the alarm system back on following suctioning. If a patient's tubing becomes disconnected while the alarm is shut off, the result can be catastrophic. A patient receiving continuous ventilatory support should never be left unattended. When the alarm sounds, it does not identify the nature of the problem but merely indicates that something is wrong. The patient should be immediately ventilated with a self-inflating bag (always available) until the situation can be corrected. If the patient can readily be ventilated without resistance, the problem is with the ventilator, tubing, or humidifier.

The excessive-pressure alarm usually indicates that the patient needs to be suctioned. A slow rise in the pressure required to deliver a constant volume may indicate decreasing pulmonary compliance (pulmonary edema due to fluid overload). A low-pressure alarm usually signifies a leak in the system. The most frequent site is the humidifier after it has been filled with sterile water and the lid has not been connected tightly. A segment of tubing may also be disconnected, particularly after the patient has been moved.

Nosocomial Infection

Patients requiring ventilatory support are often debilitated and have a lowered resistance to infection. Endotracheal tubes bypass the normal upper airway defense mechanisms. Aerosol therapy is a great source of nosocomial infection, because *Pseudomonas* and other gram-negative bacteria thrive in such hot, wet environments. For this reason, all parts of the ventilatory equipment that come in contact with the patient should be changed at least every 24 h. Meticulous attention to details of good respiratory care techniques, sterile procedures, and frequent hand washing will minimize the incidence of nosocomial infections. Sputum examination should be performed on a routine basis.

The intubated patient is no longer capable of warming and humidifying the inspired gas; therefore, heat and humidity must be continuously provided to the upper airway. The lack of humidity promotes drying and retention of secretions, which may obstruct airways and result in atelectasis and pneumonia.

Barotrauma

Barotrauma means injury as a result of pressure. Patients receiving continuous ventilatory support are subjected to high positive pressures in the lungs which may produce pneumothorax, pneumomediastinum, or subcutaneous emphysema. A common cause for pneumothorax is "ball-valving." This phenomenon occurs in an area of the lung that can accept air during inspiration but cannot expel it during expiration, because bronchial tubes are larger on inspiration and may close with expiration. As this sequence persists, air collects in this particular lung zone, pressure builds up, and rupture occurs. Pneumothorax in a patient receiving mechanical ventilation can be detected by an abrupt rise in peak-inspiratory pressure for the same tidal volume delivered. In patients with chronic airway obstruction, barotrauma frequently results from overdistention. It has been emphasized by some that there is no longer any place for the sigh in modern ventilatory management, except that a single manually activated sigh may be a useful physical therapy adjunct.

Hypotension

Positive-pressure ventilation can reduce cardiac output by decreasing venous return to the heart, particularly if the patient is hypovolemic. This adverse effect on venous return can be minimized if the expiratory phase is long enough to allow venous return during this period to compensate for the decrease that occurs during inspiration. An expiratory time that is 30 percent longer than inspiratory time will usually stabilize cardiovascular hemodynamics; however, marked hypotension may occur if the patient is hypovolemic or is receiving PEEP therapy.

Obviously, all complications cannot be prevented, but it is useful to wonder whether, if a specific complication can be successfully treated, it can also be prevented.

Bibliography

Carlon, G. C., & Klain, M. (Guest Eds.). (1984). Symposium issue: High frequency ventilation. *Crit. Care Med.* *12*(9).

Grosmaire, E. K. (1983). Use of patient positioning to improve Pa_{O_2}: A review. *Heart Lung, 12,* 650–653.

Kirby, R. R., Smith, R. A., & Desautels, D. A. (Eds.). (1985). *Mechanical ventilation.* New York: Churchill Livingstone.

Mackenzie, C. K., & Shin, B. (1985). Cardiorespiratory function before and after chest physiotherapy in mechanically ventilated patients in post-traumatic respiratory failure. *Crit. Care Med., 13,* 483–486.

Martz, K. V., Joiner, J. W., & Shepherd, R. M. (1984). *Management of the patient-ventilator system: A team approach* (2d ed). St Louis: Mosby.

part 6

Renal
Patient-Care
Problems

29

Renal Anatomy and Physiology

June L. Stark

Overview of Renal Anatomy

The kidneys are located retroperitoneally, with the upper border between T11 on the right and T12 on the left. This difference in position results from the natural displacement of the right kidney by the liver. The lower border is at approximately L3. Posteriorly, the kidney lies against the diaphragm. The kidneys are shaped like kidney beans and measure 10 to 12 cm in length, 5 to 6 cm in width, and 3 to 4 cm thick. They make up 0.4 to 0.5 percent of total body weight. The actual weight in grams can be slightly more in males than in females. A tough fibrous capsule covers the kidney and functions to limit the organ's size in edematous states.

The indentation in the side of the kidney is called the *hilus*. The hilus is the entrance site for the renal artery, lymphatics, and nerves. It also is the exit site for the renal vein, ureters, lymphatics, and nerves. The hilus leads into the renal sinus, an open space occupied mainly by the renal pelvis but containing also the major and minor calices. The renal capsule dips into the hilus and provides a protective covering for the renal sinus.

The kidney is a lobular organ; this appearance is obvious in the infant kidney. By the time a person reaches adulthood, the lobulation is usually no longer apparent. The two major layers of the kidney are the cortex and the medulla. The *cortex*, or outer layer, is normally reddish brown. The cortex receives approximately 80 percent of the kidney's blood supply and, therefore, is the site of aerobic metabolism. Positioned within the cortical region are parts of the nephron: the glomerulus and the proximal and distal tubules. On examination the outer portion of the cortex has a fine, consistent, granular appearance which is reflective of the random arrangement of the convoluted proximal

and distal tubules. The inner cortical area has a striated appearance due to the presence of the straight segments of the proximal and distal tubules plus the collecting duct and blood vessels.

The inner layer of the kidney is the *medulla*. This layer receives only 20 percent of the cardiac output and is involved in anaerobic metabolism. Contained within the medulla are the renal pyramids—fan-shaped structures which have a striated appearance created by the presence of the loops of Henle and the blood vessels. The pyramids are so positioned that their bases face the cortex and the apices, or papillae, point toward the renal pelvis. The bases of the pyramids form the corticomedullary junction, which is the point of division between the cortex and medulla. The pyramids are separated by the columns of Bertin. Each pyramid plus the surrounding cortical tissue constitutes a lobe.

At the terminal portions of the pyramids are 10 to 25 openings in which the collecting ducts merge. This area also marks the dividing point between the renal parenchyma and the major and minor calices and pelvis.

Renal Blood Supply

Renal blood flow is approximately 1200 mL/min, or 20 to 25 percent of the cardiac output. The kidneys receive this blood supply via a single renal artery. The renal artery branches off the abdominal aorta, entering the kidney at the hilus; upon reaching the hilus, it divides into two branches, which travel toward the dorsal and ventral regions of the kidney and become the interlobar arteries, which in turn follow a course through the medulla and the renal pyramids (Fig. 29-1). These arteries, upon reaching the corticomedullary junction, become the arcuate arteries. Branching into smaller vessels,

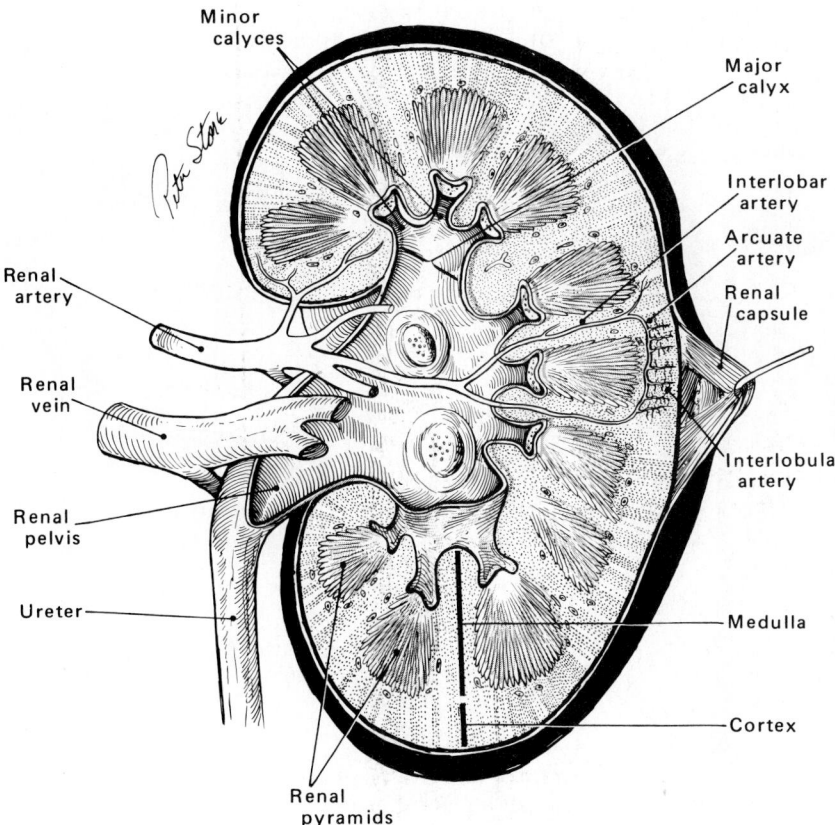

Minor calyces

Major calyx

Interlobar artery

Arcuate artery

Renal capsule

Renal artery

Renal vein

Interlobular artery

Renal pelvis

Ureter

Medulla

Cortex

Renal pyramids

Figure 29-1 A longitudinal section of the kidney showing a portion of the major arterial branches of the renal vasculature. (*From L. L. Langley, I. Telford, & J. Christensen, Dynamic Anatomy and Physiology, 5th ed., New York, McGraw-Hill, 1980.*)

the arcuate arteries eventually become the interlobar arteries, which flow through the cortical region to the outer borders of the kidney. Finally, the interlobar arteries form multiple afferent arterioles and supply the glomerulus of the nephrons (Fig. 29-2).

The glomeruli are drained by the efferent arteriole. The efferent arterioles empty the cortical nephrons and branch off into a capillary network which supplies blood flow to other tubules in that area. In the juxtamedullary glomeruli, the innermost portion of the cortex, the efferent arterioles flow into the vasa recta. It is the vasa recta that supply the tubules extending into the medullary region. The vasa recta twist and turn throughout the medulla and seem to turn back upon themselves as they follow a course which often parallels the vessel of origin.

The capillaries in the outer cortex eventually drain into the interlobar veins and empty together with the deep cortical vessels into the arcuate vein.

The renal venous system then completes its course by joining the renal vein as it leaves the kidney through the hilus.

The Nephron

The nephron is best described as the functional unit of the kidneys. One million nephrons, microscopic in size, are situated throughout the cortical and medullary layer of each kidney. The anatomic and physiologic composition of all the nephrons is essentially the same, each containing a glomerulus and tubules. The primary difference between nephrons is in their anatomic location. A majority of nephrons are positioned high in the cortical region; these are called *cortical nephrons*. These nephrons have short tubules. The nephrons positioned in the juxtamedullary region are called *juxtamedullary nephrons* and have large loops. The greater the length of the loops the greater is the sodium-reabsorbing ability of the tubule. The two types of

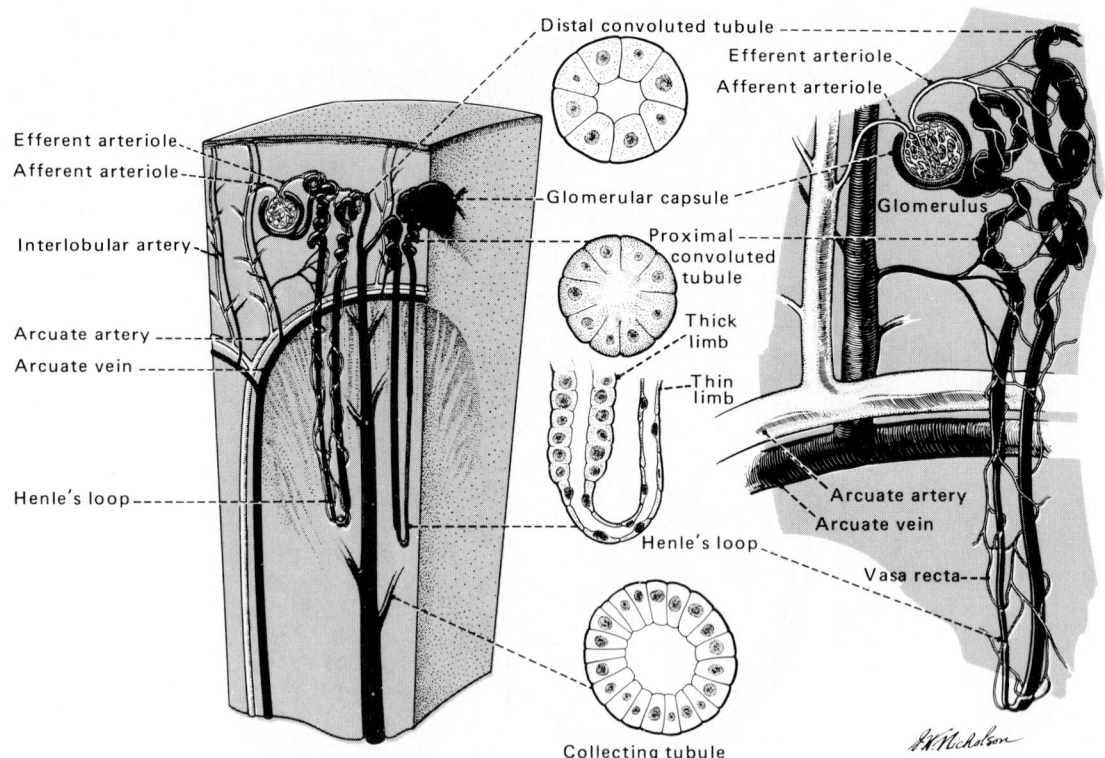

Figure 29-2 The nephron and its blood supply are shown at the sides of the figure and sections of different portions of the tubule in the center. (*From L. L. Langley, I. Telford, & J. Christensen, Dynamic Anatomy and Physiology, 5th ed., New York, McGraw-Hill, 1980.*)

nephron also differ in the sequence of their blood supply, as discussed in the preceding section (Fig. 29-2).

Glomerulus

The glomerulus, a capillary bed, arises directly from the afferent arteriole and is positioned in the glomerular capsule, or Bowman's capsule. The glomerular vessel is extremely narrow, promoting a high-pressure blood flow of 50 mmHg. The large surface area of the glomerular membranes, plus the membranes' normal semipermeability, is ideal for the passage of fluid and solute. Three cellular layers make up the glomerular membrane and contribute to its characteristic semipermeability. The innermost layer consists of endothelial cells and is followed by a middle layer of basement membrane and an outer layer of epithelial cells. The endothelial cells have fenestrations 500 to 1000 Å wide which favor the easy movement of water

and solute. The other two layers are less porous, having openings about 1500 Å thick.[1] The size of the basement membrane and epithelial pores may be one of the factors contributing to the filtration impedance of macromolecules. An additional factor determining the permeability of the glomerular membrane and the filtration capability of the molecules is the electrical charge of both membrane and molecules. The glomerular wall is negatively charged; therefore, a positive charge of a molecule will favor its passage. A negatively charged molecule such as albumin will be impeded by the negative charge found in the glomerular membrane. The loss of the normal charge of the glomerulus in disease may be a factor contributing to the proteinuria which sometimes occurs.[2] (See Fig. 29-3.)

Tubules

The tubules extend beyond Bowman's capsule. Four segments make up the tubules, each segment varying in cellular structure and function. Arising from the glomerulus is the proximal tubule. This first convoluted tubule travels in the area of its supplying glomerulus, then continues on to the cortex, pen-

etrating deeply and terminating in the outer medullary region. The entire length of the proximal tubule is composed of large epithelial cells with brush borders. The basement membrane of the

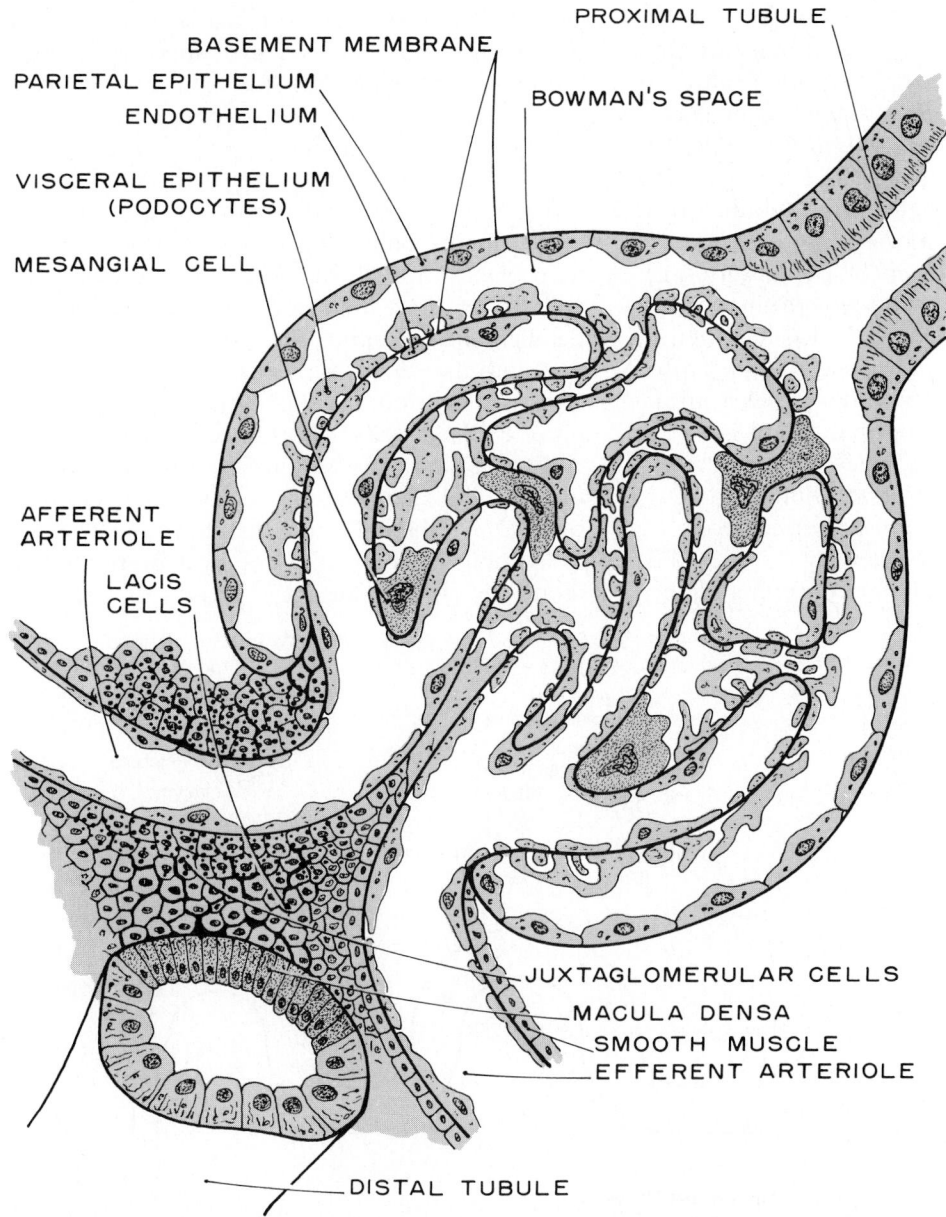

Figure 29-3   The renal corpuscle and the juxtaglomerular apparatus. The juxtaglomerular apparatus is composed of the macula densa, modified cells in the wall of the distal convoluted tubule, and the juxtaglomerular cells of the afferent arteriole near its entry point into the glomerulus. (*From S. A. Price & L. M. Wilson, Pathophysiology, New York, McGraw-Hill, 1978.*)

proximal tubule surrounds the structure in a systematic manner. The main function of this segment is reabsorption (Fig. 29-4).

At the termination site of the proximal tubule in the renal medulla, the loop of Henle begins. The loop of Henle, a U-shaped structure, has two physiologically distinct parts: the descending loop and the ascending loop. Squamous cells line the descending portion and provide the loop with its characteristic thin wall. Plasma membranes curve and are interspersed between the limb's epithelial cells. The ascending limb has cuboidal cells which increase gradually the height of the tubule.[3] The surface of this limb lacks a brush border.

The length of the loop of Henle varies in relation to the position of the glomerulus in the cortex. Nephrons with glomeruli located in the outer region of the cortex have short loops; those near the cortical-medullary border or in a juxtamedullary position have longer loops. In general, all loop sizes, short or long, when compared with one another, vary in length in the human kidney. However, the total number of shorter loops is greater than that of larger loops by 7 to 1.[4] The loop of Henle is responsible for concentrating the urine.

Next, the distal tubule is formed as the ascending loop surfaces at the cortex. This segment has both cuboidal and columnar cells. In the region forming the macula densa, the cells are tall and set close together. The distal tubule is shorter than the proximal tubule and not as convoluted; like the proximal tubule, it lacks a brush border, but it differs in other characteristics such as a larger number of mitochondria. This segment is involved with sodium and water reabsorption plus hydrogen and potassium secretion.

In the outer cortex, the collecting duct is formed as the terminal portion of two or more distal tubules joining together. The collecting duct then passes through the medulla, where it unites with other ducts to form a papillary duct. The papillary duct empties into the minor calix and then into the remaining urinary collecting system. The collecting duct is slightly granular and made up of cuboidal cells. It was once believed that the collecting duct was simply an extension of the urinary drainage system; however, current data indicate that the collecting duct functions with the distal tubule and is influenced by antidiuretic hormone and aldosterone.

Figure 29-4 Transport of water and some solutes in the proximal renal tubule. The composition of glomerular filtrate is indicated. (*From D. Maude, Kidney Physiology and Kidney Disease: An Introduction to Nephrology, Philadelphia, Lippincott, 1977.*)

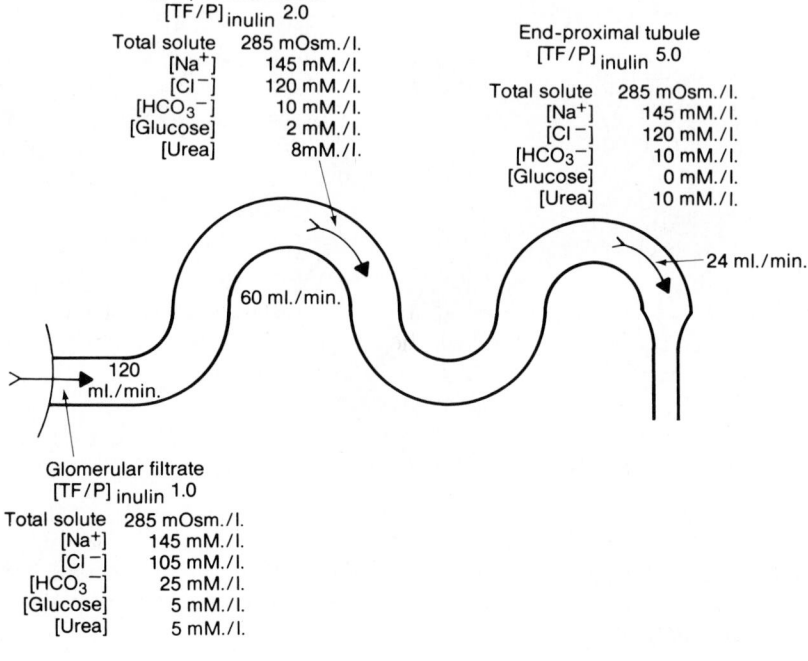

Dynamics of Fluid and Electrolyte Movement in the Nephron

A variety of processes are involved in the transfer of solute and solvent across the nephron membranes. Movement from the glomerulus to the tubules is determined by the difference in the favoring force, namely, hydrostatic pressure, and the operating forces of colloid osmotic and renal interstitial pressures. In addition, the semipermeability of the glomerular membrane favors passage. The tubular processes of transfer incorporate methods to ensure the ability to absorb, secrete, or excrete a molecule. These transfer methods may involve osmosis, passive diffusion, or active reabsorptive mechanisms.

Osmosis

Osmosis is the passive movement of water through a permeable membrane from an area of low solute concentration to an area of high solute concentration. The osmotic movement of water across the walls of the renal tubules results from prior transfer of solutes and the resulting establishment of an osmotic gradient. No active transport of water is known to occur in the kidney.

The rate of water transfer across the tubular epithelium depends on the permeability of the tubule to water and the magnitude of the osmotic gradient. With the exception of the ascending limb of the loop of Henle, the renal tubule is permeable to water throughout its length. However, the degree of water permeability of the distal tubules and collecting duct varies according to the level of antidiuretic hormone (ADH) in the blood. ADH is a hormone synthesized by specialized hypothalmic neurosecretory cells and then stored in and released from the posterior pituitary gland, or neurohypophysis. This hormone increases the permeability of the distal and collecting tubular cells to water. While ADH exerts an important effect on the distal portion of the nephron, the permeability of the proximal tubule and the loop of Henle appears to be independent of this hormone.

Osmotic forces can also act to hold increased quantities of water in the tubules and produce diuresis. For example, when large amounts of solutes such as mannitol, glucose, or any other osmotically active solute remain in tubular fluid, water is held in the tubules and an increased volume of urine is produced.

Diffusion

A few substances other than water passively diffuse from tubular fluid into the interstitial spaces of the renal parenchyma and then into the circulation. Passive diffusion occurs without the expenditure of metabolic energy, because in this type of material transfer substances move along a concentration and/or electrical gradient. Substances that carry no net electrical charge, such as glucose, will move through a freely permeable membrane along a concentration gradient from a solution that is highly concentrated to one in which the concentration is lower. However, epithelial renal tubular cells are not freely permeable to all substances, and additional factors must be considered.

When considering the transfer of ions (charged particles), both concentration and electrical gradients must be taken into account. As with neutral molecules, ions diffuse from a region of high concentration to one of lower concentration. In addition, they move along an electrical gradient. Positive ions such as sodium passively migrate from a positively charged compartment to a more negative one. Likewise, negative chloride ions move along an electrical gradient from negative to positive. When concentration and electrical gradient are oriented in opposite directions, net ionic movement will be in the direction of the larger gradient. If, however, both gradients are similarly oriented, the net gradient reflects the sum of the forces.

Active Transport

Active transport implies movement of a material against concentration and/or electrical gradients, requiring the expenditure of energy derived from cellular metabolism. Sodium is the most important substance actively transported by the kidney. Quantitatively, more sodium is actively transported (about 20,000 meq per day) than any other ionic solute. Consequently, much of the energy expended by cells of the kidneys is for sodium transport. Active transport of sodium produces important secondary results as well. Certain substances, such as chloride ions, water, and urea, said to be passively transported, actually "tag along" on the energy released from the active transport of sodium. As sodium ions are transferred from tubular fluid, the interstitial fluid becomes increasingly positive as these ions accumulate on the peritubular side of the nephron.

This electrical gradient then favors passive reabsorption of negative chloride ions. The transfer of sodium chloride out of tubular fluid creates an osmotic gradient directed from tubular to interstitial fluid which decreases the passive reabsorption of water. As water is reabsorbed, the tubular concentration of urea increases and establishes a concentration gradient for the passive reabsorption of this material. Therefore, sodium transport has consequences that extend beyond the conservation of this important ion.

The energy spent on active transport apparently is from high-energy phosphate bonds in adenosine triphosphate (ATP) and similar compounds. Energy for active transport is released when the terminal phosphate is split from ATP to form inorganic phosphate and the lower-energy compound adenosine diphosphate (ADP). New stores of ATP are generated by the metabolic processes of glycolysis and oxidative phosphorylation. Oxidative phosphorylation, a more rewarding process in terms of energy yield, requires oxygen and can be inhibited by a number of metabolic inhibitors such as cyanide and dinitrophenol. Since so much of the kidneys' metabolic energy is expended on active sodium transport, it follows that renal oxygen consumption is proportional to sodium reabsorption. When renal perfusion decreases and less sodium than normal is filtered and presented to the tubular cells for reabsorption, renal oxygen consumption also decreases.

Many cells (notably nerve and muscle) other than those of the kidney actively transport materials. While many cells actively extrude sodium ions across the entire surface of the cell membrane and are, therefore, nondirectional, or radial, in their transport characteristics, renal epithelial cells are directional, or polar. This means that the mechanism for active transport is located on only one side of the cell. Recall that the task of renal cells is to reabsorb most (about 99 percent) of the sodium ions filtered from the blood. Therefore, the flow of sodium is from tubular fluid that bathes one side of the epithelial cellular layer of the tubules to the opposite, or interstitial, side.

The mechanism for providing this energy and extruding sodium ions against an electrochemical gradient appears to be located on the peritubular side of the renal epithelial cells. Thus, renal tubular cells are unidirectional in the sense that active extrusion of sodium does not occur over the entire surface of the cells but rather is localized to the interstitial side. Obviously, if renal cells extruded sodium back into the tubular fluid as fast as it entered the cells, net sodium reabsorption could never be accomplished and the body's sodium supply would be excreted into the urine in short order.

Maximal Transport Capacity

Maximal transport capacity involves an active mechanism that allows the tubules to reabsorb certain substances in a fixed or limited amount. If the total amount of these substances exceeds this limit, the excess remains in the tubular space and is excreted in the urine. Glucose is a prime example, although maximal transport capacity can also affect the reabsorption of such substances as phosphate, vitamin C, amino acids, and sulfate.

Urine Formation

The kidney, in conjunction with hormones such as ADH and aldosterone, regulates fluid and electrolyte balance through the formation of urine. During this process of making urine, water and solutes are reabsorbed, secreted, or excreted according to the body's requirements. The unit primarily involved in this renal activity is the nephron.

Glomerular Filtration

The initial step in the formation of urine is glomerular filtration. While filtration is a passive process per se, it is dependent on physiologic processes such as adequate renal blood flow and the normal permeability of the glomerular membranes. The urine-making process begins when blood propelled by the force of the heart enters the glomerular capillaries via the afferent arteriole. The pressure of the blood in the afferent arteriole is 70 mmHg, but once the blood is inside the glomerulus, it stabilizes at 50 mmHg. This glomerular pressure force determined by cardiac functions favors the passage of ultrafiltrate. The ultrafiltrate is the fluid which passes under high pressure from the glomerular space to Bowman's capsule and onto the tubules. In addition, two forces oppose the formation of filtrate. The first force is the colloid osmotic pressure of 25 mmHg—the pressure exerted by the plasma proteins found in the glomerular blood supply. The second opposing force is the Bowman's capsule pressure of 10 mmHg, created by the tissue surrounding the glomerulus. Subtracting the factors opposing filtration from the capillary pressure shows a net filtration pressure of 15 mmHg:

Factor	Pressure (mmHg)
Capillary hydrostatic pressure	+50
Colloid osmotic pressure	−25
Bowman's capsule pressure	−10
Net filtration pressure	+15

The positive force of the net pressure encourages the fluid and solute to move across the glomerular membrane. The membrane, as mentioned earlier, has a pore size which permits the movement of water and most solute found in blood. Therefore, the filtrate contains glucose, sodium, some amino acids, and metabolic wastes (to name a few) in the same concentration found in plasma. However, the pore size restricts the movement of macromolecules such as plasma proteins, erythrocytes, white cells, and platelets. Normal filtrate as determined by membrane permeability is similar to plasma with the same specific gravity of 1.010 but is free of proteins and red blood cells.

In addition to filtration, the diffusion tendency and the electrochemical potential of an ion are also believed to be responsible for the composition of the filtrate. A portion of the glomerular membrane is composed of a gel. Water and solute diffuse easily in this substance, while the diffusibility of the larger molecule is limited or impeded. The electrochemical potential of an ion is also enhanced by an increase in the hydrostatic pressure.[5]

Tubular Processes

The tubules determine, by the processes of reabsorption, secretion, and excretion, the composition and, therefore, the concentration of the urine. This ability to precisely regulate the character of urine assures that despite wide variation in daily water and solute intake, the kidney is able to maintain internal fluids at a homeostatic volume, osmolality, and concentration. The tubules receive the plasmalike filtrate from the glomerulus. The filtrate then moves through all tubular segments, traversing the specific cell walls. The specificity of the cell walls, as previously discussed, determines the kind and degree of exchange which can take place.

The basic tubular cell is the epithelial cell; this cell type encourages transcellular transport by the properties of its membrane and its selective polarization. Between the cells are the lateral intercellular spaces and the "tight junction," which is the limited or narrow junction between a section of the cell and the intercellular space. These two anatomic structures also play a role in transport, for substances able to permeate these spaces can bypass cellular transport and move between adjoining cells. Passive ion transport uses the paracellular pathway as the major route for passage. The same principles determine solute movement in the kidney as in other organs; however, the nephron has certain limitations not found elsewhere, including its geometric shape and the relation of the small amount of filtrate to the large surface area of the nephron.[6] As a result, significant alteration can occur in the filtrate despite the short distance it travels along the renal tubules.

The urine formation process starts in the tubules, as the 125 mL of glomerular filtrate enters into the proximal tubule. At this site, 60 to 80 percent of the essential water and solutes such as glucose, phosphate, potassium, proteins, and urine acid is reabsorbed. The proximal tubule also contributes to the acid-base balance by the secretion of hydrogen ions and the preservation of bicarbonate. Its main function, however, is the maximal reabsorption of sodium chloride and water.

The specific handling of sodium by the proximal tubule requires several processes. The sodium, once moved into the luminal fluid, requires energy to move into the peritubular fluid. The energy source is Na/K-ATPase. As sodium is mobilized, other ions such as glucose and phosphate "tag along," so the energy expended for sodium transport is extended to include accompanying ions.

The contribution of the proximal tubule to acid-base regulation involves another method of sodium absorption. The reabsorption of bicarbonate promotes sodium chloride reabsorption. In addition, for every ion of hydrogen secreted in this portion of the tubule, a sodium ion is reabsorbed. Aldosterone and vasopressin are believed to have no effect in the proximal tubule. However, another hormonal effect, called the *third factor,* is believed to play a role in the regulation of sodium. This factor has not yet been identified. Lastly, a decrease in the plasma oncotic pressure participates in the movement of sodium and water into the renal interstitium. Eventually, the expansion of this space enhances the diffusion of sodium into the tubular lumen and the excretion of this ion.

After leaving the proximal tubule, the filtrate enters the loop of Henle. The loop has two segments, a descending and an ascending portion, each with separate functions in altering the filtrate. The descending loop, the thin limb, is permeable only to water, while the ascending portion, the thick limb, has an active sodium chloride (NaCL) pump and is impermeable to water. The working combination of the two segments determines the concentration or osmolality of urine from concentrated to dilute. Urine osmolality can be adjusted within a wide range from 50 to 1200 mosm/L. Another major function of the loop of Henle is the maintenance of hyperosmolar concentration in the renal medulla. These two functions, determining urine concentration and maintaining a hypertonic renal interstitium, are accomplished by the countercurrent mechanism. This mechanism is possible because of the anatomic positioning of the long descending and ascending loops in relation to the peritubular capillaries of the vasa recta. The loops act as concurrent multipliers and the capillaries as countercurrent exchanges. An isotonic glomerular filtrate of 300 mosm/L leaves the proximal tubule and enters the descending loop of the Henle. Permeable only to water, this loop assures that water is gradually drawn into a hypertonic medullary interstitium. The loss of water from the filtrate causes an increase in the osmolality. At the hairpin turn of the loop, the filtrate osmolality is dramatically increased, contributing concurrently to the formation of a hypotonic medullary interstitium. A portion of the sodium chloride is lost as the filtrate

progresses to the ascending limb of the loop of Henle. The medullary interstitium becomes more hypertonic again as its sodium concentration is increased by the pumping action at the ascending limb.[7]

A dilute filtrate reaches the distal tubule. In the distal tubule, the filtrate is altered by the presence or absence of ADH. The presence of ADH results in the formation of a concentrated urine; the absence of ADH produces the opposite effect, as dilute filtrate is excreted unchanged, creating a dilute urine with water excretion in excess of solute.

Aldosterone, a mineralocorticoid secreted from the zona glomerulosa of the adrenal cortex, acts on the distal tubule to promote sodium reabsorption. This hormone plays an additional role: its presence results in the reabsorption of sodium and the secretion of potassium, and its absence leads to the secretion of sodium and reabsorption of potassium. The factors regulating aldosterone secretion are (1) the total amount of body sodium, (2) the elevation of extracellular potassium ions, (3) the renin-angiotensin-aldosterone mechanism, and (4) the presence of adrenocorticotropic hormone.

Active regulation of the acid-base balance occurs in the distal tubule. Hydrogen ions are again secreted into the distal segment in exchange for sodium ions. These acids are then buffered by ammonia before excretion in order to avoid lowering the urinary pH to dangerous levels.

The character of the urine entering the collecting duct is a direct reflection of the state of hydration. In an adequately hydrated person, an ample amount of hypotonic filtrate is presented to the collecting duct. In addition, an antidiuretic hormone which also acts on this component of the tubule is suppressed and diuresis results.

During dehydration, ADH is secreted, increased amounts of water are absorbed, and a hypertonic urine is produced. Other secretory processes occurring in the collecting duct involve the loss of hydrogen ions and ammonia and sodium reabsorption.

To summarize, sodium and water can be reabsorbed throughout the entire tubule (allowing for the specificity of the two segments of the loop of Henle). Acid-base regulation takes place primarily in the proximal and distal tubules, with hydrogen being secreted at both sites and bicarbonate being reabsorbed only at the proximal tubule. Additionally, some hydrogen is secreted along with ammonia at the collecting duct, and potassium is secreted at the proximal and distal tubule and at the collecting duct.

Normal Renal Functions

Six normal renal functions are described in this section: the kidney contributes to homeostasis by regulation of fluid, electrolyte balance, acid-base balance, and excretion of waste products; and as a hormonal organ, it secretes erythropoietin and renin, metabolically activates vitamin D, and regulates blood pressure.

Water Regulation

The regulation of body water is accomplished via the thirst-neurohypophyseal-renal mechanism, which ensures that intake matches output. The water regulatory mechanism functions generally by stimulating the thirst mechanism to promote water intake and adjusting urinary volumes by the presence or absence of ADH and renal control.

ADH, the metabolic component of the mechanism, is synthesized in the ventromedian nucleus of the hypothalmus by specialized nerve cells. Once formed, this hormone travels down the supraoptic tracts, where it is stored in the posterior pituitary. Upon release from the posterior pituitary it travels to the distal tubule and collecting duct of the nephron. In the presence of ADH the tubular cells, in the areas identified, become highly permeable to water; thus ADH enhances water reabsorption at the terminal portions of the tubules.

The thirst center is located in the region where ADH is synthesized. The neuronal cells located at the lateral preoptic portion of the hypothalmus regulate the water intake. Despite the close proximity of the sites for ADH release and for thirst, a lesion in one area rarely affects the other; damage to ADH secretion thus often leaves the thirst mechanism intact.[8] It should be noted that in a dehydrated state the kidney can only conserve water, whereas the thirst mechanism can actively add water to the body.

An increase in plasma osmolality is the major stimulus for ADH release and the interaction of the thirst mechanism. This stimulus is so sensitive that a change in extracellular osmolality of only 1 to 2 percent will initiate a response. These changes in plasma osmolality are sensed by the osmoreceptor cells found in a distinct and separate area in the hypothalmus. The physiologic goal of ADH release is the maintenance of a normal plasma osmolality between 280 and 295 mosm/L. A serum osmolality below 280 mosm/L results in the suppression of both ADH and the thirst mechanism. The urinary response is the excretion of a maximally dilute urine. The opposite occurs as the serum osmolality climbs above 280 mosm/L. At this level increasing increments of ADH are released, up to its maximum secretion at a serum osmolality of 295 mosm/L. The renal response results in the production of an extremely concentrated urine through the reabsorption of a solute-free water. In addition, the thirst mechanism is also stimulated and, in combination with the renal response, attempts to restore a normal osmolality.

Another mechanism for ADH release is located at the stretch receptors of the carotid bodies and aorta. These sites are sensitive to changes in circulating blood volume and/or pressure. A decrease in blood volume of 7 to 15 percent, along with an increase in osmolality, is thought to stimulate ADH release.[9] As water is reabsorbed and blood volume increases, there is a further decline in ADH release. Therefore, ADH is considered to be a mechanism for protecting both the volume and the osmolality of extracellular fluid. The preservation of adequate volume takes precedence over maintaining normal osmolality; in the face of diminished circulating blood volume, water continues to be reabsorbed despite a hypotonic serum. Other nonosmotic factors which stimulate ADH release are hypoxia, pain, and stress.

The primary renal control of water balance involves two mechanisms, the countercurrent mechanism and the glomerular-tubular balance. The countercurrent mechanism was described earlier in this chapter as the renal mechanism for providing normal urinary dilution and concentration. Glomerular-tubular balance involves the phenomenon by which the amount of fluid the tubules receive via glomerular filtration is related to the amount of fluid reabsorbed or excreted by the tubules. During hypovolemia or hypotension, a decreased glomerular blood flow results in a decline in the glomerular filtration rate (GFR). The tubules respond to the decreased filtration volume by reabsorbing salt and water, thereby decreasing the amount of urine output. In this manner the kidney conserves an already diminished volume. The opposite occurs when the GFR increases, as it does in an expanded-volume situation or after the use of osmotic diuretics. In this situation, the tubules respond to the increased flow rate by allowing the production and output of large volumes of urine, thereby losing the excess fluid via renal pathways. Both glomerular-tubular responses attempt to compensate for disturbed fluid balance or to return fluid status to normal.

Electrolyte Balance

Enormous quantities of electrolytes are filtered by the kidney each day; yet only a minute fraction is actually excreted into the urine, and even that small fraction, especially in the case of sodium, is negligible. In a state of equilibrium, the amount of electrolyte excreted each day through all routes equals the amount acquired. For example, if the losses of sodium in sweat and by the intestinal route are not elevated, most of the daily intake is excreted in the urine; however, if the extrarenal losses of this ion are increased through excessive perspiration or diarrhea, renal excretion is proportionately reduced. Thus, the renal system plays a crucial role in electrolyte balance of the body fluids.

The kidneys seem best adapted for sodium regulation. Several factors, including renal perfusion, aldosterone level, and a suspected natriuretic, or third factor, are physiologic determinants of renal sodium excretion. Iatrogenic or pathophysiologic influences such as diuretics, nonreabsorbable anions in the filtrate, and intrinsic renal abnormalities also determine the balance between sodium intake and excretion. Potassium balance is also influenced by renal mechanisms, but the kidneys seem to be less sensitive to potassium balance than to sodium equilibrium.

Under normal conditions, renal perfusion and aldosterone levels are closely allied as influences

on perfusion diminish GFR. As a result, a decreased renal perfusion and an elevated aldosterone level support an increase in sodium reabsorption and excretion. Diminished renal perfusion decreases GFR, and as a result, several factors are found to support increased sodium reabsorption. First, a lowered flow rate through the tubules allows for more complete reabsorption of sodium by the active mechanism of the renal epithelial cells. Second, decreased renal blood flow results in an increased filtration fraction. Since a greater than normal fraction of the plasma perfusing the kidneys is filtered, the protein concentration of plasma leaving the glomerular capillaries and entering the postglomerular peritubular vessels is increased. The elevated oncotic pressure of peritubular plasma increases the attraction for water from tubular to peritubular fluid. Increased water reabsorption contributes to increasing tubular sodium concentration and the concentration gradient promoting its recovery. Third, decreased renal perfusion stimulates renin release from the juxtaglomerular cells of the afferent arteriole. Through the renin-angiotensin system, aldosterone secretion increases. Elevated aldosterone levels not only increase renal reabsorption of sodium, especially in the distal portion of the nephron, but also stimulate intestinal reabsorption of this ion. Thus, the effects of increased aldosterone secretion, initiated in the kidney, extend beyond the renal realm.

A natriuretic factor has yet to be isolated, but empiric evidence for such a factor and its influence on renal sodium regulation is strong. This third factor is invoked to explain the observation that increased plasma volume and hence renal perfusion stimulates sodium excretion, regardless of plasma sodium concentration. It is speculated that when plasma volume is low the level of this factor is also low, and sodium excretion diminishes. Such a mechanism would seem beneficial, in that as sodium reabsorption increases so does water reabsorption, and plasma volume is replenished. On the other hand, extracellular volume overload increases sodium excretion and decreases plasma volume. It is believed that the natriuretic factor serves to maintain plasma volume rather than plasma osmolality.

The kidneys are the primary regulators of body potassium balance, with the exception of a small amount of dietary potassium lost in the stool. In this regulatory role, the kidneys have the ability to adjust the body to wide variations in the quantity of dietary potassium. The usual western diet yields approximately 55 to 70 meq of potassium per day. This amount is first filtered and then excreted in the urine. Dietary ingestion of a large quantity of potassium (600 meq per day) can be followed by excretion of as much as ten times that amount. Conservation of potassium is also possible, but it is not as effective as sodium conservation.

Potassium excretion is influenced by a number of factors: dietary intake, high tubular flow state, aldosterone, renal sodium load, acid-base balance, and renal ammonia production. In addition, there is a diurnal pattern of potassium excretion which peaks at noon. Despite this explanation for potassium regulation at the renal site, data suggest that there is a more precise mechanism for the regulation of this ion.

Acid-Base Regulation

The kidneys share the major responsibility for acid-base regulation with the lungs, while the body's buffer system plays a minor role. From a quantitative point of view, the lungs predominate in excreting acid metabolites, but this in no way diminishes the importance of the renal contribution. Approximately 15,000 mmol of carbon dioxide is added to the body each day by cellular processes. Carbon dioxide is a unique acid in that it is volatile and is a gas amenable to excretion, in its natural form, through the lungs. While carbon dioxide does not contain hydrogen, it has an acid-forming potential and is converted to an acid when hydrated or combined with water. This reaction occurs under the influence of carbonic anhydrase (CA) as follows:

$$CO_2 + H_2O \xrightarrow{\quad CA \quad} H_2CO_3$$

The carbon dioxide molecule in the form of carbonic acid can be excreted by the kidney.

Not all the acidic products of cellular metabolism are volatile and acceptable for pulmonary excretion. Some are fixed acids that can only be excreted in solution, and this is where the kidneys contribute to acid-base balance. Fixed acids amount to about 50 to 100 mmol of hydrogen ions per day and can only be excreted through the kidneys. If the fixed and volatile acids were not excreted at the same rate at which they were produced, the body would experience an excess acid load. Thus, there is a cooperative effort between the lungs and the kidneys in maintaining the normal arterial pH of 7.35 to 7.45.

The various body buffers represent the "front-line troops" in the protection of pH. In general, the buffers combine with free hydrogen ions to prevent the acid concentration from increasing to dangerous levels and thus minimize any dramatic shift in pH. This is necessary because cell functioning and enzyme systems can tolerate only very small fluctuations in hydrogen ion concentration, reflected by a change in the pH of body fluids. Examples of important body buffers are bicarbonate (HCO_3) and carbonate acid ($H_2CO_3^-$).

The kidneys regulate acid-base balance by three mechanisms: the secretion of hydrogen ions, the reabsorption and generation of bicarbonate, and the production of ammonia. The nephron site for acid-base balance is located in the proximal and distal tubules. Approximately 80 to 90 percent of the bicarbonate is reabsorbed with sodium in the proximal tubule, but the process is completed in the distal tubule. Sodium bicarbonate is reabsorbed by exchanging with hydrogen ions secreted into the tubule. The hydrogen combines with bicarbonate to form CO_2. The CO_2 diffuses into the cell and is rehydrated to generate hydrogen and bicarbonate. At this point, hydrogen is rediffused into the tubular cell in exchange for the reabsorption of a sodium and a bicarbonate molecule. Approximately 60 percent of the reabsorbed bicarbonate is dependent on the presence of carbonic acid. Therefore, the use of a carbonic anhydrase inhibitor can lead to the excretion of alkaline urine and the creation of a metabolic acidosis.

The passive secretion of hydrogen occurs in the proximal tubules, and the active secretion occurs distally in exchange for sodium ions. Secreted hydrogen, in order to be excreted in the urine, must either be buffered or react with filtered ammonia. A variety of buffers are found in the filtrate, such as inorganic phosphate (HPO_4).

$$H^+ + HPO_4 \longrightarrow H_2PO_4$$

Ammonia (NH_3) is synthesized in the tubular cells by glutamine deamination associated with the presence of glutaminase. Once formed, the ammonia is diffused into the tubular filtrate, where it joins with a hydrogen ion to create an ammonium ion (NH_4).

$$NH_3 + H^+ \rightleftharpoons NH_4^+$$

Ammonium is excreted in the urine and accounts for more than half the secreted hydrogen ions. These buffers or uptake mechanisms interact with the hydrogen to shift the tubular filtrate pH to a less acidic reading. Control of urinary pH is essential, since a very acidic excreted urine could damage the urinary tract tissue. The pH of urine is usually 6.0; however, it may range from 4 to 8. This variation in pH occurs in response to the acid-base regulating needs of the body.

The generation or synthesis of bicarbonate occurs in the cells of the distal tubule. Carbon dioxide, either derived from cellular metabolism or obtained from venous blood, is hydrated to form carbonic acid.

$$H_2O + CO_2 \overset{CA}{\rightleftharpoons} H_2CO_3$$

Carbonic acid in the presence of carbonic anhydrase forms a hydrogen and bicarbonate ion.

$$H_2CO_3 \overset{CA}{\rightleftharpoons} H^+ + HCO_3$$

Simply, the bicarbonate is reabsorbed and the hydrogen is secreted in the urine. The complete equation is:

$$H_2O + CO_2 \overset{CA}{\rightleftharpoons} H_2CO_3 \overset{CA}{\rightleftharpoons} H^+ + HCO_3$$

The renal response to acidemia is to increase the hydrogen ion secretion at the distal tubule in association with an increase in excretion of titratable acids (HPO_{4-2}). In the proximal tubule, all the bicarbonate is absorbed. Lastly, to accommodate the need for an increase in hydrogen ion excretion, ammonia production is increased. The urinary pH may be as low as 4.4, which reflects excretion of the excess acid load.

In alkalemia, decreased hydrogen ion secretion in the distal nephron is accompanied by excess bicarbonate excretion. The measured amount of ammonia production is diminished, while the arterial pH climbs above 7.0.

Secretion of Erythropoietin

Erythropoietin is the hormonal stimulus necessary for the production and maintenance of new erythrocytes. The source of erythropoietin factor is renal tissue; however, the exact cellular source of this hormone has not been identified, although the stimulus for its release has been established as a decrease in renal oxygen supply. The specific stimulus may be hypoxia, anemia, or hypotension.[10] Upon release, erythropoietin acts on bone marrow to enhance the production of erythrocytes.

Activation of Vitamin D

The antirachitic properties of vitamin D are well known and have been recognized for many years, but certain characteristics of its biochemical transformation into an active form have been identified more recently. Vitamin D is a sterol found in plants and animals. The relatively inactive product of plants is ergosterol and that of animal tissue is 7-dehydrocholesterol. Under the influence of ultraviolet radiation, ergosterol is converted to calciferol (vitamin D_2) and 7-dehydrocholesterol is converted to cholecalciferol (vitamin D_3). Within the microsomes of liver cells, vitamin D_3 is converted to the metabolite 25-hydroxycholecalciferol (25-hydroxyvitamin D_3). Some of the 25-hydroxyvitamin D_3 circulating in blood is taken up by the kidneys and hydroxylated to 1,25-dihydroxycholecalciferol, or 1,25-dihydroxyvitamin D_3, which is the active form of the vitamin. The kidneys secrete 1,25-dihydroxyvitamin D_3 into the blood, and it is carried to the intestine, where it stimulates calcium absorption, and to the bones, where it promotes calcium mobilization.

The role of the kidneys in producing 1,25-dihydroxyvitamin D_3 has been compared to the endocrine role of the adrenal cortex. Both organs modify a blood-borne steroid into active hormones. The adrenal cortex extracts cholesterol from the plasma, transforms it into the various corticosteroids, and releases these active products back into the blood to be carried to their various target organs. The kidneys extract the steroid vitamin 25-

hydroxyvitamin D_3, convert it to 1,25-dihydroxyvitamin D_3, and release the product into the blood. Within intestinal mucosal cells, 1,25-dihydroxyvitamin D_3 stimulates production of a calcium-binding protein that has been implicated in calcium reabsorption.

The role of vitamin D metabolites in mineral metabolism of the body is complex and shared by other factors such as parathyroid hormone. There are still unanswered questions about mineral metabolism and all aspects of vitamin D metabolites in this homeostatic process, but the action of the kidneys in producing a hormone that participates in regulating calcium levels of the body is clear.[11]

Regulation of Blood Pressure

The kidneys assist regulation of the blood pressure by three major mechanisms: sodium and water regulation, angiotensin action, and renal prostaglandin secretion. The first regulatory function is accomplished by maintenance of the volume and composition of extracellular fluid, which is necessary because any alteration in plasma volume can impact on the cardiac output and systemic blood pressure. For example, a reduction of plasma volume decreases blood pressure, and expansion of plasma volume elevates blood pressure.

The renin-angiotensin-aldosterone system is a regulatory mechanism which functions to maintain systemic blood pressure and to protect against serious volume losses. The juxtaglomerular apparatus, the site responsible for renin storage and release, is made up of the juxtaglomerular granular cells and the macula densa. The juxtaglomerular cells are found within the afferent arteriole, positioned adjacent to the glomerulus; the macula densa is created by the distal tubule as it doubles back to join with the juxtaglomerular cells.

Three sources of stimulation are believed to trigger the renin-angiotensin mechanism: hypotension, hypovolemia, and hyponatremia. Other stimuli for renin release are life stressors and position change, such as moving from a lying to a sitting position. The renal center for sensing volume and pressure is located within the juxtaglomerular apparatus, and the sodium sensors are found in the macula densa. Renin, which upon release begins

the process, is stored in the juxtaglomerular cells. The site of renin's actual production is not known; however, the kidneys are believed to be responsible for its production.

Once stimulated, the juxtaglomerular cells release renin into the circulation. Renin acts on angiotensinogen, a plasma-borne substrate synthesized by the liver, by completing a proteolytic cleavage. The product of angiotensinogen cleavage is a vasoactive peptide called *angiotensin I*. Angiotensin I is converted to angiotensin II by a converting enzyme. Lung tissue is especially rich in the converting enzyme, and most of the conversion of angiotensin I occurs there. However, it has recently been determined that the conversion process may also take place in renal and liver tissue as well as in vessel walls.

Angiotensin II, once formed, is the active component of the renin mechanism. Angiotensin II functions as a potent peripheral vasoconstrictor and a stimulator of aldosterone release. As a vasoactive device, angiotensin II has a direct vasoconstrictory effect on vascular smooth muscle. This systemic vasoconstriction acts to maintain blood pressure in states of severe sodium depletion of extracellular fluid loss. The localized renal arteriolar constriction results in the renal retention of sodium and water. This volume expansion works to further elevate blood pressure. Angiotensin II may also enhance the sympathetic nervous system's activity.

The effective circulating blood volume is restored by the stimulation by angiotensin II of the zona glomerulosa cells for the release of aldosterone. Aldosterone's major effect is to increase renal tubular reabsorption of sodium at the distal and collecting ducts. Potassium and hydrogen ions are selectively secreted into the tubular fluid in exchange for the reabsorbed sodium ions. The result of the release of aldosterone is a significant expansion of plasma volume by sodium and water retention, thereby achieving elevation of systemic blood pressure.

In the healthy person the renin-angiotensin-aldosterone mechanism is stimulated to assist in adjusting for daily life activities and changes. However, in the critically ill person, this mechanism is an integral part of the compensatory response of the body (Table 29-1).

Table 29-1 Physiology of Renin-Angiotensin-Aldosterone Mechanism

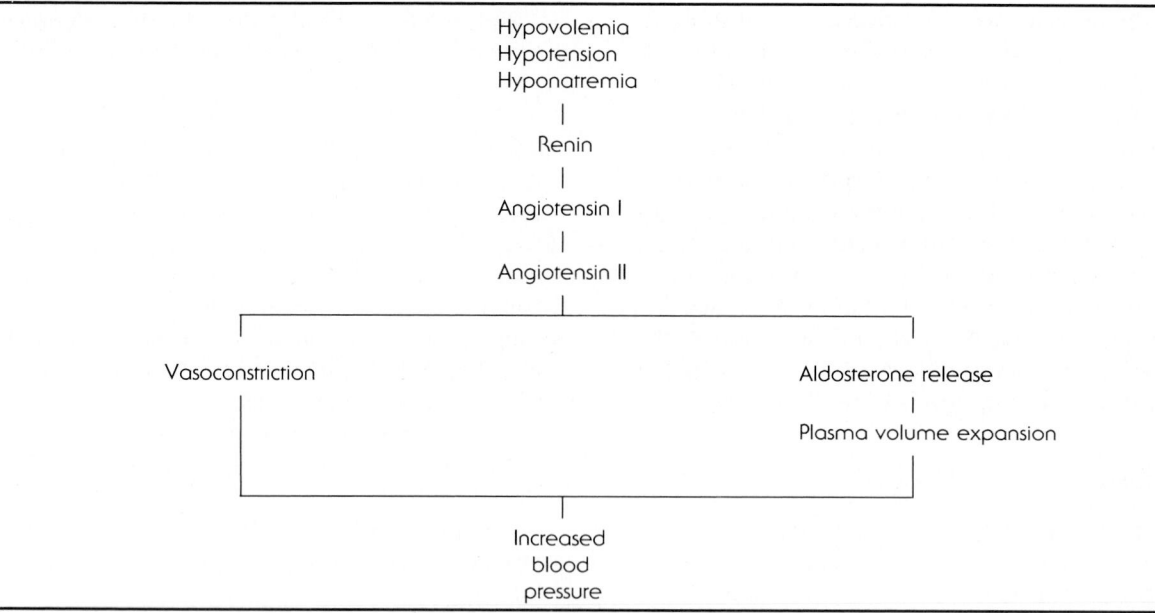

Renal Prostaglandins

Prostaglandins are unsaturated fatty acids made by most tissues in the body, including the kidneys. Five prostaglandins are recognized as originating from the kidneys, three of which are vasodilatory in nature, PGE_2, PGI_2, PGD_2; the other two prostaglandins have a vasoconstrictory role. Since a number of renal vasoconstrictors have been identified, not much attention has been paid to the prostaglandin vasoconstrictors. Instead, the prostaglandin vasodilators, particularly PGE_2, have been recognized as arterial vasodilators and inhibitors of the response of the distal tubules to ADH. The suppressed ADH response contributes to sodium and water excretion, which diminishes the effective circulatory volume.

The manner in which vasodilatory prostaglandins contribute to blood pressure is unique. These prostaglandins are secreted in conjunction with any vasoactive substance, such as angiotensin, epinephrine, norepinephrine, or bradykinin. In conjunction with other vasoactive agents, the prostaglandins function to modulate the effect of all the vasoactive substances. For example, the release of angiotensin is matched by the secretion of prostaglandin. Angiotensin creates a localized renal vasoconstrictory effect, but in the presence of prostaglandin the angiotensin effect is minimized. The vasodilatory effects of prostaglandins either restrict the degree of vasoconstriction or enhance the vasodilatory action of substances like bradykinin. To appreciate the importance of this modulatory role, one must imagine what would happen if renal prostaglandins were inhibited and vasoconstrictors like renin were secreted unopposed. Data have revealed that in this situation, administration of prostaglandin inhibitors such as aspirin, ibuprofen, or indomethacin during sustained levels of renin secretion may precipitate acute renal failure.

Excretion of Metabolic Waste Products

The excretion of body wastes and toxic substances is a primary renal function. Among the substances excreted daily are metabolic end products, excess levels of hormones, environmental waste, and pharmacologic agents. The two waste products measured for interpretation of renal function are blood urea nitrogen (BUN) and serum creatinine. Urea is a nitrogen waste product of protein metabolism which is filtered and reabsorbed along the entire nephron.[12] The BUN measurement alone is an unreliable value of renal function, because it is influenced by extrarenal factors such as dehydration, drugs, catabolic rate, and hypoperfusion states. When the extrarenal factor increases the urea nitrogen load beyond the normal excretion ability of the kidney, an elevation in BUN follows. The elevation of BUN without a corresponding rise in creatinine or a BUN rise in a 20:1 ratio to creatinine is indicative of hypovolemia, renal hypoperfusion, and increased catabolic rate. An elevation in both BUN and creatinine in a 10:1 ratio is indicative of renal disease.

Serum creatinine measurement may be described as a true assessment tool of renal function. As the waste product of muscle metabolism, creatinine is constantly produced and constantly excreted by the kidneys; the normal kidney can rid the body of daily creatinine loads. Elevations in creatinine above the normal 0.6 to 1.2 mg/dL are associated with renal disease.

References

1. Leaf, A., & Cotran, R. (1980). *Renal pathophysiology* (pp. 17–18). New York: Oxford.
2. Hosletter, T. H., & Brenner, B. M. (1983). Determinants of the glomerular filtration of macromolecules. In S. Massry & R. Glassock, *Textbook of nephrology* (pp. 1.39–1.41). Baltimore: Williams & Wilkins.
3. Zamboni, L. (1983). Anatomy and embryology of the kidney, ureter, bladder and urethra. In S. Massry & R. Glassock, *Textbook of nephrology* (p. 1.12). Baltimore: Williams & Wilkins.
4. Pitts, R. F. (1980). *Physiology of the kidney and body fluids* (p. 6). Chicago: Year Book.
5. Pitts, R. F. (1980). *Physiology of the kidney and body fluids* (p. 19). Chicago: Year Book.
6. Freidman, P. A., & Andreoli, T. E. (1983). General principles of renal tubular transport. In S. Massry & R. Glassock, *Textbook of Nephrology* (p. 1.44). Baltimore: Williams & Wilkins.
7. Stark, J. (1985). The renal system. In *Core curriculum for critical care nursing* (p. 355). Philadelphia: Saunders.
8. Berl, T., & Chiamovitz, C. (1983). The control of renal water excretion. In S. Massry & R. Glassock, *Textbook of Nephrology* (p. 3.6). Baltimore: Williams & Wilkins.
9. Fairchild, R. S. (1980). Diabetis insipidis: A review. *Critical Care Quarterly. 2*(3), 111–118.
10. Vander, A. J. (1980). *Renal physiology* (p. 6). New York: McGraw-Hill, 1980.
11. Geddes, L. E. (1981). The renal system. In M. Kinney, S. Dear, D. Packa, & D. Forman (Eds.), *AACN Desk Reference for Critical-Care Nursing.* New York: McGraw-Hill.
12. Stark, J. (1980). BUN/creatinine: Keys to kidney function. *Nursing '80, 5,* 30–38.

30 Renal System Assessment

June L. Stark

Assessment of the renal system includes a history, physical examination, laboratory data analysis, and radiologic examination. The reason for this type of assessment is to determine the presence of a renal or urinary tract disorder. Once the existence of renal system disease has been documented, the examiner attempts to establish the duration, severity, and cause of the disease.

History

Obtaining data regarding both the patient's and the family's history is the first step in the diagnostic process. The family history reveals the patient's genetic and hereditary predisposition to renal system disease. In approximately 30 percent of all azotemic patients a relation is found between the renal failure and genetic predisposition. Genetically transmitted diseases which cause or precipitate renal disease include polycystic kidneys, renal calculi, diabetes mellitus, hypertension, gout, malignant disease, hereditary nephritis, and cardiovascular disease.

The patient's history reveals the presence of and the predisposition to renal system disease. The patient may report a previous diagnosis of acute or chronic renal failure or urinary tract disease. A history of cardiovascular disease is significant, because this disease entity can impair renal function; the mechanism is a diminished cardiac output resulting in a decrease in renal perfusion. Low renal perfusion, in turn, precipitates the reabsorption of sodium and water, thus increasing the volume of total body water and diminishing the urine output. The patient, as a result, presents in an edematous state and often has oliguria.

Hypertensive disease and atherosclerosis contribute to the formation of renovascular narrowing

and structural damage to the kidney. Both these vascular changes alter renal function and may cause renal disease such as hypertensive nephritis.

Diabetes mellitus contributes to the development of several types of glomerular disease, usually presenting as nephrotic syndrome. Other renal lesions associated with diabetes are pyelonephritis, papillary necrosis, and accelerated arteriolar sclerosis.

A history of a recent upper respiratory infection, especially a streptococcal infection, is compatible with the onset of glomerular disease in 7 to 14 days. Viral infections may cause glomerular disease 1 to 3 days after infection.

A history of recurrent urinary tract infections is important to pursue, because the cause is often an abnormality in the urinary tract. The examiner should determine the diagnosis and treatment of each infection reported. Recurrent infections with the same organisms suggest that the site of infection may be either the kidney or the prostate gland, while repeated infections with different organisms often reflect a bladder infection.[1]

The patient presenting with complaints of both pulmonary and kidney-related disease must be evaluated for Goodpasture's syndrome, in which double-action antibodies attack both the lung and the kidney.

Frequently, a patient's report of an episode of renal calculi indicates a risk of recurrence. A second stone occurs in 40 to 50 percent of patients within a 5-year period and in 60 to 80 percent within 10 years.[2]

An allergic reaction as a result of hypersensitivity may cause interstitial nephritis. The patient with this disorder typically has a history of recent drug ingestion followed by the occurrence of a fever and a skin rash 1 to 3 weeks after starting the medication. Such an allergic reaction is indicated by a urinalysis that reveals hematuria, proteinuria, and pyuria. Within 1 week after the change in urinary sediment is noted, decline in renal function may appear. The medication must be discontinued in order to avoid a uremic state. The drugs most often associated with interstitial nephritis are penicillin, allopurinol, thiazide diuretics, cephalothin, sulfa drugs, and phenindione.

Pregnant patients with diabetes mellitus or hypertension are at a higher risk of toxemia and the associated alterations in renal function. A history or finding of protein in the urine during the third or fourth month of pregnancy is indicative of the onset of pre-eclampsia. Renal changes secondary to pre-eclampsia affect the glomeruli.

When the history reveals that a patient has received a renal transplant, a number of possible complications associated with transplantation should be considered by the examiner, among them acute or chronic rejection, infection, side effects of immunosuppressive drugs, and urinary leaks.

Physical Examination

The information collected during the physical examination follows a review of systems. Only the body systems providing data that contribute to an accurate diagnosis of urologic or renal involvement are discussed in this chapter. The goal, as mentioned earlier, is to document the presence and intensity of renal disease. At the same time, if renal failure exists, the extent of uremia and its impact on the patient's physical condition should be established.

General Appearance

The patient with a renal or urologic disorder often presents with malaise, fatigue, and weight loss. Excessive weight loss may be related to anorexia, nausea and vomiting associated with uremia, or the presence of chronic infection or a renal neoplasm. A flushed appearance consistent with the presence of fever usually indicates an infectious process.

Vital Signs

On physical examination, the blood pressure may vary from normal to hypo- or hypertension. Postural

blood pressure measurement is necessary, because an alteration in body water volume may be a contributing factor in an abnormal blood pressure value. Postural changes consistent with hypovolemia may result from chronic vomiting associated with uremia or from excessive urinary loss secondary to diuresis (either drug-induced or disease-related). An elevated blood pressure is associated with essential or secondary hypertensive disease or an excess of total body water that is consistent with an oliguric or anuric state.

The pulse rate may vary according to the presence of cardiovascular disease or the fluid status. Hypovolemia may be evidenced by either tachycardia or bradycardia, according to the status of the patient's compensatory mechanisms; tachycardia, however, is more common. An irregular rhythm is usually indicative of electrolyte imbalances in the renal patient.

Respiration

The respiratory rate may be normal or may be altered by acid-base imbalances or renal abnormalities that compromise pulmonary function, such as Goodpasture's syndrome and uremic lung. A severe metabolic acidosis, such as often occurs during acute and chronic renal failure, stimulates a respiratory pattern called *Kussmaul's respiration,* in which the breathing is slow, deep, and labored. The respiratory rate may also be altered by a pulmonary infection; the uremic patient is highly susceptible to infection.

Skin, Nails, and Hair

The color of the *skin* is abnormal during acute and chronic renal failure. A grayish tone and pallor are secondary to anemia, while a yellowish tinge occurs as carotenoids are retained as a result of uremia. Bruising of the skin, ecchymosis, and petechiae are common because of the enhanced capillary fragility and abnormal clotting caused by uremia. Purpuric lesions also appear in some forms of renal failure. The chronic pruritus of uremia is consistent with the appearance of scratch marks.

The texture of the skin may vary from day to day, from scaly to rough. Uremia is believed to atrophy the skin's oil and sweat glands, creating these skin conditions. A film called *uremic frost* may coat the skin's surface; it occurs as a result of the passage of urate crystals through the skin's pores.

Edema may be present in the extremities, lungs, and periorbital region because of the retention of sodium and water. Edema in the extremities is evaluated on a scale from 1+ to 4+. The examiner presses the swollen skin against a bony region with a finger. If a depression is left in the skin, the examiner subjectively scores the degree of edema. A score of 1+ is equivalent to a slight depression, while a score of 4+ indicates that the depression remains for more than 30 s.[3]

Skin changes related to specific renal factors are the butterfly facial mask accompanying lupus nephritis, the rashes associated with poststreptococcal glomerulonephritis, the purpura of Henoch-Schönlein disease, the subcutaneous nodules of polyarteritis nodosa, and the dermal vasculitis and ulcerations of Wegener's granulomatosis. Scleroderma causes a thickening of the skin, and rashes occur with acute allergic interstitial nephritis.

The *nails* may be brittle and thin and show signs of easy cracking, which reflects malnutrition resulting from renal disease. White bands across the nails are a specific symptom of protein deficiency.

Hair texture is also altered by poor nutritional intake secondary to renal disease. The hair may appear dry and lifeless, and some hair loss may be evident.

Eyes

Band keratopathy refers to white bands seen across the cornea. This sign occurs when the patient suffers from chronic hypercalcemia due to renal disease. Severe hypertension is reflected in the eyes by alterations in the optic fundi. Localized areas of hemorrhage observable on the sclera occur after episodes of uncontrolled hypertension.

Nose, Sinuses, and Mouth

Mucous membrane changes are often seen in both the nose and the mouth of patients with renal disease. Dry membranes are associated with dehydration. Swelling, redness, and ulcerations often accompany the toxic picture of uremia. Pallor may be present, indicating anemia associated with renal

failure. A uremic fetor or odor on the breath is a characteristic sign of uremia.

Ears

Nerve deafness may be indicative of toxicity of antibiotics used or specifically hereditary nephropathy. Gouty nephropathy sometimes causes gouty tophi in the ear cartilage.[4]

Neck

Neck veins become distended in response to heart failure or fluid overload, both above often coinciding with renal failure.

Systems Assessment

Pulmonary

In addition to the failure associated with fluid overload, the lungs are susceptible to a number of infections during uremia, such as pneumonia and pneumonitis. Uremia increases the patient's susceptibility to infection by impairing the immune response in the lung and suppressing the cough reflex. The patient with these two alterations in pulmonary function often presents with tenacious sputum, fever, and an irregular respiratory rate. Lung auscultation may reveal a variety of sounds, from normal to crackles, rhonchi, or wheezes.

Specific pulmonary conditions associated with renal disease are Goodpasture's syndrome and uremic lung. Goodpasture's syndrome has an insidious onset in which the patient reports a previous upper respiratory infection. Pulmonary system data include hemoptysis, orthopnea, dyspnea, crackles, or rhonchi. Neck vein distention may accompany the crackles if the cause is heart failure. Pulmonary hemorrhage may also be a cause of crackles. The presence of both congestive edema and pulmonary hemorrhage are confirmed by chest x-ray.

Uremic lung is characterized by interstitial edema and respiratory failure. The patient presents with dyspnea, labored respirations, and rales. A chest x-ray demonstrates the classic butterfly configuration or a "wet" lung indicative of failure.

Cardiovascular

The examiner may anticipate a number of cardiovascular problems, including hypertension, pericarditis, and atherosclerosis, in the presence of renal disease. Hypertension, a common problem in renal failure, is related to volume expansion, either essential in nature or secondary to hypertensive disease.

The onset of pericarditis is often coincident with an exacerbation of uremia. Chest pain, shortness of breath, and fever are the presenting signs and symptoms. Auscultation reveals a pericardial friction rub. ST elevations on the ECG consistent with an acute episode of pericarditis may appear, although in some instances the uremic patient may not display typical ECG changes.[5] Cardiac tamponade is a serious complication of pericarditis for which the nurse should be alert: the clinical signs are pulsus paradoxus, hypotension, and neck vein distention.

Various clinical signs of atherosclerosis may be present. The chronic renal failure patient may experience an acceleration of the atherosclerotic process precipitated by uremia or the process of hemodialysis. Cardiovascular disease in any form may be the result of rapid changes in vascular integrity. In addition, a hyperlipidemic state caused by uremia may contribute to cardiovascular problems.

In patients with renal failure, the congestive heart failure often resulting from fluid overload may create an S_3 heart sound. Other presenting signs and symptoms are shortness of breath, increased jugular pressure, pitting edema in the lower extremities, cold and clammy skin, further compromised urine output, and alterations in mental status. Electrolyte imbalances such as hypo- and hyperkalemia and hypo- and hypercalcemia alter normal cardiac function (see Chap. 11).

Neuromuscular

Neuromuscular symptoms in renal disease usually result from uremia or from acid-base and electrolyte imbalances. Uremia is responsible for uremic encephalopathy and peripheral neuropathy. The patient's mental status during uremic encephalopathy ranges from lethargy to coma. Seizures, diminished coordination, tremors, or asterixis may be present. Peripheral neuropathy is a segmental demyelination of the nerves progressing from the lower to the upper extremities. The specific physical findings depend on the stage of peripheral neuropathy. At the onset, the patient may experience "restless leg syndrome," which usually occurs when the patient is at rest. To relieve this aching, a restless pattern of movement is exhibited by the patient. A "burning" pain of varying intensity, beginning on the dorsal and ventral surfaces of the feet, is experienced by the patient. This syndrome can progress to foot drop and even paralysis.

Electrolyte imbalances may cause vague neuromuscular symptoms; for example, hypocalcemia may cause muscle twitching. Neurologic examinations should be supported by serum electrolyte studies.

Skeletal

The bone diseases associated with renal failure are osteomalacia and osteitis fibrosa. The patient with either of these disorders may exhibit activity intolerance and bone pain. The patient is susceptible to fractures, and radiologic examination of skull, hands, and feet reveals demineralization. The patient may have difficulty with mobility because of these problems.

Gastrointestinal

During the history taking, the patient often describes disturbances in the gastrointestinal (GI) tract such as anorexia, nausea, and vomiting. Accompanying these symptoms may be abdominal distention, stomatitis, and uremic fetor.

Peptic and stress ulcers are other potential problems often described by the patient with renal disease. Stools and vomitus should be examined for occult blood in an effort to document the presence of an ulcer. Gastric pain in the patient with renal failure may result from either an ulcer or gastritis, both of which are believed to be caused by stress factors associated with renal disease.

Uremic bowel is a condition seen in patients who have had end-stage renal disease for several years. The history reveals alternating periods of diarrhea and constipation. There may be resistance to any medication given per rectum.

An enlarged liver or spleen suggests amyloidosis. Any alteration in bowel sounds can be attributed to uremia or prolonged therapy with phosphate binders. The presence of lesions in the large or small intestine should be considered.

Genitourinary

The kidneys are palpated to determine their size and shape and to detect tenderness or masses. The right kidney is selected for examination because its lower abdominal position makes it easier to palpate than the left kidney. The patient is requested to take a deep breath, and the examiner, reaching under the rib cage, attempts to palpate the lower pole of the right kidney. Inability to locate the kidney suggests that it may be small or atrophied. Enlarged kidneys are a valuable diagnostic clue suggesting a cause such as polycystic kidney disease.

Pain indicative of renal disease is elicited by giving a firm punch over the kidney or applying pressure to the tissues in the area surrounding the kidney. If pain is present, the examiner must differentiate renal from muscle pain. Kidney pain can be reproduced by applying pressure directly over the kidney. Muscle pain is present on deep palpation of the muscles in the costovertebral angle.

The bladder is palpable only when it is distended. On percussion the full bladder produces a dull sound. Pain from the bladder is expressed during palpation in the suprapubic region.

Classically, pain originating in the anterior or posterior portion of the kidney and radiating toward the groin is characteristic of involvement of the ureter. Conditions causing ureteric colic are renal calculi or thrombus.

Pain anywhere in the urinary tract is usually accompanied by complaints of dysuria, urgency, frequency, and hesitancy of urination. The patient may also describe abnormal color of the urine, such as grossly bloody, cloudy, or orange, which indicates bilirubinuria. The patient's urination habits may change to nocturia, polyuria, incontinence, oliguria, or anuria.

Fever as the primary factor associated with the pain is suggestive of pyelonephritis (usually an acute episode) or cystitis. Enlargement of the renal pelvis in conjunction with pain is indicative of renal calculi.

Physical examination of the male genitalia may reveal a number of potential problems. Tenderness on palpation of the scrotum is indicative of epididymitis. Another cause of testicular pain is tumor. The prostate gland is examined by a bimanual technique via the rectum. Pain or enlargement of the prostate gland signifies prostatitis. Lower back pain is consistent with prostate abnormalities. The examiner should consider the prostate size variations which occur naturally with aging.

Uremia is associated with sexual dysfunction. The exact pathophysiology is unknown; however, it is suspected that hormonal or mineral deficiencies such as zinc may be responsible. Female patients experience amenorrhea and a cessation of ovulation, while the male may become impotent. Both males and females may express a decrease in libido. It should be noted that pregnancy and successful delivery, while possible, rarely occur.

Hematologic

Anemia secondary to lack of erythropoietin or frank bleeding should be evaluated in both acute and chronic renal disease. The patient may become severely anemic, with a deficiency in erythropoietin. The hematocrit is usually maintained at a value of 20% by frequent blood transfusions. The examiner must assess for symptoms of anemia in order to determine the need for treatment. Pallor, fatigue, activity intolerance, shortness of breath, and chest pain are consistent with a diagnosis of anemia.

Endocrine

The various hormones secreted daily are believed to be among the factors which contribute to the development of uremic symptoms. Parathyroid hormone is suspected of being a primary factor in the skeletal and sexual functional problems noted in uremia, described earlier in this chapter.

Sleep and Rest Patterns

An alteration in sleep and rest patterns has been associated with uremia. The patient may experience sleep apnea or sleep deprivation. The exact etiology of the sleep disturbance in renal failure is unknown, although uremic toxins are suspected. Sleep-pattern disturbances often are exacerbated on the night prior to dialysis, when the patient is most uremic. A history of the patient's sleep patterns assists in identification of inadequate rest or sleep time. The data obtained regarding sleep and rest patterns is utilized in formulating the nursing care plan.

Coping

The patient's and family's coping in relation to lifestyle changes and the demands of renal disease are assessed. Data regarding previous coping styles of the patient and family assist the nurse in anticipating the most useful coping methods for them to use in the current hospitalization. See Chap. 18 for further discussion of coping.

Data from Diagnostic Procedures

Serum Studies

Creatinine

An interpretation of the serum creatinine level provides data which directly reflect the state of renal function. This reliable correlation between serum creatinine and renal function exists because the blood level of creatinine reflects the glomerular filtration rate.

Creatinine is the product of muscle metabolism. A person's muscle mass remains relatively stable from day to day despite starvation or exercise; therefore a stable amount of creatinine is produced daily which is proportional to the amount of creatinine excreted daily. Normal renal function and glomerular filtration rate are reflected by a creatinine level of 0.67 to 1.2 mg. During renal failure, inability to excrete the daily creatinine load results in an elevation of serum creatinine.

Blood Urea Nitrogen

Blood urea nitrogen (BUN) values are used to identify extrarenal problems and, in conjunction with serum creatinine, to determine the presence of renal failure. Urea nitrogen is the end product of ingested or catabolically metabolized protein. The rate of protein metabolism varies according to the daily protein intake and the degree of catabolism caused by starvation, hematoma resorption, infection, trauma, surgery, corticosteroids, or medications.[6] In addition to variation in the rate of production, there is inconsistency in the rate of urea excretion even in the presence of normal renal function. Excessive protein metabolism may elevate serum urea levels despite a normal glomerular filtration rate. An example of this is the person who has ingested a large protein meal or the burn victim who is catabolic and who may have an elevated BUN in conjunction with normal renal function.

Dehydration or a decrease in renal perfusion causes a decrease in glomerular filtration rate. A fall in the glomerular filtration rate leads to an accumulation of urea nitrogen, while the serum creatinine does not significantly change. Extrarenal problems, excessive protein metabolism, dehydration, or low renal perfusion states elevate the BUN/serum creatinine ratio to more than 20:1.

During acute or chronic renal failure, the BUN and serum creatinine levels are both elevated in a ratio of 10:1; for example, a BUN of 100 is matched by a creatinine of 10.

Creatinine Clearance

The creatinine clearance is used to determine the presence and progression of renal disease, because the creatinine clearance provides an estimate of the percentage of functioning nephrons. A 24-h urine sample is assessed to determine the volume and the total amount of creatinine excreted. To estimate the creatinine clearance rate (Ccr), the excreted amount of creatinine (UCR) is multiplied by the urine volume per minute (V) and both values are divided by the plasma creatinine level (PCR):

$$\frac{UCR \times V}{PCR} = Ccr$$

Urinalysis

Examination of the urine provides valuable information which directs the examiner toward a diagnosis. A freshly voided midstream urine specimen—ideal for bacteriologic examination—should be provided for urine studies. To avoid precipitation and disintegration of certain casts, the urine should be studied within 30 min of collection.

Inspection

The color, clarity, and concentration of the urine are assessed by visual examination. Normal urine presents a color range from pale yellow to amber, varying according to the concentration and amount of pigment. Dilute urine appears pale yellow, while concentrated urine turns darker and deeper in color as the concentration increases. Color changes that indicate abnormalities are usually a result of three factors: an increase in the number of metabolites excreted in the urine; substances in the urine reflective of renal or urinary tract disorders; and substances of dietary or pharmacologic ingestion.

Gross hematuria, or red-colored urine, is defined as blood that is visible on inspection of the urine. The use of Hemastix or other tests for occult blood may confirm the visual assessment. A positive Hemastix reading in an essentially clear urine is described as microscopic hematuria. It should be kept in mind when assessing the urine that a small amount of blood can significantly alter the color of the urine.

Free hemoglobin and myoglobin in the urine cause a red color. Uroerythrin may appear in the urine during an acute febrile disease and may be responsible for red urine. The diagnostic dye phenolsulfonphthalein turns an alkaline urine red in color. Lastly, the metabolism of beets produces a group of pigments called *anthocyanines* which, on renal excretion, turn the urine red.

Red blood cells and heme pigments present in the urine may cause variation in the color from pink to black. Malignant melanoma is associated with the deposition of a pigment called *melanogen,* which darkens the urine to a black color. The urine of a patient with obstructive jaundice reveals a yellow, brown, or green color caused by the presence of bile salts. A dipstick may be used to reveal the bilirubin. Blue urine is produced by methylene dye and azure A. Phenazopyridine (Pyridium), the bladder analgesic, turns the urine orange. A bright yellow urine is produced by food dyes, riboflavin, and multivitamins.

Urine should appear clear on examination. A fresh specimen which is cloudy suggests the presence of epithelial cells or leukocytes in the urine. Cloudy urine is usually associated with urinary tract infection (UTI), because bacteria, even without WBCs, can cause cloudiness. A urine culture and sensitivity test on a freshly voided midstream specimen can document the existence of UTI.

Amorphous phosphate in the urine precipitates in an acid or alkaline urine causing a cloudy appearance. Mucus in the urine produces a hazy appearance, while fat produces murky urine. Red blood cells collecting in the urine cause a turbid appearance.

Odor

Urinary odors provide clues about the contents of the urine. Urinary ketones produce a sweet, fruity smell. A fishy odor is connected with excess methionine in the urine. Butyric or hexanoic acid causes a foul urinary odor, frequently compared to the odor of sweaty feet.[7]

Specific Gravity

Concentration of the urine can be estimated from the specific gravity, which indicates the density of substances dissolved in the urine. Urinary osmolality is the most accurate measurement of concentration, but serial specific gravity readings reflect the ability of the kidney to concentrate or dilute the urine.

The normal range of urinary specific gravity is from 1.003 to 1.030, corresponding to a dilute urine and concentrated urine, respectively. During the course of a day the specific gravity of the urine varies significantly, as the normal kidney responds to the body's water balance by concentrating the urine accordingly. Generally, a urine specific gravity of 1.015 to 1.022 is recognized as being in the medium range. The causes of variation from the medium range should be determined in the hospitalized patient. Falsely high specific gravity values may be produced by the presence of radiopaque dye in the urine after radiologic examinations. Large quantities of glucose or protein in the urine also lead to a high specific gravity (greater than 1.025). Other causes of an elevated specific gravity are dehydration, eclampsia, and lipoid nephrosis. Low readings may be the result of overhydration, diuretic therapy, and ingestion of coffee or alcohol. Disease processes associated with low specific gravity are hypertension, pyelonephritis, diabetes insipidus, and hypoproteinemic states.

pH

The urinary pH has a wide range of normal values, from 4.5 to 8.0, varying with the response of the kidney to changes in acid-base status and the urinary excretion of acids or alkalies.

Diagnostically, the pH reading is of minimal value. Infection with urea-splitting bacteria, either *Proteus* or *Pseudomonas,* often creates an alkaline urine; the pH in this situation may increase to more than 8.0. Moreover, some antibacterial agents do not function in an alkaline pH. A total body acidosis is suggestive of an alteration in the urine-acidifying ability of the kidney.

The normal urine is more often acidotic, because the metabolites of daily dietary ingestion are acids excreted by the kidney. However, an acid urine is guaranteed after the ingestion of large amounts of proteins or fruits. Severe diarrhea, hyperkalemia, respiratory acidosis, diabetic ketosis, and starvation all produce an acid urine. Urinary tract infection caused by *Escherichia coli* also leads to an acid urine.

Testing to determine the urine's acid-base status is essential when the pH of the urine is manipulated. Regulation of the pH is beneficial to inhibit stone formation and to suppress chronic infections. An acid urine is maintained by the administration of ammonium chloride, mandelic acid, or ascorbic acid. This measure reduces the chance that alkaline stones, either calcium phosphate or carbonate, may form. An alkaline urine is maintained by the administration of sodium bicarbonate, acetazolamide, and potassium citrate, a measure that prevents and may treat some UTIs and also restricts the development of uric acid, calcium oxalate, and cystine stones.

Protein

The urine is usually free of protein, although some people normally have a trace amount of protein in the urine. The presence of high levels of protein and albumin in the urine is suggestive of renal or urinary tract disease. However, a protein level of 150 mg to 1 g is referred to as *functional proteinuria* and is associated with nonrenal causes. Examples of conditions causing functional proteinuria are aggressive exercise, febrile states, stress, and exposure to extreme temperature changes; a reversal of any of these conditions results in reversal of the proteinuria.

A dipstick can be used to detect the presence of protein and measure trace amounts from 1+ to 4+, but more exact testing is necessary to determine the actual amount of protein. Occasionally, protein levels may increase or decrease during renal disease; therefore low levels may be misleading. A consistently elevated level of protein excretion (over 4 g per day) is associated with nephrotic syndrome, glomerulonephritis, lupus nephritis, and amyloidosis. Moderate and low levels of proteinuria, from 1 to 3.5 g, are associated with many forms of renal failure, particularly diabetic nephropathy, hypertension, polycystic disease, and chronic pyelonephritis.

Urinary tract infection may or may not be associated with proteinuria. When proteinuria occurs in UTI, the infection is usually in the upper rather than the lower urinary tract. This is because infections in the upper tract affect the kidney and glomerular function, and this is the reason for the proteinuria.

Microscopic Examination

Urinary Sediment Urinary sediment is composed of casts, cells, crystals, and a small number of miscellaneous particles. Urinary casts begin as cells or other substances and are molded in the lumen of the tubules. The specific shape of casts is determined by the area in the tubules in which the casts are formed. Some casts are straight or curved, while others are convoluted. In certain instances, casts are microproteins or serum proteins.

Cast formation is increased during acidosis and proteinuria and in highly concentrated urine. Because casts are formed in the kidney, alterations in renal function are reflective of the amount of casts formed and their type: hyaline, red cell, white cell, epithelial, granular, waxy, fatty, and renal tubular.

Hyaline casts appear in the urine more often than other casts and are composed entirely of protein. Small amounts of hyaline casts are present in normal urine. Factors which may cause the appearance of hyaline casts in the presence of normal kidney function are extremely vigorous exercise and hypovolemic states. Hyaline casts are seen during all types of renal disease, but their presence does not indicate a specific type of renal failure.[8]

Red cell casts in the urine are abnormal. Their appearance is associated with glomerulonephropathies, renal trauma, pyelonephritis, bacterial endocarditis, renal infarction, and renal vein thrombosis. When red cell casts appear in the urine, its color is brown or red-tinged.

Renal infection and/or inflammation are the cause of *white cell casts* in the urine. The types of renal disease associated with white cell casts are pyelonephritis, lupus nephritis, and interstitial nephritis.

Epithelial cell casts result from damage to the renal tubules secondary to nephrotoxic insult, allergic reactions, viral injury, ischemia, or transplant rejection. Epithelial cell casts also occur during some forms of chronic renal failure.

Normally present in small numbers in the urine, *granular casts* form from the breakdown of other cellular casts, such as white and red cell casts, or the clumping of serum proteins. In large numbers, granular casts indicate renal disease.

The substance of which *waxy casts* are composed is unknown, although it is speculated that this type of cast forms from degraded granular casts. Diseases associated with the appearance of waxy casts in the urine are chronic or acute renal failure, malignant hypertension, and renal transplant rejection.

Fatty casts, as their name suggests, contain lipoid material. The degradation of fatty substances in the tubular wall is the cause of fatty cast formation. These casts appear in the urine after tubular diseases, lipoid nephrosis, nephrotic syndrome, glomerulonephropathies, and episodes of nephrotoxicity.

Renal tubular casts are present in the urine only after tubular injury. As the tubular cells are degraded from ischemia or nephrotoxicity, they fall into the tubular space and assume the shape of the space in which the cells aggregate.

Radiologic Examination

Radiologic examination is utilized to determine the existence and extent of renal and urinary tract diseases; it reveals the renal system's structure, function, and blood supply. Among the factors considered in selecting the appropriate radiologic examination are the type of information needed to make a diagnosis, the risks of the examination, and the dependability of the examination results.

The nurse's role in patient management related to radiologic examinations is to be aware of the indications for each type of examination, the preparation for each procedure, the information regarding the tests which is necessary for patient teaching, and the risks and potential complications, in order to make assessments and adequately manage the patient after examination.

Intravenous Pyelography

The intravenous pyelogram (IVP) visualizes the kidney and urinary tract, utilizing a radiocontrast dye injection. The calices, renal pelvis, ureters, and bladder are visualized within minutes after beginning the examination. Satisfactory visualization of the urinary tract allows diagnosis of partial obstruction, renovascular hypertension, tumors, cysts, and congenital anomalies.[9] Because dilation of the renal pelvis is possible, hydronephrosis can be detected.

The contrast medium injected during an IVP has been associated with nephrotoxicity. In some high-risk patients, the dye may exacerbate or cause renal failure. Caution or perhaps avoidance of IVP dye is recommended for patients with poor renal function. The IVP dye creates a hyperosmotic state in the plasma, resulting in a diuresis which precipitates a state of dehydration. The onset of dehydration plus the nephrotoxic effects of the dye in a patient already suffering from renal failure may exacerbate the severity of the renal disease. The response described may be prevented by administering several liters of fluid prior to, during, and after the procedure; this helps to avoid the dehydration and reduces the toxicity of the dye by dilution and enhanced excretion.

The IVP is also contraindicated in the patient with multiple myeloma, diabetes mellitus, congestive heart failure, or pregnancy. The dye also promotes sickling and renal infarction in the patient with sickle cell disease.

The IVP is beneficial because it can be used cautiously in patients with glomerular filtration rates as low as 15 mg/L. Despite diminished urine flow, visualization is still possible by use of a much higher dose of the radiopaque dye. Prehydration therapy is prescribed in this situation.

Plain Film of the Abdomen

The plain film of the abdomen, or KUB (for *k*idneys, *u*reters, *b*ladder), is the first approach selected for study of the renal system because of its effectiveness and low risk to the patient. This simple x-ray of the abdomen reveals the position, size, and shape of the kidney. Renal masses and calculi also are sometimes visible on a plain film. If visualization of the desired aspects is limited or absent, another radiologic study is indicated.

The size of the kidney is diagnostically important. Bilateral kidney enlargement is consistent with an acute process. However, several chronic conditions, such as polycystic kidneys and amyloidosis, also cause kidney enlargement. Small kidneys are a sign of atrophy from long-standing chronic renal disease. The one exception to this is bilateral renal artery stenosis, which is an acute process and is reversible.[10]

Changes in size may occur in a single kidney. Conditions causing a small unilateral kidney are chronic pyelonephritis and renal artery stenosis. Unilateral enlargement occurs secondary to obstruction, acute renal vein thrombosis, or a renal mass.

As mentioned earlier, the KUB may reveal alterations in the shape of the kidneys. Renal shape is often distorted by tumors, cysts, or previous scarring from chronic infection or vascular disease.

Renal Scan

The renal scan, a radionuclide study, assesses renal perfusion and function. This study also yields information about the presence of obstruction and renal masses. This test is beneficial in determining the impact of renal ischemia caused by acute tubular necrosis or renal transplantation. The rate of uptake and excretion of the radioisotopes is measured. In the presence of acute tubular necrosis, kidneys that are visualized in 30 min are believed to have a better prognosis than those in which visualization requires a longer period.[11]

The radionuclide material is excreted in the urine, but the radiation levels of the urine are believed to be safe. However, it is recommended that the urine with the radionuclide material be discarded rather than collected in one place.

Retrograde Pyelography

During this study, catheters are passed into the ureters and a radiocontrast dye is injected. This procedure allows visualization of the ureters and the upper region of the urinary tract. Partial and complete obstruction can be diagnosed by this study. Sterile technique is utilized to eliminate the risk of retrograde infection.

Arteriography

In the renal arteriogram, radiocontrast medium is injected directly into the aorta near the bifurcation of the renal arteries or, when possible, into the renal arteries. The renal arteriogram is advantageous for visualization of the renal vasculature; it can support the existence of renovascular abnormalities such as renal artery stenosis. This study also may assist in differentiating a benign cyst from a carcinoma.

The risks associated with renal arteriograms are similar to those of IVP. The complications are believed to be connected to the radiopaque dyes used in both procedures. Other potential problems of renal arteriography are laceration of the peripheral artery and formation of hematoma, embolism, or thrombosis.

Ultrasonography

Ultrasonography is an imaging technique for both the kidneys and the bladder. This method of examination is relatively simple but provides adequate visualization of the renal system. Because of its noninvasive nature, ultrasonography is an ideal choice for patients who have allergic reactions to contrast media. Ultrasonography is also valuable in the critically ill patient who needs renal system evaluation but cannot tolerate invasive procedures.

Ultrasonography has proved beneficial in the diagnosis of the anuric patient, in whom, because glomerular filtration ceases during anuria, most of the previously described methods of examination which depend on urine flow are ineffective. Because of its effectiveness in anuric states, ultrasonography has diagnostic value for patients who have complete urinary tract or arterial obstruction. It provides accurate data about the kidney's size and shape; therefore, this examination assists in determining the presence of renal cysts, abscesses, and tumors in addition to polycystic disease. Ultrasound has proved useful in diagnosing conditions associated with renal transplantation such as lymphoceles and intra- or extrarenal hemorrhage.[12] Detecting the impact of renal trauma by ultrasound is appropriate because hemorrhage and enlargement by edema may be detected.

Hydronephrosis can be identified by ultrasound because the calices are easily visualized.

Dilation of the ureter and bladder fullness studies using ultrasound techniques are used in diagnosis of lower urinary tract problems.

Computerized Tomography

Computerized tomography (CT) provides an exact anatomic view of the kidneys, the retroperitoneal space, the bladder, and the prostate. The CT scan is often selected as the examination of choice in renal disease, and it is specifically indicated when small kidneys cannot be detected by any other methods. But other anomalies in kidney size and shape can also be detected, such as horseshoe or polycystic kidneys.

Renal Biopsy

Renal biopsy is the most invasive of all the diagnostic procedures and therefore is usually indicated only when other methods have failed to establish a diagnosis. The biopsy may be performed by an open or closed technique, the closed being more often used. Open biopsy is indicated when gross anatomic deformities exist or the diagnostic process requires a deep specimen, as when trying to determine the presence of polyarteritis nodosa or renal dense deposit disease. The kidney's position is established by fluoroscopy or ultrasonography. A posterior approach is used for inserting the biopsy needle to obtain a specimen (Tables 30-1, 30-2).

The major complication of both open and closed biopsy is localized bleeding. The nurse examines the biopsy site after the procedure for swelling and skin color changes consistent with localized bleeding. Blood pressure is taken frequently for at least 2 to 4 h after biopsy, and the hematocrit level is assessed. A small amount of bleeding is usual; however, occasionally a transfusion may be necessary. The complication specifically associated with open biopsy is wound infection.

Nuclear Magnetic Resonance

Magnetic resonance imaging (MRI) is a new imaging technique that provides information similar to that acquired from CT scan, but it does not use x-rays. This examination is special because it studies the chemical structure of intact tissues. The nucleus of

Table 30-1 Indications for Renal Biopsy

Massive proteinuria
Undetermined etiology of renal disease
Systemic disease with urinary abnormalities: lupus
  erythematosus, diabetes mellitus, Goodpasture's
  syndrome
Abnormalities in urinalysis of unknown etiology: proteinuria,
  hematuria, casts
Renal transplantation: compromised renal function of
  unknown etiology

each cell in the body emits a resonance frequency dependent on the composition of the nucleus and the strength of the magnetic field.[13] MRI operates at various frequencies and detects peaks representative of the chemical composition of each nucleus. By this means, MRI interprets the peaks representative of normal or abnormal cell function. Alterations in the peaks are suggestive of abnormalities in cell function due either to tumor growth or to metabolic alterations caused by ischemia or acid-base imbalances.

Summary

An assessment of the renal system is directed at collecting data regarding the physical and psychosocial factors affecting the patient's condition. A patient and family history must be acquired to help determine the patient's genetic risk of developing a renal disorder and factors that may contribute to the formation or increased severity of the disease. The physical examination focuses on determining the extent of uremia. Interviews conducted during the assessment process focus on the psychosocial aspects of the patient's and family's responses to the renal disease, the sleep and rest patterns, and

Table 30-2 Contraindications to Renal Biopsy

Clotting disorders
Solitary kidney
Infection: localized or systemic
Obesity
Hypertension
Suspicion of tumor
Uremia
Inability to determine kidney's position

the sexual functioning of the patient. Laboratory and radiologic examinations help verify or clarify data obtained by physical assessment. The ultimate goal is to document the presence and the extent of renal disease.

References

1. Ronald, A. R. (1983). The management of urethro-cystitis in women. *Seminars in Urology, 1*(2), 114–120.
2. Rose, D. B. (1981). *Pathophysiology of renal disease.* New York: McGraw-Hill.
3. *Renal and urologic disorders.* (1984). Nursing 84 Books. Springhouse, PA: Springhouse.
4. Morrin, P. A. F. (1983). Assessment of the patient with renal disease. In D. Z. Levine (Ed.), *Care of the renal patient* (pp. 1–15). Philadelphia: Saunders.
5. Rose, D. B. (1986). *Pathophysiology of renal disease.* New York: McGraw-Hill.
6. Stark, J. L. (1980). BUN/creatinine: Your keys to kidney function. *Nursing 80, 10*(5), 33–38.
7. Graff, L. (1983). *A handbook of routine urinalysis.* Philadelphia: Lippincott.
8. Haber, M. H. (1976). *Urinary casts: Their microscopy and clinical significance* (2d ed.). Chicago: American Society of Clinical Pathologists.
9. Stark, J. L. (1985). The renal system. In J. Alspach & S. Williams (Eds.), *Core Curriculum for Critical Care Nursing* (pp. 348–449). Philadelphia: Saunders.
10. Hennessy, W. T., Pollack, H. M., Banner, M. P., & Wein, A. J. (1981). Radiologic evaluation of anuric patients. *Urology, 18*(5), 435–445.
11. Rose, D. B. (1981). *Pathophysiology of renal disease.* New York: McGraw Hill.
12. Holmes, J. H. (1983). Diagnostic use of ultrasound for kidney and bladder. In S. G. Massey & R. J. Glasscock (Eds.), *Textbook of Nephrology* (Vol. 2, pp. 12.11–12.19). Baltimore: Williams & Wilkins.
13. Weiner, M. W., & Adam, W. R. (1985). Magnetic resonance spectroscopy for evaluation of renal function. *Seminars in Urology, 3*(1), 34–42.

31

Acute Renal Failure

June L. Stark

Acute renal failure is recognized as the most common renal problem afflicting the critically ill. Mortality rates are high at approximately 65 percent.[1] In select groups, such as trauma victims with renal failure, the mortality rate can be as high as 70 percent, but decreases to 30 percent with the use of hyperalimentation and daily dialysis.[2] Nonoliguric acute renal failure has a better prognosis, as low as 26 percent, than oliguric renal failure.

Acute renal failure can be defined as a syndrome of varying causation which results in an acute deterioration of renal function.[3] To assist in the diagnostic process, the causes are classified as prerenal, renal, or postrenal.

Postrenal Failure

Pathophysiology

Postrenal failure is associated with any condition causing obstruction to urine flow from the kidney to the urinary meatus (Table 31-1). The common causes are bladder neck, urethral, or prostatic obstruction. Because this type of acute renal failure can be rapidly reversed by surgical intervention, postrenal failure should be considered in all acute cases of cessation of urine output. Three groups are at high risk for obstruction: children, adult females, and elderly males. In children, obstruction is commonly due to congenital alterations in posterior or ureteropelvic function. In adult females, cervical cancer may obstruct urine flow adjacent to the ureterovesical junction. Lastly, the elderly male has an increased predisposition to develop either benign or malignant prostatic enlargement.

With acute bilateral obstruction, the patient presents with renal failure. The duration of the obstruction is an important factor to consider, because the potential for complications such as urinary tract infection (UTI) or pyelonephritis increases with the length of time urine flow has been impaired. The patient with bilateral obstruction usually has lower abdominal pain and associated complications, such as biochemical imbalances, related to the onset of acute renal failure.

Diagnostic determination of postrenal failure involves primarily radiologic examination, although the history, physical examination, and laboratory evaluation can provide minimal supportive data. A flat plate of the abdomen is an initial examination which can reveal kidney and renal pelvis size and the patency of the urinary drainage system. The demonstration of one patent ureter rules out the presence of bilateral obstruction. A dilated renal pelvis is the most prevalent finding in the presence of obstruction unless the patient is dehydrated. Ultrasonography reveals a dilated renal pelvis in 90 percent of patients.[4] Another benefit of this test is that it provides results even in the absence of urinary output. If the patient does not have evidence of renal failure or a serum creatinine below 3 mg/dL, intravenous pyelography (IVP) may be considered. The dye utilized during IVP has been shown to exacerbate the degree of renal failure or act as a nephrotoxic agent. During obstruction, the uptake of dye is slow or absent in the presence of coexisting renal failure. The combination of the IVP dye with a single dose of 20 to 40 mg of Lasix IV assists in visualization during mild obstruction. A renal scan may add only limited additional information to that afforded by the previously discussed tests but can be helpful in diagnosing partial obstruction.

Further diagnostic information and treatment can be obtained through urologic consultation. A cystoscopy performed by the urologist may reveal obstruction in the posterior urethra and bladder.

Table 31-1 Common Causes of Postrenal Failure

Urethral obstruction
Prostatic hypertrophy
Bladder involvement: obstruction, carcinoma, infection, or
  neurogenic problems
Ureteral obstruction resulting from renal calculi and edema
Extraureteral problems, e.g., abdominal tumor

Two kinds of pyelogram, retrograde and antegrade, provide information beyond noninvasive methods. The retrograde pyelogram is helpful during renal failure, and the antegrade is utilized when a source of obstruction cannot be bypassed. The antegrade procedure involves the passing of a catheter into the renal pelvis and, if possible, removing the obstruction.

Medical Management

Removal of the obstruction is the initial approach to postrenal failure. This must be followed by stabilization and maintenance of the patient through the postobstructive phase. The nurse needs to be aware that postobstructive diuresis usually compounds this phase. This kind of polyuria produces urine that contains electrolytes, especially sodium and potassium. A meticulous intake and output record must be maintained and correlated with daily weight. Intravenous replacement therapy follows a plan of replacing two-thirds of the previous hour's urine output plus 30 mL every hour with D$_5$/½NS. Electrolyte levels and acid-base parameters need to be obtained frequently to determine the amount of electrolyte replacement needed, and the urinary output must be monitored to ascertain the correct replacement volume. Other parameters of fluid status should be assessed every shift and whenever acute exacerbations occur. Signs of recovery include a more normal pattern of urinary output and BUN and serum creatinine levels approaching normal.

Prerenal Failure

Prerenal conditions include any pathophysiologic states which lead to diminished perfusion of the kidney without renal tubular damage. The nephrons are intact, but the decrease in blood supply causes a drop in the glomerular filtration rate which is reflected by a decrease in urine output. Conditions causing prerenal disorders are numerous and common to the critically ill. The reasons for altered renal perfusion range from hypovolemic causes to impaired cardiac function and variations in vascular dynamics (Table 31-2). Most forms of prerenal failure are easily reversible. Generally, these conditions are corrected by improving renal perfusion by volume replacement, enhanced cardiac output, and/or reversal of vasoconstriction or vasodilatation. As a result of these measures function usually resumes.

Recent laboratory and clinical investigation of prerenal failure has led to the development of specific therapies for the critically ill which attempt to reverse the diminished renal perfusion and alterations in renal hemodynamics associated with this state. Because of these findings it is necessary, for therapeutic purposes, to divide prerenal conditions into two categories, according to whether the condition places the patient at low or at high risk of an intrarenal problem. A condition which responds rapidly to therapy and is, therefore, easily reversed and places the patient at low risk is a mild form of prerenal failure.[5] A classic example of mild prerenal failure is uncomplicated dehydration. The critical-care nurse *during* this condition notices a decrease in urine output over several hours or even eventual absence of output. The nurse correlates this change in renal function with recent negative intake/output balance, weight loss, hypotension, decreased neck veins, low central venous pressure, decreased wedge pressure, dry mucous

Table 31-2 Common Causes of Prerenal Failure

Ischemic
  Hypotensive shock
  Cardiogenic shock
  Septic shock
  Hypoxic state
  Reduced cardiac output
Nephrotoxic
  Antibiotics: aminoglycosides, cephalosporins,
    amphotericin B, polymyxin B
  Contrast media
  Heavy metals: mercury, arsenic, platinum
  Endogenous: endotoxins, myoglobins, hemoglobins

membranes, and alteration in mental status, usually lethargy. Examination of recent laboratory studies reveals an elevated serum BUN and normal or slightly elevated creatinine in a greater than 20:1 ratio. A spot urine test for sodium reveals a value of 10 meq or less. All these findings support the presence of dehydration. A fluid challenge and then the initiation of volume replacement therapy with a solution comparable to the type lost (e.g., nasogastric, fistula drainage) restores urine output. In other words, low-risk or mild prerenal conditions respond to immediate treatment of the primary cause by restoration of renal function.

The prerenal conditions creating a high-risk situation are those which put the kidneys in a hypoperfused state for a prolonged period, e.g., cardiogenic shock or multiple trauma in a hemodynamically unstable patient (Table 31-3). In this situation, response to therapy is usually slow and acute tubular necrosis develops. The high-risk prerenal state is synonymous with the preventive or onset phase of acute tubular necrosis (ATN). The modes of treatment initiated during this phase as identified in the literature act to prevent ATN or to create a milder form of ATN called nonoliguria.[6–8] In experimental models, the method which actually increases renal perfusion and reverses the alteration in renal hemodynamics seen in this phase is volume expansion with a colloidal solution such as plasma.[9–11] If the use of a colloid is not appropriate, then substitution fluids such as saline or Ringer's lactate can be instituted. This therapeutic action has a central effect by improving cardiac output and thus indirectly improving renal perfusion. This effect, if sustained, may eventually alleviate the prerenal condition. If volume expansion is not

Table 31-3 Conditions Associated with High Risk of Acute Tubular Necrosis

Hemodynamic instability
  Cardiogenic shock
  Sepsis
  Hypotension
Severe multiple trauma
Prolonged surgery
Burns
Nephrotoxic drugs: aminoglycoside antibiotics, amphotericin B, cephalosporins
Rhabdomyolyis

Table 31-4 Renal Blood Flow Augmenters

Furosemide
Ethacrynic acid
Mannitol
Dopamine
Prostaglandins
Bradykinins

possible or does not prove adequate, then pharmacologic augmentation is indicated. Two types of agent are utilized for this purpose: vasodilators to improve both renal blood flow and glomerular filtration rate and diuretics to prevent potential tubular obstruction and increase urine flow (Table 31-4).

These agents are believed to augment renal blood flow, not reinstate it, and to promote the progression from a high-risk prerenal state to a nonoliguric rather than an oliguric ATN. To produce this effect dopamine is recommended at low doses (3 mg/g per min) to induce a renal vasodilatory effect, in conjunction with furosemide 100 to 200 mg q 6 to 8 h.[12] Other agents recognized as renal blood flow augmenters are mannitol, prostaglandins, bradykinins and ethacrynic acid.

Interstitial Renal Failure

Actual renal tissue damage to glomeruli, vessels, or tubules results in interstitial renal failure. Because tissue damage has been experienced by the kidneys, healing usually requires 10 days to 3 months or even 1 year. Acute tubular necrosis has been recognized as the most common cause of interstitial renal failure; therefore, the remainder of this section focuses on ATN.

Pathophysiology of ATN

Acute tubular necrosis is the most common form of acute renal failure, resulting from either nephrotoxic or ischemic injury. Antibiotics, especially aminoglycosides, are the most common causative agents.[13] The epithelial layer has the ability to regenerate, and rapid healing usually occurs over a period of 10 days to 2 weeks if other factors do not complicate the recovery period. Factors which can increase the nephrotoxic damage are hypotensive episodes, infection, and dehydration.[14,15] Current investigations of the renal hemodynamic alterations during nephrotoxicity suggest possible decreased cardiac output secondary to a systemic toxic effect.[16] The decreased cardiac output may cause primary or additional damage.

Contrast medium ranks as the second most common cause of ATN. Diabetes mellitus and chronic renal insufficiency, especially when related to multiple melanoma, place patients at the highest risk of nephrotoxicity. Large volumes of fluid administered before and after dye infusion can prevent or minimize nephrotoxicity. Heavy metals as well as endogenous toxins complete the list of common causes. Among the endogenous causes of ATN are myoglobin secondary to rhabdomyolysis, septic endotoxins, and hemoglobin posttransfusion reaction.

Ischemic injury occurs as the unresolvable high-risk prerenal condition or preventive phase progresses to the actual development of renal tubular necrosis. The implementation of therapeutic modalities to augment renal blood flow determines whether the patient will begin acute renal failure in oliguria or nonoliguria.[17,18]

Oliguria, the classic form of presentation of ATN, is associated with a mortality rate of approximately 50 percent. Mortality rates which are slightly higher, 50 to 70 percent, are seen in the trauma victim and postoperative patient.[19] Other factors that increase the mortality rate are the severity of the primary disease, the number of complications, and age more than 65 years. One of two pathophysiologic events results in the onset of oliguria: either intratubular obstruction or the backleak phenomenon.

Intratubular obstruction is the result of the sloughing off of tubular cells in response to the ischemic event and their collecting in the tubular space. To minimize the degree of intratubular obstruction, large boluses of diuretics may be administered at the onset of ATN in an effort to remove the obstructive source and restore tubular patency. This therapeutic effort is an attempt to move the patient more rapidly to the diuretic phase,[20] but this intervention is not always effective.

The backleak phenomenon is the result of "cracks" which form in the tubular wall secondary to the ischemic event. The filtrate actually leaks into the body; therefore less urine is made and oliguria results. Because the patient does not excrete water or metabolic wastes, the incidence of biochemical abnormalities is high, as exemplified by a low creatinine clearance (approximately 1 mL/min), a peak level of azotemia, and high urinary sodium levels. Hyperkalemia is more likely to become a patient problem during oliguria. The daily potassium load associated with ATN in the oliguric phase is greater than 0.5 meq/L and results from catabolism, hemolysis, tissue breakdown, or endogenous causes. Without the assistance of the kidneys in potassium excretion, levels of over 6.0 meq/L may be associated with cardiac involvement. In addition, the acidotic state which occurs during renal failure may further potentiate the hyperkalemic condition.[21] Fluid retention in this phase may be severe enough to create episodes of pulmonary edema.

Either hemodialysis or peritoneal dialysis is indicated in the above situations if the volume overload results in a risk of or actual occurrence of pulmonary edema and the hyperkalemia, acidosis, and uremia are all unmanageable by conventional methods. Another indication for dialysis is a risk of uremic complications such as pericarditis. Recently, the use of slow continuous ultrafiltration or continuous arteriovenous hemofiltration has been suggested as a therapeutic approach which may decrease the frequency of hemodialysis.[22] The oliguric phase usually lasts 10 to 16 days.

Nonoliguric ATN has a better prognosis than oliguric, with a mortality rate as low as 26 percent, and the duration is shorter, only 5 to 8 days. The nonoliguric patient excretes approximately 350 mosm of solute in the urine output. The creatinine clearance may be as high as 15 mL/min, and the urinary excretion of sodium is low. Hyperkalemia, however, remains a significant problem requiring therapeutic intervention. The pathophysiology of the nonoliguric phase is associated with less tubular damage, and signs and symptoms resemble those of the diuretic phase. The urinary output may exceed 1 L/h. Generally, these patients are easier to manage than oliguric patients, because they can excrete a large volume and some solute, so that dialysis is needed less frequently or not at all.

During the initial phases of oliguric and nonoliguric ATN, it is important to determine whether the patient is in a catabolic or noncatabolic state.

The catabolic state is associated with a significant amount of tissue breakdown. Trauma, fevers, and infections may even further complicate the catabolic condition. Laboratory values reflecting the large endogenous load of excess electrolytes and wastes reveal BUN levels greater than 30 mg/dL, serum creatinine levels greater than 2 mg/dL, serum potassium levels greater than 0.5 meq/dL, serum bicarbonate greater than 2 meq/dL, and uric acid levels greater than 1 mg/dL, all associated with catabolism. In comparison, the noncatabolic patient has lower BUN and creatinine levels approximating 10 to 20 mg/dL and 0.5 to 1.0 mg/dL respectively, which are easier to maintain.[19]

The phase which follows oliguria is the diuretic phase, while the phase following nonoliguria is recovery (Table 31-5). As one can see, nonoliguria is only one step from recovery, while the oliguric phase must proceed to a diuretic phase before it reaches recovery. This fact reinforces the claim that nonoliguria is the less severe form of acute tubular necrosis.

In the diuretic phase that follows the oliguric phase the patient makes large volumes of dilute urine. The salinity of the urine varies with the individual. A comparison of the serum and urine electrolytes, BUN, and creatinine levels clarifies for the nurse the way a patient is excreting urinary solute. Besides determining potential electrolyte imbalances and the state of metabolic waste excretion, the nurse is responsible for fluid replacement. The larger volumes of urine output associated with this phase may cause circulatory collapse unless vigorous fluid replacement is instituted. The type of fluid replaced should reflect the kind of fluid lost. Usually $D_5/\frac{1}{2}NS$ is selected, and two-thirds of the previous hour's urine output volume is replaced plus 30 mL. The 30 mL accounts for insensible losses. Potassium supplements are added to the intravenous fluids if this ion is being wasted in the urine. The diuretic phase usually lasts 48 to 72 h but can continue for as long as 7 to 12 days before normal renal function resumes.

The recovery phase follows either the diuretic or the nonoliguric phase. A gradual trend toward improvement is observed in this phase, extending over a 3- to 12-month period.[23] The BUN and creatinine, which should be checked at intervals, reveal a gradual decline. Plateaus in these values occasionally occur, only to be followed by another fall in serum BUN and creatinine levels. Eventually these levels stabilize, indicating that the kidneys have reached the final adjustment.

Medical Management of ATN

The objectives of medical therapies are:

1. Correction of fluid imbalances
2. Prevention of hyperkalemia and other life-threatening electrolyte imbalances
3. Treatment of azotemia acidosis
4. Prevention of further nephrotoxicity by altering drug therapy
5. Improvement of nutritional status
6. Avoidance and treatment of infection
7. Prevention of anemia

Medical interventions begin in the onset or prevention phase. The first step is anticipating, prior to the renal insult, which patients may be at high risk for acute renal failure. The patients falling into the category of high risk are the surgical candidates, the hemodynamically unstable, and those receiving large doses of radiologic contrast dye or nephrotoxic drugs. A prophylactic solute diuresis should be instituted in these patients at least 2 hours prior to the renal insult if not earlier.[24] During this therapy the patient receives both $D_5/\frac{1}{2}NS$, 200 mL over the first hour, then decreasing to 150 mL/h, and 20 g of mannitol. If the urinary output does not respond

Table 31-5 Phases of Acute Tubular Necrosis

Onset — — — — — — — > Oliguria — — — — — — — > Diuretic — — — — — — — > Recovery			
or			
prevention			
Onset			
or — — — — — — — > Nonoliguria — — — — — — — > Recovery			
prevention			

or if there is a threat of fluid overload, furosemide 40 to 80 mg IV can replace the mannitol dose.

The goal of this approach is to promote hydration, which helps to protect against a low blood flow and can dilute the effects of a nephrotoxic agent. It is also believed that diuretics given prior to or in the early phase of failure can prevent or reduce the severity of acute renal failure.[25] However, this belief has not been substantiated in experimental human studies. The use of diuretics can also have diagnostic value, for a urinary response indicates that a prerenal condition is present or that oliguric ATN has been converted to nonoliguric ATN. The therapeutic approach varies when the patient is experiencing a physiologic crisis associated with reduced renal perfusion; this requires the use of both volume expanders and renal blood flow augmenters.

Once the patient is diagnosed as having acute renal failure (ARF), the medical goal is to return the patient, as quickly as possible, to a homeostatic state. The idea is to avoid any condition that may again insult the kidney during its recovery period. Fluid and/or blood imbalances must be corrected. Intake and output, central venous pressure, wedge pressure, and daily weight are important parameters at this time. Once a state of fluid balance is achieved, the oliguric ARF patient is maintained on an intake of 600 mL per day plus insensible loss. The approach during nonoliguric ARF is to replace the volume or two-thirds of the urine output plus 30 mL per hour.

During both oliguric and nonoliguric ARF, electrolyte imbalances must be prevented, because they can be life-threatening (Table 31-6). This can be attempted by limiting dietary intake and trying conservative treatment such as sodium polystyrene sulfonate (Kayexalate). This conservative approach can be continued if the potassium remains below 6.0 meq/L. A potassium approaching a value of 6.5 meq/L associated with ECG changes requires active intervention. The appearance of hyponatremia has diagnostic value, because the cause of this imbalance is often the dilutional effect of fluid overload. It is an indication for the initiation of some form of dialysis. The onset of hypocalcemia and hyperphosphatemia indicates the need for 30 to 60 mL of an aluminum hydroxide gel given four to six times a day.

Dialysis is indicated in acute renal failure for:

1. Volume overload
2. Uncontrollable hyperkalemia
3. Uncontrollable acidosis
4. Symptomatic uremia
5. Pericarditis
6. BUN levels greater than 100 mg/dL

The desired outcome of control of azotemia is to keep the BUN in a range between 70 and 100 mg/dL. The onset of uremic symptoms appears to

Table 31-6 Electrolyte Imbalances in Acute Renal Failure

Imbalance	Laboratory Value	Treatment
Excess of potassium (hyperkalemia)	>5.5 meq/L	Emergency: 10 U regular insulin IV push, sodium bicarbonate 1 ampule, calcium gluconate 1 ampule Maintenance: sodium polystyrene sulfonate (kayexalate), hemodialysis
Deficiency of sodium (hyponatremia)	<130 meq/L	Correct water overload if sodium loss is present, then replace sodium gradually
Deficiency of calcium (hypocalcemia)	<8.5 mg/dL	Phosphate binders, dihydroxytachysterol (DHT), calcium PO, and dialysis
Excess of phosphates (hyperphosphatemia)	>76 mg/dL	Phosphate binders
Excess of magnesium (hypermagnesemia)	>72 to 73 mg/dL	Dialysis

occur within this range; the specific value at which the symptoms actually occur varies from patient to patient. The patient's clinical situation determines which type of dialysis is most appropriate. Patients with uncontrollable azotemia and/or electrolyte values which require rapid correction will benefit from hemodialysis. Examples of the kinds of patients often requiring hemodialysis are the severely catabolic, trauma victims, those with burns or septic conditions, and often postsurgical patients. Patients with a mild form of ATN or those who are experiencing little or no tissue breakdown often can be managed successfully with peritoneal dialysis.

The basic principles for the hemodialysis procedure are the same during acute and chronic renal failure. However, certain aspects need to be adjusted to meet the needs and tolerance levels of acute renal failure patients.

The areas of most frequent concern are:

1. Blood pressure control
2. Method of coagulation
3. Dialysate potassium levels
4. Method of correcting acidosis

The patient with acute renal failure is usually hemodynamically unstable. Therefore, an approach must be devised whereby fluid can be removed while the blood pressure is maintained. This may necessitate administering priming solution and considering albumin infusions. If the patient is unable to tolerate volume expansion, vasopressors (such as dopamine) can be used to support the blood pressure.[26]

The method used for coagulation depends on the general condition of the patient and the state of coagulation. A coagulation problem requires minimal or regional heparinization. Regional heparinization involves use of a heparin infusion on the arterial side of a vascular access, balanced by a protamine infusion on the venous side.

The amount of potassium added to the dialysate bath varies from 0 to 4 meq/L depending on the desired therapeutic effect. The prescribed amount of dialysate is determined prior to dialysis, and patients receiving digoxin need special consideration.

To control the acidosis, a bicarbonate dialysate is preferred because its effects are predictable. Either femoral catheter or AV shunt is usually selected for arteriovenous access.

Intermittent peritoneal dialysis is initiated with a temporary catheter or a Tenckoff. The advantage of a Tenckoff is that repeated dialysis can be easily initiated. Two-liter exchanges with little or no potassium are used. This procedure proves to be of low risk to the patient; it is well tolerated by the hemodynamically unstable patient and does not require significant anticoagulation therapy. Close observation of the patient's response is necessary to reassess the benefits and effectiveness of this treatment.

Other treatment concerns of the physician include the provision of nutritional therapy. A minimum of 100 g of carbohydrates must be provided. The combination of parenteral hyperalimentation and daily hemodialysis has been associated with an increased survival rate and is thought to be a factor which promotes rapid renal tubular cell healing. Hyperalimentation should include glucose and large amounts of essential and nonessential amino acids—approximately 21 g per day of each[27–29] (see Chap. 12).

Continuous arteriovenous hemofiltration (CAVH) may be utilized in acute renal failure to assist the patient in handling hyperalimentation or fluid drug boluses.[30] Another indication for CAVH is hemodynamic instability in a patient who cannot tolerate hemodialysis. CAVH in the critically ill has some advantages over hemodialysis in that it does not affect cardiac output, activate complement, or reduce leukocytes.[31] Hemodialysis, moreover, is associated with a decrease in pulmonary oxygen transport and a potential allergic reaction to the dialyzer membrane, whereas these responses appear to be absent in CAVH.[32,33]

Aseptic technique for intravenous line placement is necessary to help avoid infections, which develop in approximately 50 percent of all patients with ARF. The early removal of urinary catheters and arterial and venous lines also reduces this risk. Skin barriers and mucous membranes need to be maintained intact. If infection is suspected, antibiotics should be selected on the basis of blood culture results.

Pharmacologic agents which are primarily or partially excreted by the kidney, as well as drugs which have a nephrotoxic effect, must be dose-adjusted by the physician. Two common agents requiring adjustment are digoxin and all the aminoglycoside antibodies. Metabolic acidosis is usually treated by the administration of sodium bicarbonate IV push if the bicarbonate level drops below 10 meq/L.

Nursing Management*

Any of the following nursing diagnoses may be applicable:

Potential for acute renal failure

Altered urinary elimination pattern: oliguria, anuria, or polyuria

Fluid volume excess: oliguric phase

Potential for fluid volume deficit: diuretic or non-oliguric phase

Potential for electrolyte imbalances: hyperkalemia, hyponatremia, hyperphosphotemia, hypocalcemia, or hypermagnesemia

Potential for uremic syndrome

Potential for acid-base imbalance: metabolic acidosis

Activity intolerance: anemia and/or uremia and/or hypocalcemia

Potential for infection

Altered nutrition; less than body requirements: uremia and/or hypercatabolism

Impaired skin integrity: potential for uremia and/or malnutrition

Altered metabolism of pharmacologic agents: renal failure

Sleep pattern disturbance

Patient's lack of knowledge of disease process and treatment

Potential for ineffective coping: patient and family

Prevention

For effective prevention, the critical-care nurse must be able to identify the patient at high risk of developing ATN. The nurse needs to be aware of

*All nursing process items in this section are adapted from Stark, Reiley, & Jenuelson.

the benefits of renal perfusion in increasing cardiac output and expanding plasma volume. In addition, the indications for pharmacologic augmenters plus the dosage and method of administration must be understood. The critical-care nurse, working closely with the physician, devises and implements a plan that attempts to rescue kidney function from the hypoperfused state. If restoration is not possible, the therapies which encourage a nonoliguric ATN should be implemented.

Collaborative interventions include:

1. Correction of hypotension
2. Correction of cause of prerenal condition
3. Administration of augmenters: diuretic therapy and other hemodynamic augmenters
4. Obtaining of urine and blood specimens for laboratory analysis

Nursing interventions include:

1. Assessment and reporting of any of the findings suggestive of an impending or present prerenal condition (decreasing urine output, decreased wedge pressure)
2. Monitoring and recording of arterial and venous blood pressure and urine output

The desired outcome is detection of the high-risk patient and prevention of ATN.

Fluid Imbalance

The plan for fluid management is dependent on the patient's present fluid status. The pattern of urine output can provide a clue to help determine whether the patient is dehydrated, homeostatic, or overhydrated. For example, oliguria and anuria are associated with volume overload because the patient cannot excrete adequate urine. In polyuria the patient may be dehydrated, but only if the urinary losses have not been replaced by an equal or near equal volume. Once an imbalance is suspected, data are collected for verification of confirming symptoms.[33] The assessment criteria for dehydration are:

1. Weight loss
2. Poor skin turgor
3. Hypotension
4. Complaints of thirst
5. Dry mucous membranes
6. Minimal or absent neck vein distention

7. Low central venous pressure (CVP) or wedge pressure
8. Increased pulse rate
9. Stupor

The criteria for overhydration are:

1. Weight gain
2. Hypertension
3. Neck vein distention
4. Elevated CVP and wedge pressure
5. Edema (peripheral, ascites, periorbital)
6. Bounding pulse
7. Dyspnea, rales
8. Stupor

The data obtained via assessment lead to a nursing diagnosis of either fluid volume deficit or excess.

Collaborative interventions include:

1. Administration of fluids to correct prerenal conditions
2. Determination of plan for fluid administration
3. Determination of indicators for and type of dialysis

Nursing interventions are to:

1. Obtain daily weights: note trend in weight gain or loss and report findings.
2. Maintain intake and output records: observe trends in negative and positive balances and repo   'ngs.
3. Mai'   .1 patency of diagnostic arterial and venous monitoring lines.
4. Maintain awareness of the kinds of imbalances expected in each stage of ATN (oliguria or nonoliguria, polyuria, etc.).
5. Implement dialysis procedure as indicated by unit policy.

The goal is to reverse volume imbalances and implement methods to prevent further imbalances.

Electrolyte Imbalance

The critical-care nurse needs to be aware of the most common types of electrolyte imbalance occurring during acute renal failure: hyperkalemia, hyponatremia, hypocalcemia, hyperphosphatemia, and hypermagnesemia.

Life-threatening hyperkalemia is seen more frequently in acute than in chronic renal failure.

Knowledge of the ECG changes which occur in acute renal failure are essential. First the T waves become tall, peaked, and tented. This is followed by a wide QRS, a flattening of the P wave, and eventually asystole. The emergency medical intervention is to administer 10 U of regular insulin IV push with one ampule of 50% dextrose sodium bicarbonate and one ampule of calcium chloride or gluconate IV. This action must be immediately followed by some procedure to permanently remove potassium from the body, such as administration of sodium polystyrene sulfonate (Kayexalate) or hemodialysis treatment.[34]

Collaborative interventions are to:

1. Obtain and interpret electrolyte values daily or more frequently, if necessary.
2. Administer either drugs or dialysis to correct electrolyte imbalances.

Nursing interventions are to:

1. Observe for and report any signs or symptoms of electrolyte imbalances.
2. Interpret ECG changes.
3. Consider possible measures to maintain normal serum potassium levels.

The goal is to maintain a normal electrolyte levels.

Metabolic Acidosis

In acute renal failure the kidneys are not able to excrete the daily production of endogenous acids. The acid load produced during ATN is 1 meq/kg in repeated episodes of acidemia.

Collaborative interventions are to:

1. Measure ABGs as necessary.
2. Interpret findings.
3. Administer sodium bicarbonate for symptomatic acidosis.
4. Implement dialysis for uncontrollable acidosis.

The nursing role is to recognize signs and symptoms of acid/base imbalances and report symptoms.

The goal is to maintain an asymptomatic pH.

Anemia

Patients become anemic because of lack of erythropoietin in 20 to 30 percent of all cases. However, anemia during ATN may also result from a source of frank bleeding or other causes such as gastrointestinal bleeding, bone marrow depression, or uremic syndrome. All reasons for anemia should be considered and treated upon recognition.[35,36]

Collaborative interventions are to:

1. Obtain and interpret hematocrit and hemoglobin levels.
2. Administer iron (IM) and multivitamins.
3. Transfuse fresh blood whenever indicated.

The nursing role is to maintain awareness of the risks connected with transfusing bank blood, such as hyperkalemia, acid/base imbalances, and clotting disorders, as well as the risk of hepatitis B and non-A and non-B hepatitis to both patients and staff.

Uremia

Uremic symptoms occur when the BUN rises above 70 to 100 mg/dL and/or the glomerular filtration rate is below 10 to 15 mL/min. The uremic symptoms are better prevented, because once present, these symptoms can only be controlled, not reversed. Until renal failure is resolved, early symptoms are likely to occur.

Collaborative interventions are to:

1. Obtain and interpret BUN, creatinine, and uric acid levels.
2. Establish a plan for dialysis.
3. Assess at least daily the onset or progress of uremic symptoms.

Nursing interventions are to:

1. Be alert to the different kinds of uremic symptoms and recognize that these symptoms can be minimized by limiting the degree of azotemia.
2. Implement dialysis as ordered.

Infection

Infection is the most frequent complication of acute renal failure, occurring in 30 to 70 percent of all cases. This complication is the leading cause of death. The primary sites are the respiratory and urinary tracts and operative sites. Both gram-negative and gram-positive organisms are responsible for infections. As a result of this insult to an already compromised system, septicemia frequently occurs.

The suspected cause of the high infection rate is an impairment of the immunologic response due to the uremic state and alterations in normal skin barriers.

Collaborative interventions include:

1. Evaluation of infection at onset (blood and urine Gram's stain and culture)
2. Administration of antibiotic therapy
3. Correlation of antibiotic dosage with daily serum creatinine level
4. Avoidance of indwelling urinary catheters and other invasive procedures

Nursing interventions include:

1. Implementation of preventive measures within the nursing realm (nutrition, maintenance of skin integrity, infection control, etc.)
2. Maintenance of temperature charts, noting trend in fever spikes if they occur
3. Protection of skin and carrying out of mouth care in order to minimize breaks in normal protective barriers
4. Utilization of aseptic technique during wound and intravenous line dressing changes

The goal is prevention or early detection of infection.

Skin Care

The manifestations of uremic skin changes are dryness, itching, and bruising. Uremic frost, infections, and edema may be the end result. The changes in the texture and thickness of the skin plus other conditions previously mentioned necessitate frequent care and attention.

The nursing role is to initiate a regimen to keep skin clean, dry, and intact to prevent infection:

1. Bathe skin daily to remove waste products.
2. Apply creams or ointments.
3. Administer medications to relieve itching.
4. Use oil in bath to prevent dryness.
5. Cleanse bruises and open areas to prevent infection.
6. Monitor presence of edema.
7. Avoid tight sheets or slippers, because they may create pressure points susceptible to breakdown.

The goal is to maintain intact skin.

Nutrition

Considerations in nutritional assessment include:

1. Primary disease process (other than ARF)
2. Acute tubular cell necrosis
3. Presence of catabolism
4. Tissue breakdown
5. Vulnerability to infection
6. Fluid and electrolyte imbalances
7. Acidosis
8. Anemia

The dietary elements most often prescribed are restricted protein and a diet high in calories and essential amino acids, with at least 100 g of carbohydrate per day and restricted sodium and potassium.

Improved survival has been observed in catabolic patients receiving hyperalimentation. It is recommended that patients receive large quantities of amino acids to meet the metabolic needs. The combination of regular hyperalimentation and daily dialysis has been shown to promote rapid recovery in the patient with ATN (see Chap. 12).

Nursing interventions are to:

1. Collaborate with physician to determine nutritional replacement plan.
2. Administer hyperalimentation utilizing aseptic technique.
3. Manage hyperalimentation dosage to meet nutritional needs but minimize hyperosmololity.
4. Consider small, frequent feedings during periods of nausea and vomiting.

The goal is to promote protein sparing and to provide adequate calories and amino acids for cellular healing and reduction of the risk of infection.

Drug Administration

Dosages of pharmacologic agents which are primarily metabolized or excreted by the kidney must be regulated in impaired renal function. Adjustments become even more critical when the drug being administered has a toxic effect (nephrotoxicity, ototoxicity, or cardiotoxicity). There is only a narrow margin between drug effectiveness and safety, so the least toxic drug should be selected when possible. Examples of agents requiring dosage regulation during renal failure are diuretics (furosemide or mannitol) and aminoglycosides. Other elements, such as contrast media and myoglobin or hemoglobin pigments, require rapid removal in order to avoid nephrotoxic effects.

Collaborative interventions include:

1. Modification of drug dosages in relation to the degree of renal failure
2. Consideration of increased intervals between doses
3. Obtaining and monitoring of serum drug levels (especially the serum concentration).

Nursing interventions are to:

1. Question the orders for nephrotoxic agents to prevent further renal damage.
2. Closely observe the patient to prevent or assess toxicity due to drug accumulation.
3. Report any untoward signs, especially elevation of serum creatinine, so that the drug choice can be reconsidered, the dosage reduced, or the drug discontinued.

The goal is to minimize nephrotoxicity or cumulative effect.

Sleep Pattern Disturbance

Sleep disturbances have recently been recognized in the renal failure patient. The cause of this kind of disturbance is not known; however, it is suspected that uremia or pharmacologic agents such as testosterone may be responsible. The patient often complains of an altered sleep pattern the night before dialysis—the point when the uremic toxins are at the highest levels. This predialysis experience is also suggestive of a stress component.

The nursing role is to assess the patient's normal sleep pattern, minimize interruptions during sleep, and allow 90-min periods of uninterrupted sleep when possible.

References

1. Butkus, D. (1983). Epidemic hemorrhagic fever with renal syndrome: A broadening horizon. *Archives of Internal Medicine, 143,* 2299–2300.
2. Rainford, D. J. (1981). Nutritional management of acute renal failure. In D. D. Wright & M. Elliot (Eds.),

Parental and enteral nutrition. *Chirurgica Scandinavica, 507,* 1981, 327–329.

3. Stark, J. (1985). The renal system. In G. Alspach & S. Williams (Eds.), *Core curriculum for critical-care nursing: American Association of Critical-Care Nurses.* Philadelphia: Saunders.

4. Wilson, D. R. (1983). Obstructive uropathy. In D. Z. Levine (Ed.), *Care of the renal patient.* Philadelphia: Saunders.

5. Stark, J. (in press). Acute renal failure. In J. Stark, P. Reiley, & C. Jenuelson (Eds.), *Nursing management of renal dysfunction.* Baltimore: Aspen Corporation.

6. Diamond, J. R., & Yoburn, D. C. (1982). Nonoliguric acute renal failure. *Archives of Internal Medicine 142,* 1882–1884.

7. Anderson, R. J., Linas, S. L., Berns, A. S., Henrich, W. L., Miller, T. R., Gabow, P. A., & Schrier, R. W. (1977). Nonoliguric acute renal failure. *N. England Journal of Medicine, 296,* 1134–1138.

8. Myers, B. D., Hilberman, M., Spencer, R. J., & Jamison, R. L. (1982). Glomerular and tubular function in non-oliguric acute renal failure. *The American Journal of Medicine, 72,* 642–649.

9. Maher, J. F. (1981). Pathophysiology of renal hemodynamics. *Nephron, 27,* 215–221.

10. Hsu, C-H., & Kurtz, T. W. (1981). Renal hemodynamics in experimental acute renal failure. *Nephron, 27,* 255–259.

11. Burke, T. J., & Schrier, R. W. (1983). Ischemic acute renal failure—pathogenic steps leading to acute tubular necrosis. *Circulatory Shock, 11,* 255–259.

12. Mandal, A. K., Lightfoot, B. O., & Treat, R. C. (1983) Mechanisms of protection in acute renal failure. *Circulatory Shock, 11,* 245–253.

13. Goldstein, M. B. (1983). Acute renal failure. *Medical Clinics of North America, 67*(6), 1325–1341.

14. Mars, D. R., & Treloar, D. (1984). Acute tubular necrosis—pathophysiology and treatment. *Heart Lung, 13*(2), 194–201.

15. Kon, V., & Ichikawa, T. W. (1984). Research seminar: Physiology of acute renal failure. *The Journal of Pediatrics, 105*(3), 351–357.

16. Hsu, C-H., & Kurtz, T. W. (1981). Renal hemodynamics in experimental acute renal failure. *Nephron, 27,* 204–208.

17. Conger, J. D. (1983). Vascular abnormalities in the maintenance of acute renal failure. *Circulatory Shock, 11,* 235–244.

18. Wilson, M. F., & Brackett, D. J. (1983). Release of vasoactive hormones and circulatory changes in shock. *Circulatory Shock, 11,* 225–234.

19. Conger, J. D., & Anderson, R. J. (1983). Acute renal failure including cortical necrosis. In S. G. Massry & R. J. Glassock (Eds.), *Textbook of nephrology.* Baltimore: Williams & Wilkins.

20. Oken, D. E. (1984). Hemodynamic basis for human acute renal failure (vasomotor nephropathy). *American Journal of Medicine, 76,* 702–710.

21. Reubi, F. C., & Vorburger, C. (1976). Renal hemodynamics in acute renal failure after shock in man. *Kidney International,10,* S137–147.

22. Golper, T. A. (1985). Continuous arteriovenous hemofiltration in acute renal failure. *American Journal of Kidney Disease, 6*(6), 373–386.

23. Finn, W. J., & Chevalier, R. L. (1979). Recovery from postischemic acute renal failure in the rat. *Kidney International, 16,* 113–123.

24. Wilson, D. R. (1983). Obstructive uropathy. In D. Z. Levine (Ed.), *Care of the renal patient.* Philadelphia: Saunders.

25. Cronin, R. E. (1981). The patient with acute azotemia. In R. W. Schriev (Ed.), *Manual of nephrology* (pp. 232–258). Boston: Little, Brown.

26. Tantalo-Woods, F., & Izatt, S. (1983). Nursing care of renal patients. In D. Z. Levine (Ed.), *Care of the renal patient.* Philadelphia: Saunders.

27. Mault, J. R., Bartlett, R. H., Dechert, R. E., et al. (1982). Starvation: A major contributor to mortality in acute renal failure. *Trans. American Society for Artificial Internal Organs, 29,* 510–513.

28. Feinstein, E. I., Blumenkrantz, M. J., Helay, M., et al. (1981). Clinical and metabolic responses to parenteral nutrition in acute renal failure. *Medicine, 60,* 124–137.

29. Toback, G. F., Dodd, R. C., Maier, E. R., & Havener, L. J. (1983). Amino acid administration enhances renal protein metabolism after acute tubular necrosis. *Nephron, 33,* 238–243.

30. Kiely, M. A. (1984). Continuous arteriovenous hemofiltration. *Critical Care Nurse, 4,*(4), 39–43, 49.

31. Williams, V., & Perkins, L. (1984). Continuous ultrafiltration: A new ICU procedure for the treatment of fluid overload. *Critical Care Nurse, 4,*(4), 44–49.

32. Winkelman, C. (1985). Hemofiltration: A new technique in critical care nursing. *Heart Lung, 14*(3), 265–271.

33. Stark, J. L. (1982). How to succeed against acute renal failure. *Nursing, 12*(7), 26–33.

34. Coons, M. H. (1980). Acute tubular insufficiency: Nursing impact on recovery. *Nephrology Nurse, 2*(5), 18–23.

35. Fay, F. C., & De Tornyay, R. (1978). Experiences in clinical problem-solving: Pulling a patient through acute renal failure. *RN, 41*(11), 61–64.

36. Roberts, D. (1982). The nursing care of patients in acute renal failure. *Nursing Times, 78*(21), 896–897.

32 Chronic Renal Failure

June L. Stark
Ruth Kelleher

Chronic renal failure is a slow, progressive disorder usually continuing for years. Once chronic renal failure (CRF) develops, the disease process can be slowed but never reversed. If the patient survives for the full course of the disease, the result is end-stage renal failure. CRF has a number of causes, such as glomerulonephritis, polycystic disease, and obstructive uropathy.

Pathophysiology and Stages

During chronic renal failure, regardless of the etiology, nephron damage occurs in a progressive manner,[1] which accounts for the slow evolution of end-stage renal disease (ESRD). Damage to nephron groups eliminates their contributory role in maintaining renal function. The remaining intact nephrons compensate for the loss of functioning nephrons by doubling in size. In this state of cellular hypertrophy, the intact nephrons can accept larger blood volumes, performing larger clearances to compensate for the damaged nephrons. This compensated process is so exact that the kidney can maintain function with as much as an 80 percent nephron loss.

Four stages of chronic renal failure correlate with the degree of nephron damage experienced by the kidney: diminished renal reserve, renal insufficiency, end-stage renal failure, and uremic syndrome.

Diminished Renal Reserve

Diminished renal reserve implies a 50 percent nephron loss. Nephron compensation at this time is quite effective despite the large amount of loss. Renal function is only mildly reduced; the excretory and some regulatory functions are sufficiently maintained to preserve a homeostatic environment, and the patient is usually symptom-free. If the primary disease is hypertension, there may be an exacerbation of a once stabilized blood pressure. Chronic anemia, in association with CRF, may also present in this initial stage. Diminished renal reserve is associated with a doubling of the normal serum creatinine value of 0.6 to 1.2 mg/dL to a value of 1.2 to 2.4 mg/dL. Because a creatinine value of 1.2 mg/dL is still within the normal range, detection of renal failure by physical examination is impossible if no signs and symptoms suggest it.

Renal Insufficiency

The second stage of CRF, renal insufficiency, is synonymous with a 75 percent nephron loss. The patient demonstrates signs of impaired renal function, evidenced by mild azotemia, a slightly impaired ability to concentrate the urine, and anemia. The serum creatinine value in this stage quadruples, the level at which renal insufficiency begins being approximately 4.8 mg/dL. A primary therapeutic goal is to assist the patient to maintain this level of renal function for as long as possible. This can be accomplished by avoiding conditions which may exacerbate nephron damage: infection, dehydration, nephrotoxic drugs, and cardiac failure.

End-Stage Renal Failure

End-stage renal failure, the third stage, is the result of a 90 percent nephron loss. This stage correlates with a serum creatinine level of 10. The progression of renal deterioration is such that the stability of the internal environment can no longer be preserved. The patient is evaluated for the number of uremic symptoms present and the degree to which they interfere with the activities of daily living. The outcome of this evaluation determines how quickly the patient is considered for renal transplantation and/or dialysis.

Uremic Syndrome

The final stage of CRF, the uremic syndrome, is the systemic response of the body to the buildup of uremic waste products. All the symptoms of the uremic syndrome can be avoided by starting dialysis prior to their onset. If uremic symptoms appear, increasing the frequency or effectiveness of dialysis may minimize the symptoms. Renal transplantation eliminates most effects of the uremic syndrome.

Uremic toxins are composed of over 200 elements resulting from either accumulated metabolic wastes or excesses in hormone levels. The molecular weight of the toxins is believed to vary from small to middle-size molecules, up to a weight of 5000. The molecular weight of these elements is important because the hemodialysis membrane pore size allows for removal of small and middle-size molecules. Peritoneal dialysis is as effective as hemodialysis because the peritoneal membrane has an even larger pore size. The pore size of the hemofiltration membrane favors the movement of small particles.

Symptoms of the uremic syndrome appear in stages. Some symptoms surface during times of crisis. Early symptoms include changes in personality, increased fatigue level, malaise, nausea, and vomiting. The uremic patient develops a shortened memory span and a decreased concentration time. These changes in mental processing and ability seem to correlate with high levels of uremic toxins, and, therefore, the presence and intensity of mental alterations may vary according to the effectiveness of dialysis. Insomnia and nightmares are also associated with higher levels of urea. The untreated patient progresses from increasing levels of fatigue and drowsiness to stupor, coma, and death. The effectiveness of current treatment usually limits the mental status changes primarily to irritability and anxiety. Uremia is associated with a number of psychiatric disorders, often beginning with a personality change, and patients who have a history of personality disorders may exhibit symptoms ranging from neurosis to psychosis.

The physiologic manifestations of uremia often begin with anemia, which may be evident even in the stage of diminished renal reserve. The skin pallor accompanying anemia can be a subtle sign of renal failure.[2] Anemia is often compounded by a bleeding abnormality caused by the uremia that results from a decrease in clotting factors, an alteration in platelet aggregation, and a disorder in prothrombin consumption. All these alterations cause an increase in bleeding time and a tendency to bleed. Thrombocytopenia is another uremic complication impacting on the anemia, as is the malnutrition often experienced by the CRF patient.

The variation in skin integrity and texture and an increased susceptibility to bruising is a continuing concern of the uremic patient. Uncontrollable pruritus contributes to the patient's discomfort, and the frequently observed multiple scratch marks are a reflection of this problem. Uremic wastes excreted through the skin are believed to be the cause of pruritus. These toxins are localized to the skin and cause dryness and a thin white film known as uremic frost. Skin pigments during uremia are varied and produce a yellow-orange hue that presents as a sallow appearance when combined with the paleness created by the anemic effect. Ecchymotic areas and petechiae further complicate the skin condition.

The metabolic abnormalities experienced during uremia include carbohydrate intolerance, which presents as a pseudodiabetes and hypocalcemia resulting from inability to convert vitamin D to the activated form. Hyperlipidemia, another uremic complication, can accelerate the normal atherosclerotic process associated with aging.

Other uremic symptoms which worsen with the extent of their presence follow the early symptoms. Peripheral neuropathies, often called *restless leg syndrome,* begin with foot drop and a burning sensation in the lower extremities. If not alleviated, peripheral neuropathy may contribute to a progressive demyelinization of the distal portion of the nerves from the lower to the upper extremities which may lead to paraplegia.

The gastrointestinal system affected by chronic uremia is susceptible to both stress and peptic ulcerations. The high gastrin levels associated with uremia may be the explanation for this. *Uremic bowel* is a late syndrome that shifts the patient from the usual state of constipation to a condition of chronic diarrhea. During uremic bowel syndrome, the patient may demonstrate resistance to the effect of sodium polystyrene sulfonate (Kayexalate).

Pericarditis is a common form of cardiac involvement in uremia. The patient complains of precordial pain, usually associated with evidence of a pericardial friction rub and an effusion visualized by radiologic examination. Pleural effusion may result from uremia, and it often accompanies pericarditis. Daily dialysis is utilized to alleviate this condition. Other types of cardiac disorders associated with uremia are hyperkalemia, hypertension, premature atherosclerosis, and various types of vasculitis.[2,3]

The primary pulmonary complication of uremia, other than pleural effusion, is pulmonary edema. Another pulmonary complication is uremic lung, or uremic pneumonitis, indicated on the chest x-ray by a "butterfly" configuration.

The electrolyte imbalances characteristic of renal failure are consistent with the uremic syndrome. Hyperkalemia, hypocalcemia, hyperphosphotemia, and hypermagnesemia are among the most common disturbances.

Chronic Renal Disease Entities

Although CRF is irreversible, it is important to determine the etiology of the renal disease because the prognosis and therapeutic interventions may vary. Chronic renal disease usually begins in one portion of the nephron. For example, a glomerular disease first affects the glomerulus and gradually progresses to affect tubular function. The opposite occurs during renal disorders originating in the tubules.

Glomerular Disease

The causes of glomerulonephropathy include a variety of disorders (chronic glomerulonephritis, systemic lupus erythematosis, serum sickness, diabetic nephritis) which affect primarily the glomerulus (Table 32-1). Chronic glomerulonephritis is the most common form of chronic renal failure. Antibody-mediated mechanisms are more often responsible for pathophysiologic changes than are nonimmunologic states. Glomerular injury results from the deposition of circulating antigen-antibody

Table 32-1 Causes of Chronic Glomerulonephropathy

Multisystem disorders: Goodpasture's syndrome, systemic lupus erythematosis, Henoch-Schönlein purpura, malignant disease
Crescentic glomerulonephritis
Membranoproliferative glomerulonephritis
Membranous glomerulopathy
Infectious processes: poststreptococcal glomerulonephritis, hepatitis B, endocardtitis, sepsis

complexes. In a few instances, an antibody specific to glomerular basement membrane (anti-GBM antibody) is the cause. The degree of chronic immunologic destruction can be categorized as diffuse, focal, local, proliferative, membranous, necrotizing, or sclerotic.

Diffuse damage involves changes to some portion of all the glomeruli. When one group of glomeruli is affected and other groups are not, the damage is called *focal. Local* involvement indicates that a specific part of the glomerulus is affected. A *proliferative* response of glomerular mesangial and/or endothelial cells can ultimately alter the glomerular tuft. *Membranous* changes are those which occur in the glomerular wall, causing a thickening secondary to an immunologic reaction. The deposition of fibrinoid is characteristic of *necrotizing* glomerulonephritis. *Sclerotic* damage refers to glomerular scarring from a prior injury.

The presence of one or more deposited immune complexes contributes to the information needed to form a diagnosis. The immunoglobulins (IgG, IgA, IgM), complement (C3, C4), and fibrin are the immune complexes which have diagnostic importance. The damage to the glomerulus by the various tissue reactions described above causes cellular proliferation, leukocyte infiltration, basement membrane thickening, and sclerosis.[4] Phagocytosis and the release of enzymes occur in the area of the immune response.

The patient with glomerulonephritis may have no symptoms or may present with hypertension or abnormalities in the urine such as proteinuria or hematuria. If nephrotic syndrome is present, a gross amount of protein (more than 6 g) is found in the urine (Table 32-2).

Electron and immunofluorescent microscopy assist in the diagnostic determination of the type of glomerulonephropathy which is present. Elec-

Table 32-2 Causes of Nephrotic Syndrome

Infectious processes, bacterial and viral
Carcinomas
Systemic disease: lupus, rheumatoid arthritis, Henoch-
    Schönlein purpura, amyeloidosis
Diabetes mellitus
Myxedema
Toxins and pharmacologic agents
Other: pregnancy toxemia, renal arterial stenosis

tron microscopy may reveal morphologic changes of the glomerular capillary wall, and immunofluorescence displays the components of the immunologic system involved in the glomerular reaction. Percutaneous renal biopsy may also be used.

Hypertensive Disease

Hypertensive disease causes a rapid acceleration of the atherosclerotic process usually associated with aging. The arteriolar narrowing and possible occlusion result in diminished perfusion, tissue infarction, or ischemic atrophy to target organs, that is, the kidney, heart, and brain. Renal damage has long been recognized as occurring secondary to hypertension. A direct correlation seems to exist between the extent of renal disease and the severity of blood pressure elevation.[5] The presence of progressive hypertensive disease may cause diffusive thickening of the afferent arterioles. Other vessels, such as the interlobular arteries, exhibit thickening of the intima and "cracking" of the lamina. These nephrosclerotic changes progress to create an ischemic state which damages both glomeruli and tubules. More severe uncontrolled or malignant hypertension damages the renal arterioles even further. These types of renal damage secondary to hypertension diminish renal function to the point of end-stage renal disease.

Urinary Tract Infections

The most common complication during renal failure is infection; in fact, infection often contributes to the death of the renal failure patient. Uremia-induced immunosuppression is the primary reason for increased susceptibility to infection in these patients.

Urinary tract infection (UTI) of bacterial origin is the most common, although fungal and parasitic invaders are also possibilities. The specific site of UTI may vary from kidney to urethra. Urine is normally sterile, and when infection occurs, the invading organism is usually a fecal contaminant such as *Escherichia coli*. Factors which often predispose to the onset of UTI are bladder catheterization, urinary stasis secondary to obstruction, reflux of urine, and immunosuppression. Sexual intercourse has been suspected as a cause of infection in females. Advancing age appears to be a predisposing factor to infection in females over 60 years of age and in males with prostatic disease.

Urine culture is the primary diagnostic test for UTI. Efforts should be made to minimize contamination when obtaining a urine specimen for culture. Urethral contamination should be suspected when colony counts are below 10 mL. A colony count of more than 10^5 mL in a voided specimen is a positive result, especially if a second specimen reveals similar findings.

Symptoms of UTI are suggestive rather than diagnostic, but the confirming factor is always a positive urine culture. Dysuria, frequency, and pain in the suprapubic regions are indicative of bladder infection. These symptoms should be differentiated from symptoms of renal infection, which are flank pain, nausea, vomiting, microscopic hematuria, and fear.

Chronic Pyelonephritis

Recurrent bacterial infections were once believed to be the primary cause of chronic pyelonephritis. Many patients, however, report no history of prior infection. Further investigation has revealed that histologic changes seen in pyelonephritis are similar to those occurring with other entities, such as nephrotoxicity secondary to analgesic abuse. Chronic pyelonephritis associated with renal infection also occurs in the presence of coexisting obstruction or vesicourethral reflex. Infiltration of the renal medulla with neutrophils, lymphocytes, and mononuclear cells is the primary change noted in renal infection.

Diagnostic clues to chronic pyelonephritis are a history of infected stones, hematuria, flank pain, or vesicourethral reflex, especially in conjunction with persistent infections. Data diagnostic of chronic pyelonephritis include urine culture showing pyuria and occasional white cell casts; but a positive urine culture is not required for diagnosis. An intravenous pyelogram (IVP) reveals small kidneys, cortical scarring, and dilated and blunted calices.

Renal Cancers

Renal and urinary tract carcinomas account for 5 to 20 percent of all deaths due to cancer in the United States.[6] The tumor is initially limited to a specific area of the urinary tract or to the kidney. Within a short time after onset, metastatic spread to other sites is common. Cancer is not clinically detectable until approximately one billion cells are present. A tumor containing more than 5 billion cells is associated with systemic involvement and a poor prognosis.

Adenoma, hemangiopericytoma, hemangioma, and hamartoma are types of benign renal tumor. Renal carcinomas include nephroblastoma, adenocarcinoma, renal cell carcinoma, and sarcoma. Renal cell cancers account for 90 percent of renal carcinomas and are associated with 11,000 of the deaths due to cancer per year.[6] Males more often than females develop renal cancers, with higher incidence between the ages of 50 and 60 years. The major risk factor for renal carcinoma is believed to be cigarette smoking.

The earliest diagnostic clinical symptom of renal carcinoma is gross, painless hematuria. The hematuria may stop suddenly, or repeated episodes may follow. Flank pain, if present, is associated with diffuse disease involving nerves and muscle. The tumor is usually not palpable, but palpability in the presence of pain and hematuria suggests progressive disease.

Fever occurs in 20 percent of all patients with nausea, vomiting, anorexia, and constipation, and abdominal pain is noted in 15 percent. Systemic effects of renal carcinoma include normochromic and normocytic anemia, amyloidosis, nephrogenic hepatic disease, hypercalcemia, and hypertension. Fractures, if they occur, are suggestive of metastatic lesions.

Intravenous pyelography is indicated when suspicions of renal carcinoma arise. Distortions in the outline of the kidney are suggestive of a renal mass. An ultrasound or computerized tomographic (CT) scan may be utilized to distinguish a solid mass from a cystic tumor. Nuclear magnetic resonance (NMR) is helpful in distinguishing renal masses. Angioplasty may be used to locate and stage the tumor.

Tubulointerstitial Diseases

The tubulointerstitial diseases are a group of renal disorders affecting the tubular and/or interstitial regions of the kidney. The sources of the renal insult include bacterial, viral, or fungal agents, toxic agents, metabolic imbalances, mechanical alterations, immunologic disorders, and hereditary diseases (Table 32-3).

Despite the wide range of causes, the following approach is helpful in the diagnosis of tubulointerstitial disease. A history should be elicited dealing with drug usage, exposure to nephrotoxic agents, or frequent urinary tract infections. Urine cultures, assessment of serum electrolytes, and urinalysis also may assist in the diagnosis. Lastly, if no direct cause is ascertained from these data, a renal biopsy should be considered. Renal changes in tubulointerstitial disease are not usually specific, so the extent of information provided by biopsy may be limited.

Data Acquisition

The history, physical examination, and laboratory data are assessed to determine whether renal disease is present. If renal disease is documented, the data assist in confirming the duration and severity

---

Table 32-3 Causes of Tubulointerstitial Diseases

Infectious sources: bacteria, fungi, viruses
Immunologic disorders: Goodpasture's syndrome, lupus nephritis
Metabolic imbalances: hyperuricemia, hypercalcemia, hypokalemia
Toxins: aminoglycosides, heavy metals, radiation
Urinary tract obstruction: renal calculi, chronic infection
Drugs: analgesics
Hereditary disorders: sickle cell anemia, polycystic disease, medullary sponge kidney
Chronic transplant rejection

of the disease. These data are necessary when designing the care plan for each patient.

The history accounts for both personal and family health experiences. The goal of this portion of the data collection is to document the presence and cause of renal disease. Significant findings consistent with a positive history include (1) proteinuria and/or hematuria; (2) a previous episode of acute nephritis or nephrotic syndrome; (3) presence of lupus erythematosis, diabetes mellitus, or hypertension; (4) recurrent urinary tract infections; (5) childhood and/or adult episodes of reflux or urinary obstruction; (6) analgesic abuse; (7) anemia of unknown cause; (8) pulmonary disease (Goodpasture's syndrome); (9) recent infections (streptococcal); (10) cardiovascular disease: congestive heart failure, atherosclerosis, hypertension; and (11) renal transplant, recent surgery, toxemia of pregnancy, allergies, skin rashes, or arthralgias.

A relevant family history comprises the following genetically transmitted diseases that may be associated with renal disease: (1) renal calculi or any other renal disease; (2) diabetes mellitus; (3) gout; (4) hypertension; (5) malignant disease; (6) cardiovascular disease; (7) polycystic kidney disease; (8) hereditary nephritis; (9) medullary cystic disease; (10) sickle cell disease; and (11) a bleeding disorder or anticoagulant therapy.

Physical examination of a patient with proteinuria may reveal heart failure, hypertension, peripheral or orbital edema, a palpable kidney, or diminished hearing.[3] Isolated cases of hematuria are associated with the following findings on physical examination: flank or suprapubic tenderness, enlarged and palpable kidneys, enlarged prostate gland, malignant hypertension with or without heart murmur, skin rash, and/or diminished hearing.[3] Specific determinations made by physical examination that can be linked to a disease causing renal failure include:

Polycystic disease–large, palpable kidneys

Lupus erythematosis–butterfly-pattern facial rash, arthralgia

Urinary tract obstruction–flank or suprapubic pain, enlarged prostate, palpable tumor or kidney

Diabetes mellitus–retinopathy, neuropathy, and other signs of progressive diabetic disease

Cardiovascular disease–hypertension, heart murmurs, pulmonary failure, rales, edema

Goodpasture's disease–respiratory failure edema

Malignant disease–palpable renal masses, hypertension

Urinary tract infections–flank or suprapubic pain

Glomerulonephritis–skin rash and facial, orbital, or peripheral edema

Henoch-Schönlein purpura–fever, sore throat, heart murmur, skin rash, and arthralgias

Common tests useful in diagnosing chronic renal failure include urinalysis, urine culture, and 24-h urine test for protein and creatinine clearance; serum studies including BUN, plasma creatinine, hematocrit and hemoglobin levels, and plasma complement (C3); and such further studies as sickle cell preparation, antistreptolysin O titer, antinuclear antibody assay, and blood cultures.

Urinalysis is an important part of the assessment process because it reveals integral information about renal function. The concentration of urine indicates the extent of the remaining renal function.

Medical and Surgical Management

The ultimate goal in the early stages of chronic renal failure is to prevent or reverse any complications that can cause a further deterioration in renal function. The second line of medical management is directed at treating the uremic symptoms.

Factors which can exacerbate CRF are infection, cardiovascular disease, dehydration, obstruction, and pharmacologic agents and radiographic dyes.

Prevention of Complications

Infection

Infection in the chronically uremic patient is diagnosed by blood and urine cultures and chest and abdominal x-rays. During treatment of CRF the glomerular filtration rate (GFR) is calculated and antibiotic dosages adjusted. Tetracycline and nitrofurantoin should be avoided when the GFR falls below 40 percent of normal, because these drugs are ineffective at this GFR.[3]

Cardiovascular Disease

Anything that causes deterioration of cardiac function may result in a corresponding decline in renal function. The pathophysiologic alteration affecting renal perfusion is decreased cardiac output. Congestive heart failure and myocardial infarction are examples of pathologic factors that affect renal function. Optimizing of cardiac output by the use of digitalis and diuretics is the treatment of choice. The digitalis dosage must be adjusted to match the degree of existing renal function. Furosemide or ethecrinic acid are the diuretics of choice, in dosages several times normal.

The treatment modality for essential hypertension is the same in the presence of normal renal function as in renal disease. If the retention of sodium and water exacerbates hypertension, large doses of diuretics may be indicated. Dialysis is necessary when the patient becomes resistant to diuretic action and hypertension becomes uncontrollable.

Dehydration

Hypovolemia may alter renal blood flow, thus decreasing renal function. The expansion of vascular volume by sodium and water repletion is necessary in order to reinstate renal perfusion.

Obstruction

Obstruction, in all situations, has the potential to produce acute renal failure. The presence of obstruction in the already compromised kidney can be detrimental to future functioning. Diagnosis by radiologic examination and rapid removal of the source of obstruction is essential in order to salvage renal function.

Pharmacologic Agents and Radiographic Dyes

Pharmacologic agents may exacerbate renal failure by directly or indirectly affecting the kidney. Nephrotoxic agents such as antibiotics may directly poison the nephron. Other nephrotoxic agents accumulate in renal tissue and affect cortical and medullary functions. Renal perfusion can be reduced by diuretics, vasodilators, and digitalis. Protoglandin inhibitors, ibuprofen (Motrin), and na-

proxen (Naprosyn) exacerbate the vasoconstrictive action of the internal catecholamines and renin, thus compromising renal perfusion. The treatment of nephrotoxicity due to these causes is to decrease drug dosage, increase the intervals between or frequency of drug administration, or discontinue the drug.

The toxicity of radiographic dyes is diminished or eliminated by hydrating the patient prior to administration of the dye. After dye infusion, mannitol may be administered to further reduce the potential of nephrotoxicity.

Treatment of Uremic Symptoms

The patient who has CRF remains relatively asymptomatic until approximately 80 percent of the nephrons are lost. Symptoms of CRF appear when the GFR is 25 mL or less.

Nutrition Management

Dietary management of the patient with CRF varies according to the stage of renal failure and the nutritional needs of the patient. The dietary elements adjusted in an effort to correct any imbalances or body deficits are fluid, protein, calories, electrolytes, minerals, carbohydrates, and vitamins. During end-stage renal disease and dialysis further adjustments are made. (See Chap. 12 for further discussion of the nutritional needs of patients with CRF.)

Acidosis

Metabolic acidosis usually begins after a 50 percent nephron loss. By the time the GFR falls below 20 percent of normal the acidosis has progressed to the point at which a significant reduction in the serum bicarbonate level occurs. The patient adapts by a compensatory decrease in P_{CO_2} and pH, and a tolerance of the acidotic state. The patient in crisis experiencing an excess acid load presents with symptomatic acidosis. Treatment of acidosis is geared to correcting the primary cause and, if necessary, administering sodium bicarbonate via the oral or intravenous route. If the acidosis persists, dialysis is indicated.

Anemia

Anemia results from suppression or lack of erythropoietin production. The effect of this anemia is decreased red cell production and diminished red cell survival. The fall in hematocrit level is gradual, and the patient adapts to the decreasing hematocrit and hemoglobin levels. Prophylactic measures such as iron injections are taken to prevent symptomatic anemia.

Dialysis

As a patient with CFR approaches end stage and a creatinine of 10, a plan should be devised by the physician and the nurse for selection of an alternative form of therapy to replace kidney function. Today, the choices are quite varied, including cadaveric or family donor transplantation (discussed in Chap. 59) and several methods of dialysis. The types of dialysis that can be offered to most patients are home or in-center hemodialysis, home or in-center peritoneal dialysis, and continuous ambulatory peritoneal dialysis. The treatment alternative selected should be part of a comprehensive plan that has a total life focus.

Quality-of-Life Issues

Several factors should be considered in selecting the most appropriate form of dialysis. Regional availability has to be considered initially. Next, the selection process must consider the physical condition of the patient in order to determine which procedure can best be tolerated. Eliminating treatment alternatives according to these parameters leaves a number of alternative treatments. Among the variables that can be used to make the final choice are quality-of-life parameters. Quality-of-life measurement necessitates treating patients as individuals. Duff, in 1973, suggested that quality of life is "meaningful humanhood," which is "the capacity by the patient to love and be loved, to be independent and to be understood and to be able to participate in and plan for the future."[7] Family members closely involved in the patient's care should be given an opportunity to participate in the decision-making process. The role of the health care professional is to direct the patient and the family to the most appropriate choice by making the patient and family aware of the options, assisting in the selection of a realistic choice, and emphasizing that some treatment alternatives are more feasible than others.

The following sections include an examination of information that can assist a patient in selecting an alternative.

Hemodialysis

Uremia that is no longer manageable by conservative measures requires treatment by some form of dialysis or transplantation. Hemodialysis, the most widely used of all the renal failure treatment alternatives, has proved to be an effective method for managing end-stage renal disease. Among the indications are life-altering or life-threatening uremic symptoms and contraindications to other treatment forms (Table 32-4).

Prior to the availability of dialysis, the renal failure patient's ultimate fate was uremic coma and death. The first significant breakthrough in the development of the dialysis procedure occurred when Koff invented the artificial kidney during World War II.[8] A 15-year gap followed before hemodialysis was widely used. The regularity of the use of hemodialysis at that time depended on successfully securing an arteriovenous access. In 1960, Beldon Scribner introduced a Teflon arteriovenous shunt. The rigidity of the original Teflon graft caused damage to the vessel wall, requiring replacement of the access source every 3 to 4 weeks. The frequency of access failures led to the development of a Teflon-Silastic shunt in 1961 and

---

Table 32-4 Indications for Hemodialysis

Uremic symptoms interfering with activities of daily living: fatigue, nausea and vomiting, memory loss, shortened attention span

Uremic symptoms: life-threatening uremic pericarditis, uremic lung, uremic pleuritis, peripheral neuropathy, dialysis dementia, encephalopathy

Volume overload: potential for congestive heart failure, pulmonary edema, hypertension

Electrolyte imbalances: hyperkalemia, hypo- or hypernatremia

Symptomatic metabolic acidosis

Contraindications to peritoneal dialysis: multiple abdominal adhesions, actual or potential infection, diaphragmatic leaks

Contraindications to transplantation: chronic infection; malignant disease; immunologic incompatibilities; inability to tolerate immunosuppressive agents; cardiovascular, genitourinary, and gastrointestinal abnormalities; psychosocial problems

later an all-Silastic version. The perfecting of a long-lasting arteriovenous access guaranteed the survival of hemodialysis as a treatment for chronic renal failure.

Today, hemodialysis treatments are available to essentially everyone, even the elderly, with the specific selection criteria varying from unit to unit. The mortality rate is 5 to 10 percent in the general population and 10 percent in patients over 65 years of age. Hypertension complicated by atherosclerotic cardiac disease is no longer a contraindication to hemodialysis unless the cardiac disease has progressed to a point at which hemodialysis is not tolerated. Patients with diabetes are also accepted for this procedure despite association with the onset of cardiovascular complications, neuropathies, and the high mortality rate of 20 to 30 percent.

It is expected that the patient accepted into a hospital-based hemodialysis program will comply with the dietary restrictions and maintain circulatory access. The patient must report at least three times a week to the dialysis unit for a total of 12 to 13 h per week. The time it takes to travel to and from the hospital and the postdialysis recovery time should be included when estimating the total number of hours needed for the procedure. Knowing the exact number of hours per week needed for dialysis helps the patient plan for activities of daily living such as work and family responsibilities.

The home hemodialysis procedure demands a relatively healthy patient who is free of complications and who tolerates the hemodialysis procedure. Compliant and responsible patients are preferred who respond constructively to stressful situations. In addition, a home environment conducive to the procedure (e.g., adequate space, plumbing, and hygiene) must be available. A family member or surrogate dialyzer is needed to support the machine's operation and monitor the patient's progress. A family member who is utilized as the primary dialyzer must demonstrate the ability to learn highly technical skills.

One treatment approach is to begin hemodialysis therapy prior to the start of uremic symptoms. This approach is believed to contribute to the prevention of uremic symptoms. Intermittent treatments usually are ordered—three times a week, with each treatment lasting 3 to 4 h. The number of treatments and the length of each vary with the severity of the uremia. Stable patients often require less frequent treatments, while those with severe uremic complications may need daily hemodialysis.

Hemodialysis is a procedure that partially replaces the excretory functions of the kidney but does not replace the hormonal functions. The excretory role comprises the elimination of wastes, excess electrolytes, and water by two processes: passive diffusion and convection. Diffusion is defined as the passive movement of solutes across a semipermeable membrane from an area of high to one of low concentration. During this process, solute in the form of electrolytes, metabolic waste products, and acid-base components can be removed from or added to the blood. Several factors influence the clearance capacity or diffusion rate of the dialyzer, including the pore size of the membrane, the concentration gradient of the dialysate, and the surface area of the dialyzer. Dialysis membranes recently developed are designed for removal of small and middle-size molecules, with the upper limits of removal at a molecular weight of 3000 to 5000. There is a direct relation between the diffusion of particles and the membrane pore size. As a solute reaches the maximal pore size, there is a progressive reduction in the degree of diffusion.[9] An increase in the concentration of the dialysate bath impacts on the direction and rate of diffusion, thus enhancing the net removal of solute: the greater the surface area, the greater the rate of diffusion.

Convection, also known as *ultrafiltration,* is a process whereby water movement is encouraged by the establishment of a hydrostatic pressure force across a membrane. Although this process is primarily aimed at water movement, solute can also be transported by convection. Because of the water retention associated with chronic renal failure, the purpose of convection in this case is the removal of water. Factors affecting convection are transmembrane hydrostatic pressure, surface area, and the selective permeability of the membrane. By increasing the resistance on the blood side of the membrane, the ultrafiltration rate is increased. Using a membrane with a large surface area and a higher permeability coefficient increases the number of uremic toxins which can be removed. The removal of solute in large volumes of water across a semipermeable membrane is known as *hemofiltration.*

Knowledge of the characteristics of the semipermeable membrane is essential for understanding the outcome of the dialysis procedure. The hemodialysis membrane is selectively impermeable to plasma proteins, albumins, and red and white blood cells and affords preferred passage to solutes with a molecular weight of less, which encompasses the movement of small particles like urea. The upper range of membrane permeability (mol wt 3000 to 5000) is directed at removing midsize molecules. These midsize molecules are believed to be responsible for the uremic symptoms that are uncontrolled in the dialysis procedures; that is, removal of those molecules that have a molecular mass of 5000 daltons. Examples of midsize molecules found in high concentrations in the serum of uremic patients are glucagon (molecular weight of 3500), calcitonin (3400), gastrin (2000), and gastric inhibitory peptide (5100).[10]

The dialysis membrane is usually made of cellulose—either cuprophane, regenerated cellulose, or cellulose acetate. Earlier membranes were made of Cellophane and had a permeability selective only for small-size molecules. Newly developed membranes of polyacrylonitrile, polycarbonate, and polymethylmethacrylate are selective for midsize molecules. These membranes claim a permeability four times greater than cellulose membranes and require a special delivery system when used.[11] The hemodialysis delivery system is depicted in Fig. 32-1.

The hemodialysis delivery system consists of blood and dialysate compartments divided by the selectively permeable membrane. The blood delivery system comprises the arterial side of the access, the blood tubing entering the blood compartment, the blood compartment, the exit tubing, and the venous side of the access. The blood moves along this circuit assisted by a pump at the usual rate of 200 to 250 mL/min. The membrane or dialyzer divides the blood from the dialysate or bath compartment. Types of dialyzer include the coil, hollow fiber, and flat plate. The coil requires large priming volumes, sometimes as much as 500 mL/min. This type of dialyzer also has an unpredictable rate of ultrafiltration. The method used with the coil to enhance ultrafiltration is positive pressure on the blood compartment to increase the hydrostatic pressure and thus drive water into the dialysate.

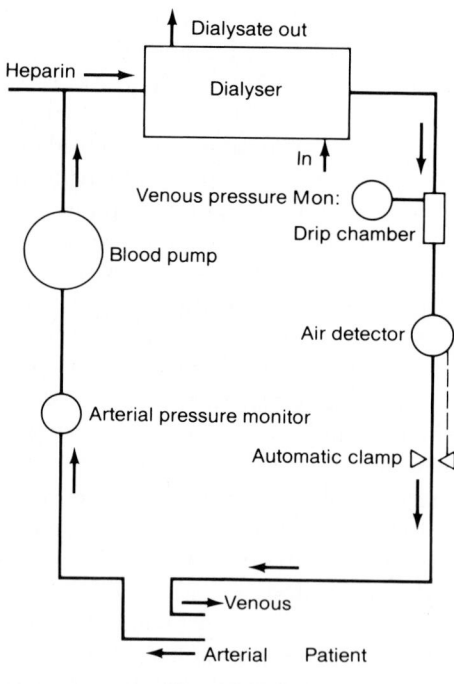

Figure 32-1 Hemodialysis delivery system. (*From D. Levine, Care of the Renal Patient, Philadelphia, W. B. Saunders, 1983.*)

The hollow fiber dialyzer uses a small circulating volume of approximately 250 mL/min. The surface area of the dialyzer is quite large. Ultrafiltration generally uses a negative pressure, although both kinds of pressure (negative and positive) can be applied. Negative pressure is applied to the venous end of the blood circuit, creating pressure on the blood compartment and thus encouraging water movement.

The dialysis delivery system pumps the dialysate past the membrane and, therefore, past the blood compartment. The exchange between blood and dialysate—that is, diffusion and convection—occur at this stage in the dialysis process.

The dialysate is formed by mixing water with an electrolyte concentration in a ratio of 1:34. The water should be sterile, because harmful substances such as pyrogens and environmental pollutants are found in untreated water. The dialysate concentrate usually contains sodium 130 to 142 meq/L, potassium 0 to 3.0 meq/L, calcium 2.5 to 4.0 meq/L, chloride 96 to 108 meq/L, and acetate 33 to 40 meq/L.

Adjustments commonly made in the dialysate involve the potassium concentration and the replacement of bicarbonate as acetate. The extent of potassium adjustment depends on whether the patient is digitalized. Potassium concentrations as high as 4 meq/L are often prescribed to prevent hypokalemia-induced digitalis toxicity. A zero-potassium bath should be avoided, because development of severe hypokalemia is possible. Using acetate to correct the metabolic acidosis has been associated with cardiovascular instability. A bicarbonate bath is an alternative to acetate and should be used in the patient with cardiovascular problems.

Vascular Access Access to the circulation for hemodialysis is by subcutaneous arteriovenous (AV) shunt or fistula and single- or double-lumen femoral catheters. The arteriovenous shunt is formed by cannulating a major artery and any adjacent vein. This type of vascular access is no longer commonly used.

Fistulas have a longer life span than AV shunts and tend to preserve the blood vessels in which they are placed. As a rule, fistulas are less restrictive than other forms of circulatory access and therefore offer greater patient freedom. The patient may experience less feeling of body image changes because this access is not visible. The fistula can be formed by the patient's vessels, which is preferred, or by a graft. Examples of graft materials are bovine carotid, woven Dacron, and umbilical vein. The surgical procedure involves anastomosis of the artery directly to the vein, utilizing most frequently a side-to-side technique. Fistulas need to mature over a 10- to 14-day period. During this period of time, the vein adapts to the high pressure of the arterial blood by dilatation and thickening of the venous wall, in preparation for the high flow of the dialysis procedure. The insertion of needles in the arterial and venous arms of the fistula permit attachments to the dialysis machine.

Complications associated with an AV fistula are infection, clotting, steal syndrome, and cardiovascular intolerance. Infection at the fistula site has direct access to the systemic circulation and can precipitate septicemia. Localized infections present as reddened, tender, warm areas over the fistula, particularly at the anastomosis or needle puncture sites. Other complications associated with infection

are endocarditis and septic emboli. Clotting sometimes causes severe pain and numbness in the affected arm; it can be confirmed by absence of the bruit and thrill of the fistula.

The steal syndrome is usually secondary to the formation of a large AV anastomosis. To accommodate the high blood flow, the vascular supply to the fistula arm is diverted from the fingers; this circulatory adjustment is typical of the steal syndrome.

Femoral or subclavian vein access is used in the patient with CRF who experiences an acute lack of circulatory access. Cannulation of either vein provides a readily available access. The length of time the catheters are allowed to remain in place varies but is often from 1 to 4 days. A complication of subclavian placement is pneumothorax. Infection, another complication, can be prevented by using aseptic technique and avoiding numerous breaks in the catheter line to obtain blood specimens. Infection is treated by removal of the catheter and initiation of antibiotic therapy. After 2 to 3 days of therapy, the line can be started at another site without the danger of infection.

Potential Problems Problems associated with hemodialysis treatment occur most often during the initial stages or during a procedure lasting more than 4 h. The incidence of dialysis-related problems (Table 32-5) is also increased during the initial treatment and in the severely uremic patient.

Early in the treatment, dysrhythmias and hypotension are common problems. Early hypotension results from the combined effect of the blood volume used to fill the extracorporeal circuit (the

Table 32-5 Hemodialysis Complications

Hypotension
Dysrhythmias
Hypoxia
Lactate accumulation
Membrane bioincompatibility
Bleeding tendency
Leukopenia
Air embolism or pulmonary embolism
Infection
Hepatitis
Disequilibrium syndrome
Muscle cramps

primer) and the rapid depletion of plasma water by ultrafiltration. In the hemodynamically unstable patient, the volume of fluid priming the dialysis delivery system should be approximately 200 to 250 mL. The desirable fluid for priming is either albumin or, in extreme situations, whole blood.[12] If necessary, vasopressors can be initiated to help maintain the blood pressure.

Extracellular osmolar changes are another major contributor to the initiation of hemodialysis-related hypotension.[13–15] Osmolar solutes are removed from the vascular and interstitial space, thus leaving these compartments in a hypotonic state, and the intracellular environment becomes hypertonic in relation to the extracellular fluid. The result is water movement from the extracellular to the intracellular compartment, with the possibility that complete extracellular volume depletion may follow.[16,17] This condition contributes to repeated episodes of hypotension throughout the hemodialysis procedure. In addition, a kind of autonomic dysfunction occurs during hemodialysis which does not allow the vessels to consistently adapt to the hypotensive state and which thus perpetuates the low pressure state.[18]

Dysrhythmias are another complication associated with the first hour of dialysis. The cause of this problem is either hypokalemia, especially in the digitalized patient, or hypoxia. To minimize the chance of rapidly developing hypokalemia, the potassium concentration of the dialysate should be maintained at 3.0 to 4.0 meq/L, a value similar to the serum value. Patients tend to tolerate a lower potassium bath and more rapid potassium removal toward the conclusion of the procedure. The cause of the early onset of dysrhythmias is hypoxia. Data indicate that hypoxia occurs with all membrane types.[19]

Three types of dialysis membrane have demonstrated a degree of bioincompatibility: cuprophane, regenerated cellulose, and cellulose acetate. When serum is exposed to these membranes, the leukocytes and platelet counts fall, suggesting membrane consumption.[20] As a result, the patient may experience hemodialysis-induced leukopenia and enhanced bleeding potential. Anticoagulation therapy also may pose problems if the correct approach is not selected or if the dosage is not carefully managed.

When critically ill patients, particularly those suffering from septic shock or hepatic failure, are treated with dialysate containing acetate or lactate, hemodynamic problems can follow.[21] These patients cannot metabolize acetate or lactate, and this leads to the accumulation of these substances and subsequent adverse reactions. Bicarbonate dialysis baths are better tolerated for the treatment of metabolic acidosis, because direct use of bicarbonate without any further metabolism is possible.

Peritoneal Dialysis

Peritoneal dialysis is available as an in-center or home treatment alternative. This procedure is offered to the majority of CRF patients, because most patient categories are included in the selection criteria. Peritoneal dialysis is a desirable alternative for those patients who cannot tolerate hemodialysis.

Patients who are usually directed to peritoneal dialysis include very young children in whom adequate vascular access is impossible and elderly patients who have cardiovascular problems. Patients who have experienced loss of all available vascular access sites for hemodialysis and those who are awaiting the maturation of an access graft also can benefit from peritoneal dialysis. Diabetic patients profit from peritoneal dialysis because vision losses and other complications exacerbated by hemodialysis are minimized by peritoneal dialysis. Some patients simply do not tolerate hemodialysis, and some, because of religious beliefs, desire to avoid the blood transfusions associated with hemodialysis emergencies. Patients awaiting renal transplantation may also be directed to peritoneal dialysis because of the financial savings it offers compared with hemodialysis.

Peritoneal dialysis treatments extend over a 10-h period three to four times per week. The amount of time consumed each week by this procedure must be taken into account in relation to the patient's responsibilities for family and employment. The patient is expected to comply with diet restrictions and maintain the prescribed body weight. The patient also must adapt to possible body image changes related to placement of the Tenckhoff catheter.

The requirements for home peritoneal dialysis are similar to those for hemodialysis. The patient's home environment must provide adequate space for the procedure. The family needs to demonstrate the ability to psychologically adapt to home dialysis treatment. Since peritoneal dialysis does not interfere with the daily routine, the family's commitment does not need to be as extensive as for hemodialysis. Most home peritoneal dialysis patients dialyze at night. Physical stability of the patient is not necessary, because the rapid hemodynamic changes associated with hemodialysis do not occur during peritoneal dialysis.

The three types of peritoneal dialysis currently in use are (1) acute or chronic, (2) automatic cycler, and (3) continuous ambulatory.

The indications for chronic peritoneal dialysis are:

1. Inability to tolerate or contraindications to hemodialysis
2. Diabetic nephropathy with vision loss and other complications
3. Cardiovascular problems in elderly patients
4. Need for maturation time for access grafts for hemodialysis
5. Absence of any access site for hemodialysis
6. Need for temporary cost-effective method of treating the uremic patient before transplantation
7. Inability or unwillingness to receive blood transfusions, as in members of certain religious bodies.

Definition and Description   Peritoneal dialysis is a procedure by which a hypertonic dialysate solution is instilled into the peritoneal cavity and solute and water are exchanged into the dialysate and removed via drainage of this solution (Fig. 32-2). The major forces encouraging solute and water removal are, respectively, diffusion and osmosis. Solute exchange by diffusion, whether removal or replacement, is governed simply by adjusting the dialysate concentration of electrolytes and acetate or lactate. The absence of a solute, such as urea, creatinine, or potassium, from the dialysate assures the loss of that solute. Osmotic forces are determined by the concentration of glucose in the dialysate, usually ranging from 1.5 to 4.25 percent. Osmotic forces can be increased for greater water removal by instilling dialysate with greater dextrose concentration (4.25%). During the administration of 4.25% dialysate the serum glucose must be

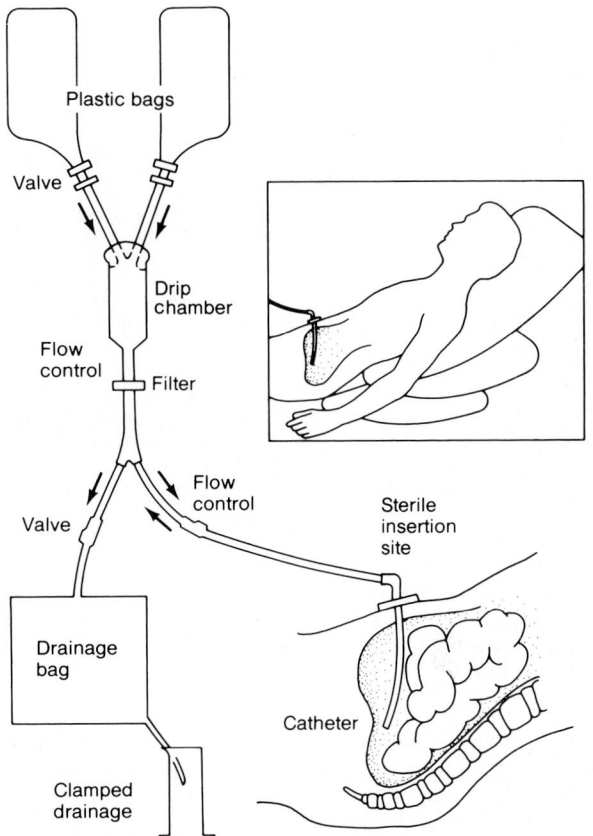

Figure 32-2 Peritoneal dialysis procedure. (*From W. Flamenbaum, & R. Hamburger, Nephrology: An Approach to the Patient with Renal Disease, Philadelphia, Lippincott, 1982.*)

monitored, because glucose can diffuse into the serum. Because hyperglycemia is a serious potential problem, a careful evaluation must be made before utilizing a 4.25% solution, especially in the diabetic patient. In addition, hydrostatic pressure leading to an ultrafiltration effect can be created by increasing the flow rate in the peritoneal capillaries up to 66 L/h.

Procedure   This form of dialysis is initiated by placement of a peritoneal catheter, either a stylet for acute dialysis or a permanent catheter for chronic peritoneal dialysis (Fig. 32-3). The stylet is inserted at the bedside, using strict sterile techniques. The actual insertion site is on the midline between the umbilicus and the symphysis pubis.

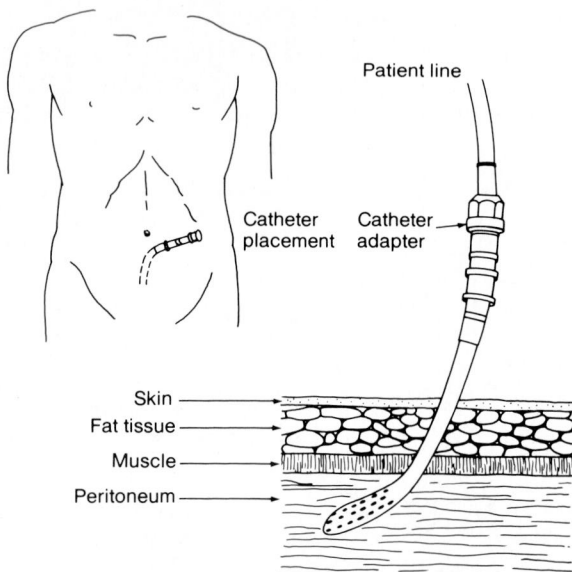

Figure 32-3   Placing the catheter into the peritoneal cavity. (*From L. Schoengrund, L. & P. Balzer, Renal Problems in Critical Care, New York, Wiley, 1985.*)

Prior to its insertion, the patient is instructed to void. The physician, utilizing firm pressure, pushes the catheter through the skin toward the peritoneal cavity. Once it is in place, 2 L of peritoneal dialysis fluid is introduced into the peritoneal cavity. The dialysate, on the first exchange, is allowed to drain immediately after administration, which permits verification of the presence of the return fluid and assessment of its consistency. The initial exchanges may be slightly blood-tinged but should clear after several exchanges. If bleeding persists or if there is gross bleeding, the physician must be notified immediately. Occasionally the application of pressure at the catheter site may stop the bleeding, but the possibility of aortic perforation must be considered. Shock is imminent in this situation, and emergency surgery is necessary. Brown-tinged returns indicate bowel perforation and usually are associated with severe pain and diarrhea. Bright yellow-tinged return suggests bladder perforation, especially when accompanied by pain and the desire to urinate. However, the presence of slightly yellow-tinged outflow may only be related to the contents of uremic wastes.

Acute peritoneal dialysis treatment usually extends for a total of 36 hourly exchanges. Each exchange comprises instillation of the dialysate, which lasts approximately 15 min; dwelling time of 20 min; and draining or outflow time of 25 min. The ideal situation is to have each exchange limited to 1 h. This time frame can be used as a guideline regarding indications for concern about increasingly lengthening times for exchanges.

The permanent peritoneal catheter is placed by the physician in the operating room or at the bedside. The original catheter, called the *Tenckhoff,* has contributed to the development of peritoneal dialysis as a chronic procedure. The permanent catheter is composed of Teflon-Silastic and is approximately 25 to 30 cm long, with two Dacron cuffs. The cuffs are placed between the intraabdominal, subcutaneous, and skin layers. The purpose of the cuffs is to stabilize the catheter and prevent seepage of dialysate and invasion of bacteria. After the catheter is in place, dialysis is started, in order to determine the presence of any problems. Bloody drainage is common, as in acute dialysis during the first few exchanges. The patient may complain of abdominal pain lasting for as long as 2 to 3 weeks after placement. After being relieved, the pain may recur after continual infusions of osmotic dialysate.

Obstruction to flow in one direction is the most common complication of chronic peritoneal dialysis. If there is an obstruction, the dialysate runs into the peritoneum easily but the flow is unable to exit. Infection frequently occurs along the exit tunnel from the extrusion of a cuff or from the bacteria on the skin. The most common organisms causing these infections are *Staphylococcus aureus* and *Staphylococcus epidermidis.* Repeated episodes of chronic peritonitis can compromise a patient's chance of continuing this procedure.

Initial signs and symptoms of peritonitis include fever and abdominal tenderness. Peritonitis is diagnosed by obtaining a white cell count of the effluent; a count of 100 white blood cells per millimeter supports the presence of peritonitis. The dialysate outflow will become cloudy with the onset of infection. The patient is treated by adding antibiotics to the dialysate and dialyzing over a 3- to 7-day period.

In situations in which the infection is not resolved by antibiotic therapy, removal of the permanent catheter may be considered. The patient is then maintained on hemodialysis for approximately

3 weeks, at which time a new permanent catheter is placed.

Other complications associated with peritoneal dialysis are hypovolemia, abdominal pain, bleeding, hyperglycemia, hypernatremia, dialysate leak, hypokalemia, dysrhythmias, respiratory distress, and interruption of dialysate outflow (Table 32-6).

The peritoneal dialysis machine known as the *automatic cycler* provides a means for the automatic infusion of dialysate. The machine regulates the inflow, dwelling, and outflow times. The advantage of automatic cycler dialysis is that it maintains a closed system, thereby limiting the chance of developing peritonitis. The machine is simple to use at home, and it is convenient because it allows dialysis during sleeping hours, which helps eliminate some of the time restrictions associated with this type of dialysis.

Continuous Ambulatory Peritoneal Dialysis Continuous ambulatory peritoneal dialysis (CAPD) is a form of self-dialysis. Patients dialyze themselves by administering 1 to 3 L of dialysate into the peritoneum through a permanent catheter. The catheter is clamped and the dialysate is allowed to remain in the abdomen for 6 to 8 h. The length of each exchange time contributes to the formation of effective dialysate clearances. This dialysis approach is a physiologic success because it replaces 10 percent of the renal function.

Most patients have a positive response to this treatment. Patients generally feel better than those on other forms of dialysis because fewer uremic symptoms are experienced. However, CAPD patients must be willing to make a psychologic commitment to the demands of 24-h treatment.

Patient selection criteria require that the peritoneum be intact and free of infection. The patient must have adequate eyesight, be able to learn technical skills, and be ready to comply with the demands of the aseptic technique and the regimen of the procedure.

Table 32-6 Peritoneal Dialysis Complications

Problem	Cause	Intervention
Hypovolemia	Increased water removal	Replace volume losses
Abdominal pain	(1) Hypertonic dialysate infusion; (2) dialysate too warm or cold; (3) infusion of more than 2 L of dialysate; (4) catheter-related discomfort	(1) Decrease toxicity of infusate; (2) warm dialysate to body temperature; (3) consider instilling a maximum of 2 L; (4) position patient for optimal comfort
Bleeding	(1) Localized to skin: puncture of major blood vessel; (2) secondary to anticoagulant theory	(1) Apply pressure, obtain surgical repair; (2) administer heparin on basis of partial thromboplastin time
Hyperglycemia	Absorption of glucose in dialysate	Consider infusing a dialysate of lower concentration; consider insulin infusions
Hypernatremia	Secondary to water loss without sodium loss	Replace volume losses with D_5W IV
Dialysate leak	Malplacement of catheter	Remove catheter, plan to replace
Hypokalemia	Infusion of dialysate free of potassium	Add potassium to dialysate
Dysrhythmias	(1) Hypokalemia; (2) hypoxia secondary to restricted lung expansion	(1) Add potassium to dialysate; (2) reposition patient for full lung expansion
Respiratory distress	Overdistention of abdomen restricting lung expansion	Limit volume of dialysate infused; reposition patient to optimize respiratory function
Interruption in dialysate outflow	(1) Fibrin or blood clot; (2) malposition of catheter; (3) obstruction by tissue flap	(1) Irrigate catheter; (2) reposition patient; (3) apply slight pressure to abdomen

The patient is involved in the procedure 24 h a day, 7 days a week. The waking-hour exchanges remain in the abdomen 6 to 8 h, while the night exchange is uninterrupted over an 8- to 12-h period. Therefore, the patient actually prepares, administers, and drains three to four peritoneal dialysis runs a day.

Continuous Arteriovenous Hemofiltration   Continuous arteriovenous hemofiltration (CAVH) is the newest form of renal replacement therapy available to the patient requiring dialysis. Hemofiltration is a process that utilizes the patient's arterial blood pressure, without the use of an external pump, to deliver blood to a low-resistance hemodialyzer primarily for water removal. Hemofiltration can be utilized in both acute and chronic renal failure as an effective method of ultrafiltration. The uremic manifestations of renal failure can be managed with CAVH when large volumes of fluid, greater than 10 L, are administered. One indication for CAVH is hypervolemia with or without renal failure in patients who are unresponsive to diuretic therapy. Examples of conditions which often become resistant to diuretic therapy are acute pulmonary edema, congestive heart failure, ascites, and chronic renal failure.

Another indication for CAVH is oliguria in patients who require large quantities of parenteral fluids, as in hyperalimentation, administration of antibiotics in fluid, and continuous administration of vasopressors. CAVH is also considered when other forms of dialysis are contraindicated, as in the hemodynamically unstable patient who is unable to tolerate hemodialysis and in whom peritoneal dialysis is contraindicated.[22,23] The contraindications to CAVH are an inability to tolerate anticoagulation and a hematocrit reading greater than 45 percent, because both these problems precipitate clotting of the hemofilter.[24]

Two general forms of hemofiltration are presently being implemented: CAVH and slow continuous ultrafiltration (SCUF). Both procedures use the same equipment; the primary difference is the smaller total volumes replaced during SCUF, making the control of uremia and electrolytes impossible with SCUF.

CAVH has distinct advantages over hemodialysis. It allows the elimination of large amounts of fluid without the osmolar changes associated with hemodialysis, thus preserving extracellular fluid (ECF) status. During hemodialysis, rapid water removal causes the ECF to become hypotonic in relation to the hypertonic environment of the cell. Extracellular fluid is drawn into the cells, creating a depleted extracellular space which contributes to repeated hypotensive episodes. The consistent process of volume removal by CAVH maintains the osmolality, and as ECF is removed the cellular water moves outward to create a repletion effect.[25] Cardiovascular stability is thus preserved with CAVH. Inappropriate autonomic function associated with hemodialysis is appropriate during hemofiltration. Therefore, the vascular response during CAVH acts to support cardiovascular stability. Another problem occurring with hemodialysis but absent with CAVH is the reduced platelet and white blood cell counts related to the contact of the patient's blood with cuprophane, cellulose acetate, or regenerated cellulose membranes. These problems with hemodialysis, which may compound the condition of the critically ill patient, can be avoided when a hemofiltration method is used.

The CAVH procedure has been proved beneficial for the critically ill patient with ARF when used in conjunction with hemodialysis. The patient is maintained on CAVH as a hemodynamically stabilizing method of volume loss and is hemodialyzed less frequently for solute removal only. This approach is better tolerated by the critically ill patient who is unable to cope with the aggressive ultrafiltration and other side effects associated with hemodialysis.[26,27]

Another advantage of CAVH is that the procedure can be managed by the critical-care nurse rather than by requiring a hemodialysis staff, which makes possible its 24-h availability.

The main disadvantage of CAVH is its limited ability to remove wastes and excess solute with minimal volume replacement. The cost is not believed to be restrictive but rather is comparable to that of hemodialysis.

Procedure   The hemodialyzer consists of a semipermeable membrane composed of a bundle of fibers approximately 0.025 m² in size surrounded by a mesh covering. The surface area of the semipermeable membrane is quite large and is conducive to the passage of water and small solutes with a molecular weight of less than 50,000.[23] At the same time, the membrane prevents the exchange of larger molecules such as red blood cells, serum proteins, and albumin. The bundle of hollow fibers and the mesh covering are housed in a plastic cylindrical filter. Arterial and venous tubing leave the filter at each end and attach to the patient's vascular access. The total volume required to prime or fill the filter and tubing is 40 mL (Fig. 32-4).

Internally, the filter is divided into blood and ultrafiltration compartments. The blood compartment houses the bundle of hollow fibers, and it is through this compartment that the patient's blood passes. The compartment between the mesh covering and the plastic cylinder is called the *ultrafiltration compartment*. As blood flows through the blood compartment driven by the patient's arterial pressure, a filtrate is made which enters the ultrafiltration compartment only to be drained via tubing to an attached filtrate collection bag. Through this process, the vascular space can be rapidly depleted. Pretreatment fluids can be administered to promote

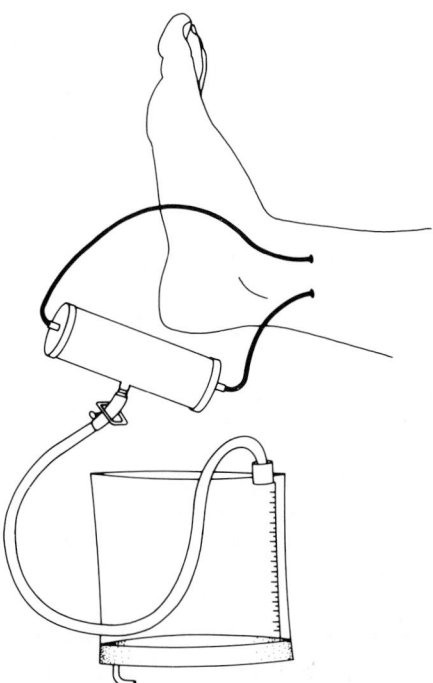

Figure 32-4 Hemofiltration system. (*From D. Levine, Care of the Renal Patient, Philadelphia, Lippincott, 1983.*)

the formation of ultrafiltrate while preventing hypotension and dehydration in the first hour. Throughout the procedure, intravenous fluids must be administered to support the ultrafiltration rate and the integrity of the vascular space.

A volume in excess of 10 L is necessary for maximal solute removal. If equal volumes of filtrate lost are replaced with a volume less than 10 L, excess solute is not removed; rather, solute in the same concentration of plasma is removed. Plasma solute levels may be stabilized with this method, but levels are never lowered.

The process of ultrafiltrate formation is facilitated by the positive hydrostatic pressure created by the arterial blood pressure. The hydrostatic pressure forces water and a small amount of solute from the blood compartment to the ultrafiltrate compartment. A negative hydrostatic pressure is present in the ultrafiltration compartment. This negative pressure exerts a pull on the blood compartment, which encourages the movement of water toward the ultrafiltration compartment. The negative pressure can be increased or decreased by changing the distance of the urinometer from the hemofilter. Moving the urinometer closer to the hemofilter decreases negative pressure and, therefore, diminishes the filtration rate, while increasing the distance between the two increases the negative pressure and enhances the rate of filtrate formation. A clamp can be placed on the ultrafiltration line to completely prevent the formation of filtrate. These two processes, hydrostatic and negative pressure, are opposed by the plasma colloid oncotic pressure. The colloid oncotic pressure exerts a pull to hold water in the vascular space. So the net pressure is the result of the forces favoring filtration and the forces opposing filtration. The total of the favoring forces must exceed the colloid oncotic pressure in order for ultrafiltration to take place.

As the blood travels along the hemofilter, more and more water is removed, thereby raising the oncotic pressure significantly as the blood moves toward the end portion of the hemofilter. Ultrafiltration is naturally greater at the arterial end of the hemofilter and decreases as the blood approaches the venous side. To minimize the effects of hyperosmolality, the blood can be prediluted by the administration of intravenous fluids. With normal blood pressure, the smallest amount of filtrate formed is 5 to 8 mL/min, but the maximum amount may exceed 1000 mL/h, placing the patient at risk for circulatory collapse.

Composition of the Ultrafiltrate The filtrate is protein- and RBC-free and contains potassium, sodium, chloride, glucose, urea, and creatinine in amounts equal to the concentrations present in the patient's plasma. Lower levels of calcium are found in the filtrate, because a percentage of this ion is bound to protein.

Arteriovenous Access A number of arteriovenous access sources may be used for CAVH, such as femoral or subclavian temporary catheters. An AV shunt or fistula cannulation may also be utilized. Factors to consider when selecting an access source are the diameter and the potential flow rate (Table 32-7) because both these can affect the success of the procedure.

Renal Transplantation

Renal transplantation is the only therapy that replaces 100 percent of renal function. The reader is referred to Chap. 59 for discussion of renal transplantation.

Nursing Management: End-Stage Renal Failure*

Many of the patient problems that arise during CRF are the same as those in acute renal failure. The difference in patient management is that the plan for CRF is part of a lifetime approach rather than a short-term plan. The nursing interventions in CRF are maintenance-oriented; in other words, interventions are directed toward maintenance of the best state of health possible for the patient. Prevention is the second focus of nursing management, in order to keep the patient safe from complications. The third focus of nursing care is adaptive, that is, helping the patient adapt to the physical and psychosocial changes that accompany CRF, which generally impact on every facet of the patient's life. Appropriate nursing interventions to meet these goals are outlined below.

---

*All nursing process items in this section are adapted from Stark, Reiley, and Jenuelson.

Table 32-7 Factors Affecting Ultrafiltration Rate

Osmolality of blood
Arterial blood pressure
Degree of negative pressure
Hydration status of blood

Nursing Diagnosis

Fluid volume excess. Etiology: inability to excrete homeostatic volumes of water via the renal route.

Goal

Maintenance of dry weight.

Collaborative Interventions

1. Establish patient's dry weight (ideal weight for individual renal failure patient).
2. Assess fluid status in relation to dry weight: normal blood pressure, absence of significant postural signs, and edema.
3. Plan desired fluid status in relation to volume intake and dialysis (patient should gain a maximum of 4 kg between dialysis procedures).
4. Treat episodes of CHF and hypertension as needed.

Nursing Interventions

1. Enforce fluid goals by restricting fluid intake.
2. Teach patient goals and methods of restricting volume with comfort, e.g., small sips of fluid or crushed ice.
3. Maintain intake and output record and obtain daily weight.
4. Assess fluid status and report changes that reflect alteration in status and the need to readjust fluid plan.
5. Manage dialysis treatments to be consistent with fluid removal goals.[1,28]

Nursing Diagnosis

Activity intolerance related to anemia. Etiology: lack or suppression of erythropoietin.

Goal

Enhanced activity tolerance.

Collaborative Interventions

1. Obtain and interpret hematocrit and hemoglobin levels periodically.
2. Establish goal for maintenance hematocrit, usually 20 in hemodialysis patients and 24 in patients suffering from angina.
3. Administer iron IM and multivitamins. Androgens are appropriate for a small group of dialysis patients.
4. Transfuse blood and blood products as indicated.

Nursing Interventions

1. Assess the degree of activity intolerance by observing the patient's mobility (sitting to standing) and tolerance of ambulation.
2. Obtain a patient history regarding activity levels.
3. Develop a plan with the patient to optimize energy level.
4. Recognize signs and symptoms of anemia.
5. Maintain awareness of risks to patient connected with transfusing bank blood and awareness of hepatitis risk to both patient and staff.

Nursing Diagnosis
Activity intolerance related to uremia. Etiology: fatigue secondary to accumulation of uremic toxins.

Goal
Increased activity tolerance.

Collaborative Interventions

1. Obtain and interpret the BUN, creatinine, and uric acid levels.
2. Establish a plan for initiating dialysis or transplantation.
3. Increase the effectiveness or frequency of dialysis treatments for removal of solute to maintain the BUN at less than 100 mg/dL and the creatinine at less than 10.
4. Assess for uremic symptoms

Nursing Interventions

1. Collaborate with dialysis nurse by sharing the patient's fluid status, cardiac status, blood pressure trends, clotting parameters, medications (vasoactive drugs or electrolyte supplements), and mental status.
2. Prepare patient and family for hemodialysis or peritoneal dialysis procedure by explaining the dynamics of the procedure.
3. Manage the hemodialysis or peritoneal dialysis and hemofiltration when appropriate.
4. Maintain awareness of the relation between elevated BUN and serum creatinine levels and the onset or exacerbation of the toxic symptoms of uremia.

Nursing Diagnosis
Impaired mobility. Etiology: chronic hypocalcemia caused by lack or absence of activated vitamin D and to hyperphosphotemia.

Goal
Maintenance of an asymptomatic hypocalcemia and hyperphosphotemia.

Collaborative Interventions

1. Obtain and interpret calcium and phosphorus levels.
2. Obtain periodic radiologic examinations.
3. Assess for signs of secondary hyperparathyroidism.
4. Administer phosphate-binding gels, forms of activated vitamin D, oral calcium, and dialysis treatments.

Nursing Interventions

1. Observe for signs of hypocalcemia (tremors, cardiac dysrhythmias, tetany).
2. Prevent tetany seizures.
3. Assess degree of mobility impairment and teach measures to promote patient safety.
4. Encourage patient to comply with medication regimen in order to prevent skeletal changes.

Nursing Diagnosis
Altered nutrition (less than body requirements). Etiology: anorexia, nausea, vomiting, altered taste sensations, and mouth ulcerations caused by uremia.

Goal
Maintenance of adequate nutritional state.

Collaborative Interventions

1. Assess nutritional needs.
2. Plan diet.

Nursing Interventions

1. Assess status of mucous membranes.
2. Provide mouth care.
3. Provide small frequent feedings with adequate calories (calorie requirement with normal level of activity is 35 kcal per kilogram of body weight).
4. Consider need for restriction of protein, sodium, and potassium.
5. Weigh patient daily and assess degree of muscle wasting; report findings to physician to determine need for changes in diet.

Nursing Diagnosis

Alteration in elimination (constipation). Etiology: (1) effect of phosphate-binding gels and (2) uremic bowel-alteration in intestinal motility caused by the toxic effect of accumulated waste products.

Goal

Maintenance of regular bowel evacuation.

Collaborative Intervention

1. Plan for dietary adjustments and pharmacologic agents.

Nursing Interventions

1. Administer and/or teach the patient to maintain a diet with increased bulk.
2. Administer (after assessment of bowel status) stool softeners or consider enemas if patient does not respond to other forms of conservative therapy.
3. Avoid magnesium-containing laxatives.
4. Observe consistency, color, and amount of stool.

Nursing Diagnosis

Sleep pattern disturbance. Etiology: possibly caused by uremia or hormonal imbalances. These are suspected of altering the quality of sleep as well as sleep respiratory patterns.[29]

Goal

Maintenance of normal sleep/rest pattern.

Nursing Interventions

1. Obtain history of patient's sleep patterns, including frequent dreaming or nightmares that may be disruptive to sleep.
2. Teach patient methods to promote sleep (warm milk prior to bed, environment conducive to rest).
3. Encourage patient to achieve at least three 90-minute sleep cycles.

Nursing Diagnosis

Sexual dysfunction related to renal failure. Etiology: uremia and its consequences are suspected of causing impotence, decreased libido, amenorrhea, and sterility.

Goal

Maintenance of satisfactory level of sexual functioning.

Collaborative Interventions

1. Plan diagnostic procedures to determine whether a reversible cause of sexual dysfunction is present.
2. Prepare patient for diagnostic tests.
3. Advise patient of methods to optimize sexuality (promote personal respect between partners; encourage recognition of individual needs for love and tenderness).
4. Consider experimental methods which may improve sexual functioning in the uremic patient (administration of zinc).

Nursing Interventions

1. Obtain history of patient's sexual functioning.
2. Provide psychologic support to the patient's spouse or significant other.

Nursing Diagnosis

Lack of knowledge of treatment alternatives for CRF.

Goal

Selection of a renal replacement therapy to enhance quality of life.

Collaborative Interventions

1. Determine what alternatives can be made available for choice by patient and family.

2. Identify the primary teacher and time period in which teaching sessions will be initiated.

Nursing Interventions

1. Acquire knowledge of treatment alternatives, patient expectations, and mortality rates.
2. Apply principles of teaching the uremic patient (shortened attention span, memory loss).
3. Reinforce learning provided.
4. Support patient and family in decision for a treatment alternative.

Nursing Diagnosis
Ineffective patient and family coping.

Goal
Effective coping with the disease process.

Nursing Interventions

1. Maintain awareness of complexities of CRF and its impact on patient and family unit, significantly or completely altering lifestyle of patient.
2. Assess stress level of patient and family.
3. Determine whether patient and/or family use productive or nonproductive coping measures.
4. Promote use of productive coping measures or help patient develop effective coping strategies.
5. Encourage patient and family to use and build support systems.
6. Provide opportunities for verbal exchange between patient, family, and nurse.

Nursing Diagnosis
Disturbance in self-concept (body image). Etiology: dialysis.

Goal
Adaptation to changes in body image.

Nursing Interventions

1. Allow patient to express feelings.
2. Encourage patient to participate in care of body parts in order to promote acceptance.
3. Assess signs of productive versus nonproductive coping.
4. Encourage maintenance of self-esteem.

Nursing Diagnosis
Lack of knowledge of CRF and dialysis procedures.

Goal
Increased knowledge of CRF and dialysis procedures.

Nursing Interventions
Instruct patient about all aspects of CRF:

1. Normal renal function and renal disease state
2. Fluid management
3. Dietary management
4. Medications (action, dosage, times)
5. Avoidance of infection
6. Rest periods to minimize fatigue
7. Skin care

and, for the dialysis patient, about

1. Dynamics of hemodialysis or peritoneal dialysis
2. Special diet and fluid allowances
3. Care of dialysis access
4. Need for weight control
5. Signs and symptoms of complications such as hypotension, bleeding, infection, and electrolyte imbalance

Nursing Diagnosis
Potential impairment of skin integrity. Etiology: uremic toxins cause changes in color, turgor, and integrity.

Goal
Maintenance of skin integrity.

Nursing Interventions

1. Assess color, texture, and turgor of skin, evidence of bruising, purpura, edema, uremic frost, infection, and presence of pruritus.
2. Plan with the patient measures to maintain skin moisture and integrity.
3. Bathe patient's skin to remove waste products, and consider adding oil to bath water to prevent dryness.
4. Apply creams or ointments.
5. Cleanse bruises and open areas to prevent infection.
6. Avoid tight sheets, slippers, or clothing, because pressure points may be created which are susceptible to breakdown.[1]

Nursing Diagnosis

Potential for infection. Etiology: alteration of immune responses and normal skin barriers caused by uremia.

Goal

Prevention of infection or its early diagnosis and treatment.

Collaborative Interventions

1. Avoidance of indwelling urinary catheters and other invasive procedures
2. Evaluation of infection at onset
3. Administration of antibiotic therapy
4. Assessment of antibiotic dosage (correlation with daily serum creatinine level)

Nursing Interventions

1. Maintenance of nutritional status
2. Protection of skin and mouth care to minimize breaks in normal protective barriers
3. Promotion of rest and of adequate sleep and wake cycles
4. Encouragement of patient to try to avoid persons with colds, influenza, or other infections
5. Utilization of aseptic techniques during dialysis procedures
6. Instruction of patient in how to care for AV site

Nursing Diagnosis

Potential for electrolyte imbalance (hyperkalemia). Etiology: accumulation of potassium ions secondary to inability to excrete potassium ions in the urine.

Goal

Maintenance of electrolyte balance.

Collaborative Interventions

1. Obtain and interpret electrolyte values.
2. Administer calcium gluconate, sodium bicarbonate, or glucose followed by sodium polystyrene sulfonate (Kayexalate) and/or hemodialysis.

Nursing Interventions

1. Observe for and report any signs or symptoms of electrolyte imbalance.
2. Interpret ECG changes.

3. Encourage patient compliance with dietary regimen in order to minimize hyperkalemic episodes.
4. Explain sodium polystyrene sulfonate and dialysis treatments to patient.

Nursing Diagnosis

Potential for metabolic acidosis. Etiology: inability of kidney to excrete hydrogen ions.

Goal

Maintenance of metabolic homeostasis.

Collaborative Interventions

1. Assess ABGs as necessary.
2. Interpret ABG levels.
3. Administer sodium bicarbonate for symptomatic acidosis and maintenance doses of bicarbonate orally.
4. Increase frequency of dialysis for uncontrollable acidosis.

Nursing Intervention

Maintain awareness of symptoms of metabolic acidosis.

References

1. Stark, J. (1985). The renal system. In J. Alspach, & S. Williams (Eds.), *Core curriculum for critical care nursing.* (pp. 348–449) Philadelphia: Saunders.
2. Schreiner, G. E. (1983). Uremia. In *Textbook of nephrology* (p. 454). Baltimore: Williams & Wilkins.
3. Rose, B. D. (1981). *Pathophysiology of renal disease.* New York: McGraw-Hill.
4. Leaf, A., & Cotran, R. S. (1985). *Renal pathophysiology* (3d ed.) (pp. 268–269). New York: Oxford.
5. Maude, D. L. (1977). *Kidney physiology and kidney disease: An introduction to nephrology.* Philadelphia: Lippincott.
6. Brosman, S. (1983). Tumors of the kidney and urinary tract. In *Textbook of nephrology* (p. 628). Baltimore: Williams & Wilkins.
7. Steele, S. M., & Harmon, V. W. (1979). *Values clarification in nursing.* New York: Appleton-Century-Crofts.
8. Freidman, E. A. (1978). *Strategy in renal failure.* New York: Wiley.

9. Schmidt, G. W., & Bach, C. (1982). Peritoneal dialysis and hemodialysis: An overview. In *Nephrology: An approach to the patient with renal disease* (p. 562). Philadelphia: Lippincott.

10. Bergstrom, J., & Furst, P. (1983). Other uremic toxins. In S. Massey, & R. Glassock (Eds.), *Textbook of nephrology* (pp. 78–79). Baltimore: Williams & Wilkins.

11. Hollomby, D. J. (1983). Introduction to hemodialysis. In *Care of the renal patient* (p. 35). Philadelphia: Saunders.

12. Freeman, R. B. (1983). Hemodialysis. In *Textbook of nephrology* (pp. 824–825). Baltimore: Williams & Wilkins.

13. Henrich, W. L., Woodard, T. D., Blachley, J. D., et al. (1980). Role of osmolality in blood pressure stability after dialysis and ultrafiltration. *Kidney International 18,* 480–488.

14. Swartz, R. D., Somermeyer, M. G., & Hsu, C. H. (1982). Preservation of plasma volume during hemodialysis depends on dialysate osmolality. *American Journal of Nephrology, 2,* 189–194.

15. Golper, T. A. (1985). Continuous arteriovenous hemofiltration in acute renal failure. *American Journal of Kidney Disease, 6*(6), 373–386.

16. Wehle, B., Asaba, H., Castenfors, J., et al. (1979). Hemodynamic changes during sequential ultrafiltration and dialysis. *Kidney International, 15,* 411–419.

17. Quellhorst, E., Schuenemarr, B., Hidebrand, U., et al. (1980). Response of the vascular system to different modification of haemofiltration and haemodialysis. *Proceedings of European Dialysis Transplant Association, 17,* 197–204.

18. Zucelli, P., Santoro, A., Sturani, A., et al. (1984). Effects of hemodialysis and hemofiltration on the automatic control of circulation. *Trans. American Society for Artificial Internal Organs, 30,* 163–167.

19. Mault, J. R., Dechart, R. E., Bartlett, R. H., et al. (1982). Oxygen consumption during hemodialysis for acute renal failure. *Trans. American Society for Artificial Internal Organs, 28,* 510–513.

20. Bohler, J., Kramer, P., Galtze, O., et al. (1983). Leukocyte counts and complement activation during pump-driven and arteriovenous haemofiltration. *Contrib. Nephrol., 36,* 15–25.

21. Aizawa, Y., Ohmori, T., Imai, K., et al. (1977). Depressant action of acetate upon the human cardiovascular system. *Clinical Nephrology, 8,* 477–480.

22. Kramer, P., et al. (1980). Management of anuric intensive care patients with arteriovenous hemofiltration. *International Journal of Artificial Organs, 3*(4), 225–229.

23. Silverstein, M., et al. (1974). Treatment of severe fluid overload by ultrafiltration. *New England Journal of Medicine, 291*(15), 747–751.

24. Keily, M. (1984). Continuous arteriovenous hemofiltration. *Critical Care Nurse, 4,* 39–43.

25. Golper, T. A. (1985). Continuous arteriovenous hemofiltration in acute renal failure. *American Journal of Kidney Disease, 6*(6), 373–386.

26. Kaplan, A., et al. (1984). Continuous arteriovenous hemofiltration: A report of six months experience. *Annals of Internal Medicine, 100*(3), 358–367.

27. Williams, V., & Perkins, L. (1984). Continuous ultrafiltration, a new ICU procedure for the treatment of fluid overload. *Critical Care Nurse, 4,* 44–49.

28. Stark, J., & Hunt, V. (1983). Helping your patient with chronic renal failure. *Nursing 83, 13*(9), 56–64.

29. Srivastara, R. (1986). Fatigue in the renal patient. *ANNA Journal, 13*(5), 246–249.

part 7

Neurologic Patient-Care Problems

33

Neurological Anatomy and Physiology

Pamela H.
Mitchell

The nervous system is at once the most fundamental and most complex of all the physiological systems. It is the primary system that allows us to interact with our environment—to function simultaneously at the most basic level of survival and the highest level of creativity. Because of its complexity in integrating multiple aspects of physical and cognitive function, knowledge of its structures is not enough. A knowledgeable approach to care of the patient with disorders of the nervous system must be built upon an understanding of the relationship between the structures damaged by the injury, disease, or pathophysiological process and the human function served by those structures. Therefore, this chapter is organized to present this information in two ways. First, an overview of the basic human functions and anatomical correlates is presented. Then the structural-functional correlates are discussed on the basis of the four gross divisions of the nervous system structures (neuroaxis approach). This organization is intended to help the reader appreciate both the vertical integration of human functions at all levels of the nervous system and the horizontal integration of higher order and reflex aspects of function within each anatomical compartment. Figure 33-1 shows the relation between the vertical (functional) and the horizontal (neuroaxis) approaches to understanding functional neuroanatomy. Such an organization is helpful, for example in focusing initial assessment parameters on those functions most at risk when the injury is at a specific location such as the thoracic spinal cord. On the other hand, understanding that a given function—perception of pain, for example—is integrated at several anatomical

Revised from a chapter in the first edition prepared by Marilyn M. Ricci.

levels helps to avoid focusing care planning on, for example, only the human responses predicted by the local area of injury.

The gross anatomical divisions of the nervous system are the *central nervous system* and the *peripheral nervous system*. The central nervous system (CNS) comprises the brain, brainstem, and spinal cord. The peripheral nervous system comprises the cranial and spinal nerves. The autonomic nervous system, which is frequently considered separately, includes parts of the central and peripheral nervous systems.

Microscopically, the nervous system consists of support structures called *neuroglial* cells and the basic nerve cell, or *neuron*. The glial cells, which serve to support, protect, and nourish the neurons, include astrocytes, oligodendroglia, microglia, and ependymal cells. The astrocytes are located between the blood vessels and neurons, restricting the passage of substances into the central nervous system. The oligodendroglia synthesize and maintain myelin. The microglia serve as phagocytes. The ependymal cells, which line the ventricular system and the central canal of the spinal cord, play a major role in cerebrospinal fluid production. The peripheral neuroglia are found in ganglia and along nerve trunks.

The *neuron* is the structural, genetic, and functional unit of the nervous system. The neuron is composed of a cell body, dendrites, and axons. The *cell bodies,* or gray matter, are located in layers on the surface of the brain, or *cortex,* and in groups deeper within the brain; cell bodies are also found in the brainstem and spinal cord and certain other locations.

Dendrites are short receptor fibers which receive impulses and conduct them to the cell body. *Axons* are the myelinated long fibers which transmit

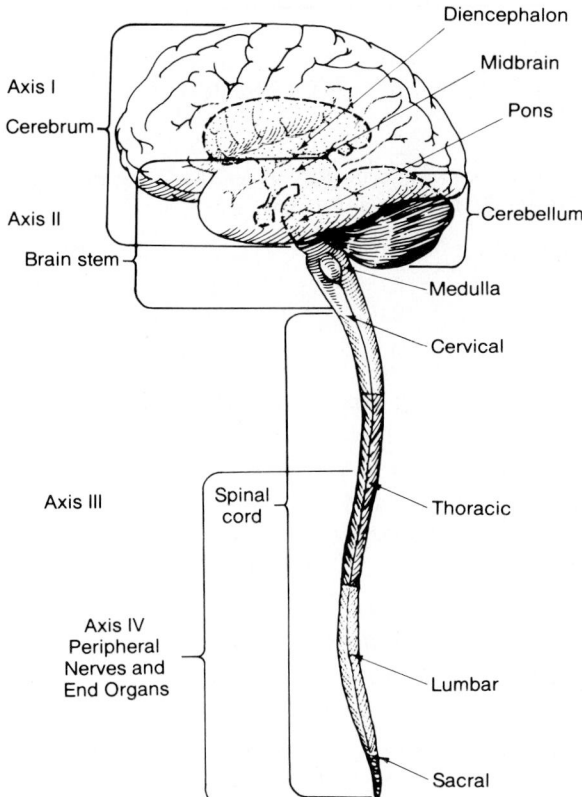

Figure 33-1 The neuraxis related to human functions. *(Adapted from L. L. Langley, I. R. Telford, and J. B. Christensen, Dynamic Anatomy and Physiology, 5th ed., McGraw-Hill, New York, 1980, p. 233.)*

impulses away from the cell body. Within the central nervous system, the axons form the white matter. The *myelin sheath* is a semifluid protein and lipid substance surrounding the axon and providing insulation. *Schwann cells* form a delicate membrane which surrounds the myelin sheath of the peripheral nerve fibers. Within the central nervous system, groups of axons with a common origin that travel alongside each other constitute a *tract*.

Vertically organized, the nervous system comprises four *functional* systems: (1) consciousness/mentation, (2) movement, (3) sensation, and (4) integrated regulation.[1] All these systems can be considered to have both reflex and higher order components. Reflex components are the sensory or receptor mechanisms and the output or effector mechanisms. The higher order components consist

of the mechanisms that interpret the incoming sensory information and integrate and initiate the motor output.

Horizontally, the nervous system can be subdivided into four axes. The *neuraxis* comprises (1) axis I: the cerebral hemispheres, which include the diencephalon and basal ganglia; (2) axis II: the brainstem and cerebellum; (3) axis III: the spinal cord; and (4) axis IV: the peripheral nerves and the end organs they innervate. Each axis contains aspects of more than one functional subsystem. For example, the cerebral hemispheres mediate arousal, mentation, higher order movement, sensation, and integrative regulatory functions.

Finally, the discussion of functional anatomy and physiology must take into account the structures that serve to protect, support, and nourish the nervous system. Disease or injury that damages these structures will have profound functional effects, often affecting the entire nervous system, not any single localized structure.

Functional Anatomy and Physiology

Basic human functions which allow us to interact normally with the environment include becoming aroused, thinking, moving, feeling, and performing such basic regulatory functions as breathing, eating, and circulating the body fluids. All these functions are organized by the nervous system and can be subsumed into four basic functions: consciousness/mentation, movement, sensation, and integrative regulation. Each of these functions is organized vertically when the nervous system structure is considered as a whole. Each requires some kind of *sensory input* and *motor output,* which is received from and transmitted to the periphery (limbs, head, viscera). In addition, each function requires mechanisms to interpret and process the information for appropriate storage or response. Such processing may occur in the spinal cord or brainstem at a lower order, or *reflex* level, or may occur in the cerebral hemispheres as a higher order type of processing. In this section, the anatomical structures are described at each level of processing for each of the four functional systems. Table 33-1 summarizes the anatomical correlates for each of these functional systems.

Table 33-1 Neuroanatomical Correlates of Fundamental Human Functions

Function	Anatomical Correlate
Consciousness	
Arousal	Reticular activating system, brainstem reticular formation, diffuse projections to thalamus and cortex, diencephalon
Self-awareness	Cerebral hemispheres
Mentation	
Memory	Limbic system, cortex; ascending activation via reticular activating system and thalamic projection system
Affect	Limbic system
Language (spoken, read, written)	Left cerebral hemisphere
Spatial perception	Right hemisphere
Problem solving	Cerebral hemispheres
Movement	
Head	
Seeing (eye movement)	Cranial nerves III, IV, VI; brainstem internuclear pathways; cerebellum
Chewing	Cranial nerves V, VII, XII
Swallowing	Cranial nerves IX, X, XII
Speaking:	
Articulating	Cranial nerves VII, IX, XII and cerebellum
Phonating	Cranial nerve X
Body	
Walking	Motor cortex, basal ganglia
Activities of daily living	Pyramidal and extrapyramidal systems, cerebellum
Coordination	Cerebellum
Sensation	
Seeing (vision)	Cranial nerve II
Smelling	Cranial nerve I
Hearing	Cranial nerve VIII
Balance	Cranial nerve VIII and posterior columns of spinal cord
Feeling	
Pain, temperature	Spinal cord: spinothalamic tracts, anterolateral tracts; cerebral hemispheres: thalamus
Touch, position	Spinal cord: posterior columns; cerebral hemisphere: sensory cortex
Discrimination, higher sensation	Cerebral hemisphere: sensory cortex
Integrative regulation	
Breathing	Motor cortex, medullary inspiratory/expiratory centers; peripheral chemoreceptors and stretch receptors; diaphragm: C3, 5; intrinsic muscles: T12, L2
Circulation	Hypothalamus; cranial nerve X, sympathetic ganglia (heart and lungs); cervical ganglia (head and upper extremities); T2, 6 (thorax); T5–10 (abdomen); T11–L2 (lower extremities and pelvis); craniosacral parasympathetic ganglia; postganglionic sympathetic, parasympathetic fibers
Temperature control	Hypothalamus; dermatomal cutaneous sympathetic and parasympathetic fibers
Ingestion/digestion	Medial temporal lobe, hypothalamus, midbrain, pons, visceral parasympathetic via cranial outflow; sacral via pelvic nerve; sympathetic via lower thoracic ganglia
Elimination	Medial frontal lobe; paracentral gyrus, hypothalamus, midbrain, pons, S2–4 pelvic, pudendal, perineal, hypogastric nerves
Sexual response	Limbic system, preoptic hypothalamus, spinal reflex centers (T11–L2, S2–4); pelvic, pudendal, perineal, and hypogastric nerves
Affect (emotional expression)	Limbic system, hypothalamus, visceral and cutaneous sympathetic and parasympathetic effectors, musculoskeletal and proprioceptive reflexes

Source: Adapted from Mitchell, Cammermyer, Ozuna, and Woods.[1]

Consciousness/Mentation

Clinical definitions of consciousness (as contrasted with metaphysical or spiritual definitions) involve two components: arousal and self-awareness. Because the component of self-awareness becomes blended with the functions of cognition, it is useful to consider the functions of consciousness and mentation (or cognition) together when discussing anatomical correlates. The *reticular activating system,* or RAS (Fig. 33-2), is the anatomical substrate for the function of arousal or behavioral activation. The RAS is a functional system composed of the reticular formation and its projections to the thalamus and cerebral hemispheres. The *reticular formation* is a group of neurons and their connecting axons located in the central core of the brainstem, ascending from the pyramids of the medulla and ending at the thalamus. These neurons project fibers to the thalamus and all areas of the cerebral cortex, functioning to alert the cerebral hemisphere to incoming stimuli. Because the reticular structures are tightly packed in the brainstem, very small lesions in the central brainstem can cause loss of arousal (or consciousness). In contrast, the diffuse nature of the projections in the cerebral hemispheres requires considerably larger lesions or bilateral lesions to disrupt arousal at the level of the hemispheres.

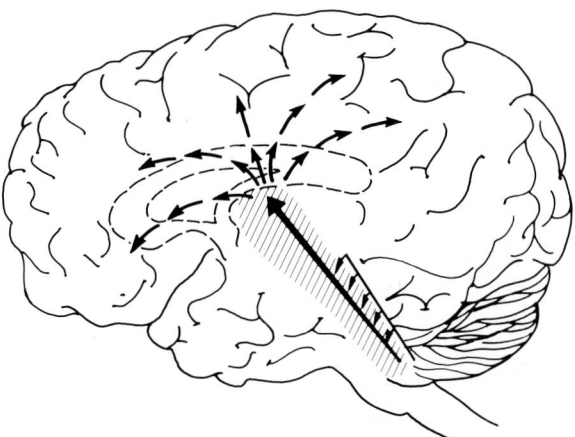

Figure 33-2   The reticular activating system. The small arrows represent multiple sensory inputs at the level of the brainstem; the large arrows are projections to the cortex. *(Redrawn from Mitchell, Cammermyer, Ozuna, & Woods.*[1]*)*

The reticular core contains the cell bodies which form the monoamines responsible for the chemical transmitters between neurons of not only the arousal system but also the motor system, pain transmission, affective states, and a number of basic vegetative responses. Norepinephrine pathways arise in the locus ceruleus (medial brainstem) and are implicated in the normal cycling between REM and non-REM sleep. Serotonin pathways begin in the raphe nucleus of the lower brainstem and are important in cycling between wake and sleep and among sleep stages.

The self-awareness component of consciousness is probably a summation of a number of mentation, or cognition, functions of the cerebral hemispheres. Although the brain functions as a whole in the complex human activities involved in human interaction with the environment, a number of anatomical areas are known to be crucial to the normal functioning of such mental activities as memory, production and understanding of language, recognition of shapes, faces, and space, and so on. These areas are contained in both surface and deep structures of the cerebral hemispheres.

Cerebral Hemispheres

The cerebral hemispheres are paired structures which are most highly developed in primates, including humans. Each hemisphere consists of gray matter (neuronal cell bodies), found primarily in the cortex and the basal ganglia, and white matter (myelinated fiber tracts), which connect the numerous functional areas of the hemispheres. *Association fibers* connect areas within the same hemisphere; transverse fibers called *commissures* connect symmetrical areas between the two hemispheres. *Projection fibers* connect the cerebral cortex with deeper brain structures, brainstem, and spinal cord. The *corpus callosum* is the commissural fiber tract that connects the two hemispheres.

The surfaces of the brain contain grooves known as *fissures* and *sulci.* The fissures (the larger grooves) serve to mark the boundaries between lobes of the brain; the sulci are smaller grooves that serve as landmarks to identify areas within lobes. The convolutions of the brain between the sulci are known as *gyri.* Figure 33-3 shows the relation of fissures, sulci, and gyri to the lobes of the hemispheres.

Figure 33-3   (*A*) Lateral view of the cerebrum. (*B*) A portion of the cortex in cross section. *(From L. L. Langley, I. R. Telford, and J. B. Christensen, Dynamic Anatomy and Physiology, 5th ed., McGraw-Hill, New York, 1980.)*

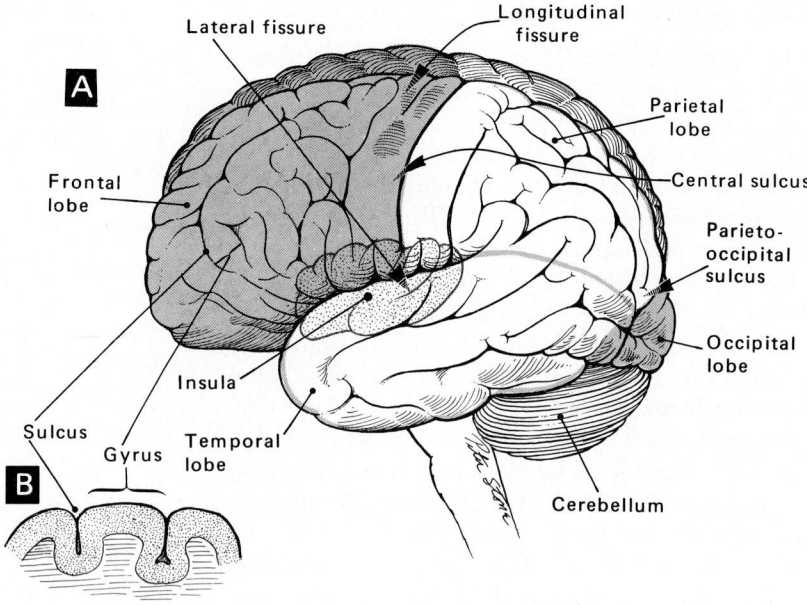

The *longitudinal fissure* separates the cerebral hemispheres. Each hemisphere is subdivided into lobes, which are separated by deep sulci or fissures. The *central sulcus (fissure of Rolando)* marks the boundaries of the frontal and parietal lobes; while the *fissure of Sylvius* separates the temporal from the parietal and frontal lobes. The *parietooccipital fissure* separates the occipital from the parietal and temporal lobes. The *limbic lobe*

(Fig. 33-4) is a paired collection of structures on the medial portion of the hemispheres. Structures commonly considered part of the limbic cortex include the cingulate gyrus, the hippocampus, the amygdala, the inferior medial frontal lobe, and the fiber tracts connecting these structures.

A number of cognitive functions with identifiable anatomical correlates are disrupted in conditions requiring critical nursing care. These func-

Figure 33-4   The limbic system. *(From D. B. Stratton, Neurophysiology, McGraw-Hill, New York, 1981, p. 310.)*

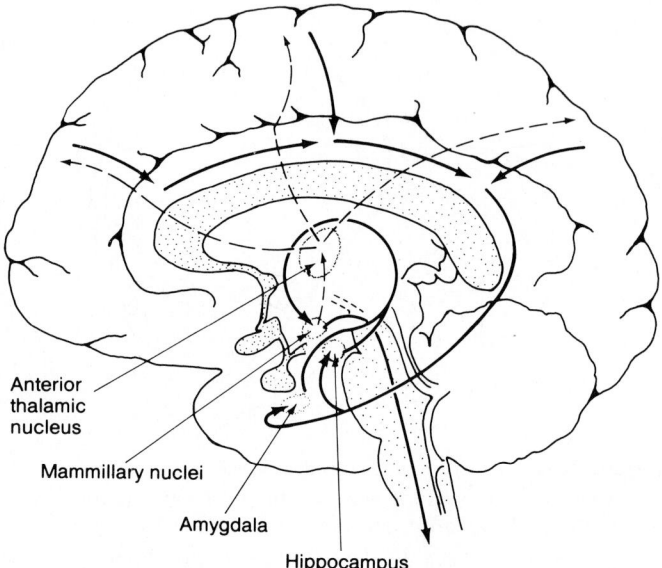

tions include memory, production and understanding of language, emotional expression, spatial perception, and generalized information processing (thinking, problem solving).

Memory

The medial temporal lobes are crucial to the storage of short-term memory and perhaps to the retrieval of longer-term memory. Damage to the hippocampal gyrus and mammillary bodies of the hypothalamus is associated with impaired storage of short-term memories. There appears to be hemispheric specialization with regard to memory functions, with the left hippocampus and medial temporal lobe being more important to storage of verbal information and the corresponding areas in the right medial hemisphere mediating memory for faces, shapes, and spatial information. No specific brain location has been shown to disrupt long-term memory, suggesting that the brain as a whole is involved in storage of long-term information.

Language

Language is a system of spoken and written symbols and involves more than just the ability to make sounds and form words. In most people, the left cerebral hemisphere is critical in the production and understanding of language. Broca's area, the third convolution (gyrus) of the frontal lobe, is important in initiating the oral movements necessary for speech. The person with lesions of Broca's area cannot easily produce words (although the ability to move the mouth is unimpaired) but can understand speech.

The areas necessary to understanding spoken language are Wernicke's area (posterior, superior left temporal lobe) and the primary auditory area in the superior temporal lobe. These areas are shown in Fig. 33-5. Comprehension of written language requires an intact visual area (posterior and medial occipital lobe) as well as intact communication with Wernicke's area.

Affect

The frontal lobes and subcortical structures of the limbic system (hippocampus, cingulate gyrus, septum, and amygdala) interact to produce affective behavior. The frontal lobes appear to act to inhibit more primitive or undifferentiated emotional responses that are integrated by the limbic system. Thus, persons with generalized brain damage or those with medial frontal lobe damage may exhibit wide swings of emotion or have difficulty modulating emotional expression.

Spatial Perception

Recognition of the relation of objects in space, of shapes, and of other persons is mediated in most people more by the right cerebral hemisphere than the left. The right parietal lobe is crucial in appreciating the three-dimensional nature of objects, locating oneself in space, and appreciating that the

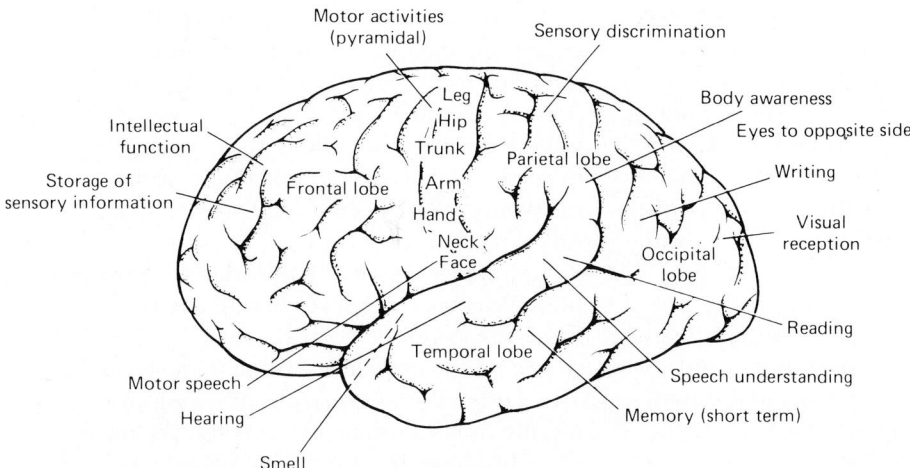

Figure 33-5 Localized functional areas of the cerebral cortex.

right side of the body is one's own. The recognition of faces is more impaired by lesions of the right hippocampus than by those of the left.

Complex Cognitive Functions

Complex cognitive functions such as problem solving, decision making, and judgment cannot be easily localized to any "center" in the brain. Each of these activities requires numerous coordinated processes of memory, recognition of pattern, and so forth. Damage to any part of the brain can impair the efficiency and quality of these operations. Thus many different lesions may result in irritability, distractibility, and difficulty in processing multiple inputs simultaneously.

Movement

The motor system is subdivided into the pyramidal and extrapyramidal systems. The pyramidal system is composed of the cells of the precentral gyrus of the frontal lobes and several tracts which descend through the internal capsule to the brainstem and spinal cord. It is the system serving voluntary muscle movement. The corticomesencephalic tract terminates in the brainstem at the motor nuclei of the oculomotor (III), trochlear (IV), and abducens (VI) cranial nerves. The corticobulbar tract terminates at the motor nuclei of the trigeminal (V), facial (VII), glossopharyngeal (IX), vagus (X), spinal accessory (XI), and hypoglossal (XII) cranial nerves. Fibers forming the corticospinal tract arise from each hemisphere, pass through the posterior limb of the internal capsule, and descend through the brainstem, and the majority cross over (*decussate*) to the opposite side of the medulla to form the lateral corticospinal tract (Fig. 33-6). These fibers terminate at the various spinal cord segments and synapse with the anterior horn cells. The fibers which do not cross descend as the anterior corticospinal tract and synapse directly with neurons in the spinal cord.

Motor impulses, which originate in the prefrontal gyrus, are transmitted by the corticospinal tract to the efferent cranial and spinal fibers and so to the periphery (Fig. 33-7). The pyramidal system primarily regulates skilled motor activities of the distal extremities and the skeletal musculature of the head and neck. The cerebral cortex has several *suppressor areas* which inhibit movements of the musculature when they are stimulated. Eye movements are influenced by suppressor areas in the frontal and occipital lobes. The motor speech area is located in the posterior-inferior aspect of the frontal lobe, with the main language center being located in the left hemisphere. Motor speech is also influenced by the facial (VII), glossopharyngeal (IX), vagus (X), and hypoglossal (XII) nerves.

The extrapyramidal system is composed of the basal ganglia and a complex network of tracts which connect the cerebral cortex, basal ganglia, cerebellum, brainstem, and spinal cord. Many circuits and feedback loops within and between the structures provide the interaction and constant influence over the parts of the cerebral cortex which give rise to the descending motor tracts, both pyramidal and extrapyramidal. The activity of the lower motor neurons of the peripheral nervous system are under the influence of the extrapyramidal system.

The extrapyramidal spinal tract either facilitates or inhibits flexor and extensor activities. The net result of extrapyramidal activity is maintenance of muscle tone; control of gross skeletal muscle activities; control of rhythmic movements, e.g., running and walking; and control of head and trunk movements related to maintaining an upright position.

The cerebellum and the related fibers which provide connections with the basal ganglia and the reticular formation coordinate muscle activities and time muscle contractions to facilitate smoothness and accuracy (synergy). Intent and performance are correlated, providing for error control. The cerebellum also provides a "braking" or damping function to enable movements to be stopped where intended. The cerebellum receives sensory input from a number of afferent fibers which assist in maintaining equilibrium and the control of spinal reflex movements (Fig. 33-7).

Impulses from visual, auditory, vestibular tactile, and proprioceptive stimuli, as well as input from the cerebral cortex, reach the cerebellum, where rapid correlation and integration take place. The cerebellum then transmits impulses which modify motor commands to voluntary muscles.

Impulses from the basal ganglia and cerebellum are first transmitted to the thalamus, where

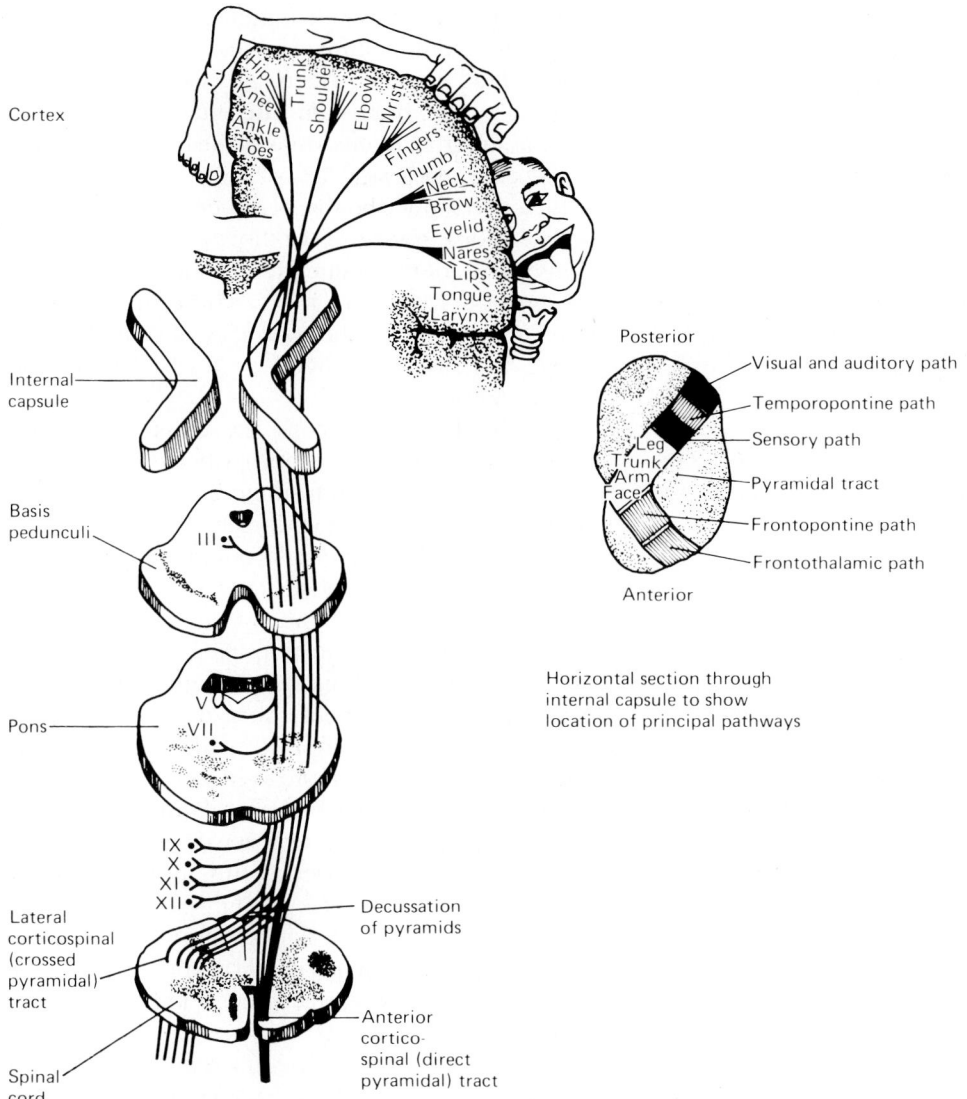

Figure 33-6 Corticospinal (pyramidal) tract. The figure drawn at the edge of the cerebral hemisphere depicts the amount of surface area on the cortex assigned to the motor function of each body part. *(From J. G. Chusid, Correlative Neuroanatomy and Functional Neurology, 17th ed., Lange, Los Altos, 1979.)*

modification and integration occur prior to transmission to the cerebral cortex. Impulses from the facilatory and inhibitory reticular nuclei are transmitted by the reticulospinal tracts to the anterior horn motor nuclei. When facilatory impulses are transmitted to extensor muscles, reciprocal impulses are transmitted to inhibit flexor muscle

activity, with the effect being extensor facilitation and flexor inhibition. When inhibitory impulses predominate, lower motor neurons transmit impulses to inhibit muscle activity. There is normally a balance of facilatory and inhibitory impulses at the lower neuron level, so that muscle tone is maintained.

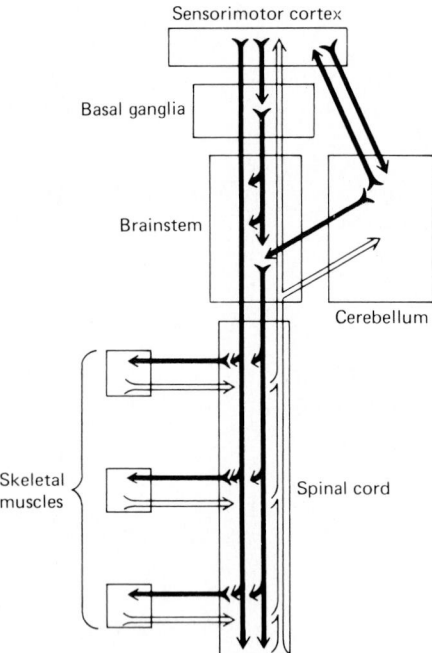

Sensorimotor cortex

Basal ganglia

Brainstem

Cerebellum

Skeletal
muscles

Spinal cord

Figure 33-7 Schematic representation of the motor system. Suprasegmental (pyramidal tract) influences are represented by the arrows connecting the motor cortex (axis I), brainstem (axis II), and spinal cord (axis III). Segmental pathways (lower motor neuron) are shown by the arrows between spinal cord and skeletal muscles (axis IV). The cerebellum (axis III) has no direct connections to cortex or spinal cord but serves to coordinate the entire system. *(From E. Henneman, in V. Mountcastle, Ed., Medical Physiology, 13th ed., Mosby, St. Louis, 1974.)*

Sensation

The sensory system consists of afferent peripheral nerves, the spinothalamic tracts and dorsal columns of the spinal cord, tracts within the brainstem, the thalamus, and the frontal, parietal, temporal, occipital, and limbic lobes.

The cranial nerves transmit highly specialized sensations to the central nervous system. The olfactory nerves transmit the sense of smell. The optic nerves receive and transmit visual input. The acoustic nerves transmit sound by the cochlear branch and the sense of equilibrium by the vestibular branch. Taste is transmitted by the glossopharyngeal and facial nerves.

The superficial sensations of crude touch, pain, and temperature of the eye and face are transmitted by the trigeminal, facial, and vagus nerves into the brainstem. The cutaneous receptors for the superficial sensations of the body are located in specific anatomical areas known as *dermatomes,* which correspond to the peripheral distribution of the sensory spinal nerve fibers. The superficial sensations are transmitted to the spinal cord by the posterior spinal nerve roots, where they synapse, pass immediately to the contralateral spinothalamic tract, and are transmitted to the thalamus and cerebral cortex.

The deep, more complex sensations of pressure, position (proprioception), vibration, fine touch, and deep pain are transmitted by the posterior spinal nerve roots to the dorsal column to ascend to the level of the medulla oblongata, where the fibers cross to the opposite side and extend to the thalamus and cerebral cortex (Fig. 33-8).

The reticular formation integrates all sensory input prior to transmission to higher levels. The stimulation of the reticular formation in the upper brainstem produces impulses which result in cortical arousal and contribute to conscious awareness.

All the lobes of the cerebral hemispheres have specific areas which receive sensory impulses and other areas which integrate this information and enable it to be understood (Fig. 33-5). The frontal lobe functions include the reception of the sense of smell, storage of information for memory, abstract thought processes, judgment, and other higher intellectual functions.

The activities of the parietal lobes consist primarily of sensory discrimination and bodily awareness for the opposite side of the body. Awareness of size, shape, and texture of objects; the relationship of body parts; two-point discrimination; and localization of other sensations are parietal lobe functions. The sensory speech center is located in the parietal lobe.

The occipital lobes are primary visual receiving and understanding areas. The temporal lobes are primarily auditory and olfactory reception areas; however, the hippocampal gyrus receives the sensory input associated with memory and bodily awareness. The limbic structures process and sort information as well as supply information for storage; therefore, learning and memory for recent events are under the influence of the limbic system.

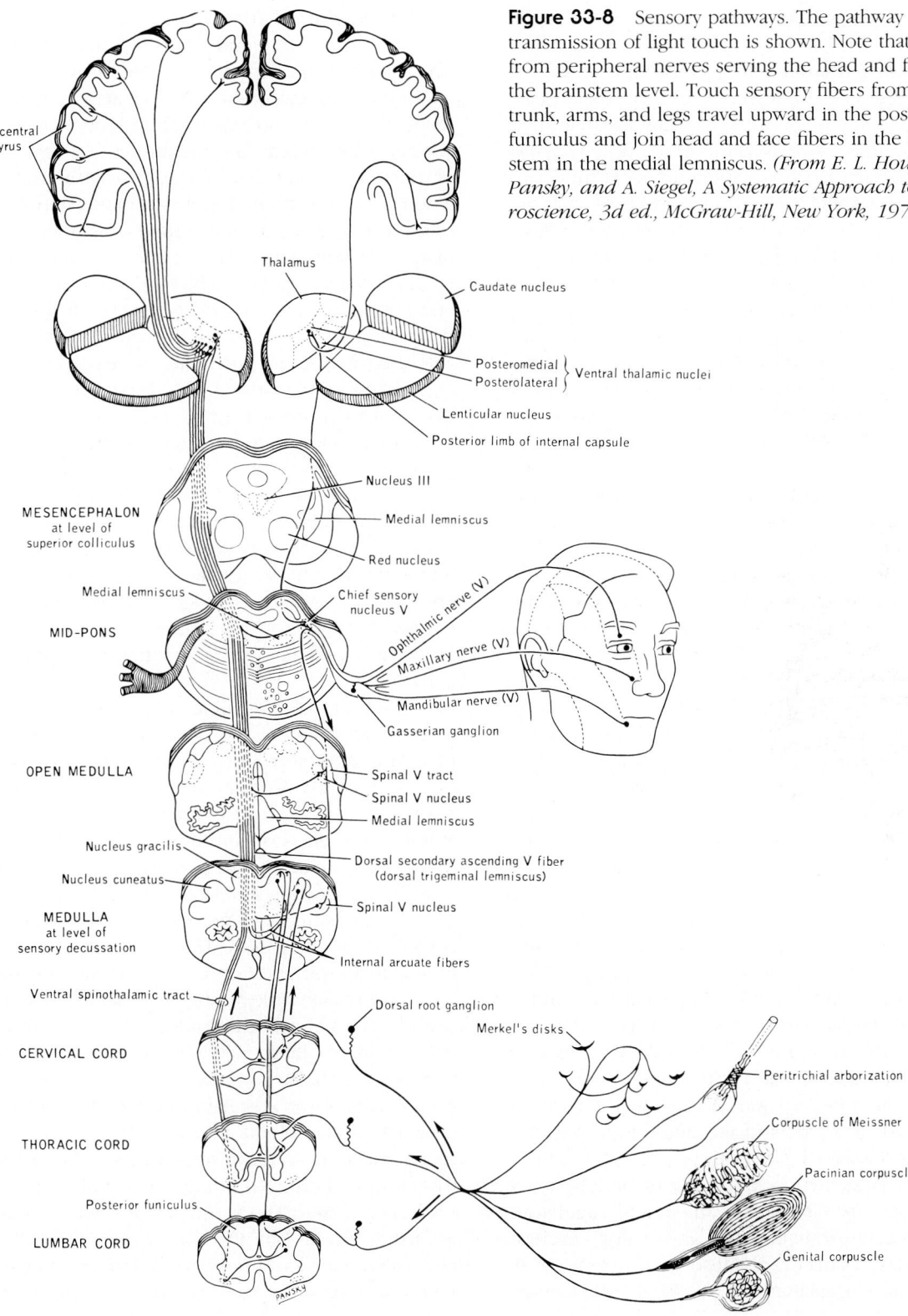

Figure 33-8 Sensory pathways. The pathway for the transmission of light touch is shown. Note that input from peripheral nerves serving the head and face is at the brainstem level. Touch sensory fibers from the trunk, arms, and legs travel upward in the posterior funiculus and join head and face fibers in the brainstem in the medial lemniscus. *(From E. L. House, B. Pansky, and A. Siegel, A Systematic Approach to Neuroscience, 3d ed., McGraw-Hill, New York, 1979.)*

Postcentral gyrus

Thalamus

Caudate nucleus

Posteromedial
Posterolateral
} Ventral thalamic nuclei

Lenticular nucleus

Posterior limb of internal capsule

MESENCEPHALON
at level of
superior colliculus

Nucleus III

Medial lemniscus

Red nucleus

Medial lemniscus

Chief sensory nucleus V

MID-PONS

Ophthalmic nerve (V)

Maxillary nerve (V)

Mandibular nerve (V)

Gasserian ganglion

OPEN MEDULLA

Spinal V tract

Spinal V nucleus

Medial lemniscus

Nucleus gracilis

Dorsal secondary ascending V fiber
(dorsal trigeminal lemniscus)

Nucleus cuneatus

Spinal V nucleus

MEDULLA
at level of
sensory decussation

Internal arcuate fibers

Ventral spinothalamic tract

Dorsal root ganglion

Merkel's disks

CERVICAL CORD

Peritrichial arborization

THORACIC CORD

Corpuscle of Meissner

Pacinian corpuscle

Posterior funiculus

LUMBAR CORD

Genital corpuscle

PANSKY

Integrative Regulation

Integrative regulation refers to the functional system that regulates basic survival functions at many levels of the nervous system. In order for mammals to adapt and survive in their environments, they must be able to carry out a large number of functions quite automatically, or without awareness. A regulatory system is one which maintains and adjusts physiological stability without conscious effort from the organism. The autonomic nervous system is usually thought of as the primary regulator in humans and other mammals. However, it is only one participant in a truly integrated process. Neurons of the regulatory system must receive sensory stimuli (from the peripheral and autonomic sensory nerves), interpret the stimuli at various reflex and conscious levels, coordinate multiple inputs, transmit motor responses to both somatic and autonomic motor systems, and provide feedback about the state of the end organ.

The basic regulatory functions include breathing, circulation, temperature control, ingestion/ digestion, elimination, and sexual and emotional expression. Sensory input to each system is via the peripheral nerves (spinal nerves, cranial nerves, or autonomic nerves). Interpretation of the sensory input occurs at several levels: spinal cord, brainstem, hypothalamus, limbic cortex, and possibly cerebellum. Motor output may be voluntary or may be reflexly controlled. The cerebral cortex mediates voluntary control, while the sympathetic and parasympathetic systems mediate reflex control. All the integrated regulatory subsystems have control at four levels: voluntary control at the cerebral cortex, central reflex control at the hypothalamus and limbic system, autonomic reflex control at the brainstem and spinal cord, and peripheral control at the end organ. Disorders that disrupt nervous system functioning at any of these levels have the potential to disturb several integrated regulatory functions. Figures 33-9 and 33-10 show the relation of the cranial nerves and the autonomic nervous system to regulatory functions.

The sympathetic and parasympathetic systems are the primary effectors of integrated regulatory activity. The hypothalamus is the major cerebral hemisphere regulator of these two systems. The anterior and medial nuclei of the hypothalamus excite parasympathetic activity, causing sweating, decrease in the rate and force of cardiac contractions, and pupil constriction. The posterior and lateral nuclei excite sympathetic activity, causing vasoconstriction, increased rate and force of cardiac contractions, increased respirations, and inhibition of peristalsis. Pupillary dilation occurs passively when parasympathetic input is removed, and vasodilatation occurs passively when sympathetic stimulation is removed. The physical expression of "fight or flight" emotion, which includes accelerated heart rate, elevated blood pressure, flushing or pallor of the skin, sweating, gooseflesh, dry mouth, and gastrointestinal disturbances, are a reflection of autonomic activities which are modulated by the hypothalamus.

The hypothalamic nuclei regulate body temperature. The parasympathetic activities of sweating and vasodilatation result in lowering the body temperature. Shivering and vasoconstriction, which are sympathetic activities, result in elevation of body temperature. The regulation of eating, drinking, emptying the urinary bladder, defecation, and sexual activity is under the influence of the hypothalamic structures and the sympathetic and parasympathetic fibers.

The supraoptic nuclei of the hypothalamus and its neuronal connections with the posterior pituitary are referred to as the *neurohypophysis* (see Chap. 36). The neurohypophysis regulates body water metabolism as a result of its production, storage, and release of antidiuretic hormone (ADH). ADH is produced by the hypothalamic nuclei and transferred to the posterior pituitary for storage. The capillaries in the supraoptic nuclei monitor the osmolality of the blood. The secretion of ADH by the posterior pituitary is either stimulated or inhibited on the basis of the existing osmolality. Increased osmolality of the body fluids and a reduction of extracellular volume, which stimulate the pressure receptors in the hypothalamus, result in the secretion of ADH by the posterior pituitary. The presence of ADH in the blood promotes increased water reabsorption from the distal convoluted tubules of the kidney, thereby limiting the volume of water lost in the urine. The return to normal osmolality is further assisted by the hypothalamic structures, since stimulation of the hypothalamus by a state of increased osmolality brings with it a feeling of thirst.

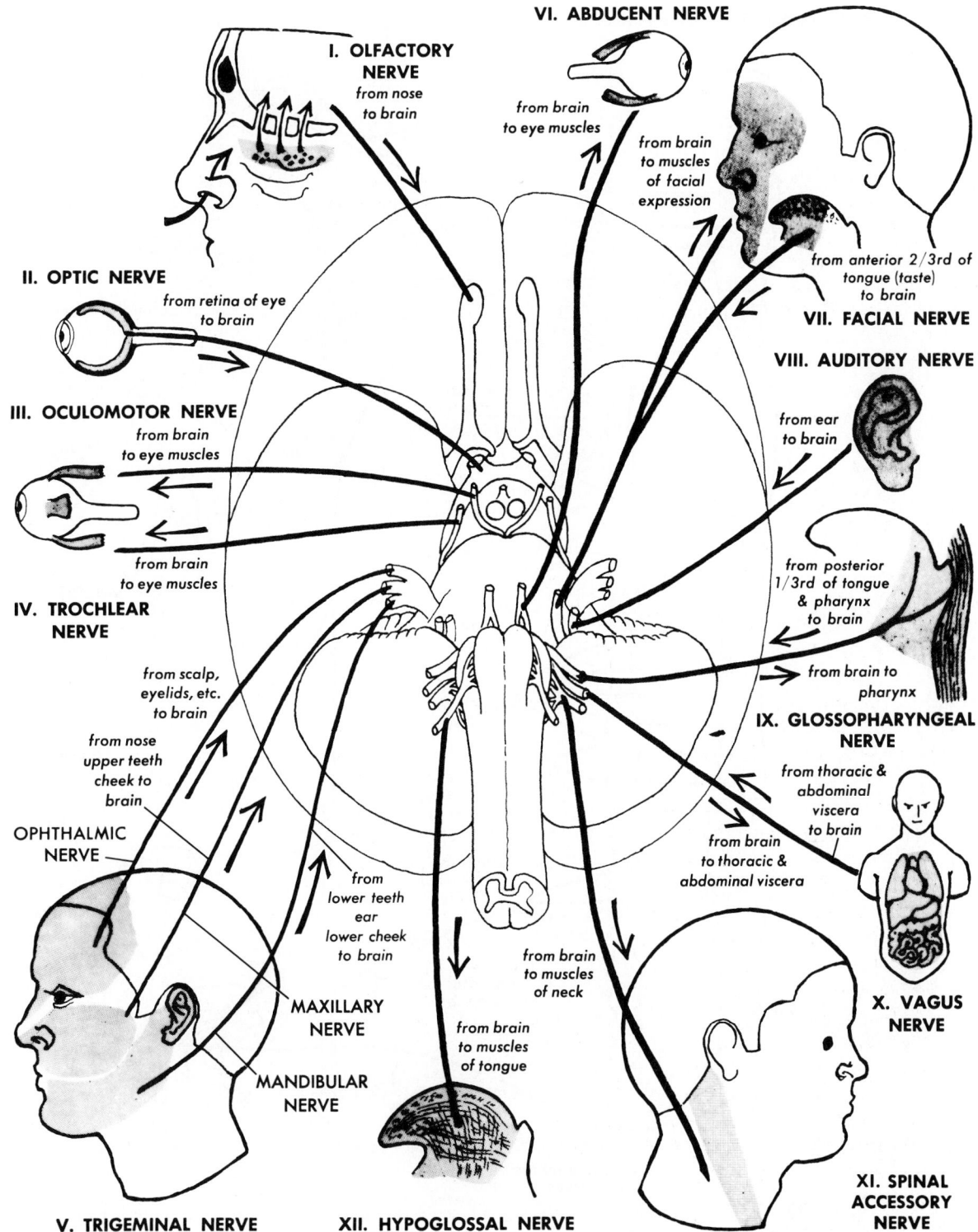

Figure 33-9 The cranial nerves. Cranial nerves I–VII and XI serve somatic motor and sensory functions. Cranial nerves IX, X, and XII provide motor and sensory input to a variety of integrated regulatory functions. *(From E. J. Reith, B. Breidenbach, and M. Lorenc, Textbook of Anatomy and Physiology, 2d ed., McGraw-Hill, New York, 1978.)*

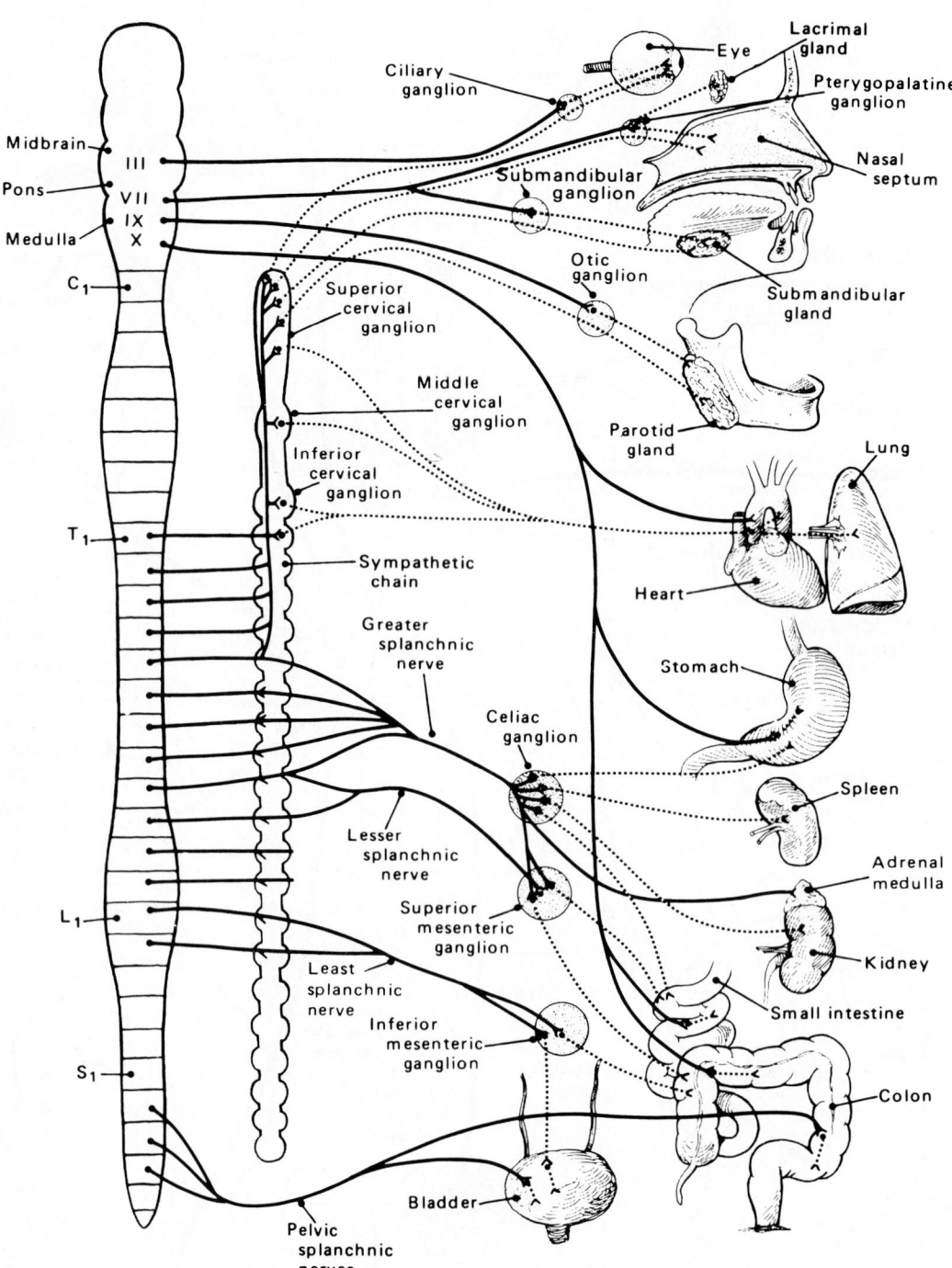

Figure 33-10 The autonomic nervous system, schematic drawing. Only one of the two sympathetic chain ganglia is shown. *(From L. L. Langley, I. R. Telford, and J. B. Christensen, Dynamic Anatomy and Physiology, 5th ed., McGraw-Hill, New York, 1980.)*

Breathing

Breathing is under the voluntary control of the abdominal and thoracic muscles via the motor cortex, with cerebellar influence on coordination of breathing. Reflex control occurs in the pons and medulla in response to changes in the pH of blood and tissues. Spinal reflexes include innervation of the phrenic nerve to the diaphragm at spinal cord levels C3 to C5 and innervation to the intercostal muscles at levels T1 through T11. The rate and rhythm of automatic breathing is regulated in the cerebral hemispheres.

Circulation

The ability to regulate heart rate and blood pressure voluntarily through biofeedback suggests that a mechanism exists for higher control of circulatory functions; however, the anatomical site for such control is unknown. Homeostatic control of blood pressure and heart rate is regulated via centers in the pons and medulla. Hypothalamus and brainstem nuclei act to regulate sympathetic and parasympathetic cardiovascular responses to a variety of stimuli. The anterior hypothalamus and parasympathetic nuclei in the brainstem act to decrease heart rate, decrease cardiac output, decrease AV bundle conduction, and perhaps constrict coronary arteries. Cranial nerve X (vagus) is the primary efferent for hypothalamic mediation of parasympathetic response.

Posterior hypothalamic nuclei, with efferents to the reticular core and to the sympathetic spinal ganglia, form the pathway for sympathetic control of circulation. Norepinephrine is the postganglionic neurotransmitter for the sympathetic system and functions to increase peripheral resistance, increase the rate and force of cardiac contraction, and increase myocardial blood flow.

Temperature Control

Thermoregulation can be cortically controlled via conscious decisions to seek warmer or cooler environments. Both the sensory and motor cortex, as well as whole brain decision processes, are involved in such control. Cerebral reflex control is centered in the hypothalamus, which is thought to function as a thermostat. Heat-losing mechanisms are regulated by the anterior hypothalamic nuclei, which stimulate parasympathetic activities such as sweating, panting, and vasodilatation. Heat production mechanisms are controlled by the posterior hypothalamus and lead to vasoconstriction, shivering, and increased metabolism.

The spinal reflexes control the autonomic functions necessary to implement hypothalamically signaled activities such as reflex constriction or dilatation of skin vessels, piloerection (gooseflesh), and increased respiration.

Ingestion/Digestion

The act of chewing and swallowing is a movement function, as discussed earlier. However, the movement of food through the alimentary tract and its digestion is a more automatic and regulatory function. This function is mostly reflex, mediated by the cranial nerves involved in chewing and swallowing and the autonomic systems of the gut. These cranial nerves include V (chewing, sensation to the inside of the mouth), VII (salivation, lip movement, taste), IX (sensation to the pharynx, upward movement of the pharynx, salivation, taste, gag reflex), X (swallowing, glottis closure, peristalsis, digestive stimulation), and XII (tongue movement). The vagus (cranial nerve X) is parasympathetic to the digestive tract and facilitates normal movement of food through the gut. The splanchnic nerves arise from the thoracic ganglia and serve as sympathetic innervation to the gut. These fibers intermingle with the parasympathetic divisions of the vagus in the autonomic plexus in the abdomen.

Elimination

Bowel and bladder evacuation are presumed to have similar anatomical correlates, although the innervation of the bowel has not been as clearly identified, particularly in terms of cerebral level controls. Cortical control of bladder evacuation is found in the medial portions of the motor and sensory cortex, as shown in Fig. 33-4. The sensory areas serve perception of the fullness of the bladder, and the motor areas allow voluntary initiation and inhibition of voiding (*micturition*). Fibers from these areas synapse with inhibitory neurons in the pons and serve to inhibit the detrusor muscle of the bladder, thus inhibiting reflex emptying of the bladder. Motor pathways from the midbrain-pontine micturition centers synapse in the interomedial gray area and the anterior horn cells of the sacral spinal cord (levels S2 through S4) and connect higher level voluntary and reflex control with spinal reflex control. Sensory input to the reflex arc at the sacral cord comes from the sensory stretch receptors in the bladder via the dorsal root of the spinal cord. The end organ is the urinary bladder, which has three muscles innervated by this system: the detrusor, the trigone, and the striated muscle of the urethra. The trigone is a triangular muscle that is continuous with the ureters. It is surrounded by the detrusor, a smooth muscle. When the detrusor contracts, it pulls away from the trigone and urine passively flows from the bladder into the urethra. Relaxation of the detrusor allows the muscle to come back together and close off the urethra. The striated muscle in the urethra serves to allow passage out of (but not into) the urethra. Parasympathetic motor output to the bladder is carried via the pelvic nerve to the detrusor muscle, sympathetic output via the inferior mesenteric ganglion to the detrusor, and voluntary motor output via the pudendal nerve to the urethra. (See Fig. 33-11.)

Lesions that interrupt this circuit in the cerebral cortex and midbrain/pons area create an uninhibited neurogenic bladder. The functional outcome is a sense of urgency and inability to postpone voiding. Lesions in the cord itself may create a reflex bladder, in which there is no sensation of fullness or voluntary control but the bladder remains able to empty reflexly when full. Lesions of the sacral cord or of the peripheral nerves serving the bladder may interrupt the reflex emptying mechanism.

The regulatory system for bowel evacuation is presumed to be similar to that for bladder evacuation with respect to cortical and midbrain/ pontine levels of voluntary and inhibitory control of the anal reflex. The internal and external anal sphincter reflexes are mediated at the spinal cord at the S2 through S4 levels. The anal sphincter is striated muscle and is served by the pudendal nerve, which is innervated from cord levels S1 through S4. The lower bowel is supplied by parasympathetic fibers from the pelvic plexus. Socially uninhibited bowel emptying can be seen in degenerative brain disorders. Reflex emptying of the bowel can be achieved in patients with spinal cord lesions above the level of the sacral reflex arcs. Lesions of the sacral cord or of the peripheral nerves serving the bowel reflex can produce a

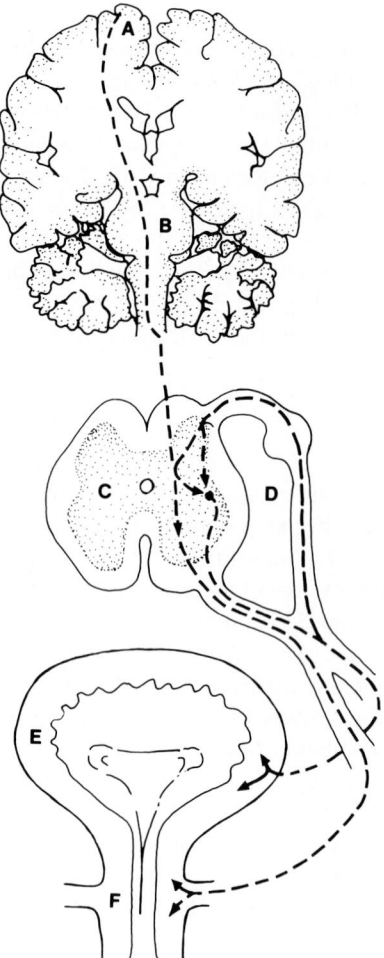

Figure 33-11 Integrated regulation of bladder: evacuation at four levels of the neuraxis. The medial frontal cortex (A) appreciates the sensation of a full bladder and works together with the pontine inhibitory center (B) to inhibit reflex bladder contractions. Spinal cord reflexes occur in the sacral cord (C), receiving sensory input from autonomic peripheral nerves (D) and sending motor signals to smooth muscle in the bladder (E) and striated muscle in the urethra (F). *(From Mitchell, Cammermyer, Ozuna, & Woods.*[1]*)*

flaccid anal sphincter and decreased colon peristalsis, with resulting constipation and overflow diarrhea.

Sexual Response

Human sexual response encompasses more than the physical act of intercourse. It consists of three phases: desire, excitement, and orgasm.[2] The desire phase is essentially a cognitive/affective response thought to be mediated by the limbic system and the preoptic nuclei of the hypothalamus. This phase can be lost in damage to the brain; conversely, it can remain as a source of sexual pleasure when spinal cord damage disconnects the physical sensations from the fantasy or cerebral aspects of sexuality.

The excitement phase is mediated by reflex vasodilatation of genital blood vessels. Arteriolar dilatation is mediated by spinal cord levels T11 through L2 and S2 to 4. The vasocongestion is primarily parasympathetic. Penile and clitoral erection and vaginal lubrication are the physical indicators of this response. The thoracolumbar area is believed to be more responsive to input from the limbic system and cortex, while the sacral centers are stimulated by tactile input to the genitals. Thus, reflex erection can be stimulated even when the higher regulatory centers are functionally disconnected by spinal cord injury, for example.

The phase of orgasm is mediated by the pudendal sensory fibers for input to the cord and motor output from the T11 through L2 levels.

Emotional Response

Emotional experience is not only a psychological state but has motor and autonomic components as well. We feel with our "guts" as much as with our minds. The limbic system (Fig. 33-4) is considered to be the major neuroanatomical correlate of emotion. The major tracts connecting portions of the limbic cortex converge on the hypothalamus, serving to activate various effector systems that serve the visceral and motor component of emotion. Stimulation of the anterior hypothalamus not only activates the parasympathetic nervous system but also reduces movement and metabolism. Depression of affect is accompanied by a whole constellation of effects involving conservation of energy and withdrawal from activity. Conversely, stimulation of the posterior hypothalamus produces energy-using defensive patterns. The affect may be anger or aggression, with much motor activity, and sympathetic visceral responses. Ordinarily there is automatic balance between activation and conservation, but it is speculated that many of the affective disorders result from a loss of the ability of the limbic system to maintain affective balance. Disorders that directly damage the limbic system or its

connections with the neocortex and hypothalamus may be expected to alter emotional control and experience.

Functional Anatomy Related to the Neuraxis

The usual approach to neuroanatomy is to describe the functions of various divisions of the nervous system. It is useful to be able to overlap both approaches described in this chapter: to know the anatomical correlates of a given human function and to know the function or level of a function mediated by each of the major axes of the nervous system.

The nervous system can be divided into four axes, which correspond to the major functional divisions shown in Fig. 33-1. To recapitulate, these are:

Axis I:–Cerebral hemispheres, including the diencephalon

Axis II:–Brainstem and cerebellum

Axis III:–Spinal cord

Axis IV:–Peripheral nerves and end innervated organs

Axis I: Cerebral Hemispheres

The cerebral hemispheres, also called the *encephalon,* are the most recent evolutionary development of the nervous system. They are the last part of the nervous system formed by the embryo and continue to develop after birth. Their major functions are to perceive and interpret incoming sensory stimuli and to initiate voluntary activity in response to such stimuli. They are also critical to the cognitive functions that allow us to learn, to plan, and to create. The cerebral hemispheres serve the most complex and highest level of information processing in the nervous system. The self-awareness component of consciousness is mediated only in the cerebral hemispheres, as is mentation. Initiation and voluntary control of movement and of integrated regulatory functions occur here, as do conscious awareness and interpretation of sensation and emotion.

For purposes of this discussion, axis I is considered to consist of the hemispheres themselves, the basal ganglia, and the diencephalon. Some authorities place the diencephalon within the hemisphere axis, and some group it with the brainstem. Because its structures contribute to complex perception and integration, it is placed in axis I in this discussion.

The cerebral hemispheres consist of the medial and lateral cerebral cortex and the connecting association fibers, as described earlier in this chapter. The limbic cortex and its connections with the neocortex, thalamus, and hypothalamus are considered part of the cerebral cortex. The limbic cortex is often called *paleocortex* ("old" cortex) in recognition of the earlier embryological development of this medial cortex and its persistence in more "primitive" levels of mammalian phylogenetic development. The term *neocortex* ("new" cortex) refers to those collections of cell bodies on the convexities or lateral surfaces of the brain. The neocortex develops somewhat later in the embryo than the limbic cortex.

The term *diencephalon* ("between brain") refers to the thalamus, hypothalamus, subthalamus, and epithalamus. These structures are collections of cell bodies through which all sensory, motor, and integrative regulatory information passes between neocortex and brainstem/spinal cord. Together, these structures serve as key relay points in perceiving and processing information before it is interpreted by higher cortical centers. The thalamus is located on either side of the third ventricle. The hypothalamus is a collection of paired nuclei (cell bodies) surrounding the inferior third ventricle and extending from the level of the optic chiasm to the midbrain.

The *basal ganglia* are paired subcortical gray structures which are located adjacent to the internal capsule (Fig. 33-12). The structures which make up the basal ganglia are the caudate nucleus, the putamen, the globus pallidus, and the amygdala. These structures, along with important connections to the substantia nigra in the brainstem and the cerebellum, are critical in the initiation and maintenance of coordinated automatic movements.

Axis II: Brainstem and Cerebellum

The brainstem consists of the midbrain, the pons, and the medulla oblongata. The midbrain is composed of fibers which connect the diencephalon with the lower brainstem and cerebellum. The substantia nigra and the red nucleus are located in the midbrain. The nuclei of cranial nerves III (oculomotor) and IV (trochlear) are located in the midbrain. The midbrain is located in the tentorial notch.

The pons lies in the front of the cerebellum. Fibers which connect to the underlying spinal cord pathways pass through the pons. The nuclei of cranial nerves V (trigeminal), VI (abducens), VII

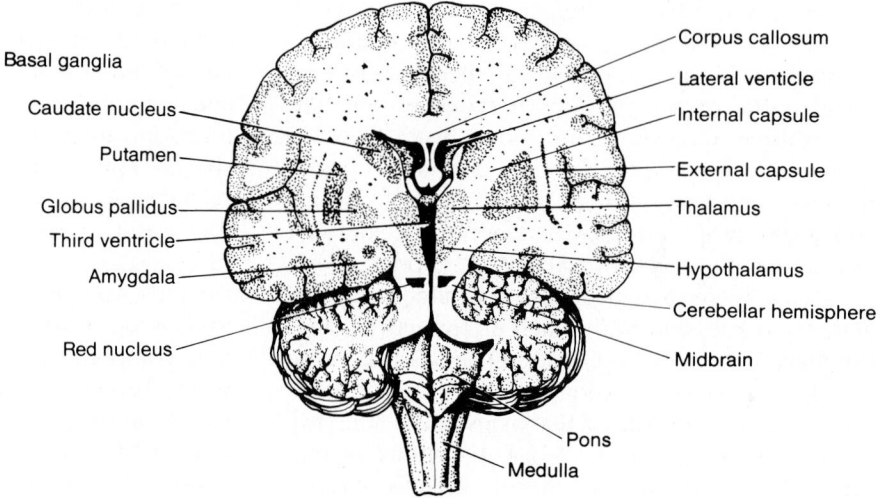

Figure 33-12   Coronal section of the cerebrum with basal ganglia, cerebellum, and posterior view of brainstem.

Basal ganglia
Caudate nucleus
Putamen
Globus pallidus
Third ventricle
Amygdala
Red nucleus

Corpus callosum
Lateral venticle
Internal capsule
External capsule
Thalamus
Hypothalamus
Cerebellar hemisphere
Midbrain
Pons
Medulla

(facial), and VIII (acoustic) are located in the pontine area.

The medulla oblongata is a pyramid-shaped structure which connects the pons with the spinal cord at the level of the foramen magnum. Tracts which connect the cerebral cortical areas with the spinal pathways cross in the medulla. The nuclei of cranial nerves IX (glossopharyngeal), X (vagus), XI (spinal accessory), and XII (hypoglossal) are located in the medulla.

The cerebellum consists of a midline portion, the *vermis,* and two lobes or hemispheres. Each cerebellar hemisphere contains an outer cortex of gray matter, a core of white fibers, and central nuclei. It is located directly below the occipital lobes and is covered by the tentorium.

The reticular formation is located in the central core of the brainstem, ascending from the medulla to the midbrain, with projections to the diencephalon and neocortex. All sensory input to the brainstem is relayed through the reticular formation, and the cell bodies for the monoamine neurotransmitters are located in the formation.

The functions served by axis II are maintenance of arousal and normal sleep-wake cycles, reflex level coordination, and integration of motor and sensory information. The cranial nerve nuclei in the midbrain, pons, and medulla serve the reflexes involved in the functions of moving the eyes, chewing, swallowing, and making sounds. Inhibitory and excitatory nuclei in the pons and medulla are part of the systems regulating breathing, circulation, and elimination. Parasympathetic output to the head, neck, and thorax is mediated from the brainstem nuclei. Finally, the coordination of voluntary movement is mediated by the cerebellum, whose only connection to the cerebral hemispheres is via the brainstem.

The brainstem is the passageway between the spinal cord and the cerebral hemispheres, and it is a relatively small structure. Therefore, the fibers relaying sensory and motor information, the primary cranial nerve, and the regulatory nuclei are closely packed together. Consequently, relatively small lesions in the brainstem can disrupt multiple functions: arousal, movement, sensation, and inhibitory control of regulatory functions. Lesions of the cerebellum affect coordination not only of movement but also of autonomic motor output. Further,

because of the proximity of the cerebellum to the vital regulatory centers in the pons, expanding lesions of the cerebellum may threaten breathing and circulation by compression of the pons.

Axis III: Spinal Cord

The spinal cord is a cylindrical structure which joins the brainstem at the level of the foramen magnum and ends at the L1–L2 vertebral level. It is called the *conus medullaris* at this distal end. The upper cervical cord segments correspond to the same vertebral level, whereas cord segments from C8 and below correspond to the vertebral level above each segment. For example, the C3 cord segment lies opposite vertebra C3, but the T1 cord segment lies above vertebra T1 (Fig. 33-13).

The spinal cord consists of central gray horns which form an H shape (Fig. 33-14). The gray matter is surrounded by columns of white matter which are fiber tracts. The size and shape of the spinal cord, the relative proportion of gray and white matter, and the configuration of the gray matter vary according to the segmental level. The cervical cord is the largest in diameter. The cervical and lumbar segments contain a greater proportion of gray than of white matter because of the larger number of neurons used to control the upper and lower extremities. The spinal cord is divided into left and right halves by a posterior sulcus and an anterior fissure. The halves are connected by commissures of gray and white matter.

The anterior, or *ventral,* horn contains the cell bodies of anterior (motor) nerve roots. The posterior, or *dorsal,* horn, contains cells on which posterior (sensory) nerve roots terminate. The lateral horn of gray matter in the thoracolumbar area contains cells which give rise to the sympathetic fibers of the autonomic nervous system. Interomedial gray matter in the cord, segments S2 through S4, give rise to parasympathetic fibers.

The white matter is subdivided into groups of tracts which ascend and descend the spinal cord. The major tracts are located posteriorly and anteriorly. The posterior tracts (*dorsal columns*) and the anterior and lateral spinothalamic tracts conduct sensory impulses upward to the thalamus and the cerebral cortex. The lateral (corticospinal, pyrami-

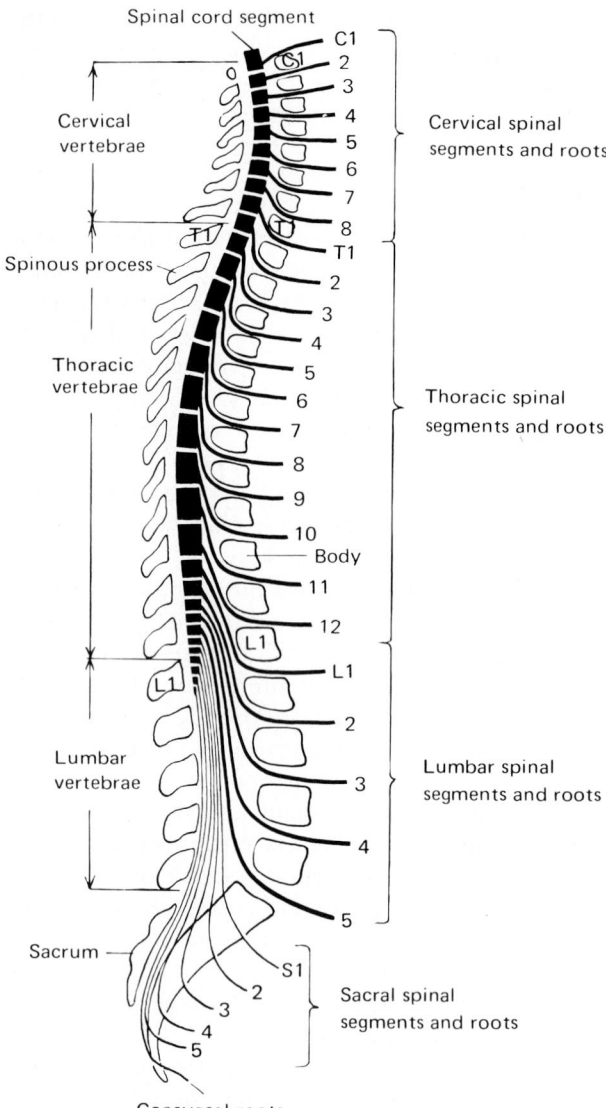

Figure 33-13   The relation of the spinal cord segments and spinal nerves to the vertebral column. *(From C. R. Noback and R. J. Demarest, The Human Nervous System, 2d ed., McGraw-Hill, New York, 1979.)*

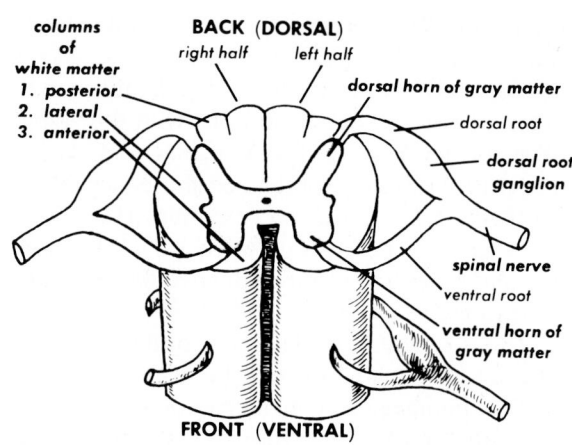

Figure 33-14   A segment of the thoracic spinal cord seen in cross section. Neurons serving the autonomic ganglia and nerves are located in the gray matter between the dorsal and ventral horns. *(From E. J. Reith, B. Breidenbach, and M. Lorenc, Textbook of Anatomy and Physiology, 2d ed., McGraw-Hill, New York, 1978.)*

dal) tracts conduct motor impulses to the anterior horn cells.

Thus, it is clear that the functions of the spinal cord are to transmit motor and sensory information between the brain and the muscles and internal organs. The major functional outcome of damage to the spinal cord is to interrupt this flow of information. Information to and from the muscle

or end organ at a given level of the spinal cord will not be impeded by damage to the cord *above* that level. In other words, the spinal reflex arc will be intact and the local reflex will be unimpaired. However, inhibitory control from the higher axes (brainstem and hemispheres) will not be received, nor can sensory information from the local level reach the cerebral hemispheres. The functional outcome of such a situation is uninhibited motor and autonomic reflexes in response to local sensory stimuli. Spasticity and autonomic dysreflexia are examples of such outcomes in the case of spinal cord injury.

Axis IV: Peripheral Nerves and End Organs

The functional unit in axis IV is the end organ (viscera, sensory receptor, or muscle), the sensory neuron and peripheral nerve transmitting information to the spinal cord and the motor neuron and motor peripheral nerve transmitting information to the end organ. Interruption at any of the three components of the functional unit will disrupt the reflex arc and disrupt the function at the level of the end organ. Like the spinal cord axis, the primary functions served are movement, sensation, and integrated regulation, but the functional outcome is loss of not only the observable or felt function but also the spinal reflex component. For example, peripheral motor neuropathy, like spinal cord injury, may result in inability to walk. However, in peripheral neuropathy, the paralysis is flaccid (disruption of the reflex), whereas in spinal cord injury the paralysis is spastic because of uninhibited reflexes. The person with spastic paralysis may be able to use the spasticity for stability during transfer to a wheelchair, whereas the person with flaccid paralysis will need to adopt a method of transfer that does not utilize weight bearing by the feet.

The peripheral nerves comprise the cranial nerves (peripheral from the brainstem), the somatic nerves (from the spinal cord), and the autonomic ganglia and postganglionic fibers.

Cranial Nerves

The cranial nerves are considered part of the peripheral nervous system. There are 12 pairs of cranial nerves (Fig. 33-9). Cranial nerves I (olfactory) and II (optic) are not typical of the remaining cranial nerves. Cranial nerves I and II extend to become tracts which connect with various structures within the cerebral hemispheres. Cranial nerves III through XII originate from the nuclei which are located either superficially or deep within the brainstem structures.

Cranial nerve I arises from the olfactory bulb and extends under the frontal lobes to penetrate the frontal and temporal lobes, where it becomes part of the limbic system.

Cranial nerve II arises from the inner retinal layer of the eye and extends posteriorly to enter the intracranial cavity. The optic nerves join at the optic chiasm, which lies above the pituitary gland. The optic tracts and radiations then extend posteriorly to areas of the occipital lobe.

Cranial nerves III (oculomotor), IV (trochlear), V (trigeminal), VI (abducens), VII (facial), VIII (acoustic), IX (glossopharyngeal), X (vagus), and XII (hypoglossal) extend peripherally to the eye muscles, face, ear, and pharynx. Cranial nerve X extends down the neck into the thorax and the abdomen. Cranial nerve XI (spinal accessory) extends to the pharynx, larynx, and muscles of the neck and shoulders (Table 33-2). Parasympathetic fibers of the autonomic nervous system extend peripherally with the oculomotor, facial, glossopharyngeal, and vagus cranial nerves.

Somatic Peripheral Nerves

Distributed along the spinal cord are 31 pairs of spinal nerves: 8 cervical, 12 thoracic, 5 lumbar, 5 sacral, and 1 coccygeal. Each segment of the spinal cord has posterior (dorsal) nerve roots with ganglia and anterior (ventral) nerve roots (Fig. 33-14), which exit the vertebrae through the intervertebral foramina and join to form the spinal nerves. The large bundle of lumbosacral nerve roots which descend from the end of the cord are referred to as the *cauda equina*. The cervical nerves exit at the corresponding vertebral level. All other spinal nerves exit one or two vertebral levels below the vertebra having the same number. The spinal nerves join peripherally to form plexuses. The cervical and brachial plexuses supply the upper extremities; the lumbar and sacral plexuses supply the lower extremities. The plexuses divide to form the various peripheral nerves. The peripheral nerves frequently have motor and sensory fibers intermingled.

Autonomic Nervous System

The autonomic nervous system receives higher level control from the hypothalamus and descending pathways within the brainstem and spinal cord. A series of ganglia and small nerve fibers constitute the peripheral portion of the system. The hypothalamus receives axons from the anterior and inferior portions of the frontal lobes. Fibers leave the hypothalamus and descend to groups of cells in the brainstem and spinal cord. The autonomic fibers are distributed with the cranial and spinal peripheral nerves to the visceral organs (Figs. 33-9 and 33-10).

The autonomic nervous system consists of the parasympathetic and sympathetic divisions. Each division differs anatomically, functionally, and pharmacologically. The peripheral autonomic fibers which originate in the cranial and sacral areas make up the parasympathetic division. Peripheral sympathetic fibers originate in the thoracic and lumbar areas (Fig. 33-10). Each visceral organ controlled by the autonomic nervous system has both parasympathetic and sympathetic innervation.

All autonomic fibers extend to synapses in ganglia after leaving their points of origin in the

Table 33-2 Summary of Cranial Nerve Functions

Number and Name	Brainstem Level	Type	Major Functions
I Olfactory	None	Sensory	Smells
II Optic	None	Sensory	Sees (central and peripheral vision)
III Oculomotor	Midbrain	Motor	Moves eyes, elevates upper eyelid
		Parasympathetic	Constricts pupil
IV Trochlear	Midbrain	Motor	Moves eyes downward and inward
V Trigeminal	Pons to cervical cord	Sensory	Feels: touch, pain, temperature Jaw and eye muscle proprioception
		Motor	Masticates
VI Abducens	Pons	Motor	Abducts the eyes
VII Facial	Pons	Motor	Closes eyelids, muscles of facial expression
		Parasympathetic	Secretes: glands of mouth and eyes
		Sensory	Tastes (anterior two-thirds of tongue)
VIII Acoustic	Pons and medulla	Sensory	
Vestibular branch			Equilibrates
Cochlear branch			Hears
IX Glossopharyngeal	Medulla	Motor Parasympathetic Sensory	Moves pharyngeal muscles Secretes saliva: parotid glands Feels: pharyngeal and posterior tongue
X Vagus	Medulla	Motor Parasympathetic Sensory	Moves pharynx and larynx Visceral activities Pharyngeal and laryngeal sensation, taste
XI Spinal accessory	Medulla	Motor	Moves: pharynx, sternocleidomastoid, and trapezius
XII Hypoglossal	Medulla	Motor	Moves tongue

central nervous system. The sympathetic preganglionic fibers extend to a chain of paired ganglia which are located along the vertebral column. The presynaptic fiber tends to be short. The postsynaptic fiber must travel the remaining distance to the organ it innervates, and it tends to be long. Sympathetic fibers are distributed to the head, neck, thorax, abdomen, and pelvic areas in conjunction with thoracolumbar spinal nerves.

Parasympathetic fibers extend to ganglia located adjacent to the organs they innervate. Thus the presynaptic fibers are long and the postsynaptic fibers short. Parasympathetic fibers are not as widely distributed as the sympathetic fibers.

The adrenal medulla, unlike other viscera, is innervated directly by presynaptic fibers. The cells of the adrenal medulla are derived from nerve tissue and constitute a modified sympathetic ganglion.

Supportive and Protective Structures of the Central Nervous System

The structures which encase, support, and protect the delicate, semisolid nervous system include the bones of the skull, the vertebral column, and the three meningeal layers.

Skull

The roof of the cranial cavity, or *calvaria,* covers the superior aspects of the brain. The calvaria consists of the frontal, the occipital, and the paired parietal and temporal bones, which are fused at suture lines. The floor of the cranial cavity consists of a group of bony structures which have many ridges and grooves (Fig. 33-15). The floor conforms to the shape of the base of the brain and is divided into three compartments: the anterior, the middle, and the posterior fossae. The anterior fossa contains the frontal lobes. The middle fossa contains parts of the temporal lobes, the upper brainstem, and the pituitary gland. The posterior fossa contains the brainstem and the cerebellar hemispheres. A number of small openings, or *foramina,* are located in the base of the skull to permit paired blood vessels and cranial nerves to enter and leave the intracranial cavity. There is also a large opening, the *foramen magnum,* where the brainstem connects to the upper cervical spinal cord.

The bones which form the cranial cavity are composed of three layers: the outer solid layer (outer table), the middle spongy layer (diploe), and the inner solid layer (inner table). The construction of the skull provides for great strength with econ-omy of weight and insulation. The thickest parts of the skull are the midfrontal and midoccipital bones; the thinnest parts are the temporal bones. The inner table, which lies over the convexity of the brain, is very smooth and contains grooves in which the branches of the middle meningeal arteries are located. The viability of the skull is maintained by thin layers of periosteum which are attached to the inner and outer tables.

Vertebral Column

The vertebral column consists of 7 cervical, 12 thoracic, 5 lumbar, 5 sacral, and 4 fused coccygeal vertebrae (Fig. 33-16). The vertebrae are joined together by multiple ligaments and intervening disks which provide flexibility and stability. The vertebral column supports the skull, forms a spinal canal which surrounds the spinal cord, and provides protection for the spinal cord, spinal nerves, and underlying structures. The spinal canal extends for the length of the vertebral column and conforms

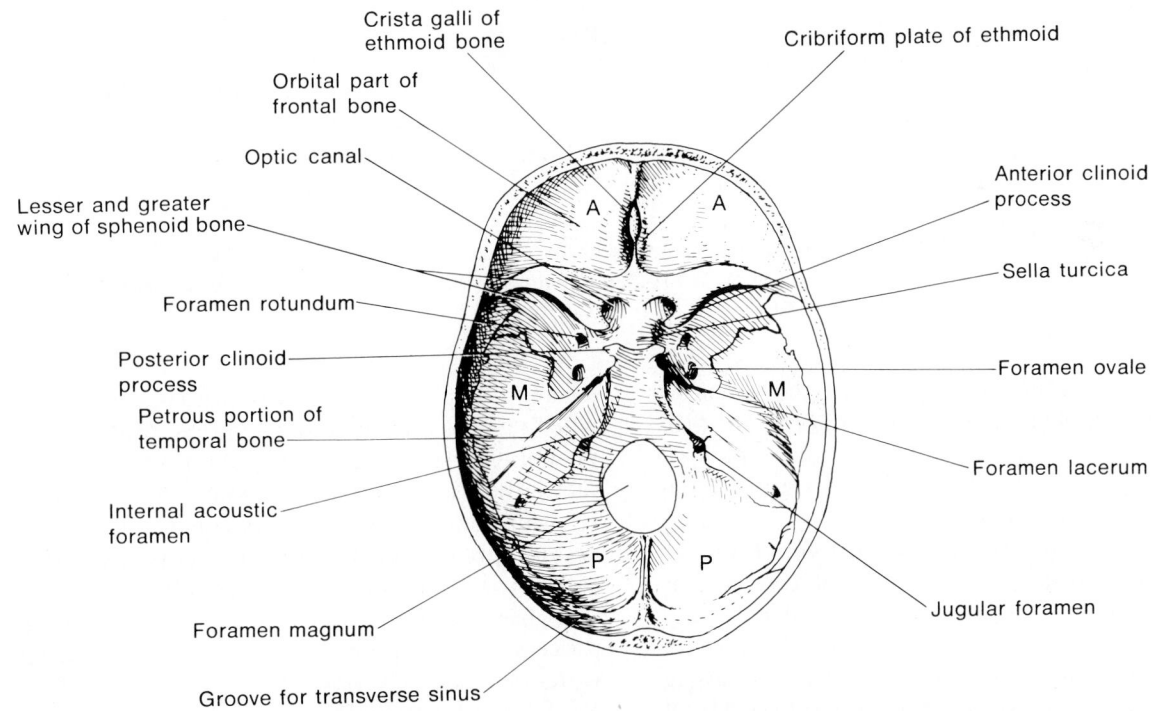

A = ANTERIOR CRANIAL FOSSA   M = MIDDLE CRANIAL FOSSA   P = POSTERIOR CRANIAL FOSSA

Figure 33-15   The bones that form the floor of the cranial cavity. *(From L. Elson, It's Your Body, McGraw-Hill, New York, 1975.)*

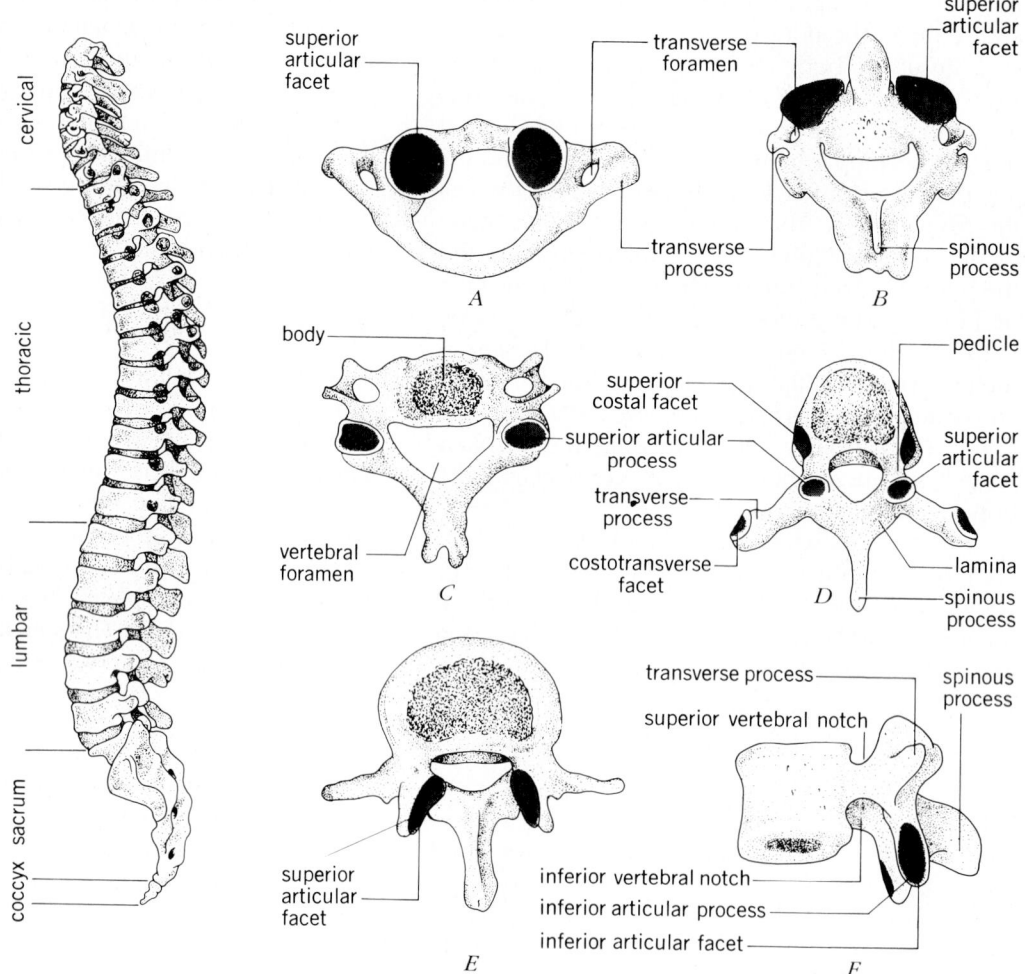

Figure 33-16   The vertebral column, with individual vertebrae: (*A*) atlas; (*B*) axis; (*C*) C4, (*D*) T6, (*E*) L3, superior view; (*F*) L3, lateral view. *(From R. M. DeCoursey, The Human Organism, 4th ed., McGraw-Hill, New York, 1974.)*

to the various spinal curvatures and to the variations in size of the spinal cord. The vertebrae are progressively larger down to the sacrum and then become smaller. The diameter of the spinal canal is greatest in the cervical region.

The first and second cervical vertebrae are highly specialized. The first cervical vertebra, or *atlas,* is joined to the base of the skull. The second cervical vertebra, or *axis,* forms a pivot around which the atlas rotates the skull. The remaining cervical, thoracic, and lumbar vertebrae have typical characteristics. Each vertebra consists of a body, a vertebral arch, and several processes for muscular and articular attachments. The vertebral body is

located anteriorly and consists of a spongy bone which gives strength and supports weight. The vertebral arch lies posterior to the body and completes the formation of the spinal canal. The arch is composed of pedicles and lamina. A spinous process projects posteriorly, and transverse processes project laterally from the vertebral arch.

Each vertebral arch has several articulating processes which permit motion between adjacent vertebrae. The vertebral notches in each pedicle form an intervertebral foramen which permits passage of the spinal nerves and associated blood vessels. Each of the transverse processes of the cervical vertebrae have foramen which form a passageway for the vertebral arteries, veins, and sympathetic nerves.

An intervertebral disk, which acts as a cushion, separates the adjacent vertebral bodies. The disk is composed of a central cartilaginous core, the *nucleus pulposus,* which is surrounded by a fibrous capsule, the *anulus fibrosus.* A series of strong, fibrous, overlapping ligaments connect the vertebrae with each other and with the cranium. The ligaments allow safe smooth movement of the head, protection from trauma, and stability and motion at the articulating processes. Additional support of the thoracic vertebrae is provided by the rib attachments.

Meninges

The brain and spinal cord are protected, supported, and surrounded by three layers of meninges (Fig. 33-17). The outer layer, or *dura mater,* consists of thick, tough connective tissue. The cranial dura forms an envelope which lines the inside and is firmly attached to the skull, serving as a periosteum. Folds of dura divide the intracranial cavity into four compartments. The horizontal dural fold which forms the roof over the posterior fossa is known as the *tentorium.* The occipital and posterior temporal lobes are located directly above the tentorium. The cerebellar hemispheres are located under the tentorium in the *infratentorial compartment.* The dural fold which separates the cerebellar hemispheres is called the *falx cerebelli.* The supratentorial compartment is divided by a midline dural fold, the *falx cerebri,* which separates the cerebral hemispheres. The cranial dural layers separate to form large venous sinuses at the junction of the dural folds.

The spinal dura is a continuation of the cranial dura. The dura surrounds the spinal cord from the foramen magnum to the level of the second sacral vertebra, where it terminates as the dural sac. The spinal dura is not attached to the vertebrae. Extensions of the dura surround the spinal nerve roots, forming dural root sleeves.

The *pia mater* is the inner vascular membrane which adheres to the surface of the brain and spinal cord. Folds of pia form part of the choroid plexus, support the superficial blood vessels which penetrate the central nervous system, and provide support for the spinal cord. Tissue bands, the *dentate*

ligaments, which attach the spinal cord to the dura, are formed by the pia. At the end of the cord, the pia forms the *filum terminale,* which merges with the dura and is attaches to the coccyx.

The *arachnoid* is the delicate, spiderweb-like membrane between the dural and pial layers. The arachnoid surrounds the surface of the brain without following its contour, surrounds the spinal cord, and extends along the roots of the cranial and spinal nerves. The combined pial and arachnoid membranes are referred to as the *leptomeninges.*

There is a potential space between the dura and the arachnoid, the *subdural space.* Vessels cross this area with little support. The space between the arachnoid and the pia mater, the *subarachnoid space,* is filled with cerebrospinal fluid. The depth of the subarachnoid space varies. The space is narrow over the convexity of the cerebral hemispheres. At the base of the brain and around the brainstem the space widens to form large cisterns. The largest cistern, the *cisterna magna,* is located between the medulla and the inferior surface of the cerebellum. A lumbar cistern located at the end of the spinal cord contains sacral nerve roots.

Tiny projections of meninges, *arachnoid granulations,* protrude into the large venous sinuses formed by the dural layers such as the *superior sagittal sinus* (Fig. 33-17). The cerebrospinal fluid which is contained in the subarachnoid space is transferred into the venous sinuses as a result of hydrostatic pressure. The arachnoid granulations are permeable and permit one-way flow of cerebrospinal fluid, plasma proteins, and serum albumin into the venous blood.

Nutritive and Metabolic Support of the Central Nervous System

The nutritional and metabolic needs of the central nervous system are met by the cerebrospinal fluid and the ventricular and circulatory systems.

Ventricular System

The ventricular system is located within the brain substance. It consists of four communicating compartments: two lateral ventricles and a third and a fourth ventricle (Fig. 33-18). Each of the lateral ventricles is a cavity within the cerebral

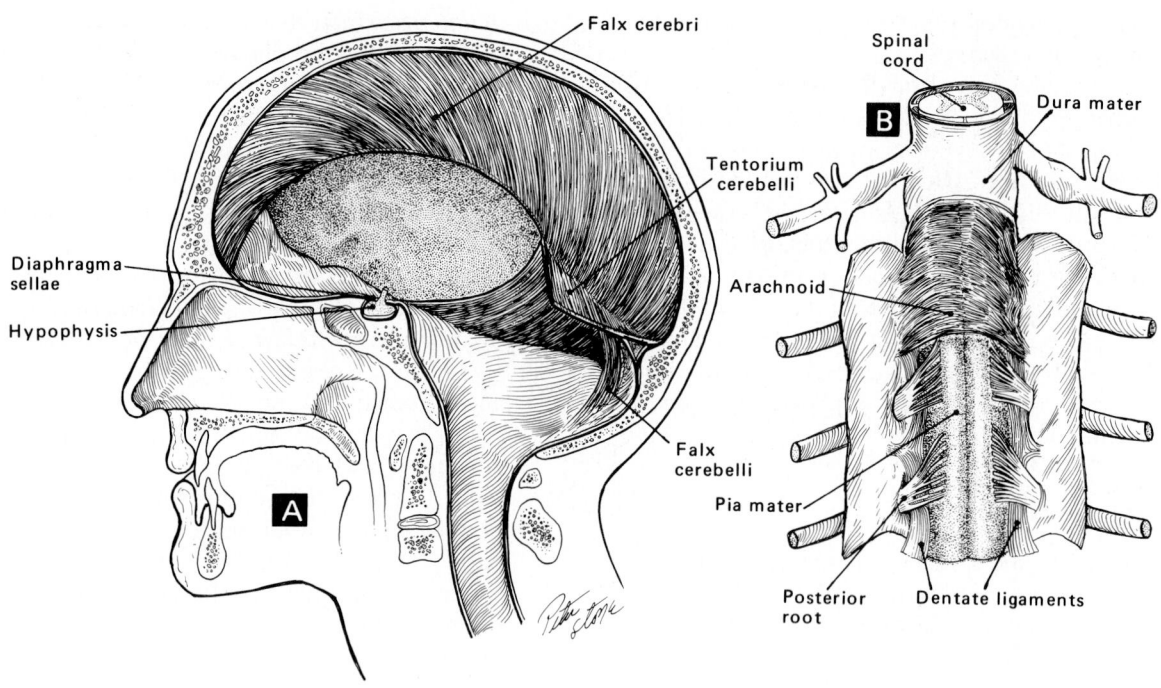

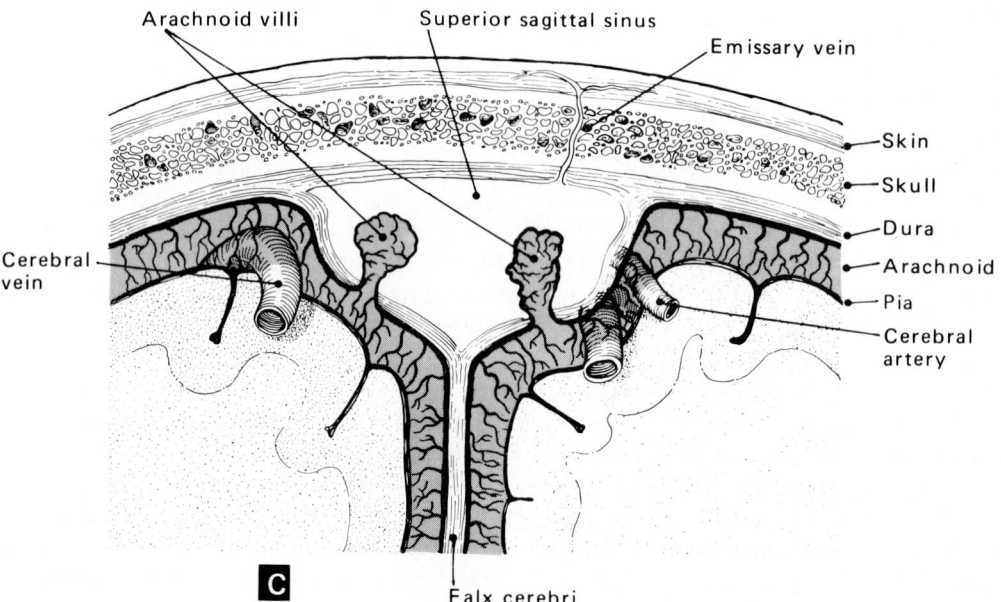

Figure 33-17   The meninges: (*A*) Extensions of the dura mater in the cranial cavity, sagittal view. (*B*) The dura and arachnoid sheath the spinal nerves at their origin. The dentate ligament separates dorsal from ventral roots and adheres to the dura. (*C*) Coronal section through the superior sagittal sinus. Note also the layers of bone between the skin and dura. *(From L. L. Langley, I. R. Telford, and J. B. Christensen, Dynamic Anatomy and Physiology, 5th ed., McGraw-Hill, New York, 1980.)*

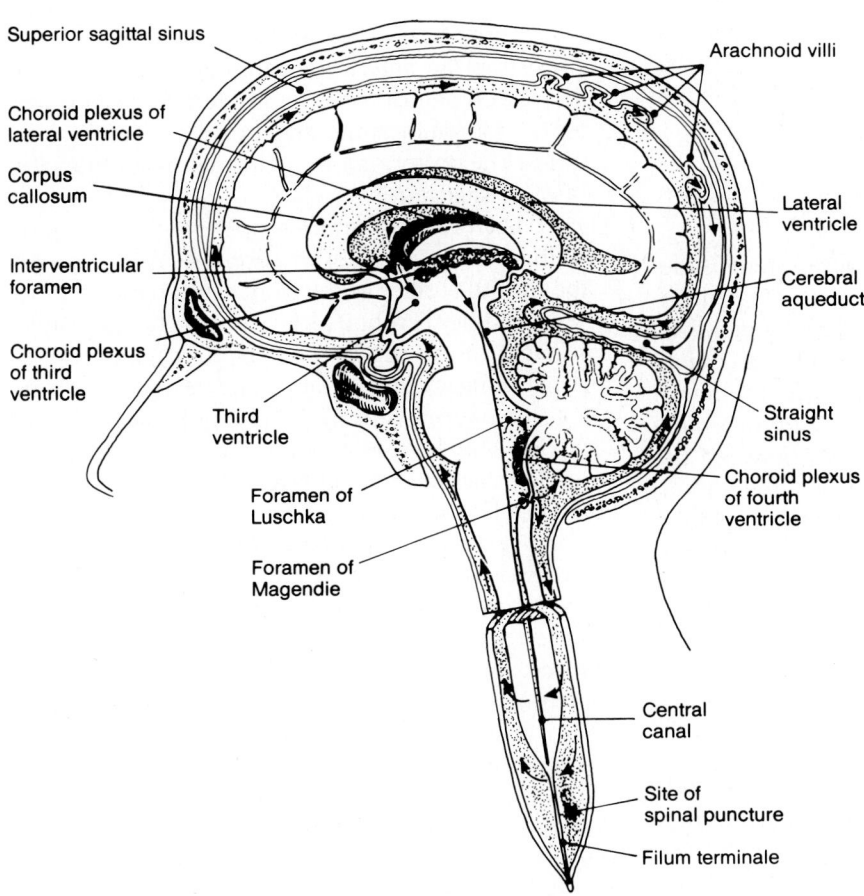

Superior sagittal sinus

Choroid plexus of
lateral ventricle

Corpus
callosum

Interventricular
foramen

Choroid plexus
of third
ventricle

Third
ventricle

Foramen of
Luschka

Foramen of
Magendie

Arachnoid villi

Lateral
ventricle

Cerebral
aqueduct

Straight
sinus

Choroid plexus
of fourth
ventricle

Central
canal

Site of
spinal puncture

Filum terminale

Figure 33-18   Lateral view of the ventricular system. Arrows show direction of flow of CSF: choroid plexus of lateral ventricles to third ventricle; through cerebral aqueduct to fourth ventricle; into subarachnoid space via foramina of Luschka and Magendie; within spinal canal and over brain; and reabsorbed in arachnoid villi of subarachnoid space of brain. *(From L. L. Langley, I. R. Telford, and J. B. Christensen, Dynamic Anatomy and Physiology, 5th ed., McGraw-Hill, 1980, p. 244.)*

hemispheres which communicates with the third ventricle by an intraventricular foramen, the *foramen of Monro*. Each lateral ventricle consists of a body and the anterior (frontal), inferior (temporal), and posterior (occipital) horns.

The third ventricle is a thin, centrally located cavity which is surrounded by the thalamic structures. The third ventricle is connected to the fourth ventricle by a narrow channel, the *aqueduct of Sylvius,* which is located in the midbrain. The fourth ventricle is an angular cavity which is located posterior to the pons and medulla and anterior to the cerebellum and extends to the central canal of the upper cervical cord. Three foramina connect the fourth ventricle with the subarachnoid spaces.

Cerebrospinal Fluid

Cerebrospinal fluid (CSF) is a clear, colorless liquid which contains a small amount of protein, glucose,

and cells and a large amount of sodium chloride. CSF provides the central nervous system with support, a cushion against trauma, and nutrition; assists in the removal of the waste products of neuronal metabolism; and assists in maintaining a relatively constant intracranial pressure. The pressure of the CSF at the lumbar cistern is 100 to 150 mmH$_2$O in the recumbent position or 0 to 10 mmHg in the cerebral ventricle.

CSF is formed principally in the lateral and third ventricles by a network of capillaries, the *choroid plexus*. Its production is a result of active transport mechanisms, the expenditure of energy, and osmotic pressure. The rate of CSF formation is estimated at 500 to 600 mL per day. The CSF circulates from the lateral ventricles through the foramen of Monro into the third ventricle, through the aqueduct of Sylvius into the fourth ventricle, and into the cranial and spinal subarachnoid spaces, where it is returned to the venous system. The total volume of CSF in the ventricular system and the subarachnoid spaces at any given time is approximately 140 mL, of which less than half is in the ventricular system.

Brain Barrier System

The activity of the central nervous system is dependent upon the physical and chemical environment. The brain barrier system is a complex network of structures which provide a stable environment by regulating the transport of chemical substances between the plasma, the cerebrospinal fluid, and the brain. A barrier exists between the bloodstream and the brain, between the bloodstream and CSF, and between CSF and the brain. The barrier system includes the capillary endothelium, the pial-glial membrane, astrocytes, ependymal cells, the choroid plexus, and the arachnoid membrane.

Circulatory System

The metabolic demands of the central nervous system for oxygen and glucose are high in comparison with other body organs. The brain consumes approximately 20 percent of the total body oxygen requirement. The oxygen is utilized for the oxidation of glucose, which is the major source of energy. The constant delivery of oxygen and glucose via the bloodstream is maintained by a complex network of arteries.

Cerebral Circulation

The brain receives its blood from the paired carotid and vertebral arteries which fill from the aortic arch. The carotid arteries supply 80 percent of the total cerebral flow, with the vertebral arteries supplying the remaining 20 percent. The internal carotid arteries supply the anterior and middle parts of the cerebral hemispheres. The vertebral arteries join to form the basilar artery. The vertebral-basilar arteries supply the posterior parts of the cerebral hemispheres, the brainstem, and the cerebellum. Blood flows from the internal carotid and vertebral-basilar arteries into a ring of anastomotic vessels, the *circle of Willis,* which is located at the base of the brain (Fig. 33-19). The circle of Willis consists of an anterior communicating artery and the paired anterior cerebral, internal carotid, posterior communicating, and posterior cerebral arteries. The posterior arteries are the major branches of the basilar artery.

Each cerebral artery supplies a specific region of the brain. The anterior cerebral arteries supply the medial surface of the frontal and parietal lobes. The middle cerebral arteries supply the lateral surfaces of the cerebral hemispheres and provide penetrating arteries to supply the deeper structures, e.g., the internal capsule, basal ganglia, and thalamic nuclei. The posterior cerebral arteries supply the medial and inferior surfaces of the occipital and temporal lobes (Fig. 33-20).

The venous drainage of the brain consists of a network of fine veins which drain into superficial and deep veins. The superficial veins pass over the surface of the brain, pass through the subarachnoid space, and empty into the venous sinuses in the margins of the dura. The paired deep cerebral veins also drain into the venous sinuses. Blood then drains into the superior and inferior sagittal sinuses, into the cavernous sinuses, through the transverse sinuses, and into the internal jugular veins. The venous sinuses are usually distended and do not collapse. Cerebral veins and sinuses do not have valves.

The vascular system regulates the resistance of the arterioles so as to maintain a constant cerebral blood flow, regardless of the pressure in the systemic arteries. This property of maintaining constant flow is known as *autoregulation*. When systemic blood pressure drops or rises precipitously outside the range of 50 to 150 mmHg mean arterial pressure, autoregulation does not compensate and cerebral blood flow passively follows systemic pressure. Autoregulation does not function well when intracranial pressure is elevated beyond 25 to 30 mmHg. Physiological factors which alter cerebral blood flow, independent of systemic blood pressure, include the partial pressure of oxygen and carbon dioxide in the plasma. Marked hypoxemia (Pa_{O_2} less than 60 mmHg) or any level of hypercarbia (Pa_{CO_2} more than 40 mmHg) causes increased cerebral bloodflow through vasodilatation of cerebral arterioles.

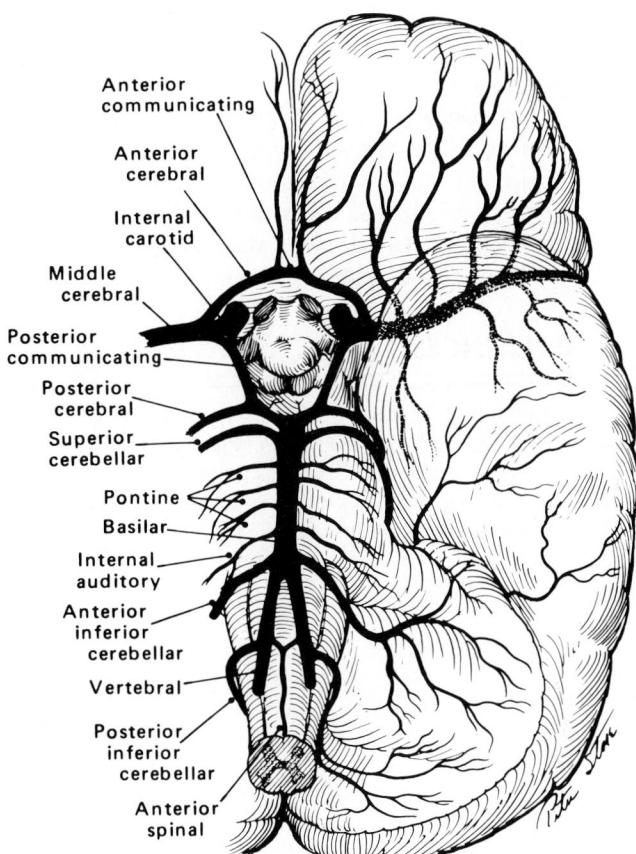

Anterior
communicating

Anterior
cerebral

Internal
carotid

Middle
cerebral

Posterior
communicating

Posterior
cerebral

Superior
cerebellar

Pontine

Basilar

Internal
auditory

Anterior
inferior
cerebellar

Vertebral

Posterior
inferior
cerebellar

Anterior
spinal

Figure 33-19   Arteries of the brain, seen from the base. The circle of Willis, at the center, joins branches of the basilar and internal carotid arteries. The vertebral arteries provide the main supply of blood to the spinal cord. *(From L. L. Langley, I. R. Telford, and J. B. Christensen, Dynamic Anatomy and Physiology, 5th ed., McGraw-Hill, New York, 1980.)*

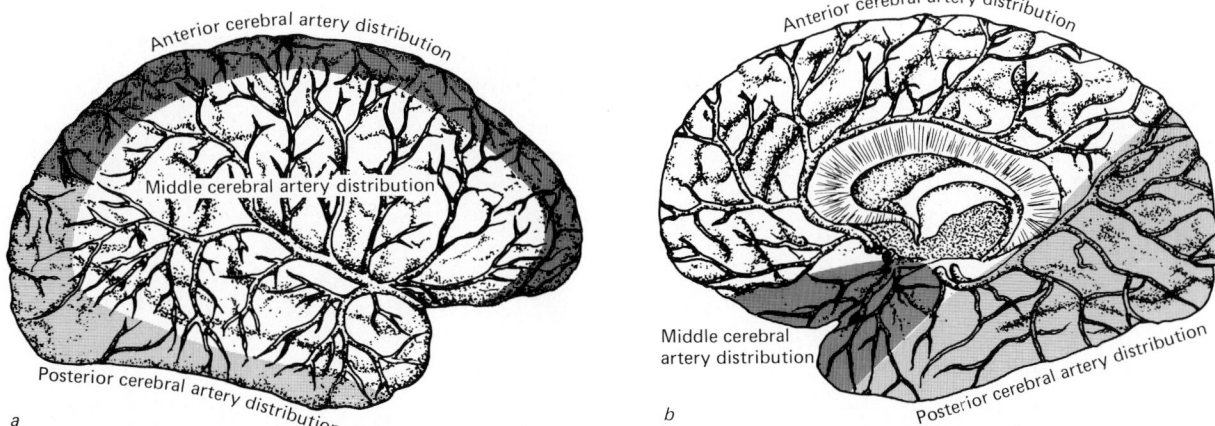

Anterior cerebral artery distribution

Middle cerebral artery distribution

Posterior cerebral artery distribution

Anterior cerebral artery distribution

Middle cerebral artery distribution

Posterior cerebral artery distribution

a

b

Figure 33-20   Distribution of the major cerebral arteries. (*a*) Lateral view. (*b*) Medial view.

Spinal Cord Circulation

The spinal cord receives its blood supply from descending branches of the vertebral arteries and multiple radicular arteries. The vertebral arteries give rise to the anterior spinal artery and the posterior spinal arteries. The radicular arteries enter the spinal canal through the intervertebral foramen and divide into anterior and posterior radicular arteries. The anterior spinal arteries join to form a single midline vessel, which is joined by anterior radicular arteries to supply the anterior and lateral parts of the spinal cord. The pair of posterior spinal arteries descends the posterior surface of the spinal cord and receives blood from the posterior radicular arteries to supply the posterior third of the spinal cord. The cervical cord segments are supplied primarily by branches of the vertebral arteries. The radicular arteries are the major source of blood supply to the thoracic and lumbar spinal cord segments.

A complex network of intradural and extradural veins provides for the venous return from the spinal cord. The distribution of the spinal veins is similar to that of the spinal arteries. Since the spinal veins have no valves, venous blood may flow directly into the systemic venous system.

REFERENCES

1. Mitchell, P. H., Cammermyer, M., Ozuna, J., & Woods, N. F. (1984). *Neurological Assessment for nursing practice.* Englewood Cliffs, N.J.: Reston.
2. Kaplan, H. (1979). *Disorders of sexual desire.* New York: Simon & Schuster.

34 Neurologic Data Acquisition

Pamela H. Mitchell

Clinician Assessment and Monitoring
History
Neurologic Examination

Technologic Assessment and Monitoring
Laboratory Studies
Radiologic Studies
Neurophysiologic Studies
Biophysical Studies
Surgical Diagnostic Procedures

References

Data regarding the neurologic status of critically ill patients are gathered for a variety of purposes. These purposes include:

1. Diagnosis of the disease producing the critical illness
2. Monitoring of psychophysiologic status to detect change (improvement or worsening)
3. Determination of the patient's ability to participate in care and treatment regimens
4. Determination of the patient's capacity to respond to demands of the care environment

Data collected for purposes 1 and 2 are used to guide medical diagnosis and intervention. Data collected for purposes 2, 3, and 4 are used to guide nursing diagnosis and intervention. Because so many areas of critical-care nursing practice and critical-care medicine are interdependent, it is important that critical-care nurses understand the purposes of medical diagnostic procedures and be skillful in using the neurologic history and examination data from both medical and nursing perspectives.

The medical history, neurologic examination, and neurodiagnostic tests are directed toward diagnosing the underlying disease and monitoring change in the pathophysiologic state. Critical-care nursing serial assessments contribute to the data used for the medical diagnosis and are crucial in monitoring change in pathophysiologic states, particularly in early detection of deteriorating status. Additionally, the nursing history, interpretation of the physical examination, and monitoring assessments are used to determine the patient's ability to respond to the demands of the physical and psychosocial environment and to participate in the care and treatment regimen.

The purpose of this chapter is to describe two major categories of data used directly or indirectly by the critical-care nurse in monitoring the status and determining nursing therapies of persons critically ill with neurologic disorders: (1) clinician assessment and monitoring of patient status, and (2) technologic assessment and monitoring. Direct clinician assessment includes history, interview, and physical examination. Technologic assessment includes invasive and noninvasive radiologic, electrophysiologic, and biomechanical medical diagnostic studies.

Clinician Assessment and Monitoring

The most common method of data acquisition regarding the patient's problem and its cause is direct interview and examination, with subsequent serial directed assessments that are compared to the baseline established at the initial examination. In neurologic disorders, the presence or absence of change in symptoms and the pattern and rapidity of change are often crucial in establishing the correct medical diagnosis. For example, the physician's differentiation of an intracranial hemorrhage from an embolic stroke is based, in part, on the worsening course associated with hemorrhage versus the static course of a completed embolic stroke.

It is the physician's responsibility to perform the initial neurologic examination to establish the baseline for medical diagnosis. It is neither necessary nor appropriate for the critical-care nursing examination to substitute for the medical examination. What is necessary is that the critical-care nurse establish a baseline against which to measure change in neurologic status for the purpose of monitoring status, evaluating changing ability to adapt to environment demands, and evaluating ability to participate in care.

Consequently, the most useful form of the examination for both physician and nurse is likely to be what is termed the *directed examination*—directed toward patients' presenting symptoms or toward detecting the most likely complications of the disorder. Such directed examination is different from the more comprehensive and detailed neurologic examination outlined in physical assessment textbooks and commonly performed by neurologists and neurosurgeons when patients come to their offices or clinics.

Frequently, critical-care nurses become skilled in directed examination and interpretation of results in terms of detection of life-threatening changes in neurologic status, as when the directed examination is used to detect potential brain herniation (a life-threatening problem). Less frequently, critical-care nurses recognize that they are carrying out a directed examination for the purpose of determining a patient's ability to tolerate environmental demands from such care activities as hygiene and position change and to determine the extent to which the patient can or should participate in care. Consequently, in this section, attention is directed to the interpretation of findings related to nursing diagnosis and monitoring as well as to interpretation that contributes to medical diagnosis and the monitoring of pathophysiologic states.

The medically focused neurologic examination detects evidence of the location and nature of neurologic disease through indirect evaluation of the *structures* of the nervous system: cerebral hemispheres (mental status), cranial nerves, motor system (including cerebellum), sensory system, and reflexes. The nursing-focused examination detects evidence of defective ability in self-care and adaptation to environmental demands by evaluating *functions* of the nervous system: consciousness, mentation, movement, sensation, and integrated regulation (see Chap. 33 for the structures that serve these functions). In the critical-care setting, because of the interdependence of medical and nursing diagnosis, it is appropriate and efficient to organize the examination and record the findings according to the medical format—that of central nervous system structures. Both interdependent and independent nursing diagnoses can be made from the data, regardless of whether they are gathered structurally or functionally (Table 34-1).

History

The history is the interview phase of data collection. The neurologic focus is used to determine whether the presenting problem is related to a nervous system disorder and to detect neurologic deficits coexisting with the primary problem that may influence care and recovery.

Because of the acute nature of many problems which precipitate admission to the critical-care setting, it is common for the history to be obtained from a variety of data sources. These data sources may include:

Ambulance or emergency medical technician (EMT) field notes and verbal report

Physician's admission history and examination

Patient, if alert enough

Table 34-1 Comparison of Structural and Functional Approaches to Neurologic Examination

Structural	Level of Neuraxis	Functional
Purpose: to determine CNS location and nature of disease or pathophysiologic state		Purpose: to determine alterations in ability to perform normal human functions and tolerate environmental demands
Mental status	Axis I	Consciousness/mentation
Cranial nerves	Axis II	Movement, sensation
Motor/cerebellar system	Axis II, III	Movement
Sensory system	Axis I–III	Sensation
Reflexes	Axis III, IV	(Included in movement/sensation)
	Axis I–IV	Integrated regulation

Family or significant other

Old medical records if this is a readmission

If the patient was transported by ambulance or medical aid unit, the EMT notes provide valuable baselines of level of consciousness, movement, and basic vegetative functions (breathing, circulation) prior to arrival in the critical-care or emergency setting. The initial physician's history should provide either brief or detailed data regarding the initial problem, rapidity of onset, precipitating and ameliorating factors, and course of symptoms. In addition, there will be at least a brief review of examination parameters: mental status, cranial nerves, motor and reflex status.

When such a physician neurologic history and notes are available, the critical-care nurse need not repeat them but rather should proceed to interview the patient or family regarding aspects of neurologic functioning that will form the data base for nursing diagnosis: namely, how the presenting problem has affected the patient's ability to:

Breathe, maintain blood pressure, eliminate wastes (integrated regulation)

Remain aroused and alert, sleep normally (consciousness)

Follow directions, respond to confusing environments, think and solve problems (mentation)

Eat, swallow, move, care for self (movement)

See, hear, protect eyes and skin, appreciate pain (sensation)

If the situation is emergent or the patient's condition is rapidly deteriorating (or has the potential to do so), the history is deferred and a directed monitoring examination is the first priority.

Neurologic Examination

As indicated earlier, the initial and subsequent monitoring examinations are not the detailed, comprehensive neurologic examination conducted in a clinic or office. Rather, the examination provides a baseline for evaluating change in neurologic status and capacity for self-care. Therefore, only selected portions of the examination in each category are needed to detect predicted or unexpected changes in status. A moderately detailed neurologic examination requires that a patient be able to follow directions. If the patient cannot, because of either confusion or decreased arousal, an approach must be used that evaluates reflex responses to stimuli, such as that described in Chap. 35 (brain herniation).

Consciousness/Mentation

This functional category assesses general behavior, level of consciousness, intellectual performance, affective behavior, and language.

General behavior is assessed by determining the appropriateness of gestures, facial expressions, attitudes toward self and others, and general appreciation of what is happening. In the intensive care setting, inappropriate responses may be related to medications, anxiety, and the sensory overload of the setting as well as to underlying neurologic disease.

The level of consciousness comprises arousal and awareness. *Arousal* is determined by responsiveness to auditory, visual, or tactile stimuli. *Awareness* is reflected in orientation to self, environment, and others in the environment. It is tested by asking the patient who and where he or she is and the day and date or month and year. Operational definitions of levels of consciousness correspond to observable responses to verbal or painful stimuli:

Awake and Alert–Opens eyes spontaneously, follows commands, oriented to self, to environment, and to others in environment

Decreased Arousal–May open eyes spontaneously or to stimuli; may follow commands; confused verbal responses

Obtunded–Opens eyes only to stimuli; may follow commands; confused or inappropriate responses to verbal stimuli

Stupor–Opens eyes to painful stimuli; appropriate motor responses to painful stimuli, confused or inappropriate verbal responses

Comatose–Does not open eyes to painful stimuli; does not follow commands; no intelligible verbal response

The specific assessment for signs of brain herniation in patients with altered consciousness is discussed in Chap. 35.

Brainstem Function

Brainstem nuclei (collections of neurons) control a variety of functions essential to control of primary survival functions: breathing, circulation, and temperature control, for example. Important protective reflexes are mediated by brainstem nuclei and their sensory and motor cranial nerves. For example, airway protection is determined by the gag and swallow reflexes; eye protection is mediated by the corneal reflex (sensory cranial nerve V) and the blink reflex (motor output through cranial nerve VII). Finally, information about the functioning of the cranial nerves originating between the midbrain and the pons provides important information regarding impending brain herniation in patients with a decreased level of consciousness (see Chap. 35).

The cranial nerves that should be repetitively assessed include III, IV, VI (extraocular movements and pupillary reflex), VII (facial symmetry), and IX, X, and XII (gag, swallow). Others are repetitively assessed when the presenting problem or subsequent consequences suggest a problem with functions mediated by those nerves. Table 34-2 summarizes clinically practical tests for each of the

Table 34-2 Clinically Practical Methods of Testing Cranial Nerve Functions and Interpretation of Problems Associated with Dysfunctions

Cranial Nerve	Function	Tested by	Interpretation of Abnormal Function
I Olfactory	Senses smells	Aromatic substance (coffee, soap), not irritants (ammonia, oil of peppermint)	*Disease:* Sphenoid ridge tumors, shearing trauma after head injury, meningeal inflammation *Functional effect:* Decreased appreciation of taste; safety hazard (cannot smell smoke, escaping gas, etc.)
II Optic	Sees	Acuity: pocket Snellen, size of headline patient can read Optic disc: fundoscopy Fields: confrontation	*Disease:* Optic nerve damage, increased intracranial pressure, field cuts indicate damage from optic radiation *Functional effects:* Safety hazard with decreased acuity, field cuts, cannot appreciate objects at sides of field; may confuse environmental cues
III Oculomotor	Moves eyes medially and up and down; constricts pupil	Extraocular movements, pupillary size and equality and symmetry of response to light shined in eyes	*Disease:* Unilateral pupillary change indicates uncal herniation; ptosis may indicate herniation, primary brainstem disorder, or Horner's syndrome *Functional effect:* Diplopia
IV Trochlear	Moves eyes down and in	Tested with III and VI	*Disease:* Paralysis of superior oblique muscle alone indicates lesion in brainstem nucleus *Functional effect:* Diplopia on upward gaze

(Continued)

Table 34-2 Clinically Practical Methods of Testing Cranial Nerve Functions and Interpretation of Problems Associated with Dysfunctions (Continued)

Cranial Nerve	Function	Tested by	Interpretation of Abnormal Function
V Trigeminal	Sensation for face, scalp, cornea and nasal and oral cavities; moves jaw	Ability to sense pinprick and cotton wisp over face; ability to clench teeth together	*Disease:* Tumor of cerebellopontine angle or acoustic neuroma, tetanus, myasthenia gravis; ALS
			Functional effects: Potential for corneal abrasion, difficulty with chewing
VI Abducens	Moves eyes medially	Tested with III and IV	*Disease:* Isolated sixth nerve paralysis associated with diabetic neuropathy, aneurysms
			Functional effect: Diplopia on medial gaze
VII Facial	Controls facial expression, also tastes (anterior two-thirds of tongue)	Ability to smile, frown, close eyes tightly; distinguish flavors—salt, sweet, sour, and bitter (front of tongue)	*Disease:* Paralysis of entire half of face indicates lesion in brainstem nucleus or peripheral nerve; weakness or paralysis of lower half of face indicates lesion in motor cortex
			Functional effects: Embarrassment over asymmetric facial appearance; some loss of clarity of speech sounds formed with lips; potential for corneal abrasion due to inability to close eye; loss of enjoyment of eating due to diminished taste
VIII Acoustic	Hears, maintains equilibrium	Ability to detect sounds in each ear; oculocephalic reflex in unconscious patients	*Disease:* Neural deafness; loss of oculocephalic reflex indicates loss of brainstem function between VIII and III, IV, VI
			Functional effects: Difficulty interpreting auditory environment; vertigo and nausea if vestibular function impaired
IX, X Glossopharyngeal, vagus	Controls gag and swallow reflexes, visceral regulation, palatal articulation	Palatal elevation, swallow and gag reflexes, glottal and palatal sounds—tested as unit	*Disease:* Brainstem lesions at level of medulla; peripheral lesions along course of nerves or muscle supplied by them
			Functional effects: Choking, aspiration, change in phonation (hoarseness) dysarthria

Table 34-2 Clinically Practical Methods of Testing Cranial Nerve Functions and Interpretation of Problems Associated with Dysfunctions (Continued)

Cranial Nerve	Function	Tested by	Interpretation of Abnormal Function
XI Spinal accesory	Shrugs shoulders, turns head	Ability to shrug shoulders, turn head against resistance	*Disease:* Supranuclear lesions from stroke, dystonias; brainstem lesions in syringomyelia; basal skull fracture, meningitis may affect the peripheral portion *Functional effects:* Pain, fatigue and deformity from hypertrophy of sternocleidomastoid; difficulty maintaining head posture with paralysis
XII Hypoglossal	Moves tongue; tastes (posterior third of tongue)	Ability to protrude tongue, push tongue against cheek; lingual sounds	*Disease:* Motor neuron disease creates wasting, cortical lesions cause spasticity *Functional effects:* Bilateral disorders—dysarthria affecting labial and lingual sounds, dysphagia due to difficulty moving bolus of food

cranial nerves and clinical problems that may be seen with abnormal findings.

The cranial nerves are peripheral nerves. Strictly speaking, cranial nerves I and II are not true nerves but rather fiber tracts of the brain itself. The true cranial nerves all arise from nuclei (collections of neurons) in the brainstem. The motor portion arises deep in the anterior brainstem in motor nuclei that are analogous to the anterior horn cells of the spinal cord. The sensory input from cranial nerves may synapse with sensory ganglia just outside the brainstem (for example, the geniculate ganglion of cranial nerve VII) or with sensory nuclei in the dorsal portion of the brainstem (cranial nerve V, for example).

The *olfactory nerve* (cranial nerve I) serves the sense of smell. *Anosmia* is the absence of the sensation of smell, and *hyposmia* is a decrease in sensitivity to smell. Decreased smell is usually associated with nasal disorders rather than neurologic problems. However, a tumor, meningitis, subarachnoid hemorrhage, or head injury can disrupt or destroy the olfactory nerve endings and thus impair smell. Hallucinations of smell may indicate lesions of the temporal lobe, where olfactory stimuli are interpreted.

The sense of smell is tested by having the patient close the eyes and occlude one nostril, then the other, and identify the scent while the examiner passes aromatic substances under the nose. Commonly used scents include coffee, cinnamon, and vanilla. Irritative substances, such as ammonia or oil of peppermint, test the response of cranial nerve V rather than cranial nerve I.

Functional problems associated with anosmia include inability to detect, by smell, warnings of environmental danger such as fire or gas leak. There may also be decreased pleasure in eating related to loss of the olfactory contribution to the taste of food.

The *optic nerve* (cranial nerve II) carries impulses from the retina to the optic chiasm. From here the impulses go to areas in the cerebral cortex where visual images are recognized and interpreted. Lesions causing disorders can occur anywhere from the eyeball to the occipital cortex. Two aspects of vision are commonly tested: visual acuity and visual fields. In addition, an ophthalmoscope is used to examine the retina, optic disk, vessels, and macula.

Visual acuity is easily tested in the critical-care unit with a newspaper or magazine. The patient, wearing glasses if they are normally worn, is asked to read with one eye at a time, covering the other with a patch. It is important to determine a patient's ability or lack of ability to read, since this will affect the ability to fully participate in the program of treatment. For example, instructions regarding activities or consent forms for procedures may be given to the patient to read. Certain cerebral disorders also may alter the ability to read and/or to interpret written items, e.g., a cerebral vascular accident.

Visual field testing uses the confrontation method. Each eye is evaluated separately as the examiner stands an arm's length from the patient. The patient is asked to close (cover with the hand) the right eye and look with the left eye at the examiner's nose. A wiggling finger is steadily brought in from the periphery until the patient sees it. The finger should be an equal distance between the examiner and the patient except temporally, when the examiner must start behind the patient. This maneuver is performed for all quadrants and then repeated with the other eye. If a defect is found, the configuration is determined by retesting and sketching the defect. Normally, the patient will see an object 60° nasally, 50° upward, 90° temporally, and 70° downward.

The *oculomotor* (cranial nerve III), *trochlear* (cranial nerve IV), and *abducens* (cranial nerve VI) nerves have similar functions and are usually examined together. These three cranial nerves act together in controlling the ocular muscles to ensure that the eyes remain parallel through all movements. In addition, the oculomotor nerve controls the muscle that elevates the upper lid and innervates the constrictor muscle of the pupil. A lesion of these nerves may produce diplopia because of weakness of the ocular muscles and deviation of the eyeball from a parallel position. Ptosis of the eyelid and sustained pupillary dilatation indicate possible problems with the oculomotor nerve. Before testing, inspect the position of the upper eyelids with the patient gazing directly at you. Observe for ptosis and for any lower lid sagging, which may indicate weakness of the orbicularis oculi muscle.

To evaluate extraocular movements, ask the patient to follow your finger through the six cardinal positions of gaze (Fig. 34-1). Pause during lateral and upward gaze to observe for nystagmus. Also observe for any deviation from normal conjugate movements and for the relation of the upper lid to the eye globe. The upper lid normally overlaps the iris slightly as the gaze moves upward from the downward position. This overlapping may not occur with hyperthyroidism.

The pupils are evaluated for size, equality, and the pupillary light reflex. Shine a light directly into one pupil and observe for constriction. This is called the *direct light response*. Again shine a light in one pupil and observe the response in the other pupil. This is called the *consensual light response*. Failure of pupillary response to light is an important sign of possible oculomotor lesions. Test accommodation and convergence by having the patient focus at a distance and then follow your finger as

Figure 34-1 Cardinal positions of gaze with corresponding cranial nerves and muscles.

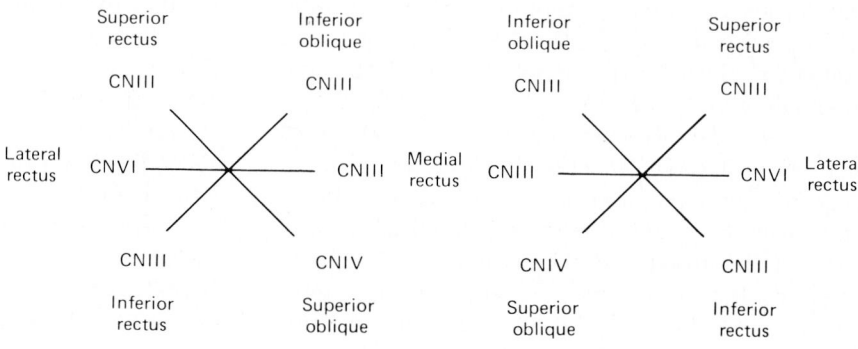

you bring it in toward the patient's nose. Note convergence of the eyes and the pupillary constriction as the pupil accommodates. Loss of the accommodation-convergence reflex may result from a lesion of cranial nerve III (oculomotor).

The ophthalmoscopic examination, not an easy task, is undertaken to add to the store of knowledge about the critical-care patient. It is not a routine part of the nursing examination. This examination should be conducted in a darkened room. The technique of using the examiner's right hand and right eye to test the patient's right eye and the examiner's left hand and left eye for the patient's left eye should be observed. The ophthalmoscope should be set at the diopter setting best suited to the examiner's needs. A setting of zero diopters is neutral (it does not converge or diverge light rays). A plus diopter (black numbers) setting is used for a farsighted patient and a minus diopter (red numbers) for the nearsighted patient. The procedure is as follows:

Place your thumb on the patient's brow and have the patient focus on a spot at a distance somewhere over your shoulder. Approach gradually from a distance of about 15 inches and a position 15° lateral to the patient's direct line of vision. Shine the light on the pupil, noting the red reflex and any lens opacities. Move in until you are touching the thumb of your opposite hand (which is on the patient's brow) with the ophthalmoscope. You should now be viewing the optic disk, which is a red-orange, smooth, round or vertically oval structure. If the disk is not yet in view, follow a blood vessel until you locate it. Observe the disk for color, shape, margin clarity, and the physiologic cup (a bright area in the center of the disk). Note the disk/physiologic cup ratio; also observe any pigmented rings or crescents around the disk. Observe the vessels for distribution in all four quadrants. Follow the vessels from the disk to the margin of the fundus, observing for occlusion, arteriolar or venous nicking, and abnormal size. Veins are normally larger and darker and pulsate; arterioles are smaller and brighter and do not pulsate (Fig. 34-2). Examine the general background, noting pigmentation appropriate to individual coloring (the darker the skin, the darker the fundus). Observe also for hemorrhages, cotton wool patches, exudates, and retinal edema. Now evaluate

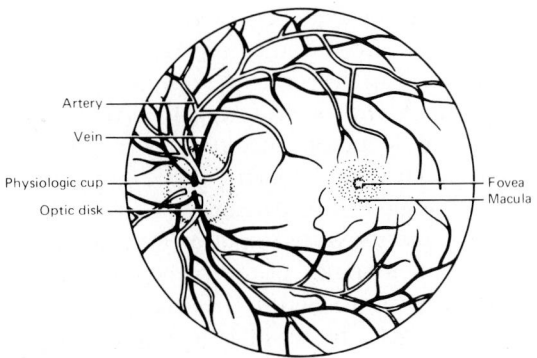

Figure 34-2   Optic disk, macula, and retinal vessels as viewed through an ophthalmoscope. *(From P. Mayfield et al., Physical Assessment: A Programmed Approach, McGraw-Hill, New York, 1980.)*

the macula and the fovea with the patient looking directly into the light. The macula is two to three disk diameters temporally from the disk and the fovea is in the center of the macula (Fig. 34-2).

The most important abnormalities which are found on fundoscopic examination are hyperemic (pinker) disks, disk atrophy (pale with blurred edges), or papilledema (choked or swollen disk). The first signs of papilledema may be the absence of retinal vein pulsation or enlargement and increase in the size of retinal veins as compared with the arterioles. Abnormal arteries may be thickened and pulsating. Optic atrophy may be the result of diseases which affect the optic nerve, such as syphilis. Papilledema, which is secondary to fairly long-standing increased intracranial pressure, may also result in optic atrophy.

Changes in visual acuity, the appearance of the optic disk, or eye movements can be indicators of expanding brain mass, as discussed in detail in Chap. 35. In addition, patients who have less emergent changes in visual acuity or eye movement may experience a number of functional problems associated with these abnormal findings.

Loss of visual acuity for either near or far distance is common, particularly as people age. Patients who are used to wearing glasses for distance may become disoriented in the intensive care unit when they cannot see clearly what is happening. Similarly, patients with dysfunction of cranial nerves III or IV may experience diplopia (double vision).

The functional consequence of diplopia may be nausea or a predisposition to sensory deprivation and disorientation.

The *trigeminal nerve* (cranial nerve V) mediates general sensation, including perception of pain, temperature, and touch for the entire face (except the angle of the jaw) and for the scalp to the vertex. It also mediates sensation for the cornea, the mucous membranes of the paranasal sinuses, and the nasal and oral cavities. The sensory divisions are the ophthalmic, the maxillary, and the mandibular. The motor portion of the nerve controls the jaw reflex and the muscles of mastication.

The trigeminal nerve is tested by determining the patient's ability to perceive pain (pinprick) and touch (cotton wisp) over the face and anterior scalp. The oral and nasal cavities are tested only if there is reason to expect problems with this nerve. The corneal reflex is tested by having the patient look up and straight ahead while the examiner approaches from the side with a fine wisp of cotton. The examiner touches the cornea lightly, avoiding the eyelashes. A less invasive way to test the ophthalmic portion of the nerve is the *lash test*. The patient's eyes may be closed or open. The examiner gently touches the eyelashes. A blink indicates that the eye protective reflex is present.

The motor portion is tested by having the patient clench the teeth while the examiner palpates the temporal and masseter muscles. The muscles should be symmetric and the examiner should not be able to open the patient's clenched jaw.

Dysfunction of the trigeminal nerve is most commonly caused by a tumor at the cerebellopontine angle, often an acoustic neuroma. Loss of the corneal reflex may indicate primary brainstem damage or brainstem compression due to brain herniation. Weakness of the jaw musculature may be due to primary neuromuscular junction disease (tetanus, botulism, myasthenia gravis) or motor neuron disease (amyotrophic lateral sclerosis).

Functional problems associated with loss of sensation to the cornea include a potential for corneal abrasion. Loss of sensation from the maxillary and mandibular divisions (local dental anesthesia is an example of a temporary loss of sensation from peripheral branches of these divisions) may produce a potential for injury to the mucous membranes of the cheek or to the tongue. Difficulty in chewing results from damage to the motor portion of the nerve.

The *facial* nerve (cranial nerve VII) innervates all the muscles of facial expression. The sensory portion mediates taste from the anterior two-thirds of the tongue and carries fibers that innervate the lacrimal, submaxillary, and sublingual glands. The motor portion is tested by having the patient look up and wrinkle the forehead (frontalis muscle); close the eyes tightly and resist the examiner's efforts to open them (orbicularis orbis muscle); and smile, whistle, and show the teeth (lower face muscles). Facial asymmetry at rest should be noted.

The sensory portion of this nerve is rarely tested as a routine part of the nursing examination. The neurologist's record of the initial examination will indicate whether the patient had presenting symptoms suggesting dysfunction of cranial nerve VII. Change in this initial symptom can be tested by having the patient protrude the tongue while the examiner touches each side with a moist applicator dipped in one of four test substances: salt, sugar, sour, or bitter. The tongue should not be withdrawn into the mouth until the substance is identified.

Facial paralysis may be due to lesions of any part of the nerve or cranial nerve nuclei. True cranial nerve facial paralysis is referred to as *peripheral* facial paralysis. Paralysis includes both the forehead and lower facial muscles. The facial "droop" following a lesion of the cerebral motor cortex involves only the lower face; it does not affect forehead wrinkling and eye closure. Tumors of the cerebellopontine angle are a common cause of progressive or permanent peripheral facial paralysis. Permanent paralysis may also be seen after removal of large acoustic neuromas (cranial nerve VIII) that also wrap around cranial nerve VII.

Functional problems associated with dysfunction of cranial nerve VII include difficulty in speaking clearly, due to inability to move the lips symmetrically, and a potential for eye injury due to incomplete closure of the eyelids. In addition, the patient may find the facial appearance embarrassing.

The acoustic nerve (cranial nerve VIII) has two divisions: the *cochlear,* which mediates hearing, and the *vestibular,* which controls balance, position, and spatial orientation.

To test the cochlear portion the examiner whispers or rubs two fingers together next to each ear and determines what the patient heard. Alternatively, a vibrating tuning fork may be held next to each ear.

If there are hearing losses, the physician may use Weber's and Rinne's tests to determine whether the loss is due to physical sound conduction or neural causes. Weber's test involves placing a vibrating tuning fork on the vertex of the skull and asking the patient whether the sound is heard equally in both ears or more to one side or the other. Equal perception is normal. Sensorineural loss in one ear will cause the sound to be perceived better in the other ear. Conversely, if there is a conduction defect (wax, fluid, or middle ear disorder), the sound will be perceived as loudest on the side of the impaired conduction. In Rinne's test, a vibrating tuning fork is held on the mastoid process behind one ear. When the patient indicates that the sound is no longer heard, the tuning fork is held directly beside the ear. The sound should still be heard beside the ear, since air conducts sound waves longer than bone. The normal air/bone conduction ratio is approximately 2:1. Sensorineural hearing loss impairs both air and bone conduction, whereas conduction defects impair only the ability to detect sound conducted through the air.

The vestibular portion of the acoustic nerve is tested in nonemergent situations by the physician if the patient has a history of vertigo or ataxia. The cold caloric test is used for this determination, if indicated. The patient is placed in the supine position, with the head tilted forward 30°. The examiner inspects the ear otoscopically to ascertain that the eardrum is intact and then introduces 5 to 10 mL of ice water into the ear canal. The normal reaction in the conscious patient is nystagmus, with the quick component to the side opposite the stimulated ear. Vertigo, nausea, and vomiting are common reactions in the conscious patient.

In the critical-care setting, the vestibular portion of the acoustic nerve is stimulated in the unconscious patient to determine the intactness of brainstem pathways between the vestibular and ocular cranial nerves. Either the oculocephalic reflex or the oculovestibular reflex may be used to stimulate the vestibular nerve.

The oculocephalic reflex, commonly referred to as the "doll's head" or "doll's eye" maneuver, is mediated afferently by the vestibular portion of cranial nerve VIII and efferently by cranial nerves III and VI. The reflex is tested by rapidly rotating the patient's head to one side and observing the eye movements (Fig. 34-3). If the reflex is intact ("doll's eyes" present), the eyes appear to remain in the initial position and then slowly turn to the direction in which the head was rotated. If the reflex is not intact ("doll's eyes" absent), the eyes will move with the head as though fixed in place. The reflex is present in all persons with intact brainstems during sleep. It cannot be elicited in the awake person because conscious fixation of the eyes overcomes the reflex. In altered consciousness the presence of the reflex indicates that the brainstem function is intact between cranial nerves VIII and III.

The oculovestibular reflex is mediated by the same set of cranial nerves. This reflex is tested as

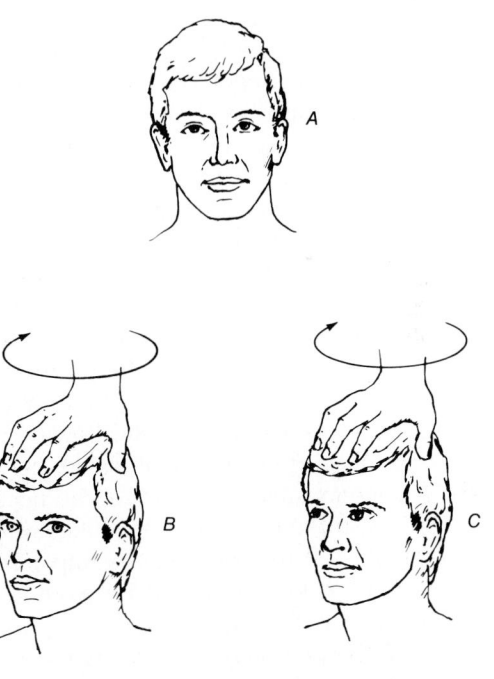

Figure 34-3   Oculocephalic reflex. *(A)* Moving the unconscious patient's head to the right *(B)* moves the eyes initially to the left if the reflex is present. If the reflex is absent *(C)*, eyes will move to the right along with the head.

described earlier with either warm or cold water in the ear canal. The oculovestibular reflex is preserved somewhat longer than the oculocephalic in brain dysfunction. Therefore, when the oculocephalic reflex is lost, the physician may wish to perform caloric stimulation to determine whether any function remains in the reflex pathway.

As described in Chap. 35, loss or change in these reflexes is an important indicator of brain herniation. From a functional perspective, loss of either the oculocephalic or the oculovestibular reflex suggests that cranial nerve function may be lost one level below as well. It should therefore be assumed that the patient does not have adequate function of cranial nerves IX and X and thus cannot protect the airway though the gag and cough reflexes.

The *glossopharyngeal and vagus nerves* (cranial nerves IX and X) are usually considered together. The glossopharyngeal mediates taste from the posterior one-third of the tongue, innervates the carotid sinus and the carotid body, and supplies general sensation to tonsillar and pharyngeal mucous membranes. The vagus nerve innervates all thoracic and abdominal visceral organs, the larynx, the pharynx, and the palate and conveys numerous sensory impulses from the walls of the digestive tract, heart, and lungs.

Clinically testable functions include the gag reflex, swallowing, and the sensation of taste. Pharyngeal function is tested by having the patient say "aah" and watching the soft palate and uvula. The soft palate should rise symmetrically and promptly. The gag reflex is tested by touching the posterior wall of the soft palate. The soft palate should contract and the uvula retract simultaneously. Swallowing is tested by giving the alert patient ice chips or water to swallow. If consciousness is impaired, the neck over the larynx is stroked to stimulate reflex swallowing of secretions. If the gag reflex is impaired in an unconscious patient, it should be assumed that swallowing is also abnormal.

The *spinal accessory nerve* (cranial nerve XI) supplies the sternocleidomastoid muscle and the upper part of the trapezius muscle. The muscles are examined for atrophy. Strength is tested by having the patient shrug the shoulders against the examiner's resistance (trapezius) and turn the head

to each side against resistance (sternocleidomastoid). The most common cause of sternocleidomastoid weakness is trauma to the neck. Weakness of this muscle may make it difficult for the patient to support the head unaided.

The *hypoglossal nerve* (cranial nerve XII) innervates the tongue musculature. It is tested by inspecting the tongue for fasciculations (fine tremors), wasting, and lack of power or mobility. The examiner observes the patient's protruded tongue for deviation and wasting. Fasciculations are best observed when the tongue is resting inside the mouth. Strength is examined by having the patient alternately push the tongue against each cheek, against the resistance of the examiner's finger. Bilateral weakness of the tongue (or paralysis) may occur in amyotrophic lateral sclerosis and in myasthenia gravis. Unilateral weakness may be associated with neck trauma, extensive neck surgery, or brainstem lesions (tumors or stroke). Difficulty in speaking clearly or in manipulating food in the mouth and swallowing may be a functional outcome of tongue weakness.

Motor Function

The motor system includes those components of the nervous system concerned with the initiation, maintenance, and control of movements of the body. Skeletal abnormalities, joint swelling or pain, decreases in range of motion, and disturbances in posture and balance are evaluated, as well as strength and mass of specific muscle groups. The abbreviated motor examination used in detecting brain herniation is described in Chap. 35.

Functional outcomes of motor system dysfunction depend upon whether the neurologic lesion is at the suprasegmental, segmental, or myoneural junction level of the motor system. Terms commonly used to describe the suprasegmental level are *upper motor neuron, corticobulbar lesion, corticospinal lesion, pyramidal lesion,* and *long tract lesion.* Terms used to describe the segmental level are *lower motor neuron, final common pathway, anterior horn cell lesion,* and *ventral horn cell lesion.* The myoneural junction is the end point of the motor segment and is included here because the functional outcome of dysfunction at this level is somewhat different from that for the spinal or peripheral portion of the motor segment. Differing functional effects of lesions at the three levels are shown in Table 34-3.

Examination of motor function includes determination of muscle strength and mass, including symmetry of strength, tone, presence of involuntary movements, coordination, gait, and balance. Gait and balance cannot be tested in the patient confined to bed; only limited aspects of coordination can be tested in such a patient. Patients with altered consciousness may be examined primarily in terms of response to simple stimuli, and only the most gross motor function can be tested.

In the alert patient who is able to follow directions, assessment of strength and mass begins with inspection of the major muscle groups of the arms, legs, and trunk for any differences in size. If differences in mass are seen or suspected, the limb girth should be measured. Reduced size of one limb may indicate segmental motor function loss.

Strength is tested on a scale of 0 to 5, defined as follows:

0. No muscle contraction
1. Flicker or trace of voluntary muscle contraction
2. Active movement with gravity eliminated
3. Active movement against gravity but not against resistance
4. Active movement against gravity and resistance but not full strength
5. Full power against examiner's resistance

Table 34-3 Clinical Signs of Disrupted Motor Function at Three Levels of the Nervous System

Level	Clinical Signs	Examples of Causative Disorders
Suprasegmental	Weakness or paralysis of voluntary movement Increased muscle stretch reflexes; reflex arc intact (after "spinal shock") Some muscle atrophy secondary to disuse EMG normal	Spinal cord lesions such as trauma, infarct, tumor, and hemorrhage
Segmental	Weakness or paralysis of voluntary movement Decreased or absent muscle stretch reflexes (reflex arc disrupted) Marked muscle atrophy secondary to denervation ($\downarrow$ trophic factors) EMG changes: fibrillation, giant polyphasic action potentials (denervation supersensitivity)	Brainstem lesions affecting cranial nuclei: tumors, infarct, hemorrhage Cerebellopontine angle tumors compressing cranial nerves Polyneuropathies such as Guillain-Barré syndrome, alcoholic polyneuropathy, diphtheritic polyneuropathy, and toxic chemical polyneuropathy
Myoneural junction	Weakness or paralysis of voluntary movement Muscle stretch reflexes intact No muscle atrophy EMG diminished: muscle able to contract when directly stimulated. Pattern of $\downarrow$ contraction varies with disorder	Chronic: myasthenia gravis (may have acute episodes of life-threatening myasthenic or cholinergic crisis); Eaton-Lambert syndrome (myasthenic symptoms associated with carcinoma) Acute: botulism, curare, succinylcholine, "nerve gas," organophosphate insecticides

Examination of the strength of the upper extremities proceeds systematically along major muscle groups, from the proximal to the distal. A number of the maneuvers used to test strength are shown in Figs. 34-4 and 34-5.

The deltoid and trapezius (abduction strength in the shoulder) are tested by having the patient push the upper arm against resistance. The biceps is tested by having the patient flex the forearm against the upper arm and resist the examiner's attempt to straighten the elbow. Wrist flexion and extension (flexor and extensor carpus radialis and carpus ulnaris) are tested by having the patient alternately flex and extend the wrist against resistance.

General strength of the proximal arm muscles is tested by having the patient close the eyes and hold both arms out, palms up. The examiner observes for downward drifting of either arm and pronation of the hand. The appearance of either is termed *pronator drift* and indicates a problem in the suprasegmental motor system. The *new* appearance of the sign in a patient with a potentially expanding lesion in the brain indicates brain shift or compression (see Chap. 35). Patients with old hemiparesis from stroke, neurosurgery, or old head injuries may demonstrate pronator drift as a continuing sign of residual neurologic deficit.

The intrinsic muscles of the hands are screened by testing finger strength and grip. Abduction of the fingers is tested by having the patient spread the fingers and thumbs and resist the examiner's attempt to push the fingers together. Grip is tested by having the patient hold the first two fingers of

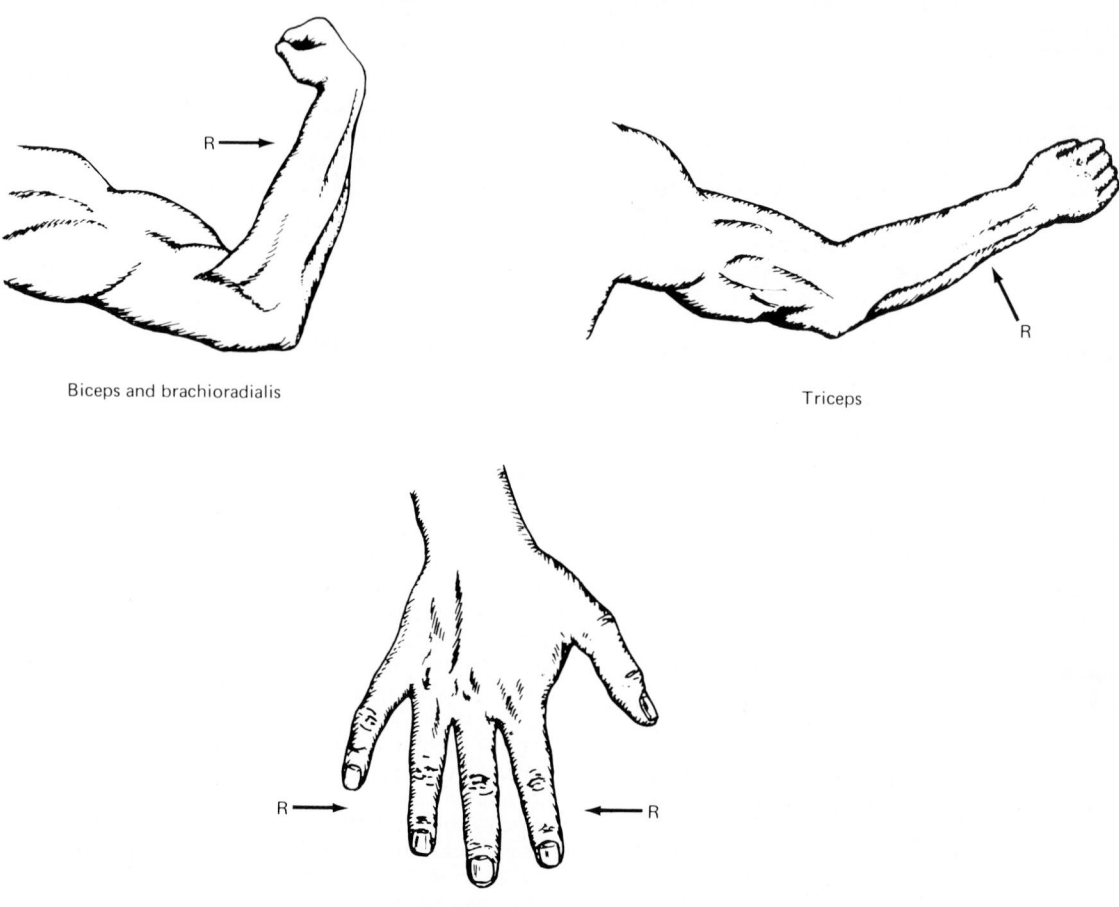

Biceps and brachioradialis

Triceps

Fingers

Figure 34-4 Examination of the upper extremities. The patient is instructed to overcome resistance which is applied by the examiner in the direction of the arrows *(R)*.

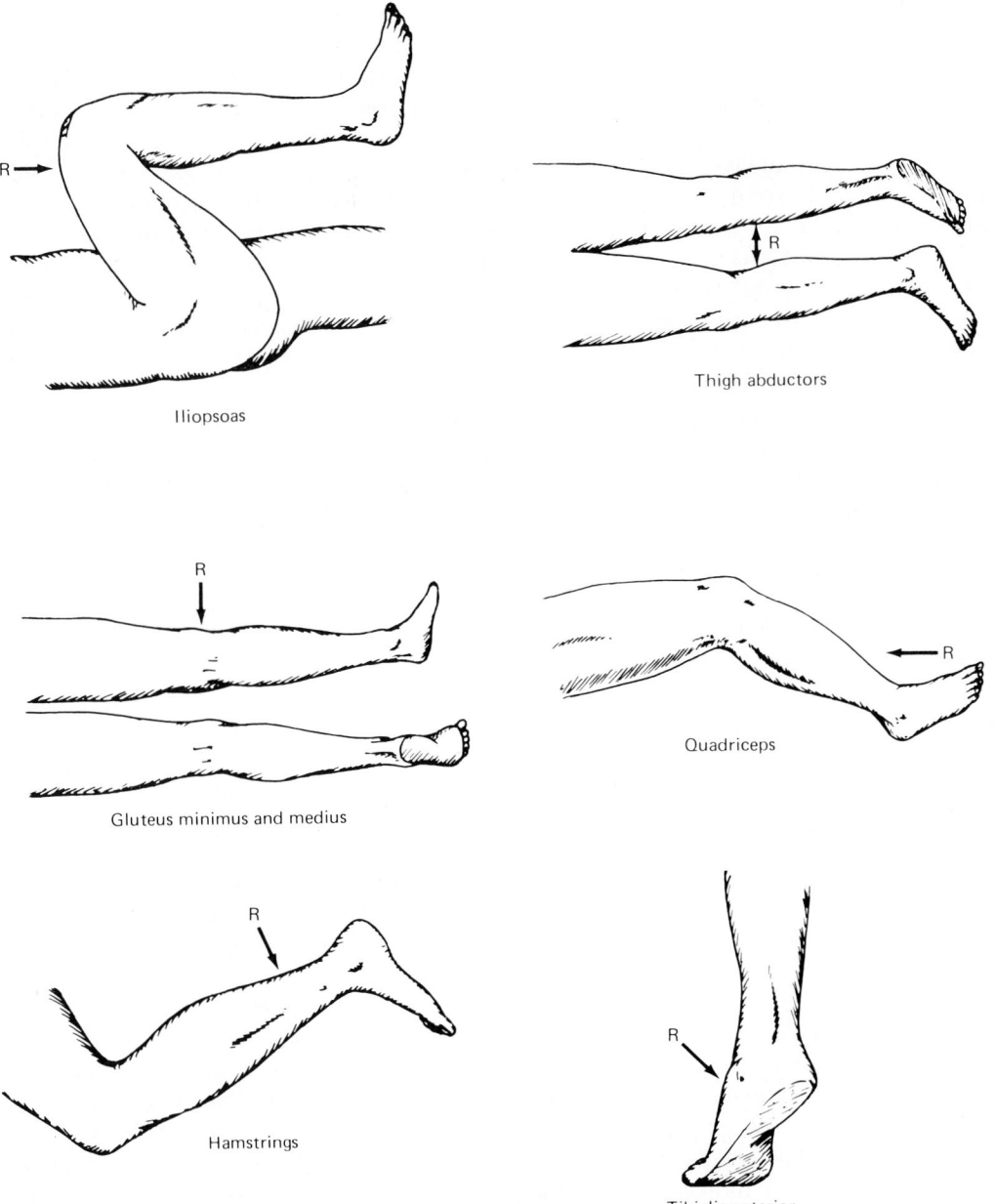

Figure 34-5   Examination of the lower extremities. The patient is instructed to overcome resistance, which is applied in the direction of the arrows (R).

the examiner's hands while the examiner attempts to pull away. Both maneuvers test the function of the intrinsic muscles and the three nerves serving the hands (the ulnar, radial, and medial nerves). If weakness exists, the physician may wish to test the muscles individually. Nurses in specialized or ex-panded roles that require such testing should consult one of the neurologic examination text-books in the references for the technique.

Trunk strength is difficult to assess directly, as the major truncal muscles are those assisting respiration. However, the examiner can note whether a sitting patient is able to maintain the erect posture. Maintaining sitting posture is a function of the strength of the paraspinal muscles. Rising to a sitting position is a function of the strength of the abdominal muscles.

The lower extremities are evaluated in the following manner (Fig. 34-5): Have the supine patient raise first one knee and then the other and resist your attempts to push the knee to the chest. This action tests the iliopsoas muscle. Have the patient extend the legs and resist your attempts to flex the knee. This tests the quadriceps. Have the patient flex the knee and resist your attempts to extend it. This tests the hamstring muscles. Have the patient dorsiflex the foot and resist your attempts to overcome the flexion. This tests the tibialis anterior muscle. Have the patient hold the knees tightly together while you attempt to open them. This tests the thigh abductor muscles. Have the patient hold the knees apart while you attempt to push them together. This tests the gluteus minimus and medius muscles. Have the patient stand on the toes. This tests flexion of the foot, while standing on the heels tests extension of the foot.

Muscle tone is tested by passively putting a limb through full range of motion. *Tone* refers to the resistance detected by the examiner. Reduced tone may be caused by diseases of the cerebellum and by lower motor neuron diseases; since normal resistance is slight, decreased tone may be difficult to detect. Increased tone is much easier to detect and is classified as spastic, resulting from upper motor neuron lesions, or rigid, as in lesions of the basal ganglia. *Spasticity* affects certain muscle groups differently. For example, with upper motor neuron lesions, the flexors in the arms and extensors in the legs are most affected. These are the antigravity muscles where most muscle spindles are located. *Rigidity,* as in Parkinson's disease, is demonstrated in the heightened tone of all flexor muscles, resulting in flexed posture.

A type of spasticity known as the *clasp knife phenomenon* is exemplified by *pyramidal spasticity,* in which resistance to a passive movement rapidly increases to a point and then suddenly gives way. For example, the patient flexes the elbow while the examiner attempts to overcome the flexion. When the flexion suddenly gives way, the patient may hit the chin.

The most common involuntary movement is the rhythmic movement known as *tremors.* Tremors resulting from diseases affecting the basal ganglia, such as Parkinson's, exist during relaxation and are called *rest tremors.* Tremors associated with cerebellar diseases are characteristically seen when the patient attempts to perform an activity.

Chorea is another type of involuntary movement and is characterized by rapid, jerky, irregular, and purposeless contractions of random muscle groups followed by immediate relaxation. The basal ganglia are affected. The best-known choreas are Huntington's and Sydenham's.

Disturbances in *coordination* can be indicative of cerebellar disorders. The following activities are useful in detecting a lack of coordination:

Have the patient pat the knee rapidly, alternating the back of the hand with the palm. Have the patient rapidly pat one hand against the palm of the other hand. Have the patient rhythmically touch the tip of the nose with the index finger with the eyes open, then closed. In cerebellar disease, the movements in these tests are slowed and nonrhythmic and may "hang." With hemiplegia, movements are just slow and stiff.

Have the patient quickly and consecutively touch the tip of the thumb to each finger of the same hand. These movements are slowed and inaccurate in cerebellar disease, whereas in certain movement disorders, such as Parkinson's disease, the movement is slowed and loses the amplitude of tapping.

Have the patient quickly and smoothly move the finger back and forth between the nose and the examiner's finger. With cerebellar disease, the hand deviates and may miss the target.

The only test of lower extremity coordination that can be performed by the bedridden patient is the heel-to-shin test. Have the patient run the heel of one foot down the shin of the other leg in a straight line while not looking. Cerebellar disease will cause irregular deviations of the heel to either side.

Since standing and walking properly require adequate muscle strength, coordination, proprioception, vestibular function, and vision, gait and stance may well have been implicitly included in the evaluation of these functions. The observation of simple walking reveals much; for example, in hemiparesis the normal rhythmic arm swinging is reduced on the side of the hemiplegia.

Gait is evaluated by having the patient walk heel to toe down a straight line and walk briskly around a chair. Cerebellar disorders cause the patient to walk with a wide base and to stagger or reel laterally. Hemiplegia causes circumduction of the leg, with a stiff knee and extended ankle, while a bilateral spastic paresis of the leg produces scissoring of the knees.

The tests for stance and gait may have to be deferred or even omitted in the patient who is quite ill or unable to ambulate. However, the critical-care nurse may have the opportunity to perform these tests and gain valuable information.

If any difficulty with coordination or gait has been noted, Romberg's test should be performed. This test differentiates cerebellar from sensory ataxia. The patient stands with feet close together and eyes first open, then closed. Increased swaying and falling occurs with closed but not open eyes in persons with an impairment of proprioception. Cerebellar disease may result in swaying but not falling with the eyes open or closed, and in unilateral vestibular disorders the patient tends to fall to the ipsilateral side.

Sensory Function

The sensory system conveys information to the central nervous system about the status of the body surface and its surrounding environment, about the position of the body and its extremities in space, and about the status of the internal organs. When evaluating the sensory system, great care must be taken to listen carefully and record accurately the patient's reporting, because sensory interpretation is extremely subjective. The patient's responses to touch and pain, temperature sensation, proprioceptive (motion and position) sensation, vibratory sensation, and cortical sensory functions are elicited on the examination. Specific patterns of sensory loss result from specific lesions; therefore, the sensory loss demonstrated may be highly diagnostic.

Superficial pain is tested by lightly pinpricking over the body in a symmetrical fashion. Particular attention should be paid to any suspected or stated area of sensory loss or deficit such as numbness or tingling. When in doubt about the reliability of the response, alternate the sharp point with the dull end of the pin. The dull end acts as a control; it does not test pain perception. If decreased sensation is found, determine the margins of the suspect area. When making a survey of the body in the absence of problems, be sure to compare each side with the other.

Deep pain is tested by squeezing the Achilles tendon, squeezing the calf muscles, and/or applying firm pressure on the sternum. Deep and superficial pain are carried in the same central pathways, and therefore lesions affecting one response will usually affect the other.

Temperature perception pathways are closely related to those for pain and usually do not need testing if pain perception is normal. Always test the temperature response if there is any impairment of pain perception. Test tubes filled with hot and cold water are used, applying them alternately over the body and asking the patient to distinguish between them.

Touch is evaluated by using a cotton wisp or a soft brush and stroking corresponding parts of the entire body. Ask the patient to respond when touch is perceived. Touch is usually intact, even with severe involvement of sensory areas, because of the many multiple pathways. If defects are found, however, determine the area of loss by defining margins. Drag the cotton wisp over the area of decreased sensation until margins of sensation can be defined; then record your findings.

Proprioception, or *motion and position sense,* is tested in every extremity by using passive motion and asking the patient to identify the position with eyes shut. Have the patient state when the movement begins and whether the extremity is up or down or how it is pointed. Position sense is best tested on the thumbs, fingers, and toes. Position sense is always lost distally first in organic lesions; so if perception is intact in the distal extremities, there is generally no need to test the more proximal portions.

Vibratory sense is tested by placing a vibrating tuning fork against any bony prominence of each extremity—ankle, toe, thumb, or wrist—and asking the patient to tell you when the vibration stops. As with position sense, vibratory perception is initially lost distally.

Cortical sensory perception can occur only if the higher cerebral centers of integration, those beyond the thalamus, are intact. The primary sensory modalities are evaluated first in order to be sure they are intact. For example, a peripheral nerve injury affecting the hand would alter perception of objects placed in the hand but not necessarily indicate a cortical deficit.

Cortical sensory perception is tested in the following ways. *Stereognosis* is the perception of objects through touch. Test each hand with the eyes closed by placing a button, key, coin, or other familiar object in the hand and asking for identification. Two-point discrimination is determined by using the points of a calibrated compass on the fingertip and asking the patient to tell you when one and two points are felt. Normally, two points can be distinguished when the points are 0.3 to 0.6 cm apart. The number of centimeters of separation required to distinguish two points is important. The average distance on the palms and soles is 1.5 cm; on the dorsum of the hand, 3 cm is average; and on the shin, 4 cm is usually necessary. Double simultaneous stimulation is the appreciation of two simultaneous touches on symmetrically opposite sides of the body. This requires normal cortical function. All the above responses are designed to test cortical sensory perception and are affected by lesions of the sensory cortex.

Reflexes

Deep tendon reflexes are best elicited by having the patient relax. The examiner then positions the limb in a manner which slightly stretches the muscle and strikes a brisk blow with a reflex hammer over the tendon insertion of the muscle. The two sides of the body are compared for equality of response. Reflexes are usually graded on a 0 to 4+ scale.

4+ Very brisk, hyperactive, and may indicate disease

3+ More brisk than average but may well be normal

2+ Average or normal response

1+ decreased response

0 No response

In addition to the deep tendon reflexes, three superficial reflexes are usually tested: the abdominal, the cremasteric responses, and the plantar.

Reflexes, generally speaking, tend to be increased in suprasegmental neuron disease and decreased in segmental disease. Table 34-4 shows the expected response, stimulus, site of stimulation, and corresponding spinal segments of commonly tested deep tendon and superficial reflexes.

Technologic Assessment and Monitoring

The physician may use a variety of radiologic, electrophysiologic, and laboratory techniques to aid in the diagnosis and monitoring of the neurologic disease process. Nursing understanding of these studies serves two purposes. First, the nurse can prepare the patient and family for what the patient will experience during the diagnostic examination and can help them understand the purpose and meaning of the tests and their findings. Second, the nurse can use the results of many of the studies to supplement physical examination findings in determining patient responses to the neurologic problem and the critical-care environment. For example, if the brainstem evoked potential examination shows intact auditory pathways for an unresponsive patient, the nurse can plan to protect the patient from noise or unguarded conversations within the patient's hearing. Table 34-5 shows diagnostic techniques often used in patients with neurologic or neurosurgical disorders.

Laboratory Studies

The most common diagnostic tests are the blood and cerebrospinal fluid analyses used in the differential diagnosis of neurologic disorders. Examination of serum electrolytes helps sort out metabolic from cerebral sources of altered consciousness, for example. Screening of urine and serum for toxic substances helps determine whether unexplained coma results from drug overdose or trauma. The majority of such studies are routine for all patients in critical-care units. Table 34-6 summarizes normal values for constituents of serum and CSF and the major neurologic implications of abnormalities.

Radiologic Studies

Only a few decades ago relatively few radiologic studies were available for diagnosing and following

Table 34-4 Spinal Segment, Stimulus/Site, and Expected Response of Deep Tendon and Superficial Reflexes

Reflex	Spinal Segment	Stimulus/Site	Expected Response Observed	Expected Response Palpated
Biceps	C5, C6	Biceps tendon	Flexion at the elbow	Contraction of biceps
Triceps	C7, C8	Triceps tendon above elbow	Extension at elbow	Contraction of triceps
Brachioradialis or supinator	C5, C6	Radius, 1–2 in above wrist	Flexion and supination of forearm	
Abdominal	T8, T9, T10 (above umbilicus) T10, T11, T12 (below umbilicus)	Abdomen; stroke the four abdominal quadrants toward the umbilicus	Contraction of abdominal muscle, and umbilicus deviates toward stimulus	
Cremasteric	L1, L2	Upper thigh; scratch inner aspect	Testicle elevates on stimulated side; absence of response suggests corticospinal tract lesion at or below L1–L2	
Patellar or knee	L2, L3, L4	Patellar tendon	Extension of knee	Contraction of quadriceps
Achilles or ankle	S1, S2	Achilles tendon	Plantar flexion at ankle	
Plantar	L4, L5, S1, S2	Lateral aspect of sole of foot from heel to ball and curving across ball	Plantar flexion of toes and foot (dorsiflexion of big toe with fanning of other toes— *Babinski response*)	

Table 34-5 Neurodiagnostic Studies Used in Critically Ill Patients

Radiologic Studies
  Skull films
  Spine series including cross-table cervical spine films
  Cranial, spinal bone scan
  Computed tomography: brain and spine
  Magnetic resonance imaging
  Myelogram
  Angiogram
  Radioisotope brain scan
  Positron emission tomography
  Air encephalogram (rare)
Laboratory Studies
  Blood studies: batteries, toxic screen, antibody titers
  Urinalysis, specific gravity

Cerebrospinal fluid analysis
Electrophoresis: blood and CSF
Neurophysiologic Studies
  Electroencephalogram
  Evoked potentials: brainstem, somatosensory, visual
  Electromyogram
Biophysical Studies
  Ultrasound studies: echoencephalogram, carotid imaging
  Oculoplethysmography
  Cerebral blood flow
Surgical Studies
  Lumbar, cisternal puncture
  Trephination
  Intracranial pressure monitoring

Table 34-6 Neurologic Implications of Abnormalities in Serum and CSF

	Average Values*		
	Cerebrospinal Fluid	Serum	Implications
Osmolarity, mosmol/L	295	295	Lethargy, confusion, seizures may be precipitated by hypo- or hyperosmolarity (<200; >350 mO/sm)
Sodium, meq/L	138	138	Low Na may be result of excess parenteral fluid administration or inappropriate ADH secretion; major electrolyte contributing to osmolarity
Potassium, meq/L	2.8	4.1	Cardiac arrhythmias and muscle weakness may occur when K is outside normal range
Calcium, meq/L	2.4	5.2	Tetany with hypocalcemia; weakness and lethargy with hypercalcemia
Magnesium, meq/L	2.7	1.9	Tremor, weakness, tetany with hypomagnesia; weakness and confusion with hypermagnesia
Chloride meq/L	124	101	Decreased in CSF with TB meningitis; decreased Na and Cl in adrenoleukodystrophies
Bicarbonate, meq/L	23	23	Patterns of blood gases, bicarbonate, pH, chloride useful in differentiating metabolic and respiratory acidosis
Carbon dioxide, mmHg	48	38 (arterial)	Lethargy, confusion, tremors with marked hypercarbia; circumoral tingling, numbness of fingers and toes with hypocarbia
Ammonia, mg/dL	30	70	Hyperammonemia found in a variety of inherited metabolic disorders; in Reye's syndrome, hepatic encephalopathy
Urea, mmol/L	4.7	5.4	High in renal failure, uremic encephalopathy
Creatinine, mg/dL	1.1	1.6	High in renal failure; high in some infantile metabolic disorders
Phosphorus, mg/dL	1.6	4.0	High in organophosphate insecticide poisoning; muscle weakness and paralysis
Total lipid, mg/dL	1.25	876	Serum lipids increased in some lipid storage diseases; low serum levels of high-density lipoproteins associated with cerebrovascular disease
Glucose, mg/dL	>45	90	Confusion, coma with hypoglycemia; coma with hyperglycemia and hyperosmolarity; decrease in CSF glucose in bacterial meningitis, TB meningitis
Lactate, meq/L	1.6	1.0	Metabolic acidosis
Total protein, mg/dL	15–50	6.5–8.4	High in CSF with tumor, infection, demyelinating disease, polyneuropathy
Gamma globulin, percent of total	3–12%	18%	CSF proportion elevated in multiple sclerosis, subacute encephalitis, Guillain Barré disease

*Average values from R. D. Adams and M. Victor, *Principles of Neurology*, McGraw-Hill, New York, 1985, p. 13.

neurologic disorders. With the advent of computer technology and very short half-life radioisotopes, the means to investigate both structures and functions of the living nervous system are increasing exponentially.

Examination of Nervous System Structures

The most common radiologic studies to show the structures of the nervous system are *plain films of skull and spine*. A variety of views of the skull and spine are used to detect fractures, in the case of trauma, or bony erosion suggestive of underlying tumors. Skull and spine films are important in ruling out fractures of the face, orbit, and spine in patients who have sustained injuries in motor vehicle accidents or other forms of trauma. Any patient who has sustained a head injury should be assumed to have an associated cervical spine injury until the latter has been ruled out by adequate films of the entire cervical spine. Table 34-7 describes nursing implications of abnormal findings on skull and spine films.

Computed tomography (CT), also known as *computed axial tomography* or *computer-assisted tomography* (CAT), of the brain and spine and *magnetic resonance imaging* (MRI), or *nuclear magnetic resonance* (NMR) are two recent technologies that have revolutionized diagnostic testing in neurologic disorders. Both technologies allow remarkably clear noninvasive visualization of brain and spinal cord structures. In many cases, the ability to see evidence of stroke, tumors, intracranial bleeding, and aneurysms enables the physician to avoid the use of invasive radiologic examinations such as angiograms or myelograms.

Computed tomography uses many thousands of x-ray beams, successively directed at horizontal "slices" of the skull or spine. With the assistance of a computer, the attenuation of the beams by the differing densities of bone, blood, and cerebral (or spinal) gray and white matter is measured and shown as a clear image of the brain (or spinal cord) in horizontal sections. Radiation exposure is approximately the same as that from a plain skull film.

Magnetic resonance imaging is actually a biophysical rather than a true radiographic technique. Rather than using ionizing radiation, MRI uses a powerful magnetic field to provide data for computer imaging of the nervous system. The patient is placed in the magnetic field, and a specific radio frequency pulse is introduced into the field. This pulse causes the hydrogen ion nuclei (protons) of tissue cells to realign their axes. When the radio frequency pulse is removed, the protons return to their original alignment and the changes in radio frequency energy that were absorbed and then emitted by the tissues are analyzed by computer. The image which is constructed is based on the fact that different energies are emitted from different types of CNS tissue.

MRI distinguishes more clearly between gray and white matter and gives better identification of white matter lesions than CT scanning. Images can be made in multiple planes (coronal, axial, and sagittal). In addition, because bone does not produce artifact in MRI, clearer images of posterior fossa and brainstem lesions can be obtained. CT scanning is superior to MRI in detecting trauma, intracranial hemorrhage, and bony abnormalities and in verifying suspected disk herniation. Movement artifact is more serious in MRI than in CT, making CT the method of choice for uncooperative or confused patients.[1,2]

No health hazards have yet been demonstrated from the magnetic field or radiofrequency pulses in persons without implanted magnetic devices.[1] Personnel and patients with magnetic implants such as postoperative clips for hemostasis, aneurysms, and intracranial bypass; cardiac pacemakers; and insulin pumps should not be near the MRI unit since the magnetic field may dislodge or interfere with the function of these devices. Table 34-8 summarizes precautions that must be taken with regard to the magnetic field of the MRI.

While plain x-ray films can be made at the bedside of critically ill patients, CT and MRI scans cannot. Therefore, the critical-care nurse may be directly involved in ensuring continuity of monitoring and care in the radiology department for the neurotrauma patient. CT scanning is much more readily available in almost all centers that have critical-care units and is the imaging technique of choice for suspected hemorrhage or trauma and in uncooperative patients. Transporting the critically ill patient to the scanner requires excellent teamwork among nursing, radiology, and often respiratory therapy personnel in managing portable monitoring equipment, maintaining ventilation during transport, restoring mechanical ventilation in the radiology department, and ensuring optimal therapeutic positioning throughout. It is essential that the critical-care nurse accompany the patient throughout the procedure.

The nurse can prepare patients who are awake for the need to lie as still as possible and should inform them that people will leave the room during

Table 34-7 Nursing Implications of Abnormal Skull and Spine X-rays

Finding	Significant Results	Nursing Implications
Skull X-rays		
Fracture	Elevation, depression	Establish baseline neurological and vital signs; head injury with associated concussion, contusion, or laceration of brain requires frequent monitoring
	Relationship to other structures (e.g., parietal occiputal)	Be alert to signs and symptoms indicating increased intracranial pressure
		Hemorrhage from blood vessels in immediate area possible, e.g., epidural hematoma from parietal fracture along meningeal artery; requires neurological assessment
		Prevent further contamination, infection
		Use loose dressings; do not try to prevent drainage
Calcifications	Tumor (glioma) Old hematoma Pineal body, choroid plexus Degenerative changes Vascular abnormalities Endocrine disorders Systemic diseases	Shifts in pineal body may be first documentation of midline shift caused by mass effect
		Listen for bruits of carotid arteries, and intracranially over eye, temporal bone
Deformities enlarged size, separating sutures	Osteitis deformans Hydrocephalus Tumor growth	Note condition of anterior fontanel; bulging may indicate increased intracranial pressure (normally closed at 18 months)
Erosion of bone	Underlying or invading tumor, e.g., erosion of sella turcica with pituitary tumor	Monitor electrolytes, intake and output, and specific gravity of urine, serum and urine osmolalities, essential in pituitary tumor
		Erosion may cause CSF leaks; check draining fluids (especially clear) for glucose with a Diastix to differentiate from mucous membrane secretions and blood
Spine X-rays		
Fracture	Level of fracture Soft tissue changes Relationship to other structures (e.g., spinal cord, nerve root level)	Immobilize suspect region
		Maintain traction
		Correlate level of injury with clinical findings; look for evidence of ascending deficits
		Take additional precautions during transfer by restricting movement and positioning
		Ensure patient safety and immobilization by safety belts, immobilization, and protecting against drops, bumps, and collisions
Subluxations	Interlocking of facets	Notify physician if patient relates sensation of change in traction, "popping," or cracking (may indicate unlocking of facets)
Congenital abnormalities	E.g., spina bifida	Monitor neurological and vital signs in comparison to baseline findings
Degenerative changes Bony erosions	E.g., arthritis Invading or underlying tumor	Report any tissue or fluid leaks

Source: AANN: *Core Curriculum for Neuroscience Nursing,* vol. 1, pp. 136–137, AANN, Park Ridge, IL, 1984.

Table 34-8 Patient Precautions in MRI Scanning

Information for the patient: The scan takes about 30 to 60 minutes and the patient must lie absolutely still, because movement will interfere with the ability of the computer to receive clear signals from the scanner. All metal objects should be removed prior to the scan (such as watch, rings, clothing with snaps, zippers, metal parts)

Contraindications to MRI scanning
  Inability to lie still
  Metal implants:

Aneurysm vascular clips	Intracranial bypass clips
Orbital prosthesis anchors	Metal ear prostheses
Cardiac pacemakers	Metal cardiac valves
Hemostatic metal clips	TENS units, insulin pumps

  Traumatic metal residuals (such as bullets, shrapnel)
Metals that are not contraindicated:
  Tantalum
  Dental alloys (tooth fillings)
  Many joint prostheses

the scanning period but will be able to see them and all the monitors. Patients having MRI scanning will hear rhythmic knocking sounds as the radio-frequency generator is turned on and off. The sounds may vary from dull to loud, like bongo drums.

Angiography and *myelography* are radiographic techniques that visualize blood vessels and the spinal canal by means of radiopaque contrast media. Their use in detecting tumors or other space-occupying lesions of the CNS has diminished with the advent of CT and MRI scanning. However, they are still valuable and have not yet been replaced in determining the patency of cerebral and spinal vessels, the presence and location of aneurysms, and the presence of obstruction to the cerebrospinal fluid flow. MRI scanning is rapidly gaining favor in detecting spinal disk herniation.[2]

In angiography, the contrast medium (radiopaque dye) is injected into the artery via a percutaneous needle or cannula, and sequential x-ray films are taken as the medium flows through the vessels. Thus, the extracranial and intracranial vessels can be visualized in the arterial, arterial-capillary, and venous phases. Patient risks include an approximate 1 percent chance of vasospasm, embolism, or thrombosis in the territory of the catheterized artery. Allergic reaction to the contrast

medium may occur, as well as hematoma or hemorrhage at the cannula or needle puncture site. Patients often experience an unpleasant sensation of warmth and burning during injection of the medium and may develop headache or nausea. A nursing care plan for cerebral angiography is shown in Table 34-9.

Digital subtraction angiography involves intravenous rather than intraarterial injection of contrast media. Digital computer processing is then used to enhance the x-ray image of the cervical and intracranial vessels. Large volumes of intravenous fluid may be used; thus this examination is contraindicated if there is concomitant cardiac failure.

Myelography involves the injection of radiopaque contrast medium into the spinal subarachnoid space in order to visualize the spinal canal and surrounding spaces. The contrast dye is injected via a spinal needle inserted percutaneously into the lumbar spinal canal. The x-ray table is tilted to move the contrast medium along the subarachnoid space. Water-based contrast (e.g., metrizamide) is lighter than CSF and will tend to move higher in the spinal canal, whereas oil-based contrast (e.g., iophendylate) is heavier than CSF and will move to the lower portion of the canal. Oil-based media are not absorbed and must be removed at the end of the procedure, while water-based media may or may not be removed. If water-based contrast is used and allowed to be absorbed, it may act as an osmotic diuretic because of its large-molecule structure. Seizures may occur if water-based contrast reaches the cranial subarachnoid space.

Radioisotope scanning of brain and cranial or spinal bone is used to visualize tumors, subdural hematomas, inflammatory masses, and some vascular lesions. Radioactive isotopes of technetium are most commonly used and are injected intravenously, with subsequent scanning of brain or bone by a gamma camera. This device detects radioisotope uptake and continuously displays its accumulation and distribution, with photographs taken at intervals. Cerebral or bone lesions that disrupt the blood-brain barrier or are highly vascular will take up more radioisotope than normal tissue. The half-life of the radioisotopes is quite short and the dosage is low; thus the radiation hazard to patient and personnel is minimal. Radiology personnel should follow normal precau-

Table 34-9 Patient Care Plan: After Cerebral Angiography

Patient Problem	Expected Outcome	Management
Circulatory compromise due to hematoma, edema, spasm, thrombosis, embolism, blood loss	Absence of neurological deterioration Absence of seizures Verbalizes changes in sensory function, e.g., temperature, tingling Absence of bleeding, swelling Distal/extremity pulses present Extremity color and temperature WNL Vital signs stable	Record condition of puncture site and distal pulses prior to and following procedure Monitor neuro/vital signs and check distal pulses and site frequently during 48 h postprocedure, e.g., q 15 min × 1 h; q 30 min × 4h; q × 4 h Be aware of changes in patient's agitation LOC (clue to B/P) Check limb size, temperature, sensory level distal to site Check pressure dressing for occlusion of artery, bleeding and swelling Apply ice pack to site immediately postprocedure, 2–4 h Minimize activity level × 24 h Position extremity to relax muscle Avoid flexion at site
Discomfort/pain at puncture site	Minimal discomfort/pain	Apply ice pack to site Position of comfort Medicate as ordered Activity to comfort level after 24 h
Compromise of adjacent structures a. Tracheal compression carotid sinus sensitivity due to carotid puncture	Absence of airway obstruction/stridor Temporal pulse present Absence of bradycardia, syncopes, hypotension	Check temporal pulse, B/P, apical pulse Observe for neck swelling, facial color, trachial deviation, and respiratory effort (stridor)
b. Brachial artery/nerve/plexus compression due to brachial/axillary puncture	Radial pulse present Arm sensation and movement present	Observe for pale, cold, pulseless hands Check radial pulses Position of comfort, usually elevated Check procedural record for sensory changes due to local anesthesia Observe arm sensation and movement
c. Femoral artery/nerve compression due to femoral puncture	Pedal pulse present Leg sensation and movement present Blood pressure stable	Check procedural record for sensory changes due to local anesthesia Measure limb size Check for absence of bleeding into thigh and abdominal cavity Check and record distal pulses Observe for sensory and movement changes Avoid hip flexion
d. Pneumothorax due to subclavian puncture	Absence of respiratory distress Breath sounds present bilaterally	Observe for respiratory distress and changes in respiratory pattern Check breath sounds
e. Spasm/compression due to vertebral artery puncture	Absence of visual deficits	Observe for visual deficits, e.g., cortical blindness, hemianopsia Provide reassurance to patient (event may be transient)
f. Renal failure due to iodine dye, femoral approach	Urinary output at least 30 mL/h	Observe intake and output × 24 h Encourage fluids, e.g., 600 mL x 8 h Adequately hydrate patient preprocedure Check renal function tests If nausea and vomiting persist, request IV therapy

Source: AANN, *Core Curriculum for Neuroscience Nursing*, vol. 1, pp. 155–156, AANN, Park Ridge, IL, 1984.

tions in handling radioactive materials. Nursing personnel in the patient's unit are not at risk for radiation hazard.

Pneumoencephalogram, or the use of air or contrast media to visualize the brain's ventricular system, is rarely performed. Prior to the advent of CT scanning, it was commonly performed to localize mass lesions in the cerebral subarachnoid and ventricular areas, with angiography being used to diagnose mass lesions in the more vascular areas. In both cases, the presence of lesions was inferred from distortion of normal anatomic features. CT scanning allows direct visualization of hemispheric lesions but is not so clear for posterior fossa lesions. The superior ability of MRI to visualize posterior fossa lesions may eliminate the need for pneumoencephalography altogether. The nursing care related to this procedure is well described in Refs. 3 and 4.

Examination of Cerebral Function

In contrast to the preceding radiologic studies, which make it possible to visualize neural structures, *positron emission tomography (PET)* makes it possible to visualize the brain as it is actively working—i.e., the metabolic functioning of various portions of the cerebral hemispheres. Radioactively marked nuclides (tracers) of substances such as oxygen, glucose, nitrogen, and carbon are inhaled or injected. These substances readily cross the blood-brain barrier and are used by metabolically active tissues. They emit positrons, which, when activated by electrons, emit gamma rays. The gamma rays are detected and their intensity measured by a computerized detector. The detector then creates a tomographic image that indicates the areas of highest metabolic activity. The half-life of the nuclides is extremely short; thus there is little exposure of staff or patients to radiation.

Differences in metabolic patterns have been found between normal brains and those of people with such disorders as Alzheimer's disease, schizophrenia, and perhaps Parkinson's disease. PET scanning has also been useful in localizing epileptic foci and in following the course of acute cerebral ischemia.[5,6] PET scanning is still largely a research tool but is quickly becoming a common diagnostic tool at specialized medical centers.

Neurophysiologic Studies

Neurophysiologic studies are based on the existence of electrical properties in functioning neural tissues. The voltage discharged from the firing of motor fibers, cortical neurons, and peripheral nerve fibers is amplified and measured. These values and patterns of electrical activity are then compared with normal patterns to help determine the location of disordered nervous system functioning.

The *electroencephalogram* (EEG) is the oldest and most widely used of the neurophysiologic studies. It is most commonly used to detect seizure activity in the brain and to measure sleep stages. In the critical-care unit, the EEG may be used to monitor status epilepticus and to verify brain death. Portable units can be brought to the bedside for monitoring in the unit. Electrodes are placed on the patient's scalp or, more rarely, subdermally. Movement of eyelids, face, or body will create artifact, and such movement should be noted on the paper recording.

EEG monitoring is increasingly used intraoperatively during a variety of neurosurgical procedures. In cerebral vascular surgery, changes in the EEG pattern provide quick evidence of compromised cortical function and ischemia. Direct recording of the cortex (electrocorticography) is often used in localizing epileptic foci during epilepsy surgery.

Evoked potentials involve computer averaging of the electrical activity evoked in the cerebral cortex and subcortical relay sites by stimulation of sense organs or peripheral nerves. Ordinarily it is not possible to distinguish the neural response to such sensory input from the background brain activity that is seen in the EEG. However, computerized averaging of the signals makes possible the enhancement of such small inputs in order to visualize distinctive waveforms for auditory, visual, and somatosensory stimuli. Normal waveforms that correspond to specific subcortical and cortical structures have been defined, as have the normal latencies (time needed to reach specified sites).[7]

Visual evoked potentials (VEP) are tested by having the patient watch a rapidly changing geometric design while the potentials are recorded from surface electrodes placed on the scalp. Visual potentials are also called *pattern reversal electrical potentials* (PREPs) or *visual evoked responses* (VERs). VERs can be recorded in the unresponsive patient by using a flashing light as the stimulus. This test is used to determine whether lesions are in the visual pathways or the visual cortex.

Auditory evoked potentials (AEPs) are also called *brainstem auditory evoked responses* (BAERs). Multiple click stimuli are presented to each ear via earphones, and the latency and shape of the waveform at the brainstem and cortical levels are evaluated. Brainstem auditory evoked potentials are preserved under anesthesia and in drug overdose and often in traumatic head injury, provided the brainstem auditory pathways are not injured. Although the presence of normal AEPs in a comatose patient does not mean the patient processes information into long-term memory at the cortex, it does mean that the pathways for hearing are intact. AEPs are used in many centers to help localize lesions and in some cases to follow the course of recovery from trauma.

Somatosensory evoked potentials (SEPs or SSEPs) are recorded from the scalp following electrical stimulation of selected peripheral nerves (usually the median, peroneal, or tibial). Once the nerve has been located, subsequent electrical stimulation is very low level and painless. Alterations in normal latency and waveform help differentiate lesions of the peripheral nerves from those of the subcortical and cortical central sensory pathways. SEPs have been found useful in following the course of recovery from spinal cord injury and are often used in helping confirm the diagnosis of multiple sclerosis.[8]

Electromyography (EMG) records the electrical activity of muscle fibers at rest and during movement. This activity can be recorded from groups of muscle fibers by electrodes placed on the surface of the skin. This type of recording is used primarily in biofeedback and relaxation training rather than for differential diagnosis of motor unit diseases. In neurodiagnostic EMG a coaxial needle is inserted into the muscle. The needle acts as an electrode and records the electrical activity of the muscle fiber. Action potentials are observed during muscle contraction, and their shape and firing rate are used to determine the presence or absence of denervation of muscle fibers, myopa-

thies, and myotonias. The frequent moving and reinsertion of the needles makes this a somewhat uncomfortable procedure for the patient.

EMG is also used for nerve conduction studies in diagnosing lesions of peripheral nerves. A peripheral nerve is stimulated electrically, and the time between action potentials at the stimulating and the recording electrodes is determined. The sensation is that of repetitive muscle twitching and sometimes mild electrical shock.

Biophysical Studies

A number of studies that may be conducted in the critical-care unit or during neurosurgery depend upon physical principles such as conduction of sound through tissue and fluid or dispersion of tracers in cerebral circulation.

Ultrasound studies use the principle that sound waves are deflected at different speeds from structures of differing densities. The *echoencephalogram,* or *echogram,* uses this principle to detect displacement of midline cranial structures as an indirect indication of mass lesions in the cranium. The ready availability of CT scanning, which can more specifically identify the location and nature of the mass lesion, has decreased the use of echograms considerably.

Carotid artery imaging by Doppler and B-mode scanners is the most common use of ultrasound in neurologic-neurosurgical patients. Doppler and B-mode scanners emit ultrasound waves, which are reflected off red blood cells, vessel walls, and muscles that surround the vessels. In Doppler scanning, the velocity of blood flow is measured from sound waves reflecting from the red blood cells. Variations in velocity are interpreted as evidence of narrowed or patent arteries. B-mode scanning combines the Doppler estimates of velocity with images created by differing reflection of ultrasound waves from the structures in the neck and the pulsations of the carotid arteries to produce an image of the lumen of vessels during blood flow. Both examinations are noninvasive. A transducer about the size of the head of an electric razor is placed on the patient's neck, over the common carotid artery. The sounds of the pulsating vessel can be clearly heard.

Oculoplethysmography is another noninvasive technique for estimating carotid flow and ultimately cerebral circulation. The ophthalmic artery is supplied by the internal carotid artery, as is the cerebral circulation. The test may be used in the diagnosis of carotid artery disease and in follow-up after carotid endarterectomy. In flow oculoplethysmography, the pulsation from the ophthalmic artery (internal carotid circulation) arriving at the eyes (detected through an eyecup-like device) and at photoelectric detectors on the ears (external carotid circulation) are compared. Any differences are considered evidence of reduced flow. Postprocedure nursing care consists in preventing or detecting corneal abrasion from the eyecup or from rubbing the eyes before the anesthetic eyedrops wear off.

Cerebral blood flow is measured by using the Fick principle to calculate the transit time of a tracer substance. Whole-brain cerebral blood flow is measured by using nitrous oxide as a tracer and measuring the time it takes for a systemic arterial blood sample to appear in the internal jugular venous circulation. Because this method gives only blood flow in the whole brain, rather than flow in different regions of the brain, it is less useful in detecting localized problems than methods of detecting regional cerebral blood flow.

Regional cerebral blood flow is most often measured in centers with large clinical research programs, as it requires elaborate detection equipment. Radioactive isotope tracers are either injected (in the carotid artery or intravenously) or inhaled and detected by external collimeters mounted around the patient's head. The flow in any given region is computed from the rate of clearance of the tracer from the brain region directly under each detector. The direct intracarotid injection gives the most accurate flow, since the radioisotope is exhaled before being recirculated to the brain. Nursing observation for hematoma or evidence of cerebral emboli (see Chapter 35) is essential after measurement of regional cerebral blood flow by direct carotid injection. Intravenous and inhalation techniques are safer and relatively noninvasive, but these procedures disperse the tracer to all body tissues and thus distort the brain clearance curve somewhat.

Surgical Diagnostic Procedures

Craniotomy is the ultimate neurosurgical diagnostic procedure to confirm what has been hypothesized from CT scan, arteriogram, EEG, etc. However, a number of minor surgical procedures may be used in the intensive-care unit to add to the diagnostic testing or to monitor the patient's progress through invasive measurement of physiologic variables.

Lumbar and cisternal puncture are invasive procedures that may be used to obtain cerebrospinal fluid for diagnostic analysis, to inject dye for myelography, to administer antibiotics or antitumor agents directly into the CSF or, more rarely, to measure intracranial pressure. If increased intracranial pressure is suspected, pressure should be measured by one of the cranial methods (see below) rather than by lumbar puncture. In existing intracranial hypertension there is a high risk of brain herniation if fluid is removed from the lumbar space, thereby creating a pressure differential between spinal and cranial cavities. Cisternal puncture is used only by experienced physicians, and only when spinal block makes it necessary to obtain CSF samples above the block or to administer medications intrathecally to the cervical spinal area. The obvious danger of cisternal puncture is inadvertent puncture of the medulla.

The most common site for lumbar puncture is at the L3–L4 vertebral interspace. The cord ends at about L1–L2 and therefore is not likely to be entered. However, in infants and young children the cord may extend to the L3–L4 interspace, so the L4–L5 interspace is recommended in children. Some patients may have a headache following lumbar puncture and will benefit from lying flat after the procedure. Nursing observation to detect brain herniation is imperative for any patient in whom there is concern about intracranial hypertension.

Skull trephination by either twist drill (small-diameter drill bit) or burr hole (larger-diameter drill bit) may be done in patients in whom extradural or subdural bleeding is suspected. While CT scanning allows the neurosurgeon to visualize hemorrhage, the radiologic procedure requires considerable time for transporting the patient and performing the scan. Many neurosurgeons feel that they can alleviate pressure on the brain more quickly by using trephination to locate and remove the clot and then transporting the patient to the operating room for location and cauterization of the bleeding vessels.

Intracranial pressure may be diagnosed and monitored by cannulation of a cerebral ventricle (ventriculostomy) or by recording the pulsations of the dura or subarachnoid space. Intracranial pressure monitoring is discussed in Chaps. 4 and 35.

References

1. Bydder, G. M., Steiner, R. E., Young, I. R., et al. (1982). Clinical NMR imaging of the brain: 140 cases. *American Journal of Roentgenology, 139,* 215.
2. Earnest, F., Baker, H. L., Kispert, D. B., & Laws, E. R. (1984). Magnetic resonance imaging vs. computed tomography: Advantages and disadvantages. *Clinical Neurosurgery, 32,* 540–573.
3. American Association of Neuroscience Nurses. (1984). *Core curriculum for neuroscience nursing* (Vol. 1). Park Ridge, IL: AANN.
4. Snyder, M. (Ed.). (1983). *A guide to neurological and neurosurgical nursing.* New York: Wiley.
5. Phelps, M. E., Schelbert, H. R., & Mazziota, J. C. (1983). Positron computed tomography for studies of myocardial and cerebral function. *Annals of Internal Medicine, 98,* 339–359.
6. Thomas, D. G. T., Gibbs, J. M., & Wise, R. J. S. (1984). Use of positron emission tomography scanning in cerebral ischemia. *Clinical Neurosurgery, 32,* 51–69.
7. Chiappa, K. H., & Ropper, A. H. (1982). Evoked potentials in clinical medicine. *New England Journal of Medicine, 306,* 1140, 1205.
8. Greenberg, R. P., & Ducker, T. B. (1982). Evoked potentials in the clinical neurosciences. *Journal of Neurosurgery, 56,* 1–18.

35

Neurologic Disorders

Pamela H. Mitchell

Neurologic and neurosurgical disorders often present a bewildering array of disease entities to practicing nurses. For the critical-care nurse, the patient presents an ever-present potential for rapid deterioration in neurologic condition. Because the central nervous system regulates all other body systems, neurologic disease and trauma can frequently complicate and initiate multisystem problems. How then, can order be brought to the confusion and mystery that so often surround "neuro" in the minds of most nurses and physicians?

Although the disorders that can affect nervous system functioning are numerous, the mechanisms by which they threaten life, their effects on the human responses that underly multisystem functioning, and their effects on the human responses that affect a person's ability to care for self are reasonably circumscribed. Thus, the concepts that critical-care clinicians must understand to provide informed care for critically ill persons with neurologic dysfunction are relatively few in number.

Therefore, this chapter is organized around two concepts: (1) the common underlying pathophysiologic states that represent major threats to life or to stable multisystem functioning and (2) the categories of human response that accompany those pathophysiologic states. Each of these categories is presented in relation to major diseases or conditions with which patients come to critical-care units.

Neuropathophysiologic States That Threaten Life

Of the numerous disorders that affect the central and peripheral nervous systems, a relatively small number are life-threatening. The three major ways in which these disorders act to threaten life are by disruption of consciousness, disruption of ventilation secondary to loss of movement but not of consciousness, and neurally induced multisystem failure. The clinical problems discussed in this chapter that disrupt consciousness are brain edema and swelling, intracranial hypertension, subarachnoid hemorrhage and cerebral vasospasm, brain herniation syndromes, and seizures and status epilepticus.

Severe motor and sensory dysfunctions that affect ventilation but not consciousness are usually caused by extracerebral disorders that affect the brainstem, spinal cord, peripheral nerves, or motor unit. Examples of such disorders include spinal cord injury, myasthenia gravis, and Guillain-Barré syndrome.

Multisystem failure follows cerebral damage to hypothalamic regulation of autonomic functions or disruption of input to the peripheral sympathetic system. Head injury, spinal cord injury, and meningoencephalitis may result in multisystem failure.

Neuropathophysiologic States That Disrupt Consciousness

Trauma, ischemia, or metabolic or infectious injury to the central nervous system is ultimately translated into a small number of pathophysiologic states that seriously threaten life. Much of the medical and nursing care of patients who are critically ill with neurologic disorders is directed at reversal, stabilization, or symptom management of these pathophysiologic states. Therefore, specific clinical problems, associated nursing diagnoses, and relevant interdependent and independent nursing interventions are discussed for each category of pathophysiologic state.

Clinical problem is used in Carpenito's terminology to mean a physiologic or pathophysiologic disturbance of functioning that is managed collaboratively by nursing and one or more other disciplines (one usually medicine).[1] *Collaborative* or *interdependent interventions* are those which require the protocol or "order" of another discipline to initiate but require considerable nursing judgment to execute. A *nursing diagnosis* is the statement of a health problem or pathophysiologic state for which intervention may be independently managed by nursing. Many current statements of nursing diagnoses applicable to critically ill patients overlap with statements of clinical problems or pathophysiologic states as defined above. These are included and identified when appropriate in this chapter.

Brain Swelling

Brain swelling is a generalized pathophysiologic process that has the potential to disrupt consciousness. Almost any severe insult to the cerebral hemispheres may disrupt vasomotor regulation, cellular metabolism, or the integrity of cell membranes sufficiently to affect the autoregulation of blood flow to the brain or the amount of water in the gray and white matter.[2] *Brain swelling* is a net increase in *any* of the brain fluid compartments (intravascular, intracellular, or extracellular), while *brain edema* is defined as a net increase in the intracellular or extracellular *water content* of the brain.[3,4] The two most common sources of brain swelling are (1) an increase in the intravascular volume, or *hyperemia,* and (2) an increase in extracellular or intracellular water volume, or *edema.*[5]

Brain swelling due to hyperemia is most commonly seen in the first hours following head injury but may also occur in the first hours following craniotomy if manipulation of the cerebral vessels results in vasomotor paralysis. Hyperemic brain swelling thus represents a temporary failure of autoregulation. The term *autoregulation* refers to the ability of the blood vessels to maintain a constant flow to an organ (in this case, the brain) despite considerable fluctuation in systemic blood pressure. Cerebral arterioles continually constrict or dilate in response to fluctuations in blood pressure in order to maintain constant cerebral blood flow. Trauma or surgical manipulation may disrupt this vasomotor stability. The excess fluid in the cerebral cavity is contained entirely within the cerebral vessels and does not represent excess brain water, as in brain edema.

Brain swelling secondary to hyperemia is evident on CT scan as an increase in overall density (blood being read as denser than brain tissue) and is found in as many as 70 to 90 percent of patients with acute head injury.[6–8] Clinically, rapid and massive brain swelling may be manifested as intracranial hypertension (increased intracranial pressure).

A similar process has been seen in the initial hours following experimental spinal cord injury, with initial vasoconstriction and subsequent vasomotor paralysis.[9] The volume of the spinal cord is increased by virtue of an increase in the volume of blood contained in the intramedullary vessels, just as the volume of blood in the cranial vessels increases the overall volume of the cranial cavity. The functional effects of spinal cord swelling are manifested in changes in motor and sensory function rather than changes in consciousness.

As indicated earlier, central nervous system edema is a state reflecting a net increase in the water content of the CNS. The water is found either between neurons (extracellular, interstitial) or within neurons (intracellular). Neural edema has been divided into three classes: vasogenic, cytotoxic, and interstitial (hydrocephalic).[3,10,11]

Vasogenic edema is the most common of the brain edemas and results from disruption of the blood-brain barrier. The barrier between the systemic blood (in capillaries) and brain tissue is formed by the tight junctions of the endothelial cells that line the capillaries. Normally, only water and very small molecules pass through these junctions into the brain interstitial spaces. In brain injury, it is thought that the tight junctions may open, owing to endothelial cell shrinkage, or that cytoplasmic transport of protein molecules across the endothelial cells increases.[3,9] The end result is an increase in water content between cells as the hydrostatic pressure in the capillaries causes fluid to flow passively across the capillary membrane and into the interstitium of the brain. White matter accumulates more of the fluid than gray matter because it is less resistant to flow. Reabsorption takes place primarily via the glial cells of the white matter. The disorders in which vasogenic edema is most commonly seen include trauma, tumors, heavy metal encephalopathies, and infectious processes such as meningitis and abscesses.

Cytotoxic edema is an intracellular process, most commonly seen in disorders in which the intracellular sodium-potassium pump fails. The cell thus loses the ability to maintain an osmotic gradient vis-à-vis the extracellular fluid, and water passively flows into the cell to restore osmotic equilibrium. Astrocytes, which constitute a large percentage of the brain cells in the white matter, are the primary site of cytotoxic edema. In addition, endothelial cells exhibit an increased permeability to water and add a component of vasogenic edema to the picture. Hypoxia, ischemia, Reye's syndrome, hypoosmolality, and a variety of neuronal poisons are all conditions in which cytotoxic edema may occur.

Because edema-based brain swelling reflects an overall increase in water, CT scan will show *decreased* density, since water is seen by the x-rays as less dense than either blood or brain. Most commonly, the area of decreased density surrounds a focal lesion (tumor, hematoma, etc.), but it may also be diffuse.

Interstitial, or hydrocephalic, edema is seen only as a long-term consequence of obstructive hydrocephalus and is not of primary concern in the critical-care setting. It is believed to be due to diffusion of ventricular fluid into the spaces around the cerebral ventricles secondary to the hydrostatic pressure of increasing fluid in the obstructed ventricles.[10]

The net result of either hyperemic brain swelling or brain edema may be intracranial hypertension due to a net increase in the volume of either blood or water in the intracranial cavity. Therefore the associated nursing diagnoses and medical management are discussed later, with that clinical problem. However, it is useful to differentiate the source of the intracranial hypertension as either hyperemia or edema.

Brain swelling due to hyperemia may occur within minutes or hours of injury to the CNS, whereas brain swelling due to edema is a slower process, commonly manifested in 24 to 72 h following trauma or surgery. While both hyperemia and edema may be clinically manifested by changes in level of consciousness or by intracranial hyper-

tension, the time course and CT findings help differentiate the source of the clinical symptoms. This differentiation becomes important in medical therapy, since the treatment of edema involves removing water while the treatment of hyperemia is intended to constrict vessels.

Hyperemia and edema of the spinal cord are believed to contribute to secondary injury by interfering with adequate blood flow to the cord. The associated problems and nursing diagnoses vary with the level of the spinal cord affected and are discussed later with disorders that affect ventilation and multisystem dysfunction.

Intracranial Hypertension

Many textbooks describe signs of transtentorial herniation as if they were also signs of increased intracranial pressure. While rapidly increasing intracranial pressure may cause transtentorial herniation, it need not do so and furthermore cannot do so by itself. The purpose of this section is to separate what is known about increased intracranial pressure from its potentially life-threatening outcome in transtentorial herniation.

Pathophysiology   The neurocranium, or braincase, contains three basic substances—brain tissue, blood, and cerebrospinal fluid—within a nearly inexpandable cranial cavity. Expansion of the volume of any one of these three elements requires adjustment of the volumes of the other two in order to maintain intracranial pressure at a steady level. This principle is known as the Monro-Kellie doctrine. Experimental work with nonhuman primates has demonstrated that there is considerably more compensatory reserve in the intracranial cavity than was previously believed. Up to a point, expansion of any of the three elements can be compensated for by contraction of the other two components of the intracranial space.

When an intracranial mass expands or when cerebrospinal fluid (CSF) flow is blocked and fluid accumulates, some CSF will be expressed from the cranial cavity to accommodate the expanded volume. Intracranial pressure (ICP) remains nearly constant as long as the volume of CSF or intravascular blood displaced is nearly equal to the volume of tissue or fluid added to the cranial compartment. This effect is illustrated in the flat portion of the

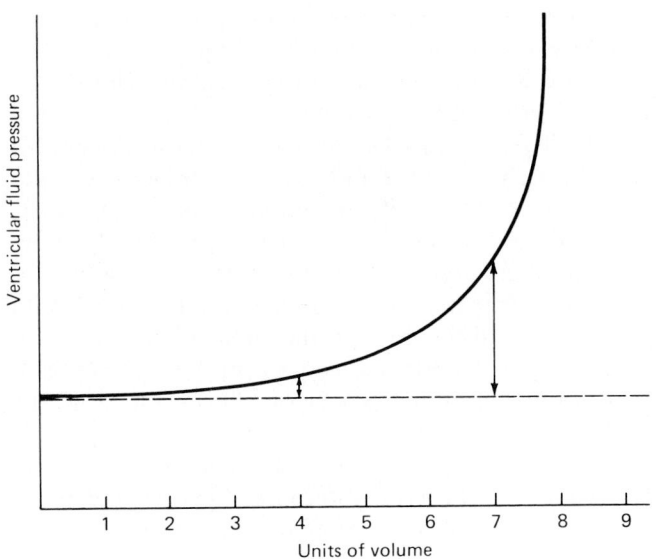

Figure 35-1   Intracranial volume-pressure curve. Note that for the addition of any given unit of volume (abscissa) a markedly different rise in pressure occurs, depending on location (flat or steep portion) on the curve. Thus adding one unit of volume at the second arrow results in nearly four times the increase in pressure from the same volume at the first arrow.

volume-pressure curve shown in Fig. 35-1. In this flat portion, additions to intracranial volume do not result in appreciable changes in pressure.

Displacement of intracranial fluid volume can occur in three ways: decrease in rate of formation of CSF, slight increase in rate of CSF reabsorption, and displacement of CSF into the spinal sac. In slowly growing brain masses, these compensatory mechanisms may be sufficient to maintain nearly normal ICP for some time.

Eventually, however, the limits of volume displacement are reached; volume is added at a rate greater than displacement, and ICP rises. Note on the steep portion of the volume-pressure curve that continued additions to volume result in disproportionately greater rises in pressure. This relation of change in pressure to change in volume ($\Delta P/\Delta V$) is termed *elastance*. Elastance is the inverse of *compliance* ($\Delta V/\Delta P$), a term used to describe pressure-volume relationships in the lung. In the case of intracranial pressure, high elastance (synonymous with low compliance) implies a large change in pressure with a small change in volume. Any disorder which increases brain mass, decreases absorption of CSF, or blocks the flow of CSF increases intracranial pressure. Common examples of these disorders are summarized in Table 35-1.

Increase in Brain Mass   The most obvious example of an increase in brain mass is an intra-cranial tumor. Most tumors are relatively slow-growing and thus increase ICP at relatively slow rates. Generally it is only late in the course of tumor growth that cranial contents are so displaced that ICP rises rapidly. Tumor growth or brain displacement may obstruct CSF pathways and thus create more rapid rise in ICP.

Hemorrhage, either into the brain substance or subdural and epidural layers, acts as a mass lesion. Although the hemorrhage is not brain tissue, the effect is the same as expansion of the brain tissue itself. The growing mass of blood acts as a

Table 35-1   Causes of Intracranial Hypertension

Functional Cause	Examples of Disorders
Increase in brain mass	Hyperemic brain swelling
	Edematous brain swelling
	Cerebral tumor
	Intracranial, extradural, and intradural hemorrhage
Decrease in CSF reabsorption	Subarachnoid hemorrhage
	Meningitis
Blockage of CSF circulation	Cerebral tumor
	Brain herniation
	Chronic hydrocephalus
	Normal-pressure hydrocephalus
	Ventricular tumor

rapidly expanding lesion, creating volume-pressure curves like the classic one shown in Fig. 35-1.

Subdural hematomas are of two types, acute and chronic. Acute subdural hematomas may result from head trauma, bleed relatively rapidly from dural-cortical bridging veins, and result in acute brain herniation. Chronic subdural hematoma is more often associated with lesser or even unremarkable blows to the head, bleeds at a slower rate, and grows more from the coalescence of fibrous membranes and breakdown products of blood. It acts more like a slow-growing tumor in terms of ICP changes.

Head injury per se does not always cause increased ICP. If the trauma results in hematoma, intracranial hemorrhage, significant brain swelling, or alterations in CSF pathways, the result may be increased intracranial pressure. However, a certain percentage of patients have diffuse brain injury with or without intracranial hypertension. This percentage may be as high as 60 to 70 percent of patients in highly specialized neurosurgical critical-care units. The number of patients with diffuse brain injury who do not have increased intracranial pressure varies from 30 to 50 percent, depending upon the level of ICP accepted as the upper limit of normal and the specialized nature of the critical-care unit from which the study comes. Many of these patients are comatose and exhibit signs of brainstem dysfunction attributable to their injury rather than to increased intracranial pressure.[8]

Another cause of increasing brain volume affecting ICP is brain swelling. If the whole brain is hyperemic or if a portion of the brain (for example around a tumor, infarct, or contusion) is rapidly becoming edematous, compensatory volume displacement may be insufficient to maintain normal ICP. Reye's syndrome, a metabolic disorder of children, is a classic example of massive cytotoxic and vasogenic brain edema with concomitant intracranial hypertension. Other examples include hypoxic-ischemic brain edema and edema following massive hemispheric infarction.

Alteration in CSF Absorption and Flow The volume of CSF can increase by three means: increase in production, decrease in absorption, or blockage of flow. Increase in production can occur with tumors of the choroid plexus, which are relatively

rare. In the populations seen in critical care, decrease in absorption and blockage of flow are the most common factors in CSF volume change.

Cerebrospinal fluid is produced in the choroid plexus of the lateral ventricles, flows downward through the third and fourth ventricles, exits the ventricles through the foramen of Magendie, is collected in the cisterns at the base of the brain, and then circulates upward to be reabsorbed over the convexities of the brain. Cerebrospinal fluid also circulates through the subarachnoid space of the spinal cord, passing to and from the basal cisterns. This movement of CSF is shown in Fig. 35-2.

Any disorder which affects the meninges can alter reabsorption. Infections such as meningitis can alter CSF reabsorption by covering the meninges with exudate. More commonly, the breakdown of fibrin and blood products after subarachnoid hemorrhage "coats" the meninges and prevents reabsorption. Since the CSF can still circulate (i.e., the pathways are not blocked) but cannot be reabsorbed, cranial volumes of CSF increase secondary to malabsorption. This condition is called *communicating hydrocephalus.* Up to 20 percent of patients with subarachnoid hemorrhage have communicating hydrocephalus at least temporarily. Only about 10 percent require permanent shunt procedures to control ICP. It has recently been recognized that changes in ICP previously attributed to hydrocephalus may actually be due to a combination of hydrocephalus and vasospasm.

Blockage of CSF pathways produces *noncommunicating hydrocephalus.* The most common blockage of CSF pathways related to brain herniation occurs at the aqueduct of Sylvius (Fig. 35-2). As the brain herniates over the tentorium, the outflow from the third to the fourth ventricle is blocked. Herniation of cerebellar tonsils into the foramen magnum can block the basal cisterns. When elastance is high (when the patient is on the steep part of the volume-pressure curve), even temporary obstruction to CSF flow at the basal cisterns or at the entry to the spinal subarachnoid space may leave sufficient CSF in the cranial cavity to precipitate an increase in ICP.

Increase in Cerebral Blood Volume The volume of blood in the normal brain is regulated in

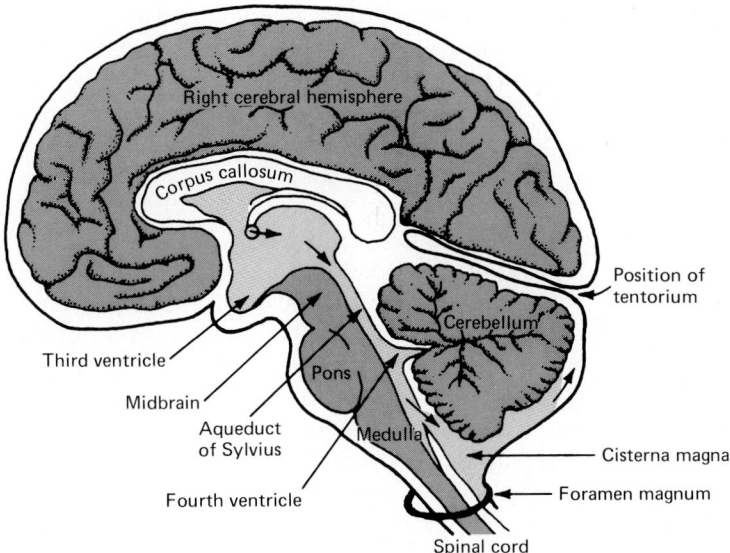

Figure 35-2   Normal flow of cerebrospinal fluid. Cerebrospinal fluid is formed in the choroid plexus and flows caudally through the lateral to fourth ventricles. It exits the ventricular system at the cisterna magna and flows up over the surface of the brain, to be reabsorbed over the convexities. A large portion of the CSF is held in the spinal dural sac as well.

such a way that it is relatively constant despite changes in arterial blood pressure through a fairly wide range (mean arterial pressures from 50 to 170 mmHg). Consequently, in normal circumstances, cerebral blood volume contributes little to ICP. However, in the injured brain and in the brain in which tissue or CSF volumes are already increased, small changes in cerebral blood volume may lead to large changes in ICP.

Causes of altered cerebral blood volume may be (1) vasodilatation, (2) passive transmission of arterial blood pressure if autoregulation is lost, and (3) decrease in venous outflow.

Hyperemic brain swelling is a persistent state of vasodilatation that increases overall blood volume in the brain. Transient dilatation of cerebral resistance vessels occurs markedly with hypercapnia (almost on a millimeter by millimeter basis), with hypoxemia (Pa_{O_2} less than 50 mmHg), and if the patient is exposed to volatile anesthetics such as halothane or nitrous oxide. Arterial pulsations are transmitted to the cerebral cavity most forcibly when mean arterial pressure exceeds 170 mmHg. Such pressures may be reached in normal persons while straining at stool and in the afterphase of the Valsalva maneuver. When intracranial pressure exceeds about 30 mmHg, autoregulation of cerebral blood volume is lost. Then arterial pressure is passively transmitted to the cerebral circulation.

With continuous ICP monitoring at such times, one finds greater amplitude of ICP pulse pressure and more marked arterial waveforms (dicrotic notch). There is evidence that such arterial pulsations produce a "water hammer" effect on brain cells, which may account for the permanent brain damage seen in such conditions as chronic hydrocephalus.

Finally, cerebral blood volume is increased if venous return is obstructed. This can happen with increases in intrathoracic pressure, as during the Valsalva maneuver or during positive end-expiratory pressure (PEEP) in respiratory therapy. Flexion of the neck and extreme head rotation have been demonstrated to obstruct the internal jugular vein and potentially compress basal CSF cisterns.

Measurement of Intracranial Pressure   Intracranial pressure monitoring research has demonstrated repeatedly that the presence of increased ICP cannot be reliably inferred from clinical signs and symptoms. In a patient at risk for intracranial hypertension, the only reliable means to determine whether it exists is to actually measure the ICP continuously.

There are many means of measuring ICP. The oldest and least reliable is single measurement of CSF pressure in the spinal sac during lumbar or cisternal puncture. Not only are single measurements useless in determining ongoing intracranial dynamics, but also any disorder which blocks free flow of CSF from cranial to spinal cavity invalidates the spinal pressure as a reliable estimate of intracranial pressure.

Pioneering work in the 1960s which monitored intraventricular pressure continuously in over 100 patients with space-occupying lesions has led to ICP monitoring becoming commonplace in many critical-care units throughout the world. ICP may be measured by direct cannulation of a cerebral ventricle (usually a lateral ventricle), by pulsations in the subarachnoid space (via a "screw" or "bolt" threaded into the skull), or by pulsations of the dura (epidural transducer). (See Chapter 4.) Pulsations of the CSF or of the meninges are then converted to electrical signals and displayed in graph, computer, or digital format. These three common methods of ICP measurement (ventricular, subarachnoid, and epidural) are highly correlated linearly, although the actual values obtained tend to be lower with epidural recording.

In addition to continuous electronic monitoring, some institutions utilize external ventriculostomy shunts as indices of ICP. An intraventricular cannula is connected to a pressure reservoir external to the patient, and CSF is continuously drained against positive pressure. For example, if the surgeon wishes to maintain ICP at about 10 cmH₂O (about 8 mmHg), the pressure reservoir is set 10 cm above the zero ICP reference point (usually taken at the external auditory meatus). Whenever pressure inside the ventricle reaches or exceeds 10 cmH₂O, CSF drains into the reservoir. A manometer can be set up in such a system for intermittent measurement of ventricular fluid pressure. It must be emphasized that any manometer system must be considered as only an indication of ICP. Manometers damp the rapid oscillations of ICP which are normally seen with heart rate and respiration. At rapid oscillation the pressure measured in a manometer is likely to be falsely low by an undefined amount.

Ideally, ICP is expressed in millimeters of mercury to facilitate calculation of perfusion pressure. It will be recalled that cerebral perfusion pressure (CPP) reflects the mean arterial blood pressure (MABP) minus the mean intracranial pressure (MICP):

$$CPP = MABP - MICP$$

Normal ICP is generally accepted as 0 to 10 mmHg. Miller and colleagues make a strong case for using 10 mmHg as the upper limit of normal.[12] They cite numbers of patients with high elastance whose resting ICP was between 10 and 15 mmHg. In other words, though the resting ICP remained relatively "normal," addition of a small volume of fluid precipitated a marked rise in ICP. ICP values of 20 mmHg and over are uniformly regarded as elevated. Values greater than 40 mmHg are considered markedly elevated. Note that with an ICP of 40 mmHg and an MABP of 90 mmHg, CPP would be only 50 mmHg, barely adequate to sustain neuronal perfusion. Ranges of ICP are shown in Table 35-2. CPP normally ranges from 70 to 90 mmHg, with EEG changes evident experimentally when CPP drops below 45 mmHg.[13] There is increasing clinical evidence that the level of CPP is the best predictor of outcome in severe head injuries and that uniformly poor outcomes are associated with CPP of less than 40 mmHg.[14,15] Most clinicians attempt to maintain a CPP no lower than 50 to 60 mmHg.

Medical Therapy of Intracranial Hypertension
There is no single therapy for intracranial hypertension. The ideal medical therapy would be to remove the cause of the increased ICP. When this cause is a mass lesion or a tumor that blocks CSF flow, such surgical therapy is definitive. Unfortunately, the majority of patients with intracranial hypertension in critical-care settings do not have such lesions. Large series of head injury cases from specialized critical-care settings in several countries indicate that patients with surgically treatable lesions make up 25 to 58 percent of all head-injured patients.[6,12,16,17]

For those patients who do not have surgically remediable lesions, the aim of medical therapy is

Table 35-2 Ranges of Intracranial Pressure (Supratentorial Cavity)

	mmHg	mmH₂O
Normal	0–10	0–136
Possibly elevated	11–15	150–204
Elevated	>15	>200
Moderately elevated	>20	>270
Markedly elevated	>40	>500

to control intracranial hypertension and maintain adequate cerebral perfusion in order to protect the brain from secondary injury. Secondary injury is neuronal ischemia or hypoxia beyond that induced by the primary brain insult. Medical therapies can be categorized as pharmacologic, mechanical, or systemic. These therapies and their proposed mechanisms of function are summarized in Table 35-3. The pharmacologic and mechanical measures used to control ICP have multisystem effects. Consequently, careful attention must be paid to the fluid and electrolye, respiratory, and cardiac status of the patient in whom these therapies are used.

Pharmacologic therapies consist of hyperosmotic agents, steroids, sedatives, and muscle-para-lyzing and anesthetic agents. Hyperosmotic agents such as mannitol and glycerol act to draw fluid out of brain tissue by increasing the osmolality of the blood. Such agents depend upon an intact blood-brain barrier to prevent diffusion of the large molecules into the brain itself. Agents such as urea can cross the blood-brain barrier, equilibrate with brain interstitial fluid, and thus cause a rebound increase in ICP some hours after administration. The lesser ability of mannitol to diffuse across membranes is the factor behind the relatively low incidence of rebound effect in its use.[18] The usual dose is 0.5 to 1.0 g/kg, given as a bolus. The concomitant use of furosemide (Lasix) potentiates the duration of effect of mannitol. Repeated use of

Table 35-3 Medical Therapies Commonly Used in Uncontrolled Intracranial Hypertension

Medical Therapy	Proposed Mechanism	Nursing Responsibility
ICP >20–25 mmHg for >5 min		
Hyperventilation	Vasoconstriction: reduced cerebral vasodilatation and thus cerebral blood volume	Maintain Pa_{CO_2} of 20–25 mmHg; may hyperinflate prior to noxious stimuli
Drain CSF against positive pressure (10–20 cmH$_2$O)	Reduced CSF volume	Maintain positive pressure to avoid ventricular collapse; prevent infection with aseptic technique
Osmotic diuretics (mannitol, sometimes urea, glycerol); loop diuretics (furosemide)	Reduced brain water (may affect CSF formation)	Monitor serum osmolality; do not give if >350 mosmol. Monitor electrolytes, particularly Na and K. Monitor intake and output
ICP Still >20–25 mmHg Despite Above		
Sedation: diazepam (Valium), morphine (dose and combination vary with physician preference)	Reduced response to environmental stimuli; morphine may affect cerebral metabolism	Monitor respiration (sedation depresses rate if patient not receiving controlled ventilation). Monitor blood pressure (BP), maintain normotension. Pupillary response may be constricted by morphine
Muscle paralyzing agents (pancuronium)	Decreased motor response; prevents Valsalva, isometric muscle contractions that increase BP; prevents posturing	Protect patient from assumption that lack of movement means lack of hearing; protect eyes; prevent immobility complications. Careful observation of pupillary changes (dilatation), which may be only sign of seizures, herniation
Anesthetic agents: short-acting barbiturates, lidocaine	Decreased cerebral metabolism. Topical lidocaine reduces cough response to suctioning	Barbiturates: monitor cardiac output, BP, maintain normotension, temperature (therapy induces poikilothermia), output; may monitor EEG; only evidence of seizures is sudden pupillary dilatation. Lidocaine in bolus may induce seizures

mannitol can lead to continuously elevated serum osmolality, with attendant risk of seizures, renal failure, and serious fluid and electrolyte imbalance. Consequently, urine output, serum electrolytes, and osmolality must be monitored frequently in patients receiving mannitol. Serum osmolality should be maintained below 320 mosmol.

Corticosteroids, particularly dexamethasone (Decadron) and methylprednisolone (Solumedrol), are frequently given to control ICP. While the efficacy of corticosteroids on the edema surrounding tumors is well established, there is no similar evidence for the value of corticosteroids in brain edema secondary to head injury. Prospective double-blind studies have not shown any differences in outcome or level of ICP in patients treated with placebo, low-dose steroids, or high-dose steroids.[19-21] Some argue, however, that the high doses used in clinical studies (up to 3.0 mg/kg of dexamethasone) are not high enough to demonstrate the effect seen in laboratory studies.[22] Although steroids are often implicated as the cause of gastrointestinal bleeding in head trauma patients, the incidence of gastrointestinal bleeding, hyperglycemia, and infection has not been demonstrated to be greater in steroid-treated patients than in those given placebo.[19,20,22]

Sedating agents such as morphine sulfate and benzodiazepines (chiefly diazepam) are often given to reduce responsiveness to environmental stimuli and thereby maintain ICP at a more even level. It is also thought that morphine may exert a direct effect on cerebral metabolism and thereby on cerebral blood volume. Muscle-paralyzing agents are intended to reduce decerebrate posturing and other sustained muscle contractions that serve to increase blood pressure and thus increase cerebral blood flow in the nonautoregulating brain. The most common agent used is pancuronium (Pavulon), because of its relatively short duration of action and thus ease of reversal. Because all muscles are paralyzed, including those of respiration, this drug is used only in mechanically ventilated patients. It is crucial to remember that this drug is not a CNS sedative; a patient will *appear* unresponsive because motor output is lost but may be completely aware of what is occurring in the environment.

Anesthetic agents often used in the control of ICP include barbiturates and lidocaine. Barbiturate coma has fluctuating popularity in controlling intracranial hypertension that has been unresponsive to other therapies. Decreased mortality has been shown in some uncontrolled studies in patients with uncontrollable ICP treated with pentobarbital or thiopentone. However, recent controlled studies comparing high-dose barbiturates to similar treatment without barbiturates have not shown any difference in long-term outcome in either head injury or postcardiac arrest.[24-26] A variety of short- and long-acting barbiturates are used, with the aim of maintaining serum levels at about 3 to 5 mg/dL. The mechanism of action in head injury is not clear. Current hypotheses include a direct vasoconstrictive effect on cerebral vessels, reduction of cerebral blood flow secondary to decreased cerebral metabolism, and amelioration of cerebral edema. Barbiturate coma requires complete supportive care of the comatose, ventilated patient. In addition, monitoring of arterial blood pressure, cardiac output, and pulmonary wedge pressure is needed in view of the systemic effects of barbiturates on cardiac output and blood pressure. Hypotension (due to reduced cardiac output) is a serious potential problem with this therapy, since it can compromise CPP.

Lidocaine is often used topically to reduce the ICP response to suctioning and has also been found to reduce ICP over a sustained time when given in intravenous boluses.[27] Like all anesthetics, lidocaine has the potential to induce seizures and depress respirations and cardiac rhythms. Consequently, these parameters must be monitored when lidocaine is used on a prn basis.

Mechanical therapies include the use of hyperventilation and drainage of CSF. Assisted ventilation, with hyperventilation to maintain Pa_{CO_2} at around 20 to 25 mmHg, is commonly used to control ICP. It should be recalled that increases in Pa_{CO_2} act as potent vasodilators and thus increase cerebral blood volume. Conversely, a decrease in Pa_{CO_2}, as in hyperventilation, acts to constrict cerebral vessels.

Continuous or intermittent drainage of CSF is particularly indicated when the cause of intracranial hypertension is increased production or blocked circulation of CSF. It is of little value in hyperemic brain swelling or in edema. Indeed, in such cases, drainage of CSF may lead to ventricular collapse and loss of all opportunity to monitor ventricular fluid pressure. CSF drainage does not change the shape of the volume-pressure curve—i.e., does not change elastance.[28] Absolute pressure can be reduced, thus improving cerebral perfusion pressure temporarily. Drainage against positive pressure is safest to prevent ventricular collapse. Rapid removal of CSF and ventricular collapse can cause the brain to pull away from the dura, rupturing bridging veins and perhaps adding subdural hematoma to the patient's problems.

Systemic support refers to general medical therapies that maintain blood pressure and adequate ventilation. Since cerebral perfusion pressure is clearly the *key* factor in survival and ultimate outcome in patients with severe head injuries, it is critical to maintain adequate systemic blood pressure. In patients with normal CT scans at admission who ultimately develop intracranial hypertension, abnormally low blood pressure is one of the few predictive factors.[8,28,29] Medical therapies for patients with arrhythmias, hypotension, and adult respiratory distress syndrome are discussed in Chaps. 11, 7, and 27, respectively.

Nursing Diagnoses Associated with Intracranial Hypertension   Intracranial hypertension is a clinical problem that coexists with a number of medical diagnoses (Table 35-1). Nursing implementation of the medical therapies described above requires considerable independent knowledge and judgment. For example, when intracranial pressure is rising, the nurse must decide whether to give or withhold mannitol on the basis of knowledge of the osmolality. Management of the blood pressure and prevention of infection are part of the judgment nurses use in caring for patients in barbiturate coma. In addition, nurses have been trying to find a nursing diagnosis that indicates the complexity of the independent nursing judgment and management required in the care of patients with intracranial hypertension.

A number of diagnostic labels have been proposed for nursing diagnoses associated with the clinical problem of intracranial hypertension, including potential for secondary brain injury, de-creased cerebral perfusion pressure, alteration in cerebral tissue perfusion, and decreased intracranial adaptive capacity.[30,31] The diagnosis *decreased intracranial adaptive capacity* is used in this chapter because it can be defined in terms of clinically recognizable indicators and can be managed independently by nurses. Decreased cerebral perfusion pressure is itself an indicator for this diagnosis; altered cerebral tissue perfusion cannot be verified clinically; and potential for secondary brain injury is a clinical problem that encompasses more than just intracranial hypertension.

Decreased intracranial adaptive capacity is caused by the failure of normal intracranial compensatory mechanisms and is manifested by repeated disproportionate increases in ICP in response to a variety of noxious and other stimuli. Thus, the patient with intracranial hypertension whose ICP is increased 5 to 10 mmHg for 3 min or longer with turning, suctioning, or verbal stimuli is manifesting decreased intracranial adaptive capacity. The intracranial system is unable to compensate for the transient increases in cerebral blood volume, systemic blood pressure, or trapped CSF that accompany these activities, and thus ICP increases markedly with small changes in input to the system. Nursing management of patients with this diagnosis has two major goals: to reduce adaptive demand and to increase adaptive capacity. Activities that accomplish these goals are described below.

Not every patient with intracranial hypertension has decreased adaptive capacity, nor is it desirable to wait until those with the diagnosis have marked and potentially harmful increases in ICP with ordinary care activities. Therefore it is useful to identify patients at high risk for the diagnosis and institute nursing management that decreases adaptive demands and increases adaptive capacity.

Patients with any disorder that is associated with intracranial hypertension (Table 35-1) are potentially at risk for decreased intracranial adaptive capacity. Those with CT evidence of hyperemic brain swelling or edema with decreased or absent visualization of ventricles are at even higher risk. In the face of trauma or cerebral disorders that produce brain swelling, the absence of visible ventricles and compression of the basal cisterns both indicate loss of the major intracranial compensatory mechanism—the CSF ventricular and spinal spaces that increase CSF capacity. The presence of hypotension adds to the risk factors.

If ICP is not monitored electronically, it must be assumed that patients with the above risk factors have high potential for both the clinical problem, intracranial hypertension, and the nursing diagnosis, decreased intracranial adaptive capacity. If the patient has an ICP monitor, the clinical problem of intracranial hypertension will be evident, and several pieces of clinical data more easily identify the patient who is at high risk for the nursing diagnosis of decreased intracranial adaptive capacity. These risk factors have been identified from clinical research and include repeated large and sustained increases in ICP in response to a nursing maneuver (>10 mmHg for >3 min), abnormal volumetric challenge response, or any two of the following: ICP >20 mmHg, CPP <30 mmHg, wide-amplitude ICP tracing.[31]

A single disproportionate response to a nursing care activity or environmental demand is somewhat predictive of further such increases.[31] Volumetric challenges may be either a roughly reversible challenge such as brief bilateral compression of the external jugular veins (reduces venous return, thus leaving more blood in the cranial vessels) or controlled addition of a small bolus of saline to the ventricles. A noticeable increase in ICP in response to bilateral compression or an ICP increase that is at least twice the volume of fluid injected is considered abnormal. Volumetric challenges are usually under supervision of the patient's physician and thus provide additional but not integral information related to the nursing diagnosis.

Nursing Management of Decreased Intracranial Adaptive Capacity   As noted earlier, the goals of nursing interventions for the diagnosis, decreased intracranial adaptive capacity, are to reduce adaptive demands (activities that increase cerebral blood volume or CSF volume) and increase adaptive capacity (activities that improve cerebral compliance). Concomitant with these independent activities are those involved in collaboratively managing the medical therapies for the basic clinical problem

of intracranial hypertension. The outlines below summarize nursing care for both the nursing diagnoses and the clinical problems in patients with intracranial hypertension, then further expand on the nursing interventions according to precipitating factor and mechanisms involved.

Nursing Diagnosis
Decreased intracranial adaptive capacity related to inadequate or failure of normal compensatory mechanisms

Defining Characteristics
Repeated disproportionate rises in ICP with environmental stimuli

Clinical Indicator
Repeated sharp increases in ICP with stimuli ($\geq$10 mmHg, $\geq$3 min). Risk factors: ICP $\geq$20 mmHg, CPP <30 mmHg; wide-amplitude ICP trace; high elastance or low compliance

Anticipated Outcome
Absence of sustained (>3-min) increases in ICP following nursing care activities; CPP maintained at >50 mmHg

Goals

1. Reduce demand on intracranial adaptive capacity: space activities, turn slowly, etc.
2. Increase adaptive capacity: position patient's head for maximum venous return, use medical therapies such as sedation or osmotic diuretics prior to known noxious stimuli.

Nursing Interventions
Precipitating activity: Passive or active turning in bed. *Mechanisms:* Decreased venous outflow secondary to head flexion or rotation; increased BP with Valsalva; arousal response:

1. Maintain patient's head and neck in neutral position throughout turn.
2. Use turning sheet or turning bed for exceptionally labile patients.
3. Premedicate with prn sedation or muscle relaxants in labile patients.

Precipitating factor: Decerebrate or decorticate posturing. *Mechanism:* Increased BP secondary to isometric muscle contraction:

1. Use slow, sustained movements.
2. Premedicate with pancuronium or muscle relaxants prior to movement.

Precipating activity: Head rotation or flexion. *Mechanisms:* Decreased venous outflow, possibly transient occlusion of CSF outflow to spinal sac:

1. Maintain patient's head in neutral position with small pillows.
2. Do not allow head to flex during patient positioning.
3. Cervical collar may be useful.

Precipitating factor: Bowel evacuation. *Mechanisms:* Increased intrathoracic pressure and BP secondary to Valsalva; in conscious patients, isometric muscle contractions involved in using bedpan:

1. Prevent constipation: use stool softeners, adequate fluids, prn suppositories.

Precipitating factor: Coughing. *Mechanism:* Increased intrathoracic pressure and BP; stimulated by suctioning, endotracheal tube, PEEP:

1. Firmly secure endotracheal tube to prevent movement in trachea.
2. Minimize suction time (<15 s).
3. Maintain head-up position (15 to 30°) to increase venous outflow.
4. Use lidocaine prn endotracheally prior to suctioning in particularly labile patients; pancuronium may be used also.

Precipitating factor: Sensory stimuli (touch, conversation, noise). *Mechanism:* Possibly increased or decreased ICP; increase may be secondary to arousal or startle response; mechanism of decrease not clear:

1. Approach all patients as if they hear and process sensory stimuli.
2. Warn patient prior to touching; stroke slowly and firmly.
3. Minimize loud noises in environment.
4. Use stimuli that are associated with decreased ICP for the individual patient.

Nursing Diagnosis

Alteration in comfort, headache, related to CSF pulsations and effect of mass lesion on pain-sensitive dural structures

Defining Characteristics

Restlessness, verbalization of head pain

Nursing Interventions

1. Decrease adaptive demands as described above to minimize transient increases.
2. Medicate with nonnarcotic analgesics on regular basis.
3. Maintain patient in head-up position.

Collaborative Clinical Problem

Potential for inadequate cerebral perfusion related to decreased adaptive capacity

Defining Characteristics

CPP ≤50 mmHg even transiently with given environmental stimuli; highest risk in patients with systemic hypotension and intracranial hypertension

Nursing Interventions

1. Monitor ICP and systemic arterial blood pressure (SABP).
2. Reduce demands on intracranial system as above.

Collaborative Clinical Problem

Potential for transtentorial brain herniation related to decreased adaptive capacity

Defining Characteristics

Rapid, persistent increase in ICP despite usual efforts to control, sudden expansion of intracranial mass, evident by CT or ultrasound; highest risk in patients with active intracranial bleeding

Nursing Interventions

1. Monitor ICP and SABP.
2. Monitor for signs of brain herniation (changes in level of consciousness, pupil equality, motor signs).

Nursing activities that represent adaptive demands are those which have been systematically identified as influencing ICP: prone position; turning in bed; endotracheal suctioning; use of bedpan; rapid shift in position; head rotation; conversation about prognosis, pain, and condition; and cumulative nursing care activity, regardless of nature.[31,32] Modifications of nursing care relevant to patients at risk for decreased intracranial adaptive capacity can be inferred from the mechanisms influencing ICP.

Nursing activities which increase cerebral blood volume should be avoided. Any activity which increases systemic arterial pressure may increase cerebral blood volume when autoregulation has failed. In the injured brain, this failure of autoregulation may occur at a point far below the limits in the normal brain. Activities known to increase MABP include coughing, Valsalva maneuver, and isometric muscle contractions. Frequent decerebrate posturing is particularly troublesome in this regard. Any tactile stimulus in the course of care may stimulate such posturing, and pancuronium (Pavulon) or phenothiazines (Thorazine) may be necessary to reduce it.

Cerebral blood volume can also be increased by obstruction to venous outflow. Head rotation obstructs jugular venous return, as does the Valsalva maneuver. Moderate elevation of the head (15 to 30°) improves venous outflow and can be shown to decrease ICP. When patients are turned, special care should be paid to the position of the head to avoid forward, backward, and lateral neck flexion and head rotation.

Prone position probably increases ICP by a combination of both abdominal compression and jugular compression from head rotation. Fortunately, with assisted ventilation and mechanical aids to prevent skin breakdown, the use of the prone position is not crucial for the critically ill patient.

Suctioning can produce hypoxemia, leading to vasodilatation and increased blood pressure related to coughing. Although suctioning is often noted to increase ICP, careful attention to minimizing the suction period (10 to 15 s), use of intermittent suction, and pretreatment with lidocaine can prevent many of the increases seen with uncontrolled suction.[33,34]

Positioning the patient to prevent obstruction of CSF flow is important. While CSF flow obstruction due to a pathologic condition is beyond the control of the nurse, the body position of the patient can create transient obstruction to CSF flow. Head rotation and neck flexion and extension not only obstruct venous outflow but probably briefly obstruct free passage of CSF between cranial and spinal dural sacs. In the patient with high elastance, even small amounts of CSF trapped in the cranial cavity can increase ICP. The supine position is most likely to create forward neck flexion, whereas lateral positions with the head in neutral position allow free flow of CSF into the spinal sac.

The mechanisms underlying increases and decreases in ICP seen with turning the patient in bed are not clear. Obstruction of CSF flow between cranial and spinal sacs, blood pressure waves secondary to rapid movement, and stimulation of decerebrate posturing are among the possibilities. Not all patients have an increase in ICP with turning. Patients with decreased adaptive capacity manifested by response to other maneuvers are at highest risk. Several groups have shown minimal ICP and CPP response to turning in patients with a baseline ICP below 15 mmHg and in those who have no increase with the initial turn in a sequence.[31] Cumulative effects of nursing activities are not demonstrated consistently in nursing studies. It is likely that the patients who demonstrate a cumulative increase in ICP with a series of nursing care activities are those with decreased adaptive capacity, and that such a cumulative increase is not seen with all patients.

Independent nursing interventions are aimed primarily at decreasing adaptive demands by modifying procedures such as turning and suctioning, but some specific activities can be used to increase adaptive capacity. In patients with communicating hydrocephalus, the elevated head position or side-lying position may increase adaptive capacity by improving venous return or CSF flow. Careful timing of medical pharmacologic therapies such as mannitol may increase compliance before a known noxious stimulus occurs and may also increase adaptive capacity. Finally, there is some evidence that interpersonal activities such as stroking and soothing verbal communication reduce ICP, at least in some children. The mechanism is unknown, but it may be speculated that such activities improve intracranial adaptive capacity.

These nursing management measures are designed to minimize or prevent frequent transient increases in ICP in the patient with intracranial hypertension. Despite careful nursing management, it is possible for the intracranial pressure to rise steeply in response to basic pathophysiologic processes. In such cases it is necessary to use the medical protocol to reduce ICP and maintain CPP. Nursing measures should never be substituted for the medical protocol in such situations.

Subarachnoid Hemorrhage and Cerebral Vasospasm

Another pathophysiologic state that is a source of sudden or gradual deterioration in level of consciousness or general neurologic function is cerebral vasospasm following subarachnoid hemorrhage. Subarachnoid hemorrhage may occur spontaneously in persons with uncontrolled hypertension or it may result from head trauma that ruptures cerebral arterioles, particularly in the vertebrobasilar system, or from rupture of saccular aneurysms in the intracranial circulation, particularly in the circle of Willis.

Vasospasm is defined in this context as a narrowing of the arteries of the circle of Willis and its major branches that is verified by angiography. Since angiography is not routinely performed in patients with subarachnoid hemorrhage without neurologic deficit, the true overall incidence is unknown. However, a number of reports are available documenting vasospasm in patients with subarachnoid hemorrhage who develop new neurologic deficits and who have not had fresh bleeding from their aneurysm. These reports suggest that the incidence of neurologic deficit attributable to vasospasm in aneurysm patients ranges from 21 to 50 percent.[35-37] The extent of symptomatic vasospasm in posttraumatic subarachnoid hemorrhage is difficult to determine, because the initial injury often substantially impairs consciousness and neurologic function. Some angiographic series are available, however, and the incidence of angiographic vasospasm has been estimated at 20 percent or more in this population as well.[17]

Cerebral vasospasm is more common following subarachnoid hemorrhage in patients with in-

tracranial hypertension, severe initial neurologic deficits, and large collections of blood in the basilar cisterns on CT scan. The presence of intraventricular hemorrhage is not predictive of vasospasm.[35,37,38] For reasons not yet clearly understood, the presence of blood in the subarachnoid space stimulates intense constriction of cerebral vessels. Over time, this constriction is postulated to result in inadequate cellular respiration of the vessel, a subsequent inflammatory reaction, impairment of the normal regulation of muscle relaxation by Ca^{2+}, swelling of the intima, and endothelial damage. A variety of vasoactive substances, such as serotonin, prostaglandins, and catecholamines, have been postulated to act as initiators of the vasoconstriction. The subsequent intimal swelling is believed to contribute to ischemia by increasing vessel resistance and decreasing blood flow. The end result of sustained vasospasm is reduction of flow to brain cells in the distribution of the involved artery, ischemia, and ultimately cerebral infarction.

Cerebral vasospasm is most likely to occur 4 to 12 days after the subarachnoid hemorrhage and should be suspected in any patient with ruptured aneurysm or head trauma who begins to deteriorate neurologically. A CT scan can quickly rule out fresh bleeding or acute communicating hydrocephalus as the source of new changes in consciousness.

Medical management of subarachnoid hemorrhage from aneurysm varies considerably from region to region. Some neurosurgeons restrict fluid intake, induce systemic hypotension, and delay surgical repair of the aneurysm as long as possible to allow time for reduction of brain swelling, while others operate early to reduce the chance of rerupture of the aneurysm. The antifibrinolytic agent aminocaproic acid (Amicar) is used by some physicians to prevent clot lysis and thus rerupture of the aneurysm while waiting for surgery. While antifibrinolytics have been shown to result in a lower incidence of rebleeding, they are also associated with a higher likelihood of vasospasm and with other complications related to abnormal clotting, such as deep-vein thrombosis and pulmonary embolism.[36] Fluid restrictions, which are often instituted in the belief that they will prevent brain swelling, probably aggravate cerebral ischemia if vasospasm occurs and do little to prevent cerebral edema. Given the current ability to monitor ICP, hemodynamic status, and CPP, most authorities no longer recommend fluid restrictions in neurosurgical patients.[17]

Nursing management in this clinical problem is collaborative with medical management. The clinical problem is the potential for vasospasm and permanent neurologic deficit. The desired outcome is early detection of vasospasm and improvement of cerebral perfusion. Initial action consists of knowledgeable monitoring of clinical status, particularly for subtle changes in level of consciousness and motor or reflex status. A protocol should be in effect that allows for rapid CT scanning to rule out fresh bleeding and institution of hypervolemic and hypertensive therapy. Nursing monitoring of neurologic, hemodynamic, respiratory, and ICP status is crucial in titrating this therapy to the point of neurologic improvement without inducing pulmonary edema.

A number of therapies are aimed at preventing vasospasm or at reducing ischemia if vasospasm has occurred. Calcium channel blockers such as nimodepine and nifedipine are being investigated for their ability to prevent vasospasm.[36,37] Once vasospasm has occurred, hypervolemic and hypertensive therapy is directed at increasing CPP in the hope of improving cerebral microcirculation in the ischemic area. Intracranial pressure is monitored and reduced if necessary via ventricular drainage and osmotic diuresis. Intravascular volume is expanded with intravenous crystalloids and colloids to maintain a pulmonary artery wedge pressure of approximately 18 to 20 mmHg, with recommended hematocrit reading of 30 to 40 percent. If the neurologic status does not improve, controlled hypertension is induced with vasopressors, raising the blood pressure to the level that will effect improvement in neurologic status or until the systolic pressure is in the range of 180 to 200 mmHg. Bradycardia and diuresis may occur reflexly with this regimen and are managed with atropine to maintain the heart rate at 80 to 120 beats per minute.

Brain Herniation Syndromes

Observation for brain herniation syndromes is undoubtedly the most commonly taught neurologic assessment procedure in nursing. Yet the pathophysiology and nature of what the nurse is attempting to prevent are often left unclear. Brain herniation is usually discussed under increased intracranial pressure, without a clear distinction between the two. Syndromes of central and uncal herniation are addressed as if they were one, and cerebellar herniation is rarely described at all. The following presentation is an attempt to clarify the situation. The widely accepted Plum and Posner classification of herniation syndromes is used here to place syndromes in categories by functional anatomy.[39]

Herniation refers to the protrusion of an organ through a natural or accidental opening in the wall of its cavity. In the brain, herniation is the protrusion of a portion of the brain through the openings or linings of the cranial cavity. Although the incisure or notch of the tentorium (Fig. 35-3) is the best known of these natural openings, herniation can also occur under the falx cerebri and through the foramen magnum. Three distinctive syndromes may result: (1) that of cingulate lobe herniation, which involves movement laterally under the falx cerebri; (2) the syndrome of central or uncal transtentorial herniation (through the incisure); and (3) the syndrome of cerebellar hernia-

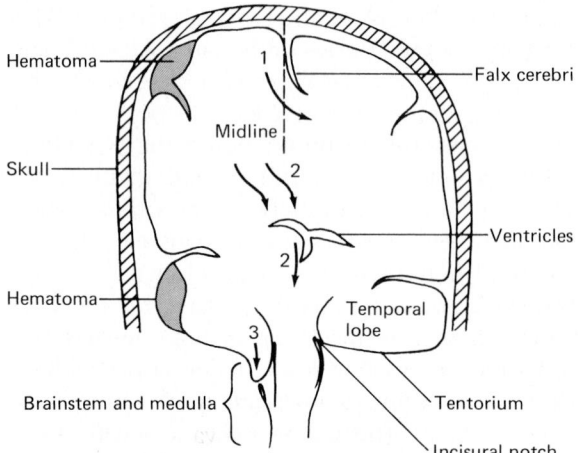

Figure 35-3   Three types of supratentorial herniation. Cingulate herniation (1) occurs when the falx cerebri is displaced. Central herniation (2) is the downward movement of the brain, displacing the ventricles. Uncal herniation (3) involves compression of the midbrain and brainstem by the herniating tip of the temporal lobe. (*After H. Moidel et al., eds., Nursing Care of the Patient with Medical-Surgical Disorders, 2d ed., McGraw-Hill, New York, 1976, p. 866.*)

tion, which takes place either upward through the incisure or downward through the foramen magnum.

Each of these involves displacement of brain through or around openings in the lining of the cranial cavity. Each produces a distinctive syndrome by virtue of displacement, distortion, or necrosis of specific brain tissue.

Transtentorial Herniation   For all practical purposes, cingulate herniation can be considered with transtentorial syndromes, since any condition which creates cingulate herniation is likely to produce transtentorial herniation also. The unifying and essential feature of cingulate-tentorial syndromes is the rostral-caudal, or literally "head-to-tail," nature of their progression. They are caused by any of a variety of expanding mass lesions above the tentorium. Anything which acts as a mass in the relatively closed cranial cavity and which is growing will eventually push aside and distort brain tissue. Eventually, the expanding brain will seek a relief valve by herniating through the few openings available—around the falx, through the tentorium, or through the foramen magnum. The numerous conditions which can lead to an increase in brain mass and brain herniation are listed in Table 35-4. The most obvious is a brain tumor. Similarly, the clot from an intracerebral hemorrhage acts as a mass, and as an expanding one if hemorrhage continues. General or local brain edema also increases the mass of the brain. Trauma, contusions, thrombotic and embolic stroke, hypoxia, and metabolic and infectious processes can create areas of focal or general edema.

While many of the conditions listed in Table 35-4 may lead to increased intracranial pressure, it is important to remember that intracranial hypertension in itself does not inevitably lead to herniation unless the cause of the elevated pressure is also a cause of mass effect (for example, massive brain edema). Herniation may also be secondary to intracranial hypertension if pressure is rising very rapidly or if there are pressure differentials between supratentorial and infratentorial compartments.

Astute observation of changing neurologic function can not only aid in early detection of progressing herniation but also help the experi-

Table 35-4 Symptoms of Brainstem Compression Caused by Brain Herniation

Symptoms	Cause of Brain Herniation
Diminished consciousness; coma (with inability to communicate and to protect airway)	Head injury, e.g. confusion leading to subdural or epidural hematoma; intracranial hemorrhage
Respiratory alkalosis/acidosis from impaired breathing patterns	Cerebral edema from head trauma, tumor, metabolic or fluid-electrolyte disturbance (e.g., Reye's syndrome)
Decerebrate/decorticate rigidity	
Intracranial hypertension (may coexist)	

enced clinician determine the area of brain still functioning. This last is crucial to detecting further deterioration once consciousness has been lost. It is also central to protecting the patient against complications resulting from absent defenses, such as gag and corneal reflexes.

The purposes of assessment in conditions which place the patient at high risk for brain herniation are (1) to detect progressing brain herniation, (2) to determine the level of brain functioning, and (3) to determine the extent of protective care required. Although Chap. 33 provides a review of general neuroanatomy and physiology, pertinent functional neuroanatomy is presented here to aid in understanding how signs and symptoms relate to the brain function impaired. Although all nurses know the general signs of herniation ("neurocheck"), there is frequently an overreliance on signs of brainstem dysfunction (pupils) through failure to appreciate the rostal-caudal nature of herniation.

Because of the widespread influence of the ascending reticular activating system, changes in the level of consciousness are the earliest and often most subtle signs of progressing brain dysfunction. In central and transtentorial herniation, changes in respiratory pattern and motor function closely follow alterations in consciousness. Conjugate eye movements, equal pupil size, and pupil reactivity change when brain function is disrupted at the level of the midbrain (the midbrain is at approximately the same level as the tentorial incisure).

The rostral-caudal pattern of brain herniation generally progresses through five categories of brain function. Inspection of Fig. 35-4 shows that these functions correspond roughly to anatomic levels of the brain. In order to determine whether the patient is getting better or worse and at what level the brain is functioning, the practitioner must routinely evaluate all five categories. The categories of brain function, in descending order, are level of consciousness, motor function, respiratory patterns, eye function (movements and pupillary reaction), and vital signs.

Level of Consciousness   Consciousness, arousability, and orientation to self and environment are governed by the reticular activating system (RAS). This system originates in the brainstem and ascends to influence the cerebral cortex (see Chap. 33). Because it is widespread, disturbances at many levels affect consciousness. Although changes in level of consciousness clearly indicate that brain function is disrupted, knowing the level of disruption requires information from the other assessment parameters, particularly motor function and eye movements. Nevertheless, a change in consciousness is a clear indication that brain function is further disrupted.

Many schemes have been proposed to quantitate consciousness and to construct a terminology consistent among medical centers. Probably the most useful measure is a very simple one, the *Glasgow coma scale*. It was devised to systematically record neurologic function in a multi-institutional study of the outcomes of head injury. In the coma scale, consciousness is evaluated with respect to three kinds of response to stimuli: eye opening, verbal response, and motor response (Table 35-5). A sample assessment record is shown in Fig. 35-5.

The kind of stimulus required and response obtained are rough measures of arousability. If a verbal stimulus does not produce measurable response (eye opening, verbal response, obeying command), a painful stimulus is employed. Points can be assigned to each level of response and a coma score obtained. Provided that instruction is given, a high degree of interrater reliability can be achieved by various levels of staff assessing the same patient. Any change of two points or more on the total coma score is likely to represent a real improvement or deterioration.[40] A number of publications are available for instructing staff on use of the scale.[41–43]

When recorded in conjunction with data regarding respiratory pattern, symmetry and type of motor response, pupillary response, and eye movements, the coma scale allows one to see graphically any progression toward brain herniation and to judge the level at which the brain is functioning. This last not only allows the physician to better diagnose the nature of the disorder causing pro-

Figure 35-4   Categories of brain function that may be affected by brain herniation as it reaches the levels shown. *(Courtesy of George McNeil).*

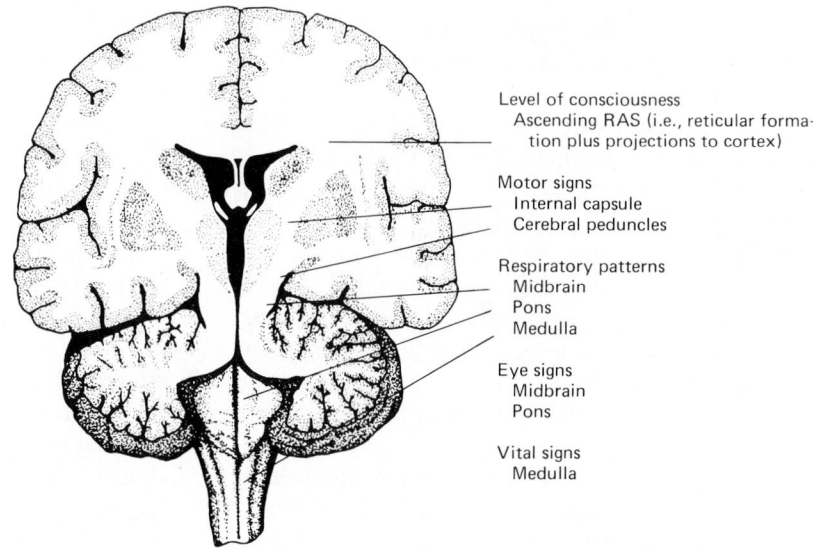

Level of consciousness
  Ascending RAS (i.e., reticular formation plus projections to cortex)

Motor signs
  Internal capsule
  Cerebral peduncles

Respiratory patterns
  Midbrain
  Pons
  Medulla

Eye signs
  Midbrain
  Pons

Vital signs
  Medulla

Table 35-5 Glasgow Coma Scale

Category of Response	Appropriate Stimulus	Response	Score
Eyes open	Approach to the bedside	*Spontaneous*	4
	Verbal command	*To speech.* Eyes open to name or to command	3
	Pain (pressure on the proximal nail bed)*	*To pain.* Does not open eyes to previous stimuli but does to pain	2
		None. Does not open eyes to any stimulus	1
Best verbal response	Maximum arousal. Painful stimulus may be needed	*Oriented.* Converses; knows who he or she is and where, year and month	
		Confused. Converses but disoriented in one or more spheres	4
		Inappropriate words. Without sustained conversation; words disorganized or inappropriate (for example, cursing)	3
		Incomprehensible. Makes sounds (moaning, for example) but no recognizable words	2
		None. No sound even with painful stimuli	1
Best motor response	Verbal command (for example: "Raise your arm; hold up two fingers")	*Obeys command*	6
	Pain (pressure on proximal nail bed)	*Localizes pain.* Does not obey but "finds" offending stimulus and attempts to remove it	5
		Flexion-withdrawal.† Flexes arm in response to pain, without abnormal flexion posture	
		Abnormal flexion. Flexes arm at elbow and pronates, making a fist	3
		Abnormal extension. Extends arm at elbow, usually adducts and internally rotates arm at shoulder	2
		None	1

*Produces least interrater variability.
†Added to the original scale by many centers.

gressive brain dysfunction but also allows the nurse and physician to recognize early the need to protect functions dependent upon brainstem reflexes such as coughing, gagging, and swallowing.

Motor Function Evaluation of motor response brought the most consistent ratings in testing the reliability of the Glasgow coma scale. However, best motor response to stimulation is only one aspect of motor function which must be considered in determining whether brain function is worsening.

Motor function should be evaluated serially and systematically in relation to the following areas: type of response to verbal or painful stimuli, tone and strength, symmetry of response, and presence of pathologic reflexes.

The ability to obey a command to perform a motor act is one measure of how well consciousness and voluntary movement are integrated. Impairment of consciousness (operationally defined as inability to follow a motor command) requires use of a painful stimulus. A variety of painful stimuli are employed to elicit motor response, but the

Neurological Assessment Record

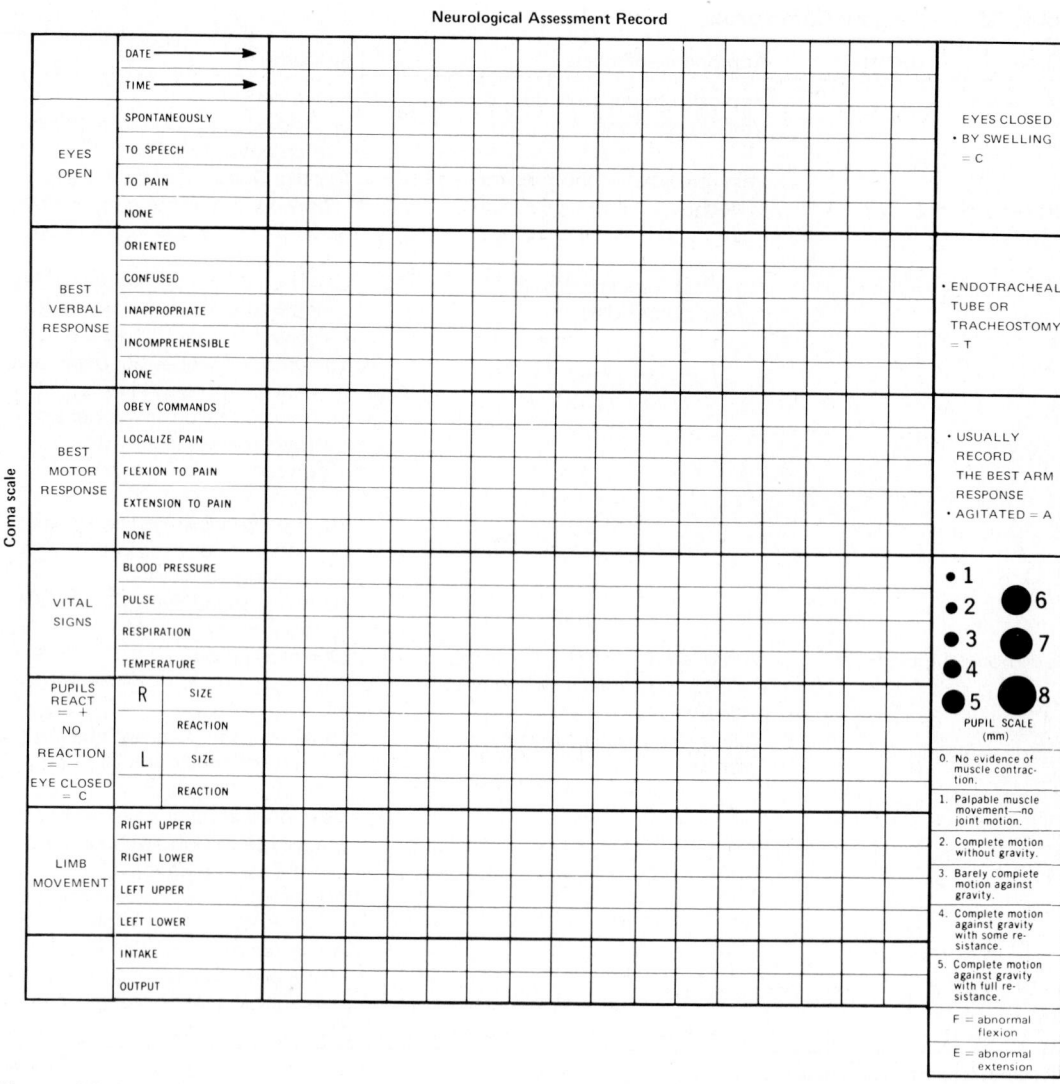

Figure 35-5 Neurologic assessment record employing the Glasgow coma scale (reduced from original size). A suggested operational definition of coma is a score of 7 or less (no eye opening, no comprehensible verbal response, no motor response to command). Dysphasic patients cannot be scored on the verbal section; a note is made on the observation record of dysphasia or mechanical impediment to speech, such as endotracheal tube or tracheostomy.

Glasgow group found pressure applied to the proximal nail bed to provide the most reproducible motor response.

A number of terms have evolved to describe motor response, some related to the "appropriateness" of response to pain, others to the presumed anatomic deficit causing abnormal reflex response (for example, *decerebrate* and *decorticate*). Such terms are open to a range of subjective interpretation and are not as helpful in identifying a rostral-caudal pattern of deterioration as the operationally defined responses of the Glasgow coma scale. The coma scale defines "best" motor response in relation to consciousness per se. Response on both sides of the body (symmetry of response) must also be compared.

The type of stimulus applied (verbal, then painful if there is no response to verbal) and the nature of the response are noted. At the highest level of integration, the patient follows a verbal command, for example, "Hold out both arms." With some impairment of consciousness, a painful stimulus may need to be applied. If there are functioning motor tracts (corticospinal and corticobulbar), the patient will attempt to remove the painful stimulus. Pathologic motor responses are evident in flexion and extension at the elbow in response to painful stimuli. These responses imply functional disconnection of the inhibiting influences of the cerebral cortex on motor tract synapses deep in the hemisphere and midbrain. Appearance of these abnormal postural reflexes spontaneously or in response to pain indicate that transtentorial herniation is impending or may already have occurred. *Decerebrate* and *decorticate posture* (or simply *posturing*) are terms commonly used in reference to these pathologic postural reflexes.

The appearance of an extensor plantar reflex (Babinski sign) implies dysfunction of the corticospinal tract anywhere from the cortex to the anterior horn cell in the spinal cord. While the appearance of this abnormal reflex does not help localize the dysfunction, it does indicate deterioration of brain function in the patient at risk for herniation.

Strength and tone of muscles must be evaluated in conjunction with type of motor response. Motor fibers are fairly widely distributed at the cortex but converge into a relatively tight bundle deep in the hemisphere. Because fibers from the upper extremities are lateral in the corticospinal bundle until they reach the internal capsule, pressure from an expanding hemispheric lesion may cause subtle weakness before consciousness is markedly impaired. Such weakness tends to affect the proximal rather than distal muscles of the upper extremity. Thus simply testing strength of hand grip may not detect early onset of weakness. Pronator drift is a subtle early sign of proximal weakness. It can be noted by asking the patient to hold out both arms with palms up (thus simultaneously testing ability to obey commands). If drift (and therefore proximal weakness) is present, the affected arm drifts downward slightly, with the wrist and hand pronating. Such a finding implies dysfunction of motor tracts in the opposite hemisphere. If the patient cannot follow commands, both arms may be lifted simultaneously and then dropped. The weaker one will fall to the bed more rapidly. Absence of spontaneous movement on one side of the body also implies disruption of motor tracts in the opposite hemisphere.

Weakness or paralysis may become bilateral when herniation has progressed to the midbrain level for anatomic reasons. The cerebral peduncles, which carry corticospinal tract fibers, join the brainstem at the midbrain. The fibers course downward in the lateral aspects of the brainstem before they cross in the pyramid of the medulla and continue down the spinal cord to innervate the side of the body opposite to the hemisphere in which they arose.

An expanding mass which has distorted tissue sufficiently may push the midbrain across the midline, compressing structures between the midbrain and the tentorium on the side opposite the expanding mass. This will be disclosed by the appearance of bilateral decerebrate posturing and ocular abnormalities in a patient who has previously had unilateral signs. If herniation cannot be reversed at this point in adults, it is likely to be irreversible.

Abnormal postural and cutaneous reflexes may become bilateral with distortion of the brain higher in the hemispheres. The level of brain function cannot be identified and subsequent irreversibility of herniations estimated from signs of a single system alone. Table 35-6 summarizes the constellation of findings at three levels of brain function and the implications for reversibility.

Respiratory Patterns Plum and Posner carefully documented the correlations between patterns of respiration and level of brain function.[39] These are useful in detecting decrease in level of brain function with brain herniation (Fig. 35-6).

Cheyne-Stokes respiration is characterized by a pattern of crescendo-decrescendo breathing followed by apnea. This pattern represents disturbance of deep-hemispheric function bilaterally and is differentiated from periodic apnea of brainstem origin by the regularity of the hyperpneic-apneic pattern. Cheyne-Stokes breathing occurs physiologically because of abnormally increased central ventilatory response to carbon dioxide (hyperpneic

Table 35-6 Transtentorial Herniation Syndromes at Various Brain Levels

Cortex, Hemisphere: Signs of Early Brain Shift*	Diencephalon: Signs of Later Brain Shift†	Midbrain: Signs of Herniation‡
Subtle changes in consciousness: Increased stimulus required to elicit eye opening, verbal response Ability to follow commands usually intact	Decreased consciousness: Painful stimulus required for arousal Does not follow commands	Unresponsive to verbal stimuli Abnormal posturing to painful stimuli
Motor changes: Unilateral pronator drift Gegenhalten (increased tone) may be present	Motor changes (usually unilateral): Increased tone May be hemiplegic; may show motor change ipsilateral to lesion if brain has shifted across midline	Abnormal motor posturing Flexor/extensor posturing May show motor change
Eye signs: Pupils equal, reactive to light, and accommodation (PERLA) intact; extraocular movements (EOM) intact Respirations unremarkable	Eye signs: PERLA and EOM intact to "doll's eye" maneuver Spontaneous "roving" disconjugate gaze may occur Respirations may be Cheyne-Stokes or hyperventilatory	Eye signs: Pupils unequal, unresponsive to light unilaterally or bilaterally Loss of oculocephalic reflex unilaterally or bilaterally Respirations hyperventilatory

*Reversible if mass lesion can be treated.
†Reversible.
‡May be reversible if herniation does not proceed to pons.

phase). The hyperventilation reduces arterial carbon dioxide to the point where breathing is no longer stimulated and apnea results. Arterial partial pressure of carbon dioxide, building during apnea, finally exceeds the respiratory stimulation threshold and restarts the oscillating cycle. The overreaction involved in this control of breathing has been compared to the overcompensation of the drunk

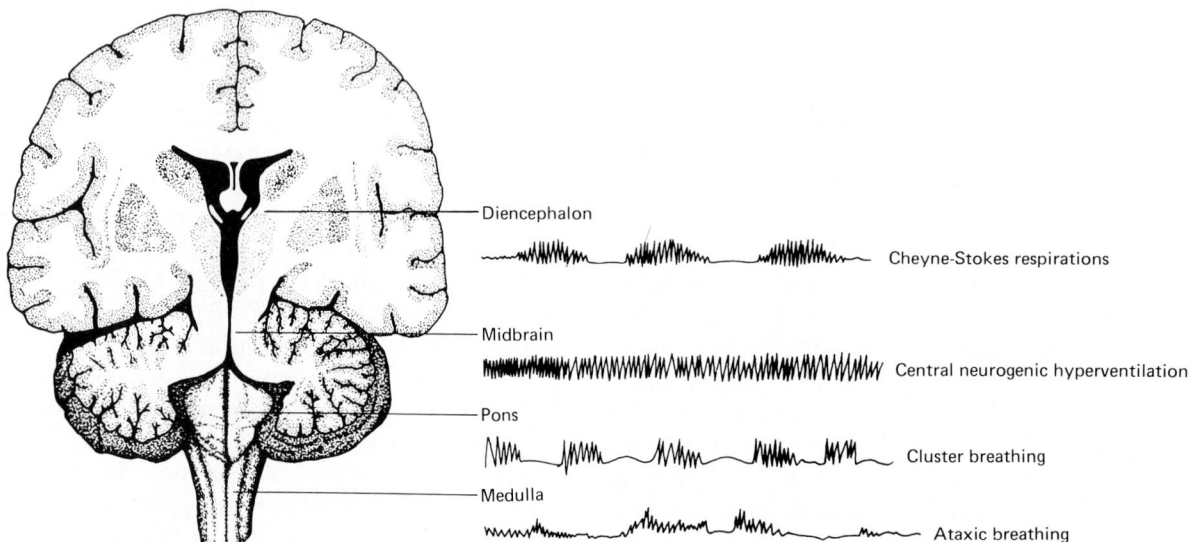

Diencephalon — Cheyne-Stokes respirations

Midbrain — Central neurogenic hyperventilation

Pons — Cluster breathing

Medulla — Ataxic breathing

Figure 35-6   Respiratory patterns correlated with brain function level. As the influence of higher areas is removed through ischemia or compression, characteristic breathing patterns are found. *(After Plum and Posner).*[39]

driver for the normal variations of movement of the car.

Metabolic disorders usually affect all parts of the nervous system equally and are the most common cause of the bilateral hemisphere dysfunction manifested by Cheyne-Stokes respiration. Such respiration is also seen in patients with bilateral cerebral infarct or hypertensive encephalopathy (implying bilateral lesions) and during non-REM sleep in some persons with chronic respiratory disease and some with prolonged circulation time (cardiac failure). However, the appearance of Cheyne-Stokes respiration in a patient at risk for transtentorial herniation signals deteriorating brain function and imminent herniation. Because the appearance of this pattern seems to require bilateral dysfunction of the internal capsules, simultaneous changes in motor functions would be expected.

The manner in which a focal mass lesion can cause bilateral deep hemisphere dysfunction leading to Cheyne-Stokes respiration can be inferred from Fig. 35-3. Expansion of the right hemisphere lesion and surrounding edema may initially compress structures in that hemisphere and produce focal findings on the opposite side of the body. Further expansion leads to additional swelling and eventually movement of brain tissue from one hemisphere across the midline with subsequent downward displacement of structures in both hemispheres.

Other abnormal breathing patterns occur with brainstem and medullary dysfunction. These patterns are useful in determining whether neurologic status is deteriorating or improving once consciousness is lost. They must be used along with other signs of midbrain and brainstem functioning.

Central neurogenic hyperventilation is a pattern of deep, regular, and rapid hyperpnea. It occurs with dysfunction of the *tegmentum,* or central portion of the brainstem, usually between the lower midbrain and pons. Since arterial oxygen tension is normal in patients with "true" central neurogenic hyperventilation, the physiologic explanation must be an abnormally low threshold for stimulation by carbon dioxide.

Pontine-medullary breathing patterns include *ataxic* breathing (sometimes called *Biot's respiration*) and *cluster* breathing (Fig. 35-6). Both are forms of periodic breathing, with frequent periods of apnea. Reciprocal firing of inspiratory and expiratory neurons in the medulla is impaired. Since the medulla is well below the tentorium, such patterns occur only in well-established herniation and portend a poor prognosis. Posterior fossa lesions which create herniation of brainstem and posterior fossa contents *upward* through the tentorium may produce ataxic breathing. Rapidly expanding posterior fossa lesions leading to herniation of cerebellar tonsils into the foramen magnum are more likely to produce respiratory arrest. Posterior fossa lesions include those of the cerebellum, the fourth ventricle, and the area where the cerebellar fibers join the pons.

Eye Signs Pupillary reaction and ocular motility are important clues to the state of brain structures at the level of the tentorium. The IIId cranial nerve controls pupillary reactivity and elevation of the eyelid. Its nucleus is in the midbrain. The nerve itself courses between the posterior cerebral and superior cerebellar arteries and passes out of the brainstem through the incisure. Consequently, pressure from a herniating temporal lobe can produce unilateral pupillary dilatation and/or ptosis before the midbrain is compressed sufficiently to alter ocular motility. The parasympathetic fibers of cranial nerve III are in the outermost portion of the nerve bundle. Paralysis of these parasympathetically mediated functions (pupillary constriction and eyelid elevation) follows compression of the nerve against the incisure or the posterior cerebral artery. The appearance of unilateral pupillary dilatation in a patient with head trauma or suspected mass lesion is a definitive sign that herniation is occurring and constitutes a neurosurgical emergency. In patients who are in therapeutic barbiturate coma or paralyzed with pancuronium, pupillary dilatation will be the *only* sign of herniation.

The pupillary light reflex is mediated by parasympathetic fibers which constrict the pupil when light stimulates the optic nerve. The reflex can be interrupted by structural damage at several points. The points include the optic nerve, diencephalic nuclei (pretectal), midbrain nuclei (Edinger-Westphal), the IIId cranial nerve itself, and the ciliary ganglion (just dorsal to the eye). In tentorial herniation, damage to the IIId cranial nerve at the incisure or compression of the midbrain are the most likely reasons pupils lose their reactivity to light. Preservation of the light reflex in coma is an important clue that the cause is metabolic (for example, drug overdose or uremia) rather than structural. A strong light and magnifying glass may be necessary to determine with certainty that the pupillary light reflex is or is not present.

Ocular motility is controlled by brainstem structures. Thus eye movements provide important clues to the level at which the brain is functioning. When consciousness is depressed, changes in eye movements may provide the only clues that brain function is deteriorating because of transtentorial herniation. Symmetry of eye movements and presence or absence of oculocephalic reflexes are evaluated; these eye movements not only provide clues as to the level of brain functioning but also yield information regarding the patient's ability to protect the airway and vital functions such as respiration.

Eye movement is controlled by cranial nerves III, IV, and VI. Even in the unconscious patient, in whom voluntary control of eye movement cannot be tested, there may be spontaneous roving eye movement. In general, if brainstem function is intact, these eye movements will be conjugate and full, indicating that all three of the cranial nerves are functioning. Cranial nerve III controls all eye movement except lateral movement and downward movement when the orbit is rotated internally. (In patients lacking voluntary control the function of the IVth cranial nerve can rarely be observed.) Although the IIId cranial nerve is the same nerve which controls pupillary constriction and eyelid elevation, changes involving movement of the eye are apt to occur later than those controlling pupils and eyelid elevation. Consequently, changes in pupil size may be observed before the onset of disconjugate gaze. Although disconjugate gaze is evidence of abnormally functioning brainstem structures, in the comatose patient it cannot help localize damage; instead, the oculocephalic reflex is employed.

The oculocephalic reflex, commonly referred to as *doll's eye phenomenon,* is mediated afferently by the VIIIth cranial nerve and efferently by the IIId and VIth cranial nerves. This reflex may be tested by rapidly rotating the head to one side and observing the eye movements. If the reflex is intact, when the head is rotated the eyes appear to remain in the initial position and then slowly turn in the direction to which the head is rotated. If the reflex is not intact, the eyes move with the head as though fixed in place (see Chap. 34 for demonstration of the reflex).

The term *doll's-eye* refers to old-fashioned dolls with eyes mounted on a swivel. When the head of such a doll is rotated, the eyes do not rotate immediately with the head; hence the term *doll's eyes present.* In modern dolls the eyes are not mounted on a swivel, and the eyes rotate as the doll's head is turned. This eye movement is equivalent to what clinicians mean by *doll's eyes absent.*

The oculocephalic reflex is elicited by head movement that moves fluid in the semicircular canal, stimulating the vestibular portion of the VIIIth cranial nerve. The vestibular impulses pass through the brainstem to the nuclei of the IIId and VIth cranial nerves, thus eliciting the eye movement seen. The neural connections are shown in Fig. 35-7. The reflex is present in all persons with intact brainstems during sleep. In an awake person the reflex cannot be elicited because the eyes will be fixed upon objects and the reflex overcome. In altered states of consciousness the presence of the reflex indicates that the brainstem function is intact between cranial nerves VIII and III.

The oculovestibular reflex is mediated by the same set of cranial nerves. It is stimulated directly by irrigation of the ear with either hot or cold fluid, a procedure commonly called *caloric stimulation.* Although the two reflexes utilize the same afferent

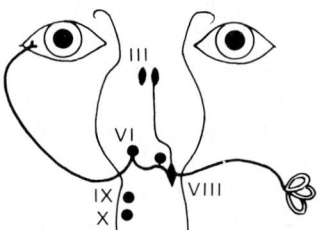

Figure 35-7 Protective reflexes: anatomic relation of ocular movements (cranial nerves III and VI) to swallow, gag, and cough reflexes (cranial nerves IX and X). Cranial nerve VIII is the afferent limb of the oculocephalic reflex.

and efferent pathways, the oculovestibular reflex is preserved somewhat longer in brain dysfunction than the oculocephalic reflex. Thus when the oculocephalic reflex is absent, the physician may wish to use caloric stimulation to determine whether the reflex pathway has indeed been lost.

Testing the oculocephalic and oculovestibular reflexes appears to have prognostic value for comatose patients who have suffered structural brain damage and for patients who have suffered metabolic brain damage other than barbiturate overdosage. In large studies of brain-injured patients and patients in metabolic coma, investigators found that the absence of oculovestibular reflexes for periods longer than 24 h correlated strongly with either death or vegetative existence.[17,44] It must be emphasized that this correlation does not apply to patients with a drug overdose, particularly barbiturate overdose. These substances depress the entire central nervous system but do not appear to cause irreversible metabolic damage. Thus the absence of oculovestibular reflexes in these patients does not in itself imply a poor prognosis.

Tests of eye movement symmetry and oculocephalic reflexes have two major uses by critical-care nurses: (1) to detect further rostral-caudal deterioration in patients who have lost consciousness and (2) to determine the need for protective care of the airway.

In the patient who is already unresponsive to verbal and painful stimuli, the appearance of disconjugate eye movements or the change from present to absent oculocephalic reflexes indicates that the brain is functioning at a lower anatomic level than before. Cranial nerves III and VI are at the level of the tentorium, and VIII is nearly at the level of the medulla. Consequently, disappearance of oculocephalic reflexes or a sudden asymmetry of eye movement in response to head rotation indicates that brainstem function is seriously compromised and that tentorial herniation is occurring. Furthermore, it warns that the airway is in imminent danger. As shown in Fig. 35-7, cranial nerves IX and X are innervated just caudal to cranial nerve VIII. These cranial nerves are important in the cough and gag reflexes. Thus impairment of intrinsic airway protection is predicted by loss of brain function just rostral to the pons. The absence of oculocephalic reflexes or change in their function thus indicates the need for endotracheal intubation and for particular attention to suctioning and pooling of secretions in the patient's airway.

Vital Signs   Vital signs—blood pressure, pulse, respiratory rate—are frequently listed among high-priority observations in the critically ill neurologic patient. However, as Fig. 35-4 clearly indicates, the structures which mediate these functions are low in the brainstem and the medulla. Consequently, sustained major change in these functions occurs late in the process of transtentorial herniation. Reliance upon changes in vital signs to *detect* impending herniation is unwise, because these changes occur too late to protect the patient and prevent herniation. Fluctuating vital signs may well reflect fluctuating levels of intracranial pressure.

Blood pressure is mediated at a reflex level in the medulla. Although the classic Cushing triad is often referred to as a sign of increasing intracranial pressure and/or impending transtentorial herniation, it really is a sign of imminent death. The classic triad consists of increasing systolic blood pressure, decreasing diastolic blood pressure, and bradycardia. The mechanism for this triad of symptoms appears to be ischemia and pressure upon medullary brain structures. Although there may well be gradual increases in systolic blood pressure in patients with herniation and fluctuating periods of bradycardia, the presence of the triad is the terminal event in both experimental and clinical studies of the phenomenon. Waiting for the triad to appear before doing anything is waiting much too long! As indicated earlier in this chapter, respiratory patterns can provide clues to the level of brain still functioning, but absolute respiratory rate is both notoriously inaccurate and not particularly helpful.

Uncal Herniation   Herniation of the *uncus,* or medial portion of the temporal lobe, may occur in connection with central herniation or by itself with intracranial or epidural lesions of the temporal lobe (Fig. 35-3). Epidural hematoma from a lacerated middle meningeal artery often produces classic uncal herniation, whereas a unilateral intracerebral hematoma may produce a combined central-uncal herniation as the expanding hemisphere pushes the uncus over the tentorial incisure.

The major difference in clinical presentation of central and uncal syndromes is the point at which pupillary changes occur relative to change in consciousness and movement. Because the uncus is at the level of the tentorium, pure uncal herniation may present with rapid changes in motor function and pupillary equality nearly simultaneous with deterioration of consciousness. Although differentiating the type of syndrome is not critical to evaluating impending herniation, the nurse should be alert to patients particularly at risk for the uncal syndrome and be prepared to mobilize neurosurgical help immediately upon change in neurologic status. Such patients include those with linear skull fractures of the temporal bone (high risk of lacerating the middle meningeal artery) and those postcraniotomy patients who have had temporal lobe surgery, with subsequent risk of postoperative localized edema.

Cerebellar Herniation Not only can the brain be displaced downward through the tentorial incisure but also, as already mentioned, the contents of the posterior fossa can herniate upward through the incisure. The posterior fossa contains largely the cerebellum, the nerve trunks connecting the cerebellum to the pons, and the cranial nerves which exit the brainstem at the pons. Downward displacement drives the structures toward the foramen magnum. Abrupt herniation into the foramen magnum impinges upon the medulla and is fatal.

Because the cerebellum lies just posterior to pontine-medullary structures mediating respiration, expansion of posterior fossa contents may be heralded by ataxic respirations or apnea. Upward herniation of posterior fossa contents may compress the brainstem at the midbrain, thus impairing consciousness, pupillary reflexes, and eye movements. Pupils are likely to be constricted and nonreactive because of compression of ocular sympathetic pathways as they pass through the pons as well as compression of parasympathetic fibers of the IIId cranial nerve itself. The upward-herniating subtentorial brain accounts for direct compression of the IIId cranial nerve.

Patients at high risk for acute upward herniation are those with potential *rapidly* expanding lesions: cerebellar hemorrhage and occipital skull fracture with attendant risk of epidural or subdural bleeding. Patients with cerebellar abscesses and tumors are ultimately at risk for herniation if the disease process is not arrested. However, such lesions are usually expanding slowly, and the brain can compensate for the relative compression ischemia for a remarkably long time. In contrast, in rapidly expanding lesions the process is too rapid for the brain to compensate for the attendant ischemia and compression.

Management of the Clinical Problem, Potential for Brain Herniation Potential for brain herniation is a clinical problem, managed collaboratively by nursing and medicine. The problem may be managed at the level of primary prevention by any concerned health professional or layperson. Early detection of the problem is a major goal of intensive-care monitoring by both physicians and nurses. Physicians carry primary responsibility for definitive therapy of treatable lesions that are precipitating brain herniation (for example, expanding epidural hematoma). Both physicians and nurses have collaborative responsibilities in maintaining and monitoring the pharmacologic and supportive therapy regimens that reduce brain mass in nonsurgical conditions causing brain herniation.

It behooves all critical-care personnel to take an active part in community education aimed at primary prevention. Head trauma sustained in motorcycle, bicycle, automobile, and home accidents accounts for a substantial portion of the patients in any intensive or trauma unit who are at risk for brain herniation. Uncontrolled hypertension is the primary cause of intracerebral and cerebellar hemorrhage. All health personnel have a role in educating the public regarding proper use of helmets on bicycles and motorcycles and seat belts in automobiles. The National High Blood Pressure Education Program has identified a major role for nurses in both education and early detection of hypertension.

The preceding discussion has been aimed largely at secondary prevention, or the early detection of an existing disorder, which prevents further complications. If herniation can be detected before it has become irreversible, the opportunity for effective medical therapy is greatly enhanced. Computed tomography (CT scan) is frequently used upon admission or upon appearance of focal or diffuse brain damage signs to determine whether a mass lesion exists. In some cases echoencephalography may be performed at the bedside to detect brain shift.

If a mass lesion is found to be the cause of deteriorating neurologic function, removal of the mass becomes the major aim of medical care. For example, evacuation of a subdural hematoma or evacuation and ligation of the bleeding artery in epidural hematoma removes the expanding mass lesion and allows the brain to assume its normal relationships. Hypertonic agents such as mannitol and urea may be given prior to emergency craniotomy in the hope of shrinking a swollen brain and "buying time" to get the patient to the operating room. If herniation is secondary to focal or general cerebral edema, removal of the cause becomes more difficult. In such cases, symptomatic treatment of the edema and resultant increased intracranial pressure may be pursued until the brain's healing processes have reversed the edema. It must be emphasized that the use of such agents as mannitol, urea, glycerol, corticosteroids, and barbiturates is aimed at controlling intracranial pressure secondary to swelling and edema and is not primary therapy of the brain injury itself. The controversy surrounding the efficacy of corticosteroids and barbiturates was discussed earlier, under "Intracranial Hypertension."

In severe brain swelling, surgical decompression may be used in the hope that herniation will be reversed or averted long enough for reparative processes to shrink the swollen brain. A flap of bone is removed and the dura may be incised to allow the expanding brain a place to expand other than through the tentorium. Needless to say, care must be taken not to place external pressure on the surgical dressing over the exposed dura mater.

Nursing monitoring for the clinical problem of potential for brain herniation has been described above. Several nursing diagnoses associated with this problem are common to many brain-injured patients. Chief among these are complete physical immobility related to coma and potential for injury related to inability to protect cornea, airway, and skin. Nursing interventions for these diagnoses are basic to care of the immobilized, unresponsive patient and are outlined in the section on head injury under "Neurotrauma," later in this chapter.

Seizures

By definition, generalized seizures and focal seizures that become general affect the functioning of the whole brain and thereby disrupt consciousness. A generalized seizure is the result of uncontrolled neuronal discharge in the brain. In a seizure, neurons begin to discharge uninhibitedly, recruit other nearby neurons, and thus excite a "storm" of electrical activity in the brain. The discharge may arise from deep in the central core of the brain, immediately disrupting consciousness through excess activity in the reticular activating system. Other generalized seizures may arise from focal areas of hyperactive neurons, whose uncontrolled discharge spreads to central structures and becomes general. Both the typical *grand mal,* or major motor seizure, and *petit mal,* or "absence attacks" of children, are generalized seizures. Electroencephalography during such a seizure shows excessive electrical activity over the entire brain. Clinically, consciousness is disrupted in both types of seizure, but excess motor activity is characteristic of grand mal episodes, while arrest of motor activity (but not loss of tone) is characteristic of the typical petit mal of childhood. In addition, the typical EEG pattern, although general in both, is quite different in petit mal and in grand mal.

Most seizures are idiopathic, that is, without identifiable cause. However, in a critical-care setting, they are likely to stem directly from an identifiable disorder which primarily or secondarily affects the patient's brain. Metabolic disorders, by altering the acid-base and fluid environment of the brain, effectively lower membrane potential and thus the threshold for seizures. Both hypertonicity and hypotonicity of brain fluid can lead to seizures by altering the normal electrochemical balance on each side of the cell membrane. Trauma can predispose the patient to seizures. The underlying cause is not so likely to be cortical scar formation in the early stages, for healing and thus scar formation have not yet taken place. More likely, the lactic acidosis and respiratory alkalosis secondary to neurogenic hyperventilation alter the electrochemical balance of brain cells. Tumors and subdural hematomas directly irritate the brain tissue, leading to increased cell firing. Correction by the physician of the underlying structural, metabolic, or respiratory problems is the most effective treatment for such seizures. However, particularly in an injured brain, seizures beget seizures. Thus, most clinicians elect to control seizures with anticonvulsants while pursuing the underlying causes in the critically ill patient.

The primary clinical problem associated with seizures in critically ill patients is potential for secondary brain damage related to uncontrolled seizures. This is a clinical problem that must be managed collaboratively by nurses, physicians, and sometimes respiratory therapists. The metabolic requirement of brain cells during epileptic discharge far exceeds that of resting or normally active brain cells. Even focal seizures (epileptic discharge confined to a small area of the brain) increase overall cerebral metabolism, and generalized seizures increase cerebral metabolic requirements severalfold. Most often, cerebral blood flow increases sufficiently to deliver oxygen and substrate to the cells. Therefore investigators now believe that the primary cause of cell death is breakdown of internal cellular metabolic machinery.[45] The major goal of care is absence of neuronal damage, and the expected outcomes are detection of generalized seizures and rapid control of generalized seizures. Management to achieve these outcomes consists of (1) monitoring for signs of focal or generalized seizures, (2) institution of predetermined protocols to manage seizures if they occur, and (3) nursing measures to protect the patient from physical injury during a seizure.

Monitoring to detect focal and generalized seizures is made more difficult in many intensive-care neurologic patients at high risk for focal and generalized seizures because the protocols for management of brain swelling, intracranial hypertension, and respiratory insufficiency mask motor manifestations of seizures. Thus, patients who are artificially ventilated and paralyzed with pancuronium have little or no motor response to focal or generalized motor seizures. Depending upon the serum level of pancuronium, these patients may show only minor twitching or only a sudden marked increase in level of ICP (secondary to increase in cerebral blood flow to meet the flow needs of excessive cellular activity) and sudden dilatation of pupils. The attending physician may elect continuous EEG monitoring to detect recurrent seizure activity in such patients.

Because the injured brain is more vulnerable to secondary injury from excessive neuronal activity, seizures must be stopped rapidly. The pharmcologic protocol used most commonly includes a short-acting benzodiazepine (diazepam or lorazepam) to stop the seizure, followed by a loading dose and then maintenance doses of a longer-acting anticonvulsant (most commonly phenytoin or phenobarbital). Dosages and nursing observations are discussed under "Status Epilepticus."

Nursing management is collaborative in monitoring and carrying out the drug protocol in the event of seizures. Further nursing intervention is required for the nursing diagnosis of potential for physical injury, which is present in any patient suffering generalized seizures. Goals of care are to maintain an adequate airway and prevent aspiration and to prevent injury to soft tissues and bones. Interventions to protect the airway include positioning the patient in the lateral position, use of an oral airway or endotracheal tube, and oropharyngeal suctioning to keep the mouth free of secretions that could be aspirated. Bone and soft tissue injury can be prevented by taping pillows or commercially available pads to the bed rails and loosening any limb restraints that may be in place. Injury to teeth is best prevented by *avoiding* the use of padded tongue blades.

Status Epilepticus   A patient who is having seizures from any acute or chronic cause may develop status epilepticus, but it is more common in those with epilepsy whose brain cells have become regulated by anticonvulsants. The sudden withdrawal of these, either deliberately or by forgetting medication, renders all the brain cells hyperexcitable, thus leading to seizure activity among epileptic foci cells. Neurochemical changes in the cellular fluid around these cells then render neighboring cells more excitable and lead to generalized seizures.

Grand mal status epilepticus is an absolute emergency! Continual seizures prevent brain cells from restoring metabolic processes between firing. Patients in grand mal status epilepticus whose seizures cannot be controlled die of brain exhaustion with definite evidence of metabolic and structural neuronal death. Investigators have demonstrated that prevention of muscular activity during continual seizures in baboons neither protected the brain nor prevented death.[45,46] Electroencephalography demonstrated that continual seizure activity occurred even though the motor manifestations were prevented by curare and even though respirations and blood pressure were supported. In both baboons and rats, neuronal damage was greatest in the neocortex and hippocampus.

In addition to the protective care described above, critical-care nurses should be prepared to institute anticonvulsant therapy for a patient in status epilepticus. The time necessary for a physician to arrive, evaluate the situation, and initiate therapy may be sufficient for large numbers of brain cells to be irreparably damaged. Therefore, the nurse should be able to (1) recognize status epilepticus and (2) initiate a standard protocol determined in advance by the critical-care staff. A typical protocol is shown in Table 35-7.

Table 35-7 Protocol for Management of Status Epilepticus

1. Obtain adequate airway.
2. Establish diagnosis: 15 to 20 min of generalized motor seizure or 20 to 30 min of overlapping seizures without regaining consciousness.
3. Establish intravenous line.
4. Draw blood for laboratory studies: glucose, electrolytes, CBC, calcium, BUN, toxicology screen, liver enzymes, anticonvulsant serum levels.
5. Administer anticonvulsant therapy:
   a. Benzodiazepine:
      Diazepam (Valium)—*Children:* 0.25–0.4 mg/kg IV over 2 min; 5–10 mg maximum; repeated at 15 min if needed, not to exceed 30 mg total. *Adults:* 5–10 mg over 5–10 min, repeated at 15 min if needed, not to exceed 30 mg total. Be prepared for mechanical ventilation in the event of respiratory arrest.
      Alternative drug: Lorazepam (Ativan)—*Children:* 0.05 mg/kg at 1 mL/min; repeated at 15 min if needed to total of three doses. *Adults:* 4–8 mg IV over 2 min; repeated at 10 mi if needed. Be prepared for respiratory arrest.
   b. Phenytoin (Dilantin):
      Initial dose: *Children:* 15–20 mg/kg at 1–3 mg/kg per minute. *Adults:* 20 mg/kg no faster than 50 mg/min. Monitor ECG.
      Stop drug if ST segment widens.
      Maintenance dose: 250 mg IV q 4 h to total of 1 g in first 24 h.
6. If seizures are not stopped with initial one or two drugs, phenobarbital IV, paraldehyde IV, barbiturate, or general anesthesia may be considered.

A typical generalized seizure lasts 20 to 40 s, with recovery of consciousness within 30 min. Generalized status epilepticus is thus defined as seizure activity that exceeds usual time. Specifically, status epilepticus is a single seizure lasting longer than 15 to 20 min, or a series of seizures over 20 to 30 min in which the patient fails to regain consciousness between seizures.

Treatment of generalized status epilepticus follows the same steps involved in any emergency: attention to airway and breathing, steps to diagnose the underlying cause, protective care while the seizures persist, and definitive treatment. Establishment of an adequate airway is, as always, of prime importance. At the same time, oxygen should be administered by prongs or mask. If the patient does not have an artificial airway already in place, one should position the patient on his or her side and insert an oral airway. An endotracheal tube may ultimately be required if the seizures prove difficult to control.

Because most status epilepticus seen in a critical-care unit is a symptom of an underlying structural or metabolic pathology, determination of the primary cause is crucial in long-term therapy. If an intravenous line is not already established in the patient, one should be established as soon as airway patency is attended to. At this time, blood should be drawn for laboratory tests, including blood glucose, serum osmolality, and serum electrolytes. It is often the case that correction of the underlying metabolic deficit (for example, hypoglycemia or hyperosmolality) will end the seizures.

Among the drugs used to control repetitive seizures, the initial drug of choice is most commonly diazepam (Valium), given intravenously. Diazepam may be given to adults in doses of 5 to 10 mg over 5 to 10 min, repeating as necessary at 15-min intervals but not exceeding 30 mg for a total dose. In children, the dose should be 0.25 to 0.4 mg/kg over 2 min with a maximum of 5 to 10 mg per bolus and 30 mg per episode.[47,48] Alternatively, 5 mg/min may be administered by intravenous drip, using nonabsorptive tubing.[49] Diazepam is a short-acting anticonvulsant with a rapid onset of action. Large doses can depress, or even arrest, respirations. Therefore, a slow rate of administration is crucial, and equipment to manually ventilate the patient should be readily available if needed.

Lorazepam (Ativan) is a benzodiazepine that is often used instead of diazepam. It has a longer duration of action and somewhat less sedating activity. Respiratory depression and respiratory arrest are potential side effects, just as with diazepam.[50]

Following the initial dose of benzodiazepine to rapidly control the seizures, phenytoin (Dilantin) is given for longer-term anticonvulsant effect. It is preferable to phenobarbital in persons with central nervous system disorders because it has much less sedating effect in large doses than phenobarbital. Phenytoin is given initially as an intravenous loading dose (15 to 20 mg/kg for both children and adults) at a rate no greater than 50 mg/min in adults and 3 mg/min per kilogram in children. The maximum dose in 24 h is 1 g. Phenytoin crystallizes when standing in solution and therefore should be given intravenously in a bolus, directly into the cannula, rather than mixed in a hanging solution. It is never appropriate to give phenytoin intramuscularly; tissue absorption and therefore serum levels are unpredictable by this route, and crystallization in tissues has been demonstrated.

Phenytoin has potentially dangerous side effects on cardiac rhythm, particularly in elderly patients and in those with heart disease. Therefore, the ECG should be monitored when phenytoin is used in status epilepticus. Indications for immediate discontinuance of the drug are hypotension, widening of the QRS complex, prolongation of the PR or QT intervals, and depression of T waves.

If a benzodiazepine and phenytoin are not successful in controlling the seizures, amobarbital or phenobarbital are often given intravenously, in a dose of 5 to 10 mg/kg and a rate of 30 mg/min in children and 9 mg/kg at 50 mg/min in adults, with total dose not to exceed 1 g for either. Potential side effects to be monitored include sedation, hypotension, respiratory depression, and cardiac arrest.

Paraldehyde may be added if these drugs fail to control the seizures. Rectal paraldehyde is no longer recommended, as the rate of absorption is unpredictable. Intravenous paraldehyde is given in a solution of 4 mL of paraldehyde in 100 mL of normal saline at 3.75 mL per kilogram of solution (0.15 mL per kilogram of the drug) over 60 min, to a total not to exceed 100 to 125 mL of solution. Paraldehyde dissolves plastics and therefore must be mixed and administered in glass containers. It will deteriorate to acetic acid upon exposure to the air, so must be mixed fresh for each administration. Pulmonary edema and hepatic and renal toxicity are potential side effects.

If all else fails, general anesthesia may be used to stop the seizures. Such therapy requires continuous EEG monitoring to determine whether the brain seizure activity has ceased. Some investigators have used high-dose barbiturate anesthesia (pentobarbital) and hypothermia as an alternative to volatile gas anesthesia;[51] care of patients so treated also requires continuous EEG monitoring but is otherwise identical to that for patients with uncontrollable ICP under barbiturate coma.

Neuropathophysiologic States That Disrupt Ventilation But Not Consciousness

The disorders commonly seen that may produce respiratory problems include high cervical spinal cord injury, polyneuropathies (such as Guillain-Barré syndrome), and motor unit disorders, such as myasthenia gravis, botulism, and tetanus. In these the respiratory problem is secondary to loss of motor function rather than to loss of consciousness and ability voluntarily to protect the airway.

These three types of disorder disrupt human functioning in all basic aspects of self-care except mentation and consciousness. Survival and the quality of life after recovery are vitally dependent upon skilled and knowledgeable nursing care.

Motor loss from extracerebral causes can threaten life if it involves sensory or motor reflexes that protect the airway or if innervation of respiratory musculature is depressed or lost. Thus, relevant nursing diagnoses include (1) ineffective airway clearance related to loss of airway protective reflexes and (2) ineffective breathing patterns related to paralysis or weakness of respiratory muscles.

Ineffective Airway Clearance Due to Loss of Airway Protective Reflexes

The gag, swallowing, and cough reflexes that protect the airway are integrated in the brainstem, at the medullary segment. Cranial nerves IX, X, and XII are the peripheral nerves carrying motor and sensory fibers to and from the structures involved in these functions. Table 35-8 summarizes the anatomic structures involved.

Evaluation of Airway Protection Since airway protection is dependent upon those reflexes which serve gag, cough, and swallowing, assessment of the adequacy of these functions is important. In contrast to the patient with cerebral involvement who is at risk for inadequate airway protection, the patient with extracerebral motor problems is usually conscious. Consequently, the nurse can utilize evaluation of speech, facial movement, and head and shoulder movement to assess closely related cranial nerve function. Finally, the nurse must know which patients are at risk for loss of airway protection and evaluate potential loss of protection in light of general motor functioning.

Patients who are at risk for airway problems and who may be seen in critical care include those with myasthenia gravis (particularly after thymectomy, during intercurrent illness, or in myasthenic or cholinergic crisis), those with polyneuropathy involving upper extremities and/or cranial nerves, those with poliomyelitis (involving brainstem motor neurons), and those with brainstem stroke or contusion. The last group of patients may be unconscious if the reticular activating system is involved. Cranial nerves IX, X, and XII are most crucially involved in protecting the airway. Evaluation of the function of adjacent cranial nerves helps detect potential problems before aspiration has occurred. Table 35-8 describes cranial nerves in relation to the functions served.

Important questions to consider in evaluating lower cranial nerve function are the following: (1) Is the quality of speech changing or becoming nasal, slurred, or "thick-tongued"? (2) Is the volume of speech decreasing? In regard to swallowing: (1) Is food or fluid coming back through the nose (indicating palatal weakness)? (2) Is there choking on nonviscous substances such as water? (3) Can the patient swallow his or her own saliva? (4) Is there pooling of secretions in the mouth of the conscious person? In testing swallowing, it should be remembered that water is the most difficult substance to swallow—more difficult than saliva. Therefore, if the nurse is concerned that the patient may aspirate the test substance, ice chips rather than water should be used.

In ascending polyneuropathies, upper extremity function and movement of head and neck may be affected before the cranial nerves serving airway protection. Therefore changes in the strength and symmetry of head turning, neck flexion, and extension are important cues to evaluate swallow, gag, and cough more frequently in patients with such changes. These evaluations of cranial nerve function are not relevant to the patient with cervical spine injury (unless there is associated head injury), because any spinal cord injury compatible with life is below the cranial nerves.

In myasthenia gravis, changes in muscular function may occur very rapidly, within minutes. Therefore, for these patients airway protection and respiratory status must be evaluated frequently. Any slurring or nasality of speech or increased ptosis of eyelids serves as a cue to evaluate swallowing and cough and vital capacity as often as every 5 min if changes are occurring rapidly.[52] Such variables are summarized in Table 35-9.

Of the disorders used as examples in this section, only brainstem stroke and contusion are

Table 35-8 Nerve Fibers and Skeletal Muscles Involved in Protecting the Airway

Function	Afferent Fibers, Cranial Nerve No.	Efferent Fibers, Cranial Nerve No.	Muscle(s)
Gag	IX (glossopharyngeal)	IX, X (vagus)	Stylopharyngeus, soft palate, pharynx
Swallow	IX (posterior ⅓ of tongue; pharynx, larynx)	X	Pharynx, soft palate
	X (epiglottal taste buds)	XII (hypoglossal)	Tongue
Cough	X (pharynx, larynx, trachea, bronchial tree)	X, to respiratory center (medulla) and then to periphery via:	Soft palate, larynx, glottis
		(1) Phrenic nerve (C4–C5)	Diaphragm
		(2) Intercostal nerves (T1–T11)	Intercostal

Table 35-9 Critical Evaluation in Myasthenia Gravis

Vital capacity	Maximum expiratory volume following maximum inspiration, measured in liters by spirometer
Swallowing	Measured subjectively by asking the patient to identify the type of substance or diet thought possible to swallow at the time: 0—nothing 3—pureed soft 1—saliva 4—soft 2—liquids 5—regular diet
Ptosis	Documented according to the following scale (with the patient looking straight ahead): 1—Unable to open eye, none of iris visible 2—Lids open, some of lowermost iris visible 3—Lower half of pupil visible 4—All of pupil visible, none of uppermost iris visible 5—All of pupil visible, some of uppermost iris visible
Diplopia	Measured subjectively by asking the patient to move eyes through their extreme range of motion and identify positions in which diplopia is experienced.

Source: M. Blount, A. Kinney, and N. Luttrell, Myasthenia Gravis and the Guillain-Barré Syndrome, in D. L. Nikas (Ed.), *The Critically Ill Neurosurgical Patient,* Churchill-Livingstone, New York, 1982.

stable lesions. Once the initial damage has occurred, symptoms tend to remain the same or diminish. The other disorders (polyneuropathies and disorders of neuromuscular transmission) may become progressively worse and often involve respiratory musculature as well. In these disorders, potential for ineffective airway clearance and potential for ineffective breathing pattern must be evaluated together. They should be evaluated as frequently as the vital signs. Any deterioration occurring in any of the functions is an important cue to increase the frequency of evaluation. The nurse *must intervene* if the patient cannot swallow saliva, if gag and/or cough reflex is markedly diminished or lost, if food and fluid regurgitates through the nose, or if vital capacity is less than one-third of predicted (about 600 cm³ in the "average" adult). The combination of bulbar dysfunction and decreased vital capacity puts the patient at particular risk of both aspiration and respiratory failure.

Collaborative management consists of placement of a cuffed endotracheal or tracheostomy tube (depending upon anticipated length of dysfunction) to prevent aspiration of saliva and a nasogastric, esophageal, or gastric feeding tube. Reintroduction of oral feeding requires careful nursing monitoring.

Ineffective Breathing Patterns Due to Dysfunction of Respiratory Musculature

Decreased movement of air due to disordered respiratory musculature may be life-threatening.

Muscles important to breathing are the diaphragm and the intercostal muscles. In health, the diaphragm is the primary muscle of inspiration. The internal and external intercostal muscles assist in deep inspiration. Expiration is a passive process. The motor neurons of the diaphragm receive impulses from the phrenic nerve, which emerges from spinal nerve C4, with some input from C3 and C5. Spinal nerves T1 to T11 innervate the intercostal muscles.

Thus, spinal cord lesions at C5 and above will affect both diaphragmatic and intercostal musculature. Lesions below C5 will allow diaphragmatic movement but paralyze the intercostals. During the period of spinal shock, a patient with a lesion of the midthoracic region is able to voluntarily depress the diaphragm and thus take a breath. The ability to inspire maximally is lost because of paralysis of the intercostal muscles. When reflexes return, spasticity of the intercostal muscles aids in maximal chest expansion.

Respiratory musculature can also be affected by peripheral polyneuropathies, which impair both voluntary and reflex movement by demyelination of the motor component of the reflex arc. Myasthenia gravis and other disorders of neuromuscular transmission interfere with respiratory movement by blocking transmission at the myoneural junction. The intense muscular spasms of tetanus can also interfere with respiration by preventing full expansion of the chest.

Evaluation of Respiratory Function   In patients at risk for ineffective breathing patterns due to respiratory musculature failure, function can be evaluated by measuring vital capacity serially, measuring blood gas values, and observing respiratory effort. Secondary clues to impending respiratory distress are increasing anxiety and fear of going to sleep. Patients at risk include those with spinal cord lesions above T6, those with polyneuropathies with trunk and upper extremity weakness, and those with generalized myasthenia gravis, particularly those who are postoperative patients or have intercurrent illness.

Since spinal cord sensory roots follow skin dermatomes, and since most traumatic lesions of the cord involve both motor and sensory pathways, the level of cord injury can be roughly estimated by mapping sensory dermatome levels. Figure 35-8 depicts schematically important dermatome levels in the quadruped human. The figure is shown in quadruped fashion to aid in appreciation of the extension of sacral and thoracic dermatomes along arms and legs.

Critical dermatomes in terms of functional outcome are shown. T1 extends from about the level of the scapula along the arm and is the upper limit of the intercostal nerves. T4 is approximately at the nipple line. Patients with lesions slightly below T4 will probably have adequate voluntary respiratory function, while those with lesions at T4 and above require frequent evaluation of respiratory function and may need ventilatory assistance. The functional significance of other dermatomes is discussed later under multisystem problems. Although most of the severe polyneuropathies involve greater motor than sensory loss, sensory dermatomes may be of some value in determining the level of peripheral nerve loss in symmetric polyneuropathy. Sensory dermatome evaluation is of no value in disorders of neuromuscular transmission (such as myasthenia gravis), since the disturbance is entirely at the neuromotor junction.

Although there are much more sophisticated measures of pulmonary function available, bedside evaluation of vital capacity remains an important tool in serially evaluating respiratory status in neurologic disorders. The bedside spirometer is easily used with the conscious patient and provides an immediate measure, without the time lag inherent in blood gas measurement. A single measurement of vital capacity is not as useful as a series, compared with the predicted normal for a person that size. Continually decreasing vital capacity indicates a patient who is losing respiratory muscle function and may need respiratory assistance. As a rule of thumb, patients with vital capacity below one-third of normal (or below 600 cm^3) require assisted ventilation. Decreasing tidal volumes or vital capacity in a patient with spinal cord injury indicates extension of the injury (because of edema or bleeding into the cord). Such decreases may be expected in a patient with ascending polyneuropathy or worsening myasthenia gravis.

Measurement of partial pressure of dissolved gases in the blood is important in evaluating the overall respiratory status of patients with severe motor disorders but is not to be relied upon in determining the need for assisted ventilation in disorders characterized by rapid deterioration. For example, in myasthenia gravis, a patient may move from intact respiratory status to complete loss of voluntary respiratory effort in 20 min. Although polyneuropathies such as Guillain-Barré syndrome have a somewhat slower time course, waiting for

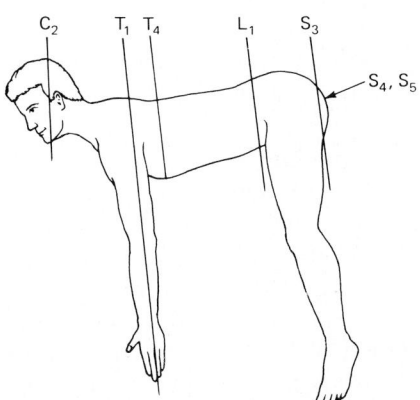

Figure 35-8   Representation of demarcating sensory dermatomes in the quadruped human. The figure is shown in quadruped fashion to illustrate the extension along the arms and legs of the dermatomes dividing the thoracic and lumbar spine. Knowledge of dermatome levels in mapping the extent of sensory loss can help predict the functional deficits and abilities of the patient. (*Redrawn from H. Patton et al. (eds.), Introduction to Basic Neurology, Saunders, Philadelphia, 1977, p. 176.*)

the determination of arterial blood gases may delay respiratory assistance unnecessarily. Blood gas values may be more appropriately used to guide decisions regarding respiratory assistance in more stable lesions such as spinal cord injury. Secondary evaluative cues may be helpful. The nurse may observe respiratory effort or a patient's anxiety about going to sleep. Such secondary cues should cause the nurse to initiate measurement of vital capacity and blood gases and to increase the frequency of evaluation.

Management of ineffective breathing pattern is collaborative among physicians, nurses, and respiratory therapists. The expected outcomes are (1) early detection of ineffective breathing pattern, (2) maintenance of adequate oxygenation with mechanical ventilation, and (3) restoration of effective breathing patterns without mechanical ventilation in patients whose lesions allow independent breathing.

Monitoring is the primary management strategy for early detection of insufficient respiratory effort and is described above. Assisted or controlled ventilation with a mechanical respirator is generally necessary when vital capacity is less than 33 percent of expected or when blood gases are abnormal.

Care of patients on assisted ventilation is described in Chap. 8. Secondary nursing diagnoses that apply to patients with neurologically induced respiratory muscle failure include fear or anxiety related to ineffective breathing, complete physical immobility, and impaired verbal communication related to presence of endotracheal tube.

Although the pathologic processes which create extracranial life-threatening motor dysfunction are quite different, they all have the potential to create a severely immobilized person who is fully alert and aware of what is happening. The patient with Guillain-Barré syndrome lives with paralysis creeping upward rather rapidly; the patient with tetanus experiences growing stiffness, culminating in suffocating muscular spasm; the person with myasthenia never knows whether the next dose of medication can be swallowed, or worse, whether breath will come the next hour. Finally, the patient with a cervical spine injury is transformed suddenly from a healthy active person to a person who cannot even breathe. Coupled with these devastating changes in body image and function are the frightening sights and sounds of critical care. Many of these patients have only the ceiling or floor to look at and can only imagine the worst about what is happening.

The reactions of most persons with acute, life-threatening illnesses follow a similar pattern: fear, denial, anger, depression, and resolution. In the critical-care setting one is most likely to see alternating fear, anger, and denial. While few patients deny that they cannot move at the moment, most deny that this situation will be permanent. Such denial probably has both physiologic and psychological protective value in the critical-care stage. It is appropriate to support the patient's hope for complete recovery in such disorders as Guillain-Barré syndrome and diphtheritic polyneuropathy, as this is consistent with the natural history of the disorders. False hope should not be offered the patient with an apparent complete spinal cord injury; neither should the patient be forced to abandon denial of severity of injury. With modern rehabilitative techniques, most persons with spinal cord injuries can expect to lead an independent life. A study of the attitudes of nurses toward spinal cord-injured patients suggests that critical-care nurses were the most pessimistic compared to intermediate care and rehabilitation nurses.[53] This pessimism probably reflects exposure to these patients during their bleakest time and may make it difficult for critical-care nurses to offer sincere hope to them.

Coupled with the abrupt change in lifestyle and the reasonable fears which the patient has regarding survival is the difficulty of communicating inherent in tracheostomy and assisted ventilation. It is crucial to invent some means of communication which allows more than yes and no answers whenever possible. If the patient has any strength in the mouth, a letter board and mouthstick can be used to point out phrases and individual letters. Some patients have been able to use Morse code through eye blinks or small finger taps.

Fear can express itself in both anger and incessant requests for nurse attention. Firm limits regarding what the nurse can and cannot do and when may help provide a sense of security for the patient, *provided* the nurse is consistent in letting the patient know what to expect and consistently follows through. It is important to remember that increased anxiety can reflect respiratory insufficiency as well as psychological response to injury.

Patients with severe extracranial motor dysfunction may spend long periods in critical care if ventilatory assistance is required. Consequently, the axiom that rehabilitation begins in critical care is certainly true with these patients. Skin care to prevent pressure sores, passive range of motion to prevent contractures, and attention to psychological needs are second only to measures to preserve life.

Impaired Gas Exchange Due to Pulmonary Embolism

In addition to the direct effect of motor loss on respiratory musculature, patients immobilized from motor disorders are at increased risk for pulmonary embolism from deep vein thrombosis. Although there is disagreement in the literature regarding the incidence of deep-vein thrombosis in spinal cord–injured patients and others with neurologically induced immobility, studies which report a low incidence rely on clinical signs rather than the more accurate plethysmography or ^{125}I-labeled fibrinogen studies to detect thrombosis. Clinical signs have been shown to miss both thrombosis and pulmonary embolism in the most widely studied groups, postoperative and postmyocardial infarction patients. The few studies published which use appropriate techniques to detect thrombosis show an incidence that ranges from zero in patients with spinal fracture but no paralysis to as high as 75 to 100 percent in paralyzed spinal cord–injured persons.[54,55] The rate of pulmonary embolism in spinal cord–injured patients has been shown to be as high as 9 or 10 percent, with up to 3 percent mortality.[54–57] Management of pulmonary embolism is a collaborative problem, involving the ventilation/perfusion mismatch engendered by the embolism. See Chap. 27 for discussion of medical therapy for pulmonary embolism.

Multisystem Dysfunction and Failure

Since the central nervous system integrates the input to the autonomic nervous system at both the cerebral and spinal cord levels, general injury to the diencephalon, brainstem, or spinal cord can interfere with autonomic and endocrine regulation of multiple body systems.

Cerebral regulation of the autonomic and endocrine systems occurs at the level of the diencephalon, with the hypothalamus the major integrator of input to the pituitary releasing hormones and to the preganglionic level of the sympathetic nervous system. Regulation of temperature, metabolic rate, blood pressure, and fluid balance all have important hypothalamic and pituitary inputs. Cranial regulation of the parasympathetic nervous system occurs in the brainstem.

Thus, patients with diffuse damage from head injury, intracranial hemorrhage, global hypoxia, or massive cerebral edema are all at risk for multisystem dysfunction secondary to abnormal cranial regulation of vegetative functions. The clinical problems stemming from disordered endocrine and autonomic control that may be manifested in such patients include hyperosmolar and hypoosmolar states, hyperthermia, catabolic state, coagulation disorders, and ventilation/perfusion mismatch (shunt).

The most common source of hyperosmolar and hypoosmolar states is inappropriate management of parenteral fluids.[58] However, diabetes insipidus (DI) and syndrome of inappropriate antidiuretic hormone (SIADH) are potential neuropathologic causes of the fluid and electrolyte imbalance problems that may be seen in patients with diffuse head injury, diencephalic stroke, or parasellar tumors or in those who have had pituitary surgery. DI results from the inability to produce antidiuretic hormone (ADH), with resultant polyuria and, if untreated, subsequent dehydration, hemoconcentration, and hypovolemia. DI is characterized by urine output in excess of fluid intake, hypotonic urine (specific gravity 1.001 to 1.005 and urine osmolality 50 to 150 mosmol/kg), and normal or increased serum sodium.[58,59] The conscious patient will experience excessive thirst. Nonketotic hyperglycemia is a second source of a hyperosmolar state, with subsequent osmotic diuresis. It may be seen in patients with occult diabetes but more commonly is the result of excessive mannitol, high-protein tube feedings, or corticosteroids. The common treatment of a hyperosmolar state includes replacement of urinary losses plus insensible losses with dextrose and water, rather than saline. Vasopressin may be necessary to control the diuresis.

In contrast, SIADH is caused by excessive production of ADH, resulting in low urine output compared with fluid intake, hypertonic urine (increased urinary sodium, urine osmolality higher than serum osmolality, and decreased serum sodium and serum osmolality of <280 mosmol/kg).[58] Treatment of the hypoosmolar state consists of fluid restriction titrated by monitoring of urinary sodium and serum osmolality. Some advocate rapid correction with hypertonic saline.[60]

Careful nursing monitoring of fluid balance, electrolytes (both urine and serum), and osmolality is essential in the prevention or early detection of iatrogenic sources of fluid-electrolyte imbalance in these patients. The majority of patients with neurologic disorders in critical-care units are comatose or too confused to express their thirst and thus meet their own fluid intake needs. Therefore, only careful monitoring and analysis of intake and output and urine and serum electrolytes will prevent serious fluid imbalance.

Hyperthermia is a second problem that may stem from failure of CNS regulatory mechanisms in patients with severe head injuries, hypothalamic stroke, or hypothalamic damage from any source. Infection must be ruled out before assuming that fever in neurologic and neurosurgical patients is of hypothalamic origin. Respiratory and urinary tract infections are the most common sources of fever in neurologic patients.

Patients undergoing therapeutic barbiturate coma may become *poikilothermic*—i.e., take on the temperature of the environment—because of the action of barbiturates on central temperature regulation.[61] Therefore, it may be necessary to use artificial warming or cooling to maintain the patient's core temperature at 33 to 39°C.[61]

Controversy exists regarding the extent to which neural trauma induces a catabolic state compared with trauma from all causes. The bulk of evidence suggests that patients with head trauma, at least in the first week after injury, increase their metabolism to a greater degree than is seen after surgery or non-CNS trauma. The net effect is high nitrogen excretion in the urine, extremely high caloric need, and rapid muscle wasting when caloric needs cannot be met nutritionally.

The catabolic state is a collaborative problem and is best managed by close teamwork of nutritionists, physicians, and nurses. Ordinary parenteral fluids cannot deliver more than about 600 kcal per day, far short of the estimated 3500 kcal needed to maintain body weight during hypermetabolism after head injury. Therefore the goal of nutritional regimens in severely head-injured patients is to provide calories via dextrose in water intravenously for as short a time as possible, advancing to enteral feedings via nasogastric tube as soon as the patient has adequate bowel tones. If enteral feeding is not possible, parenteral alimentation is necessary. A common nutritional goal is 3500 kcal per day, with 20 g of nitrogen per day. Caloric needs increase in the presence of fever and continuous spontaneous movement. Corticosteroids used in the treatment of intracranial pressure also increase nitrogen excretion and impair cellular response to insulin. The most rational nutritional regimen is tailored to the metabolic needs of the individual patient and coordinated by a skilled nutritionist.[62,63]

Coagulation disorders, specifically disseminated intravascular coagulopathy (DIC), may occur in any multiply injured patient, including those with head and spinal cord injury as part of their multiple trauma. The incidence of abnormal coagulation increases markedly with the severity of head injury, although not every patient with abnormal coagulation develops DIC.[17] Heparin is the treatment of choice in DIC, as outlined in Chap. 43. However, neurosurgical DIC patients receiving heparin must be monitored exceptionally carefully because of the possibility of precipitating an intracranial hemorrhage.

Ventilation/perfusion mismatch, or shunt, is a common finding in patients following head injury, massive cerebral ischemia, and intracranial hemorrhage.[64] There is continuing discussion regarding the comparative extent to which this reflects central impaired regulation of sympathetic input to the pulmonary vasculature rather than systemic problems that influence the pulmonary disorder.

There is experimental evidence that severe CNS injury can create massive sympathetic nervous system discharge, leading to constriction of pulmonary vessels, increased hydrostatic pressure in the pulmonary vasculature, subsequent extravasation of fluid into the interstitium and alveoli, and finally, pulmonary edema or adult respiratory distress syndrome (ARDS). Although frank neurogenic pulmonary edema is rarely seen, the presence of some degree of shunt in a large proportion of head-injured patients has led a number of researchers to propose that neural as well as systemic factors are responsible.

In addition, neurally injured patients are frequently in coma and thus unable to protect the airway from aspiration of oral and gastric secretions; may have concomitant chest trauma or multiple fractures that predispose them to fat embolism; and are at high risk for pulmonary embolism from deep-vein thrombosis. Treatment of ARDS and pulmonary emboli is discussed in Chap. 27. Positive end-expiratory pressure (PEEP) is a common therapy in ARDS and other pulmonary disorders. It has the potential to increase ICP in high-risk patients because of the effect on intrathoracic pressure. However, a number of recent investigations have shown that PEEP can be used safely in neurosurgical patients if the head is kept elevated at 30° and PEEP is maintained at about 10 cmH$_2$O.[23]

Multisystem failure may also occur following injury or disease of the spinal cord, which is a primary integrator of peripheral autonomic nervous system function. The following discussion of multisystem problems is most pertinent to acute spinal cord injury. Since polyneuropathies may also have an autonomic neuropathy component, it is applicable to patients with polyneuropathies as well.

Functions which may be compromised by acute spinal cord injury and polyneuropathy include cardiovascular reflexes, temperature control, gastrointestinal motility, elimination, and integumentary function. The effects on the respiratory system have already been discussed. Multisystem effects are summarized in Table 35-10.

The cardiovascular effects result primarily from loss of sympathetic outflow below the level of injury. A period of spinal shock occurs for some time after injury, in which somatic and autonomic reflex activity is lost. Although autonomic demyelination is not the rule in polyneuropathy, it can occur and present similar systemic problems.

Most visceral innervation is from the sympathetic outflow. The efferents leave the spinal cord in the thoracolumbar spine, between T1 and L1 to 2. Heart, lungs, tracheobronchial tree, viscera, peripheral blood vessels, bowel, and bladder all receive their sympathetic innervation from the thoracolumbar sympathetic ganglia. Parasympathetic innervation of these organs is from the vagus (medulla) and, that of the bladder, rectum, and penis from the pelvic plexus (sacral spinal nerves). Consequently, any lesion of the thoracic or cervical cord will interrupt cardiovascular function and the function of most of the viscera. The higher the lesion, the more autonomic function is disrupted.

The viscera will not cease functioning entirely, because they also receive parasympathetic input. However, the parasympathetic input is unbalanced and will tend toward quiescence. For example, paralytic ileus occurs because motility depends upon the balance of sympathetic and parasympathetic activity. Cardiac and lung function do not cease, because of intrinsic rhythmicity in the heart and because vagal input is still intact. However, bradycardia and arrhythmias may occur because the vagal influence is unopposed. In addition, with a cervical lesion, hypotension may occur because there is no sympathetic outflow to maintain peripheral vascular resistance. Cardiovascular reflexes which adjust blood pressure to postural changes are impaired in such cases, and hypotension may manifest itself whenever the patient's position is changed, even from side to side. Finally, added to the risk of deep vein thrombosis due to immobility is that from decreased peripheral vascular tone and thus increased tendency to stasis of blood. Absence of muscle tone impairs venous return and contributes to both hypotension and venous thrombosis.

Monitoring of cardiac rate and rhythm should be instituted in patients with cervical cord injury to detect serious arrhythmias or bradycardia that would impair cardiac output. Hypotension is usually time-limited and self-regulating. However, if associated injuries are causing bleeding or sequestration of fluid in third spaces, cautious volumetric and colloid replacement may be used. Care must be exercised not to put the patient into pulmonary edema through overzealous fluid replacement.

Difficulties with temperature regulation are related to loss of peripheral vasodilatation and constriction. Again, the higher the lesion, the less ability the patient has to regulate temperature by constriction and dilatation of skin vessels. The patient becomes *poikilothermic,* that is, takes on the temperature of the environment. Instead of being able to regulate the core temperature through

Table 35-10 Relation of Brainstem and Spinal Segments to Critical Functions in Acute and Long-Term Spinal Disorders

Muscles	Brainstem or Spinal Segment	Dermatome Reference Points	Acute Dysfunctions	Functional Ability If Lesion Persists
Soft palate, pharyngeal, tongue	Medulla (CN IX, X, XII	—	↓ gag, swallow leading to choking, aspiration	Swallowing with retraining if reflex returns; may need permanent esophagostomy
All below trapezius, sternocleidomastoid	C2	Back of head	Total loss of respiration and movement from shoulder down (such patients now survive with speedy prehospital care)	Requires permanent respirator; can shrug shoulders, turn head (CN XI), and use all cranial nerves
Diaphragm	C3, 4, 5	Ear, neck, clavicle to wrist	↓ or absent diaphragmatic as well as intercostal respiratory effort, high risk of hypotension, hypothermia, ileus, atonic bladder, skin breakdown	Can move head, shrug shoulders, breathe with intercostals (after reflexes return); experimental use of phrenic nerve stimulation
Deltoid, biceps	C6	Lateral third of arm, shoulder to thumb	↓ respiratory function (diaphragm intact, without intercostals); risk for hypotension, hypothermia, ileus, atonic bladder, skin breakdown	Can move head, shoulders; breathe independently but with ↓ reserve; flex elbow, feed self with prosthesis; use electric wheelchair
Latissimus, serratus, pectoralis, radial wrist extensors	C7	Doral midarm to 1st/2d digits (dorsal and palmar)	↓ respiratory function (without intercostals); risk for hypotension, hypothermia, atonic bladder, ileus, skin breakdown	Some rolling over; can flex elbow, feed self with hand devices; sit up; self-propel adapted wheelchair
Triceps, finger extensors and flexors	C8	Medial third of arm including digits 3 and 4	↓ respiratory function; risk of hypotension, hypothermia, ileus, atonic bladder, skin breakdown	Can feed self with devices, roll over, sit up, transfer, dress, toilet, move in bed unassisted
Hand intrinsics, ulnar, wrist, and fingers	T1	Midpectoral (T4 at nipple line)	↓ respiratory function; risk of hypotension, hypothermia, ileus, atonic bladder, skin breaddown	Independent eating, moving in bed, toilet, use of wheelchair, respiratory reserve

(Continued)

Table 35-10 Relation of Brainstem and Spinal Segments to Critical Functions in Acute and Long-Term Spinal Disorders (Continued)

Muscles	Brainstem or Spinal Segment	Dermatome Reference Points	Acute Dysfunctions	Functional Ability If Lesion Persists
Upper intercostals, upper back	T6	Two segments below nipple, three segments above umbilicus (T10)	Ileus, atonic bladder, skin breakdown; low risk of hypotension and hypothermia	Normal respiratory reserve; independent in all of above; can stand with bracing
Abdominals, thoracic extensors	T12	Between umbilicus (T10) and inguinal fold (L1)	Atonic bladder, fecal retention	Can ambulate with bracing; reflex bowel and bladder (true of all lesions above sacral cord)

Note: All patients with lesions above T6 have high risk for hypotension and hypothermia/hyperthermia because of interruption in sympathetic outflow. These same persons are at increased risk for autonomic hyperreflexia in the rehabilitation period. All lesions above the lumbar level carry high potential of paralytic ileus; all persons with lesions above sacral cord have atonic bladder and anal sphincter during the acute phase. Lesions above the sacrum convert to reflex, and bladder and bowel are uninhibited when reflexes return. Those with sacral lesions are most apt to retain atonic bladder and bowel secondary to absent reflexes.

vasodilatation to lose heat through the skin or vasoconstriction to conserve heat, the vessels of the patient in spinal shock remain dilated. Most commonly, the functional result is that body temperature drops, particularly in air-conditioned units. However, in extremely warm weather, hyperthermia may result because the patient can neither sweat below the level of the lesion nor further dilate skin vessels. The patient's environment must be regulated to maintain core temperature. If hypothermia is serious, it may be necessary to monitor core temperature by tympanic membrane or esophageal temperature. Usually rectal or oral electronic measurements are sufficient, however, to indicate trends in temperature. In no case should touch or skin temperature be relied upon to monitor the patient's temperature. The patient may be warmed by blankets, by increasing the room temperature, or by electrical heating devices or may be kept cool by fans or other cooling devices. It is imperative to remember that the patient cannot feel the latter devices and cannot sense when there is danger of thermal or cold injury.

Loss of gastrointestinal motility may manifest itself in paralytic ileus. The nurse should not wait for distention and vomiting before assessing gastrointestinal function. Any patient with a sensory level above T8 (output to the splanchnic plexus) is at risk for decreased gastric motility. As Fig. 35-8

shows, L1 is just above the inguinal crease. Thus patients with lesions between the inguinal fold and umbilicus (and above) should be evaluated for ileus.

Bowel sounds should be assessed regularly and low nasogastric suction begun if they are decreased or absent. Gastrointestinal bleeding from stress ulcers occurs in up to 20 percent of patients. Pain may be absent, and tarry stools may be the only manifestation.

Bowel and bladder evacuation are impaired by a variety of lesions above the sacral cord. Most sympathetic and parasympathetic input is from the lumbar and sacral plexuses. Therefore almost any cord injury or polyneuropathy affecting the lower extremities can be expected to involve the bowel and bladder. Until reflexes return, the bladder will fill and distend just as the bowel does. Periodic release of urine with intermittent or continuous catheterization will be necessary. Nasogastric suction and intravenous feeding will be required until bowel sounds return. If feces are present in the rectum, manual removal or gentle enemas may be needed until rectal reflexes return. The presence of rectal reflexes can be determined by inserting a gloved finger into the rectum. The rectal sphincter will contract on the finger if the reflex is present.

Finally, the integument is at high risk for breakdown in the paralyzed patient. Loss of sympathetic tone, diminished trophic influence of motor nerves, and paralysis combine in a paralyzed limb or body to bring about a more rapid breakdown of skin under pressure. Studies in both animals and humans have demonstrated histologic evidence of tissue destruction within 1 to 2 h of sustained pressure in normal tissue; this time is shortened by as much as half in paralyzed tissue. In the person with either segmental or suprasegmental motor loss, mechanical devices which vary pressure over body surfaces and frequent change of position are imperative from the moment of admission. Skin breakdown can occur in the severely immobilized myasthenia gravis patient as well but is not so rapid as in disorders of the central or peripheral nerves. Sepsis secondary to pressure sores was the major cause of death in spinal cord injury prior to the development of modern spinal cord injury centers. It remains one of the major sources of disability and hospitalization.

Human Responses to Neural Disorders That Alter Consciousness, Ventilation, and Multisystem Regulation

The preceding portions of this chapter have been focused on pathophysiologic states common to many neural disorders and the clinical problems and nursing diagnoses common to these states. The remaining section of the chapter is organized around neurologic diseases and disorders that are frequently seen in critical-care patients. Since so many of the human responses are common to multiple disorders, relevant nursing diagnoses and clinical problems are presented in outlines, with cross-referencing to the first description of appropriate protocols and nursing interventions. Five categories of disorder account for the majority of patients with nervous system disease in critical-care units: neurotrauma, cerebrovascular disorders, neurosurgical procedures, infectious disorders, and autoimmune and neurotoxic disorders.

Neurotrauma

Head and spinal cord injuries are the primary kinds of neurotrauma that result in hospitalization in critical-care units. The annual incidence of head and spinal cord injury is estimated at 1 million cases, with nearly 5 billion dollars spent yearly on acute and chronic care of persons so injured.

Since both head and spinal cord injury stem from motor vehicle accidents and falls, such as those in diving, skiing, and skateboarding, such neurotrauma is largely preventable.[65] All health professionals share a responsibility for community and individual education regarding means to prevent such accidents. Legislation and personal decisions regarding the use of seat belts, automobile air bags, proper sports training and techniques, and alcohol-free driving are all means of reducing the number of head and spinal cord injuries in the United States.

Alteration in Consciousness and Multisystem Regulation Related to Head Injury

Head injury is a catch-all term for a large number of medical diagnoses related to trauma involving the skull and brain. A common operational definition requires a blow to the head and altered consciousness, no matter how brief. Minor head injuries are considered to be those in which the loss of consciousness is less than 20 min and in which the Glasgow coma score is 13 to 15. Major, or severe, head injuries are operationally defined as those with Glasgow coma scores of 8 or less. (Several combinations of responses are possible but commonly these patients open their eyes only to pain, do not follow directions, may have abnormal movements, and utter no comprehensible sounds or only inappropriate words.)

Head injury serious enough to require critical care results from a blow to the head, often delivered at high speed. There may be focal injury consisting of contusions and hematomas at the site of the blow, the opposite side of the brain (*contrecoup injury*), and where the brain hits the rough projections on the underside of the skull. Rupture of small and large vessels may result in subdural and epidural hematomas, which act as mass lesions, and subarachnoid hemorrhage, which releases blood into the cerebrospinal fluid. In addition, the dissipation of energy throughout the brain tissue often results in diffuse tearing of nerve fibers. Such widespread diffuse damage is often associated with a long-term vegetative state and is now known to be the source of what used to be called primary brainstem damage.

Pathophysiologic responses to these structural injuries include brain swelling and edema, increased intracranial pressure, and transtentorial herniation. Focal or generalized motor seizures may develop as early sequelae (during the first week) or late sequelae (up to 2 years after injury) to the injury. Hypothalamic damage or ischemic responses to intracranial hypertension may initiate alterations in temperature regulation, coagulation disorders, cardiac arrhythmias, hyper- and hypoosmolar states, and increased metabolism.[66,67]

Clinical Problems and Nursing Diagnoses Associated with Severe Head Injury

The outline that follows summarizes the medical protocols and nursing diagnoses commonly applicable to patients with acute head injury.[63,64]

Collaborative Clinical Problem

Potential for brain swelling and intracranial hypertension

Common Medical Protocol

Hyperventilation, corticosteroids, mannitol

Nursing Diagnosis

Potential for decreased intracranial adaptive capacity

Nursing Interventions

1. Monitor for disproportionate change in ICP with activity. Assess electrolytes, osmolality.
2. Position patient carefully.
3. Institute drug protocols to decrease ICP prior to nursing activities.

Collaborative Clinical Problem

Potential for brain herniation

Common Medical Protocol

Surgical decompression; hypertonic agents

Nursing Intervention

1. Monitor and assess neurologic status, particularly level of consciousness.

Collaborative Clinical Problem

Potential for hypermetabolism (alteration in nutrition, less than body requirements)

Common Medical Protocol

Tube feeding; hyperalimentation if needed

Nursing Interventions

1. Monitor bowel sounds and institute enteral feeding as soon as they return.
2. Coordinate nutritionist referral as needed.
3. Monitor osmolarity, electrolytes.

Collaborative Clinical Problem

Potential for hypo- or hyperosmolar state

Common Medical Protocol

(See text under "Multisystem Dysfunction and Failure.")

Nursing Intervention

1. Monitor electrolytes, osmolarity, urine specific gravity.

Collaborative Clinical Problem

Potential for hypo- or hyperosmolar state

Common Medical Protocol

(See text under "Multisystem Dysfunction and Failure")

Nursing Intervention

1. Monitor blood gases, respiratory status.

Nursing Diagnosis

Complete physical immobility related to coma

Nursing Interventions

1. Change patient's position frequently, with careful monitoring of ICP response.
2. Give passive range-of-motion exercises.
3. Use antiembolic stockings or pneumatic compression boots to prevent thrombosis.
4. Monitor bowel activity and prevent constipation.

Nursing Diagnosis

Potential for injury related to coma: skin breakdown, corneal abrasion

Nursing Intervention

1. Change patient's position frequently.
2. Give good skin care.

3. If patient cannot close eyes, use eyedrops q 1 to 2 h, patch eyes periodically.

Nursing Diagnosis
Potential for injury related to hyperarousal

Nursing Interventions

1. Pad bed rails.
2. Use sheepskin-type bedding to prevent sheet burns.

Nursing Diagnosis
Potential for altered family processes related to severity of injury

Nursing Interventions

1. Provide information as appropriate.
2. Facilitate family contacts with physician and social worker.
3. Assure family it is permissible to take time for themselves if indicated.
4. Facilitate family-patient interaction.

Alteration in Ventilation and Multisystem Regulation Related to Spinal Cord Injury

Spinal cord injury resulting from dislocated fracture, contusion, or direct injury to the cord may result in functional transection of the spinal cord at any level, with concomitant multisystem dysfunction during the initial phase of spinal shock. Injuries at C6 and above impair ventilation by disrupting neural input to the diaphragm. Injuries between C6 and T11 impair the ventilatory function of the intercostal muscles.

The overall incidence of spinal cord injury is estimated at 3 per 100,000 persons annually, with 72 percent of new injuries occurring in males in the 15- to 24-year age group. The overwhelming preponderance of spinal cord injuries in this group is the result of motorcycle and automobile accidents. The second most susceptible group is elderly adults, with the injuries resulting from falls.

In experimental studies of the pathologic changes occurring from blows to the spinal cord, there is an initial phase of 15 to 30 min in which neurons and vessels appear normal, followed by a massive release of vasoactive neurochemicals with subsequent cord swelling and then ischemia. Eventually neurons in the cord die and are replaced by glial cells or by cavities.[9] The degree to which cell death occurs determines the completeness of the functional transection of the cord. Sensory and reflex input from intact cord distal to the injury cannot reach the brain, and motor and autonomic output from the brain and brainstem cannot reach the periphery past the injured area. The effects of functional transection on ventilation and multisystem function are described fully in the earlier section "Multisystem Dysfunction and Failure."

Initial management of acute spinal cord injury is collaborative, involving emergency medical technicians, emergency room nurses, and physicians. The primary goal of management in the field and upon arrival at the acute care hospital is to *minimize the extent of spinal cord trauma.*[67] The primary intervention is immobilization and stabilization of the fracture and spinal cord.

Although critical-care nurses are not often the first to receive the newly spinal-injured patient, they should understand the principles of movement and transfer of such patients from the moment of injury, which are crucial to prevention of further damage to spine or cord. Nothing is more tragic than for a patient to come to the hospital with a fractured spine and with moving extremities and to leave paraplegic or quadriplegic after inexpert transfer from bed to x-ray to bed.

At the scene of the accident or at the first contact with the patient, the possibility of a spinal injury must always be kept in mind. *Patients with head injury, particularly if unconscious, must be presumed to have cervical spine injury until proved otherwise by an x-ray which visualizes all eight cervical vertebrae.* Approximately 10 to 15 percent of head-injured patients have associated cervical spine injuries. In the conscious patient, reported pain over any portion of the spine, parathesias or decreased sensation in the trunk or extremities, or difficulty in moving extremities is presumptive evidence of spinal injury. The patient should be transported as if spinal injury were present until this is definitively ruled out by x-ray. Until x-rays have been taken and read, the patient should remain on the emergency vehicle stretcher. Each additional transfer of the patient with an unstable fracture increases the chances of cord compression.

Any patient with a suspected spinal injury must be transported supine on a hard, flat surface. The hard surface is sufficient in itself to immobilize the thoracic and lumbar spine. In suspected cervical spine injury, the head must be in neutral position, with lateral immobilization by sandbags and preferably a stiff cervical collar. Wide tape or cloth extending over the forehead and to the spine board will serve to prevent forward flexion. The major objective of neck immobilization is to *prevent flexion, extension, and rotation of the cervical spine.* Figure 35-9 shows one method of manually immobilizing the neck while producing maximum visualization of all cervical vertebrae during x-ray.

Transfer of the patient from one surface to another should not be started until a person skilled and trained in such transfers is present to act as team leader. A patient with an unstable fracture will never be harmed by remaining on an emergency vehicle stretcher but may be permanently paralyzed

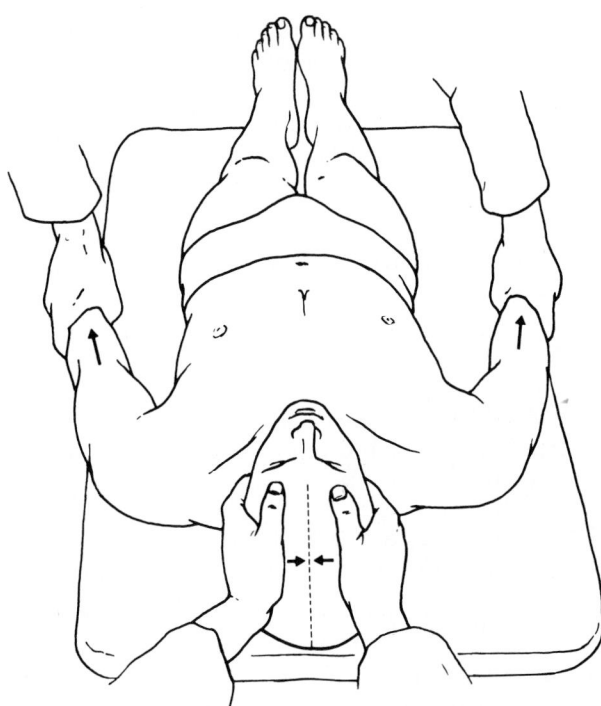

Figure 35-9 A method of immobilizing the head and exerting gentle manual traction during x-ray of a patient with suspected cervical spine injury. *(Drawing by Shirley Baty in Emergency Medicine, 9(12):100, 1977.)*

by improper transfer from it to an emergency room or nursing unit bed. Transfer of the patient with cervical spine injury requires at least four persons: three to support the body and maintain perfect alignment with the head, which is immobilized by the fourth person. The best method of stabilizing the head is to use a cervical traction halter. One hand exerts a gentle cephalad pull on the ties of the halter and the other is used under the occiput to support the head and neck in neutral alignment. Transfer of the patient with thoracic or lumbar injury is similar but does not require traction and immobilization of the neck.

If there is an unstable fracture or fracture dislocation, the neurosurgeon or orthopedic surgeon usually applies skeletal traction in the form of skull tongs. The patient in skeletal traction is then maintained on the nursing unit in a standard bed, Stryker frame, or kinetic bed. Cleansing of the insertion sites daily or twice daily and application of antibiotic ointment are useful in preventing local infection around the tongs.

Ongoing medical management varies considerably according to physician preference. Many physicians give a bolus of dexamethasone (Decadron) or methylprednisolone (Solu-Medrol) as soon after injury as possible, on the theory that the use of steroids may reduce cord damage secondary to swelling. While there is evidence of reduced swelling and improved neurologic function following steroids in experimental animal models of acute spinal cord injury, the only controlled trial in humans did not show any dose-related efficacy of methylprednisolone in altering neurologic disability.[68] Naloxone and thyroid stimulating hormone (TSH) have both shown good results in animal models, but their efficacy in humans has not been reported.[69] A number of other experimental techniques such as perfusion of the cord with hypothermic solutions, myelotomy, and osmotic diuretics have been tried in an attempt to reduce the secondary cord injury from swelling. No controlled trials have been conducted to adequately evaluate these therapies.

Low-dose heparin, aspirin, dipyridamole (Persantine), and calf compression have all been recommended to prevent deep-vein thrombosis and pulmonary embolism.[55,57] However, no adequately controlled trials have been conducted to satisfactorily answer the question of whether the risk of heparinization is justified, given the relatively low rate of morbidity and mortality even in the face of a high rate of deep-vein thrombosis in these patients.[57] Gastric suction and intermittent or continuous catheterization are routinely ordered in managing paralytic ileus and neurogenic bladder.

Nursing management is collaborative with medicine in minimizing the extent of cord damage, preventing multisystem complications, and monitoring for extension of the injury. The clinical problems faced by the spinal cord–injured patient relative to the level of cord injury, discussed earlier under "Multisystem Dysfunction and Failure," are summarized in Table 35-10; the primary potential nursing diagnoses can be inferred from that table and comprise the following:

Ineffective breathing related to respiratory muscle dysfunction

Impaired gas exchange related to pulmonary embolism (from deep-vein thrombosis)

Multisystem dysfunction related to spinal shock: positional hypotension, bradycardia, paralytic ileus, atonic bladder with urinary retention, poikilothermia

Complete self-care deficit related to level of paralysis

Impairment of skin integrity related to immobility and decreased trophic factors in paralyzed tissue

Grief response related to abrupt change in lifestyle

Nursing intervention comprises both monitoring and specific actions for common problems. Monitoring is critical in early detection of extension of injury or development of multisystem failure. Knowledge of the level of spinal injury from the x-ray findings plus mapping of sensory dermatomes and motor ability will enable the nurse to focus observation on those problems most likely to occur for each patient. Table 35-10 is a guide to predicting those problems.

Sensory level can best be mapped by beginning in areas which are known to be anesthetic and moving upward, asking the patient to indicate when a pricking pin feels sharper. This level should

be marked on the skin to note a baseline and aid in determining whether the level of injury is extending. Swelling and intracord hemorrhage in the first hours after injury may extend the level of damage both up and down the cord. Muscle testing uses the 0 to 5 scale described in Chap. 34, with zero indicating no flicker of contraction and 5 indicating full resistive strength. Testing of shoulder shrug, raising arms, flexing and extending elbows, dorsiflexing and extending wrists, pinch strength of thumb and index finger, and abdominals; hip, knee, and ankle extension and flexion; and anal reflex are the minimum necessary to adequately monitor change in motor function following spinal cord injury.[70]

Clinical Problems and Nursing Diagnoses Associated with Acute Spinal Cord Injury

Specific actions related to multisystem dysfunctions, described earlier in the section of that name, are outlined below.

Collaborative Clinical Problem

Potential for ineffective breathing pattern with cervical or high thoracic injury

Common Medical Protocol

Assisted ventilation if needed; respiratory therapy

Nursing Interventions

1. Monitor respirations, blood gases, and vital capacity.
2. Assist patient in coughing.
3. Give deep breathing exercises.

Collaborative Clinical Problem

Potential for impaired gas exchange secondary to pulmonary embolism

Common Medical Protocol

May or may not use prophylactic low-dose heparin

Nursing Interventions

1. Apply antiembolic stockings.
2. Monitor for sudden change in respiratory status.

Collaborative Clinical Problem

Potential for secondary injury due to displacement or fracture

Common Medical Protocol

May include immobilization, frame bed, traction, cervical tongs, etc.; may use steroids to prevent cord edema

Nursing Intervention

1. Give scrupulous attention to maintaining alignment of neck and back during transfer or turning.

Collaborative Clinical Problem

Potential for multisystem dysfunction related to spinal shock

Common Medical Protocol

Nasogastric decompression for ileus, urinary catheter for atonic bladder

Nursing Interventions

1. Monitor for return of bowel sounds.
2. Use intermittent or continuous catheter.
3. Monitor for hypotension and bradycardia, particularly that stimulated by positioning change or suctioning.
4. Monitor temperature, maintaining environment that keeps patient normothermic.

Nursing Diagnosis

Potential for alteration in skin integrity related to immobility and paralysis

Nursing Interventions

1. Change patient's position q 2 h and inspect all skin surfaces.
2. Use kinetic bed if possible to help prevent skin breakdown and atelectasis.
3. Assure adequate nutrition.

Nursing Diagnosis

Potential alteration in comfort related to immobility, paresthesia, inability to scratch self

Nursing Interventions

1. Assist patient in scratching, etc., as needed.
2. Give pain medication as needed for incisional pain if laminectomy or spinal fusion is done.
3. Change patient's position frequently.
4. Provide diversional activities if appropriate.

Nursing Diagnosis

Potential grief response to sudden change in lifestyle

Nursing Interventions

1. Listen to patient's expressions of anger or denial.
2. Focus on short-term goals and achievements.
3. Provide as much control for patient as possible in choices about ongoing care.

Cerebrovascular Disorders

The majority of cerebrovascular disorders, transient ischemic attacks, and strokes do not result in a need for care in the intensive-care unit. However, massive hemispheric stroke, intracerebral hemorrhage, aneurysmal subarachnoid hemorrhage, and some brainstem strokes can impair consciousness or ventilation sufficiently to require intensive nursing care. Further, current therapies for vasospasm secondary to subarachnoid hemorrhage require intensive technological monitoring. Concentration of all stroke patients in critical-stroke units has not been found to have any advantages over having a knowledgeable stroke team available to patients on the general units.[71]

Cerebrovascular accident, or stroke, is not a single entity but rather a category of cerebrovascular disease that results in sudden or rapidly progressive nonconvulsive neurologic deficit. Stroke is the third leading cause of death in the United States, second only to coronary artery disease and cancer. In 1984, over 2 million Americans suffered stroke, with 155,000 deaths. Over half of all patients hospitalized for neurologic disease have had acute strokes.

Cerebrovascular accidents or strokes are characterized by progressive or abrupt focal neurologic deficits that result from ischemia or infarction of the brain tissue supplied by a particular cerebral artery and its branches. The specific neurologic deficits depend on the function of the portion of the brain supplied by that arterial distribution. The internal carotid and its branches supply the anterior portion of the brain, including most of the cerebral cortex. The structures supplied by the carotid and its major branches include the frontal lobes, motor cortex, sensory cortex, auditory cortex, and optic radiations. Branches of the anterior circulation penetrate into the medial surface of the brain and supply the hippocampus, basal ganglia, and internal capsule (radiations of the motor fibers from motor cortex to brainstem). Thus, ischemia or infarction of the anterior distribution of the cerebral blood supply can impair the functions of movement, sensation, speech, cognition, and vision, depending upon which brain area is infarcted. Consciousness is not commonly altered in anterior circulation stroke unless there is bilateral hemispheric damage, hemorrhage into the intracerebral ventricles, or brain shift and swelling from large intracerebral hemorrhage or infarct.

The vertebral arteries provide the posterior circulation of the brain, which supplies the brainstem, medial surface of the occipital lobe, diencephalon, and cerebellum. Ischemia or infarction of this distribution can affect the functions of visual perception, movement (via brainstem motor tracts or cerebellar control of coordination), cranial nerves, or control of breathing. Consciousness is generally preserved unless there is infarction of the reticular formation in the pons or midbrain, pressure on the brainstem from cerebellar hemorrhage and swelling, or subarachnoid hemorrhage into the basal cisterns.

Ischemia and infarction may occur in the cerebral circulation from occlusive emboli and thrombi, from rupture of microaneurysms into the brain parenchyma (hypertensive intracerebral hemorrhage), or from rupture of saccular (Berry) aneurysms into the subarachnoid space (subarachnoid hemorrhage). Strokes from any cause become life-threatening if they alter consciousness or ventilation. Therefore, the following discussion of nursing diagnoses and clinical problems in stroke relates only to those life-threatening problems likely to be seen in critical care.

Alteration in Consciousness Related to Intracerebral Infarct or Hemorrhage

Strokes from emboli or thrombi rarely cause coma unless an entire hemisphere is infarcted and massive swelling ensues.[72] However, intracerebral hemorrhage from the anterior or posterior circulation often causes coma. Posterior circulation hemorrhage into the diencephalon creates coma by direct effects on the reticular activating system, whereas anterior circulation hemorrhages are more likely to alter consciousness as a result of brain shift from mass effect or secondary swelling. Cerebellar hem-

orrhage (posterior circulation) may cause coma by direct compression of the brainstem from the expanding mass or by upward herniation of the cerebellum through the tentorium.

Medical management of intracerebral or intracerebellar hemorrhage consists of definitive diagnosis of hemorrhage versus large infarct by CT or magnetic resonance scan, supportive therapy to prevent secondary brain injury, and, if surgically feasible, evacuation of the hematoma. Evacuation of hemorrhages into the basal ganglia and of cerebellar hemorrhage is often accompanied by rapid clinical improvement. Hemorrhage into the third ventricle may require ventricular shunting. Hemorrhage into the midbrain-upper pons is manifested by both coma and absence of spontaneous breathing or markedly abnormal breathing patterns and is not benefited by surgical therapy.

Nursing management of patients with completed hemorrhagic stroke that impairs consciousness is nearly identical to that for the patient with impaired consciousness from any other disorder affecting the cerebral hemispheres. The primary potential nursing diagnoses and collaborative clinical problems include:

Brain herniation (transtentorial for intracerebral hemorrhage, upward for cerebellar hemorrhage)

Ineffective airway clearance

Intracranial hypertension

Complete self-care deficit

Complete physical immobility, with potential for multiple secondary injury: skin breakdown, atelectasis, corneal abrasion, deep-vein thrombosis, renal calculi

Multisystem dysregulation: hyper- or hypoosmolarity, poikilothermia, cardiac arrhythmias

Relevant nursing management is summarized in the earlier section on head injury, under "Clinical Problems and Nursing Diagnoses Associated with Severe Head Injury."

Alteration in Ventilation and Movement Related to Brainstem Stroke

The posterior cerebral circulation supplies the brainstem, which in turn regulates the function of the cranial nerves and basic vegetative functions, such as swallowing, breathing, and control of blood pressure. Further, all motor and sensory fibers pass through the brainstem enroute to the cortex from the periphery.

The majority of brainstem strokes impair one or more focal neurologic functions but do not threaten life. However, when airway protection, automatic control of breathing, or the muscles of respiration are impaired, the patient requires ventilatory support and critical-care nursing. Infarction or hemorrhage of the caudal anterior pons (basis pontis) spares the reticular formation but impairs all the cranial nerve nuclei from IX through XII, interrupts all motor output, and produces what is known as the *locked-in syndrome.* The patient is fully alert but unable to speak or move except for the eyes. Nursing diagnoses for such patients include:

Ineffective airway clearance related to paralysis of palate and pharynx

Potential for inadequate gas exchange related to paralysis of intrinsic muscles of respiration (phrenic nerve may remain intact)

Complete physical immobility related to flaccid paralysis of lower face and total body, with potential for multiple secondary complications: skin breakdown, atelectasis, subluxation of shoulders, renal calculi, constipation or impaction, urinary tract infection

Complete self-care deficit

Potential for inadequate nutrition related to inability to swallow

Inadequate verbal communication related to paralysis of speech structures

Fear related to inability to communicate alertness

Alteration in Consciousness and Multisystem Regulation Related to Subarachnoid Hemorrhage

Subarachnoid hemorrhage and cerebral vasospasm were discussed earlier under "Neuropathophysiologic States That Disrupt Consciousness." Subarachnoid hemorrhage is classified as a type of stroke and most often occurs following rupture of saccular (Berry) aneurysms in relatively young people. A smaller number of subarachnoid hemorrhages occur when vessels rupture into the subarachnoid space in head trauma or in older people with hypertension, presumably from microaneurysmal rupture into the subarachnoid space rather than into the brain parenchyma. The severity of neurologic deficit following aneurysm rupture is somewhat indicative of prognosis and surgical risk. The grading system of Hunt and Hess is commonly used to quantify such risk and deficits:[73]

0	Unruptured aneurysm
I	Asymptomatic or minimal headache, slight nuchal rigidity
Ia	Fully alert, no meningeal signs, but fixed neurologic deficit
II	Moderate to severe headache, nuchal rigidity, perhaps cranial nerve palsy but no other neurologic deficit
III	Drowsiness, confusion, or mild focal neurologic deficit
IV	Stupor, moderate to severe hemiparesis, perhaps early decerebration, vegetative disturbances
V	Decerebrate rigidity, vegetative dysfunction, deep coma

Several mechanisms have been proposed to account for the changes in level of consciousness noted with subarachnoid hemorrhage. Initially there is a sharp increase in intracranial pressure, which may account for changes in consciousness with rupture. Sustained coma usually indicates extensive bleeding into the brain parenchyma or ventricles. Changes in level of consciousness several days after the initial rupture may indicate rerupture of the clot, cerebral vasospasm, or increasing ICP secondary to communicating hydrocephalus.

A number of disturbances in integrated regulatory functions (vegetative functions) occur in patients with subarachnoid hemorrhage, including cardiac arrhythmias, hyper- and hypoosmolality, and sometimes unexplained fever. Since the majority of saccular aneurysms occur in the circle of Willis, it is postulated that the sudden ejection of blood under high pressure directly injures the hypothalamus or that the accumulation of blood in the basal cisterns interferes with hypothalamic function.

Medical management of subarachnoid hemorrhage varies widely in physician preference. Control of hypertension in patients with hypertensive hemorrhage is crucial to prevent further episodes. In patients with saccular aneurysms, the goal is to prevent secondary brain injury following the initial bleeding and to obliterate the aneurysm to prevent rebleeding. Achieving this goal is complicated by two factors: the state of the injured brain following initial rupture and the fact that about 20 percent of aneurysm patients have multiple aneurysms.

There is considerable controversy among neurosurgeons regarding the best timing for surgery to obliterate aneurysms and the supportive therapy to prevent rebleeding and vasospasm prior to surgery. Early surgery (within the first few days following hemorrhage) markedly reduces the incidence of rebleeding but is technically difficult, and some believe it may increase the severity of neurologic deficit. Late surgery, with antifibrinolytic agents to reduce the incidence of rebleeding, carries a higher incidence of deficits from cerebral vasospasm.[36,74]

Despite the variety of medical and surgical therapies attempted in aneurysmal subarachnoid hemorrhage, the mortality and morbidity remain high, with deaths within 3 months ranging from 40 to 50 percent.

Nursing management is collaborative with medical management in monitoring for rebleeding (peak incidence 7 to 15 days) and vasospasm (4 to 7 days after bleeding), supporting systemic physiologic function, and preventing secondary brain injury. In centers that use hypervolemic and hypertensive therapy to prevent vasospasm, nursing monitoring and knowledgeable titration of fluid volume and hypertensive therapy to neurologic status is crucial. Nursing has primary responsibility for creating an environment that minimizes rebleeding. Typical aneurysm precautions are designed to prevent emotionally or physically induced sudden increases in blood pressure that could rupture the newly formed clot or additional aneurysms.[75]

Clinical Problems and Nursing Diagnoses Associated with Aneurysmal Subarachnoid Hemorrhage

Nursing diagnoses and clinical problems that may arise in patients with aneurysmal subarachnoid hemorrhage are summarized in the following outline.

Collaborative Clinical Problem
Potential for rebleeding from aneurysm

Common Medical Protocol
May use antifibrinolytic agents, e.g., ϵ-aminocaproic acid (Amicar)

Nursing Interventions

1. Monitor for deep-vein thrombosis.
2. Take aneurysm precautions: quiet environment, no straining, no emotional upsets or other sources of rapid increases in blood pressure.
3. Monitor blood pressure, maintain normotension.

Collaborative Clinical Problem
Potential for vasospasm

Common Medical Protocol
Hypervolemic and hypertensive therapy; may add vasopressors

Nursing Interventions

1. Monitor neurologic status, particularly level of consciousness.
2. Monitor ICP and institute protocols to reduce ICP if needed.
3. Monitor hemodynamic status, titrating volume expansion to maintain pulmonary wedge pressure of 18 to 20 mmHg, hematocrit reading of 30 to 40 percent.
4. If neurologic status is not improved, add vasopressors according to protocol to increase blood pressure, titrated to point of neurologic improvement.

Nursing Diagnosis
Alteration in consciousness with resulting self-care deficit related to neurologic grade (see text for grading system)

Nursing Intervention

1. Encourage patient participation in self-care (feeding, hygiene) as ability permits, but caution against straining and isometric muscle contraction, which increase blood pressure.

Neurosurgical Procedures

In most critical-care units, the majority of patients with nervous system disorders are likely to be there for monitoring following neurosurgical procedures. It is common for patients to be closely observed in intensive care for 24 h or so after craniotomy, carotid endarterectomy, cervical laminectomy, and hypophysectomy. The primary complications being monitored for include brain swelling, intracranial or intracord bleeding, ventilatory insufficiency, and fluid and electrolyte imbalance following pituitary surgery. The potential nursing diagnoses are discussed below in relation to the category of neurosurgical procedure. Relevent nursing observations and management are discussed earlier in this chapter in the sections on head injury and spinal cord injury, under "Neurotrauma."

Supratentorial Craniotomy

Supratentorial craniotomy refers to all neurosurgical procedures in the cranium above the level of the tentorium. Craniotomy may be performed to remove intracranial tumors, hematomas, arteriovenous malformations, epileptic foci, or clip aneurysms in the anterior circulation or to create focal lesions in the thalamus. The primary complications that may ensue are intracerebral bleeding and brain swelling, either of which may result in intracranial hypertension, altered consciousness or, if severe, transtentorial brain herniation. Focal deficits may also occur related to ischemia or infarction of the areas involved in the surgical procedure.

Therefore, the primary potential clinical problems for which these patients are at risk include intracranial hypertension secondary to brain swelling (24 to 72 h after surgery) and transtentorial brain herniation secondary to intracranial bleeding (first 24 h). The potential concomitant nursing diagnoses are decreased consciousness with resultant self-care deficit and physical immobility, skin breakdown related to lack of position change during surgery, and alteration in comfort (headache related to craniotomy).

Primary management consists of careful monitoring of neurologic status as described under "Brain Herniation Syndromes" and often monitoring of intracranial pressure (described under "Intracranial Hypertension"). Dexamethasone is commonly given to control postoperative brain edema, and antiembolic stockings are used to prevent deep-vein thrombosis. Atelectasis is a potential problem, as with all postoperative patients, and preventive management is complicated by the detrimental effect of coughing on intracranial pressure. Deep breathing alone will maintain open alveoli, and it is unnecessary to stimulate these patients to cough.

Infratentorial Craniotomy

Craniotomy in the posterior fossa (below the tentorium) is used to remove acoustic neuromas and other tumors of the brainstem, cranial nerves, or cerebellopontine angle and cerebellar tumors and hemorrhages. The primary complications stem from the potential for swelling or bleeding in a small space that is immediately adjacent to the brainstem structures that control airway protection, breathing, motor coordination, and multiple cranial nerve functions.

The potential clinical problems that must be monitored for include respiratory arrest secondary to medullary compression or tonsillar herniation, decreased consciousness secondary to upward herniation, and aspiration secondary to loss of gag reflex. Concomitant potential nursing diagnoses include corneal injury related to loss of corneal reflex, inadequate verbal communication related to dysarthria, and self-care deficit related to ataxia or dysmetria. There must be careful monitoring of respirations and level of consciousness and serial assessment of cranial nerve functioning (particularly corneal, gag, swallow, and articulation). The onset of hiccups is an ominous sign of medullary involvement.

Patient positioning is designed to protect the surgical site and avoid flexion and extension of the neck, which might increase pressure in the posterior circulation and brainstem. The patient should be turned like a log, with support to the head and neck. Coughing and Valsalva maneuver should be avoided to prevent sudden increases in systemic blood pressure. Suctioning, if necessary to remove oral secretions, should be gentle and should avoid stimulating the cough reflex. Deep breathing is sufficient to prevent atelectasis. Aspiration can be prevented by scrupulous oral hygiene and careful testing of gag and swallow reflexes prior to allowing oral feeding.

Cerebrovascular Surgery

Vascular procedures involving the cerebral circulation may involve both vascular and neurologic surgeons. Patients thought to benefit from cerebrovascular surgery are those with transient ischemic attacks who have demonstrable stenosis of the carotid artery or its major branches. Most authorities recommend against surgery when stenosis is not symptomatic. When the stenosis is in the extracranial carotid circulation, endarterectomy is the procedure of choice, with the surgical objective of restoring normal flow and removing the plaque, which is a source of emboli. The ultimate goal is prevention of a completed stroke (or additional strokes if one has already occurred).

The major potential clinical problems are embolic stroke during or following surgery, oozing or frank hemorrhage at the incision site on the artery secondary to preoperative and intraoperative heparinization, respiratory distress due to hematoma or edema at the operative site, and peripheral cranial nerve injury. Nursing monitoring is directed to early detection of incipient stroke, inadequate airway (from hematoma compressing trachea), and cranial nerve injury. Serial neurologic examination, involving comparison with preoperative status, is essential. Stroke is best detected by recurrent examination of movement, speech, visual fields, and sensation contralateral to the side of the surgery. Hematoma at the operative site can be detected by observing the neck for swelling and tracheal deviation and by listening for stridor and labored respirations. Cranial nerve assessment should focus on those nerves which traverse the neck, such as the recurrent laryngeal, vagus, accessory, and hypoglossal. Speech clarity, swallowing, head and shoulder strength, facial symmetry, and pulse rate are important parameters for serial assessment.

Intracranial-extracranial (IC-EC) bypass surgery is sometimes used to bypass the stenosis when it is in an intracranial vessel and therefore inaccessible for endarterectomy. Most commonly, the superficial temporal artery is anastomosed to the middle cerebral artery, using microsurgical techniques. A recent multicenter randomized trial showed no benefit of this surgery over conservative medical therapy. However, many of these procedures continue to be done, and a number of surgeons still believe there is a subset of patients who benefit from it.[76]

Potential clinical problems include cerebral ischemia secondary to vasospasm and lost patency of the anastomosis, hemorrhage at the anastomosis secondary to preoperative heparinization, and seizures secondary to exposure of the cortex. Nursing monitoring for cerebral ischemia has been described earlier. Monitoring of blood pressure and maintenance of normotension are important, to prevent loss of patency of the anastamosis and perhaps also to prevent spasm, as is frequent monitoring of the pulse at the anastamosis site, to detect early signs of loss of patency. The patient should not lie on the operative site or use restrictive eyeglasses or head bands, to avoid compressing the anastamosis.[77]

Infectious Disorders

Central nervous system infections that may require intensive nursing care include generalized inflammation of the cortex, white matter, and meninges (encephalitis); generalized infection or inflammation of the meninges alone (meningitis); and focal infection of the brain (brain abscess).

Encephalitis

Encephalitis is an acute inflammation of the brain proper (cortex, white matter, and meninges) that is most commonly viral. Because viruses must reproduce *within* the host's cells, viruses that gain access to the CNS have the potential to create serious, irreparable damage to brain tissue. The most common cause of viral encephalitis is herpes simplex type 1 (estimated at 100 to 1000 cases annually in the United States). Other causative viruses include arboviruses (eastern and western equine and St. Louis encephalitis, also called *sleeping sickness,* and a variety of togaviruses seen only in Asia and the Pacific); enteroviruses (polio virus, echovirus, coxsackie virus); other herpes viruses which cause encephalitis only in immunocompromised hosts (Epstein-Barr virus, cytomagolovirus, and varicella-zoster virus); and a variety of other systemic viruses, the most important of which are the viruses of rabies, mumps, and measles. More rarely, bacterial, fungal, and protozoan infections may invade the brain and cause encephalitis.

The viruses or other causative organisms gain access to the brain via the bloodstream or peripheral nerves, particularly in patients who are rendered susceptible by immunosuppressive therapy, immunodeficiency diseases (AIDS, combined immunodeficiency of children), systemic debilitation, or an immune system stressed by other infectious disease. A nonexudative inflammation occurs, often with degeneration and destruction of neurons by the invading virus, demyelination, and subsequent necrosis, hemorrhage, and cavitation. Infectious organisms vary in their capacity for tissue destruction.

The symptoms reflect the involvement of the whole brain, and particularly the predilection of the viruses for the temporal lobe. Behavioral changes, including personality change, delirium, uninhibited behavior, and restlessness, are common, occurring in up to 85 percent of patients. Dysphasia occurs in 67 percent, seizures in 67 percent, autonomic dysfunction in 60 percent, and movement problems, particularly ataxia, in 40 percent. There may be localized motor deficits (hemiparesis, cranial nerve deficits) in as many as 85 percent.[78]

Medical therapy of encephalitis depends upon clear diagnosis of the causative agent. Brain biopsy is frequently necessary to specifically identify the virus, and initial treatment is based on presumptive diagnosis, pending serologic testing. There are no specific therapies for the majority of viruses that cause encephalitis, and primary prevention of such viral infections as poliomyelitis, measles, and mumps by immunization is the only viable approach. In the event of encephalitis from these agents, supportive therapy that maintains vital functions and protects the patient from injury while the body's immune functions attempt to destroy the virus is all that can be offered.

In recent years, specific antiviral therapies have been developed for herpes simplex type 1; acyclovir sodium, 30 mg/kg daily, is the drug of choice. Even with this drug, mortality remains high (28 percent, compared with 54 percent before the advent of acyclovir). Acyclovir has been found to achieve a better rate of survival than vidarabine and a lower incidence of neurologic residual deficits (62 percent with deficits treated with acyclovir versus 87 percent with vidarabine).[79] Clearly, even when treated, herpes encephalitis has a high mortality and morbidity rate. Mortality is also high in eastern equine encephalitis (more than 50 percent), with a high incidence of neurologic sequelae; these are lower in western equine and St. Louis encephalitis (3 percent and 2 to 20 percent, respectively, depending upon age).[78]

Meningitis

Meningitis is an inflammation of the leptomeninges that does not invade the brain parenchyma. Some infections involve both the meninges and the parenchyma; such a disorder is classified as *meningoencephalitis*. Meningitis can be caused by viruses, in which case it is called *aseptic meningitis;* or by bacteria—*purulent meningitis.*

The most common viruses causing aseptic meningitis are enteroviruses: coxsackie virus and echovirus. Prior to the development of an adequate vaccine, poliovirus was the most common cause of meningitis and encephalitis. Aseptic meningitis may have a sudden onset or may follow a prodromal phase of "flu," fever, sore throat, and gastrointestinal symptoms. Fever, drowsiness, frontal headache, stiff neck, and perhaps paresthesias are common. No specific therapy is available, but recovery is usually complete, and patients with aseptic meningitis are not seen in critical-care units. Purulent meningitis, however, may produce serious and life-threatening symptoms, particularly if the cranial nerves protecting the airway are involved and if acute brain swelling (and thus increased ICP) occurs.

Organisms gain access to the meninges via the bloodstream in systemic bacteremia; directly when the dura has been torn by injury; by nasopharyngeal venules that communicate with the meninges; and by direct spread from adjacent foci of infection as in sinusitis or brain abscess. Bacterial meningitis is preceded by upper respiratory tract infection, otitis media, or pneumonia in the majority of cases attributed to *Haemophilus influenzae, Neisseria meningitidis,* and *Streptococcus pneumoniae.* Gram-negative bacillary meningitis (*Escherichia coli, Enterobacter, Klebsiella, Proteus, Serratia,* and *Pseudomonas*) is usually seen only in immunosuppressed patients, infants, and patients with advanced cancer. Meningococcal meningitis (*N. meningitidis*) occurs in outbreaks in crowded situations and is the only meningitis to require fecal and oral precautions prior to adequate antibiotic levels, as well as prophylactic treatment of contacts.

As with encephalitis, specific medical therapy depends upon identification of the causative organism. Fortunately, therapy for bacterial diseases is better developed than that for viral disorders, and early specific treatment often results in resolution of the meningitis with little or no neurologic residual. Large doses of antibiotics are given intravenously, to ensure an adequate level in the CNS. Penicillin G is the antibiotic of choice for the majority of organisms, with chloramphenicol as a second choice. Gram-negative organisms may require chloramphenicol or aminoglycosides. Intrathecal administration is sometimes necessary.[77]

Brain Abscess

Brain abscess is a localized area of bacterial encephalitis, usually caused by direct extension of bacteria from infected sinuses or mastoids or of organisms that have entered the brain from a traumatic wound or via the bloodstream in septicemia, bacterial endocarditis, or lung abscess. Because they are localized and act as space-occupying lesions, brain abscesses mimic tumors or hematomas. Diagnosis is usually made on the basis of epidemiologic evidence for a source of infection and a characteristic ring around the abscess on CT scan. Medical therapy is initially conservative, with antibiotics appropriate to the suspected or confirmed organism. If the abscess is encapsulated, craniotomy may be performed to drain it.

Clinical Problems and Nursing Diagnoses

Although the initiating organisms and thus the specific drug therapy differ, the potential human responses common to all three infectious processes described are (1) alterations in consciousness, behavioral control, movement, and multisystem regulation and (2) injury related to coma and seizures. Because the whole brain is involved, the potential disruption in function is widespread, as in acute head injury.

Alterations in consciousness may range from decreased arousal to hyperarousal. Because all three pathologic processes have the potential to either increase intracranial pressure or act like a mass lesion, potential brain herniation is a clinical problem common to all.

Nursing management has a strong monitoring component, including monitoring to detect signs of brain herniation; monitoring intracranial pressure and adaptive capacity (see "Nursing Diagnoses," under "Intracranial Hypertension," earlier in the chapter); monitoring for signs of cranial nerve dysfunction, particularly as it affects airway and eye protection and protection from injury during seizures; and monitoring for multisystem regulatory problems such as SIADH, DIC, and septic shock.

Management relevent to airway protection, protection from injury, and multisystem failure is discussed under "Neurotrauma," as is the care for the patient with decreased arousal. Nursing care related to seizures is discussed under "Seizures," earlier in this chapter.

Hyperarousal is a common manifestation of meningeal and brain parenchymal irritation. The patient with abnormally increased arousal has a high potential for injury from random movements, for nutritional deficit related to increased caloric expenditure, and for skin breakdown due to rubbing on sheets. Common interventions consist of padding the bed with bolsters and lining it with sheepskin to prevent skin abrasions and bruises. The patient who no longer needs intravenous lines or monitoring lines but still requires close observation to prevent injury may be moved to an intermediate care unit, with a floor bed used to avoid falls. Caloric intake is increased via tube feeding or oral feeding, and all staff should take special care to continually orient the patient to the environment and to maintain as quiet and nonstimulating an environment as possible.

Autoimmune and Neurotoxic Disorders

Several disorders of autoimmune and neurotoxic origin alter ventilation and movement without impairing consciousness and may be sufficiently severe to require intensive care. Myasthenia gravis, Guillain-Barré syndrome, and multiple sclerosis with respiratory involvement are all disorders in which the body is believed to direct its immune processes, normally used to combat foreign tissue, against its own nervous system. The body makes antibodies to muscle acetylcholine receptors in the case of myasthenia gravis, against central myelin in multiple sclerosis, and against peripheral nerve myelin in Guillain-Barré syndrome.

Neurotoxic disorders include those, such as botulism and tetanus, which result from endogenous neurotoxins produced by invasion or ingestion of anaerobic organisms and those resulting from exogenous toxins such as organophosphates.

Guillain-Barré syndrome is a disorder of the peripheral nerves in which the myelin degenerates, presumably in response to autoimmune processes following a viral infection. It is generally characterized by ascending motor, more than sensory, loss and becomes life-threatening if it involves the muscles of respiration and the peripheral portion of the cranial nerves that protect the airway. Consciousness is fully preserved in Guillain-Barré patients, but they may be able to communicate with others only by moving the eyes. Generally the Schwann cells regenerate and restore the myelin over several weeks; thus full recovery is possible. Expert nursing care is critical to prevent secondary complications that interfere with that recovery. Nursing diagnoses and nursing care are essentially the same as for a patient with high cervical cord injury, except that the paralysis is flaccid (rather than becoming spastic after spinal shock) and the patient often has sensory function and may thus be in considerable discomfort from the immobility.

Myasthenia gravis and the neurotoxic disorders are primarily disorders of the myoneural junction. The nerve terminal of the motor axon releases packets of acetylcholine, or *quanta*. These quanta bind to receptors on the membrane of the muscle fiber and create end-plate potentials, which eventually summate and produce an action potential and contraction of the muscle fiber. Deficits in firing may occur because too little acetylcholine is released (as is thought to occur in botulism); because acetylcholinesterase clearance in the synaptic cleft is inhibited with resultant fatigue of the receptors (as in organophosphate poisoning); or because receptor sites are too few (as is thought to be the case in myasethenia gravis) or are occupied by another neurochemical. The end result of these differing pathologic processes is the same: muscular weakness or paralysis, which becomes worse with repetitive stimulation, and depression of reflexes.

Myasthenia Gravis

Myasthenia gravis is a disorder that challenges both patient and professional staff when control is unstable. It can be highly unpredictable and may rapidly become unstable, thus requiring astute nursing monitoring. While patients suffering from ascending polyneuropathy (Guillain-Barré syndrome) may increasingly lose function over a period of days, the patient in myasthenic or cholinergic crisis may lose ability to protect the airway in *less than one hour.* Furthermore, it is often difficult to determine whether increasing weakness is secondary to too little medication (myasthenic state) or too much medication (cholinergic state).

Clinically, the patient with myasthenia experiences increasing weakness with continued effort and weakness of specific muscle groups. Some patients have weakness only of the extraocular muscles, with continual or intermittent diplopia and ptosis. Others may have primarily head and upper extremity weakness, and still others may have involvement of all extremities as well as the head and neck.

The onset is bimodal, with women more often affected between 20 and 30 years and men between 50 and 60 years. Spontaneous remissions occur, although remission is more likely following thymectomy in young women. The critical-care nurse is most likely to care for a person with myasthenia who has lost or is at high risk of losing the ability to protect the airway because of myasthenic crisis (severe weakness with decreasing response to medication), cholinergic crisis (severe weakness plus cholinergic signs due to overdosage with medication), or thymectomy. Myasthenic crisis may be directly related to increased demands upon the patient's system, such as severe illness or surgical procedures unrelated to the myasthenia, or may be of unknown cause.

Anticholinesterase drugs are the mostly commonly used treatment for myasthenia (Table 35-11); pyridostigmine bromide (Mestinon) is the most widely used. Neostigmine (Prostigmin) is shorter-acting and less used for maintenance; however, it can be given parenterally and may be used more often in acute situations. Edrophonium chloride (Tensilon) is an extremely short-acting anticholinesterase used diagnostically. All anticholinesterase agents act to prevent acetylcholinesterase from chemically breaking acetylcholine in the synaptic cleft into acetate and choline. Such chemical breakdown of the acetylcholine ends depolarization of the muscle membrane and allows the muscle to repolarize and thus be ready for another action potential. Since the number of receptor sites is

Table 35-11 Time of Action of Selected Drugs for Myasthenia Gravis

Drug	Onset	Peak	Duration
Edrophonium (Tensilon; used diagnostically only)	30 s	30–60 s	4–5 min
Neostigmine (Prostigmin)	30 min	1–2 h	2–3 h
Pyridostigmine (Mestinon)	30 min	1–2 h	2–4 h
Parenteral neostigmine	10–15 min	30 min	2–3 h

reduced in myasthenia, prolongation of depolarization allows somewhat longer firing of fewer fibers and thus increased muscle contraction. Obviously, excessive prolongation of depolarization can result in *increased* weakness if further nerve impulses are unable to initiate further action potentials; consequently, muscle weakness can result from too much anticholinesterase medication as well as from too little. While the drug treatment of myasthenia may dramatically improve the patient's ability to carry on daily tasks, it does not alter the basic disorder. Plasmapheresis, the exchange of the patient's plasma for plasmalike solution, temporarily affects the disease process by removing autoantibodies.

While patients in the neurology units of a hospital may be well enough to administer their own anticholinesterase drugs, those in critical care most often must rely upon the nurse for this. It cannot be overemphasized that timing is crucial. A delay of 15 to 20 min can make the difference between a patient who has sufficient strength to swallow the medication and one who does not. Any patient at risk or in crisis has the potential for rapid changes in condition and rapid changes in strength. Since excess medication is one cause of increasing weakness, the nurse is frequently in the position of having to decide whether increasing weakness is from too little or too much medication. If it is from too much, the next dose must be omitted. Unfortunately, the clinical presentation of myasthenic and cholinergic crisis are so similar that even the most experienced clinicians may have difficulty making this differentiation.

While both situations produce increasing weakness in the patient, the timing of such weakness is one clue to the cause. Weakness due to myasthenia is apt to come at about the time of onset of action of the medication, whereas weakness due to excess medication usually occurs within the duration of action of the drug. These times are given in Table 35-11. The presence of abdominal cramps, salivation, diarrhea, and muscle fasciculations accompanied by increased weakness are also highly suggestive of cholinergic (drug excess) rather than myasthenic state. If the increasing weakness is clearly drug-related, the next dose must be omitted to prevent precipitation of life-threatening cholinergic crisis. However, it is often difficult to tell whether the weakness is related to too much or too little anticholinesterase drug. In such cases, the physician will often elect to perform an edrophonium test. If weakness is due to excess drug, the weakness will become even worse and often be associated with cramping with the addition of edrophonium, whereas the clinical condition will improve if the weakness is secondary to too little anticholinesterase. Because edrophonium is a rapid-acting, short-duration drug, both worsening and improvement in condition are transient. The nurse must be prepared to administer atropine sulfate to reverse the anticholinesterase effect and to suction or even ventilate the patient if the edrophonium test precipitates a cholinergic crisis. However, used judiciously, the test can often prevent crisis by distinguishing between the two states before dysphagia and bulbar weakness are pronounced.

Prevention of Neurotoxic Disorders

The life-threatening motor problems caused by tetanus, botulism, and diphtheritic neuropathy are totally preventable by prevention of the basic disorders. Table 35-12 summarizes the sites of action, critical-care problems, and management of these disorders in relation to the endotoxins which attack the nervous system. It is evident that once the endotoxin has been made in the body, there is little in the way of definitive treatment. Expert nursing care is the key to the survival of patients until the endotoxin ceases being formed and the body can heal itself. How much better for the patient to have been appropriately immunized or for the food to have been properly prepared in the first place!

Table 35-12 Comparison of Sites of Action, Critical Problems, and Management of Movement Problems Caused by Endotoxins

Endotoxin	Site of Action	Effect	Management
Tetanus: tetanospasmin made by *Clostridium tetani*	Local effect on muscle. Major effect is to interfere with spinal inhibitory neurons	Sustained muscle contraction; rigidity, stiffness progressing to paroxysmal spasms without loss of consciousness. Death may occur from apnea, suffocation, secondary spasm of glottal muscles and respiratory muscles. Circulatory collapse possible	Single-dose antitoxin (no effect on established symptoms but prevents further endotoxin). Tracheostomy if having spasms; minimal manipulation, sedation, minimal stimulation; nursing care crucial in maintaining quiet environment. Constant monitoring. Curare if spasms uncontrollable; requires total life support
Diphtheritic neuropathy: endotoxin from *Corynebacterium diphtheriae*	Membrane of Schwann cell of proximal peripheral nerve and dorsal root ganglion. Demyelination occurs	Weakness, paralysis of muscles affecting cranial nerves 1–2 weeks after infection; spinal peripheral nerves about 7–10 weeks after infection. Usually descending weakness of bulbar muscles, arms, legs	Symptomatic; antitoxin ineffective once neuropathy established (affects about 20% of patients). Expert nursing care; detection of bulbar symptoms early; tracheostomy if necessary. Prognosis good for recovery if well supported in acute phase
Botulism: botulins toxin from *Clostridium botulinum*	Neuromuscular junction; inteferes with release of acetycholine	Weakness, paralysis of bulbar, systemic, and smooth muscles	Expert supportive nursing care; may require complete respiratory, alimental support; symptoms may fluctuate, requiring frequent evaluation

Both diphtheria and tetanus are completely preventable by appropriate immunization in childhood, with booster doses for tetanus at 10-year intervals. Toxoid boosters may be given to persons previously immunized and exposed to diphtheria and to those who sustain a contaminated injury (tetanus).

Botulism most commonly occurs following the ingestion of food containing botulinus toxin. Improperly cooked home-canned foods are the most common source. The best prevention for botulism is to follow canning directions carefully, especially for nonacid foods. Many recommend boiling home-canned nonacid foods prior to eating as an additional precaution.

Nursing Diagnoses

Nursing management of patients with polyneuropathies and of those with autoimmune and neurotoxic disorders of the myoneural junction is quite similar, even though the pathologic conditions differ. The primary potential nursing diagnoses are:

Inadequate airway clearance

Inadequate breathing pattern

Complete immobility and total self-care deficit

Fear and anxiety related to decreasing ability to breathe and fear of dying

Inadequate nutrition related to inability to swallow safely

Discomfort related to preservation of sensation with total immobility

Pain related to severe muscle spasms in tetanus

Nursing monitoring and management relevant to these problems was discussed earlier under "Neuropathophysiologic States That Disrupt Ventilation but Not Consciousness."

References

1. Carpenito, L. J. (1983). *Nursing diagnosis: Application to clinical practice.* Philadelphia: Lippincott.

2. Jordan, R. C. (1983). Pathophysiology of brain injury. *Critical Care Quarterly, 5,(4),* 1–11.

3. Klatzo, I. (1985). Brain oedema following brain ischaemia and the influence of therapy. *British Journal of Anaesthesia, 57,* 18–22.

4. Langfitt, T. W. (1983). CT, NMR and emission tomography in the diagnosis and management of brain swelling and intracranial hypertension. In S. Ishii et al. (Eds.), *Intracranial pressure V* (pp. 54–62). Berlin: Springer.

5. Miller, J. D. (1985). Head injury and brain ischaemia. *British Journal of Anesthesia, 57,* 120–130.

6. Gennarelli, T. A., Spielman, G., Langfitt, T. W., et al. (1982). Influence of the type of intracranial lesion on outcome from severe head injury. *Journal of Neurosurgery, 56,* 26–32.

7. Langfitt, T. W., & Gennarelli, T. A. (1982). Can the outcome from head injury be improved? *Journal of Neurosurgery, 56,* 19–25.

8. Narayan, R. K., Kishore, P.R.S., Becker, D. P., et al. (1982). Intracranial pressure: To monitor or not to monitor? *Journal of Neurosurgery, 56,* 650–659.

9. Collins, W. F. (1983). A review and update of experiment and clinical studies of spinal cord injury. *Paraplegia, 21,* 204–219.

10. Fishman, R. A. (1975). Brain edema. *New England Journal of Medicine, 293,* 706–711.

11. Fishman, R. A., & Rhan, P. A. (1980). Metabolic basis of brain edema. *Advances in Neurology, 28,* 207–215.

12. Miller, J. D., et al. (1977). Significance of intracranial hypertension in severe head injury. *Journal of Neurosurgery, 47,* 503–517.

13. Graham, D. (1985). The pathology of brain ischaemia and possibilities for therapeutic intervention. *British Journal of Anesthesia, 57,* 3–17.

14. McGraw, C. P., & O'Conner, C. (1986). Analysis of the intracranial responses to mannitol and furosemide. In J. D. Miller et al. (Eds.), *Intracranial pressure VI* (pp. 601–604). Berlin: Springer.

15. Tsutsumi, H., et al. (1986). The relationship between intracranial pressure, cerebral perfusion pressure and outcome in head injured patients: The critical level of CPP. In J. D. Miller et al. (Eds.), *Intracranial pressure VI* (pp. 661–666). Berlin: Springer.

16. Marshall, L. F., Smith, R. W., & Shapiro, H. M. (1979). The outcome with aggressive treatment in severe head injuries. Part 1: The significance of intracranial pressure monitoring. *Journal of Neurosurgery, 50,* 20–25.

17. Jennett, B., & Teasdale, G. (1981). *The management of head injuries.* Philadelphia: Davis.

18. Pollay, M., Fullenwider, C., Roberts, P. A., & Stevens, F. A. (1983). Effect of mannitol and furosemide on blood-brain osmotic gradients and intracranial pressure. *Journal of Neurosurgery, 59,* 945–950.

19. Cooper, P. R., et al. (1979). Dexamethasone and severe head injury: A prospective double-blind study. *Journal of Neurosurgery, 51,* 307–316.

20. Kaktis, J., & Pitts, L. H. (1980). Complications associated with megadose steroids in head-injured patients. *Journal of Neurosurgical Nursing, 12,* 166–171.

21. Pitts, L. H., & Kaktis, J. (1980). The effect of megadose steroids on ICP in traumatic coma. In K. Shulman et al. (Eds.), *Intracranial pressure IV* (pp. 638–642). Berlin: Springer.

22. Braughler, J. M., & Hall, E. D. (1985). Current applications of "high-dose" steroid therapy for CNS injury. *Journal of Neurosurgery, 62,* 806–810.

23. Cooper, K. R., et al. (1985). Safe use of PEEP in patients with severe head injury. *Journal of Neurosurgery, 63,* 552–555.

24. Brain Resuscitation Clinical Trial I Study Group. (1986). Randomized clinical trial of thiopental loading in comatose survivors of cardiac arrest. *New England Journal of Medicine, 314,* 397–403.

25. Ward, J. D., Becker, D. P., Miller, J. D., et al. (1985). Failure of prophylactic barbiturate coma in the treatment of severe head injury. *Journal of Neurosurgery, 62,* 383–388.

26. Yano, M., Ikeda, Y., Kobayashi, S., et al. (1986). The outcome with barbiturate therapy in severe head injuries. In J. D. Miller et al. (Eds.), *Intracranial pressure VI* (pp. 769–773). Berlin: Springer.

27. Bedford, R. F., Parsing, J. A., Poberski, L., & Butler, A. (1980). Lidocaine or thiopental for rapid control of intracranial hypertension. *Anesthesia and Analgesia, 59,* 435–437.

28. Henneman, E. A. (1986). Brain resuscitation. *Heart and Lung, 15,* 3–11.

28a. Miller, J. D. (1975). Volume and pressure in the

craniospinal axis. *Clinical Neurosurgery, 22,* 76–105.

29. Selig, J. M., Klauber, M. R., Toole, B. M., & Bowers-Marshall, S. (1986). Increased ICP and systemic hypotension during the first 72 hours following severe head injury. In J. D. Miller et al. (Eds.), *Intracranial pressure VI* (pp. 675–679). Berlin: Springer.

30. American Nurses Association and American Association of Neuroscience Nurses. (1986). *Neuroscience nursing practice: Process and outcome criteria for selected diagnoses.* Kansas City: ANA.

31. Mitchell, P. H. (1986). Intracranial hypertension: Influence of nursing care activities. *Nursing Clinics of North America, 21,* 563–576.

32. Magnaes, B. (1976). Body position and cerebrospinal fluid pressure. Part 1: Clinical studies on the effect of rapid postural changes. *Journal of Neurosurgery, 44,* 687–697.

33. Metcalf, C., & Mitchell, P. H. (1987). The effects of pre- and post-suctioning treatment on intracranial pressure: Hyperoxygenation versus combined hyperinflation and hyperoxygenation [Abstract]. *Heart and Lung, 16,* 372–328.

34. Parsons, L. C., & Shogan, J. S. O. (1984). The effect of endotracheal tube suction/manual hyperventilation procedure on patients with severe closed head injuries. *Heart and Lung, 13,* 372.

35. Chyatte, D., & Sundt, T. M. (1984). Cerebral vasospasm after subarachnoid hemorrhage. *Mayo Clinic Proceedings, 59,* 498–505.

36. Allen, G. S. (1984). Cerebral arterial spasm. *Clinical Neurosurgery, 22,* 70–77.

37. Jackson, L. O. (1986). Cerebral vasospasm after an intracranial aneurysmal subarachnoid hemorrhage: A nursing perspective. *Heart and Lung, 15,* 14–20.

38. Voldby, B., & Enevoldsen, E. M. (1982). Intracranial pressure changes following aneurysm rupture. *Journal of Neurosurgery, 56,* 186–196.

39. Plum, F., & Posner, J. B. (1980). *The diagnosis of stupor and coma* (2d ed.). New York: Davis.

40. Teasdale, G., Knill-Jones, R., & Van der Sande, J. (1978). Observer variability in assessing impaired consciousness and coma. *Journal of Neurology, Neurosurgery and Psychiatry, 41,* 603–610.

41. Jones, C. (1979). Glasgow coma scale. *American Journal of Nursing. 79,* 1551–1553.

42. Teasdale, G. (1975). Acute impairment of brain function. 1. Assessing the "conscious level." *Nursing Times, 71,* 914–917.

43. Teasdale, G. and Galbraith, S. (1975). Acute impairment of brain function. 2. Observation record. *Nursing Times, 71,* 972–973.

44. Born, J. D., Albert, A., Hans, P., & Bonnal, J. (1985). Relative prognostic value of best motor response and brain stem reflexes in patients with severe head injury. *Neurosurgery, 16,* 595–601.

45. Simon, R. P. (1985). Physiologic consequences of status epilepticus. *Epilepsia, 26(Suppl. 1),* 558–566.

46. Nevander, G., Ingvar, M., Auer, R., & Siesjo, B. K. (1984). Irreversible neuronal damage after short periods of status epilepticus. *Acta Physiologica Scandinavica, 120,* 155–157.

47. Brodoff, A. S. (1983). Intervening to stop status epilepticus. *Patient Care, 17(7),* 153–160.

48. Lovely, M. P., & Ozuna, J. (1982). Status epilepticus. In D. L. Nikas (Ed.), *The critically ill neurosurgical patient.* New York: Churchill-Livingstone.

49. Bell, H. E., & Bertino, J. S. (1984). Constant diazepam infusion in the treatment of continuous seizure activity. *Drug Intelligence and Clinical Pharmacy, 18,* 965–970.

50. Lacey, D. J., Singer, W. D., Horwitz, S. J., & Gilmore, H. (1986). Lorazapam therapy of status epilepticus in children and adolescents. *The Journal of Pediatrics, 108,* 771–774.

51. Orlowski, J. P., Erenberg, G., Leuders, H., & Cruse, R. (1984), Hypothermia and barbiturate coma for refractory status epilepticus. *Critical Care Medicine, 12,* 367–372.

52. Blount, M., Kinney, A. B., & Luttrell, N. (1982). Myasthenia gravis and the Guillain-Barré syndrome. In D. L. Nikas (Ed.), *The critically ill neurosurgical patient.* New York: Churchill-Livingstone.

53. Leinart, B. (1979) Attitudes of nurses toward spinal cord injury patients. *ARN (Journal of the Association of Rehabilitation Nurses), 4(1),* 7–9.

54. Chu, D. A., Ahn, J. H., Ragnarsson, K. T., et al. (1985). Deep venous thrombosis: Diagnosis in spinal cord injured patients. *Archives of Physical Medicine and Rehabilitation, 66,* 365–368.

55. Myllynen, P., Kammonen, M., Rokkanen, P., et al. (1985). Deep venous thrombosis and pulmonary embolism in patients with acute spinal cord injury: A comparison with nonparalyzed patients immobilized due to spinal fractures. *Journal of Trauma, 25,* 541–543.

56. Cerrato, D., Ariano, C., & Fiacchino, F. (1978). Deep vein thrombosis and low-dose heparin prophylaxis in neurosurgical patients. *Journal of Neurosurgery, 49,* 378–381.

57. Sugarman, B. (1985). Medical complications of spinal cord injury. *Quarterly Journal of Medicine* (New Series 54), *213,* 3–18.

58. Saul, T. G. (1983). Intensive care of the brain-injured patient. *Critical Care Quarterly, 5(4),* 82–89.

59. Raimond, J., & Taylor, J. W. (1986). *Neurological*

emergencies: Effective nursing care. Rockville, MD: Aspen.

60. Doczi, T., Tarjanyi, J., Huszka, E., et al. (1982). Syndrome of inappropriate secretion of antidiuretic hormone (SIADH) after head injury. *Neurosurgery, 19,* 685–688.

61. Shapiro, H. M. (1985). Barbiturates in brain ischaemia. *British Journal of Anesthesia, 57,* 82–95.

62. Deutschman, S. S., Konstantinides, F. N., Raup, S., et al. (1986). Physiological and metabolic response to isolated closed head injury. *Journal of Neurosurgery, 64,* 89–98.

63. Robertson, C. S., Clifton, G. L., & Goodman, J. C. (1985). Steroid administration and nitrogen excretion in the head-injured patient. *Journal of Neurosurgery, 63,* 714–718.

64. Sanford, S. (1982). Respiratory complications of intracranial disorders. In D. L. Nikas (Ed.), *The critically ill neurosurgical patient.* New York: Churchill-Livingstone.

65. McGuire, A. (1986). Issues in the prevention of neurotrauma. *Nursing Clinics of North America, 21,* 549–554.

66. Gardner, D. (1986). Acute management of the head-injured adult. *Nursing Clinics of North America, 21,* 555–562.

67. Nikas, D. L. (1986). Resuscitation of patients with central nervous system trauma. *Nursing Clinics of North America, 21(4),* 693–704.

68. Bracken, M. B., Shepard, M. J., Hellenbrand, K. G., et al. (1985). Methylprednisolone and neurological function 1 year after spinal cord injury. *Journal of Neurosurgery, 63,* 704–713.

69. Bar-Or, D. (1985, May). Naloxone—new applications. *Trauma Quarterly, 3(2),* 25–31.

70. Metcalf, J. A. (1986). Acute phase management of persons with spinal cord injury: A nursing diagnosis perspective. *Nursing Clinics of North America, 21,* 589–598.

71. Norris, J. W., & Hachinski, V. (1985). Acute stroke units: A reappraisal. *Current Concepts of Cerebrovascular Disease (Stroke), 20(6),* 31–33.

72. Miller, V. T., & Hart, R. G. (1987). Heparin anticoagulation in acute brain ischemia. *Current Concepts in Cerebrovascular Disease (Stroke), 22(2),* 7–11.

73. Hunt, W. E., & Hess, R. M. (1968). Surgical risk as related to time of intervention in the repair of intracranial aneurysms. *Journal of Neurosurgery, 28,* 14–20.

74. Adams, H. P., Kassell, N. F., Torner, J. C., et al. (1981). Early management of aneurysmal subarachnoid hemorrhage: A report of the cooperative aneurysm study. *Journal of Neurosurgery, 54,* 141–145.

75. Lee, K. (1980). Aneurysm precautions: A physiologic basis for minimizing rebleeding. *Heart and Lung, 9,* 336–343.

76. Goldring, S., Zervas, N., & Langfitt, T. (1987). The extracranial-intracranial bypass study: A report of the committee appointed by the American Association of Neurological Surgeons to examine the study. *New England Journal of Medicine, 316,* 817–820.

77. American Association of Neuroscience Nurses. (1984). *Core curriculum for neuroscience nursing (Vol. II).* Chicago: AANN.

78. Hirsch, M. S. (1985). Acute viral central nervous system diseases. In E. Rubenstein & D. D. Federman (Eds.), *Scientific American Medicine,* Section 7, XXVII, 1–5.

79. Simon, H. B. (1986). Immunizations and chemotherapy for viral infections. In E. Rubenstein, D. P. Federman (Eds.), *Scientific American Medicine,* Section 7, XXXIII, 12–15.

part

8

Endocrine Patient-Care Problems

36 Endocrine Anatomy and Physiology

Sarah J. Sanford

Functional integrity of the human organism requires that activities of all body systems be adjusted to correlate with changes in the demands posed by the external and internal environments. Delicate physiologic balance must be achieved and maintained, and complex processes must be precisely regulated. The endocrine system, closely interacting with the nervous system, is responsible for many vital adjustments in physiologic integration. Mechanisms in that integration overlap; those of the nervous system are discussed in Chap. 33. Integration by the endocrine system is effected through the secretion of hormones into the circulation, which are then carried to various body tissues.

In this chapter the structural and functional categories of hormones as well as the mechanisms by which they exert their effects are discussed as background for a discussion of the anatomy and physiology of the various glands of the endocrine system.

It is almost impossible to exaggerate the importance of the endocrine glands. Each of the glands is capable of exerting a specific effect, and at times this effect is profound with regard to physiologic influence on body tissues. As an interacting system, the endocrine glands are responsible for the regulation of complex processes including growth and development, reproduction, metabolism, and the stress response. In addition, they play vital roles in the establishment and maintenance of fluid and electrolyte, acid-base, and energy balance. The nature of their regulation and maintenance of homeostasis is multifaceted and widespread. A list of the glands and their locations is given in Table 36-1.

Hormones: The Physiologic Effectors

The endocrine system performs its vital functions through hormones that can be categorized according to structural and functional properties.

Structural Categories

Hormones fall into one of the following four structural categories: amines, steroids, polypeptides, and prostaglandins.[1,2]

Amines
The amines include the catecholamines norepinephrine and epinephrine. Norepinephrine is formed by hydroxylation and decarboxylation of the amino acids phenylalanine and tyrosine. The enzymes necessary for this conversion are present in adrenergic nerve endings. However, conversion of norepinephrine to epinephrine involves methylation of the former by enzymes found only in the adrenal medulla. Thus, release of norepinephrine occurs at adrenergic nerve endings, while both epinephrine and norepinephrine, but predominantly epinephrine, are released from the adrenal medulla.[1,2]

Steroids
Steroid hormones include the glucocorticoids, mineralocorticoids, and sex hormones (androgens and estrogens). They are synthesized and secreted by both the adrenal cortex and the gonads. All steroid hormones are derivatives of cholesterol. The cells in which synthesis occurs as well as the biochemical pathways employed are similar.[1] The actual structure formed is determined by sequential action of

Table 36-1 Location and Function of the Endocrine Glands

Gland	Location	Function
Pituitary (hypophysis)	Cranial cavity (pituitary fossa)	
Anterior lobe (adenohypophysis)		Functional integrity and responsiveness of thyroid gland via TSH, adrenal cortex via ACTH, gonads via FSH, LH
		Lactogenesis via prolactin
		Anabolism, growth via GH
Posterior lobe (neurohypophysis)		Milk ejection via oxytocin
		Maintenance of free water balance via ADH
Thyroid	Neck—either side of trachea	Control of metabolic rate via T_4, T_3, vital to growth
Parathyroids	Neck—embedded in thyroid	Maintenance of serum calcium level via PTH
Adrenals	Upper poles of kidneys (retroperitoneal space)	
Adrenal cortex	Outer layer of gland	Maintenance of physiologic stress response, catabolism, hyperglycemia via glucocorticoids
		Maintenance of extracellular fluid volume via mineralocorticoids
		Secondary masculinization via adrenal androgens
Adrenal medulla	Interior portion of gland	Augmentation of sympathetic nervous system "fight or flight" response via catecholamines
Endocrine pancreas (islets of Langerhans)	Abdomen—pancreas	Glucose uptake, energy storage via insulin
		Glucose release, energy substrate mobilization via glucagon
Pineal	Cranial cavity (below third ventricle)	Believed to be part of time clock for puberty via inhibition of gonadotropins (FSH, LH); natural darkness-induced hypnotic, sedative effects via melatonin
Thymus	Mediastinum	Development, maturation of T cells via thymosin

catalytic enzyme systems present in each of the respective glands. Deficiencies of any of these enzyme systems can result in the production of abnormally high quantities of other, similar structures that are not subject to the normal physiologic control mechanisms. Such deficiencies therefore produce a wide variety of manifestations, all of which are attributable to aberrant steroid activity.

In the adrenal cortex, enzymes result in the synthesis of physiologically significant amounts of two glucocorticoids (cortisol and corticosterone), one mineralocorticoid (aldosterone), and one androgen. Small amounts of several androgens, estrogens, and other structurally similar sex hormones are also secreted. The gonads (testes in the male and ovaries in the female) contain enzyme systems capable of synthesis of androgens, and in the ovary, androgens are further acted upon to become estrogens.

Polypeptides

Polypeptide hormones include those secreted by the endocrine pancreas, the thyroid, and the anterior pituitary. These hormones have in common varying numbers and combinations of amino acids arranged in chainlike structures. All are synthesized within the cells of the glands which secrete them under the direction of messenger ribonucleic acid (mRNA).[2] In the case of the thyroid hormones, tetraiodothyronine (T_4) and triiodothyronine (T_3) iodine molecules are also incorporated.

Prostaglandins

Unlike the three structural categories just discussed, these hormones are not primarily synthesized or secreted by a specific structure. Rather, they are synthesized by a wide variety of tissues and are frequently referred to as *tissue hormones*. Tissues in which prostaglandins are synthesized include the seminal vesicles, kidneys, lungs, iris, brain, and thymus. They are composed of a series of closely related unsaturated fatty acids containing a cyclopentane ring. Three categories of prostaglandin have been defined on the basis of the configuration of their cyclopentane rings: group A prostaglandins (PGA), group E prostaglandins (PGE), and group F prostaglandins (PGF). Although prostaglandins are similar to other hormones in that they enter the bloodstream, they do so in minuscule amounts and probably exert their major effects by diffusing to cells adjacent to those from which they are secreted.[3]

This group of hormones has diverse physiologic effects, generally of an extremely potent nature. Group A prostaglandins are thought to result in relaxation of smooth muscle fibers in the walls of arteries and arterioles. They therefore produce an immediate decrease in blood pressure with simultaneous increases in the blood flow of the regions in close proximity to the cells from which they are released, one of these regions being the kidney. Prostaglandins in the E group have been implicated as mediators in hematopoietic, inflammatory, and gastrointestinal processes, including platelet aggregation, fever, and the regulation of hydrochloric acid secretion. Group F prostaglandins apparently affect contraction of smooth muscle in the uterus and bowel. Compounds in this group have been found to induce labor and accelerate delivery as well as play an essential role in the maintenance of normal peristalsis.[3]

Mechanisms of Action

Once secreted, hormones enter the circulation and exert their influence upon *target organ tissues,* or tissues that contain specific receptors capable of reacting with the particular structure of the hormone involved. Upon reaction of a target cell receptor with a hormone, one of two mechanisms is initiated: cAMP activation or the intracellular mechanism.

cAMP Activation: The "Second Messenger"

The "second messenger" mechanism of hormonal action involves formation of adenosine 3',5'-monophosphate, or *cyclic AMP* (cAMP), from intracellular adenosine triphosphate (ATP). Conversion of ATP is possible because the combination of the hormone with the target-cell receptor liberates a catalytic enzyme, *adenyl cyclase.* Adenyl cyclase then converts ATP to cAMP. Once formed, cAMP directs the target cell to perform its specialized function.[2]

In this mechanism, the hormone serves as the first messenger, presumably delivering a biochemical message from the endocrine gland to the target organ. The second message is then delivered to cAMP and is the message responsible for the actual response on the part of the cell. Recent research indicates that adenyl cyclase activation may be effected by prostaglandins. They are known to both facilitate and antagonize activation of adenyl cyclase in tissue cells. Through selective adenyl cyclase activation, prostaglandins are believed to play a role in the regulation of cellular cAMP content and thus mediate the cellular response to hormones acting by this mechanism.

Three hormones that affect cellular function via the second messenger mechanism include epinephrine, glucagon, and parathormone. Activation of cAMP in the cells of bronchiolar smooth muscle, hepatic cells, and the cells of bones results in relaxation and bronchiolar dilatation, breakdown of hepatic glycogen (and an elevation in blood glucose), and release of ionized calcium from bones, respectively. Characteristic of this mechanism is a rapid tissue response, due in part to the fact that hormone receptors are located on or within the target cell membranes and thus are readily exposed to circulating hormones. Hormones activating cAMP also tend to exert a profound impact on target cells.[2]

Some pharmacologic agents are known to exert their effect by alteration of the second messenger mechanism of hormone response. One of these is aminophylline. This substance prolongs epinephrine-induced bronchiolar dilatation by inhibiting phosphodiesterase, the enzyme that normally results in breakdown of cAMP. A second agent is aspirin. Current research indicates that the antiinflammatory and anticoagulant properties of aspirin are probably due at least in part to prevention of group E prostaglandin synthesis. As a result of decreased PGE, alteration in cellular cAMP content occurs, presumably limiting cellular responsiveness.

Intracellular Mechanism

The second mechanism of hormone action is the intracellular mechanism. Hormones exerting their effect via this mechanism must be lipid-soluble and able to traverse cell membranes, because receptors are located within cellular boundaries. Once within the cell, the hormone is transferred to the cell nucleus, where the hormone-receptor complex directs alterations in the synthesis of mRNA and subsequently of specific proteins. Both the traversal of cellular membranes and the alteration of mRNA synthesis require a longer time frame than is required for cAMP activation. Therefore, while no less profound in impact, hormones acting via the intracellular mechanism require days to weeks both to reach peak effect and to subside. Steroid and thyroid hormones are examples of hormones exerting their impact by this mechanism.[1] Schematic representations of both these mechanisms are presented in Fig. 36-1.

Functional Categories

Dividing the endocrine hormones into functional categories facilitates their organization.

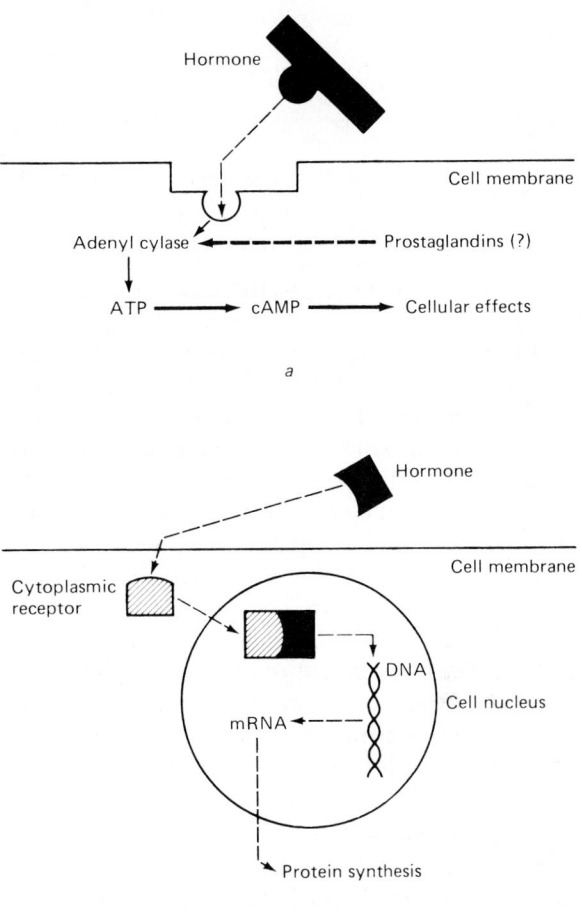

Figure 36-1   Mechanisms of hormone action. (*a*) The "second messenger," cAMP activation. (*b*) Intracellular mechanism.

Releasing and Inhibiting Hormones

The releasing and inhibiting hormones are a group of hormones that are synthesized by the hypothalamus. They and the hormones secreted by the posterior pituitary gland are unique in being synthesized within the central nervous system rather than in the gland from which they are secreted. The only target for releasing and inhibiting hormones is the anterior pituitary, and for each of the hormones secreted by the anterior pituitary there is thought to be both a releasing and inhibiting hormone secreted by the hypothalamus; however, only eight have been identified:

1. Corticotropin releasing hormone (CRH)

2. Thyrotropin releasing hormone (TRH)
3. Growth hormone releasing hormone (GRH)
4. Growth hormone inhibiting hormone (GIH)
5. Follicle stimulating hormone releasing hormone (FRH)
6. Luteinizing hormone releasing hormone (LRH)
7. Prolactin releasing hormone (PRH)
8. Prolactin inhibiting hormone (PIH)

As their names imply, these hormones either stimulate or inhibit the secretion of the hormones of the anterior pituitary. With the exception of FRH and LRH, each is discussed in conjunction with the hormone it directly affects in the section that follows. FRH and LRH affect secretion of the gonads, the testes in the male and ovaries in the female. These glands, which are responsible for maintenance of reproductive capability, are not associated with acute or critical illness and therefore are not discussed.

Secretion of the releasing and inhibiting hormones is regulated by diffuse interaction within the central nervous system and also by the condition of the blood perfusing the hypothalamus through the negative feedback mechanism described below.

Tropic Hormones

By definition, tropic hormones increase the size and secretion rates of other endocrine glands. These hormones are secreted only by the anterior pituitary. From there they enter the general circulation to be carried to target endocrine glands. Control of their secretion is directly influenced by hypothalamic secretion of releasing and inhibiting hormones. It is also affected by the blood levels of the hormones secreted by their target glands. As the blood level of a target gland hormone increases, the secretion rate of the anterior pituitary tropic hormones decreases; thus target gland hormones exert negative feedback upon further tropic hormone release. Negative feedback also operates at the hypothalamic level with regard to the secretion of releasing hormones.[4] Each of the tropic hormones is discussed in detail in the section dealing with the anterior pituitary that follows.

Peripheral Hormones

The hormones with which we are most familiar are those which act directly upon peripheral tissues.

With the exception of the two hormones secreted by the posterior pituitary, peripheral hormones are gland-specific in origin in that they are secreted by the gland in which their synthesis occurs. Their targets are perfused by the general circulation and are defined by the presence of receptors capable of responding to the particular structure of the hormone.

Control over the secretion rates of these hormones is twofold. Nervous system influence is prominent. The autonomic nervous system directly affects the release of some peripheral hormones (e.g., catecholamines); the hypothalamus directly affects the release of others (e.g., oxytocin and antidiuretic hormone) and indirectly affects the release of still others via secretion of releasing hormones (e.g., prolactin, growth hormone, and all the pituitary tropic hormones, which then increase the secretion of target glands). In addition, blood-borne or humoral conditions directly stimulate release of still other peripheral hormones. Insulin and glucagon are two examples; they are secreted, respectively, in response to elevations or insufficient levels of blood glucose. A summary of the hormonal relationships between the hypothalamus, pituitary, and peripheral hormones is presented in Table 36-2.

Endocrine Glands

Pituitary (Hypophysis)

The pituitary gland is an almond-sized organ located deep in the pituitary fossa of the sella turcica. It is protected not only by surrounding bone but also by a layer of dura known as the *pituitary diaphragm.* Off the upper aspect there is a cylindrical projection, the *pituitary stalk,* that joins the gland to the hypothalamus.[1,2]

Because of the wide variety of the pituitary hormones and the profound influence they exert, the pituitary is frequently referred to as the *master gland.* It is composed of three lobes (the anterior, the intermediate, and the posterior), each of which functions independently with regard to hormones secreted.[5]

The anterior and intermediate lobes microscopically resemble other endocrine tissue. Func-

Table 36-2 Hormonal Relationships between the Hypothalamus, Pituitary, and Peripheral Hormones

Hypothalamic Hormones		Pituitary Tropic Hormone	Peripheral Hormone
Releasing	**Inhibiting**		
Growth hormone releasing hormone (GRH)	Growth hormone inhibiting hormone (GIF)	—	Growth hormone
Prolactin releasing hormone (PRH)	Prolactin inhibiting hormone (PIH)	—	Prolactin
Corticotropin releasing hormone (CRF)	—	Adrenocorticotropic hormone (ACTH)	Adrenal steroids
Follicle stimulating hormone releasing hormone (FRH)	—	Follicle stimulating hormone (FSH)	Gonadal steroids
Luteinizing hormone releasing hormone (LRH)	—	Luteinizing hormone (LH)	Gonadal steroids
Thyrotropin releasing hormone (TRH)	—	Thyroid stimulating hormone (TSH)	Thyroid hormones
—	—	—	Oxytocin
—	—	—	Antidiuretic hormone (ADH)
—	—	—	Melanotropins (melanocyte stimulating hormones, MSHs)

tionally, they are connected to the hypothalamus by a portal capillary network *(portal-hypophyseal tract)* in the pituitary stalk. Axons from hypothalamic secretory cells terminate near the origin of this network, and it is into these capillaries that hypothalamic releasing and inhibiting hormones are released to be transported to the anterior pituitary.[5]

The posterior lobe of the pituitary microscopically resembles nervous system tissue. The posterior lobe, unlike the anterior and intermediate lobes, is functionally linked to the hypothalamus by a tract of nerve fibers. Transmission of neural impulses down this tract is the mechanism by which the secretion of posterior pituitary hormones is influenced by the hypothalamus.[6] An illustration of the anatomic hypothalamic-pituitary relationship is presented in Fig. 36-2.

Anterior Pituitary (Adenohypophysis)

Histologically, the anterior pituitary is composed of three types of granular secretory cells, connective tissue, and a dense vascular network. In terms of their reaction to dyes, the secretory cells consist of acidophils—those whose granules readily stain with acid dyes; basophils—those whose granules readily stain with basic dyes; and chromophobes—those which do not readily stain with either type of dye

(from the Greek *chroma,* meaning "color," and the Latin *phobos,* meaning "fearing"). Acidophils secrete the two anterior pituitary peripheral hormones prolactin and growth hormone. Basophils secrete the four anterior pituitary tropic hormones. Chromophobes are probably "burned out" acidophils or basophils and no longer function in a secretory capacity.[5]

The vascular network of the anterior pituitary enters the gland as a continuation of the portal capillary network in the pituitary stalk. After extensive winding among the secretory cells, it empties into the general circulation. The dense circulatory nature of the anterior pituitary provides the anatomic basis for the high degree of interaction between the hypothalamus and the anterior pituitary. Functionally, it provides not only a means of bathing the anterior pituitary secretory cells in blood which contains releasing and inhibiting hormones from the hypothalamus but also a readily accessible means of delivering anterior pituitary hormones to the general circulation.

Tropic Hormones of the Anterior Pituitary Four of the six hormones secreted by the anterior pituitary are tropic hormones: thyroid stimulating hormone (TSH); adrenocorticotropic hormone

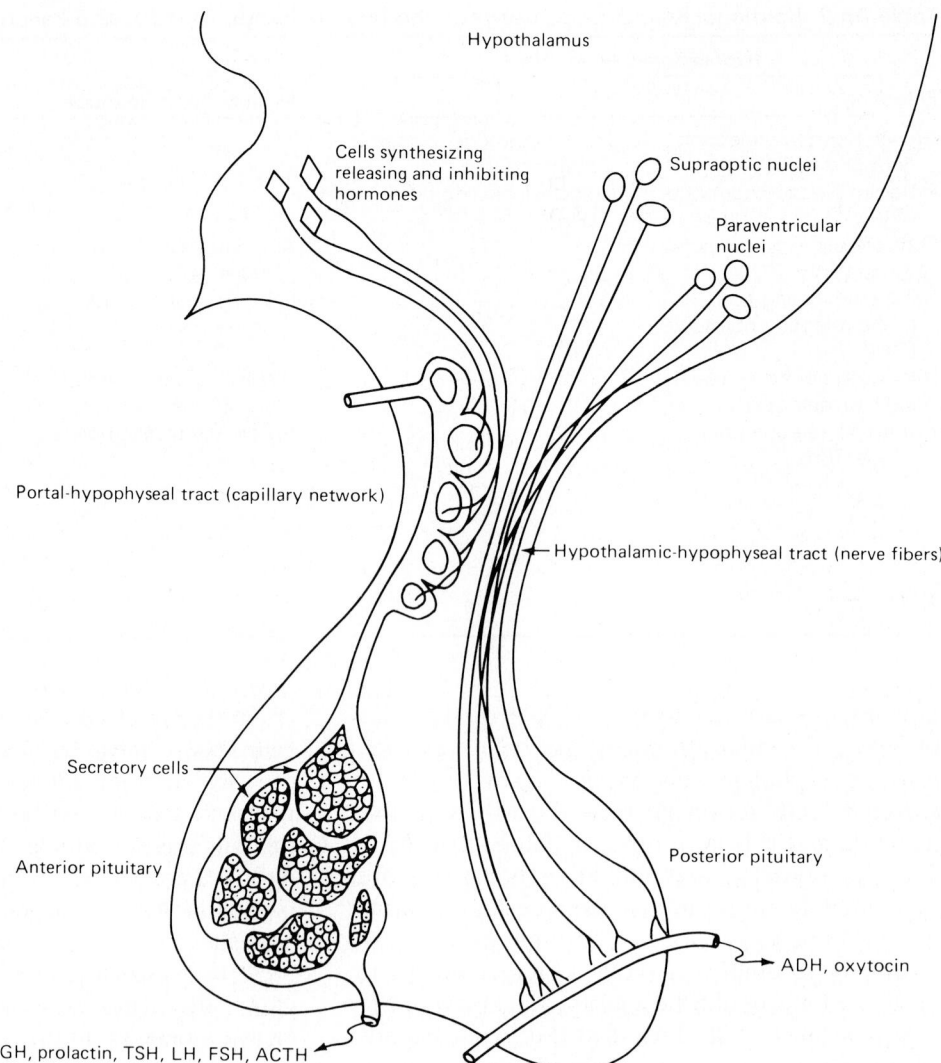

Figure 36-2 Anatomic basis of hypothalamic-pituitary relationships.

(ACTH); and the gonadotropins, follicle stimulating hormone (FSH) and luteinizing hormone (LH), also called interstitial cell stimulating hormone (ICSH) in males. Prolactin is no longer considered a gonadotropin and is discussed under "Peripheral Hormones of the Anterior Pituitary," below.[7]

Thyroid-stimulating hormone is necessary for appropriate thyroid gland function. Without it the thyroid gland atrophies. If it is present in excessive quantities, gland enlargement or goiter formation occurs.

Neural influences regulate TSH secretion via TRH from the hypothalamus. In addition, negative feedback to both the anterior pituitary and hypothalamus produced by high circulating blood levels of thyroid hormones regulates TSH secretion. Changes in the internal and external environment can therefore produce appropriate adjustments in the rate of thyroid secretion.[7]

The function of the adrenal cortex is dependent upon *adrenocorticotropic hormone (ACTH)*. Without this anterior pituitary tropic hormone, the adrenal gland atrophies and becomes incapable of synthesizing and secreting adequate quantities of glucocorticoids and mineralocorticoids. Insufficient ACTH also results in a progressive decline in adrenal responsiveness to itself, a situation which requires repeated exposure to increasing levels of ACTH to restore normal responsiveness.[7]

Neither baseline adrenal cortical secretion of glucocorticoids nor the increased secretion necessary in stress situations can occur in the absence of ACTH. Basal output of glucocorticoids is dependent upon a diurnal pattern of ACTH secretion. Peak secretion occurs consistently during one part of the day, most commonly in the morning, while lowest secretion levels occur 12 h before (and after) each peak. While the time clock mechanism directing this pattern is not fully understood, it is known to be directed by the hypothalamus via release of corticotropin releasing hormone (CRH). Stress in the form of physical, chemical, or emotional trauma superimposes bursts of ACTH secretion upon the underlying diurnal pattern of secretion. These bursts are also affected by hypothalamic release of CRH.[7]

Negative feedback at both the hypothalamus and anterior pituitary is produced by high circulating levels of glucocorticoids, regardless of whether the source of these glucocorticoids is internal or external. Significant danger exists when prolonged therapeutic doses of glucocorticoids are abruptly stopped. Decreased ACTH secretion induced by negative feedback has resulted in both adrenal atrophy and decreased responsiveness to ACTH. Return of responsiveness is slow, and meanwhile adequate levels of glucocorticoids cannot be synthesized or secreted by the adrenal cortex. Gradual withdrawal of exogenous glucocorticoids is therefore necessary to provide the time needed for normal adrenal gland function and responsiveness to return.

The two remaining tropic hormones secreted by the anterior pituitary are the gonadotropins *follicle stimulating hormone (FSH)* and *luteinizing hormone (LH)*. Both these hormones are necessary to prevent atrophy of the gonads, ovaries in the female and testes in the male. Reproductive capability is dependent upon their secretion as well. FSH is necessary for the maintenance of spermatogenic capability by the cells of the testes and is responsible for the early growth of the ovarian follicles in the ovary. LH is responsible for maintaining the synthesis and secretory capacity of testicular Leydig cells with regard to testosterone.

In females LH directs the final maturation of the ovarian follicles, including development of their capacity for estrogen secretion. In addition, possibly interacting with FSH, LH is necessary for ovulation, formation and maintenance of the corpus luteum, and subsequent synthesis and secretion of progesterone[7] (see "Gonads," below.)

Secretion patterns of the gonadotropins are influenced by hypothalamic secretion of follicle stimulating hormone releasing hormone and luteinizing hormone releasing hormone and involves cyclic sequences. Complete discussion of these sequences with regard to gonadotropin secretion is beyond the scope of this chapter, and the reader is referred to the literature. Negative feedback is exerted at the level of the hypothalamus by high circulating levels of the target gland hormones, namely, estrogen and testosterone, leading to inhibition of anterior pituitary secretion of FSH and LH, respectively.

Peripheral Hormones of the Anterior Pituitary
Two hormones that exert their effect directly on peripheral tissues are secreted by the acidophils of the anterior pituitary: prolactin and growth hormone (GH). *Prolactin* has been categorized as a gonadotropin and has been referred to as *luteotropic hormone* (LH) because it has been found to maintain the corpus luteum of many laboratory animals, specifically rodents. However, LH, *not* prolactin, performs this function in mammals, including humans. Thus classification of prolactin as a gonadotropin is misleading, since its primary target is not an endocrine gland but rather the alveolar cells of the breasts.[7]

Prolactin is a lactogenic hormone; that is, it prepares milk and effects its synthesis by the mammary alveolar cells. However, this requires prior estrogen and progesterone preparation, or "priming." The function of prolactin in males is unknown.[7]

Except during pregnancy, secretion of prolactin is tonically suppressed by prolactin inhibiting hormone (PIH) from the hypothalamus. When pregnancy occurs, hypothalamic secretion of prolactin releasing hormone (PRH) exceeds that of PIH, and as a result prolactin secretion increases. Peak prolactin secretion occurs at delivery; secretion then falls to nonpregnant levels roughly 8 days later. While suckling produces increases in its secretion rate, the degree of increase progressively declines in females nursing for more than 3 months.[7]

Growth hormone (GH) is a peripheral tissue hormone with widespread physiologic activity. It is a protein anabolic hormone; that is, it promotes tissue synthesis and is thus essential for healing and repair. Mechanisms by which it exerts its anabolic effects include acceleration of intracellular amino acid transport, stimulation of intracellular mRNA-mediated amino acid synthesis, and stimulation of production of a peptide substance known as *somatomedin* in the liver and kidneys. Somatomedin facilitates chondrogenesis, or cartilage formation, and plasma levels of this substance have been found to correlate more closely with tissue synthesis rates than with plasma growth hormone levels.[7]

Tissues particularly high in protein content, such as cartilage and muscle, are profoundly influenced by GH. Bones are also affected and, like muscle and cartilage, increase in mass under the influence of growth hormone. Linear growth of long bones occurs between the epiphyseal growth plates at each end. There, chondrogenesis produces a matrix structure that later serves as the site of bony calcification. Growth hormone facilitates chondrogenesis and thus promotes long-bone lengthening until fusion or closure of the epiphyseal plates occurs. This closure roughly corresponds to the termination of puberty, at which time total stature has been achieved.

Secretion of GH occurs as a result of hypothalamic secretion of GRH. GH secretion, like that of ACTH, follows a diurnal pattern of fluctuation that is determined by a hypothalamic time clock. This time clock produces periods in which GRH secretion predominates, alternating with periods in which GIH is dominant.[7] Peak GH secretion is usually at night and is associated with both the onset and occurrences of nonrapid eye movement (non-REM) sleep.

Superimposed upon the diurnal GH secretion pattern are wide fluctuations. These fluctuations are also a function of the hypothalamus. Stimuli responsible for some of these include conditions such as fasting, hypoglycemia, or strenuous exercise in which there is an insufficient availability of substances capable of supplying cellular energy. Conditions in which there are high circulating levels of amino acids, as following a large (especially protein-rich) meal, also result in GH secretion.[7] Physiologically these stimuli are appropriate in that growth hormone secretion mobilizes free fatty acids and thus creates a readily available energy pool to reverse any insufficiency. At the same time, it facilitates amino acid transport into cells to be used for tissue synthesis rather than fuel and in effect protects, or "spares," amino acids from undergoing hepatic gluconeogenesis. Other stimuli for the secretion of growth hormone include stress and the presence of glucagon. The latter is discussed in detail under "Endocrine Pancreas," later in this chapter. A schematic representation of hypothalamic–anterior pituitary hormonal interrelationships is shown in Fig. 36-3.

Posterior Pituitary (Neurohypophysis)

The posterior pituitary is composed of modified nervous system cells incapable of synthesis of the two hormones, oxytocin and antidiuretic hormone (ADH), secreted by this gland. Both these hormones are synthesized within cell bodies of the hypothalamus, specifically in the supraoptic and paraventricular nuclei. Axons of these cells combine and form the *hypothalamic-hypophyseal nerve tract,* which functionally connects the hypothalamus to the posterior pituitary (Fig. 36-2). Once synthesized, the hormones are bound into small pouches or vesicles, which are transported down the axons (axoplasm transport) to the posterior pituitary. Secretion of these hormones occurs in response to neural impulses from the hypothalamus. Both oxytocin and ADH are peripheral hormones.[6]

Oxytocin   The major physiologic effect of oxytocin is milk ejection from the secretory ducts of the breast. It does not influence milk synthesis, which is dependent instead upon the actions of estrogen, progesterone, and prolactin. Milk ejection is a reflex that is initiated by stimulation of touch receptors around the nipple. As a result of nipple stimulation, impulses are generated which are then transmitted to the supraoptic and paraventricular nuclei of the hypothalamus. The posterior pituitary is stimulated and oxytocin is released. The milk-ejection reflex can also be initiated by genital stimulation and by strong emotions.[6]

Oxytocin also causes contraction of uterine smooth muscle and is secreted during labor as a result of transmission of impulses generated by

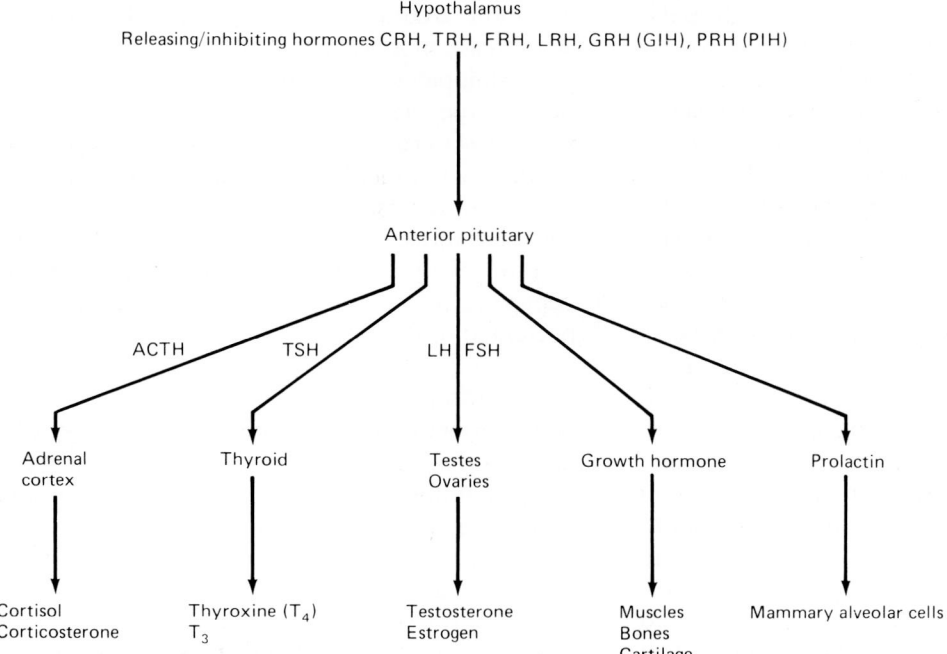

Hypothalamus
Releasing/inhibiting hormones CRH, TRH, FRH, LRH, GRH (GIH), PRH (PIH)

Anterior pituitary

ACTH   TSH   LH | FSH

Adrenal   Thyroid   Testes   Growth hormone   Prolactin
cortex   Ovaries

Cortisol   Thyroxine (T$_4$)   Testosterone   Muscles   Mammary alveolar cells
Corticosterone   T$_3$ Estrogen   Bones
                                Cartilage

Figure 36-3 Hormonal interrelations between the hypothalamus and anterior pituitary.

touch receptors in the birth canal. As in the milk-ejection reflex, these impulses reach the hypothalamus and effect oxytocin release.[6] It may also play a role in the initiation of labor; however, this process involves many complex mechanisms, and the precise role of oxytocin has yet to be defined.

Antidiuretic Hormone (ADH) Antidiuretic hormone is also known as *vasopressin* and *arginine vasopressin*. Its principal action is to conserve or retain free water or effect antidiuresis. It acts upon the distal tubules and collecting ducts of the kidney, where it produces an increase in permeability, thus allowing water to freely follow the osmotic gradient out of the tubules into the surrounding hypertonic interstitium.[6] As water leaves the collecting tubules, less urine volume remains, urine concentration increases, and, since water is retained in excess of solute, the osmotic tonicity of body fluids decreases and they become more dilute.

When ADH secretion is low, collecting tubule permeability does not allow water to leave the tubular lumen; therefore, urine volume increases while concentration decreases. In this situation, urine is hypotonic in comparison to the body fluids,

a net loss of water occurs, and the osmotic pressure of the body fluids is increased. In large amounts, ADH also constricts arteriolar smooth muscle and consequently elevates arterial blood pressure, although the hypertensive action of ADH is minor compared with its effect on body free water balance.[6]

Secretion of ADH is dictated by the hypothalamus. There, receptor cells alter their rate of impulse generation and transmission to the posterior pituitary in the face of changes in body fluid tonicity or osmolarity. These cells, known as *osmoreceptors*, shrink when body fluid tonicity is increased or hyperosmolarity exists, because of intracellular water loss to the surrounding (abnormally) hypertonic interstitium.[6] The result is secretion of ADH, maximal retention of water, and a decrease in osmolarity which contribute to the production of low volumes of highly concentrated urine.

In contrast, situations in which excess free water is present cause osmoreceptor cells to swell because of water influx from a hypotonic environment. As a result, impulse transmission to the posterior pituitary decreases, effecting suppression of ADH secretion. Water is unable to escape the tubular lumen and therefore contributes to the production of large volumes of dilute urine.

In addition to the osmotic feedback regulatory mechanism just described, regulation of ADH is also affected by the status of the extracellular fluid (ECF) volume. Stretch receptors within the vascular system, specifically in the atria and pulmonary vasculature, respond to ECF volume changes by altering their rate of impulse transmission to the hypothalamus. When ECF volume is decreased, ADH secretion is increased. The opposite occurs in the case of ECF volume overload. These receptors provide the prime volume-based mediation of ADH secretion and are extremely sensitive.[6] They are known to produce an increase in ADH secretion in response to change in body position from recumbent to upright. Presumably this effect occurs because an overall decrease in ECF volume is perceived because of decreased venous return due to blood pooling in the lower extremities, even though the ECF volume has not changed. In situations in which a loss of ECF volume is of sufficient magnitude to produce a decrease in blood pressure, other volume receptors also become involved in the regulation of ADH secretion. These receptors, in

the aortic arch and carotid sinuses, also produce an increase in ADH.[6,8]

Multiple stimuli other than osmolarity and ECF volume increase ADH secretion. These include pain, emotional or physiologic stress, sympathetic nervous system activation, and a variety of pharmacologic agents including anesthetics, morphine, and barbiturates in large doses. Alcohol, on the other hand, decreases ADH secretion.[6] A schematic depiction of stimuli affecting ADH secretion is presented in Fig. 36-4.

Intermediate Pituitary

The intermediate lobe of the pituitary is normally quiescent in humans. The majority of the cells composing the intermediate lobe are angular and nonsecreting, and some basophils are present. Two peripheral hormones are synthesized in the basophils. Both are *melanotropins,* or melanocyte stimulating hormones (MSH)—so named because they disperse melanin (pigment) granules known as *melanocytes* in the cells of the skin. The function of MSHs in humans is uncertain, but pituitary tumors can produce hyperpigmentation, presumably because increased MSHs excessively stimulate melanocytes.[8]

Figure 36-4   Stimuli affecting ADH secretion.

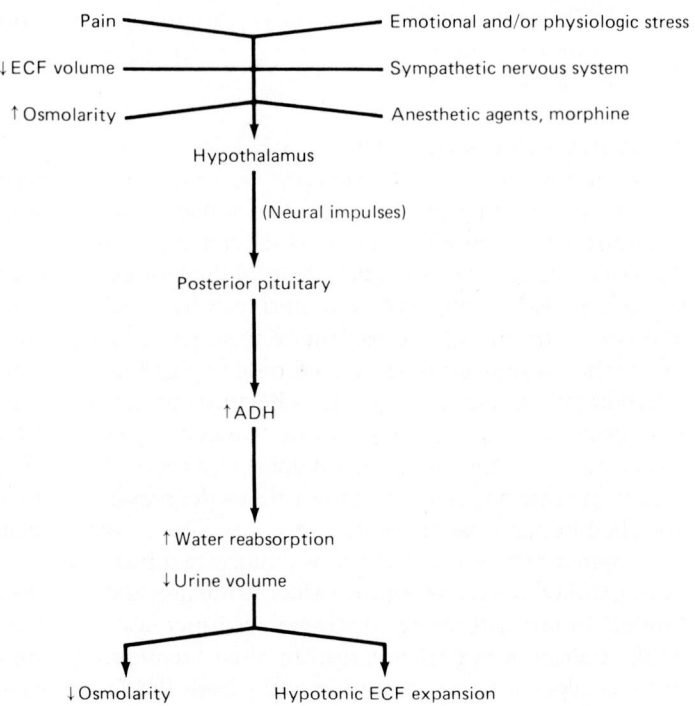

Thyroid

The thyroid gland is composed of two lobes located on either side of the upper trachea. Connecting these lobes is an isthmus, or bridge, that lies anterior to the larynx. Microscopically the thyroid gland is composed of follicles or small, closed sacs defining central cavities; parafollicular cells distributed on the outer aspects of the follicles; and a rich vascular network. The follicles are responsible for the synthesis of iodine-containing thyroid hormones—actually two hormones with similar structures: thyroxine, or tetraiodothyronine (T_4), which contains four iodine molecules, and triiodothyronine (T_3), which contains three iodine molecules. These hormones are responsible for metabolic regulation of body tissues at the levels necessary for optimum performance of normal functions. Parafollicular cells synthesize a hormone, thyrocalcitonin or calcitonin, that plays a role in regulation of serum calcium level and produces a calcium-lowering effect. The high degree of vascularity of the thyroid is responsible for a rate of blood flow that is among the highest of all the organs in the body on a gram-for-gram basis.[9] This large blood flow is necessary for synthesis of thyroxine and T_3. Plasma iodine levels are generally low (about 0.3 μg per 100 mL). Normal rates of thyroid hormone synthesis require that the gland pick up 120 μg each day; therefore blood flow through the gland must be high if hormone synthesis is to occur at normal rates.

Thyroxine (Tetraiodothyronine, T_4) and Triiodothyronine (T_3)

Both T_4 and T_3 act by the intracellular mechanism of hormone action.[1] They are calorigenic in that they increase metabolic rate and stimulate oxygen consumption by most of the cells of the body. In addition, they affect carbohydrate and lipid metabolism by increasing the rate of carbohydrate absorption from the gastrointestinal tract and stimulating cholesterol synthesis. Thyroid hormones also play a vital role in growth and maturation by increasing the metabolic rate to the levels necessary to promote tissue synthesis. They are also necessary in order for growth hormone to be secreted. Finally, thyroid hormones are necessary for the development and maintenance of the nervous system. In the peripheral nerves, thyroid hormone regulates the reaction time of reflexes. In the central nervous system, thyroid hormones are necessary for functional development and maintenance.[9] Their precise role in this regard is not known, but apparently thyroid hormones have a unique relationship with the catecholamines. They are mutually synergistic, and thyroid hormones potentiate catecholamine effects. Since catecholamines are neurotransmitters, this thyroid-catecholamine relationship may be one of the mechanisms involved in thyroid-dependent nervous system maturation and function.[8]

Thyroid hormone secretion is under the influence of the hypothalamus via thyrotropin releasing hormone (TRH) and subsequent alteration of the secretion rate of TSH. Day-to-day control of thyroid hormone secretion is primarily a function of negative feedback exerted upon TSH and to a lesser extent TRH secretion related to circulating levels of T_4 and T_3. A drop in body temperature or exposure to cold, as perceived by the hypothalamus, increases thyroid secretion, although not markedly. Certain hormones, namely, catecholamines and ADH, exert a direct stimulatory effect on the thyroid and therefore increase the release of T_4 and T_3.[8] A schematic depiction of control of thyroid secretion is shown in Fig. 36-5.

Thyrocalcitonin (Calcitonin)

The exact physiologic role of thyrocalcitonin is unknown, and it may be relatively inactive in adult

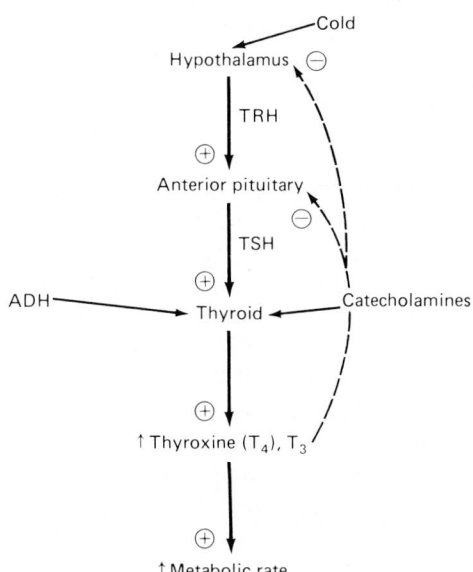

Figure 36-5 Stimuli affecting thyroid hormone secretion.

humans. The serum ionized calcium level is lowered under its influence because it inhibits bone breakdown (resorption) and decreases formation of the active form of vitamin D (1,25-dihydroxycholecalciferol), which is necessary for absorption of calcium from the intestine.[10] Secretion of thyrocalcitonin occurs in response to elevations in the serum concentrations of ionized calcium; a direct effect on the gland is postulated because thyrocalcitonin secretion is unaffected by TSH. However, adequate ionized calcium is vital in many important physiologic processes, and regulation of its concentration is dominated by the action of parathormone from the parathyroid, which acts to increase serum levels.[8]

Parathyroids

There are two to six parathyroid glands, with identical functions. They can be found in many locations but most commonly are embedded in the posterior aspect of the thyroid gland. The secretory cells of the parathyroids are known as *chief cells* and they secrete parathormone (PTH), a hormone essential for survival.[8]

This hormone acts to increase the serum level of ionized calcium, a vital mineral which must be in adequate supply if blood coagulation, normal contraction by cardiac and skeletal muscle, and the maintenance of nerve excitability are to be assured. Parathormone secretion occurs when the blood perfusing the parathyroid glands contains insufficient levels of ionized calcium, resulting in a direct stimulatory effect on the gland. Parathormone then increases ionized calcium by exerting a direct resorptive or mobilizing influence on bones and effecting active transport of calcium into the ECF. In addition, it stimulates both renal reabsorption of calcium and renal production of 1,25-dihydroxycholecalciferol, or active vitamin D, which is necessary for calcium absorption from the intestines.[10] A general reciprocal relationship exists between ionized calcium and phosphate ions, and parathormone tends to decrease serum phosphate levels by increasing their excretion by the kidney.[8]

Adrenals

There are two adrenal glands, each distinct and functioning independently. The outer layer is the adrenal cortex; it surrounds the adrenal medulla, which composes the gland's interior. The adrenal glands are located at the upper poles of each kidney in the retroperitoneal space.[8]

Adrenal Cortex

The adrenal cortex secretes three steroids: (1) glucocorticoids, steroids which produce effects on metabolism as well as play a role in a multitude of other important functions; (2) a mineralocorticoid, which is essential to the maintenance of sodium balance and therefore ECF volume; and (3) sex hormones, predominantly androgens, which exert minor effects on secondary sex characteristics. These three steroids synthesized by the adrenal cortex are structurally similar. Even though the secretion of these steroids in physiologic amounts produces distinct effects, when they are secreted in abnormally elevated amounts, their effects may overlap.[11]

Glucocorticoids Two glucocorticoids, cortisol and corticosterone, are secreted by the adrenal cortex. Direct metabolic effects of these hormones include increased protein breakdown in all but hepatic cells, impaired peripheral tissue utilization of insulin and thus glucose, and increase in hepatic glucose output by increasing gluconeogenesis and glycogenesis simultaneously with increasing production of glucose-6-phosphatase, an enzyme which rapidly converts glycogen to glucose. The result of these actions is hyperglycemia, catabolism, and a pronounced tendency to development of a negative nitrogen balance. The glucocorticoids also increase plasma lipids and in the presence of insufficient insulin influence ketone body formation[11] (see "Insulin," below). Needless to say, diabetes is more pronounced in the presence of these hormones.

Glucocorticoids exert a multitude of *permissive actions;* that is, actions that must be present for many other physiologic events to occur. The effectiveness of glucagon in hypoglycemic states depends upon their presence, as does the metabolic response to catecholamines (see "Adrenal Medulla" and "Glucagon," below). The action of norepinephrine on vascular smooth muscle and of ADH on the collecting tubules of the kidney also requires the presence of glucocorticoids. The glucocorticoids also have permissive effects on the maintenance of normal excitability in the central nervous system as well as in the myocardium.[8]

The action of glucocorticoids in the presence of stress is critical. Apart from their permissive role with regard to catecholamines, however, the mechanism by which they produce physiologic resistance to stress is unclear. Adrenalectomized animals supplied with maintenance levels of glucocorticoids but without increases in glucocorticoids in the presence of stress die when exposed to even minor insults. That glucocorticoids are essential for survival under stress is unquestioned.[8]

Glucocorticoids also produce an antiinflammatory effect when supplied in amounts greater than normally secreted. They inhibit the release of histamine and other kinins and thus limit the physiologic cascade of events involved in the inflammatory response. They increase splenic sequestration of two types of leukocytes, the eosinophils and basophils, and thus decrease their levels in the circulating blood. They may also exert a protective effect against bacterial toxins by a mechanism that involves stabilization of the membranes containing lysosomes (autolytic enzymes) within all body cells. Since toxins are known to affect release of these enzymes and in that way lead to cellular autolysis, this action facilitates the maintenance of cellular integrity.[8] However, glucocorticoids can mask symptoms of potentially serious or fatal bacterial invasion, so their use is not without danger.

Both basal secretion of glucocorticoids and the increased secretion provoked by stress are dependent upon ACTH from the anterior pituitary and thus CRH from the hypothalamus.[11] The reader is referred to the detailed discussion of ACTH under "Anterior Pituitary Tropic Hormones," earlier in this chapter. A schematic representation of the hypothalamic-pituitary-adrenal relationship, or "axis," with regard to glucocorticoid secretion is presented in Fig. 36-6.

Mineralocorticoids *Aldosterone* is the primary mineralocorticoid secreted by the adrenal cortex, although small amounts of others are also secreted. It is a vital hormone in that it serves to maintain adequate ECF volume through its action in promoting sodium resorption from the urine and, to a lesser extent, from sweat, saliva, and gastric secretions. Its primary site of action is the renal tubular network, where it directs exchange of sodium ions in the tubular lumen for either potassium or hydrogen ions from the tubular cells.

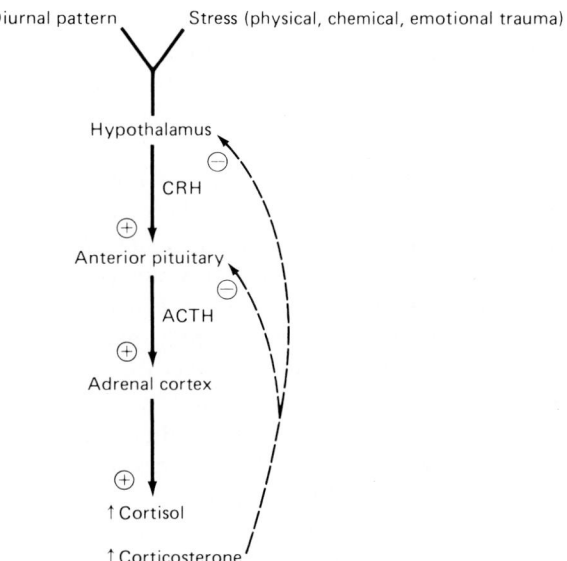

Figure 36-6 Hypothalamic-pituitary-adrenocortical axis in glucocorticoid secretion.

Aldosterone-mediated reabsorption of sodium is therefore associated with moderate urinary loss of potassium and hydrogen.[8]

Three types of regulation are involved in aldosterone secretion. ACTH from the anterior pituitary plays a role, although the amount of ACTH necessary to increase aldosterone secretion is considerably larger than that required to produce maximal glucocorticoid secretion. In addition, the effect of ACTH is transient, and even in the presence of prolonged ACTH-induced increases, aldosterone secretion declines after about 2 days.[11]

A second regulatory mechanism in the secretion of aldosterone involves direct stimulation of the adrenal cortex. A rise in serum potassium, a fall in serum sodium, or an increase in the ratio of serum potassium to serum sodium (which is normally very low) also increase aldosterone secretion.[11]

However, the primary regulatory mechanism for aldosterone secretion is the *renin-angiotensin mechanism*. Renin is secreted from renal juxtaglomerular cells in response to a decrease in ECF or intraarterial volume as perceived by stretch receptors in renal afferent arterioles. This secretion results in catalytic formation of angiotensin I, which is then rapidly converted to angiotensin II by an enzyme circulating in the blood. Angiotensin II directly stimulates adrenocortical cells to produce aldosterone. The aldesterone-induced ECF volume expansion that results inhibits further renin secretion, in effect shutting off the stimulus.[8,11]

Adrenal Androgens   Several steroids with sex hormone activity are secreted by the adrenal cortex; however, only one, the androgen *dehydroepiandrosterone,* is produced in significant physiologic amounts. Like other androgens, it exerts a masculinizing effect and promotes protein anabolism and growth. The adrenal androgen has about one-fifth the potency of the most active androgen, testosterone, produced by the testes. Another adrenal androgen, *androstenedione,* is converted to estrogen in the circulation. The adrenal gland may also secrete small amounts of some estrogens. The secretion of adrenal androgens is controlled by ACTH, not by the gonadotropins.[8]

Adrenal Medulla

The adrenal medulla is located in the interior aspect of the adrenal gland and secretes two catecholamines, epinephrine and norepinephrine (proportionately more epinephrine). The adrenal medulla is perhaps most appropriately viewed as an extension of the sympathetic nervous system, because norepinephrine is the transmitter at all adrenergic nerve endings and epinephrine is capable of producing adrenergic effects in all tissues with adrenergic receptors. In addition, both catecholamines are neurotransmitters throughout the central nervous system. Secretion of adrenal medullary catecholamines is predominantly under the control of the sympathetic nervous system.[8]

Increased secretion of catecholamines serves a critical role in the physiologic preparation to meet or cope with emergency situations. Adrenomedullary secretion in such circumstances reinforces the sympathetic response. Stimuli known to evoke sympathoadrenal discharge include hypoxemia, hypoglycemia, cold, hemorrhage, and emotional stresses provoked by situations of a frightening or unfamiliar nature.[12] A schematic depiction of factors producing sympathoadrenal catecholamine secretion is shown in Fig. 36-7.

Epinephrine relaxes bronchiolar smooth muscle, producing bronchodilatation and facilitation of maximum ventilation. Both catecholamines in-

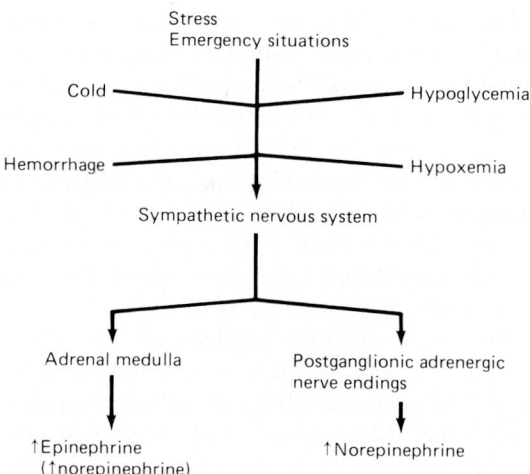

Figure 36-7   Control of catecholamine secretion.

crease the force and rate of myocardial contraction, i.e., exert positive ionotropic and chronotropic effects. They also increase the velocity and overall excitability of myocardial impulse conduction. Norepinephrine produces vasoconstriction (in the presence of glucocorticoids) in most if not all organs, but epinephrine counteracts this effect, producing vasodilatation in skeletal muscles, the central nervous system, the myocardium, and the liver.[12] In the presence of both, total peripheral resistance to blood flow is decreased, but many "nonvital" organs experience decreased oxygen delivery because of decreased perfusion.

Metabolic effects of the catecholamines are profound. Both exert a marked calorigenic effect and greatly increase metabolic rate. The mechanisms involved in the catecholamine-induced increase in metabolic rate are not precisely known but are thought to involve increased glycogenolysis in skeletal muscle (producing hyperglycemia) and increased hepatic oxidation of lactic acid. Lactic acid production is a function of norepinephrine-induced vasoconstriction and decreased oxygen delivery to "nonvital" cells, with their subsequent dependence upon anaerobic metabolism. Epinephrine is more potent than norepinephrine with regard to metabolic effects.[12]

Another metabolic effect of catecholamines is free fatty acid mobilization from adipose tissue, physiologically appropriate in that overall elevation in metabolic rate requires increased availability of maximum energy sources.[12] Free fatty acids are necessary despite hyperglycemia because norepinephrine inhibits insulin secretion and therefore limits glucose uptake by many body cells (see "Insulin," below).

Finally, epinephrine and norepinephrine act as central nervous system activators. Both alertness and attentiveness are increased by the presence of catecholamines. In addition, epinephrine is thought to be responsible for production of anxiety and fear.[8]

Endocrine Pancreas

The endocrine component of the pancreas is small but mighty. It constitutes about 2 percent of the total pancreatic mass and is composed of clusters of endocrine cells called *islets of Langerhans* or *pancreatic islets*. The cells in the islets are classified in three categories on the basis of their granulation and staining properties: alpha, or A, cells; beta, or B, cells; and delta, or D, cells. Alpha cells constitute about one-fifth of the islet cells and secrete glucagon. Beta cells compose the majority of the islet cells, about 75 percent, and secrete insulin. The delta cells make up the remainder of the islet cells and secrete a polypeptide substance known as *somatostatin*.[8] The precise physiologic role of somatostatin is not known, but it inhibits secretion of insulin and of glucagon from beta and alpha cells, respectively.

Insulin and glucagon play important roles in the regulation of carbohydrates, protein, and fat metabolism. Insulin is anabolic in that it increases storage of glucose, fatty acids, and amino acids. Glucagon is catabolic in that it mobilizes glucose and breaks down or converts stored fat and protein into utilizable energy sources.[13] These two hormones are therefore antagonists, and appropriately, their secretion patterns are generally reciprocal.

The overall status of energy stores at any given time is reflected by the ratio of insulin to glucagon. In normal states, where a balanced diet is being consumed, the insulin/glucagon (I/G) ratio is 2.3:1, indicative of a net storage tendency, establishment of a positive nitrogen balance, and anabolism.[13] In fed (or overfed) states, an increase in insulin results in elevation of the I/G ratio, anabolism, and weight gain. In contrast, fasting produces an increase in glucagon and consequently a decreased I/G ratio, catabolism, and weight loss.

Insulin

Insulin increases glucose uptake in all body tissues except the pancreatic beta islet cells, brain, renal tubules, intestinal mucosa, and red blood cells. The mechanism involves facilitation of glucose transport across cellular membranes. Insulin also produces increases in free fatty acid and protein synthesis, an action which is accomplished by preventing the action of enzymes necessary for their breakdown and also increasing amino acid transport into cells. Finally, it decreases hepatic glucose output and stimulates glycogenesis in the liver and skeletal muscle.[8]

Regulation of insulin secretion is primarily a function of a feedback mechanism exerted by blood glucose concentration directly on the pancreas. Glucose entry into beta islet cells is not affected by insulin; thus changes in glucose levels are rapidly sensed by these cells. When blood glucose levels are low, so is insulin secretion. When blood glucose levels increase, insulin secretion by the beta cells also increases. The subsequent decrease in blood glucose thus removes the stimulus that initiated increased insulin secretion. This feedback mechanism normally operates with great precision and results in a close parallel between the blood glucose and insulin levels.[8]

By a mechanism yet to be defined, the presence in the serum of some amino and keto acids also increases insulin secretion. That these substances increase insulin secretion is physiologically appropriate in that insulin increases synthesis of both protein and fat and thus serves to "protect" amino acids from being used as cellular energy sources. When keto acids are present in the serum, free fatty acids have already been burned, reflecting fat breakdown and catabolism, both of which are reversed by insulin.[8]

The degree of insulin secretion in response to intravenously infused glucose and amino acids is less than that produced by oral ingestion of the same substances, as a result of the action of a hormone secreted by the intestinal mucosa and known as *gastric inhibitory peptide* (GIP). In the presence of glucose or fat in the gastrointestinal tract, secretion of GIP is increased. GIP then affects beta cell stimulation, resulting in increased insulin secretion. Other substances secreted by the gastrointestinal tract that produce similar effects include cholecystokinin, secretin, gastrin, and mucosal glucagon, although GIP is thought to be the primary "gut factor" normally involved.[13] Glucagon is discussed in detail in the section that immediately follows.

Free catecholamines (primarily epinephrine) as well as sympathetic stimulation prevent insulin secretion. Other inhibitory effects on insulin secretion are produced by thiazide diuretics, diazoxide, and somatostatin.[8] As discussed in other sections, several hormones, including glucocorticoids and growth hormone, impair insulin effect.

Glucagon

Most of the glucagon is secreted by the alpha islet cells, although as noted, it is also released by mucosal cells of the gastrointestinal tract. Glucagon is a catabolic hormone that exerts its influence by increasing hepatic glycogenolysis and gluconeogenesis and promoting fat breakdown. Blood glucose is elevated in its presence, and because it involves alpha cell cAMP activation, its effect is rapid. When secreted, glucagon also produces an increase in insulin secretion.[8] Although seemingly inappropriate, this effect is physiologically logical, because insulin facilitates tissue uptake of the released energy sources. Glucagon in large quantities also exerts an inotropic effect on the myocardium, but this effect is minor in comparison with its role in metabolism.

A variety of stimuli affect alpha cell glucagon secretion, such as sympathetic nervous system activation, glucocorticoids, and exercise. Large amounts of amino acids also stimulate glucagon secretion. Because amino acids also stimulate insulin, glucagon secretion is necessary in this situation to assure blood glucose adequacy while these substances are used in tissue synthesis.[13] In this way, glucagon facilitates the protein-sparing and the storage effects of insulin.

Glucagon secreted in response to orally ingested amino acids is similar to insulin in that it is greater than that produced by intravenous administration of the same substances. Presence of protein in the gastrointestinal tract stimulates the secretion of cholecystokinin and gastrin from mucosal cells,

and both these substances increase glucagon secretion from the alpha cells as well as from the intestinal mucosal cells.[13]

Glucagon secretion is inhibited by hyperglycemia. However, this inhibition is dependent upon insulin. Apparently, alpha cells are unable to react to elevated blood glucose levels unless insulin first promotes alpha cell pickup of glucose. When blood glucose levels are low, increased secretion of glucagon produces increased blood glucose simultaneously with increased insulin. The subsequent presence of both hormones produces a negative feedback action on further alpha cell secretion. Glucagon secretion is also decreased by somatostatin.[8] A schematic representation of the bihormonal endocrine pancreas control of energy metabolism is presented in Fig. 36-8.

Pineal

The pineal gland (*epiphysis*) is located at the midline of the cranial cavity just under the third ventricle. It is primarily composed of nervous system tissue, although some secretory cells are present. During infancy the pineal is large, but by the time puberty occurs it has undergone involution and its size is approximately that of a small grape.[8]

In humans the function of the pineal is not understood. It produces melatonin, a hormone that inhibits the effect of gonadotropins and, in rodents, produces changes in pigmentation of the skin. Some believe that melatonin secretion occurs prior to puberty when the gland is large and that the gonadotropin inhibition plays a role in delaying the onset of puberty until the time deemed appropriate by the hypothalamus.[8] It is *not* thought to be related to skin pigmentation in humans; however, its effect on skin has not been precisely defined. Some pituitary tumors do produce hyperpigmentation, but this is thought to occur as a function of excess levels of melanocyte stimulating hormone (MSH) or other chemically similar tropins from the intermediate and anterior lobes (see "Intermediate Pituitary," above). Increased melatonin secretion is not known to be an effect of MSH.[8]

Secretion of melatonin in humans is a direct function of the nervous system and is associated with light and darkness. Light receptors in the retina initiate nervous system impulse generation and

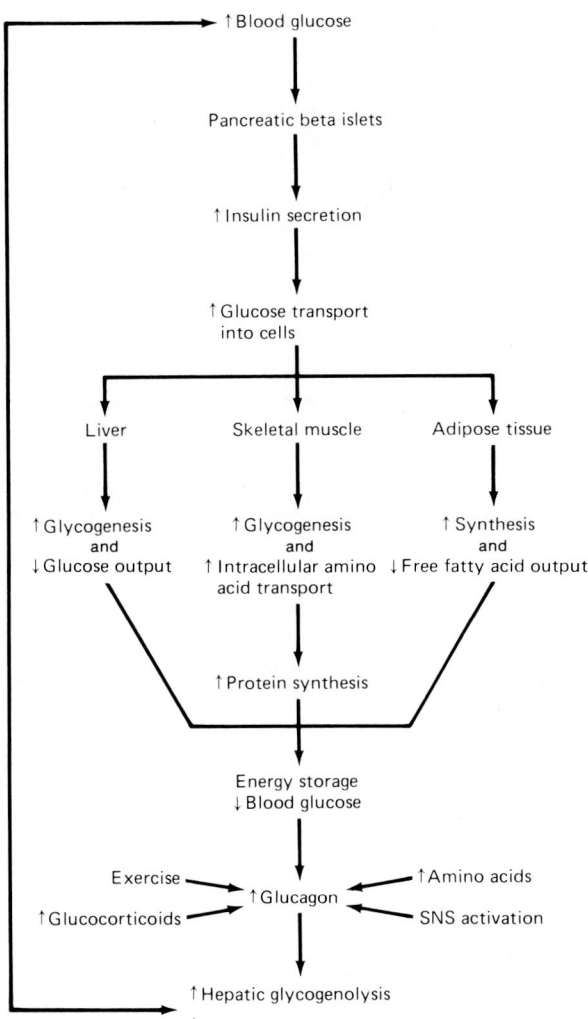

Figure 36-8   Bihormonal control of energy metabolism by the endocrine pancreas.

transmission to the pineal gland. As a result, plasma concentrations of melatonin are consistently high in dark environments and dramatically decreased in those with an abundance of light. Recent research suggests that melatonin decreases self-reported alertness and increases sleepiness. Its overall effect is significant, short-acting sedation.[14]

Thymus

The thymus is located in the mediastinum and is the primary central organ of the lymphatic system. It is a single structure composed of two lobes. Its largest dimensions are seen at puberty. From then

on it begins to involute and may be essentially absent in old age, having been replaced by fat.[8]

The function of the thymus is still in the process of being defined. It is known to be vital in the development of the immune defense mechanism, a function that is essentially completed early in life and thus unaffected by later involution. Soon after birth it affects maturation of fetal lymphocytes. After their maturation, these lymphocytes leave the thymus and accumulate in the spleen, lymph nodes, and other lymphatic tissue.[8]

The thymus is considered an endocrine gland because soon after birth it secretes a hormone known as *thymosin*. This hormone results in development and maturation of plasma immune cells, *T cells,* or *T lymphocytes,* from nonspecific lymphocytes. T cells play a vital role in cellular immunity throughout the body (see Chap. 44). They are present in just about all body cells, and when they encounter foreign antigens (proteins) on cells such as those from another person or cells associated with viruses, they become "activated" and produce *lymphokins,* which are capable of protein destruction and thus foreign cell destruction.[15] It is T cell activation that produces rejection of transplanted tissue and provides the major defense against viral invasion.

Thymosin administration has been known to enhance immune defenses, presumably by increasing the number or activity of T cells. Its use in immunosuppressed patients such as those undergoing chemotherapy or radiation therapy for malignant disease may provide a means of increasing resistance to systemic infections. It may also prove to be helpful in the body's defense against malignant processes in that tumor cells are known to contain some foreign antigens.[15] Theoretically, if T cells could be sufficiently activated, they could effect destruction of these cells.

References

1. Clark, J., et al. (1985). Mechanisms of steroid hormone action. In J. Wilson & D. Foster (Eds.), *Williams textbook of endocrinology* (7th ed. pp. 33–75). Philadelphia: Saunders.
2. Roth, J. (1985). Mechanism of action of peptide hormones and catecholamines. In J. Wilson & D. Foster (Eds.), *Williams textbook of endocrinology* (7th ed. pp. 76–122). Philadelphia: Saunders.

3. Lee, J., & Katayama, S. (1985). Prostaglandins, thromboxanes, and leukotrienes. In J. Wilson & D. Foster (Eds.), *Williams textbook of endocrinology* (7th ed. pp. 1345–1362). Philadelphia: Saunders.

4. Wilson, J. (1983). Principles of endocrinology. In R. Petersdorf et al. (Eds.), *Harrison's principles of internal medicine* (10th ed. pp. 580–586). New York: McGraw-Hill.

5. Daughaday, W. (1981). The adenohypophysis. In R. Williams (Ed.), *Williams textbook of endocrinology* (6th ed. pp. 73–114). Philadelphia: Saunders.

6. Culpepper, R., et al. (1985). The posterior pituitary and water metabolism. In J. Wilson & D. Foster (Eds.), *Williams textbook of endocrinology* (7th ed. pp. 614–652). Philadelphia: Saunders.

7. Daughaday, W. (1985). The anterior pituitary. In J. Wilson & D. Foster (Eds.), *Williams textbook of endocrinology* (7th ed. pp. 568–613). Philadelphia: Saunders.

8. Ganong, W. F. (1985). *Review of medical physiology* (12th ed.). Los Altos, CA: Lange.

9. Ingbar, S. (1985). The thyroid gland. In J. Wilson & D. Foster (Eds.), *Williams textbook of endocrinology* (7th ed. pp. 682–815). Philadelphia: Saunders.

10. Aurbach, G., et al. (1985). Parathyroid hormone, calcitonin, and the calciferols. In J. Wilson & D. Foster (Eds.), *Williams textbook of endocrinology* (7th ed. pp. 1137–1217). Philadelphia: Saunders.

11. Bondy, P. (1985). Disorders of the adrenal cortex. In J. Wilson & D. Foster (Eds.), *Williams textbook of endocrinology* (7th ed. pp. 816–890). Philadelphia: Saunders.

12. Landsberg, L. (1985). Catecholamines and the adrenal medulla. In J. Wilson & D. Foster (Eds.), *Williams textbook of endocrinology* (7th ed. pp. 891–965). Philadelphia: Saunders.

13. Cryer, P. (1985). Glucose homeostasis and hypoglycemia. In J. Wilson & D. Foster (Eds.), *Williams textbook of endocrinology* (7th ed. pp. 989–1017). Philadelphia: Saunders.

14. Lieberman, H., et al. (1984). Effects of melatonin on human mood and performance. *Brain Research, 323,* 201–207.

15. Gilliland, B. (1983). Introduction to clinical immunology. In R. Petersdorf et al. (Eds.), *Harrison's principles of internal medicine* (10th ed. pp. 344–353). New York: McGraw-Hill.

37

Endocrine Data Acquisition

Sarah J. Sanford

Evaluation of endocrine function requires comprehensive data collection and interpretation. The interactive and overlapping nature of endocrine glands makes differential determination of alterations in specific glandular responses, secretion patterns, and consequences extremely complex. Compounding the complexity is, for all intents and purposes, the inability to visualize the glands themselves. Recognition of altered glandular structure and function, therefore, functionally depends upon understanding the diffuse and delicate balance between and among the various glands and all other body systems.

Endocrine dysfunction classically involves two types of disorders: those associated with hyperfunction and those of hypofunction. *Hyperfunction* refers to elevated secretion patterns and is associated with clinical findings indicating increased hormone activity on target tissues. In contrast, *hypofunction* is associated with insufficient secretion of hormone, and symptoms reflect the target tissue impact of deficient hormone levels. Because of the interrelated nature of the endocrine system, both hyper- and hyposecretory syndromes can reflect dysfunction of a particular gland, altered secretion of the gland's tropic hormones, and/or alteration in the gland's physiologic stimuli.

When disorder of a specific gland results in secretion abnormalities, *primary dysfunction* is said to exist. When disease alters either a gland's tropic hormone secretion or its physiologic stimulators or inhibitors, the resultant alteration of the gland's secretion constitutes *secondary dysfunction*. In secondary dysfunction there is no causative disease in the gland per se, even though anatomic changes—typically atrophy, hypertrophy, hypoplasia, or hyperplasia—may be present.[1]

Assessment of the Endocrine System

Assessment of endocrine function is perhaps one of the most formidable challenges in nursing practice. The effects of endocrine dysfunction are pervasive and multidimensional. For example, hypertension may reflect the presence of a pheochromocytoma, while hypotension may signal acute adrenal crisis. Tachycardia may be the result of hyperthyroid crisis, while bradycardia may reflect either hypothyroid status or, in adrenocortical insufficiency, hyperkalemia.

In the critical-care setting, recognition of endocrine dysfunction is essential, not only because the potential consequences of inadequate treatment may be severe and life-threatening, as in endocrine emergencies, but also because most states are reversible with immediate corrective therapy.

History

Gathering the history begins with a full account of why treatment has been sought or is being rendered. It is necessary to ascertain the nature and timing of the onset of symptoms; to determine the location, duration, quality, and severity of those symptoms; and to identify any aggravating or alleviating factors. Data regarding potential correlations between the timing of symptoms and sleep or activity, emotional state, and nutritional intake should be gathered. Both prescribed and over-the-counter pharmacologic agents, as well as previous medical and surgical treatment for current symptoms, need to be noted.

More general information is also needed. Has there been an alteration in body proportions or weight? Has either thirst or appetite increased or decreased? Has the volume or frequency of urination changed? Responses to such questions can provide distinguishing data to differentiate endocrine disorders from one another. Similarly, distinguishing data may include information regarding a history of nausea, vomiting, constipation, diarrhea, or abdominal pain.[2]

Energy levels should also be described. Have there been changes, and if so, are such changes continuous or intermittent? Is sleep effective and does it restore energy? Weakness and fatigue associated with endocrine dysfunction characteristically increase in severity toward the end of the day, with the exception of thyroid disorders, which tend to produce continuous manifestations.[2] Muscle tremors, palpitations, headaches, and/or visual disturbances may reflect excessive thyroid effect but may also signal the presence of pheochromocytoma. Intolerance to heat and insomnia suggest hyperthyroid function, while cold intolerance and somnolence may reflect either hypothyroid function or adrenocortical insufficiency.

Because some endocrine disorders have hereditary tendencies, any family history of diabetes, thyroid disorders, hypertension, cardiac or renal disease, or cancer needs to be noted. General or routine use of over-the-counter pharmacologic agents as well as all prescribed agents should also be included. Finally, it is necessary to be alert to clues indicating use of street or illicit drugs. The effects of many of these drugs can mimic both thyroid and adrenal imbalance.[2]

Endocrine dysfunction seen in the critical-care setting is most commonly acute and of an emergent nature. Fortunately, life-threatening physiologic compromise of a purely endocrine nature is relatively rare. It is because of this relative rarity that specific attention needs to be directed at what might be otherwise considered nonspecific findings. Table 37-1 outlines examples of findings often associated with chronic and acute endocrine dysfunctions.[3] It is important to remember, however, that virtually all findings listed in Table 37-1 have a variety of potential origins. Their significance, therefore, can be determined only in the context of data from the history and physical examination.

Physical Examination

The diffuse nature of the endocrine system virtually mandates the use of a systematic approach in physical examination. The approach discussed generally follows a head-to-toe framework.

Vital Signs

Measurement of heart and respiratory rate, blood pressure, and temperature is the first step in the physical examination. Both apical and radial recording of pulse is necessary. Tachycardia (either with or without tachyarrythmias)—typically atrial fibrillation and/or paroxysmal atrial tachycardia— may reflect the effect of elevated thyroid hormone on the heart. Slowed pulse rates may reflect hypothyroid function.[4]

The character and rate of respirations should be described. Rapid, deep Kussmaul respirations are a hallmark finding in diabetic ketoacidosis, as is a sweetish, acetone-like breath odor.

Blood pressure should be measured in both arms and checked for postural changes. Hypertension, with a widened pulse pressure, commonly accompanies hyperthyroidism.[4] Elevated blood pressure is also a fairly frequent clinical finding in the adrenal disorders—Cushing's syndrome, hyperaldosteronism, and pheochromocytoma. In the latter, however, hypertension is often paroxysmal in nature and is frequently associated with ingestion of caffeine or nicotine, anxiety and stress, or situations in which external abdominal pressure is applied, as in deep palpation and postural changes (see "Abdomen," below).

In contrast, hypotension, frequently with postural exaggeration, often occurs in adrenocortical insufficiency as a result of depressed catecholamine vasoactivity, renal sodium loss, and extracellular volume depletion.[5] A similar but often less pronounced finding may also occur in high-flow urinary states. In diabetes insipidus, for example, renal sodium loss is exaggerated by the high urinary flow state and results in extracellular volume depletion and sustained as well as postural hypotension.[6] Hyperglycemic osmolar diuresis associated with both diabetic ketoacidosis and nonketotic hyperosmolar states may also lead to extracellular volume

Table 37-1 Nonspecific Findings in Endocrine Dysfunction

Finding	Potential Endocrine Dysfunction
Abdominal cramps and distention	Diabetic ketoacidosis, nonketotic hyperglycemic hyperosmolar coma, adrenocortical insufficiency
Anorexia	Adrenocortical insufficiency, diabetic ketoacidosis
Agitation	Hyperthyroidism, hypoparathyroidism due to hypocalcemia
Blurred vision	Pituitary tumor, hypoglycemia, pheochromocytoma
Confusion	Hypoglycemia, hyperthyroidism, hypothyroidism, hypoparathyroidism due to hypocalcemia
Constipation	Hypothyroidism, pheochromocytoma, hyperparathyroidism due to hypercalcemia
Diaphoresis	Hypoglycemia (cold and clammy), hyperthyroidism (warm and flushed), pheochromocytoma
Dry skin	Diabetic ketoacidosis, nonketotic hyperglycemic hyperosmolar coma, adrenocortical insufficiency, hypothyroidism
Edema	Hypothyroidism (ascites-like), hyperthyroidism (anasarca-like), Cushing's syndrome
Fever	Hyperthyroidism, adrenocortical insufficiency
Headache	Hypoglycemia, adrenocortical insufficiency, pheochromocytoma (usually associated with palpitations)
Nausea and vomiting	Same as for abdominal cramps; also hyperthyroidism
Palpitations	Hyperthyroidism, pheochromocytoma
Tachycardia	Hypoglycemia (acute, rapidly evolving), hyperthyroidism, pheochromocytoma
"Internal tremors"	Hypoglycemia
Tremors	Hyperthyroidism, pheochromoctyoma
Weakness	Hypoglycemia, adrenocortical insufficiency, hypothyroidism

depletion and thus to both sustained and postural hypotension.

Elevations in temperature may accompany both hyperthyroid states and adrenocortical insufficiency.[5] Hypothermia, on the other hand, is characteristic of severe myxedema and is also frequently a finding in diabetic ketoacidosis.[7]

General Observation

As the physical examination is initiated, it is important to be alert to gross or obvious signs of endocrine dysfunction. Disproportionate size of body parts, abnormal body size, or unusual facial features may reflect abnormal endocrine function. In gigantism, excessive growth hormone before epiphyseal closure of the long bones results in a very tall stature. Following long-bone growth plate closure, excessive growth hormone produces acromegaly, a syndrome manifested by enlargement of the nose, jaw, tongue, and soft tissues of the hands and feet.[8] In hypothyroid states, mucopolysaccharide infiltration may result in facial swelling and puffiness around the eyes. Features also tend to look coarse, and eyebrows frequently appear thinned and sparse.

Cushing's syndrome, with its associated excessive levels of glucocorticoids, is accompanied by a specific pattern and type of obesity. In the face, trunk, and cervicodorsal and supraclavicular regions, fatty accumulations produce the characteristic moon face, buffalo hump, and pendulous abdomen. Typically, limbs are thin.[5,9]

Skin

In assessing skin it is important to remember that normal pigmentation reflects racial and ethnic backgrounds. It is characteristically greater on the face, the backs of the hands, the areolae, and the genitalia. In addition, all pigmentation intensifies during pregnancy.

In endocrine dysfunction, pigmentation is often intensified; moderate to significant hyperpigmentation may be an indication of either diabetes mellitus or adrenocortical insufficiency. Amber to yellow tinges can indicate myxedema and may look much like jaundice. To differentiate jaundice from the pigmentation associated with hypothyroidism it is necessary to inspect the sclerae, for only jaundice produces yellowing of the sclerae.[10]

All lesions should be evaluated; distribution, location, shape, and color should be noted. Petechiae, excessive bruising, evidence of poor wound healing, and/or purple striae ("stretch marks"), especially on the abdomen, may indicate Cushing's syndrome. Areas of cracking superimposed on dry scaly skin often accompany hypothyroidism, while hyperthyroidism is characteristically associated with silky smooth, flushed-appearing skin with diaphoresis.[10]

Evaluation of hair may also suggest endocrine dysfunction. Coarse, dry hair, especially with evidence of hair loss, frequently accompanies hypothyroid states, while in hyperthyroid states hair tends to feel smooth, soft, and fine. Unusual hair loss may also signal chronic adrenocortical insufficiency and pituitary or parathyroid disorders.

In women, excessive hair or hair in abnormal locations is known as *hirsutism*. It suggests either Cushing's syndrome or the presence of excessive adrenal androgens. Characteristically, hirsutism is manifested by development of a mustache and hair on the chest and abdomen.[5]

The condition of the nails can also provide data regarding endocrine function. Pitting or nails of unusual shape may reflect hypoparathyrodism, while nails separated from nail beds, a condition known as *onycholysis,* is a frequent finding in hyperthyroidism. Thickened, brittle, and friable nails may indicate hypothyroidism. Pigmented, darkened nails may signal adrenocortical insufficiency.

Finally, skin turgor needs to be assessed. Poor turgor may reflect dehydration, a feature not infrequently associated with diabetes insipidus, diabetic ketoacidosis, and nonketotic hyperglycemic hyperosmolar states. In contrast, edema may occur in thyroid disorders. In acute and severe hyperthyroid states and in thyrotoxic crisis, edema results from hypervolemic, hyperdynamic cardiac failure. Even though the glomerular filtration rate exceeds normal values, it is still decreased relative to overall volume; thus pulmonary edema and anasarca may occur.[4] Similarly, in hypothyroid states, decreased glomerular filtration may result in ascites-type fluid accumulation.[11]

Head

Facial expression should be evaluated. A flat or dull expression, especially coupled with coarse features and puffy eyes, as previously noted, suggests hypothyroidism. In contrast, an overly alert to anxious expression may reflect hyperthyroidism.[4]

Retracted upper eyelids with protruding eyeballs are hallmarks of *exophthalmos.* Also known as *bilateral proptosis,* this bulging of the eyeballs gives the appearance of continuous staring. It is thought to occur as a result of immunoglobulin G (IgG)-mediated changes in the mucopolysaccharide tissue of the retroorbital glands.[12] Exophthalmos is virtually diagnostic of Graves' disease, a specific form of hyperthyroidism.

Visual field defects or cranial nerve dysfunction may indicate a pituitary tumor (see Chap. 34 for assessment procedures). If blurred double vision or diplopia is reported, cranial nerve dysfunction should be suspected, although hypoglycemia and pheochromocytoma may also result in blurred vision.

At all times the eyes should remain parallel to each other, that is, conjugate gaze should be maintained. Similarly, eye movements should remain smooth. Nystagmus or rapid, jerky movements should be noted. Finally, the patient should be asked to raise the eyebrows, close the eyes tightly, puff the cheeks, show the teeth, frown, and smile. Muscle contraction on both sides of the face should be equal; asymmetry should be noted.[13]

A nasal speculum is used to check the patency of the nasal canals or nares. Signs of inflammation, such as reddened mucous membranes and discharge, may indicate infection, a common accompaniment of Cushing's syndrome. Excessive nasal hair may also reflect Cushing's. Highly inflamed nasal passages should be investigated, for they may reflect inhalation of cocaine, an agent whose effects can mimic endocrine dysfunction.

The lips and tongue should be evaluated for symmetry and color. An enlarged tongue may indicate myxedema; asymmetry may reflect a pituitary lesion.[12,14] Malformed or pitted teeth commonly occur in hypoparathyroidism. As previously noted, an acetone or fruity odor of the breath is associated with diabetes mellitus.

Neck

In evaluation of the neck for data on endocrine function, the focus is on the thyroid gland. Unlike its counterparts in the endocrine system, the thyroid gland itself is at least indirectly visible.

For assessment of the thyroid, the patient should be upright. With the neck in normal position, it should be inspected for signs of thyroid enlargement (goiter) or asymmetry. The same inspection should be performed with the neck somewhat extended. The patient should also be observed while swallowing; upward midline movement should be visible. Any reported difficulty with swallowing or hoarseness should be noted.

Before palpating the thyroid, it is important to remember that the thyroid is usually not palpable unless the patient has a very thin neck. Thus, when either lobes or nodules can be easily felt, further examination is necessary. To palpate the thyroid gland, begin by having the patient flex the neck slightly to relieve tension on the sternocleidomastoid muscles. Changes in the isthmus can be palpated by placing the index and middle fingers just below the cricoid cartilage on one side. Ask the patient, still with neck flexed, to turn the head slightly to the side being palpated and swallow. Repeat the procedure for the other side. Changes in the lobes of the gland can be detected by displacing the thyroid cartilage slightly to first one side and then the other. With the cartilage thus displaced, the space between the sternocleidomastoid and cartilage can be palpated.[13]

The thyroid should be auscultated when enlargement or nodules are suspected from either inspection or palpation. With a stethoscope, listen to first one lobe and then the other. A soft, rushing sound, or *bruit,* may indicate hyperthyroidism and increased blood flow through an already highly vascular gland. To distinguish a bruit from a venous hum, ask the patient to stop breathing momentarily; then, while compressing the jugular vein on the same side as the lobe being auscultated, listen to first one lobe and then the other. Compression of the jugular will remove a venous hum but not a bruit.[13]

Abdomen

With the patient in a supine position, observe for contour, striae, bulges, and discolorations. Normal abdominal contour is flat; a protuberant contour occurs in obesity and may reflect hypothyroidism or Cushing's syndrome. Striae, or stretch marks, often accompany obesity and occur as a result of stretching of the skin. Typically, young or new striae are bright pink or blue in color while long-standing ones tend to be silvery pink. Striae of a somewhat vivid purplish color are fairly common in Cushing's syndrome.[15]

Bowel sounds should be auscultated and frequency, pitch, and duration noted. Normal bowel tones characteristically occur 5 to 35 times a minute, are low-pitched, and last roughly 1 to 5 seconds.[16] Decreased or absent bowel tones are common in hypothyroidism and pheochromocytoma, while hyperactive, high-pitched sounds are a common feature in hyperthyroidism.[12]

Abdominal percussion can provide useful data regarding endocrine function. An enlarged liver may reflect the effect of fatty infiltration as a result of poorly controlled diabetes. Dullness and bulging in the flanks can reflect ascitic fluid accumulation, as in hypothyroidism.[12]

All four quadrants of the abdomen should be palpated to ascertain the presence of tenderness, masses, or enlarged organs. As previously noted, an enlarged liver may reflect poorly controlled diabetes. Upper abdominal tenderness, sometimes severe, accompanies acute pancreatitis and may signal the onset of acute diabetes. A mass on the upper pole of the kidneys may be a pheochromocytoma. If however, the patient has a history of paroxysmal hypertension, headache, dulled to absent bowel tones, and/or findings associated with hypermetabolic states, deep abdominal palpation should *not* be performed. Pressure on the adrenal medulla and/or the tumor itself can result in a sudden burst of catecholamines into the circulation.

Diagnostic Procedures

A vast arsenal of diagnostic tools exists to assess endocrine function. For example, radioimmunoassay (RIA) allows direct measurement of even minuscule amounts of hormone; computerized tomography (CT) scans allow the next best thing to direct visualization to determine size and structure in selected tissues; and advances in ultrasonography now allow differentiation of structural abnormalities.

Laboratory Studies

Laboratory studies utilized to assess endocrine function fall into three primary categories: measurement of serum or plasma hormone levels, measurement of urine levels of a hormone or its metabolite, and measurement of hormonal reserve and regulation through stimulation and suppression.[11] Typically, abnormalities in standard laboratory screens provide the stimulus for utilization of tests from one or more of these categories. For example, a decreased alkaline phosphatase in a blood chemistry may prompt RIA measurement of serum triiodothyronine (T_3) to rule out hypothyroidism. Similarily, hypochloremia noted in a rou-

tine electrolyte screen may prompt 24-h measurement of urinary aldosterone to determine whether primary hyperaldosteronism is present. Elevated BUN and creatinine levels in a blood chemistry may lead to an ACTH stimulation test to evaluate adrenal function. Tables 37-2, 37-3, and 37-4 list electrolyte, blood chemistry, and hematologic changes in endocrine dysfunction.

Pituitary Function

Pituitary function is most commonly assessed by measuring the plasma levels of hormones, typically in concert with stimulation of hypothalamic releasing hormones or after suppression of target tissue hormones. Assessment of anterior pituitary function thus involves measurements relating to adrenocorticotropic hormone (ACTH), thyroid stimulating hormone (TSH), luteinizing and follicle stimulating hormones (LH and FSH), growth hormone (GH), and prolactin (PRL). Antidiuretic hormone (ADH) and oxytocin are measured to evaluate posterior pituitary function.

Hyperpituitarism most commonly is reflected by excessive secretion of one or more anterior pituitary hormones. Elevations usually involve, in order of most to least frequent, PRL (normally inhibited), GH, ACTH, and rarely, TSH, FSH, or LH. Hypopituitarism, on the other hand, most commonly reflects decreased levels of GH. Less often, FSH, LH, TSH, or ACTH levels and PRL levels are decreased. Panhypopituitarism and deficiency of all anterior pituitary hormones may occur but is extremely rare and usually accompanies glandular

Table 37-2 Electrolyte Changes in Endocrine Dysfunction

Electrolyte	Increased in:	Decreased in:
Sodium	Cushing's syndrome, diabetes insipidus, nonketotic hyperglycemic hyperosmolar states, primary hyperaldosteronism	Adrenal hypofunction, chronic primary adrenocortical insufficiency, hypothyroidism
Potassium	Adrenal hypofunction	Cushing's syndrome, primary aldosteronism
Chloride	Hyperparathyroidism	Primary hyperaldosteronism, adrenal hypofunction
Calcium	Hyperparathyroidism, adrenal hypofunction, hyperthyroidism	Hypoparathyroidism, Cushing's syndrome
Magnesium	Adrenal hypofunction, end-stage diabetic acidosis	Hyperparathyroidism, hyperthyroidism, primary hyperaldosteronism
Phosphate	Hypoparathyroidism, acromegaly	Hyperparathyroidism

Table 37-3 Blood Chemistry Changes in Endocrine Dysfunction

Constituent	Increased in:	Decreased in:
Total protein	Diabetic acidosis, hypothyroidism	Chronic uncontrolled diabetes mellitus, hyperthyroidism
Albumin	Diabetic acidosis, hypothyroidism	Hyperthyroidism
SGOT	Hypothyroidism, diabetic acidosis	
Alkaline phosphatase	Acromegaly, hyperparathyroidism, hyperthyroidism	Hypothyroidism
Lactic dehydrogenase	Hypothyroidism, severe diabetic acidosis	
Blood urea nitrogen	Adrenal hypofunction, uncontrolled diabetes mellitus	Acromegaly
Creatinine	Adrenal hypofunction, uncontrolled diabetes mellitus	
Cholesterol	Hypothyroidism	Hyperthyroidism
Bicarbonate	Cushing's syndrome	Adrenal hypofunction
Glucose	Diabetes mellitus, Cushing's syndrome, acromegaly, hyperpituitarism (GH, ACTH), hyperthyroidism, pheochromocytoma	Insulinoma, adrenal hypofunction, hypopituitarism (GH, ACTH), hypothyroidism

destruction such as occurs in hemorrhage into a tumor or glandular infarction.[14]

Radioimmunoassays are available to measure plasma hormone levels of all anterior pituitary hormones; however, absolute values are often misleading because of variable diurnal secretion patterns and differing metabolic pathways. Thus, where stimulation or suppression tests are available, they are almost always done in conjunction with RIA measurements. Table 37-5 provides normal values of anterior pituitary hormones along with the stimulation or suppression tests most commonly utilized to detect anterior pituitary dysfunction.[17]

Laboratory evaluation of posterior pituitary function focuses on antidiuretic hormone (ADH). Oxytocin, the other hormone released by the posterior pituitary gland, is normally absent from the circulation. It is released reflexly upon nipple stimulation and results in milk ejection from the secretory ducts of the breast (see also Chap. 36).

Table 37-4 Hematologic Changes in Endocrine Dysfunction

Parameter	Increased in:	Decreased in:
Hematocrit reading	Adrenal hypofunction, Cushing's syndrome, diabetic acidosis, pheochromocytoma	
Hemoglobin	Cushing's syndrome, pheochromocytoma	Ectopic ACTH syndrome, hypopituitarism, hypothyroidism
Red blood cells	Pituitary tumors	Adrenal hypofunction
White blood cells		
Neutrophils	Cushing's syndrome, diabetic acidosis, hyperthyroidism	Adrenal hypofunction
Eosinophils	Adrenal hypofunction, hyperthyroidism, anterior pituitary hypofunction	Cushing's syndrome, diabetic acidosis
Basophils	Hypothyroidism, anterior pituitary hypofunction	Hyperthyroidism
Lymphocytes	Adrenal hypofunction, hyperthyroidism	Cushing's syndrome, diabetic acidosis

Table 37-5 Evaluation of Anterior Pituitary Hormones

Hormone	Normal Value	Stimulation Test/Normal Value	Suppression Test/ Normal Value

GH	Adult
	  Male, 0–5 ng/mL
	  Female, 0–10 ng/mL
	  Child, 0–16 ng/mL
		Arginine stimulation:
		  Male: GH rise to >10 ng/mL
		  Female: GH rise to > 15 ng/mL
		  Child: GH rise to > 48 ng/mL
			Glucose loading: GH suppression to < 3 ng/mL

ACTH	Fasting: 20–100 pg/mL Nonfasting: 10–50 pg/mL	None	None

TSH	0–10 μIU/mL	Thyrotropin releasing factor: peak rise in TSH in 15–30 min
		  Female: peak value 16–26 μIU/mL from base of 6 μIU/mL
		  Male: slightly lower
			None

PRL	Fasting
	  Female: 6–30 ng/mL
	  Male 5–18 ng/mL
		None	None

LH	Female
	  Follicular phase: 5–30 mIU/mL
	  Ovulatory phase: 75–150 mIU/mL
	  Luteal phase: 3–40 mIU/mL
	  Postmenopausal: 30–200 mIU/mL
	Male: 6–30 mIU/mL
	Child: 4–20 mIU/mL
		None	None

FSH	Female
	  Follicular phase: 5–20 mIU/mL
	  Ovulatory phase: 4–35 mIU/mL
	  Luteal phase: 2–11 mIU/mL
	  Postmenopausal: 40–200 mIU/mL
	Male: 5–20 mIU/mL
	Child: up to 12 mIU/mL
		None	None

Direct measurements of serum and urine ADH are possible but are rarely utilized. Instead, evaluation of ADH centers on serum osmolality and water deprivation or loading tests. Table 37-6 summarizes values and findings for the assessment of ADH.

Thyroid Function

Radioimmunassays and stimulation and suppression tests are utilized to assess thyroid function. Generally levels of triiodothyronine (T_3) are more useful than those of thyronine or tetraiodothyronine (T_4), because most T_4 is closely bound in the circulation to thyroxine-binding globulin (TBG), and only the nonbound, or free, T_4 exerts clinical effects.[12] T_3 is derived from T_4, is more potent, and binds with less affinity than T_4. The T_3 RIA is highly specific and allows measurement of both bound and free T_3; thus this test is considered a sensitive indicator of thyroid function.

Free levels of serum T_3 and T_4 are also vital in thyroid evaluation. They are usually measured simultaneously. Because nonbound or free hormone levels both influence and are influenced by anterior pituitary feedback mechanisms, which result in negative or positive influence on TSH secretion, adjustment for changes in protein levels, and thus protein-binding concentrations, is in essence automatic. Thus, measurement of free hormone levels is a valuable indicator of thyroid function[12] (see also Chap. 36).

Indirect information regarding free T_4 levels can also be gained from a T_3 resin uptake study. This measurement quantifies available protein-binding sites for T_4, that is, those not occupied by T_3. A mathematical formula can be applied, in concert with T_4 RIA, to determine free T_4 levels with correction for TBG variations and abnormalities.[2] Table 37-7 summarizes normal laboratory values and findings in thyroid evaluation.

Table 37-6 Assessment of ADH

Parameter	Normal Value	Increased in:	Decreased in:
Serum ADH	1–5 pg/mL	SIADH, hyperthyroidism, adrenal insufficiency, hemorrhage or shock, stress, pain	Diabetes insipidus, metastatic disease, viral infection, neurologic trauma
Serum osmolality	275–295 mosmol/kg	Diabetes insipdus, ketotic and nonketotic hyperglycemic states, hypercalcemia	SIADH, excessive water intake
Water-loading test	>80% of water excreted within 5 h; urine osmolality falls to <100 mosmol/L		SIADH: <40% excretion
Water-deprivation test	Urine flow decreased to <0.5 mL/min; urine osmolality >800 mosmol/L	Diabetes insipidus: increased urine volumes, decreased concentration	

Parathyroid Function

Radioimmunoassay measurement of serum parathormone (PTH) is a fundamental part of parathyroid evaluation. It is necessary, however, to simultaneously measure serum calcium and phosphorus levels, as normal parathyroid secretion of PTH is controlled via negative and positive feedback mechanisms involving the serum levels of both these substances (see also Chap. 36).

PTH levels can also be assessed by evaluating tubular reabsorption of phosphates. Because PTH inhibits tubular reabsorption of phosphorus, changes

Table 37-7 Laboratory Values and Findings in Thyroid Evaluation

Parameter	Normal Value	Increased in:	Decreased in:
Serum thyroxine (T_4)	5–13 µg/dL	Thyrotoxicosis, acute thyroiditis, pregnancy	Hypothyroidism, chronic debilitating illness
Serum triiodothyronine (T_3)	Neonate: 134–146 ng/dL 1–2 yrs: 116–132 ng/dL 3–10 yrs: 131–141 ng/dL 11–19 yrs: 129 ng/dL Adult: 90–230 ng/dL	Thyrotoxicosis, Hashimoto's thyroiditis	Severe acute illness, trauma, malnutrition
T_3 resin uptake	25–35 T_3 binding	Thyrotoxicosis, protein malnutrition	Hypothyroidism
Serum TSH	0–10 µIU/mL	Primary hypothyroidism	Secondary hypothyroidism, (anterior pituitary hypofunctional), thyrotoxicosis
Thyroid (T_3) supression	TSH falls to below baseline: T_4 falls to <50% of baseline	Primary hyperthyroidism: failure to suppress (e.g., multinodular goiter)	
TSH stimulation	Normal response in primary hyperthyroidism, hypothyroidism from deficient (but not absent) pituitary or hypothalamic function; see also Table 37-5		No response to TRH: secondary hypothyroidism from pituitary hypofunction, hyperthyroidism from autonomous gland (e.g., toxic goiter); subnormal response to TRH: treated Grave's disease, multinodular goiter

in reabsorption rate can be compared with normal or borderline serum calcium and phosphate levels to detect abnormal parathyroid function.[18] Urinary calcium also changes in the presence of parathyroid dysfunction. Table 37-8 summarizes laboratory findings utilized to evaluate parathyroid function.

Adrenocortical Function

Both RIA measurement of blood and urine hormone levels and stimulation and suppression tests are utilized to evaluate function of the adrenal cortex. Determinations of plasma and urinary cortisol levels are usually ordered for suspected adrenal dysfunction, but suppression and stimulation studies are characteristically necessary for diagnosis. Serum aldosterone is also often measured, but because normal values are typically low and difficult to quantify accurately, urine aldosterone levels are commonly utilized as well. Typically, 24-h specimens are analyzed to decrease the impact of diurnal variations, postural changes, and variations due to sodium and potassium levels.

Urinary studies are also utilized to evaluate overall adrenocortical hormone output. These include measurement of 17-hydroxycorticosteroids (17-OHCS), 17-ketogenic steroids (17-KGS), and 17-ketosteroids (17-KS). Measurement of 17-OHCS provides information regarding glucocorticoid secretion and to a lesser extent aldosterone output, as does the 17-KGS test. The former tends to directly reflect cortisol; the latter reflects more the less abundant glucocorticoids. Because the 17-KGS reflects almost all the adrenocorticoids, it is often utilized to provide a general overview of adrenocortical function. The 17-KS test is utilized less frequently. It measures the metabolites of adrenal androgens, but the most potent adrenal androgen, testosterone, is not a 17-KS. Thus, this test provides only a rough estimate of adrenal androgenic activity, and if abnormal adrenal androgen function is suspected, plasma testosterone must be simultaneously measured.[2,5]

Measurements of serum ACTH are often utilized in tandem with urinary and plasma cortisol levels to evaluate adrenocortical function. When abnormality is suspected, the urinary and plasma cortisol may be measured before and after administration of a measured dose of ACTH to determine the secretory capacity of the adrenal cortex.

Table 37-8 Laboratory Values and Findings in Parathyroid Evaluation

Parameter	Normal Value	Increased in:	Decreased in:
Serum PTH	163–347 pg/Eg/mL (depends on serum calcium)	Hyperparathyroidism, parathyroid and nonparathyroid PTH-secreting tumors (lung, breast, kidney)	Parathyroid trauma, inadvertent parathyroidectomy as in thyroid surgery
Serum calcium	Children: to 12 mg/dL Adults: 8.9–10.1 mg/dL or 4.5–5.5 meq/L	Hyperparathyroidism, metastatic bone tumors, nonparathyroid PTH-secreting tumors (lung, breast, kidney)	Hypoparathyroidism, alcoholism, chronic renal disease, malabsorption syndrome
Serum phosphates	Children: to 7 mg/dL or 4.1 meq/L during periods of rapid bone growth Adults: 2.5–4.5 mg/dL or 1.8–2.6 meq/L	Hypoparathyroidism, nonendocrine hypocalcemia, renal insufficiency or failure	Hyperparathyroidism, non endocrine hypercalcemia
Urine calcium	1+ to 2+; negative to moderately positive	Concentrated urine, hyperparathyroidism, osteoporosis, renal tubular acidosis, hyperthyroidism, vitamin D intoxication	Dilute urine, hypoparathyroidism, vitamin D deficiency
Tubular reabsorption of phosphate	Absorption of 80% or more of phosphate		Primary hyperparathyroidism, hypercalcemia from PTH-secreting malignant tumor, renal defects

When adrenocortical hyperfunction is suspected a metyrapone suppression test may be used to evaluate the role of the pituitary gland. Metyrapone is an adrenal inhibitor that prevents the final step in cortisol synthesis. With normal pituitary function, metyrapone administration lowers serum cortisol and, as a result of negative feedback, should lead to increased pituitary ACTH secretion. The dexamethasone suppression test is utilized similarly to evaluate pituitary feedback mechanisms. Since dexamethasone supresses pituitary ACTH production, the plasma cortisol level should drop after administration of this agent.[2,19]

Suppression and stimulation tests are also used to evaluate adrenocortical aldosterone secretion. The aldosterone stimulation test involves administration of furosemide. Normally, the resultant diuresis triggers alteration in the serum sodium/potassium ratio and juxtaglomerular perfusion pressure, changes that normally stimulate renin formation and therefore aldosterone secretion (see Chap. 36). The aldosterone suppression test involves administration of spironolactone, a potent mineralocorticoid antagonist. Large doses of this agent will normalize hypokalemia due to hyperaldosteronism.[2,20] Table 37-9 summarizes laboratory values and findings in adrenocortical evaluation.

Adrenomedullary Function

Laboratory evaluation of the adrenal medulla involves direct measurement of plasma and urine catecholamines. Urinary vanillylmandelic acid (VMA) is also measured, but because VMA is a catecholamine metabolite, its level in the urine is increased by emotional and physiologic stress as well as strenuous exercise and is therefore somewhat nonspecific.[2,20] Table 37-10 summarizes laboratory values and findings utilized in evaluation of the adrenal medulla.

Endocrine Pancreas Function

Most laboratory studies involved in evaluation of the endocrine pancreas focus on either direct or indirect measurement of glucose in blood or urine. Common tests used to measure serum glucose include random samples after fasting and 2 h after eating a meal (postprandial). Glucose tolerance tests are also commonly performed when diabetes is suspected. This test provides what may be the most sensitive and accurate evaluation of carbohydrate metabolism. In glucose tolerance testing, a loading dose of glucose is orally administered after 3 days of a high-carbohydrate diet and an overnight fast. For the next 3 h plasma and urine glucose levels are monitored at frequent intervals to assess insulin secretion and glucose metabolism.[2,20]

In persons known to be diabetic, the glycosylated hemoglobin test may be performed to help assess average glucose levels over time. Normally, glucose molecules gradually attach to hemoglobin A within erythrocytes; the process of attachment is known as *glycosylation*. Since the life span of erythrocytes is 120 days, measurement of glycosylated hemoglobin provides data regarding average glucose levels over the life span of the erythrocytes.[2]

In hypoglycemia, RIA measurement of serum insulin is almost always performed along with measurements of glucose levels and the two correlated. These data can help differentiate between possible glucocorticoid deficiency, hepatic disease, and hypoglycemia due to insulinoma or hyperplasia of the pancreatic islet cells.

Urinary tests for glucose include copper reduction (Clinitest) and glucose oxidase (Tes-Tape, Clinistix) procedures. They are commonly used for self-testing purposes. Both types of test produce standardized color reactions either by reduction of copper in a hot alkaline solution with subsequent formation of a colored precipitate or by sequential enzymatic oxidation of glucose. Copper reduction tests may yield false positives for glucose, because other substances can stimulate chemical reduction of cupric ions. Glucose oxidase tests are generally more accurate for glucose, because reagent strips are impregnated with specific enzymes. Similarly, strips impregnated with sodium nitroprusside, an agent specific for acetoacetic acid, allow self-testing for urinary ketones.[2] Table 37-11 summarizes laboratory values and findings used to assess function of the endocrine pancreas.

Radiographic and Nuclear Imaging

Radiographic and nuclear imaging tests used in endocrine evaluation include x-rays, computerized tomography (CT), arteriography, ultrasonography, and nuclear isotope studies.[2] Generally, one or more of these procedures are utilized to confirm

Table 37-9 Laboratory Values and Findings in Adrenocortical Evaluation

Parameter	Normal Value	Increased in:	Decreased in:
Plasma cortisol	8 A.M.: 7–28 μ/dL 4 P.M.: 2–18 μ/dL	Adrenocortical hyperfunction, obesity, stress, pregnancy, diabetes mellitus	Adrenocortical hypofunction, hypopituitarism
Plasma ACTH	8 A.M.: 20–100 pg/mL 4 P.M.: 10–50 pg/mL	Primary adrenal insufficiency, stress, pituitary neoplasm	Hypopituitarism, adrenal hyperfunction (via negative feedback)
Serum aldosterone	A.M. recumbent: 3–10 ng/dL A.M.: upright: 4–30 ng/dL (Normal values greatly increase with low-sodium diet)	Primary and secondary hyperaldosteronism, nephrotic syndrome, severe stress	Adrenal hypofunction, hypothyroidism
Urinary 17-hydroxycorticosteroids	Female: 2–10 mg/24 h Male: 3–12 mg/24 h	Adrenal hyperfunction, adrenal cancer, hyperpituitarism, hyperthyroidism	Adrenal hypofunction, hypopituitarism, hypothyroidism
Urinary 17-ketosteroids	1–11 yrs: 0.1–3 mg/24 h 11–14 yrs: 2–12 mg/24 h Adult female: 4–17 mg/24 h Adult male: 6–21 mg/24 h (Normally decline after age 60).	Adrenocortical hyperfunction or cancer, adrenogenital syndrome, testicular or ovarian neoplasm	Adrenal hypofunction, hypogonadism, hypopituitarism
Urinary 17-ketogenic steroids	1–11 yrs: 0.1–4 mg/24 h 11–14 yrs: 2–9 mg/24 h Adult female: 2–15 mg/24 h Adult male: 4–22 mg/24 h	Adrenocortical hyperfunction or cancer, adrenogenital syndrome	Adrenal hypofunction, hypopituitarism
Urine aldosterone	2–16 mg/24 h	Primary and secondary aldosteronism, severe stress	Adrenal hypofunction
ACTH stimulation (ACTH infusion)	8-h infusion: twofold to fourfold increase in plasma cortisol, 17-KS, 17-OHCS over baseline. Screening test: plasma cortisol doubles within 60 min after intravenous ACTH	Pituitary insufficiency with secondary adrenal insufficiency, adrenocortical hyperplasia	Delayed response: chronic adrenal suppression due to iatrogenic steroid therapy. No response: adrenal insufficiency
Metyrapone suppression	Compound S-(plasma cortisol and urinary metabolites) baseline: <1 μg/dL After metyrapone: >7 μg/dL (or twofold to fourfold increase in urinary 17-OHCS); plasma cortisol: A.M.: 7–18 μg/dL P.M.: 2–9 μg/dL	Cushing's disease, pituitary-dependent adrenal hyperplasia	With normal baseline cortisol: Cushing's due to adrenal carcinoma, autonomous adrenal function, adrenogenital syndrome. With low baseline cortisol: pituitary failure, hypothalamic failure
Dexamethasone suppression	Overnight screening: A.M. plasma cortisol <5 μg/dL	Cushing's syndrome	
Aldosterone stimulation (furosemide)	Urine aldosterone increases twofold to threefold: plasma aldosterone increases twofold to fivefold	Primary aldosteronism	Hypoaldosteronism
Aldosterone suppression (spironolactone)	>50 % decrease in aldosterone secretion	Little or no suppression: primary aldosteronism	

Table 37-10 Laboratory Values and Findings in Adrenomedullary Evaluation

Parameter	Normal Value	Increased in:
Plasma catecholamine fractionation	Supine, resting: Epinephrine: 0–150 ng/L Norepinephrine: 103–193 ng/L Standing: Epinephrine: 0–150 ng/L Norepinephrine: 293–489 ng/L	Pheochromocytoma (>1000 ng/mL), neuroblastoma, ganglioneuroblastoma
Urinary vanillylmandelic acid	1–2 yrs: <2 mg/24 h 12–14 yrs: <5 mg/24 h Adult: 0.7–8.8 mg/24 h	Pheochromocytoma, neuroblastoma, ganglioblastoma, physiologic and emotional stress, muscle disorders

Decreases in parameters not found in any pathologic condition.

suspected anatomic glandular changes such as hypo- or hyperplasia, cysts, neoplasms, or glandular destruction.

Thyroid gland evaluation may frequently involve a nuclear isotope study, nuclear scan, and/or ultrasonography. Measuring the thyroid uptake of radioactive iodine (^{131}I uptake) can provide data to help distinguish between thyrotoxicosis factitia and subacute thyroiditis or to distinguish hypofunctioning toxic adenoma from thyrotoxicosis. The test involves external monitoring of radioactivity to measure the accumulation of ^{131}I in the thyroid 2,

Table 37-11 Laboratory Values and Findings in Endocrine Pancreas Evaluation

Parameter	Normal Value	Increased in:	Decreased in:
Plasma glucose	Fasting: 70–100 μg/dL; 2 h postprandial: <145 μg/dL	Diabetes mellitus, adrenal hyperfunction (Cushing's syndrome), acromegaly, stress	Hypoglycemia, hyperinsulinism, adrenocortical insufficiency, malnutrition, alcoholism
Glucose tolerance	Plasma glucose at 30 min: <160 μg/mL, normal at 2 h; no urine sugar	Glycosuria or prolonged elevation suggests diabetes	
Serum insulin	4–24 μIU/mL	Insulinoma, insulin resistance	Diabetes mellitus, obesity
Glycosylated hemoglobin	<7.8%	Hyperglycemia, poorly controlled diabetes mellitus	Hemolytic states due to hemoglobin loss as opposed to decreased production
Urine copper reduction (Clinitest)	Negative	Color changes indicate glycosuria in diabetes mellitus, adrenal and thyroid dysfunction	
Urine glucose oxidase (Tes-Tape, Clinistix)	Negative	Color changes indicate glycosuria in diabetes mellitus, adrenal and thyroid dysfunction	
Urine ketone	Negative	Color changes indicate ketonuria and reliably reflect serum ketone levels; ketonuria occurs in uncontrolled diabetes mellitus and starvation.	

6, and 24 h after oral ingestion of a measured dose of [131]I. Thyroid scans performed after injection of radioactively tagged iodine can provide data not only about glandular size and the uniformity of iodine uptake but also about overall metabolic function of the gland. Gray-black regions on the scan, known also as *hot spots,* indicate hyperfunction, while white regions, or *cold spots,* indicate hypofunction of the gland. Such cold spots are often associated with malignant, nonsecreting thyroid tumors.[12] Ultrasonography may be utilized to distinguish between anatomic abnormalities in the thyroid gland, for example, a cyst versus a tumor.

Ultrasonography is also performed as part of parathyroid gland evaluation. Normal glands appear on the sonogram as solid masses; their echo patterns are of somewhat less amplitude than the surrounding thyroid tissue. Glandular enlargement due to tumors or hyperplasia can be detected through ultrasound evaluation of the parathyroid.[2]

Pancreatic ultrasound as well as CT scans are useful in evaluation of altered pancreatic function. Ultrasonography can reveal altered size, contour, and texture of the pancreas such as frequently occur with pancreatic tumors, cysts and pseudocysts, or pancreatitis. Similar data regarding size and shape of the pancreas can be obtained with a CT scan.

CT scans of the pituitary have almost replaced x-rays, historically used to view the sella turcica, to infer the presence of a pituitary tumor. They are also useful in adrenal evaluation. Small, hard to locate tumors of the adrenal glands such as adenomas, carcinomas, and pheochromocytomas are often discernible by CT scan.

Adrenal arteriography and adrenal vein catheterization with blood sampling are also useful in adrenal evaluation. Abnormal adrenal vasculature may be discovered in the former, suggesting adrenal adenoma, pheochromocytoma, or adrenal hyperplasia. An elevated cortisol level in blood drawn from the adrenal vein on one side strongly suggests a unilateral secreting tumor as the cause of Cushing's syndrome, while an elevated cortisol level in samples from the adrenal veins on both sides suggests bilateral adrenal hyperplasia.[2,12] Similarly, a markedly elevated level of plasma catecholamines in the blood drawn from the adrenal vein on only one side suggests a unilateral pheochromocytoma, while an elevated level in the blood from the adrenal veins on both sides suggests bilateral pheochromocytomas.[2,21]

References

1. Federman, D. (1981). General principles of endocrinology. In R. Williams (Ed.), *Williams textbook of endocrinology* (6th ed. pp. 1–14). Philadelphia: Saunders.

2. Kee, J., et al. (1984). Fundamental endocrine facts. In H. Hamilton (Ed.), *Endocrine disorders* (pp. 9–21). Springhouse, PA: Nursing 84 Books.

3. Bacchus, H. (1984). *Metabolic and endocrine emergencies* (2d ed.). Baltimore: University Park Press.

4. Ingbar, S. (1985). The thyroid gland. In J. Wilson & D. Foster (Eds.), *Williams textbook of endocrinology* (7th ed. pp. 682–815). Philadelphia: Saunders.

5. Bondy, P. (1985). Disorders of the adrenal cortex. In J. Wilson & D. Foster (Eds.), *Williams textbook of endocrinology* (7th ed. pp. 816–890). Philadelphia: Saunders.

6. Culpepper, R., et al. (1985). The posterior pituitary and water metabolism. In J. Wilson & D. Foster (Eds.), *Williams textbook of endocrinology* (7th ed. pp. 614–652). Philadelphia: Saunders.

7. Unger, R. (1985). Diabetes mellitus. In J. Wilson & D. Foster (Eds.), *Williams textbook of endocrinology* (7th ed. pp. 1018–1080). Philadelphia: Saunders.

8. Daughaday, W. (1985). The anterior pituitary. In J. Wilson & D. Foster (Eds.), *Williams textbook of endocrinology* (7th ed. pp. 568–613). Philadelphia: Saunders.

9. Liddle, G. (1981). The adrenals. In R. Williams (Ed.), *Williams textbook of endocrinology* (6th ed. pp. 249–292). Philadelphia: Saunders.

10. Fitzpatrick, T., & Haynes, H. (1983). Interpretation of alterations in the skin. In R. Petersdorf et al. (Eds.), *Harrison's principles of internal medicine* (10th ed. pp. 2249–2254). New York: McGraw-Hill.

11. Bacchus, H. (1984). *Metabolic and endocrine emergencies* (2d ed.) Baltimore: University Park Press.

12. Ingbar, S., & Woeber, K. (1983). Diseases of the thyroid. In R. Petersdorf, et al. (Eds.), *Harrison's principles of internal medicine* (10th ed. pp. 614–633). New York: McGraw-Hill.

13. Bates, B. (1974). *A guide to physical examination.* Philadelphia: Lippincott.

14. Kohler, P. (1983). Diseases of the hypothalamus and anterior pituitary. In R. Petersdorf et al. (Eds.), *Harrison's principles of internal medicine* (10th ed. pp. 587–603). New York: McGraw-Hill.

15. Williams, G., & Dluhy, R. (1983). Diseases of the

adrenal cortex. In R. Petersdorf et al. (Eds.), *Harrison's principles of internal medicine* (10th ed. pp. 634–656). New York: McGraw-Hill.

16. Ganong, W. (1985). *Review of medical physiology* (12th ed. pp. 394–420. Los Altos, CA: Lange.

17. Buross-Herlihy, J., et al. (1984). Disorders of the pituitary gland. In H. Hamilton (Ed.), *Endocrine disorders* (pp. 46–62). Springhouse, PA: Nursing 84 Books.

18. Aurbach, G., et al. (1981). Parathyroid hormone, calcitonin, and the califerols. In R. Williams (Ed.), *Williams textbook of endocrinology* (6th ed. pp. 922–1031). Philadelphia: Saunders.

19. Williams, G., & Dluhy, R. (1983). Diseases of the adrenal cortex. In R. Petersdorf, et al. (Eds.), *Harrison's principles of internal medicine* (10th ed. pp. 634–656). New York: McGraw-Hill.

20. Griffin, J. (1985). Dynamic tests of endocrine function. In J. Wilson & D. Foster (Eds.), *Williams textbook of endocrinology* (7th ed. pp. 147–154). Philadelphia: Saunders.

21. Landsberg, L., & Young, J. (1983). Pheochromocytoma. In R. Petersdorf et al. (Eds.), *Harrison's principles of internal medicine* (10th ed. pp. 657–660). New York: McGraw-Hill.

38

Diabetic Disorders and Patient Care

Beverly S. McKenna

Diabetes mellitus affects an estimated 5.5 million people in the United States. It is a chronic condition characterized by decreased insulin secretion or resistance to insulin in peripheral tissues. Common manifestations include abnormalities in carbohydrate, fat, and protein metabolism. Diabetes is not just one disease; rather, it is a genetically heterogeneous group of disorders that have in common glucose intolerance. Both genetic and environmental conditions have been implicated in the etiology of diabetes.

In 1979, five classifications for diabetes mellitus were established by the National Diabetes Data Group and endorsed by the American Diabetes Association (Table 38-1).

Type I, or insulin-dependent diabetes mellitus (IDDM), includes those disorders historically referred to as *juvenile, ketosis-prone,* or *brittle* diabetes. Those affected are typically young, lean, and dependent on exogenous insulin to prevent ketoacidosis and death. While the precise causation is unclear, pancreatic beta islet cell damage due to viral illness, toxic chemicals, or autoimmune processes have been implicated.[1] Genetic predisposition may also be involved; there is an association between type I diabetes and specific HLA antigens on chromosome 6.[1] Roughly 10 to 20 percent of all diabetic patients fall into the type I category.

Type II, or non-insulin-dependent diabetes mellitus (NIDDM), includes disorders traditionally referred to as *adult* or *maturity onset* or *ketosis-resistant* diabetes. Those affected are usually over 40 and obese and do not consistently need insulin to prevent or control hyperglycemia. Unless exposed to significant stress, such as occurs with infectious processes, type II diabetic patients are not prone to ketosis, because very small amounts of insulin will prevent ketogenesis even in the presence of hyperglycemia (see Chap. 36).

Endogenous insulin levels are abnormal in type II diabetes; in some cases they may be elevated. In addition, there is thought to be a decrease in either tissue or hepatic sensitivity to insulin, abnormal insulin binding to cell receptors, an altered number of cell receptors, or an intracellular postreceptor defect.[2] While the etiology of type II diabetes has not been precisely described, a genetic predisposition in combination with environmental factors is thought to be involved. Those with type II diabetes make up 80 to 90 percent of all diabetic persons.

Stress may contribute to the development of both type I and type II diabetes. In the presence of a physical or emotional threat, the physiologic stress response results in secretion of hormones which are counterregulatory to normal control mechanisms for carbohydrate and fat metabolism. Epinephrine, cortisol and other glucocorticoids, growth hormone, and glucagon all induce hyperglycemia and catabolism (see Chap. 36). Over time, susceptible persons may develop diabetes as a function of system exhaustion.

The three other types of diabetes mellitus include diabetes associated with other conditions or syndromes, impaired glucose tolerance, and gestational diabetes in pregnancy. Diabetes associated with other conditions and syndromes occurs in pancreatic or other endocrine disease, as well as with administration of pharmacologic agents such as phenytoin, steroids, or birth control pills, presumably because all impair glucose metabolism. Impaired glucose tolerance is a condition in which the fasting glucose fluctuates between normal and only slightly elevated (<140 mg/dL). Gestational

Table 38-1 Types of Diabetes Mellitus

New Names	Old Names	Clinical Characteristics	Diagnostic Criteria
		Clinical Categories	
Type I: insulin-dependent diabetes mellitus (IDDM)	Juvenile diabetes (JD), juvenile-onset diabetes (JOD), ketosis-prone diabetes, brittle diabetes	Patients have little or no endogenous insulin and need injections to preserve life. New patients may be of any age but are usually young; they often have islet-cell antibodies. Scientists believe causes may be genetic, environmental, or acquired, probably involving abnormal immune responses	**Diabetes Mellitus in Nonpregnant Adults:** **Either A.** Classic symptoms of diabetes—e.g., polyuria, polydipsia, ketonuria, rapid weight loss **or B.** Elevated fasting glucose on more than one occasion (mg/dL): Venous W.B.* ≥ 120 Capillary W.B. ≥ 120 **or C.** Fasting glucose less than B above, but sustained elevated glucose during the OGTT† on more than one occasion. Both the 2-h sample and some other sample taken between administration of the 75-g glucose dose and 2 h later must meet the following criteria (mg/dL): Venous W.B. ≥ 180 Capillary W.B. ≥ 200
Type II: non-insulin-dependent diabetes mellitus (NIDDM)	Adult-onset diabetes (AOD), maturity-onset diabetes (MOD), ketosis-resistant diabetes, stable diabetes, maturity-onset diabetes of youth (MODY)	Except during infection or other stress, patients rarely develop ketosis. They vary in amount of endogenous insulin and may need injections to avoid hyperglycemia. New patients may be of any age but are usually over 40. Most are obese. NIDDM is thought to be caused by genetic susceptibility plus environmental factors	**Diabetes Mellitus in Children:** **Either A.** Classic symptoms of diabetes—e.g., polyuria, polydipsia, ketonuria, rapid weight loss **or B.** In asymptomatic individuals, both an elevated fasting glucose and a sustained elevated glucose during the OGTT on more than one occasion. Both the 2-h sample and some other sample taken between administration of the glucose dose (75 g/kg ideal body weight, up to a maximum of 75 g) and 2 h later must meet the following criteria (mg/dL):
Diabetes mellitus associated with other conditions or syndromes	Secondary diabetes	These patient's diabetes is accompanied by conditions known or suspected to cause the disease, including pancreatic or hormonal disease, drug or chemical toxicity, abnormal insulin receptors, or certain genetic syndromes	Fasting: Venous W.B. ≥ 120 Capillary W.B. ≥ 120 2-Hour OGTT and an intervening value: Venous W.B. ≥ 180 Capillary W.B. ≥ 200
Impaired glucose tolerance (IGT) Type a: non-obese Type b: obese	Asymptomatic diabetes, chemical diabetes, subclinical diabetes, borderline diabetes, latent diabetes	Glucose levels are between those of normal people and diabetics. Patients have above-normal susceptibility to atherosclerotic disease. Renal and retinal complications generally do not become significant	**IGT in Nonpregnant Adults (mg/dL):** Fasting Venous W.B. ≥ 120 Capillary W.B. ≥ 120 ½-, 1-, or 1½-h OGTT: Venous W.B. ≥ 180 Capillary W.B. ≥ 200 2-Hour OGTT: Venous W.B. 120–180 Capillary W.B. 140–200

(Continued)

Table 38-1 Types of Diabetes Mellitus (Continued)

New Names	Old Names	Clinical Characteristics	Diagnostic Criteria	
		Clinical Categories		

Gestational dia-betes (GDM)	Gestational diabetes	This classification is retained for women whose diabetes begins (or is recognized) during pregnancy. They have an above-normal risk of perinatal complications. Their glucose intolerance may be transitory, but it frequently recurs	**IGT in Children (mg/dL):**
			Fasting
			    Venous W.B.
			    Capillary W.B.
			2-Hour OGTT:
			    Venous W.B.
			    Capillary W.B.
			GDM:
			Two or more of the following, after a 100-g glucose dose, must be met or exceeded:
				
				<120
				<120
				and
				>120
				>120

				Venous or Capillary W.B. (mg/dL)
			Fasting 1 h 2 h 3 h	90 170 145 125
		Statistical Risk		

Previous abnormality of glucose tolerance (prevAGT)	Latent diabetes, prediabetes	Despite a history of hyperglycemia, these patients now have normal glucose metabolism. Among them are some former obese diabetics whose weight loss has eliminated glucose intolerance	**Normal Glucose Levels in Nonpregnant Adults (mg/dL):**
			Fasting:
			    Venous W.B.
			    Capillary W.B.
			½-, 1-, or 1½-hour OGTT:
			    Venous W.B.
			    Capillary W.B.
			2-Hour OGTT:
			    Venous W.B.
			    Capillary W.B.
				
				<100
				<100
				
				<180
				<200
				
				<120
				<140

Potential abnormality of glucose tolerance (PotAGT)	Potential diabetes, prediabetes	Even though they've never had glucose intolerance, these patients are judged relatively likely to become diabetic. Included are persons with diabetic close kin or evidence of islet-cell antibodies, mothers of babies who weighed more than 9 lbs. at birth, Pima indians, and the obese	**Normal Glucose Levels in Children (mg/dL):**
			Fasting
			    Venous W.B.
			    Capillary W.B.
			2-Hour OGTT
			    Venous W.B.
			    Capillary W.B.
				
				<115
				<115
				
				<120
				<140

*W.B. = whole blood.
† OGTT = oral glucose tolerance test.
Source: Ames Division, Miles Laboratories, Inc., Elkhart, Ind; *Diabetes,* vol. 28, Dec. 1979.

diabetes is a result of the increased hormonal and glucose load associated with pregnancy. Its occurrence not only increases perinatal complications but also predisposes those affected to residual and subsequent alterations in glucose metabolism. Half the women experiencing gestational diabetes develop serious glucose intolerance within 15 years.[1]

Pathophysiology of Diabetes Mellitus

Common to all types of diabetes is either a relative or an absolute lack of insulin and therefore inability to respond to glucose stimulation. Without insulin, glucose cannot be used by cells, that is, cellular "starvation" occurs despite an elevated serum glucose. Compensatory secretion of catabolic hormones is stimulated in an attempt to meet cellular energy needs. As a result, elevations in intravascular blood sugar and hyperglycemia are aggravated and cellular starvation continues (see Chap. 36).

Systemic effects of sustained hyperglycemia reflect direct effects of persistent alterations in carbohydrate metabolism. Sustained, increased circulating levels of glucose cause sorbitol to accumulate in Schwann cells in the nervous system. The resultant myelin damage leads to the development of neuropathies.[3] Attachment of glucose to proteins in the capillary basement membranes of the eyes and kidneys leads to retinopathy and nephropathy as a result of thickening and damage to the membranes themselves. Altered carbohydrate and fat metabolism in diabetes accelerates progression of arteriosclerotic changes in both large and small vessels. Increased incidence of fatty plaques and increased prevalence of advanced lesions with calcified, ulcerated, or occluded vessels lead to arterial and cardiovascular compromise.[4]

Cardiovascular disease accounts for roughly 70 percent of deaths in the diabetic population.[5] Large and small vessel changes occur more frequently and at an earlier age in the presence of diabetes. Both type I and type II diabetes predispose to acute myocardial infarction; however, in NIDDM, only women have a higher risk. While insulin therapy in NIDDM only questionably protects against increased mortality, poor blood glucose control before and during hospitalization increases the mortality rate from acute myocardial infarction (MI).[6] Blood glucose levels above 300 mg/dL at the time of hospitalization for acute myocardial infarction have been found to be associated with a poor prognosis.[6]

In IDDM silent MIs are common. Diabetic neuropathies can block the sensation of pain; therefore cardiac ischemia and damage can occur in the absence of symptoms. In addition, coronary vessel sclerosis can lead to arrhythmias such as sinoatrial and atrioventricular blocks.[6]

Adding to the complexity, hospitalization is in itself stressful. Blood sugar may increase as a result of the physiologic response to stress. Blood glucose control is often difficult. In addition, for controlled or overcontrolled diabetic patients, hypoglycemia is a special risk. Precipitous or significant decreases in blood sugar may extend a preexisting or evolving infarct or even cause an infarct in susceptible persons.[6]

All diabetic persons are predisposed to infections. Hyperglycemia alters resistance by impairing phagocytosis and slowing granulocytic activity.[7] Gram-positive organisms (*Candida, Staphlococcus*) tend to grow better at high sugar concentrations, whereas gram-negative organisms are usually inhibited at a blood sugar greater than 400 mg/dL.[3] Gram-positive organisms may be enhanced by the uncontrolled glucose concentration in diabetic persons; the most common manifestations include urinary tract and skin infections. Fever associated with the infectious response can aggravate hyperglycemia by stimulating adrenal medullary secretion of epinephrine and adrenal cortical secretion of cortisol.[7] Not surprisingly, infections are often the precipitating events for hyperglycemic states such as nonketotic hyperglycemic hyperosmolar coma or diabetic ketoacidosis.

Insulin Therapy

The goal of insulin therapy in diabetes mellitus is to normalize metabolism, control serum glucose, and prevent ketogenesis (see Chap. 36). Hormone extracted from porcine and beef pancreatic tissue or genetically engineered synthetic human insulin preparations are utilized. Synthetic human insulin has no unique advantage over purified porcine preparations except perhaps that it is available in inexhaustible supply. Typically, insulin is administered subcutaneously or intramuscularly. Available preparations vary in onset of action, peak effect, and duration of action (Table 38-2).

Recently improved methods for self-monitoring of blood sugar have allowed utilization of small open-loop insulin pumps for the management of diabetes. Capillary blood sugar results are used to titrate delivery rates of fixed, predetermined doses of insulin. In addition, bolus doses can be administered just prior to meals.

Closed-loop systems designed to mimic normal pancreatic secretion of insulin, that is, fluctuations of secretion in response to changes in glucose levels are being used in research settings. Currently, however, these systems are too large to be suitable for home use.

Table 38-2 Time Course of Action of Insulin Preparations

Insulin Preparation	Onset of Action	Peak Action, h	Duration of Action, h	Time Hypoglycemia Is Most Likely to Occur
Short-acting				
Regular Iletin II (crystalline-zinc)	15–30 min	2–4	5–7	2–4 h after lightest meal (usually between mid morning and noon if insulin is taken before breakfast)
Actrapid	30 min	2½–5	8	
Velosulin	30 min	2–5	8	
Humilin R	30 min	2–5	8	
Intermediate-acting				
Lente	1–2 h	6–12	18–24	Before meals, 8–10 h after insulin administration (midafternoon or before evening meal if insulin is taken before breakfast)
NPH	1–2 h	6–12	18–24	
Monotard	2½ h	7–15	18–24	
Humulin N	1–2 h	6–12	14–24	
Long-acting				
Ultralente	4–6 h	18–24	32–36	18–24 h after insulin administration (between 2 A.M. and breakfast if insulin is taken before breakfast)
PZ I	6–8 h	16–24	24–36 +	

Source: Adapted from R. T. Spencer et al., *Clinical pharmacology & nursing management,* in Beyers, M. and Dudas, S. (Eds.), *The Clinical Practice of Medical-Surgical Nursing.* Boston: Little, Brown, 1984.

Pancreatic islet cell transplantations are also being performed, but with limited success. Such transplants do, however, offer hope for preventing the myriad vascular, renal, and ocular complications associated with diabetes. To date, these complications have persisted despite amelioration of many of the metabolic abnormalities associated with diabetes.[7]

Acute and critical illness in persons with insulin-dependent diabetes mellitus can significantly alter insulin requirements and result in a need to provide supplements of regular insulin. Sliding-scale doses of regular insulin are added every 4 to 6 h or more often, on the basis of blood glucose levels. Since regular insulin does not precipitate in standard intravenous solutions, supplemental regular insulin is usually administered intravenously, because absorption and circulatory uptake can be unpredictable with subcutaneous and intramuscular administration. Use of open-loop insulin pumps is usually suspended during acute illness. Once the crisis is over or alertness returns, open-loop pumps are often reinstituted.

Patients with type II diabetes mellitus who have not required insulin prior to illness may need exogenous insulin for a short time to control hyperglycemia. Purified insulins are generally used to decrease the likelihood of antibody production and development of insulin resistance in the event exogenous insulin is required at a later time. Similarly, purified insulins are used in newly diagnosed type I diabetes to prolong the so-called honeymoon period before development of antibody-induced complications associated with selected forms of exogenous insulin.[8]

Impurities in insulin preparations are thought to be responsible for the local reactions, lipodystrophy, and allergic responses that for years have plagued insulin-dependent diabetic patients. Historically, insulin preparations have contained 25 parts per million of impurities; current purified preparations contain less than 10 parts per million.[8] The purified insulins, especially porcine insulin, are considered the least immunogenic.

Diagnostic Aids

Initial diagnosis of diabetes is rarely made in the critical-care setting. Acute or critical illness, however, in a patient with either undiagnosed or known diabetes, often results in hyperglycemic emergencies and mandates frequent, accurate monitoring of the rapid and profound changes in serum glucose levels.

Blood Glucose Determination

Laboratory determinations of serum glucose are a necessity in acute and critical illness. Bedside blood glucose tests are also necessary and offer additional advantages in critical illness because they provide accurate, easy, and rapid results. Many products for such tests are available: Dextrostix, Chemstrip, and Visidex are three of the most common. All have been found to have a close correlation with laboratory values when correct technique is used. These products consist of strips, impregnated with enzymes, that change color according to the glucose content of blood obtained from a finger-stick sample. Comparison of the strips with a color chart yields value ranges for blood glucose. Meters that read the glucose reagent strip and give a numerical value are also available.

Blood glucose levels over the preceding 6 weeks to 3 months can be assessed by a laboratory test known as glycosylated hemoglobin A_1 or A_1C assay. By measuring the amount of glucose attached to hemoglobin (the major protein in erythrocytes) as a proportion of the serum concentration of glucose, the degree of serum glucose control can be objectively evaluated (see also Chap. 37). Glycosylated hemoglobin A_1 or A_1C measurements are uniquely valuable because they are unaffected by short-term blood sugar fluctuations over the preceding hours or days.[2]

Urine Testing

Variability in the renal threshold for glucosuria affects the usefulness of urine testing in acute diabetes management. Factors such as chronically increased blood sugar, increased age, and heart and renal failure are all known to increase the renal threshold for glucose excretion. Values as high as 300 mg/dL may be reflected as normal in some cases.[3] In the critically ill, urine testing is used only if blood glucose determinations are not available. In such instances only fresh urine, either from a catheter or a second-voided specimen, should be used.

Medications being taken should be considered in selecting a method of urine testing. Both false-positive and false-negative results have been recorded when ascorbic acid, acetylsalicylic acid, cephalosporins, l-dopa, and probenecid are being taken. False readings are also likely when ketone bodies and sugars other than glucose are present in the urine.[4]

There are numerous urine glucose tests on the market. Various peculiarities need to be highlighted:

Clinitest–A copper reduction test which offers results in percentages from 1 to 10. It is performed either by a five-drop or a two-drop method. The two-drop method is generally more accurate. With high levels of urine sugar, the boiling reaction must be carefully watched. A "pass-through" phenomenon may occur as the reaction rapidly progresses through all the chart colors and then just as rapidly fades.[4] The final result may be incorrectly interpreted as lower than it actually is. This pass-through should be read as greater than 5 percent if using the five-drop method or greater than 10 percent if the two-drop method is used.

Diastix–An oxidase dipstick specific for glucose. (A dipstick with an acetone test is also available; this is known as *Keto-diastix*. It is important to be aware that high urine ketones inhibit the glucose reaction and can produce a falsely low glucose reading.[4]

Chemstrip uG–A two-color oxidase dipstick. The results, in percentages, range from 0 to 5. As with Diastix, high ketone levels in the sample may produce a falsely low glucose reading.

Tes-Tape–A roll of paper impregnated with reactive material. The results are in percentages ranging from 0.1 to 2. It is important to be aware that high doses of acetylsalicylic acid or ascorbic acid can produce false-negative glucose readings. When either substance interferes with the sugar test, sugar migrates up the strip of green above a yellow area. The reading is taken from the green strip.[4]

The most valuable urine testing in the critical-care setting is for ketones. Several products are available:

Acetest–A white tablet. One drop of urine is placed on the tablet and the color change is read after 30 s. Readings for urinary ketones are classified as small, moderate, or large.

Ketostix—A dipstick. The reading must be made precisely 15 s after dipping the strip into the urine sample. Results are grouped into classifications of small, moderate, or large ketones.

Chemstrip uK—A dipstick which provides results after 2 min. The range is from negative to 3+.

Diabetic Coma

All diabetic comas are life-threatening emergencies. Reversal requires prompt and appropriate therapy. There are three types of diabetic coma: (1) hypoglycemic coma resulting from administration of excessive insulin or other hypoglycemic agents; (2) hyperglycemic coma due to ketoacidosis (diabetic ketoacidosis, DKA), which is associated with severe insulin deficiency; and (3) coma due to mild to moderate insulin deficiency, referred to as nonketotic hyperglycemic hyperosmolar coma (NHHC).

Comas in diabetes can reflect a multitude of precipitating events. Because a patient is diabetic, loss of consciousness should not automatically be attributed to a diabetic emergency. Assessment should address potential causes of coma of both diabetic and nondiabetic origin. A memory aid has been devised to help remember common possibilities:[3]

*A*lcohol

*E*pilepsy

*I*nsulin: too much or too little

*O*pium and narcotics

*U*remia

*T*rauma to the head

*I*nfection of the central nervous system

*C*ardiovascular accident

*S*hock

Hyperglycemic Ketoacidotic Coma

Coma due to diabetic ketoacidosis (DKA) is the most common type of diabetic hyperglycemic coma.

It is also the most common cause of hospitalization for diabetic patients below the age of 20: 14 percent of all diabetes-related hospital admissions are for DKA.[7] Nationally the mortality associated with DKA ranges from 2 to 18 percent; the highest mortality occurs in the elderly population.[7]

Hyperglycemic ketoacidosis most commonly occurs in type I diabetic persons who are dependent upon exogenous insulin to maintain normal glucose levels. Usually the precipitating event in diabetic ketoacidosis is infection, but trauma, surgery, nonadherence to regimen, inadequate dosage of exogenous insulin, or severe emotional stress can all precipitate DKA. Recently DKA has been seen in insulin pump users who rely solely on checks of capillary blood glucose to adjust insulin dosages. Failure to test also for the presence of circulating ketones leads to vulnerability to DKA if insulin leakage or other pump malfunction results in inadequate insulin infusion.

Pathophysiology

Diabetic ketoacidosis is a life-threatening event that is manifested by hyperglycemia, ketosis, dehydration, electrolyte imbalance, and acidosis. Survival depends on prompt recognition and rapid treatment.

The pathophysiology of DKA is outlined in Fig. 38-1. Relative or absolute deficiency of insulin precludes a normal response to glucose stimulation. Cells literally starve despite abundant serum glucose. Inability to use available glucose for the energy requirements of cellular work results in secretion of catabolic stress hormones (epinephrine, glucagon, growth hormone, glucocorticoids), which further elevate the serum glucose. Hyperglycemia escalates, and in addition, breakdown of amino acids and fats is triggered.

The rapid rate of fat breakdown and ketone excretion invariably exceed the capability of normal ketone excretory pathways. When the pathways become overloaded, ketones accumulate in the blood. With continued insufficient insulin, ketogenic and gluconeogenic metabolic pathways predominate.[7]

When the blood sugar exceeds the renal threshold, glucosuria occurs. Excess ketones are also excreted in the urine. Osmotic diuresis ensues and with it loss of sodium, potassium, and body

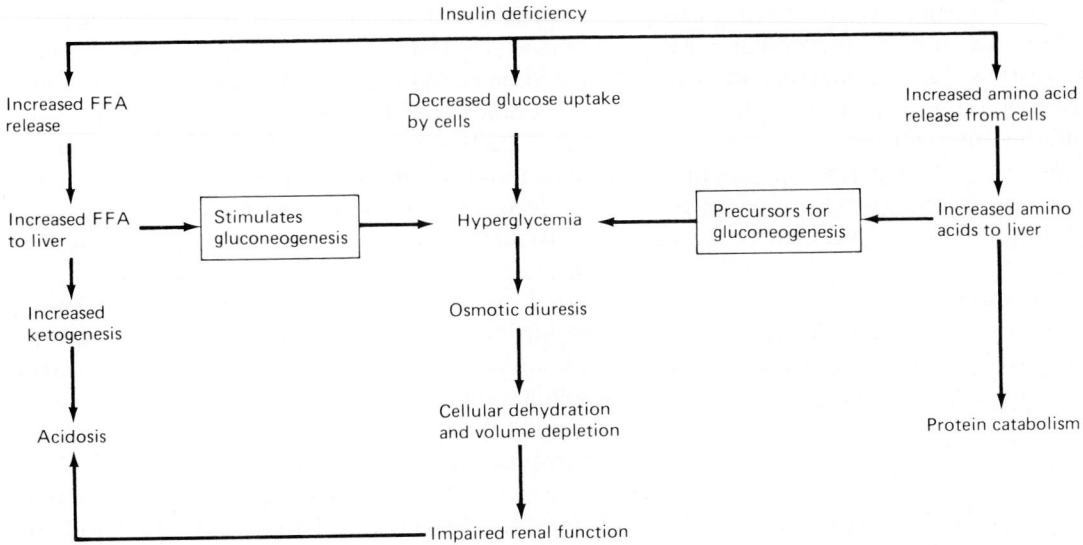

Figure 38-1   Metabolic consequences of insulin deficiency. FFA = free fatty acids. *(From Thomas G. Skillman, Diabetic ketoacidosis, Heart & Lung, 7:594–602, 1978.)*

water. Dehydration and extracellular volume depletion rapidly develop.

Adaptive mechanisms fail as DKA progresses. With high serum glucose levels, a hyperosmolar state ensues and perpetuates the existing renal loss of water and electrolytes. Intracellular dehydration and hypovolemia become pronounced. As ketones are increasingly produced, blood pH drops, resulting in a potential for profound metabolic acidosis. Respiratory compensation in the form of rapid, deep (Kussmaul) respirations attempts to rid the body of excess hydrogen ions. The breath has a characteristic "fruity" acetone odor. As the vicious circle continues, muscle weakness and decreased ventilatory ability make respiratory compensation less and less effective. With severe acidosis and pH levels below 7.0, compensation fails and respirations tend to slow. Coma and death then follow.[9]

Clinical Findings

Initial laboratory tests for suspected DKA include those for blood sugar, serum acetone, arterial blood gases, electrolytes, serum osmolality, BUN, hematocrit, WBC, urine sugar, and ketones. Typical findings include glucosuria of 2 percent, moderate to large ketones in the urine, elevated blood glucose (over 250 mg/dL, usually 250 to 800 mg/dL), varying degrees of (serum) hyperkalemia, a low arterial pH, and low CO_2 levels, indicating a depleted alkaline reserve.[9] Although the mechanism is not understood, serum amylase is also commonly elevated in DKA, and in this situation elevated amylase should not be considered an indicator of acute pancreatitis.[9]

Neurologic status can vary from alert to deep coma, depending on the progression of the ketoacidotic state. Fortunately, with general community awareness and increased patient education and monitoring, most patients are conscious when first seen. Upon admission there is typically a history of polydipsia, polyuria, weight loss, and weakness for several days.

As ketoacidosis develops, and often before urinary ketones are present, nausea and vomiting frequently occur. Severe abdominal pain can result from sodium and extracellular fluid loss. These abdominal signs are often mistakenly interpreted, with elevated WBC values, as evidence of an acute surgical abdominal condition.[3] With rehydration, abdominal pain often disappears and WBC values frequently normalize.

Dehydration and extracellular volume depletion are manifested by a flushed face, tachycardia, sustained and postural hypotension, and decreased pulse pressure. Serum hyperkalemia may be pronounced and may result in peaked T waves on the electrocardiogram. The elevation in serum potassium occurs at the expense of intracellular potassium content, as intracellular potassium ions are replaced by hydrogen ions as part of the compensatory acid-buffering mechanisms.

Because of severe dehydration, lung sounds may be clear even in the presence of severe pneumonia.[9] With rehydration, rales may be heard and infiltrate may appear in the radiographic examination. Dehydration can also cause pleuritic pain and friction rubs; both usually disappear upon rehydration.[7] In DKA, hypothermia is common. If fever is present an underlying infection should be strongly suspected.

Medical Therapy

The medical goals in the treatment of DKA are to correct acidosis, restore fluid and electrolyte balance, avoid complications, and identify and treat the precipitating cause.

Fluid replacement is a priority to avoid hypovolemic shock, the most common cause of death in DKA. Usually the fluid deficit is 4 to 6 L.[3] Initially, to rapidly replace the depleted circulating volume, isotonic saline is given at a rate of 500 to 1000 mL/h for the first 2 to 3 h; infusion rates are then slowed to 250 to 500 mL/h thereafter. In severe cases plasma and other volume expanders may also be administered. When urine flow is reestablished at a rate greater than 50 mL/h, intravenous infusion rates are generally decreased to 125 to 250 mL/h.[3]

As acidosis is corrected, serum potassium levels fall. Therefore, when admission potassium values are either low or normal, potassium phosphate is added to the initial intravenous solutions. Once urinary output is established, potassium replacement typically involves administration of 80 to 160 meq during the initial 8 to 12 h of treatment. Intracellularly, phosphate acts as a buffer in much the same way as the bicarbonate-carbonic acid system. Phosphate depletion can occur in the presence of severe or prolonged acidosis and activation of cellular buffering mechanisms. Therefore, potassium phosphate is the preparation of choice for potassium replacement. Reversal of phosphate depletion enhances buffering and facilitates oxygen transport to tissues. If phosphate is given too rapidly, however, hypocalcemia may result. Iatrogenically induced tetany has occurred.[3]

If the blood pH is 7 or less or blood bicarbonate is below 9 meq/L, 1 to 2 ampules of sodium bicarbonate (44 meq bicarbonate per ampule) may be administered in a hypotonic (45% saline) solution.[9] Bicarbonate is not, however, routinely administered in DKA because of the danger of paradoxical cerebral spinal fluid acidosis associated with too rapid correction of systemic acidosis. Bicarbonate alters the oxygen dissociation curve, that is, it increases the affinity of oxygen for hemoglobin, thus decreasing its affinity for tissues. Bicarbonate also reacts with hydrogen ions in extracellular fluid. The resultant formation of carbon dioxide, which freely penetrates the blood-brain barrier, increases the potential for progressive cerebral spinal fluid acidosis; bicarbonate cannot penetrate the blood-brain barrier.[3] Coupled with reduced cerebral blood flow, these effects may precipitate significant and paradoxical cerebral spinal fluid acidosis.[9]

Insulin therapy is essential in the treatment of DKA. Insulin corrects acidosis by decreasing hepatic gluconeogenesis and inhibiting lipolysis. It also reduces hyperosmolality by decreasing hyperglycemia and promoting peripheral cellular utilization of glucose.[3] Prior to 1982, large doses of insulin were used to treat DKA. Current evidence suggests, however, that the desired effects can be achieved by administering smaller, more frequent, or even continuous doses of insulin. Exact doses of insulin are based on body weight. A typical loading dose is approximately 10 U of regular insulin IV followed by 5 to 10 U/h by continuous infusion. Intramuscular administration usually involves a somewhat larger initial loading dose, typically 20 U, followed by 10 U/h. Such regimens usually reduce the serum glucose at a rate of about 75 to 100 mg/dL per hour.[3] Intramuscular administration has been found consistently successful provided severe circulatory decompensation is not present. In addition, IM administration has been associated with a lower incidence of precipitous drops in blood glucose and potassium levels than IV administration.[3]

Nursing Management

In the critical-care setting, nursing management of patients with diabetic ketoacidosis must be directed toward managing real and potential fluid and electrolyte imbalance; administering insulin to aid in restoration of normal carbohydrate, fat, and protein metabolism; and prompt recognition and treatment of systemic manifestations. Applicable nursing diagnoses are discussed in the following sections.

Nursing Diagnosis

Actual fluid volume deficit related to abnormal fluid loss from osmotic diuresis.

Interventions

Nursing management begins with early identification of patients at risk for actual fluid volume deficit related to abnormal fluid loss from hyperglycemia-induced osmotic diuresis. In DKA pronounced osmotic diuresis may lead to rapid development of both dehydration (intracellular fluid loss) and extracellular fluid volume depletion. All patients with a history of diabetes who are experiencing acute or critical illness are vulnerable. Those unable to perceive or respond to thirst and those being given tube feedings and parenteral hyperalimentation are even more vulnerable (see also the nursing diagnosis "Alterations in Nutrition," below).

Ongoing assessment centers on hydration status and prevention of complications. Fluid volume deficit related to abnormal fluid loss leads to signs of dehydration. Skin turgor is decreased and mucus membranes are often parched and cracked. Extreme thirst and history of rapid weight loss are typically present.

Meticulous recordings of body weight and intake and output are necessary to accurately follow trends. Postural or sustained blood pressure decreases, especially with tachycardia, may indicate impending shock, developing as a result of fluid shifts that occur in response to volume depletion.

With treatment, fluid overload may result if fluid replenishment is too rapid. Underlying cardiac compromise exaggerates these risks. Vital signs, continuous cardiac monitoring, and auscultation of the heart and lungs need to be performed frequently to guide fluid management.[7] Monitoring should include assessment of central venous pressure, preferably by indwelling catheter, and vigilance for neck vein distention, developing peripheral edema, cardiac arrhythmias, and rales.

Dehydration increases the risk of hyperviscosity, abnormalities of platelet function, and in-creased clotting factors, all of which contribute to a tendency to hypercoagulation.[7] The risk of thromboembolism can be reduced by taking action to prevent stasis of blood, e.g., assuring adequate hydration, providing antiembolic stockings, and performing range of motion exercises of extremities.

Nursing Diagnosis

Impaired gas exchange related to metabolic acidosis with compensatory respiratory alkalosis.

Interventions

Kussmaul respirations are a classic finding in DKA and represent a compensatory mechanism to rid the body of excess hydrogen ions in metabolic acidosis. The degree of acidosis can be assessed by monitoring blood pH, serum CO_2 and bicarbonate, and urine ketones. Other parameters to be regularly assessed include progression or regression of Kussmaul respirations, acetone or "fruity" breath, and level of consciousness.

Serial respiratory auscultation should be performed, with special attention to the adequacy of pulmonary excursion and the nature of breath sounds. A pulmonary friction rub may be present secondary to dehydration. As rehydration progresses, vigilance must be maintained to detect signs of rales and retained secretions. If dehydration and extracellular volume depletion have been pronounced, breath sound deterioration may accompany volume restoration. Even severe pulmonary infectious processes may not be reflected in breath sounds until fluid volume has been restored.

Nursing Diagnosis

Electrolyte imbalance related to acidosis and osmotic diuresis.

Interventions

Acidosis and osmotic diuresis precipitate potassium and phosphate imbalance in DKA. Ongoing assessments therefore must include careful monitoring of parenteral infusions and monitoring for signs of electrolyte imbalance.

Initially, serum potassium may be either normal or high, because of the combined effects of acidosis and dehydration. With treatment and rehydration, serum potassium may decrease rapidly as potassium returns to the intracellular compartment. Hyperkalemia is manifested by a weak, slow, and often thready pulse. Other findings include flaccid paralysis and flattened P waves, tented T waves, a widened QRS interval, and a prolonged PR interval on the electrocardiographic tracing.

The nursing assessment should include monitoring for hypokalemia beginning 4 to 6 h after insulin therapy has been instituted. Signs and symptoms associated with hypokalemia include muscle weakness, hypotension, anorexia, irritability, paresthesias, and electrocardiographic findings including peaked P waves, flattened T waves, and the appearance of U waves. Electrolyte imbalance in hyperglycemic states can be profound, especially potassium fluctuations. Cardiac dysrhythmias are likely, and continuous ECG monitoring is indicated.

As noted, potassium phosphate is the agent of choice for potassium replacement in DKA because of the coexisting potential for phosphate depletion. However, if phosphate infusion is too rapid, a reciprocal drop in serum calcium may result in development of symptomatic hypocalcemia. Signs and symptoms of hypocalcemia include parathesias, numbness and tingling around the mouth and in the fingers, muscle cramps, positive Chvostek and Trousseau signs, and, in severe cases, tetany and convulsions[7,10] (see also Chap. 36).

Nursing Diagnosis

Altered (decreased) nutrition, less than body requirements, related to illness, inability to use glucose normally, decreased level of consciousness, and inability to take oral supplement.

Ongoing assessment, with meticulous monitoring of caloric intake and insulin therapy, is necessary for diabetic patients experiencing acute illness. Characteristically, control of blood glucose is complex, because illness alters both nutritional needs and oral intake. If nutritional needs are met by providing either enteral or parenteral supplements, special attention is needed to prevent acute complications of diabetes. The high glucose load in these solutions not only increases the risk of hyperglycemia and ketosis but also may result in a marked increase in serum osmolality, osmotic diuresis, dehydration, and extracellular fluid depletion. Insulin dosages need adjustment in patients with type I diabetes. Insulin must often be initiated

for patients with type II diabetes receiving enteral or parenteral feedings.

Interventions

Nursing interventions should include at least hourly bedside blood sugar monitoring, urine ketone testing, and assessment of the effectiveness of insulin. Glucose-containing solutions are utilized when the blood sugar decreases to the 250 to 300 mg/dL range. At that point, the nursing assessment should specifically include observation for signs and symptoms of hypoglycemia (see "Hypoglycemic Coma," below).

When patients regain alertness and bowel tones return, oral intake is resumed. Clear liquids are provided for the first 8 to 12 h, followed by gradual initiation of solid foods. Approximately 12 h after the ability to tolerate solid food has been assured, intermediate insulin preparations are begun. Regular insulin is then used for supplemental coverage. Observations for hypoglycemia should be based on knowledge of the peak and duration of action of the insulin preparation being used.

Insulin resistance, although not common, can occur. If the blood glucose is not decreasing despite increasingly large doses of insulin, resistance may be responsible. Often, however, insulin resistance is suspected when the basis for difficulty in controlling the blood glucose is uneven delivery of intravenous doses due to adherence of insulin to intravenous solution containers and tubing. As much as 20 percent of the insulin dosage can be compromised in such situations. A nursing intervention to minimize insulin loss includes infusing 25 to 50 mL of IV solution containing at least 25 U of insulin through the tubing before starting the continuous infusion. Because of the tendency of insulin to gravitate to both glass and plastic in solution containers, solutions should be rotated hourly. If true insulin resistance is found to be present, glucocorticords may be ordered to limit antibody reaction.[3]

Nursing Diagnosis

Potential for impaired bowel evacuation related to hypokalemia.

Interventions

Hypokalemia-induced paralytic ileus often accompanies DKA.[11] The nursing assessment therefore should focus on intestinal motility. Bowel sounds should be auscultated at least every 2 h. In the presence of coma with gastric distention or vomiting, a nasogastric tube should be placed. Patients should be given nothing by mouth until nausea has subsided and bowel sounds have returned.

Nursing Diagnosis
Potential for infection related to diabetes.

Interventions
Nursing interventions focus on prevention and/or treatment of infections. Diabetic patients commonly have underlying neuropathies and peripheral vascular compromise. Local infections may progress with few or no symptoms. Peripheral vascular compromise also increases risk of breakdown of tissue and slows healing once tissue disruption occurs. When this is present, documentation of wound assessment should include presence of erythema, fluctuation of margins, drainage, and odor. Monitoring for signs and symptoms of systemic sepsis should be continuous. Initially, an increase in white blood cells may be due to a dehydrated state caused by increased adrenocortical activity and is usually an unreliable index for the presence of infection. Infections are a major cause of mortality and morbidity for the diabetic patient. If not prevented, they must be carefully monitored once they occur.

Nursing Diagnosis
Alterations in thought processes related to acidosis and dehydration.

Interventions
As discussed under "Medical Therapy," excessive use of sodium bicarbonate to correct extracellular fluid acidosis in DKA may paradoxically increase the spinal fluid acidosis and exaggerate existing alterations in level of consciousness. Bicarbonate also shifts the oxygen dissociation curve and therefore limits oxygen availability to tissues. Thus, in addition to administration of prescribed oxygen therapy, monitoring for signs of cyanosis is important. Similarly, increasing lethargy after treatment with bicarbonate should prompt investigation.

Cerebral edema can occur, especially in younger patients, when restoration of blood sugar or pH to normal is too rapid. Cerebral edema,

which is detected by frequent monitoring of level of consciousness, should be suspected whenever deterioration of consciousness occurs *after* treatment has been initiated.

Acidosis and dehydration may impair learning and concentration skills for 48 to 72 h after a DKA crisis. Ability to concentrate, follow instructions, or engage in conversation must be monitored to assess learning readiness. Until mental recovery occurs, patient teaching should be postponed. Typically, extensive teaching is done after transfer from the critical-care unit.

When patients are discharged from the critical-care unit, the transfer summary should include information regarding the duration of diabetes, usual management, concurrent illnesses, history of the crisis event, how the patient recognized and responded to the impending crisis, and identification of family members or significant others who are available to assist with care during hospitalization and at home.

Patient Goals and Desired Outcomes
The treatment plan is successful if fluid intake approximates output and body weight returns to normal. Additionally, laboratory findings for serum glucose, electrolytes and acid/base balance will be within normal limits. Maintenance of oral nutritional intake to meet metabolic requirements will be reestablished, and gastrointestinal motility will return to normal. The patient will be awake and alert, and symptoms of impaired thought processes will be relieved.

Hypoglycemic Coma
The most common of all diabetic comas is hypoglycemic coma. While it most frequently affects patients with type I or type II diabetes, it may occur in patients with any form of diabetes. Hypoglycemia is usually associated with a drop in blood glucose level to less than 50 mg/dL. It occurs when the diet-exercise-medication balance is disrupted, as when there is too little food, too much exercise, or too much medication.[2] The symptoms come on suddenly and if left untreated result in coma.

Pathophysiology
Hypoglycemia, also known as *insulin shock,* occurs when inadequate supplies of circulating glucose

are available to meet tissue glucose demands. Insufficient levels of glucose stimulate the physiologic stress response and activate the sympathetic nervous system. In hypoglycemia, the physiologic stress response and sympathetic activation are compensatory. Epinephrine secretion results in hepatic gluconeogenesis. Glucocorticoid secretion (primarily cortisol) and growth hormone secretion also elevate blood glucose. These responses occur not only in absolute hypoglycemia (blood glucose levels at 50 mg/dL or less), but also when there is a rapid drop in blood sugar even with serum glucose levels greater than those typically associated with hypoglycemia.

Not uncommonly, hypoglycemia occurs because administered doses of insulin or oral hypoglycemic agents are too high relative to caloric intake. Skipping meals, weight loss programs, or increased exercise or exertion shortly after a dose of insulin may result in hypoglycemia. Altered tissue absorption of insulin may also precipitate hypoglycemia, as may renal disease and completion or termination of pregnancy.[5]

Symptoms of hypoglycemia are variable from person to person, but each person usually experiences the same one or two symptoms with each episode. In elderly persons, hypoglycemic symptoms are typically more pronounced and occur at higher blood glucose levels than in the young.

Hypoglycemia in patients taking oral hypoglycemic agents is usually severe and prolonged because these agents characteristically have a long half-life.[2] Patients who take insulin or oral hypoglycemic agents may precipitate hypoglycemia by ingesting alcohol and blocking gluconeogenesis. Frequently, people with uncoordinated behavior and mental deterioration are mistakenly thought to be intoxicated, and treatment may be dangerously

delayed until the onset of frank coma. Similarly, hypoglycemia may be missed in patients with autonomic neuropathy or those taking beta-blocking drugs (e.g., propranolol). In both situations, the adrenergic response to hypoglycemia is prevented and diagnosis depends on recognition of the cerebral signs and symptoms (blurred vision, confusion, headache, nervousness) of hypoglycemia.[8]

Nocturnal hypoglycemic episodes are thought to be involved in a phenomenom known as the *Somogyi effect*. In this phenomenon glycosuria, sometimes accompanied by mild ketonuria, is present in the morning. It is thought that during the night, brief and relatively asymptomatic periods of hypoglycemia stimulate compensatory secretion of epinephrine, glucocorticoids, glucagon, and growth hormone[12] (see Fig. 38-2). The subject may be unaware of hypoglycemic episodes, but if asked, will commonly report sleep disturbances, fatigue, and headache. Urine ketones may be present and morning blood glucose levels may be quite high as a result of catabolic hormone secretion. Typically, this rebound lasts for 12 to 72 h. Treatment with higher doses of insulin only aggravates the problem by increasing both the likelihood and the severity of nocturnal hypoglycemic episodes. Treatment therefore more commonly involves decreasing the insulin dose and adding additional protein to the diet, typically in a nighttime snack.

The Somogyi effect is more likely to occur during acute illness, because illness is associated with more, and more frequent, fluctuations in insulin needs. Surgery, renal insufficiency, and enhanced sensitivity to insulin following pregnancy also increase susceptibility to the Somogyi effect.

Another form of morning hyperglycemia, and one which is often confused with the Somogyi effect, is known as the *dawn phenomenon*. This

Figure 38-2 The Somogyi phenomenon. Hypoglycemia triggers release of stress hormones (epinephrine, glucagon, cortisol, and growth hormone). These hormones increase blood glucose, causing hyperglycemia. If hyperglycemia brings about an increase in insulin, the result again is hypoglycemia.

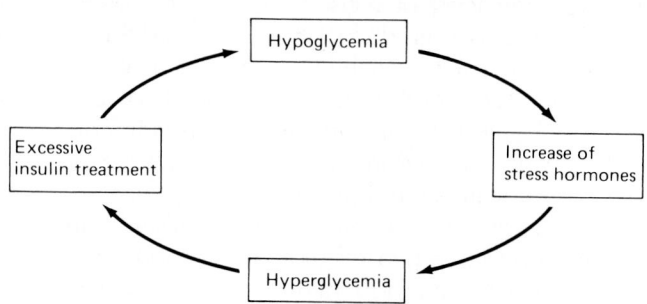

phenomenon occurs in both type I and type II diabetes.[13] In contrast to the Somogyi effect, the dawn phenomenon involves an abrupt increase in plasma glucose (and thus insulin requirements) between 5 A.M. and 9 A.M. without a preceding hypoglycemic episode. It is thought that hyperglycemia in the dawn phenomenon is due to accelerated insulin clearance, increased tissue sensitivity to insulin and to nocturnal surges of growth hormone, or the diurnal early morning surge of cortisol[3] (see also Chap. 36.) Increasing the morning dosage of insulin to treat the dawn phenomenon increases the chance of hypoglycemia during the day. Instead, doses of intermediate-acting insulin are either added or increased in the evening. In this way, nocturnal glycemic instability can be avoided.[3]

In the presence of early morning hyperglycemia, differentiation between the Somogyi effect and the dawn phenomenon may be difficult. To differentiate them, before-meal and 3 A.M. blood glucose levels must be measured on several successive days.

Clinical Findings

The brain relies on readily available glucose for fuel, whereas the peripheral tissues can utilize other energy sources.[3] Thus, many of the symptoms of hypoglycemia reflect cerebral cellular malfunction. Without adequate glucose, CNS changes include headache, dizziness, blurred vision or diplopia, mental confusion, personality changes, irritability, seizures, and a decreasing level of consciousness.[3] Other clinical findings in hypoglycemia reflect the effect of catecholamines. Initially, symptoms include tachycardia, anxiety, trembling, and diaphoresis. Patients typically describe feeling shaky, hungry, cold and clammy, and nervous. Often numbness and tingling in and around the lips and finger tips are also described. If adequate blood glucose levels are not rapidly restored, the severity of the symptoms increases. Catecholamine-induced vasoconstriction can lead to angina pectoris, premature ventricular ectopic beats, myocardial ischemia, and even infarction in patients with preexisting coronary compromise.

Medical Therapy

The aim of treatment in hypoglycemic states is to restore the plasma glucose to normal. If the patient is conscious, immediate ingestion of a rapidly absorbed form of glucose-containing food or liquid is needed. Examples include Lifesavers (eight or more), orange juice (6 to 8 oz), raisins (3 tablespoons), or a sugar-containing soft drink (one 12-oz can).

Glucagon 0.5 to 2 mg IM may be given and repeated 20 min later if there is no response to the first injection.[3] In patients prone to hypoglycemic reactions, family members may be taught to administer glucagon to increase glycogenolysis and increase circulating glucose levels.

If hypoglycemia is suspected in the acute care setting, blood samples for glucose determination are immediately obtained. Treatment is initiated, however, without waiting for results. An ampule of 50% glucose is administered by intravenous push. A continuous infusion of 50% glucose is then administered until consciousness returns or the blood glucose level is more than 200 mg/dL. Occasionally, even after vigorous glucose administration and elevation of blood sugar levels to 200 mg/dL or more, consciousness does not return. In such instances severe or prolonged hypoglycemia may have resulted in cerebral damage; neurologic compromise may persist for extended periods and may even be permanent.[3] Typically, patients can be rapidly stabilized unless the hypoglycemia is complicated by cardiovascular, renal, or liver disease.

Nursing Management

Nursing intervention for patients experiencing hypoglycemia focuses on administering substances to elevate the plasma glucose and educating both patients and families regarding prevention and treatment. Applicable nursing diagnoses and interventions in hypoglycemia are discussed below.

Nursing Diagnosis

Altered nutrition (less than requirements) related to too much insulin, increased exercise, illness, and/or skipped or delayed meals.

Nursing assessment centers on the manifestations of an acute insufficiency in the level of circulating blood glucose. Alterations in CNS function may be manifested as a decreasing level of consciousness with confusion, stupor, or frank coma. Seizures may occur, and headache, irritability, diplopia, and personality changes are common.

Cardiovascular findings include tachycardia with peripheral vasoconstriction due to the stress response–induced surge in catecholamine secretion. In patients with a history of myocardial compromise, continuous electrocardiographic monitoring is indicated, because both angina and premature ventricular contractions may occur during hypoglycemic events. The burst of catecholamines is also thought to be the basis for complaints of shakiness, hunger, nervousness, trembling, and the typical cold, clammy diaphoresis.

Interventions

Nursing interventions focus on obtaining a blood sample and immediately administering glucose supplements. Typically, supplements are provided until preevent consciousness returns or blood glucose exceeds 200 mg/dL. Whether supplements are provided orally or intravenously, frequent and serial bedside blood sugar finger tests should be performed to monitor patient response to therapy.

If blood glucose exceeds 200 mg/dL but preevent level of consciousness does not return, there may be residual neurologic compromise. Nursing interventions in such instances should include frequent serial neurologic assessments and specific evaluation to assure adequacy of basic protective reflexes, including the gag, swallow, and cough reflexes. If these responses are compromised, measures must be instituted to protect the airway. Seizure precautions should also be instituted (see also Chap. 35).

Nursing Diagnosis

Knowledge deficit related to prevention and treatment of hypoglycemia.

Over 50 percent of diabetic patients fail to follow their prescribed diet. Lack of education regarding needed alterations in nutritional intake or insulin dose in the presence of lifestyle changes is common, as is lack of knowledge regarding the medical and dietary goals of treatment.

Dietary approaches differ for type I and type II diabetes. Hypoglycemia is more common in the insulin-dependent diabetic population. Patients with type I diabetes must ingest calories at times that correspond to the onset and duration of action associated with the particular agent(s) involved in their individual regime. Those with type I diabetes

thus need consistency in intake of carbohydrates, protein, and fat. They are encouraged to eat meals and snacks at regular times. Increased food intake is prescribed before unusual exercise.

In contrast, for those with non-insulin-dependent diabetes (type II), the diet is designed to achieve and maintain ideal body weight. Snacks, especially at night, are discouraged. A decrease in calories is known to protect or improve the function of beta cells. Where indicated, weight loss is beneficial, because the number of insulin-binding receptors on the target cells increases in relation to overall cell size; thus more efficient entry utilization of glucose is promoted.[14]

Interventions

Nursing interventions begin with ensuring that the patient understands clearly the prescribed diabetic diet. Reinforcement of dietary goals is needed. Similarly, education is needed to facilitate establishment of appropriate dietary patterns while maintaining individual preferences. A dietary consultation is indicated especially if economic, social, or ethnic factors are extensively linked to dietary practices. Education may also be necessary to assure that ongoing monitoring of blood glucose is accurate. Since patients commonly experience the same one or two symptoms with the onset of hypoglycemia, bedside blood sugar finger tests should be utilized to identify the glucose levels at which symptoms first appear. In this way patients can be assisted to recognize early the development of hypoglycemia and will be better able to intervene rapidly to prevent severe incidents.

At the point of transfer from the critical-care unit, information regarding the patient's understanding of applicable medical and dietary goals, methods of monitoring blood glucose, and recognition of early signs and symptoms of hypoglycemia needs to be conveyed to nursing staff who will be providing care. Similarly, the presence of sensory deficits that impair the patient's ability to comply with treatment requirements needs to be reviewed. Finally, support systems need to be reviewed with nursing staff who will be working with the patient. Involvement of family and significant others in patient education can strengthen the foundation of the teaching plan to prevent recurrence of hypoglycemia.

Patient Goals and Desired Outcomes

The treatment plan is successful if blood glucose returns to normal limits, the patient demonstrates knowledge of the symptoms of evolving hypoglycemia and is able to describe appropriate responses, dietary strategies are understood and practiced, and a plan is devised to ensure that the treatment regimen fits into the patient's lifestyle.

Nonketotic Hyperglycemic Hyperosmolar Coma

Nonketotic hyperglycemic hyperosmolar coma (NHHC) most commonly occurs in older patients with type II diabetes. It may, however, also occur in undiagnosed diabetes. It occurs with equal frequency in men and women and about one-sixth as often as diabetic ketoacidosis. It is life-threatening and is associated with a mortality rate of over 50 percent, no doubt at least in part because its onset characteristically includes extended periods of uncontrolled hyperglycemia. Thus physiologic crisis often exists before medical help is sought.

Pathophysiology

NHHC is characterized by marked hyperglycemia without significant ketosis and by severe dehydration, hyperosmolality, and alteration in level of consciousness.[15] The pathophysiology of NHHC is outlined in Fig. 38-3. A precipitating event combined with a decreased insulin reserve almost always initiates it. The event may be ingestion of a hyperglycemia-inducing agent (hyperalimentation, insulin-inhibiting drugs), acute exacerbation of chronic disease (typically renal or cardiovascular), or anything that provokes a stress response. The hyperglycemia that occurs is potentiated by a decreased insulin reserve and stress-induced catecholamine and glucocorticoid secretion.[15] Inability to produce enough insulin to assure transport of glucose into cells becomes pronounced, and blood glucose continues to rise. Decreased hepatocellular glucose utilization leads to increased glycogenolysis and gluconeogenesis. Endogenous hepatic glucose production can supply up to 1000 g a day.[11]

Hyperglycemia is more pronounced in NHHC than in diabetic ketoacidosis. Values are typically between 600 and 2500 mg/dL. As many as 85 percent of patients with NHHC have been found to have renal insufficiency, with renal thresholds for glucose excretion higher than normal.[11] The elevated renal threshold may partly explain the marked hyperglycemia commonly seen in NHHC at the point when treatment is sought. When glucosuria occurs, pronounced osmotic diuresis is initiated. Significant depletion of free water and electrolytes soon follows.

Severe dehydration, characterized by a 15 to 25 percent depletion of body water, leads to hemoconcentration.[11] Extracellular fluid depletion becomes pronounced, and with it renal perfusion decreases and prerenal azotemia develops. Blood glucose levels rise further as a function of decreased urinary glucose excretion.

Normally, elevations in plasma osmolality lead to posterior pituitary secretion of antidiuretic hormone (ADH) and maximal water retention. In NHHC, however, glucose-induced hyperosmolality in the distal and collecting tubules counteracts the ADH effect in the kidneys and water balance can no longer be maintained (see Chap. 36, also "Diabetes Insipidus" in Chap. 39).

The initial hyponatremia reflects the effects of the high-flow urinary state, urinary sodium losses, and dilution of serum sodium as a result of water shifts from the intracellular to the extracellular compartment. Over time, however, water loss exceeds sodium loss and hypernatremia develops. The combination of hypernatremia and hyperglycemia dramatically increases plasma osmolality. In NHHC, the osmolality frequently exceeds 350 mosm/kg.[2]

Decreased renal perfusion stimulates aldosterone secretion by the adrenal cortex (see Chap. 36). Sodium is maximally reabsorbed. Because sodium is reabsorbed in exchange for potassium, depletion of total body potassium becomes pronounced.

In contrast to DKA, NHHC is characterized by absence of significant ketosis. It has been suggested that although available insulin is inadequate to control blood glucose, it is sufficient to prevent or inhibit lipolysis. The ability of insulin to inhibit lipolysis is believed to be 10 times greater than its ability to promote glucose uptake.[10] It has also been suggested that a defect in hepatic ketogenesis or possibly a circulating antiketogenic substance may be present in NHHC.[3]

Figure 38-3 Pathophysiology of nonketotic hyperglycemic hyperosmolar coma. *(Adapted from Grace[15])*

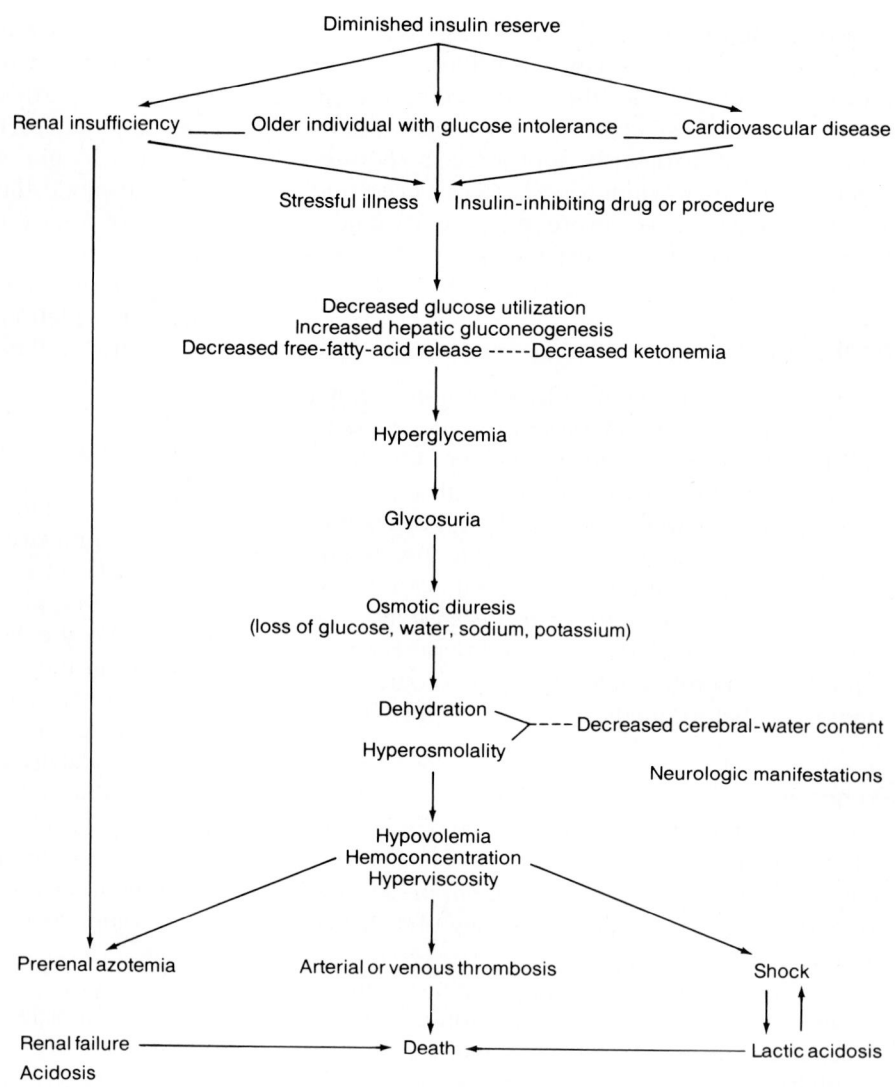

The characteristics of the types of diabetic coma are compared in Table 38-3; it is often difficult to differentiate between them.

Clinical Findings

The onset of NHHC is insidious, developing typically over a period of days or weeks. Usually symptoms include polyuria, polydipsia, weight loss, fever, tachycardia, dry mucous membranes, poor skin turgor, shallow respirations, soft eyeballs, and deterioration in mental status.[11,15] All patients develop some disturbance in consciousness, manifestations ranging from lethargy to frank coma. Reduced intake of fluid is common, especially in elderly, bedridden patients. Obtundation, impaired sense of thirst or inaccessibility to fluids, and gastrointestinal upset are also typical.

Abnormal neurologic findings are common. NHHC is often mistaken for a cerebrovascular accident.[15] Approximately 25 percent of patients with NHHC experience some form of seizure, usually of a focal motor type. These seizures commonly disappear with hydration.[15] Sensory deficits and/or hemiparesis may also occur.

Medical Therapy

The medical goals of treatment for NHHC are to correct fluid and electrolyte imbalance, normalize

Table 38-3 Characteristics of Diabetic Comas

	DKA	NHHC	Hypoglycemia
General	Acidotic, dehydrated, rarely comatose	Dehydrated, not acidotic, frequently comatose	Hydrated, not acidotic, frequently comatose
Age	Younger persons	Usually elderly	All ages
Type of diabetes	Type I	Type II	Types I and II
Precipitating events	Infection, stress	Infection, steroids, diuretics	Exercise without increased food, decreased food intake, too much insulin, drugs
Laboratory tests			
Blood sugar, mg/dL	<800	>800	<50 mg/dL
Plasma ketones	Present	Absent	Absent
Serum potassium	Normal or high	Normal or low	Normal
Serum bicarbonate, meq	<10	>16	Normal
Blood pH	<7.35	Normal	Normal
Serum osmolality, mosm/kg	<300	>350	Normal
Dehydration	Variable (total body water loss 5–15%)	Severe (total body water loss 15–25%)	Normal
Symptoms at onset Nutrition	Extreme thirst, weight loss, polyuria	Extreme thirst, weakness, polyuria	Hunger
GI system and skin	Abdominal discomfort		Diaphoresis, skin cool
Neurologic system	Drowsiness or lethargy		Impaired vision, nervous and shaky
Usual preventing symptoms Respiration	Kussmaul, acetone breath	Normal	Normal
CV system	Blood pressure normal, tachycardia, hypothermia	BP normal, tachycardia, hyperthermia	BP normal, tachycardia, hypothermia
	ECG changes with elevated serum potassium	ECG changes with lowered serum potassium	
GI system	Nausea and vomiting		
Skin	Hot flushed dry skin, parched mucous membranes	Normal; parched mucous memberanes	Diaphoretic; normal mucous membranes
Neurologic system	Headache, drowsiness, lethargy, coma	Coma (30%), impaired consciousness (50%), aphasia, hemisensory defect, seizures, hemiparesis, + Babinksi	Headache, irritability, personality change, numbness or tingling of lips or fingertips, slurred speech, staggering gait
Prodromal time	One day	Several days	Minutes to hours
Mortality	Rare, 1–10%	20–50%	? Rare

Source: Adapted from G. P. Kozak and A. R. Rolla, Diabetic comas, in Kozak.[3]

metabolism, and identify and treat the precipitating cause(s). Fluid and electrolyte replacement is a high priority. Usually, half the estimated water deficit is replaced during the first 12 h, with the remainder supplied over the next 24 h.[15] Both hypotonic and isotonic fluids are utilized and are titrated according to central venous or other hemodynamic parameters.[15] Potassium is added to infusions on the basis of serum values. In patients with preexisting cardiovascular or renal compromise, somewhat slower fluid replacement is necessary to avoid overload and cardiac decompensation.

Despite the fact that hyperglycemia tends to be far more pronounced in NHHC, insulin is administered in somewhat smaller amounts than in DKA. In NHHC patients usually secrete some endogenous insulin and may be very sensitive to exogenous doses. When the blood glucose falls to 250 or 300 mg/dL and osmolality decreases to roughly 310 mosm/kg, glucose-containing infusions are initiated to decrease the chance of treatment-induced hypoglycemia.

Dehydration and hemoconcentration in NHHC increase the potential for arterial or venous thrombosis. Early prophylactic heparin therapy may be instituted.

After an NHHC crisis, many patients can be controlled with oral medication or diet alone. Recurrences however, are not uncommon, especially in those with significant impairment of renal function. Proper education regarding diet, medications, and procedures for periodic home checks of blood glucose are needed to help prevent recurrence.

Nursing Management

In the critical-care setting, nursing interventions involved in providing care for patients with non-ketotic hyperglycemic hyperosmolar coma must be directed toward management of dehydration, hyperglycemia, and altered central nervous system function. Frequent multisystem assessments must include special emphasis on cardiac, respiratory, renal, neurologic, and gastrointestinal function.

Most of the applicable nursing diagnoses in NHHC are the same as those in DKA. Three additional diagnoses and their related interventions are discussed in the following paragraphs.

Nursing Diagnosis

Actual fluid volume deficit related to osmotic diuresis.

Patients at risk for actual fluid volume deficit related to osmotic diuresis in NHHC include older adults with type II non-insulin-dependent diabetes and those with underlying cardiac and/or renal insufficiency.

Interventions

As in DKA, ongoing assessment in NHHC centers on hydration and prevention of complications (see also "Nursing Management" in section on DKA). Special attention must be directed, however, to the cardiac and renal systems. Renal assessment includes careful monitoring of intake and output and serum creatinine levels. With increasing age and microvascular changes, the renal threshold may be raised and the kidney may not filter excess glucose, thus making urine tests for sugar invalid. The kidney's ability to degrade insulin may result in a decreased requirement for insulin.

Often it is the older adult with underlying cardiac insufficiency who experiences NHHC. The underlying cardiac compromise increases the risk of overload with fluid replenishment. Frequent monitoring of vital signs and auscultation of the heart and lungs, as well as continuous cardiac monitoring, are needed to guide fluid management (see also "Nursing Management" in section on DKA).

Nursing Diagnosis

Potential for injury related to seizure or coma.

Seizures, usually focal, occur in about 25 percent of patients with NHHC. Their pathogenesis remains uncertain, but focal organic cerebral lesions have been found on x-ray and on postmortem examination. The fluid, electrolyte, and metabolic abnormalities involved in NHHC are thought to enhance seizure activity in these lesions. With treatment and return of normal osmolality, seizures tend to resolve.[15] If NHHC recurs, seizures often also recur.

Interventions

Nursing interventions include frequent serial neurologic assessment. Seizure precautions are instituted. Anticonvulsive drugs are commonly not used, because such agents are generally ineffective in NHHC and because of concern regarding inhibition of insulin release and potential for worsening the patient's condition, particularly with the use of phenytoin (Dilantin).[15]

Nursing Diagnosis

Knowledge deficit related to health maintenance and prevention of NHHC.

Interventions

Impaired learning ability from dehydration coupled with the shortness of the stay in the critical-care unit dictates that extensive teaching be postponed until the patient has been transferred from the critical-care unit. At that time the transfer summary should include information regarding the duration of the patient's disease, management of the diabetes, concurrent illnesses, history of the crisis event (including how the patient recognized it and responded), and a description of family and social support systems.

Patient Goals and Desired Outcomes

The treatment plan is successful if fluid intake approximates output and vital signs are maintained within the patient's normal range, laboratory findings for blood glucose and electrolytes return to normal, and the patient demonstrates a knowledge base adequate for self-care.

References

1. Guthrie, D., & Guthrie, R. (1983). The disease process of diabetes mellitus. *Nursing Clinics of North America, 18*(4), 617–631.

2. Rifkin, H. (Ed.). (1984). *The physician's guide to type II diabetes (NIDDM): diagnoses and treatment.* New York: American Diabetes Association.

3. Kozak, G. (Ed.). (1984). *Clinical diabetes mellitus.* Philadelphia: Saunders.

4. Guthrie, D., & Guthrie, R. (1982). *Nursing management of diabetes mellitus.* St. Louis: Mosby.

5. Beyers, M., & Dudas, S. (1984). *The clinical practice of medical-surgical nursing.* Boston: Little, Brown.

6. Rytter, L. (1985). Prevalence and mortality of acute MI in patients with DM. *Diabetes Care 8*(3), 230–234.

7. Ellenberg, M., & Rifkin, H. (Eds.). (1983). *Diabetes mellitus—Theory and practice.* New York: Medical Examination Publishing.

8. Price, M. (1983). Insulin and oral hypoglycemia agents. *Nursing Clinics of North America, 18*(4), 687–705.

9. Karam, J. (1985). Diabetes mellitus, hypoglycemia and lipoprotein disorders. In M. A. Krupp & M. J. Chatton (Eds.), *Current medical diagnoses and treatment.* Los Altos, CA: Lange.

10. Stroot, V., Lee, C., & Schaper, C. (1982). *Fluid and electrolyte: A practical approach.* Philadelphia: Davis.

11. Kenner, C., Guzzetta, C., & Montgomery-Dossey, B. (1985). *Critical care nursing—body-mind-spirit.* Boston: Little, Brown.

12. Hite, A., & Humphrey, J. (1984). How to spot the vicious cycle of insulin rebound. *RN*, pp. 46–47.

13. Bolli, G., & Gerich, J. (1984). The dawn phenomenon—a common occurrence in both non-insulin dependent and insulin dependent diabetes mellitus. *New England Journal of Medicine, 310* (12), 746–749.

14. Heins, J. (1983). Dietary management in diabetes mellitus. *Nursing Clinics of North America, 18*(4), 631–643.

15. Grace, T. (1985). Hyperosmolar non-ketotic diabetic coma. *American Family Practitioner, 32*(2), 119–125.

39

Endocrine Crises and Patient Care

Sarah J. Sanford

Endocrine crises, while rare, are frequently dramatic. When they occur, either as primary pathologic events or in conjunction with other critical illnesses, prompt recognition and intervention is vital to assure optimal patient outcomes.

In this chapter, seven conditions are discussed: diabetes insipidus, syndrome of inappropriate antidiuretic hormone secretion, hyperthyroid or thyrotoxic crisis, hypothyroid crisis or myxedema coma, hypoparathyroidism, acute adrenal insufficiency (Addison's disease), and pheochromocytoma. Pathophysiology, medical therapies, and nursing diagnoses and interventions are discussed for each condition. While some background anatomy and physiology and specific data acquisition information are integrated into the discussion of each condition, the reader is also referred to Chaps. 36 and 37.

Diabetes Insipidus

Diabetes insipidus (DI) is characterized by insufficient antidiuretic hormone (ADH, vasopressin). Normally, ADH secretion is dictated by the hypothalamus. There, receptor cells known as *osmoreceptors* alter impulse generation to the posterior pituitary in response to changes in body tonicity or osmolality. In the presence of increased tonicity, or hyperosmolality, osmoreceptors shrink as intracellular water shifts out of the cell to the (abnormally) hypertonic interstitium. Impulses generated by osmoreceptors shrinkage lead to release of ADH from the posterior pituitary. ADH then results in maximal free water retention, low volumes of highly concentrated urine, and a decrease in plasma osmolality.[1]

Not uncommonly, insufficiency of ADH is neurogenic in origin. Errant sensing of water overload may occur in cerebral inflammatory conditions and cerebral edema. Direct damage to the hypothalamus, the hypothalamic-hypophyseal tract, or the posterior pituitary may also produce DI, as may acute traumatic head injury, craniotomy, cerebral infarct, and metastatic or sarcoid lesions.[2]

Diabetes insipidus may also be nephrogenic in origin. In contrast to neurogenic DI, nephrogenic DI may result from decreased renal responsiveness to ADH, with no alteration in synthesis or release of the hormone per se.

Pharmacologically induced DI also occurs. Lithium and demeclocycline decrease renal responsiveness to ADH, while phenytoin inhibits ADH secretion.

Clinically, DI presents with polyuria. There is excessive loss of large volumes of hypotonic, dilute urine. Volumes approaching 10 to 12 L per day are not uncommon. The excessive urinary free water loss depletes total body water and sets the stage for dramatic potential increases in body osmolality. Fortunately, in the presence of an adequate thirst mechanism and ability to obtain and ingest fluids, the likelihood of significant fluid imbalance is small, although thirst, polydipsia, and nocturia are nonetheless significant and distressing.

Permanent severe polyuria is rare. In order for it to occur, 85 percent of the posterior pituitary secretory capacity must be lost. More commonly, DI is a result of surgery or injury to the hypothalamus or pituitary, and polyuria characteristically lasts for 1 to 5 or 6 days.[3]

Patients who are unable to respond to thirst or for whom perception of thirst is diminished, face significant vulnerability to dangerous and potentially lethal hyperosmolality in the presence of DI. Depressed levels of consciousness are frequent in patients unable to perceive or respond to thirst. In such patients, tube feedings or parenteral hyperalimentation may be instituted to meet nutritional needs. Unfortunately, these interventions can potentiate the existing risk of severe water deficit resulting from insufficient ADH, because many of the solutions used are extremely hypertonic (see "Nursing Management," below).

Medical Therapies

The medical goal in treatment of DI is maintenance of normal water balance and osmolality. Fluid and hormonal replacement therapy are the mainstays of medical treatment. Fluid therapy usually involves intravenous infusions of hypotonic solutions at volumes titrated to match urinary output. Oral fluids are encouraged.

Desmopressin (DDAVP), vasopressin tannate (Pitressin tannate) in oil, and aqueous vasopressin (Pitressin) are the three commonly used hormonal replacement agents. *Desmopressin* is a synthetic form of antidiuretic hormone that has become increasingly popular because it creates less smooth muscle excitation and subsequent abdominal cramping and hypertensive effects than natural hormones. It is supplied in 2.5-mL vials which contain 100 μg desmopressin per mL; a daily dose ranges from 5 to 20 μg. Desmopressin is administered intranasally, using a calibrated catheter supplied with each vial. Generally, the dose is adjusted to control polyuria for 12-h periods. Side effects are rare but include headache, abdominal cramps, and nausea.[4]

Vasopressin tannate in oil was for many years the primary treatment for DI. It is a long-acting combination of lysine and vasopressin suspended in peanut oil. It is supplied in 1-mL vials, each of which contains 5 U of active hormone. Vigorous shaking of the ampule is required to assure adequate suspension of the active drug. It is administered either intramuscularly or subcutaneously. Generally, a dose of 2 to 5 U is used. Sometimes one or two doses are sufficient, since the duration of action can be as long as 72 h. The most common side effects can be attributed to the smooth muscle effects of vasopressin and include abdominal and menstrual-like cramps, nausea, and blood pressure elevation.[4]

Vasopressin tannate in oil is used with caution in patients with coronary artery disease, because it may result in myocardial ischemia. Susceptibility to both water intoxication and hyponatremia is greater with vasopressin tannate use because of its long duration of action. Repeated doses are generally given only when polyuria recurs.[4]

Aqueous vasopressin is a water-soluble pituitary extract containing 20 U/mL of arginine and lysine vasopressin. It is usually administered in doses of 5 to 10 U subcutaneously. Its onset of action occurs in about 1 h, and it has a duration of 3 to 4 h.[4] It can also be administered by slow intravenous drip, but if it is, an infusion control device, electrocardiographic monitoring, and frequent recording of vital signs are recommended. Side effects and precautions are similar to those of vasopressin tannate in oil.

Nursing Management

Diabetes insipidus in the critical-care setting most commonly accompanies cerebral insult, whether iatrogenic as a complication of surgical procedures or resulting from traumatic injuries or inflammatory processes. Nursing care must combine interventions designed to manage the effects of real and potential neurologic compromise with those needed to manage the effects of insufficient ADH. The reader is referred to Chap. 35 for discussion of nursing care for patients with neurologic disorders.

The primary nursing diagnosis in diabetes insipidus is actual or potential fluid volume deficit related to excessive fluid loss. An additional nursing diagnosis, sleep pattern disturbance related to polydipsia and nocturia, is applicable in awake, ambulatory patients.

Nursing Diagnosis

Actual or potential fluid volume deficit related to excessive urinary fluid loss.

Nursing management begins with early identification of patients at risk for actual or potential fluid volume deficit related to excessive urinary fluid loss. All patients unable to perceive or respond to thirst are vulnerable. That vulnerability is exaggerated by tube feedings, parenteral hyperalimentation, and either a history of or current administration of lithium, demeclocycline, or phenytoin, because, as noted earlier, the first two agents decrease renal responsiveness to ADH, while the third inhibits ADH secretion. In addition, any patient with a history of ongoing vasopressin replacement therapy is at risk.

Ongoing assessment centers on hydration status. Meticulous recording of body weight and of intake and output are necessary for accurate determination of trends. Urine specific gravity and plasma and urine osmolality should be recorded consistently. In early untreated DI, urine volumes can approach 2 L/h and body weight can decrease dramatically, up to 3 percent, without adequate fluid replacement. Characteristically, urine specific gravity is less than 1.003 and urine osmolality less than 500 mosm/kg. In contrast, plasma osmolality exceeds 295 mosm/kg. Laboratory studies reveal hemoconcentration and hypernatremia.

Physical examination of the patient with fluid volume deficit related to excessive urinary loss reveals signs of water deficit or dehydration. Skin turgor is decreased, and mucous membranes may appear dry and even cracked. If the condition is prolonged or untreated, signs of extracellular fluid volume depletion also appear. Postural or orthostatic hypotension progresses to sustained hypotension; tachycardia also occurs and may indicate impending hypovolemic shock.

Interventions

Nursing interventions include administration of fluids (oral and intravenous) and pharmacologic replacement agents. Typically, both fluid and pharmacologic replacement agents are titrated around urine output. During the replacement process, continued vigilance needs to be directed at hydration status. Water intoxication and fluid overload can occur as a complication of aggressive replacement therapy, especially when the longer-acting vasopressin tannate in oil is used.

Patients receiving tube feedings or parenteral hyperalimentation pose additional nursing challenges. Many of the solutions used are extremely hypertonic. Enteric preparations can produce an osmotic fluid gradient into the gastrointestinal tract, with a net inward flow of body water. This water influx produces gastrointestinal distention, one of the most powerful stimuli to increased motility.

Diarrhea is likely, and with it exaggerated free water loss and the potential for further increases in osmolality. Nursing interventions for patients receiving enteral alimentation include addition of supplemental water to hypertonic preparations to decrease the potential for significant osmotic influx of water into the gastrointestinal tract. Controlling the rate of administration of enteral solutions to avoid rapid delivery of large volumes may also decrease gastrointestinal distention and the likelihood of diarrhea.

Parenteral hyperalimentation involves infusion of a large glucose load, potential hyperglycemia, spilling of glucose into the urine, and initiation of osmotic diuresis. The resultant large volumes of urine lead to loss of both sodium and water, but proportionately more water. If the condition is allowed to progress, extracellular volume and water depletion compound the initial hyperosmolar state. With patients receiving parenteral hyperalimentation, even optimal vasopressin replacement may be inadequate. Free water availability is decreased, and body water that is available follows the strongest osmotic gradient. The presence of high levels of renal tubular glucose results in physiologic competition for water between the tubular and interstitial spaces. In these situations additional nursing interventions must be directed at monitoring and managing serum and urine glucose levels.

Finally, nursing interventions should be directed at preserving and promoting skin integrity and moist mucous membranes. Frequent adjustments in position, massage, and supplemental padding for bony pressure points should all be utilized. Providing ice chips if the patient can take them or swabbing the mouth with glycerin may be helpful.

Nursing Diagnosis

Sleep pattern disturbance related to polyuria and nocturia.

Interventions

Polyuria and nocturia interfere with obtaining uninterrupted sleep and rest. Nursing interventions should center on ensuring that sleep and rest periods are not unnecessarily interrupted (see Chap. 14). In addition, efforts to conserve patient energy should be instituted. Assistance with self-care activities and frequent rest periods are needed. Finally, appealing fluids should be easily accessible, as well as toilet facilities.

Patient Goals and Outcome Criteria

The treatment plan is successful if fluid intake approximates output and vital signs; hemodynamic parameters and body weight are maintained within the patient's normal range; laboratory findings for plasma and urine osmolality, electrolytes, and urine specific gravity are within normal ranges; symptoms of dehydration are relieved; and skin and mucous membranes are intact.

Syndrome of Inappropriate ADH

The syndrome of inappropriate ADH (SIADH) has also been referred to as *cerebral salt wasting* or *pulmonary salt wasting*. It is characterized by aberrant or sustained ADH effect with hypotonic expansion of body fluids. In SIADH, ingested or supplied water is not excreted. With hypotonic volume expansion, glomerular filtration increases. Urinary sodium excretion is increased and leads to a progressive decline in body sodium. The result is a varying degree of absolute body sodium depletion, water retention, and a consequent marked decrease in serum sodium.[1]

SIADH occurs in many situations. Water retention and hyponatremia may appear postoperatively as a result of the stimulatory effect of many anesthetic agents on ADH coupled with the physiologic stress response elicited by surgery, another stimulant to ADH secretion. Positive pressure ventilation may also promote increased ADH secretion through alteration of the pressure relationships involved in pulmonary volume-sensing mechanisms (see Chap. 36).

In congestive heart failure, cirrhosis of the liver, and nephrosis, interstitial sodium shifts and edema are often compounded by water retention. While prolongation of the half-life of ADH due to diminished metabolism and excretion by the liver and kidneys undoubtedly plays a role, a normally functioning osmoreceptor mechanism should be capable of correcting the (excess) water-induced decrease in osmolality. The fact that it does not consistently do so has resulted in speculation that

the volume-sensing mechanism has been "fooled" and is overriding osmotic regulation. In these states, overall extracellular fluid volume may be perceived as decreased when the actual basis of the disorder is cardiac inefficiency and third space and/or peritoneal fluid shifting. In these situations, ADH secretion is "inappropriate" and exaggerates and complicates the initial disease.[5–7]

Cerebral disease may also lead to inappropriate secretion of ADH. Intracranial lesions are thought to produce this effect by one of three possible mechanisms: (1) allowing "escape" of the hormone because of structural damage to the posterior pituitary; (2) producing an irritated focus that stimulates the posterior pituitary to release ADH; and/or (3) stimulation of the sympathetic nervous system due to cerebral hypoxia.

Intrathoracic disease may also interfere with ADH secretion. In these situations it is thought that neural pathways that normally translate and transmit messages regarding body fluid volume to the hypothalamus are disrupted. Normal suppression of ADH secretion fails to occur, and ADH secretion is inappropriately increased. Intrathoracic metastatic lesions may also lead to SIADH by secreting ADH, as in bronchogenic cancer.[1] Prostatic and pancreatic cancers can also secrete ectopic ADH.

Medical Therapies

When SIADH occurs as a result of malignant disease, surgical resection, radiation, or chemotherapy is utilized. In SIADH associated with intracranial, pulmonary, myocardial, and hepatic or renal disease, treatment is directed at specific precipitating pathologic processes. Regardless of cause, and even if the syndrome is thought to be transient, as after surgery or with positive pressure ventilation, the goal of medical interventions is to normalize free water balance.

Free water intake is severely restricted, and overall fluid intake is based on urine output plus insensible loss. Demeclocycline or lithium may be administered to inhibit renal ADH effects and phenytoin to inhibit ADH secretion. In severe hyponatremic states, hypertonic sodium chloride infusions, intravenous furosemide, or osmotic diuretics such as urea or mannitol may be used to promote water excretion.[8]

Nursing Management

Nursing therapies in providing care for patients with SIADH center on the goal of restoring fluid and electrolyte balance. The reader is referred to chapters addressing patient care for patients with cardiac, pulmonary, renal, and hepatic disorders for specific and related interventions utilized when compromises of these systems occur in conjunction with SIADH. The primary nursing diagnosis in SIADH, actual or potential fluid overload, is discussed below.

Nursing Diagnosis

Actual or potential fluid overload related to insufficient excretion of free water.

Nursing management begins with identification of patients at risk: postoperative patients; those receiving positive pressure ventilation; those with central nervous system disorders (skull fractures, contusions, cerebral vascular accidents, neoplasms, or infections); those with congestive heart failure, cirrhosis, or nephrosis; and those with pulmonary disorders (pneumonia, asthma, cystic fibrosis, or neoplasms).

Ongoing assessment focuses on the status of fluid and electrolyte balance. Deliberate and sequential evaluation involves careful monitoring of intake and output, consistent recording of daily weights, and monitoring of urine specific gravity, plasma osmolality, and serum sodium. Generally, unless the condition is complicated by cirrhosis or nephrosis, extracellular volume in SIADH is adequate and blood pressure is fairly normal, with minimal if any postural or orthostatic changes. Weight is increased, urine specific gravity is elevated, and urine volumes are decreased. Dilutional hyponatremia and decreased plasma osmolality are present.

The physical examination reveals absence of edema despite weight gain, because the bulk of the fluid excess occurs intracellularly. Early in the course of SIADH, neurologic signs of water intoxication are subtle and include a decrease in level of consciousness, headache, fatigue, and weakness. Later there may be personality changes, confusion, irritability, a sense of impending doom, restlessness, sluggish deep tendon reflexes, and seizures. Anorexia, nausea, and vomiting, reflecting the effect of hyponatremia on the gastrointestinal tract, may also be present.

Interventions

Nursing interventions include administration of fluids (oral and intravenous), electrolyte supplements, and diuretics and management of the neurologic and gastrointestinal effects of water intoxication. Because fluid intake is restricted, neither carafes of water nor ice chips should be left at the bedside; infusion control devices should be utilized for intravenous lines. The patient and visitors should be instructed as to the nature and purpose of fluid restrictions. Similarly, the basis for behavioral changes should be explained. Frequent reorientation of the patient may be required.

Constipation may occur as a result of the combined effects of restricted fluid intake, decreased activity, and decreased gastrointestinal motility related to hyponatremia. Enemas, if needed, should not be of the tap-water type because of the risk of water absorption.

With confusion, weakness, and the potential for seizure activity, safety measures should be instituted. Side rails should be kept up and padded if hyponatremia is severe; the bed should be kept in the lowest position, and the patient should not get up unattended.

Finally, nursing care should be provided to limit the effects of immobilization. Frequent position changes, deep breathing, aggressive skin care, and graduated activity need to be instituted.

Patient Goals and Outcome Criteria

The treatment plan is successful if fluid intake approximates output and body weight returns to normal. Additionally, laboratory findings for serum sodium, plasma osmolality, and urine specific gravity will be within normal limits, and signs of water intoxication will be relieved. The patient will be alert and oriented, and deep tendon reflexes and gastrointestinal motility will return to normal.

Hyperthyroid Crisis

Hyperthyroid crisis (thyrotoxic crisis or thyroid storm) is an emergency hypermetabolic state which occurs in untreated or inadequately treated patients with hyperthyroidism. It is precipitated by febrile illness (typically pulmonary infections), physiologic stress such as occurs in traumatic injury, surgery, diabetic ketoacidosis, or toxemia of pregnancy, and severe psychologic trauma. The mechanism behind the shift from hyperthyroidism to thyrotoxic crisis is unclear.

Hyperthyroidism without crisis occurs when excessive amounts of thyroid hormones (thyroxine, or T_4, and triiodothyronine) in the circulation affect peripheral tissues (see Chaps. 36 and 37). The most common cause of hyperthyroidism is Graves' disease, a condition which involves production of antibodies to thyroid tissue. In Graves' disease the mechanism by which antibodies are produced is not understood, but their effect is thyroid inflammation, diffuse enlargement and hyperplasia of the gland, and exophthalmic goiter. Thyroid hormone–induced increases in metabolic rate promote development of a negative nitrogen balance because of protein and fat catabolism to meet increased energy needs. Characteristics of Graves' disease include weight loss and heat intolerance, both of which reflect the effect of increased metabolic rate. *Exophthalmos,* or bulging ocular orbits, is a hallmark of Graves' disease and is thought to reflect antibody action on periorbital tissue, although the precise mechanism has yet to be explained.[9]

Other causes of hyperthyroidism include hyperfunctioning thyroid adenomas (often called *hot nodules*), toxic multinodular goiter, early granulomatous thyroiditis, TSH-producing pituitary adenomas, secreting thyroid carcinomas, and ingestion of excessive amounts of thyroid hormone. In all these conditions, as well as in Graves' disease, hyperthyroidism can lead to clinical findings that include nervousness and tremors, warm pink skin, hyperthermia, increased pulse and pulse pressure, and increased urine output. Potentiation of catecholamines in neurotransmission with increased excitability of peripheral reflexes is probably the basis for the nervousness and tremors. Warm, pink skin reflects activation of heat-dissipating mechanisms (vasodilatation), necessary because the increased metabolic rate produces hyperthermia. Pulse rate and pressure and increased urine output reflect compensatory increases in cardiac output and glomerular filtration.

Since heart failure is present whenever the cardiac output (regardless of actual volume) is unable to maintain adequate tissue perfusion, high-output cardiac failure may occur if compensatory increases in cardiac output are inadequate. Hyperthyroid persons are vulnerable to liver failure because of chronic depletion of hepatic glycogen stores in an attempt to meet the increased metabolic needs. Such glycogen depletion increases susceptibility to hepatic injury and degeneration.[10]

Thyrotoxic crisis has in the past been thought to occur as a result of a sudden increase in circulating thyroid hormone, presumably due to exacerbation of underlying hyperthyroidism. Laboratory studies during thyrotoxic crises have not, however, revealed levels of thyroid hormones significantly greater than those characteristic of the hyperthyroid state. It may be that an abrupt but transient release precipitates thyrotoxic crisis.[9]

An alternate precipitatory theory is the basis for the alternate name *decompensated thyrotoxicosis* often applied to thyrotoxic crisis. According to this hypothesis, crisis occurs when peripheral tissues are no longer able to respond to elevated circulating levels of thyroid hormones. Catecholamines are potentiated by thyroid hormones, and prolonged adrenergic influence could certainly predispose tissues to decompensation.[9] In crisis states, cardiac exhaustion is a prominent feature and heat can no longer be effectively dissipated. In light of the fact that thyrotoxic crisis often occurs with or shortly after febrile illness and physiologic stress reactions, the decompensation theory for the shifting of hyperthyroidism to a crisis state seems plausible.

Clinical findings in thyrotoxic crisis are similar to but far more exaggerated than those of hyperthyroidism. Hyperthermia can be extreme and cardiac and gastrointestinal decompensation pronounced. Tachycardia is marked and unrelenting and is frequently accompanied by congestive failure and angina. Hyperdefecation and vomiting are also common.

Medical Therapies

Treatment for hyperthyroidism is either ablative (radioactive iodine or surgery) or nonablative (antithyroid pharmacologic agents). Ablative procedures are typically used in Graves' disease, toxic goiters, and neoplasms of the thyroid; nonablative therapies may also be used on an ongoing basis. In the presence of thyrotoxic crisis, antithyroid agents are increased and provided along with other interventions to support vital functions.

Two thionamides, propylthiouracil (PTU) and methimazole (MMI), are used in the treatment of hyperthyroidism. These agents block organification of iodine, thus decreasing formation of thyroid hormones. PTU is administered orally, initially 100 mg three times a day. As levels of thyroid hormone normalize, the dose is decreased to 50 to 200 mg daily in equally divided doses. MMI is approximately 10 times as potent as PTU, and the usual starting dose is 10 mg three times a day. MMI has a longer half-life than PTU; thus, once normal levels of thyroid hormone are achieved, one dose of 5 to 10 mg daily often suffices.[11]

In thyrotoxic crisis, PTU is believed to be preferable to MMI because it has the unique effect of blocking peripheral conversion of thyroxine to T_3 (see Chap. 36). PTU is administered orally, by nasogastric tube if necessary, 300 mg q 6 h. In conjunction with PTU, iodine is also administered to inhibit thyroid hormone release. Saturated solution of potassium iodide (SSKI) contains approximately 50 mg of iodine per drop; in crisis states it is given orally, 10 drops q 8 h, beginning shortly after the first dose of PTU. As an alternative, sodium iodide may be given intravenously 1 to 2 g per day.[11]

Since thyroid hormones have a prolonged half-life, blocking synthesis and release of new hormone is not sufficient in crisis states; the effects of circulating hormone must also be decreased. Sympatholytic agents, most commonly propranolol (Inderal) in doses of 1 to 3 mg IV or 20 to 40 mg PO q 2 to 4 h, are indicated unless there is a history of asthma or congestive failure independent of the thyrotoxic state.[11] Reserpine or guanethidine may also be used.

Because endogenous corticosteroids are metabolized faster in the hypermetabolic state, glucocorticoids are administered to enhance general physiologic support in thyrotoxic crisis. Glucocorticords may also be needed to prevent or overcome adrenal insufficiency in the presence of a severe and prolonged stress response. Hydrocortisone, 100 mg IV q 4 to 6 h, or its equivalent is typically ordered.

Digitalis preparations are often used to relieve congestive failure and antipyretics to control body temperature. High-calorie nutritional support, frequently with supplemental vitamin B, is provided, as is intravenous fluid therapy. Levels for both caloric and fluid intake are significantly above normal levels because of the need to respond to extreme hypermetabolism.

Nursing Management

Nursing care in thyrotoxic crisis must combine interventions addressing precipitating factors with those necessary because of the profound hypermetabolic emergency state. Frequent multisystem evaluation is necessary, including cardiac, respiratory, neurologic, and gastrointestinal assessments.

Applicable nursing diagnoses and interventions in thyrotoxic crisis are discussed in the following paragraphs.

Nursing Diagnosis

Altered nutrition: potential for less than body requirements, related to hypermetabolism.

Focused assessment addresses nutritional and metabolic status. Appetite is typically increased, as is caloric consumption, but weight loss is nonetheless present. Mild hyperdefecation often occurs and reflects autonomic hyperactivity and the effect of thyroid hormones on intestinal motility.

Reflective of catabolism, anthropometric measurements frequently fall at 90 percent of reference levels or below for midarm circumference, midarm muscle circumference, and triceps skin fold thickness. Muscle weakness is present, and muscle wasting is often visible. Rapid protein turnover leads to soft, fine hair and friable nails; frequently the free margin of the nails is lifted from its base *(onycholysis)*.

Serum proteins, particularly albumin, may be decreased. Other hematologic findings may include neutropenia, lymphocytosis, anemia, and increased red cell mass due to the excess demand for oxygen.[9]

Interventions

Nursing interventions include administration of glucose-rich infusions and monitoring for appropriate glucose metabolism. Serum and urinary glucose must be monitored. Hyperglycemia may occur as a result of increased glycogenolysis, impaired insulin secretion, and insulin resistance related to glucocorticoids and the physiologic stress response.

Daily weights should be monitored and caloric consumption carefully recorded. If oral intake is possible, frequent high-calorie supplements should be provided; visitors should be encouraged to supply favorite foods and beverages. A dietary consultation should be obtained to assure well-balanced, nutritionally sound meals.

In administering pharmacologic agents, hypermetabolism should be constantly considered. Because of the greatly increased metabolic rate, drug turnover and degradation will be accelerated; above-normal dosages given at shorter intervals than usual may be required.

Nursing Diagnosis

Impaired thermal regulation related to insufficient heat dissipation.

In thyrotoxic crisis hypermetabolism is pronounced and tissue decompensation, most notably cardiac exhaustion, impairs effective heat dissipation. Flushed, moist skin is common and heat intolerance profound. Fever may approach 106°F, and even minor infections can trigger excessively high fevers.

Interventions

Nursing interventions center on fever reduction. Antipyretic agents, usually acetominaphen, are administered. Aspirin is not recommended in thyrotoxic crisis, because it displaces thyroid hormone from its carrier protein, thus increasing free hormone levels. Hypothermal blankets, tepid baths, and ice packs over major vessels are also utilized.

Nursing Diagnosis

Sleep pattern disturbance related to insomnia.

Elevated thyroid hormone levels directly impair sleep. Insomnia is a frequent complaint. Non-REM and REM sleep debts may develop as a result of inability to obtain adequate sleep. Non-REM sleep debts result in physical fatigue and malaise; in

thyrotoxic crisis these effects no doubt exaggerate the effects of muscle weakness. REM debts may create disorientation, suspiciousness, and withdrawal; paranoia and even hallucinations may occur in severe deprivation (see Chap. 14).

Interventions

Nursing therapies center on minimizing fatigue by providing frequent uninterrupted rest periods. Attention must also be given to promoting a restful environment, enhancing patient comfort and promoting relaxation through back rubs and position changes, and ensuring patient privacy.

Nursing Diagnosis

Altered cardiac output related to excessive demand.

Thyroid hormones increase metabolic rate and stimulate oxygen consumption throughout the body. Demand on cardiac function is thus increased in hyperthyroid states. Thyroid hormones also directly affect the myocardium. Palpitations, tachycardia and tachyarrhythmias (typically atrial fibrillation and paroxysmal atrial tachycardia), systolic hypertension, and increased pulse pressure are common findings. In thyrotoxic crisis these findings are often accompanied by angina and signal impending myocardial failure and decompensation.[9] Acute pulmonary edema and anasarca may develop. In the elderly, as well as those patients with preexisting cardiovascular disease, signs of cardiovascular compromise may dominate the clinical presentation in thyrotoxic crisis.

Interventions

Nursing interventions include administration of agents to control cardiac arrhythmias, although frequently rhythm disturbances are refractory until the effects of thyroid hormones have been blocked. Sympatholytic agents are also administered. Their effects must be monitored carefully, especially when there is a history of asthma or congestive heart failure. Ongoing cardiac assessment requires dynamic monitoring of heart rate and rhythm and frequent blood pressure recordings.

Nursing Diagnosis

Impaired gas exchange related to dyspnea.

Elevated thyroid hormone levels increase peripheral tissue oxygen consumption. That increased demand, coupled with intercostal muscle weakness and resultant dyspnea, produces the potential for impaired gas exchange. In thyrotoxic crisis, increased oxygen demand is further exaggerated by extreme hypermetabolism. Additional respiratory compromise occurs as a result of cardiac failure with pulmonary edema. Respiratory failure may occur.

Interventions

Nursing interventions include serial assessments of pulmonary function. Arterial blood gases should be monitored and breath sounds auscultated regularly. Patient activity needs to be paced to conserve energy and allow for rest periods.

Nursing Diagnosis

Sensory/perceptual alterations: overload related to hypersensitivity to the environment.

Increased thyroid hormone levels and potentiation of catecholamines result in exaggerated adrenergic activity. Hypersensitivity to the environment is manifested by exaggerated alertness, inability to relax, and frequently overreaction to almost all stimuli. In thyrotoxic crisis, hypersensitivity is pronounced; patients frequently have a decreased attention span, agitation, and nervousness. REM sleep deprivation may compound symptoms by adding suspiciousness and paranoia. Delirium and emotional lability may progress to psychosis.[8]

Interventions

Nursing interventions center on providing structure, consistency, and simplicity in care activities. The scope of the environment should be limited; a private room is desirable. Efforts need to be addressed to controlling extraneous and sudden noises; unfamiliar sounds should be explained.

Frequent, even repetitive, reassurances and calm explanations are needed. Safety measures should be instituted if there is delirium: side rails should be kept up and the bed maintained in the lowest position. The patient should not be allowed to get up without assistance.

Patient Goals and Outcome Criteria

The treatment plan is successful if vital signs stabilize to the patient's normal range and body temperature

normalizes, sinus tachycardia is reversed, the patient is awake and oriented, and symptoms of hypersensitivity to the environment are relieved. Laboratory values for serum glucose and electrolytes will return to normal, and body weight will stabilize.

Hypothyroid Crisis

Hypothyroid crisis, also known as *myxedema coma,* is the extreme of hypothyroidism and represents a life-threatening emergency. It may be precipitated by infection, trauma, critical illness, exposure to cold, or administration of sedatives, anesthetics, narcotics, or psychotropic drugs at dosages or frequencies beyond the ability of the hypothyroid patient to metabolize. It may also occur as a result of insufficient thyroid hormone replacement after thyroidectomy or ablative therapy, traumatic injury to the thyroid gland, or chronic or autoimmune thyroiditis. Finally, it may be triggered in preexisting hypothyroidism by dysfunction of the hypothalamic-pituitary axis due to pituitary infarction, hypophysectomy, pituitary irradiation, or head injury.

In hypothyroidism without crisis, the effect of insufficient thyroid hormone levels is reflected in the clinical findings. There is decreased metabolic rate, weight gain, and intolerance of cold. Reflexes and mentation are frequently slowed. Cutaneous accumulations of water and protein-polysaccharide compounds occur as a result of slowed metabolism and protein synthesis. A puffy appearance and a nonpitting edema provide the basis for referring to adult hypothyroidism as myxedema.

With the onset of myxedema coma, all symptoms of hypothyroidism are exaggerated. Hypothermia is so pronounced that thermometer malfunction is often suspected. Hypercarbia and hypoventilation are common and probably reflect the effects of reduced ventilatory capacity, due to interstitial accumulations of mucopolysaccharides, lesions in the respiratory muscles, and decreased responsiveness in the central nervous system respiratory center.[9] Hypotension and bradycardia are severe as a result of decreased myocardial contractility. Level of consciousness is significantly depressed, and frank coma may exist. Hypoglycemia occurs, probably reflecting the effect of decreased caloric intake in the obtunded state, decreased gluconeogenesis due to hypometabolism, and decreased glucocorticoid effect in the presence of insufficient thyroid hormone.[9] Mild to severe dilutional hyponatremia also accompanies myxedema coma. It occurs as a result of a decreased glomerular filtration rate with consequent decreased clearance of free water. Superimposed SIADH may also contribute to the increase in total body water.[9]

Medical Therapies

When myxedema coma is suspected, diagnostic tests include serum thyroid hormones, TSH, and T_3 resin uptake. Treatment, however, is initiated immediately, without waiting for results, because of the extreme, life-threatening nature of the crisis.

Thyroxine (T_4) (Synthroid, levothyroxine) is the drug of choice for hormone replacement in myxedema crisis. It is given intravenously (2 μg/kg over 5 to 10 min), followed by 100 μg IV on a daily basis. This dose may be decreased in the presence of cardiac disease. Oral administration of thyroid hormone replacement is inappropriate in myxedema crisis because of the likelihood of ileus and poor gastrointestinal absorption. As clinical improvement begins, the IV dose is gradually adjusted downward and oral replacement is resumed.[12]

Glucocorticoid support is also provided. Typically a bolus of hydrocortisone 100 mg (or its equivalent) is administered intravenously, followed by a continuous infusion of 10 mg/h. The goal of glucocorticoid administration is to provide optimal physiologic support for the ongoing stress response and for concurrent adrenal insufficiency, often an accompanying disorder. Pharmacologic doses are not used, however, because such doses inhibit peripheral conversion of thyroid hormone and thus impede efforts to reestablish adequate peripheral hormone response.[9,12]

Respiratory acidosis and hypercarbia are treated by intubation and mechanical ventilation. Hypotension is treated by volume expansion, hormone replacement, and glucocorticoids, as noted. Pressor agents are usually avoided because of the risk of cardiac arrhythmias and myocardial decompensation with increased peripheral resistance. Intravenous glucose-containing fluids are administered on the basis of serum glucose values. Hypotonic solutions and free water are avoided, however, because of the risk of exacerbation of the hyponatremia.[12]

Nursing Management

Nursing care in myxedema coma involves interventions directed at reversal of the precipitating event in addition to those required by the multisystem dysfunction due to the acute thyroid hormone deficiency. Frequent nursing evaluations are required and focus on cardiac, respiratory, and neurologic function as well as hydration and metabolic status.

The applicable nursing diagnoses and interventions in myxedema coma are discussed below.

Nursing Diagnosis

Impaired gas exchange related to decreased ventilatory capacity.

Interventions

Focused assessment addresses adequacy of ventilation and oxygenation. Initially, mechanical ventilatory support is often needed to control respiratory acidosis. Serial pulmonary auscultation to ensure optimal ventilation of all lung fields and monitoring of arterial blood gases are required. Later, as mechanical assistance is no longer required, serial monitoring of lung sounds and blood gases is even more important, as are frequent repositioning and encouragement of deep breathing. Decreased ventilatory capacity as a result of interstitial accumulations of mucopolysaccharides and compromised respiratory musculature combine with decreased responsiveness of the central nervous system respiratory center to produce continuing vulnerability to respiratory insufficiency as the crisis state is reversed and peripheral oxygen demands increase.

Pharmacologic agents with a potential for respiratory depression are to be avoided. If they are absolutely necessary, the dose should be carefully considered because of delayed metabolism and degradation of agents in the myxedematous state.

Nursing Diagnosis
Altered thermal regulation.

Interventions
Hypothermia is profound in myxedema coma as a result of severe hypometabolism. Generally, the lower the temperature the worse the prognosis. Nursing interventions to raise body temperature are needed. It is essential, however, that efforts be gradual and passive. Rapid rewarming can result in excessive or sudden demand on an already compromised and depressed myocardium by increasing peripheral oxygen requirements and decreasing vascular tone. Room temperature should be increased (75°F) and extra blankets provided. Warming lights and externally warmed blankets may also be utilized. Core body temperature needs to be monitored frequently.

Nursing Diagnosis
Altered cardiac output related to depressed myocardial function.

Insufficient thyroid hormone results in decreased myocardial contractility. Hypotension and bradycardia may be severe. Thus, focused assessment centers on the adequacy of cardiovascular function. Continuous electrocardiographic and hemodynamic monitoring is indicated. The ECG is likely to show low voltage and prolongation of the QT interval. Clinically, heart sounds may be distant and pericardial effusion may occur. Chest x-rays typically reveal cardiomegaly.[8]

Interventions
Nursing interventions include consistent serial monitoring of cardiovascular response as thyroid hormone replacement is provided and body temperature is increased. Hormone replacement and correction of hypothermia may increase myocardial demand and precipitate tachyarrhythmias, ischemia with angina, and congestive failure. Hypotension, as noted previously, is usually treated with volume expansion, glucocorticoid support, and thyroid hormone replacement. Pressor agents are generally avoided because of the risk of arrhythmias, excessive stimulation of the depressed myocardium, and the risk of increased peripheral resistance. Admin-

istration of intravenous fluids is discussed in the section that immediately follows.

Nursing Diagnosis
Impaired elimination, urinary and gastrointestinal.

Insufficient thyroid hormone in myxedema coma leads to depressed cardiovascular function, decreased glomerular filtration, and impaired free water clearance. Congestive failure may alter intrathoracic pressure relationships and result in concurrent SIADH, with aggravation of total body water excess. Focused assessment thus centers on evaluation of cardiac and respiratory status as discussed, and in addition, serial evaluation of hydration.

Deliberate and sequential assessment involves careful monitoring of intake and output, consistent recording of daily weights, and monitoring of urine specific gravity, plasma osmolality, and serum sodium. Clinically, physical examination reveals weight gain without edema, because the bulk of fluid excess is free water and thus is distributed intracellularly.

Monitoring for actual or potential water intoxication includes evaluation of neurologic status. Complaints of headache, fatigue, and weakness and a deteriorating level of consciousness are associated with early water intoxication. In myxedema coma, however, these signs may be obscured by the existing depressed level of consciousness. The same is true of the sluggish deep tendon reflexes, confusion, agitation and restlessness, and sense of impending doom that accompany pronounced water intoxication.

Interventions
Seizures may occur in severe hyponatremia; thus nursing interventions should be directed to ensuring patient safety. Padding of side rails and keeping the side rails up and the bed in the lowest position are also indicated. Other measures needed as a result of the comatose state include vigorous skin care, frequent repositioning, and provision of padding over bony pressure points.

Nursing interventions also include careful administration of fluid as well as diuretics and glucose. The treatment goal is to reverse dilutional hyponatremia; thus fluid orders involve restriction of free water. If seizures are present or hyponatremia is severe, hypertonic sodium chloride solutions with concurrent furosemide may be utilized. Osmotic diuretics are generally not indicated in myxedema coma, because the mobilization of excessive free water from the intracellular space poses too great a risk for cardiac decompensation. Infusion control devices are helpful to ensure appropriate fluid delivery.

If the patient is capable of ingesting oral fluids, the nature and purpose of water restrictions should be explained. While occasional ice chips may be provided, they must be counted in overall intake and output figures, and water-containing carafes should not be left at the bedside. Frequent mouth care can help the patient tolerate water restrictions.

Glucose-containing infusions are used to supply calories. Because of the extreme hypometabolic state, nutritional requirements tend to be low. Nonetheless, because hypoglycemia often occurs in myxedema coma, nursing interventions should include monitoring of serum glucose.

As the patient improves and oral nutritional intake is considered, the potential for impaired bowel function must be continually considered. Constipation, abdominal distention, and paralytic ileus may occur in extreme hypothyroid states. Nursing interventions should include assessment of gastrointestinal function. Bowel sounds should be auscultated, and serial measurements of abdominal girth may be indicated. If constipation occurs, enemas may be necessary; tap-water enemas, however, should not be used because of the potential for free water absorption from the colon. When the patient is allowed to eat, low-calorie, well-balanced meals high in roughage should be supplied.

Patient Goals and Outcome Criteria

The treatment plan is successful if vital signs return to normal and adequate oxygenation and ventilation are assured. Blood gases will normalize, dilutional hyponatremia will be reversed, and serum sodium levels and plasma osmolality will be within normal ranges. Body weight will stabilize, and body temperature will remain within the normal range. The patient will be awake, oriented, and able to perform activities of daily living without undue fatigue. Finally, urinary output will approximate fluid intake,

and oral nutritional intake and bowel function will return to the patient's baseline patterns.

Hypoparathyroidism

Hypoparathyroidism is characterized by insufficient parathormone. Absence of parathormone may have lethal effects, because levels of serum ionized calcium fall dramatically. The resultant alterations in neuromuscular excitability may seriously compromise cardiac, respiratory, and skeletal muscle function.

Normally, parathyroid secretion of parathormone occurs by a continuous feedback mechanism involving the level of serum ionized calcium. When blood perfusing the parathyroid glands contains insufficient amounts of ionized calcium, the glands are directly stimulated to secrete parathormone. The effect of the hormone is to raise the serum level of ionized calcium by exerting a resorptive or calcium-mobilizing effect on bones, effecting active transport of calcium into the extracellular fluid, stimulating renal reabsorption of calcium, and stimulating renal production of 1,25 dihydroxycholecalciferol or active vitamin D, which is necessary for calcium absorption from the gastrointestinal tract.[1]

Hypoparathyroidism may be a result of ischemia, damage to or inadvertent removal of parathyroid tissue during neck surgery for thyroid or other disorders, or damage to the gland from neoplasms, autoimmune processes, or infiltrative diseases. Hypomagnesemia (as in chronic alcoholism and malabsorption syndromes) may also result in insufficient amounts of parathormone, because decreased magnesium levels interfere with parathyroid secretion. Chronic forms of hypoparathyroidism include idiopathic hypoparathyroidism, for which a cause has not been specifically identified, and pseudohypoparathyroidism, a genetic disorder characterized by peripheral resistance to the actions of parathormone.[13]

Insufficient parathormone results in increased renal calcium loss and decreased renal phosphate excretion; generally there is a reciprocal relationship between serum ionized calcium and phosphate levels. Along with the ensuing hypocalcemia, mild metabolic alkalosis also develops as a result of decreased bicarbonate excretion. Other effects of insufficient parathormone exaggerate the impact of increased renal calcium excretion and include a decrease in bone resorption, vitamin D activation, and gastrointestinal calcium absorption.

Clinically the findings associated with hypoparathyroidism reflect the impact of hypocalcemia. Even minor reductions in serum calcium increase neuromuscular excitability and result in muscle tremors and cramps. Numbness and tingling in the extremities and circumoral area may occur.

With severe reductions in serum calcium, tetany, or muscle twitching and spasm without effective contraction, and generalized tonic-clonic seizures may develop. A positive *Chvostek's sign,* or unilateral twitching and muscle spasm of the upper lip in response to a supramandibular finger tap over the parotid gland, and a positive *Trousseau's sign,* or carpopedal spasm in response to inflation of a blood pressure cuff, are two hallmarks. Diarrhea, abdominal cramps, and biliary colic are also common. Spasm in the bronchial and laryngeal musculature may produce laryngeal stridor, wheezes, and labored breathing. In an extreme form, tetany of the respiratory musculature results in respiratory arrest.

Hypocalcemia also directly impairs cardiac function. Bradycardia with first- and second-degree blocks may progress to cardiac arrest. Myocardial contractility is also decreased, and this decrease may lead to a decrease in cardiac output and blood pressure. Electrocardiographic changes include prolongation of the ST and QT intervals.[9]

Prothrombin levels may also decrease as a result of hypocalcemia, leading, rarely, to bleeding abnormalities in hypoparathyroidism.

Medical Therapies

In chronic hypoparathyroidism, supplemental oral calcium and vitamin D are required. Many calcium supplements are available: calcium lactate (8 g equals 1 g calcium), calcium gluconate (10 g equals 1 g calcium), or calcium carbonate (2.5 g equals 1 g calcium). Generally, 1 to 3 g of calcium is the daily dosage.[14]

Vitamin D supplement is provided either by administering 50,000 to 100,000 IU of vitamin D daily or by using a daily dosage of 0.25 to 0.50 μg

of 1,25-dihydroxyvitamin D. The latter is preferred in documented hypoparathyroidism because of impaired conversion of vitamin D to the active form in the presence of insufficient parathormone.[14]

In acute hypoparathyroid states manifested by significant hypocalcemia, signs of pronounced neuromuscular excitability, and cardiac or respiratory compromise, calcium is provided intravenously. Typically, calcium gluconate, 10 mL of a 10% solution, is infused over 10 min. Sustained infusions involving 10 to 15 mg/kg over 4 to 8 h may also be used. Serial monitoring of serum calcium is a fundamental element of medical treatment.[14]

Nursing Management

Hypoparathyroidism in the critical-care setting is most commonly associated with previous surgical procedures involving the neck or ablative treatment involving the thyroid. It often occurs in the immediate postoperative period but may also develop after a significant length of time. Nursing management thus begins with identification of patients at risk and recognition of the fact that a history of surgical procedures involving the thyroid or parathyroid glands or of ablative procedures such as radioactive iodine treatment for thyroid disorders creates a potential for hypoparathyroidism.

The paragraphs that follow discuss the applicable nursing diagnoses and interventions.

Nursing Diagnosis
Alteration in cardiac output: decrease.

Hypocalcemia in hypoparathyroidism produces profound effects on the myocardium. Focused nursing assessment thus centers on evaluation of cardiovascular status. Dynamic electrocardiographic monitoring is needed to detect and evaluate changes in the ST and QT intervals, heart rate, and rhythm. Hemodynamic monitoring may be indicated to evaluate cardiac output in severe hypocalcemia. Vital signs should be assessed serially at a frequency appropriate to the patient's condition. Because hypocalcemia causes insensitivity to the cardiac glycoside digitalis, it is important to continue serial cardiovascular assessments after serum calcium levels begin to rise, to ensure prevention or at least early detection of digitalis intoxication. Intake and output and daily weights should be monitored as part of the evaluation of cardiovascular function.

Interventions

Nursing interventions include administration of fluids and calcium replacement preparations. Infusion control devices may be indicated to ensure intravenous fluid delivery at a rate consistent with myocardial status and blood pressure and to ensure an appropriate rate of administration of calcium preparations. Overly rapid infusion of calcium solutions can enhance the effect of cardiac glycosides and may result in cardiac arrest. Finally, regular assessment of the patency of intravenous lines is needed, because calcium extravasation can produce tissue necrosis.

Nursing Diagnosis

Impaired mobility related to increased neuromuscular excitability.

Increased neuromuscular excitability with a likelihood of spasm, tetany, and cramping accompany hypoparathyroidism-induced hypocalcemia. Focused nursing assessment involves evaluation of neuromuscular status. Serial checking for positive Chvostek's and Trousseau's signs is indicated, as well as determination of the presence of paresthesias, numbness, or tingling.

Interventions

Nursing interventions in the presence of impaired mobility related to increased neuromuscular excitability include efforts to prevent spasm and tetany and increase activity tolerance. Assistance with moving and repositioning should be provided gently and at a pace determined by the patient. Positions that might promote or aggravate muscle spasm by putting pressure on motor nerves should be avoided: the legs should not be crossed, and care should be taken to prevent overcompression of the arms when the patient is in the side-lying position. Moist heat will sometimes prevent spasms, and passive or limited active range of motion exercises may decrease the discomfort associated with numbness and tingling. Finally, providing frequent opportunities for rest and graduating demands during activity periods are important in order to avoid unnecessary fatigue.

Tonic-clonic and grand mal seizure activity may occur with profound hypocalcemia and require that safety measures be instituted: side rails should be padded and kept in the upright position and the bed should be kept in the lowest position. Anticonvulsant medications should be immediately available, as should emergency resuscitative equipment.

Nursing Diagnosis

Potential for ineffective airflow related to respiratory tetany.

The impact of hypocalcemia-induced neuromuscular excitability on respiratory musculature is in some ways similar to its effect on skeletal muscle. Spasm can progress to tetany and preclude effective contraction. In the respiratory musculature, such changes are manifested by stridor (sometimes loud), crowing noises, wheezes, labored breathing, and a choking sensation. Without intervention tetany may develop and result in cessation of airflow.

Interventions

Nursing interventions begin with focused assessment to assure adequacy of oxygenation and ventilation. Breath sounds should be auscultated and arterial blood gases monitored. With dyspnea, patients are frequently more comfortable with the head of the bed elevated. Wheezing and stridor should alert all care givers to prepare for a potential respiratory emergency; a tracheostomy tray and resuscitation equipment should be immediately available.

Nursing Diagnosis

Alterations in thought processes or moods.

Hypocalcemia is often associated with mood changes and apathy; withdrawal, sadness, and anger are not uncommon.

Interventions

Nursing interventions include frequent and repetitive reassurances as to the temporary nature and basis of these changes. Providing an accepting, quiet environment and anticipating comfort needs can be helpful in promoting effective patient coping. Maintaining low-level lights and limiting and explaining extraneous and unfamiliar stimuli also may help.

Patient Goals and Outcome Criteria

The treatment plan for hypoparathyroidism is successful if the serum ionized calcium returns to normal range, cardiac output returns to the patient's baseline, and digitalis toxicity has been prevented. Adequate airflow and oxygenation will be maintained, blood gases will return to the patient's baseline, and labored breathing will be relieved. Signs of neuromuscular hyperexcitability will be reversed, and the patient will be free from injury and from mental changes associated with hypocalcemia.

Acute Adrenal Insufficiency

Adrenal insufficiency, or *Addison's disease,* refers to a condition in which function of the adrenal cortex is impaired and, as a result, insufficient glucocorticoids (cortisol and corticosterone) and mineralocorticords (aldosterone) are secreted. Adrenal androgen secretion is also insufficient in Addison's disease, but because the adrenal cortex is a secondary source of these hormones, only a few fairly insignificant effects result provided that testicular and ovarian function are normal.

Chronic adrenal insufficiency is characterized as either primary or secondary. Primary chronic adrenal insufficiency occurs with bilateral atrophy of the glands, autoimmune disorders, and tuberculosis. Less common causes include histoplasmosis, metastatic disease, amyloidosis, and vascular compromise of the adrenal gland. Secondary chronic adrenal insufficiency involves disorders of the hypothalamic-pituitary axis and resultant impaired secretion of corticotropin releasing hormone (CRH) and/or adrenocorticotropic hormone (ACTH)[9,15] (see Chap. 36). Addisonian or adrenal crisis is an emergency life-threatening state characterized by either an absolute or a relative deficiency of cortisol and aldosterone. In chronic adrenal insufficiency, Addisonian crisis may be precipitated by inadequate hormone replacement in times of acute stress. It may also result from damage to the adrenal cortex following infections (meningococcal, staphylococcal, pneumococcal, streptococcal, or those involving *Haemophilus influenza*); or it may be part of hemorrhagic disorders, leukemias, or anticoagulant therapy; or it may be a result of adrenal vein thrombosis.

Iatrogenic acute adrenal crisis may occur also in patients maintained on pharmacologic doses of glucocorticoids for reasons unrelated to adrenal function. Prolonged administration of exogenous glucocorticoids leads to suppression of hypothalamic CRH and pituitary ACTH secretion, resulting in adrenal atrophy and latent adrenal insufficiency. Exposure to stress in patients with such conditions creates a potential for acute adrenal crisis.[9]

Because of the diverse and pervasive effects of adrenocortical hormones, acute adrenal crisis is associated with dramatic findings. Glucocorticoid deficiency leads to water retention, significantly depressed to absent ability to maintain blood glucose levels without regular caloric intake (as in fasting), and failure to respond to norepinephrine from adrenergic nerve endings, which produces vulnerability to vascular dilatation and hemodynamic collapse in the presence of hypovolemia. Mineralocorticoid deficiency compounds the problem by allowing excessive renal sodium excretion, extracellular volume depletion, and potassium retention. Clinically, the findings include hyponatremia, hypoglycemia, hypotension, hypovolemia, and hyperkalemia.[1] Hyperthermia may also be present but does not always occur and is poorly understood.

Medical Therapies

Chronic adrenal insufficiency is treated with oral replacement of glucocorticoids. Mineralocorticoid replacement may also be used but is not always necessary, because glucocorticoids exert some mineralocorticoid effects and, in combination with an elevated salt intake, may suffice.

Commonly used glucocorticoid replacement regimens include either hydrocortisone (10 to 20 mg in the morning and 10 mg in the evening) or cortisone acetate (12.5 to 25 mg in the morning and 12.5 mg in the evening). Equivalent doses of prednisone, prednisolone, or dexamethasone may also be used. If symptoms are difficult to control, dexamethasone may be preferred because of its longer half-life and thus more sustained effects.[16]

If mineralocorticoid replacement is needed, fludrocortisone 0.1 to 0.2 mg is given orally, once a day. If glucocorticoid replacement is provided by the use of dexamethasone, prednisone, or prednisolone, mineralocorticoid supplement is more frequently required, because these glucocorticoids have minimal sodium-retaining properties compared with hydrocortisone or cortisone acetate. When the latter agents are utilized, a liberal salt intake, with further increases during periods associated with excessive diaphoresis or when there is vomiting or diarrhea, may avoid the need for mineralocorticoid replacement.[16]

In the presence of superimposed acute illness, especially involving fever or potential extracellular volume depletion as with vomiting or diarrhea, replacement doses of glucocorticoids are at least doubled. Vomiting within an hour after ingestion of the replacement dose is considered to cancel the dose and readministration is required. In severe illness, the replacement dose of glucocorticoids may need to be more than doubled.[9,16]

Adrenal crisis requires supraphysiologic doses of replacement glucocorticoids and rapid volume restoration. Blood samples are obtained for measurement of glucose, electrolytes, and cortisol, but treatment is initiated immediately without waiting for results if there is clinical suspicion of adrenal crisis. An intravenous bolus of 100 mg of hydrocortisone succinate, hydrocortisone phosphate, or an equivalent is followed by either repeat doses every 6 to 8 h or continuous infusion. Intravenous mineralocorticoid preparations are not available, but large doses of hydrocortisone coupled with volume restoration generally correct hypotension. If hypotension remains a problem even with glucocorticoid and fluid replacement, volume expanders may be used.[16]

Fluid replacement in adrenal crisis should be aggressive. Glucose-containing physiologic saline is the solution of choice at the outset. There may be a deficit of several liters, and fluid replacement must be rapid. Typically, the first liter is infused within 60 min, followed by 1 to 2 L over the ensuing 4 to 8 h.[9]

Nursing Management

Nursing management of patients with acute adrenal insufficiency begins with recognition of those at risk for crisis. Patients with known chronic Addison's disease may easily develop adrenal crisis during the stress associated with critical illness. Patients with a history of ongoing glucocorticoid therapy even for reasons unrelated to adrenal cortical function may experience adrenal atrophy or latent adrenal insufficiency and thus be vulnerable to stress-induced adrenal crisis. Overwhelming sepsis, especially involving menningococci, staphlococci, pneumococci, streptococci, or *Haemophilus influenzae,* may precipitate adrenal crisis, as may hemorrhagic disorders and leukemic crisis. Finally, intense and prolonged critical illness has been known to trigger adrenal crisis even in patients without a history of adrenal insufficiency. In this situation excessive stress-induced hypothalamic secretion of CRH and pituitary secretion of ACTH result in overstimulation of the adrenal cortex. Glandular decompensation results and is often accompanied by internal decompensation, hemorrhage, and glandular destruction.

The applicable nursing diagnoses and interventions are discussed below.

Nursing Diagnosis
Actual fluid volume deficit.

Insufficient mineralocorticoid activity in adrenal crisis leads to excessive renal sodium excretion and extracellular volume deficiency. Ongoing nursing assessment must center on evaluation of hydration status. Deliberate and sequential assessment includes careful monitoring of intake and output, consistent recording of daily weights, and monitoring for adequacy of central and peripheral perfusion. Blood pressure and heart rate should be monitored closely and serially at a frequency appropriate for the patient's condition. Postural changes in both parameters should also be evaluated. Continuous electrocardiographic monitoring is indicated; a shortened PR interval may result from insufficient glucocorticoids.[1] Hemodynamic monitoring may provide useful data regarding cardiac output, atrial filling pressure, and peripheral vascular resistance, all of which are decreased in acute adrenal crisis as a result of decreased vascular tone (glucocorticoid insufficiency) and hypovolemia (mineralocorticoid insufficiency).

Interventions
Nursing interventions include administration of glucocorticoid and volume replacements. As deficiencies are corrected, all ongoing assessments need to be performed frequently. Fluid replacement

must be rapid; if not carefully administered and monitored, it may result in cardiovascular overload.

Improvement is usually dramatic and rapid unless there is coexistent severe complicating illness. As the patient is stabilized, glucocorticoid dosages are decreased and changed to the oral route. Similarly, oral fluid intake is encouraged. At that point, the patient should be encouraged to consume food and fluids high in sodium. Oral fludrocortisone may also be administered.

Nursing Diagnosis

Mental or sensory alterations and need for stress reduction.

Insufficiency of glucocorticoids markedly decreases tolerance for all forms of stress. In addition, distinct central nervous system alterations occur in adrenal insufficiency. Although the basis is not well understood, distinct personality changes, which are reversed only by administration of glucocorticoids, commonly occur. These changes include irritability, apprehension, and fear and inability to concentrate. The impact of the changes is often exaggerated by concomitant and consistent increases in sensitivity to olfactory and gustatory stimuli.

Interventions

Nursing interventions include efforts to reduce exposure to stress and provide care in a way that conveys acceptance of and sensitivity to mental and sensory alterations. Extraneous stimuli may be limited by placing the patient in a private room. The impact of excessive olfactory sensitivity may be decreased by assuring adequate room ventilation. Care givers should avoid using perfumes, lotions, powders, or after-shave lotions, as even faint odors may seem overpowering and irritating to the patient.

Undisturbed rest periods and frequent, calm explanations should be provided. Care routines, unit noises, unfamiliar equipment, and uncertainty regarding the outcome are all legitimate reasons for fear and apprehension. Reassurance and support should be offered frequently and consistently.

Nursing Diagnosis

Impaired thermal regulation.

Hyperthermia frequently accompanies acute adrenal insufficiency; occasionally periods of hypothermia follow periods of fever. The mechanism behind such thermal changes in adrenal crisis is not understood. Nonetheless, nursing interventions need to be directed at maintaining a stable body temperature during hormone and fluid replacement.

Interventions

For hyperthermia, tepid baths and ice packs over major vessels may help reduce fever. Only clothing and bed linens needed for privacy should be used, and room temperature and ventilation should be maintained at a low comfort range (62 to 65°F). Cooling blankets and antipyretic agents such as aspirin or acetaminophen may also be used.

In the presence of hypothermia, extra bed linens and blankets should be provided. Room temperature should be increased to 75°F. Over-bed warming lights and externally heated blankets may also be helpful.

Patient Goals and Outcome Criteria

The treatment plan is successful if vital signs, hemodynamic parameters, and electrocardiographic tracings return to the patient's normal baselines; serum electrolytes, specifically serum sodium and potassium, as well as serum glucose, are within normal ranges; mental and personality changes are relieved; and body temperature is stabilized at a normal value.

Pheochromocytoma

A *pheochromocytoma* is a chromaffin tissue tumor that secretes epinephrine and norepinephrine. The tumor may be a single or multiple growth, either in isolation or diffusely spread wherever chromaffin tissue is present.

Chromaffin tissue is widespread in utero. After birth, however, most cells degenerate and disappear. The chromaffin tissue that remains is found predominantly in the adrenal medulla but also occurs less often in the paraspinous ganglionic regions of the abdomen and pelvis. The vast majority (95 percent) of pheochromocytomas occur in the adrenal medulla, the remainder in the abdomen and pelvis.[9]

The adrenal medulla is perhaps best characterized as an extension of the sympathetic nervous system. Its secretion of epinephrine and norepinephrine normally occurs with sympathetic activation. Physiologically glandular catecholamine secretion serves to reinforce the sympathetic "flight or fight" response. The medulla secretes both catecholamines, but proportionally more epinephrine than norepinephrine. The physiologic effects of both catecholamines are widespread and profound (see Chap. 36).

Secretion by pheochromocytomas results from sympathetic nervous system activation, but unlike the normally functioning adrenal medulla, pheochromocytomas secrete epinephrine and norepinephrine autonomously as well. Although the tumors are not consistent, they typically secrete both catecholamines. When hyperglycemia and hypermetabolism are prominent features, epinephrine is probably the more plentiful catecholamine. In situations characterized by hypertension of a fairly sustained nature, norepinephrine is likely to be the predominant catecholamine in the tumor.

Classically, pheochromocytoma is associated with paroxysmal and labile hypertensive episodes. One mechanism postulated for these episodes describes bursts of epinephrine from the tumors as the initiating event. The resultant decrease in peripheral resistance, coupled with hypovolemia (see below), dramatically reduces blood pressure and leads to sympathetic activation. The subsequent release of norepinephrine from vascular adrenergic nerve endings leads to vasoconstriction and hypertension. Presumably, the initiating burst of epinephrine depletes the tumor's epinephrine content, and despite both adrenomedullary and tumor stimulation with sympathetic activation, norepinephrine-mediated vasoconstriction dominates while synthesis and replenishment of tumor epinephrine content is restored. This mechanism is consistent with other findings associated with hypertensive episodes. Dizziness, fainting, syncopal episodes, flushing, warmth, and palpitations probably reflect the effects of epinephrine-induced peripheral vasodilatation and myocardial stimulation.[9,17]

Tachyarrhythmias, angina, cardiomegaly, and catecholamine myocardiopathy all occur with pheochromocytomas and are thought to reflect the effect of excessive catecholamines on the heart. Congestive heart failure from cardiomyopathy may result.

Hyperglycemia and hypermetabolism reflect the metabolic consequences of excessive catecholamine levels, effects which undoubtedly contribute to the polyuria and subsequent hypovolemia associated with pheochromocytoma. Diaphoresis that is often profuse no doubt also contributes to hypovolemia. Weight loss, weakness, and fatigue are common with pheochromocytomas and reflect the effect of the general catabolic condition. Anorexia and nausea, common gastrointestinal responses to sympathetic nervous system activation, further aggravate these findings.[17]

Headache almost always accompanies hypertensive events with pheochromocytomas. Although the mechanism is not clear, other central nervous system manifestations are associated with pheochromocytomas as well, including tremulousness, anxiety, agitation, and, infrequently, psychosis.[17]

Medical Therapies

Definitive treatment of pheochromocytoma requires excision of the tumor(s). Prior to surgery, however, specific preparation is required. Generally, the goals of presurgical treatment are to reduce or eliminate hypertension and/or hypertensive attacks and their associated symptoms and to institute adrenergic blockade to prevent precipitation of an extreme crisis state as a result of bursts of catecholamine secretion from the tumor(s) under the influence of anesthesia and surgical manipulation.

Depending upon whether the tumor is believed to be secreting predominantly norepinephrine or epinephrine, pharmacologic agents that primarily provide either alpha-adrenergic or beta-adrenergic blockade are used.

Traditionally, phenoxybenzamine, a noncompetitive inhibitor of norepinephrine, has been the agent of choice to provide alpha-adrenergic inhibition. Although the faster-acting agent prazosin has also been used, it tends to be associated with a greater incidence of symptomatic postural hypotension.

Typically, the initial dosage of phenoxybenzamine is 10 mg administered every 12 h. Every 2 days thereafter the dosage is increased by 10 mg a day to achieve a recumbent, resting blood pressure that is within normal range and is not associated with symptomatic postural hypotension. That dosage is then continued for approximately one week in an attempt to allow time for readjustment of alpha-adrenergic receptors. Because of the tendency to high levels of norepinephrine with untreated pheochromocytomas, alpha-adrenergic receptors tend to become undersensitized. With treatment, it is hoped that normal responsiveness can be reestablished in preparation for surgical removal of the tumor(s). If catecholamine myocardiopathy has led to heart failure, longer preparatory phenoxybenzamine treatment may be utilized in an attempt to optimize myocardial function preoperatively.[18]

When alpha-adrenergic blocking is not effective in controlling hypertension or when medication side effects limit the usefulness of such blocking, a norepinephrine synthesis blocker such as metyrosine may be tried. This agent inhibits the enzyme tyrosine hydroxylase and has been found to reduce the synthesis of norepinephrine to less than half the pretreatment rate. The initial dosage of 250 mg twice a day is gradually increased, according to patient tolerance, to up to 500 mg four times per day. Metyrosine depletes levodopa and dopamine in the central nervous system, however, and side effects tend to be pronounced. Excessive sedative effects and parkinsonian symptoms are frequently reported and often disabling.[18]

Tumors that secrete large amounts of epinephrine tend to be associated with a high incidence of tachyarrhythmias. Beta-adrenergic blocking may also be a part of surgical preparation for patients with such symptoms. Agents commonly utilized include propranolol and metoprolol. Dosage is typically adjusted to maintain a resting heart rate of 100 beats per minute or less.[18]

Nursing Management

Most commonly, patients with pheochromocytoma are encountered in the critical-care setting, either for severe hypertensive crises or for postoperative care following excision of the tumor(s). Occasionally, patients are also admitted for monitoring or evaluation of undiagnosed hypertension or syncope. In these patients the possibility of pheochromocytoma is often considered only after all other potential causes have been ruled out.

When the cause of hypertension is not clear, obtaining a urine sample to be sent for analysis for catecholamines and their by-products (vanillylmandelic acid, or VMA) is a simple and relatively inexpensive way to obtain useful diagnostic data (see Chap. 37). If hypertension is episodic, obtaining such a sample during or shortly after blood pressure elevations is crucial. Because 24-h levels of urinary catecholamine metabolites have a wide range of normal, bursts of secretion may be masked in the typical 24-h sample. Sometimes correlation of the urinary content of catecholamine by-products with clinical findings gives the only laboratory clue to the presence of a pheochromocytoma.

The paragraphs that follow present the applicable nursing diagnoses and appropriate interventions.

Nursing Diagnosis

Alteration in tissue perfusion related to catecholamine effects.

Epinephrine and norepinephrine exert profound effects on peripheral circulation in both direct and indirect ways. Norepinephrine produces pronounced peripheral vasoconstriction and with it increased systemic vascular resistance, increased cardiac workload, and peripheral ischemia. Epinephrine, on the other hand, produces vasodilatation and decreased peripheral resistance. With untreated pheochromocytomas, either sustained or episodic hypertension may occur. In addition, pronounced hypotension, exaggerated by postural and position changes, may also occur as a result of epinephrine-induced vasodilatation and varying degrees of hypovolemia. Thus, in the periphery, either sustained ischemia or alternating periods of vasoconstriction and vasodilatation may be found.

Additional indirect effects on tissue perfusion may result from the action of catecholamines on the myocardium. Both catecholamines increase heart rate, epinephrine to a much greater extent than norepinephrine. In addition, catecholamine myocardiopathy may lead to a decrease in cardiac output and potential congestive heart failure.

Nursing management of patients with pheochromocytoma begins with focused assessments of cardiovascular effectiveness and hydration status. Serial monitoring should include vital signs, checks for postural changes in blood pressure and heart rate, and continuous electrocardiographic monitoring. In the presence of sustained hypertension or severe episodic attacks, indwelling arterial monitoring may be utilized and requires careful serial monitoring. Intake and output and daily weights should be recorded, as should urine specific gravity, and tissue turgor should be assessed. Lung sounds also should be auscultated to monitor for rales and developing congestive failure.

Continual cognizance of the risk of myocardial ischemia or infarction and cerebral vascular accidents is needed with either sustained or episodic hypertension. Thus ongoing assessments should also include evaluation of chest pain and neurologic function and serial monitoring of orientation, level of consciousness, peripheral strength, and presence and symmetry of reflexes and motor function.

Interventions

Primary nursing interventions involve administration of fluid (oral and intravenous) and medications for adrenergic blocking. Alterations in cardiovascular function and fluid balance as fluid and drugs are administered should be recorded. Symptomatic postural hypotension with syncope and fainting may accompany administration of adrenergic blocking agents; and existing congestive heart failure or a predisposition to it may be aggravated by overly rapid correction of hypovolemia.

Postoperatively, undersensitized alpha-adrenergic receptors may predispose previously hypertensive patients to profound hypotension in the presence of even minor degrees of hypovolemia. Volume expanders, isotonic fluids, and blood products must be administered carefully to ensure support for circulating volume without producing undue demand on the heart.

Nursing Diagnosis

Alteration in nutrition: potential for less than body requirements.

Catecholamines increase metabolic rate, although epinephrine exerts somewhat more profound effects than norepinephrine. Excessive levels of catecholamines, as with untreated pheochromocytomas and especially those which secrete predominantly epinephrine, result in a general catabolic state and weight loss. Compounding the catabolic condition are catecholamine-induced gastrointestinal responses which impair both ability to eat and interest in eating. Under the influence of catecholamines, sphincters throughout the gastrointestinal tract close and blood flow to the tract decreases.[1] The resulting ischemia and spasm produce nausea, vomiting, and anorexia.

Interventions

Nursing interventions center on the need to increase caloric intake and reverse the effects of catabolism. Glucose-containing infusions may be necessary for patients unable to tolerate oral food intake. In such instances, serum and urinary glucose should be monitored. Preoperatively, hyperglycemia is likely as a result of catecholamine-induced increases in glycogenolysis and insulin resistance. When glucose-rich solutions are used, hyperglycemia can become pronounced and require insulin supplement. Control of serum glucose is also important to prevent the additive effect of osmotic duresis on the potential for fluid depletion secondary to the often profuse diaphoresis (see below) and polyuria.

Postoperatively there is a risk of hypoglycemia. Sudden decreases in levels of circulating catecholamines can decrease glycogenolysis. With removal of catecholamine-induced insulin resistance, blood glucose may fall significantly. Tachycardia, cold clammy skin, diplopia, or complaints of shakiness or "internal" tremors should prompt evaluation of serum glucose.

For patients able to eat, frequent small meals and high-calorie snacks should be provided. Efforts should be made to obtain favorite foods, either from the dietary department or by having family and friends bring them in. A dietary consultation may also be helpful to ensure adequate intake of vitamins and minerals and appropriate calorie intake. Intake and serial calorie counts should be carefully recorded.

Nursing Diagnosis

Alterations in comfort related to the potential for an exaggerated stress response.

Untreated pheochromocytomas secrete catecholamines autonomously as well as in conjunction with sympathetic nervous system activation. With bursts of catecholamine secretion, hypertension is often accompanied by palpitations, severe headaches, profuse diaphoresis, and sometimes intense anxiety and fear *(panic syndrome)*.

Interventions

The patient's immediate environment should be kept as quiet and restful as possible. Explanations and reassurances should be offered frequently and consistently. Keeping lights dimmed during hypertensive attacks and providing analgesics will help decrease the discomfort of headaches. Offering frequent assistance with hygiene and keeping the room cool and well ventilated may also help to relieve discomfort from diaphoresis during hypertensive periods. Additional blankets and bed clothing should be provided after hypertensive attacks to prevent chills from diaphoresis.

Nursing interventions must also be directed at eliminating stimuli known to evoke autonomous tumor secretion. Both nicotine and caffeine have been found capable of precipitating catecholamine discharge from pheochromocytomas; smoking, chewing tobacco, and drinking caffeine-containing substances (coffee, tea, cola drinks) should therefore be discouraged. Sudden or pronounced changes in activity level or position, especially assumption of a posture that compresses the abdomen, should be avoided to decrease the risk of stimulating catecholamine release from pheochromocytomas. Activities should be graduated and moderate and significant exertion prevented. Position changes should be made gradually, and positions requiring the patient to bend over or draw the knees upward should be avoided. Abdominal palpation should not be performed if pheochromocytoma is suspected. Potentially constricting or tight clothing or restraints should not be utilized.

The Valsalva maneuver should also be avoided, as it has been known to precipitate tumor secretion. Patients need to be taught how to move about in bed without holding their breath; assistance should be provided in changing position and getting up. Stool softeners, dietary roughage, and adequate fluids may help minimize effort associated with bowel evacuation.

Patient Goals and Outcome Criteria

Preoperatively, the treatment plan is successful if adrenergic blocking maintains blood pressure within normal range and the resting heart rate is 100 beats per minute or less, without symptomatic postural hypotension. Additionally, symptoms of acute congestive heart failure will be relieved and hypovolemia corrected, and blood glucose will remain within the normal range. Headaches and profuse diaphoresis, if not prevented, will be associated with significantly less discomfort. Myocardial ischemia or infarction and cerebrovascular accidents will be prevented.

Postoperatively, vital signs will return to normal range without adrenergic blocking, hypoglycemia will be avoided, and serum glucose will remain within normal range. Body weight will stabilize, appetite and gastrointestinal function will return to normal, and the incisional wound will heal.

References

1. Ganong, W. (1985). *Review of medical physiology* (12th ed.), Los Altos, CA: Lange.
2. Culpepper, R., et al. (1985). The posterior pituitary and water metabolism. In J. Wilson & D. Foster (Eds.), *Williams textbook of endocrinology* (7th ed., pp. 614–652). Philadelphia: Saunders.
3. Buross-Herlihy, J., & Garofano, C. (1984). The posterior pituitary and water metabolism. In H. Hamilton (Ed.), *Endocrine disorders* (pp. 46–71). Springhouse, PA: Nursing 84 Books.
4. Solomon, R. (1985). Diabetes insipidus. In R. Rakel (Ed.), *Conn's current therapy* (pp. 488–489). Philadelphia: Saunders.
5. Braunwald, E. (1983). Edema. In R. Petersdorf et al. (Eds.), In *Harrison's principles of internal medicine* (10th ed., pp. 167–170). New York: McGraw-Hill.
6. Levinsky, N. (1983). Fluids and electrolytes. In R. Petersdorf et al. (Eds.), *Harrison's principles of internal medicine* (10th ed., pp. 220–229). New York: McGraw-Hill.
7. Glickman, R., & Isselback, K. (1983). Abdominal swelling and ascites. In R. Petersdorf et al. (Eds.), *Harrison's principles of internal medicine* (10th ed., pp. 209–211). New York: McGraw-Hill.
8. Alspach, J., & Williams, S. (1985). *Core curriculum for critical care nursing* (3d ed.). Philadelphia: Saunders.
9. Bacchus, H. (1984). *Metabolic and endocrine emergencies* (2d ed.). Baltimore: University Park Press.
10. Ingbar, S., & Woeber, K. (1983). Diseases of the thyroid. In R. Petersdorf et al. (Eds.), *Harrison's principles of internal medicine* (10th ed., pp. 614–633). New York: McGraw-Hill.

11. Cooper, D., & Wood, L. (1985). Hyperthyroidism. In R. Rakel (Ed.), *Conn's current therapy* (pp. 501–506). Philadelphia: Saunders.

12. Kolodny, J., & Larsen, P. (1985). Hyperthyroidism. In R. Rakel (Ed.), *Conn's current therapy* (pp. 507–510). Philadelphia: Saunders.

13. Aurbach, G., et al. (1985). Parathyroid hormone, calcitonin, and the calciferols. In J. Wilson & D. Foster (Eds.), *Williams textbook of endocrinology* (7th ed., pp. 1137–1217). Philadelphia: Saunders.

14. Bilezikian, J. (1985). Hyper and hypoparathyroidism. In R. Rakel (Ed.), *Conn's current therapy* (pp. 491–493). Philadelphia: Saunders.

15. Bondy, P. (1985). Disorders of the adrenal cortex. In J. Wilson & D. Foster (Eds.), *Williams textbook of endocrinology* (7th ed., pp. 816–890). Philadelphia: Saunders.

16. Dexter, R. (1985). Adrenocortical insufficiency. In R. Rakel (Ed.), *Conn's current therapy* (pp. 481–482). Philadelphia: Saunders.

17. Landsberg, L., & Young, J. (1985). Catecholamines and the adrenal medulla. In J. Wilson & D. Foster (Eds.), *Williams textbook of endocrinology* (7th ed., pp. 891–965). Philadelphia: Saunders.

18. Sisson, J., & Thompson, N. (1985). Pheochromocytoma. In R. Rakel (Ed.), *Conn's current therapy* (pp. 513–515). Philadelphia: Saunders.

part 9

Hematologic
Patient-Care
Problems

40

Hematologic Anatomy and Physiology

Brenda S. Jackson
Mary Brewer
Jones

As multicellular organisms evolved, cells lost their direct contact with the external environment. A means of transporting nutrients and wastes between the interior and exterior environments gradually took form. The pump and conduits are the heart and blood vessels; the medium for carrying nutrients and wastes is, of course, the blood, consisting of a fluid in which cells and other substances are suspended. This *blood circulatory system* restores a kind of interface between the external and internal environments for essential functions.

The *hematopoietic system* includes blood-forming organs as well as blood-circulating organs. The blood-forming organs consist of the bone marrow, liver, spleen, thymus gland, and lymph nodes. During the years of early childhood, all the bones are filled with blood-forming red marrow, whereas in the adult the red marrow is found mainly in the ribs, the sternum, and the bodies of the vertebrae, which are therefore the major centers of erythropoietic (red cell) and granulopoietic (white cell) activity.

This chapter focuses on the physiologic characteristics and unique contributions of the various constituents of the hematopoietic system to homeostasis.

Functions of the Hematopoietic System

The primary physiologic functions of the hematopoietic system are respiration, nutrition, and excretion. Blood carries the respiratory gases (oxygen and carbon dioxide), nutrients, and wastes, providing transport between the hematopoietic tissues, the connective tissues, and other tissues and organs of the body. In its travels it distributes heat and

flows through specialized sensors which selectively react to such variables as osmotic pressure, pH, temperature, and the level of certain hormones. Thus other functions in which blood participates are temperature regulation and fluid and acid-base balance. The hematopoietic system also participates in defense: the blood contains cells and substances that attack infectious organisms and other foreign antigens. Through the process of hemostasis, blood participates in a mechanism which controls escape of the blood from the vascular compartment.

Blood: Composition and Characteristics

Blood is actually a fluid "connective tissue" containing circulating cells and a pale yellow liquid, called *plasma,* which constitutes approximately 55 percent of the total blood volume. Plasma represents part of the extracellular fluid of the body. The other 45 percent of the blood volume consists of solid suspended particles, cells making up most of this solid material. The ratio of red blood cells to blood plasma is expressed as the *hematocrit reading.* The normal hematocrit reading is approximately 40 percent for the adult female and 45 percent for the adult male. These values have a wide range and can be influenced by many factors. The hematocrit reading can serve as a valuable guide, especially useful in the assessment of the patient's hydration status. For example, it can be used in monitoring the patient response to aggressive fluid replacement in the treatment of an acute burn. As with most laboratory studies, it is best used in conjunction with other tests, so that several parameters can be monitored and compared in a comprehensive and serial manner.

Color, Specific Gravity, Osmotic Pressure, and pH

Color

The color of normal blood varies with the state of hemoglobin oxygenation. Arterial blood is normally bright red, reflecting the high oxygen saturation of the hemoglobin molecule contained within the red blood cells. Venous blood is a darker red, because much of the oxygen has been removed from the hemoglobin and given up to the tissues.

Specific Gravity

Blood normally has a specific gravity that ranges between 1.048 and 1.066, averaging about 1.055. *Specific gravity* is the ratio of the weight of a certain volume of a substance to the weight of an equal volume of water. The specific gravity of blood depends largely on the number of red blood cells present. Blood is three to four times more viscous than water. The viscosity of a liquid is due to the mutual attraction of its molecules, the molecules thereby tending to offer resistance to the flow of the liquid. The degree of viscosity of blood is a clinical consideration because the greater the viscosity, the more slowly blood flows through blood vessels and the greater is the force required to propel it through the circulatory system. Conditions which increase the viscosity of the blood, such as dehydration and polycythemia (increase in the number of red blood cells), decrease blood flow and can actually make circulation quite sluggish.

Osmotic Pressure

The osmotic pressure of plasma averages 300 mosm per kilogram of H_2O (equivalent to a 0.9% NaCl solution), mainly owing to the presence of various salts, waste products, glucose, and other crystalloids dissolved in the plasma. Plasma proteins also contribute to osmotic pressure, in particular the plasma protein albumin. Because the composition of the blood undergoes continual small changes, the osmotic pressure varies slightly. The change in composition is due to the passage of water and dissolved nutrients and the various waste products which continually pass in and out of the blood. The osmotic pressure is maintained within physiologic limits by the kidneys.

pH (Hydrogen Ion Concentration)

The pH of the blood is of great importance to homeostasis and can facilitate or retard the action of the many enzyme systems within the body. Optimum activity of enzymes requires that the pH of the blood remain within a relatively narrow range. In health this normal range is approximately 7.36 to 7.44, which is slightly alkaline. Various mechanisms related to the buffering capacity of the blood are involved in maintaining the constancy of the range within acceptable limits.

Blood Volume

The blood in the human body represents approximately 8 percent of the body weight. (The blood and the tissue fluid constitute almost 20 percent of the total body weight.) It is estimated that there is about 5 L of blood in the adult male and 3.5 to 4.5 L in the adult female, with normal increases in the pregnant state. Assuming normal renal function, this amount is relatively constant and is not increased or decreased markedly or for any length of time by drinking fluid, by injections, or by hemorrhage. When a person drinks a large quantity of water, the water is rather rapidly removed from the blood by the tissues or is eliminated by the kidneys. Keeping the amount of blood in the vascular compartment constant is of great importance, since without a minimum amount, adequate circulation is impaired and life is endangered.

Distribution of Blood

Of the 4500 mL of blood in the systemic circuit, about 18 percent (800 mL) is in the arteries and 6 percent (300 mL) in the capillaries. The remaining 76 percent (about 3400 mL) is in the venules and veins. Approximately 500 mL of the blood volume is in the pumonary circulation, of which about 24 percent (120 mL) is in the arteries. About 50 percent (250 mL) is in the capillaries and 30 percent (150 mL) in the veins and venules. The veins act as the body's capacitance, or reservoir, system. They have the ability to accommodate a large extra volume of blood with minimal increase in intravascular venous pressure.

Effects of Acute Blood Loss

For a period of time after an acute blood loss, hemoglobin values and plasma protein concentrations may remain normal. But because of the protective process known as *autotransfusion,* a decrease in intravascular pressure allows protein-free fluid to enter the circulation from the interstitial spaces. Initially, arteriolar vasoconstriction maintains *systemic pressure* (the pushing force of the blood). As blood loss continues, the fall in the systemic blood pressure coupled with the increasing concentration of plasma protein causes the plasma oncotic pressure to dominate and to draw fluid from cells and the interstitial spaces.

After 2 or 3 h, sufficient amounts of interstitial fluid enter the vascular compartment to dilute the blood, so that both the hemoglobin value and the plasma protein value fall. Over the next 24 h, as the circulating blood volume is restored, the decline in the plasma protein and hemoglobin values continues. Should this sequence of events occur without fluid replacement, a state of relative interstitial and intracellular dehydration will result.

Between 2 and 4 days after the blood loss, normal plasma protein concentration is restored. Hemoglobin values are normalized much more slowly, depending upon the quantity of blood lost and the availability of the body's iron stores, which are requisite to hemoglobin synthesis. In a healthy adult it is estimated that approximately 20 days is required for hemoglobin levels to become normal after a blood loss of 200 mL.

The clinical implication of this information is that hemoglobin and hematocrit values obtained soon after a hemorrhage may not yet reflect the severity of the blood loss. After autotransfusion has begun, however, the lowering of the two values reflects the movement of the interstitial fluid into the vascular compartment or the quantity of infused intravenous crystalloids and colloids. All these variables must be considered in relation to the time of hemorrhage for accurate evaluation of the hemoglobin and hematocrit values.

Plasma

As indicated earlier, plasma constitutes 55 percent of the blood volume. It is composed of serum and fibrinogen. If whole blood is withdrawn into a test tube and allowed to clot, after a period of time the clot will withdraw from the sides of the tube. The fluid expressed from the clot is called *serum.* Serum is primarily plasma minus the plasma protein fibrinogen.

Blood plasma is an extremely complex fluid containing large quantities of organic and inorganic substances. The yellowish color of plasma is due to the presence of bile pigments. The solutes which make up the largest percentage of total plasma weight are the plasma proteins. Except in hepatic failure or prolonged malnutrition, plasma proteins tend to be the most constant constituent of blood.

Site of Plasma Protein Synthesis

The parenchymal liver cell, the *hepatocyte,* is the main site of protein synthesis, with the exception of immunoglobulins, which are synthesized by lymphocytes. The hepatocyte is also the site of synthesis of the trace proteins in the plasma which constitute the coagulation factors essential to clot formation.

The Plasma Proteins

Approximately 6 to 8 percent of the plasma weight is made up of protein substances: albumin, serum globulins, fibrinogen, prothrombin, and plasminogen.

Serum Albumin

Serum albumin, the largest of the plasma proteins, plays an important part in the regulation of intravascular plasma volume. Since little protein escapes from blood vessels, there is far more inside than outside them. This difference in protein concentration sets up an osmotic pressure, tending to bring fluid in from the interstitial space. At the arteriolar end of a capillary bed this pressure is less than the blood pressure, so there is a net movement of fluid out of blood vessels. With the drop in blood pressure at the venous end of the capillary bed, the net movement of fluid is no longer outward but inward, in accordance with the osmotic pressure created by the plasma proteins.

If this dynamic relationship is deranged as a result of a decrease in plasma proteins, for instance, in hypoalbuminemia, more fluid leaves the vessel at the arterial end than reenters at the venous end, and the result is interstitial edema.

Pathologic conditions associated with abnormally low serum protein levels include liver disorders, in which protein decline is the result of inadequate synthesis, and the nephrotic syndrome, in which the problem is the loss of large quantities of plasma proteins through the kidney.

Serum Globulins

Serum globulins can be subdivided into alpha, beta, and gamma fractions. The alpha fraction is associated with the transport of steroids, lipids, and bilirubin. The beta fraction is associated with iron and copper transport and transport of the beta-lipoproteins. Immunoglobins are discussed later, in the section, "Leukocytes and the Immune Process." Fibrinogen, prothrombin, and plasminogen are discussed under "Coagulation and Coagulation Factors," later in this chapter.

Hematopoiesis

Hematopoiesis is a process of self-renewal. It involves the production and maintenance of physiologic levels of the blood and bone marrow cells. The process includes cellular proliferation, division of immature hematopoietic stem cells, and ultimately, the differentiation of the stem cells into mature cell types. Cells produced by the organs of the hematopoietic system include erythrocytes (red blood cells); neutrophils, lymphocytes, monocytes, eosinophils, and basophils (white blood cells, or leukocytes); platelets; and plasma cells. Most of these cell types are illustrated in Fig. 40-1, and their normal values are listed in Table 40-1.

Blood Cell Origins and Development

In postnatal human life, erythrocytes, granular leukocytes or granulocytes, and monocytes, in addition to megakaryocytes (platelet precursors), are produced in the bone marrow or myeloid tissue. However, the lymphocyte (a type of leukocyte) is produced in lymphoid tissue and the thymus gland, as well as in the bone marrow.

Several lines of indirect but convincing evidence point to the existence in human bone marrow of a pluripotent hematopoietic stem cell precursor capable of differentiating into erythroid, granulocytic, monocytic, megakaryocytic, and certain lymphoid cell lines. This pluripotent cell may give rise to a more restricted, multipotential marrow stem cell, which in turn produces the restricted precursor for erythrocytes, granulocytes, monocytes, and platelets.[1]

Research with experimental animals has demonstrated the presence of such multipotential stem cells. Evidence in humans for such a cell is derived from certain myeloproliferative disorders such as polycythemia vera, myelofibrosis with myeloid metaplasia, and chronic myelogenous leukemia, in which one precursor cell gives rise to the abnormal erythrocytes, granulocytes, and platelets but not to lymphocytes, marrow fibroblasts, and other cell lines.

Stem cells are a dormant reserve; they are present in small numbers in blood and bone marrow. Their turnover depends upon the needs of the body. Indirect evidence suggests that the structure of the stem cell is quite similar to that of the lymphocyte. The parent cell is described as resembling a large lymphocyte which contains a large nucleus with one or more nucleoli and with considerable basophilic cytoplasm.

Hematopoietic Principle

Mature erythrocytes are generated from precursor stem cells under the influence of the growth factor, burst-promoting activity (BPA), and the glycoprotein hormone erythropoietin.[2] Erythropoietin is manufactured in the kidney and is secreted in response to hypoxia and anemia. Erythropoietin levels appear to increase at a central venous O_2 tension of 30 mmHg (normal = 38 mmHg). This tension corresponds to a mean hemoglobin concentration of 9.2 ± 1.6 g/dL. There is a direct relation between the degree of hypoxia and the degree of marrow stimulation.[1]

Differentiation to the granulocyte-macrophage lineage requires the two humoral growth factors, granulocyte-macrophage colony-stimulating factor (GM-CSF) and granulocyte colony-stimulating factor (G-CSF). Granulocytopoiesis is stimulated by

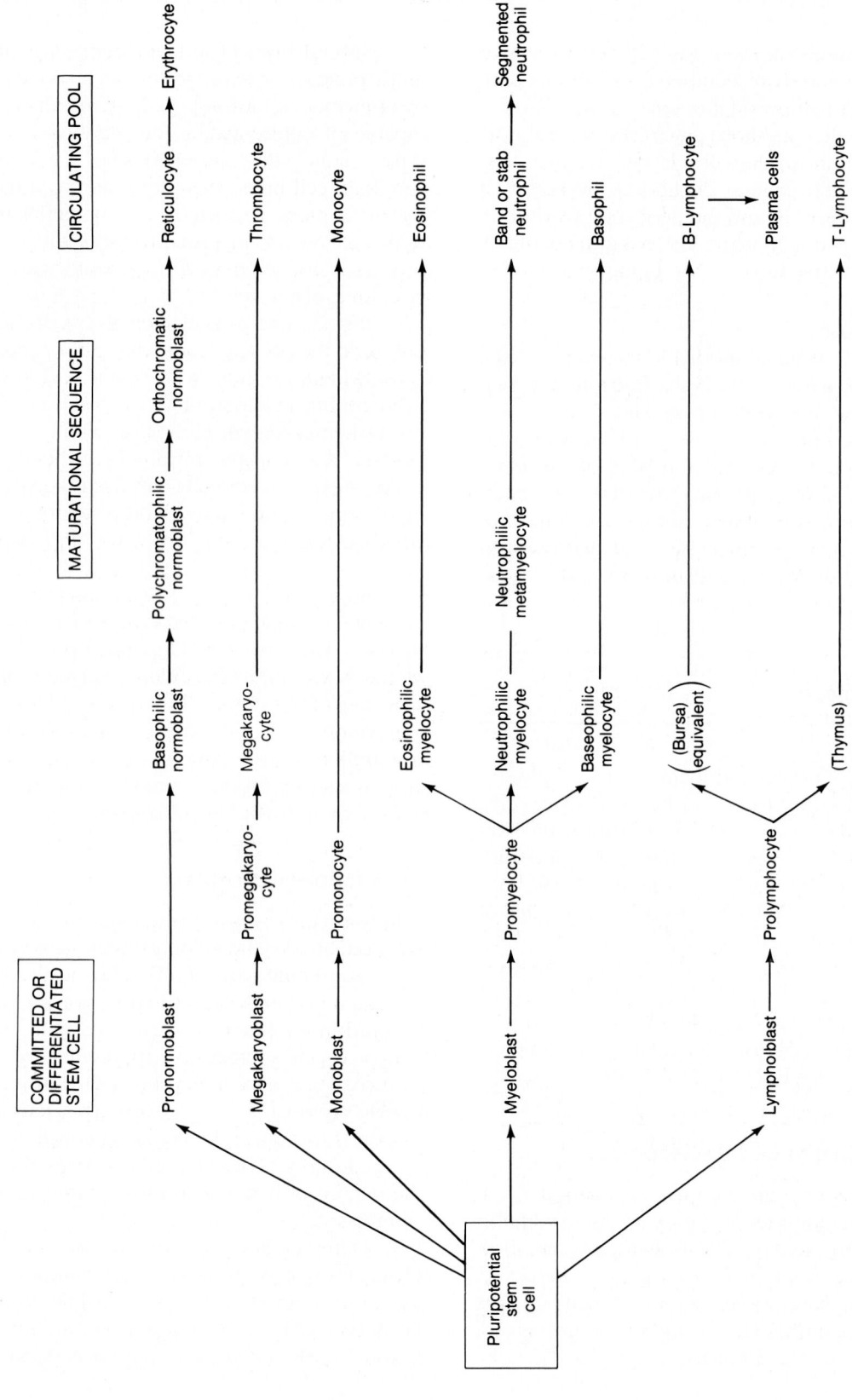

Figure 40-1 Theory of formation and maturation of blood cells (hematopoiesis). *(From S. A. Price and L. M. Wilson, Pathophysiology, 3d ed., McGraw-Hill, New York, 1986, p. 181.)*

neutropenia. Megakaryocytopoiesis and platelet production appear to be regulated, in part, by a humoral substance called *thrombopoietin* and are stimulated by thrombocytopenia.[2]

For all cell lines, proliferation and differentiation are precisely regulated so that mature cell production equals mature cell loss. This requires the production of an average of about 150 million red cells and 120 million granulocytes during every minute of life.

Blood Cells

Erythrocytes (Red Blood Cells)

Normal human erythrocytes are extremely flexible and elastic biconcave disks without nuclei. The primary component of the erythrocyte is hemoglobin, whose function is the transport of oxygen and carbon dioxide. Red blood cells (RBCs) are capable of traveling at high speeds and under increasing pressure, and can bend and twist as they pass through the tiny capillaries. This assumption of an elongated shape exposes more surface area for the exchange of oxygen and carbon dioxide.

Although RBCs contain no nucleus, they are capable of maintaining hemoglobin in the functional state, but they are unable to maintain their structural integrity or to reproduce. Despite the fact that they are not true cells, since they are without a nucleus, they are metabolically quite active. It is estimated that erythrocytes consume 1.5 to 2.2 mmol of glucose per liter of blood every hour. This metabolic activity is required to pump out sodium and pump in potassium against an electrochemical gradient and to reduce the methemoglobin to hemoglobin.

Transport of Oxygen

The main function of the erythrocytes is respiration. This function is accomplished by the unique presence of the hemoglobin pigment in the RBC. The iron-containing protein hemoglobin binds with oxygen in the lungs and transports it from the lungs to the tissue. Globin is a simple protein which is attached to heme, the iron-containing pigment.

Normally, there is about 15 g of hemoglobin per 100 mL of blood. The affinity of hemoglobin for oxygen is modified by several factors. As the blood pH falls, this affinity also falls, causing more oxygen to be released to the tissues. Increasing the intracellular concentration of certain organic phosphates, especially 2,3-diphosphoglycerate (2,3-DPG), also decreases the affinity of hemoglobin for oxygen and results in oxygen delivery to the tissues. Hypoxia increases the production of 2,3-DPG in the cell, and this creates an environment in which oxygen delivery to the tissues is increased. Fetal hemoglobin does not bind 2,3-DPG, and as a result, has a high affinity for oxygen. This mechanism is beneficial, maximizing the amount of oxygen picked up in the low-oxygen environment in utero.

Life Span and Removal of Erythrocytes

Erythrocyte formation is one of the most active anabolic processes in the body. In the human adult, about 2×10^{11} erythrocytes are replaced by the bone marrow every 24 h. Each milliliter of blood contains approximately 5 billion erythrocytes, and since their average life span is normally about 120 days, $\frac{1}{120}$ of the circulating cells (about 25 g) must be removed every day from the circulation. This 120-day life span represents the interval between a cell's delivery from the bone marrow and its ultimate destruction. The process of elimination results in the daily destruction of almost 1 percent of the total RBCs in the body.

Clinical Significance of Red Blood Cell Maturity

When bone marrow produces RBCs at a very rapid rate in response to body demands, many of the released cells are not mature. The degree of immaturity and the number of cells present in the bloodstream at any one time reflect the stress that is being placed upon the system. When demands for production are great, the percentage of circulating immature erythrocytes (*reticulocytes*) may rise as much as 30 to 50 percent above normal. Should the demand continue or increase, a cell type which is even more immature, the *normoblast,* may appear in large numbers. In some of the serious anemias the number of normoblasts may be as high as 5 to 20 percent of all circulating RBCs. Cells of still greater immaturity, the erythrocyte precursors such as proerythroblasts, may also appear in the circulating blood. This information has diagnostic significance in the determination of the various types of anemias. In general, classic abnor-

Table 40-1 Average Range of Normal Blood Values Measured at Different Ages

Component	Preterm	Full Term	2 days	7 days	14 days	2 mo
Hemoglobin, g/100 mL	13–18	13.7–20	18–21.2	19.6	13–20	13.3
RBC/mm³, in millions	5–6	5–6	5.3–5.6	5.3	5–5.1	4.5
Nucleated RBC, %	5–15	1–5	1–2	0*		
Hematocrit, g/100 mL	45–55	43–65	56.1	52.7	30–66	38.9
WBC/mm³, in thousands	15	9–38	21–22	5–21	5–21	5–21
Neutrophils, %	40–80	40–80	55	40	36–40	36–40
Eosinophils, %	2–3	2–3	5	5	2–3*	
Lymphocytes, %	30–31	30–31	20	20	48–53	48–53
Monocytes, %	6–12	6–12	15	15	8–9	
Immature WBC, %	Over 10	3–10	5	0*		
Platelets/mm³, in thousands	50–300	100–350	400	400	300–400	300–400
Reticulocytes, %	Up to 10	4–6	3	3	0.5–1.6†	

*Not normally found in the circulating blood after this age.
†Remains approximately the same for succeeding age levels.
Source: P. Green and L. Cooper in G. Scipien et al. (eds.), *Comprehensive Pediatric Nursing,* 3d ed., New York, McGraw-Hill, 1986, pp. 986–987.

malities are associated with specific types of anemia. See Table 40-1 for normal RBC values at various ages. Figure 40-1 depicts the various erythrocyte precursors.

Leukocytes (White Blood Cells)

The leukocytes are the body's primary defense against extraneous substances. They are larger than red blood cells and are nucleated. Leukocytes are classified on the basis of the unique structure of various types of leukocyte and the affinity of each type for a certain dye (Fig. 40-1). *Polymorphonuclear leukocytes* (PMNs), sometimes shortened to "polys," include those WBCs which have a granular appearance because of the presence of various cytoplasmic granules. These granular leukocytes, or *granulocytes,* are of three types: neutrophils, eosinophils, and basophils. Nongranular leukocytes are of two types: monocytes and lymphocytes. Table 40-1 shows the normal values for each type of WBC at various ages and for male and female adults.

Although leukocytes are less numerous than RBCs, this group of blood cells contains a variety of cells which are specialized for different functions. As mentioned, the primary function of the WBCs is to provide the required humoral and cellular response to invading infectious organisms and foreign antigens. This function is accomplished in part by a process called *phagocytosis*. Through this process the neutrophils and monocytes ingest and destroy invading organisms and foreign particles. Although the leukocytes are transported via the circulating blood to all parts of the body, phagocytosis actually occurs within the interstitial fluid.

Neutrophils

Neutrophils are the most numerous of the granulocytes. They make up 60 to 70 percent of the total number of WBCs in the peripheral blood of adults and 18 to 40 percent in infants.

The nuclei of neutrophils stain deeply with neutral dye. The nuclei are irregular and often have shapes which look like the letters E, Z, and S. Delicate filaments separate segments of the cell, making it appear that there are several nuclei. These filaments have length but no breadth. A *segmented* neutrophil has at least two of its lobes separated by such filaments. A *band* neutrophil has either a strand of nuclear material that is thicker than one of these filaments connecting the lobes or a U-shaped nucleus of uniform thickness. The number of lobes in normal neutrophils ranges from two to five. This description is given as a basis for a later discussion of various findings in different clinical situations.

Segmented neutrophils make up, on average, 56 percent of total leukocytes, band neutrophils 3 percent. A *shift to the left* occurs when there is an increased number of bands and fewer mature

Table 40-1 Average Range of Normal Blood Values Measured at Different Ages (Continued)

3 mo	6 mo	1 yr	2 yr	4 yr	8–12 yr	Adult Male	Adult Female
9.5–14	10.5–14	11–12.2	11.6–13	12.6–13	11–19	14–18	12–16
13–4.5	4.6	4.6–4.7	4.7–4.8	4.7–4.8	4.8–5.1	5.4	4.8
28–41	33–42	32–40	34–40	36–44	39–47	42–52	37–47
6–18	1–15	4.5–13.5	9–12	8–10	8	5–10	5–10
30–35	30–45	40–50	40–50	50–55	55–60	35–70	35–70
						2–3	2–3
55–63	48–60	48–53	48–50	40–48	30–39	30–35	30–35
7	5	5	5–8	5–8	5–8	5–8	5–8
360	250–350†					250–350	250–350
						0.5–1.6	0.5–1.6

*Not normally found in the circulating blood after this age.
†Remains approximately the same for succeeding age levels.
Source: P. Green and L. Cooper in G. Scipien et al. (eds.), *Comprehensive Pediatric Nursing*, 3d ed., New York, McGraw-Hill, 1986, pp. 986–987.

neutrophils in the blood, as well as a lower than average number of lobes in segmented cells.

An increase in the number of circulating neutrophils, called *neutrophilia,* is associated with any inflammatory process. Neutrophils are attracted to areas of inflammation and bacterial proliferation by *chemotaxis.* Chemotaxis occurs in response to the liberation of serum chemicals called *chemotaxins.* This reaction is quite complex and may involve chemotactic stimuli derived from the activated complement system, from bacteria or bacterial products, and from lymphocytes. Neutrophils themselves may release chemotactic substances.

Neutrophilia can be expected to occur in association with any activity or process which increases the level of epinephrine, ACTH, or adrenal corticoids in the bloodstream. Such diverse conditions as foreign protein injection, excessive exercise, blood loss, and excessive fatigue all result in an increase in circulating neutrophils. The vasodilatory effects of epinephrine and the resultant increase in blood flow through capillary beds flush out sequestered leukocytes. Rapid blood flow through the capillaries mobilizes these granular leukocytes, making them available for response to any insulted body tissue.

Eosinophils

The mature eosinophil constitutes 2 to 4 percent of the total number of leukocytes in the adult peripheral circulation. The cell is slightly larger than the mature neutrophil, and the nucleus occupies a relatively smaller volume of the cell. The function of eosinophils is thought to be detoxification of foreign proteins, but this is still under investigation. During an allergic attack the total number of circulating eosinophils increases, collecting at the site of antigen-antibody reaction. Eosinophils are present in large numbers in the mucosa of the intestinal tract and also in the tissues of the lungs. Both these locations are points of entry of foreign proteins into the body. The number and function of eosinophils are depressed by the administration of glucocorticoids.

With respect to their phagocytic activity, eosinophils are referred to as *microphages.* These WBCs are thought to be active in the phagocytosis of the causative organism of trichinosis, the trichinae parasite. The suggested function of the eosinophil is the detoxification of the protein substances secreted by these organisms.

Basophils

A third type of leukocyte with specific granules is the basophil. Basophils are not phagocytic cells per se but are similar to mast cells, which are located outside many of the body's capillaries. Mast cells liberate heparin into the bloodstream. Endogenously secreted heparin is considered important in preventing blood clot formation or growth; they are also active in accelerating the removal of fat particles from the bloodstream after a fatty meal. Basophils have a high content of heparin, seratonin, and histamine and play an important role in acute systemic allergic reactions. When the basophil undergoes degranulation during an anaphylactic reaction, it liberates heparin, seratonin, and histamine in the process.

Although normally the total number of basophils is relatively low, this number may increase in asthma as well as in association with myeloproliferative disorders such as tuberculosis; during estrogen administration; in carcinoma; after splenectomy; in inflammatory bowel disease; and in hypothyroidism. A slight elevation is maintained in states of chronic inflammation. Inflammation has a coagulant effect upon RBCs, and it is theorized that the increase in basophils is in response to the body's need for more heparin to prevent RBC loss in coagulation.

Monocytes

Monocytes are regarded as mobile components of the reticuloendothelial system (RES). Most of the RES is composed of fixed cells lining sinusoids in the lymph nodes, liver, and bone marrow. Mature monocytes are released into the circulation and are carried to their sites of function.

Monocytes are the largest of the nongranular leukocytes, but they have relatively few cytoplasmic granules. Upon release into the bloodstream, they are transformed into mature forms known as *macrophages*. Macrophages are capable of phagocytizing large foreign particles and cell fragments. They even have the capacity to engulf whole red blood cells and the malarial parasite. An important function of the macrophage is to phagocytize necrotic tissue in chronic infections.

Both the microphage (eosinophil) and the macrophage contain large quantities of lysosomal enzymes which are both proteolytic and lipolytic. In addition, these phagocytes contain substances which are bactericidal; that is, they are capable of destroying bacteria before they can multiply and destroy the phagocytic cell.

In the process of combating infection and clearing necrotic debris, the phagocytes themselves eventually die. The accumulation of the dead pha-

gocytes and the necrotic process result in the production of material commonly known as *pus*. Containing the infectious process and preventing its dissemination are vital components of the defense function of these cells.

Monocytes have demonstrated a unique sensitivity in studies with corticosteroids in vitro. After brief exposure to low concentrations of hydrocortisone, monocytes show impaired random movement, chemotaxis, and bactericidal activity.

Lymphocytes

Lymphocytes are mononuclear leukocytes which originate and first differentiate in the primary lymphoid structures of the bone marrow and thymus gland and then are distributed to the secondary lymphoid tissue of the lymph nodes, spleen, Peyer's patches in the liver, and intestines. They have a relatively large nucleus and scanty nongranular cytoplasm.

These cells make up about 20 to 35 percent of the total leukocytes in the normal adult and approximately 40 to 70 percent of the leukocytes in infants.

Leukocytosis

The term *leukocytosis* refers to an absolute increase in the concentration of white blood cells in the peripheral blood. This definition does not distinguish the degree of immaturity or the cell type, both of which are important considerations. The normal range for the concentration of WBCs is 5000 to 10,000 per cubic millimeter in the healthy adult. A total white blood cell count above 10,000 to 12,000 per cubic millimeter constitutes leukocytosis. *Granulocytosis* refers to an increase in the number of circulating granulocytes and is calculated as the product of the total leukocyte count and the percentage of granulocytes in the differential count. The upper limit of normal for the absolute number of granulocytes is 8000 per cubic millimeter.

Various types of nonpathologic stimuli such as exercise, sudden emotional surges, or administration of epinephrine may produce an increase in the circulating granulocytes to as much as two to three times normal. These acute reactions result from the release of the granulocytes from maturation-storage pools in the bone marrow.

Pathologic stimuli which produce granulocytosis include infections, inflammation, invasive tumors, and myeloproliferative disease. The mechanism producing the increase in granulocytes may be increased proliferation, prolongation of survival time, shift of this type of white blood cell from storage to the circulating pool, or any combination of these factors. The observed response in terms of cell type tends to be quite specific to the inciting stimulus. In certain granulomatous disorders, monocytes respond; in allergic and parasitic conditions it is the eosinophils that increase. Basophilic leukocytes are associated with hypersensitivity reactions. If the stimulus or stress on the system continues over a period of time, immature forms of these cell types may be seen—a clue to the magnitude of the disorder.

Pyogenic bacteria in particular induce *neutrophilia,* or *neutrophilic leukocytosis* (an increase in the absolute count of neutrophils). Typically this type of infection is localized such as appendicitis, salpingitis, or otitis media. In general, it is believed that the more pathogenic the agent, the higher the resulting neutrophil count. In fact, the height of the leukocytosis is frequently used as an index of a patient's resistance potential. As indicated earlier, a *shift to the left* refers to a neutrophilic leukocytosis in which there is an increase in young or immature forms and in segmented forms of neutrophils. The greater the shift to the left, the more severe the infection. There is also an increase in the number of bands as well as a lower average number of lobes in the segmented cells. A *shift to the right* refers to an increase in mature, hypersegmented polymorphonuclear leukocytes. This type of shift, unlike the shift to the left with its infectious etiology, is associated with pernicious anemia and chronic morphine addiction. It has been reported that in early chronic granulocytic leukemia, it is occasionally possible to see both types of shift simultaneously, i.e., a right and a left shift.

Leukocytes and the Immune Process

Traditionally the concept of immunity was almost synonymous with resistance to infectious disease. A person fortunate enough to have survived an acute infection was considered to have developed an *immunity,* i.e., a resistance against future episodes of that particular infection.

The concept of immunity has broadened in recent years to include noninfectious agents. Through the immune process, an immune attack is organized against a foreign protein or tissue but not against a person's own or genetically identical tissue. The immune system is extremely sensitive in its ability to recognize even slight differences between what is "self," or native to the organism, and what is foreign, or "nonself."

In the immune process, immunocytes work synergistically with phagocytes to maintain the integrity of the whole organism against invading organisms. Immunocytes are classified morphologically as lymphocytes, plasma cells, and their precursor cells.

The precursor of the lymphocyte is believed to be the multipotential, primitive stem cell that also gives rise to the common progenitor cell of the myeloid, erythroid, and megakaryocytic cell lines. Lymphoid precursor cells travel to specific sites and then differentiate into cells capable of either expressing cell-mediated immune responses or secreting immunoglobulins. The lymphocytes responsible for cell-mediated immunity differentiate in the thymus gland. The resulting cell type is defined as a *thymus-dependent lymphocyte,* or *T cell.* The site of formation of lymphocytes with the potential to differentiate into antibody-producing cells (*plasma cells*) has not been definitively identified. In chickens it is the bursa of Fabricius, and for this reason lymphocytes from the "bursa-equivalent" organ in humans are called *B cells.* These lymphocytes are produced in hematopoietic tissue, primarily the bone marrow.

Lymphocytes participate in the process of immunity in several unique ways. It is this cell type that gives specificity to the attack by phagocytes upon foreign antigenic material. The memory of such specificity is also a function of these immunocytes, so that future defenses against a known antigenic agent are more rapidly mobilized. The immune response is described in detail in Chap. 44.

Plasma cells are B lymphocytes which have undergone differentiation into large, metabolically active cells after stimulation by antigens. These cells produce immunoglobulins on the endoplasmic reticulum. Usually, each plasma cell produces only one class of immunoglobulin. Plasma cells are found predominantly in the lymph nodes, spleen, and bone marrow, not circulating in peripheral blood.

Occasionally plasma cells undergo neoplastic transformation and produce abnormal amounts of immune globulins. These dyscrasias can cause monoclonal production of single types of immunoglobulin or polyclonal production of multiple types of immunoglobulin which circulate freely. In multiple myeloma (a malignant proliferation of plasma cells), abnormal amounts of immunoglobulin are produced, as well as an osteoclast activating factor which causes destructive and painful bone lesions. The immunoglobulins produced in plasma cell dyscrasias may not function properly in the immune response, so that even if their relative amounts are increased, the subject may have an impaired response to antigens and therefore be prone to develop infections.

Platelets

Platelets are the smallest of the formed elements of the blood. They are minute biconvex disks about 2 to 3 μm in diameter. Platelets are formed by the cytoplasmic division of megakaryocytes. *Megakaryocytes* are extremely large cells of the hematopoietic series present in the adult in the bone marrow, lung, and spleen. The separation of the individual platelets from the parent cell is an orderly process involving the formation and fusion of small cytoplasmic vesicles to form the platelet membrane. It is estimated that each megakaryocyte is capable of producing more than a thousand platelets. Figure 40-1 depicts platelet precursors.

Platelets normally have a life span of 7 to 14 days. Approximately 10 to 15 percent of circulating platelets are continually being consumed in repairing the small vascular injuries which occur as part of daily life.

The platelet count for a normal adult ranges from 150,000 to 400,000 per mm³, with slightly higher levels being found in arterial blood. In general there is no sex-linked difference in platelet counts, although variations in the normal range are associated with the menstrual cycle and with pregnancy. A slight increase in platelet count is reported

to occur at the time of ovulation, followed by a progressive decrease in the 14 days preceding menstruation. A second rapid increase occurs after the onset of menses. Platelet counts do not appear to change significantly during pregnancy.

Variables Affecting Quantity and Quality

The rate of platelet production and the level of circulating platelets are believed to be controlled by a humoral factor called *thrombopoietin* or *thrombopoiesis-stimulating factor*. The origin and nature of this factor are not known at this time. It has been demonstrated that chronic thrombocytopenia may well be the result of the deficiency of a factor which is normally present in the plasma and which is necessary for the maturation of megakaryocytes and therefore normal platelet production. In this connection, it is now believed that the clinical value of using fresh whole blood in correcting platelet deficiencies versus platelet replacement or supplement is predicated upon the fact that the transfusion provides thrombopoietin.

The level of circulating catecholamines has been documented to have a profound effect on platelet levels. Administration of adrenalin produces an immediate 20 to 50 percent increase in the platelet count. This response is thought to be the result of platelet mobilization from the splenic pool. However, since an increase in the platelet count, which is normally associated with exercise, has been demonstrated to occur in patients after splenectomy, it is now believed that the lung also releases platelets into the circulation. Regardless of the type of stimulus, i.e., exercise or catecholamines, the platelet count returns to normal within 30 min after the initial rise. The biochemical effects of exercise are reported to be associated with adenosine diphosphate (ADP)–induced platelet aggregation and platelet adhesion. Platelets effect most of their hemostatic function by aggregation and adhesion. *Aggregation* refers to platelets attaching to one another. *Adhesion* is the attachment of platelets to nonplatelet surfaces, e.g., blood vessel walls or foreign surfaces.

Other variables are known to influence the quantity and quality of circulating platelets. Altitude, hypoxia, and smoking may influence both the number and the characteristics of platelets. A significant increase in platelet number is produced by high altitudes, and in animal studies even short-term hypoxia produces thrombocytosis. Studies have suggested that smoking may not only shorten the life of platelets but also may produce hyper-aggregability of these cell fragments. A large number of disease states as well as various drugs are also associated with adverse effects upon platelet number and function.

Role in Hemostasis

Platelets are often referred to as *thrombocytes* because of the primary role which platelets play in hemostasis. Platelets contribute to hemostasis in two distinct ways: they participate in the hemostatic mechanism physically by occluding rents and tears in small vessels by the formation of platelet plugs, and they are involved in the coagulation process by their biochemical activities.

During the process of coagulation the platelets respond to collagen and thrombin by the *release reaction,* during which the platelets release intracellular constituents (e.g., ADP, adenosine triphosphate, serotonin, catecholamines, potassium, calcium, and platelet factor 4) into the surrounding plasma. This is not a passive process but is energy-dependent and is accomplished by the cell's contractile mechanism. The release reaction is considered to be a secretory function which resembles secretory processes observed in other cell systems, as in the adrenal gland. The functioning of platelets in hemostasis is measured in the standard tests summarized in Table 40-2.

Relative and Absolute Thrombocytopenia

To be considered normal, platelets must be qualitatively or functionally adequate and must be present in adequate numbers. An artificial thrombocytopenia, a clinical state in which laboratory values reflect normal or near normal platelet levels, may exist if the platelets are functionally abnormal. This possibility must always be considered should unexplained bleeding (oozing) or petechiae occur in the presence of normal platelet levels.

Characteristics

The mature platelet is a complex structure and is quite active metabolically, although, like the erythrocyte, it contains no nucleus. Protein makes up about 52 to 60 percent of the dry weight of thrombocytes and approximately 10 percent of their net weight. Some of the protein is bound in the form of enzymes, while the remainder is incorporated in structural components of the cell. A number of different platelet proteins have been identified. Two of these are of particular importance in hemostasis. One is fibrinogen, normally considered to be only a plasma protein, which represents between 10 and 13 percent of the soluble protein fraction present in platelets. Fibrinogen, as is discussed later, undergoes physical and chemical changes to form the fibrin threads of the clot. With respect to platelet function, fibrinogen is an essential cofactor for ADP-induced platelet aggregation besides being involved in other platelet activities.

Another platelet protein active in hemostasis and having unique contractile properties is called *thrombostenin.* Platelets have occasionally been referred to as *muscle cells.* Thrombostenin is believed to be active in the consolidation phase of the hemostatic plug formation, which is characterized by active contraction of the platelet mass. Ninety percent of the total amount of platelet thrombostenin is contained in the cytoplasm, while the remainder is located on the surface of the platelet.

Platelet Coagulation Factors

Platelets contain other substances which are active in blood coagulation and which are unique to thrombocytes. These are indicated in the literature by arabic numbers rather than by the roman numerals that are used to indicate the plasma coagulation factors. There are four platelet factors, factors 1 through 4. Factor 1 is now known to be the same as plasma coagulation factor V but is contained within the platelets.

Fibrinogen-activating factor, which accelerates the clotting of fibrinogen by thrombin, was formerly designated factor 2. It is not released or enhanced by aggregation.

Platelet factor 3 is a phospholipid-like activity present in platelets which becomes available when platelets aggregate. This activity can develop even when the release reaction does not occur. Although its presence is not sufficient to initiate clotting, platelet factor 3 is necessary for clotting in the intrinsic system.

Table 40-2 Coagulation Studies

Study	Purpose	Normal Values	Clinical Significance
Bleeding time	Measures platelet and vascular function	2–9½ min	Prolonged in thrombocytopenia, thrombocytopathy, von Willebrand's disease, aspirin ingestion, anticoagulant therapy, and uremia
Platelet count	Assesses platelet concentration	150,000–400,000/mm^3	Decreased in ITP and bone marrow malignancies, drugs, especially chemotherapeutic agents, may cause prolonged bleeding. Elevated in early myeloproliferative disorders; after splenectomy, may predispose to later thrombotic episodes
Clot reaction	Assesses platelet adequacy to form fibrin clot	Clot retracts to one-half size in 1 h, firm clot in 24 h if undisturbed	Poor clot retraction in thrombocytopenia and polycythemia; lysis of clot in fibrinolysis
Lee-White clotting time (coagulation)	Assesses coagulation mechanism—time required for solid clot on exposure to glass	6–12 min	Relatively insensitive test. Prolonged with severe deficiencies of coagulation factors, in excessive anticoagulant therapy, and with selected antibiotics. Decreased with corticosteroid therapy
Prothrombin time (PT)	Measures extrinsic and common coagulation pathway	11–16 s	Prolonged in deficiencies of factors VII and X and fibrinogen, excess dicumarol therapy, severe liver disease and DIC, and vitamin K deficiency
Activated partial thromboplastin time (APTT)	Measures intrinsic and common coagulation pathway	26–42 s	Prolonged in deficiencies of factors VIII to XII and fibrinogen, with circulating anticoagulant therapy, in liver disease and DIC, and in vitamin K deficiency. Shortened in malignancies (except liver)
Thrombin time (TT) or thrombin clotting time	Measures fibrinogen to fibrin formation	10–13 s	Prolonged with low fibrinogen levels, inhibitors, DIC and liver disease, anticoagulant therapy, and in dysproteinemias
Thromboplastin generation test (TGT)	Measures ability to form thromboplastin	12 s or less	Prolonged in thrombocytopenia, with deficiencies of factors VIII to XII, and with circulating anticoagulants

Table 40-2 Coagulation Studies (Continued)

Study	Purpose	Normal Values	Clinical Significance
Capillary fragility test, tourniquet test, Rumpel-Leede test	Tests vascular fragility and platelet function	Occasional or no petechiae after 5 min of 70- to 90-mm pressure with blood pressure cuff	Increased petechiae with thrombocytopenia, thrombasthenia, and vasculitis
Platelet aggregation test	Tests platelet function	Platelets aggregate within a specified time when exposed to substances such as ADP, collagen, epinephrine	Decreased or absent aggregation in thrombasthenia, aspirin ingestion, myeloproliferative disorders, severe liver disease, dysproteinemias, von Willebrand's disease

Source: S. A. Price and L. M. Wilson, *Pathophysiology: Clinical Concepts of Disease Processes,* 3d ed., New York, McGraw-Hill, 1986, p. 221.

Platelet factor 4 is known for its heparin-neutralizing activity. It is a glycoprotein which is released from platelets which have been aggregated. Several procoagulant activities are associated with this factor, and it is suggested that it is an extremely potent and specific triggering agent in vivo, in addition to being active in platelet aggregation and in coagulation.

Coagulation factor XIII is an intracellular constituent of platelets. Platelets contain approximately 30 to 50 percent of the total amount of this factor.

Bleeding Associated with Platelets

Thrombocytopenia (quantitative platelet deficiency) is one of the most common causes of hemorrhagic diatheses. This condition is characterized clinically by petechiae and ecchymoses of the skin and mucous membranes. Bleeding produced by platelet deficiency differs from that observed in disorders of plasma coagulation factors in that platelet-associated bleeding results in petechiae of the skin and mucous membranes and a tendency to internal (cerebral and gastrointestinal), menorrhagic, epistaxic, gingival, and tongue bleeding. The petechiae are more numerous over dependent areas of the body because of increased venous pressure. If these grow and become confluent, large ecchymoses will occur, but petechiae still tend to be present at the margins. Coagulopathies of non-platelet etiology tend to involve hemorrhages into skin, muscle, and joints in contrast to the more superficial areas of petechial involvement. A general tendency to bleeding occurs with or without pe-

techiae when platelet levels fall below 100,000 per cubic millimeter.

Coagulation

The process of visible coagulation and fibrin clot formation represents the end result of an intricate series of reactions that involve a number of different factors present in the blood and tissues. These substances influence the clotting mechanism either by promoting clotting with procoagulants, or by retarding or inhibiting clotting with anticoagulants; some even function in the removal of the clot once it is formed. Coagulation function can be measured by the standard tests reviewed in Table 40-3.

Nomenclature

Within the circulating blood there are certain trace proteins known collectively as *clotting factors* or *procoagulants.* These proteins directly participate in the coagulation process. Over the years considerable misunderstanding and confusion has developed concerning their identification and description. During one era, descriptive names such as *fibrinogen, thrombin,* and *prothrombin* were used. Later, functional names such as *labile* and *stable factors* were adopted to describe these proteins. Then there was a period during which the surnames of the kindreds in which the hereditary defects were initially observed were used to identify the clotting factors (Hageman, Stuart, Fletcher, and so

Table 40-3 Fibrinolysis Tests

Study	Purpose	Normal Values	Clinical Significance
Euglobin lysis time	Measures activity of systemic fibrinolysis, measured from clot formation to clot lysis	90 min to 6 h	Decreased time in fibrinolysis, streptokinase infusion, cancer of the prostate, shock
Fibrin degradation products (FDP) or fibrin split products (FSP)	Direct indication of fibrinolysis	Less than 10 μg/mL	Increased time in DIC and fibrinolysis

on). To compound the problem, not infrequently several names were being used simultaneously to describe the same substance.

In an attempt to remedy the problem, an international committee established a nomenclature of blood clotting factors (Table 40-4). Roman numerals are now used to identify the various factors in the order of their discovery. (This numerical sequence in no way suggests their order of reaction and participation in the coagulation process.) In addition to the roman numerals, a shorthand abbreviation, a subscript letter *a*, is used

Table 40-4 International Nomenclature for Blood Coagulation Factors

Factor	Synonyms
I	Fibrinogen
II	Prothrombin, prethrombin
III	Tissue factor, tissue thromboplastin
IV	Calcium
V	Proaccelerin, labile factor, Ac globulin
(VI)	Not assigned
VII	Proconvertin, SPCA, stable factor, autoprothrombin I
VIII	Antihemophilic globulin (AHG), antihemophilic factor (AHF), antihemophilic factor A, platelet cofactor I
IX	Plasma thromboplastin component (PTC), Christmas factor, antihemophilic factor B, autoprothrombin II, platelet cofactor II
X	Stuart-Prower factor, Stuart factor, autoprothrombin III
XII	Plasma thromboplastin antecedent (PTA), antihemophilic factor C
XII	Hageman factor
XIII	Fibrin-stabilizing factor, fibrinase, Laki-Lorand factor

Note: Activated factors are designated by a (a subscript letter) after the roman numeral.
Source: W. J. Williams et al., *Hematology*, 3d ed., New York, McGraw-Hill, 1983, p. 1202.

to indicate the active forms of each factor. For example, conversion of factor X to its active form is written $X{-}{-}{-}{-}{-}X_a$. It is worth mentioning again that the platelet factors which are active in clotting are indicated by arabic numerals to distinguish them from the coagulation factors.

Intrinsic and Extrinsic Pathways

The interaction of the coagulation factors which evolve to a final common pathway of clot formation has been described in terms of two chains or cascades of actions. In effect, these are alternative modes of activating factor X. In the *intrinsic* pathway, all the procoagulants necessary for clot formation are contained within the circulating blood. This system is activated when factor XII contacts an abnormal surface. In turn, factors XI, IX, VIII, X, II, and I are activated. The *extrinsic* system requires the release of factor III from the endothelial cells or other tissue extracts before activation can occur. The extrinsic system is activated when the tissue factor contacts factor VII, producing sequential activation of factors X, V, II, and I.

Whether the inciting stimulus occurs when the blood comes in contact with an abnormal surface (the intrinsic system) or when factor III gains access to the bloodstream (the extrinsic system), the final result is the same—the production of large amounts of thrombin followed by the transformation of fibrinogen to fibrin. Figure 40-2 depicts this sequential reaction.

Coagulation Factors

Factor I (Fibrinogen)

Fibrinogen is the protein converted into fibrin by the action of the proteolytic enzyme thrombin. The

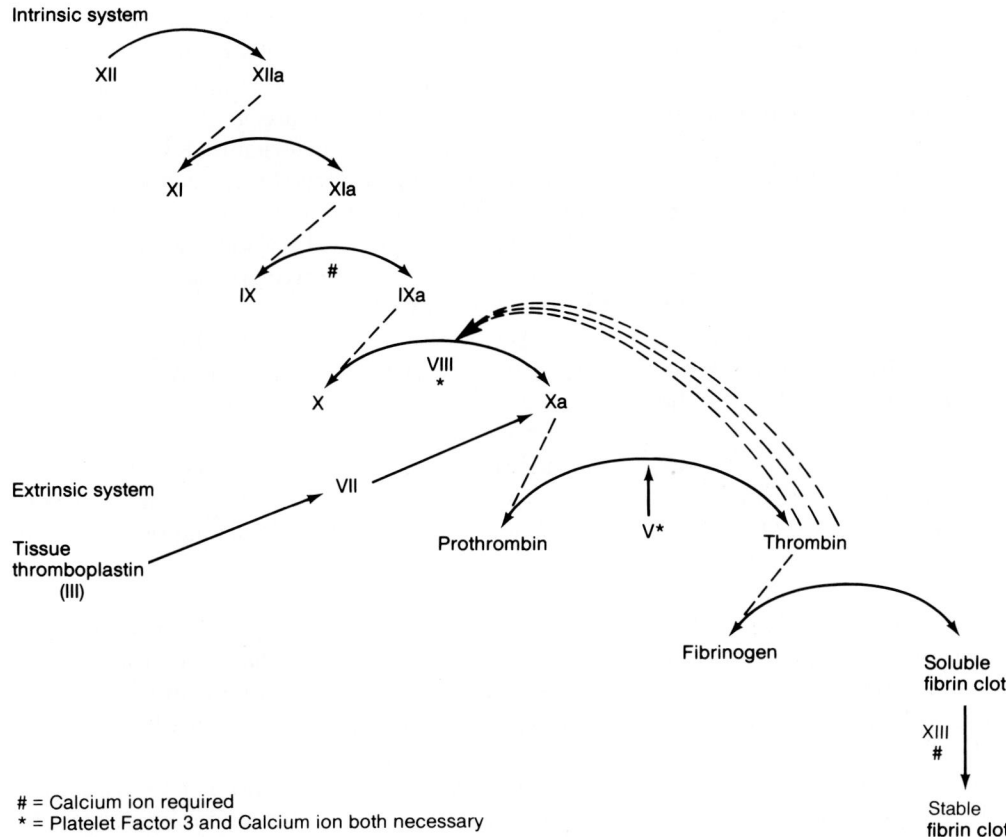

= Calcium ion required
* = Platelet Factor 3 and Calcium ion both necessary

Figures 40-2   The sequence of coagulation. *(From C. M. Hudak, B. Gallo, and J. Lohr, eds., Critical Care Nursing, 4th ed., Lippincott, Philadelphia, 1986, p. 234.)*

resulting fibrin strands form the microstructure of the hemostatic plug. When fibrin is mixed with thrombin, two peptides are split off, resulting in a fibrin monomer which then undergoes continuous polymerization and depolymerization in the bloodstream. The rapid turnover of fibrinogen in the bloodstream suggests that this process of polymerization and depolymerization occurs normally and continually in the bloodstream as weil as taking place at the endothelial surface of blood vessels when they are traumatized.

Fibrinogen is a relatively insoluble glycoprotein synthesized by the parenchymal cells in the liver. It is normally found in the bloodstream, in the lymph, and in many tissues. Approximately 75 percent of the total body pool is present in the circulating blood. This clotting factor is thought to

be essential in normal platelet function and in the process of wound healing.

In health, the concentration of fibrinogen in the blood remains relatively constant. Normal values of fibrinogen range from 200 to 400 mg per 100 mL of blood. It is produced by the liver and catabolized at about the same rate. The overall mechanism of fibrinogen catabolism is still under study.

Various disease states may increase fibrinogen metabolism. These include conditions such as cirrhosis, multiple myeloma, and nephrosis. In fact, virtually any disorder associated with stress, inflammation, or tissue necrosis may produce hyperfibrinogenemia. This response develops within a matter of hours and is the major factor leading to acceleration of the erythrocyte sedimentation rate (ESR) sometimes shortened to "sed rate." Normal increases in fibrinogen are associated with pregnancy as well as with the administration of anovulatory drugs; they are also associated with hypermetabolic states.

Depressed fibrinogen levels are associated with hypothyroidism. Large amounts of circulating tissue thromboplastin may produce a severe depression of fibrinogen. Tissue thromboplastin is a procoagulant material which interacts with fibrinogen to form the microstructure of the fibrin clot. *Fibrinogenopenia,* also known as *hypofibrinogenemia* or *defibrination,* is associated with the entry into the bloodstream of fragments of various body tissues which are particularly rich in tissue thromboplastin. These areas include the lungs and prostatic and cerebral tissues, in addition to fragments of placenta which happen to gain access to the maternal circulation. Regardless of the source, when such tissue enters the circulation, large quantities of fibrinogen are consumed in the formation of fibrin clots. A consumption coagulopathy is produced, since platelets and other clotting factors are also depleted in the process of disseminated intravascular clotting. The magnitude of the coagulation response is directly related to the quantity of the entering tissue thromboplastin and also to the ability of the reticuloendothelial system to cope with the imposed stress.

Factor II (Prothrombin)

Prothrombin, the inactive precursor of thrombin, is constantly present in the blood in excess of clotting requirements. Even with a 50 percent reduction in the blood volume, blood can clot normally.

Prothrombin is one of four vitamin K-dependent factors; that is, the hepatocyte requires the presence of vitamin K for prothrombin synthesis. (The other three factors which are dependent upon the presence of vitamin K are factors VII, IX, and X, with some reports that factor XI may also be vitamin K-dependent.) It is suggested that vitamin K acts as a rate regulator for the assembly of the prothrombin molecule and may be responsible for the calcium binding sites. When vitamin K is deficient, regardless of the cause, a marked decrease in prothrombin occurs.

Vitamin K is not stored in the body but is synthesized by bacteria which are part of the normal intestinal flora. Should this flora be disturbed, as when certain antibiotics are given, a decrease in prothrombin results. Since vitamin K is a fat-soluble vitamin, bile salts produced by the liver are required for its absorption from the intestinal tract. Diseases which interfere with fat absorption, such as obstructive jaundice and steatorrhea, may produce impaired vitamin K absorption.

Severe liver disease may also produce the same type of deficiency as vitamin K deficiency because the liver cells, in this case, are unable to utilize vitamin K sufficiently to make prothrombin in adequate quantities. Coumarin-type anticoagulants, when present in therapeutic blood levels, may also alter the level of circulating prothrombin.

Factor III (Tissue Thromboplastin)

Homogenates of normal tissues are known to markedly accelerate blood coagulation. Factor III functions by interacting with factor VII in the extrinsic pathway. The active principle and its biochemistry have not been definitively described.

Although factor III is thought to arise from virtually any body tissue, the brain, lung, prostate, and placental tissue are particularly rich sources of tissue thromboplastin.

Factor IV (Calcium)

Factor IV is found in the blood in normal concentrations of 9 to 11 mg/mL. Approximately 50 percent is present in the ionized state (Ca^{2+}). Only small quantities of Ca^{2+} are required for normal functioning of the coagulation mechanism; therefore, calcium deficiency as a cause of a coagulopathy is quite rare. Occasionally coagulopathy is associated with a large quantity of blood replacement after a severe hemorrhage. The numerous transfusions with citrated blood produce a relative hypocalcemia as a result of the combination of the ionized calcium with ethylenediaminetetraacetic acid (EDTA), oxalate, citrate, fluoride, and ion-exchange resins. These are irreversible reactions which make calcium unavailable for participation in the coagulation mechanism.

Hyperglobulinemia and dysglobulinemia associated with sarcoidosis and myeloma may also result in abnormal binding of calcium. In these situations the calcium binds to the abnormal globulins, resulting in a hemostatic defect. The point to be emphasized in both these conditions is that they produce a relative calcium deficiency even though laboratory reports indicate a normal calcium level or even hypercalcemia. Despite the normal calcium level, the calcium is not available for the coagulation process.

Factor V (Labile Factor, Ac Globulin, Proaccelerin)

Factor V occurs in the plasma of all normal persons. It is synthesized in the liver and is a labile, water-soluble globulin. It is totally consumed in the process of coagulation and is not found in serum. Factor V is essential in the formation of prothrombin in the common pathway (Fig. 40-2). The extrinsic and intrinsic thromboplastic products appear to react with factor V in the presence of calcium (Ca^{2+}).

A congenital deficiency of factor V results from an autosomal recessive trait that is not sex-linked but is manifested when the trait is inherited from both parents. The deficiency is characterized by parahemophilia, in which there is a tendency to bleeding from vascular areas of the body (e.g., the mucous membranes) and to epistaxis, menorrhagia, and the like.

Acquired factor V deficiency may occur in severe liver disease (hepatocellular) or from circulating anticoagulants. Increased fibrinolysis (lysis of fibrin clots) may also produce factor V deficiency.

Factor V_a (activated factor V) was formerly known as factor VI.

Factor VII (Stable Factor, Proconvertin)

Factor VII is one of the vitamin K–dependent factors produced by the liver. Factor VII is active only in the presence of factor III (the extrinsic system) and when activated, reacts with factor III and calcium to activate factor X.

Factor VIII (Antihemophilic Factor)

Factor VIII is a trace protein that is involved in the intrinsic pathway of coagulation. Despite extensive study, the production site of this factor has yet to be established. Factor VIII has two major activities:

procoagulant activity and maintenance of a normal bleeding time. Procoagulant activity is deficient in classic hemophilia, and both activities are deficient in von Willebrand's disease.

Factor VIII is normally present in excess of need. Although it is required for thromboplastin generation, it has been determined that this process can proceed even when factor VIII is present at only 40 percent of normal concentrations. Significant impairment of the coagulation mechanism does not occur until the concentration has dropped to between 10 and 20 percent of normal.

Circulating levels of factor VIII are reported to increase after vigorous exercise, following epinephrine administration, and in certain metabolic states such as pregnancy.

Factor IX (Plasma Thromboplastin)

Factor IX is also known as *Christmas factor, antihemophilic factor B,* and *plasma thromboplastin component* (PTC). This factor plays an essential role in the intrinsic pathway of coagulation. It is present in both serum and plasma. Plasma levels of factor IX are depressed by the pharmacologic activity of coumarin drugs, although not as significantly as those of factors VII and X.

Clinically, abnormalities of factor IX are associated with the sex-linked recessive condition of hemophilia B, or Christmas disease. Like factor VII, it is also associated with hemorrhagic disease of the newborn.

Factor IX is vitamin K–dependent. Plasma levels decrease with vitamin K deficiency, advanced hepatocellular disease, and prolonged anti–vitamin K therapy.

Factor X (Stuart-Prower Factor)

Factor X is also known as *autoprothrombin*. It is a glycoprotein which is found both in the plasma and in the serum. Factor X forms the final common pathway through which the products of both the extrinsic and intrinsic system proceed as they form the terminal thromboplastic substances necessary for the conversion of prothrombin to thrombin. This reaction requires the presence of Ca^{2+} and factor V.

Deficiency of factor X is primarily seen as a hereditary disorder produced by an incompletely recessive autosomal trait. An acquired deficiency is seen in liver disease and vitamin K deficiency.

Factor XI (Plasma Thromboplastin Antecedent)

Factor XI, plasma thromboplastin antecedent (PTA) or antihemophilic factor, also appears to be essential in the intrinsic pathway. A deficiency of this factor is probably inherited as a simple autosomal recessive trait that leads to a mild hemophilia-like state following trauma or surgery. Plasma levels of this factor are frequently diminished in liver disease, but proof of hepatic biosynthesis of this protein has yet to be established.

Factor XII (Hageman Factor)

Factor XII is maintained in an inactive state in normal blood by the action of coagulation inhibitors. Factor XII reacts with factor XI to form an active prothromboplastic substance initiating the intrinsic pathway of coagulation. A deficiency of factor XII does not usually produce a hemorrhagic state, but it is associated with a prolonged venous clotting time, a long partial thromboplastin time, and an abnormal thromboplastin generation test. Clinically it is transmitted as an autosomal recessive or dominant trait.

There is evidence to suggest that activated factor XII (XII$_a$) serves as a surface-sensitive trigger mechanism that translates the stimuli of injury into diverse physiologic processes associated with hemostasis and fibrinolysis, humoral and cellular defense, and inflammation and wound healing.

Factor XIII (Fibrin Stabilizing Factor)

Fibrin stabilizing factor is a glycoprotein with as much as 50 percent of the amount present in the platelets and 50 percent in other circulating blood elements. Clinical evidence suggests that the quantity that is associated with the platelets is actually synthesized by the megakaryocyte rather than being adsorbed from the plasma. Factor XIII acts in the common pathway of coagulation, where it forms a stabilizing covalent bond within fibrin strands.

Although deficiency of factor XIII occurs in many patients with liver disease, direct evidence for biosynthesis is lacking. Its deficiency in liver disease suggests that factor XIII may be activated by the liver or that the liver may produce an

inhibitor of the factor. Hereditary deficiencies of factor XIII (and fibrinogen) are frequently associated with abnormal scar formation, wound dehiscence, postcircumcision bleeding, and bleeding from the umbilical stump.

Mechanisms of Coagulation

Over the years the sequence of reactions resulting in blood coagulation has been considered to be of the nature of an enzyme-substrate reaction. According to this theory, each clotting factor functions as an enzyme which, upon activation, proceeds in a stepwise fashion in amplifying the reaction by activation of many times its own weight in substrate. In the process of activation, there is a net gain response in which a single molecule of an activated enzyme (clotting factor) converts not just one but perhaps thousands of specific substrate molecules into active enzymes. A chain reaction, in a *cascade* or waterfall effect, occurs in which activation of a single proenzyme molecule may lead to the explosive generation of the entire clotting mechanism. Figure 40-2 depicts this reaction.

This cascade theory of the coagulation mechanism is still accepted but with minor alterations. It has been reported that at least three of the reactions do not appear to follow the typical enzyme-substrate format. The following reactions are believed to result in the formation of a complex in contrast to the serial activation of a single enzyme substrate: the reaction involving factor III (tissue factor), factor VII, and calcium; the reaction involving activated factor IX, factor VIII, phospholipid, and calcium; and the reaction involving activated factor X, factor V, phospholipid, and calcium. In the formation of a complex, the product of the reaction is a mixture of several of the reactants. The current concept of the coagulation mechanism comprises both enzymatic conversion of the protein clotting factors and the formation of complexes (physical combination of reactants).

Positive Feedback

In addition to acting upon their primary substrate, some of the clotting factors are capable of activating other inactive clotting factors. For example, thrombin, in addition to acting upon fibrinogen, has the ability to activate factors V and VIII. Thrombin may also act upon and destroy platelets. Because of this ability to act upon these other factors, including platelets, as soon as a small amount of thrombin is formed, the clotting mechanism becomes autocatalytic (self-activating). A large amount of thrombin, once formed, can then rapidly activate even more platelets, degrading even more of the clotting factors V and VIII and ultimately producing even more fibrin. Freely circulating thrombin can have a significant influence on the acceleration of the coagulation process because of this multiple activity.

Kallikrein, a substance which results from the activity of activated factor XII, and plasmin both have multiple effects on the coagulation mechanism. Plasmin is considered under "Fibrinolytic Forces," below. See Fig. 40-2 for cascade sequence and feedback effects.

Implications of the Cascade Theory

The theoretical basis for the cascade theory of coagulation is based upon the enzymatic activation of the various inactive clotting factors and the biologic-amplifier effect of this process. Although subscribed to for a number of years, the theoretical basis for this hypothesis has been based largely upon in vitro studies. Considerable research has yet to be done to establish the precise in vivo mechanism(s). The reader is encouraged to keep this point in mind and to evaluate future research in terms of whether the design is based on in vitro or in vivo study. Until disproved or qualified by new research findings, the cascade theory deserves mention and consideration for its physiologic implications.

System Antagonists

The delicate balance that exists in health between clot formation and clot lysis is maintained by a number of factors and forces. Homeostasis of the hemostatic mechanism is maintained by a system of naturally occurring anticoagulant forces and factors, the procoagulant activity of thrombin, and the lysis of formed clots by the fibrinolytic system. In fact, when one considers the proposed biologic amplifier effect of enzyme activation and the positive feedback or autocatalytic effects of thrombin out-

lined in Fig. 40-2, one might well ask why episodes of exaggerated clotting do not occur. It is the precise interaction of these forces that maintains a system of checks and balances.

Coagulant Force

Thrombin is the most powerful coagulant force in the body. It has been reported that there is enough prothrombin in 10 mL of blood to clot 2500 mL of plasma in 15 s. Considering that the average adult male typically has about 5 L of blood within the circulatory system, the significance of these figures can be appreciated. Obviously, the factors and forces in the body which prevent abnormal clotting must be very effective.

Anticoagulant Forces

The anticoagulant forces normally present and active in the body include the following factors which serve as a system of checks and balances against the powerful procoagulant force of thrombin:

1. Smoothness of normal vascular endothelium
2. A monomolecular layer of negatively charged proteins which are described as repelling the positively charged clotting factors
3. Blood flow velocity, which promotes dispersion of activated clotting factors that fail to be contained within the clot
4. Fibrin threads of the clot, which are thought to absorb 85 to 90 percent of all activated thrombin, containing it within the clot
5. Antithrombin III, a plasma protein which is believed to inactivate that thrombin which fails to be contained within or adsorbed to the clot
6. Heparin, produced by mast cells located primarily in the lungs and the liver, in addition to that produced by basophils; normally produced in minute quantities, but considered important in the ongoing maintenance of homeostasis
7. The functional capacity of the liver to both produce and filter activated clotting factors which fail to be contained within the clot

In addition to the specific factors and forces mentioned, natural inhibitors of coagulation are thought to be present and effective against every step in the process of coagulation.

Fibrinolytic Forces

Plasma contains two complex enzyme systems which function in hemostasis. In addition to the coagulation system, there is a system that is responsible for removal of the clot after its function has been accomplished and the integrity of the blood vessel has been restored. Once the vessel has been repaired and loss of blood is no longer a threat, restoration of distal blood flow is critical.

The fibrinolytic system is one of the most important defense mechanisms of the body. The activity of this system is mediated by the enzyme *plasmin,* which is capable of digesting fibrinogen and fibrin. The specific effect of the fibrin lysis is the production of *fibrin split products* (FSP), also known as *fibrin degradation products* (FDP). The presence of FSP is determined by a very sensitive laboratory test which can be used to monitor the abnormal activity of the fibrinolytic system (Table 40-3). Normally FSP should not be present in the circulation.

Plasminogen is normally present in the plasma but is kept in check by a system of activators and inhibitors. Plasma plasminogen activators can be found in trace amounts in all body fluids, in urine, and in most tissues. In body cells, the activators are proteolytic enzymes found in lysosomes, whereas in blood vessels the activator tends to be located in the endothelial lining. In general, the activators are a heterogenous group of proteins which react with plasminogen to produce plasmin. The activator concentrated in the endothelial lining of blood vessels is readily soluble and diffusible and is available for release in response to a variety of vasoactive stimuli, especially vasodilatation. It is this mechanism that provides for local concentration of the activator at the site of trauma or inflammation in time of need. Two plasminogen activators, urokinase and streptokinase, are commercially available for the treatment of thrombosis.

The activity of plasmin, called *fibrinolysis,* is considerably greater at all times within the microcirculation. It is assumed that it is this high level of activity, as compared with that of the systemic circulation, that maintains the patency of the capillary beds. The larger vessels, since they contain a lower concentration of endothelial cells, therefore contain a lower concentration of plasminogen activator. This situation suggests that the larger vessels are not as well prepared to deal effectively with fibrin deposition and thrombus formation. In fact, this lower level of fibrinolytic activity may be considered to somewhat predispose the larger vessels to the growth of clots, once they are formed.

Normally, when clots are formed, there is a certain amount of plasminogen and plasminogen activator incorporated within the clot. It is also assumed that some plasminogen activator diffuses into the formed clot, providing an opportunity for the larger vessels to benefit from the circulating plasminogen activator. Whether the presence of the activator within the clot is due to the process of diffusion, absorption, or incorporation, once inside, plasmin activity mediates the progressive lysis of the clot.

Certain physiologic states are associated with transient increases of plasminogen activator above basal levels. These include intense exercise, sudden fright, and procedures such as electroshock and pneumoencephalography. Levels of plasma plasminogen are also increased by hypoglycemia, after administration of insulin and anabolic steroids, and following extensive surgery on the heart and lungs. Certain diseases such as prostatic cancer, cirrhosis of the liver, and various infections are also associated with elevated levels of plasminogen.

Plasma contains a large amount of antiplasmin activity. In fact it is estimated that there is a sufficient quantity of these substances to inactivate 10 times the quantity of available plasmin in the plasma. This activity is believed to reside in the activity of two α-globulin components. Platelets are also known to contain some antiplasmin activity.

Anticoagulant Effects of Plasmin Activity

Fibrinolysis and coagulation are both normal components of the hemostatic response to vascular injury. Although both thrombin and plasmin have the capacity to act on fibrinogen, they act on different sites. The digestion of fibrinogen by plasmin produces fragments which are potent anticoagulants. They function in several ways: one fragment (X) may be acted upon by thrombin to form a fragile fibrin clot. This reaction occurs slowly, delaying the formation of a clot. Other fragments (Y, D, and E) do not form a clot, but the fragments inhibit fibrin polymerization and thrombin activity. Normally this does not create a problem, but in

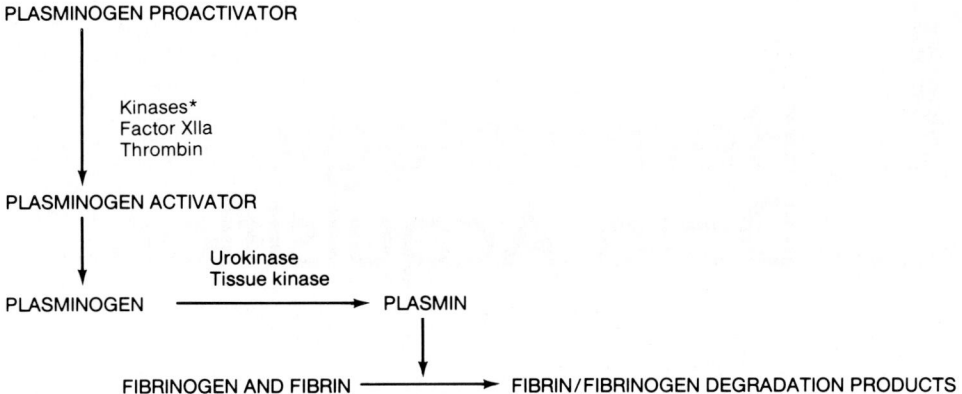

PLASMINOGEN PROACTIVATOR

Kinases*
Factor XIIa
Thrombin

PLASMINOGEN ACTIVATOR

Urokinase
Tissue kinase

PLASMINOGEN ⟶ PLASMIN

FIBRINOGEN AND FIBRIN ⟶ FIBRIN/FIBRINOGEN DEGRADATION PRODUCTS

*Includes: streptokinase, staphylokinase, tissue kinase

Figure 40-3 The fibrinolytic system. *(From S. A. Price and L. M. Wilson, Pathophysiology, 3d ed., McGraw-Hill, New York, 1986, p. 218.)*

situations of excessive clotting and clot lysis, these events aggravate a consumption coagulopathy. Figure 40-3 illustrates the action of plasmin and the generation of plasmin split products.

Hemostasis

Normally, blood is in a liquid state circulating throughout the vascular compartment. Whenever a blood vessel loses its integrity and allows the liquid blood to escape, clotting is initiated. Blood changes from its liquid state to a solid gel. The events in hemostasis include:

1. Vascular spasm
2. Stickiness of the endothelial surfaces
3. Formation of the platelet plug
4. Formation of the blood clot (activation of plasma coagulation factors)
5. Clot retraction
6. Fibrous repair of the injured vessel wall
7. Clot lysis

Several of the events listed are closely interrelated functionally and are simultaneous; others occur in a sequential fashion.

A few seconds after the blood vessel is injured and integrity is lost, platelets adhere to the margin and stick to the exposed subendothelial fibers, usually collagen, forming a loose mesh. This mechanism, in addition to vasospasm, reduces blood loss. Platelets release potent chemicals which facilitate the process and which also attract more platelets. One of these chemicals is a thromboplastic substance essential to the coagulation mechanism. In the process the platelets extrude a contractile protein which draws together the threads of fibrin, producing retraction of the clot. Platelets and red blood cells are trapped within the clot, as are plasminogen and plasminogen activator, substances which will ultimately produce plasmin, which lyses the clot. Within 30 to 60 min serum is expressed from the clot; it is estimated that after a few hours fibroblasts begin to invade the clot, initiating a fibrous organization. Complete fibrous organization of the clot into fibrous tissue requires approximately 7 to 10 days. This very effective mechanism prevents blood loss in arterioles, venules, and the capillaries of the microcirculation, but immediate mechanical action, e.g., pressure or a ligature, is required to stop blood loss in medium- to large-size arteries and veins.

References

1. Rifkind, R. J., Bank, A., Marks, P. A., Kaplan, K. L., Ellison, R. R., & Lindenbaum, J. (1986). *Fundamentals of hematology* (3d ed.), Chicago: Year Book.
2. Williams, W. J., Beutler, E., Erslev, A. J., & Lichtman, M. A. (1983). *Hematology* (3d ed.). New York: McGraw-Hill.

41

Hematologic Data Acquisition

Brenda S. Jackson

This chapter discusses assessment of the patient with possible hematologic dysfunction. Since the signs and symptoms of hematologic problems may be manifested in many organ systems, careful attention must be paid to subtle clues in the patient's history and review of systems before physical assessment is initiated. Pertinent findings in the history and physical assessment and appropriate diagnostic procedures are presented.

In most critical-care settings, with the possible exception of the emergency department, the patient's initial history and physical examination are completed prior to admission to the critical-care unit. When the patient is too ill to talk, family members or significant others are questioned to gather additional information about the patient's history, the onset of the present illness, and other relevant data. Various members of the health care team may gather important supplemental data throughout the duration of the illness.

Patient Assessment

History

During the initial interview with the hematologic patient, certain predetermined facts related to the current illness are collected such as when symptoms began and whether they occurred abruptly or gradually, the course of events, duration and frequency of episodes, character and location of symptoms, precipitating and relieving factors, and other associated data. Presence of allergies, current medications (both prescribed and over-the-counter), past medical history, and family history are equally important. Even though primary hematologic diseases are relatively uncommon, the patient's medical history and family history may indicate a long-

standing personal or family problem that was previously unrecognized. For example, a history of pallor, fatigue, and dyspnea on exertion may indicate chronic anemia. A family history of unusual bleeding such as frequent epistaxis, easy bruising, bleeding after circumcision, or excessive bleeding from small cuts may indicate a genetic basis for the hematologic problem. Particular note should be made of spontaneous bleeding episodes or those which do not seem to be related to any specific trauma. Previous treatment with blood components should also be noted in the history.

The patient should be questioned regarding bleeding after injuries, dental extractions, and surgery. In women a thorough menstrual and obstetric history should be obtained. A number of diseases can affect the hematologic system. A history of liver disease, systemic lupus erythematosis, or other collagen vascular diseases (e.g., Marfan's syndrome and osteogenesis imperfecta, which are hereditary connective tissue diseases), uremia, and hematologic malignant disease should be noted. (See Table 41-1 for terminology associated with bleeding patterns.)

Many severe infections are also associated with bleeding manifestations. Typhoid, subacute bacterial endocarditis, meningococcemia, septicemias, and childhood viral infections (measles and chickenpox) can cause bleeding problems.[1] Parasitic infections such as malaria and leishmaniasis and mycotic infections such as acute histoplasmosis can also trigger bleeding episodes.[2]

Careful attention should be given to eliciting a thorough medication history. Many prescription and over-the-counter medications can interfere with hemostasis. Aspirin impairs the formation of platelet plugs and therefore prolongs bleeding time. The nonsteroidal anti-inflammatory agents phenylbuta-

Table 41-1 Terminology of Bleeding Patterns

Epistaxis	Hemorrhage from the nose
Hemarthrosis	Effusion of blood into a joint cavity
Hemoglobinuria	Presence of extracellular hemoglobin in the urine
Hemoptysis	Expectoration of bloody sputum
Melena	Black vomitus resulting from action of digestive juices on free blood in the intestinal tract
Menorrhagia	Excessive menstrual bleeding
Hematochezia	Passage of stools containing blood

zone and indomethacin can interfere with normal coagulation, as can dipyridamole, clofibrate, antihistamines, certain tranquilizers, penicillin, β-lactam antibiotics, heparin, and coumarin.[1] Alcohol and drug abuse are also important factors; alcohol may decrease platelet count and increase bleeding time, and drug abuse may result in higher required doses of anticoagulants.

Many chemotherapeutic agents given to treat malignant disease affect the bone marrow and therefore may alter normal coagulation processes. Patients with malignant disease are particularly prone to develop bleeding problems.

A nutrition history may be useful, as malnutrition may be a factor in the development of hematologic problems. Diets which are lacking in iron, protein, or essential vitamins can affect the integrity of vascular walls, the synthesis of plasma proteins, and the development of cellular components of the blood. Scurvy, which results from vitamin C deficiency, is characterized by hemorrhagic manifestations. Vitamin K is necessary for the formation of the coagulation protein prothrombin, hence vitamin K deficiency results in prolonged clotting times.

Physical Examination

A thorough physical examination of the patient should be conducted on admission. Since manifestations of hematologic problems evolve over time in many organ systems, daily physical assessment is also needed. Particular emphasis should be placed on examining those organs and systems in which signs and symptoms of hematologic problems are most likely to occur. The skin and mucous membranes, conjunctivae, liver, spleen, neuromuscular system, and joints should be assessed at frequent intervals during acute bleeding episodes.

Vital signs should be assessed frequently. Elevated temperatures may indicate infection or underlying inflammatory processes that have an impact on the hematologic system. Alterations in the pulse rate, blood pressure, or respiratory rate may indicate the body's attempt to adapt to hematologic stressors such as anemia and bleeding.

The skin and mucous membranes reveal important clues to hematologic functioning. Color variations, the presence of lesions, the character of wounds, turgor, and hair distribution should be noted. The color of the nail beds, mucous membranes, and palmar creases can serve as a guide to hemoglobin levels, but conjunctival blood vessel patterns and color may be a more reliable index. Pallor can be a useful guideline in evaluating anemia, but it must be remembered that skin color is determined by pigment and temperature as well as capillary blood flow. The pinkness of palmar creases usually disappears at hemoglobin levels of less than 7 g/100 mL. Cyanosis is indicative of extreme problems. Cyanosis is noted when hemoglobin is reduced to 5 g/100 mL, methemoglobin to 1.5 to 2.0 g/100 mL, or sulfhemoglobin to 0.5 g/100 mL. The skin and mucous membranes should be examined by daylight or other natural lighting for accurate determination of color changes and particularly for the presence of jaundice, because artificial lighting can distort color perception. For jaundice to be detected the bilirubin must be 2 to 3 mg/100 mL.

Examination of the skin and mucous membranes may also reveal lesions characteristic of specific bleeding problems (Table 41-2). Petechiae are usually seen in dependent areas. Ecchymoses may be seen around venipuncture sites or areas where other invasive procedures were performed. The mucous membranes of the mouth may show pallor or other changes due to hematologic problems. Changes in the surface of the tongue, monilial superinfection, gingival hypertrophy, glossitis, and ulcerations should be reported.

Examination of the ears, eyes, nose, and throat may reveal lesions indicating bleeding problems. Ophthalmascopic examination is important to evaluate the condition of retinal vessels and to detect the presence of retinal hemorrhages or exudates.

Table 41-2 Skin Lesions Associated with Hematologic Problems

Lesion or Condition	Description
Petechia	Small purplish, hemorrhagic spot that does not blanch with pressure; usually 1—3 mm in diameter
Ecchymosis	Variable-size macular, irregularly formed hemorrhagic area of the skin with color varying from blue-black to yellow-green; does not blanch with pressure
Purpura	Condition characterized by hemorrhages into the skin, mucous membranes, or other organs, producing skin lesions which do not disappear with pressure
Telangiectasis	Hyperemic spot due to capillary or small artery dilatation; small angioma with a tendency to hemorrhage
Spider nevus	Branched growth of dilated capillaries resembling a spider
Angioma	Form of usually benign tumor consisting principally of blood or lymph vessels
Hematoma	Blood-filled tumor

Changes in auditory or visual acuity may indicate hemorrhagic phenomena that are not obvious to the naked eye.

Palpation of lymph nodes in the head and neck region may reveal lymphadenopathy due to inflammation, infection, or malignant disease. Posterior auricular, occipital, preauricular, parotid, tonsillar, submental, submaxillary, cervical, and supraclavicular nodes may be involved in these processes. Localized or generalized lymphadenopathy should be described.

Assessment of the respiratory system of the patient with hematologic problems includes the usual observations of rate and depth of respiration and diaphragmatic excursion, palpation for vocal fremitus, and auscultation for adventitious breath sounds. Cardiovascular assessment includes observation of the point of maximal impulse (PMI), auscultation of normal heart sounds, murmurs, gallop rhythms, and irregular rhythms. Pericardial friction rubs and muffling of cardiac sounds are of particular importance and should be reported immediately, because they may indicate bleeding in

the mediastinum. Peripheral vascular assessment should include observation for distended neck veins, edema, and signs of phlebitis or other unusual vascular markings.

During abdominal assessment the presence of distention, masses, ascites, organ enlargement (hepatomegaly or splenomegaly), and tenderness should be noted. Auscultation for presence or absence of bowel sounds and presence of bruits should precede palpation and percussion of abdominal contents, since manipulation of these organs may distort normal peristalsis and therefore alter bowel sounds. Diarrhea, melena, or cramping should be noted in the patient's history. Stomach contents obtained by nasogastric suction, feces, and substances draining from abdominal wounds should be routinely tested for occult blood.

The genitourinary system should be assessed for signs of inflammation, swelling, lesions, tenderness, and continence. The urine should be tested for occult blood. The urine in hematuria may range from slightly smoky to bright red in color. Hemoglobinuria, with urine usually of port wine color, can result from intravascular or extravascular hemolysis.

Neurologic function should be carefully monitored. A variety of hematologic abnormalities may be reflected by neurologic signs and symptoms. Cranial nerve function and pupillary reactions should be tested, as well as motor function and spinal reflexes. Changes in mentation such as general malaise, drowsiness, weakness, vertigo, and headache may portend impending neurologic disaster due to hemorrhage. Sensory disturbances, including paresthesias and numbness or pain, may indicate hematoma impinging on peripheral nerves.

Tenderness, stiffness, or pain in bones and joints may indicate hematologic problems ranging from soreness over active hematopoietic areas to hemorrhage into joint capsules or hemolytic sickle cell crisis.

In summary, all patients with suspected hematologic problems should have a thorough physical examination. The signs and symptoms of hematologic disorders may be present in all organ systems. Since the magnitude of these disorders may evolve over time, repeated assessments are necessary to detect changes in the patient's condition.

Hematologic Diagnostic Procedures

Laboratory Tests

The basic diagnostic tests for hematologic functioning are the complete blood count (CBC) and differential blood count. The CBC includes an actual count of circulating red blood cells (RBCs), white blood cells (WBCs), and platelets in addition to the hemoglobin and hematocrit levels. The differential count is a measure of the total WBC count and the number of cells in each subcategory: neutrophils (granulocytes or polymorphonucleocytes), lymphocytes, monocytes, eosinophils, and basophils. An increase in WBC count, or leukocytosis, may indicate infection or leukemia but may also be a result of normal responses to stress or trauma. Decreased WBC counts, or leukopenia, can result from bone marrow failure, dietary insufficiency, various autoimmune processes, or overwhelming infection.

The red blood cell count is the actual number of circulating RBCs in 1 mm³ of blood. A decreased RBC count of less than 10 percent of normal indicates anemia due to hemorrhage, hemolysis, dietary problems, genetic abnormalities, or drug toxicity. RBC counts may be elevated in persons with chronic hypoxia, adaptation to high altitudes, or polycythemia vera (a neoplastic process in red cell formation). Other measures of RBCs include mean corpuscular volume (MCV, the size of a single red blood cell), mean corpuscular hemoglobin (MCH, the average amount of hemoglobin in a single RBC), and mean corpuscular hemoglobin concentration (MCHC, the average concentration of hemoglobin in a single RBC).

Hemoglobin (Hb) assessment measures the amount of hemoglobin in peripheral blood. Changes in hemoglobin level may reflect changes in plasma volume such as those in overhydration and dehydration. The hematocrit (Hct) reading reflects the percentage of red blood cells in the total blood volume. Hematocrit levels may also indicate changes in plasma volumes.

Reticulocytes (immature red blood cells) may be measured during a complete blood count. The reticulocyte count shows bone marrow production of new RBCs. Reticulocyte counts are normally elevated in anemia as a physiologic compensation. In patients with otherwise normal CBCs, an elevated reticulocyte count may indicate polycythemia vera.

An estimate of the platelet count may be given in a CBC. A more definitive count is usually performed during coagulation studies. Diminished platelets may indicate marrow failure or consumption coagulopathy. Elevated platelet counts may occur in myeloproliferative disorders such as polycythemia vera, leukemias, and multiple myeloma.

Table 41-3 gives the normal values for the CBC and the clinical implications of the values.

The erythrocyte sedimentation rate (ESR) is a measure of the speed at which erythrocytes settle when an anticoagulant has been added to the blood sample. The sedimentation rate is increased in a variety of conditions such as pregnancy, cancer, and infection. It may be decreased in liver disease. The ESR has neither disease nor organ specificity, so it is useful only as a general screening test. It may be used to follow the progress of diseases such as rheumatic fever in which a gradually decreasing ESR indicates improvement in the patient's condition.

When indicated, additional diagnostic tests may be performed to determine whether specific disorders of hemoglobin are present. A number of hemoglobin variants have been identified. Some of these variants are due to genetic traits which lead to hematologic diseases, including sickle cell disease, thalassemia, and various other hemolytic anemias.

The hemoglobin measured in the CBC reflects the total amount of hemoglobin in peripheral blood. In anemic states more discrete tests determine the cause and specific treatment for the problem. Total serum iron (60 to 190 µg/dL) and total iron binding capacity (TIBC; 250 to 420 µg/dL) are decreased in iron deficiency anemia.[3] Chronic illnesses, including infections and neoplasms, can cause iron deficiency anemia, as can insufficient iron intake, malabsorption syndromes, and loss of blood.[3] Serum ferritin levels may be measured to validate the diagnosis of iron deficiency anemia. Serum ferritin is the chief iron storage protein in the body; its amount reflects reticuloendothelial storage of iron. In iron deficiency anemia, serum ferritin levels are decreased. Normal serum ferritin levels in adult males range from 20 to 300 ng/mL; adult female levels range from 20 to 120 ng/mL. In other disease states, such as acute and chronic liver disease, hemosiderosis, leukemias, Hodgkin's disease, and infections, serum ferritin levels may be increased.[4]

Table 41-3 Complete Blood Count, Normal Values

Parameter	Normal Values	Clinical Implications
RBCs, millions per mm³	Males: 5.4 Females: 4.8	Decreased in anemia and hemorrhage, increased in chronic hypoxia
MCV, μm³	81–96	Increased in macrocytic anemia, decreased in microcytic anemia
MCH, pg/RBC	27–31	
MCHC, g/dL (%)	32–36	Decreased in hypochromic cells
Hemoglobin, g/100 mL	Males: 14–18 Females: 12–16	Decreased in anemia, increased in chronic hypoxia
Hematocrit, g/100 mL	Males: 42–52 Females: 37–47	Same as preceding
WBCs, thousands per mm³	Males: 5–10 Females: 5–10	Increased in infection and leukemias, decreased in bone marrow failure
Differential, % of WBCs		
Neutrophils	38–70	Increased in infection, stress, trauma, and myelocytic leukemia, decreased in aplastic anemia and myelotoxic drug ingestion
Eosinophils	1–5	Increased in allergy, autoimmune diseases, eczema, and parasitic infections; decreased in adrenal steroid production increases
Lymphocytes	15–45	Increased in bacterial viral infections, multiple myeloma, mononucleosis, lymphocytic leukemia; decreased in immune deficiency states, antineoplastic drug use, and some forms of sepsis
Monocytes	1–8	Increased in viral infection (mononucleosis) and bacterial and parasitic infections, collagen diseases, myelocytic leukemia, lymphomas, and multiple myeloma
Basophils	0–1	Increased in granulocytic and basophilic leukemia, myeloid metaplasia, and inflammation, after radiation, in polycythemia vera, and in chronic hemolytic anemias; decreased in acute allergic reactions, hyperthyroidism, stress reactions, and hypersensitivity reactions and after prolonged steroid therapy
Reticulocyte count, % of RBCs	0.5–2	Decreased in marrow failure, increased in polycythemia vera
Platelets, thousands per mm³	150–400	Decreased in marrow failure and hypersplenism, accelerated destruction, DIC, and hemorrhage; increased in compensation for hemorrhage, in polycythemia vera, and in leukemia, after splenectomy, and in malignant diseases

An additional test that may be performed to differentiate types of anemia is the osmotic fragility test of RBCs. Fragility is tested by placing RBCs in varying concentrations of NaCl solution. Fragility is increased in some hereditary anemias, acquired hemolytic anemia, and hemolytic anemias associated with malignant lymphoma, leukemia, carcinoma, pregnancy, cirrhosis, and infections. It is decreased in iron deficiency anemia, thalassemia, sickle cell anemia, nutritional megaloblastic anemia, and liver disease and after splenectomy.[4]

The presence of specific hemoglobinopathies can be determined by other tests. These hemoglobinopathies are usually genetic in origin and result in chronic hemolytic anemias. Hemoglobin electrophoresis is used to determine the presence of sickle cell anemia. The presence of Heinz bodies in RBCs when examined on a smear indicates glucose-6-phosphate dehydrogenase (G-6-PD) deficiency.

The most commonly performed tests of blood coagulation are the prothrombin time (PT), partial thromboplastin time (PTT), platelet count, and assay for fibrin split products (FSP). Assays for other individual clotting factors may also be performed after initial clotting tests to facilitate replacement therapy with appropriate factors. Calcium (factor IV) is measured during electrolyte testing. While calcium deficits are not commonly the cause of clotting abnormalities, in critically ill patients who have received numerous blood transfusions calcium levels may be of concern. EDTA, a preservative used in banked blood, binds calcium so that it is not available in its ionized form to participate in normal coagulation processes.

Table 41-4 Basic Coagulation Studies

Test	Normal Values	Clinical Implications
Prothrombin time	11–12.5 s (85–100%)	Increased in deficiencies of factors V, VII, and X and fibrinogen, dicumarol therapy, severe liver disease, DIC, and vitamin K deficiency
(Activated) partial thrombo-plastin time	26–42 s	Increased in deficiencies of factors VIII–XII and fibrinogen, with anticoagulation therapy, in liver disease and DIC, and in vitamin K deficiency
Platelet count	150,000–400,000	Decreased in idiopathic thrombocytopenia purpura and malignant disease of the bone marrow and during chemotherapy; increased in pyeloproliferative disorders such as polycythemia vera and after splenectomy
Fibrin split products	< 10 μg/mL	Increased in DIC and fibrinolysis
Calcium (IV)	9–11 mg/dL	Decreased in massive transfusions with banked blood (EDTA)

These basic coagulation tests are further described in Table 41-4. Further information on clotting studies is given in Chaps. 40 and 43.

Additional diagnostic tests are often required to evaluate the source and impact of hematologic problems. When patients have discolored urine, urine hemoglobin levels should be measured. Normally there is no hemoglobin in urine. The amount of hemoglobin present in urine, therefore, can be used to assess the presence and extent of hemolysis from various causes.

Other Diagnostic Procedures

X-rays can be used to assess the extent of blood accumulation during hemorrhages in the chest, abdomen, or head. Radionucleotide scans can be used to assess the function of the liver and spleen in patients with hepatomegaly or splenomegaly.

When severe hematologic problems are present, bone marrow aspiration may assist in the diagnosis. Since the formed elements of the blood are generated in the bone marrow, a description of the cells present in the marrow is often necessary to accurately diagnose blood dyscrasias and delineate appropriate treatment.

References

1. Rifkind, R. A., et al. (1986). *Fundamentals of hematology* (3d ed., p. 174). Chicago: Year Book.
2. Beck, W. S. (Ed.). (1985). *Hematology* 4th ed. (p. 469). Cambridge, MA: MIT.
3. Griffin, J. P. (1986). *Hematology and immunology concepts for nurses.* Norwalk, CT: Appleton Century Crofts.
4. Wallach, J. (1983). *Interpretation of pediatric tests.* Boston: Little, Brown.

42 Hyperviscosity and Anemias

Brenda S. Jackson

This chapter reviews two hematopoietic disorders, hyperviscosity syndromes and anemias, which may be seen by critical-care practitioners. Pathophysiologic processes are presented, as well as clinical findings and medical and nursing therapies.

The care of patients with hematologic dysfunctions requires a team approach. Even though the specific roles and capabilities of team members may vary from institution to institution, the complexity of the patient's needs and the potential for rapid changes in the condition demand that the critical-care nurse pay particular attention to subtle but potentially significant changes. As the primary care giver in critical-care settings, the nurse has a unique opportunity to continually assess the patient and detect the signs and symptoms in various organ systems that may indicate impending hematologic emergencies.

Hyperviscosity Syndromes

Pathophysiology

Viscosity refers to the relative resistance of a fluid to flow, that is, the state of stickiness or adherence of particles within the fluid to each other. In the blood, viscosity is usually determined by plasma protein concentration, red cell mass, and deformability of red cells. *Hyperviscosity,* then, is an exaggeration of the adhesion of particles in a fluid which results in increased resistance. In the blood this may be a result of increased concentrations of plasma proteins, increased red cell percentage of whole blood (hematocrit readings), or deformed erthyrocytes such as sickle cells. This phenomenon is seen in various malignant diseases, anemias, and inflammatory diseases.[1] Malignant diseases such as multiple myeloma, Waldenström's macroglobulin-

emia, leukemia, and polycythemia rubra vera may be the source of the marked elevation in plasma protein concentration leading to hyperviscosity syndrome.

In hyperviscosity syndrome cardiac output is compromised and perfusion of all organ systems may be impaired because of reduced regional blood flow. The increased protein mass that causes hyperviscosity increases oncotic pressure, which in turn disturbs normal pressure/flow relations. The microcirculation of highly vascular organs is particularly at risk.

Viscosity is determined by comparing the flow of the fluid in question to that of water, as represented in the following formula:

$$\text{Viscosity} = \frac{\text{rate of descent of a volume V of the test sample}}{\text{rate of descent of the same volume of water}}$$

Table 42-1 lists the viscosity values of various blood components in centipoises (cp).

Etiology

The patients most likely to present with hyperviscosity syndrome are those with hematologic neoplastic or immunologic neoplastic processes (Table 42-2). Waldenström's (primary) macroglobulinemia is a relatively rare neoplasm of B lymphocytes and plasmacytic cells resulting in production of large amounts of monoclonal IgM (macroglobulin). It is a slowly progressive disease, usually diagnosed in the fifth to sixth decade; 60 percent of the victims are male.

Multiple myeloma is a malignant disease of plasma cells that involves the bone marrow and may involve other tissues as well. Myeloma has an equal incidence in men and women, with diagnosis

Table 42-1 Normal Viscosity of Blood Components

Component	Viscosity, cp
Blood	3.6–5.4
Plasma	1.9–2.3
Serum	1.4–1.8
Water as standard	1

at a mean age of 62 years. There is a higher incidence in blacks. Massive elevations of the immunoglobulins IgG or IgA may cause hyperviscosity. The causes of multiple myeloma and macroglobulinemia are unknown.

Polycythemia rubra vera is a chronic myeloproliferative disorder that involves primarily erythrocytes but may also include thrombocytes and leukocytes. It is typically diagnosed in late middle age. In polycythemia there is a sustained increase in the level of erythropoiesis in the bone marrow, resulting in increased red cell mass (over 55 percent) and hemoglobin concentration (greater than 18 g/100 mL). A relative polycythemia may be the result of water deprivation, fluid and electrolyte disorders, and plasma loss due to burns. Hypoxia can also cause polycythemia through compensatory release of erythropoietin by the kidneys. Other disorders, such as hemangioblastoma, hepatoma, uterine fibroid tumors, renal disease, and hormonal imbalances due to androgen administration, may

also cause a relative polycythemia.[2] In polycythemia vera the total blood volume may be several times greater than normal, resulting in severe tissue and organ congestion. Clinical manifestations include headaches, pruritus, dyspnea, hemorrhage, plethora, paresthesias, thrombosis, hypermetabolism, night sweats, weight loss, splenomegaly, and hyperviscosity syndrome. Polycythemia vera is considered to be a malignant process similar to leukemia.

Hyperviscosity syndrome is a medical emergency which may present with manifestations in multiple organ systems due to disruptions in the microcirculation. The exact mechanism of circulatory disruption is not clear, but alterations in platelet function and interaction with other coagulation factors may be underlying problems, in addition to laminar flow problems related to viscosity itself.

Clinical and Diagnostic Findings

Patients with hyperviscosity syndrome may present with neurologic signs and symptoms ranging from headache, dizziness, paresis, hearing loss, blurred vision, and loss of vision to coma, congestive heart failure, bleeding diathesis, and renal failure. Ocular changes are often prominent. On ophthalmoscopic examination, distention and tortuosity of retinal veins, local areas of beading and dilatation creating a "string of sausages" appearance, and flame-shaped

Table 42-2 Causes of Hyperviscosity

Pathophysiology	Underlying Condition
Increased plasma proteins	
Hyperfibrinogenemia	Hodgkin's disease, inflammatory syndromes
Increased immunoglobulins	
Monoclonal (IgG)	Primary macroglobulinemia (Waldenström's), multiple myeloma, cryoglobulinemia
Polyclonal (IgA)	Disorders with circulating immune complexes
Increased red cell mass	Polycythemia rubra vera, erythrocytosis
Abnormalities in deformability of red blood cells (drepanocytes)	Sickle cell disease, thalassemia
Relative hyperviscosity	Hypoxemia, water deprivation, plasma loss due to burns, fluid and electrolyte disorders, renal disease, androgen administration, hemangioblastoma, hepatoma, uterine fibroid tumors

hemorrhages are common findings. Conjunctival tissues may also be engorged, with dilated and tortuous vessels and marked sludging of red cells readily apparent.

Laboratory findings may include marked elevations in the various formed elements in the complete blood count, elevation of blood proteins on electrophoresis, and elevated viscosity of more than 1.8 cp. Many patients do not have overt signs and symptoms until the viscosity reaches 4 to 5 cp, however. There is great variability in viscosity levels and onset of clinical manifestations among patients, influenced by hydration status, age, and other preexisting problems.

Medical and Surgical Interventions

The treatment of the underlying disease process resulting in hyperviscosity varies. Generally, myeloma, polycythemia vera, and Waldenström's macroglobulinemia are managed on a chronic basis by chemotherapy and other supportive modalities. None of these processes are curable by medical regimens, so hyperviscosity syndrome may recur. When hyperviscosity occurs, it is considered a medical emergency. Removal of excess plasma proteins by plasmapheresis, using a cell separator, is a rapid and effective means of treating the syndrome. This improves the congestive heart failure, the retinopathy, the bleeding diathesis, and the central nervous system symptoms. Plasmapheresis may also be employed on a chronic outpatient basis to manage disease processes predisposing to hyperviscosity syndrome.

Plasmapheresis is a method for selective removal of blood components, consisting in removal of blood from the patient, centrifugation to remove the plasma, and return of the packed red cells to the patient. In acute situations 3 to 4 L of blood may be processed over 1 to 2 days. In polycythemia vera, treatment may consist of phlebotomy rather than pheresis to reduce blood volume as well as concentration of erythrocytes and other elements.

Plasmapheresis is a safe procedure; however, hypotension and bradycardia may result from rapid changes in blood volume. Vital signs should be monitored frequently during the procedure. Hypovolemia can result if the amounts of plasma removed are not carefully balanced with fluid replacement therapy, usually in the form of Ringer's lactate solution. Patients with a hemoglobin level of 9 g/100mL may be given a transfusion prior to plasmapheresis to prevent these problems. Intensive plasmapheresis at a rate of 1 L per day may lead to significant depletion of albumin and platelets. Serum albumin may need to be replaced at the beginning of treatment to prevent these problems. Platelet packs may be needed, but platelets usually recover rapidly.

Hypocalcemia can occur during plasmapheresis, because a great deal of calcium is lost in the plasma which is removed and additional amounts are inactivated by the acid-citrate-dextrose (ACD) solutions used for anticoagulation. The patient should be carefully monitored for signs of neuromuscular irritability, tetany, and prolongation of the QT interval on the electrocardiogram. Early clinical signs of hypocalcemia include tingling in the fingers and circumoral region and muscular cramps. If calcium gluconate is administered, the patient must be carefully monitored for ventricular arrhythmias and possible cardiac arrest caused by overzealous replacement and resulting in hypercalcemia.

Emotional and supportive care during the crisis and therapy periods are essential. Pain is usually experienced by the patient only when the needles for pheresis (usually 16-gauge) are inserted. Immobilization during the period of plasmapheresis can lead to discomfort and boredom. The staff should provide for frequent repositioning and diversion. Efforts should be made to provide continuity of care during the procedure. If possible, frequent family visits should be allowed in an effort to decrease anxiety.

Following plasmapheresis, pressure dressings are applied to the needle puncture sites. The sites should be frequently checked to assess for bleeding, and areas distal to the sites should be assessed for adequacy of perfusion. During the treatment, vital signs and heart and breath sounds should be monitored frequently, as should the ECG, jugular venous pressure, and mental status, to assess the patient's response to therapeutic intervention.

Nursing Interventions

Care of the patient suffering from hyperviscosity syndrome varies with the organ systems involved and the degree of compromise. A thorough assessment of the patient's physiologic and psychologic needs will dictate the plan of care. The patient who is conscious will probably be extremely weak and will tire easily, so nursing activities should be planned to conserve the patient's energy. Optimal nutrition should be encouraged. Apprehension and anxiety can be reduced by explaining all procedures and tests and honestly answering the questions of the patient and family. The patient should be encouraged to verbalize feelings, since a sense of well-being is important in securing cooperation with treatment regimes.

Pertinent nursing diagnoses associated with the care of patients with hyperviscosity syndrome include potential fluid volume deficit related to rapid fluid loss during plasmapheresis, potential for injury related to hypocalcemia caused by plasmapheresis, altered level of consciousness related to poor cerebral perfusion, and altered tissue perfusion related to sluggish microcirculation. Fluid and electrolyte imbalances may also contribute to alterations in consciousness. Alterations in cardiac output and anxiety related to fear of the unknown are also pertinent. Suggested nursing interventions are outlined below.

Nursing Diagnosis

Decreased cardiac output related to decreased venous return and increased blood viscosity.

Interventions

1. Monitor ECG, vital signs, peripheral pulses, and hemodynamic parameters frequently.
2. Assess for skin color, warmth, turgor, and edema.
3. Assess jugular vein distention.
4. Evaluate heart and breath sounds and report shortness of breath, cough, or frothy sputum.
5. Record weight and fluid intake and output daily.
6. Assess for mental status changes: restlessness, headache, etc.
7. Keep head of bed elevated.
8. Promote a restful environment.
9. Provide good skin care.
10. Reposition patient frequently.

Nursing Diagnosis

Alteration in tisue perfusion related to sluggish microcirculation.

Interventions

1. Monitor changes in mentation, vital signs, and laboratory results such as arterial blood gases, complete blood count, electrolytes, BUN, creatinine, and cardiac enzymes.
2. Observe for signs and symptoms of congestive heart failure and signs of pulmonary emboli (chest pain, cyanosis, respiratory distress, hemoptysis, diaphoresis, hypoxia, anxiety, restlessness).
3. Note complaints of nausea or vomiting.
4. Auscultate bowel sounds.
5. Assess visual, personality, and sensorimotor changes (headache, dizziness, altered mental status).
6. Report chest pain.
7. Record weight and fluid intake and output daily.
8. Assess extremities for skin texture, edema, ulcerations, capillary refill, presence or absence of pulses.
9. Monitor blood count and clotting time.
10. Provide small, easily digested meals and fluids as tolerated.
11. Encourage rest after meals.
12. Promote a quiet, restful environment.
13. Reposition patient frequently and observe skin integrity.
14. Carry out active or passive range of motion exercises.
15. Promote circulation in the extremities and avoid stasis by having the patient elevate the legs when sitting and avoid leg crossing, by using antithromboembolic hose or Ace bandages on the patient's legs, and by avoiding leg massage and use of the knee-jointed Gatch bed.
16. Use an air mattress, sheepskin, and/or padding as indicated and provide a cradle to protect the extremities from the weight of the bedclothes.
17. Keep the head of the bed elevated.

Nursing Diagnosis

Potential anxiety related to fear of the unknown.

Interventions

1. Accept the patient as he or she is.
2. Acknowledge the fears, explain procedures to the patient and family, and answer questions honestly.

3. Provide opportunities for the patient and family to ventilate feelings.
4. Stay with the patient when possible and maintain a calm, confident manner.
5. Minimize environmental stimuli and provide a consistent and nonthreatening environment.
6. Monitor physical responses, e.g., changes in vital signs, restlessness, irritability, insomnia, voice changes, narrowed perception, withdrawal, and preoccupation with feelings of impending doom.
7. Identify the defense mechanisms of the patient and family and assess their normal coping skills.

Nursing Diagnosis
Potential fluid volume deficit related to plasmapheresis.

Interventions

1. Weigh patient before and after treatment.
2. Monitor fluid intake and output.
3. Assess vital signs frequently, including orthostatic pressure changes.
4. Review results of laboratory tests.
5. Assess skin turgor and dryness, also oral mucous membranes.
6. Assess for thirst and provide frequent oral care.
7. Monitor changes in mental status.

Nursing Diagnosis
Potential injury related to hypocalcemia produced by plasmapheresis.

Interventions

1. Monitor patient for signs of tetany (tingling in the fingers and circumoral area).
2. Observe ECG for prolonged QT interval.
3. Monitor laboratory test values.

Nursing Diagnosis
Alteration in thought processes related to fluid and electrolyte imbalance or sluggish microcirculatory flow.

Interventions

1. Monitor changes in mentation, vital signs, laboratory results, and fluid intake and output.
2. Provide safe environment, with sides of bed raised, restraint only when absolutely necessary.

3. Reorient patient to environment frequently and explain all procedures.

Anemia

Pathophysiology and Clinical Findings

Anemia is the most common condition resulting from hematopoietic disease. It is characterized by a reduction in circulating red blood cells or hemoglobin or both. The normal hemoglobin concentration is 13 to 14 g per 100 mL of blood in males and 11 to 12 g/100 mL in females. The normal hematocrit reading for males is 47 ± 5 mL per 100 mL and for females, 42 ± 5 mL per 100 mL.

The general effects of anemia can be attributed to a reduction in oxygen-carrying capacity, but the varied clinical manifestations are related to the specific cause and the pathophysiology involved. Hypoxia has profound effects on all organ systems, but the neurologic system and cardiovascular system are particularly vulnerable. Excessive blood loss can cause anemia by reducing the amount of circulating red blood cells and hemoglobin available for oxygen delivery in tissues. Three different types of anemia which may be encountered in critically ill patients are discussed in this section: the aplastic, hemolytic, and sickle cell varieties.

Tissue hypoxia occurs when oxygen is unavailable or insufficient on the cellular level for required metabolic activity. Many of the clinical manifestations of anemia are related to compensatory mechanisms which are activated in an attempt to preserve the oxygenation of vital tissues. At the cellular level, there is an increased synthesis of 2,3-diphosphoglycerate (2,3-DPG), which shifts the oxygen dissociation curve so that more oxygen is released to the tissues at a higher oxygen tension. Another compensatory mechanism is the use of all potential collateral and capillary channels to increase tissue perfusion to vital areas at the expense of nonvital donor areas. The major donor areas for redistribution of the blood are the skin and kidneys. Vasoconstriction and deoxygenated hemoglobin contribute to the clinical finding of pallor in anemic persons. Even though the kidneys are vital organs, under normal circumstances the oxygen supply is far in excess of demands, so that even in severe anemia, with renal blood flow reduced by almost

50 percent, renal function may be only mildly or moderately reduced. The benefit of reductions in blood flow to the skin and kidneys is seen in the enhanced supply to the myocardium, brain, and muscles.

Compensatory increases in cardiac output may result in increases in myocardial oxygen demand. Cardiac output does not measurably increase in chronic anemias until the hemoglobin levels approach 7 g/100 mL. In acute anemia there may not be time for physiologic adjustments, so the symptoms may be much more prominent. The signs of compensatory cardiac activity include tachycardia, flow murmurs (usually systolic), and orthostatic hypotension. The normal heart can sustain hyperactivity (hyperdynamic state) for prolonged periods of time; however, high output failure and ischemic pain (angina) may occur if coronary oxygen demands are not met or if there is preexisting coronary disease. An increased respiratory rate occurs also in an attempt to increase oxygenation. This accounts for tachypnea, exertional dyspnea, and orthopnea in the anemic patient.

In chronic anemia the blood volume is usually normal because of increased plasma volume. In acute anemia, particularly in the face of large volume blood loss, both volume and blood component replacement may be necessary to sustain life. Patients encountered in critical-care areas may have chronic or acute anemia, or both concurrently. An example of the type of patient who presents with both types of anemia is the alcoholic patient who is admitted with bleeding esophageal varices. Chronic anemia should be suspected in any patient who is malnourished. Patients with anemia from any source are vulnerable to impaired wound healing in addition to failure in vital organ systems.

The final compensatory mechanism for anemia is an increase in the rate of erythrocyte (red blood cell, or RBC) production, as indicated by an increased reticulocyte count. Reticulocytes are immature red blood cells which contain networks of filaments and granules; they normally constitute about 1 percent of the circulating RBCs. Increased erythrocyte production is stimulated by erythropoietin, a hormone produced by the kidney in physiologic response to hypoxia. When the bone marrow is functionally responsive, with resultant increased bone marrow activity, the patient may

complain of generalized aches and pains or sternal tenderness.

When compensatory mechanisms are unable to correct the tissue hypoxia, symptoms may occur such as angina pectoris, intermittent claudication, and night cramps due to muscle hypoxia and local lactic acidosis. Neurologic symptoms may be prominent. The patient may complain of headache, lightheadedness, roaring in the ears (due to increased cardiac output), faintness, irritability, restlessness, and/or depression.

Aplastic Anemia

The bone marrow is responsible for the production of granulocytes, platelets, and erythrocytes. Aplastic anemia is a deficiency disorder brought about by failure of hematopoietic stem cells. The deficiency is usually accompanied by granulocytopenia (a reduction in leukocytes) and thrombocytopenia (a reduction in platelets), resulting in pancytopenia.

Aplastic anemia is a rare disorder with an incidence of approximately four cases per million population.[2] In 50 percent of the cases it is not possible to identify a specific cause, and the process is labeled *idiopathic*. In the other 50 percent, aplastic anemia may follow exposure to certain drugs, chemicals, viruses, or other environmental agents (Table 42-3). The actual process whereby the microenvironment of the bone marrow is disturbed and results in direct injury to stem cells is not known. Supression of hematopoietic processes by the immune system, metabolic derangements during cellular differentiation, and genetic anomalies probably account for many of the stem cell changes resulting in aplastic anemia.

The clinical severity of aplastic anemia varies from insidious and gradual in onset, as in idiopathic cases, to rapid, as in exposure to myelotoxins or radiation. Patients usually present with progressive lassitude, fatigue, and dyspnea due to poor tissue oxygenation and with decreased ability to fight infections. Bruising and nosebleeds resulting from thrombocytopenia may occur, as well as general pallor, petchiae, or purpura. Splenomegaly and lymphadenopathy are usually not found. Blood tests reveal decreased cell and platelet counts. The diagnosis is confirmed by bone marrow biopsy, which will show moderate to severe hypocellularity with fatty replacement. The remaining hemato-

Table 42-3 Potential Causes of Aplastic Anemia

Drugs
   Chloramphenicol
   Phenylbutazone
   Diphenylhydantoin
   Mephenytoin
   Gold compounds
   Tolbutamide
   Sulfonamides
   Prophylthiouracil and methimazole
   Quinacrine
   Chlorpromazine
   Alkylating agents
   Antimetabolites
Toxic chemicals
   Benzene insecticides (DDT); organic solvents
      trinitrotoluene and toluene (glue fumes)
Infections
   Tuberculosis, viruses
Immune processes
   Humoral
   Cellular
Diseases
   Hepatitis
   Paroxysmal nocturnal hemoglobinuria
Environmental agent
   Radiation
Genetic factors
   Diamond-Blackfan syndrome
   Fanconi's anemia
   Dyskeratosis congenita

poietic cells are usually normal. Tests of hemostasis are usually normal except for bleeding time, capillary fragility, and clot retraction, all of which reflect low platelet count.

The prognosis for patients with aplastic anemia varies. The overall mortality in adults is about 65 to 75 percent, with a median survival of 3 months. Patients who develop aplastic anemia after exposure to marrow toxins generally do better than those with idiopathic processes. The more severe the pancytopenia and marrow aplasia the worse the prognosis. Generally, the prognosis is slightly better for children with acquired aplastic anemia than for adults.

Medical and Surgical Interventions   The medical management of aplastic anemia involves discontinuation of possibly toxic medications and removal from exposure to toxic agents in the environment. Additionally, supportive care such as transfusion of blood components, administration of corticosteroids and androgens to help stimulate remaining bone marrow function, prevention of and/or treatment of infection, splenectomy when indicated, and bone marrow transplantation may be required. Bone marrow transplantation is the treatment of choice in patients with severe forms of the disease.

In the hospital setting, reverse isolation consisting of reduced patient exposure to crowds or visitors, thorough hand washing with antiseptic soap before all personal contact, and use of face masks should be instituted. Strict use of gowns and gloves and large protective devices such as "life islands" may be used in some facilities. Laminar airflow systems which direct air away from the patient may also be used. Most infections in these patients are endogenous and originate on the skin or in the gastrointestinal tracts of the patients, but care should still be taken to avoid introduction of pathogens in the environment. Certainly the patient should not be exposed to visitors or staff members who have communicable diseases. The rigor of isolation is determined by the amount of granulocyte suppression present in the patient.

Bone marrow transplantation is the treatment of choice for patients under the age of 40 years who have severe aplastic anemia and who have an HLA-identical sibling who is willing to serve as a donor. All patients with severe aplastic anemia at appropriate ages should be cross-matched for HLA with all family members in an attempt to find a suitable donor. Transplantation is usually carried out as soon as possible, because early bone marrow transplantation minimizes the risk of graft rejection, and the patient should be in the best physical condition possible as well as free from infection.[3] Blood transfusions may be withheld in patients awaiting bone marrow transplantation to avoid potential graft failure due to heightened immune response. The rationale for bone marrow transplantation in aplastic patients is to provide normal hemotopoietic stem cells to restore the patient to health. In severe aplastic anemia, the cure rate may be 70 to 80 percent with allogenic transplantation (HLA-matched family member).[4]

Hemolytic Anemia

Hemolytic anemia occurs when there is an increased rate of destruction of erythrocytes, resulting in a shortened red blood cell life span (less than 120 days). Hemolytic anemia may be congenital or acquired. Hemolytic processes can be further classified according to whether the hemolysis is predominantly intravascular or extravascular. Extravascular hemolysis occurs predominantly in the reticuloendothelial system of the liver or spleen, where defective or old red cells are removed from circulation and then destroyed. Most forms of hemolysis are extravascular.

Inherited abnormal hemoglobin, defective erythrocyte glycolysis (glucose-6-phosphate, or G6PD, deficiency; pyruvate kinase deficiency; sickle cell disease; and thalassemia), membrane abnormalities, immune and autoimmune processes, infection, and red cell trauma are the usual factors producing hemolytic anemia. The forms of hemolytic anemia and their causes are listed in Table 42-4. Clinical manifestations may be highly variable, ranging from a mild anemia to a severe fulminating hemolytic process. Any stressful situation may aggravate or accelerate the hemolytic anemia, although specific physiologic mechanisms for such an effect are yet to be identified. Infections, surgery, trauma, pregnancy, and psychologic stress are particularly noteworthy stressors.

The severity of the hemolytic anemia is determined by the rate of red blood cell destruction and the bone marrow's capacity for erythroid production. When red cells are lysed, free hemoglobin is released into the circulation. The hemoglobin released in the plasma is degraded to substances which bind to haptoglobin. These hemoglobin-haptoglobin complexes are then removed by the reticuloendothelial system. When haptoglobin binding capacity is exceeded, the breakdown products (alpha and beta dimers) pass into the glomerular filtrate and cause hemoglobinuria. Patients with severe hemolysis may also develop pigmented gallstones and exhibit jaundice. Hepatomegaly and splenomegaly may be present. An additional clinically important consequence of hemolysis is that erythrocytic membrane particles released into the plasma can act as potent stimuli for disseminated intravascular coagulation.[5] The oxygen-carrying capacity of the patient with hemolytic anemia is impaired, and this leads to fatigue and other compensatory cardiovascular responses previously discussed.

The laboratory findings in hemolytic anemia vary somewhat with the etiology. The hematocrit reading and hemoglobin are variably decreased. The reticulocyte count is elevated when the bone marrow is appropriately responding. Other tests such as the direct and indirect Coombs tests, which measure antibodies such as IgG on red blood cells and the presence of free serum antibodies, respectively, are performed when immune reactions are in question. Other laboratory tests are related to diagnosis-specific causes that go beyond the scope of this text.

Medical and Surgical Interventions   The management of hemolytic anemia is related to the specific cause and severity of the problem. When oxygen-carrying capacity is severely impaired, transfusions are given. Not surprisingly, patients with immune-mediated hemolytic anemia are difficult to cross-match. In immune-mediated hemolytic processes, steroids and other immunosuppressive drugs may be administered. In hereditary conditions the care is largely supportive. In several hereditary conditions, genetic counseling of family members may serve as a preventive measure. In the future, genetic engineering may provide a means of cure for hereditary hemolytic disorders.

Splenectomy may be performed in cases where extravascular hemolysis in the spleen is the major problem. This encompasses a wide variety of disorders characterized by splenomegaly and hemolysis, such as hepatic cirrhosis, lymphoma, Gaucher's disease, connective tissue disorders, Felty's syndrome, sarcoidosis, and tuberculosis.[5]

Management of hemolytic anemia is largely supportive. The underlying cause must be identified and treated if possible. Improvement of tissue oxygenation and support of cardiovascular function are critical goals. Patients who have sustained trauma or who have undergone surgery must be carefully managed, since wound healing is delayed and there is a propensity to infection in anemic patients.

Skin care is important in these patients to prevent trauma and infection. In jaundiced patients pruritus can be quite distressing. Soap should be avoided in bathing these patients because of its drying effects, and soothing, emollient lotions should be used to ease discomfort from itching.

Table 42-4 Potential Causes of Hemolytic Anemia

Immune-mediated
  Cold agglutinin disease
  Warm antibody processes
    ABO incompatibility, delayed transfusion reaction, anti-Kell and Duffy reactions
  Autoimmune diseases: systemic lupus erythematosis, thrombotic thrombocytopenia
    purpura
  Paroxysmal nocturnal hemoglobinuria (complement-mediated)
Inherited
  Sickle cell disease
  G6PD deficiency
  Elliptocytosis
  Spherocytosis-pyropoikilocytosis
  Alpha and beta lipoproteinemias
  Pyruvate kinase deficiency
Trauma to erythrocytes
  Severe burns
  Prosthetic valves
  Cardiopulmonary bypass
  Microangiopathic hemolysis (damaged arteriolar endothelium or fibrin deposition,
    disseminated intravascular coagulation, vascular disorders, other vasculititides)
Infectious agents
  Falciparum malaria
  Cholera
  Sepsis (*Clostridia, E. coli*)
  Mucoplasma pneumoniae
  Infectious mononucleosis
Drug-related
  Penicillin
  Alpha-methyldopa
  Levodopa
  Quinidine
  Quinine
  Phenacetin
  Sulfonamides
  Aspirin
  Nitrites (butyl and isobutyl)
  Vitamin K derivatives
  Chloramphenicol
  Thiazide diuretics
  Dapsone
Other
  Snake and spider venoms
  Hypersplenism
  Lead exposure
Overdose of lipid emulsion
Freshwater drowning
Saltwater drowning
Liver disease

Sickle Cell Anemia

Sickle cell disease is a form of hereditary hemolytic anemia. It represents the most common abnormality of the hemoglobin molecule. The gene for sickle cell is inherited as an autosomal dominant. It occurs in about 10 percent of the American black population. The homozygous condition is referred to as *sickle cell disease* or *sickle cell anemia.* Sickle cell trait is usually asymptomatic, whereas sickle cell anemia causes chronic hemolysis and acute, episodic vasoocclusive crises (*sickle cell crisis*) which can lead to organ failure. Sickle cell crisis accounts for most of the mortality and morbidity of this condition.

Erythrocytes carrying the hemoglobin S of sickle cell anemia become deformed and sickle-shaped when oxygen concentrations are reduced, pH decreases, or the concentration of 2,3-diphosphoglycerate (DPG) increases. Sickled cells cause alterations in blood viscosity by impairing flow; therefore occlusions of small vessels in multiple organs may occur when the circulation contains a large number of sickled cells. Any factor that precipitates hypoxemia, acidosis, high 2,3-DPG levels, or red cell dehydration can cause sickling of the affected red cells.

Sickling is usually reversible if oxygenation is restored. Patients with sickle cell anemia, however, carry varying numbers of irreversibly sickled cells. When these abnormal cells are removed by the reticuloendothelial system, hemolysis with varying degrees of anemia results.

The clinical appearance of patients with sickle cell anemia is consistent with that of other patients with anemia. Jaundice may be present because of extensive hemolysis. Physical and sexual development are frequently retarded. Cholelithiasis is common in these patients.

Patients with sickle cell anemia are susceptible to infections because of splenic dysfunction and complement system abnormalities. An additional problem that can inhibit the ability to fight infections may be the presence of substances that inhibit polymorphonuclear leukocyte migration during crisis periods.[5]

Sickle cell crisis is a potentially life-threatening complication caused by painful vascular occlusions in many organ systems, such as the kidney, liver, spleen, musculoskeletal system, lungs, eyes, corpus cavernosum of the penis, uterus, and brain. The rate of stroke is high in patients with sickle cell anemia.

Aplastic crises with temporary but total arrest of erythropoiesis, resulting in rapid fall in hemoglobin and hematocrit levels, and absence of reticulocytes from the peripheral blood may occur as well. Blood transfusions are vital in the management of the patient with sickle cell anemia during aplastic crisis.

Additional physical problems that the patient with sickle cell anemia experiences are related to relentless vasoocclusive episodes that may occur throughout the life span. Chronic leg ulcers constitute a difficult problem, particularly since ability to fight infection is impaired. Of particular concern to critical-care nurses are the possibility of extensive vascular impairment in the kidneys, which can lead to hematuria or papillary necrosis and ultimately renal failure, and pulmonary vascular occlusions, which can lead to infarctions that alter blood flow and promote hypoxia. Supplemental oxygen therapy is important in sickle cell anemia to maintain arterial oxygen levels within the normal range to prevent further sickling.

Medical and Surgical Interventions   The management of patients with sickle cell anemia is directed at maintaining hemostasis in an attempt to prevent and manage sickling and aplastic crisis. Supportive care includes administration of blood transfusions as needed, providing supplemental oxygen, and avoiding dehydration and acid-base derangements. Prevention and aggressive management of infections is vital, since these patients have an impaired ability to fight infection. The patient experiencing sickle cell crisis requires aggressive management of the severe pain which occurs because of disseminated vascular occlusions in multiple organs.

The management of patients with sickle cell anemia who require surgery or care for intercurrent illness is complicated by the fact that the multisystem effects of sickle cell anemia must be taken into account when planning care of the concurrent illness. Patients who are going to have elective surgery may require serial blood transfusions prior to surgery to increase the concentration of circulating normal hemoglobin preoperatively, in an attempt to prevent sickle cell crisis in the perioperative period. Particular attention should be directed toward assessing neurologic, renal, cardiopulmonary, and gastrointestinal function postoperatively. The stress of surgery may precipitate problems with the sickling process.

In long-term management of sickle cell anemia and trait, genetic counseling is important. Patients with sickle cell anemia frequently survive into the reproductive years. Pregnancy presents risks to the patient and fetus because of previously discussed problems with vasoocclusion and hemolysis. These patients need to be counseled regarding the risk of transmitting the defective gene to their offspring. The major need for counseling is with persons who have asymptomatic sickle cell trait. When two persons with sickle cell trait have children, there is the possibility of one-fourth of their children having sickle cell trait and one-half having sickle cell anemia.

Nursing Interventions

Pertinent nursing diagnoses in patients with anemia are identified with the specific pathophysiology in mind. All anemic patients share the same potential problems in altered cardiac output, altered tissue perfusion, impaired gas exchange, decreased activity tolerance, and potential for injury from poor wound healing and transfusion reactions. Other potential nursing diagnoses relate to type-specific concerns such as pruritus, knowledge deficit, thrombophlebitis, maintenance of acid-base and fluid balance, nutritional alterations, pain, impairment of skin integrity, and potential ineffective coping. General nursing diagnoses and interventions for the anemic patient are outlined below.

Nursing Diagnosis
Increased or decreased cardiac output due to compensatory mechanisms for tissue hypoxia.

Interventions

1. Monitor vital signs and peripheral pulses, hemodynamic parameters, and ECG frequently.
2. Assess for skin color, warmth, turgor, and edema.
3. Assess jugular distention.
4. Assess heart and breath sounds and report shortness of breath, cough, or frothy sputum.
5. Record weight and fluid intake and output daily.
6. Assess for mental status changes, restlessness, headache, etc.
7. Keep head of bed elevated.
8. Promote restful environment.
9. Provide good skin care.
10. Reposition patient frequently.

Nursing Diagnosis
Potential injury related to decreased ability to fight infection.

Interventions

1. Note risk factors for occurrence of infection.
2. Observe for signs of infection at sites of insertion of invasive lines, sutures, or wounds.
3. Observe for signs and symptoms of sepsis: fever, chills, diaphoresis, altered level of consciousness.
4. Monitor laboratory results: WBC, blood and other cultures.
5. Stress proper hand washing by all personnel.
6. Maintain aseptic technique when inserting invasive lines.
7. Cleanse wounds daily or prn with Betadine or appropriate solutions.
8. Change dressings as needed.
9. Monitor visitors and care givers to protect compromised host.
10. Provide for isolation as needed.

Nursing Diagnosis
Potential injury related to transfusion reaction or thrombophlebitis.

Interventions

1. Monitor patient carefully during infusion of blood products, observing for mentation changes, flank pain, hematuria, urticaria, or pruritus.
2. Administer prescribed medications such as diphenhydramine (Benadryl).
3. Assess IV insertion sites for erythema, induration, or pain and rotate IV sites every 72 h or per hospital policy.
4. Change IV dressing aseptically per hospital policy.

Nursing Diagnosis
Alteration in comfort related to pruritus.

Interventions

1. Avoid use of soap or other drying or irritant substances on the skin; use emollient lotions.
2. Urge patient not to scratch pruritic areas, and apply topical medications as prescribed.

Nursing Diagnosis
Activity intolerance related to potential tissue hypoxia.

Interventions

1. Assess ability of patient to move about and degree of assistance required.
2. Assess treatment-related factors such as medication side effects.
3. Plan care with rest periods between activities.
4. Protect patient from injury by assisting with activities as indicated.
5. Take comfort measures and administer pain relief measures if needed.
6. Encourage patient to participate in planning of activities when feasible.
7. Provide restful environment.
8. Assist patient to learn appropriate safety measures.
9. Provide for progressive increase of activity as tolerated.

References

1. Sultan, C., Gouault-Heilmann, M., & Imbert, M. (1985). *Manual of hematology.* New York: Wiley.
2. Griffin, J. (1986). *Hematology and immunology concepts for nursing.* Norwalk, CT: Appleton-Century-Crofts.
3. Gordon-Smith, E. C. (1985). Aplastic anemia and allied disorders. *Current therapy in hematology-oncology* (pp. 3–4). Saint Louis: Mosby.
4. Santos, G. W. (1985). Bone marrow transplantation. *Current therapy in hematology-oncology.* Saint Louis: Mosby.
5. Staff. (1982, December). IV Anemia: Hemolysis, hematology. *Scientific American,* p. 5–31.

43 Coagulopathies

Brenda S. Jackson
Mary Brewer Jones

Pathophysiology and Clinical and Diagnostic Findings

This chapter focuses on disorders of hemostasis which the nurse may encounter in critically ill patients. Defects in hemostasis may be due to abnormalities of platelets, plasma coagulation factors, or damage to the vascular endothelium. Coagulopathies may be inherited or acquired. Hemophilia and von Willebrand's disease are inherited disorders which are, fortunately, relatively rare. Acquired coagulation disorders are more common. Thrombocytopenia, vitamin K deficiency, and disseminated intravascular coagulation (DIC) are acquired disorders most frequently seen in critically ill patients.

The normal mechanisms of coagulation are activated as a means of repairing injured blood vessels. When blood vessels are damaged, vascular spasm usually ensues at the site of injury, a platelet plug is formed, the clotting cascade is initiated, and a fibrous organization of various blood proteins results in a blood clot to stop blood flow. Similarly, to reopen the clogged vessel and reestablish normal circulation, a fibrinolytic system in the blood plasma is activated to dissolve the clot at a later time when tissue repair has begun. Normally, blood clotting is localized to the area of injury. Rapid blood flow dilutes activated clotting factors, and these circulating factors are cleared by the liver and the reticuloendothelial system.

There are two systems within the clotting mechanism: the intrinsic and extrinsic pathways. The intrinsic pathway is activated when damage to the vessel endothelial wall exposes collagen to circulating platelets and clotting factors. For normal hemostasis to occur, the platelet system must be intact. A sufficient number of normally functioning platelets is necessary for the first phase of hemostasis. A platelet plug forms in two stages following injury to the vessel wall. The initial response is platelet adhesion; the second stage is platelet aggregation, or thrombus formation. Platelet adhesion requires the platelet surface glycoprotein GP-lb and the presence of another glycoprotein, the von Willebrand factor, on the injured vessel wall. After initial contact with the injured vessel surface, platelets change shape and release substances into the vessel wall which play a role in repair of the injured area. Substances released by the platelets into blood plasma promote vasoconstriction and recruit additional platelets to form a thrombus. Fibrinogen is necessary for platelet aggregation. Thrombin, ADP, collagen, epinephrine, and serotonin are substances which can also initiate changes in platelet shape and trigger subsequent release of platelet constituents into the surrounding area. Patients with platelet deficiencies (less than 150,000 to 350,000 per microliter) or abnormal platelet function cannot form normal platelet plugs and, as a result, have prominent skin and mucosal bleeding.[1]

The numerous clotting factors normally present in the plasma are discussed in Chap. 40. When the intrinsic clotting pathway is activated by exposing collagen in the vascular endothelium to circulating clotting factors, factors XII, XI, IX, and VIII interact and then stimulate the final common pathway, composed of factors V and X and calcium, leading to the final stage of activation of prothrombin to thrombin and fibrinogen to fibrin to form the actual clot matrix.

The extrinsic pathway of coagulation is initiated when a tissue factor, thromboplastin (factor III), is released into the circulation. Factor VII is also required in the extrinsic pathway. The extrinsic pathway then activates the same final common pathway to activation of prothrombin to thrombin and fibrinogen to fibrin, leading to formation of a clot matrix. The normal coagulation system is a sophisticated and complicated enzyme substrate reaction. It is not as important to remember every distinct step in the process as it is to keep in mind that normally coagulant, anticoagulant, and fibrinolytic forces are balanced so that intravascular clotting beyond the site of actual tissue trauma does not take place. Naturally occurring anticoagulant forces include heparin, produced by mast cells in the lungs and liver; antithrombin III; adequate blood flow; the reticuloendothelial system (which clears activated clotting factors); and the fibrinolytic system.

The fibrinolytic system consists of plasma proteins: plasminogen, plasminogen activators, and antiplasmins. Plasminogen is produced by the liver and converted by activated factor XII (factor XII$_a$), thrombin, and plasminogen activators to plasmin, which is a proteolytic enzyme. Plasmin digests fibrin and factors V and VIII. Polypeptide chains cleaved from intact fibrinogen are called *fibrin split products* (FSP) or *fibrin degradation products* (FDP). The FSP bind to fibrin and prevent polymerization or extension of the fibrous matrix of the clot; they can also inhibit platelet aggregation and therefore can serve as anticoagulants. Tissue plasminogen activator (TPA) is thought to be present in the vascular wall, particularly in veins. It is released in response to exercise, certain drugs, and hypercoagulability.[2] During thrombolysis, free plasmin is inactivated by antiplasmin in the blood to prevent a systemic fibrinolytic state. In normal persons the process of fibrinolysis, phagocytosis, revascularization, reestablishment of intact vascular endothelial lining, and stabilization is completed in about 10 days after injury.[3]

A summary of factors that may activate the coagulation pathways is shown in Table 43-1. It will be noted that damage to the vascular endothelium may activate both the intrinsic and extrinsic pathways.[4]

Disseminated Intravascular Coagulation

Acquired clotting disorders are the most common coagulopathies encountered in clinical practice. DIC is a major threat to critically ill patients, because it can be activated by diverse disease states. The syndrome is always secondary to acute or chronic injury or disease. Clinically DIC is a paradoxical condition characterized by both profuse bleeding and thrombosis. The true incidence of DIC is unknown because of inadequacies in reporting, but Spero and colleagues noted a 10 percent incidence of DIC in a retrospective chart audit in a hospital.[5] Hewitt and Davies reported an incidence of 0.1 percent in hospitalized patients, or 1:1000.[6]

In DIC there is massive activation of the coagulation system which extends beyond local tissue injury and results in overwhelmed body defenses. Despite the vigorous treatment used in DIC, the mortality rate remains greater than 50 percent.

The pathogenesis of DIC is complex. The basis of the disorder is thought to be excessive proteolysis of fibrinogen and fibrin by thrombin and plasmin in the systemic circulation, which results in fibrin deposition in the microvasculature, consumption of clotting factors and platelets, and activation of the fibrinolytic system.[7] Fibrin split products, which are anticoagulants, are produced as a result of this process. If the reticuloendothelial system is impaired or overwhelmed by the volume of FSP, they are not cleared adequately from the circulation and can potentiate the state of anticoagulation that already exists in DIC. Factors which trigger DIC can be grouped as (1) conditions that introduce tissue factors (procoagulants) into the

Table 43-1 Clinical States That Activate Coagulation

Intrinsic Pathway	Extrinsic Pathway	Common Pathway
Anoxia, acidosis, heat stroke, viremia, antigen-antibody complexes that denude vascular endothelium, damaged vascular endothelial walls	Massive tissue trauma, burns, surgery, septicemia, breakdown of tumor cells, tears in vascular endothelial walls	Snake venom, amniotic fluid embolism, acute pancreatitis

Table 43-2 Factors Which Can Trigger DIC

Factors	Associated Conditions
Introduction of tissue factors into the circulation	Tissue necrosis, hemolysis, crush injury, neoplasm (especially pancreatic carcinoma and promyelocytic leukemia) fat embolism, snake bite, abruptio placentae, retained dead fetus, septic abortion, amniotic fluid embolism
Damage to vascular endothelium	Aneurysm, heat stroke, hemolytic-uremic syndromes, sickle cell anemia, acute glomerulonephritis, microangiopathic hemolytic anemia, Rocky Mountain spotted fever, hemangioma, major surgery (especially cardiothoracic), endotoxins, near drowning, antigen-antibody reactions (transfusion mismatch), antigen-antibody complexes (systemic lupus erythematosis), anoxia, cyanotic heart disease, ARDS, organ transplant rejection
Stagnant blood flow	Shock, acidosis, cardiac arrest and CPR, Kasabach-Merritt syndrome (carvernous hemangioma)
Infectious agents	Bacterial (gram-negative meningococcemia) and viral diseases (arboviruses, varicella, variola, rubella), parasitic infections (malaria, kala-azar); mycotic infection (histoplasmosis), rickettsial disease

circulation, (2) damage to the vascular endothelial surfaces, (3) conditions that contribute to stagnant blood flow, and (4) various infectious agents.[8] These factors can activate both clotting pathways. A summary of conditions related to these factors is presented in Table 43-2.

Procoagulant potency, duration of exposure, speed and route of entry of procoagulants into the circulation, quality of perfusion, and acid-base balance determine the severity of DIC. An additional problem area in many critically ill patients is the functional capability of the reticuloendothelial system (RES). Normally the RES removes fibrin and activated clotting factors, endotoxins, and FSP from the circulation. Dysfunction of the RES resulting from liver failure or shock may result in an inability to clear these factors, leading to hypercoagulability and DIC. Steroid therapy may also impair the function of the RES.

DIC may be present as a chronic or acute syndrome accompanying many illnesses. Chronic subacute DIC may be associated with various chronic underlying systemic diseases such as malignant disorders, promyelocytic leukemia, retained dead fetus, hemangioma, and aortic aneurysm. Connective tissue diseases and chronic renal disease also predispose patients to chronic DIC. Thrombotic manifestations may be prominent in chronic DIC, including persistent thrombophlebitis. The chronic form of DIC is probably more common than the acute form. Severity fluctuates with time. Chronic DIC is often asymptomatic but documented by abnormal laboratory findings. Critical-care nurses should be alert to patients at risk for chronic DIC when performing patient assessment. The added stress of critical illness may favor development of fulminant acute DIC.

Clinically the patient with acute DIC usually presents with bleeding from multiple sites such as points of venipuncture, suture lines, gums, the genitourinary tract, and the gastrointestinal tract. Petechiae and ecchymoses may be present. Acral cyanosis with infarction of the digits and tip of the nose may be noted. Organ failure such as renal insufficiency, sudden-onset cardiac failure, and strokelike symptoms and convulsions may be encountered; they are due to widespread fibrin deposits in the microvasculature of multiple organ systems. Shock of any kind may either precipitate or be a sign of DIC. Persistent acral cyanosis or the development of gangrene is highly suggestive of DIC.

Critical-care nurses should be particularly thorough in assessing patients who are at high risk for acute DIC. The skin and mucous membranes and all secretions should be observed at regular intervals for obvious and occult bleeding. Patients with shock, crush injuries, septicemia, or extracorporeal circulation should be monitored carefully to detect the development of DIC.

The cardinal sign of DIC is an elevated level of FSP. Fibrinogen levels are usually low but may be normal in some cases. Other laboratory tests may be used to further substantiate the diagnosis of DIC, including platelet count, prothrombin time, and partial thromboplastin time. Factors V and VIII may be normal or grossly decreased. A summary of diagnostic findings for DIC is presented in Table 43-3.

The presence of *schistocytes* (fragmented RBCs) indicates fibrin deposition in small vessels and thrombotic phenomena. A microangiopathic hemolytic anemia may therefore occur in DIC.

It may be difficult to distinguish DIC from primary fibrinolysis, which is a relatively rare phenomenon. In primary fibrinolysis platelet counts are normal, however, and the plasma paracoagulation test, which provides evidence of circulating fibrin monomers, is negative.

Thrombocytopenia and Platelet Dysfunction

Decreased production of platelets and platelet dysfunction may arise from a variety of factors. Drugs such as thiazide diuretics, estrogens, cytotoxic agents, interferon, gold, ethanol, and sulfonamides may suppress platelet production. Table 43-4 lists drugs that interfere with platelet production. In some cases the mechanisms for drug-associated thrombocytopenias are not known.

Irradiation of bone marrow, aplastic anemia, leukemias, myeloproliferative disorders, metastatic carcinoma, and vitamin B_{12} or folate deficiencies may also cause thrombocytopenia. Some persons may have hereditary thrombocytopenias. Increased destruction of platelets can be caused by autoimmune processes such as thrombocytopenic purpura and systemic lupus erythematosis, other antigen-antibody reactions, and hypersplenism, extracorporeal circulation, and prosthetic cardiac valves.

Platelet dysfunction may also occur. *Congenital* defects may occur in platelet adhesiveness,

Table 43-3 Laboratory Findings in DIC

Fibrin split products	Increased
Platelet count	Decreased
Partial thromboplastin time	Prolonged
Prothrombin time	Prolonged
Fibrinogen	Usually decreased
Factors V and VIII	Usually decreased
Schistocytosis	Present

platelet secretion, or platelet factor 3 (procoagulant activity). *Acquired* platelet dysfunction may be found in uremia, myeloproliferative disorders, dysproteinemias, and liver disease and as a result of drug ingestion (dextrans, aspirin, and dipyridamole).

When thrombocytopenia or platelet dysfunction exists, patients may exhibit petechiae, purpura, or confluent ecchymoses as well as oozing from mucous membranes in the nose, mouth, uterus, and gastrointestinal, genitourinary, and respiratory tracts. When platelet counts are greater than 40,000 per cubic millimeter but less than 150,000 per cubic millimeter, bleeding occurs after injuries or surgery, but spontaneous bleeding is uncommon. With platelet counts less than 40,000 per cubic millimeter, there may be spontaneous bleeding. Severe, spontaneous bleeding may occur any time the platelet count falls below 10,000 per cubic millimeter.[7]

Liver Disease

Liver disease is one of the most common causes of coagulopathies. Critical-care nurses must be particularly alert for the possibility of underlying liver disease when patients have a history of alcohol abuse. Bleeding in liver disease can result from decreased synthesis of clotting factors and increased proteolytic activity because of impaired reticuloendothelial cells in the liver. Alcohol ingestion suppresses plasma protein production and platelet function.

In severe liver disease, coagulation test results are usually abnormal, showing low fibrinogen level, prolonged prothrombin time, normal or prolonged partial thromboplastin time, and prolonged thrombin time. All clotting factors except VIII are typically reduced.

Vitamin K Deficiency

Vitamin K is a fat-soluble vitamin which is not stored in the body. It is a vitamin which is essential in the formation of prothrombin and clotting factors VII, IX, and X. Vitamin K is present in many plant and animal sources, so a balanced diet should provide adequate intake. It is also normally synthesized by bacterial flora in the intestinal tract. Vitamin K deficiency is rare in healthy people, but it may be found in people with inadequate diets and those

Table 43-4 Drug Causes of Thrombocytopenia

Analgesics
  Aspirin   Oxyphenbutazone
  Indomethacin   Phenylbutazone
  (acetaminophen, antipyrine, sodium salicylate, fenoprofen, ibuprofen)
Antimicrobials
  Sulfonamide antibiotics   Isoniazid
  Sulfamethoxazole   Rifampicin
  Chloramphenicol   Paraaminosalicylic acid
  Nitrofurantoin   Trimethoprim
  (penicillin, ampicillin, methicillin, cephalothin, lincomycin, novobiocin, streptomycin, pentamidine, oxytetracycline)
Sulfonamide derivatives
  Furosemide   Diazoxide
  Chlorthalidone   Chlorpropamide
  Chlorothiazide   Tolbutamide
  Hydrochlorothiazide   Clopamide
  Acetazolamide
Cinchona alkaloids
  Quinine
  Quinidine
Sedatives, hypnotics, antidepressants, analeptics
  Allylisopropylacetylurea   Carbamazepine
  Diphenylhydantoin   Centalun
  (allylisopropylbarbiturate, butabarbitone, clonazepam, diazepam, paramethadione, meprobamate, primidone, ethyl-
    phenylthydantoin, ethyl-allylacetylurea, thioridazine, imipramine, desipramine, sodium valproate)
Other chemotherapeutic agents
  Ethanol   Arsenical antiluetics
  Estrogens   Chloroquine
  Heroin abuse   Hydroxychloroquine
  Heparin   Gold salts
  Alpha methyldopa   Mercurial diuretics
  Digitoxin   Pertussis vaccine
  Stibophen   D-Penicillamine
  (chlorphenramine, antazoline, disulfiram, hexapropymate, iopanoic acid, prochlorperazine, propylthiouracil,
    spironolactone, cimetidine, levodopa, topical podophyllin)

Note: Parentheses enclose drugs rarely reported to cause thrombocytopenia.
Source: Modified from M. Rosove, Bleeding disorders, in W. Hocking (Ed.), *Practical Hematology*, Wiley, New York 1983, p. 85.

receiving total parenteral nutrition without vitamin K supplements, in intestinal obstruction and malabsorption syndromes, in liver disease, and in people being treated with certain drugs. Coumarin blocks vitamin K utilization. Some broad-spectrum antibiotics also interfere with vitamin K activity by disrupting intestinal flora that normally synthesize it; vitamin K deficiency may develop within 1 to 3 weeks after intestinal synthesis is inhibited.

Patients with liver disease may be unable to utilize vitamin K in the synthesis of vitamin K–dependent clotting factors. Inadequate production of bile salts can impair digestion of food sources of this vitamin, since it is fat-soluble. Ingestion of large amounts of vitamin E, another fat-soluble vitamin, may antagonize the action of vitamin K in synthetic processes.

Prothrombin time and partial thromboplastin time are abnormal in vitamin K deficiency. Parenteral administration of vitamin K often corrects these abnormal laboratory values within 12 to 24 h.

Hemophilia

Hemophilia A is a genetic disease characterized by a deficiency of factor VIII procoagulant molecule complexes. Subcategories of hemophilia A have been identified, but generally the term refers to deficiency of factor VIII:C,* a relatively common (1:10,000) sex-linked recessive trait. In 30 percent of the cases, however, no family history can be elicited, leading to the assumption that random mutation may also be a causative factor.[7] The clinical manifestations of hemophilia vary. Platelet plug formation is normal. Onset of bleeding is usually delayed for several hours or days after injury but may persist for several days or weeks. The defect results in an inability to maintain hemostasis. Bruising, ecchymoses, and deep subcutaneous and intramuscular hematomas are frequent, but petechiae and purpura do not occur. Bleeding can be a particular problem after dental work, but any organ may be the site of bleeding. Bleeding into joints may cause serious chronic disability. Spontaneous bleeding may occur, but it is rare in mild cases. Exsanguination may follow injury or surgery without proper treatment.

Hemophilia should be suspected when the sex of the patient, family history, age of onset (early childhood), and type of bleeding are consistent with the typical picture of hemophilia. Blood analysis establishing low levels of factor VIII:C is diagnostic of the defect. Platelet function, platelet count, bleeding time, and prothrombin time are normal. The partial thromboplastin time is prolonged.

Von Willebrand's Disease

Like hemophilia, von Willebrand's disease is a relatively common hereditary coagulopathy. It is usually transmitted as an autosomal dominant trait with varying expression and penetrance. In rare instances it may be inherited as an autosomal recessive character. It affects both sexes equally, with no racial or ethnic preference. Mild cases may not be identified, so the incidence is difficult to estimate. It is the most common congenital bleeding disorder diagnosed in adulthood. The underlying defect in von Willebrand's disease is in vascular endothelial cells, which are either unable to pro-

duce factor VIII:RAg or produce molecules that cannot polymerize into VIII:vWF. This leads to decreased amounts of factor VIII:C and impaired interaction between platelet glycoprotein and the subendothelium of blood vessels during the clotting process, so that primary hemostatic mechanisms related to platelet adhesion are impaired. Factor VIII is essential for normal function of the intrinsic pathway. In this syndrome, bleeding time is characteristically prolonged. There are also other abnormalities in the factor VIII complex. Platelet aggregation with ADP, epinephrine, and collagen is usually normal in von Willebrand's disease.

Clinically, patients with von Willebrand's disease present with localized bleeding problems. Often the patient reports a family history of excessive bleeding after trauma or surgery or in childbirth. In severe form bleeding tendencies are usually identified in childhood, but less severe expression may not be obvious before adulthood. Skin and mucosal hemorrhages are the most common expressions of the disorder. Spontaneous bleeding should be reported. With injuries, bleeding typically starts within seconds and may continue for hours. Once hemostasis has been achieved it can usually be sustained. In women, menorrhagia is common, and severe postpartum bleeding occurs in about 30 percent of cases. Since the condition is an inherited trait, neonates should be assessed for possible coagulopathy.

Von Willebrand's disease is characterized by prolonged bleeding time, normal platelet count, decreased platelet adhesiveness, and reduced factors VIII:C and VIII:R.

Medical and Surgical Therapies

The goal of medical treatment of coagulopathies is maintenance of hemostasis. Underlying deficiencies are treated with replacement therapy; in acquired coagulopathies, the primary disease is treated, if possible, as a means of correcting the coagulopathy. Specific therapies for each of the previously discussed coagulopathies are addressed below.

Disseminated Intravascular Coagulation

The treatment of DIC is as complex as the pathophysiology of the disorder. Since DIC is a secondary

---

*Factor VIII is a complex of subfactors, each identified by a letter or letters. Factor VIII:C causes classic hemophilia A when deficient. Factor VIII:vWF is von Willebrand's factor and, when deficient, causes von Willebrand's disease. Factors VIII:C and VIII:vWF normally circulate as a complex. Factor VIII:Ag is an antigen associated with factor VIII:C. Another subfactor in the factor VIII complex is factor VIII:R (or the antigen form, factor VIII:RAg).

process, the ultimate goal is to treat the primary disease state that creates the factors triggering it. If there is significant bleeding, blood lost is replaced and plasma given to replace clotting factors. When shock and resultant metabolic abnormalities are present, they must be treated aggressively. Acidosis creates an environment favoring clotting. Fresh-frozen plasma is given, since it contains all the clotting factors. Initially 10 mL/kg is given. Platelet concentrates are given to correct thrombocytopenia. Cryoprecipitate may be used to treat severe hypofibrinogenemia. When large vessel and microvascular thrombosis leading to end-organ damage occurs, heparin is also given. The presence of schistocytes in the peripheral blood smear is indicative of these processes. In many patients, plasmin action may be increased while thrombin action has ceased; heparin is of no benefit when thrombin action is not a factor.

Heparin is useful in the early course of major hemolytic transfusion reaction to deter development of DIC, as well as in Kasabach-Merritt syndrome (giant cavernous hemangioma), some snake bites, and amniotic fluid embolism. It appears to be useful also in removing fibrin in situations where thrombosis, thromboembolism, or necrosis is the primary complication of DIC and in the treatment of the chronic DIC of malignant disease. Heparin plus platelet transfusion is sometimes used along with chemotherapy in induction therapy for acute promyelocytic leukemia, because the incidence of DIC is so high in patients with promyelocytic leukemia. Heparin is not useful in DIC associated with abruptio placenta, aortic aneurysm, hemorrhagic shock, or postcardiopulmonary bypass.[7] Heparin dosage is usually regulated so that the PTT is prolonged to 2½ times normal. A bolus of heparin of 10,000 units or more is given initially, followed by intermittent or continuous intravenous infusion. Platelets and clotting factor replacements are also given when heparin is used. The effect of replacement therapy may be short-lived, however, in the face of continued consumption.

Treatment for DIC must be tailored to the clinical manifestations in the patient, laboratory findings, and underlying disease processes. Acidosis must be corrected for therapy to be successful. The best index of successful therapy is reduction or cessation of bleeding. It may take additional time for the platelet count to return to normal after bleeding has stopped and other clotting factors are normalizing.

ε-Aminocaproic acid (EACA; Amicar) is a fibrinolytic inhibitor substance which blocks the accumulation of fibrin degradation products and thus protects hemostatic plugs. Bleeding usually ceases rapidly after administration of EACA, but vascular channels remain thrombosed, which can be dangerous if the patient has not been previously treated with heparin. Fibrinolytic inhibitors should be used cautiously in patents with DIC. In DIC the fibrinolysis is typically limited to the microvasculature, and it is a physiologic response to deposition of thrombin. Lysis in the macrocirculation is characteristic of systemic hyperfibrinolysis, possibly as a result of activators released from endothelial cells. It is difficult to distinguish between DIC and systemic hyperfibrinolysis, since the abnormal laboratory values are similar. In isolated primary fibrinolysis there is a shortened euglobulin lysis time without thrombocytopenia. Fibrinolytic inhibitors such as EACA are useful in the treatment of systemic fibrinolysis associated with prolonged cardiopulmonary bypass, cyanotic heart disease, and prostatic carcinoma.[9]

The variations in treatment for DIC are summarized in Table 43-5.

Thrombocytopenia and Platelet Dysfunction

Treatment of the patient with thrombocytopenia and/or platelet dysfunction is largely supportive. Platelet infusions are given to support levels for adequate hemostasis. If platelet destruction is a result of an autoimmune process, steroids may be used. Splenectomy is performed in refractory cases of thrombocytopenia. Medications that interfere with platelet activity and suppress platelet production should be given with caution in patients with thrombocytopenia and platelet dysfunction.

Liver Disease

Patients with coagulopathies resulting from liver disease present treatment difficulties that depend on the severity of hepatocellular dysfunction. Clotting factor synthesis is usually impaired. Fibrinogen levels are normal until the liver disease is far advanced. Thrombocytopenia may result from portal hypertension and associated hypersplenism.

Table 43-5 Treatment of Acute, Severe Disseminated Intravascular Coagulation

Treatment	Rationale	Details	Goals
Life-support measures	Self-evident	Fluids, blood, respiratory care, pressors, etc.	Maintain cardiac output, gas exchange, electrolyte balance, etc.
Treatment of underlying disorder	Correct the cause of DIC	Dependent upon primary diagnosis	Inhibit or block complicating pathologic mechanism of DIC, in parallel with response (if any) of disorder
Antithrombotic agents	Block microthrombus formation	Therapeutic doses of heparin by continuous intravenous infusion; monitor by plasma fibrinogen concentration; continue as long as predisposing clinical state persists	Prevent fibrin formation; tip balance within microcirculation toward physiologic fibrinolysis; allow reperfusion of skin, kidneys, brain
Transfusion	Reestablish normal hemostatic potential once thrombosis is blocked by heparin	Infuse platelets and cryoprecipitate for fibrinogen and factors V and VIII; repeat as indicated by laboratory and clinical observation	Increase platelet count and plasma fibrinogen to 50% of normal, if consumption blocked; diminish and stop bleeding during interval of hours to several days
Fibrinolytic inhibitors	Block accumulation of degradation products in blood; protect hemostatic plugs	ε-Aminocaproic acid, loading dose 4–6 g, then 1 g every 1 or 2 h for limited duration (up to 48 h)	Rapid cessation of bleeding keeping vascular channels occluded with thrombus; dangerous if thrombotic process not previously treated with heparin

Source: Williams et al.,[9] p. 1439.

When patients with liver disease develop bleeding complications, factor replacement is used, since the underlying disease process is often incurable. Fresh-frozen plasma, cryoprecipitate, and platelet transfusions are administered if necessary. Vitamin K is also given parenterally. Malabsorption of vitamin K is common in liver disease.

Vitamin K Deficiency

In vitamin K deficiency the underlying condition is treated and vitamin K supplements are given either orally or intravenously. A 10-mg dose of vitamin K given intravenously will correct the coagulation defect in 24 to 48 h. Doses of up to 50 mg IV may be administered for more rapid reversal. Response to therapy is monitored by following serial prothrombin times 24 h after administration. A poor prognosis is related to prothrombin times greater than 1½ times normal which do not respond to

vitamin K therapy. When dietary intake of vitamin K is not feasible, as in patients receiving long-term nasogastric suction or total parenteral nutrition and those with malabsorption syndromes from various causes, vitamin K supplements should be given. Patients who are capable of eating should be instructed about the necessity of consuming a balanced diet, including green leafy vegetables and vegetable oils rich in vitamin K. Drugs which block vitamin K use in the synthesis of clotting factors (e.g., warfarin) must be monitored carefully. Patients who are receiving antibiotics which destroy intestinal flora that normally synthesize vitamin K should also be monitored to detect vitamin K deficiency.

Hemophilia

Local measures such as application of pressure and cold are used in patients with hemophilia who are experiencing bleeding episodes. Factor replacement therapy is given to temporarily correct the deficiency of factor VIII. Antihemophilic factor (AHF) is a concentrate of factor VIII. In emergency situations or for surgery AHF must be given every 10 to 12 h because of its short duration of action and the need to bring levels up to 80 to 100 percent of normal. Factor VIII activity disappears rapidly after transfusion, having a half-life of 12 h, so repeated infusions are required until bleeding stops. The amount given depends on the severity of bleeding. Patients who have sustained severe blood loss are given transfusions of whole blood for volume replacement. Cryoprecipitate is used to treat bleeding episodes in some medical centers, but it is not recommended because of unreliable factor VIII concentrations and because it carries a risk of transmission of hepatitis B. It is used primarily in patients with milder forms of hemophilia who do not require frequent replacement therapy. Some hemophilic patients develop antibodies to factor VIII over time. In patients with low titers of factor VIII antibodies, major and life-threatening hemorrhages are treated with massive doses of factor VIII from animal sources (bovine and porcine) and use of unactivated prothrombin complex concentrates (Konyne, Proplex) or activated prothrombin complex concentrates (FEIBA, Autoplex). Most hemophilic patients who have had transfusions show evidence of hepatitis B surface antigens and/or antibodies when tested. Acquired immunodeficiency syndrome has been recognized in some hemophilic patients who have had multiple transfusions.

Von Willebrand's Disease

Patients with von Willebrand's disease who are experiencing bleeding episodes are treated with local measures and factor replacement therapy. Transfusions of normal plasma have a sustained effect on factor VIII levels in patients with von Willebrand's disease, unlike those with hemophilia. Cryoprecipitate is used because it contains factor VIII and von Willebrand factor plus fibrinogen and fibronectin. It must be administered every 4 h as long as bleeding continues. Serial bleeding times are assessed to judge the effectiveness of therapy. The arginine vasopressin analogue desmopressin (DDAVP) is reported to be effective in treating mild

to moderate classic von Willebrand's disease; it apparently stimulates endothelial cell production of von Willebrand factor.

Nursing Diagnoses and Interventions

Patients with coagulopathies have complex problems which require cooperative interventions by the medical and nursing teams. Although the etiology and pathophysiology of a patient's problems vary and therefore require individual attention, certain nursing diagnoses related to actual or potential injury, inadequate tissue perfusion, altered cardiac output, anxiety, altered comfort, and ineffective patient and/or family coping are common to all patients with coagulation disorders.

Nursing Diagnosis
Potential for injury related to altered clotting mechanisms

Nursing Interventions
Prevent further bleeding and trauma:

1. Pad side rails and sharp objects in the environment. Use air mattress, sheepskin, or other devices to prevent pressure areas. Use bed cradle and padding to protect extremities.
2. Avoid constrictive clothing or appliances such as restraints.
3. Clean skin carefully.
4. Turn patient frequently and support with pillows to avoid development of pressure areas.
5. Shave patient only if absolutely necessary and then use electric razor.
6. Use cotton gauze and cotton swabs or Toothettes for oral hygiene. Provide frequent oral rinses with nonirritants such as normal saline.
7. Avoid rectal temperature taking, suppositories, enemas, and vaginal douches. Avoid bladder catheterization if at all possible.
8. Monitor vital signs frequently for signs of hemorrhage or shock.
9. Check BP by cuff only as necessary. Avoid cuff overinflation and rotate cuff to different extremities. Avoid prolonged tourniquet use.
10. Use local pressure over bleeding sites when possible or apply cold compresses.
11. Avoid needle punctures if possible. Use small-bore needles. Avoid IM injections. Obtain blood

specimens through central lines when possible. Apply pressure over puncture sites for 3 to 5 min.

12. Avoid use of adhesive tape. Remove tape and bandages gently.

13. Suction carefully and only when absolutely necessary.

14. Assess patient frequently for signs and symptoms of bleeding. Note oozing from mucous membranes and puncture sites, lesions of the skin and mucous membranes, changes in vital signs or mental status, abdominal distention, hematemesis, hematuria, and hemoptysis. Report pad count for menstruating or postpartum patients. Assess all body secretions for occult blood.

15. Monitor laboratory findings.

Nursing Diagnosis
Potential for decreased cardiac output related to volume loss from hemorrhage

Nursing Interventions

1. Monitor vital signs and other hemodynamic parameters frequently.

2. Assess mental status and neurologic function, fatigue, weakness, or orthopnea.

3. Check intake and output hourly. Weigh patient daily.

4. Monitor cardiac rhythm continuously.

5. Administer transfusions and repacement therapy as ordered.

6. Monitor medication regimen.

7. Promote restful and quiet environment.

Nursing Diagnosis
Alteration in tissue perfusion (cerebral, cardiopulmonary, renal, gastrointestinal, and peripheral) related to sluggish or diminished blood flow

Nursing Interventions

1. Observe for skin color, temperature, and lesions. Report acral cyanosis or gangrene of the digits or tip of nose.

2. Assess peripheral vascular function by checking pulses, capillary refill, calf tenderness (Homan's sign), and peripheral edema.

3. Check vital signs frequently. Monitor cardiac rhythm and hemodynamic parameters. Assess neurologic status, urinary output, bowel sounds, abdominal distention, and complaints of nausea and vomiting.

4. Monitor laboratory studies and coagulation profile.

5. Monitor intake and output.

6. Provide adequate nutrition. Give small, easily digested foods as tolerated.

7. Provide a quiet, restful environment.

8. Give passive range-of-motion exercises if patient is unable to move.

9. Reposition patient frequently to avoid pressure areas. Avoid the use of the knee frame; elevate the entire extremity as needed. Use air mattress, sheepskins, padding, and bed cradle to protect extremities.

10. Avoid massage of extremities.

Nursing Diagnosis
Alteration in comfort related to bleeding into tissues and diagnostic procedures

Nursing Interventions

1. Assess patient for pain. Instruct patient to report pain as soon as it develops.

2. Allow patient to verbalize feelings about pain.

3. Use heat and cold for relief as indicated.

4. Avoid massage. Reposition patient frequently.

5. Provide a quiet and calm environment.

6. Assist patient with relaxation techniques, guided imagery, therapeutic touch, and breathing skills.

7. Tell patient when a procedure will hurt.

8. Remain with patient during procedures to provide psychological support, or allow family or significant other to remain with patient.

9. Be alert to changes in pain presentation that may indicate new problem areas.

10. Administer analgesics as indicated.

Nursing Diagnosis
Anxiety related to fear of the unknown (patient and family)

Nursing Interventions

1. Assess anxiety level and coping mechanisms used.

2. Establish a therapeutic relationship: encourage patient and family to acknowledge feelings.
3. Give accurate information and do not give false reassurance.
4. Be available to the patient and family for listening and talking.
5. Accept the patient and family as they are.
6. Stay with the patient who is in a state of panic. Maintain a calm, confident manner. Speak in brief sentences, using language familiar to the patient and family.
7. Provide consistent, nonthreatening environment. Minimize stimuli. Allow supportive family members or significant other to remain with patient whenever possible.
8. Involve the patient and family in planning and providing care when possible.

Nursing Diagnosis
Ineffective coping (patient and family) related to the stress of serious illness

Nursing Interventions

1. Assess ability of patient and family to understand the situation.
2. Identify previous coping mechanisms and support effective coping behaviors.
3. Treat the patient and family with courtesy and respect. Listen to their concerns.
4. Explain events in clear, simple terms. Answer questions honestly.
5. Be nonjudgmental.
6. Encourage verbalization of fears and anxieties.
7. Encourage open communication between patient and family and the health care team.

8. Assist in dealing with change in body image.
9. Provide quiet environment. Provide for continuity of care when possible.
10. Allow supportive family member or significant other to remain with patient whenever possible.
11. Arrange referral to other health care professionals or clergy as necessary.

References

1. Rand, J. H., Fruchtman, S. M., & Aledort, L. M. (1985). Hemorrhagic disorders in pregnancy. In S. H. Cherry, R. L. Bukowitz, & N. G. Kose (Eds.), *Rovinsky and Guttmacher's medical, surgical, and gynecologic complications of pregnancy* (3d ed.). Baltimore: Williams & Wilkins.
2. Russell, J. C. (1983). Prophylaxis of postoperative deep vein thrombosis and pulmonary embolism. Collective review. *Surgery, Gynecology and Obstetrics, 157,* 89–102.
3. Marder, V. J., & Francis, C. W. (1983). Clinical aspects of fibrinolysis. In Williams, W. J., et al. (Eds.), *Hematology* (3d ed.). New York: McGraw-Hill.
4. Hubner, C. (1986). Altered clotting. In Carrieri, V. K., Lindsey, A. M., & West, C. M., *Pathophysiological phenomena in nursing: Human responses to illness* (pp. 370–371). Philadelphia: Saunders.
5. Spero, J. A., Lewis, J. H., & Haseba, U. (1980). Disseminated intravascular coagulation: Findings in 346 patients. *Thrombosis and Haemostasis, 43,* 28–33.
6. Hewitt, P., & Davies, S. (1983). The current state of DIC. *Intensive Care Medicine, 9* (5), 249–52.
7. Rifkind, R. A., et al. (1986). *Fundamentals of hematology* (3d ed.). Chicago: Yearbook.
8. Beck, W. S. (Ed.). (1985). *Hematology* (4th ed., p. 469). Cambridge, MA: MIT.
9. Williams, W. J., et al. (1983). *Hematology* (3d ed.). New York: McGraw-Hill.

part 10

Immunologic Patient-Care Problems

44 Immunologic Anatomy and Physiology

Sister Mary
Rebecca Fidler

Introduction

The purpose of any human defense is survival. This defense can be as subtle as the destruction of an invading microorganism or as overt as a protective reflex. The body has to protect against exogenous (external) as well as endogenous (internal) threats to its integrity. Historically these defense mechanisms were called *vis medicatrix naturae* ("the healing force of nature"). They are normally efficient in protecting and maintaining the body's integrity against foreign substances and restoring it when damage occurs.

The body employs not only natural defenses but acquired, adaptive defenses as well. *Natural defenses* are nonspecific mechanisms either present at birth or developing in the course of natural maturation. Among the natural defenses are anatomic and chemical barriers that keep potentially harmful substances out of the body. If these should fail, inflammation and nonspecific phagocytosis quickly remove the substances from the body periphery by effectively diluting, neutralizing, or destroying them. Natural defenses also include genetic differences in susceptibility or sensitivity and the effect of age, interferon, natural antibodies, body pH, and body temperature.

If the natural defenses allow a foreign substance to invade and subsist in the body, an *acquired* adaptive mechanism is called into action. This is the *immune response,* which, unlike natural defenses, recognizes and destroys the foreign substance (Fig. 44-1). The lymphoreticular system is responsible for this specific reaction and for preventing repeated challenge by the same type of substance through immunologic memory. The maintenance of these defenses is the topic of this chapter. A homeostatic equilibrium is needed between natural and acquired host responses. If this equilibrium is lost, interventions are needed to enhance or depress the response as necessary. They must be based on knowledge of the processes involved.

The Role of Nursing in Immunology

At present nursing textbooks offer scant documentation of ways to maintain human defense systems. The reasons for this are multiple. First, immunology has only recently become a medical science, and its importance in nursing practice is now being recognized. Immunopathologic mechanisms have been clinically defined within the past 15 to 20 years, but therapy to enhance or suppress immune mechanisms is only now becoming common. Second, while skin care has always been part of nursing, care to maintain other epithelial surfaces may or may not have been given adequate concern in the clinical setting. For instance, the role of urethral secretions in the prevention of ascending bladder and kidney infections has been documented in the past decade. Observations about the importance of proper breathing and humidity in the prevention of alveolar mucous plugs have been given new meaning by what is known about immune defenses. The same can be said for the consequences of loss of air conditioning or ciliary action in the patient who has a tracheostomy or is on a respirator.

Sterile techniques have a long history in nursing but were instituted to prevent infection when the first line of defense had been compromised by injury, such as surgery or trauma. While these are still important, nursing activities have been placed in a broader context of transplantation, congenital and acquired immune deficiencies, hypersensitivity, autoimmunity, cancer, and immunosuppression. This requires an expanded knowledge base for nursing practice.

1172

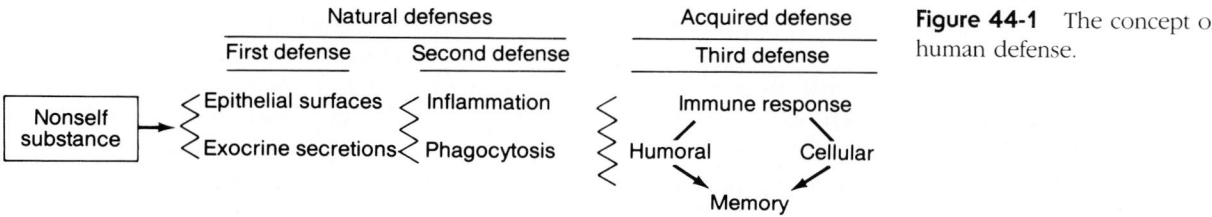

Figure 44-1 The concept of human defense.

Infections and the Compromised Host

Soon after birth a human comes in contact with many microorganisms which colonize the epithelial surfaces and are ultimately referred to as *normal flora* or *endogenous microbes*. Most of the infections which gained prominence in the past were exogenous microbes not normally found surviving on the human body surfaces. For many years only exogenous organisms were considered a threat to human existence, and fear of these organisms enabled scientists to find ways to conquer them through vaccines, antibiotics, and other means. Indeed, immunology as a medical science had its origin in efforts to deliberately establish resistance to pathogenic microbes. Technologic and pharmacologic advances have largely solved the problem of exogenous pathogenic organisms and in so doing have helped create a milieu conducive to superinfections from endogenous organisms. These organisms easily colonize epithelial surfaces and are so adaptable that they have become resistant to modern drugs. Thus, antibiotics and vaccines have shifted the balance of power in favor of adapted endogenous organisms, a situation which has little effect on the healthy person but may be devastating and lethal to the compromised host.

A *compromised host* is a person who, because of disease, age, therapy, or stress, has inadequate defense mechanisms against normally harmless microorganisms. An *infectious disease* is a complex interaction of the host with an infecting organism. Though a few infections occur as a direct result of the microorganism or its by-products, most infections are a result of variation in the defenses of the host. An environment most conducive to infection is one in which virulent antibiotic-resistant populations of endogenous microorganisms colonize the surfaces of a compromised host. This best describes the situation found in hospitals, and since the patient in a critical-care unit is often a compromised host, the interventions chosen must be aimed at not allowing the defenses to become further compromised.

New knowledge of how surgical techniques, anesthetics, medications, emotional states, and so on affect the immune response will change attitudes toward maintaining defense mechanisms in the critically ill as well as in healthy persons. The nursing profession is currently producing scholars with a sufficient knowledge base in immunology to be able to clarify the significant relationships between nursing and the maintenance of defense systems. As a result, the role of nursing in maintaining defense mechanisms will rapidly expand.

Epithelial Surfaces—First Line of Defense

The first concern in defense is to maintain the integrity of the body surfaces. This includes the skin; oral, anal, vaginal, gastrointestinal, respiratory, and urinary epithelium; and the lining of the external ear as well as the conjunctiva and cornea of the eye. These surfaces are epithelial in nature and prevent penetration by both anatomic structure and chemical secretion. Although all these surfaces are epithelial, they vary from region to region as to their type and function. Recently, it has been recognized that epithelial cells have receptors for the attachment of certain antigenic determinants. These receptors are important in maintaining normal flora and also help to explain the preferential attachment of certain microbes or chemicals to particular areas.

The antibody known as *secretory IgA* is produced by local submucosal plasma cells and is probably one of our most important defense mechanisms. IgA function has not been fully appreciated because of its role in prevention rather than response. Secretory IgA has been found in most exocrine secretions of the human body and may be critical in preventing the attachment of potential pathogens to epithelial cells.

For many pathogens, the first step in the initiation of infection is attachment to a receptor on an epithelial cell. The virulence of a particular organism may be determined by its ability to attach to such a receptor. The host defense against the attachment is apparently accomplished nonspecifically by pH, motility, flow of mucus and other secretions, cilia, desquamation, and the preferential coverage of receptor sites by normal endogenous flora. IgA enhances these natural defense mechanisms by binding to antigens and preventing their attachment to epithelial surfaces. Thus, these potential invaders are eliminated from the body.

Skin and Its Appendages

The epidermal layer of skin is a stratified squamous epithelium with a pH of about 5. It is dry and constantly exfoliates its outer surface and regenerates its basal cell layer. Exfoliation will ultimately slough any bacteria or chemicals which penetrate the outer layers of intact integument. The normal flora which can exist in this acidic, dry lipid environment are mainly staphylococci, corynebacteria, and propionibacteria. These particular organisms make survival of other microbes difficult by splitting the lipids of the epidermis into bactericidal unsaturated fatty acids (oleic acids). Mechanisms such as these keep the size of the inoculum of invading agents at a low level, allowing other body defenses to destroy alien agents promptly when injury or a break in the epithelium occurs. Sweat, sebaceous glands, and mammary glands produce secretions whose flow, osmolality, pH, cellular components, and IgA militate against infection. Mammary secretions after childbirth contain many chemical and cellular components which not only defend the infant against infections and allergic reactions but also contribute to the maturation of the infant's intestinal mucosa and the immune system. This is a host defense maturation mechanism.

Respiratory Epithelium

The anatomic structure of the respiratory tract and its epithelium plays a major role in maintaining a healthy respiratory system. The ciliated, mucus-secreting epithelium lining the nose, sinuses, larynx, and trachea warm, moisturize, and cleanse the air prior to its reaching the functional level of the alveolar spaces where exchange occurs. The bony structure of the nasal cavity, with its turbinates (conchae), controls the flow patterns of air so that it swirls and deposits particles of dust, microorganisms, or foreign substances upon the mucoid ciliated epithelium, where they will adhere to the mucus and be transported by the ciliated movement to the exterior of the body.

The respiratory tract is usually sterile below the larynx. Ciliated simple columnar epithelium lines this area. Progressing toward the interior of the lung, the epithelium changes gradually to cuboidal and finally to squamous in the alveoli. Mucus is not secreted below the bronchioles. Cilia progressively decrease in number from the trachea to the bronchioles and are not found in the alveolar areas. Mucociliary transportation of inhaled particles toward the oropharynx, together with coughing and sneezing, helps eliminate organisms from these areas. Deep breathing and proper coughing help prevent infection in a similar manner. Small quantities of microorganisms are usually aspirated during sleep but are readily phagocytosed by alveolar macrophages or physically removed by ciliary action.

Gastrointestinal Mucosa

The oropharynx is lined with a nonkeratinized squamous stratified epithelium. This is similar anatomically to skin but does not produce keratin. Epithelial glands, which include the parotid, sublingual, and submandibular glands, produce saliva. This secretion contains water, lysozyme, mucus, secretory IgA, enzymes, and cells. These collectively keep bacterial quantity in the mouth to a minimum and create a fluid flow which makes it difficult for chemicals and foreign agents to be absorbed. The lining changes from squamous to cuboidal to columnar as it descends from the oral cavity to the esophagus to the stomach.

The gastric mucosa produces hydrochloric acid, gastric juice, and mucus. The low pH of the gastric contents does not permit survival of most microorganisms. The intestinal mucosa is lined with simple columnar epithelium and produces many intestinal juices, enzymes, and hormones, as well as secretory IgA, mucus, and various other products.

Specific regional features, together with the epithelial receptor attachment of normal flora, peristaltic motility, and exfoliation, help eliminate millions of foreign agents daily by defecation.

The intestine is heavily inhabited by symbiotic-type bacteria which benefit the host in vital digestive assimilative functions, and these microbes compete with pathogenic organisms for epithelial receptors.

Genitourinary Mucosa

Anatomic differences in male and female exemplify the role of structure in infection. The male urethra is long and serves both the urinary and reproductive systems. Seminal fluid and urine maintain adequate flow through the system and add secretions which are nonconducive to the survival of foreign substances. Prostatic secretions are antibacterial in much the same way as other glandular secretions. Infections of the bladder are rare in the male, even when the system is partially obstructed—unless catheterization has occurred.

The female, on the other hand, has a short urethra, which serves only the urinary system. Bladder infections are more common in women than in men. The urinary tracts of both sexes are lined with transitional epithelium which is capable of secreting mucus, the enzyme lysozyme, secretory IgA, and other antimicrobial and antiviral substances. The peristaltic motility of the ureters, acidity of the urine, and reflexes of the bladder create a unidirectional flow which eliminates many microorganisms daily in the urine. The reproductive system of the female is defended by the acidity of its epithelial barrier as well as by its secretions.

Epithelium as a Barrier—Summary

Epithelium is an effective barrier between the body's internal and external environments. When epithelium is healthy, few microorganisms are able to attach and/or penetrate the internal environment. Only when this first line of defense fails is there a need for others (Fig. 44-1).

In summary, healthy epithelial surfaces are extremely difficult to penetrate for several reasons:

1. Because of their structure and pH
2. Because the inoculum is kept small by continual elimination

3. Because both bacterial attachment to epithelial receptors and secretory IgA prevent attachment of pathogenic organisms
4. Because of local production of chemical antimicrobial and antiviral agents

Inflammation, Phagocytosis, and Other Nonspecific Defenses—Second Line of Defense

If the first line of defense fails and foreign substances penetrate body tissues, an inflammatory response is evoked. The reaction to cellular injury is a local vascular response characterized by increased blood flow, the release of chemotactic chemicals, migration of cells, and exudation. All these are detrimental to the viability of injurious agents.

Inflammation

Inflammation is nonspecific and is initiated by any cellular injury. Presumably it is a vascular response, but phlogistic (inflammatory) substances arise from various sources, even the autonomic nervous system. Damaged tissue may release such enzymes as histamine, serotonin, prostaglandins, lysosomal enzymes, clotting factors, kinins, complement fragments, and immune factors, which also initiate inflammation.

The signs and symptoms of inflammation are well known and universally experienced. The five classic signs (heat, pain, redness, swelling, and loss of function) are the result of functional changes in blood flow through the injured area. The cause of these vascular changes is unclear. Histamine release is known to initiate the process and is followed by a sequential change in the physiology of the localized area. Prostaglandins and kinins are also powerful vasodilators.

Inflammation not only helps in the destruction of injurious agents but also prepares the area for and must precede the healing process. It is important to the maintenance of life, but it may also be destructive. Loss of homeostatic control of this process may lead to serious illness and even death.

Phagocytosis

Nonspecific phagocytosis ("cell eating") is the process by which injured cells and antigens are removed from an area. Two general cell types, polymorpho-nuclear cells and macrophages, are capable of nonspecific phagocytosis.

Polymorphonuclear Phagocytosis

Polymorphonuclear cells are particularly important in preventing infectious disease at this particular phase of the host response. Polymorphonuclear neutrophils and, to a lesser degree, eosinophils are principally concerned with the phagocytosis of bacteria. Once phagocytosed, the bacteria are usually killed and digested by lysosomal enzymes and other cell products. These two cell types, along with basophils, constitute a group of cells called *granulocytes,* and all differentiate from a common precursor cell. The process of destroying bacteria involves chemotaxis, opsonization, phagocytosis, and killing. *Chemotaxis* is the chemical attraction of phagocytes to the injured area. The chemotactic chemical is thought to be activated by the inflam-matory response. An *opsonin* is an antibody which attaches to receptors on phagocytic cells. It causes the organism to adhere to the surface of the

phagocyte and thus increases the possibility of phagocytosis. Phagocytosis may occur in the ab-sence of opsonins when a microbe is trapped between the surface of two cells, one of which must be a phagocyte (Fig. 44-2). Once the organism is inside the phagocyte, it becomes membrane-bound and is called a *phagosome.*

Neutrophils have two basic types of granules within their cytoplasm. The primary granules con-tain arginine-rich protein, myeloperoxidase, acid phosphatase, sulfated mucopolysaccharides, and other enzymes normally found in lysosomes. The secondary type is smaller and contains alkaline phosphatase, aminopeptidase, and lysozyme but is not a true lysosome. Mature neutrophils have both types, and the numbers of the secondary type increase with maturity. Both are important in the bacterial killing and digestion of ingested materials. Neutrophils are controlled by cellular by-products and are eliminated through mucosal surfaces.

The lysosomal hydrolytic enzymes are re-leased into the phagosome, with subsequent death and degradation of the ingested organism. Neutro-

Figure 44-2 Phagocytosis. Neutrophils and monocytes ingest particles by causing cytoplasm to flow around them and then bring them within an envelope of cell membrane, the pha-gosome. The digestive enzymes of the lyso-somes are then released into the phagolyso-some. *(From S. A. Price and L. M. Wilson, Eds., Pathophysiology: Clinical Concepts of Disease Processes, McGraw-Hill, New York, 1978.)*

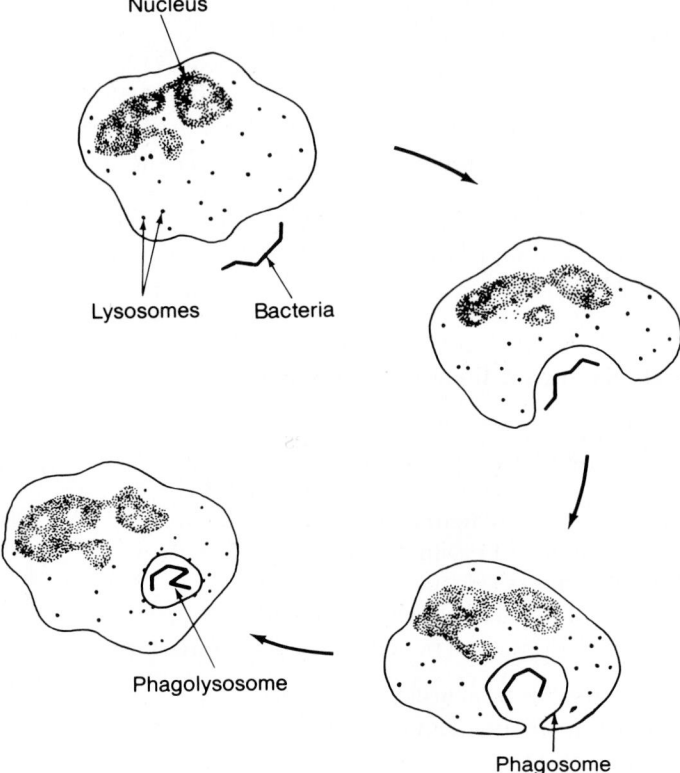

Nucleus

Lysosomes   Bacteria

Phagolysosome

Phagosome

phil phagocytosis is rapid and is initiated within minutes after microbial penetration or injury has occurred. The neutrophil usually dies in the process and forms a significant portion of purulent exudates.[1]

The main contribution of neutrophils to the defense of the host is in fighting bacterial infections. Neutropenia places a subject at high risk of developing bacterial infections. However, neutrophil counts may be normal despite the inability of host cells to kill the bacteria after phagocytosis. Acute infections have a tendency to impair the bactericidal capacity of neutrophils, because immature forms (juvenile, stab, etc.) are present in increased numbers. Patients with burns also show similar signs. Defects in neutrophil chemotaxis are also commonly seen in diabetes mellitus, cirrhosis, and rheumatoid arthritis. Drugs may affect the killing of bacteria by diminishing the numbers or the functioning of neutrophils. In certain conditions, this may render a person susceptible to recurrent pyogenic infections.[1]

Eosinophilic Phagocytosis

Eosinophils mature in the bone marrow and have a circulating half-life of about 30 min and a tissue half-life of 12 days. They are eliminated through mucosal surfaces of the respiratory and gastrointestinal tracts. They have many granules in their cytoplasm containing acid phosphatase and peroxidase and have a crystalline core (eosinophilic basic protein) which is toxic to parasites as well as to normal host cells of the tracheal epithelium.[1] The main functions of eosinophils are:

1. To ingest immune complexes
2. To limit the degree of inflammation through an antagonistic effect of aryl sulfatase B upon Slow-Reactive Substance of Anaphylaxis (SRS-A)
3. To release eosinophilic basic protein (EBP), injurious to tissue and parasites
4. To participate in antibody-mediated cytotoxicity reactions

Eosinophils are regulated by products of other cells such as T lymphocytes, mast cells, and complement factors. They are associated with allergic and parasitic disease.[1]

Macrophage Phagocytosis

Macrophages are large mononuclear phagocytic cells. They represent a separate cell line differen-

tiated from the bone marrow stem cell. They are characterized by their ability to ingest debris as well as foreign materials, unlike neutrophils, which are unable to ingest large particles (such as cells), so that their contribution is usually limited to the phagocytosis of invading bacteria. Macrophages are not terminal cells like the granulocytes but are longer-lived and participate in many facets of the immune responses as well as in nonspecific phagocytosis. When foreign material is ingested by macrophages, the material is recognized as nonself, processed, and presented to lymphocytes for destruction.

As monocytes leave the vascular system, they mature into macrophages. In tissues, they are termed *alveolar macrophages* (lung) or *Kupffer cells* (liver); in spleen, lymph node, peritoneum, mammary secretions, and elsewhere they are termed *macrophages*.[2] Chemotaxis is less apparent for these cells than it is for neutrophils. Macrophages arrive at the locally injured area later in the sequence than neutrophils, have a longer life span, and are slower, larger, and more adaptable. They secrete large quantities of *lysozyme,* a protein enzyme liberated from lysosomes of phagocytic cells that lyses bacterial cell walls; it is found in tears and saliva and in nasal, mammary, and other secretions. Bacteria, viruses, cells, debris, and other particles are phagocytosed by macrophages (Fig. 44-3). Macrophages also play an important role in immune responses, described later in this chapter.

Phagocytosis may occur prior to or simultaneously with the inflammatory process; it is increased by the inflammatory response and greatly enhanced by the immune response, although phagocytosis is not dependent on these processes.

Macrophages, when activated by a foreign substance, cell, or organism, secrete monokines, one of which is interleukin-1 (IL-1), which functions to alert lymphocytes to the presence of a foreign antigen and activate them.[2]

Additional Nonspecific Defenses

Pyrogen

Fever is the body's response to trauma or infection. It is caused by the release from host cells of a substance called *pyrogen.*

Neutrophils produce five times more pyrogen than macrophages and are thus important in febrile

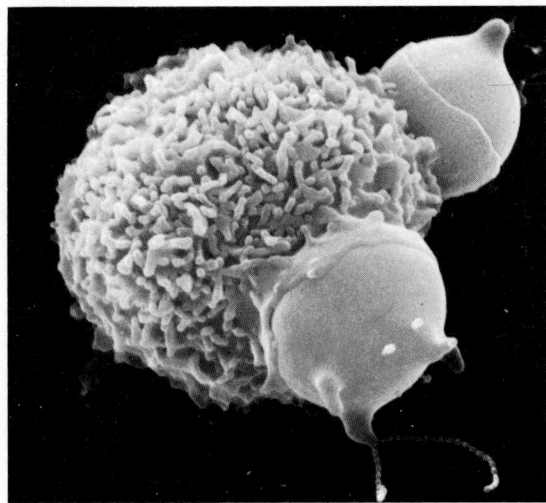

Figure 44-3   Mouse macrophage ingesting erythrocytes. The macrophage periphery extends like a collar over the erythrocytes. *(From L. Weiss and R. Greep, Eds., Histology, 4th ed., McGraw-Hill, New York, 1977.)*

conditions. However, the importance of macrophages in the febrile response, as shown in a study of fever in agranulocytosis, is quite significant. IL-1 secreted by macrophages is known to produce fever and proliferation of lymphocytes and fibroblasts and to promote production of prostaglandins and collagenase.[3]

The increase in temperature subsequent to the appearance of pyrogen is a nonspecific response which may have an inhibitory effect on bacterial multiplication and may change enzyme reactivities and diffusion, which are at least partly temperature-dependent.

Interferon

Interferon comprises a group of large glycoproteins produced by any human cell when appropriately stimulated. It was first recognized as a nonspecific mechanism to protect host cells from viral infections prior to the start of a specific immune response. Once it is synthesized, it diffuses to other cells and binds on their surface receptors. This attachment triggers production of the cells' synthesizing machinery for viral reproduction. These protein inhibitors remain inactive until the cell is infected by a virus particle.

It now appears that interferon production can be stimulated not only by virus but also by macroorganisms with an intracellular phase in their growth cycle, bacterial endotoxins, nonspecific mitogens, complex polysaccharides, double-stranded RNA, and cytokines produced by other cells. It also has become clear that interferon can do more than inhibit viral infection. Interferon produced by T cells, called *gamma interferon* (γ-INF), also inhibits division of both normal and malignant cells, enhances the cytotoxic ability of macrophages, and stimulates the activities of cytotoxic T lymphocytes.

These actions make it logical to use interferon in the treatment of malignant disease. It has been shown that interferon is capable of preventing the spread of osteogenic sarcoma and inhibiting multiple myeloma, breast cancer, melanoma, and certain types of leukemia and lymphoma. Most persons treated with interferon have been in advanced stages of disease; the use of interferon in the early stages of disease would seem even more promising. Even when interferon fails to produce regression of cancer, it may be beneficial to the cancer patient, who is likely to have immune mechanisms in a suppressed state, by inhibiting otherwise fatal viral infections.

Interferon may also be effective therapy in neonatal and adult pericarditis and myocarditis caused by Coxsackie B virus, as well as in transplant recipients.

Harmful effects have also been documented, such as bone marrow suppression, altered liver function, fever, chills, and loss of appetite. These effects are reversed when interferon therapy is discontinued.[1]

Inflammation, Phagocytosis, and Other Nonspecific Defenses—Summary

When epithelial surfaces fail to prevent penetration of foreign substances, the inflammatory process is initiated. Inflammation, a nonspecific process, is necessary before repair can begin; however, it can also be troublesome if uncontrolled. Neutrophils are most effective in the phagocytosis of bacteria. Macrophages are required, however, for effective phagocytosis of cells and debris.

In a serious inflammation, pyrogens are released by host cells into the blood. These may aid the body by raising its temperature and so inhibiting bacterial multiplication and regulating enzymatic reactions.

Interferon is produced by many cell types and appears to play a variety of roles ranging from blockade of viral reproduction to regulating the intensity of the immune response. Natural responses do not require specificity or human leukocyte antigens (HLA) restriction; therefore they do not confer upon the host cells either memory or immunity.

Acquired Host Defenses—Third Line of Defense

Immune Defenses and Biologic Self

Immune defenses are acquired defenses. They are set in motion when natural defenses fail. Immune defenses are based on the precept that self molecules are to be protected and nonself molecules destroyed (Fig. 44-4). When nonself substances are recognized by the reticuloendothelial system, the immune response is evoked. Molecules of the self fail to produce immune reactions because of a natural tolerance produced during fetal development.[4] The word *immunity* is derived from the Latin *immunitas* ("exempt" or "free from") and indicates safety or freedom from invading or transplanted nonself molecules.

Differences between individuals within a species, as well as those between species, start at the level of molecular structure. An individual's particular structure of proteins and other body materials is specified during genetic transcription of DNA.

Although, within a species, the proteins of one body are similar in structure to those of another, there are small differences in composition and shape which give uniqueness to each individual. This uniqueness is what is meant by *biologic self.*

Nonself is that which is specified by a different set of chromosomes. Constituents of the self may be called *native;* nonself substances are called *foreign* or *alien,* or *antigenic.*[5] Both self and nonself substances may carry macromolecules known as *antigens* on their surface, but only nonself material (above a certain size) is antigenic, that is, evokes an immune response.

Exogenous material such as microorganisms or transplanted cells or tissues is given its structure by an alien genetic code. Endogenous material may become antigenic subtly, through an error in the genetic code—that is, a *mutation*—or by physical change of its structure. Another way is through attachment of native protein (*carrier molecule*) to an introduced molecule too small by itself to be antigenic. The carrier molecule, together with the *hapten,* as the small molecule is called, is foreign-appearing to the lymphoreticular system.[5]

Still another source of nonself endogenous substances is native material that has become situated in an abnormal (ectopic) location. The body includes various inviolable compartments. Materials inside cells do not mix indiscriminately with those outside cells. Neither do certain molecules from various organs. The body, therefore, may treat materials or molecules that are out of place just as it does foreign material.[5]

It would seem, therefore, that to be recognized as part of the biological self, a substance must

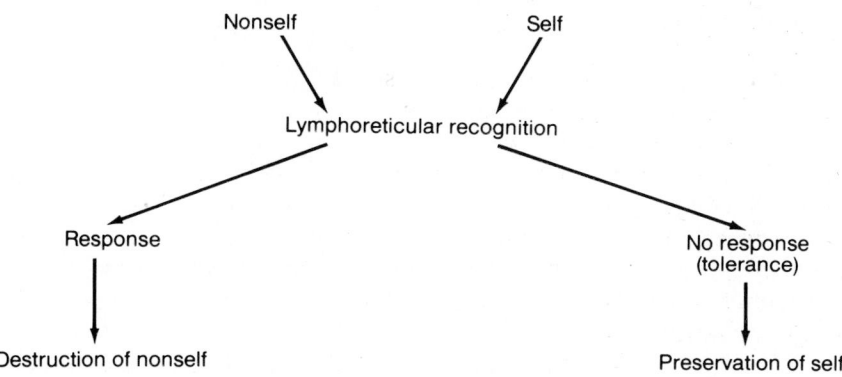

Figure 44-4 Preservation of the self by the lymphoreticular system.

be specified by the body's genome in an unmutated form, must be unchanged in structure, and must be in its normal position within the body.[5]

One of the main mysteries of immunity is how the body distinguishes between nonself and the antigen of its own cells. When antigenic challenge produces a depressed response or none, a state of *tolerance* is said to exist. The natural tolerance enjoyed by cells of the body is theorized to be a condition in which responsive cell clones have been eliminated or inactivated by antigens present during fetal development. (A *clone* is a group of cells descendant from a single parent cell.) Presentation of antigen to an animal at a time when its immune system is immature often results in an artificially induced tolerance toward the antigen when the animal is challenged with it after maturity.

The most active time for immune mechanisms seems to be shortly after birth, when the infant is exposed to a new environment and receives the greatest antigenic stimulation of its life. A substantial amount of immunity is acquired during childhood as a consequence of experience with small doses of the same organism or with cross-reacting antigens (antigens on harmless substances that closely match antigens or pathogens). Opsonizing antibody develops within a few weeks as a result of exposure to various naturally occurring environmental antigens. The newborn infant depends on passive immunity conferred by the mother's milk for prevention of allergies and also assistance in the development of immunocompetence. After about 6 or 7 years the child has a mature immune system.

A normal person seems never to be too old or too young to develop resistance mechanisms against nonself antigens, but the ability to respond appropriately is quantitatively less efficient in the very young and in old age and is altered by the level of wellness.

Specificity is essential to immune defenses. An immune response after exposure to antigen confers immunity for that agent alone, because it produces antibodies and sensitized cells able to recognize, react with, and neutralize only the offending antigen.

The first encounter with nonself antigen stimulates a primary response. A second exposure, months or even years later, elicits a much more intense secondary response. The ability of certain lymphoreticular cells to recall prior experience with the antigen is called *immunologic memory* and is characteristic of the acquired immune response.

Immune system defenses are said to be either active or passive. *Active defense* occurs when the body participates by manufacturing cells and mediators which destroy the agent. *Passive defense* occurs when the cells or mediators are merely transferred from someone already immune to the antigen to a person lacking such immunity.

The Lymphoreticular System

The lymphoreticular system includes all the cells and structures associated with recognition of, response to, and memory of antigen. Included are primary and secondary lymphoid tissue, lymphatic cells, and a network of phagocytic cells within lymphatic as well as other organs that engulf and process nonself materials (Fig. 44-5). Understanding of this system grew out of an earlier concept called the *reticuloendothelial system,* thought to consist mainly of a group of organs whose vascular sinuses were lined with phagocytic cells. Lymphoid tissue is now known to play a major role in immunity.[1]

Functions of the Immune System

The term *defense system* designates collectively all organs, tissues, cells, and functions which aid in

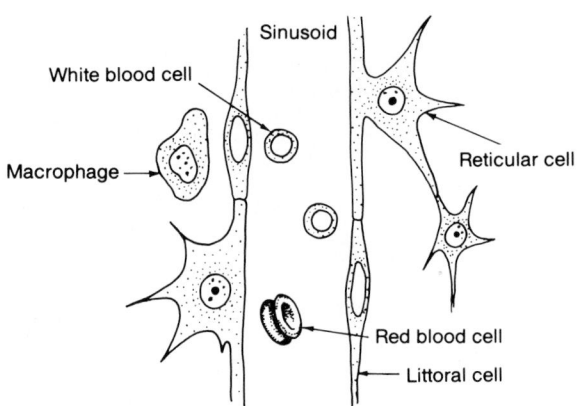

Figure 44-5   The reticuloendothelial elements purify blood, lymph, and tissue fluid.

maintaining a healthy body free from nonself organisms or molecules. Thus, cells capable of phagocytosis, cells which produce antibodies, cells which produce bioactive immune cytokines, lymph vessels, organ sinusoids, diffuse lymphoid tissue, and lymphoid organs all belong to this defense system.

The lymphoreticular system, an integral part of the defense system, extends throughout the body, in order to cover all possible surfaces, routes, and avenues of possible attack by foreign agents. Components of the lymphoreticular (or reticuloendothelial) system are encountered in all lymphoid structures and macrophages and in reticular cells, all of which are phagocytic, forming a reticular network or line of venous and lymph sinusoids (Fig. 44-5).

Healthy defense involves both natural and acquired defense. Natural defense involves epithelial surface functions, inflammation, and nonspecific phagocytosis. These natural functions include preventing a nonself molecule from violating the human body and/or destroying it. If the molecule gains entrance, rapid containment, destruction, and removal are mediated by a vascular response (inflammation) combined with nonspecific phagocytosis and sequentially followed by a cellular response of repairing any damage which may have resulted. No specificity is required, no remembering, thus no immunity is acquired as a result of natural defenses.

Acquired immune defense, however, is quite complicated, has a specificity requirement, and confers memory—i.e., immunity from nonself organisms, cells, and materials—by the following processes:

Surveillance (patrolling) and *recognition* of nonself molecules within the human body. This includes the ability to process, concentrate and present the enemy to the lymphatic cells.

Activation of differentiating populations (clones) of specialized regulator and effector cells in response to surveillance and recognition.

Specific *destruction* and *removal* of the selected nonself material.

Cellular memory, which allows recall should this specific nonself material again invade the body.

Immunogenetics

Self is determined genetically and is defined as anything synthesized by a person's own particular genetic blueprint (DNA code). In humans, a portion of chromosome 6 contains a group of genes which determine the major histocompatibility (MHC) antigens of the individual. These self antigens are called *human leukocyte antigens* (HLA) because they were first discovered on white blood cell surfaces. Self antigens, despite some variation in quantity and location, are on or in the surface membrane of virtually all body cells.[1]

Each individual receives one set of self antigens from each parent on each of four gene loci (HLA-A, B, C, and D and D-related). These are inherited according to mendelian laws, with a person's genotype determined by one paternal and one maternal haplotype.[1] The HLA antigens are inherited codominantly; thus all eight are expressed unless homozygosity exists. Identical twins have an identical set of HLA antigens, while close relatives and siblings share some of these antigens.

HLA antigens were originally identified as antigens which evoked rejection of transplanted organs. They are now recognized as important in regulation of the immune response, as well as conferring resistance and/or susceptibility to a growing list of diseases. Almost 100 different HLA antigens have been identified; they are divided into three classes on the basis of their tissue distribution and function.

Class I antigens include HLA-A, HLA-B, and HLA-C and serve as determinants for immune recognition of self and elimination of virus-infected cells. Additionally, they may serve as components of graft rejection. Class I antigens are found on virtually all body cells. Class II antigens (also called Ia) include HLA-D and D-related and have a restricted distribution.[1]

Class II HLA antigens are found chiefly on cells of the immune system (B lymphocytes and macrophages) and act as communication receptors in initiation and regulation of the immune response. Interestingly, these class II antigens are also found on Kupffer, Langerhans, and dendritic cells, endothelial cells, spermatozoa, ovarian interstitial cells, activated T cells, and activated myeloid cells. They may serve as differentiation antigens. Gamma interferon is a powerful inducer of HLA-D and D-related (D/DR) expression, which may foster the recognition of self antigens on certain tissues. Class II antigens are involved in many levels of immune interaction. HLA-D/DR antigens must be shared between macrophages and T cells in order for effective collaboration between T helper and B lymphocytes in immune regulation to occur, and they are important for antigen presentation. Class II antigens have been detected during kidney graft rejection, and they may play a role in graft-versus-host disease occurring after bone marrow transplants. Recently, it has been suggested the class II HLA type of compatibility may play a significant role in graft survival[1] (see Chap. 59).

Class III antigens include certain complement proteins such as factors B and C4 and are presently poorly described.[1]

Closely associated with the MHC genes on chromosome 6 are a group of immune response genes (Ir genes). They determine the responsiveness of a person's immune system and cells to a particular antigen. The Ir genes may function with and require recognition of class II HLA antigens.[1]

The Ir genes code for class II antigens, controlling fine specificity of the response involving thymus-dependent antigens. HLA class II antigens may be products of the Ir genes and, together, may determine a person's responsiveness to foreign antigens.[1]

The MHC antigens have also been associated with the risk of developing certain diseases, such as ankylosing spondylitis, related to HLA-B27; myasthenia gravis, related to HLA-A1, B8, and DR3; and psoriasis, related to HLA-CW6, BW37, and BW17.

Lymphoid and Reticular Organs

Organs and tissues in which lymphocytes are produced, mature, and/or reside are called *lymphoid organs* (Fig. 44-6). Lymphoid organs have a physiologic rather than an anatomic relationship. Those organs in which lymphocytes are produced and mature are said to be *central,* or *primary,* while those in which mature lymphocytes reside and function are said to be *peripheral* or *secondary.* The thymus and the human equivalent of the avian bursa of Fabricius (thought to be bone marrow) are considered central or primary lymphoid organs. They are necessary for the generation and matu-

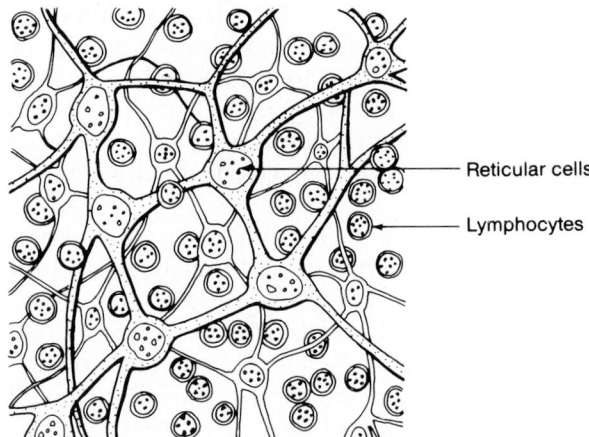

Figure 44-6 Lymphoid tissue.

ration of two functionally distinct populations of competent lymphocytes, the T (thymus-dependent) and the B (bursa-dependent) cells. Peripheral, or secondary, lymphoid structures include lymph nodes and vessels, spleen, and gut-associated lymphoid tissues (lamina propria, Peyer's patches, tonsils, and vermiform appendix). These peripheral lymphoid structures are responsible for the recognition and processing of, responding to, and subsequent destruction of nonself (antigen)-threatening molecules through a series of reactions called the *immune response.*

Thymus

The thymus gland is an encapsulated, bilobed lymphoepithelial structure located in the anterior superior mediastinum immediately beneath the sternum. The largest relative size of the thymus is reached at puberty, after which the gland involutes into an inconspicuous, small fatty structure persisting throughout adult life. It is lobulated, with each lobe containing a cortex and a medulla. Entodermal epithelium budding off the pharynx gives rise during fetal development to the reticular cells of the thymus.

The cortex contains densely packed small lymphocytes called *thymocytes.* The medulla is less dense and contains degenerating, concentrically arranged epithelial cells called *thymic corpuscles of Hassall.* Their precise significance is currently unknown.

The main function of the thymus gland is the production and maturation of a pool of circulating thymus-derived T lymphocytes. These T cells migrate to other lymphoid organs and seed into thymus-dependent zones. Additionally, the thymus is thought to produce a hormone called *thymosin,* which influences lymphocyte production as well as development of immunologically competent T cells capable of recognizing nonself antigens while remaining tolerant of self antigens. Thymosin is thought to play a major role in T cell maturation, immunologic self-tolerance, enhancement of graft-versus-host (GVH) reactions, and development of T cell surface markers. The thymus is required for production of eosinophils and is influenced by gonadal, adrenal, and thyroid hormones. Mast stem cells are found in the thymus, and an enlarged thymus is a consistent finding in myasthenia gravis, although the significance of this relationship remains unknown.

The thymus gland develops in humans during the eighth week of gestation, with both thymocytes and Hassall's corpuscles appearing at this time.[4] The thymus continues to be an important source of lymphocytes throughout life, despite adipose tissue replacement of thymocytes and epithelial reticular cells. Interestingly, Hassall's corpuscles persist even in old age.

Bone Marrow

An actively hematopoietic myeloid tissue found in certain marrow cavities of bone is called *red bone marrow.* In the adult, red bone marrow is found mainly in flat bones (sternum, skull, vertebrae, ilium, ribs, and proximal epiphyses of some of the long bones).

Bone marrow contains a stroma of reticular fibers, phagocytic reticular cells, adipose tissue, blood vessels (large sinusoids), and parenchyma-free cells (all developmental stages of platelets and red and white blood cells).

Three phases of hematopoiesis have been identified in intrauterine life, and in all three, mesenchymal cells differentiate into basophilic stem cells called *hemocytoblasts.* Hemocytoblasts proliferate actively and differentiate into the various cellular elements of peripheral blood. The first phase occurs in the wall of the yolk sac during the third gestational week of human development. The mesenchymal cells differentiate into hematoblasts, then into erythroblasts, and finally give rise to primitive nucleated red cells.[4] The second phase of hematopoiesis occurs in the sixth week of human gestation within the liver and spleen. In this phase, the hemocytoblasts differentiate into erythroblasts, leukoblasts, and megakaryoblasts.[4] Hepatic erythropoiesis continues through fetal life, normally disappearing at about the time of birth.[4] The spleen, however, continues lymphopoiesis postnatally. During this phase also, the thymus begins producing mature thymocytes. The third phase involves lymph nodes and marrow. Myeloid tissue (bone marrow) appears in the third fetal month, giving rise to hemocytoblasts, which differentiate into all future cellular elements of adult human blood. Lymph nodes develop late in fetal life and produce lymphocytes along with the spleen. This lymphopoiesis normally continues throughout life. Bone marrow in humans is considered a central lymphoid structure. It is necessary for the maturation of the B lymphocyte population. In birds, the gut-associated bursa of Fabricius has been identified as the site of B cell differentiation. In humans, as indicated earlier, the bursa equivalent is thought to be bone marrow, although this has not been verified.

Lymph Nodes

Lymph nodes are small, bean-shaped peripheral lymphoid structures occurring throughout the body and interconnected by a set of lymphatic vessels (Fig. 44-7). Lymph circulates through a lymph node, and the vessels eventually drain into large lymphatic ducts which empty into the venous portion of the vascular system. This system of nodes, vessels, and lymph is collectively called the *lymphatic system* and is responsible for filtering and cleansing the interstitial fluid of the body as well as producing and circulating lymphocytes. Lymph nodes vary in number and frequently occur in groups or chains in the head, neck, axilla, groin, and abdominal mesentery. Open-ended lymphatic capillaries arise in the interstitial spaces and drain the intercellular spaces of excess intercellular fluid and its products. This fluid is transported by afferent lymphatic vessels to regional lymph nodes, where the lymph enters a subcapsular sinus in the cortex of the node and percolates through the cortical and sinusoidal spaces to the medullary sinus, where it leaves the

Figure 44-7 The lymph system.

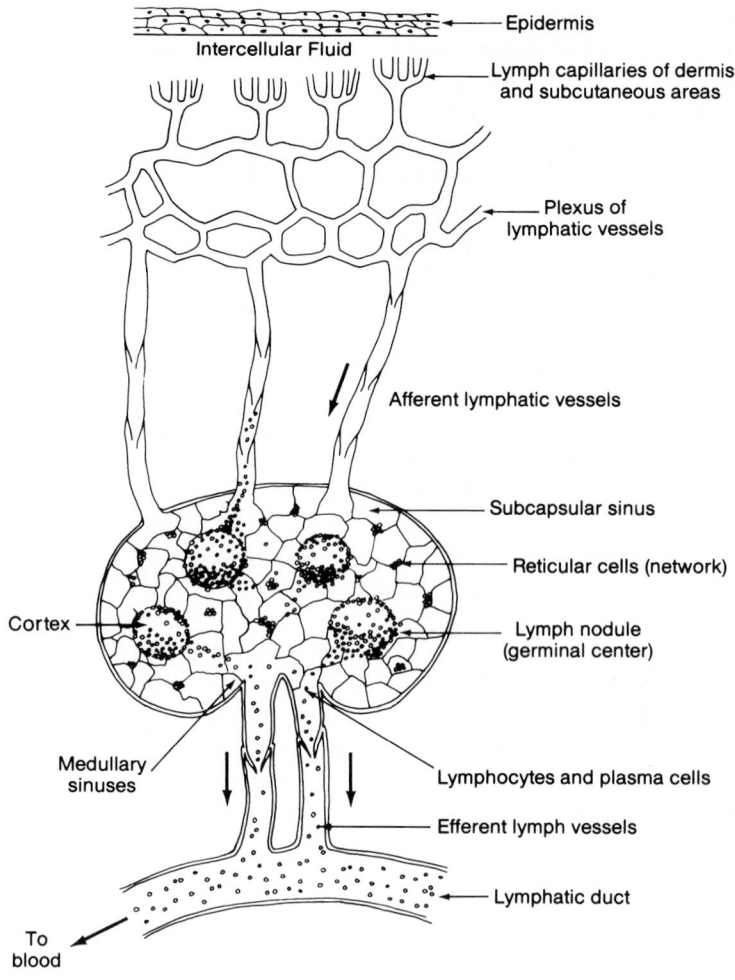

Epidermis

Intercellular Fluid

Lymph capillaries of dermis and subcutaneous areas

Plexus of lymphatic vessels

Afferent lymphatic vessels

Subcapsular sinus

Reticular cells (network)

Lymph nodule (germinal center)

Cortex

Medullary sinuses

Lymphocytes and plasma cells

Efferent lymph vessels

Lymphatic duct

To blood

node along with lymphatic cells via the efferent lymphatic vessel (Fig. 44-7).

A typical lymph node is surrounded by a dense fibrous capsule which blends with the surrounding connective tissue. The lymph node has a stroma of reticular connective tissue, the spaces of which are filled with densely packed lymphocytes except for the portions called *sinuses*. Each node has a cortex and a medulla. The cortex contains the typical lymph (follicle) nodule, which houses germinal centers that become active during an immune response. Diffuse masses of lymphocytes are found between the germinal centers. The medulla is composed of thick cords of densely packed lymphocytes, extending from the cortex into the medulla. The rest of the node is occupied by sinuses,

which permit the streaming and filtering of the lymph.[6]

These sinuses begin as subcapsular sinuses which are continuous with the cortical sinuses, themselves continuous with wide medullary sinuses. These sinuses are lined with reticular and littoral cells capable of phagocytosis.[6] Recirculating lymphocytes, as well as those produced by the lymph node, are added to the lymph as it percolates through the node. This anatomic arrangement permits slow flow and purification of the intercellular fluid, so that cleansed lymph leaves the node. Lymph nodes become enlarged and tender when actively involved in an immune response such as fighting an infection or when nonself material is being drained into the node from the interstitial spaces.

A predominantly B lymphocyte zone is located in the follicles. A T cell zone is found surrounding the follicles in the medullary cords (paracortical region). The medulla contains many B cell–derived plasma cells which actively synthesize specific antibodies[1] (Fig. 44-8). Thus the lymphatic system prevents local edema, phagocytically rids (filters) the interstitial fluid of any debris or foreign nonself antigens, and produces and circulates lymphocytes and lymphatic fluid.

Spleen

The spleen is a peripheral lymphoid organ which filters and purifies the blood of foreign material, dead cells, and debris. In addition to performing general immune functions, it degrades (breaks down) erythrocytes, produces monocytes, and serves as a blood reservoir. The spleen is the largest lymphatic organ in the body. Located intraperitoneally and surrounded by a muscular fibrous capsule, the spleen is filled with reticular connective tissue and venous sinuses lined with phagocytic cells. Portions of the reticular tissue are packed with lymphocytes called *white pulp* (containing the splenic corpuscles). The splenic corpuscles contain the germinal centers. The venous sinusoid areas are filled with blood instead of lymph and are collectively called the *red pulp*. The central artery is surrounded by lymphocytes and, as it leaves the white pulp, becomes ensheathed with reticular cells

and then branches into terminal capillaries opening into the red pulp.[6]

The marginal zones are areas of diffuse lymphatic tissues which trap blood-borne antigens and are important in the immunologic functioning of the spleen. In the white pulp, the T lymphocytes form the periarterial sheath while the B lymphocytes are concentrated in the germinal centers and marginal zones (Fig. 44-9). The white pulp occupies the greatest volume of the spleen but diminishes in size and activity with age, while the red pulp then becomes more prominent. The spleen is not hematopoietic in the normal adult; however, since it possessed this function during fetal life, the adult spleen may undergo myeloid metaplasia and actually produce blood in certain pathologic conditions.

Blood enters the spleen at the hilus via the splenic artery and branches into a splenic arterial system along the capsular trabeculae. As these arteries are reduced to small size, they leave the stroma, enter the splenic parenchyma, and become central arterioles, which branch into capillaries (*penicilli*) that supply both the white and the red pulp. As the capillaries traverse the white pulp, they become ensheathed and transport the blood to the venous sinusoids lined with phagocytic littoral (reticular) cells. The venous sinuses empty into pulp veins, which unite to form trabecular veins, leaving the splenic hilus as the splenic vein. The spleen has little or no afferent lymphatics; a few efferent lymphatics may be present in the capsule, trabeculae, and white pulp.

Splenic function in humans is not well understood. In most cases the spleen can be removed without harm to adults; but in some persons splenectomy may result in death. Other lymphoid organs can and usually do assume the functions of the spleen when needed. The white pulp germinal centers are an important source of lymphocytes. The spleen separates plasma from blood cells and stores the cells and platelets in the red pulp. It also monitors and regulates red blood cell volume, need, and destruction. The spleen may produce hormones that cause bone marrow to produce or release monocytes and/or eosinophils into general circulation. Immunologically, the spleen has tremendous potential for clearance of foreign molecules from the blood. These blood-borne antigens

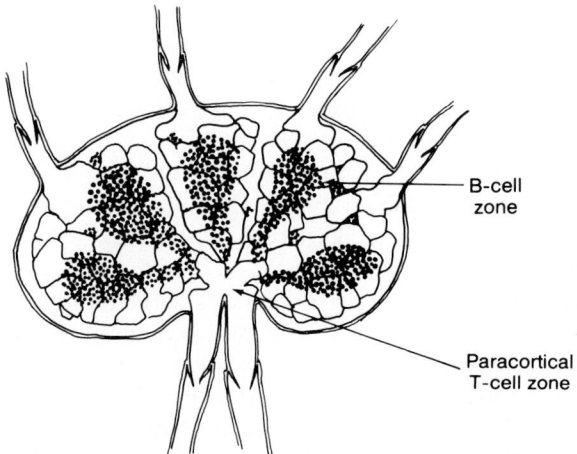

Figure 44-8 Lymph node with T and B cell zones.

B-cell zone

Paracortical T-cell zone

Figure 44-9 The splenic lymph system. Inset: A splenic corpuscle (white pulp).

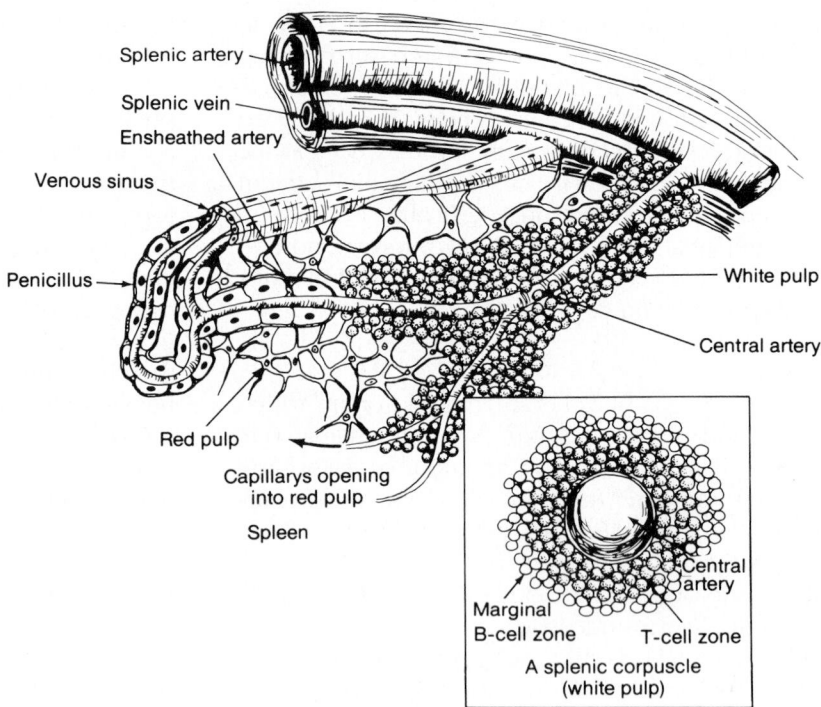

Splenic artery
Splenic vein
Ensheathed artery
Venous sinus
Penicillus
White pulp
Central artery
Red pulp
Capillarys opening into red pulp
Spleen
Central artery
Marginal B-cell zone
T-cell zone
A splenic corpuscle (white pulp)

are recognized, trapped, and processed in the spleen, activating its resident T and B cells, which respond by proliferating, differentiating, and producing effector cells and antibodies that destroy these foreign molecules and thus protect the organism.[1]

Liver

The liver is an endodermally derived organ budding off from the foregut. It is not a lymphoid organ, but early in embryonic development it is hematopoietic in function. The bone marrow assumes this function in the adult, and the liver takes on many new functions.[4] The liver produces bile, complement, and coagulation factors; conjugates bilirubin; is involved in carbohydrate and lipid metabolism; and functions as a lymphoreticular organ. The blood returning from the small intestine (including absorbed materials) is delivered to the liver via the portal vein, where it is allowed to percolate through its sinusoids, which are lined with fixed macrophages (phagocytic cells). These cells are mesodermally derived and constitute the lymphoreticular portion of the liver.[4]

The liver is an important phagocytic organ receiving intestinally derived antigen directly from the portal circulation and systemic antigen from the celiac artery. In either case it acts as a filter, with hepatic phagocytes rendering bacterial and food- or gut-derived antigens nonimmunogenic. Conversely, the spleen and lymph node macrophages serve to enhance immunogenicity.[7]

Loss of the liver filtration function will affect routes of immunization and enhance the immune response. The liver is responsible for clearing large complement-fixing immune complexes from the portal and systemic circulation via sinusoidal phagocytosis. The spleen usually filters out and clears smaller non-complement-fixing complexes. The loss of phagocytic liver function allows these complexes to accumulate in the plasma and may or may not result in immune complex disease. Endotoxins are phagocytized and detoxified by the liver and are known to increase significantly in conditions of impaired liver function.

The liver synthesizes many immunologically active plasma proteins. The best examples are alpha fetoprotein (AFP), B alpha globulin, and complement factors. Alpha fetoprotein is produced by the endodermal cells of the liver and is normally present during fetal development and not present after birth. Increased concentrations are often seen in liver diseases which initiate hepatic regeneration, such as neoplasia or hyperplasia. AFP functions as a suppressor of immune function. B alpha globulins are a group of serum proteins with immunoregulatory effects; they are increased during pregnancy, cancer, and liver disease and inhibit T cell function, complement, and coagulation systems. They may play a role in regulating K cell function.[2] Various complement components produced by liver cells are reduced during impaired liver function.

Chronic liver disease usually results in alterations in the humoral immune response such as hypergammaglobulinemia, increased viral antibody titer, increased IgA (in alcohol-related disease), production of IgM instead of IgG in the secondary response, and depressed function of T helper cells (in primary biliary cirrhosis).

Thymus-independent antigens, which involve only B cells, show increased immune responses in chronic liver disease. Thymus-dependent antigens, which involve T cells, macrophages, and B cells, show a significant reduction in both primary and secondary response in chronic liver disease.

Patients with chronic liver disease also reflect alterations in the cell-mediated response by a de-crease in the ratio of T4+ to T8+ cells, failure to develop a skin test hypersensitivity reaction to common bacterial and viral antigens (anergy), reduction in mature T lymphocytes, increase in immature T cells, decrease in effector cytotoxicity, and depressed macrophage function.

Lymphocyte Circulation Patterns

Bone marrow is the place of origin of all lymphoid cells. They differentiate and mature under the influence of primary (central) lymphoid organs and thus must circulate from their place of origin to the thymus and human bursa-equivalent areas. After maturing to immunocompetent cells under thymic and bursal influence, these naive or antigen-unprimed T and B lymphocytes circulate by way of the blood and lymphatics to the secondary (peripheral) lymphoid organs (Fig. 44-10).

Most bone marrow small lymphocytes are recent postmitotic cells showing different stages of maturation. After division, about 30 percent of these cells become B cells. These unprimed B cells migrate preferentially to the spleen rather than to the lymph nodes.

The precursor T lymphocytes, which also arise in the bone marrow, circulate in the blood to the thymus. It should be noted that the bone marrow contains stem cells and precursor T and B lympho-

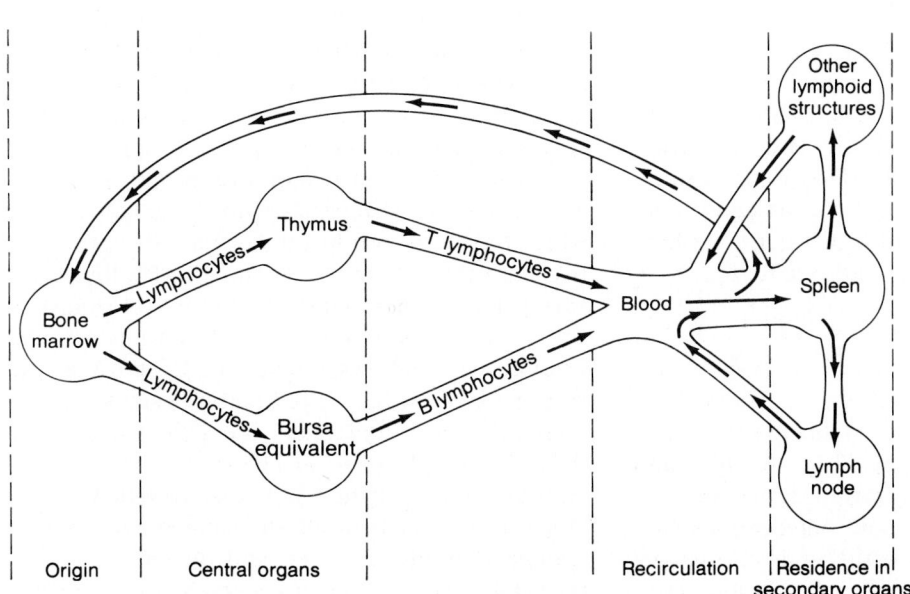

Figure 44-10 Lymphocyte development and circulation patterns.

cytes as well as mature recirculating immunocompetent lymphocytes.

Immunocompetent unprimed T cells then migrate from the thymus to the lymph nodes of the spleen or other peripheral lymphoid organs to provide a population of nonrecirculating, short-lived T cells—short-lived unless primed by encounter with an antigen, which converts them to a long-lived antigen-specific recirculating pool of T memory cells.

The recirculating lymphocyte pool travels from the blood to the lymph nodes to the lymphatic vessels and back to the blood. The transit time for recirculating T and B cells is 18 to 30 h, with B cells requiring a little longer than T cells. Recirculating competent T and B lymphocytes patrol or act to survey the entire body for invading antigens.

Both T and B cells enter the spleen through the marginal zone of the white pulp and migrate to the splenic red pulp, where they reenter the blood via the splenic vein. This circuit requires about 5 to 6 h to be completed.

Antigen-Antibody

The antigen-antibody concept must be understood in order to grasp the meaning of immune defense mechanisms. Antigens are macromolecules (large molecules) that provoke an immune response. Self antigens are found on the surface as well as within the walls of all types of cells. Host, nonhost, bacterial, viral, and plant cells have self antigens associated with their cell membranes and walls.

Antigens usually have a molecular weight of 10,000 or more. Smaller molecules are not ordinarily antigenic. However, as described earlier, haptens (half-antigens) are able to attach themselves to human body proteins, making a larger complex that will provoke an immune response:

Hapten + native protein = hapten protein complex
         Carrier   Complete antigen

Any substance with the ability to produce an immune response (humoral, cellular, or both) when introduced into the human body is called an *immunogen,* or *antigen.*[1] Antigenicity is not an inherent property of a molecule but depends on many factors such as the way the molecule gains entrance into the host and its own quantity and quality, as well as the host's genetic system. The molecule must have the quality of foreignness (i.e., be recognized as nonself), and it usually is large, chemically complex, and administered in such a manner that it will or can be recognized by the T lymphocyte. The parts of the antigen molecule which determine the specificity of antigen-antibody reactions are called *antigenic determinants.*

The most important characteristic of immunogens is their ability to initiate recognition and induction of cellular immunity by thymus-derived T lymphocytes, something that haptens are unable to do. These antigens are called *thymus-dependent antigens.*

Certain types of antigen molecules may be immunogenic without apparent participation of T lymphocytes. These trigger B lymphocytes without T help. They are thus designated *thymus-independent antigens.* The antigens usually induce production of an IgM class of antibody and do not confer immunity. Activation of T cell responses depends on Ir genes within the major histocompatibility complex. This apparently is not a requirement for B cell activation by haptens. Haptens are attached to self proteins; thus, they may initiate an immune response against self (autoimmunity).[1]

Many drugs are haptogenic and, in certain persons, may bring about drug allergies. Genetic differences ensure that the proteins of each person are different; thus only certain protein structures are capable of or will allow combination with a particular hapten. When this combination occurs, sensitivity to the drug ensues.

Antibodies are proteins secreted by plasma cells which differentiate from B lymphocytes in response to the presence of foreign antigen. These antibodies react specifically with the antigen against which they were produced. An antibody consists of two light chains (about 220 amino acids long) and two heavy chains (about 430 amino acids long).

The V-region end of both chains is quite variable, which allows for antigen identification; the rest of the chain (C region) within a single class is constant.[3] The four chains are held together by disulfide bridges (Fig. 44-11).[3] It has been shown experimentally that the outer portion of the V region (Fab) attaches specifically to antigen, forming an antigen-antibody complex, and that the C region (Fc) of the two heavy chains attaches nonspecifically

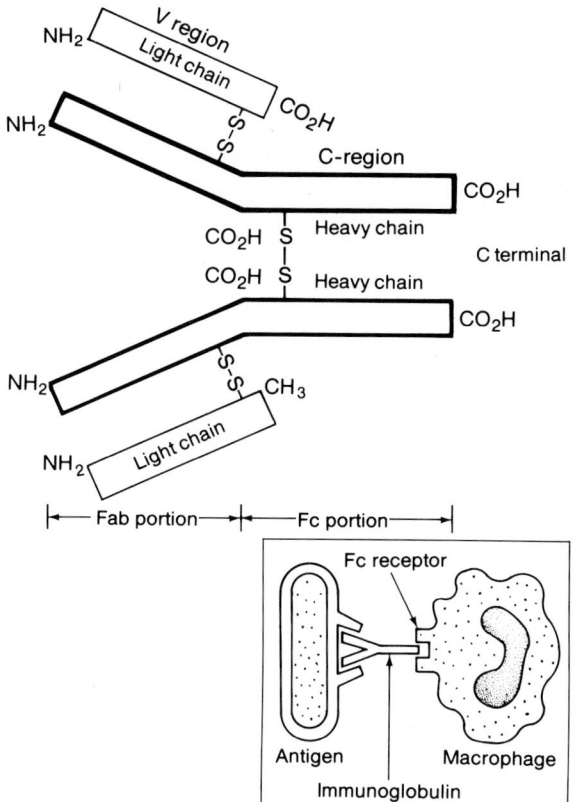

Figure 44-11 Structure of immunoglobulin. The Fab portion is variable and confers specificity for antigen attachment. The Fc portion is constant and will attach to any cell with an Fc receptor (note inset).

to any cell which has an Fc receptor on its surface, such as a macrophage.[3]

H-chain amino acid sequences are different for each antibody type; thus, H chain designates the antibody classification and perhaps some of its specific biologic functions.[3] Antibody is properly called *immunoglobulin,* since it is found in the globulin fraction of the serum. There are five classes of human immunoglobulin, abbreviated IgG, IgM, IgE, IgD, and IgA. Their specific characteristics and differences are indicated in Table 44-1.

Antibodies may be natural or acquired. *Natural* antibodies are usually of the IgM type and are present in the sera of normal persons who have had no known contact with the particular antigen against which they are directed. Their formation is most likely due to contact with cross-reacting an-

tigens of normal flora, killed organisms in food, and other normally available environmental agents. *Acquired* antibodies arise as part of the humoral response of active immunity to a foreign antigen.

Role of Complement

*Complement** is a term applied to a group of nonspecific proteins that circulate in an inactive form in the blood of all warm-blooded animals. Although they are found in the globulin fraction of serum, they are not immunoglobulins and therefore are not increased during immunization. Complement proteins are involved in nonimmune reactions as well as in the immune response, and they function in a nonspecific way in both cases. The complement lyses cells by fixing to any cell to which IgM or IgG has become attached. The antibody thus guides the attack to specific targets, sparing other cells.

Complement Activation
The fraction known as C1 is primarily synthesized by intestinal epithelium, while C2 and C4 are produced by macrophages; C3, C6, and C9 by the liver; and C5 and C8 by the spleen. The cascade of complement reactions is usually set off by an encounter of complement with IgG or IgM linked to antigen-antibody complex. This encounter and the resultant binding of complement to such a complex is called *complement fixation.* Basically, the complement sequence occurs in three major phases (Fig. 44-12). First is the production of C3-splitting enzyme, known as *C3 convertase;* second is the actual activation of C3. The third phase is the activation of the remaining complement proteins (terminal component) in what is called the *terminal sequence.*

C1q fixes to the antigen-antibody complex, which starts a series of reactions leading to the production of C3 convertase (C1,4b,2a) and inactive fragments (C2b, and C4a). C3 is thus activated by the convertase to produce biologically significant components C3b and C3a. One function of C3b is

---

*The nomenclature for the classic components of complement uses numbers preceded by C (e.g., C1, C2). The subsequent small letters (e.g., C1q, C2a) denote subunits. Complexes are denoted by sequential numbers separated by commas (e.g., C5,6,7).

Table 44-1 Properties of the Five Major Classes of Human Immunoglobulin

Property	IgG	IgA	IgM	IgD	IgE
Antibody activity	Major antibody in serum	External secretions	Formed to new antigens	Found on the surface of B lymphocytes	Histamine release
	Antibacterial antitoxins	Body surface protection	Important in primary response	Serves mainly as an antigen receptor	Subsurface protection
	Important in secondary response	Prevents surface attachment of organisms	Natural antibodies	May function in controlling lymphocyte activation, suppression, or differentiation	Responsible for type I anaphylactic reactions
Compliment fixing	All but one of four subclasses	No	Yes	?	No
Placental transfer	Yes	No	No	No	No
Location	Serum and intercellular fluids	Serum exocrine secretions, intestinal secretions, milk	Serum	Serum	Intercellular fluids and serum

to attach itself to phagocytes, facilitating phagocytosis like an opsonin. C3 works as a blood vessel dilator and as a chemotactic agent for neutrophils. An additional C3 fraction (C1,4b,2a,3b) subsequently activates C5; this marks the third stage in complement activation. The rest of the components, C6 to C9, combine to form a complex C1,2,3,4,5,6,7,8,9, which initiates membrane lesions leading to cell lysis. Two C5 fragments are active in the inflammatory response; C5a, like C3, acts as a vasodilator and chemotactic substance. Another chemotactic substance is formed by a second C5,6 fragment, which combines with C6 and C7, becoming C5,6,7.

The complement system is capable of being activated by other than antigen-antibody complexes (Fig. 44-12). This "alternate" pathway is especially important. It is considered to be a primitive antibody-independent mechanism for augmenting the body's defenses against bacteria, fungi, certain viruses, virus-infected cells, and malignant cells.[8] Proteins of the alternative pathway are properdin C3 and factors B,D,H, and I. Factors B and D are initiators of this pathway, whereas factors I and H and properdin (P) function as regulators. The

"alternate" pathway is given positive feedback by continuous formation of C3b via C3b,Bb ("alternate" C3 convertase). Obviously, this feedback must be homeostatically controlled or massive complement activation through amplification would occur every time C3 was split or fixed. C3b inhibitors, factor H and factor I, interrupt the feedback cycle essential to the alternative pathway.[1,8] The action of these two control proteins prevents the depletion of factor B and C3 in plasma. Properdin stabilizes "alternate" C3 convertase; thus it was previously referred to as the properdin pathway.

Lymphocyte Populations

Many different populations of specialized lymphocytes are required to defend against the infinite number of potential nonself antigens. Each group seems genetically determined to respond to a group of physically related antigens.

All lymphocytes have a similar light-microscopic structure but differ significantly in function, receptors, and maturational origins. A maturational division into T and B lymphocytes allows for two

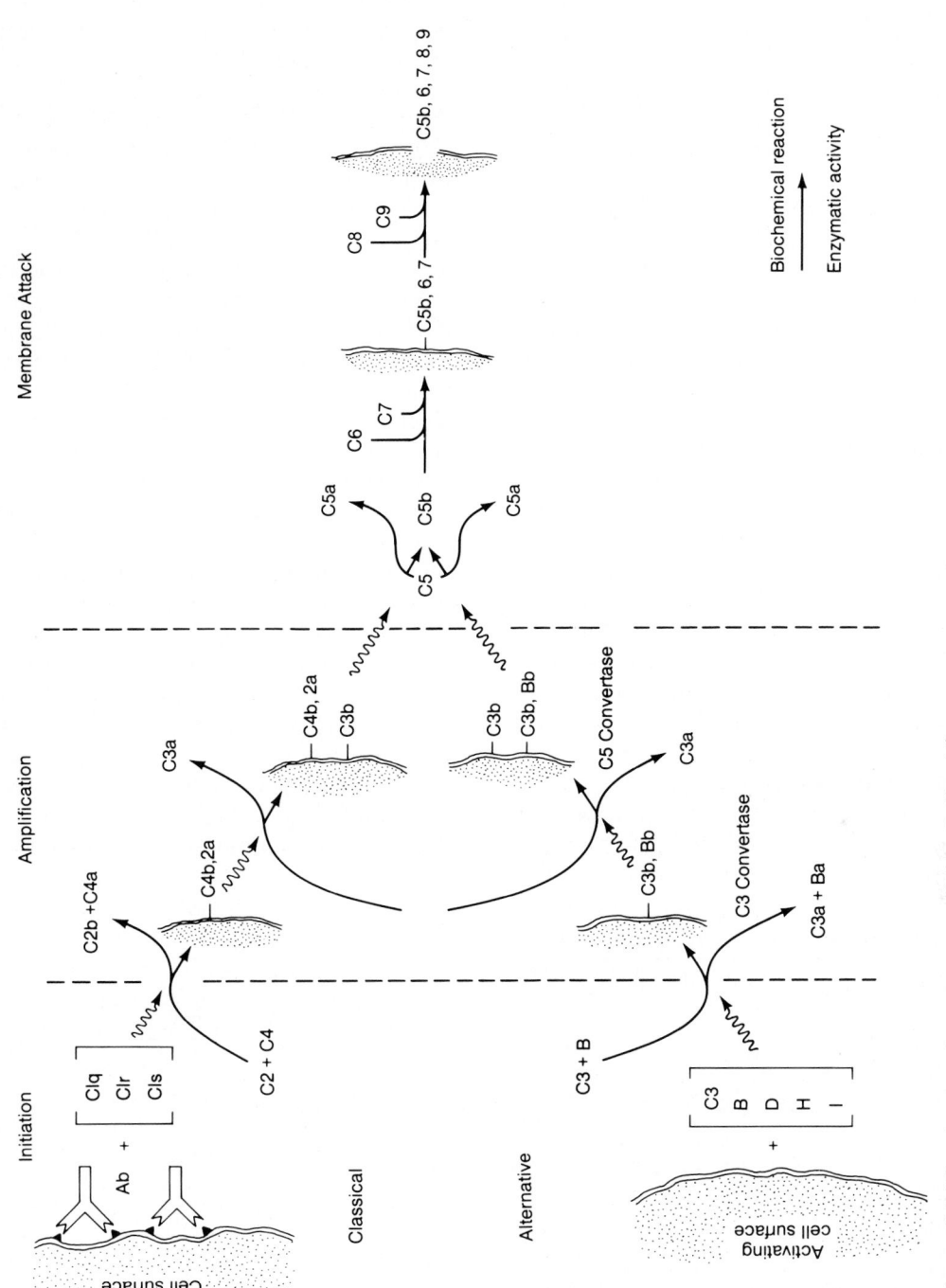

Figure 44-12 The complement system. *(From Bellanti.[1])*

distinctively functional lymphocyte populations, each group genetically programmed via cell membrane–associated receptors to respond to a variety of antigens. In general, a distinct lymphocyte population expresses common as well as specific antigenic determinants (receptor binding sites). Lymphocyte populations are activated only when an antigen can bind to its specific antigenic receptor (Table 44-2).

Various immunologic parameters have been utilized in the past to define different lymphocyte populations. Only recently have scientists been able to delineate precise lymphocyte differentiation by using monoclonal antibodies, developed by the use of a hybridization technique, as a tool. Monoclonal antibodies are different from the usual polyclonal antibodies in that they can identify a single cellular receptor rather than a group of receptors; thus subpopulations within a group of morphologically similar cells, such as the lymphocyte, can be identified. The availability of lymphocyte monoclonal antiserum has allowed analysis of both normal and malignant lymphoid cells, giving important insights into lymphocyte differentiation and the origins of leukemias.[9] Clearly there are many subsets of both T and B lymphocytes, differing in function as well as in surface receptors (markers).

T Cell Lymphocyte Populations

Many subsets of thymus-derived lymphocytes are known to exist. Bone marrow prothymocytes migrate to the thymus and, under its influence, mature through various stages to become immunologically competent unprimed T lymphocytes. During this process, eleven different receptors are synthesized, degraded, and/or remodeled. Monoclonal antiserum is available for each receptor and allows for analysis of specific T cell populations (Fig. 44-13). As illustrated, after maturing in the thymic environment, two distinct subpopulations of T cells emerge to home or seed into the peripheral lymphoid structures. These are designated *T helper* (T_4) and *T suppressor* (T_8) cells, because of their regulatory effects on the intensity of the immune response. Regulatory T lymphocytes govern the outcome of antigen triggering and control the differentiation or activation of cytotoxic effector cells and their products (*lymphokines*). As can be seen in Fig. 44-13, T helper and T suppressor cells share certain antigenic receptors but differ in that the T helper cells have a T_4 receptor while T suppressor cells have a T_8 receptor. This receptor difference allows for different functions which upgrade (help) or downgrade (suppress) the intensity of the immune response.[10,11]

Effector T lymphocytes are responsible for actual destruction of nonself antigens. These include lymphokine-producing T cells and cytotoxic (killer) T cells.

Another type of effector lymphocyte is the natural killer (NK) cell, a large granular lymphocyte which lyses neoplastic cells, virus-infected cells,

Table 44-2 Surface Receptors on Immune Response Cells

Cell Type	HLA Class I	HLA Class II	Receptors* OKT/Leu	Surface Ig	SRBC	FC IgG	FC IgM	C3b	Viral
T cells	+	†		−	+			−	Measles
T helper	+	†	OKT 4/Leu 3	−	+			−	+
T suppressor	+	†	OTK 8/Leu 2	−	+	+		−	+
Cytotoxic	+	−	OKT 8/5	−	+	+	+	+	+
NK cell	+	−	OKT 10/OKM 1	−	+	−	+	−	
DHR cell	+	−	OKT 4	−	+	−	−	−	
B cells	+	+		+	−	+	+	+	Epstein-Barr +
Macrophages	+	+	OKM 1	−	−	+	+	+	

*Leu and OKT antigens are determined by commercial nonclonal antibodies. OKT and OKM designations are available through Ortho Pharmaceutical Co., Raritan, NJ; Leu designations are available through Becton-Dickinson, Mountainview, CA.
†T Lymphocytes are positive for class II HLA antigens only when activated by antigen.
Source: Adapted from Aisenberg[9] and Bellanti.[1]

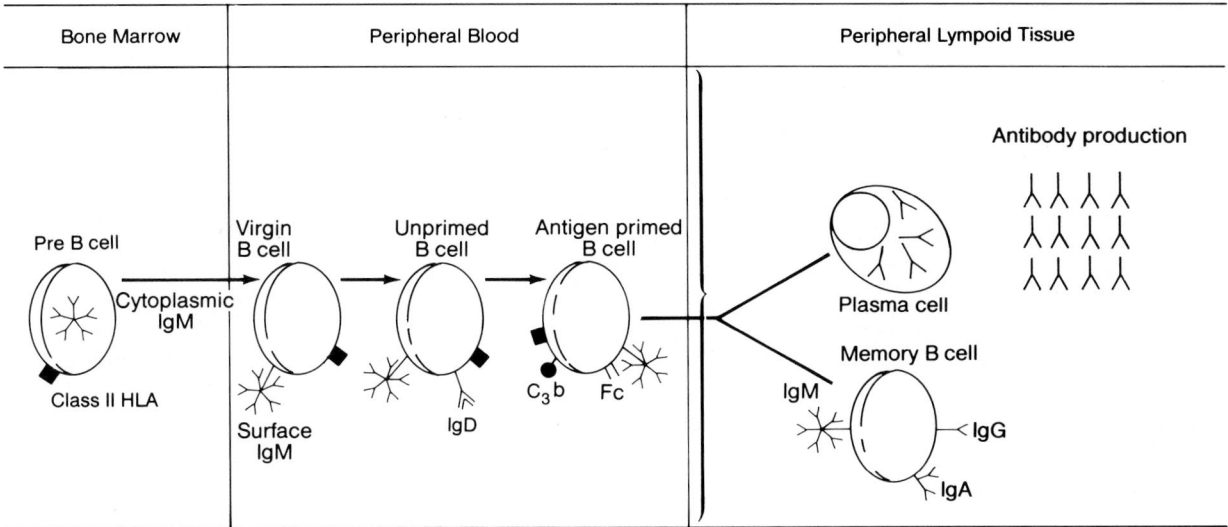

Figure 44-13 Stages of human T lymphocyte differentiation as determined by monoclonal antibodies. *(Adapted from Bishop[11] and Bellanti.[1])*

and fetal cells.[12] Unlike T cells, NK cells do not require sharing of major histocompatibility antigen for lysing. NK cells are nonadherent, nonphagocytic, and thymus-independent but function like killer cells and share the T cell marker (T_{10}) and OKM1 monocyte/macrophage marker. NK cell activity is augmented by interferon and retinoic acid and is believed to be important in immune surveillance (Table 44-3).[12]

Cytotoxic T cells (killer cells) are activated T cells which attack antigens by direct contact. They are T_8+ cells and originate from T suppressor cells.[1]

The T_4+ cell (helper cell) also gives rise to an effector lymphocyte, which produces lymphokines and other mediators that initiate localized delayed hypersensitivity reactions (DHR) and inflammation.

Lymphokines are soluble bioamines produced by lymphocytes; soluble products of macrophages are called *monokines*. These soluble products allow chemical communication between cells of the immune response and are called *interleukins*. Lymphokines identified in the past were designated by their function as cytotoxic factor, macrophage activating factor (MAF), macrophage inhibiting factor (MIF), mitogenic factor, interferon, transfer factor, etc. More recent terms are interleukin-1 (IL-1) and interleukin-2 (IL-2), and these are replacing the former names. Interleukin-1 is a monokine produced by an antigen-activated macrophage. It activates the T cell to expand into antigen-sensitized

Table 44-3 Distinguishing Features of Effector Cells

Effector Cell	Method of Cytotoxicity	Antigen-Specific	HLA-Restricted
Cytotoxic T (T_8+ cells)	Direct contact with antigen	+	+
K Cell (T cell)	Antibody-dependent, cell-mediated cytotoxicity	+	−
NK cell	Natural; FC receptor bearing cell enhanced by lymphokines	−	−

Adapted from Bellanti.[1]

Table 44-4 Monokines

Name	Other Names	Origin	Effect
Interleukin-1 (IL-1)	Lymphocyte activating factor (LAF), mitogenic factor (MF)	Antigen-stimulated macrophages (class II HLA-dependent)	Enhances thymocyte proliferation; T helper cell activator; induces IL-2 production by T cells
Prostaglandin E_2 (PGE$_2$)		Antigen-activated macrophages and other sources	Activates suppressor T cells and thus downgrades the immune response; depresses IL-2 production, thus suppressing helper function; also affects smooth muscle
Tumor necrosis factor (TNF)		Antigen-activated macrophage	Platelet aggregation and electrolyte shifts, hemorrhagic necrosis of tumors

clones and induces T_4+ cells to produce IL-2 (Tables 44-4 and 44-5).[10,13]

T memory cells, which differentiate from antigen-activated T cells, are long-lived cells that recognize antigen upon reexposure and confer immunity to a specific antigen.[13]

T cells are responsible for cell-mediated immune (CMI) responses and the regulation of B cell

Table 44-5 Lymphokines

Name	Other Names	Origin	Effect
Interleukin-2 (IL-2)	T cell growth factor (TCGF)	Activated T helper cells; induced by IL-1	Enhances natural killer cells; enhances cellular immunity via cytotoxic effect or function; induces INF production by T suppressor cells
Lymphotoxin (LT)		Activated T cells	Direct cell lysis
Colony-stimulating growth factor (CSGF)	Macrophage-activating factor (MAF)	Activated T cells and macrophages	Required for differentiation of cells into granulocytes and monocyte colonies
B cell growth factor (BCGF)		T helper cells	B cell proliferation
B cell differentiation factor (BCDF)	T cell replacement factor (TRF)	T helper cells	B cell differentiation into plasma cell secreting antibody
Interferon (immune) (INF)	Type 2	Leukocytes, probably T cells and NK cells (induced by IL-2)	Suppresses B cells; enhances cellular immunity by activating NK cells, cytotoxic lymphocytes, T lymphocytes, and macrophages; may be toxic to normal cells

proliferation and maturation into antibody-secreting plasma cells. Thus thymus-dependent T cells regulate (enhance or suppress) the humoral immune response and participate in the elimination of foreign antigen via the cellular immune response.[10,13]

B Cell Lymphocyte Populations

B lymphocytes are responsible for the humoral (antibody-mediated) immune response. B cell proliferation and differentiation are quantified by the interaction of T helper and T suppressor cells. Effectors in the humoral response are specific antibodies which circulate in the body fluids, bind with antigen, and destroy it. B cells do not have to be physically present at the antigen site for destruction to occur; thus, B cells are responsible for antibody-mediated immune protection. B cells differentiate from a pre-B cell found in the bone marrow (Fig. 44-14) to become unprimed B cells. When activated by antigen plus T helper cells, they become a primed B cell clone and differentiate into plasma antibody-secreting cells or B memory cells. The stages of differentiation can be deter-

mined by receptors on their surfaces. Plasma cells remain fixed in lymphoreticular organs, while B memory cells, B primed cells, and B unprimed cells circulate in the body fluids and seed into peripheral lymphoid organs.[10,11,13]

Accessory Cells and Molecules

Macrophages

Macrophages are important not only in recognizing and processing antigen (afferent limb) and thus initiating the immune response but also in a variety of regulatory (central limb) and effector (efferent limb) mechanisms dealing with destruction and degradation of both the antigen and the resultant tissue debris. Macrophages produce antigen-specific and nonspecific mediators called *monokines* that influence T lymphocytes (Table 44-4). The monokine IL-1 induces T helper cells to produce IL-2 lymphokines, B cell growth factor (BCGF), B cell differentiating factor (BCDF), and macrophage-activating factor (MAF). IL-1 and IL-2 synergistically act to induce proliferation of T cells. BCGF and BCDF are signals for B cell growth and differentia-

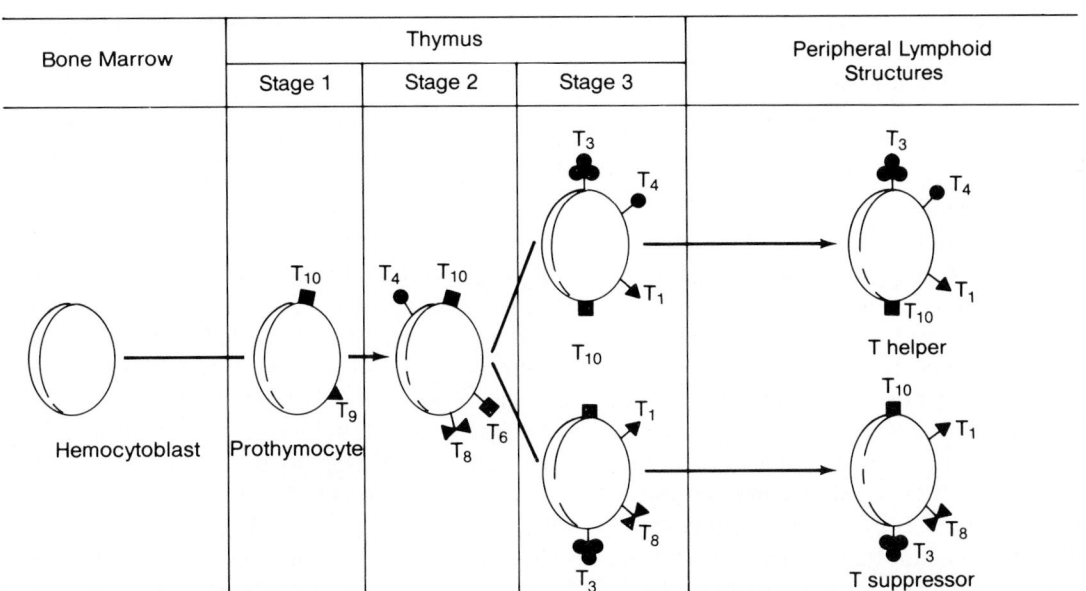

| Bone Marrow | Thymus | | | Peripheral Lymphoid Structures |
| | Stage 1 | Stage 2 | Stage 3 | |

Figure 44-14 Human B lymphocyte differentiation. B lymphocytes activated by antigen and T cells help loose surface IgD gain receptors for B cell growth factor and B cell differentiation factor produced by activated T helper cells. Memory cells circulate in peripheral blood; plasma cells do not. (*Adapted from Bishop.*[11])

tion to plasma antibody-secreting cells. MAF activates macrophages to produce prostaglandin E_2 (PGE$_2$). PGE$_2$ exerts a suppressor effect on normal immune responses by activating suppressor function, thus downgrading the humoral response while enhancing cytotoxic lymphocyte and natural killer function. Macrophages, then, have both specific and nonspecific roles in all limbs of the immune response.[10,13]

Immunoglobulin

Antibodies function by specific binding to the antigen that promoted their synthesis, forming antigen-antibody complexes which can then be phagocytically destroyed. Antibodies can also act as immune regulators. High concentrations of immunoglobulin tend to bind antigenic determinants on cell surfaces and cover the antigenic site. This blocks the receptor and renders it inaccessible to destruction by activated lymphocytes. A low titer of antibody appears to interfere with interaction and cooperation between T helper and B cells, however. The formation of antigen-antibody complexes triggers activation or production of T suppressor cell function, thus depressing the immune response. Clinically, antibodies are implicated in enhanced graft tolerance, abrogation of graft-versus-host disease, and tumor enhancement and/or destruction, and they modulate autoimmune reactions as well.[1,10,13]

Immune Interferon

Immune interferon (gamma INF) produced by T suppressor cells is antiviral and has antiproliferative functions. It acts as a second signal with antigen to regulate the quality of the immune response. It can affect a variety of immune cells at various stages and levels of the immune response. Lymphokine effectiveness is dependent on gamma INF. Gamma INF immunoenhances by augmentation of cytotoxic functions or diminution of helper functions.[1,10]

Thus, gamma INF has been shown to decrease antibody production by T cell inhibition, enhance accessory cell functions and their enzyme production, increase IL-2 receptors on T cells, increase Ia/DR class II HLA antigen expression, increase FC-dependent phagocytosis of macrophages, and enhance cytotoxic T cell activities.[1,10]

In general, it can be said that gamma INF suppresses T$_4$+ function and enhances T cell effector functions. However, these reactions vary according to the type of interferon and the stage of therapy.[1,10]

The Immune Response

Macrophages, T lymphocytes, and B lymphocytes cooperate to control the immune response.[10] The precise mechanisms involved are quite complex and still not fully understood (Fig. 44-15 A–D).

The essential elements are recognition and presentation of antigen to T cells, specific destruction of the antigen, and protection against repeated challenge by the antigen through immunologic memory.

It is clinically useful to divide the immune response into three physiologically dependent limbs: the afferent limb, the central limb, and the efferent limb. This classification into three phases has practical application in diagnosis and treatment. In assessing the immune response, tests for defects in the afferent, central, or efferent limb of the response are often conducted. Likewise, many drugs and therapies are directed primarily at a particular activity or cell type within a particular limb.

The Afferent Limb

The afferent limb of the immune response recognizes and processes antigens. It involves macrophages and T and B lymphocytes. The antigen is recognized by the macrophage, activated, and presented to appropriate unprimed lymphocytes. Soluble antigens can activate B cells in a direct manner and do not require HLA recognition. Thymus-dependent antigens require an HLA class restriction for B cell activation (Fig. 44-15, A). T cells require activation by a specific recognition of antigen plus self MHC genes. T helper cells recognize antigen when class II HLA antigens are present and identical on both the macrophage and the T cell. T suppressor cells recognize antigen only in the presence of class I HLA molecules. This HLA restriction is necessary for activation and differentiation of T cells and prevents free circulating antigen from activating them. The macrophage is required to present antigen in conjunction with MHC HLA genes suitable

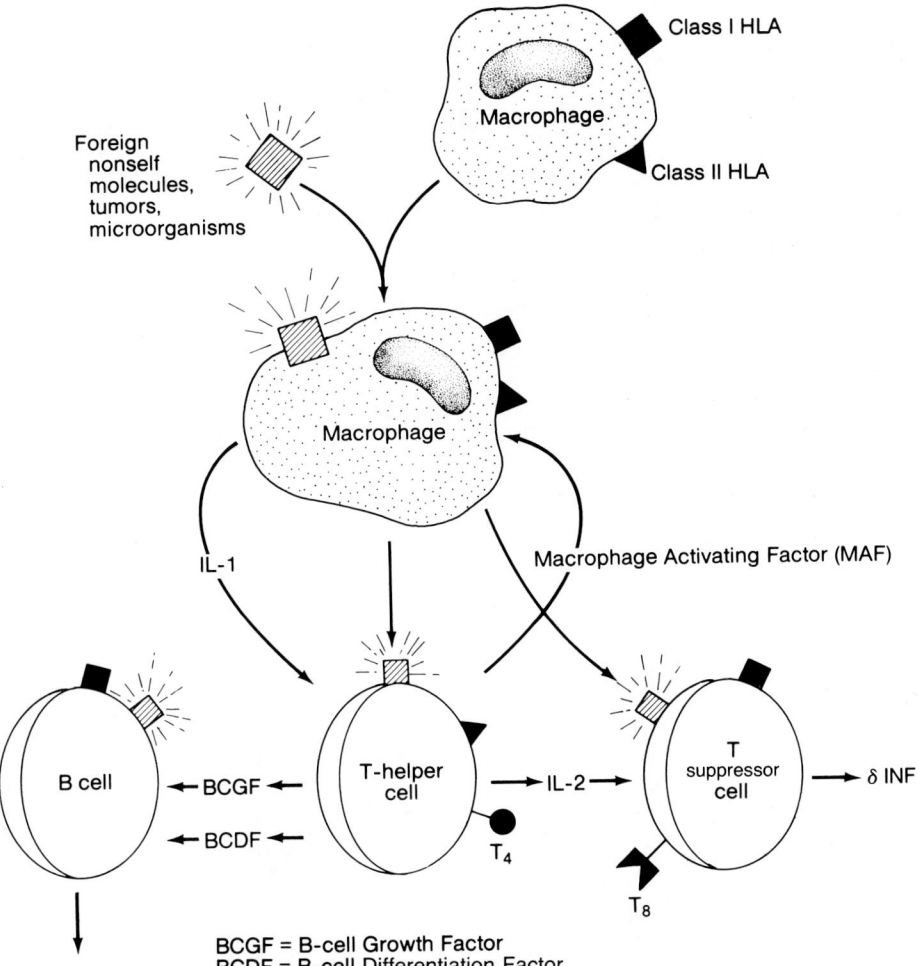

Figure 44-15   Summary of the immune response. *A.* The role of macrophages in recognizing, processing, and initiating the immune response: the monokine interleukin-1 (IL-1) plus antigen initiation of T lymphocyte cloning.   (*Continued*)

for recognition by the T cell receptor. Macrophages also secrete the IL-1 necessary for T cell activation and proliferation.

The Central Limb

The second, or central, limb includes all events that are necessary for preparation of an effective immune response to antigen, including cell cooperation, cloning, and production of effector and memory cells and their cytokines. Process antigens are molecularly changed for recognition by lym-

phocytes. This recognition by the lymphocytes causes them to bind the antigen to their surface via receptors and enlarge and proliferate into a distinct clone of cells with specific information about that particular antigen. The HLA restriction ensures specificity. Interleukin-2, B cell growth and differentiation factors, macroactivating factor, gamma interferon, and other cytokines are produced in this limb of the response. These lymphokines allow for regulation and modulation and ensure an appropriate response.

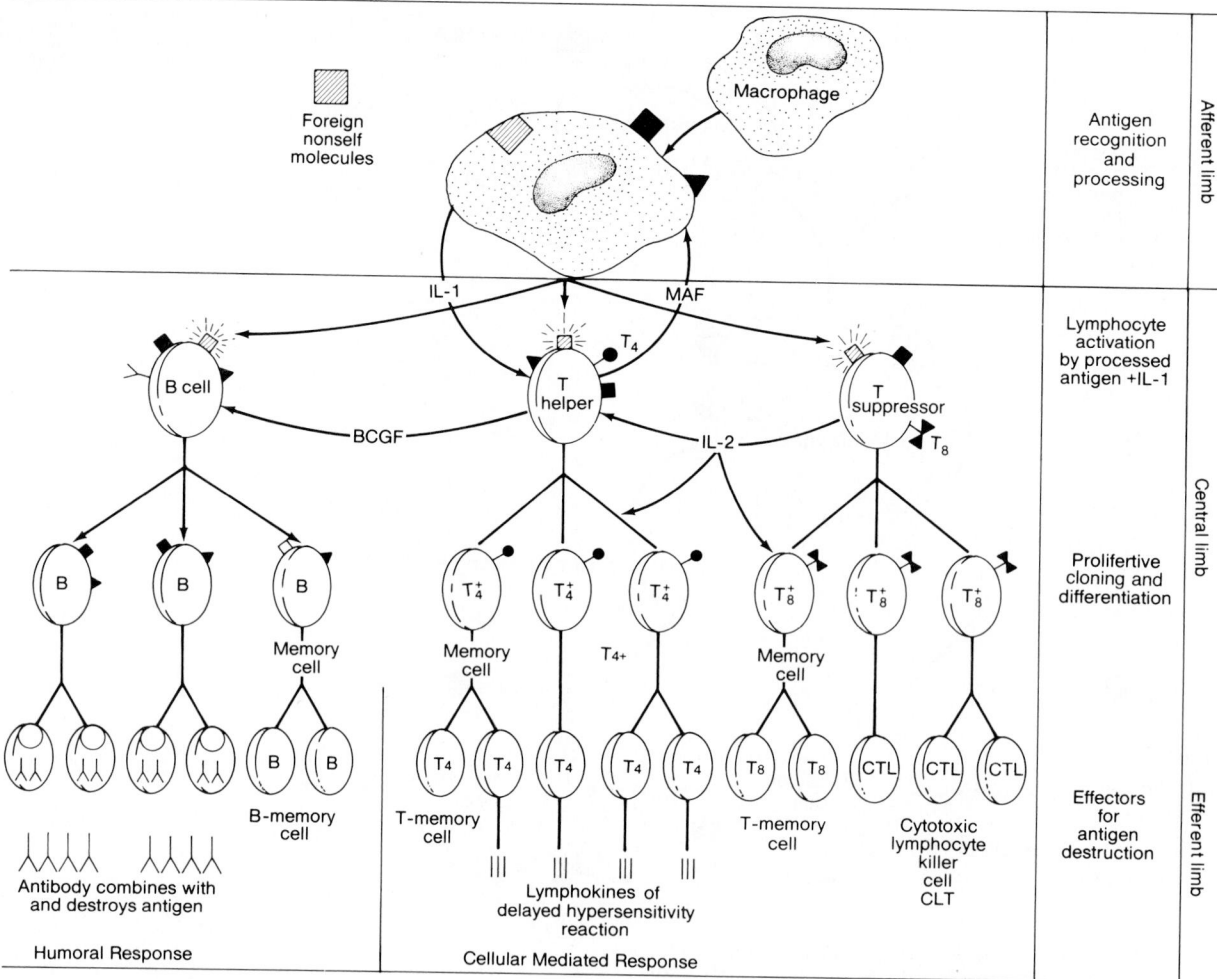

Figure 44-15 (*Continued*) *B.* Activation cloning, differentiation, and synthesis of effectors by regulatory T helper and T suppressor cells and their lymphokines. This culminates in a dual effector destruction, i.e., antibody-mediated and cell-mediated responses.

The Efferent Limb

The efferent limb is a dual-type response to ensure destruction and removal of the offending antigen. It involves interactions among T lymphocytes, B lymphocytes, macrophages, and their respective cytokines. This dual system allows antigen to be destroyed by either circulating antibody or cytotoxic T cells, or both. Basically T cell and B cell interaction results in an antibody-mediated (humoral) response, while interaction between T cells culminates in a cell-mediated response.

Humoral Immunity The humoral response is initiated by antigen binding to receptors on B lymphocytes. This leads to B cell activation, proliferative cloning, and subsequent differentiation to antibody-secreting plasma cells. This proliferation and differentiation require T help. T helper cells are genetically committed to provide the lymphokines essential for B cell proliferation and differentiation. The immunoglobulin produced is specific for the sensitizing antigen. The response is humoral in the sense that plasma cells located in secondary

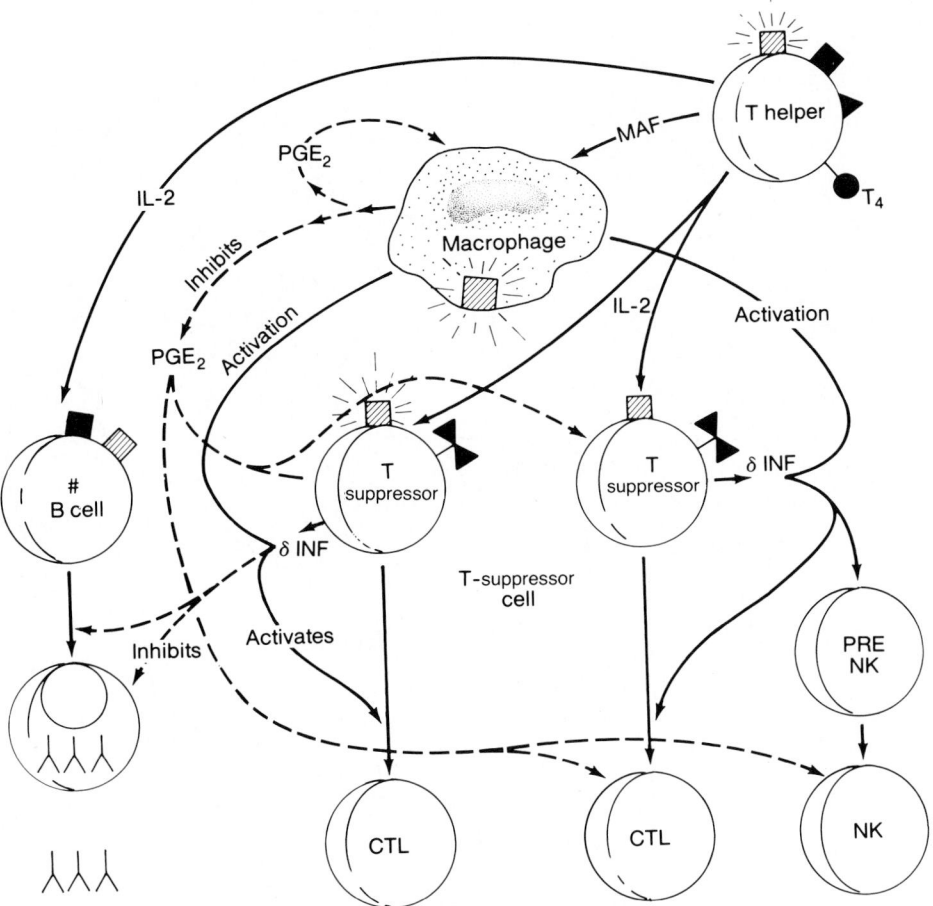

Figure 44-15 (Continued)   *C.* The lymphokine interferon (γ-INF) produced by T suppressor cells activates the macrophage to produce the monokine prostaglandin E₂ (PGE₂); enhances differentiation and activation of cytotoxic T lymphocytes and natural killer cells; and activates T₈+ cells (suppressor) to downgrade antibody production.

lymphoid structures remain there, and only the antibody they produce circulates in the plasma and other body fluids; hence this type of immunity can be passively transferred in serum. When the antibody comes in contact with the antigen, a specific binding occurs, forming an antigen-antibody complex. The complex is subsequently selectively destroyed by either lysis or precipitation of the complex, followed by nonspecific phagocytosis and degradation by activated macrophages. The reaction is immediate, since antibody is preformed before encountering the antigen.[1,10,13]

Defects in B lymphocytes reflect quantitative changes in their numbers and/or functional ability. A deficiency of B cells results in an inability to produce antibody. Persons with this humoral immune deficiency are particularly susceptible to extracellular bacterial infections such as those caused by *Hemophilus, Pneumococcus, Staphylococcus,* and *Streptococcus.* Antibodies provide one of the main mechanisms for defense against viruses. However, since viruses are intracellular organisms, cell-mediated immunity is more important in the eradication of established viral infections. Excesses

Figure 44-15 (Continued) *D.* Macrophage PGE₂-initiated T suppressor functions to downgrade the immune response by T suppressor cell lymphokines.

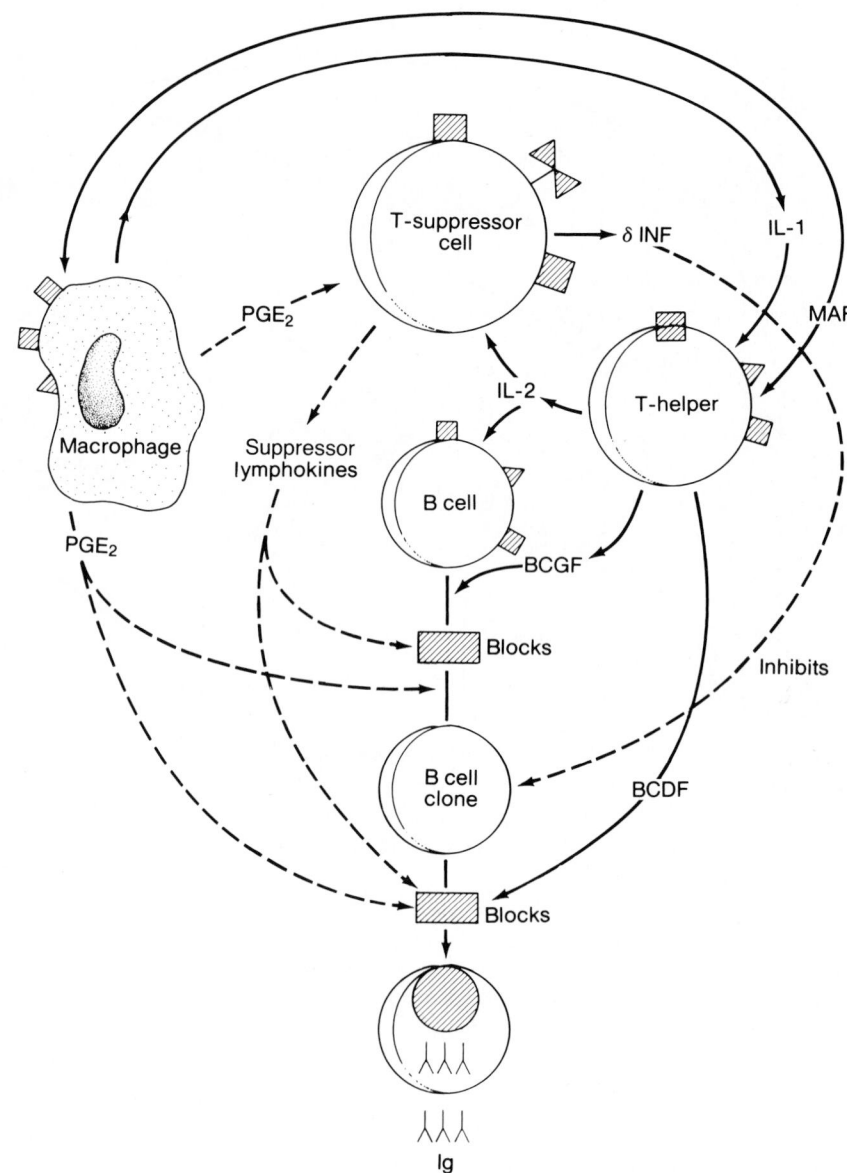

of B cells result in increased quantities of the antibodies associated with certain autoimmune disorders.[1,3]

Cell-Mediated Immunity   Cell-mediated immunity (CMI) is mediated by cytotoxic cells which function at the site of the reaction (Fig. 44-15, B). This type of immunity can be passively transferred by one person to another only by cells. The T lymphocyte recognizes an activated antigen on the surface of macrophages and responds by enlarging and then proliferating a clone of sensitized T lymphocytes which migrates throughout the body and accumulates at the actual location of the antigen. The cells destroy the alien macromolecule by direct participation of the cytotoxic T cell as well as by secretion of lymphokines. Unlike antibody, which is immediate, this is a delayed reaction which allows time for the synthesis of cytokines and migration of cytotoxic cells. Lymphokines have many different functions and act on different kinds of cells, including macrophages, lymphocytes, neutrophils, eosinophils, and tissue cells[1,3,10,13] (Table 44-5).

Cell-mediated immunity dominates in most cases of intracellular infection as well as in graft rejection, graft-versus-host disease, and immune defense against neoplasia.

Defects in T lymphocytes are suggested by recurrent infections of fungal, viral, and intracellular organisms. Serum antibody levels are usually low, transplanted grafts are compatible, rare types of neoplasia may be present, and delayed hypersensitivity reactions are absent or diminished in T cell deficiencies. Many viruses cause a lymphopenia in humans, and this often leads to severe or fatal bacterial and fungal infections.[1,3]

The normal immune response reflects a T helper/T suppressor cell ratio of approximately 2:1. Changes in this ratio cause the regulatory functions of these cells to change and result in immunopathologic disorders. A deficiency of T helper cells and/or excess of T suppressor cells render the immunodeficient person susceptible to virus-related disease and other infections. An excess of T helper cells and/or deficiency of T suppressor cells renders the person susceptible to allergies, certain lymphoid malignant diseases, myelomas, and certain autoimmune disorders.[1,2,10]

Most antigens evoke the sensitization and proliferation of both T and B cells. However, in any given situation, one or the other (humoral or cellular) type of destruction dominates as determined by the antigenic receptors on the T and B lymphocytes. In addition to the production of antibodies and cytotoxic T cells, longer-lived T and B memory lymphocytes are produced, conferring immunity to most but not all antigens.

References

1. Bellanti, J. A. (1985). *Immunology III.* Philadelphia: Saunders.
2. *Nurses' clinical library. (1985). Immune disorders.* Nursing 85 Books. Springhouse, PA: Springhouse.
3. Sites, D. P., et al. (Eds.). (1985). *Basic and clinical immunology* (5th ed.). Los Altos, CA: Lange.
4. Sadler, T. W. (1985). *Langman's medical embryology* (5th ed.). Baltimore: Williams & Wilkins.
5. Bickley, H. C. (1980). *Practical concepts in human disease* (2d ed.). Baltimore: Williams & Wilkens.
6. Elias, H., and Pauley, J. E. (1966). *Human microanatomy* (3d ed.). Philadelphia: Davis.
7. Leeson, C. R., et al. (1985). *Textbook of histology* (5th ed.). Philadelphia: Saunders.
8. Day, N. K. (1985, May). Complement deficiencies. In *Clinical immunology today* (No. 14). New York: World Health Communications.
9. Aisenberg, A. C. (1981). Current concepts in immunology. *New England Journal of Medicine, 304* (6), 331–336.
10. Gupta, S. (1984, September). Interactions between cellular and humoral immunity. In *Clinical Immunology Today* (No. 10). New York: World Health Communications.
11. Bishop, C. (1984). Immunoassays in hematology: Cell surface antigens. *Journal of Medical Technology, 1,* 41–45.
12. Lopez, C. (1985, March). Natural killer cell functions. In *Clinical Immunology Today* (No. 13): New York: World Health Communications.
13. Jaret, P. (1986). Our immune system: The wars within. *National Geographic, 169* (6), 702–734.

45

Immunologic Data Acquisition

Sister Mary
Rebecca Fidler
Marjorie S. Morgan

General Immune Assessment
History and Physical Examination
Skin Tests
Lymphocye Transformation and HLA Typing

Specific Immune Components
Blood Tests
Urine Assay

Other Procedures
Biopsy
Lymphangiography
Radionuclide Imaging
Magnetic Resonance Imaging
Cytogenetic Techniques

References

If the body can largely protect itself from external and internal threats, what then is the role of health care intervention? To answer this question, the limits of human adaptation must be considered. Clinical experience supports the observation that self-regulation and self-repair have definite limitations. A person cannot be expected to adapt to self-regulation when the capacity to respond has not developed or has been lost after initially developing. The overwhelming effect of hyperimmune responses has to be countered to achieve a level of wellness consistent with individual independence. Conversely, in hypoimmune situations, enhancement of the body's immune response is necessary, and the person must be protected from existing and potential injurious agents during this incompetent period.

In the face of these interventions, it is most important to allow self-mechanisms to function at their highest capability. Time alone may provide this chance of self-regulation, and health providers must be careful to choose proper timing and sequencing of interventions to maximize the self-defense mechanisms. Vaccinating a child before the child is able to respond immunologically will not achieve immunity and may cause harm. Preventing inflammation may also prevent repair and increase scarring.

Interventions should support normal defense mechanisms in a timed sequence, for the wrong timing may preclude the restoration of self-regulation. Sometimes therapeutic agents replace rather than support the physiologic self-protective process. The human body has ample reserve for adapting and restoring health. The human capacity for modification of structure and function is high and far exceeds our expectations at times.

Only a portion of the liver cells, for example, function at a given time; the other cells are in a resting reserve. The same can be said of the kidney when it is filtering or of the cells of the immune system when challenged by antigens. However, if the kidney or liver cells are injured, this tends to reduce the resting reserve as well as the resting time for single healthy cells. If this process of cellular injury is allowed to continue, gradually all reserve is lost and a state of continuous fatigue may result in cells which are unable to divide. With kinetically mitotic cells such as epithelium and lymphocytes, replacement of reserve is probable, but the ability to restore lost cells seems to dissipate with age and immune experience, which also increase the chances of inappropriate responses. Thus susceptibility to neoplasia, autoimmune diseases, and common pathogenic organisms often increases in elderly or unhealthy persons.

A new and different homeostatic level is achieved in an ill person. A particular mode of treatment used in the ill state produces more potent and varied results than in the well state. Elevated temperatures may be lowered by cold application and/or aspirin, but these have no overt effect on a normal temperature. Vitamins will correct a vitamin deficiency but generally have no overt effect on the normal person. Likewise immune therapy may not have an effect when there is no immune disease.

The cells of the human body exist in mutual interdependence despite generous provisions of reserve. The integrity of the organism as a whole rests on the integrity of its individual elements, and the elements in turn are useless except as parts of an organized whole.

Assessment of a person for immune defects is often difficult because of subtle changes, the delay that often occurs between antigen exposure and the onset of symptoms, and the commonality of these symptoms in various immune and other pathologic situations. The fact is that immunology is such a new science that its diagnostics and therapeutics are just developing. Many of the newer diagnostic assays are still available only in large facilities or research centers.

Nursing assessment of the immune system is becoming increasingly important in providing data upon which to base nursing interventions and predictors for interventions and therapies. The nurse must assess not only the physical imbalances but the total needs of the individual patient. The nurse has the role of assisting each patient to achieve a new homeostatic state, maximizing the wisdom of the body and minimizing the detrimental external environmental influences. This is not to regulate the actions of the patient but to positively control what is affecting the integration of the therapy/body/mind relationship.

Testing of immune function involves clinical laboratories, radiology department, and other specialty areas. Knowledge of the specific immune alteration is essential for effective diagnosis, prognosis, and therapy. Clinically, general testing is usually approached by attempting to establish which part of the response is quantitatively altered.[1] Dividing the response into three physiologic limbs, (afferent, central, and efferent) is clinically most useful for this approach (Table 45-1; see also Chap. 44).

Host resistance, an older term for *immune competence,* refers to the ability of an individual organism to resist a threat from another organism or altered self. Immune competence is often equated with health in that a person with an intact functional immune system is able treavoid infections and other pathologic conditions.

The measurement of immune competence is most important and requires most exactitude in certain congenital immunodeficiency disorders. An inaccurate or delayed assessment of the precise deficiency can result in a fatal outcome. Measurement of immune competence has many applications in critical care, but in most cases immune dysfunction is secondary to other disease. The role of immunity is less precise in the secondary immune disorders than in congenital (primary) immune situations.[2] Nevertheless, immune status is an important facet of many critical-care conditions and plays an important role in the practical management of patient care through attempts to manipulate the immune response to benefit the patient. In organ transplantation, for example, the recipient's immune response is suppressed to prevent the organ from being rejected. In neoplastic disease, which seems to create its own suppression, the malignant process avoids immune destruction. In addition to disease processes, many therapies themselves alter a patient's immune status and must be considered as problems in the critically ill.

The human body is somewhat compartmentalized despite its functional and interdependent wholeness; therefore differences in immune competence may vary in different parts of the body. Some tests measure general immune competence, which reflects the immune status of the body as a whole, while others reflect a local response or anergy, which will not be detected in tests for general competence. The response in a lymph node may be different from the response of the lymphocytes circulating in the bloodstream. Also, there are immunologic privileged sites which show little, if any, immune response because of their anatomic nature. The anterior chamber of the eye does not allow penetration of lymphocytes or antibodies, so corneal transplants are rather successful. The central nervous system has no efferent lymphatics; therefore a person's neural specific antigens are not exposed to the immune system. Enhanced tumor growth may occur in an area of the body which receives local radiotherapy. These are examples reflecting local immune mechanisms and alterations.[1]

Table 45-1 Immune Response Functions of the Physiologic Limbs

Physiologic Limb	Immune Response Functions
Afferent	Ability to recognize and process new antigens
Central	Ability to produce clones, leukotrienes, lymphokines, and monokines; regulation of intensity of response
Efferent	Memory (ability to recall previously encountered antigens); functional ability of effector cells and their biologic mediators to effectively neutralize and remove antigen

Normal defense mechanisms protect against well-recognized pathogens and also enable a normal person to live and coexist with the many species of microbes inhabiting the body. The human body serves as a natural host for nonpathogenic viruses, rickettsia, bacteria, yeast, fungi, protozoans, and helminths. In the immunodeficient patient, these normally harmless organisms may establish invasive and lethal infections; thus any of them may be potential pathogens.[2] When a parasite is allowed to enter a host, there are two possible outcomes: either the parasite wins and causes transitory illness or death of the host, or the host wins, with death and removal of the parasite and the host returning to health. The encounter usually confers immunity to subsequent infection. With the immunocompromised patient this is no longer valid; immune memory may be lost and immune cells may be missing or decreased, or perhaps present but nonfunctional. This places the challenge upon nursing and medicine to find ways of protecting these patients and maximizing immune knowledge and responses to benefit the critically ill.

Acquisition of data related to immunity involves many different types of methodology. The type of information needed will be suggested by the answers to the following questions with regard to a patient's defense:[1]

1. Can the patient's body recognize and process a new antigen, i.e., demonstrate a primary immune response?
2. Can the patient's body recognize previously encountered antigens (demonstrate a secondary immune response), i.e., is there evidence of recall or memory?
3. Did the patient have an intact and competent immune system at birth or prior to the present situation?
4. Does the patient have quantitatively adequate numbers and ratios of mature lymphoreticular cells?
5. Does the patient have functionally competent lymphoreticular cells?
6. What is the specific defect? Is it a cell type or subcell type which is defective, or is the defect maturational or developmental?
7. What is the ontogeny (origin and stage of development) of the defective cell type?

8. Does the patient have a genetic predisposition to immune defects?

These questions address two types of immune assessment: the general functional immune defense of the patient and the specific immune defects of a component within the lymphoreticular system itself. General testing is mainly in vivo, while specific component defects are usually confirmed by in vitro laboratory testing.[7]

This chapter aims to assist the nurse in acquiring and understanding objective and subjective data related to the immune system. The critical-care nurse needs this knowledge to identify antecedent conditions and behaviors which promote health and to plan interventions as needed to prevent tertiary illness in the patient. Data acquisition is conveniently divided for clarity into general and specific testing.

General Immune Assessment

History and Physical Examination

Nursing management relies on accurate assessment and collection of objective data. An extensive health history of the patient as well as the family is imperative. This should be followed by a comprehensive physical assessment. The patient will often be unable to give information; then previous health records and the patient's family will have to be the informational sources. A correct diagnosis may often be reached because the critical-care nurse suspected an immune alteration or simply asked the right question.

The history should consider factors which influence the immune system; for example, age is important in immunologic disease—the elderly and the very young are at risk. The newborn, however, are protected by maternal antibody for about 3 months; only then will immune imbalance become symptomatic. Occupation, fatigue, nutrition, stress, and lifestyle may all influence the patient's immune status. Inquiry into any changes in body weight, appetite, and elimination should be included, as well as a detailed medication and immunization history.[2]

Detailed examination of the condition of the skin and mucous membranes is an integral part of the physical examination. Eruptions and skin changes often reflect internal body conditions. Swellings, color, vasculations, papules, spots (petechiae, purpura), ulcers, and abscesses should be noted.[3,4] Table 45-2 lists diseases associated with a variety of skin lesions.

Vital statistics and weight should be recorded. The patient should be checked for fever, chills, pain, productive cough, and abnormal secretions. All regional lymph nodes, liver, and spleen are examined and palpated.[4]

Other data to be sought include a genetic history, previous hospitalization, surgery, blood or blood product transfusions, special therapies, home remedies, pets, nutritional status, and home conditions. Does the patient still have tonsils, appendix, and spleen? What is the history of allergies or autoimmune problems? All body systems should be reviewed, with particular emphasis on evaluation of skin and mucous membranes, noting temperature, moisture, and turgor. The examination also includes ausculation for respiratory, cardiac, and abdominal problems which may indicate infection.[4]

If data from the history and physical examination indicate that the immune status is altered, diagnostic and confirming data must be obtained. However, in critical care, the primary reason for admission may be a disorder that creates a potential for secondary immune defects rather than primary immune defects. It is also important to keep in mind that inflammation is a generalized response to all injury and is dependent upon cells and factors also integral to the immune response. When a person's immune system is suppressed, the symptoms of even acute life-threatening infections may be subtle and difficult to assess. The nurse must assess immune status frequently in order to avoid or prevent infection and immunopathologic conditions.

Clues which often indicate immune defects are infections which recur or which are a result of unusual organisms (opportunistic). Normal children may have many infections a year, but certain types of recurring infection (pneumonia, meningitis, osteomyelitis, or septicemia) should create suspicion of immune disorder.[4]

Skin Tests

General immune competence is usually measured by in vivo skin tests. The type of antigen utilized can differentiate humoral from cellular immune status as well as evaluate the functional limbs of the immune response. Skin tests utilized in this manner are meant to answer the question, "Can this person respond immunologically and can he or she respond appropriately?" A careful history is helpful in evaluating the patient's response to these test antigens.[1,2]

Skin testing for immune competence falls into two categories: testing the response to a new antigen and testing immune recognition (memory) of prior antigenic exposure (recall response).[1,2]

The ability to respond to a new antigen requires the ability to recognize the antigen and present it to other lymphoreticular cells (afferent limb). Cloning, with subsequent production of monokines and lymphokines, cellular communication, and cooperation (central limb) and production of effector antibodies and cells (efferent limb) are also necessary to achieve a positive response to a new antigen. The ability of a person to respond to a new antigen reflects competence of all aspects of immunity. A failure to respond (*anergy*), however, does not give information as to which limb of the immune response is defective.[1,2,5]

Skin testing with an antigen of which the patient has had prior experience measures immune recall or memory. A positive response to a previously encountered antigen measures the central memory and efferent limbs of the response. If the response is negative, one assumes the person has a loss of memory cells or function and that the immunity of the efferent limb of the response is defective. This is true only when there is certainty that the person has previously had a primary immune response to the antigen[1,2,5] (Table 45-3).

Dinitrochlorobenzene (DNCB) is useful as a new antigen, since it is not found naturally in the environment but is synthesized in the organic laboratory, and 95 percent of the normal population are reactive. The recall response to antigens is best evaluated by a panel of test antigens to which there is reasonable assurance that the patient has had previous exposure.[1,2,5]

Table 45-2 Cutaneous Signs Associated with Neoplastic Disorders

Possibly Associated Disorder	Disease or Syndrome	Cutaneous Sign
Thyroid and breast cancer	Cowden's disease	Cobblestone appearance, flat wart-like papules
Premalignant GI polyps, colon cancer	Gardner's syndrome	Deforming epidermoid cysts
Intussusception polyps	Peutz-Jeghers syndrome	Pigmented papules on mucosa of lips and nose, fingertips, and nails
GI and stomach polyps and cancer	Cronkhite-Canada syndrome	Cutaneous and muscosal hyperpigmentation
GI tract multiple carcinoma	Torre's syndrome	Sebaceous gland tumors of trunk
Esophageal and lung	Howel-Evans syndrome (tylosis)	Palmoplantar hyperkeratosis
Thyroid and GI pheochromocytomas	Multiple mucosal neuroma syndrome	White nodules on lips and tongue
Pheochromocytomas, Schwann cell tumors	von Recklinghausen's disease	Multiple mucosal neuromas (neurofibromatosis)
Congenital deficiencies	Immunodeficiency syndrome, hormone-secreting tumors	Telangiectasia
Oat cell carcinoma	Ectopic ACTH syndrome	Hyperprigmentation, muscle weakness
Appendix and small bowel	Carcinoid syndrome	Upper trunk flushing and cyanotic flushing
Alpha cell, pancreatic glucagon secreting tumor	Glucagonoma syndrome	Necrolytic (eczematous) migratory erythema
GI tumor, endocrinopathy, porphyria	Hypertrichosis lanuginosa	Lanugo hair on face, neck, trunk (malignant down), with painful swollen tongue
Adenocarcinoma of the stomach	Acanthosis nigricans	Hyperpigmented velvety flexural areas
Stomach, female organs	Leser-Trelat sign	Multiple seborrheic keratosis
Myelogenous (granulocytic) leukemia	Chloroma	Odd green-appearing tumor, often periorbital
Paraneoplastic acrokeratosis	Bazex's syndrome	Dystrophic nails, hyperkeratotic palms, and psoriasiform facial eruptions
Pre-intraepidermal squamous cell carcinoma	Bowen's disease	Scaly lesions resembling psoriasis
Plasma cell dyscrasia, mainly multiple myeloma	Primary amyloidosis	Pinch purpura, macroglossia, periorbital lesions
Acute myelocytic leukemia	Sweet's syndrome	Red-tender vesicular plaques on face, upper trunk, extremities
AIDS, or acquired immune deficiency	Kaposi's sarcoma	Coalescing red-brown or purple papules on feet and lower legs
AIDS, early	Infectious disorders	Oral or esophageal candidiasis
Leukema, lymphoma	Infectious disorders	Herpes zoster
Lung, GI, breast	Dermatomyositis	Heliotrope rash, Grotton's papules, inflammation of skin and muscle
Heart disease, metastatic lung lesion	Digital clubbing	Subperiosteal new bone formation
Tumors of the pancreas, lung prostate gland, or hematopoietic system	Coagulopathies	Purpura, hemorrhage, thrombosis
Tick bites, Lyme disease, cancer (nonspecific)	Figure-eight erythema	Red areas of skin forming various shapes
Bullous pemphigoid cancer	Blistering diseases	Erupting blisters, usually in the elderly
Hypersensitivity	Psoriasiform dermatitis	Silver-gray, crusty, exfoliating lesions on extremities, joints, and trunk

Source: Adapted from Thiers.[3]

Table 45-3 Antigens Often Used to Assess General Immune Competence

Type of Response	Humoral Response	Cellular Response
Primary Response (new antigen)	Tetanus toxoid or Flagellin	Dinitrochlorobenzene (DNCB) or Allografts
Recall Responses (previously encountered antigen)	Diphtheria toxoid or *Proteus*	TB (PPD) or Streptokinase dornase or Mumps antigen or *Candida albicans*

Lymphocyte Transformation and HLA Typing

Transformation tests evaluate lymphocyte competency without injection of antigens into the patient's skin. These in vitro tests eliminate the risk of adverse effects but can still accurately assess the ability of lymphocytes to recognize and respond to antigens.

The mitogen assay, using nonspecific plant lectins, evaluates the mitotic response of T and B lymphocytes to a foreign antigen. The mitogens phytohemagglutinin (PHA) and concanavalin A stimulate T lymphocytes preferentially, whereas pokeweed mitogen stimulates primarily B lymphocytes, T lymphocytes only to a lesser extent. In the mitogen assay, a purified culture of lymphocytes from the patient's blood is incubated with a nonspecific mitogen for 72 h—the interval during which the greatest effect on deoxyribonucleic acid (DNA) synthesis usually occurs. The culture is then labeled with tritiated thymidine, which is incorporated into the newly formed DNA of dividing cells. The uptake of radioactive thymidine can be measured by a liquid scintillation spectrophotometer in counts per minute (cpm), which parallels the rate of mitosis. Lymphocyte responsiveness, or the extent of mitosis, is then reported as a stimulation index, determined by dividing the cpm of the stimulated culture by the cpm of a control culture.[2,5,6]

Human Leukocyte Antigen

Human leukocyte antigen (HLA) is a polymorphic system of antigens located on virtually all nucleated human cells. These HLA antigens are known to determine transplantation (histocompatibility) antigens, immune response genes (Ir genes), and some components of complement. This system controls transplant survival or rejection and has a role in regulating immune responsiveness as well as the development of susceptibility to certain diseases. In humans, the HLA system is located on the short arm of the autosomal chromosome 6 pair at five identified loci designated A, B, C, D, and DR (D-related). The D locus is closest to the centromere of the chromosome, with B, C, and A, in that order, to the right of the D locus.[2,5]

Each of these loci is multiallelic (about 90 different alleles are possible), which means that a large number of alleles are possible at each locus, each defining a different antigen. However, only one allele can define a given antigen at one locus on one chromosome. Each person, therefore, has five alleles inherited from the mother and five from the father. Each person is characterized by his or her alleles, defined as the haplotypes, or phenotype, of the individual. This haplotype is inherited as a unit on the chromosome 6 from each parent; thus each person has two HLA haplotypes constituting the phenotype.[2,5]

The HLA nomenclature was standardized by the World Health Organization (WHO) in 1976. WHO assigns new specificities to the system and changes the status of antigens from provisional (or workshop, *w*) to full specificities. The locus is assigned a capital letter, A, B, C, D, or DR. Each antigen specificity assigned to a locus is given a specific number; thus, A7 and B27 are antigen specificities at locus A and locus B, respectively. Aw32 indicates locus A antigen specificity 32, which is provisional (*w*)—i.e., has not met all WHO requirements.[5]

The phenotype is used to report a person's HLA type. It is written in alphabetical order by locus, with the loci separated by semicolons. Example:

Phenotype Individual I:–A1,28; B5,27; Cw1,w3; Dw2,w7; DR1,7

Phenotype Individual II:–A10, ; B7,14; Cw1,w2; Dw5,w9; DR1,4

Note that individual II is homozygous for the A10 locus, therefore a blank space is left. Haplotypes can be determined by family studies. The particular genotype designation can be assigned when haplotypes are known. Haplotypes are written in alphabetical order by locus, with the loci separated by a slash. Example:

A1,B5,Cw1,Dw2,DR1/A10,B7,Cw3,Dw5,DR2

Tissue typing (HLA typing) identifies the HLA haplotypes and uses microcytotoxicity assays and/or the mixed lymphocyte culture technique.

Microcytotoxicity Test

The microcytotoxicity test (MCT) is a serologic assay based on the fact that an alloantibody against a particular HLA antigen will lyse cells expressing that antigen on its surface in the presence of rabbit complement. Utilizing a dye specific for dead cells, a percentage quantitation of cells bearing that surface antigen is possible. Lymphocytes are used as the target cell in MCT, for they express large amounts of surface HLA antigens and are easily obtained from individual patients and remain stable in storage for long periods of time.[2,5]

Antibodies to HLA surface antigens do not occur naturally in humans and cannot be produced by immunization of animals. They are found by screening sera from humans who have been immunized by multiple blood transfusions or previous tissue transplants or from multiparous women immunized by the paternal expressed HLA antigens of the fetus. It would be possible to obtain HLA antigens by injecting humans with leukocytes, but this is not legal in the United States.

Rabbit complement will attach to any antigen-antibody complex and trigger activation of the classical complement cascade with subsequent cell membrane lysis. A supravital dye is then added to this system. Live cells are able to prevent the entrance of this dye; thus only cells whose membranes are disrupted will take up the dye. After 200 to 300 single cells are counted, the percentage of live or dead cells is calculated; 30 to 40 percent dead cells is usually taken to indicate that an antigen-antibody reaction has taken place.

Mixed Lymphocyte Culture Test

The mixed lymphocyte culture (MLC) test determines lymphocyte competence to respond to foreign histocompatibility antigens and is useful in matching transplant recipients and donors. In this assay, the recipient's lymphocytes are cultured with the donor's for 5 days to test compatibility. (In the one-way MLC test, one group of lymphocytes is pretreated with irradiation or mitomycin C, so that they cannot divide but can still stimulate the other group of lymphocytes.) After the culture is labeled with radioactive thymidine, the stimulation index is reported.[2,5,6]

The MLC technique is currently used mainly to detect D locus antigens. Presently, D locus antibody is unavailable. This assay is based on the fact that a person's live immunocompetent lymphocytes can recognize antigen differences at the D locus. This antigenic stimulation is observed by a subsequent series of lymphocyte mitotic divisions. If the lymphocytes from a donor share the same D locus as the lymphocytes from the recipient, there is little cell division, thus little incorporation of radioactive thymidine. If the D locus of the donor differs from that of the recipient, there is stimulation and increased incorporation of radioactive thymidine.[2,5,6]

Primed Lymphocyte Typing

Primed lymphocyte typing (PLT) is the same technique as MLC but utilizes primed lymphocytes, which respond much more rapidly than unprimed cells.

MLC and PLT techniques are used to define HLA-D antigens and are therefore employed in finding suitable transplant donors. These tests are used to assess and monitor genetic and acquired immunodeficiency states; for histocompatibility typing of tissue transplant recipients and donors; to detect exposure to various pathogens, such as those causing malaria, hepatitis, and mycoplasmal pneumonia; to test for paternity; and to type platelets and granulocytes for transfusions.[2,5,6]

Specific Immune Components

The laboratory methods most commonly used to confirm specific immune defects include quantitative and qualitative cell counting, agglutination, precipitation, immunodiffusion and immunoelectrophoresis, radioimmunoassay (RIA), enzyme-linked immunosorbent assay (ELISA), complement fixation, histochemical and cytogenetic techniques, and the more recent monoclonal antibody assays.

Blood Tests

Serum Protein, Albumin, and Globulin

Plasma contains approximately 100 different proteins. Serum, unlike plasma, is deficient in proteins utilized in the clotting process, such as fibrinogen. Many of these proteins exist in such minute amounts that they cannot be quantitatively measured except in terms of their enzymatic or transport function.[7] Most are produced by the liver, a major exception being immunoglobulins, which are synthesized by B lymphoprogeny plasma cells in the lymph nodes, spleen, and bone marrow.

Proteins (*peptides*) are synthesized from building blocks called *amino acids*. Two amino acids constitute a *dipeptide* and three amino acids a *tripeptide;* chains of amino acids form *polypeptides.* Complex proteins are usually described by the nature of their nonprotein portion; thus, there are glycoproteins, lipoproteins, hemoglobin, etc. Additionally, there are transport proteins, coagulation proteins, protein enzymes, and hormones circulating in the blood plasma.[7,8]

The plasma proteins were previously measured by their solubility and separation, employing precipitation with ammonium sulfate or alcohol. Later they were identified and measured by electrophoresis, which was able to separate six serum and seven plasma groups. This separation is possible because in an electrical field, different proteins (according to electrical charge) move independently toward either a positive or a negative pole. The seven plasma protein groups identified by electrophoresis are albumin; alpha 1, alpha 2, beta 1, beta 2, and gamma globulins; and fibrinogen.[7,8]

Electrophoresis measurements of total protein and albumin are often performed as screening tests for immune disorders. Plasma proteins usually remain in the vascular system and are, because of their molecular weight, too large to be transported to the tissues. Albumin makes up approximately 60 percent of the total plasma protein and serves as a vital contributor to the osmotic pressure of the vascular system, thus controlling the distribution of water between blood plasma and the tissues. Albumin also serves as a nonspecific transport protein

for bilirubin, aspirin, antibiotics, etc. and it is utilized to build tissue proteins.

Globulins, particularly immunoglobulins, found in the gamma globulin fraction on electrophoretic separation, provide an important humoral mechanism of human defense against nonself agents. Globulins constitute most of the other (nonalbumin) 40 percent of the total protein.[7]

Total Protein and the Albumin/Globulin Ratio

Clinically, plasma proteins are important in relation to water balance and protein metabolism. There are many different kinds of plasma proteins, most of which are important but present in minute amounts. Therefore, measurement of the total protein (TP) by itself is often of little value. However, the ratio of albumin to globulin (A/G ratio) is altered in many disease states. Measurement of the total serum protein and the albumin and subtraction of the albumin value from the TP gives the quantity of globulin. Thus, calculation of the A/G ratio serves as a screening test for diseases that increase or decrease the albumin/globulin ratio (Table 45-4). Abnormalities discovered from A/G ratio determinations are further studied by electrophoresis, immunoelectrophoresis, or other techniques.[7,8]

Immunoglobulins Immunoglobulins (Ig) are produced by B cell–derived plasma cells and are commonly called *antibodies.* They are formed in response to antigen and are specific for the offending antigen. Antibodies migrate in the gamma globulin band during electrophoresis into predestined classes IgM, IgG, IgE, IgA, IgD (Table 45-5).[2,5]

Decreases in the level of gamma globulin are usually associated with B cell disorders, as seen in persons with an inability to synthesize antibody (agammaglobulinemia), hypogammaglobulinemia, or a lack of T_4 helper cells, all of which may result in a change in the immunoglobulin level. Increased gamma globulin usually is associated with B cell dyscrasia such as multiple myeloma, macroglobulinemia, or deficiency of T_8 suppressor cells (Table 45-4).

Evaluation of the immunoglobulin in a patient's serum is useful in identifying abnormal globulins (cryoglobulins, macroglobulins, and those produced against a particular microorganism, indicating infections).[2,5]

Table 45-4 Conditions Which Affect Albumin and Globulin Values

	Increases	Decreases
Total protein (normal: infant, 4.7–7.4 g/dL; adult, 6.0–8.3 g/dL)	Multiple myeloma, macroglobulin-emia, sarcoidosis, dehydration	Hodgkin's disease, renal disease, ulcerative colitis, severe burns, water intoxication, cirrhosis
Albumin (normal: 3.5–5.5 g/dL)	Dehydration	Water intoxication, nutritional deficiency (protein starvation), liver disease, kidney disease, bowel disease (colitis, sprue), burns
Globulins (normal: 1.5–3.7 g/dL)	AIDS, leukemia, Hodgkin's disease, multiple myeloma, macroglobulinemia, infections, autoimmune disease	Agammaglobulinema, severe combined immunodeficiency syndrome
A/G ratio (normal: 1.5:1–2.5:1; average 2.1)	Macroglobulinemia, multiple myeloma, infections, hepatitis, autoimmune disease, sarcoidosis	Dehydration

Source: Adapted from Byrne, J. C. et al. (1986), *Laboratory Tests: Implications for Nurses and Allied Health Professionals* (2d ed.), Reading, MA: Addison-Wesley.

A monoclonal electrophoretic pattern occurs when a single class of antibody is increased and the others decreased, as in multiple myeloma, plasma cell dyscrasias, macroglobulinemia, and amyloidosis and with the presence of cold agglutinins.[7,8]

Polyclonal electrophoretic patterns of antibody show an increase in more than one class of Ig or in all classes. This is often seen in chronic infections, chronic liver disease (hepatitis and cirrhosis), autoimmune disease, infectious mononucleosis, and other diseases.[7,8]

Table 45-5 Immunoglobulins: Structure and Function

Property	IgG	IgA	IgM	IgD	IgE
Sedimentation coefficient	6–7 S	Monomeric: 7–10 S Dimeric: 14 S	19 S	7–8 S	8 S
Activity	Major antibody in serum and other extracellular fluids	External secretions, surface protection, antiviral	Formed to new antigens; stays in vascular system; antibacterial lysis	Predominant type on B lymphocytes	Histamine release, subsurface protein
Complement fixing	All but one of four subclasses	No	Yes	No	No
Placental transfer	Yes	No	No	No	No
Hypersensitivity types involved	II, III	?	II	?	I, anaphylaxis
Usual form and special structure	Monomeric	Dimeric or monomeric secretory component, J chain	Pentameric, J chain	Monomeric	Monomeric
Mol. weight (thousands)	150	150–300	900	180	200
Serum concentration (mg/dL)	1200	200	120	3	0.02
Serum half-life (days)	23	6	5	2–8	1–5

Serum Protein Electrophoresis and Immunoelectrophoresis Electrophoresis is a procedure which separates electrically charged serum proteins into their various component types and allows for their identification by migration toward a positive or negative pole in an electrical field, as discussed earlier. To recapitulate, this movement separates the proteins into distinct bands, identified as albumin; alpha 1 (α_1), alpha 2 (α_2), beta 1 (β_1), beta 2 (β_2), and gamma (γ) globulins; and fibrinogen.[7,8]

Albumin, the largest quantity of serum total protein, is responsible for 75 percent of the osmotic pressure of the blood and combines with many drugs, pigments, etc., for transport purposes. Albumin is produced by the liver. In normal conditions it cannot be transported across endothelium because of its large molecular size and thus stays in the blood plasma compartment.[7]

Globulins constitute a group of several types of serum protein. The gamma globulin band is composed of lipoprotein, transcortin (cortisol transport), thyroid-binding globulin, antitrypsin, and acid glycoprotein. The alpha 2 globulin band includes ceruloplasmin (copper transport), haptoglobulin (binds free hemogloblin), glycoproteins, lactic acid dehydrogenase, cholinesterase, alkaline phosphatase, and macroglobulins. The beta globulin band contains complement, plasminogen, hemopexin (binds heme), transferrin (iron transport), and β-lipoprotein.[7,8]

The gamma globulin band contains the five classes of immunoglobulin which can be further separated by immunoelectrophoresis. A summary of changes occurring in electrophoretic patterns in various disease states is given in Table 45-6.

Uric Acid

Uric acid is the waste product of purine metabolism. Purines (adenine and guanine) are important substrates for nucleic acid (DNA and RNA) synthesis as well as for ATP, cAMP, AMP, and GTP. Purine-rich foods are those with a high cell (nucleus) content such as liver, fish, eggs, legumes, mushrooms, spinach, sweetbreads, and pancreas. Coffee, tea, and cocoa, which contain xanthines, are, in themselves, high in purines.[7,8]

Uric acid is rather insoluble, and if it is produced faster than it can be excreted, it tends to supersaturate body fluids and crystallize in the kidney and urinary tract. Likewise, uric acid will, if too concentrated, crystallize and form tophi (deposits) in cartilage and other tissues around joints, particularly the big toe joint, resulting in gout. Uric acid concentrations in the serum and urine depend on the rate of purine synthesis and degradation, dietary intake of purine-rich foods, and renal function. The quantity of uric acid excreted is governed by its rate of formation versus the ability of the kidneys to filter and excrete the product.[7,8]

Severe renal disease is the most frequent cause of secondary hyperuricemia; faulty purine metabolism (primary hyperuricemia) is less frequent. An increase in uric acid occurs in many lymphoproliferative disorders, because of rapid destruction of cells and degradation of their nuclear protein into uric acid (Table 45-7).[7,8]

Coombs' Test (Antiglobulin Test)

Human antibodies, when injected into a nonhuman species (rabbit or horse) will elicit the production of antihuman immunoglobulin designated *Coombs' serum, or antiglobulin serum.* This serum is used to screen for the presence and quantity of human immunoglobulin in certain patient situations. Two types of antiglobulin testing exist, the direct and indirect. Originally this test was called direct because it was a one-step test performed on infant cord blood to determine whether the infant's erythrocytes were coated with maternal anti-Rh antibodies. The indirect Coombs tested the serum of the mother for the presence of circulating anti-Rh antibody. Both were means of diagnosing erythroblastosis fetalis. The direct test is now designated *direct antiglobulin test* and the indirect test is called *antibody screening test* (Fig. 45-1).[7,8]

Direct Coombs' Test (Direct Antiglobulin Test) This test detects human IgG attached to circulating red blood cells. Antihuman globulin (Coombs' serum) is added directly to washed erythrocytes from a patient and observed for agglutination. Coombs' serum can be used to detect either IgG or complement.[7,8]

Indirect Coombs' Test (Antibody Screening Test) Unexpected circulating human antibodies may cause severe problems for a developing fetus or a person receiving blood transfusions. The purpose of anti-

Table 45-6 Electrophoretic Protein Fraction Changes in Various Diseases

Condition	Total Protein	Albumin	α_1-Globulin	α_2-Globulin	β-Globulin	γ-Globulin
Acute infection		Decreased		Increased		
Asthma, allergies with poor response to therapy		Decreased		Increased		Decreased
Carcinomatosis		Decreased	Increased	Increased		
Chronic infection		Decreased				Increased
Cryoglobulinemia						Increased
Dehydration	Increased	Increased	Increased	Increased	Increased	Increased
Diabetes mellitus		Decreased	Increased	Increased	Increased	
Glomerulonephritis	Decreased	Decreased	Increased			
Hepatic cirrhosis	Decreased	Decreased				Increased
Hepatitis, viral		Decreased	Decreased	Decreased	Increased	Increased
Hodgkin's disease	Decreased	Decreased		Increased		Increased
Hypogammaglobulinemia	Decreased					Decreased
Leukemia, myelogenous		Decreased				Increased
Lupus erythematosus		Decreased		Increased		Increased
Lymphoma and lymphatic leukemia	Decreased	Decreased				Decreased
Macroglobulinemia	Increased	Decreased			Increased	Increased
Malabsorption, starvation	Decreased	Decreased	Decreased	Decreased	Decreased	Decreased
Myeloma	Increased	Decreased				Increased
Myasthenia		Decreased				Increased
Myxedema		Decreased		Increased		Increased
Nephrosis	Decreased	Decreased		Increased		Decreased
Rheumatic fever		Decreased		Increased		
Rheumatoid arthritis		Decreased		Increased		Increased
Sarcoidosis	Increased	Decreased		Increased	Increased	Increased
Sclerodema	Decreased	Decreased	Decreased	Decreased	Decreased	Decreased
Ulcerative colitis, exudative enteropathies	Decreased	Decreased	Increased	Increased	Decreased	Decreased

Source: From Byrne, J. C. et al. (1986), *Laboratory Tests: Implications for Nurses and Allied Health Professionals* (2d ed.), Reading, MA: Addison-Wesley.

Table 45-7 Uric Acid, Levels in Various Pathologic Conditions

(Normal uric acid: male 2.1–7.5 mg/dL, female 2.0–6.6 mg/dL)

Increased uric acid (hyperuricemia)
    Destruction of breakdown of tissue (leukemia, polycythemia, pneumonia)
    Uremia (lack of urinary secretion)
    Diabetic acidoses (reabsorption of uric acid)
    Ingestion of toxins (alcohol, diuretics)
    Genetic diseases: glycogen storage disease, hyperlipoproteinemia
Decreased uric acid (hypouricemia)
    Uricosuric drug ingestion (allopurinol, aspirin, probenecid, corticosteroids)
    Wilson's disease
    Fanconi syndrome
    Xanthine oxidase deficiency
    Acromegaly

Source: Adapted from Byrne, J. C. et al. (1986), *Laboratory Tests: Implications for Nurses and Allied Health Professionals* (2d ed.), Reading, MA: Addison-Wesley.

body screening is to assess blood donors and recipients for all possible unexpected antibodies, using Coombs' serum and appropriate red blood cells as antigens.[7,8]

Coombs' testing is performed to verify that an immune response has occurred. This response may be typical (to a foreign antigen) or atypical (to a self-antigen). The indirect and direct Coombs tests are useful in transfusing blood, in diagnosing acquired hemolytic anemia and erythroblastosis fetalis, and in detecting in utero fetal infections.[7,8]

Cold Agglutinins

Cold agglutinins (antimycoplasmic antibodies) are antibodies of the IgM type which react with a person's own red blood cells at temperatures between 0 and 20°C, causing them to agglutinate. This

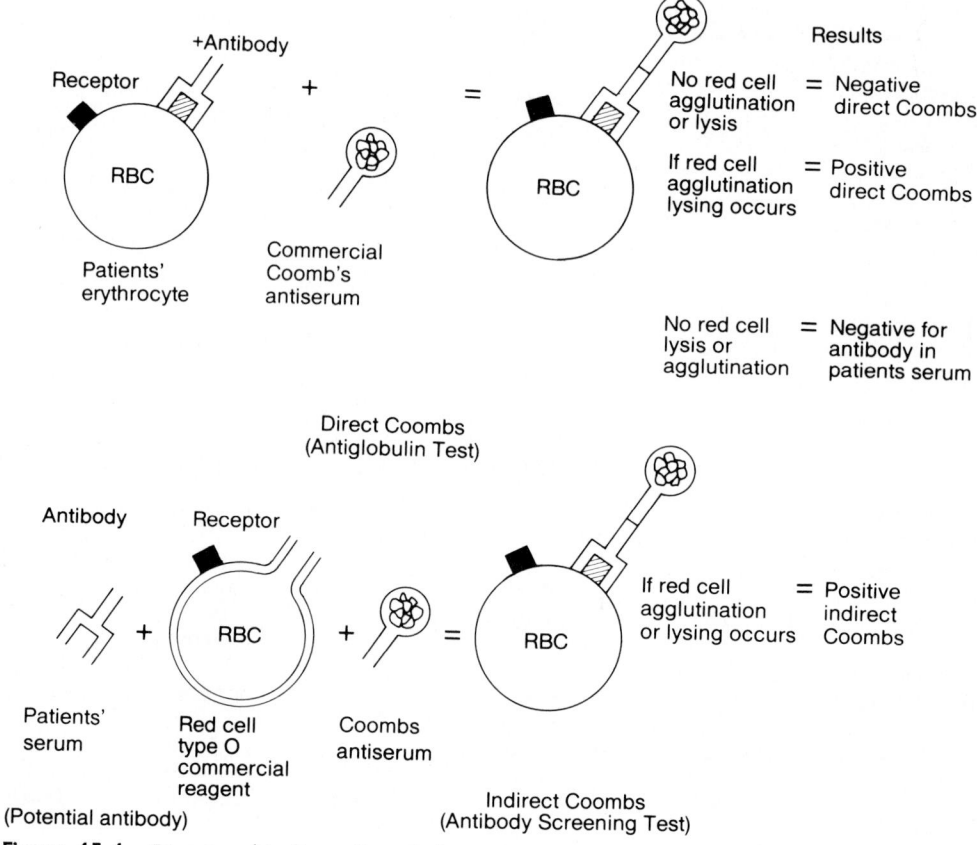

Figure 45-1 Direct and indirect Coombs' test.

agglutination is reversed when the cells are warmed to a temperature of 37°C or above; however, the antibody will remain on the red cell surface, allowing hemolysis and development of transient or chronic hemolytic anemia.[6–8]

Cold agglutinins are known to be present in many conditions. They may occur as primary phenomena or maybe secondary to infections or lymphoma. In mycoplasmal pneumonia (atypical pneumonia), cold agglutinins are present in one-half to two-thirds of all patients in the first week of acute infection, even before antimycoplasmal antibodies can be detected by complement fixation or metabolic inhibition tests. Infectious mononucleosis and certain viral infections are also associated with the presence of cold agglutinins. Other diseases in which cold agglutinins are present include cytomegalic viral disease, hemolytic anemia, multiple myeloma, Raynaud's phenomenon, and scleroderma. Cold agglutinins may also be found infrequently in pregnancy. In addition, lymphoreticular malignant disease is associated with chronically elevated cold agglutinin titers.[6–8] In all these conditions, symptoms are related to the body temperature of the patient. If the patient becomes cold, such problems as vascular purpura, Raynaud's phenomenon, hemolysis, and hemoglobinuria may result.

The cold agglutinin test is used primarily to provide evidence for mycoplasmal pneumonia, although it may also be used to provide evidence for other diseases. Normal persons have cold agglutinin titers below 1:32.

A blood specimen obtained for cold agglutinins should be immediately transported to the laboratory and kept at body temperature (37°C). The specimen should not be refrigerated. Cold agglutinin antibodies, if exposed to cold temperatures, will coat the red blood cells and give a false-negative result when the serum is tested.

With the exception of mycoplasmal pneumonia, cold agglutinin titers of 1:32 or over are not confirmatory evidence of any pathologic condition. Even in mycoplasmal pneumonia, the test is of limited value when only one titer is obtained—sequential titers over time are more valuable. A definite pattern occurs in mycoplasmal pneumonia. Titers are positive usually at 7 days, peak to titers above 1:32 in 4 weeks, and are usually absent in 4 months. When sequential titers verify this pattern and clinical evidence of pneumonia is present, the diagnosis of mycoplasmal pneumonia is supported. This test is not highly sensitive: only one-half to two-thirds of patients with mycoplasmal pneumonia exhibit cold agglutinin titers.[6–8]

High cold agglutinin titers, in the thousands or millions, can occur in idiopathic cold agglutinin disease which precedes the development of lymphoma. Patients with very high titers are more susceptible to intravascular agglutination, which causes significant clinical problems.[6,7]

Cryoglobulins

Cryoglobulins are abnormal serum globulins usually related to immune disease. Cryoglobulins precipitate out at a low temperature (4°C) and redissolve when warmed. They differ from cold agglutinins in that they do not bind to red blood cells and do not cause their agglutination. Cryoglobulins are usually immune-type complexes and exist as three basic types. Type I, a single monoclonal antibody precipitating at cold temperatures, is found in multiple myeloma, macroglobulinemia, and chronic lymphatic leukemia. Type II is mixed, in that a monoclonal-type antibody directed against polyclonal immunoglobulin is present; it is associated with rheumatoid arthritis and Sjögren's syndrome. Type III, a mixed polyclonal variety of cryoglobulin, is associated with many autoimmune diseases, viral infections, liver disease, poststreptococcal disease, and a few parasitic infections.[6–8]

Patients with circulating cryoglobulins are subject to pain and to cold, cyanotic fingers and toes when exposed to cold temperatures (Raynaud's-like syndrome).

Patients are tested for cryoglobulins when immune disease is suspected with Raynaud's symptoms. Lipids in serum make it difficult to detect precipitates forming at low temperatures, so patients should fast 6 to 8 h prior to testing. Also, blood specimens to be tested for cryoglobulins (as for cold agglutinins) should be maintained at 37°C and delivered immediately to the laboratory. If the blood is not kept at body temperature until it clots, the cryoglobulins will be lost, giving a false-negative result.[6,7]

Fetal Antigen Tests

Carcinoembryonic Antigen Carcinoembryonic antigen (CEA) is known to be present in the first two trimesters of fetal life but absent at birth. The appearance of this antigen later in life is sometimes indicative of the presence of an endoderm-derived tumor. CEA is detected by the use of radiolabeled antibodies in radioimmunoassay. It is found in 70 percent of patients with colon carcinoma, 35 percent of patients with breast carcinoma, and 90 percent of patients with cancer of the pancreas.[6-8]

CEA is presently used not as a diagnostic aid but to monitor for recurrence of colon cancer. Surgical removal of the tumor results in a decrease in serum CEA levels, while recurrence results in an increase. CEA is sometimes elevated in groups of people other than those with adenocarcinoma, especially persons with nonmalignant inflammatory diseases, particularly gastrointestinal, such as diverticulitis, regional enteritis, and ulcerative colitis. These inflammatory conditions, as well as biliary obstruction, chronic heavy smoking, and alcoholic hepatitis, are known to cause increased levels of CEA.[6-8]

Levels of CEA above 40 ng/mL usually indicate malignant disease, although these levels may also occur in the nonmalignant conditions referred to above. The value of the test is relative: if the patient has an above-normal level before resection of a colon tumor and this level drops 2 to 18 days after surgical removal, then an increase in levels in subsequent months is likely to be indicative of tumor regrowth.

Alpha Fetoprotein Alpha fetoprotein (AFP) is a protein produced primarily by embryonal and fetal hepatocytes, which can be transported across the placental barrier. It is found in fetal and maternal serum as well as in amniotic fluid. It begins to decrease prior to birth from peak levels of 4000 to 5000 ng/mL to 0 to 40 ng/mL.[6-8]

For unknown reasons, AFP is reactivated in some malignant processes and in immunologic disorders such as ataxia-telangiectasia. It is also elevated in the blood and amniotic fluid of pregnant women whose fetuses have neurologic malformations. Radioimmunoassay provides quantitative analysis of AFP. High levels of AFP at 16 to 18 weeks of gestation is indicative of neural tube defects such as spina bifida or anencephaly.[6-8]

AFP is used as a diagnostic tool as well as a monitor for the progression or regression of malignant conditions such as hepatomas, embryonal carcinomas, and malignant teratomas of the ovary and testes. In addition, elevated levels are indicators of nonmalignant conditions such as viral hepatitis and ataxia-telangiectasia, but the usefulness of AFP as a diagnostic aid for these conditions has not been established.[6-8]

Acquired Immune Deficiency Syndrome Tests

Acquired immune deficiency syndrome (AIDS) is characterized by a diminished cell-mediated immunity. The cause is theorized to be an oncogenic virus, the human T cell lymphotropic virus III (HTLV-III), which selectively infects and destroys T_4 (helper) cells. Thus, the basic defect in AIDS is loss of T_4 cells and their helper function, defective T cell cytotoxicity, and defects of macrophage function, resulting in quantitative changes in both humoral and cellular immunity (Table 45-8).[9-11]

HTLV-III antibody tests are currently being performed to screen for infection with HTLV-III virus and possible AIDS. All types of HTLV (HTLV-I, HTLV-II, and HTLV-III) contain three major structural genes termed *Gag, Pol,* and *Env.* The Gag gene codes for core antigens, the Env for surface glycoproteins in the envelope, and the Pol for reverse transcriptase and endonuclease. The most important for laboratory testing are the Gag and Env. Exposure to the virus results in production of antibody mainly against Env antigens.[9,10]

Test procedures used to detect antibodies are immunofluorescence, immunoprecipitation, Western blotting, and enzyme-linked immunosorbent assay, or ELISA (the most commonly used). ELISA techniques utilize the current FDA-licensed products. HTLV-III antigen is produced by growing the virus in a T lymphocytic cell line called H9/HTLV-III. This cell line is sensitive to infection by the virus but resistant to lysis. The virus is isolated from the culture and inactivated (HTLV-III antigen, commercially available). Patient serum is added to the HTLV-III antigen; if antibody is present, it will bind to the virus. The complex is visualized by antihuman IgG conjugated with horseradish peroxidase and a substrate which gives a yellow-orange color pro-

Table 45-8 Humoral and Cellular Immunity in AIDS

Humoral Immunity	Cellular Immunity
Factors Increased	
Circulating anti-HTLV-III antibody	None—all cell-mediated are depressed
Alpha interferon	
Alpha 1 thymosin	
Beta 2 macroglobulin	
Immunoglobulins IgA and IgG	
Immune complexes	
Suppressor factors	
Factors Decreased	
Gamma interferon	Lymphokine production T_4/T_8 ratio inverted
Thymosin	Expression of IL 2 receptors
	Number and function of T_4 (helper) cells
	Reaction to mitogens
	Mixed lymphocyte reactivity (MLC)
Other Factors	
Polyclonal B lymphocytes activated	Lymphopenia
	Skin-testing anergy
anti-Lymphocytic antibodies present	Normal or decreased number of T_8 (suppressor) cells

Source: Adapted from Lewandowski.[9]

portional to the antibody bound to the virus. The intensity of color is read on a colorimeter at 492 nm absorbency and compared with a known negative control.[9,10]

Care must be taken in evaluating ELISA for HTLV-III antibody. The H9 cell line is also known to be positive for various HLA antigens, including DR4. Multigravid females often show a positive test because of cross reactivity of HLA antigens.

Immune Complex Assays

Every human cell has on its surface or within it a variety of antigenic determinants. Some of these are shared with other cells of the body and are called *self-antigens* or *histocompatibility antigens* of the HLA type. Some are specific to an organ or to a tissue, while others are specific to cells and cell subtypes. When a person's own immune system produces antibodies against these, two variations of autoimmune diseases are observed clinically: organ-specific and non-organ-specific. Organ-specific disease (e.g., thyroiditis, gastritis, adrenalitis) is associated with lymphocytic invasion of the target organ and subsequent destruction of the parenchy-

mal cells. Non-organ-specific disease (e.g., systemic lupus erythematosis) is associated with lesions because of deposition of immune complexes (type III hypersensitivity); the lesions occur anywhere in the body and are not confined to any particular organ.[12]

There is a tendency for more than one type of organ-specific antibody to occur in the same person. These are not cross-reacting antibodies but have different organ specificities. Autoimmune thyroiditis and pernicious anemia share such a relationship. Persons with immune thyroiditis demonstrate antithyroglobulin which will not react with gastric parietal cells, and concomitantly parietal cell antibodies which will not react with thyroid tissue. Autoimmunity shows a familial pattern as well. The fact that organ-specific antibodies exist concomitantly with symptoms does not answer the question of whether they are the cause or the effect. The role T cells and cell-mediated immunity play in the development of autoimmune disease suggests that autoantibody may be an outcome, at least in some of these disorders. Organ-specific antibodies, then, are quite different from the autoantibodies formed against soluble components, which result in the formation of immune complex (type III) hypersensitivity, as in systemic lupus erythrematosis or rheumatoid arthritis. Methods utilized to demonstrate organ-specific antibody are indirect immunofluorescence, radioimmunoassay, agglutination, and more recently, immunoperoxidase techniques that use monoclonal antibody[12-15] (Table 45-9).

Immune complexes are the product of the interactions of antigen with antibody and are normally formed during an immune response. The presence of these complexes is often necessary before antigen can be destroyed. If they are produced faster than they can be cleared by the lymphoreticular system, immune complex disease may occur.

Many disorders result from circulating antigen-antibody immune complexes—for example, postinfectious syndromes, serum sickness, drug sensitivity, rheumatoid arthritis, and systemic lupus erythematosus (SLE). Immune complexes can develop when a certain ratio of antigen reacts with antibody of isotypes IgG1, 2, or 3 or IgM in tissues. These disorders occur when the antigen is deposited in tissues, as in type III hypersensitivity reactions; the immune complexes fix complement and activate the complement cascade. The subsequent complement-mediated activity leads to inflammation, with local tissue necrosis. In the blood, soluble circulating immune complexes may also activate complement and eventually cause damage, usually in the renal glomeruli and in the aorta and other large blood vessels.[2,5,12,15]

Histologic examination of tissue obtained by biopsy generally detects immune complexes. However, since tissue biopsies cannot provide information about the titers of complexes still in circulation, serum assays, which detect circulating immune complexes indirectly, may be required. Because of the inherent variability of these complexes, several serum test methods may be appropriate, using complement, rheumatoid factor (RF), or cellular substrates (such as Raji cells; see below) as reagents.

Table 45-9 Comparison of Organ-Specific and Non-Organ-Specific Autoimmune Diseases

Organ-specific (e.g. thyroiditis, gastritis, adrenalitis)	Non-organ-specific (e.g. systemic lupus erythematosus)
Antigen available to lymphoid system only in low concentration	Antigen accessible at higher concentrations
Antibodies and lesions organ-specific	Antibodies and lesions non-organ-specific
Clinical and serologic overlap of thyroiditis, gastritis, and adrenalitis	Overlap of SLE, rheumatoid arthritis, and other connective tissue disorders
Familial tendency to organ-specific autoimmunity	Familial connective tissue abnormalities in immunoglobulin synthesis in relatives
Lymphoid invasion, parenchymal destruction by + cell-mediated hypersensitivity and + antibodies	Lesions due to deposition of antigen-antibody complexes
Therapy aimed at controlling metabolic deficit	Therapy aimed at inhibiting inflammation and antibody synthesis
Tendency to cancer in organ	Tendency to lymphoreticular neoplasia
Organ-specific antibodies evoked by antigens in normal animals with complete Freund's adjuvant	No antibodies produced in animals with comparable stimulation
Experimental lesions produced with antigen in Freund's adjuvant	Diseases and autoantibodies arising spontaneously in certain animals (e.g., NZB mice and hybrids and some dogs) or after injection of parental lymphoid tissue into F1 hybrids

Source: Adapted from Riott.[25]

Since most immune complex assays have not been standardized, more than one test may be required to achieve accurate results. This is not surprising, because of the dynamic nature of the formation of immune complexes. The purpose of immune complex assay is to demonstrate the presence of circulating immune complexes and to assist in estimating the severity of the disease.

The presence of detectable immune complexes in serum has etiologic importance in many autoimmune diseases, such as SLE and rheumatoid arthritis. However, for definitive diagnosis, the presence of these complexes must be considered together with the results of other studies. For example, in SLE, immune complexes are associated with high titers of antinuclear antibodies and circulating antinative deoxyribonucleic acid antibodies.[2,5]

Because of their filtering function, renal glomeruli seem most vulnerable to immune complex deposition, although blood vessel walls and the choroid plexus (vascular folds in the ventricles of the brain) may also be affected. Renal biopsy to detect immune complexes can provide conclusive evidence for immune complex (type III) glomerulonephritis, differentiating this from other types of glomerulonephritis.[2,5]

In the *Raji test,* immune complexes are identified by their ability to interact with cell receptor on a cultured lymphoblastoid B cell line containing complement factor 3 (C3) receptors but lacking surface immunoglobulins. These Raji cells are mixed with the sera suspected of containing circulating immune complexes. If present, the complexes will bind to the Raji cell surface. This binding can be estimated by adding a radiolabeled antiimmunoglobulin without interference of the usual surface immunoglobulin found on B cells.[6,7,8]

T and B Lymphocyte Counts

Cells designated as mononuclear include several populations of lymphocytes (T, B, K and null) as well as monocytes. These cells cannot be differentiated on the basis of structure alone but are identified by their membrane receptors. The different classes of lymphocyte cells are determined quantitatively by cell separation technique. First mononuclear cells have to be separated from other cellular elements of blood by the use of Ficoll-Hypaque density gradients. The whole blood is layered over a density gradient of Ficoll-Hypaque and centrifuged. The granulocytes and erythrocytes form a sediment at the bottom of the tube, and lymphocytes, monocytes, and platelets form a band at the Ficoll-plasma interface. This procedure recovers approximately 80 percent of the lymphocytes.[6,7,8,13]

After washing, the mononuclear layer is ready for quantitation of the various types of mononuclear cells such as the T, B, K, and null lymphocytes and macrophages[6,8] (Table 45-10).

Total Count   Total lymphocyte counts are calculated from the white blood cell and blood differential count and reported in lymphocytes per cubic millimeter of blood.

T Count   T lymphocyte counts are determined by the ability of the lymphocytes to spontaneously make rosettes (E rosettes) with sheep red blood cells (SRBC) at 4°C. This is a property not shared with B lymphocytes or other lymphocytes. The rosettes are quite unstable, and accuracy depends on the experience and technical skill of the laboratory worker.

The mechanism of E rosetting is not totally understood but depends on receptors and antigen recognition by the T lymphocyte. The T lymphocyte can also be identified by immunofluorescence, using specific anti–T cell serum. T cells make up 60 to 85 percent of all peripheral blood lymphocytes.[6]

Table 45-10 Normal Values for Lymphocytes and Subclasses of Lymphocytes

Lymphocytes: 65 to 75 percent of total peripheral blood lymphocytes

"Active" E rosette cells: 20 to 30 percent of total peripheral blood mononuclear cells

B lymphocytes: 10 to 20 percent of total peripheral blood lymphocytes

K lymphocytes: 5 to 20 percent of total peripheral blood lymphocytes

Null lymphocytes: 5 to 20 percent of total peripheral blood lymphocytes

Total lymphocyte count: 4000 per cubic millimeter of blood (higher in children)

B cell count: 270 to 640 per cubic millimeter of blood

T_8 (suppressor cells): 20 percent of T cells

T_4 (helper cells): 75 percent of T cells

B Count   B lymphocytes have immunoglobulin on their surface, which is easily detected by direct immunofluorescence at 4°C; thus the number of B cells in the circulation can be assessed by measuring the proportion and absolute number of circulating lymphocytes that have surface Ig. B lymphocytes also have detectable receptors for complement, as well as a receptor for the Fc region of immunoglobulin. These markers are absent in typical T cells.[2,5,6]

Other Lymphocytes   The remainder of the lymphocyte population may be either K cells or null lymphocytes. K cells express both complement and Fc receptors but no IgG. Null cells are a population with no detectable markers. K cell assays exist but are not at present routinely used; null cells are determined by subtracting the sum of T, B, and K lymphocytes from 100 percent, the total number of lymphocytes.[2,5]

T and B cell determinations are made for two purposes. First, they are used for diagnosing primary and secondary immune deficiencies. Knowing the type of lymphocyte that is lacking helps predict probable complications facing the patient and forms the basis for an approach to correct or compensate for the deficiency. Second, they are used to distinguish between benign and malignant lymphocytic proliferative diseases. The most readily recognized abnormalities are those due to an abnormal proliferation of lymphoid cells in diseases such as leukemia. Most chronic leukemias are of the B cell type, while acute lymphoblastic leukemia is thought to be T cell–derived.[14,16–18]

T and B cell increases and decreases must be confirmed by signs and symptoms and by the history. Just as with any other laboratory values, they are used as data which may help confirm the suspected. B cells are found to be increased in such conditions as chronic lymphocytic leukemia (thought to be a B cell malignant disease), multiple myeloma, Waldenström's macroglobulinemia, and Di George's syndrome (a congenital T cell deficiency); they are decreased in acute lymphocytic leukemia and certain congenital and acquired immunoglobulin deficiency diseases. In other immunoglobulin deficiencies, especially when only one class of immunoglobulin is deficient, B cells are normal.[14,16–18]

T cells are sometimes found to be increased in infectious mononucleosis and more frequently in multiple myeloma and acute lymphocytic leukemia. They are decreased in congenital T cell-deficiency diseases such as Di George's syndrome, Nezelof's syndrome, and Wiskott-Aldrich syndrome, also in certain B cell proliferative disorders such as chronic lymphocytic leukemia, Waldenström's macroglobulinemia, and Burkitt's lymphoma.[14,16–18]

Even normal levels of T or B cells do not necessarily mean that a person has a competent immune system. In certain selective immunoglobulin deficiency diseases, for example, there may be adequate numbers of B cells but they do not differentiate into plasma cells capable of producing the immunoglobulins necessary to mount an immune response. T cells may be present in adequate numbers and yet may not be functionally competent. Therefore, the information obtained by lymphocyte determinations can be interpreted as supportive evidence for or against a specific disease but is usually not by itself diagnostic of these conditions. Since all lymphocyte counts depend on lymphocyte viability, specimens must be sent to the laboratory immediately.

The percentage and proportions of T and B cells can change rapidly because of stress, surgery, or health status and also because of chemotherapy, steroid therapy, or x-ray; T and B cell counts should therefore not be performed on a person who has recently received these therapies. However, occasionally the T and B cell counts are determined in these situations and compared with baseline data (prior to treatment) to assess the effect of a therapy or progression of the disease process.[2,5]

The accuracy of lymphocyte population assays depends on delicate technical skills of the laboratory technician as well as freedom from interfering immunoglobulins, such as the autologous antilymphocyte antibodies sometimes seen in autoimmune disease. If antilymphocyte antibodies are suspected, as in systemic lupus erythematosis, the laboratory should be informed, so as to make alterations in the procedure to allow for shedding of the adsorbed autoantibody.

Monoclonal Antibody Assays

For years, antibodies and antigens have played a major role in the diagnosis of many pathologic conditions. Radioimmunoassays and other immunologic tests are used extensively to detect and quantitate bacterial, fungal, and viral products, tumor-specific antigens, immune globulins, histocompatibility (HLA) types, and drugs. These tests, however, have always been rather nonspecific and unpredictable because of the polyclonal nature of available antiserum, antigenic impurity, cross reactivity, and lack of knowledge regarding the immune mechanisms.[13]

In 1975, Kohler and Milstein conferred immortality on the B cell by hybridizing (fusing) it with a neoplastic syngeneic plasma cell line (myeloma cell).[19] When such cell hybrids (hybridomas) are grown in continuous culture, many are found to produce monoclonal antibodies that are specific for a single antigenic determinant. This exact specificity makes them excellent markers for the identification of individual tissues and cell types.[13]

Both direct and indirect immunofluorescence assays have successfully utilized monoclonal antibodies. However, clinical use of a histochemical immunoperoxidase technique using monoclonal antibodies is increasing because of its specific, yet permanent, stably colored product and the fact that it can be observed with an ordinary light microscope, eliminating the need for special equipment.[13]

Markers for specific cell types, hormones, enzymes, drugs, and other proteins have rapidly developed within the past 5 years in the form of monoclonal antibodies directed against specific antigenic determinants within or on the cell surface. Hybridoma-produced monoclonal antibodies also currently make it possible to identify specific regulatory and effector cells in the various T and B cell subsets of the immune system.[13]

Thus, monoclonal antibodies are not only making it possible to unravel the intricate and delicate maturation and regulation of the immune response but are clarifying the etiology of many previously elusive immunopathologic conditions. Use of most monoclonal antibodies is still classified as a research tool but will no doubt find many clinical applications in the diagnosis of immune, autoimmune, and neoplastic conditions. These antibodies offer hope as specific therapeutic agents in the treatment of these conditions.

Several T and B cell assays are commercially available. Some of these assays utilize monoclonal and polyclonal antibodies coupled to microbeads which serve as cell-labeling agents. The beads form color-coded rosettes easily identified by conventional light microscopy. Other techniques characterize T and B cells in the peripheral blood by direct and indirect immunofluorescence techniques with appropriate monoclonal and fluorescein-conjugated antibodies. Monoclonal antibodies for tumor antigens, hormones, and other protein markers in tissue samples are also available. The immunoperoxidase technique using the appropriate antibody is employed to assay for these markers. While most of these assays have not yet been approved for clinical diagnostic or therapeutic procedures, their specificity and potential for clinical evaluation and therapy of immune and neoplastic disorders assuredly mandates their replacing the polyclonal specificity of antisera now being used in clinical assays.[13]

Immunopathology often requires knowledge of the presence and quantity of specific cell types as well as their ability to function. The proportion of certain subpopulations is crucial in maintaining immunologic balance and health. The development, by hybridoma technology, of monoclonal-type antibodies that react with a specific antigenic determinant has been a major breakthrough in immune testing and will undoubtedly confirm or change existing theories, assays, methods, and therapies. Cells communicate via chemical mediators which bind to and affect these various determinants (receptors). Lymphocytes, macrophages, and other human cells, as discussed in Chap. 44, have many types of antigenic determinants and receptors on their surfaces.[14,19]

Antigenic determinants are those structures on the surface of or within a cell which, when recognized, provoke an immune response. *Receptors* are those molecular structures and configurations at a cell's surface which are able to receive and bind humoral mediators (such as antibodies, lymphokines, and prostaglandins), which in turn produce a change in the cell's behavior (function).[14]

Until 1975, most laboratory assays used polyclonal antisera which contained several antibodies directed against many determinants; thus they usually did not produce highly specific results and gave many false-negative and false-positive results. Monoclonal assays, however, employ an antibody produced against a single determinant; this allows for specific identification when the procedure is performed accurately. These determinants are referred to as *cell markers* and are currently being produced and investigated at a rapid pace.[14,19]

Studies of the thymus utilizing monoclonal antibodies has confirmed what was theorized for many years: that the thymic environment induces the maturation of lymphocytic stem cells to mature functional unprimed T helper and T suppressor cell populations found in the secondary lymphoid T cell compartment [blood, gut associated lymphoid tissue (G.A.L.T.), lymph node, spleen, etc.].[14]

Cell markers are used to identify determinants on normal cell populations as well as abnormal cell populations. They are sometimes used as controls and sometimes as test targets for the presence of abnormal markers. Therefore, knowledge of the normal percentage of the lymphocyte subpopulations is important for comparison in disease states. The normal helper/suppressor ratio is approximately 2:1.[2,5]

T_4/T_8 ratios, or helper/suppressor ratios are particularly helpful in that an increase in T_4 cells or a decrease in T_8 cells shifts the homeostatic balance toward a hyperimmune (hypersensitivity) state, while a decrease in T_4 or an increase in T_8 cells will shift the immunological balance toward a hypoimmune or immune deficiency (anergic) state (Fig. 45-2).[11,13]

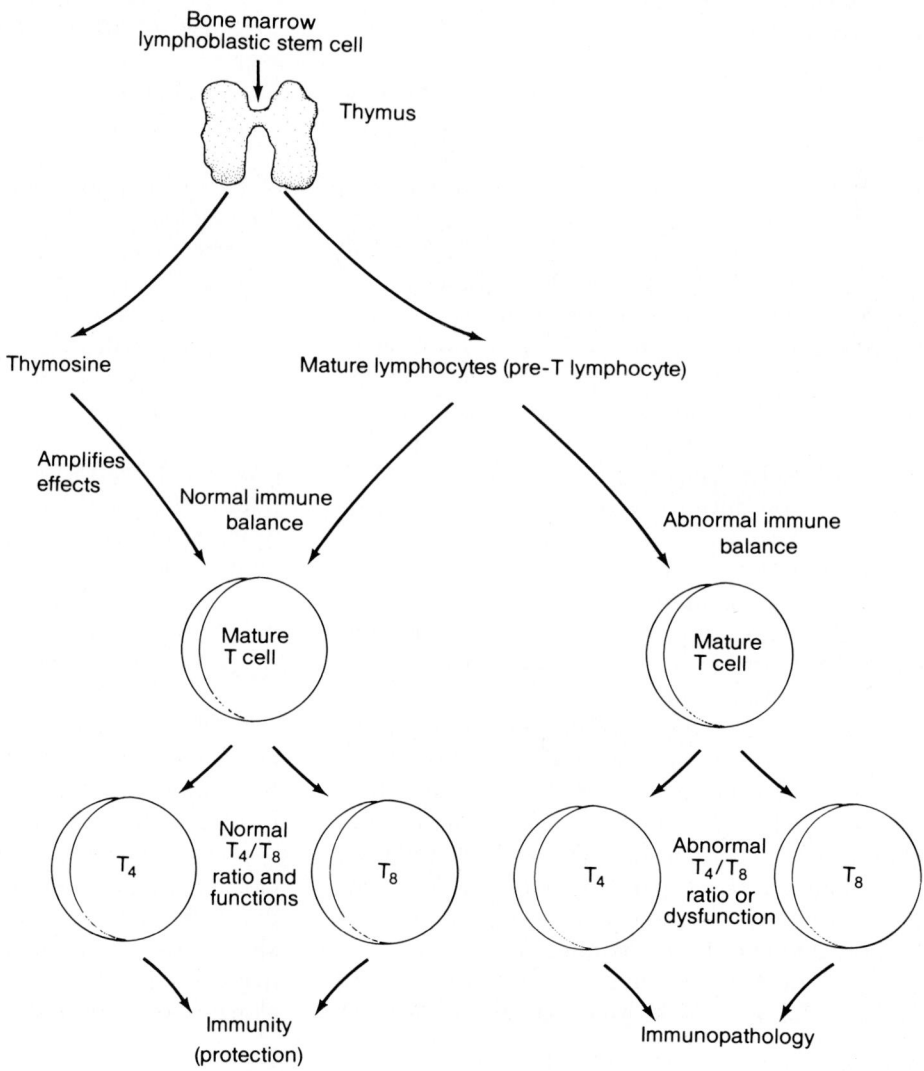

Figure 45-2 Functions of thymus in immune homeostasis.

Table 45-11 Immunoregulatory Imbalance: Monoclonal Antibody T Cell Subset Phenotyping in Human Disease

Disease	Ig +	T_3 +	T_4 +	T_5 +	T_8 +	T_4/T_8	T_4/T_5
Autoimmune disease		↓			↓	↑	
SLE, active		↓	↔	NA	↓	↓	NA
inactive		↓	↔	NA	↓	↓	NA
Sjögren's syndrome		↓	NA	NA	↓	↑	NA
Juvenile rheumatoid arthritis, active		↔	↓	NA	↑	↓	NA
inactive		↔	↔	NA	↔	↔	NA
Multiple sclerosis		↓	↔	↓	NA	NA	4:1
Viral-associated (infected)	↑	↑	↓	↑	NA	NA	
Acquired immune deficiency disease			↓				1:2
Infectious mononucleosis	↑	↑	↓	↑	NA	NA	1:2
Normal healthy adults (4000 lymphocytes per cubic millimeter)	11 ± 4	67 ± 10	44 ± 8	18 ± 6	$22 +$	1.9 ± 0.2	2:1

Key: ↑ = increased; ↓ = decreased; ↔ = no change; NA = assayed.
T_4 + = T helper; T_8 + = T suppressor ($T_{5/8}$ +); T_5 + = T suppressor and cytotoxic subsets; T_3 + = all mature lymphocytes; Ig + = immunoglobulin receptor B cells; (T_5 + Ig +) = phenotype T cell in chronic graft-versus-host disease and in immunodeficiency.
Source: Adapted from C. Morimoto et al., in Haynes and Eisenbarth.[13]

Monoclonal Antibody T Cell Phenotyping The importance of T cell-subset phenotyping in clinical disorders of T lymphocytes has recently been emphasized[13,16–18,20] (Table 45-11). Utilizing monoclonal antibodies, the researchers cited have not only advanced the knowledge of T cell ontogeny (Table 45-12) but have also demonstrated immunoregulatory imbalances in mature T lymphocyte subsets and initiated standards leading toward confirmation of the diagnosis of diseases which before could only be assumed to involve imbalances. Their work also suggests the role viral infections may play in acquired immune deficiency.

Mechanisms operative in autoimmunity have been difficult to establish because of the various kinds of autoantibodies and symptoms displayed by patients. Evidence to support a decreased number of T_8 cells with resultant B cell hyperactivity in serum lupus erythematosis (SLE) is accumulating. Further, it seems that active, exacerbated SLE shows an imbalance in immune regulation which returns toward normal when the disease becomes inactive. The same pattern is found in active versus inactive multiple sclerosis, although the immune defects are different.

Sjögren's syndrome is a chronic inflammatory, systemic, autoimmune disease involving exocrine glands. Clinically, it is characterized by xerostomia (dry mouth), xerophthalmia (dry eyes, lack of tearing), hypergammaglobulinemia, RA factor, and

Table 45-12 T Cell Maturational Markers

T Cell Marker	Monoclonal Anti-T Antibody	Type of Cell/Cells Possessing Marker Ratio, %			Commercial Nomenclature
		T_1 Thymocytes	T Cells	B Cells	
T_1	Anti-T_1	+ (10)	+	0	OKT 1, Leu 16
T_3	Anti-T_3	+ (10)	+	0	OKT 3, Leu 4 (helper)
T_4 (helper)	Anti-T_4	75	60	0	OKT 4, Leu 3a/3b (helper)
T_5	Anti-T_5	80	25	0	OKT 5
T_8 (suppressor)	Anti-T_8	80	30	0	OKT 8, Leu 2a/2b
T_6	Anti-T_6	70	0	0	OKT 6
T_9	Anti-T_9	10	0	0	OKT 9
T_{10}	Anti-T_{10}	95	5	10	OKT 10
T_{11}	Anti-T_{11}	100	100	10	OKT 11, Leu 5

OKT = Ortho Pharmaceutical Company; Leu = Becton-Dickinson Company.
Source: C. Marimoto et al., in Haynes and Eisenbarth.[13]

antibody to extractable nuclear antigen (ENA). This likewise points to B cell hyperactivity. There is also a demonstrated difference in the population of T cell subsets in the glands as compared with the peripheral blood lymphocytes in Sjögren's.

Infectious mononucleosis (IM) is associated with selective infection of B cells by the Epstein-Barr virus. There is a proliferation of activated T lymphocytes, presumably stimulated by the virally infected B cell or by the virus itself. The virus usually causes the production of multiple autoantibodies which can produce secondary disease, but in some cases the patient exhibits agammaglobulinemia, suggesting loss of immune regulation. More recently, it has been suggested that a specific T cell (T_5 +) plus Ig + phenotype is both activated and increased. This phenotype is also present in patients with chronic graft-versus-host disease and naturally occurring immunodeficiency states.[11,13]

Immunoregulation relies on a discrete balance of T cell subsets which interact to maintain a normal and appropriate immune response. An excessive number of suppressor cells results in immunodeficiency, while loss or inactivation of these cells produces heterogeneous autoimmune disorders. A balance of helper and suppressor T cells is required for a normal immune response. An excess of either cell type can change the intensity as well as the outcome of the response.

Autoimmunity is one form of hypersensitivity in which the immune response is misdirected against the body's own tissues. Increasing evidence seems to support T suppressor cell function for prevention of certain autoimmune diseases. Loss of T_8 cells allows the T_4 cells to be unregulated, and this results in augmented production of antibody against self-antigens (i.e., autoimmune disease).[15,16]

In multiple myeloma, a single abnormal clone of plasma cells can result in a single type of immunoglobulin which subsequently inhibits totally the production of other types of antibodies. In this manner, hypersensitivity reactions can lead to immunodeficiency.

Lymphocyte Marker Assays in Lymphoproliferative Disease A normal immune response requires a balance between the regulatory activities of several interacting cell types. Particularly important is the T helper/T suppressor ratio. It has become increasingly evident that various levels of lymphocyte differentiation can be defined by using highly specific monoclonal antibodies. This allows analysis of both normal and malignant cell populations. Monoclonal antibody is employed in many types of immunoassays, but direct and indirect immunofluorescence, microcytotoxicity, and immunoperoxidase techniques are the most frequently employed. Monoclonal antibodies offer the advantage of reacting with a single antigenic site, and thus their reactivities can be precisely defined. Table 45-13 gives a rather incomplete listing of T and B cell markers currently available in larger laboratories and research centers. Most are still considered investigational. They can be ordered separately or as lymphocyte subset panels.[14] It should be noted that T cell and B cell assays are currently being standardized, and values may differ from one laboratory to another, depending on the test technique (Table 45-10).

Pan–T Cell Marker This is a marker present on nearly 100 percent of mature T cells but absent on non-T cells. It is more precisely restricted to T cells with the E rosette marker, which is usually absent on immature T cells.[14] The purpose of the pan–T cell marker assay is to quantitate mature T cells in immune disease. It is not currently recommended for differentiation of lymphoproliferative diseases.

T Helper/Inducer Subset Marker This marker, designated T_4, anti-Leu 3, and OKT 4, is present on the surface of T helper cells. The T_4 marker is usually present on T cell lymphoblastic lymphomas, Sézary syndrome cells, and the T cells of mycosis fungoides. It is usually absent on T cell acute lymphoblastic leukemia. The purpose of this assay is to characterize, in conjunction with markers for T suppressor cells, certain autoimmune or immunoregulatory disorders; to detect immune deficiency states such as AIDS; and to differentiate T cell acute lymphoblastic leukemia (ALL) from T cell lymphomas and other lymphoproliferative disorders.[16]

T Suppressor/Cytotoxic Subset Marker This marker, designated T_8, anti-Leu 2, or OKT 8, is present on the surface of T suppressor cells. T_8 is found on a few ALL and lymphoma T cells. This

Table 45-13 Lymphocyte Marker Assays

Assay	Purposes
Pan–T cell marker	To measure mature T cells in immune dysfunction
T helper/inducer subset marker	To identify and characterize the proportion of T helper cells in autoimmune or immunoregulatory disorders; to detect immunodeficiency disorders, such as AIDS; and to differentiate T cell acute lymphoblastic leukemia from T cell lymphomas and other lymphoproliferative disorders
T suppressor/cytotoxic subset marker	To identify and characterize the proportion of T suppressor cells in autoimmune and immunoregulatory disorders and to characterize lymphoproliferative disorders
T cell E rosette receptor	To differentiate lymphoproliferative disorders of T cell origin, such as T cell lymphocytic leukemia and lymphoblastic lymphoma, from those of non-T cell origin
Pan-B (B-1) marker	To differentiate lymphoproliferative disorders of B cell origin, such as B cell chronic lymphocytic leukemia, from those of T cell origin
Pan-B (BA-1) marker	To identify B cell lymphoproliferative disorders such as B cell chronic lymphocytic leukemia
CALLA (common acute lymphocytic leukemia antigen) marker	To identify bone marrow regeneration and to identify non-T cell acute lymphocytic leukemia
Lymphocytic subset panel (B, pan-T, T helper/inducer, T suppressor/cytotoxic, and T helper/T suppressor ratio	To evaluate immunodeficiencies; to identify immunoregulation associated with autoimmune disorders; and to characterize lymphoid malignant disease
Lymphocytic leukemia marker panel; includes T cell markers (E rosette receptor and Leu-9), B cell markers (B-1 and BA-1), and CALLA	To characterize lymphocytic leukemias as T, B, non-T, or non-B, regardless of the stage of differentiation of the malignant cells

Source: Reprinted with permission from Wheat, B., Fidler, R. Nurse's Reference Library, *Diagnostics*, 2d ed, 1986. Springhouse Corporation, All Rights Reserved.

assay is done to detect immune deficiency states by the reduction in the potentially cytotoxic lymphocytes and to characterize certain autoimmune and immunoregulatory disorders by the T_4/T_8 ratio.[14]

T Cell E Rosette Receptor The E rosette receptor (a receptor binding sheep red blood cells) is found on all primed T cells, 95 percent of thymocytes, and some null cells. It is present on the surface of most T cells, ALL cells, lymphoblastic

lymphomas, chronic lymphatic leukemia, and Sézary cells. It is absent on ALL non-T cells. This test is useful in discriminating lymphoproliferative disorders of T cell origin from those of non-T cell origin.[14]

T Cell Leu 9 Marker This surface antigen is present on 85 to 100 percent of peripheral T cells and most non-T and non-B lymphocytes. It appears on T cell ALL and T cell lymphomas. It is absent on common ALL, null cell ALL, and B cell ALL. The T cell Leu 9 marker is used to quantitate mature lymphocyte populations when immune deficiency or immunoregulatory diseases are suspected.[14]

Pan-B (B-1) Marker This antigen is found on the surface of mature B cells in peripheral lymphoid organs and bone marrow. B-1 is also found on B cell chronic lymphocytic leukemia and non-T ALL, including about 50 percent of the common acute lymphocytic leukemias. B-1 is absent on T cells, monocytes, granulocytes, and their tumors. The pan-B marker differentiates lymphoproliferative disorders of B cell origin from those of T cell origin.[14]

Pan-B (BA-1) Marker BA-1 antigen is found on B cells in peripheral blood, B cell chronic lymphatic leukemia, pre-B ALL, and some non-T and non-B ALL. It is thought to appear before B-1 in the differentiation sequence. It is absent on normal and malignant T cells, monocytes, and ALL and identifies B cell lymphoproliferative disorders.[14]

CALLA (Common Acute Lymphocytic Leukemia Antigen) Marker This antigen is absent on normal mature peripheral lymphocytes. Normal bone marrow contains a few cells bearing the CALLA antigen; when bone marrow is regenerating, the cells increase in number. CALLA is present on cells in 70 percent of non-T ALL and usually predicts a less aggressive course. It is also present in about half the patients with chronic myelogeneous leukemia blast crisis. This correlates well with the enzyme TdT. The CALLA marker denotes bone marrow regeneration and helps to identify non-T cell ALL.[14]

Lymphocytic Subset Panel This panel includes B, pan-T, T helper/inducer, T suppressor/cytotoxic, and T helper/T suppressor markers. The panel is used to evaluate immune deficiencies, to identify immunoregulatory abnormalities associated with autoimmune disorders, and to assist in the characterization of lymphoid malignant diseases.[14]

Lymphocytic Leukemia Marker Panel This panel includes T cell markers (E rosette receptor and Leu-9), B cell markers (B-1 and BA-1), and CALLA for identifying lymphocytic leukemia.[14]

Terminal Deoxynucleotidyl Transferase Terminal deoxynucleotidyl transferase (TdT) is an important enzyme marker in lymphoid cell differentiation. TdT is an enzyme (DNA polymerase) found in immature lymphocytes of either pre-T or pre-B cell lines. Mature and mitogen-stimulated cells show no detectable activity. TdT is present in lymphoid cells of the bone marrow and in cortical thymocytes; its activity is measured by incubating small radiolabeled nucleotides in a suitable buffer. If TdT is present, it will catalyze the polymerization of these small nucleotides into larger radiolabeled nucleotides (Fig. 45-3).[20] The extent of polymerization is directly related to the presence of TdT, and by measuring the radioactive acid–insoluble product, the TdT level may be determined on cells of blood, bone marrow, or CSF.

In adults, TdT-positive cells make up less than 2 percent of marrow cells. They are virtually absent in normal peripheral blood. TdT-positive cells appear in bone marrow and peripheral blood in over 90 percent of ALL patients.[20] They are absent in the CSF of ALL patients in remission but are present in central nervous system relapse. The enzyme is also found in blast cells of 33 percent of all patients with chronic myelogenous leukemia in blast crisis. Patients with TdT-positive blast cells respond better than those whose blast cells are TdT-negative in that they seem to respond more favorably to vincristine and prednisone.[20]

TdT is found during normal proliferation of prelymphocytes in the bone marrow of children; thus blood may be the sample of choice in children.

It must be kept in mind that TdT levels cannot be strictly correlated with morphology, since 10 percent of pediatric patients with acute myelogenous leukemia have TdT-positive cells, and non-Hodgkin's-lymphoma lymphocytes can also be TdT-positive. In addition, bone marrow regeneration, idiopathic thrombocytopenia purpura, and neuroblastoma may cause TdT-positive marrow.[20]

The purpose of TdT assay is to identify immature lymphocytes (blasts) and tumor cells of lymphatic origin in adults; such an assay may also be useful in detecting ALL relapse.

Other Tests for Lymphoproliferative Disorders

Leukocyte Alkaline Phosphatase Stain Leukocyte alkaline phosphatase (LAP), an enzyme found in 40

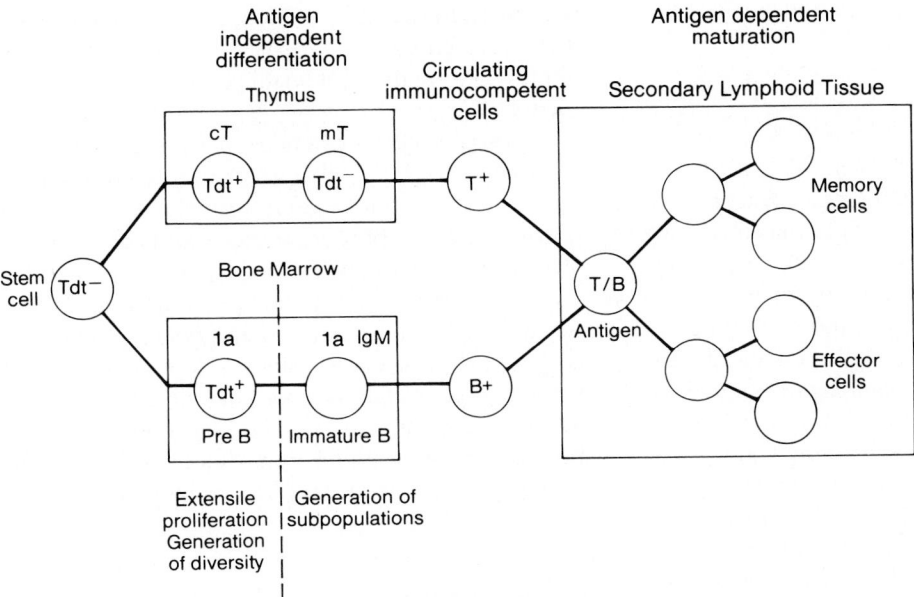

Figure 45-3 Differentiation and maturation of human B and T cells. Tdt = terminal deoxynucleotidyl transferase; cT = cortical T cell surface antigen; mT = mature T cell surface antigen. The early replicating cells in the thymus and bone marrow are in the majority. Thymocytes are educated to recognize self-MHC haplotype. Tolerance to self-antigens is induced in the immature B and T cells within the primary lymphoid organs. Ia+ and pre-B cell precursors are Tdt-positive; the Tdt enzyme may be involved as one of the mechanisms controlling the generation of diversity. (*Adapted from Riott.*[25])

to 100 percent of all normal neutrophils, is tested by specific staining. LAP is decreased in chronic myelogenous leukemia and increased by stress, infections, chronic inflammatory disease, and Hodgkin's and other hematologic disorders. Thus it is useful in differentiating chronic myelogenous leukemia from other disorders[7] (Table 45-14).

Nitroblue Tetrazolium Reduction Test Normal neutrophil metabolism converts nitroblue tetrazolium (NBT; a colorless dye) to a blue dye (lysosomol enzyme), which is readily observable and measurable. In chronic granulomatous disease, neutrophil metabolism is abnormal and there is a decrease or absence of the NBT reaction. Neutrophilic func-

Table 45-14 Neutrophil Function Test Values

Normal	Decreased	Increased
	LAP Test	
40–100% neutrophils; positive for alkaline phosphatase	Chronic myelogenous leukemia, aplastic anemia, infectious mononucleosis	Hodgkin's disease, polycythemia vera, leukemoid reaction
	NBT Test	
10% positive NBT in bacterial-disease—free persons	Chronic granulomatous disease: loss of bactericidal ability of neutrophils, negative NBT	Bacterial diseases: 45% positive neutrophils

tional phagocytic and bactericidal ability is evaluated by the NBT test[6] (Table 45-14).

Urine Assay

Bence Jones Protein

Bence Jones proteins are light-chain fractions of antibodies from a single clone of plasma cells. They are usually demonstrated in the urine of persons with gammopathies such as multiple myeloma.

There are various types of monoclonal gammopathies; Bence Jones, or L (light)-chain, disease is only one. These abnormal gammaglobulins result from uncontrolled proliferation of a single clone of antibody-producing cell, with consequent elevation in the serum levels of that particular type of antibody or, in the case of Bence Jones protein, of that particular portion of antibody. All the classes of immunoglobulin as well as light chains are known to be elevated in multiple myeloma, while in Waldenström's macroglobulinemia only the IgM is found in excessive levels. These monoclonal gammopathies are associated with a gamma or beta spike in the electrophoretic pattern. Immunoelectrophoresis is performed to determine the specific class of immunoglobulin or chain present in excess.[6-8]

Bence Jones protein is present in the urine of about half the patients with multiple myeloma. Of these, approximately 30 percent have other monoclonal gammopathies as well. Bence Jones kappa (κ) or lambda (λ) chains are present in the serum as well as the urine. Only 10 to 20 percent of myeloma patients exhibit Bence Jones or light-chain disease alone, and in those, the only detectable paraproteins are found in the urine.

Bence Jones proteins can be detected in several ways. The classic method is to heat the urine to the boiling point; if it contains Bence Jones proteins, there will be turbidity at 40 to 60°C, clearing at the boiling point, and a recurrence of turbidity when the urine cools again to between 40 and 60°C (Bradshaw's test).[6] Another method of detecting these abnormal L chains is urine immunoelectrophoresis. This technique is more often used, since it picks up as many as one-third of the cases missed by the heating method. An abnormal peak at the alpha 2 globulin area indicates excess Bence Jones proteins. Serum electrophoresis is less successful in detecting Bence Jones proteins, since they are such small molecules that they are rapidly filtered out by the glomeruli or are rapidly metabolized.[6-8]

The detection of Bence Jones proteins is useful for diagnosing and characterizing multiple myeloma. Generally, it is used to make a conclusive diagnosis when there are other symptoms of myeloma such as anemia and bone pain.

The Bence Jones protein test can give a false-negative result in a urine which is not freshly voided or properly preserved. Since a less concentrated urine may give a false-negative result, it is important to use a first morning voided specimen. It should be taken to the laboratory as soon as possible to prevent deterioration and loss of light chains.[6-8]

Other Procedures

Biopsy

Bone Marrow Biopsy

In adult human bones there are two types of marrow, yellow and red. Yellow bone marrow is composed mostly of fat, while red bone marrow is composed of hematopoietic cells both differentiated and undifferentiated and serves as the progenitor of the elements of the blood formed in maturity. The fetus and infant have red bone marrow in all medullary canals and spaces throughout the skeletal system. As the bones develop the bone marrow becomes more yellow and less red, so that by adulthood, red bone marrow is found only in the spongy areas of long bones and the medullary spaces of short irregular and flat bones.[21]

Bone and bone marrow studies are often indicated in hematologic as well as in immunologic disease, as the two share many components and functions. If adequate specimens are to be obtained, the areas in which samples of red bone marrow can be obtained must be known. The most common bone marrow assays are carried out by bone biopsy and bone marrow aspiration.[21]

Bone Biopsy   *Bone biopsy* is the excision of a small area of bone for histologic examination. This procedure is indicated in patients in whom a suspected abnormal area is revealed by palpation or radiologic studies. Such a biopsy makes it possible to diagnose the abnormality as well as to differentiate between malignant and benign conditons.[4,21]

Bone biopsy can be a local procedure (*drill biopsy*) or a surgical procedure (*open biopsy*). The drill biopsy utilizes a needle with a trocar; the trocar is removed and a core of bone is obtained. This is retrieved from the needle and placed in 10% formalin. In open biopsy, a larger piece of bone is removed and sent to the laboratory for immediate analysis to determine whether further surgery is indicated.[4,21]

Conditions diagnosed by bone biopsy are benign and malignant bone and cartilaginous tumors; tumors arising from bone marrow which spread into bone; vascular tumors; tumorlike lesions (cysts, dysplasia, etc); and metastatic disease (from other primary sites such as the lungs, breast, or prostate).[4,21]

Bone Marrow Aspiration

Bone marrow specimens must be obtained from red bone marrow; thus in the adult, special sites assure a good sample with minimal effort. Bone marrow aspiration is usually a local procedure, which uses a needle with trocar. If the fluid portion of the marrow alone is sufficient, an aspiration biopsy is obtained. If a core of marrow is needed, a needle biopsy is done. Occasionally, both are required.[4,21]

Bone marrow is hematopoietic in function, that is, it is the normal adult source of all formed elements of the blood (red cells, white cells, and platelets). Imbalance of these cells in the peripheral blood often indicates study of the bone marrow in order to accurately diagnose the condition.[4,21]

Anemias, lympho- and myeloproliferative disease, and thrombocytopenia are all confirmed by bone marrow studies. Staging of malignant disease and the monitoring of chemo- and radiotherapy are also possible from bone marrow studies and are indicated in some situations. Strict sterile procedures are required for bone or bone marrow aspiration and biopsy. Any invasive procedure places the patient at risk for infection, but when the immune system is imbalanced and the patient immunocompromised, such procedures can result in fatal infection. In a patient who has a primary immune deficiency, bone marrow invasion (or any invasive procedure) is contraindicated.[4]

Preferred sites for bone marrow aspiration are the sternum, posterior superior iliac spine, lumbar vertebra spinous process (third or fourth), and metaphysis (end) of the tibia. The sternum involves the greatest risk, because of its anatomic relation to many vital structures, but it is the most commonly preferred site because of its accessibility and the ease and assured success of the procedure. The tibia is best for infants (birth to 12 months); the vertebral spine is chosen when multiple aspirations are needed.[4]

A portion of the aspirated bone marrow is smeared on cover slips (usually by a laboratory technician), and the rest is placed in Zenkers' acetic acid fixative with proper identification of the patient and date. Specimens and requisition are immediately sent to the pathology laboratory. Care should be taken to avoid contamination of the aspiration site and bleeding. A patient who is immunocompromised should be observed frequently and carefully for signs of local and systemic infection. Immunocompromised patients may have serious infection with only mild symptoms, because of the lack of functional cells and/or amplifying systems.[4,21]

Liver Biopsy

Liver biopsy is a local or general surgical procedure performed to diagnose both primary and secondary hepatic disease. It is performed infrequently and only in cases where other noninvasive procedures have failed to give a confirmed diagnosis. Liver biopsy is helpful in the diagnosis of primary and metastatic liver disease.[21]

The Menghini needle allows the physician to limit the depth of penetration by setting the needle flange. The preferred site is the right eighth intercostal space just superior to the ninth rib between the anterior and posterior axillary lines. Anatomically, the intercostal nerve and vessels are located below each rib; therefore, placing the needle just above the rib will avoid damage or injury to these structures. Since the needle must penetrate the skin and superfical fascia before reaching the liver, it is necessary to clear it by injecting 2 mL of sterile normal saline. Once this is done, the liver can be penetrated to obtain the biopsy. The patient must lie very still and is asked to avoid taking a breath at the exact moment of liver penetration and removal of the biopsy sample.[21]

The specimen is placed in 10% formalin and sent to the laboratory immediately. Patients with liver disease often have a bleeding tendency and thus should have liver biopsy only after bleeding and clotting tests have been made. After biopsy in these patients, the nurse should check for signs of shock four times per hour at first, then twice an hour for the next 24 h.[4,21]

Because the needle often passes through the recesses of the pleural cavity, the patient should be observed for possible pneumothorax. Pain is normal and is controlled with mild analgesics. Infection is always a threat, and the nurse should be alert for signs of bile peritonitis.[21]

Lymph Node Biopsy

A biopsy of a lymph node may be obtained by needle or by surgical excision; the latter is the more frequent and the preferred method. Lymph node biopsy is used when nodes are palpable in order to discern the cause of enlargement. Infections, inflammation, and lymphoproliferative disease all have associated enlarged lymph nodes. The nodes are usually tender to palpation when infection is the cause and not tender in lymphoproliferative disease.[4,21] Lymph node biopsy is also important in distinguishing benign from malignant tumors, in the staging of lymphoproliferative disease, and as evidence of metastatic spread to draining nodes from a primary neoplastic site. In addition, it has prognostic value.[21]

In certain viral infections (e.g., cat-scratch fever) and other abscess-forming infections, lymph node excision and biopsies are contraindicated, as they often complicate the disease. Histologic study of lymph nodes may confirm T cell deficiency and B cell deficiency as well as other immunodeficiency states by demonstrating the depletion of T and B cell histologic zones within the node.

Lymphangiography

Radiographic examination of the lymphatic system is called *lymphangiography*. A blue, oil-based contrast medium is injected intradermally into the finger web or toe web. The lipid will drain into the open lymphatic capillaries and reach the lymph vessels in about half an hour. The vessels are visibly outlined by the blue medium. At this point a local incision is made and a lymphatic vessel cannulated for pump infusion of the contrast medium.[4,22,23]

The blue contrast medium remains in the nodes for up to 6 months, and monitoring of the progression of the disease is possible by subsequent x-rays. It usually takes about 1 to 2 h to obtain a lymphangiogram. This procedure is indicated in patients with excessively swollen extremities, lymphoma, or metastatic disease.[4]

Since cannulation of lymph vessels is extremely difficult, the patient is usually fluoroscopically observed until the dye reaches the thoracic duct. For the lower extremity, which is more common, infusion is then stopped, the cannula is removed, and the incision is sutured and surgically attended. X-rays are then taken and repeated in 3 to 4 h.[4,21–23]

Patients hypersensitive to iodine or those with severe renal, hepatic, cardiac, or pulmonary disease should not undergo lymphangiography. Pulmonary lipid embolization, edema (particularly of the extremities), pain, and infections are frequent complications of this procedure, and patients who have undergone it should be monitored for these subsequent complications.[4,22,23]

Blockage of the lymph channels and lack of opacification of nodes indicate metastatic involvement of the lymph nodes. The presence of large foamy and nonhomogeneous nodes usually indicates lymphoma. Lymphangiography also allows for staging of lymphoma as to the number of nodes involved and the area, as well as the regional expansion of the disease (i.e., above or below the diaphragm or both).[4,22,23]

Radionuclide Imaging

Radiopharmaceuticals

The radiopharmaceuticals used in radionuclide imaging procedures are nontoxic radioactive chemical agents complexed to a metabolic substance. Their usefulness depends on the ability of the radioactive complex to be rapidly and traceably incorporated into a particular type of cell or organ structure (Table 45-15). Radiopharmaceuticals fall into one of the following six groups:[22,23]

Table 45-15 Uptake Patterns of Radiopharmaceuticals

Organ	Radionuclides Most Commonly Utilized	Uptake Pattern
Bone	^{99m}Tc methylene diphosphonate (MDP medionate) or ^{99m}Tc hydroxydiphosphonate (HDP-oxidronate)	Localizes in areas of increased osteogenesis
Liver/spleen/bone marrow	^{99m}Tc sulfur colloid	Phagocytosed by fixed reticular cells (shows structure)
Liver	^{131}I rose bengal or ^{99m}Tc-labeled 1-iminodiacetic acid (IDA)	Removed by hepatocytes and excreted in GI tract (shows function)
Tumor/abscess or inflammation	^{67}Ga citrate	Mechanism unknown but concentrates in the lesions; bound to transferrin and in tumors is concentrated in lysosome-like structures; also localizes in lactoferrin found in neutrophils

Source: Modified from Meschan and Ott.[23]

1. Those which give an image of the organ and its structure
2. Those which allow organ flow studies showing the rate of perfusion and distribution within an organ
3. Those which measure how well an organ performs its function
4. Those which make possible the localization of an organ or of material such as placenta or an effusion
5. Those which accumulate abnormally in tissues such as tumors or inflammatory exudate
6. Those which make possible the determination, from a sample of blood, urine, or feces, of the dilution (volume), clearance, absorption, or rate of metabolism of the agent

The main problems with using in vivo radioisotopes for imaging have been the length of their radioactive decay time, the invasiveness of the procedures, and the general threat they pose when not handled carefully and appropriately. Their major advantages are their specific imaging and their ability to show physiologic (functional) as well as morphologic defects. Additionally, they are more accurate diagnostically and more rapid than ordinary x-rays.[22,23]

Critically ill patients who are actually or potentially immunocompromised may require organ imaging for morphologic or for functional studies. Imaging procedures may be directed to any organ, but for the immunocompromised patient they most commonly involve bone, bone marrow, liver, spleen, and/or lymphatic organs.

Types of Radionuclide Scan

Tumor and Inflammation Imaging Procedures
Tumor scanning is performed to differentiate malignant from benign lesions and to determine the extent of invasion of known malignant tumors for the purposes of therapy and follow-up.

Gallium-67 citrate is a screening medium often used in multiclinical diagnosis because of its ability to localize in pyogenic abscesses and acute pyogenic inflammatory regions. Its use is indicated as a means of identifying infections and regions of primary or metastatic disease; for staging Hodgkin's disease and lymphomas; to differentiate a benign from a malignant tumor; and for following a patient's response to therapy (radiation and/or chemotherapy). Gallium is bound to the protein transferrin. It finds its way into the cells and concentrates in lysosomes of the cytoplasm. In infection, gallium binds to lactoferrin found in neutrophils, which logically suggests that tumor cells which concentrate gallium must have a high level of lactoferrin.[22,23]

Liver Scan Liver scanning is performed to demonstrate gross anatomic changes of the liver or to evaluate biliary patency. It may be done by computed tomography (CT), ultrasound, or nuclear colloid radiopharmaceutical imaging with nuclear colloids such as ^{131}I rose bengal, ^{99m}Tc sulfur colloids, or ^{99m}Tc-labeled iminodiacetic acid (IDA). ^{131}I rose bengal and IDA are taken up by the polygonal hepatic cells and excreted into the gastrointestinal tract. Colloids, when given intravenously, are distributed macroscopically in a uniform manner within the liver by being phagocytosed by the Kupffer cells which line the sinusoids and make up approximately 40 percent of the liver. ^{99m}Tc sulfur colloid is taken up not only by the liver but also by the spleen and bone marrow, especially when hepatic blood flow is decreased.[22,23]

IDA is used to aid in the differential diagnosis of jaundice; ^{99m}Tc colloids reveal displacement, destruction, or blood flow characteristics of the sinusoids and liver structure. Computed tomography reveals the different tissue densities of liver structures, while ultrasonography reveals changes in the architecture of the liver stroma.

Liver nuclear images cannot give a tissue diagnosis, but CT and ultrasonography can characterize a lesion. In order to cut costs and increase efficiency, nuclear imaging is used for intitial screening and is followed by ultrasonography to confirm and characterize. The more expensive computed tomography is used only when other scans are inconclusive.[22,23]

Bone Scan   Bone-seeking radionuclides include ^{99m}Tc-labeled phosphate compounds, ^{18}F, ^{85m}Sr, and ^{87m}Sr. All accumulate in bone lesions, allowing visualization via blood flow long before lytic destruction occurs. Bone-seeking nuclides are particularly helpful in imaging skeletal structure in bone metastasis and other bony lesions, since other radiographs become positive only after 30 to 50 percent decalcification has occurred.[22,23]

Bone scans are used for bone pain of undetermined origin, for metastatic cancer, for cancer staging, and for following the effects of therapy. The imaging may be total or regional, depending on the situation.

Bone Marrow Scan   Bone marrow scan is used to demonstrate the anatomy and physiology of the bone marrow. Since iron is the core of the hemoglobin molecule, radioactive iron is employed, which incorporates into the areas of red bone marrow. Hematopoiesis generally can be estimated from the quantity of the labeling.

Radiocolloids may also be used to demonstrate the structure and distribution of bone marrow. Bone marrow–seeking colloids are phagocytosed and visualized in the marrow reticular cells. Bone marrow scans are useful in demonstrating metastatic sites and in the study of anemia and polycythemia.[22,23]

Magnetic Resonance Imaging

Magnetic resonance imaging (MRI) detects abnormalities by directing magnetic and radio waves at body tissue to determine the response. MRI relies on the natural magnetic properties of atoms in the body and uses superconducting or resistance magnets to create electromagnetic echoes, which are relayed to a computer.[23]

When a body or organ is placed in a strong magnetic field and radio waves are passed through the field, there is a movement of hydrogen nuclei, at particular frequencies of that field. This movement is recorded by a detector and relayed to a computer, which visualizes it and makes a cross-sectional picture of the organ or body which resembles CT imaging but has better quality.[23]

The only disadvantage of MRI is that persons with claustrophobic and similar tendencies cannot be subjected to this type of imaging. Additionally, MRI is noisy and tends to frighten even normal persons. The magnetic field will displace small clips and sutures of metal and convert cardiac pacemakers from fixed to demand mode; this excludes patients with pacemakers from MRI testing. The disadvantages, except for the phobia, can be controlled by careful screening and patient teaching.

The test requires 1 to 2 h, depending on the part to be visualized. The advantages are that MRI is a noninvasive procedure, uses no x-rays, and gives a three-dimensional visualization of the human anatomy as well as functional information. It images soft tissue in great anatomic detail, which may distinguish between healthy and pathologic tissues.[21,23]

Cytogenetic Techniques

Since the discovery of the Philadelphia chromosome (Ph^1) in 1960 and its association with chronic myelogenous leukemia (CML), cytogenetics has

Table 45-16 Cytogenetic Abnormalities in Lymphomas

Type of Lymphoma (Non-Hodgkin's)	Chromosomal Abnormality
Burkitt's (chromosome 8)	t(8;14) (80% of patients); t(2;8) or t(8;22) (20% of patients)
Small-cell lymphoblastic	t(8;14)
Small-cell lymphocytic	+12 addition
Diffuse large-cell lymphocytic	t(11;14)
Follicular (all types)	t(14;18)

Source: Modified from Whang-Peng and Knutsen.[24]

gained importance in the diagnosis and differentiation of malignant disease. Chromosome banding, especially high-resolution chromosome banding, has shown that 90 percent of all patients with neoplasms have chromosome abnormalities (some of which are specific) and thus has given new meaning to the study of leukemias and other malignant diseases by the use of cytogenetic techniques.[24]

The diagnosis of CML is not verifiable until the Ph[1] chromosome is identified and the disease subclassified. The abnormality has a unicellular origin, i.e., it is derived from a stem cell common to the myeloid series. Approximately 85 percent of patients with typical CML syndrome have the Ph[1] chromosome.[24]

Trisomy 12 is the most frequent chromosome abnormality in CML. Abnormalities of chromosome 8 are the most commonly seen in acute nonlymphatic leukemia (ANLL), followed by monosomy 7 and abnormalities of chromosomes 9, 21, X, Y, and 17. Chromosome studies have made possible subclassification of ANLL, earlier diagnosis and treatment, and better recovery.[24]

In acute lymphatic leukemia, the bone marrow often has coexistent cells which have and cells which do not have the Philadelphia chromosome; the Ph[1]-positive cells disappear from the bone marrow during remission. This is not the case in CML, which presents many translocations, e.g., t(4;11), t(8;14), and t(1;19).[24]

Treatment can be life-saving when diagnosis is accurate and swift, and this can often be achieved with the use of cytogenetic studies. The preleukemic state can also be detected by chromosomal studies of bone marrow and peripheral blood; the abnormalities parallel those of ANLL and include monosomy 5 and 7 (most common deletions), trisomy 8, and Ph[1] chromosome. Diagnosis of the preleukemic state can improve patients' chances for survival. Chromosomal studies are also useful in establishing an accurate diagnosis in lymphoma[24] (Table 45-16).

In summary, cytogenetic studies can be lifesaving, as they often permit precise subclassification of hematologic malignant diseases, earlier treatment, and a better prognosis.

References

1. Castro, J. E. (1973). *Immunology for surgeons.* Baltimore: University Park Press.
2. Sites, D. P., et al. (Eds.). (1985). *Basic and clinical immunology* (5th ed.). Los Altos, CA: Lange.
3. Thiers, B. H. (1986). Dermatologic manifestations of internal cancer. *CA-A Cancer Journal for Clinicians, 36,* 3.
4. Nurse's Clinical Library. (1985). *Immune disorders.* Nursing 85 Books. Springhouse, PA: Springhouse.
5. Bellanti, J. A. (1985). *Immunology III.* Philadelphia: Saunders.
6. Wheat, B., & Fidler, R. (1986). *Diagnostics* (2d ed.). Nurses Reference Library. Springhouse, PA: Springhouse.
7. Byrne, J. C., et al. (1986). *Laboratory tests: Implications for nurses and allied health professionals* (2d ed.). Reading, MA: Addison-Wesley.
8. Widmann, F. K. (1983). *Clinical interpretation of laboratory tests* (9th ed.). Philadelphia: Davis.
9. Lewandowski, A. J. (1986). Immunopathogensis of AIDS. *Journal of Medical Technology, 3* (3), 145–147.
10. Siegal, F. P. (1984, No. 10, September). AIDS update. *Clinical Immunology Today.* New York: World Health Communications.
11. Fahey, John L., et al. (1985, No. 13, March). Assessment of cellular immune parameters in disease. *Clinical*

Immunology Today. (pp. 3–9). New York: World Health Communications.

12. Kimberly, R. P. (1985, No. 14, May). Immune complex diseases. *Clinical Immunology Today* (pp. 8, 9, 10). New York: World Health Communications.

13. Haynes, B. F., & Eisenbarth, G. S. (1983). *Monoclonal antibodies.* New York: Academic Press.

14. Bishop, C. (1984). Immunoassays in Hematology: Cell surface antigens. *Journal of Medical Technology, 1,* 1.

15. Karr, C. K. (1986). Autoimmunity now and then. *Journal of Medical Technology, 3* (5), 276–278.

16. Aisenberg, A. C. (1981). Current concepts in immunology: Cell surface markers in lymphoproliferative disease. *New England Journal of Medicine, 304* (6), 331–335.

17. Aisenberg, A. C., et al. (1983). Monoclonal studies in non-Hodgkins' lymphoma. *Blood, 61* (3), 469–475.

18. Sallan, S. E., et al. (1980). Prognostic implications in childhood acute lymphoblastic leukemia: Cell surface antigens. *Blood, 55* (3), 395–401.

19. Kohler, G., & Milstein, C. (1975). Continuous cultures of fused cells secreting antibody of predefined specificity. *Nature, 256,* 495.

20. Bollum, F. J. (1979). Terminal deoxynucleotidyl transferase as a hematopoietic cell marker. *Blood, 54* (6), 1203–1214.

21. Nurses' Clinical Library. (1985). *Neoplastic Disorders.* Nursing 85 Books. Springhouse, PA: Springhouse.

22. Sodee, B. D., & Early, P. S. (1981). *Mosby's manual of nuclear medicine procedures* (3d ed.). St. Louis, MO: Mosby.

23. Meschan, I., & Ott, D. J. (1984). *Introduction to diagnostic imaging.* Philadelphia: Saunders.

24. Whang-Peng, J., & Knutsen, T. (1986). Cytogenetics: Methods and findings in hematologic disease. *Laboratory Management, 24* (4), 19–26.

25. Riott, I. M. (1982). *Essential immunology* (5th ed.). Oxford, England: Blackwell Scientific Publications.

46 Hypersensitivity and Anaphylaxis

Sister Mary
Rebecca Fidler
Mary Frances
Keen

Types of Immunopathologic Reaction

The immune response is a mechanism normally protecting the human against nonself. As discussed in Chap. 44, the response is intricately controlled by genetic makeup, but sometimes factors controlling the response are missing, and this disrupts the balance and results in potential or actual immune disease. This chapter discusses the hyperactive aspect of this loss of homeostasis.

The efferent limb of the immune response presents itself as either cell- or antibody-mediated. So, too, immunopathologic states may be conveniently divided into cell-mediated and humoral pathologic states. Imbalance of the homeostatic mechanisms modulating immune responses results in hypo- or hyperimmune states (Fig. 46-1).

Hyperimmune states are recognized by the presence of allergies and other immunologic injury. Conversely, hypoimmune persons demonstrate anergy, increased susceptibility to common infections, increased severity and difficulty in controlling infections, and a lack of response to both new and recall antigens.

When the immune response is exaggerated beyond a purely protective effect or is directed inappropriately toward a material that is not potentially harmful, the subject is said to be *hypersensitive*. *Allergy* is defined as an altered state of immune reactivity. The terms *hypersensitivity* and *allergy* are now used interchangeably by most health workers.

A classification of hyperimmune pathologic mechanisms on the basis of humoral and cell types of immunity was proposed by Coombs and Gell.[1] Immune injuries of types I, II, and III are antibody-mediated; type IV injury is mediated by sensitized lymphocytes and their products in the absence of antibodies or complement. This classification is for convenience and understanding; clinical manifes-

tations of loss in immune regulation may express one or more types of reaction. Table 46-1 compares these four immunopathologic types. They differ significantly in time sequence, location, antibody type, and mediators. Classifications listing other types have been proposed but are not included in this discussion.[1,2,3]

Type I: Anaphylactic Reaction

Type I reactions occur immediately after exposure as a result of interactions between mast cells, IgE antibody, and a specific antigen. This interaction results in the release of mast cell granules. IgE is nonspecifically fixed to the surface of mast cells via Fc receptors, leaving the variable portion for specific antigen attachment. When the specific allergen attaches to the IgE, the mast cell degranulates and releases histamine and leukotrienes, progenitors of slow-reacting substance of anaphylaxis (SRS-A), and other vasoactive products which mediate a hyperimmune type of reaction. IgE circulates in the body fluids, but it is also found fixed to mast cells in the subcutaneous tissues of the body. This is usually a local protective response to environmental antigens, but some persons seem to have certain HLA combinations or Ir genes which predispose them to hyperimmune sensitivity and result in overt expression of the anaphylactic-type reaction. Recently it has been suggested but not confirmed that since during early development environmental antigens that do not bind to mast cells induce IgA synthesis, perhaps persons hypersensitive to these antigens have a primary IgA deficiency state and produce IgE-mediated responses to them as an adaptive response.[2,3]

Mast cells are found surrounding small veins in the submucosal and subcutaneous areas of the body which most frequently encounter environ-

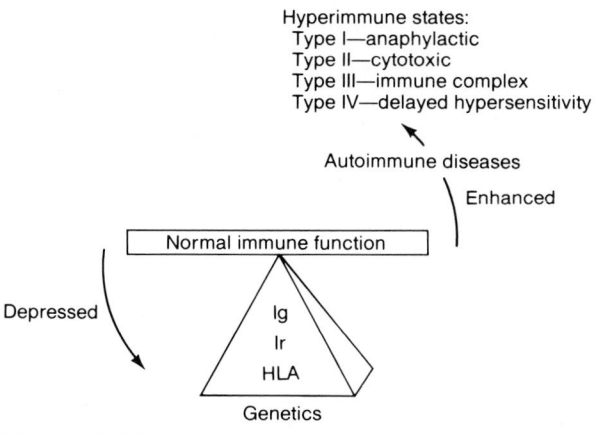

Figure 46-1 Concept of immunopathology.

mental antigens; they are known as *basophils* when circulating in the blood. Their morphology is easily discernible because of the large basophilic-staining granules within the cytoplasm. These granules contain histamine, serotonin, and other vasoactive amines capable of producing anaphylactic-type responses.[2,3]

Cell membranes are actively involved in intercellular communication in order to maintain physiologic homeostasis within the total individual. This is especially evident in the mechanisms of anaphylaxis. Sometimes the phospholipids stored in cell membranes are termed *local hormones* because of their localized effect as opposed to a systemic effect.

The *eicosanoids* are a family of 20-carbon vasoactive substances derived from arachidonic acid, which is itself synthesized from the essential fatty acid linoleic acid. Animal tissues cannot produce linoleic acid, hence it must be ingested from a vegetable source in the diet. Linoleic acid is converted to arachidonic acid by a series of metabolic reactions, and the arachidonic acid is then stored in the phospholipids of the cell membrane until needed.[4]

Upon activation, arachidonic acid is released from storage by the enzyme phospholipase A_2. Once released, the arachidonic acid may be converted into a variety of bioactive products, with the ultimate product determined mainly by the type of cell involved. These substances are produced by one of two major pathways, the cyclooxygenase and the lipoxygenase[4] (Fig. 46-2).

In the first pathway, the enzyme cyclooxygenase inserts several oxygen atoms to produce a key intermediate which can be converted into any of a number of vasoactive compounds known as the *prostaglandins* (so named because they were first identified in prostate gland secretions). On the basis of differences in structure and biologic activity, the prostaglandins (PG) fall into four major categories. The E and F series of prostaglandins (PGE and PGF) cause increased vasodilatation and permeability. They also have pronounced, and opposite, effects on smooth muscle, with PGE causing relaxation while PGF causes contraction. A third prostaglandin class (PGAs, also called *thromboxane*) is synthesized predominantly in platelets and causes vasoconstriction and platelet aggregation upon release. The fourth prostaglandin class, the prostacyclins (PGI), are produced by blood vessel walls and oppose the action of thromboxanes by inhibiting platelet aggregation. Thus the prostaglandins are important mediators of homeostasis, since thromboxane release is crucial for clot formation

Table **46-1** Comparison of Four Hypersensitivity Reactions

Type of reaction	Location	Time between antigen exposure and reaction	Observable signs	Mechanism of or effect of injury	Antibody type involved	Complement involved	Other factors
Type I Anaphylactic (systemic)	Vascular system, mucous membranes Smooth muscle	5–15 min	Respiratory distress and obstruction, cardiovascular shock	Mast cell release of histamine, SRS-A, and other pharmacologic agents	IgE		Strong familial predisposition
Atopic (chronic)	Skin, mucous membranes	5–15 min	Skin eruptions, bronchospasm, airway obstruction, abdominal pain, nausea, diarrhea, edema	Same	IgE	None	May be related to IgA deficiency
Type II Cytotoxic	Any tissue, but usually vascular system or kidney	Minutes	Deficiency of target cell type, e.g., anemia, thrombocytopenia, leukopenia, and vascular purpura	Lysis of target cells due to haptens being adsorbed on native cells	IgG or IgM	C1–C9 (C fixing)	Associated with autoimmune disease; K cell antibody-dependent cytotoxicity may be involved

Type	Location/Tissue	Time	Associated diseases	Mechanism	Antibody	Complement	Comments
Type III Complex-mediated	Systemic type: vascular system. Local type (Arthus): extravascular, e.g., skin, mucous membrane, joint	Minutes; 2–5 h	Glomerulonephritis, arthritis, polyarteritis nodosa	Anaphylatoxin and neutrophil release of necrotizing lysosomal enzymes which produce local ischemic necrosis at location of antigen-antibody and complement complex	IgG	C3, C5, C567, C8, C9: anaphylatoxins	Associated with autoimmune disease
Type IV Delayed	Any tissue	Maximum 24–48 h delayed	Contact dermatitis, poison ivy, tuberculin reaction, graft rejection, allergic reactions to infection, graft-versus host disease	Lymphokine release and subsequent lymphocyte-mediated cytolysis; cell-mediated via lymphocytes and macrophages	None	None	Associated with autoimmune disease; K cell cytotoxicity may be involved

Source: Adapted from R. A. Coombs and P. G. H. Gell, in Gell, Coombs, and Lackman.[1]

Figure 46-2   Arachidonic acid pathways in anaphylaxis. *(Adapted from Martin, Mayes, and Rodwell.[4])*

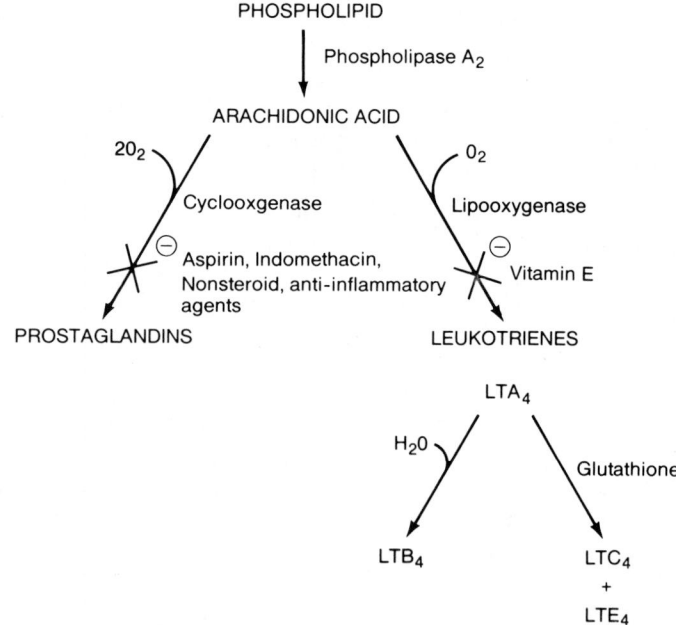

following injury, while the prostacyclins allow eventual dissolution of the clot.[4]

Leukocytes synthesize from arachidonic acid a different class of pharmacologically active compounds, the leukotrienes (LT). The leukotrienes are made from arachidonic acid by the lipoxygenase pathway, which proceeds through the key intermediate leukotriene A_4 (LTA_4). The enzyme-catalyzed addition of a water molecule to LTA_4 yields LTB_4, which has a potent effect on neutrophil adhesion to postcapillary venules. Enzyme-mediated reaction of LTA_4 with glutathione (the guardian of the cellular oxidation-reduction balance) yields the leukotrienes LTC_4 and LTE_4; all three of these leukotrienes increase vascular permeability. A mixture of these three leukotrienes (also known as *SRS-A,* or *slow-reacting substance of anaphylaxis*) results in an anaphylactic reaction, since it is a more potent constrictor of the bronchial airway musculature than histamine.[4]

Various sorts of drugs may inhibit key enzymes in these pathways to halt the formation of these pharmacologically active compounds. Steroids are believed to interfere with the phospholipase A_2–catalyzed release of arachidonic acid, hence stopping the production of all its bioactive derivatives. Aspirin, indomethacin, and other nonsteroid anti-inflammatory agents inhibit the cyclooxygenase

enzyme, thus halting the production of the prostaglandins, prostacyclins, and thromboxanes. These agents decrease the inflammation caused by the PG-induced increase in vascular permeability but may result in increased bleeding time, since thromboxane-mediated vasoconstriction and platelet aggregation are also inhibited.[4]

The type of anaphylaxis expressed clinically depends on the route of antigen access, the target organ, and the person's genetic makeup. *Systemic anaphylaxis* usually occurs when the antigen dose is large and given rapidly by intravenous, intramuscular, or subcutaneous injection. It is a generalized reaction causing contraction of smooth muscle, increased vascular permeability, hypotension, incoagulability of blood, and decreased heart rate and complement levels. Hypersensitive persons may develop circulatory shock and respiratory difficulties within minutes after intravenous injection of drugs or insect venom. In extremely sensitive persons, even small amounts of antigen on the skin or in the air may cause severe systemic anaphylaxis. To summarize, systemic anaphylaxis involves the entire body, may lead to cardiovascular shock, and may be rapidly fatal.

Cutaneous anaphylaxis has the same mechanism as systemic anaphylaxis but is a localized reaction due to skin-fixing IgE and is manifested in the skin or mucous membranes. The symptoms include many lesions occurring in the skin, gastrointestinal tract, or nasal mucosa, reaching a maximum within 15 to 20 min after exposure to the antigen.[2,3,5]

In either type of anaphylaxis, mast cells release their mediators through lytic or nonlytic means. The nonlytic type involves IgE, antigen, and mast cells as previously described, with subsequent degranulation. Lytic reactions are mediated by IgG or IgM, which combine on the surface of mast cells along with complement. Complement involvement results in membrane lesions and finally cell lysis, with the release of mast cell granules.

An association of certain HLA-type persons with allergic sensitivity, elevated titer of IgE, and decreased suppressor T cells has been found. The precise role of genetics in allergy, however, is still to be explained.

Atopic allergy refers to human allergies to natural environmental antigens. The mechanism is essentially the same as that in systemic and cutaneous anaphylaxis. Sometimes type I reactions are categorized under the general heading of atopy. Atopic allergies include hay fever, allergic rhinitis, asthma, hives, serous otitis media, nasal polyps, dermatitis, eczema, food allergies, and the like. Atopy is controlled by Ir genes, the degree of environmental exposure to potential allergens, and autonomic neural and physiologic mechanisms of a nonimmune nature.[2,3,5]

A fact which complicates the diagnosis of type I reactions is that any stimulus which releases histamine will mimic this type of immune injury. This nonimmune release of histamine is called an *anaphylactoid reaction*. Morphine, polymyxin B, iodinated contrast materials, and curare, among others substances, are examples of nonimmune agents which release histamine from mast cells and produce anaphylactoid reactions. In urticaria pigmentosa, which presents a large mast cell population, these drugs can be fatal because of massive histamine release. Complement fragments (*anaphylatoxin*) are also able to produce these effects when complement is activated by either the classic or the nonimmune phenomenon (alternate pathway). Clinically, however, it is difficult to distinguish anaphylaxis from anaphylactoid-type reactions.

Type II: Cytotoxic Reaction

Cytotoxic hypersensitivity involves the combination of the Fab portion of antibody with antigenic receptors on membranes of cells. Haptens, combined with or adsorbed on the surface of native cells with which the antibody combines, give the same net effect. Complement is usually but not always required for cytotoxic reactions. Cell lysis occurs if a cell is the antigen and IgG the antibody; the cell is removed by phagocytosis and a deficiency of the cell type results. Cytotoxic reactions occur most frequently in the vascular system; thus the target cells for type II hypersensitivity are usually red blood cells (anemia), white blood cells (leukopenia), platelets (thrombocytopenia), or endothelium (vascular purpura). Cytotoxic reactions may, however, involve any cell type in a specific tissue. The immunoglobulin involved in the vascular reaction may be either IgG or IgM; however, tissue cytotoxicity would require IgG because of its small size and its ability to cross membrane barriers.[2,3,5]

Tissue cytotoxicity may occur in almost any tissue, but the kidneys, because of their blood-filtering function, are quite vulnerable to type II as well as type III reactions. Many haptogenic drugs and substances are excreted via the kidney; this adds to the risk of their being adsorbed on the glomerular cell membrane. The glomerular basement membrane (GBM) seems particularly vulnerable. The introduction of heterologous antiserum can induce nephrotoxic serum nephritis. This type of injury is seen in renal transplant recipients who receive antilymphocyte serum (ALS). Goodpasture's syndrome and many other autoimmune diseases such as scleroderma, systemic lupus erythematous (SLE), and polyarteritis nodosa all exhibit some cytotoxic phenomena. The presence of antiglomerular basement membrane antibody (GBA) is diagnostic of renal-type cytotoxic injury.[2,3,5]

Cytotoxic injury can affect transplanted kidneys in patients with GBA already present in their serum. Potential transplant recipients should be evaluated for the presence of GBA before transplantation is carried out. In Goodpasture's syndrome the GBAs are able to attack not only glomeruli but lung basement membranes, with subsequent life-threatening pulmonary hemorrhage. Lung and kidney basement membranes seem to share like or similar antigens.[2,3,5]

To summarize, cytotoxic injury usually occurs in the vascular system, causing a lysis of specific target cells because of the combination of IgG or IgM with antigenic determinants or haptens adsorbed on the surface of these cells. Complement is fixed to the IgM complex and the target cells are selectively destroyed, producing a cell deficiency. IgG-mediated toxic reactions cause them to be phagocytosed by macrophages and subsequently degraded, thus producing a deficiency. Examples of cytotoxic injury include erythroblastosis fetalis, transfusion incompatibility reactions, hemolytic anemia, thrombocytopenia, leukopenia, drug reactions, and certain autoimmune disorders.

Type III: Complex-Mediated Reaction

Immunologic injury in immune complex disease is secondary to precipitation and localization of antigen-antibody complexes, which, when soluble antigen combines with specific antibody, form insoluble complexes localizing around small blood vessels. In the vascular system they tend to become trapped in blood vessel walls. The antigen-antibody complexes fix and activate the complement cascade. Activated complement subsequently releases phlogistic fragments C3a, C3b, C5a, C567, etc. (see Chap. 44 and Fig. 44-12), which chemotaxically attract neutrophils and mediate an inflammatory reaction. Release of lysosomal enzymes and arachidonic acid metabolites (leukotrienes) from accumulated neutrophils causes destruction of the elastic lamina of arteries, the basement membrane of the kidney, and the walls of small vessels. The usual lesion is an ischemic necrosis of the area in which the toxin is deposited. It is important to note that there is usually no specificity for the tissue in which the complex localizes; rather, it is shed from the areas of the original infection or pathologic condition, complexed with antibody in the circulating fluids, and physically deposited in an area as it circulates. The complex is trapped in these areas and elicits an inflammatory reaction in that particular location.

Immune complexes also appear to play a role in maintaining normal hemostasis. Circulating IgA/antigen complexes are found after ingestion of certain foods. They also help in regulating the cooperation between the humoral and cell-mediated reactions to the threat of nonself. Therefore it is important to distinguish helpful immune complexes from those causing immunopathologic conditions.[2,3,5]

Immune complexes precipitate in the kidney as random irregular deposits of inflammation and may be distinguished from the cytotoxic-type nephritis in which the presence of GBA reacts in a smooth linear pattern along the basement membranes.[2,3]

Ordinarily the reticuloendothelial system clears immune complexes from the body fluids. When this does not happen, toxic complex disease occurs. Lack of proper clearance may be due to excessive amounts of complex or to defects in immune phagocytosis.

Basically, two types of immune complex disease need consideration: an extravascular reaction (*Arthus reaction*) and an intravascular type (*serum sickness*).[2,3,5]

Arthus reaction was originally described as a result of placing antigen-antibody complexes in the skin, which caused edema, erythema, and hemorrhage within a few hours. The lesion was characterized by elapsed time (2 to 5 h), accumulation of neutrophils, and changes in vascular permeability, culminating in a localized ischemic thrombosis. Typical Arthus reactions, which are distributed in vessels throughout the human body, describe the pathogenesis of polyarteritis nodosa. Similar lesions in articulating joints of the body (arthritis) or in the kidney (glomerulonephritis) have been confirmed.[2,3,5]

Serum sickness is the formation of immune complexes in the bloodstream. It consists of vasculitis, arthritis, and glomerulonephritis and has the same mechanism as the Arthus reaction. It is usually associated with drug reactions and transplant recipients receiving ALS. Serum sickness may be caused by immune antibody production in response to either an exogenous or endogenous antigen, passive transfer of antibody or antigen, or the injection of preformed antigen-antibody complexes. Arthus reactions most often occur when there is an excess of antibody, whereas serum sickness is more often associated with an excess of antigen. Regardless of which is in excess, both form toxic complexes which produce necrotic injury.[2,3,5]

Many diseases in their latent form have been associated with immune complex formation. Infections (bacterial, viral, and parasitic), disseminated malignant disease, autoimmune disorders, drug reactions, and many other diseases have lesions caused by deposition of toxic complexes. Whether the complexes are primary or secondary to the condition is not always discernible. Most immune complex disorders, however, are associated with an immune response with an excess of either antibody or soluble antigens.

Several factors seem to influence the deposition of immune complexes. The size of the complex, which is determined by the relative antigen antibody ratio, is important. Acidity of antibody may affect the size and stability of the complex. Vasoactive amines, clearing of complexes by phagocytic cells, hemodynamic factors, blood flow, constrictions, and bifurcation all conceivably contribute to or influence the localization process.

In humans the antigen in the immune complex is usually not known, but the result of its presence is quite consistent. IgG and IgM are the usual types of antibody involved. Complement fixation with activation of the complement cascade and release of anaphylatoxins is essential. The pathologic lesions, however, are a result of neutrophil release of necrotizing lysosomal enzymes, which produce a local ischemic thrombosis. When this involves organs or organ systems, the damage may be life-threatening.

Type IV: Delayed Reaction

Types I, II, and III immune injuries are all *immediate humoral* reactions. Type IV, considered in this section, is *cell-mediated* and is called *delayed*.[2,3,5,6] Cell-mediated immune responses (CMI) are, as discussed earlier, carried out chiefly by sensitized T lymphocytes. These cells destroy antigen by direct or indirect means in the absence of either antibody or complement. Direct destruction requires actual physical contact of T lymphocytes with antigen and may be cytolytic or cytostable in nature. Indirect toxicity is produced via mediators (lymphokines and monokines) released from lymphocytes which induce local lesions characterized by infiltration with macrophages and lymphocytes and a chronic inflammatory exudate. In either type, direct or indirect, the response is maximal 48 to 72 h after antigen exposure.

Cell-mediated immunity involves cooperation between T lymphocytes and macrophages. Macrophages as well as T lymphocytes are capable of direct cytotoxicity. Macrophages contain numerous cytoplasmic lysosomes containing a variety of hydrolytic enzymes capable of degrading proteins, lipids, and nucleic acids. From a functional point of view, macrophages are of prime importance in all limbs of the immune response, are radioresistant, and are able to survive in an adverse environment. The macrophage is always a prime mover in host defense, yet its function is often overlooked because of the prominence of lymphocytes.[2,5,6]

The exact mechanism of delayed hypersensitivity is still uncertain. It is characterized by infiltration of mononuclear cells 24 to 72 h after antigen exposure at the antigen site. Most of the infiltrating cells are not sensitized by the antigen but are recruited into the area by a small number of sensitized T lymphocytes. These few sensitized cells release lymphokines, which influence cell migration, differentiation, cloning, and patterns of nonsensitized mononuclear cells. The most common example of delayed hypersensitivity is the tuberculin skin test. Intradermal injection of old tuberculin produces erythema, induration, and possible necrosis of the area in approximately 24 to 48 h in persons previously sensitized by the tuberculin antigen. This differs from the Arthus reaction in both time (2 to 5 h) and type of cellular infiltration (neutrophils). Neither antibody nor complement is required in type IV reactions.[2,3,5]

Contact Allergies

Many contact allergies are type IV delayed reactions. Poison ivy sensitivity is a classic example; however, many cosmetics, clothing, tapes, jewelry, soaps, and chemicals normally in contact with the skin may produce injury in the predisposed person. These haptogenic substances must be lipid-soluble in order to penetrate the skin and then must be chemically capable of combining with body proteins in order to be antigenic. When these situations occur in a previously exposed, sensitive person, contact dermatitis, or delayed hypersensitivity reaction, can occur. Delayed reactions must be differentiated from Arthus-type reactions—something readily accomplished since delayed hypersensitivity reaction requires 48 to 72 h to develop, and mononuclear cells instead of neutrophils infiltrate. Symptoms are redness, induration, vesiculation, and discomfort, all reaching a maximum in 48 to 72 h after exposure. Rupture of the vesicles may spread the antigen to new areas of skin and prolong the reaction.[2,3]

Transplants

Transplantations of foreign tissue have promoted an intense study of cellular immune responses. Genetic control of transplants via HLA antigens has been readily determined. If a person has a skin graft from a donor with genetic disparity, vascularization and acceptance of the graft will usually occur within 6 to 7 days. After about 1 week, signs of graft rejection begin to appear, with mononuclear cells infiltrating and the graft becoming blanched, white, and edematous (9 to 10 days). Gradually the graft turns brownish, indicating thrombosis of vessels, and finally it dries and/or sloughs off 11 to 14 days after grafting. This is called *primary*, or *first set, rejection.*[2,3]

If a second skin flap from the same donor is again grafted to the same recipient, the graft fails to become vascularized and a more rapid and vigorous rejection ensues. The *secondary*, or *second set, rejection* then occurs within 4 to 5 days. Extreme care should therefore be taken to avoid sensitizing the transplant recipient with any kind of donor cells. Antibodies may also affect transplanted tissue toward either acceptance or rejection.[2,3]

Sometimes antibodies produced against the graft will in fact enhance the "take" by blocking the actions of sensitized T cells. The mechanism of immunologic enhancement is not fully agreed upon but appears to be cytolytic or phagocytic removal of sensitized lymphocytes. Conversely, specific antibody directed against the graft, if injected into the graft site, will cause ischemic necrosis and rejection of the graft. Enhancement was first observed and described when attempts were made to destroy tumors by injection of antiserum prepared against tumor antigens; this therapy, disappointingly, resulted in enhanced tumor growth.[2,3]

Infection

Infection is related to delayed hypersensitivity. Although antibodies provide the main mechanism for defense against viral penetration, cell-mediated immunity is required for dealing with established viral infections. IgA seems particularly important in preventing virus attachment to epithelial cells, which is the first step in the infectious process. Failure of these mechanisms or lack of them may cause a person to become a chronic virus carrier; this is particularly likely with poliomyelitis and hepatitis A viruses.

When one looks at cell-mediated defects with respect to viral agents, it becomes clear that a lack of T lymphocytes allows frequently recurring viral infections. Virus-infected cells may change the surface antigens of the cell; this renders them recognizable as nonself and brings about their destruction by T cell cytotoxicity. Activated macrophages are also important in removing virus-infected body cells. Certain chronic human viral infections are associated with lymphopenia, though the precise manner in which the lymphocytes disappear is unclear. Lack of lymphocytes renders the subjects susceptible to opportunistic and antibiotic-resistant infections.[2,3,5]

Certain viruses, such as the poliomyelitis virus, are released from an infected cell and destroyed by a specific antibody. Most, however (e.g., human immunodeficiency virus), spread from cell to cell and persist despite a high titer of the specific antibody. A cell-mediated response is required to destroy established viral infections, but antibody and interferon are important in preventing their penetration and spread.[2,3,5]

Bacterial infections are resisted by many mechanisms. Those bacteria which attach to epithelial cells but do not penetrate do not usually provoke an immune response. Entrance of bacteria is effectively prevented by epithelial structures and their functional activities. If these fail, extracellular-type bacteria are usually nonspecifically phagocytosed by neutrophils and the intracellular types by macrophages. Both cells have the capability of destroying phagocytosed material, and this is a way of eliminating bacteria which obtain entrance into the mucosa or subcutaneous areas of the body. If bacteria are too numerous or are allowed to multiply faster than phagocytosis can remove them, the bacteria tend to release antigens into the body fluids, provoking the immune response. The majority of the antigens to which humans are exposed seem to be those of exogenous infective organisms.

Natural antibodies support this statement, since they are commonly directed toward microorganisms. It has long been recognized that extracellular-type bacteria are usually destroyed by humoral antibodies, while intracellular types require destruction by sensitized T lymphocytes. Fungal organisms are destroyed in the same way as other organisms. Competition between normal flora and other organisms is quite important in preventing fungal disease and opportunistic infections, as are environmental moisture, warmth, and acidity.[2,3,5]

Most fungal diseases are countered by cell-mediated immunity, and they often render the subject anergic. *Candida albicans* (a yeast) is commonly found in T lymphocyte–deficient persons. Candida infection in such persons is difficult to prevent and control and is a prime example of the ability of a fungus to induce immune suppression.

Chronic parasitic disease likewise induces immune injury. Many worm infestations are characterized by eosinophilia, IgE antibody formation, and an atopic response. Diarrhea in *Ascaris* infestation has an allergic basis. Unusual opportunistic protozoa such as *Pneumocystis carinii* (a lung protozoan) and *Giardia lamblia* (an intestinal protozoan) often infect and produce disease in the immunodeficiency syndromes.[5]

Immunopathologic conditions may be secondary to infections. The release of a soluble bacterial antigen into blood in which a specific antibody is already circulating may produce an immune complex disease. Gram-negative bacteria produce endotoxins which, by activating the "alternative" complement pathway, may be one cause of septic shock. Disseminated intravascular coagulation (DIC) may also be caused in some cases by these immune complex lesions. Chronic bacterial infections may also cause a localized immune complex disease.[2,3]

Iatrogenic Conditions

Iatrogenic drug-induced hyperimmunologic injury is common in the clinical area; stopping the offending drug will usually stop the symptoms. Most drugs function as haptens, which combine with body proteins on the surface of cells. Genetic factors and combining affinity help determine the outcome of drug-induced injury. What is apparent, however, is that an immune response to a drug does not necessarily ensure that an allergic reaction will occur.[2,3,5]

Many factors homeostatically controlling the balance between defense and immune disease are still unidentified. Some blood dyscrasias are iatrogenically induced, and many of these present as type II cytotoxic, type III complex, or type IV delayed hypersensitivity reactions.[2,3,5]

Autoimmune Disease

Inappropriate immune responses often, but not always, result in injury. Autoimmunity (from *auto*, meaning "self") may fit best into this category, for the immune response is misdirected toward self antigens. It is believed that autoallergic mechanisms may underlie most chronic disease processes, from rheumatoid arthritis to pernicious anemia. Autoantibodies usually arise in response to intracellular antigens which are not normally exposed to the immune system, such as inner layers of cell membranes, nuclear membranes, nucleoprotein, nucleic acids, and cytoplasmic structures such as mitochondria; or they arise in response to haptens, viruses, and the like. Autoimmune diseases present an odd combination of decreased suppressor T cells and complement with an excess of autoantibody. Most autoimmune lesions are infiltrated with lymphocytes, plasma cells, and macrophages. This describes type IV reactions, but because of the excess immunoglobulins and their known involvement in certain cytotoxic and immune complex diseases, the autoimmune diseases are considered humoral reactions. Experimental studies with New Zealand Black (NZB) mice seem to indicate that there is a defect in suppressor T cells and that a viral etiology is more than speculation. NZB mice spontaneously develop antoimmune disease and are an important animal model for study of these conditions. Neither suppressor T cell deficiency nor viral causation has been confirmed in human autoimmunity, but much evidence supports their role in its etiology.[2,3,6]

Two basic types of autoimmune disease are seen clinically: that which involves a single organ (as in Hashimoto's thyroiditis) and that which involves multiple organs (as in SLE). Controlled cooperation between T cells, B cells, and macrophages must occur to give an appropriate immune response. The summation of suppressor and helper T cell activity results in appropriate types and quantities of antibodies produced by the B cell progeny. If suppressor T lymphocytes are lacking, then helper T cells will dominate B cell differentiation and function and may result in overproduction of autoantibodies. This imbalance is characterized by excessive activity on the part of B cell progeny and a deficiency of suppressor T cell activity.[2,3,6]

A genetic basis for autoimmunity has been of increased interest since a relation has been shown between certain HLA types and the propensity to develop autoimmune disease. Whether these control genes are actually HLA or from the nearby Ir region is yet to be determined; but it appears that genetic factors, probably the Ir genes, lymphocyte surface antigens, and viral receptors, may be involved separately or in concert in the development of autoimmune reactions.[2,3,6]

Theoretically there is loss of homeostatic equilibrium between suppressor and helper T cells when B cell activity is allowed to dominate or is enhanced and suppressor T cell activity is decreased, resulting in autoimmune disease. This imbalance may occur as a consequence of Ir genes in which viral and environmental mechanisms are acting together or independently. The influence of thymic hormones may be important, since in animal models they seem to be diminished in autoimmunity and when therapeutically administered to the affected animal, they improve its condition.[2,3,6]

Medical and Surgical Interventions

Priorities in the therapy of a patient with an anaphylactoid reaction include:

Maintenance of a Patent Airway–Bronchospasms and angioedema may be severe and block the airway. The insertion of an oral airway or an endotracheal tube, or in severe cases a tracheostomy, may be necessary. CPR may need to be initiated.

Prevention of Antigen Spread–This is accomplished by application of a tourniquet proximal to the injection site if the offending antigen was injected into an extremity.

Peripheral Vasoconstriction and Bronchodilatation–For this purpose, epinephrine, 1:1000 strength, 0.2 to 0.5 mL subcutaneously, may be given every 5 to 10 min according to hospital protocol or physician's prescription until signs of anaphylaxis disappear. Epinephrine may also be given by continuous infusion. Diphenhydramine hydrochloride (Benadryl), 5 to 100 mg IM, or cimetidine (Tagamet), 600 mg IV, may also be given to block the effects of histamine.

With severe anaphylaxis, hypovolemic shock may occur because of the loss of intravascular fluid into the interstitial spaces. Chapter 7 contains an in-depth discussion of shock states and their treatment. To prevent and correct anaphylactoid shock, two measures should be taken immediately:

Administration of IV Volume Expanders–The type of solution used depends upon the patient's serum electrolyte levels. However, most patients receive a combination of fluids and plasma expanders (plasma, dextran, albumin). Plasma expanders are preferred over glucose solutions for anaphylactoid shock because the molecules are larger and remain in the vascular bed for a longer time.

Administration of Vasopressors to Raise the Blood Pressure–Drugs which stimulate both alpha and beta receptors include norepinephrine, levarterenol bitartrate (Levophed), metaraminol bitartrate (Aramine), dopamine (Intropin), and dobutamine (Dobutrex). IV infusion rates and patient hemodynamic parameters must be carefully monitored to maintain the desired pressure.

Supplemental therapy may include the administration of aminophylline to relax bronchial spasms and corticosteroids (Solu-Cortef) to prevent protracted laryngeal edema and suppress the inflammatory response.[7] Despite the considerable anxiety the patient may suffer, sedatives are avoided because of their tendency to depress respiration.

Long-term treatment of the patient with extrinsic allergies is aimed at artificially producing a state of tolerance to the offending antigen. Desensitization is the process of injecting small amounts of antigen, gradually increasing the amount over a period of time. This is effective in desensitizing some patients by producing immunologic competition between IgG and IgE, since both are able to bind the antigen and thus reduce allergic symptoms. Hyposensitization is the use of a specific antibody to reduce symptoms by blocking the release of mast cell granules. Sometimes an effective response to small doses of antigen is successful in inducing tolerance even though neither desensitization nor hyposensitization may be demonstrated.

Antihistamines may also be used on a long-term basis in the treatment of a patient with allergies. Common side effects include dryness of the oral mucous membranes, nausea, dizziness, blurred vision, and drowsiness.

Large-volume plasmapheresis has recently been used in conjunction with immunosuppression to treat type II cytotoxic injury. This tends to decrease circulating target cell antibody and prevent further cell lysis—an intervention similar to that involved in the use of exchange transfusions for erythroblastotic infants. (See Chap. 42 for further information on plasmapheresis and implications for nursing interventions.) Immunosuppression used alone has little effect, since glomerular basement membrane antibodies persist for a few weeks to 2 years, the titer gradually diminishing with time.

Nephrectomy has sometimes been performed to treat Goodpasture's syndrome and prevent pulmonary hemorrhage, but it is a harsh treatment with little effect. In cases of cytotoxic deficiencies of blood components, replacement therapy is used to eliminate the symptoms.

Nursing Interventions

For the patient in anaphylactic shock, with ineffective breathing patterns and altered cardiac output, the primary nursing interventions are surveillance and protection of vital functions. *Surveillance* in the critical-care situation is defined as the application of behavioral and cognitive processes in the systematic collection of information used to make judgments and predictions about a patient's life status. The behavioral component of surveillance involves the collection of information, while the cognitive component includes the evaluative or judgmental aspect. Data must be analyzed to determine the range of probabilities and to isolate those factors which are influencing a given situation.[8]

Data collection, reporting, and recording for the patient in anaphylactic shock should include vital signs, hemodynamic measures, urinary output, ECG readings, breath sounds, and review of laboratory test results (e.g., arterial blood gases, electrolytes). Collaborative nursing functions include the administration of drugs, fluid replacement, and oxygen as indicated to correct the altered cardiac output and ineffective breathing patterns.

Following the acute stage, the nurse should facilitate adequate rest by decreasing stimuli in the environment as much as possible. Nursing activities should be carefully organized to maximize sleep and rest periods for the patient. During the recovery phase, it is also essential that the nurse describe what has happened to the patient and discuss methods for prevention.

Prevention is primarily aimed at the identification and elimination or reduction of offending allergens. Smoke, fumes, dust, and aerosols should be avoided in the environment of patients with atopic respiratory problems. Animal danders, feathers, molds, and house dust are also frequently troublesome to these and other atopic persons. Aspirin and isoproterenol abuse, as well as ozone production from electrostatic air filters, have recently been demonstrated to act as asthmatic stimulants. Many other environmental agents and common habits probably serve as allergens and could be controlled if they were recognized.

Dry skin promotes itching associated with atopic dermatitis; thus proper skin care and topical lubricants are required to keep the patient from scratching. Secondary infections may be reduced by eliminating irritating fabrics, by bathing frequently with mild soap, and by keeping the hands and fingernails particularly clean. The nurse should observe for any secondary contact dermatitis, which in hypersensitive persons is commonly due to topical antibiotics or antihistamines.

Since persons with a history of known allergies are more likely to be reactive to other antigens, patients should be instructed to make their allergies known to all health care providers. High-risk persons should wear a medical-alert bracelet or tag at all times indicating known allergies. For persons allergic to insect stings, commercially prepared emergency sting kits should be readily available. The patient should be instructed in applying the tourniquet and self-injecting the subcutaneous epinephrine.[9]

Other preventive measures include instructing the asthmatic patient to avoid dehydration, since this condition enhances the formation of mucous plugs and further impairs alveolar ventilation. Patients may also need assistance in dealing with anxiety. While the dyspnea associated with asthma is widely recognized as eliciting fear, the rhinitis, itching, and urticaria associated with other allergies are also stressful. Empathy with these persons and conveying understanding for their problems and feelings may well affect the outcome of any therapy. Specific interventions for decreasing patient anxiety are further discussed in Chap. 47.

References

1. Gell, P. G. H., Coombs, R. R. A., & Lackman, P. J. (Eds.). (1975). *Clinical aspects of immunology.* Oxford: Blackwell.

2. Bellanti, J. A. (1985). *Immunology III.* Philadelphia: Saunders.

3. Sites, D. P., Stobo, J. D., & Wells, V. (1987). *Basic and clinical immunology* (6th ed.). Los Altos, CA: Appleton and Lange.

4. Martin, D. W., Mayes, P. A., & Rodwell, V. W. (1983). *Harper's review of biochemistry* (19th ed.), pp. 214–217. Los Altos, CA: Lange Medical Publications.

5. Bergeron, D. A. (1986). The laboratory evaluation of AIDS. *Journal of Medical Technology, 3*(3), 152–155.

6. Karr, C. K. (1986). Autoimmunity: Now and then. *Journal of Medical Technology, 3*(5), 276–278.

7. Phipps, W. J., Long, B. C., & Woods, N. F. (1987). *Medical-surgical nursing: Concepts and clinical practice* (p. 271). St. Louis: Mosby.

8. Dougherty, C. M., & Molen, M. T. (1985). Surveillance. In G. M. Bulechek & J. C. McCloskey (Eds.), *Nursing interventions: Treatments for nursing diagnoses* (pp. 301–305). Philadelphia: Saunders.

9. Lewis, S. M., & Collier, I. C. (1983). *Medical-surgical nursing: Assessment and management of clinical problems.* New York: McGraw-Hill.

47

The Immunocompromised Patient

Sister Mary
Rebecca Fidler
Mary Frances
Keen

A normal, functionally balanced immune system, complex as it is, effectively protects the self from nonself molecules. When a system imbalance occurs, the system changes quantitatively to over- or underreact to nonself stimuli. A clear understanding of a normal immune response is necessary to understand these quantitatively inappropriate responses whose consequences are immune disorders.

Functional deficiency of the immune response can be either congenital or acquired. *Congenital immune deficiencies* are those conditions which are associated with a genetic malfunction or defect. *Acquired immunodeficiency* is due to an environmental rather than a genetic cause. Deficiencies are generally named according to the component which is decreased; thus stem cell, T lymphocyte, B lymphocyte, immunoglobulin, and complement component deficiencies and phagocytic defects have been designated. More recently, functional deficiencies have been described, such as a deficiency in antigen processing (afferent limb defect), lack of lymphocyte communication (central limb defect), and effector cell deficiency (efferent limb defect). Most hypoimmune states are still designated T cell, B cell, or stem cell deficiencies, but in the clinical situation a functional defect is usually observed and treated accordingly.[1]

When the human body is unable to defend itself against nonself, the potential to sustain life is threatened. The deficiency may be due to lack of certain cell types such as stem cells, T lymphocytes, or B lymphocytes; absence of a primary lymphoid organ required for lymphocyte maturation such as the thymus; or present but nonfunctional cell types. The basic defect may result in failure to recognize a foreign threat, inability to recall past immune encounters, and/or inability to secrete antibody or lymphokines. Regardless of the basic defect, immunodeficiency results in recurrent infections, lesions of the skin and mucous membrane, and increased risk of neoplastic disease.[2]

The availability of monoclonal antibodies continues to restructure the understanding of immune deficiency syndromes. Past categorization of immunodeficiencies according to their missing components, such as T and B cells, stem cell, or complement, has become too simplistic, for the deficiency may be related to missing subgroups or even a defective or dysfunctional enzyme which is responsible for the inability to recognize, process, respond to, or destroy a threatening, invading, live, or inert nonself molecule.[3,4]

Primary congenital deficiencies are rare and may affect specific and/or nonspecific human defenses. Congenital defects are usually recognized during the first 2 years of life and are suspected when recurrent infections become apparent. In general, if an infant is born without a thymus, the result is impaired cellular immune defense. If the missing component is the bursa-equivalent (B cell) component, humoral immunity is impaired. If the defect is of stem cell origin, both cellular and humoral defenses are lost. Nonspecific immune defects are related to complement and other biologic amplification systems.[1,2]

Four major effector systems interact to defend humans against constant assault from nonself agents: humoral immunity (B cell antibody-mediated defense), cellular immunity (T cell defense), phagocytosis, and complement (see Chap. 44 for an indepth discussion of these concepts). Chronic and recurrent infections with usual and unusual organisms which fail to respond to treatment are suggestive of immunodeficiency. Skin rash, chronic diarrhea, recurrent abscess, osteomyelitis, growth failure, and hepatosplenomegaly further suggest immune defects. The type of infection often gives clues about the type of deficiency. Recurrent infections by extracellular organisms are common with defective humoral immunity. When cell-mediated responses are deficient, fungal, protozoal, and viral organisms are the usual infectious agents. Infection by rare organisms is characteristic of chronic granulomatous disease and combined defects. Phagocytic defects allow superficial skin infections and/or septicemia by normal nonpathogenic skin flora (pyogenic bacteria). Complement deficiencies also allow pyogenic infections.[1,2] Lymphocyte defects in primary immune deficiency syndromes are listed in Table 47-1.

Congenital Humoral Defects

Congenital humoral immune defects are perhaps the most frequent. They are characterized by inability to produce quantitatively and qualitatively functional antibodies. B cells are usually deficient or dysfunctional, allowing extracellular bacteria to infect and cause uninhibited disease.

X-Linked Agammaglobulin of Bruton

This disease is due to lack of immunoglobulin synthesis caused by deficiency of B cells. Serum immunoglobulins are absent, and severe recurrent infections begin in the infant as soon as maternal

Table 47-1 Lymphocyte Defects in Selected Primary Immune Deficiency Syndromes

Deficiency Syndrome	Affected Lymphocyte Populations		Mode of Inheritance
	B Cells	T Cells	
Disorders Mainly Affecting B Cells			
Congenital hypogammaglobulinemia (Bruton type)	Yes	No	X-linked
Congenital hypogammaglobulinemia	Yes	No	AR
Immunodeficiency with excess gamma-M globulin	Yes	No	X-linked
Common variable immunodeficiency	Yes	Yes*	?, familial
IgA deficiency	Yes	No	Sporadic, AR, AD
IgM deficiency	Yes	No	Sporadic
IgG and IgG subclass deficiencies	Yes	No	Sporadic, AR
Disorders Mainly Affecting T Cells			
Di George syndrome	No	Yes	Sporadic, familial
Chronic mucocutaneous candidiasis	No	Yes	Sporadic, AR
Combined B Cell and T Cell Deficiencies			
Severe combined immunodeficiency	Yes	Yes	X-linked, AR
Immunodeficiency with abnormal immunoglobulins (Nezelof's syndrome)	Yes	Yes	Familial, X-linked, AR
Immunodeficiency with short-limbed dwarfism	Yes	Yes	AR
Immune Deficiency—Enzyme Deficiency Syndromes			
Ecto-5'-nucleotidase† deficiency	Yes	No	X-linked, AR, sporadic
Adenosine deaminase deficiency	Yes	Yes	AR
Nucleoside phosphorylase deficiency	No	Yes	AR
Biotin-dependent carboxylase deficiency	Yes*	Yes*	Sporadic
Complex Immunodeficiences			
Wiskott-Aldrich syndrome	Yes	Yes	X-linked
Ataxia-telangiectasia	Yes*	Yes	AR
Immunodeficiency with thymoma	Yes	Yes	Sporadic
X-linked lymphoproliferative syndrome	Yes*	Yes*	X-linked
Acquired immunodeficiency syndrome	No	Yes	Sporadic

AR = autosomal recessive; ? = undetermined; AD = autosomal dominant.
*Defect is variable or selective.
†Ecto-5'-nucleotidase is a marker for mature B cells.
Source: Bellanti.[2]

passive immunity dissipates (approximately 5 to 8 months of age). Extracellular bacteria such as *Streptococcus, Staphylococcus, Haemophilus,* and *Pneumococcus* cause recurrent pneumonia, bronchitis, otitis media, and other skin and/or mucous membrane infections. The basic defect appears to be maturational arrest at the pre–B cell stage, with lack of mature B cells resulting in loss of potential antibody-secreting plasma cells. T cells and T cell functions are normal, with delayed hypersensitivity reactions and allograft rejection potential unimpaired. Secondary lymphoid structures show depleted B cell–dependent germinal centers and zones. Plasma cells are not observed, and the tonsils are poorly developed. Inability to form specific antibodies to bacteria and viruses is the paramount problem in Bruton-type agammaglobulinemia.[1,2]

Interesting, yet perplexing, is the accompanying autoimmune disease seen in patients with this condition. Rheumatoid arthritis, dermatomyositis, lupus erythematosis (SLE), and vasculitis are common, because of an intact cell-mediated immune response. Defense against intracellular infections is present despite the inability to produce antibodies. Hepatitis virus, echovirus, and poliovirus, however, escape this protection and often cause hepatic and neurologic disease. The fact that this disease is X-linked recessive restricts it to male infants.

Common Variable Immunodeficiency

This syndrome is a common group of immunodeficienies characterized by persistent diminished antibody production which allows recurrent bacterial infections. Both sexes are equally affected. Most patients have adequate numbers of mature B cells, with normal to hyperplastic B cell–dependent areas within the secondary lymphoid organs. The basic defect appears to be the inability of B cells to mature into antibody-secreting plasma cells despite adequate T helper function. Autoimmune disease (rheumatoid arthritis, pernicious anemia, and hemolytic anemia), giardiasis, and lymphoreticular malignant disease often accompany this type of deficiency. Dysfunction of or absence of interleukin-2 (IL-2) may play a role in the pathophysiology.[1,2]

IgA Deficiency

In IgA deficiency, there is an absence of both plasma and secretory IgA. Often this defect is without symptoms, but when symptoms are present, the defect may present as recurrent viral and bacterial sinopulmonary infections. Allergies and autoimmunity are common complications, probably because of the role of IgA as a mucosal defense against foreign antigens. The actual etiology of IgA deficiency is not known; anti-IgA antibody, IgA-specific T suppressor cells, inadequate T helper cells, and the absence of IgA-secreting plasma cells have all been suggested. Diarrhea, malabsorption associated with allergy and autoimmune disease, and bacterial infections of the respiratory, genitourinary, and gastrointestinal tracts are common in primary IgA deficiency.[1,2]

Congenital T Cell Defects

Di George's Syndrome

Thymic and parathyroid hypoplasia (third and fourth pharyngeal pouch defect), presenting as a deficiency of T cells with increased B cells and hypocalcemia, was first described by Di George. T cell deficiency usually affects B cell function, because of a lack of T helper function. Persons born with this defect have little defense against fungi and intracellular organisms and are quite prone to opportunistic infections such as *Candida albicans* (yeast) and *Pneumocystis carinii.* Live viral vaccines as well as common childhood viral diseases such as chickenpox are severe and can be fatal in Di George's syndrome victims.[1,2]

Nezelof's Syndrome

Nezelof's syndrome is a combined dysfunction of T cells and immunoglobulins. Normal levels of antibody are present but not functional. Nezelof's is inherited as an autosomal recessive or X-linked recessive or an undefined familial defect. T cell numbers are decreased and cell-mediated response to antigens is depressed. The exact immunologic defect is yet to be identified.[1,2]

Congenital Combined Immune Defects

Combined immunodeficiency states are due to defective T and B cell immunity. Complete defects, such as severe combined immunodeficiency disease, and partial defects, as in ataxia-telangiectasia, are two variations. Infants with these defects lack competent T cells or B cells and are thus unable to mount a cell-mediated immune response or make antibody for a humoral response. These patients are susceptible to graft-versus-host reactions when any adult (competent) white cells are infused intentionally (therapy) or unintentionally (during gestation or at birth via maternal infusion).[1,2]

Severe Combined Immunodeficiency Disease (SCID)

Both T and B cell–mediated immunity are absent in SCID. The result is an inability to protect against any type of microorganism, and survival beyond 1 year is rare. Many infants die before diagnosis can be established, which accounts for the lack of data on incidence. The defect is congenital, and two recessive types have been described: an X-linked and an autosomal (Swiss) type. Histocompatible bone marrow transplant is an effective but difficult therapy. If diagnosis is made and bone marrow transplant carried out quickly and successfully, these infants can develop normally.[1,2]

The cause appears to be a stem cell defect with resultant absence of T and B cells. The possibility of a primary lymphoid tissue maturational defect (thymus or bursa equivalent) has been suggested. Enzyme deficiencies in the purine metabolic pathway have been described in SCID which suggest defective nucleic acid synthesis.[1,2]

Infants with SCID fail to grow and exhibit chronic diarrhea, pneumonia, otitis media, sepsis, and persistent oral yeast infections. They are particularly susceptible to yeast, cytomegalovirus, and *Pneumocystis carinii* infection. Vaccination with live or attenuated virus may cause severe disease or may be fatal. Any invasive procedure places these infants at high risk of fatal infection and must be done only when absolutely necessary and with extreme caution.

Ataxia-Telangiectasia

Ataxia-telangiectasia (AT) is a combined primary immunodeficiency in which both humoral and cellular immunity are impaired. Cerebellar ataxia and mucosal telangiectasia of skin and eyes are symptoms associated with this combined defect. Ataxia-telangiectasia is considered to be a hereditary syndrome (autosomal or inborn error) which creates a lack of endonucleases, depressing the ability of the cells to repair damaged DNA and thus favoring neoplastic transformation. T cells are decreased in number and impaired in subclass function, and immunoglobulins IgA, IgE, and IgG are commonly reduced. This accounts for the symptoms of recurrent upper respiratory tract infections, growth failure, gonadal hypoplasia, lymphomas, slight mental defects, and insulin-dependent diabetes. Ten percent of all AT patients die of cancer. Elevated levels of alpha fetoprotein and carcinoembryonic antigens suggest a primary defect in tissue differentiation, but these could also be consistent with a defect in endonucleases.[1,2]

Enzyme-Mediated Immune Defects

Primary immunodeficiency is occasionally associated with genetic biochemical errors. Usually, these involve enzymes essential to purine nucleotide metabolism, as in ataxia-telangiectasia. Clinically, the symptoms are similar to those of other immunodeficiencies, but there is a real need to diagnose and differentiate these defects from the others for effective therapy. Adenosine deaminase deficiency inhibits both T and B lymphocyte function by accumulation of deoxyadenosine, a potent lymphotoxin. Nucleotide phosphorylase deficiency results in poor purine nucleotide phosphorylase enzymatic activity, causing severe T lymphocyte dysfunction with deoxyguanosine accumulating as a T cell toxin. The third enzyme-provoked immunodeficiency is the absence of biotin-dependent carboxylase. Biotin is essential for cytotoxic T cell response, and lack of biotin accounts for the resultant selective IgA deficiency, poor response (anergy) to vaccine (pneumococcal) skin testing, and lowered T cell counts. Definitive diagnosis is determined by the presence of an abnormal amino acid pattern in the urine which is corrected by oral biotin (10 mg per day).[2]

Phagocytic Defects

Phagocytic defects occur when there is an inadequate number or dysfunction of phagocytic cells. Neutrophils, eosinophils, macrophages, and/or fixed histiocytes are the major phagocytic cells, and decreased numbers or dysfunction of one of these cell types can produce immunodeficiency.[1,2] A reduction in the number of neutrophils (neutropenia) or macrophages, their inability to migrate (chemotaxic defects), or their inability to ingest and kill nonself agents all qualify as phagocytic defects. Neutrophils function efficiently in the phagocytosis and degradation of bacteria, thus preventing extracellular infections. Macrophages function in phagocytosing and degrading entire cells which are infected, viral, foreign, dead, or transformed. They also have the responsibility for processing nonself molecules, presenting the activated antigen to T helper cells, and producing monokines (IL-1 and tumor necrosis factor), which play major roles in the regulation of the efferent limb of the immune response. These cells are also necessary for removal of necrotic tissue so that repair can occur.[1,2]

Congenital defects of phagocytes include Job's, Chédiak-Higashi, and "lazy leukocyte" syndromes (neutrophil chemotaxic defects). Chronic granulomatous disease affects the ability of phagocytes to kill and degrade ingested bacteria and is usually an X-linked trait. The defect is impaired oxygen-dependent superoxide and hydrogen peroxide formation resulting from absence of the necessary enzymes. In granulomatous disease, the microorganism can be phagocytosed but not killed or degraded. Phagocytic cell function may also be adversely affected by drugs and disease. Table 47-2 lists current tests evaluating phagocytic functions.

Complement Defects

The complement system is a major amplification system of immunity, augmenting the activity of antibodies, phagocytes, and the inflammatory process. It consists of nine protein factors C1 to C9, regulator proteins, and several inhibitors that interact on the surface of a cell at the location of antigenic determinants. The system is dependent on activation (complement fixation) of C1 by immunoglobulin, which sets into motion a cascade of events that activates and cleaves the nine factors to culminate in destruction of the cell membrane (lysis). In the process, many complement fragments are cleaved which have biologic activities such as opsonization, cytoadherence, and phagocytosis (C1a, C4a, and C3b), anaphylatoxins (C3a and C5a), chemotaxis (C5a), and other nonlytic functions. Classic

Table 47-2 Tests for Evaluation of Phagocytic Dysfunction

Test	Comment
Quantitative nitroblue tetrazolium (NBT)	Used for diagnosis of chronic granulomatous disease and for detection of carrier state
Quantitative intracellular killing curve	Used for diagnosis of chronic granulomatous disease. Can be performed by the use of organisms isolated from the patient
Chemotaxis	Abnormal in a variety of disorders associated with frequent bacterial infection. Does not provide a specific diagnosis. Performed by the use of a Boyden chamber utilizing a microscopic or radioactive technique. Roebuck skin window provides a qualitative result in vivo.
Random migration	Abnormal in "lazy leukocyte" syndrome. Tests nonchemotactic migration of leukocytes
Chemiluminescence	Abnormal in chronic granulomatous disease and myeloperoxidase deficiency

Source: Adapted from Sites, Stobo, and Wells,[1] p. 343.

pathway activation of complement is regulated by C1q inhibitor, which binds C1q and prevents its attachment to the Fc region of antibody. C1 esterase inhibitor binds C1r and C1s and prevents their activation. C4-binding protein facilitates inactivation of C4 by another regulatory protein, C3b inactivator. In the alternative activation pathway, factor D regulates the cleavage of C3b-bound factor B and bound C3b. C3b and factor B, if unregulated, would soon be depleted, but depletion is blocked by factor H, a serum globulin which cleaves Bb from C3b Bb complex, and by factor I, an enzyme that degrades unbound C3b.[1,2,6]

Congenital complement deficiencies involving any or all of the complement factors and inhibitors have been observed. Numerous diseases have been associated with deficiencies of complement components and inhibitors. Deficiencies involving early complement components show an increase in immune complex (type III) diseases and their associated pathology. The patients are also vulnerable to infection as a result of losing the phagocytic and bacterial enhancing activity afforded by complement fragments. The etiology of complement deficiencies is still questionable as related to defective structural or regulator genes of the HLA loci.[6] A summary of congenital complement deficiencies and their inheritance, symptoms, and associated syndromes is presented in Table 47-3.

These conditions, since they are congenital, appear early in life. Correct diagnosis is imperative, because improper treatment can be fatal, while proper treatment may sometimes correct the defect. Bone marrow transplants and live vaccines may save a life; they may also initiate graft-versus-host disease or lead to a serious or lethal infectious disease.

Acquired Immune Defects

Most patients in critical-care areas are immunocompromised to some extent. Acquired immune deficiencies are more common than congenital types and are likely to be the type most often encountered. Study of the congenital defects, however, has led to greater understanding of the diagnosis and classification of the acquired types. Acquired deficiencies may be primary, that is, occurring later in life because of a specific defect, but most are

Table 47-3 Congenital Complement Deficiencies

Deficiency	Mode of Inheritance and Symptoms	Associations
C1 esterase inhibitor (rare)	Autosomal dominant; classic pathway; acute inflammatory edema of extremities, skin, larynx, and GI tract; often fatal	Hereditary angioneurotic edema
Factor I	Severe infections; septicemia, meningitis, etc.; C3 depletion	Little or no C3 (since C3 is usually inhibited by factor I; it is depleted) See C3 below
C5	Recurrent bacterial infections, autoimmune disease (SLE)	Impaired chemotaxis and cytolysis
C3 (rare)	Autosomal codominant; recurrent skin and chronic infections; frequently fatal	Opsonization, phagocytosis, chemotaxis, and lytic defects
C1q	Recognition unit for classic pathway; severe recurrent infections; usually fatal	SCID, autoimmune disease, multiple myeloma, SLE
C1r	C1s; activation renal disease and recurrent chronic infections; autosomal recessive trait; inability to clear immune complexes	Vascular disease, chronic glomerulonephritis, lupus lesions
C2 (common)	May be none	Vascular and renal diseases, skin rashes, recurrent infection, malignant diseases

secondary to other conditions such as stress, malnutrition, disease, injury, chemotherapy, or immunosuppression. Secondary immune deficiencies may disappear when the primary disease is corrected.[1,2]

Acquired hypoimmune conditions occur when a person who once had normal immune function loses, either progressively or suddenly, the ability to recognize and respond to foreign materials. Acquired immune deficiency is associated with aging, stress, and iatrogenic therapy and is also secondary to certain disease states. Many therapeutic iatrogenic agents such as x-rays, drugs, surgery, and antisera are likely to produce a hypoimmune state. Cancer and infections also reduce immunologic responsiveness. This anergy may be transient or persistent.

Acquired Immunodeficiency Syndrome (AIDS)

Acquired immunodeficiency syndrome is an entirely new disease, currently epidemic, eventually always fatal, and thus far minimally controllable. It is a T_4 cell immunodeficiency (cell-mediated defect) in a previously healthy adult associated with rare opportunistic infections and malignant diseases. The typical AIDS patient has an abnormal T_4/T_8 ratio because of a decreased T_4 helper cell population. AIDS is more common in males than females. The high-risk groups are homosexual males with a history of multiple partners, persons with multiple and frequent heterosexual contact, drug abusers using and sharing IV injection paraphenalia, and persons needing multiple blood transfusions such as hemophiliacs.[7,8]

The agent believed to cause AIDS is a retrovirus, the human T cell lymphotrophic virus (HTLV-III), known to infect T helper (T_4) cells. Other viral agents frequently isolated from AIDS patients include herpes virus, hepatitis B virus, cytomegalovirus, Epstein-Barr virus, and adenovirus.

Certain sexual practices within the homosexual population may result in the deposition of semen and sperm into the colon, which is actually an ectopic placement of motile haploid germ cells. Additionally, many homosexuals have severe trauma to the colon and are continually exposed to foreign cells, antigens, and microorganisms via the sexual partner. Moreover, sperm possess and express not only class I HLA antigens but also like B cells,

macrophages, reticular cells, activated T cells, and class II HLA antigens. Class II HLA antigens are involved in regulating many levels of immune networking and may serve as differentiating antigens for immune cells. Researchers have suggested that gamma interferon induces DR (class II HLA) expression, and this enhanced expression may increase autoimmune risk by allowing recognition of self antigens. While these facts may help explain AIDS in homosexuals, they are not an adequate explanation for other high-risk groups.[7,10]

All adult AIDS victims previously demonstrated a normal immune system; therefore, the deficiency is acquired. Those who then fall prey to AIDS are those commonly burdened by multiple infections (viral and other) or multiple exposures to allogeneic cells (foreign human cells) such as sperm, whole blood, or blood products, which can in themselves cause immunologic imbalance. Infants are vulnerable in that they are born with an immature immune system. The fact that AIDS appeared abruptly in 1981 supports the infective agent hypothesis rather than a response to allogeneic cells.

Concurrent infections and syndromes are found in patients with AIDS. *Pneumocystis carinii* is a protozoan which caused pneumonia only rarely prior to 1981. Today, however, in persons with AIDS, it is a common pathogen. Kaposi's sarcoma also is frequently seen in sexually active immunodeficient homosexual males. This disease until recently was rarely observed, and only in elderly men of Mediterranean descent. Dark blue to purple-brown lesions, usually on the extremities, weight loss, fever, night sweats, and fatigue are the signs and symptoms observed in persons with Kaposi's sarcoma. Chronic (*Candida*) yeast infections are common and severe, often causing chronic esophagitis.[11] A summary of clinical findings in AIDS patients is presented in Table 47-4.

A retrovirus called *lymphadenopathy-associated virus* (LAV) was recently isolated in Paris from a patient with symptoms of AIDS. Around the same time Dr. Robert Gallo, a researcher at the National Institutes of Health in Washington, isolated a retrovirus from cells in American AIDS victims.[9] Dr. Gallo called this virus *human T cell lymphotropic virus* type III (HTLV-III). It has subsequently been shown that LAV and HTLV-III are probably the same virus. *Human immunodeficiency virus* (HIV) is an acceptable alternative name. While other viruses have frequently been isolated form the cells of AIDS patients, HTLV-III is different in that it preferentially infects, reproduces within, and kills T_4 lymphocytes, thus accounting for the immune defect demonstrated in AIDS.[10]

These same researchers found a T cell line in which HTLV-III could be grown without killing the cell and thus made available large quantities of HTLV-III for study, allowing the development of techniques and assays for diagnostic purposes. Enzyme-linked immunosorbent assay (ELISA) is now widely used to screen serum for the presence of anti-HTLV-III antibodies. The ELISA is almost 100 percent positive in AIDS patients and high in healthy members of high-risk groups; it is 80 percent positive in intravenous drug users and 60 percent positive in sexually active homosexuals. ELISA is *not,* however, a test for AIDS but screens only for prior infection and antibody response to the HTLV-III virus.[7] HTLV-III appears to be at least AIDS-associated. However, the presence of HTLV-III antibodies could be a result of AIDS (opportunistic infection) rather than its cause. HTLV-III infection requires direct transfer of contaminated body secretions from one individual to another through intimate contact or direct transfusion. This virus seems able to infect only a few human cell types, such as activated T_4 (helper) lymphocytes, certain B lymphocytes, and certain cells of the central nervous system. HTLV-III virus seems to have a special affinity for neurons and may cause neurologic disease. In fact, the behavioral changes observed in AIDS patients such as depression, withdrawal, persistent headaches, and lack of concentration may be signs of virus-infected neurons.[7]

HTLV-III is a *retrovirus,* that is, a virus whose genetic material, RNA, is transcribed into DNA by reverse transcriptase, an enzyme which reverses the transcription of DNA to RNA. This viral DNA becomes incorporated into the human genetic DNA of the cell nucleus and reproduces itself, using the cell's machinery and energy to produce many new infectious viral particles. Retroviruses are a family of medium-size enveloped RNA viruses of vertebrates consisting of three subfamilies, Oncovirinae (A,B, and C), Spumavirinae (foamy virus group),

Table 47-4 Signs and Symptoms in Acquired Immunodeficiency Syndrome

Wasting with lymphadenopathy
Decrease of gamma interferon
Lymphopenia (T cell)
Decreased T_4/T_8 ratio
T_4 deficiency (HTLV-III destruction)
Loss of immune memory, anergy to a variety of antigens such as mumps and *Candida*
Inability to recognize new antigens (DNZB)
Increase in soluble suppressor factors
Increase in number of B cells and associated hypergammaglobulinema (usually IgG or IgA)
Increase in circulating immune complexes
Decrease in lymphokines
Failure of B cells to respond to antigenic stimulation (they are already activated), e.g., negative to pokeweed mitogen
Malignant disease, e.g., Kaposi's sarcoma, lymphoma, Hodgkin's cALL
Oportunistic infections:
  Protozoan
    Pneumocystis carinii (pneumonia)
    Toxoplasma gondii
    Cryptosporidium (enteritis)
    Giardia lamblia
    Endamoeba histolytica
  Viral
    Cytomegalovirus*
    Herpes simplex virus
    Epstein-Barr virus
    Varicella virus
    Retrovirus (HTLV-1, HTLV-III)
    Adenovirus
  Bacterial
    Mycobacterium avium (intercellular tuberculosis)
    Salmonella
    Listeria
    Chlamydia
    Neisseria
  Fungal/yeast
    Candida (esophageal)
    Aspergillus
    Cryptococcus neoformans (meningitis)
    Nocardia

*Often the terminal event.

and Lentivirinae (slow viruses). Oncovirinae type C are best known for their ability to produce tumors.[8,9] Current information suggests that HTLV-III is a type C oncovirus that is exogenously acquired or a slow virus that causes inflammatory cytolytic and chronic disease in vitro.

Recent information suggests that HTLV-III may share a nucleotide sequence homology with visna virus.[11] The virus is well known for slow, persistent cellular and tissue phenomena in keeping with clinical observations associated with AIDS; in fact, sheep (brain) subtype visna virus is named for the Icelandic word for "wasting." Retroviruses are oncogenic, having acquired their human oncogenes through repeated integration with host chromosomes. The Epstein-Barr virus, cytomegalovirus (CMV), adenoviruses, and hepatitis B virus may interact with HTLV-III to enhance immunosuppression or recombine genetically. However, the main pathogenic threat of HTLV-III as a human oncogenetic virus is the fact that it has the ability to persist within the host's immune cells.[11]

AIDS is primarily diagnosed by clinical evaluation of the patient showing severe immunodeficiency and a group of opportunistic infections. Laboratory data serve to further evaluate and follow the condition (Table 47-4). One depressing fact is that once HTLV-III infection and integration into human DNA occurs, elimination of the viral blueprint through therapy is precluded. Therapy is limited to protecting uninfected cells against the virus by using antiviral drugs and natural interferons. Despite the demonstration of antibody against HTLV-III in the serum of AIDS and potential AIDS victims, the antibody is unable to effectively eliminate or neutralize the virus. Only after 6 months of infection is the antibody detectable; this complicates the identification of carriers. The time lag between infection and detection allows depletion of T_4 cells and development of acquired immune deficiency. Once infected, the victim becomes an HTLV-III carrier even in the absence of disease symptoms.[7]

AIDS-related Complex (ARC) is a condition caused by the human immunodeficiency virus in which the patient has a set of specific clinical symptoms and tests positive for the AIDS infection. The symptoms of ARC are less severe than those of classic AIDS; they may include loss of appetite, weight loss, fever, night sweats, diarrhea, fatigue, low resistance to infection, or swollen lymph nodes.[7,10]

The AIDS epidemic presents a complex challenge to health care workers.[7] Its evasive etiology and fatal consequences only complicate the matter of caring for a population of persons already stigmatized by society, i.e., homosexuals and drug abusers. AIDS, although a serious medical and health threat, presents political, social, and ethical dilemmas which must be solved if these patients are to receive proper care and new cases are to be prevented.

Immunodeficiencies Secondary to Other Conditions

A summary of the features of immunodeficiency secondary to a variety of other conditions is given in Table 47-5. The mechanisms involved are discussed in the following paragraphs.

Aging

The age of a person affects the ability to respond immunologically. The very young and the old are in an immunodepressed condition and thus are more susceptible to injurious agents. The immunocompetence of young children is not fully developed. In elderly persons the gradual loss of immune memory, unprimed T and B cells, loss of immune reserve, and perhaps the influence of primary lymphoid organs depress immune capacity, rendering them more susceptible to health problems. A readily observable increase in infections, autoimmunity, and malignant disease occurs with age. The very young are immunologically immature; they receive their initial resistance from passive immunity via placental transfer of maternal IgG and the mother's milk, which is rich in IgA, competent lymphocytes, and macrophages.[1,2]

Malnutrition

Malnutrition is also an important cause of hypoimmune states, particularly where protein deficiency exists. T lymphocyte deficiencies and their responses are the primary defect in malnutrition. Immunoglobulin levels appear high. Thymus and lymph node atrophy, lymphopenia, and diminished cell-mediated immunity reactions are all present in the malnourished. Complement components are also absent, with consequently reduced opsonic activity. Thus the malnourished person is more susceptible to fungal, viral, and intracellular bacterial infections. Hyperalimentation, however, may itself produce a transient period of anergy and may be a complicating problem for the already immunodeficient person.[1,2]

Irradiation

Lymphocytes are radiosensitive; thus x-ray may destroy T and B lymphocytes. Recirculating T cells

Table 47-5 Features of Secondary Immunodeficiency

Clinical Setting	T Cell	B Cell	Phagocytosis	Complement	Comments
Infection					
Rubella (congenital)	May have decreased T cells, PHA, MLC	May have hypogammaglobulinemia or selective immunodeficiencies; no response to rubella immunization; decreased response to multiple antigens	Normal	Normal	Defects vary with severity of disease
Measles	Transient suppression of delayed hypersensitivity; decreased PHA	Normal immunoglobulins; normal antibody response	Normal	Normal	Similar effect may be seen with measles immunization
Leprosy	Decreased delayed hypersensitivity; decreased response to M. leprae; decreased PHA, T cells	Decreased B cells in some, increased in others; increased antibody	Unknown	Unknown	Immunologic deficiency greater in lepromatous form
Tuberculosis	Decreased delayed hypersensitivity; decreased T cells; decreased MIF	Immunoglobulins normal	Unknown	Unknown	Severe infection may be associated with anergy
Coccidioidomycosis	Decreased delayed hypersensitivity; lymphocyte blastogenesis, MIF to coccidioidal antigen	Normal	Unknown	Unknown	Usually specific decreased immunity; generalized depression may be present
Chronic infection	Usually normal	Increased immunoglobulins	Decreased chemotaxis	Increased components	Increased autoantibody
Acute viral infection	Lymphopenia; decreased T cells; decreased PHA in some; depressed helper/suppress-cell ratio	Normal	Normal	Normal	Defect may vary with severity of illness.
Cytomegalovirus	Specific unresponsiveness to cytomegalovirus	Elevated IgM, IgA	Unknown	Unknown	
Multiple or repeated viral infection	Decreased T cells, PHA, MLC, helper cells	Elevated immunoglobulins, IgA, antibody to virus	Unknown	Unknown	Occurs in selected homosexuals; cause unknown
Malignant Neoplastic Disease					
Hodgkin's disease	Suppression of delayed hypersensitivity; decreased PHA: serum factors suppress T cells	Immunoglobulins normal to increased; decreased antibody response to certain antigens	Frequent pneumococcal and H influenzae infection; decreased chemotaxis	Unknown	Some abnormalities may be due to treatment or splenectomy

(Continued)

Table 47-5 (Continued) Features of Secondary Immunodeficiency

Clinical Setting	T Cell	B Cell	Phagocytosis	Complement	Comments
Malignant Neoplastic Disease					
Acute leukemia	Decreased delayed hypersensitivity, PHA	Variable immunoglobulin levels	Normal	Unknown	Some abnormalities due to treatment
Chronic leukemia	Serum factors inhibit PHA	Variable immunoglobulin levels	Normal	Unknown	Some abnormalities due to treatment
Nonlymphoid cancer	Variable decrease in delayed hypersensitivity; suppression of PHA, MLC, T cells; immunosuppressive factors	Variable immunoglobulin levels	Normal	Some tumors associated with decreased components	Some abnormalities of T cells related to severity of disease, others to immunosuppression or irradiation
Myeloma	Increased suppressor T cells (? macrophages)	Impaired antibody response; decreased immunoglobulins	Normal		Decreased complement components
Autoimmune Disease					
Systemic lupus erythematosus (SLE)	Decreased delayed hypersensitivity; decreased T cells, PHA, MLC: decreased suppressor cells in animal models and in humans	Immunoglobulins usually elevated; increased antibody titers to multiple antigens	Normal	Certain congenital complement deficiencies (C1q, C1r, etc.) associated with SLE: secondary complement deficiencies frequent	Some T cell defects may be secondary to treatment
Rheumatoid arthritis	Decreased delayed hypersensitivity; decreased PHA, MLC	Immunoglobulin levels usually increased; normal antibody response to antigens	Normal	Increase in complement levels	Some patients with hypogammaglobulinemia have arthritis
Chronic active hepatitis	Decreased delayed hypersensitivity; decreased lymphocyte cytotoxicity; decreased T cells; mitogen response normal to decreased	Immunoglobulin increased	Unknown	Decreased values in some patients	Steroids increase some abnormalities

Table 47-5 (Continued) Features of Secondary Immunodeficiency

Clinical Setting	T Cell	B Cell	Phagocytosis	Complement	Comments
Protein-Losing States					
Nephrotic syndrome	Normal	Decreased IgG; IgM and IgA may be decreased; antibody response decreased	Unknown	Normal in idiopathic lipid nephrosis, may be decreased in other forms	
Protein-losing enteropathy	Decreased delayed hypersensitivity; decreased T cells, PHA, MLC	Hypogammaglobulinemia frequent	Unknown	Unknown	
Other Disorders					
Diabetes	Decreased PHA; MLC normal	Normal	Decreased chemotaxis; poor bacterial ingestion	Unknown	
Alcoholic cirrhosis	Decreased PHA	Unknown	Abnormal chemotaxis	Some components decreased	
Malnutrition	Lymphopenia; decreased T cells; decreased delayed hypersensitivity	Immunoglobulins normal; normal antibody response	Abnormal bacterial killing	Decreased CH_{50}	
Burns	Decreased delayed hypersensitivity; lymphopenia	Decrease in all immunoglobulins; normal antibody response	Decreased phagocytic function; decreased chemotaxis		
Sarcoidosis	Decreased delayed hypersensitivity; decreased PHA: inhibitory plasma factor	Increased immunoglobulins; normal antibody response	Unknown	Unknown	
Splenectomy	Normal	Immunoglobulins normal; decreased antibody response to whole organisms; normal antibody response to purified antigens	Normal	Normal	Tuftsin deficiency found in some patients
Sickle cell disease	Normal in most; some have mild T cell impairment	IgM may be decreased; decreased antibody response to whole organisms with normal response to purified antigens	Decreased phagocytosis; decreased opsonization; defect in properdin	Some defects in alternative pathway described	Some immunologic abnormalities may be related to zinc deficiency

(Continued)

Table 47-5 (Continued) Features of Secondary Immunodeficiency

Clinical Setting	T Cell	B Cell	Phagocytosis	Complement	Comments
Other Disorders					
Uremia	Decreased delayed hypersensitivity; serum blocking factors suppress PHA, MLC	Immunoglobulins normal; normal antibody response	Normal	Levels may be reduced in certain diseases	
Aging	Decreased delayed hypersensitivity; decreased mitogen response; decreased T cells; suppressor T cells variably abnormal	Increased IgG (IgA in some); increased B cells; decreased IgG response to certain antigens	Unknown	Unknown	Increased autoantibodies
Subacute sclerosing panencephalitis	Specific unresponsiveness to measles antigen; blocking factor present in some	Increased antibody to measles	Unknown	Unknown	
Down's syndrome	Decreased lymphocyte response to PHA	Impaired primary and secondary antibody responses	Unknown	Unknown	Increased susceptiblity to infection
Newborn and premature infants	Increased suppressor cells	Diminished IgM, IgA; impaired ability to form antibody to a variety of antigens	Decreased killing	Decreased complement factors; abnormal chemotaxis	Decreased placental transfer of IgG in the premature
Immunosuppressive Treatment					
Corticosteroids	Transient decrease due to sequestration	Transient decrease; late: reduced immunoglobulin synthesis	Inhibits release of lysosomal enzymes, decreases phagocytosis of IgG-coated particles	No effect	Actions of steroids differ in humans and mice
Cytotoxic drugs (alkylating agents, antimetabolites)	Variable decrease in numbers and functions; responses suppressed or enhanced	Variable decrease in numbers and function (primary antibody responses impaired)	Decreased production of neutrophils and monocytes	No effect	Effects depend upon multiple factors
Antithymocyte globulin	Decrease in T cell numbers and functions	Unknown (some T cell–dependent reactions impaired)	Unknown	Unknown	Activity against other cells (e.g., platelets)

Table 47-5 (Continued) Features of Secondary Immunodeficiency

Clinical Setting	T Cell	B Cell	Phagocytosis	Complement	Comments
Immunosup-pressive Treat-ment					
Radiation	Decrease in T cell numbers and functions (may be prolonged)	Impaired antibody production	Transient decrease in blood monocytes	Unknown	Total nodal irradiation produces long-lasting immunosuppression
Cyclosporins	No change in T cell number; profound depression of allograft rejection reaction	Inhibition of T cell–dependent antibody responses	Unknown	Unknown	
Phenytoin, penicilla-mine	Unknown	IgA deficiency, hypogammoglobulinemia	Unknown	Unknown	May or may not be reversible
Anesthesia	Inhibits function	Inconclusive	Reduced phagocytosis	Unknown	Effect may last for weeks

PHA = phytohemagglutinin stimulation of lymphocytes; MLC = mixed lymphocyte culture (allogeneic cell stimulation of lymphocytes); CH_{50} = amount of complement to lyse 50% of cells; MIF = macrophage inhibiting factor.
Source: Sites, Stobo, and Wells,[1] pp. 348–350.

seem more sensitive than B cells, while macrophages, plasma cells, and B memory cells are somewhat radioresistant. Radiation therapy for cancer may reduce peripheral blood T lymphocytes for periods of up to 1 year, varying with dose, type, and area of irradiation. Patients in this situation should be made aware of their decreased resistance. They are susceptible to sudden devastating infections; therefore, mild infections of any sort should be treated early in their course.[1,2]

Drugs

Cytotoxic drugs may suppress the immune response; indeed, they are often given to accomplish that end. Immunosuppression and/or chemotherapy affect immune competence, but it is often difficult to determine just how they affect a person who already has a reduction in immune responsiveness. Lymphopenia usually becomes greater in the presence of chemotherapy. If a person is already deficient in T lymphocytes prior to chemotherapy, little effect is seen in either T or B cells. However, with prolonged chemotherapy (4 to 6 months), T lymphocyte levels begin to drop and B cells tend to increase. Some persons receiving chemotherapy have significant changes in T and B cell counts or

T and B cell ratios. After chemotherapy-induced T cell deficiency occurs, approximately 3 months is required for the patient to return to normal T cell levels and functioning. Chemotherapy seems to have little effect, if any, on humoral immune functions.[1,2]

In transplantation, immunosuppression is specifically aimed at producing anergy so that a foreign graft may be accepted and tolerated. Therapies which suppress T cell function without affecting the B cell function would be ideal, since graft rejection is primarily the responsibility of T cells and macrophages. Heterologous antilymphocyte serum (ALS) selectively removes lymphocytes and suppresses immune function. Antilymphocyte serum can be produced and has been used in clinical transplant recipients. Its efficiency and safety are still under study. Lack of precise understanding of how it works precludes indiscriminate use as a therapeutic agent to prolong the acceptance of grafts.

Stress and Immunity

Important relations of corticosteroids, personality, and stress to immune responses have recently been emphasized. All three of these have a definite effect on host defenses. They have in common a high level of plasma adrenal hormones, which reduce the inflammatory response, cause lymphopenia by depleting B lymphocytes, and cause T lymphocytes to sequester in the bone marrow. Circulating patterns of neutrophils and monocytes are altered, and chemotaxic responses are decreased. These events have occurred in animals that are handled in a rough manner, are given ether, or have undergone surgery. Increased levels of endogenously produced steroids have been found in humans with tuberculosis, myocardial infarction, leukemia, and diabetes and in those with high social readjustment rating scores and those experiencing bereavement. The stress of cold may cause an increase in plasma corticosteroids at three times the normal level.[1,2,10]

Stress, with its release of endogenous steroids, is apparently an important factor in the development of infections. This not only applies to healthy persons but is particularly important for those persons in a clinical setting in which stress levels are usually high. The host compromised as a result of disease, therapy, and age has long been a concern of health professionals. Nurses have recently become aware that stress modulation may be a way of promoting host defenses and preventing infection. The nurse, therefore, has the obligation of promoting factors and initiating interventions to reduce stress in order to enhance human resistance to infectious agents.

Medical and Surgical Interventions

Medical-surgical therapies for the immunocompromised patient may be directed at treating the cause, whether that cause is congenital or acquired, or at treating the symptoms and preventing complications of the disease. Unfortunately, because of limited understanding of the complexities of the immune system, the most successful therapies are directed at treating symptoms and preventing complications. Many of the therapies available for treatment of the immunocompromised state itself are considered experimental or are available only on a limited basis at selected medical centers.

Primary Immunodeficiencies

Primary immunodeficiencies may be treated with specific replacement therapy. When B cell defi-

ciency is present, gamma globulin or fresh-frozen plasma may be given at monthly intervals. Gamma globulin is frequently administered as a prophylactic measure against viral diseases such as hepatitis in doses of 0.02 to 0.06 mL per kilogram of body weight; however, in the patient with an immunodeficiency, much larger doses (0.66 to 1.3 mL per kilogram of body weight) must be given intramuscularly.[12] Obviously, these larger volumes are more painful and frequently not well tolerated. Plasma therapy is better tolerated and has the advantage of including the five immunoglobulins. Ironically, homologous serum hepatitis and transfusion reactions are potential risks with plasma therapy.

Replacement therapy for T cell–mediated immune deficiencies is more complex. Transfer factor, also known as *dialyzable leukocyte extract,* confers specific immunity from the donor to the immunocompromised recipient. The factor is extracted from the lymphocytes of humans who have demonstrated delayed hypersensitivity and is then injected into the recipient with negative skin tests. The recipient's lymphocytes become sensitized and confer cell-mediated immunity when the procedure is successful. Transfer factor has been used experimentally on a limited basis for the treatment of resistant infections such as mucocutaneous candidiasis.

Isolated thymic hormones used in clinical trials include thymine and thymosin (serum thymic factor). These agents are being tested for their ability to restore cell-mediated immunity in patients with acquired and congenital T lymphocyte defects and in those with autoimmune disease.[13] Thymic hormones have been effective in some instances in which the T cell precursors are already present.

Bone marrow transplants may also be used to treat T cell–mediated immune deficiencies in cases where an HLA-identical donor is available. Before transplantation takes place, the recipient must undergo intensive immunosuppression in the hope of assuring a successful transplant. Immunosuppression is usually accomplished by the use of total body irradiation and immunosuppressive chemotherapy. The combination of a primary immunodeficiency with an induced immunosuppressed state obviously places the patient in double jeopardy for the development of a life-threatening infection.

While immunosuppression is used to prevent graft rejection, the newly grafted immunocompetent cells may recognize the recipient's antigens as foreign, resulting in graft-versus-host disease. Many immunodeficient patients who develop GVHD die from the complication or its accompanying infections. Bone marrow transplantation is discussed further in Chap. 48.

Secondary Immunodeficiencies

Treatment of secondary immunodeficiencies consists primarily in treatment of the underlying condition that has affected the immune response. For example, correction of malnutrition or the removal of immunosuppressive drugs from a drug regimen where possible should result in the eventual return of appropriate immune function.

Other medical therapies are frequently directed at treatment of an infectious process and the symptoms associated with that infection. Interferons have been demonstrated to inhibit viral protein synthesis at the gene level by interfering with the translation of messenger RNA. The actions of interferons are pathogen-nonspecific and have been used in the treatment of various types of viruses and intracellular parasites in immunosuppressed patients.

Infections suspected to be bacterial are commonly treated with a combination of intravenous broad-spectrum antibiotics. Frequently a penicillin derivative (Carbenicillin or Ticarcillin), an aminoglycoside (Garamycin or Tobramycin), and cefazolin sodium (Ancef, Kefzol) are given in combination until the infecting organism is identified and a more specific antibiotic can be prescribed.

The drug of choice for treatment of systemic fungal infections is amphotericin B, despite its considerable side effects and toxic properties (Table 47-6). The required dosage is administered slowly, and the patient is observed closely during infusion.

Ketoconazole (Nizoral) is a newer drug, administered orally, that is effective in the treatment of fungal infections. However, the recommended dosage for systemic infections is 400 mg daily for a minimum of 6 months. Poor response and recurrence of clinical symptoms are often related to an erratic dose regimen. Toxicity appears to be minimal; pruritus, minor gastrointestinal intolerance, and liver function abnormalities have been reported.[14]

Interstitial pneumonia is a frequent complication in immunosuppressed patients. Cytomegalovirus, herpesvirus, and *Pneumocystitis carinii* are common causes and are treated with broad-spectrum antibiotics, acyclovir (Zovirax), and sulfame-

Table 47-6 Amphotericin B Side Effects and Interventions

Side Effects	Interventions
Systemic reactions during infusion (chills, fever, aching, nausea, vomiting)	Monitor vital signs 30 min for 4 h; observe closely. Premedicate with aspirin or acetominophen, diphenhydramine (Benadryl), or promethazine (Phenergan) and/or prochlorperazine (Compazine)
Phlebitis and inflammation at IV infusion size	Check IV site frequently for leakage. Use pediatric scalp vein (most distal vein possible); alternate veins; alternate-day dosage schedule if possible. Add heparin and/or hydrocortisone (Solu-Cortef) to the infusion
Nephrotoxicity	Monitor intake and output; observe for changes in urine output or appearance. Monitor with biweekly BUN or serum creatinine levels; withhold drug and report if BUN exceeds 50 mg/dL or serum creatinine exceeds 3 mg/dL
Hypokalemia	Observe for and report signs of hypokalemia; monitor K+ levels; administer oral potassium as ordered
Cytotoxicity	Assess for tinnitus, vertigo, hearing loss

thoxazole-trimethoprim (Bactrim, Septra).[12] Even with treatment, interstitial pneumonias are often fatal as a result of progressive pulmonary infiltration.

If an infection fails to respond to appropriate therapy, granulocyte transfusions may be given. Granulocytes are collected by means of leukapheresis from ABO-compatible, HLA-matched donors; donors are often related family members. The patient receiving a granulocyte transfusion must be carefully monitored for the common reactions of fever and shaking chills and for potential anaphylactic responses. Patients may also experience pulmonary symptoms of fluid overload or white cell sequestration in the lungs if the granulocytes are transfused too rapidly.[15]

Obviously, the treatment and prevention of AIDS is the greatest challenge facing the health care professional today. Azidothymidine (AZT) is currently approved for use with AIDS patients who have survived at least one bout of *Pneumocystis carinii* pneumonia, and at the time of this writing, AZT is being tested in patients with earlier stages of AIDS. AZT is a reverse transcriptase inhibitor which blocks replication of the AIDS virus; consequently, some immune function is restored by sparing T_4 cells, and the life of the AIDS patient is maintained. Compounds such as gamma interferon and interleukin-2 assist in bolstering the immune response. However, to date, there are no data demonstrating that the improvements in immune function actually cure AIDS.

Development of a vaccine for AIDS seems unlikely because of the nature of HTLV-III. The human HTLV-III antibodies produced in response to the virus are unsuccessful in destroying the virus. In addition, the binding site on the virus is capable of structurally changing through antigenic drift, a process common among influenza and cold viruses. Only a broad-spectrum vaccine would be capable of recognizing the variants.

Nursing Interventions

Nursing strategies are most importantly directed at the immunosuppressed patient's potential for infection. Infections may be prevented by decreasing the patient's exposure to exogenous organisms and by reducing the numbers of normal endogenous organisms. Measures aimed at decreasing the patient's exposure to exogenous organisms include

1. Improvements in hand-washing techniques. Hand washing is considered the most important barrier to the transmission of infection. All hospital personnel must use meticulous hand-washing techniques. Visitors must also be instructed to wash their hands before entering the patient's room.
2. Prohibition of flowers and plants in the patient's room. The standing water, as well as the plants themselves, provides an ideal reservoir for organisms.
3. Elimination of fresh produce such as lettuce from the diets of patients who are severely neutropenic (500 WBC or less per cubic millimeter).
4. Assessment of the need for protective isolation, use of a laminar airflow unit, or complete sterile isolation in "life islands" if available.
5. Improvements in the sterilization and maintenance of equipment, particularly respiratory equipment.
6. Cohort nursing of patients. With this type of nursing assignment, a limited number of nurses care for a limited number of patients on the unit. Primary nursing and case management, as opposed to team nursing or functional nursing, are examples of this type of patient assignment. Cohort nursing also limits the number of exposed patients should an infectious outbreak occur.

Measures aimed at reducing the number of normal endogenous organisms include:

1. Avoidance of indwelling urinary catheters, one of the major sources of infection in the hospitalized patient, if possible.
2. Avoidance of any unnecessary breaks in the integrity of the skin because of the immunodeficient patient's susceptibility to local or systemic infections. Manipulative and invasive procedures such as venipunctures, IV catheter injections, dental work, bronchoscopy, liver biopsy, IV pyelography, and barium enemas should be limited and kept to a minimum. The patient should be ambulated or, if on bed rest, turned every 1 to 2 h to prevent decubitus ulcers and the loss of skin integrity. Rectal temperature taking should be avoided because of the risk of causing rectal abrasions which could provide access for local infections or abscesses.

3. Meticulous care of any necessary invasive lines. Specific recommendations for site and line care frequently vary with the institution; however, it is accepted practice to use sterile technique in inserting lines and changing site dressings, to clean the site with an antimicrobial agent, and to apply an occlusive dressing. For short IV catheters, site care and tubing change should be performed every 24 h. The catheter should remain in place no longer than 72 h and preferably for only 48 h. Solutions should be changed at least every 24 h.[17]

4. Instruction of the patient about the need for good personal hygiene. Skin care with adequate lubrication is essential to prevent breakdown.

5. Scrupulous mouth care to prevent stomatitis. Nonabrasive toothpaste should be used, and the mouth should be rinsed periodically with saline.

New recommendations for the prevention of HIV transmission in health-care settings have been provided by the Centers for Disease Control (CDC).[18] These guidelines suggest the use of universal infection control precautions for *all* patients since medical history and examination cannot reliably identify all HIV infected patients. The CDC recommends routine barrier precautions to prevent skin and mucous membrane exposure when contact with blood or other body fluids is anticipated, and especially during all invasive procedures. (See Table 47-7). In the critical-care unit and other situations when the need for resuscitation is predictable, mouthpieces, resuscitation bags, and other ventilation devices should be readily available. Specimens of blood and other body fluids from *all* patients should be considered infective and placed in well-constructed containers with secure lids; contamination of the outside of the container should be avoided. Following these guidelines eliminates the need for infective warning labels on specimens. Hands and other skin surfaces should be washed immediately after contamination with blood and other body fluids and immediately after gloves are removed. Adherence to universal blood and body fluid precautions recommended for all patients will minimize the risk of transmitting HIV and other blood borne pathogens from patients to health-care workers and from health-care workers to patients during invasive procedures.[18].

Another major nursing goal is early detection

Table 47-7 Universal Precautions to Prevent Transmission of HIV in Health-Care Settings

Masks Indicated for personnel having direct, sustained contact with a patient who is intubated, being suctioned, or coughing extensively.

Gowns Recommended for staff if soiling of clothing with blood or other body fluids is anticipated.

Gloves Recommended for staff during contact with blood, other body fluids, mucous membranes or surfaces soiled with the same; recommended during venipuncture and other vascular access procedures.

Goggles Recommended during endotracheal intubation, bronchoscopy, endoscopy, or dental work or in situations where splattering with blood or body secretions is possible.

Needles/Syringes Disposable only; discard in rigid, puncture-resistant containers; do not recap or break in hand or use needle-cutting devices.

Specimens Consider all specimens infective; clean outside of contaminated specimen container with disinfectant such as 1:10 household bleach in water.

Source: Centers for Disease Control.[18]

of existing or developing infections. Because immunosuppressed patients have the potential to develop sepsis, vital signs and hemodynamic parameters should be monitored frequently. A hyperdynamic state may represent an early stage of sepsis. Low blood pressure, tachycardia, chills, subnormal temperature, or temperature spikes may likewise be indicative of sepsis.

The critical-care nurse must keep in mind that temperature patterns may differ from normal because of the immunosuppressed state of the patient. A small increase in temperature may be of much greater significance than the same increase in a patient with normal immune functioning. For example, a temperature of 101°F can be the sign of a dangerous infection in an immunosuppressed patient. Since white cells are necessary for the usual temperature elevation associated with infection, the infection will be in a more advanced stage in the immunosuppressed patient before the temperature is able to reach 101°F. The patient may also have a dangerous infection without any elevation in temperature if the white cells are severely depressed. Likewise, control of fever with antipyretics may impair a significant indicator of the infection's course. Without leukocytosis as a marker of infection, temperature curves are of prime importance and should not be obliterated with antipyretics.

In addition, the lungs should be auscultated for abnormal breath sounds that may occur with respiratory infections. Secretions should be examined for changes in color or consistency, and the patient should be questioned about symptoms of cough or sore throat. Pulmonary toilet, coughing, and deep breathing are essential for preventive care.

The nose, mouth, and perineal areas should be inspected daily for disruptions in integrity. White cell and neutrophil counts should be monitored daily for changes, and the results of all cultures should be monitored and additional cultures taken as necessary.

Another important potential nursing diagnosis in the immunosuppressed patient is alteration in nutrition. The causes may be related to either excess intake due to high caloric requirements during infection or inadequate intake due to stomatitis or esophagitis. A high-protein, high-calorie diet is essential for the immunosuppressed patient, and the critical-care nurse plays an important role in assessing nutritional needs and developing creative interventions for meeting those needs (see Chap. 12).

When oral intake is contraindicated, enteral feedings are preferred over parenteral feedings, since the latter offer another invasive line and possible portal of entry for organisms. If the gastrointestinal tract is incompetent, total parenteral nutrition may be administered to supply the needed calories, amino acids, and nutrients. Nursing interventions related to this procedure include astute assessments for complications of hyperosmolality and infection.

Knowledge deficit is defined as lack of the specific information necessary for the patient to make informed choices regarding his or her condition, therapies, and treatment plan. The knowledge deficit may be caused by lack of exposure, misinterpretation of information, unfamiliarity with information resources, or, as is particularly the case with immune system dysfunctions, lack of appropriate information resources for the patient to access.

While knowledge deficits are a concern with any health care problem, a deficit can almost certainly be anticipated in a patient with an immune system dysfunction. The fact that the immune system cannot be easily visualized or demonstrated with the use of diagrams makes immune system dysfunction difficult to comprehend and accept. The use of analogies to the defense system may be helpful.

Interventions appropriate for the correction of a knowledge deficit include the following:

1. Assess the patient's readiness to learn and learning needs.
2. Establish teaching priorities in conjunction with the patient.
3. Identify the content to be included, develop objectives, and identify teaching materials. Learning may be facilitated by providing written information for the patient to refer to as necessary.
4. Pace and time the learning sessions to the individual's needs. Begin with information the patient already knows and progress to unfamiliar information. Teaching may need to be done in a different or unusual sequence. Information causing the greatest anxiety to the patient may need to be dealt with first if the anxiety is interfering with the learning process.
5. Provide the patient with the opportunity to take an active part in the learning process and incorporate opportunities for feedback and evaluation of learning.

The real knowledge deficit on the patient's part combined with the health care profession's limited understanding of the immune system, the lack of specific known treatments or cures, the loneliness imposed by protective isolation, and the chronicity and usually poor prognosis of the diseases may manifest itself as anxiety.

Anxiety in the patient with AIDS may have multiple causes. A sense of powerlessness may result from the devastations of the disease process; altered body image may result from weight loss, visible lesions, and other changes in personal appearance; loss of employment and increasing dependency on others may result in declining self-esteem. Fear of potential or actual stigmatization and guilt from exposing family or significant others to a devastating disease may culminate in intense psychologic reactions to AIDS.[18]

Interventions aimed at decreasing anxiety include encouraging patients to acknowledge and verbalize their fears, with positive regard expressed through verbal and nonverbal communication. Mutual goal setting which establishes small accomplishments can promote increased feelings of independence and self-esteem. Accurate information should be provided, and the patient should not be grandly reassured that "everything will be all right." Explanations of isolation precautions are imperative to reassure the patient of his or her own protection against oportunistic infections. Anxiety-provoking stimuli in the environment and unnecessary isolation should be minimized. Distractions suitable to the physical condition of the patient may be designed to assist in reducing the level of anxiety.

Interventions directed at decreasing patient anxiety may also include the use of relaxation training. Scandrett and Uecker classify relaxation techniques in two basic categories: externally oriented and internally oriented techniques.[19] Externally oriented techniques include progressive muscle relaxation, biofeedback, and hypnosis. Internally oriented techniques include autogenic relaxation, meditation, and self-hypnosis. Most relaxation training programs begin with such progressive muscle relaxation exercises as those listed in Table 47-8.

Table 47-8 Progressive Muscle Relaxation: Instructions to Patient

Hand Tighten the dominant hand into a fist. Release fist. Tighten the nondominant hand into a fist. Release fist. (Check for relaxed state.)

Upper and Lower Arm Bend elbow of the dominant arm and point it to the ceiling, tensing both upper and lower arm. Repeat with the nondominant arm. Release. (Check for relaxation.)

Forehead Raise eyebrows toward top of head. Release eyebrows.

Eyes and Nose Squint your eyes and wrinkle your nose.

Mouth Purse your lips into a little round "O" and push out in an accentuated "kiss." Release. (Check for relaxation.)

Neck Hyperextend your head, grit your teeth, and make a wide smile.

Upper Back Try to touch your shoulder blades, arching your back.

Abdomen Pull in your abdomen. Release abdominal muscles.

Buttocks Tighten your buttocks. Release. (Check for relaxation.)

Thigh Raise your dominant leg about 6 in from the floor and tighten your upper leg.

Calf Pull your dominant foot toward your head. Pull your nondominant foot toward your head.

Foot Point your dominant foot away and curl your toes. Point your nondominant foot away and curl your toes. Release. (Check for relaxation.)

Source: Scandrett and Uecker.[19]

References

1. Sites, D. P., Stobo, J. D., & Wells, J. V. (1987). *Basic and clinical immunology* (6th ed.). Los Altos, CA: Appleton and Lange.
2. Bellanti, J. A. (1985). *Immunology III*. Philadelphia: Saunders.
3. Bishop, C. (1984). Immunoassays in hematology. *Journal of Medical Technology, 1,* 41–45.
4. Aisenbach, A. C. (1981). Current concepts in immunology. *New England Journal of Medicine, 304*(6), 331–336.
5. Westbrook, C. A. & Golomb, H. M. (1985), No. 16, November). Immune defects and infectious complications in hairy cell leukemia. *Clinical Immunology Today,* pp. 1–3.
6. Day, N. K. (1985, No. 14, May). Complement deficiencies. *Clinical Immunology Today.*
7. Krim, M. (1985). "AIDS: The challenge to science and medicine. In C. Levine & J. Bernel (Eds.), *AIDS, the emerging ethical dilemma. Institute and Society Ethics and Life Science,* A Hastings Center Report.
8. Siegal, F. P. (1984, No. 10, September). AIDS update. *Clinical Immunology Today.*
9. Gallo, R. C., Salahuddin, S. Z., et al. (1984). Frequent detection and isolation of cytopathic retroviruses (HTLV-III) from patients with AIDS and at risk for AIDS. *Science,* vol. 224, 500–503.
10. Lewandowski, A. J. (1986). The immunopathogenesis of AIDS. *Journal of Medical Technology, 3,* 145–149.
11. Griffin, J. T. (1986). The virology of AIDS, *Journal of Medical Technology, 3,* 149–151.
12. Govoni, L. E., & Hayes, J. B. (1985). *Drugs and nursing implications.* Norwalk, CT: Appleton-Century-Crofts.
13. Nurse's clinical library. (1985). *Immune disorders.* Springhouse, PA: Springhouse.
14. Phipps, W. J., Long, B. C., & Woods, N. C. (1987). *Medical-surgical nursing: Concepts and clinical practice.* St. Louis: Mosby.
15. Vredevoe, D. L., et al. (1981). *Concepts of oncology nursing.* Englewood Cliffs, NJ: Prentice-Hall.
16. Finkbeiner, A., Hancock, E., & Scheide, S. (1986). AIDS: Just the facts. *Johns Hopkins Magazine, 38,* 22–24.
17. Millar, S., Sampson, L. K., & Soukup, M. (1985). *AACN procedure manual for critical care.* Philadelphia: Saunders.
18. Centers for Disease Control (1987). Recommendations for prevention of HIV transmission in health-care settings, *Morbidity and Mortality Weekly Report,* Aug. 21, 1987, *36*(25), Atlanta: CDC. HHS Pub. No. (CDC) 87-8017.
19. Scandrett, S., & Uecker, S. (1985). Relaxation training. In G. M. Bulechek & J. C. McCloskey, *Nursing interventions: Treatments for nursing diagnoses* p. 22. Philadelphia: Saunders.

48 Acute Lymphoproliferative Oncological Disorders

Sister Mary Rebecca Fidler
Mary Frances Keen

Some of the most feared and aggressive human malignant diseases involve uncontrolled growth of cells responsible for normal human immunity; i.e., lymphocytes and their subgroups, macrophages and myeloid cells. These account for about 8 to 10 percent of all cancer. Clinically, they are important because they are often life-threatening and are feared childhood diseases. The cause of these oncological disorders is unknown, but high-risk groups are children and others with immunologic defects, immunosuppressed persons, and those exposed to carcinogens and infections—conditions which cause persistent mitotic stimulation of normal hematopoietic cells.

In well-differentiated malignant disease, cancer cells function much like normal cells. They may synthesize and secrete excessive antibody (B cell malignant disease), resulting in the so-called gammopathies, or produce lymphoproliferative disorders (lymphomas and leukemias) which rapidly kill the patient by overpopulation of one cell type at the expense of other normal, vital cell types. This chapter describes the acute lymphoproliferative oncological disorders most commonly seen in critical-care units, including lymphomas, leukemias, and the plasma cell dyscrasias.[1,2] Figure 48-1 gives an overview of the cell origins of hematologic proliferative disorders.

Types of Lymphoproliferative Disease

Lymphomas and lymphatic leukemias are malignant proliferations of lymphocytes. A review of the oncological patterns of T and B lymphocytes helps in understanding the clinical classification and behavior of these soft tumors. Leukemias arise from stem cells in the bone marrow, are usually blood-borne, and frequently spread to involve other anatomic sites. Lymphomas present as a tumor mass, often arising in lymph nodes or other lymphatic tissues, which spreads into and populates the peripheral vascular system.[1-4]

Lymphomas are basically described as either Hodgkin's (cell origin unknown) or non-Hodgkin's (the lymphocyte is the cell of origin).[5,6] Leukemias are classified by cell type, e.g., granulocytic, monocytic, lymphocytic, etc.

The techniques described in Chap. 45 for recognition of cell type assist in identifying and classifying lymphomas and leukemias; often they can be precisely defined and classified according to cell origin by the use of specific monoclonal antiserum. This technique not only allows for designation as B cells, T cells, or macrophages but often identifies as well their specific subtypes (such as T helper, T suppressor) or early development precursor types (such as T_{10}, T_1, T_6 antigen cells). Knowing the particular cell of origin in any malignant disease is vital for decisions about clinical management, therapy, and prognosis. The Lukes and Collins classification, for example, resulted in studies suggesting a better prognosis for patients with B cell lymphomas compared with those with T cell lymphomas.[7]

Lymphomas

Lymphomas are neoplasms of lymphoid tissue. The cells of origin may be lymphocytes or macrophages or their precursors. Lymphomas are lethal unless effectively treated. Hodgkin's lymphoma is a different disease from the non-Hodgkin's lymphoma. Hodgkin's has a distinct morphologic characteristic, the Reed-Sternberg (RS) giant cell, as well as an inflammatory cell component. The non-Hodgkin's

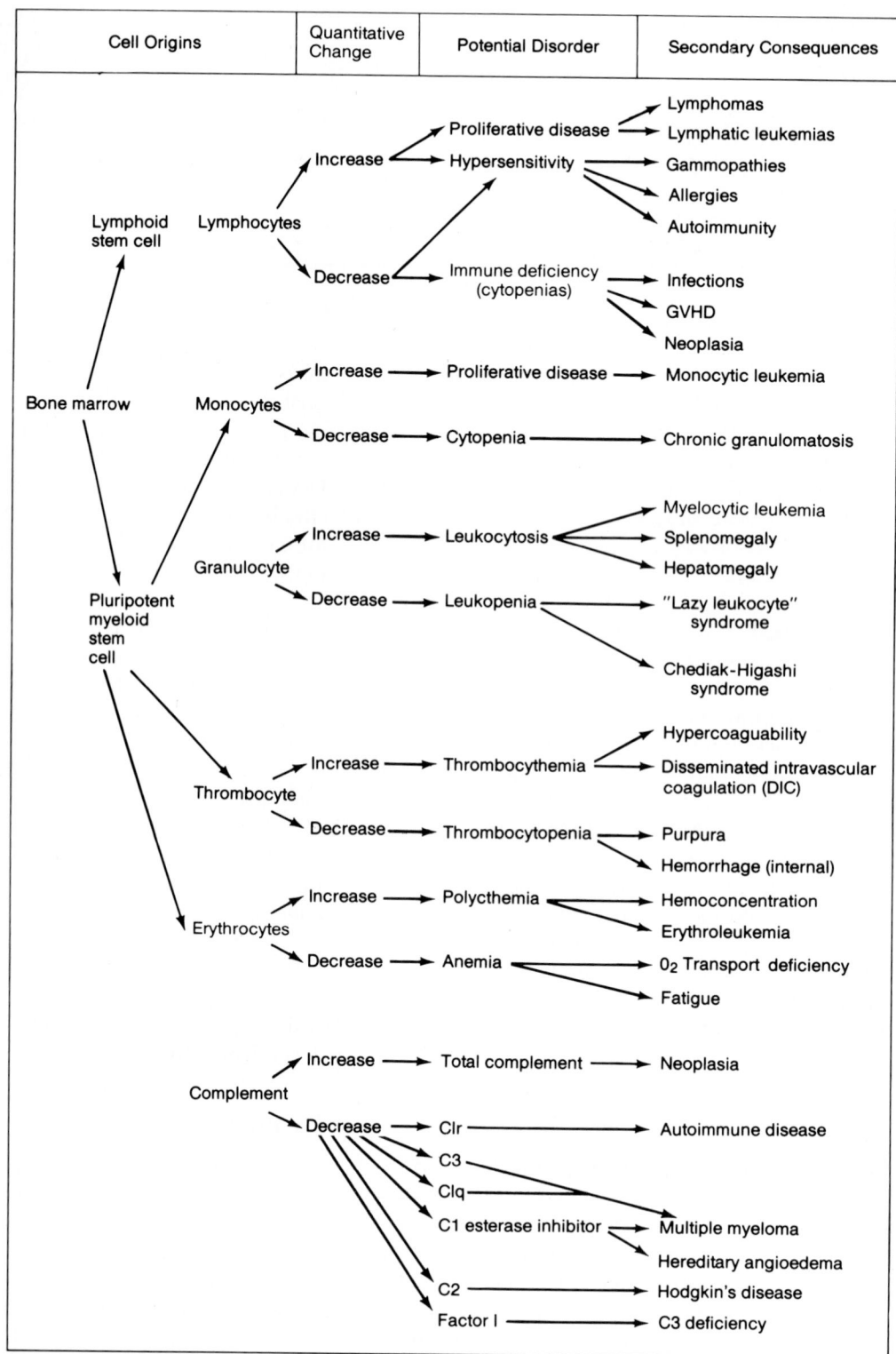

Figure 48-1 Cell origins of hematologic proliferative disorders.

lymphomas are known to be of lymphocytic origin and do not exhibit RS cells.[5,6,8] (See Fig. 48-2.)

Local or generalized enlarged, painless lymph nodes are usually the first signs of lymphomas. Later, lymphoma patients often exhibit splenomegaly and/or hepatomegaly. The course of the disease is unpredictable as it spreads from lymphoid tissue to new anatomic lymphoid areas.[1,2] Enlarged nodes are also found in many infectious and inflammatory situations, and such conditions must be differentiated from lymphoma. Infection and/or inflammatory conditions exhibit tenderness on nodal palpation, while lymphomatous nodes are painless.[1,2]

Lymphomas spread from their site of origin to other nodes and eventually involve the spleen,

liver, and bone marrow. Very rarely, they take a different course, present a leukemic peripheral blood picture, and then disseminate to involve the lymph system and nodes.

Non-Hodgkin's Lymphoma

Non-Hodgkin's lymphoma (NHL) occurs in various forms and arises from many different cell types, making classification rather complex. Rappaport classified non-Hodgkin's lymphomas as either diffuse or nodular on the basis of the stained cytologic characteristics of the lymphoma cell and the anatomic growth pattern of the disease, while Lukes and Collins differentiated them on the basis of the immunologic characteristics of lymphoid cells; i.e.,

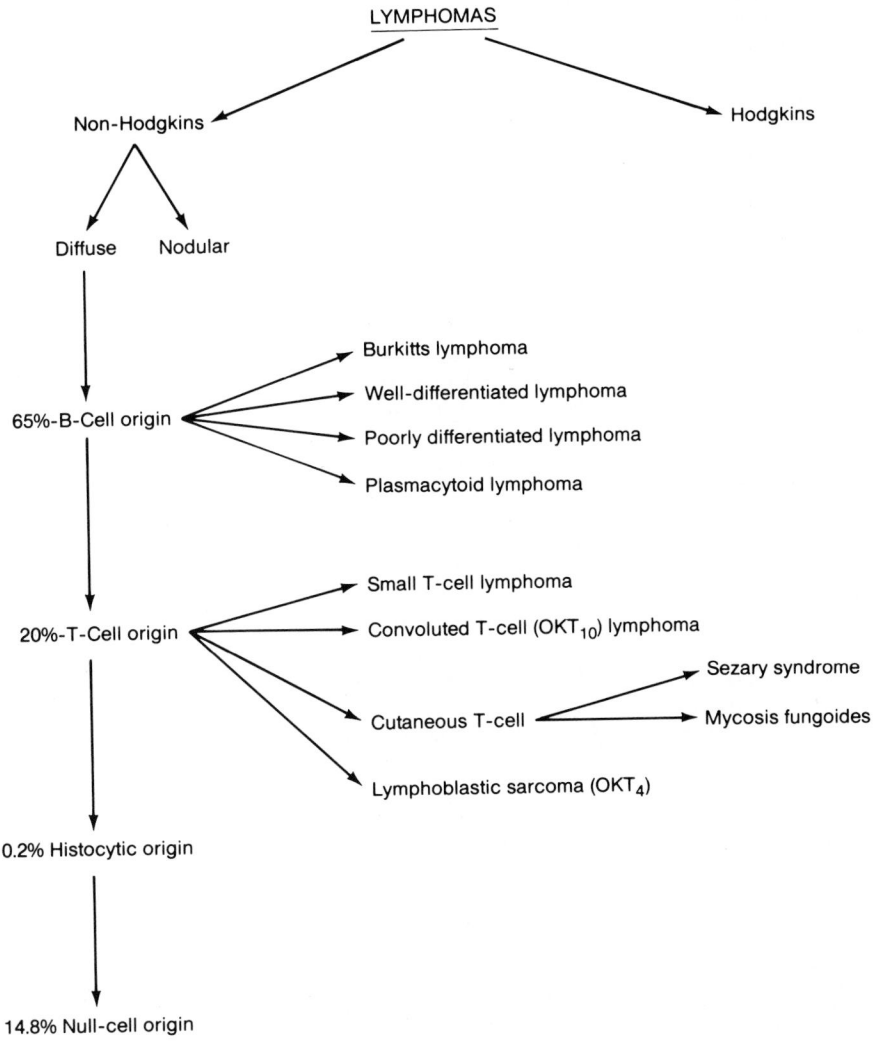

Figure 48-2   Types of clinical lymphoma.

T or B cell lymphomas or of histiocytic origin.[7] The Lukes and Collins classification recognizes distinct histologic subgroups of the Rappaport classification of diffuse non-Hodgkin's lymphomas. Both classifications have merit, but neither is wholly satisfactory. The availability of monoclonal antibodies has initiated a new approach in attempting to unify classification for clinical use[5] (Table 48-1). The pathologic classification of NHL places lymphomas in ten distinct subgroups according to morphology, clinical features, and diagnosis. This should eliminate current confusion and inability to compare clinical lymphoma data. The immunologic nature of the lymphoma cells in these ten types is yet to be fully understood but will undoubtedly have a major impact upon future classification, therapy, and prognosis. This pathologic classification also allows the identification of convoluted T cell lymphoma (lymphoblastic) as a distinct disease of T cell origin with convoluted nuclei occurring in young male patients with large mediastinal masses.[5,8] About 50 percent of non-Hodgkin's lymphomas are of the nodular form distinguished by identifiable clusters (follicles) of malignant cells within the lymph node. These nodules do not destroy the normal lymph node structure, as the cortex and medulla are still discernible. Sometimes these nodules become sub- or even extracapsular and may

Table 48-1 Pathologic Classifications of Non-Hodgkin's Lymphomas

Rappaport Classfication	Working Classification of Non-Hodgkin's Lymphomas for Clinical Use	Lukes and Collins Classification
	Low grade:	
Diffuse lymphocytic, well differentiated	ML, small lymphocytic	Small lymphocytic and plasma-cytoid lymphocytic
Nodular, poorly differentiated lymphocytic	ML, follicular, predominantly small cleaved cell	Small cleaved FCC, follicular only or follicular and diffuse
Nodular, mixed lymphocytic-histiocytic	ML, follicular, mixed small cleaved and large cell	Small cleaved FCC, follicular; large cleaved FCC, follicular
	Intermediate grade:	
Nodular histiocytic	ML, follicular, predominantly large cell	Large cleaved and/or non-cleaved FCC, follicular
Diffuse lymphocytic, poorly differentiated	ML, diffuse small cleaved cell	Small cleaved FCC, diffuse
Diffuse mixed lymphocytic-histiocytic	ML, diffuse, mixed small and large cell	Small cleaved, large cleaved, or large noncleaved FCC, diffuse
Diffuse histiocytic	ML, diffuse large cell	Large cleaved or noncleaved FCC, diffuse
	High grade:	
Diffuse histiocytic	ML, large cell immunoblastic	Immunoblastic sarcoma, T cell or B cell type
Lymphoblastic convoluted/non-convoluted	ML, lymphoblastic	Convoluted T cell
Undifferentiated, Burkitt's and non-Burkitt's	ML, small noncleaved cell	Small noncleaved FCC
	Miscellaneous: Composite Mycosis fungoides Histiocytic Extramedullary plasmacy-toma Unclassifiable	

Key: ML, malignant lymphoma; FCC, follicular center cell.
Source: Modified from the National Cancer Institute-sponsored study of the classifications of non-Hodgkin's lymphomas (Ultmann and Jacobs[5]).

be confused with inflammatory or infectious hyperplasia. Diffuse lymphomas, however, infiltrate the entire node in an unidentifiable pattern and destroy the normal architecture of the node. The cytologic features of the cells in both types are similar, and therefore the diffuse form was thought to be an advanced form of the nodular; but this has not been documented.[5,8] Nodular lymphomas occur primarily in persons over the age of 20, affect males and females equally, and have a better prognosis than the diffuse types.[5,8]

The Burkitt's and non-Burkitt's lymphoma cells bear little morphologic resemblance to normal lymphocytes or macrophages and are thus called *undifferentiated*. The Burkitt's type is related to the Epstein-Barr virus (EBV) and has a high mitotic rate, considerable cell death, and actively phagocytic macrophages. Burkitt's lymphomas primarily affect children or young adults and only rarely arise in lymph nodes. In Africa, where this tumor is endemic, the disease usually appears in the maxillary or mandibular region, whereas abdominal tumors are more common in the American form of Burkitt's lymphoma. The non-Burkitt's undifferentiated lymphomas affect adults (mean age 34), are harder to treat, and have no known viral relation to EBV.[8]

Malignant lymphomas were believed by Lukes and Collins to arise from normal components of the immune system, and thus they classified them as being of T cell, B cell, or histiocytic origin and defined subgroups of T helper, suppressor, etc. Most lymphomas (65 percent) are of B cell origin, 20 percent are of T cell origin, less than 1 percent are histiocytic, and 14 percent are undefined as to cell origin.[5,7,8]

B cell lymphomas include (1) small lymphocytic diffuse type, (2) well-differentiated lymphocytic lymphoma, (3) Burkitt's lymphoma, (4) immunoblastic sarcoma of B cells, and (5) plasmacytoid lymphocytic lymphoma (with secretion of antibody).[1,2,5,8]

T cell lymphomas are less frequent, and currently four types are known: (1) small lymphocytic T cell lymphoma, (2) convoluted T cell lymphoma (OKT_{10}), (3) cutaneous T cell lymphoma (mycosis fungoides and Sézary syndrome; OKT_4), and (4) immunoblastic sarcoma of T cells. Histiocytic lymphoma is thought to arise from macrophages and is extremely rare. Undefined lympho-

mas include those which cannot be classified as T, B, or histiocytic and are assumed to be primitive forms of these cells (of "null cell" origin).[1,2,5,8]

The cause of non-Hodgkin's lymphomas is unknown, but they are postulated to develop when there is a deficit in immunoregulation in the face of a persistent stimulus for lymphocyte proliferation. Persons with congenital immunodeficiencies, transplant recipients, persons with autoimmune disease, immunosuppressed persons, and those with infections are at greater risk of developing lymphomas.[1,2,5,8]

Most lymphomas arise from B cell proliferation. Theoretically, this could occur when T_8 suppressor cells are abnormal or T_4 helper lymphokines are promoting B cell growth (B cell growth factor, BCGF). In the case of Burkitt's lymphoma, EBV acts to cause B cell proliferation; T cells then regulate and control this proliferation, resulting in either no disease or infectious mononucleosis. A genetic defect in T regulation of this process allows a sustained, unlimited proliferation of B cells which produces the lymphoma.

Chromosomal aberrations are frequent in lymphomas. They involve especially translocations of the chromosome 14, which may be the locus of control over B cell proliferative processes or the carrier of the structural genes that code for immunoglobulin heavy chains.[5,9]

Non-Hodgkin's lymphomas are usually seen in 50- to 60-year-old persons. Lymphoblastic and undifferentiated lymphomas are the two most common types. These respond well to appropriate therapy, and approximately half are curable.

Hodgkin's Disease

Hodgkin's disease is characterized by Reed-Sternberg cells mixed with an inflammatory component of cells. It spreads in a predictable manner from one lymph node to the adjacent groups and never disseminates to become blood-borne (leukemic). There are, however, several variations of Hodgkin's disease, often complicating diagnosis.[6]

Hodgkin's disease usually begins in a single node or chain of nodes but may occasionally be present within the thymus or spleen. In this case, it spreads within the region of origin with a soft, uniform, fish-flesh appearance similar to non-Hodgkin's diffuse lymphomas.[6]

The etiology of Hodgkin's disease is unknown. The origin of Reed-Sternberg cells and the inflammatory component lead one to suspect the presence of an infectious agent. The fact that Hodgkin's affects two distinct age groups (the 15 to 34 age groups and the 45- to 60-year-olds) suggests a dual origin. In the younger group it is thought to be related to delayed infection by a common agent such as EBV. The person with this type of Hodgkin's has a high titer of EBV capsule antibody. Viral etiology is not suspected in the older age group. It is generally agreed that the Reed-Sternberg cells represent the malignant cells, but there is no agreement as to whether they derive from T cells, B cells, or macrophages. These patients, however, have impaired T cell–mediated immunity, with cutaneous anergy and increased susceptibility to fungal and opportunistic infection. Reed-Sternberg cells are positive for two macrophage-associated enzymes (acid phosphatase and nonspecific esterase). Monoclonal antibody assays suggest reticular cell origin.[5,6]

General clinical observations in patients with Hodgkin's disease show a painless enlarged lymph node or group of nodes with subsequent lymphatic spread, fever, night sweats, weight loss, pruritus, and anemia. Hodgkin's is classified, according to extent of involvement, in stages I through IV[5] (Table 48-2).

Table 48-2 Hodgkin's Disease: Ann Arbor Modification of Rye Staging System (1971)

Stage 1 Involvement of a single lymph-node region (I) or of a single extralymphatic organ or site (I_E).

Stage II Involvement of two or more lymph-node regions on the same side of the diaphragm (II) or localized involvement of an extralymphatic organ or site and of one or more lymph-node regions on the same side of the diaphragm (II_E).

Stage III Involvement of lymph-node regions on both sides of the diaphragm (III), which may also be accompanied by localized involvement of an extralymphatic organ or site (III_E) or by involvement of the spleen (III_S) or both (III_{SE}).

Stage IV Diffuse or disseminated involvement of one or more extralymphatic organs or tissues with or without associated lymph-node enlargement. Reasons for classifying the patient as stage IV should be identified.

Note: In Hodgkin's disease, all patients are subclassified A or B to indicate the absence or presence, respectively, of unexplained weight loss of more than 10 percent of body weight, unexplained fever with temperatures above 38°C, and night sweats.
Source: Ultmann and Jacobs,[5] p. 68.

Leukemias

Leukemias are malignant tumors of white blood cell precursors. They are characterized by diffuse replacement of bone marrow with proliferating leukemia cells, which spread to the peripheral blood and infiltrate the liver, spleen, lymph nodes, and other sites. Anemia, bleeding, coagulation disorders, and loss of normal white blood cells are the usual causes of death. Leukemia is classified according to maturity and white blood cell origin. If the malignant clone of cells is of lymphocytic origin, it is called *lymphocytic leukemia.* If the clone is granulocytic in origin, it is called *granulocytic* or *myelogenous leukemia.* If the cells are immature (blastic), the disease is referred to as *acute;* if they are mature or stable, the disease is considered *chronic.*

The major types of Leukemia (Table 48-3) are acute lymphatic leukemia (ALL), chronic lymphatic leukemia (CLL), acute myelogenous leukemia (AML), chronic myelogenous leukemia (CML), and a few unusual types such as hairy cell, monocytic, and erythrocytic leukemia. In leukemia, early signs include a low white blood cell count which later becomes very high—in the 200,000 to 500,000 per cubic millimeter range. Acute leukemia is rapidly fatal when untreated; the chronic form permits a longer untreated survival (2 to 6 years). Viral disease (low white cell count) and acute inflammatory disorders (leukemoid, high white cell count) often present a picture similar to leukemia and must be ruled out as causes of change in the blood profile.[10–13]

The production and availability of monoclonal antibodies has made possible further classification according to specific cell origin. Even the maturation stage of a particular cell line at which the aberrant cell occurs is, in some cases, possible to detect using commercially available monospecific antibodies. This also adds to the complexity of the existing leukemia classification system. For example, leukemia of null cell origin is referred to as *common ALL,* or cALL[1,2,10,11] (Table 48-3).

As can be discerned from the above discussion, hematologic disease and immunopathology are often closely associated because they share a physiologic and developmental (phylogenetic/oncological) component. Loss of functional homeo-

Table 48-3 Summary of Major Leukemia Types and Comparisons

Type of Leukemia	Cell Origin	Age Group	Sex preference	Percent of All Leukemias	Percent of Type	Identifying or Distinguishing Factors	Prognosis
ALL	Lymphoblast null cell, pre-B or pre-T cell	1–15; peaks at age 4 (child); 80% of all childhood leukemias	Male	60% acute	40% of acute	TdT*	Surviving 5-years: 90% (children), 50% (adults)
AML	Myeloblasts, monoblasts, granulocytes	15–39; children but also adults	Male		60% of acute		Poor prognosis
CLL	Small lymphocyte B cells (usually), T cells (rarely)	Over 60 (adults), rare in children	Male 2:1	40% chronic	66% of chronic	Hard to distinguish from lymphocytic lymphoma	Survival time many years; complications of anemia and thrombocytopenia with survival approx. 2 years
CML	Myelocytes, granulocytes, monocytes	Over 40 (adults), rare in children	Male		33% of chronic	Philadelphia chromosome (Ph₁)	3–6 months to 4 years +

*TdT = Terminal deoxynucleotidyl transferase marker for primitive lymphoid cells.

1277

stasis within the hematologic (hematopoietic) system will affect one or more of its functions, i.e., immunity, oxygenation, and/or intra- and extravascular clotting. This is observed in patients as potential for infection and/or immune disease, anemia, polycythemia, and bleeding disorders (Fig. 48-1). Chapters 40 to 43 discuss the hematologic perspective.

Chromosomal changes are probably present in all leukemic types and may be a necessary prerequisite for initiation of the leukemia process.[9] The Philadelphia chromosome, t(22 +; 9 −),* observed in CML, is the best known example. Acute myelogenous leukemia presents translocation between chromosomes 8 and 21: t(8−; 21+) and between chromosomes 15 and 17: t(15+; 17−). Many other translocations and monosomy and trisomy variations have also been described in the literature. The discovery and understanding of oncogenes has created renewed interest in the association between chromosomal changes and the initiation of a leukemic cell.[9] In Burkitt's lymphoma, a t(8−; 14+) chromosome aberration is often present, and an oncogene has been mapped close to the broken area on chromosome 8. When chromosome 8 breaks, the translocation shifts the oncogene to chromosome 14. The Philadelphia chromosome represents a translocation of the cellular oncogene present on chromosome 9 to chromosome 22.[9]

Leukemic transformation can occur at any maturational phase of cell differentiation; sometimes it may be the undifferentiated myeloid stem cells or clearly mature differentiated cell types. In lymphatic leukemia, the cell origin is the lymphoblast, T lymphocyte, B lymphocyte, or macrophage. In myelogenous leukemia it may be the myeloid blast cell which dominates the blood picture.[10]

Acute Leukemia

Acute lymphatic leukemia is characterized by the absence of mature white cells and an overabundance of immature forms. Normally, when stem cells divide, one of the daughter cells matures and is functionally committed while the other remains as

---

*t = translocation between chromosome 22 and chromosome 9; + indicates chromosome getting the new genetic material, − indicates chromosome losing the genetic material.

an uncommitted stem cell retaining the pluripotentiality needed in normal hematopoiesis. The normal ratio of functional cells to uncommitted cells is 1:1. This ratio is altered in acute leukemia, because leukemia is essentially an interruption of the cell differentiation process, causing the proportion of stem cells to increase.[10–13]

Chronic Leukemia

Chronic leukemia is not due to a maturational block, as evidenced by the fact that the stem cells continue to differentiate and form colonies of mature, committed cell types. The evidence seems to support a failure of the leukemic stem cell to respond functionally to regulator growth factors, so the cells look mature but have a functional impairment. This results in a long generation cycle of nonfunctional cells which tend to accumulate and exist for too long a period. It has been suggested that the translocation of an oncogene close to genes which could act as promoters may turn them on and initiate the leukemic process.[10–13]

The actual specific cause of leukemia is, however, presently unknown. Persons at increased risk are those exposed to and/or associated with human T cell leukemia virus (HTLV), ionizing radiation, or chemical carcinogens (benzene and oxidants).[1,2]

Hairy Cell Leukemia

Hairy cell leukemia (HCL) is a lymphoid malignant disease characterized by distinctive "hairy cells" in the blood and bone marrow accompanied by splenomegaly and varying degrees of pancytopenia. Splenectomy effects remission in 50 percent of patients, but the hairy cells persist; the other 50 percent of patients may relapse, with a worsening, degrading cytopenia. Recently, alpha interferon therapy has given excellent results in hairy cell leukemia. Infection from unusual pathogens is the major cause of death in these patients, suggesting immune defects. The hairy cells are thought to be of B cell origin and are attributed to a cell matured beyond the pre-B cell stage (CLL defect) but preceding the actual maturation to a secretory plasma cell (multiple myeloma defect).[10–13] (Refer back to Chap. 44, Fig. 44-14.)

In hairy cell leukemia immunoglobulin levels are normal. T cell subsets show an inverted T_4/T_8 ratio (normal = 1.8; HCL = 0.8 to 0.9). An increase in normal T_8 (suppressor) cells is postulated. T_4 helper cells are normal in both function and numbers. Quantitative increase in neutrophils, a decrease in monocytes (normal = 442 per microliter, HCL = 74 per microliter), and a decrease of natural killer cells and their cytotoxic functions are all readily demonstrated in persons with hairy cell leukemia.[1,2]

Plasma Cell Dyscrasias

Uncontrolled proliferation of plasma cells occurs when a cell involved in immunoglobulin synthesis becomes malignantly transformed. This results in gammopathies and peripheral blood infiltration by plasma cells. These are really B cell neoplasms but are differentiated to the extent that they are able to secrete abnormal monoclonal immunoglobulins. Table 48-4 presents a classification of plasma cell dyscrasias.

There are five potential types of dyscrasia; IgG, IgM, IgA, IgD, and IgE. The plasma cell monoclone can produce a complete antibody, heavy chains, or light chains only of a single class. Usually, the immunoglobulin has a high molecular weight,

Table 48-4 Classification of Plasma Cell Dyscrasias

Malignant monoclonal gammopathy
  Multiple myeloma
  Waldenström's macroglobulinemia
  Solitary plasmacytoma
  Amyloidosis
  Heavy-chain diseases
  Malignant lymphoma
  Chronic lymphocytic leukemia
Secondary monoclonal gammopathy
  Cancer (nonlymphoreticular)
  Monocytic leukemia
  Hepatobiliary disease
  Rheumatoid disorders
  Chronic inflammatory states
  Cold agglutinin syndrome
  Benign hyperglobulinemic purpura of Waldenström
  Papular mucinosis
  Immunodeficiency
  Gaucher's disease
Benign monoclonal gammopathy
  Transient
  Persistent
  Drug-associated

Source: Sites et al.[1], p. 388.

restricting it to the circulatory system, and each is unique. It may damage the glomerulus and appear in the urine (proteinuria). Bence Jones proteins are small enough to be excreted in the urine without frank glomerular damage. Common to all plasma cell dyscrasias is the appearance of excessive levels of serum or urine immunoglobulins (complete or incomplete). They are therefore often referred to as *gammopathies, dysproteinemias,* or *paraproteinemias.* Only the more common types of gammopathy, multiple myeloma (plasma cell myeloma) and Waldenström's macroglobulinemia, are described here (Table 48-5).

Multiple Myeloma

The more common gammopathy is an uncontrolled abnormal proliferation of plasma cells called *multiple myeloma* (MM). It starts within the bone marrow, then infiltrates into other osseous tissue, and eventually spreads to the peripheral blood and other sites. These cells, though abnormal, are sufficiently differentiated to be able to synthesize and secrete antibody or parts of antibody. Multiple myeloma patients are usually diagnosed by the demonstration of an increased level of one immunoglobulin class and Bence Jones proteins in the urine. Immunoglobulin G is the most commonly seen, followed by IgA and rarely the other three types, IgM, IgD, and IgE.[1,2,14]

Osteolytic lesions, hypercalcemia, pathologic fractures, abnormal and excessive immunoglobulins in plasma and/or urine, renal damage, and infection are the usual clinical findings. Paradoxically, MM is associated with severe deficiency of normal immunoglobin-secreting cells and their precursors. These findings, the first symptoms to appear, are unfortunately present in other conditions. Persons with long-standing chronic infections such as pneumonitis, tuberculosis, or osteomyelitis are at high risk for developing MM, but the cause is still unknown. Persistent B cell antigenic stimulation has been suggested as an antecedent condition to plasma cell dyscrasia.[1,2,14]

Myeloma cells produce an osteoclast-activating factor (OAF) which results in the focal lytic lesions of compact bone observed on x-ray as punched-out defects. In advanced disease, the myeloma cells infiltrate the peripheral blood, spleen, liver, kidneys, lungs, and lymph nodes as well as

Table 48-5 Comparison of Waldenström's Macroglobulinemia and Multiple Myeloma

Feature	Macroglobulinemia	Myltiple Myeloma
Recurrent bacterial infections		+ + +
Bone pain		+ + +
Lytic bone lesions		+ + +
Bleeding from mucosal areas	+ + +	+
Hepatosplenomegaly	+ + +	+
Lymphadenopathy	+ + +	+
Neuropathy		+
Visual changes	+ + +	+
Abnormalities in optic fundus	+ + +	+
Anemia	+ +	+ + +
Leukopenia		+
Thrombocytopenia		+
Hypercalcemia		+ +
Serum hyperviscosity	+ + +	+
Renal insufficiency		+ +

+−+ + + = degree of frequency.
Source: Sites at al.[1], p. 391.

other soft tissues. The vertebral column is the bone region most often affected, followed by the skull, pelvis, femur, clavicle, and scapula, although any bone region may be involved. Pain is a problem in most patients, because of tumorous infiltrations of vertebrae, with subsequent pathologic fractures, nerve root compression, and frank nerve root involvement. Systemic amyloidosis occasionally accompanies MM and complicates the primary disease with widespread deposits of amyloid. Myeloma is also associated with deficient T helper cell function and virtual absence of T_8 suppressor cell function, as well as a number of rather elusive immunoregulatory defects.[1,2,14]

Lymphokine regulation may play a role in MM. Lymphocytic interferon therapy has resulted in complete healing of the osteolytic lesions in some patients with MM. This would suggest that the lymphocyte-lymphokine network may be involved. There is also some evidence that non–T suppressor cells may play a role in the etiology. The effector cell, thought to be doing the suppressing, is the so-called large granular leukocyte or natural killer cell which inhibits proliferation and differentiation of B cells. Complement C1q deficiency is also common in this disease.[1,2,14]

Multiple myeloma usually is diagnosed from radiologic and blood assays and confirmed by biopsy. Hypercalcemia accompanies the lytic lesions of bone resorption. High calcium levels account for the weakness, confusion, polyuria, osteoporosis, and pain which often cause the patient to seek medical assistance. These are followed by progressing recurrent infections due to decrease of humoral immunity and loss of normal antibody production. Cellular immunity appears unaffected. Renal disease, occurring in about half the cases, is due to the toxic nature of Bence Jones proteins, glomerular damage by abnormally high levels of protein (plasma hyperviscosity), and high urinary calcium. Clinical findings most often observed are pain, recurrent bacterial infections, muscle weakness, pathologic fractures, anemia, and renal disease. Rates of survival and cure are poor, partly because of the advanced stage of the disease at the time of diagnosis. The actual cause of death is usually infection or renal failure.[1,2,14]

Two variants of multiple myeloma are solitary myeloma and a nonsecretory myeloma. Solitary lesions occur in bone and take on most of the characteristics of MM; they are thought to be an early, localized form of the disease. However, in the solitary form, extraosseous lesions remain localized and can be surgically excised with cure resulting. The nonsecretory type of the disease lacks the secretion of abnormal immunoglobulin.

Allogeneic and snygeneic bone marrow transplants have been successful in a few cases of MM. The graft usually seeds the bone marrow and brings remission, but in most patients the MM recurs. The most successful bone marrow transplant has resulted in a 1-year remission with 3-year survival. Clinical use of lymphokines may be the future direction for treatment of this disease.[1,2,14]

Waldenström's Macroglobulinemia

This monoclonal gammopathy is similar to MM except that it usually produces an IgM-type immunoglobulin (large antibody) and presents itself as a diffuse leukemia. IgA and IgG immunoglobulins may also be present. Patients with Waldenström's disease, unlike MM patients, produce a monoclonal abnormal antibody which infiltrates the lymphocytic tissues, resembling lymphocytic leukemia. The lytic bone lesions are not present. Renal involvement is infrequent despite the presence of Bence Jones protein. This gammopathy usually appears after the age of 70 with complaints of fatigue, weakness, and loss of weight. Hepatosplenomegaly may be present. Plasma hyperviscosity, with resultant headache, dizziness, visual problems, hemorrhage, and other exudative problems, is common. Cold agglutinins and cryoglobulins are often present and create a Raynaud's-like syndrome on exposure to cool temperatures. Macroglobulinemia is difficult to differentiate from lymphoma, since both are of B cell origin (see Chap. 42). Survival with appropriate treatment is 2 to 5 years.[1,2]

Medical and Surgical Interventions

Chemotherapy

The drugs employed in cancer chemotherapy generally have the potential for interfering with cellular function and replication. While the drugs affect both normal cells and cancer cells, the replication characteristics of the cancer cells usually make them more vulnerable to the effects of the drugs. Maximum therapeutic response with minimal toxicity to the patient is the major aim in cancer chemotherapy and a primary factor in evaluation of the therapeutic potential and usefulness of any drug.

The selection of specific drugs is also dependent upon the cytokinetic characteristics of the tumor. The length of time required for the cell to complete one mitotic cycle and the phase of the cycle which the drug affects are important components in the decision.[15] The various chemotherapeutic agents are classified as cell cycle phase–specific or cell cycle phase–nonspecific. Agents that are phase–specific act on replicating cells during a sensitive phase of the cell cycle; they are selectively more potent if administered when a large portion of the cancerous cells are passing through that phase. Since only a certain percentage of cells are replicating at any one time, the cell cycle phases also assist in determining the optimal time interval between doses.

An effective drug in a single dose usually kills 20 to 99 percent of the cells. This is important in considering chemotherapy protocols requiring long-term administration. Since a single dose of chemotherapy does not have the capacity to kill 100 percent of the cancer cells, multiple doses of multiple drugs at various time intervals may be necessary to achieve the maximal therapeutic response.

Cancer chemotherapeutic drugs may be classified as alkylating agents, antimetabolites, antibiotics, vinca alkaloids, hormones, and miscellaneous. An understanding of the general characteristics of the drugs in terms of mode of action, administration, common side effects, and toxicity is essential to providing nursing care.

Alkylating Agents

Alkylating agents cause breaks in the DNA molecule and cross linking, thus interfering with replication and transcription. When the cell attempts to divide, it dies. This is similar to the effect of ionizing radiation; alkylating agents have been called *radiomimetics*. The drugs as a group are cell cycle phase–nonspecific. Important drugs in this category used in the treatment of leukemias and lymphomas include nitrogen mustard cyclophosphamide (Cytoxan), and chlorambucil.[15,16] Major side effects and implications for care are indicated in Table 48-6.

Antimetabolites

Antimetabolites are similar in structure to the essential metabolites needed for replication. Because

Table 48-6 Alkylating Agents

Agent	Dose and Administration	Pharmacologic Factors	Significant Side Effects and Toxicity	Nursing Interventions	Use
Mechlorethamine hydrochloride (Mustargen, nitrogen mustard, HN$_2$)	*Intravenous:* 0.4 mg/kg once or 0.1–0.2 mg/kg for 2 days (dose dependent on patient's bone marrow reserve); 4-week rest period before second dose. *Intracavitary:* 0.2–0.4 mg/kg; change patient's position every 15 min for 1 h after dose for uniform distribution. Drug causes blistering (*vesicant*); administer in rapidly running saline IV solution (prepare and use immediately, decomposes quickly); use gloves	Rapid cellular interaction, inactivated in blood within 5 min	Bone marrow suppression (nadir 7–12 days after first dose); severe nausea, vomiting, diarrhea; alopecia; sterility; birth defects	Avoid extravasation of IV, assess signs and symptoms, protect against infection and bleeding, check blood counts, administer antiemetics (sedation if needed), maintain hydration, adjust dit, assist coping with hair loss, offer sexual counseling	Hodgkin's disease, lymphomas
Melphalan (Alkeran, L-phenylalanine mustard, L-PAM)	*Oral:* 6 mg daily for 2–3 weeks, then withdrawn for 4–5 weeks	Generally slow-acting	Bone marrow suppression (nadir unpredictable), immunosuppression, nausea, sterility	Assess signs and symptoms, protect against infection and bleeding, check blood counts, administer antiemetics, offer sexual counseling	Multiple myeloma
Busulfan (Myleran)	*Oral:* 4–10 mg per day until WBC count is 15,000/mm^3, then rest, maintenance at 2–4 mg per day	Rapid-acting; renal excretion	Bone marrow suppression, pulmonary toxicity	Assess for signs and symptoms of bone marrow suppression and pulmonary dysfunction, protect against infection and bleeding, check blood counts (especially platelet count and granulocyte level)	Chronic myelocytic leukemia

1282

Table 48-6 (Continued) Alkylating Agents

Agent	Dose and Administration	Pharmacologic Factors	Significant Side Effects and Toxicity	Nursing Interventions	Use
Chlorambucil (Leukeran)	*Oral:* 0.1–0.2 mg/kg daily in single or divided doses for 3–4 weeks, then maintenance at 0.03–0.1 mg/kg daily	Slow-acting	Minimal prolonged use: immunosuppression, bone marrow suppression	Assess signs and symptoms, protect against infection and bleeding, check blood counts	Chronic lymphocytic leukemia
Cyclophosphamide (Cytoxan, Ctx)	*Oral:* 1–5 mg/kg daily in divided doses; *intravenous:* 20–30 mk/kg IV push in rapidly running IV solution	Must be activated by liver; renal excretion	Bone marrow suppression, immunosuppression, nausea, vomiting, alopecia, hemorrhagic cystitis, sterility, birth defects	Assess for signs and symptoms, especially of cystitis; protect against infection and bleeding; check blood counts; administer antiemetics; assist in coping with hair loss; maintain hydration: must have high fluid output (optional GU irrigation for patients receiving high dose)	Multiple myeloma, lymphomas

Source: Adapted from Vredevoe et al., pp. 88–92.[15]

the antimetabolites appear to be metabolites, they are able to enter the cell and inhibit the enzymes involved in nuclear acid synthesis. By competing with or substituting for metabolites, they disrupt the cell's normal metabolic pathways, and the cell cannot function or replicate properly. The antimetabolites are cell cycle phase–specific, with the exception of 5-fluorouracil. Important drugs in this category include methotrexate, cytarabine, thioguanine, and mercaptopurine.[15,16] Major side effects and implications for nursing care are indicated in Table 48-7.

Antibiotics

Antineoplastic antibiotics are natural products of the soil fungus *Streptomyces*. They directly bind to

DNA and thus inhibit DNA and RNA synthesis. Antibiotics are cell cycle phase–nonspecific. Important drugs in this category include doxorubicin, daunorubicin, and bleomycin.[16] Major side effects and implications for nursing care are presented in Table 48-8.

Vinca Alkaloids

The periwinkle plant is the source of vincristine and vinblastine, two important antineoplastic drugs. These plant alkaloids bind to microtubular proteins during mitosis, thus leading to mitotic arrest. Vinca alkaloids are cell cycle phase–specific.[16] Major side effects and implications for care are indicated in Table 48-9.

Table 48-7 Antimetabolites

Agent	Dose and Administration	Pharmacologic Factors	Significant Side Effects and Toxicity	Nursing Interventions	Use
Cytarabine (Cytosar, cytosine arabinoside, ARA-C)	*Intravenous:* 100 mg/m² IV push q 12 h for 5–7 days or constant infusion over 2–3 days. *Intrathecal:* 5–75 mg/m² q 3–7 days. Refrigerate unconstituted solution	Rapid-acting; minor renal excretion	Bone marrow suppression (nadir 12–14 days after dose), nausea, vomiting, diarrhea, stomatitis, hepatitis (may occur within 1 week), birth defects	Assess for signs and especially of hepatitic symptoms, dysfunction; protect against infection and bleeding; check blood counts; administer antidiarrheal agents, antiemetics; maintain hydration; adjust diet; give frequent mouth care with assessment	Acute lymphocytic leukemia
Methotrexate (amethopterin, MTX)	*Intravenous:* 25–50 mg/m² per week; high dose (e.g., over 500 mg/m²) must be followed by 10–20 mg citrovorum factor IV or orally q 6 h (dose dependent on renal function and plasma methotrexate level). *Oral:* 10–30 mg/m² twice a week. *Intrathecal:* 6–12 mg/m² (dissolved in 10 mL saline or artificial CSF) twice weekly or monthly for maintenance	Renal excretion; citrovorum factor (Leucovorin) "rescues" cells from cytotoxicity by providing cofactors for DNA synthesis	Bone marrow suppression, stomatitis, severe diarrhea, hepatic toxicity, birth defects; renal toxicity with high doses; neurotoxicity (acute and chronic) with intrathecal administation	Assess for signs and especially of hepatitic symptoms, dysfunction; protect against infection and bleeding; check blood counts; administer antidiarrheal agents; maintain hydration; adjust diet; give frequent mouth care with assessment. *For high doses:* make sure citrovorum factor ("rescue") has been given; maintain intravenous hydration (3000 mL/m² per day); monitor intake and output; check that drug levels are assessed	Acute lymphocytic leukemia, non-Hodgkin's lymphoma

Table 48-7 (Continued) Antimetabolites

Agent	Dose and Administration	Pharmacologic Factors	Significant Side Effects and Toxicity	Nursing Interventions	Use
Methotrexate (amethopterin, MTX)				and renal function tests performed; keep urine alkaline to augment renal clearance (acetazolamide, sodium bicarbonate). *For intrathecal administration:* assess for signs and symptoms of neurotoxicity (nausea, vomiting, headache, dementia)	
6-Mercaptopurine (6MP, Purinethol)	*Oral:* 1.5–2.5 mg/kg daily in single or divided doses (dose must be reduced ¼–⅓ when given with allopurinol)	Metabolized by xanthine oxidase; allopurinol (a xanthine oxidase inhibitor) inhibits drug breakdown. Renal excretion	Bone marrow suppression, nausea and vomiting, hepatic dysfunction	Assess for signs and especially of hepatic symptoms, dysfunction and jaundice; protect against infection and bleeding; check blood counts; administer antiemetics; adjust diet	Acute lymphocytic leukemia, chronic myelocytic leukemia, non-Hodgkin's lymphoma
Thioguanine (TG, 6-thioguanine, 6-TG)	*Oral:* 2 mg/kg per day (dose alteration with allopurinol not needed)	Incomplete oral absorption, rapid renal excretion	Bone marrow suppression (may be delayed), nausea, vomiting, hepatic dysfunction, stomatitis	Assess for signs and symptoms, especially of hepatic dysfunction; protect against infection and bleeding; check blood counts; administer antiemetics; adjust diet; give frequent mouth care with assessment	Acute myelocytic leukemia

Source: Adapted from Vredevoe et al., pp. 94–100.[15]

Table 48-8 Antibiotics

Agent	Dose and Administration	Pharmacologic Factors	Significant Side Effects and Toxicity	Nursing Interventions	Use
Doxorubicin hydrochloride (Adriamycin, ADR)	*Intravenous:* 60–75 mg/m² q 3 weeks, 550 mg/m² total dose limit (450 mg/m² maximum dose if risk of cardiac toxicity). Vesicant	Activated by liver; biliary excretion; increases sensitivity to radiation	Severe bone marrow suppression, alopecia, nausea, severe vomiting, stomatitis, cardiac toxicity, red-colored urine (harmless), recall phenomenon (skin reaction due to prior radiotherapy)	Avoid IV extravasation; assess for signs and symptoms of cardiac toxicity, arrythmias, dyspnea, edema; protect against infection and bleeding; check blood counts; assist in coping with hair loss; administer antiemetics; adjust diet; give frequent mouth care with assessment; inform patient of urine change; assess skin in previously irradiated sites	Lymphomas, leukemia, Hodgkin's disease
Daunorubicin hydrochloride (cerubidin, daunamycin, DNR)	*Intravenous:* 60 mg/m² for 1–3 days q 3–4 weeks	Same as doxorubicin	Same as doxorubicin	Same as doxorubicin	Acute leukemia
Bleomycin sulfate (Blenoxane)	*Intravenous:* 10–20 U/m². *Intramuscular:* 10–20 U/m². *Subcutaneous:* 10–20 U/m². Total dose accumulation over 400 units associated with increased toxicity	Rapid-acting; renal excretion	Pulmonary toxicity (pneumonitis, pulmonary fibrosis); skin reactions (hyperpigmentation, ulceration, erythema); stomatitis; alopecia; nausea and vomiting; anaphylaxis; fever	Assess for signs and symptoms of respiratory distress (especially dyspnea, rales); assess skin carefully; give frequent mouth care with assessment; assist in coping with hair loss; administer antiemetics; adjust diet. Give test dose (1 mg) and observe for anaphylaxis: fever, hypotension, wheezing (take temperature, administer antipyretics)	Lymphomas, Hodgkin's disease

Source: Adapted from Vredevoe et al., pp. 100–104.[15]

Table 48-9 Vinca Alkaloids

Agent	Dose and Administration	Pharmacologic Factors	Significant Side Effects and Toxicity	Nursing Interventions	Use
Vinblastine sulfate (Velban, VLB)	*Intravenous:* initial dose 2.5 mg/m², subsequent doses individualized, given at 7-day intervals; maximum dose not over 18.5 mg/m². Vesticant	Metabolized by liver; slow biliary and renal excretion; crosses blood-brain barrier	Bone marrow suppression (nadir 5–10 weeks after dose), nausea, vomiting, alopecia, neuropathy (rare)	Avoid IV extravasation, assess signs and symptoms; protect against infection and bleeding, check blood counts (especially granulocyte count), administer antiemetics, assist in coping with hair loss	Hodgkin's disease
Vincristine sulfate (Oncovin, VCR)	*Intravenous:* 0.01–0.05 mg/kg per week. Vesicant	Metabolized by liver; slow biliary and renal excretion	Peripheral neuropathy, autonomic neuropathy (severe constipation, paralytic ileus)	Avoid IV extravasation; assess for signs and symptoms of neurotoxicity: depression of Achilles' tendon reflex (earliest sign), paresthesias in fingers and toes, inability to perform fine motor skills, weakness; assess bowel habits, administer stool softeners, cathartics, and enemas as needed	Acute lymphocytic leukemia, Hodgkin's disease, lymphomas, multiple myeloma

Source: Adapted from Vredevoe et al., pp. 93–94.[15]

Hormones

Exogenous hormones affect the growth pattern of hormonally sensitive tumors. Estrogens, antiestrogens, progestational agents, androgens, and adrenocortiosteroids have all been used in cancer chemotherapy.[15] However, only adrenocorticosteroids are used in the treatment of leukemias and lymphomas. They are commonly used as a component of combination chemotherapy; however, their use is controversial and their mechanism of action is not well understood.[15] Major side effects and implications for care are presented in Table 48-10.

Miscellaneous Drugs

The miscellaneous drugs do not fit into any other category. Many of these drugs may be considered experimental, and their mechanisms of actions and side effects are not as well understood as those of drugs that have been used for many years. Important drugs in this category are procarbazine, hydroxy-

Table 48-10 Adrenocorticosteroid Hormone

Agent	Dose and Administration	Pharmacologic Factors	Significant Side Effects and Toxicity	Nursing Interventions	Use
Prednisone (pred, PDN)	*Oral:* 15–100 mg on alternate days, taken with milk, food, antacid; gradual withdrawal if taken for prolonged period, not necessary for short, high-dose course	Metabolized by liver; renal excretion	*All steroids* (prolonged high doses). Fluid retention, hypertension, hypokalemia, diabetes, immunosuppression, gastrointestinal bleeding, potassium loss	*All steroids* monitor daily weight; note edema; monitor blood pressure; assess for signs and symptoms of hypokalemia; give potassium replacement (e.g., bananas); observe for evidence of GI bleeding	Leukemia, lymphomas, multiple myeloma, CNS metastases, hypercalcemia

Source: Adapted from Vredevoe et al., pp. 105–110.[15]

urea, and asparaginase. See Table 48-11 for comparisons, side effects, and implications for nursing care.

Immunotherapy

Cancer immunotherapy involves the introduction of substances into the body in the hope of stimulating the immune system to attack cancer cells. This new type of treatment, still under investigation, is called *biologic response modifiers* (BRM) and is aimed at stimulation of the body's antitumor responses. Three categories of substances currently included among BRMs are immunomodulators, cytokines, and monoclonal antibodies.

Immunomodulators are natural or synthetic products that enhance the immune responses of cytotoxicity of macrophages and natural killer cells. BCG, lentinan, levamisole, and bestatin are examples of these agents.

Cytokines are hormonelike molecules produced by normal cells of the body in response to endogenous or exogenous stimuli. The three types of cytokine are *lymphokines* (produced by lymphocytes, e.g., interleukin-2 and alpha and gamma interferons); *monokines* (produced by monocytes, e.g., tumor necrosis factor and interleukin-1); and *lymphotoxins.*

Monoclonal antibodies are used to regulate growth factors or to block cell surface receptors to molecules regulating tumor growth.

Interleukin-2, although not currently used for treatment of leukemia or lymphoma, the primary subjects of this chapter, deserves mention and has specific relevance for critical-care nurses because of its toxicity and severe side effects that bring the patient to the critical-care unit.

Interleukin-2 (IL-2) is used to activate killer lymphocytes. These lymphokine-activated killer (LAK) cells have been demonstrated to mediate the lysis of fresh tumor target cells but not of fresh normal cells. Clinical trials are under way to study the effectiveness of IL-2 administered alone and in combination with prepared LAK in patients with advanced metastatic cancer of the liver, kidney, or colon. Significant tumor shrinkage has been demonstrated also in three patients with melanoma who received large doses of IL-2 alone.[17]

Side effects of the administration of large doses of IL-2 include fever, chills, nausea and vomiting, diarrhea, extreme weight gain due to excessive and potentially dangerous fluid retention and extravasation, and marked esoinophilia. Central nervous system toxicity may result in confusion, disorientation, combativeness, and increased anxiety.[18]

Table 48-11 Miscellaneous and Experimental Agents

Agent	Dose and Administration	Pharmacologic Factors	Significant Side Effects and Toxicity	Nursing Interventions	Use
Procarbazine (Matulane, proc)	*Oral:* 2–4 mg/kg daily for 1 week, then 4–6 mk/kg daily until WBC count is less than 4000 or maximum response obtained; discontinue until bone marrow recovers, then 1–2 mg/kg daily	Rapid-acting; renal excretion; crosses blood-brain barrier; MAO inhibitor; cell cycle phase–nonspecific	Bone marrow suppression and immuno-suppression; nausea and vomiting; central nervous system toxicity: depression, restlessness, psychosis, somnolence, ataxia, convulsions; birth defects; hemolytic anemia	Assess signs and symptoms; protect against bleeding and infection; check blood counts; administer antiemetics; assess mental status for confusion, depression, and drowsiness; warm patient to avoid barbiturates, antihistamines, alcohol, narcotics, sedative antihypotensive agents, sympathomimetic tricyclic antidepressant drugs, ripe bananas, and cheese; provide information for contraception	Lymphomas, Hodgkin's disease
Hydroxyurea (Hydrea, O-urea)	*Oral:* 20–30 mk/kg per day or 80 mg/kg every 3 days	Metabolized by liver; renal excretion; inhibits DNA synthesis; cell cycle phase–specific	Bone marrow suppression, nausea, vomiting, stomatitis, skin reactions, alopecia	Assess signs and symptoms, protect against infection and bleeding, check blood counts, administer antiemetics, give frequent mouth care with assessment, observe skin closely, assist in coping with hair loss	Chronic myelocytic leukemia
L-Asparaginase (Elspar, L-ASP)	*Intravenous:* 1000 IU/kg per day for 10 days when used in combination therapy. *Intramuscular:* 6000 IU/m² every third day until remission	Excreted via reticuloendothelial system; destroys extracellular L-asparagine; cell cycle phase–nonspecific	Anaphylaxis, hepatic toxicity, pancreatitis, coagulopathy, CNS disturbances (hallucinations, depression)	Observe carefully for anaphylaxis (be preapred with emergency supplies); test dose in patient with prior exposure to drug	Acute lymphocytic leukemia, non-Hodgkin's lymphoma

Source: Adapted from Vredevoe et al., pp. 92, 111–114.[15]

The cardiovascular effects of IL-2 relate to the extreme weight gain due to extravasation of fluid into the extravascular space, which results in peripheral edema, abdominal ascites, and later in the course of fluid accumulation, pulmonary interstitial edema.[18] Respiratory distress may require intubation and ventilation. Hypotension is also commonly associated with IL-2 administration, because of reduction in systemic vascular resistance. Management of hypotension may require colloid solutions to restore central venous pressure, and a vasopressor such as dopamine may be required to maintain blood pressure. Aggressive fluid replacement is not indicated, as this could lead to further fluid extravasation.[18]

The ideal immunotherapy for cancer would be prophylactic, but to date, vaccines to prevent cancer have been unsuccessful. Thus accepted immunotherapy at this time is considered therapeutic and given only to persons with clinical evidence of malignant disease.

Of importance in the treatment of patients with leukemias or lymphomas is the use of transfer factor and thymosin. Both these agents are discussed in Chap. 47.

Bone Marrow Transplantation

Transplantation is considered when the patient's disease is refractory to conventional therapy and the transplant is the only hope for a cure. Bone marrow is transplanted primarily to reconstitute hematologic and immunologic function in patients who have leukemias, immunologic deficiencies, or congenital or acquired regenerative anemias.[19]

In order to increase the likelihood of a transplant being successful, the recipient must be matched with a compatible donor. Compatibility is determined on the basis of human leukocyte antigen (HLA) typing and mixed lymphocyte culture (MLC) results. The types of bone marrow transplant are syngeneic, HLA-matched allogeneic, HLA-mismatched allogeneic, and autologous.

Syngeneic transplants are those in which donor and recipient are identical twins; successful transplantation is assured. *HLA-matched allogeneic transplants* are those between compatible sibling or nonsibling donor and recipients.

HLA-mismatched donor and recipient transplants have become possible in recent years with the development of the lectin separation technique. The technique removes harmful mature T lymphocytes from the donor's marrow by agglutination with soybean lectin in a test tube. Lectin separation permits HLA–half-matched parents to be donors. With *autologous transplants,* the patient's own marrow is frozen and stored for reinfusion after chemotherapy and radiation treatments to destroy the underlying malignant growth are completed.[19]

When a compatible donor is identified, the recipient is admitted to the hospital for the purpose of immunosuppression prior to the procedure. Protection from the patient's own normal flora is also important, since the necessary degree of induced immunosuppression is severe. The patient should be admitted to a laminar airflow room; all items in the room should be cleaned with a germicidal agent. The patient should be bathed twice a day with an agent such as chlorhexidine (Hibiclens); and sterile clothing and sheets should be used. The patient's GI tract should be sterilized with nonabsorbable IV antibiotics, and female patients should receive antibacterial and antifungal agents intravaginally.

Following the procedure to eliminate normal flora, the patient undergoes immunosuppression. Immunosuppression reduces the incidence of graft rejection, removes malignant cells, and prepares bone marrow spaces for engraftment. A typical regimen includes total body irradiation (TBI) for 4 days followed by intravenous chemotherapy for 2 days. TBI is high-dose radiation given in fractionated doses (total 1320 rads). Specific chemotherapeutic agents that are commonly used include cyclophosphamide (Cytoxan), procarbazine (Matulane), and human antilymphocyte globulin.

The bone marrow for transplantation is obtained by multiple aspirations from the donor's posterior and anterior iliac crests. After the marrow has been filtered and mixed with heparinized saline, it is transferred to blood bags and transfused into the recipient over several hours via a specialized catheter in a peripheral vein. The transplant itself closely resembles a simple blood transfusion.[20]

Successful engraftment is signified by the development of erthrocytes, leukocytes, and platelets in the marrow. The white blood cell differential should indicate an increase in polymorphonucleocytes, or mature granulocytes, thus indicating that the marrow is functioning normally. These signs should appear 10 to 30 days after transplantation.[21]

The critical period for a patient who has received a bone marrow transplant is the 2 to 4 weeks after transplantation. During this time the patient is susceptible to infection, bleeding, and graft-versus-host disease (GVHD). Care of the patient susceptible to infection is discussed in Chap. 47, and care of the patient with bleeding disorders is discussed later in this chapter and in Chap. 43.

In graft-versus-host disease, the newly grafted immunocompetent cells recognize the recipient's antigens as foreign. The disease primarily affects the skin, gastrointestinal tract, and liver. GVHD may present in acute or chronic form. The earliest sign of acute GVHD is a faint red maculopapular rash occurring 7 to 14 days after transplantation, usually beginning on the face, palms, and soles of the feet and spreading to the trunk and extremities. The skin may become dry and peel or may progress to blistering.[21]

At this time the disease may stop or progress to chronic GVHD. Chronic GVHD, however, can develop without being preceded by the acute form. In chronic GVHD, which may occur 2 to 12 months after transplantation, the skin becomes firm and inelastic and may be ulcerated. Gastrointestinal involvement presents as guaiac-positive diarrhea, anorexia, nausea, vomiting, abdominal pain, and severe malabsorption. GVHD of the liver presents with hepatosplenomegaly, jaundice, and pruritus.

Systemic treatment of GVHD is aimed at reducing the number of donor lymphocytes. GVHD may first be treated with high-dose steroids; if the disease does not improve, antithymocyte globulin may then be administered. Nonsystemic treatments are aimed at alleviating the numerous manifestations of the disease.

Nursing Diagnoses and Interventions

Potential for Infection

The severe leukopenia that results from cancer chemotherapy leaves the patient at great risk of developing infection. This potential for infection is usually the most life-threatening complication of chemotherapy. Nursing interventions related to an increased potential for infection are discussed in Chap. 47. The goal of nursing care for the leukemic patient is prevention of nosocomial and/or iatrogenic infections.

Potential for Injury Related to Thrombocytopenia

Thrombocytopenia with its accompanying risk of bleeding is the second most life-threatening complication of chemotherapy. The nursing responsibilities include assessment to detect bleeding as it occurs in order to minimize the blood loss and prevention of bleeding by taking necessary precautions.

Assessment includes frequent observations for signs of bleeding from any body orifice or mucous membrane including the eyes, ears, nose, mouth, urethra, vagina, and anus. Catheters, IV sites, and nasogastric tubes should also be checked for signs of bleeding. Stools, urine, vomitus, and nasogastric drainage should be tested for blood. Any blood loss that occurs should be measured as accurately as possible by counting and weighing dressings, sanitary pads, or bed pads. Hematocrit and hemoglobin levels should be monitored in addition to platelet counts, prothrombin time, PTT, fibrin split products, and bleeding time.

Internal bleeding will not be as easily detected as external bleeding. The respiratory system should be assessed every 1 to 2 h for any signs of difficulty, including wheezing, stridor, tachypnea, cyanosis, and hemoptysis. Bleeding into the abdominal cavity may be detected by measuring abdominal girth every shift. Cerebral hemorrhage may be determined by assessing the patient for changes in mental status in addition to signs of confusion, lethargy, coma, or seizures.

The patient should also be assessed frequently for changes in pulse and blood pressure. When there is hemorrhage, the patient's pulse will increase before the blood pressure falls appreciably. The color and temperature of the extremities and the presence of peripheral pulses should also be assessed in addition to the presence of petechiae, purpura, and ecchymoses. If these signs are present, close observation for changes in color or size is warranted.

In addition to assessing for signs of bleeding, the critical-care nurse is responsible for preventing bleeding whenever possible. The patient should be protected from bruising and hematomas by padding the bed rails with blankets; by care in lifting, turning, moving, and ambulating the patient; and by padding of bony prominences or use of an alternating pressure mattress.

Intramuscular injections should be avoided whenever possible. If an injection is necessary, a small-gauge needle should be used and the medications should be injected slowly. Following the injection, pressure should be applied for 10 min; ice should then be applied for 30 min, and the site should be examined every 10 to 15 min for bleeding.[16] Rectal temperatures and suppositories should also be avoided, and the patient should be instructed to use an electric shaver in place of a razor.

Bleeding gums are a common problem. The gums may be protected by having the patient use a soft toothbrush, WaterPik, or Toothette. Some patients may be able to use only oral solutions. Currently, a normal saline or hydrogen peroxide solution appears to be most effective. In addition, patients should avoid reinserting ill-fitting dentures and should eliminate fibrous and highly spiced food from the diet.[22]

Alteration in Nutrition: Less than Body Requirements

Alteration in nutrition in the cancer patient is frequently related to the nausea, vomiting, stomatitis, and diarrhea that may accompany chemotherapy. The nausea and vomiting which occur after chemotherapy are not easily controlled by the common antiemetics; therefore, it is imperative that the critical-care nurse assist the patient to achieve adequate nutritional intake during those times when nausea and vomiting are not present. A complete assessment of dietary patterns is essential to identify total daily intake, foods most difficult to tolerate, favorite foods before onset of the illness or chemotherapy, and time periods when nausea is at a minimum.

A dietary plan for the patient may include change in seasonings, smaller portions, increased frequency of meals or snacks, timing of meals to coincide with periods when nausea is at a minimum, and favorite foods ordered out or brought from home. Since high-protein intake is important and aversion to meat is a common problem for patients receiving chemotherapy, alternatives to meat should be explored. Commercial food supplements may be used, or homemade blenderized, high-calorie, high-protein drinks with ice cream as a base may be prepared. Intravenous supplements may be essential to meet caloric and protein requirements and to prevent cachexia.

Stomatitis usually develops about 2 weeks after the start of chemotherapy at the same time that bone marrow suppression occurs. An important principle in the prevention and treatment of stomatitis is to provide mouth care every 4 h. After 6 h without mouth care, the oral mucosa begins to deteriorate. A normal saline or hydrogen peroxide solution is recommended for mouth care. Lemon juice changes the pH of the saliva and may be damaging to the teeth, and glycerin is drying to the lips and oral mucosa.[23] Viscous lidocaine (Xylocaine) may be prescribed as a mouthwash before meals to provide local anesthesia to the oral mucosa, and bland foods of moderate temperature and soft consistency in small portions may facilitate intake.

Diarrhea or abdominal cramps may be indicative of hypermotility due to mucosal damage throughout the gastrointestinal tract. In the most severe cases, ulceration, bleeding, and perforation may result. With diarrhea, it is important to record the frequency, amount, and consistency of stools. Meticulous perianal care should be provided because of the risk of infection. A bland or low-residue diet may be helpful, and drugs to decrease GI motility may be prescribed. For other patients, bowel rest must be obtained by the use of a liquid diet or total intravenous replacement.

Body Image Disturbance

The classic definition of *body image* includes both the postural model of the body and also the perceptions, attitudes, emotions, and personality reactions of the individual in relation to his or her body.[24] Body image develops as a result of topologic, behavioral, and somatic bodily experiences, interacting with cultural and environmental variables and the attitudes of parents, society, the peer group, and significant others. The way in which these variables interact to create a body image depends upon a person's developmental stage. As a person's body image becomes more clearly delineated with maturity, an illness or handicap may become more difficult to incorporate into that image.[25]

Patients with cancer may have an abstract perception of their bodies being attacked by the unseen and uncontrollable cancer cells, or they may have a very concrete indicator of change as demonstrated by severe weight loss and/or alopecia.

Assessment of the patient with a disturbance in body image should include determining the patient's feelings about self before and since the condition occurred; the value placed on beauty, self-control, wholeness, and activity and the value given to others' reactions; the meaning of the body part affected; the knowledge and awareness of the extent of the condition; and the mechanisms used in adapting to the condition and its implications.[26]

Nursing intervention to help patients with a threat to or change in body image involves helping to reintegrate their self-view and self-esteem in relation to the condition. Strategies which may be helpful in achieving this outcome include:[27]

1. Visiting the patient frequently and recognizing him or her as someone who is worthwhile.
2. Providing opportunities for listening to concerns and questions.
3. Acknowledging and accepting feelings of dependency, grief, and hostility.
4. Providing accurate information as desired or requested.
5. Encouraging the patient to make decisions and to identify and accept his or her own strengths as well as inadequacies.
6. Setting limits on maladaptive behavior, while assisting the patient to identify positive behaviors that will aid in recovery.
7. Assisting significant others to cope with the patient's changes in appearance.
8. Discussing the availability of support groups or therapy as indicated.

References

1. Sites, D. P., Stobo, J. D., & Wells, J. V. (1987). *Basic and clinical immunology* (6th ed.). Los Altos, CA: Appleton and Lange.
2. Bellanti, J. (1985). *Immunology III.* Philadelphia: Saunders.
3. Nurses' Clinical Library. (1985). *Neoplastic disorders.* Springhouse, PA: Springhouse.
4. Nurses' Clinical Library. (1985). *Immune disorders.* Springhouse, PA: Springhouse.
5. Ultmann, J. E., & Jacobs, R. H. (1985). The non-Hodgkin's lymphoma. *Ca-A Cancer Journal for Clinicians, 35,* 66–87. New York: American Cancer Society.
6. Lacher, M. J. (1985). Hodgkins disease: Historical perspective, current status and future directions. *Ca-A Cancer Journal for Clinicians, 35.* 88–94, New York: American Cancer Society.
7. Lukes, R. J., & Collins, R. D. (1975). New approaches to the classification of the lymphomata. *British Journal of Cancer 31*(Suppl. II), 1–28.
8. Aisenberg, A. C., et al. (1983). Monoclonal antibody studies in non-Hodgkin's lymphoma. *Blood, 61,* 469–475.
9. Whang-Pereg, J., & Turid, K. (1986). Cytogenetic methods in hematologic disease. *Lab Management, 24,* 19–26.
10. Schroff, R. W., et al. (1982). Immunologic classification of lymphatic leukemias based on monoclonal antibody-defined cell surface antigens. *Blood, 59,* 207–215.
11. Aisenberg, A. C. (1981). Cell surface markers in lymphoproliferative disease. *New England Journal of Medicine, 304,* 331–335.
12. Bishop, C. (1984). Immunoassay in hematology. *Journal of Medical Technology, 1,* 41–45.
13. Sallan, S. E., et al. (1980). Cell surface antigens: Prognostic implications in childhood acute lymphoblastic leukemia. *Blood, 55,* 395–401.
14. Ozer, H. (1985, May, no. 14). Immunoregulatory defects in multiple myeloma. *Clinical Immunology Today,* pp. 1–3.
15. Vredevoe, D. L., et al. (1981). *Concepts of oncology nursing.* Englewood Cliffs, NJ: Prentice-Hall.
16. Burns, N. (1982). *Nursing and cancer.* Philadelphia: Saunders.
17. Rosenberg, S. A., & Lotze, M. (1986). Cancer immunotherapy using interleukin-2 and interleukin-2 activated lymphocytes. *Annual Review of Immunology,* 4: 681–709.
18. Jassak, P., & Sticklin, L. (1986). Interleukin-2: An overview. *Oncology Nursing Forum, 13*(6), 17–22.
19. Nucher, R., et al. (1984). Bone marrow transplantation. *American Journal of Nursing, 84:* 764.
20. Nucher, R., et al. (1984). Bone marrow transplantation: The procedure. *American Journal of Nursing, 84:* 768–769.
21. Nucher, R., et al. (June, 1984). Bone marrow transplantation: Complications. *American Journal of Nursing, 84,* 770–772.

22. Griffin, J. (June 1986). Be prepared for the bleeding patient. *Nursing, 16*: 34–40.

23. Daeffler, R. (December 1980). Oral hygiene measures for patients with cancer, II. *Cancer Nursing, 3*: 427–432.

24. Kolb, L. (1959). Disturbances in body image. In *American Handbook of Psychiatry* (vol. 1, p. 750). New York: Basic Books.

25. Brown, M. A. (1977). The nursing process and distortions or changes in body image. In F. L. Bowes (Ed.) *Distortions in body image in illness and disability* (pp. 7–9). New York: Wiley.

26. Murray, R., & Zentner, J. (1985). *Nursing assessment and health promotion through the life span* (pp. 441–442). Englewood Cliffs, NJ: Prentice-Hall.

27. Doenges, M., & Moorhouse, M. (1985). *Nurses pocket guide: Nursing diagnoses and interventions* (pp. 220–224). Philadelphia: Davis.

part

11

Gastrointestinal Patient-Care Problems

49

Anatomy and Physiology of the Gastrointestinal System

Patricia Kallweit Kaldor

Anatomy

From its earliest embryologic state, the gastrointestinal (GI) tract emerged as a simple system. By a natural, yet dramatic, sequence of embryologic foldings, the primitive foregut, midgut, and hindgut evolved into a continuous muscular tube modified along its length by diverse secretory glands. Each segment of the basic tube—be it esophagus, stomach, small intestine, or colon—is anatomically specialized for a unique physiologic role.

The alimentary tract holds a unique position among body systems. Food and water are taken in, processed, absorbed, and delivered in an orderly, efficient sequence of physical and biochemical events. In a coordinated response, the digestive secretions of the salivary glands, the pancreas, the liver, and the gallbladder contribute to the conversion of food and water into metabolic energy and substrates.

This chapter is designed to follow an orderly anatomic course down the alimentary tract (Fig. 49-1). Beginning at the mouth and terminating at the colon, the anatomy of each organ is discussed for its unique contribution to gastrointestinal physiology. Structure and function are critically reviewed.

The extrinsic glands are discussed as they are encountered along the digestive tract. The liver and the pancreas are each presented in two parts. The exocrine pancreas and the biliary system are discussed in the context of their digestive functions, separately from the endocrine pancreas and the remaining hepatic functions.

Histologic Layers

Before beginning the anatomic descent down the alimentary tract, a review of basic gastrointestinal histology will be helpful. With few exceptions, all the tubular portions of the alimentary canal have the same histologic structure (Fig. 49-2); significant differences are noted.

The histologic layers of the digestive tube may be outlined as follows (proceeding from the innermost outward):

I. Mucosa
   A. Epithelium
   B. Lamina propria
   C. Muscularis mucosae
II. Submucosa
III. Muscularis externa
   A. Inner circular fibers
   B. Outer longitudinal fibers
IV. Serosa or adventitia

Mucosa

The mucosa is composed of three sublayers. From the inside outward they are the epithelial layer, the lamina propria, and the muscularis mucosae.

The *epithelium* varies throughout the tube. Squamous epithelium lines the mouth and the anus, while columnar epithelium is found everywhere else. The common columnar epithelium is often modified to better meet the needs of the individual organs.

The *lamina propria* is loosely arranged connective tissue support, often rich in capillaries. The *muscularis mucosae* is smooth muscle only. It receives sympathetic innervation and is responsible for local mucosal foldings.

Submucosa

This second major layer of the gut wall contains dense connective tissue fibers, blood vessels, and nerve fibers. Meissner's plexus is a collection of parasympathetic nerves found in this layer. Fibers

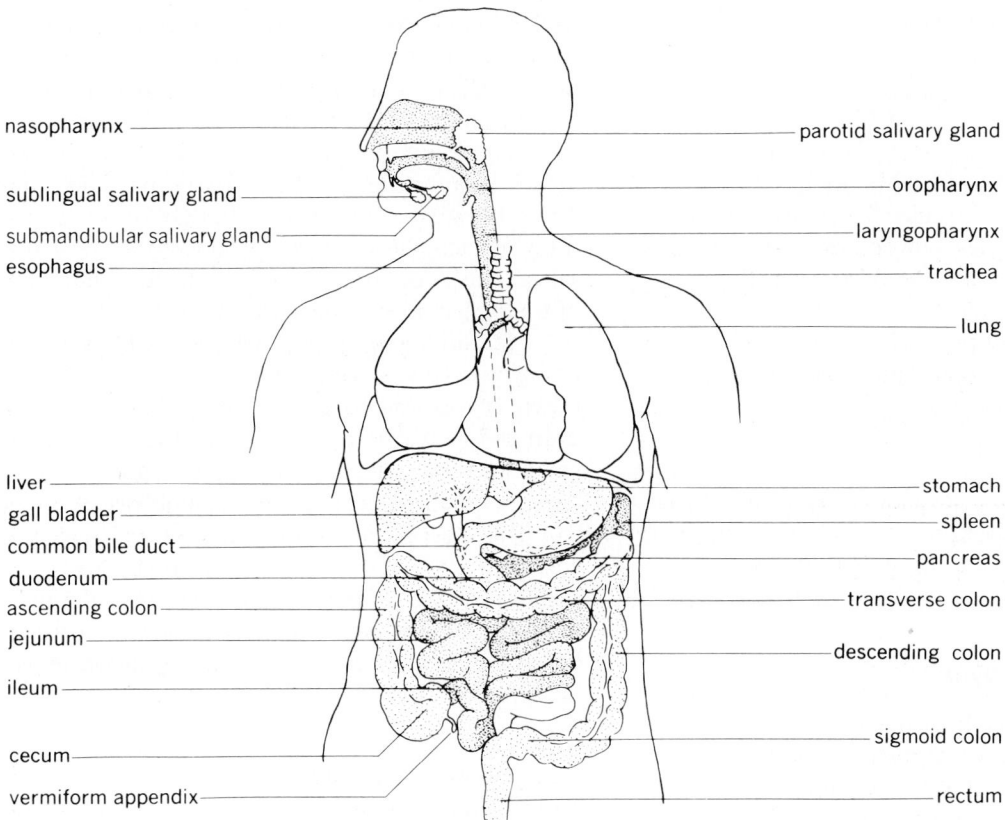

Figure 49-1   General topography of the digestive tract. *(From R. M. DeCoursey, The Human Organism, McGraw-Hill, New York, 1974.)*

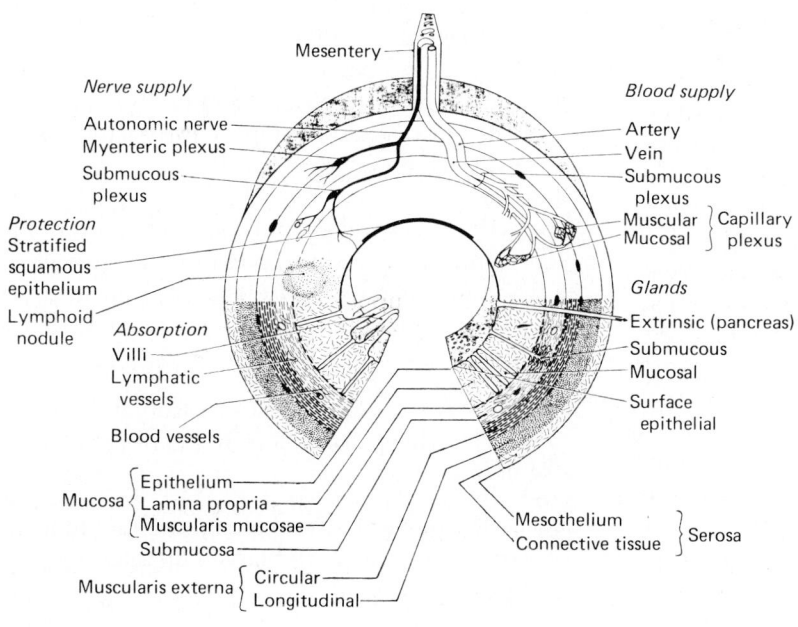

Figure 49-2   Histology of the gastrointestinal tract. *(Adapted from R. Passmore and J. S. Robson, A Companion to Medical Studies, vol. 1, Blackwell, Oxford, 1971.)*

from this plexus stimulate the secretions of mucosal glands.

Muscularis Externa

This is the major muscular layer of the wall. Normally it is composed of smooth muscle, arranged as an inner circular layer and an outer longitudinal layer. The myenteric nerve plexus (Auerbach's plexus) is located between these two layers. It is responsible for muscular contractions of the wall. The esophagus, stomach, and colon have significant variations of the muscularis externa; they are discussed later.

Serosa or Adventitia

This is the outermost layer of the gut wall. It may be continuous with the surrounding connective tissue as the adventitia, or it may be completely separate. If separate, it is named the *serosa.*

Mouth and Oropharynx

The alimentary tract begins with the mouth and oropharynx. The oral cavity includes the lips, cheeks, gums, palate, tongue, teeth, and salivary glands. Its main functions are ingestion, mastication, salivation, and the first stage of deglutition (swallowing).

Tongue

The tongue is a highly muscular organ. It is important for normal speech and for initiation of mastication and deglutition.

The lingual surface is covered with a specialized, durable squamous epithelium. This is further modified by visible clusters of cells called *papillae.* Within these papillae, specialized sensory cells, or *taste buds,* are found: the circumvallate, the foliate, and the fungiform papillae are mentioned by name because they contain the majority of the taste buds. Branches of the vagus nerve, along with two other cranial nerves, innervate the taste buds and mediate taste sensation.

Salivary Glands

A person secretes between 0.5 and 1 L of saliva per day. The composition is 99 percent water and 1 percent glycoprotein (*mucin*) and amylase.

Salivary secretion is regulated by nervous innervation alone. There are pressure receptors as well as chemoreceptors which stimulate salivary secretion. Both the parasympathetic and sympathetic nervous systems are involved, mainly via the afferent fibers of the vagus nerve.

There are three major pairs of salivary glands in the mouth: the parotid, the submaxillary, and the sublingual (Fig. 49-1). Though histologically distinct, each pair of glands produces the substance saliva. This aqueous secretion facilitates the mixing of food early in the digestive process.

In addition, these glands synthesize an α-amylase. This enzymatic protein causes the breakdown of polysaccharides to disaccharides. Thus, even before carbohydrates reach the stomach or small intestine, their digestion has begun.

Normally, saliva has an alkaline pH of about 7.0. This keeps the saliva saturated with calcium and prevents loss of calcium from the teeth. In addition, saliva is rich in the secretory immunoglobulin IgA, which plays an important role in control of oral bacterial growth and again promotes healthy dentition.

Mastication and Deglutition

The mechanics of mastication involve biting off and chewing with the teeth; mixing the food bolus with mucins, amylase, and other glandular secretions, mainly by the actions of the tongue; and finally the backward propulsion of the bolus toward the oropharynx as deglutition or swallowing is initiated.

The reflex of deglutition requires 25 muscles, lasts 1 to 2 s, and begins as the food bolus reaches the oropharynx. The process can be thought of as an organized cascade of steps, each giving rise to the next (Fig. 49-3):

Step 1–The backward propulsion of the food bolus stimulates pressure receptors in the wall of the oropharynx. These afferent signals go to the "swallowing center" in the medulla of the brain.

Step 2–The soft palate elevates to seal off the nasal cavity. This protects it from the reflux of food and liquids.

Step 3–The central "swallowing center" inhibits respiration while the larynx elevates and the glottis closes.

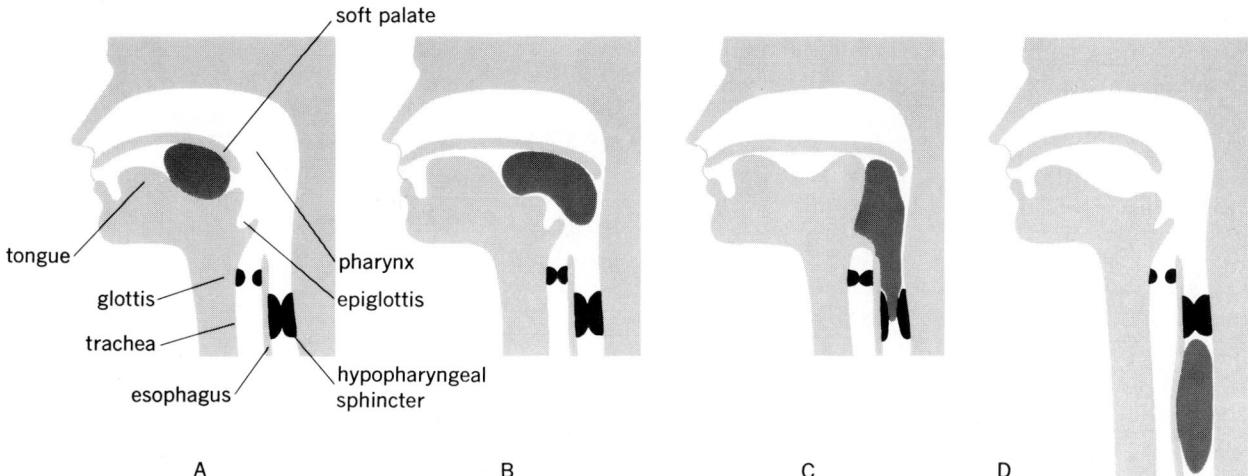

Figure 49-3   Movement of a bolus of food through the pharynx and upper esophagus during swallowing. *(From A. J. Vander, J. H. Sherman, and D. Luciano, Human Physiology, McGraw-Hill, New York, 1975.)*

Step 4–The central nervous system signals contraction of the upper esophageal sphincter, causing opening of the esophageal orifice. The food bolus then passes into the esophagus.

Step 5–Once in the esophagus, food passes into the stomach by peristaltic contractions.

Esophagus

The primary role of the esophagus is to act as a conduit for the passage of food and liquid from the mouth to the stomach. For the 25-cm length of the esophagus, no absorption takes place and only residual carbohydrate digestion from salivary amylase occurs. Clearly, the unique role of the esophagus depends upon wall motility and the competence of its upper and lower sphincters.

Gross Anatomy

Anatomically, the esophagus is primarily located within the thoracic cavity. It is crossed anteriorly by the left bronchus. At the same level, it is also in close proximity to the aortic arch.

The arterial supply to the esophagus delivers separate vessels to each section of the organ. Thus the upper third, the middle third, and the lower third are independent.

Another outstanding anatomic feature of the esophagus is the venous drainage. There are two major sets of vessels: one a large plexus on the surface, the other deeper within the esophageal wall. These two vascular groups come together below the diaphragm and merge with veins draining the stomach. Since the venous system of the stomach ultimately drains into the liver, the veins of the stomach, and therefore of the esophagus, are subject to increased pressure and flow if normal hepatic circulation is obstructed. Thus, if a patient develops portal hypertension (elevation of pressure in the portal vein secondary to obstructed flow) from whatever cause (e.g., cirrhosis), blood flow will be shunted to the esophageal veins, causing massive dilatation of these vessels. These veins, known as *esophageal varices,* carry tremendous quantities of blood under very elevated pressures. They are prone to rupture easily. Massive hemorrhage from ruptured esophageal varices is a major complication and a potential cause of death for patients with portal hypertension.

Histology

Histologically, the mucosa of the esophageal lumen contains squamous epithelium. It is poorly modified for food absorption and has only rare mucous-producing glands throughout its wall. No major digestive enzymes are secreted by the esophagus.

Unlike the other gastrointestinal organs, the upper third of the esophagus contains only skeletal muscle in the muscularis externa; the lower two-thirds has only smooth muscle. The outer muscle layer of the esophagus runs longitudinally. This evolutionary change facilitates the voluntary aspect of swallowing.

Stomach

Unlike the esophagus, the stomach provides several major digestive functions in addition to mechanical mixing and transport of food. This organ produces important digestive secretions. It has a small but recognizable role in selected absorptive activities and provides a reservoir for partially digested food. Chyme is retained in the stomach until it is sufficiently altered, both physically and chemically, to permit further digestion in the first part of the small intestine, the duodenum.

The stomach has a much greater secretory capacity than the esophagus. The hormones, acid, mucus, water, and electrolytes secreted by the stomach mix and interact while chyme is retained in the stomach.

In the stomach itself, little absorption of foodstuffs occurs. Most of the particles are large and ionically charged, making their diffusion across the cell membrane difficult. Because of the stomach's acid environment, substances which are weak acids convert to their noncharged, nonionic form. Under these conditions, they are easily absorbed. Thus a weak acid, such as acetylsalicylic acid (aspirin), is rapidly absorbed in the stomach. Though most alcohol absorption occurs in the small intestine, some occurs in the stomach as well.

Beyond its role in digestion, the stomach also has some antibacterial function. The acidity of the stomach is partially responsible for this phenomenon, but certain aspects remain to be explained. This mild antibacterial control helps to keep the environment of the small intestine sterile.

Gross Anatomy
The stomach is located at the distal end of the esophagus. It is divided into five regions (Fig. 49-4):

1. The *cardia* is the part adjacent to the esophagus.
2. The *fundus* rises above the cardia and merges with the main part of the stomach.

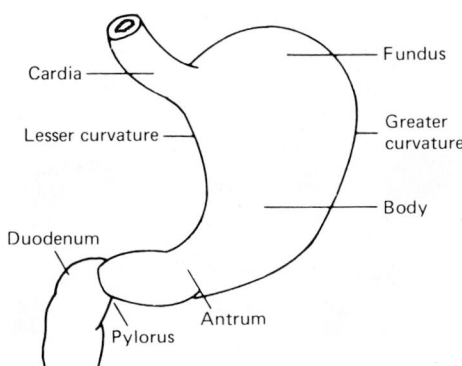

Figure 49-4 Gross anatomy of the stomach. *(Adapted from W. F. Ganong, Review of Medical Physiology, 8th ed., Lange, Los Altos, CA, 1977.)*

3. The major portion of the stomach is the *body*.
4. That area of the stomach immediately before the pylorus is the *antrum*.
5. The *pylorus* is the muscular sphincter between the stomach and the duodenum.

On gross inspection of the stomach, one finds muscular walls thrown into multiple folds, or *rugae*. These folds increase the actual surface area of the organ, and together with the muscular nature of the organ, allow for greater expansion of the stomach. The usual capacity is 1 to 1.5 L.

The major arterial blood supply of the stomach arises from the celiac artery directly off the aorta. Sympathetic nerve fibers from the celiac plexus and parasympathetic fibers, principally from the vagus nerve, innervate the stomach. Parasympathetic tone predominates.

Histology
Histologically, the mucosal surface of the stomach is lined with columnar epithelium. Most importantly, this surface itself is a continuous flow of involutions and convolutions forming deep gastric pits. The gastric pits are important because they increase the overall surface area and because they house the many secretory glands of the stomach. Note also that the muscularis externa of the stomach differs from other gastrointestinal organs. It has an additional layer of muscle. This third layer is arranged in an oblique fashion and forms the innermost fibers of the muscularis externa.

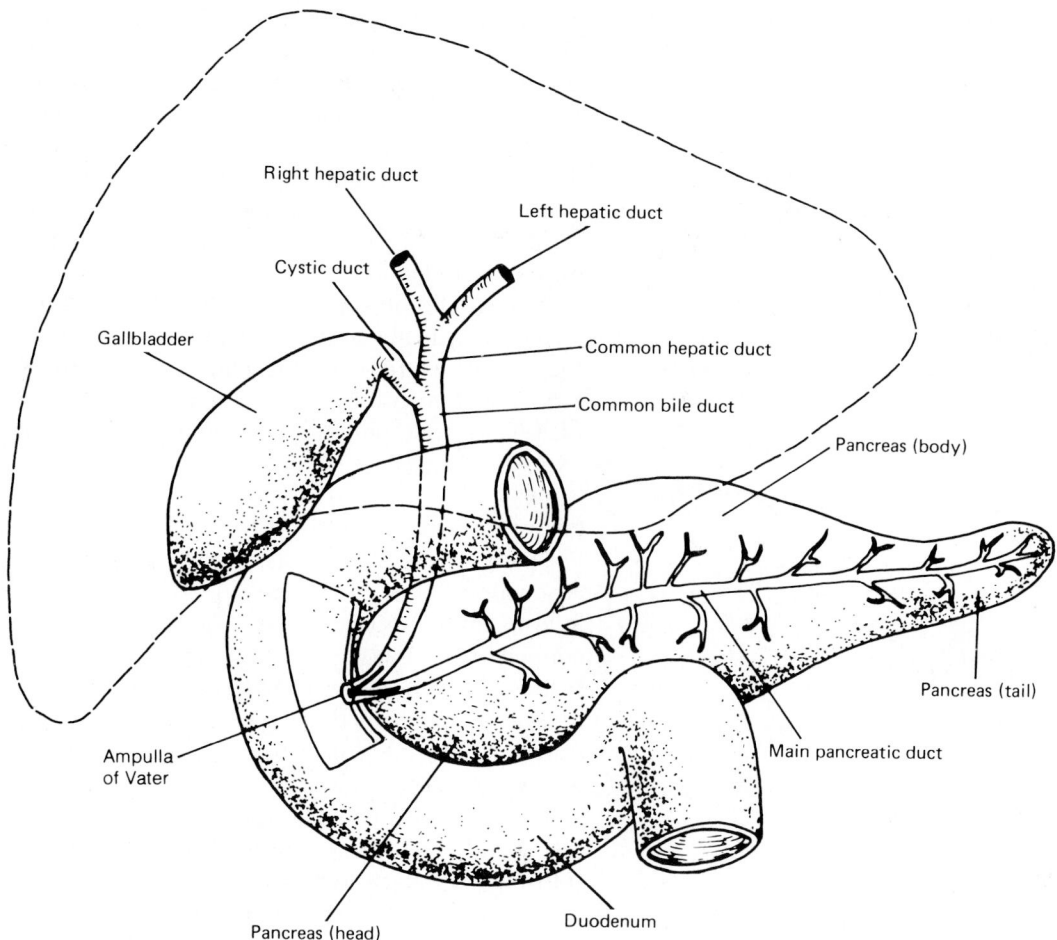

Figure 49-5 Connecting ducts of the liver, gallbladder, and pancreas.

Exocrine Pancreas and Biliary System

In order to facilitate the study of intestinal digestion and absorption, a short anatomic digression is helpful. Rather than descending the alimentary tract in its strict anatomic outline, the discussion focuses on the structure and function of the exocrine pancreas* and the biliary system. Understanding the contributions of these two auxiliary systems is critical to subsequent discussion of gastrointestinal physiology.

Only that part of the pancreas and the liver relevant to digestion are presented here. Further along in the chapter, the other diversified functions of the liver and pancreas are outlined and discussed.

Gross Anatomy of the Exocrine Pancreas

The pancreas is a large gland, with both endocrine and exocrine activity. It is located retroperitoneally (posterior to the peritoneum) within the abdominal cavity. It is divided into a head, a body, and a tail. The head lies within the C-shaped portion of the duodenum. The body or main portion of the gland is posterior to the stomach (Fig. 49-5). The tail extends to the spleen. Unlike the liver and the

---

*Glands are considered *endocrine* if the hormones they synthesize are secreted directly into the blood. They are called *exocrine* if they secrete hormones into a nonvascular system of ducts.

other abdominal organs, the pancreas has no defined protective external capsule.

The arterial blood supply of the pancreas is rich and comes principally from the celiac and superior mesenteric arteries. Sympathetic nerves from the celiac plexus and parasympathetic fibers from the vagus nerve innervate the organ.

Histology of the Exocrine Pancreas

The overall microscopic structure of the whole gland is complex (Fig. 49-6). The principal component is a system of lobules separated by connective tissue septa. Within this multilobulated structure, small grapelike glands called *acinar glands* are found. They are accompanied by a partner system of collecting ducts. These ducts branch into an almost endless array of small ductules. The ductules, in turn, merge to form larger ducts which eventually coalesce and form the major pancreatic duct of Wirsung. The duct of Wirsung then empties into the duodenum.

It should be kept in mind that this combined system of acinar glands and connecting ducts belongs only to the exocrine pancreas. The microscopic anatomy of the endocrine pancreas is completely separate and has no connection with the exocrine duct gland system.

Biliary System

For the purpose of understanding fat digestion and absorption in the intestine, the discussion now focuses on the biliary system. This vast network of connecting channels and ducts involves the gallbladder as well as the biliary passages of the liver. Among its many functions, the liver synthesizes and transports the bile salts and bile pigments needed for fat digestion.

From both an anatomic and a functional level, the liver is extremely complex. However, for the purposes of the present discussion, only the biliary component of the liver is included here. Again it should be remembered that this is only a small part of a complex organ. Further along in the chapter, liver structure and function are presented.

Bile is synthesized by the liver cell, or *hepatocyte.* Then it is secreted into *bile canaliculi* or ductules which lie adjacent to the liver cells. The bile canaliculi have many orders of branching and eventually merge to form the right and left hepatic ducts within the liver. After exiting from the liver, these two ducts join and become the common hepatic duct. The cystic duct, a continuation of the gallbladder normally about 4 cm long that carries bile from the gallbladder, joins the common hepatic duct and becomes the common bile duct. The common bile duct and the major pancreatic duct merge at the ampulla of Vater and enter the small intestine through the duodenal papilla (Fig. 49-5).

The *gallbladder* is responsible for the storage and concentration of bile. Located on the undersurface of the right lobe of the liver, the adult

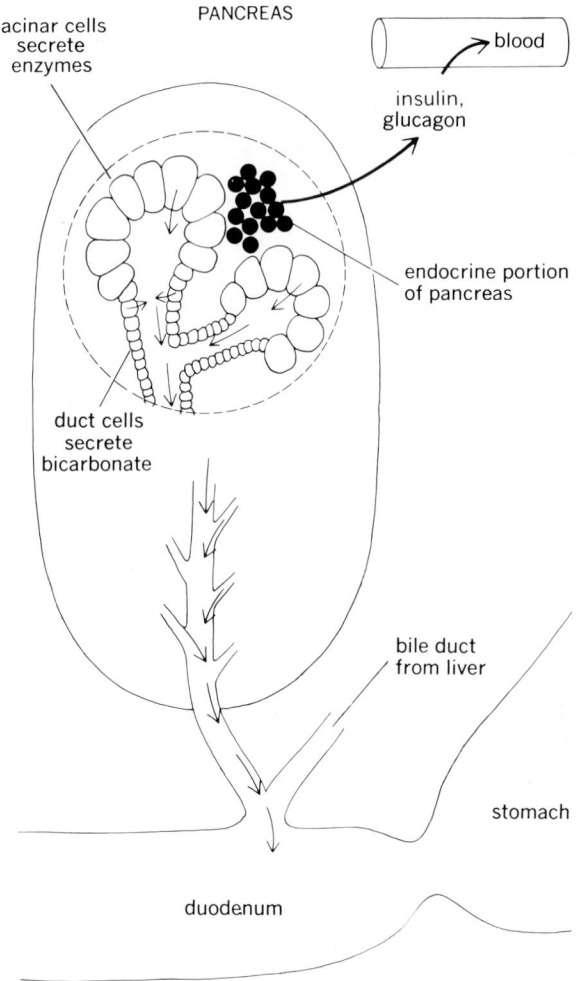

Figure 49-6 Endocrine and exocrine structure of the pancreas. *(From A. J. Vander, J. H. Sherman, and D. Luciano, Human Physiology, McGraw-Hill, New York, 1975.)*

gallbladder has a capacity of 30 to 50 mL. Between meals, bile reaches the gallbladder from the liver by way of the interconnecting duct system.

Like the duodenal papilla, the common bile duct also has a muscular sphincter surrounding its orifice. As the sphincter opens and closes, it determines the amount of bile that will pass through from the gallbladder and liver. Note that unlike the common bile duct, the pancreatic duct has no separate muscular sphincter. Hypothetically, this anatomic difference may make the pancreas more susceptible to bile reflux under certain circumstances. As a result, subsequent inflammation and pancreatitis may occur.

The arterial blood supply of the gallbladder comes from the cystic artery. Most frequently this is a branch off the right hepatic artery. Venous drainage is via the cystic vein into the portal vein.

Histologically, the gallbladder mucosa is remarkable for the many invaginations which characterize its surface. The crypts or pockets formed are of variable depth and during disease states are favored spots for bacterial retention and multiplication. Normally bile is sterile.

In addition to the storage facility of the gallbladder, rapid absorption of water and certain electrolytes occurs there as well. Consequently, the bile found in the gallbladder is more concentrated than that found within the bile ducts of the liver. Occasionally these shifts in bile concentration, coupled with other incompletely understood mechanisms, cause precipitation of bile components with resultant formation of gallstones.

Small Intestine

The small intestine comprises some 3 m of tubing coiled within the abdominal cavity. It extends from the stomach to the ileocecal valve, where the colon, or large intestine, begins.

Together the three parts of the small intestine—the duodenum, the jejunum, and the ileum—are responsible for most digestion and absorption. Almost all food types, as well as water and vitamins, are processed and absorbed before they reach the large intestine.

Mechanical transit of intestinal material, though less important than in other gastrointestinal organs, is still a specialized function of the small intestine.

A mixing action predominates as the most important motor activity.

Like other GI organs, the small intestine has a secretory role. But again, its unique contribution to gastrointestinal function is digestion and absorption, not secretion.

Gross Anatomy

The first and the shortest segment of the small intestine is the duodenum. Normally about 20 cm long, the duodenum is critical because of its hormonal secretions; because of its anatomic proximity to the connecting ducts of the liver, gallbladder, and pancreas; and because of its unfortunate predisposition to ulcerative disease.

Continuing after the duodenum is the jejunum. Anatomically the jejunum is defined as beginning at the ligament of Trietz.

The remainder of the small intestine, the ileum, terminates at the ileocecal valve. In addition to its role in routine nutrient absorption, the ileum also absorbs vitamin B_{12} and bile salts. Together the jejunum and the ileum usually measure 2 to 3 m in length.

Because of the important absorptive capacity of the small bowel, adequate blood supply to this organ is critical. As a result, even at rest, the small bowel has a blood flow of 1 L/min, or one-fifth of the total resting cardiac output.

The sole arterial blood supply of the ileum and jejunum is the superior mesenteric artery. The duodenum is supplied by several different vessels. Because of this anatomic difference, occlusion of the superior mesenteric artery may lead to infarction and death of the entire ileum and jejunum. However, the duodenum, with multiple blood sources, is less likely to suffer the same catastrophic event if part of its arterial supply is cut off.

The venous drainage of the small intestine is noteworthy because, as mentioned before, it is part of the enterohepatic circulation. All venous blood leaving the intestine, rich in absorbed food and vitamin nutrients, passes through the liver before reaching the heart. In the liver the hepatocytes extract what they need and detoxify noxious products. Venous blood then continues to the heart.

Both branches of the autonomic nervous system innervate the small intestine. Extrinsic fibers meet in the various plexuses within the intestinal wall. Reflex pathways also contribute to overall functioning.

The lymphatic system of the small bowel is important because of its central role in fat absorption. In the ileum large collections of lymph nodules, called *Peyer's patches,* are grouped together within the intestinal wall.

Histology

The microanatomy of the small bowel is specifically designed to maximize the absorptive functions of this organ. The inner surface of the entire intestine is folded, thus increasing the absorptive surface area for the first time. The surface of each fingerlike projection thus formed is itself covered with multiple small invaginations and projections called *villi.*

The surface area has increased for the second time. Finally, each villus consists of epithelial cells, each of which is covered with thousands of hairlike projections called *microvilli.* The absorbing surface has been increased for a third time. The net result of this multiplication system is that the surface area of the small intestine is almost 30 times greater than that defined by the original luminal surface alone (Fig. 49-7).

The villus is the main structural unit of the small bowel. It is constantly in motion, following rhythmic contractions within the muscle layer of the wall. The contractions alter the length, and therefore the surface area, of the villus. Thousands of microvilli, anchored in the surface epithelial cells, cover the surface of each villus. The microvilli

Figure 49-7 Structure of small intestine villus. *(From A. J. Vander, J. H. Sherman, and D. Luciano, Human Physiology, Mc-Graw-Hill, New York, 1975.)*

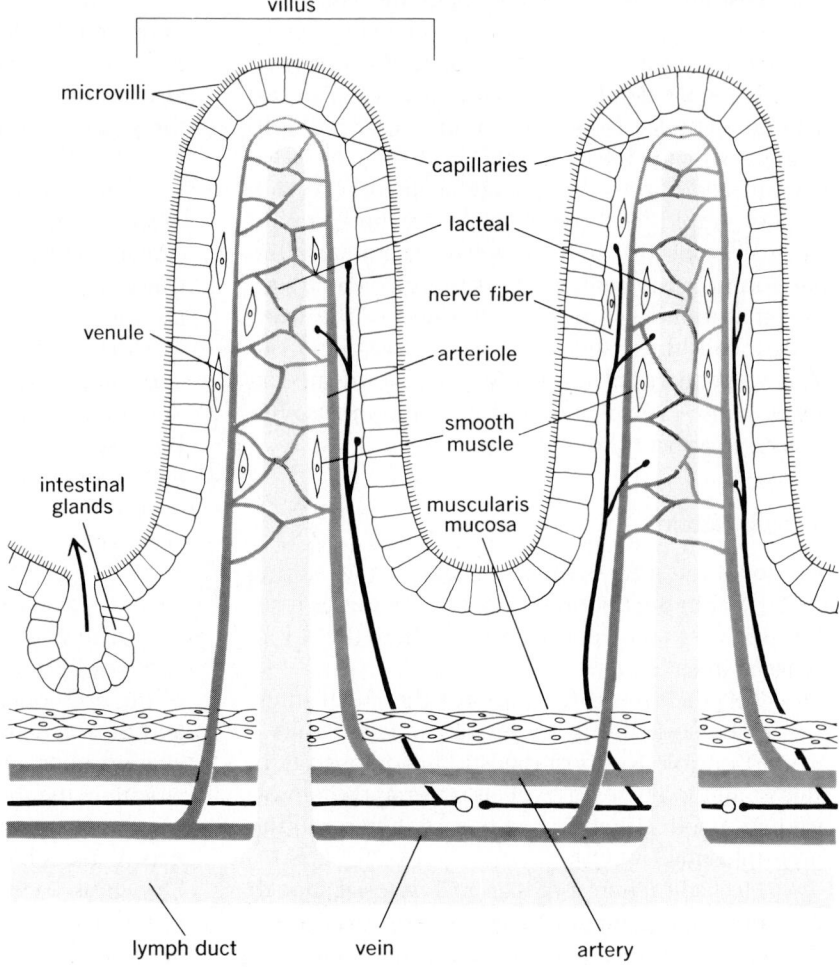

themselves contain certain enzymes needed for further nutrient digestion. In the center of the villus are found the artery, vein, nerve, and lymph vessel, or lacteal (Fig. 49-7).

The intestinal lining cells have one of the most rapid turnover rates in the body. New cells from the base of the villus migrate up to the top and replace old, worn cells that are sloughed off into the intestinal lumen. The entire intestinal epithelium is replaced every 36 h. The mechanisms controlling this enormous mitotic and migratory activity are complex and as yet incompletely understood.

Large Intestine

Just as the mouth gives entrance to the gastrointestinal tract, the colon provides an exit. When digested materials reach the colon and are expelled, the circuit is completed.

The colon, some 150 cm long, carries intestinal contents to the end of the gastrointestinal tract. Together with its terminal portions, the rectum and the anus, the colon is responsible for mucus secretion and water and electrolyte absorption. The colon houses the natural bowel flora that is important to particular metabolic pathways and that under certain conditions can lead to life-threatening infections.

The final result of all colonic function is the production of stool. Normally, stool is one-quarter solid and three-quarters liquid. Its brownish color is attributed to the products of hemoglobin degradation. Its characteristic odor results from certain bacterial metabolites, especially the amine compounds. The bulk of the stool is composed of cellulose and indigestible fibers, bacteria, degenerated cellular debris, fat, and inorganic material.

Gross Anatomy

The large intestine begins just distal to the iliocecal valve. The cecum is the blind pouch which begins the colon (Fig. 49-8). The vermiform appendix is a small outpouching off the cecum. The major part of the colon is divided anatomically into four divisions: the ascending, the transverse, the descending, and the sigmoid, or S-shaped, colon. Following the sigmoid colon are the rectum and the anus.

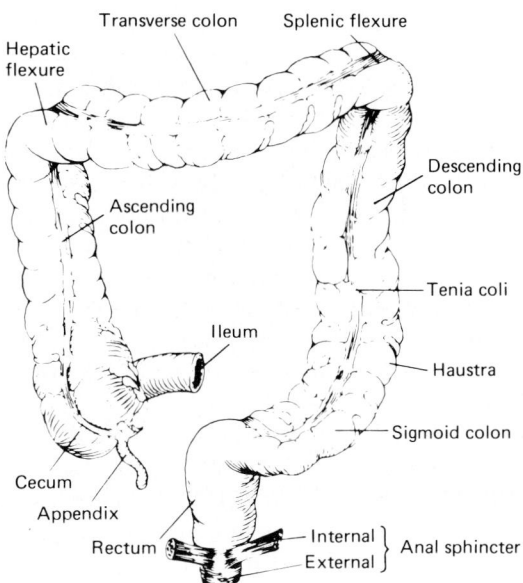

Figure 49-8   The human colon. *(Adapted from W. F. Ganong, Review of Medical Physiology, 8th ed., Lange, Los Altos, 1977.)*

The muscular iliocecal valve separates the small and large bowel. At the distal end of the large bowel are two other regulating sphincters, the internal and the external anal sphincters. They play an important role in regulating defecation.

Grossly, the colon is a wider-diameter tube than the small intestine. Inspection of the colon reveals an outer longitudinal muscle layer separated into three fiber tracts. The three muscular bundles eventually fan out at the rectum and form a complete muscle coat. These longitudinal bands, called *teniae coli*, are shorter than the colon itself. This difference in length, coupled with the contractions of the inner muscle layer, causes outpouchings of the colonic wall called *haustra*. The haustra and the teniae give the colon its unique gross appearance (Fig. 49-8).

The internal anal sphincter is a continuation of the inner muscle layer. It is under involuntary control. The external sphincter is a separate skeletal muscle. Unlike the internal sphincter, it is not an extension of the smooth muscle in the colonic wall. It extends the entire length of the anus and is under voluntary control.

The colonic blood supply originates from the superior and inferior mesenteric arteries. The venous system parallels the arterial system and is noteworthy because of the plexus of veins formed around the anus. This plexus, like the one at the base of the esophagus, may become tortuous and dilated. The resulting hemorrhoids are a frequent development in many people. They are of special interest and concern in patients with portal hypertension. Just as esophageal varices are prone to rupture when blood is shunted away from the liver, so too are the varices of the rectal plexus. The incidence of life-threatening hemorrhage from rectal varices is significantly lower than that from esophageal varices, however.

The nervous innervation of the colon, like that of the other gastrointestinal organs, contains both parasympathetic and sympathetic fibers. Parasympathetic input has variable consequences, and the overall impact is not clearly worked out. Sympathetic fibers apparently have more effect on colonic vasculature than on colonic muscle tone. Again, the exact role of this adrenergic stimulus is not clear.

Histology

The microscopic anatomy of the colon is less specialized than the details seen in the small intestine. There are relatively fewer foldings of the mucosa, and there are no villi or microvilli in the colon.

Columnar cells line the colonic mucosa, but as one approaches the anus, a more rugged stratified squamous epithelium covers the surface. Mucus-producing glands are found throughout the colon. Their viscous secretions are important lubricants for passage of fecal material.

Endocrine Pancreas

Microscopic inspection of pancreatic tissue reveals an intricate network of acinar glands and their connecting duct system. This system is pertinent to the *exocrine* function of the gland and eventually connects with the small intestine lumen.

The endocrine pancreas does not participate in this system. Instead, small islands of endocrine tissue are scattered throughout the gland (Fig. 49-6). These islands are called *islets of Langerhans*. The endocrine pancreas constitutes 1 to 2 percent of total pancreatic weight. Normally the adult pancreas has 1 to 2 million islets. Though they are found throughout the gland, the tail of the pancreas has a higher concentration of islets than the body or head.

Liver

The liver, the largest gland in the human body, occupies an esteemed and essential role in body physiology. To even begin to understand hepatic structure and function, one must concentrate and focus on the detailed microscopic anatomy, the unique vascular circuits, and the endless, always interconnecting channels found throughout the hepatic parenchyma.

The goal here is to present certain salient features of the liver as they relate to unique hepatic functions. For the reader who wishes more detailed and specialized discussions, the medical literature is replete with books devoted solely to the liver.

The liver represents one-fiftieth of total body weight in the adult. Functionally, this organ has five interrelated yet anatomically definable components:

The parenchymal liver cell, or hepatocyte, is responsible for the major synthetic and storage functions of the organ.

A well-developed and extensive *reticuloendothelial system* throughout the liver provides an effective body-defense barrier against foreign intrusion. In fact, the defense system of the liver constitutes some 60 percent of the total body reticuloendothelial system.

The *hepatic biliary system* is responsible for the synthesis and transport of the bile salts and pigments to the gallbladder. The details of hepatic bile metabolism have already been presented in the context of fat digestion and absorption.

A vast *circulatory system* pervades the liver. One of the few organs with a dual blood supply, the liver must care for its own well-being and simultaneously deal with the metabolic end products of almost the entire gastrointestinal system and spleen.

The *connective tissue reticulum* of the liver provides the structural support for all the other components. A healthy hepatic reticulum promotes an environment for hepatocyte regeneration in cases of disease and injury. With absent or damaged connective tissue stroma, the normal liver architecture cannot be sustained and hepatic function becomes deranged.

The biliary system has already been discussed. Four other areas of hepatic function remain for discussion: the vascular system, the hepatocytes, the reticuloendothelial system, and the connective tissue stroma.

Before detailing the individual hepatic components, the gross and microscopic anatomy of the liver are considered. From that foundation, each element is then discussed with emphasis on important structural and functional relationships.

The liver is located in the right upper quadrant of the abdomen. Gross inspection reveals four incompletely separated lobes. The largest is the right lobe, followed in size by the left lobe. Two additional smaller lobes, the caudate and the quadrate, are also discernible. The entire organ is encapsulated by a thin connective tissue covering, Glisson's capsule.

The liver is attached to, and therefore moves with, the diaphragm. The porta hepatis is that area of the liver in which the hepatic artery, the portal vein, and the common bile duct emerge from it.

Histology

Historically, several different but not mutually exclusive models have been offered to describe the microscopic anatomy of the liver. Each of the models stresses different hepatic structures as the focal point of a functional unit. All the models are correct; they merely present varying perspectives on the same question. Conscious that these various models exist, this chapter presents the *classic model* of microscopic liver anatomy.

The classic lobule theory describes the functional units of the liver as hexagonal areas poorly demarcated by connective tissue septa (Fig. 49-9). The hexagon is more reproducibly outlined by a triad of structures at each of its six corners. The three structures, collectively referred to as a *portal triad,* are terminal branches of the hepatic artery, the portal vein, and the common bile duct. The center of the hexagon, or lobule, is marked by the central vein, the smallest division of the hepatic veins. Radiating from the central vein out to the portal area are rows of hepatocytes.

Vascular System

The overall circulatory anatomy provides a dual blood supply to the liver. The hepatic artery, a vessel directly off the celiac trunk, carries fully oxygenated blood to the liver. The portal vein, carrying approximately 80 percent of the hepatic blood supply, is formed by the union of the splenic vein and the superior mesenteric vein. Portal blood

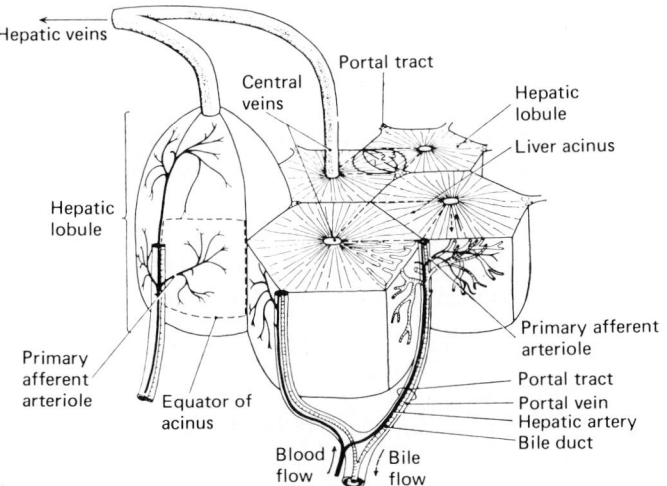

Figure 49-9   The classic hepatic lobule. *(Adapted from R. Passmore and J. S. Robson, A Companion to Medical Studies, vol. 1, Blackwell, Oxford, 1971.)*

is venous blood from the gastrointestinal tract, spleen, and pancreas. Though less well oxygenated than blood in the hepatic artery, it is rich in absorbed nutrients and metabolic products from the alimentary tract.

After entering the liver at the porta hepatis, the hepatic artery and portal vein branch out into increasingly smaller tributaries which pervade the entire liver parenchyma (Fig. 49-10). Anatomically, these vessels travel together and at one level of branching actually mingle their blood in the specialized hepatic capillary, or *sinusoid*. At the sinusoid hepatocytes absorb what they need. The sinusoids then begin a reverse order of branching. The smallest and first order of branching is the central vein. From the central vein, branching continuously gets larger until finally the right and left hepatic veins emerge from the liver and empty into the inferior vena cava.

In summary, oxygenated blood in the hepatic artery and nutrient-rich venous blood in the portal vein enter the liver through the porta hepatis. Traveling together, this artery and vein arborize into successively smaller branches. Within the specialized hepatic capillary or sinusoid, mixing of arterial and venous blood occurs. The hepatocytes extract needed substrates. The central veins begin to reconstitute the venous system and eventually

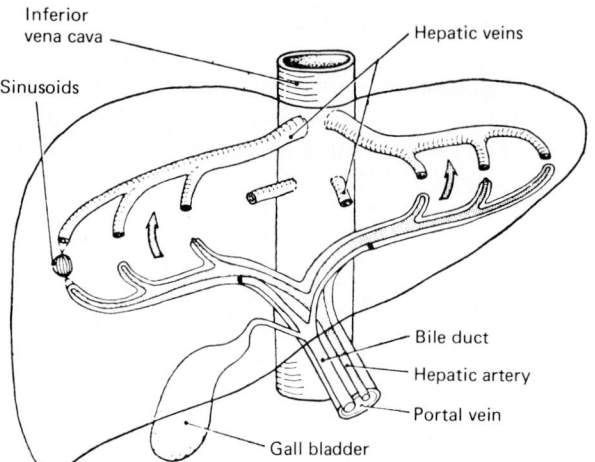

Figure 49-10   Hepatic circulation. *(Adapted from R. Passmore and J. S. Robson, A Companion to Medical Studies, vol. 1, Blackwell, Oxford, 1971.)*

develop into the hepatic veins. Blood then returns directly to the inferior vena cava.

The tremendous number of vascular structures in the liver and the almost 1.5 L of blood flow per minute that it receives make the liver an unlikely place for tissue destruction from infarction. Trauma and/or lacerations involving the liver, however, may cause massive blood loss, shock, and death.

Portal hypertension may be defined as an elevated pressure in the portal vein. It may result from any number of causes. The common denominator for all these conditions demands that there be pre- or postsinusoidal obstruction to blood flow. Ascites will more commonly develop with postsinusoidal obstruction, however.

In the case of cirrhosis of the liver, the hepatic parenchyma is replaced by fibrous nodules of scar tissue. These areas of abnormal architecture disrupt the normal blood flow and, in essence, cause obstruction to flow. As the obstruction occurs, pressure in the portal vein increases. In an attempt to decrease pressure, blood flow is shunted back to the right ventricle by way of developing systemic collaterals. Increased vascular marking may be seen on the abdominal wall when collaterals involving the periumbilical veins develop. The collaterals involving the venous plexuses of the esophagus and the rectum cause esophageal varices and hemorrhoids, respectively. Rupture of these delicate and massively distended varices may cause death by exsanguination.

Another distinguishing feature of hepatic blood flow is the specialized capillary bed encountered in the liver. Venous blood from the gastrointestinal tract, having already passed through one capillary network, is then filtered through the sinusoidal bed of the liver. Here at this second "capillary stop" the liver extracts needed substances from the rich venous blood. Likewise, products may be removed and detoxified, or newly synthesized compounds may be given up by the liver to the blood. It is an economical and efficient means of maximizing the various metabolic functions performed by the liver.

Hepatocytes

The liver cell itself is polyhedral in shape. Hepatocytes constitute almost 80 percent of the total cell population within the human liver. Each hepatocyte is rich in intracellular organelles and enzymes. The span of diversified biochemical interactions occurring in the liver is extensive, but space prevents an adequate discussion here.

The hepatocytes are arranged like spokes radiating out from the central vein to the portal triads. They are organized as rows of cells supported by a meshwork of fine connective tissue. Two important anatomic relationships deserve emphasis.

First is the close proximity of the hepatocyte to the bile ductules. Every hepatocyte, on at least one of its sides, lies adjacent to a bile ductule (Fig. 49-11). The liver cell synthesizes bile and secretes it into the bile canaliculus. Communal surface area is therefore critical to an effective system of synthesis and transport.

The second point to note is the physical relation of the hepatocyte to the sinusoid. Here again, every hepatocyte is in direct apposition to a sinusoid on at least one of its surfaces. As the bile ductule is the conduit for bile transport from the hepatocyte, the sinusoid is the transport vessel for all other hepatic metabolites. Maximal areas of contact are essential to the survival of the system.

Reticuloendothelial System

The hepatic sinusoid is important not only for its role in the transport of metabolites but also for its part in the reticuloendothelial system of the liver. The sinusoids are distinct from other capillaries in several ways. Most noticeable is the presence of phagocytic cells along the lining of the vessel. These specialized cells, called *Kupffer cells,* are active phagocytes rich in lysosomes (Fig. 49-11). They ingest foreign matter, degenerated red blood cells, bacteria, and other metabolic degradation products. These Kupffer cells make up 60 percent of the total body reticuloendothelial system.

Connective Tissue Framework

Covering the surface of the liver and extending throughout the organ is a vast network of connective tissue. Though difficult to physically delineate, the resulting framework is essential to normal hepatic activity. Glisson's capsule envelops the entire liver. Major areas of reticulum support are found around the structures of the portal triads and between rows of parenchymal cells.

The connective tissue component of the liver is important for another reason as well. The liver parenchyma has no pain fibers of its own. When a patient reports tenderness involving the liver, the pain actually results from stimulated pain-stretch receptors triggered by distention of the hepatic capsule.

In addition to providing structure for normal activity, the connective tissue elements take on new importance when the liver is diseased. If the injury has been so extensive as to destroy the underlying framework, regeneration of parenchymal cells is retarded. The newly generated cells are arranged haphazardly and do not follow the original carefully built hepatic architecture. Hepatocytes may lose their proximity to sinusoids and bile canaliculi, thus decreasing the effectiveness of the liver's activities. Furthermore, normal vascular connections may be interrupted by injury-induced proliferation of connective tissue, or cirrhosis. Postsinusoidal obstruction and portal hypertension may result.

Even from this brief outline and discussion of hepatic function one can see why so many investigators have dedicated years of study to the liver. Its intricate histologic and physiologic characteristics require full concentration if one is to understand them. Even to the pathologist, accustomed to examining and inspecting the minute

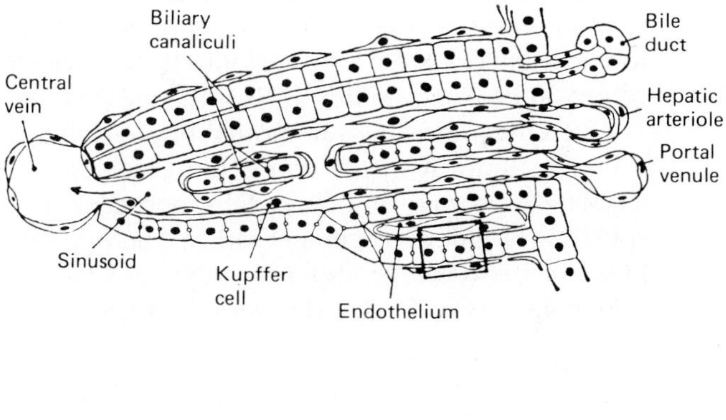

Figure 49-11   The anatomic relation of hepatocytes, sinusoids, and biliary canaliculi. *(Adapted from R. Passmore and J. S. Robson, A Companion to Medical Studies, vol. 1, Blackwell, Oxford, 1971.)*

intricacies of this organ, the liver remains a mystery. As Stanley Robbins has written: "Beneath the deceptively bland glistening capsule of Glisson that envelops the liver lurks a bewildering host of functional and structural details."

Physiology

Regulation of Hunger and Thirst

Hunger

The desire or need for food is called *hunger*. It is a complex sensation involving many variables. Though much still remains to be learned about hunger, research has demonstrated and time has supported several important concepts.

Two nuclei or groups of cells within the hypothalamus have been shown to mediate hunger and satiety. The ventromedial group, referred to as the *appetite center,* causes increased food intake when stimulated. The ventrolateral cell group, or *satiety center,* inhibits food ingestion when stimulated.

Normally, these two centers interact. When a person is satiated, the ventrolateral nucleus inhibits the ventromedial nucleus; in a hunger state the reverse occurs. Experimentally, destruction of the satiety center leads to severe obesity if available food is not restricted. Likewise, destruction of the appetite center produces marked anorexia and weight loss if corrective intervention is not initiated.

Attempts to explain the careful balance between these regulatory nuclei are varied. Though the theories range from blood glucose concentrations to hypothalamic temperature levels, no satisfactory explanation has been found. The reader is referred to a more detailed source for added information.

Thirst

Analogous to hunger, thirst can be defined as a need or desire for liquid. Interestingly, the sensation of thirst can be satisfied simply by moistening mucous membranes, even if no net change in body fluids occurs.

The kidney is intimately involved in the regulation of body water. Via volume and osmoreceptors throughout the body, the kidney receives its appropriate signals. The role of antidiuretic hormone secreted by the hypothalamus adds yet another fine control to the renal circuit.

Like that of its solid counterpart, the mechanism of thirst is incompletely understood. Here, too, specialized centers in the hypothalamus seem to be part of a neural circuit that stimulates or inhibits drinking. Again, the reader is referred to a more in-depth text for further discussion.

Esophageal Function

Esophageal Motility

Along the esophagus, a series of rhythmic contractions called *peristaltic waves* propel the food bolus downward. A wave consists of a contracting and a relaxing phase. Each peristaltic movement lasts some 5 s and travels toward the stomach at about 3 cm/s. Normal transit time from the top of the esophagus to the stomach is 9 to 10 s.

The role of the upper esophageal sphincter or hypopharyngeal sphincter has been discussed. It is this specialized muscular area of the esophagus which contracts when stimulated by the central nervous system and permits relaxation of the esophageal opening. The food bolus thus passes into the esophagus and down toward the stomach.

The lower esophageal sphincter (LES), also called the *gastroesophageal sphincter,* helps to maintain the correct direction of flow as digested materials pass into the stomach. This sphincter, unlike the upper esophageal sphincter, is not identifiable by gross or histologic inspection. It is only through manometric (pressure) studies that the role of a sphincter has been assigned to this distal part of the esophagus.

Normally the lower esophageal sphincter is closed when swallowing is not occurring. Once the sphincter opens, food passes into the stomach and the sphincter again contracts and closes. In this fashion, the esophageal mucosa is protected from the acid environment of the stomach. Esophageal reflux of food and liquids is also discouraged.

Though anatomically most of the esophagus is in the thoracic cavity above the diaphragm, a small 3-cm portion is below the diaphragm. This special anatomic arrangement utilizes the pressure gradient between the thoracic cavity and the abdominal cavity to further discourage gastric reflux.

Under normal circumstances, intraabdominal pressure exceeds intrathoracic pressure. The thoracic esophagus and the abdominal esophagus maintain the level of pressure within their respective anatomic cavities. Since the pressure at the gastroesophageal sphincter can and does increase with increases in intraabdominal pressure, sufficient tone can be generated at the LES to prevent reflux into the esophagus.

If, however, the LES is anatomically displaced by massive ascites or a growing fetus, then the distal esophagus, indeed the entire esophagus, is within the thoracic cavity. Corresponding increases in intraabdominal pressure are not transmitted to the lower esophagus. The LES is unable to generate sufficient pressure, and gastric reflux may occur.

Apparently, then, there is at least a double safeguard against acid reflux: first, the sphincter quality of the LES and its ability to contract and relax; and second, the pressure gradient between the thoracic and the abdominal cavities. Although the gastroesophageal junction is below the diaphragm, in the cavity of higher pressure, with a competent sphincter reflux back into the esophagus should be adequately controlled.

Esophageal Regulation

The controls regulating the esophageal sphincters are varied. The upper sphincter opens and closes principally on signals from the central nervous system. Once the trachea is protected by closure of the glottis, the brain signals the upper sphincter to contract and thus permits entrance of food into the esophagus. Note that for the upper sphincter, contraction opens the entrance while relaxation closes it.

Unlike its upper counterpart, the lower esophageal sphincter is influenced by an enormous number of factors. The list continues to grow, and the actual mechanism for many of these controls is still speculative. Two basic groups of controls are known. One is hormone-mediated, and the other depends on nervous innervation. A few of the more common ones are presented.

The vagus is the primary nerve regulating lower esophageal sphincter tone and pressure. Though it is responsible, in part, for creating the normal resting tone of the sphincter, its major function is to relax the sphincter during swallowing.

Governed by the myenteric plexus, vagal mediation helps propagate esophageal peristalsis and therefore passage of food into the stomach.

Certain circulating hormones are intricately involved in maintaining the baseline sphincter tone. Though there is still some question about their exact mechanism of action, much progress has already been made in this field.

Gastrin, a hormone secreted by the pyloric glands in the stomach, has many functions. For the discussion here, it is enough to know that gastrin stimulates the secretion of hydrochloric acid (HCl) by the stomach; this acidifies the stomach contents and enhances digestion.

In order to prevent reflux into the esophagus, with possible mucosal damage from the acidity, lower esophageal sphincter tone must increase and narrow the opening. What causes the sphincter tone to increase is not completely understood. Early experiments suggested that LES tone increased because of direct stimulation by gastrin. It seemed reasonable that as gastrin caused secretion of HCl for food digestion in the stomach, it also caused increased lower esophageal sphincter pressure which prevented reflux and damage to the esophagus. However, later research refutes this role of gastrin and proposes that in physiologic doses gastrin may play only a small role in LES pressure (Sleisenger and Fordtran, 1983).

Two other hormones, secretin and cholecystokinin (CCK), secreted by the duodenum oppose the action of gastrin and in pharmacologic, but not in physiologic, doses decrease lower esophageal sphincter pressure. In addition, they both retard the actual secretion of gastrin.

Secretin and CCK are secreted by the small intestine just after the chyme (partially digested food) leaves the stomach. By that time, the partially digested food is farther from the gastroesophageal opening and is therefore less likely to reflux. In addition, stomach acidity has been buffered by pancreatic and duodenal bicarbonate, again making damage to the esophagus less likely. Since at this stage in digestion the esophagus is less vulnerable to harmful reflux, the lower sphincter does not need to be as tightly closed as before.

Lower esophageal sphincter tone is also affected by certain food types. Since fats, proteins, and starches stimulate the secretion of certain hormones, their method of intervention can be considered hormonal. Fats, for example, decrease lower esophageal sphincter tone. The speculative mechanism involves secretion of CCK, which in turn retards the production of gastrin. The proposed, but not proved, direct effect of CCK in reducing lower esophageal sphincter pressure, as well as its indirect effect in lowering gastrin and thereby altering sphincter pressure, is potentially responsible for the net change in sphincter tone.

Cigarette smoke and alcohol lower sphincter pressure, whereas caffeine raises it. It has even been shown that some of the prostaglandin compounds affect tone and pressure.

Lastly, antacids have a role in regulating the lower esophageal sphincter. Antacids buffer stomach acidity and raise the pH (make it more alkaline). High pH stimulates the secretion of gastrin, and as indicated, gastrin seems to be related to increased sphincter tone. Perhaps patients with symptomatic esophageal reflux receive a dual benefit from treatment with antacids: the acid is neutralized and sphincter tone is increased.

Gastric Secretions

Gastric Glands

There are some 15 million glands in the many glandular structures in the stomach wall. Grouped by location and function, they are the cardiac, the gastric (or fundic), and the pyloric glands.

The *cardiac glands,* as their name suggests, are located near the cardia of the stomach. They are responsible for mucus secretion only.

At the distal end of the stomach the *pyloric glands* are found, just before the pyloric sphincter. Like their counterparts in the cardia, these glands are mucus secretors; however, the pyloric glands also synthesize the hormone gastrin.

The *gastric,* or *fundic, glands* located in the body of the stomach secrete many different substances (Fig. 49-12). Their ability to produce more diversified products is a result of a more varied cell type in their epithelial layer. The *neck mucous cell* is found in the uppermost part of the gastric gland. It secretes mucus. The *parietal cell* is found in the middle of the gland. This cell secretes HCl and intrinsic factor, a substance necessary for the oral absorption of vitamin B_{12}. The final cell type,

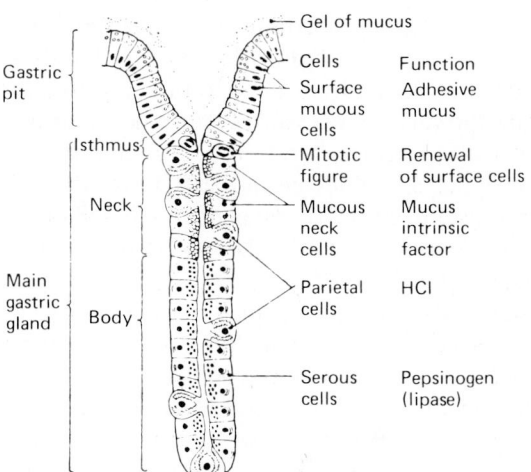

Figure 49-12 Histology of the gastric glands. *(Adapted from R. Passmore and J. S. Robson, A Companion to Medical Studies, vol. 1, Blackwell, Oxford, 1971.)*

located deepest within the gastric gland, is the *chief cell.* The specialization of this cell allows it to secrete other enzymes. The most well known of these is pepsinogen.

The secretory function of the stomach can be conceptualized as two fundamental groups: the acid and the nonacid secretions.

Acid Secretion

The parietal cell, located in the pit of the gastric gland, is solely responsible for secretion of HCl. The amount of HCl secreted is directly proportional to the parietal cell mass. Normally, almost 2 L of HCl is secreted per day.

The internal environment of the parietal cell is composed of normal cellular matrix and the various electrolytes—Na^+, K^+, Cl^-, and so on. Each cell is rich with large adenosine 5-triphosphate (ATP)–producing mitochondria, which supply the needed energy for HCl synthesis.

The secretion of the HCl requires active ionic transport rather than passive diffusion of H^+ and Cl^-. As a consequence, large amounts of energy in the form of ATP are required. Appropriately, the parietal cell contains many large mitochondria.

Why active transport rather than passive diffusion? Since H^+ and Cl^- are pumped against an unfavorable concentration and pH gradient, a specialized transport system must be used. Both H^+ and Cl^- are actively transported, and separate ion pumps are believed to be responsible. Note that the hydrogen ion concentration in the stomach lumen is almost 3 million times greater than the concentration in the blood.

Despite years of study, many of the details surrounding HCl secretion are unclear. Several simultaneous reactions occur within the parietal cell which generate and replenish the needed stores of ionic substrates.

The source of hydrogen ions (H^+) is believed to be the ionization of water (H_2O):

$$H_2O \rightleftarrows H^+ + OH^-$$

Coincidental with this, an enzyme in the parietal cell, carbonic anhydrase, catalyzes the reaction of carbon dioxide (CO_2) and water (H_2O) to make carbonic acid (H_2CO_3):

$$CO_2 + H_2O \rightleftarrows H_2CO_3$$

The carbonic acid is further broken down into a bicarbonate ion (HCO_3^-) and a hydrogen ion (H^+):

$$H_2CO_3 \rightleftarrows H^+ + HCO_3^-$$

For each H^+ ion that is actively transported across the cell membrane into the stomach lumen, one HCO_3^- ion diffuses (not actively transported) back into the bloodstream. Since this is a 1:1 exchange, as the stomach contents become more acid, the venous blood leaving the stomach after a meal becomes more alkalotic.

Normally, there are no significant changes in body pH with meals because the pancreas and duodenum secrete HCO_3^- into the intestinal lumen and neutralize the pH. An important point to keep in mind, however, is that measurable pH shifts can occur in patients with large amounts of vomiting. With prolonged vomiting, and therefore loss of H^+ greater than loss of HCO_3^-, patients may become alkalotic.

In summary, H^+ ions are derived from the ionization of H_2O. Both H^+ and Cl^- are actively transported across the cell membrane into the stomach lumen. For each H^+ ion that is transported into the lumen, one HCO_3^- ion diffuses back into the blood (Fig. 49-13).

Nonacid Secretion

Intrinsic Factor   To finish discussing the secretions of the parietal cell, mention should be made of the nonacid substances that are secreted. *Intrinsic factor* is a glycoprotein necessary for the oral absorption of vitamin B_{12}. Though the mechanism is incompletely understood, it is believed that cyanocobalamin (vitamin B_{12}) binds to intrinsic factor. This complex travels to the distal ileum (third part of the small intestine) and binds to another receptor on the surface of the ileal mucosa. Once attached, the vitamin B_{12}, through an as yet unknown mechanism, is absorbed.

A person without intrinsic factor cannot absorb oral vitamin B_{12}. With gastrectomy (removal of the stomach), a patient will lose parietal cells

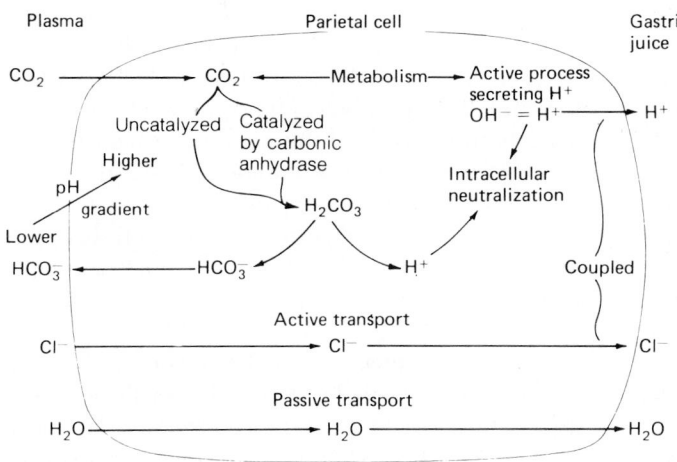

Figure 49-13   Proposed mechanism of HCO_3 secretion within the parietal cell of the stomach. *(Adapted from H. W. Davenport, Physiology of the Digestive Tract, 5th ed., Year Book, Chicago, 1982.)*

and therefore not produce intrinsic factor. Vitamin B_{12} must be replaced parenterally.

The example of gastrectomy causing lack of intrinsic factor is quite obvious. More subtle causes are at work in atrophic gastritis, a condition that reduces parietal cell mass so that decreased and finally inadequate amounts of intrinsic factor are synthesized. Pernicious anemia, a not uncommon disease, is idiopathic gastric atrophy with absence of intrinsic factor, resulting in B_{12} deficiency and anemia. Other causes of decreased vitamin B_{12} absorption not strictly related to the absence of intrinsic factor exist but are not discussed here.

Pepsinogen *Pepsinogen,* a nonacid substance, is secreted by the chief cells of the gastric glands. In its initial form, this proteolytic enzyme is inactive. It is activated only when the stomach pH becomes sufficiently acidic. In this acid environment part of the original molecule is hydrolyzed, and the remaining active form, known as *pepsin,* cleaves amino acid bonds within protein chains. Maximal activity of pepsin occurs in a pH range between 1 and 3. Once the intestinal contents are neutralized by pancreatic and duodenal bicarbonate, pepsin loses its enzymatic activity.

Pepsin initiates the first major step in protein digestion. Whole proteins are broken down into small polypeptide fragments. As the digestive process continues, these newly formed fragments play a role in regulating gastric motility and secretion.

Gastrin The other major nonacid compound to consider is *gastrin.* In recent years this hormone has been intensively studied and is believed to be one of the major controlling factors in gastric acid secretion. Gastrin is secreted primarily by the cells of the pyloric glands in the antrum of the stomach. However, small amounts have also been found in the upper part of the duodenum and in certain cells of the pancreas. Structurally, gastrin is a peptide of 17 amino acids. The four amino acids at the carboxyl terminal end are believed to be the active agents regulating acid control.

Understanding of the role of gastrin in the overall functioning of the gastrointestinal tract is growing by leaps and bounds. Here the discussion covers only the major functions of this versatile hormone.

Gastrin's principal role is to stimulate secretion of HCl by parietal cells. Gastrin actually comes into physical contact with a receptor on the parietal cell surface. In an as yet unknown way, this contact propagates the secretion of HCl. Beyond its role as regulator of gastric acid, gastrin, in pharmacologic doses, increases lower esophageal sphincter tone and also enhances gastric motility.

Below is a partial list of other varied responses which are thought to be actions of gastrin. Gastrin is believed to stimulate:

1. Growth of the gastric fundic mucosa
2. Secretion of pepsinogen
3. Secretion of gastric intrinsic factor
4. Secretion of pancreatic bicarbonate and pancreatic digestive enzymes
5. Insulin release from pancreatic islets
6. Secretion of bicarbonate from Brunner's glands in the duodenum
7. Hepatic secretion of biliary bicarbonate
8. Intestinal motility
9. Rhythmic contractions of the stomach and gallbladder

Gastrin is believed to inhibit:

1. Gastric emptying
2. Secretion of secretin
3. Gastric resting tone
4. Secretion of cholecystokinin
5. Sodium absorption from the ileum
6. Ileocecal valve resting tone

Regulation of Gastric Secretions

The regulation of gastric acid is as complex as the intricate molecular reactions responsible for HCl secretion. Like the control mechanisms for the lower esophageal sphincter, the regulation of acid secretion is both nerve- and hormone-mediated. In vivo, the humoral and the neural mechanisms are so intermingled that it would be difficult to explore them separately, and this discussion treats them simultaneously. Regulation of pepsinogen secretion virtually parallels HCl output and is included here as well.

The Cephalic Phase The first phase of acid secretion, the cephalic phase, begins when one sees, smells, tastes, or even thinks about an appetizing meal. Thus, HCl is secreted even before food reaches the stomach. This phase of acid control is via parasympathetic input delivered by the vagus nerve. In part, the vagus directly stimulates acid secretion by the gastric glands. In addition, the vagus increases gastrin production by the pyloric glands in the antrum. This added gastrin augments acid output. Note that antrectomy (removal of the antrum) does not totally obliterate acid secretion. This supports the evidence that the vagus directly stimulates the gastric glands themselves; acid secretion is not mediated by gastrin alone.

Vagal impulses are increased by hunger, hypoglycemia, and anger, as well as by pleasant gustatory stimulation. Measurable reduction in vagal tone is found with hyperglycemia, an overdistended stomach, and certain drugs, especially the anticholinergic agents.

The Gastric Phase   The second phase of acid secretion, the gastric phase, occurs, as its name implies, when food reaches the stomach. Though vagal input is still present, the predominant regulatory factors during the gastric phase are humoral. Alcohol and coffee (because of peptides, not caffeine) have also been shown to increase HCl secretion during this phase.

The hormone of note in acid regulation is gastrin. Though gastrin increases pepsinogen secretion as well, it does so to a lesser degree. It should be remembered that during the cephalic phase, some gastrin is secreted; however, the gastric phase is responsible for the major outflow of this hormone. The secretion of gastrin is stimulated by antral distention, by polypeptide fragments in the antrum, and by an alkaline pH in the stomach. Simultaneous secretion of pepsinogen increases the amount of polypeptide fragments, thus adding indirectly to the stimulus for gastrin secretion.

Gastrin secretion employs a feedback mechanism on itself. As gastrin is secreted, HCl is poured out, lowering the pH of the gastric contents. When the pH becomes sufficiently low, and therefore the H^+ ion concentration sufficiently high, gastrin secretion decreases.

The Intestinal Phase   The final step of acid control, the intestinal phase, begins as chyme enters the duodenum. When polypeptide fragments reach the antrum, gastric acid secretion increases. Though it

is not well understood why, this mechanism continues to work even when the vagus nerve is not intact.

The intestinal phase has more inhibitory influence on gastric acid secretion than either of the earlier phases. If the pH within the duodenum is 2.5 or less, acid output markedly drops off. Likewise, fat in the duodenum also decreases acid production. CCK and secretin, two duodenal hormones, exert an inhibitory effect on gastrin and thereby decrease acid output. Since CCK is stimulated by fat in the duodenum, there is some question as to the exact mechanism causing the acid reduction. Does fat directly inhibit acid? Or does CCK, stimulated by the presence of fat, inhibit acid? Or both?

In summary, control of gastric acid secretion has three major components: the cephalic phase, mediated principally by the vagus nerve; the gastric phase, influenced primarily by the hormonal effects of gastrin; and finally, the intestinal phase, mainly an inhibitory stage which reduces acid output as chyme leaves the stomach and enters the small intestine.

Gastric Motility

In the stomach, food continues its physical and chemical breakdown. The partially digested food must be physically degraded into particles small enough to pass through the pyloric canal into the duodenum. Similarly, at the molecular level, gastric contents must be adequately mixed to ensure optimal enzyme exposure. Clearly, then, motility plays a central role in the stomach's contribution to digestion.

The movement of the stomach is both active and passive. Initially, as food enters the stomach, the passive phase of gastric motility occurs. This is *receptive relaxation*. It is a reflex initiated by earlier movements of the pharynx and the esophagus. As noted earlier, the usual reservoir capacity of the stomach is between 1 and 1.5 L. During receptive relaxation, volumes as high as 6 L have been recorded!

The true activity of the stomach, that which mixes food and forces it through the pylorus, combines peristaltic contractions across the body of the stomach with strong contractions of the terminal antral segment.

The stomach has an intrinsic electrical pacemaker. These trigger cells are responsible for initiating electrical depolarization and subsequent muscular peristalsis. Initially, the electrical and muscular activity travel in the outer muscle layer. Soon they spread to the inner muscle layer and sweep across the body of the stomach toward the antrum. Normally, the frequency of contractions is three per minute. The initial rate of speed is only about 1 cm/s. However, as the antrum is approached, the peristaltic waves travel faster and may reach speeds in the range of 3 to 4 cm/s.

Slow, weak muscular contractions are the rule early in digestion. It is only after about 1 h of digestive activity that the speed and the intensity of the waves increase. When contractions reach the antrum, they have enough force to push small amounts of chyme ahead of them. Digested food accumulates in the antrum, and antral pressure rises and actually overcomes the pressure in the open pyloric canal. Small amounts of viscous chyme are able to squeeze through into the duodenum.

However, like the antrum, the pylorus contracts as well. While contracted, the pyloric canal is closed; chyme is not able to pass through. The antrum, contracting against a closed pylorus, cannot generate enough pressure to push food into the duodenum. Instead, the chyme is forced backward into the stomach. It is this retropulsion of chyme into the stomach when the pylorus is closed that accounts for the active mixing quality of gastric motion.

Regulation

Several factors control gastric motility. All the influences, whether mechanical, chemical, or neural, interact to produce optimal mixing of food in the stomach before it is passed along to the small intestine for absorption.

Significant abnormalities of gastric motility often lead to malabsorptive states. Though food may reach its destined site of absorption in the small intestine, if it has been improperly or incompletely processed in the stomach, normal absorption will not occur.

The stomach has been called the "handmaiden" of the small intestine. If one considers the stomach as such, perhaps it is easier to understand the control mechanisms of gastric emptying.

Basically the stomach alters partially digested food for absorption within the small intestine. If chyme is adequately prepared, gastric motility increases and chyme passes through the pylorus. On the other hand, the stomach attempts to detain gastric contents by decreasing gastric motility and gastric emptying when chyme is incompletely processed. Similarly, if the duodenum is incapable of accepting more chyme, the stomach will attempt to delay further emptying.

Gastric Influences   The principal gastric factors affecting motility are tension within the stomach wall and gastrin. Tension builds within the stomach walls as the volume of food increases. In an attempt to decrease wall tension, gastric emptying speeds up.

Gastrin, the hormone which causes increased secretion of hydrochloric acid, also enhances antral motility. Acid is for digestion, and mixing promotes digestion. Reasonably, gastrin affects them both in a complementary manner. It should be remembered also that gastrin is related to increased LES pressure. Thus during peak gastric motility, esophageal reflux is discouraged.

Intestinal Influences   Duodenal distention signals the stomach to slow gastric unloading. If the duodenum is unable to keep pace with the rate of emptying, incomplete interaction of hormones results and chyme is inadequately prepared for transit further along in the small intestine. Similarly, if chyme reaching the duodenum is too acidic or too hypertonic, gastric emptying is inhibited. This checkpoint, called the *enterogastric reflex,* is partially mediated by the vagus nerve.

Fat in the duodenum stimulates the secretion of cholecystokinin, which in itself directly delays gastric motility. Fats leave the stomach more slowly than proteins and proteins more slowly than carbohydrates.

Receptors to HCl, fatty acids, and osmotic stimuli have been postulated to exist in the duodenum and jejunum. By unknown mechanisms, perhaps humoral or neural, these receptors affect gastric emptying. The controls regulating gastric motility seem designed to maximize the unique role of each organ along the gastrointestinal tract, with the checkpoints optimally providing a most economical and practical method for food ingestion, digestion, and absorption.

The Vomiting Reflex

Vomiting is initiated in the medulla of the brain. Mechanically, the partially digested food material in the stomach is forced back up through the esophagus into the mouth. Often the process is associated with common signs and symptoms of sympathetic nervous discharge, e.g., tachycardia and sweating.

Incoming signals to the medulla arise from various body sensory receptors. The more common emetic stimulants involve mechanical stimulation of the posterior oropharynx, increased intracranial pressure, overdistention of the stomach or duodenum, pain, or ingestion of certain chemical compounds.

Mechanically, five steps are involved:

1. A deep inspiration is followed by closure of the glottis.
2. The soft palate rises.
3. The abdominal muscles contract and increase intraabdominal and intragastric pressure.
4. The gastroesophageal sphincter (LES) relaxes.
5. Elevated intragastric pressure forces the food back through the esophagus, opens the upper esophageal sphincter, and forces food into the mouth.

As mentioned earlier, prolonged vomiting may lead to severe electrolyte and pH imbalances and, of course, dehydration.

Pancreatic Secretions (Exocrine)

Two major products are secreted by the exocrine pancreas: digestive enzymes and bicarbonate fluid. The acinar glands produce enzymes while the lining cells of the ducts secrete the bicarbonate-rich pancreatic juice. The combined output of enzymatic and bicarbonate secretions approaches 2 L/day. The actual proportion of the two components is determined by the nature of the food ingested.

Bicarbonates

In addition to providing the service of carrier conduit for the glandular secretions, the ductal epithelium or lining cells produce a bicarbonate-rich fluid. Unlike the glandular cells, these duct cells have few of the intracellular organelles needed for synthetic functions. Instead they are rich in the enzyme carbonic anhydrase. Like the parietal cells of the stomach, also rich in carbonic anhydrase, the pancreatic duct cells secrete bicarbonate.

Within the duct lumen, the alkaline secretion of the duct cells mixes with the enzymatic secretion of the acinar cells. What eventually reaches the major pancreatic duct, and therefore the small intestine, is a pancreatic juice rich in HCO_3^- and enzymes.

The mechanism of HCO_3^- secretion by the exocrine pancreas is analogous to the secretion of HCl by the stomach. However, in the case of the pancreas, it is HCO_3^- and not H^+ that is pumped into the intestinal lumen. Here, as in the stomach, and for similar reasons of unfavorable osmotic gradients, the process requires active transport, not simple diffusion. Just as the stomach alkalinizes venous blood during secretion of HCl, so the pancreas acidifies it because of HCO_3^- secretion.

Pancreatic Enzymes

The acinus, or gland part, of the exocrine pancreas contains many secretory cells. These cells, rich in specialized intracellular organelles, are responsible for enzyme synthesis and packaging. *Zymogen granules,* large microscopic droplets within each cell, are storage particles laden with digestive enzymes.

The acinar cells secrete their enzymatic products into the duct system. Eventually, after many orders of ductules and ducts merge, the resulting major pancreatic duct empties into the duodenum.

The secretions of the acinar glands are a composite of enzymes, water, and salts. The successful digestion of fat, carbohydrate, and protein depends on the presence of these products. If the gland is unable to produce sufficient enzymes because of disease, or if the enzymes are unable to enter the small intestine because of anatomic obstruction, malabsorption in varying degrees may result. However, the pancreas has a tremendous reserve. Normal digestion can occur even if enzymatic secretion has been reduced to 10 percent of normal.

Pancreatic juice contains three basic groups of enzymes: amylytic (carbohydrate breakdown), proteolytic (protein breakdown), and lipolytic (fat breakdown).

Amylytic Of the amylytic group, α-amylase is the principal component. This enzyme, like salivary α-amylase, is responsible for hydrolysis of carbohydrates. The principal end products are glucose and maltose, a disaccharide of two glucose molecules. Pancreatic amylase is active in its original form and, unlike salivary amylase, is able to digest raw as well as cooked starches.

Proteolytic Trypsinogen, chymotrypsinogen, and procarboxypeptidase are the major proteolytic enzymes, or rather proenzymes. Each of these three must be altered before it becomes biochemically active.

Trypsinogen is converted to trypsin by the action of secretin. In addition, the trypsin thus formed acts as a self-catalyst so that trypsin activates trypsinogen. Trypsin cleaves amino acid bonds in the interior of protein chains.

Chymotrypsinogen is activated to chymotrypsin by trypsin. Its biochemical function, like that of trypsin, is to cleave only interior amino acid bonds and thus add to the growing pool of small polypeptides and single amino acids in the intestine.

Procarboxypeptidase, unlike the other two proteolytic enzymes, cleaves terminal amino acids and produces amino acids with free carboxyl ends. Procarboxypeptidase is converted to its active form by secretin and probably by trypsin.

Lipolytic The lipolytic enzymes, principally pancreatic lipase and phospholipase A, are important in early stages of fat digestion.

Lipase degrades triglycerides to free fatty acids and monoglycerides. Active in its original form, it requires the presence of bile salts to stabilize the fat-water interface of the intestinal contents. Phospholipase A is responsible for the hydrolysis of lecithin, a complex lipid, to lysolecithin.

Two additional pancreatic enzymes, nuclease and deoxyribonuclease, do not fall into any of the groups described but deserve mention. As their names suggest, these enzymes are involved in the degradation of nucleotides within DNA and RNA molecules.

Regulation

The secretory mechanisms of the exocrine pancreas are controlled by humoral and neural factors. As with the stomach, the regulatory aspects of exocrine secretion have a cephalic, a gastric, and an intestinal phase.

The cephalic phase, as before, is stimulated by pleasant olfactory, visual, and gustatory aspects of a meal. Mediation is principally through the vagus nerve. Pancreatic juice secreted during the cephalic phase is rich in enzymes and contains only small amounts of HCO_3^-.

The gastric and intestinal phases of control are closely interwoven. The composition of gastric contents delivered to the duodenum decides whether secretin or cholecystokinin will be secreted by the duodenum. These two hormones then dictate how much and what kind (enzyme-rich or HCO_3^--rich) of pancreatic juice will be secreted. When high concentrations of amino acids and/or free fatty acids reach the duodenum, CCK is stimulated. CCK fosters secretion of pancreatic juice rich in digestive enzymes and poor in HCO_3^-.

This design is a reasonable one to serve the ends of digestion. When chyme rich in undigested proteins and fats is the stimulus, further digestion must occur. The pancreas, via stimulation by CCK, causes secretion of an enzyme-rich pancreatic juice. (Although carbohydrates are a stimulant to pancreatic secretion, they are far less potent than either proteins or fats.)

Acid is one of the most important influences during the gastric phase of regulation. High acidity (low pH) in the duodenum stimulates production of secretin. Secretin, in turn, stimulates the output of HCO_3^- and water from the pancreas. Thus pancreatic juice, resulting from acid stimulus and secretin mediation, is rich in HCO_3^- and low in enzyme content. Once again, these actions and reactions are coordinated to serve digestion.

Bile Metabolism and Function

Bile production occurs continuously within the hepatocyte. After synthesis, bile is secreted into the canaliculi. The rate of synthesis approaches 0.6 mL/min in an average adult, with a total of 15 mL of bile being secreted for every kilogram of body weight. The rate of synthesis and secretion are controlled primarily by the amount of blood flow reaching the liver.

The major constituents of bile include bile acids and bile salts (principally sodium cholate and chenodeoxycholate) and pigments (most notably bilirubin), cholesterol, phospholipids (especially lecithin), alkaline phosphatase, electrolytes, and water.

Bile Salts

Bile salts are cholesterol derivatives. Together with lecithin they prevent the precipitation of cholesterol as cholesterol stones in the gallbladder. Bile salts are bipolar compounds, that is, they have a water-soluble and a fat-soluble end. Cholesterol and lecithin are fat-soluble molecules. In the gallbladder, bile salts interact with the water phase of the bile, leaving their fat-soluble end free to mix with cholesterol and/or lecithin. The particles thus formed are called *micelles*. Eventually the micelles become saturated with cholesterol. At this point of super-saturation, cholesterol precipitates out in the bile and cholesterol stones are formed. The ratio of bile salts and lecithin to cholesterol is the basis of stone formation in the gallbladder. If the proportion of cholesterol in the bile increases (without a con-current increase in bile salts or lecithin), stone formation is favored; likewise, if the bile concen-tration of salts and lecithin decreases, stones will form.

Bile salts are also important because of their role in fat digestion and absorption. Once in the small intestine, bile salts mix with fat to form micelles. As will be explained later, these water-stable complexes facilitate lipid (fat) absorption. In addition, bile salts are needed to activate pancreatic lipase, an enzyme needed for breakdown of tri-glycerides. In short, normal fat digestion and ab-sorption are not possible without bile salts. If obstruction prevents the entrance of bile salts into the intestine, fat malabsorption and steatorrhea (fatty stools) result.

Normally, bile salts are not lost in the stools. Instead they are reabsorbed in the terminal part of the ileum (third part of the small intestine) and returned, via the venous system, to the liver, where they are taken up by the liver cell and used again. All but some 2 to 3 percent of bile salts is reutilized in this way.

Bile salts are recycled via the enterohepatic circulation. This vascular circuit, unique to the gastrointestinal tract, drains venous blood from all the alimentary organs and returns it to the liver. In passing through the liver, the venous blood meets a second set of capillaries. At the level of these specialized capillaries, the liver sequesters what it needs for synthetic and detoxifying functions and returns the blood to the heart. This type of anatomic percolator is found only in the liver and in the vascular circuit of the anterior lobe of the pituitary gland.

Bile Pigments

Bilirubin and other bile pigments are products of hemoglobin degradation. Plasma bilirubin is bound to the protein albumin as it is delivered to the hepatocyte. However, only free bilirubin is able to enter the liver cell. Inside it binds to a hepatic protein carrier, thereby preventing escape back into the circulation. Bilirubin then reacts with two mol-ecules of glucuronic acid via the enzyme glucuronyl transferase. The new water-soluble compound, bil-irubin glucuronide, is then actively secreted into the bile canaliculus.

Once bile pigments are mixed in the bile and delivered to the small intestine, they are degraded by normal bowel flora. Subsequent pigments de-rived from the continued degradation are respon-sible for the normal color of stool. Therefore, with extrahepatic biliary obstruction and consequent absence of bile within the small intestine, stool color will turn from brown to grey—the acholic (without bile) stool.

In normal concentration, bile pigments do not form pigment stones. However, in disease states such as the hemolytic anemias, where there is an increased amount of bilirubin reaching the liver, the concentration of bile pigments increases and so-called pigment or bilirubinate stones precipitate out in the gallbladder. Cholesterol stones make up 90 percent of gallstones. The remaining 10 percent are pigment stones.

Regulation

The regulation of bile secretion into the small intestine is a function of the neural and hormonal effects influencing the muscular sphincters of the biliary system and the contractility of the gallbladder.

In what might be called the cephalic phase of bile secretion, vagal stimulation received by the hepatocytes stimulates increased bile secretion and subsequent bile outflow. The sphincter of Oddi is normally in a partially opened state between meals. As a result, there is a constant trickle of bile into the small intestine.

When food reaches the duodenum, a more active phase of bile regulation begins. As mentioned previously, fats and polypeptides are strong stimulants for secretion of cholecystokinin. CCK, in turn, is the major hormonal stimulus for gallbladder contraction. With food present within the stomach or duodenum, the sphincter of Oddi relaxes. As the gallbladder contracts, increased bile passes through the relaxed sphincter into the intestine. Between meals, when the stimulus for CCK decreases, the gallbladder does not contract. The sphincter adopts a contracted pose, and the bile, always in continuous flow, travels from the liver to the gallbladder. There it is stored and concentrated until the gallbladder is stimulated to empty.

Since there are no absolute stop valves on hepatic bile production, there is always a flow of hepatic bile arriving directly at the intestine. Hepatic bile contains more water and HCO_3^- than bile from the gallbladder. It is more alkaline and therefore important to the small intestine if a large acid load arrives at the duodenum. Precisely because of these differences, secretin (stimulated by increased acid) causes preferential stimulation of hepatic bile flow rather than contraction of the gallbladder. Likewise, gastrin, a strong stimulant of gastric acid, indirectly increases hepatic bile flow by enhancing the production of secretin. Furthermore, gastrin has its own direct effect on the liver and increases hepatic outflow of HCO_3^--rich bile.

In summary, cholecystokinin is secreted in response to fat and protein in the duodenum. Fats need bile salts for digestion. Fat and protein need enzymes for digestion. CCK causes release of pancreatic digestive enzymes as well as contraction of the gallbladder with resultant release of concentrated bile.

Secretin is stimulated by the arrival of an acid load at the duodenum. The acid contents need a diluting buffer to prevent duodenal mucosal damage and to protect pH-sensitive digestive enzymes. Secretin causes outflow of pancreatic bicarbonate. In addition, secretin provides preferential flow of dilute alkaline hepatic bile into the small intestine. For both CCK and secretin, the response is an appropriate answer to the stimulus.

Intestinal Function

Secretions

The role of the small intestine as a secretory organ has only recently come under extensive study. Relatively little is known about the regulation of intestinal secretions. Some evidence suggests that the intestinal mucosa, stimulated by hydrochloric acid and food products, releases into the blood a hormone, enterocrinin, which brings about increased production of digestive enzymes within the intestinal mucosa. Presumably, neural mechanisms also help control the secretion of this digestive juice. The lining epithelium of the small intestine is modified with numerous goblet, or mucus-producing, cells. This mucous secretion and the CCK and secretin synthesized by the duodenal mucosa are the major secretory contributions of the small bowel. Note that CCK and secretin are synthesized by the duodenal mucosa, but they are secreted directly into the blood, not into the intestinal lumen.

One other important component should also be mentioned. Within the duodenal wall there is a collection of glands, *Brunner's glands,* which secrete an HCO_3^--rich fluid. Like pancreatic HCO_3^-, the secretion of Brunner's glands helps to neutralize the acid gastric contents and protect the duodenal mucosa. Again like pancreatic HCO_3^-, Brunner's glands are stimulated by acid in the duodenum, by secretin, and by gastrin.

Motility

Like each of the organs before it, the small intestine has its own specialized type of motility. Since this organ is designed to digest and absorb chyme, it follows that the principal form of movement should promote mixing and facilitate contact with the absorbing surface. *Segmentation,* the unique motion of the small intestine, achieves precisely these two objectives. However, since the small bowel must deliver the intestinal contents to the colon, a propulsive motion must exist as well. Weak peristaltic waves can be demonstrated throughout the small bowel. Each one contributes to the forward propulsion of chyme toward the colon.

In the duodenum, near the entrance of the common bile duct, an intrinsic electrical pacemaker is found in the longitudinal muscle of the wall. The impulse travels from duodenum to ileum. Importantly, the strength, the frequency, and the speed of the impulse decrease as they get farther from the duodenum. This temporal prolongation allows increased time for digestion and absorption.

Segmentation contractions follow the intrinsic pacemaker rhythm but involve only rings of muscle around the small intestine. As one area relaxes, another contracts all along the intestine, thus creating a "sausage links" effect. This action mixes; it does not propel intestinal contents.

Weak peristaltic waves of contraction, preceded by relaxation, slowly propel chyme toward the colon. Usually they are short waves and do not involve the entire length of the small bowel. Distention of the bowel at any point triggers this sequence of events. It is called the *myenteric reflex*.

As chyme approaches the large intestine, ileal contractions increase. The ileocecal valve, normally in a closed position, relaxes and allows chyme to flow into the colon. This *gastroileal reflex* regulates passage of chyme from the small intestine to the large intestine.

Both segmentation and peristalsis require intact intrinsic (that is, within the intestinal wall) neural structures. For segmentation to occur, the duodenal pacemaker must discharge its impulse.

With peristalsis the pressure receptors in the bowel wall respond to the sense of increased distention. The myenteric reflex is stimulated. For the reflex to complete itself, the nerve plexus in the intestinal wall must be intact. Generally, sympathetic stimulation causes decreased intestinal motility while parasympathetic input increases activity. CCK promotes enhanced motility, but glucagon and secretin slow intestinal action.

Absorption

The discussion has followed the path of ingested foods as they traveled from the mouth down the esophagus and through the stomach and collected pancreatic and hepatic digestive secretions at the ampulla of Vater. Now we turn to the major issues of digestion and absorption within the small intestine.

Before reaching the ileum, most foodstuffs, with certain notable exceptions, have been absorbed. Because of the small bowel's tremendous absorbing surface, almost 50 percent of the bowel may be removed without producing clinical malabsorption. In addition to the fats, carbohydrates, and proteins absorbed in the small intestine, water and electrolytes are significantly absorbed as well (Fig. 49-14).

Carbohydrates   Carbohydrates or starches constitute a substantial part of the average North American diet. Consumption varies from 200 to 800 g per day. The majority of carbohydrates are ingested as polysaccharides. Only small amounts of the common disaccharides lactose and sucrose are consumed daily.

In the mouth, salivary amylase begins to digest carbohydrates. Some 50 percent of starches, mostly in the form of polysaccharides, are hydrolyzed to disaccharides. This continues to a lesser degree as the food bolus moves down the esophagus. In the stomach, no significant starch digestion occurs, since the acid environment inactivates amylase. (The optimal pH for starch digestion is 6.7.)

Once in the small intestine, pancreatic amylase continues the process. The most common disaccharide formed is maltose. Absorption of disaccharides is not feasible because of their size. Therefore, in order for carbohydrate absorption to occur, monosaccharides must be generated. The microvilli of the small intestine contain special enzymes—lactase, maltase, sucrase, and so on—which split the specific disaccharides into monosaccharides. Lactose intolerance is a disease resulting from absence of the enzyme lactase. Consequently, patients with this disorder are unable to absorb lactose, and they suffer from diarrhea and abdominal complaints if lactose is not removed from their diets.

Once formed, the simple sugars—glucose, galactose, and fructose—are absorbed relatively easily because of their smaller size. Most sugars are absorbed before reaching the last portion of the ileum. Both glucose and galactose require active transport across the intestinal membrane into the blood. Their absorption is therefore coupled to

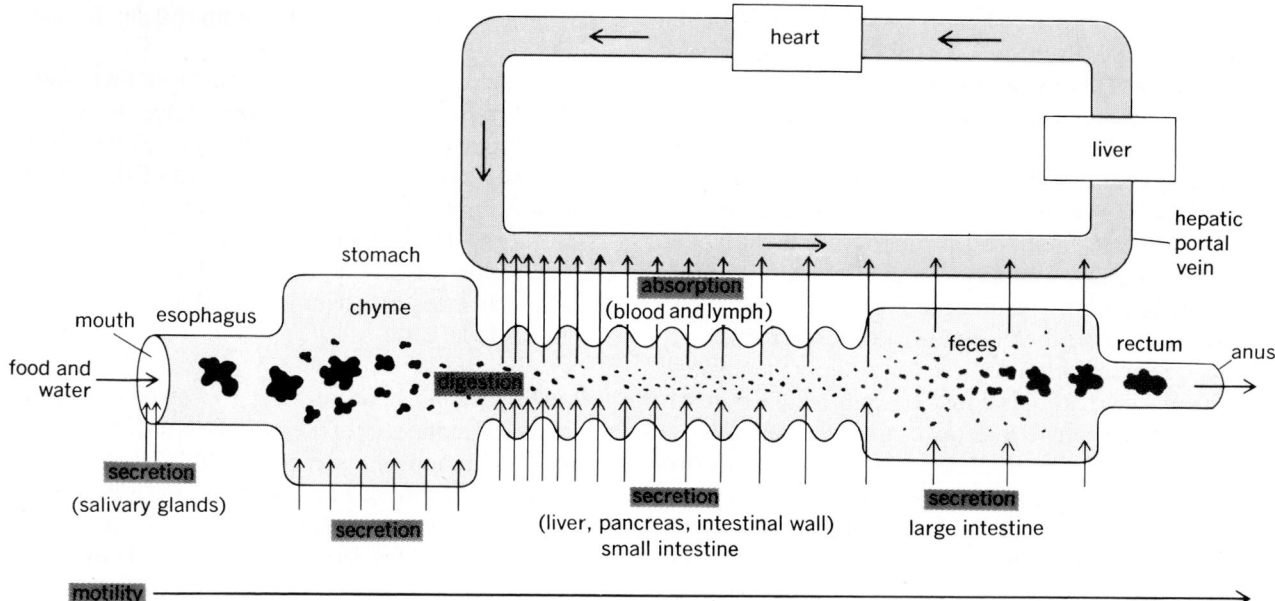

Figure 49-14   Summary of gastrointestinal activity involving motility, secretion, and absorption. *(From A. J. Vander, J. H. Sherman, and D. Luciano, Human Physiology, McGraw-Hill, New York, 1975.)*

Na^+ transport and is directly proportional to the Na^+ concentration in the intestinal lumen. Fructose, however, passively diffuses through the membrane into the blood.

Now in the venous blood, the absorbed sugars are transported to the liver. In the specialized hepatic capillaries, the hepatocytes utilize the sugars either for immediate energy, for storage as glycogen, or as metabolic intermediates in other hepatic biochemical pathways.

In summary, ingested polysaccharides are hydrolyzed to disaccharides by *salivary α-amylase* by the time they reach the stomach. In the stomach no significant change occurs. Within the small intestine *pancreatic α-amylase* continues the generation of disaccharides. *Sugar-splitting enzymes* of the intestinal microvilli cleave disaccharides to monosaccharides. These simple sugars are absorbed across the intestinal membrane into the venous blood either by active transport (glucose and galactose) or by passive diffusion (fructose). The venous blood, rich in absorbed carbohydrate, returns to the liver for appropriate utilization and storage.

Proteins   A daily protein intake of 50 g, under normal healthy conditions, is considered adequate for the average adult. This quantity provides the needed essential amino acids and meets the demands of ordinary protein synthesis and degradation. The diet of most adults in the United States averages about 200 g of protein per day.

Unlike the carbohydrate group, protein is not altered until it reaches the stomach. There the acid pH hydrolyzes certain amino acid bonds, and gastric pepsin, activated by the acid, cleaves internal peptide bonds forming amino acid fragments or polypeptides.

In the duodenum, pepsin is inactivated because of the increased alkalinity. However, the pancreatic proteolytic enzymes trypsin and chymotrypsin (optimal pH 7.8) continue to cleave internal bonds. Carboxypeptidase, also from the pancreas, initiates removal of terminal amino acids. The protein pool is composed of peptide fragments and rare free amino acids.

Like the disaccharides of carbohydrate digestion, the polypeptide fragments are too large to be absorbed across the mucosal surface. Again the intestinal microvilli supply specialized enzymes—dipeptidases, aminopeptidases, and so on—which split polypeptides into free amino acid components. Single amino acids, like simple sugars, can be absorbed. Investigative studies indicate that dipeptides with short side chains may also be absorbed intact and are hydrolyzed to free amino acids within the cell.

Amino acid absorption is highly specific, with unique mechanisms for neutral, acidic, and basic amino acids. The molecular structure of the compound determines, in part, whether active transport and Na^+ coupling or passive diffusion are needed for absorption. Most amino acid absorption occurs in the duodenum and the jejunum.

Like the products of starch metabolism, protein building blocks are also returned to the liver. Once there, the amino acids are degraded by the liver into their two organic parts, carbon and nitrogen (ammonia). Free ammonia is toxic to the human body in abnormal amounts. Therefore, the liver uses the free ammonia to form the waste product urea. This urea then travels to the kidney and is excreted in the urine, thus disposing of a toxic product. If, however, because of significant hepatic damage, the liver is unable to synthesize urea, free ammonia will accumulate and reach toxic levels. This phenomenon, the liver's inability to handle a nitrogen (ammonia) load, is in part the basis for hepatic encephalopathy, a condition seen not infrequently with severe liver disease.

The above series of metabolic events is the rationale for a protein-restricted diet in patients with hepatic encephalopathy or in those patients in whom it is likely to develop. Likewise, gastrointestinal bleeding, with resultant blood (composed of protein and therefore amino acids) in the gut lumen, also predisposes selected patients with liver disease to hepatic encephalopathy. With an increased amino acid load presented to the small intestine, increased amino acid absorption occurs. The liver receives an increased load of free ammonia. Since its synthetic ability to make urea is subnormal, the concentration of free ammonia in the blood rises and clinical encephalopathy may result.

Fats The fat content of the daily adult diet varies greatly. The biochemical form most commonly ingested is the triglyceride or neutral fat. Cholesterol and the complex phospholipids also add significantly to the daily lipid intake. Normally, stool contains only 5 percent of the daily dietary fat intake. But even this small proportion comes from bacterial metabolism rather than from dietary fats alone.

The overall digestion and absorption of lipids is slightly more complex than the mechanisms involved in carbohydrate and protein metabolism. The additional steps required arise chiefly from the size and solubility characteristics of the lipids.

No fat digestion occurs before the fat reaches the duodenum. Fat arrives at the duodenum mainly as triglycerides, cholesterol, and phospholipids. Pancreatic lipase is the enzyme responsible for the first step of fat digestion.

Triglycerides are fat-soluble. Enzymatic lipase is water-soluble. Therefore, in an aqueous solution such as intestinal fluid, triglycerides will lump together, forming large droplets. Because of their water insolubility, they will not mix with the water milieu. Lipase, being water-soluble, will mix with the water. Bile salts are required in order to bring water-soluble lipase in contact with fat-soluble triglycerides.

Bile salts, coming from the liver and primarily the gallbladder, enter the duodenum when a fatty stimulus is present. These salts contain both a water-soluble and a fat-soluble portion. As a result, they can bring together the two otherwise opposing elements.

The large lipid droplets, having been stabilized by the bile salts, now come in contact with lipase. The action of this enzyme, together with normal intestinal motility, causes much mixing and breaking apart of the large fat droplets. This process, called *emulsification,* provides increased numbers of small fat particles and thereby increases the overall surface area in which lipase can act. Lipase is responsible for degrading triglycerides (TG) primarily to monoglycerides (MG) and free fatty acids (FFA) (Fig. 49-15).

Step 1: Emulsification

Triglycerides as large fat droplets $\xrightarrow[\text{lipase}]{\text{bile salts}}$

smaller droplets $\xrightarrow[\text{lipase}]{\text{bile salts}}$ FFA + monoglycerides

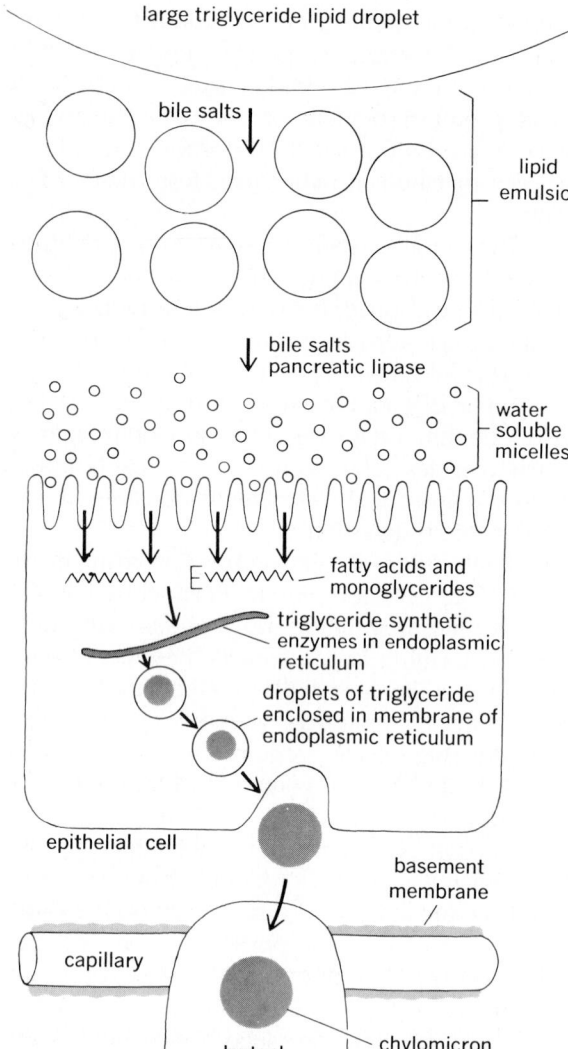

Figure 49-15 Summary of fat absorption across the walls of the small intestine. *(From A. J. Vander, J. H. Sherman, and D. Luciano, Human Physiology, Mc-Graw-Hill, New York, 1975.)*

The FFA and monoglycerides thus formed combine with varying proportions of cholesterol and phospholipid. This new combination of fatty molecules is again acted upon by bile salts. The new particle, now stabilized and water-soluble, is called a *micelle*. It is from the micellar form that FFA and monoglycerides are absorbed across the intestinal mucosa.

Step 2: Micelle formation

FFA + MG + cholesterol

$$+ \text{ phospholipid } \xrightarrow{\text{bile salts}} \text{micelle}$$

When the micelle is in close proximity to the mucosal surface, passive absorption of the FFA occurs. Depending on the length of the FFA, absorption will take place directly into the blood (for FFA less than 10 to 12 carbons long) or, as is more often the case, the FFA (longer than 12 carbons) will be resynthesized to a triglyceride within the intestinal cell (Fig. 49-16).

Once resynthesized, the triglyceride is coated with cholesterol and phospholipid. This new complex, called a *chylomicron,* is then picked up by the lacteal or lymph vessel of the intestinal villus and carried to sites of fat storage (adipose tissue) throughout the body. Thus most free fatty acids travel as triglycerides in chylomicrons via the lymph, not via the blood.

Note that bile salts remain behind within the intestinal lumen when the free fatty acid diffuses

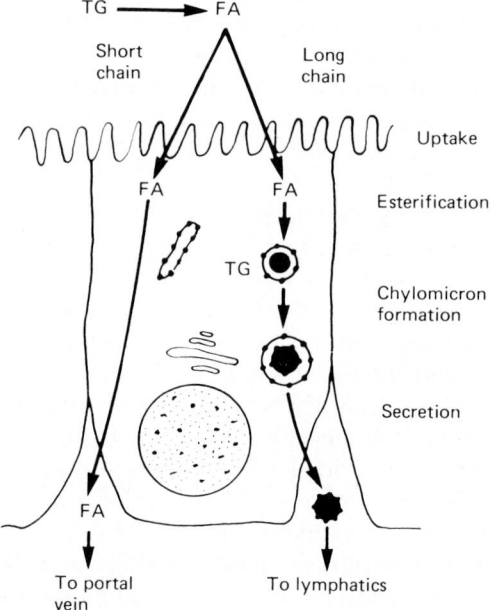

Figure 49-16 Differential absorption of short- and long-chain fatty acids across the small intestine wall. *(Adapted from W. F. Ganong, Review of Medical Physiology, 8th ed., Lange, Los Altos, 1977.)*

into the intestinal cell. Reabsorption of these salts takes place in the terminal ileum. They are reabsorbed directly into the blood and are then recycled in the enterohepatic circulation. The greater part of the triglyceride absorption via lacteals takes place in the jejunum, not in the terminal ileum.

Water, Electrolytes, and Vitamins   As much as 10 L of fluid enters the gastrointestinal tract each day. Usually, only about 2 L is exogenous. Amazingly, the remaining 8 L comes from gastrointestinal secretions! Contributions from the stomach, pancreas, liver, gallbladder, and small and large intestines accumulate to an impressive sum.

The usual fluid volume lost in stool is only 100 to 200 mL per day. Consequently, the remaining volume must be reabsorbed by the gastrointestinal tract.

From the stomach to the colon, the mucosal surface is adapted for water reabsorption. Though the stomach really contributes relatively little to volume control, it still attempts to achieve isotonicity with the plasma.

The duodenum, on the other hand, is the place of great fluid shifts. All contents leaving the duodenum are isotonic as they pass on to the jejunum. That implies absorption of osmotically active particles (sugars, amino acids) and/or secretion of buffering fluids to dilute the intestinal contents.

The colon, another major site of water absorption, is discussed more thoroughly further along in this section.

Electrolyte shifts within the gastrointestinal tract are important to overall function. The role of the Na^+ ion in carbohydrate and protein metabolism makes it evident that significant electrolyte imbalances may pose serious limitations on the normal absorptive functions of the bowel.

Normally, Na^+ is actively reabsorbed in the small intestine and water passively follows. Chloride is absorbed in the ileum, while HCO_3^- is secreted into the lumen. K^+ is absorbed as well as secreted by colonic mucosa.

Vitamins, with the exception of B_{12}, are absorbed in the upper part of the small bowel. The B_{12}-intrinsic factor complex is absorbed in the terminal ileum. Water-soluble vitamins do not require any special enzymes or mechanisms for absorption.

Fat-soluble vitamins A, D, E, and K require that normal enzymes and bile salts for routine fat absorption be present. If fat malabsorption occurs, the fat-soluble vitamins are not absorbed.

Iron, though not a vitamin, is important to the balance of hemoglobin synthesis and degradation. Iron is normally easily absorbed in the upper small intestine. It does, however, require active transport.

Colonic Function

Motility

The colon, unlike the small intestine, does not move intestinal contents along rapidly. Instead, the colonic motions permit mixing and molding of stool followed by slow exit from the anus. Since the colon has a relatively small absorptive surface area, slowed transit along its course permits the needed absorption of water and electrolytes.

Chyme reaching the colon is in liquid form. The large intestine must be able to absorb sufficient amounts of water to produce solid stools. It should be remembered that some 9 L of fluid enters the gastrointestinal tract each day. Of that total volume, 1 L reaches the colon. Since only 150 mL of fluid is lost in the stools each day, the colon must absorb between 800 and 900 mL of liquid a day.

The motion accountable for mixing and molding is segmentation. Like segmentation in the small intestine, colonic segmentation corresponds to contraction of the inner muscle layer and changes in the haustral configurations. Segmentation occurs simultaneously in various parts of the bowel in a rather uncoordinated pattern. Again, this lack of coordination slows colonic motility and facilitates absorption.

Propulsive motions of the colon are supplied by weak peristaltic contractions occurring along its length. However, this relaxation and contraction of relatively short segments of bowel provides only minimal forward motion. Indeed, there is even some evidence that antiperistaltic waves exist and cancel out the forward distance gained! This is yet another mechanism by which colonic transit is slowed and absorption enhanced.

These short peristaltic waves would be inadequate as the sole source of forward propulsion in the colon. As a consequence, another more assertive type of movement takes place. Normally, during a 24-h period, the colon experiences three or four stronger, more extensive peristaltic contractions. These peristaltic rushes cause what is known as *mass movements* down the colon. As much as one-third of the bowel may be traversed with one of these rushes. Interestingly, human beings are not aware of their presence.

There is little definitive information about the control mechanisms of colonic motility. The outcome of autonomic input is not straightforward, and laboratory experiments report variable responses. More recently, hormonal control via prostaglandins, 5-hydroxytryptamine, and/or CCK has been suggested. The *gastrocolonic reflex* is a central neural circuit which signals colonic activity as chyme distends the stomach.

Defecation is a reflex initiated by increased tension in the rectal wall. If this pressor stimulus is not inhibited, the normal act of defecation occurs.

The underlying mechanism of defecation involves contraction of the distal colon and rectum, causing increased rectal pressure and shortening of the rectum. As pressure mounts within the rectum, the involuntary internal anal sphincter and the voluntary external anal sphincter relax and stool is able to pass through.

If the urge to defecate is ignored, the walls of the rectum eventually relax and intraluminal pressure decreases and obliterates the desire to defecate. When another mass movement delivers additional stool to the rectum, pressure again increases and the urge to defecate returns.

Humans are able to assist the basic mechanisms involved in evacuation by initiating the Valsalva maneuver. With deep inspiration, descent of the diaphragm and closure of the glottis increase both intraabdominal and intrathoracic pressure. This greater pressure is transmitted to the intestine and aids in evacuation.

While straining facilitates defecation, it has potentially dangerous consequences for cardiorespiratory function. As intrathoracic pressure increases, there is an initial abrupt rise in arterial blood pressure and peripheral venous pressure.

Immediately following that, a marked decrease in cardiac output develops because of poor venous return to the heart. The decreased output causes a marked reduction in arterial blood pressure. Consequently, many patients, but especially those with cerebral vascular disease and/or coronary artery disease, are at greater risk for life-threatening events if allowed to strain during defecation.

Diarrhea is abnormal evacuation from the colon, usually excessive in frequency and more liquid than solid. Diseases which induce diarrhea are plentiful and varied. However, despite the commonplace nature of this disturbance, the underlying causative mechanism (or mechanisms) are not obvious.

Many theories have been offered. Some focus on abnormal colonic irritability and increased motility; others support defects of water reabsorption and inability to reabsorb nutrients along the bowel. More recently, excessive gut secretions mediated by cyclic adenosine 5-monophosphate have been implicated as the primary abnormality.

Indeed, the answer is not readily apparent. Nevertheless, diarrhea, from whatever cause, is important to clinical medicine. It poses a vivid and annoying threat to body hydration, pH stability, and electrolyte balance.

At the other end of the spectrum, constipation, or abnormally infrequent bowel movements, does not instigate the wide range of metabolic instability that is produced by diarrhea. Its major clinical significance is as a presenting symptom of possible underlying bowel disease, e.g., colonic carcinoma.

Secretion and Absorption

Unlike the stomach and small intestine, the colon does not produce an abundance of diversified secretions. The major secretory product in the large bowel is mucus. The goblet cells along the mucosal surface secrete a viscous fluid which mixes with the forming stool and assists its mechanical passage toward the anus.

The colon is also responsible for secretion of K^+ and HCO_3^- into the intestinal lumen. Potassium is secreted into a favorable electrochemical gradient, and active transport is not required. Both K^+ and HCO_3^- can suffer dangerous shifts if normal colonic activity is hampered. Adequate K^+ replacement and careful management of pH changes are central to the eventual well-being of patients with chronic or acute diarrheal diseases.

The major absorptive processes occurring in the colon are active Na^+ reabsorption accompanied by passive flow of water and active Cl^- absorption coupled to HCO_3^- secretion. Close to 900 mL of fluid must be reabsorbed daily if body fluid balance is to be maintained. Anything which alters the normal colonic motility or the mucosal surface threatens to alter the sodium-water regulation in the colon. Likewise, if chyme reaches the colon poorly processed because of abnormalities of the upper tract, the colon may be unable to handle the increased load. Thus even a normal large intestine, if associated with a diseased small bowel or stomach or the effects of gastrointestinal surgery, may not be able to complete the reabsorption process and adequately maintain body fluid balance.

Flora

The colon distinguishes itself as a storehouse for various types of bacteria. The sluggish motility of the colon makes it a lush breeding ground for multiplying organisms. Enteric (intestinal) bacteria, especially *Escherichia coli,* are found in abundance throughout the colon. Other gram-negative rods, anaerobic species, and certain gas-producing organisms are present as well.

Certain of the colonic florae are responsible for vitamin production. Vitamin K, essential to hepatic synthesis of blood clotting factors II, VII, IX, and X, is produced by certain flora of the large bowel. In addition, several B vitamins and folic acid are derived from bacterial metabolism.

Bacterial organisms are partially responsible for gas found in the intestine. Though 60 to 70 percent of the flatus passed comes from swallowed air, the remaining portion is contributed by bacterial fermentation. At any given time, the normal colon contains as much as 100 cm³ of gas.

Pancreatic Secretions (Endocrine)

The islet of the pancreas has three main cell types, each responsible for secretion of specific products. The α cell produces glucagon. The polypeptide insulin is secreted by the β cells. The third cell type is the $\delta1$ cell. Its secretory contributions are controversial and still under investigation. Unlike the exocrine pancreas, the hormones of the endocrine pancreas, by definition, are secreted directly into the blood and not into a system of ducts.

Entire books have been written describing the detailed roles of insulin and glucagon. Since the primary concern here is basic gastrointestinal structure and function, discussion of the intricate biochemical workings of these two hormones will be left for another section. For the purposes here, it is sufficient to remember that insulin and glucagon are essential to the biochemical fate of fats, proteins, and especially of carbohydrates.

Hepatic Synthesis

The liver is responsible for the synthesis of clotting factors II, V, VII, IX, and X. It is needed for the conversion and inactivation of certain steroid hormones and many medications. It is critical for carbohydrate synthesis and storage. Hepatic synthesis of plasma proteins such as albumin is fundamental to successful maintenance of body fluid balance.

Simply stated, the liver, or more specifically, the hepatocyte, is responsible for a host of anabolic and catabolic processes that are essential to life.

Blood Supply and Innervation of the GI System

Arterial Blood Supply

The arterial blood supply to the GI tract originates at the aorta and follows through the aortic arch, thoracic arch, and abdominal aorta to the celiac artery and the superior and inferior mesenteric arteries. Branches of the celiac artery supply major portions of the GI tract as follows: left gastric (supplies stomach, esophagus), hepatic to right gastric (supplies stomach), gastroduodenal (supplies stomach, duodenum), cystic (supplies gallbladder), and splenic (supplies stomach, pancreas, and spleen). The superior mesenteric artery supplies the jejunum, ileum, cecum, ascending colon, and part of the transverse colon. The inferior mesenteric artery supplies the transverse, descending, and sigmoid colon as well as the rectum.

Portal Vein System

All venous drainage from the GI tract and liver passes through the portal vein system. The main branches that bring blood to the portal vein include the gastric (returns blood from the stomach and esophagus), the splenic (returns blood from the stomach, esophagus, duodenum, pancreas, and gallbladder), the superior mesenteric (returns blood from the small intestine, ascending and transverse colon), and the inferior mesenteric (returns blood from the descending and sigmoid colon and rectum). The portal vein subdivides into liver sinusoids, which then unite with branches from the hepatic artery to form the hepatic vein, which empties into the inferior vena cava. The portal vein system is physiologically significant in that it delivers partially metabolized digestive products to the liver sinusoids for further metabolism. Liver dysfunction, then, can cause portal venous hypertension, resulting in ascites and incomplete metabolism of the products of digestion.

Innervation

The extrinsic nerves of the autonomic nervous system are located outside the wall of the GI tract and include parasympathetic (vagus and sacral) and sympathetic fibers. The sympathetic system consists of vertebral ganglia situated on either side of the vertebral trunk, terminating in all organs of the GI tract. Neurostimuli from postganglionic fibers include epinephrine, norepinephrine, and dopamine. Intrinsic nerves of the autonomic nervous system are located inside the wall of the GI tract and are extensions from the extrinsic nerves.

Bibliography

Alspach, J. G., & Williams, S. M. (1985). *Core curriculum for critical care nursing*. Philadelphia: Saunders.

Anthony, C. P., & Thibodeau, G. A. (1983). *Textbook of anatomy and physiology* (11th ed.). St. Louis: Mosby.

Davenport, H. W. (1982). *Physiology of the digestive tract* (5th ed.). Chicago: Year Book.

Guyton, A. C. (1986). *Textbook of medical physiology* (7th ed.). Philadelphia: Saunders.

Robbins, S. L. (1979). *Pathologic basis of disease* (2d ed.). Philadelphia: Saunders.

Schiff, L. (1982). *Diseases of the liver* (5th ed.). Philadelphia: Lippincott.

Sleisenger, M., & Fordtran, J. (1983). *Gastrointestinal disease* (3d ed.). Philadelphia: Saunders.

Spiro, H. M. (1983). *Clinical gastroenterology* (3d ed.). New York: Macmillan.

Williamson, R., & Chir, M. (1978). Intestinal adaptation, I and II. *New England Journal of Medicine, 298,* 1398–1402 and 1444–1450.

50

Gastrointestinal Data Acquisition

Patricia Kallweit
Kaldor

Clinical Assessment
History
Physical Examination of Abdomen and Rectum

Diagnostic Studies

There are three steps in the gastrointestinal data collection process: history taking and physical examination (which together constitute the clinical assessment) and integration of the findings of diagnostic studies.

Clinical Assessment

History

The gastrointestinal history includes nonspecific problems or complaints, symptoms associated with eating, symptoms associated with bowel habits and/or function, other GI symptoms, medications, diet, and past medical history. General signs and symptoms include poor nourishment states, easy fatigability, change in weight, and change in appetite.

Symptoms associated with eating are pain, nausea and vomiting, difficulty in swallowing, and regurgitation or heartburn. The type of pain should be described as to location, nature, duration, intensity, character, aggravating or relieving factors, and associated symptoms. If nausea or vomiting occur, information relating to frequency, timing, aggravating or relieving factors, description of vomitus, and relation to pain should be obtained. Any difficulty in swallowing should be differentiated as to whether it occurs with liquids, solids, or both.

Symptoms relating to stools, constipation, and/or diarrhea are important as they describe bowel habits and/or function. The frequency, amount, nature, and appearance of stools (blood, melena, fat, undigested food) should be noted. If either constipation or diarrhea occurs, the duration, frequency of stool, and aggravating or relieving factors should be noted as well as the patient's use of laxatives, enemas, or other medication.

Other signs of GI problems include easy bruising or bleeding, dark or orange urine, pruritus, and positional shortness of breath. The use of medications, including prescriptions and over-the-counter drugs, should be ascertained, as well as alcohol use.

The patient's medical history should include current and significant past GI illnesses. Certainly peptic ulcer disease, GI hemorrhage, hepatic disease, pancreatitis, abdominal trauma or GI surgery, and previous hospitalizations are important to note. Anemia, chronic diseases, allergic states, exposure to any contagions, occupational history, and stress factors are also important.

Physical Examination of Abdomen and Rectum

Some of the abdominal and rectal disorders indicated by physical assessment findings are shown in Table 50-1.

Abdomen

Examination of the abdomen should be performed with the comfort of the patient foremost in the mind of the examiner. If the patient has any abdominal pain or is apprehensive about the examination, or if the examiner does not carefully explain what is to be done, the examination may not yield full information regarding the state of the abdomen. Prerequisite to the examination is knowledge of the anatomy of the abdomen and an awareness of the proper techniques of examination. Figure 50-1 demonstrates the division of the abdomen into nine areas to show the underlying anatomy. The nine areas and their representative organs are:

1. *Epigastric*–duodenum, pancreas, aorta
2. *Umbilical*–omentum, mesentery, jejunum, and ileum
3. *Pubic* or *hypogastric*–ileum, bladder, pregnant uterus

Table 50-1 Physical Assessment Findings of the Abdomen and Rectum Related to the Critical-Care Patient

Disorders	Inspection	Percussion	Palpation	Auscultation
Acute surgical abdomen, peritonitis	Body posture and facial expression evidencing pain		Rebound tenderness; boardlike, rigid abdomen; guarding against palpation	
Ascites	Distended abdomen; bulging flanks in supine position	Shifting dullness; possible area of tympany at top of abdominal curve (due to air-filled gut rising above fluid)		
Ileus	Abdominal distention; possible vomiting		Generalized tenderness, possibly localizing	Bowel sounds are diminished or absent; when present, may be high-pitched
Impaction	Absence of bowel movements for several days; possible slight abdominal distention	Possibly increased dullness in lower colon	Hard fecal mass	
Hemorrhoids	Bright red rectal bleeding; visible "tags" around anal sphincter (external)		If thrombosed, internal hemorrhoids may be palpated	

4. *Right hypochondriac*–gallbladder, right lobe of liver, part of right kidney, adrenal
5. *Left hypochondriac*–stomach, spleen, upper pole of left kidney, adrenal
6. *Right lumbar*–ascending colon, lower half of right kidney
7. *Left lumbar*–descending colon, lower half of left kidney
8. *Right inguinal*–cecum, appendix, right ureter, right ovary or spermatic cord
9. *Left inguinal*–sigmoid colon, left ovary or spermatic cord

Figure 50-2 shows the more common division into four quadrants:

RUQ (right upper quadrant)–liver and gallbladder, duodenum, portion of right kidney, adrenal, portions of ascending and transverse colon

LUQ (left upper quadrant)–left lobe of liver, spleen, stomach, portion of left kidney, adrenal, portions of transverse and descending colon

RLQ (right lower quadrant)–lower pole of right kidney, cecum and appendix, ovary or right spermatic cord, uterus (if enlarged)

LLQ (left lower quadrant)–lower pole of left kidney, sigmoid colon, portion of descending colon, ovary or left spermatic cord, uterus (if enlarged)

The order of examination of the abdomen differs from that of other systems in that auscultation follows inspection. This alteration in the examination sequence is justified because palpation and percussion may alter the frequency and quality of bowel sounds. The patient should have an empty bladder and be in a comfortable supine position draped from the nipples up and from the pubis down. The knees may be flexed over a pillow for comfort and increased abdominal muscle relaxation. The arms should be placed at the side or over the chest. The examiner should have warm hands and a warm stethoscope. The patient is approached slowly, explaining the intent, with constant awareness of the patient's reactions and facial expressions. The examiner will need a stethoscope and tangential lighting.

Inspection During inspection of the abdomen, the skin is observed for scars, rashes, and lesions,

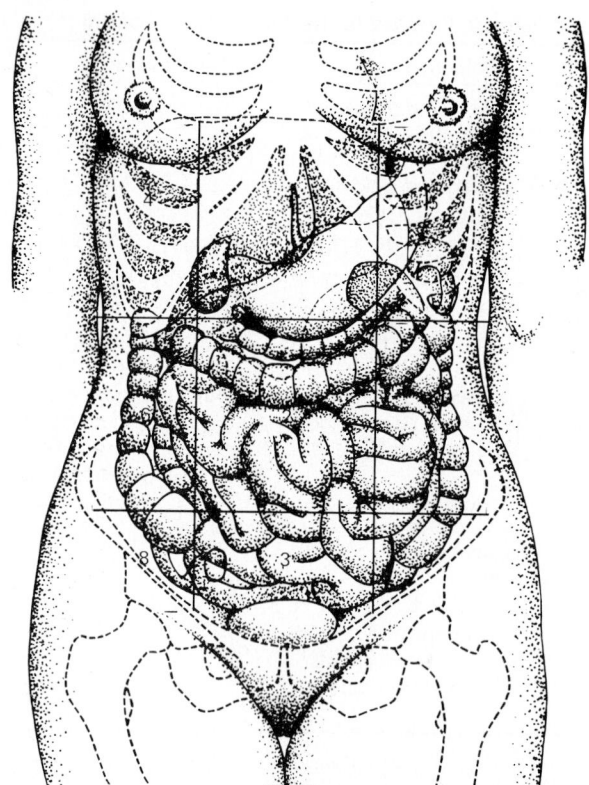

Figure 50-1   The nine regions. *(From A. H. Robins, G. I. Series of the Abdomen, pt. 1, Physical Examination of the Abdomen, A. H. Robins, Richmond, VA, 1969.)*

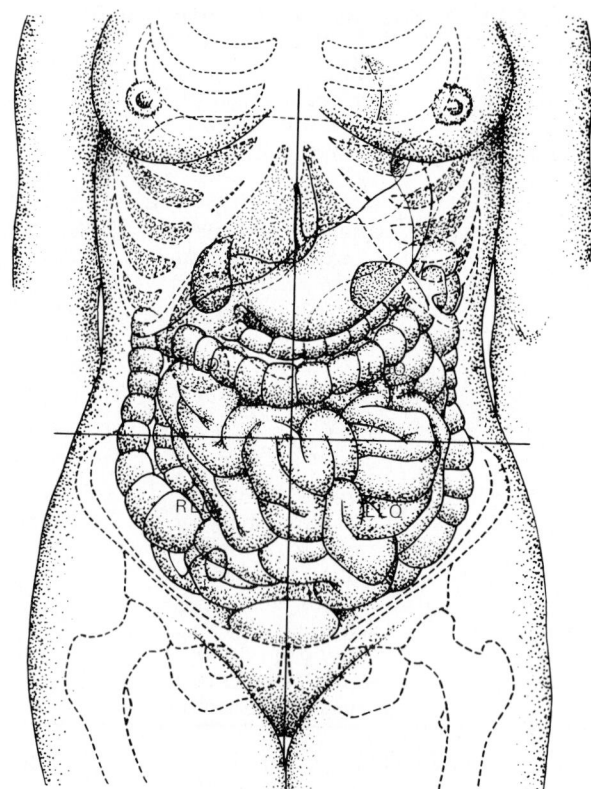

Figure 50-2   The four quadrants of the abdomen. *(From A. H. Robins, G. I. Series of the Abdomen, pt. 1, Physical Examination of the Abdomen, A. H. Robins, Richmond, VA, 1969.)*

and their appearance, location, size, and shape are recorded. The presence of dilated veins could be indicative of inferior vena cava obstruction. Striae, or stretch marks, result from prolonged stretching of the skin. New striae are pink or blue in color, while older ones are silvery. The abdominal contour is usually flat, rounded, protuberant (as in obesity), or scaphoid (as in the emaciated patient). The umbilicus is usually located in the center of the abdomen. Any obvious asymmetry of the abdomen may be an important finding and should be assessed in greater detail. All observations should be made from above as well as from the side. If supraumbilical fullness is noted, it may indicate a mass in the stomach, upper colon, liver, or pancreas, while fullness below the umbilicus may indicate pregnancy, a full bladder, or a mass in the colon, uterus, or ovaries. Careful note should be made of any

such findings as to size, shape, location, and so on. Peristalsis may be observed by using tangential lighting and viewing the abdomen from the side. It is usually possible to detect peristalsis in thin people but not in persons with obese abdomens. Peristaltic movements may also be observed with intestinal obstruction. The pulsations which are usually visible in the epigastric area are normal aortic pulsations.

Auscultation   Auscultation of the abdomen is performed using the diaphragm of the stethoscope and placing it lightly over each of the four abdominal quadrants. The bowel sounds will be heard normally at a frequency of 5 to 34 clicks and gurgles per minute. Bowel sounds may be very loud (borborygmi) when the patient is hungry. This is the familiar stomach growling. Increased sounds may be heard with diarrhea or early intestinal obstruction, while absence of sound is indicative of paralytic ileus, peritonitis, or following abdominal surgery.

The examiner also auscultates for vascular sounds such as systolic bruits, venous hums, and rubs. The stethoscope is placed over the renal artery, abdominal aorta, and iliac arteries to listen for systolic bruits. A bruit is the sound of turbulence from partially obstructed arterial blood flow. Friction rubs are rare, but when present, they sound like rubbing sandpaper and are indicative of peritoneal irritation. Venous hums are also rare, but when heard, they present as a continous humming sound. Figure 50-3 indicates sources of diagnostic noises which may be heard during abdominal auscultation.

Percussion   Percussion is a useful technique for general orientation to the abdomen for identification of gas, air, and fluid in the abdominal cavity and/or organs and for measurement of the liver. This part of the examination begins with a general orientation to the abdomen by lightly percussing all quadrants and determining the areas of tympany and dullness. Tympany is usually found over the stomach, gut, and any other air-filled viscera. Percussion in the left lower anterior rib cage area will reveal the gastric air bubble. Dullness is heard over

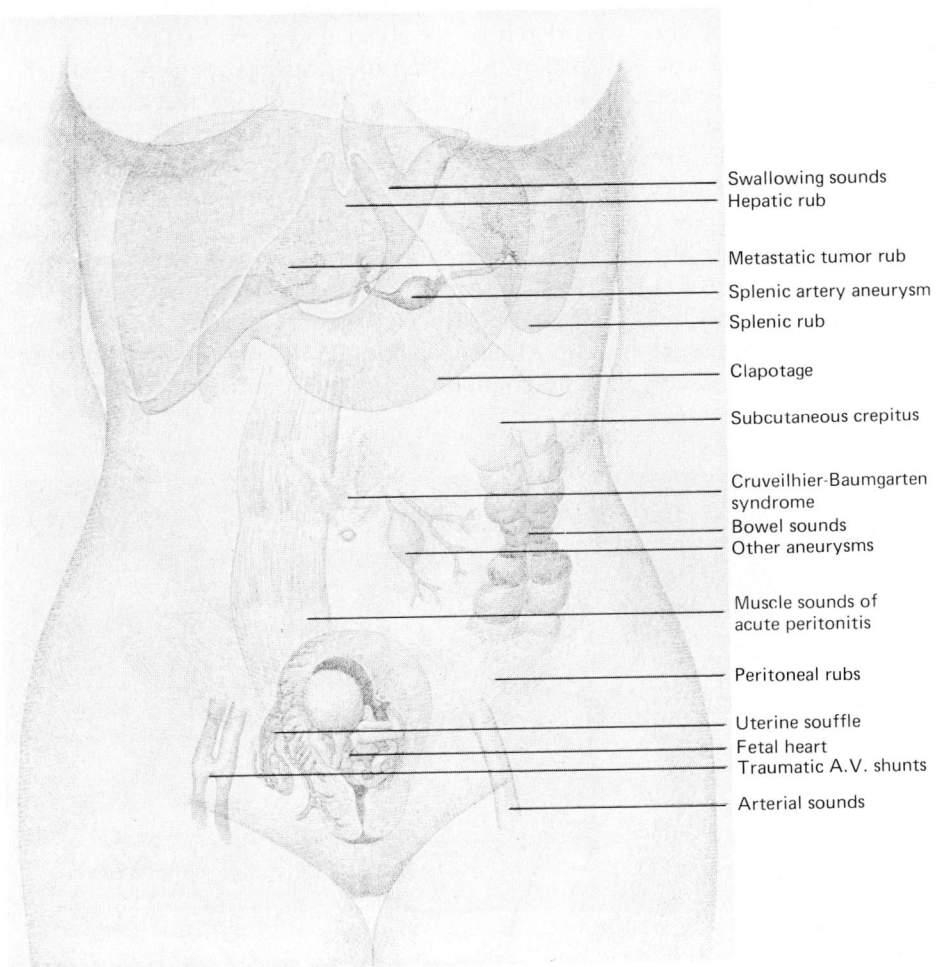

Swallowing sounds
Hepatic rub

Metastatic tumor rub

Splenic artery aneurysm

Splenic rub

Clapotage

Subcutaneous crepitus

Cruveilhier-Baumgarten syndrome

Bowel sounds
Other aneurysms

Muscle sounds of acute peritonitis

Peritoneal rubs

Uterine souffle
Fetal heart
Traumatic A.V. shunts

Arterial sounds

Figure 50-3   Sources of diagnostic sounds to be considered during a routine abdominal auscultation. *(From A. H. Robins, G. I. Series of the Abdomen, pt. 4, Physical Examination of the Abdomen, A. H. Robins, Richmond, VA, 1969.)*

the liver, spleen, a full bladder, pregnant uterus, and the like. Dullness is also heard over fluid, and therefore, the technique of percussion is quite useful in determining the amount of free fluid present in the abdominal cavity. Percussion for shifting dullness is the technique used for detecting free fluid. For this purpose, with the patient initially supine, the examiner percusses from midline to first one side then the other. The point where dullness begins is marked on each side. The patient then is rolled to one side, then the other, and percussion is used in the same manner, with the line of dullness marked. The area between the two lines indicates the amount of free fluid (Fig. 50-4).

Liver size is determined through percussion also. The abdomen is percussed upward along the right midclavicular line from a point just below the umbilicus to determine the lower border of liver dullness, then downward on the midclavicular line from lung resonance to liver dullness. This identifies the upper border of the liver. The normal liver size is 6 to 12 cm. There are, however, normal livers which extend as low as the right lower quadrant.

Often the spleen cannot be identified by percussion, but it is located near the 10th rib just posterior to the midaxillary line (Fig. 50-1). If the spleen is enlarged, it may be detected by percussing the lowest interspace in the left anterior axillary line. The normal sound in this area is tympanic. The examiner should have the patient take a deep breath before percussing. If the spleen is of normal size, the percussion sound will remain tympanic. If the spleen is enlarged, a dull note will be elicited.

Palpation   Light and deep palpation are utilized in examining the abdomen. Before attempting deep palpation, the examiner should employ light palpation, using light, firm pressure and moving smoothly to feel all quadrants. Areas of tenderness and increased resistance can be identified during light palpation. The technique of light palpation involves placing the entire palm and extended closed fingers of the hand on the surface of the abdomen and pressing gently with the fingertips to a depth of about 1 cm (Fig. 50-5). Patient participation by having the ticklish patient place a hand over the palpating hand during the examination will generally decrease the feeling of ticklishness. To determine areas of tenderness, the tips of the fingers are pressed gently into the abdomen and then withdrawn suddenly (Fig. 50-6). The transient pain which results is called *rebound tenderness*. This pressure is always applied in an area remote from the suspected area of tenderness.

Deep palpation is usually required to delineate abdominal organs or masses, and should be

Figure 50-4   Technique for percussing for shifting dullness. *(From A. H. Robins, G. I. Series of the Abdomen, pt. 3, Physical Examination of the Abdomen, A. H. Robins, Richmond, VA, 1969.)*

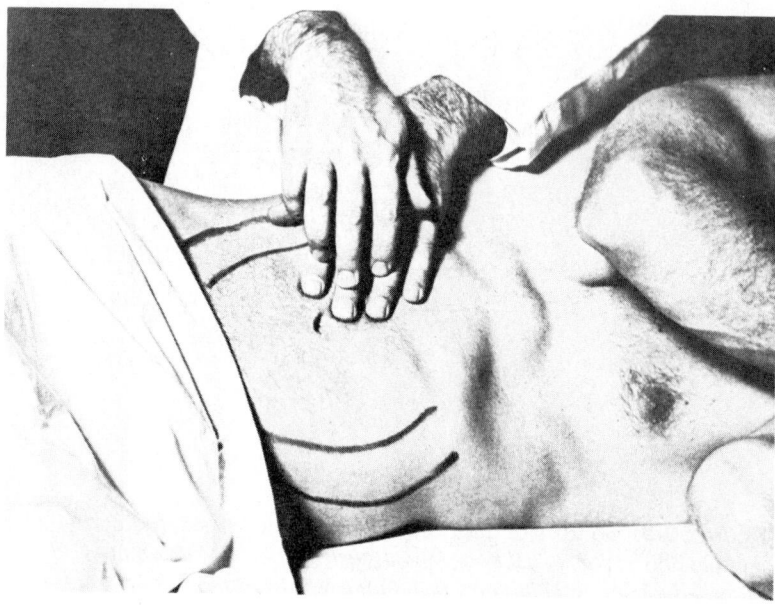

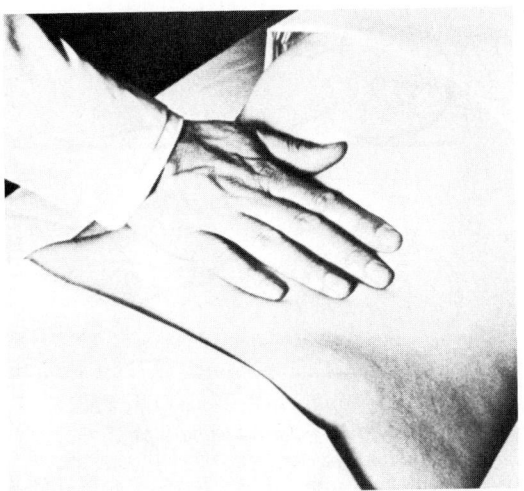

Figure 50-5 Light palpation. *(From A. H. Robins, G. I. Series of the Abdomen, pt. 2, Physical Examination of the Abdomen, A. H. Robins, Richmond, VA, 1969.)*

performed carefully, especially if abdominal disease or injury is present or suspected. Deep palpation is performed by pressing the entire palmar surface of the hand with approximated fingers into the abdomen to a depth of 4 to 5 cm. This may be done with only one hand or with the fingertips of the other hand pressing on the distal joint of the examining hand for increased tactile awareness of the examining fingers, as demonstrated in Fig. 50-7. If on the initial deep palpation a mass is felt, it should be determined whether it is an intraabdominal mass or an intramural mass. Having the supine patient raise the head during palpation will give the examiner this information. The intraabdominal mass will move away from the examiner's hand, while the intramural mass will be more readily palpable (Fig. 50-8).

Next the femoral arteries are palpated. Diminished or absent femoral pulses could indicate common iliac artery thrombosis or dissecting aortic aneurysm. Next is the left upper quadrant, which

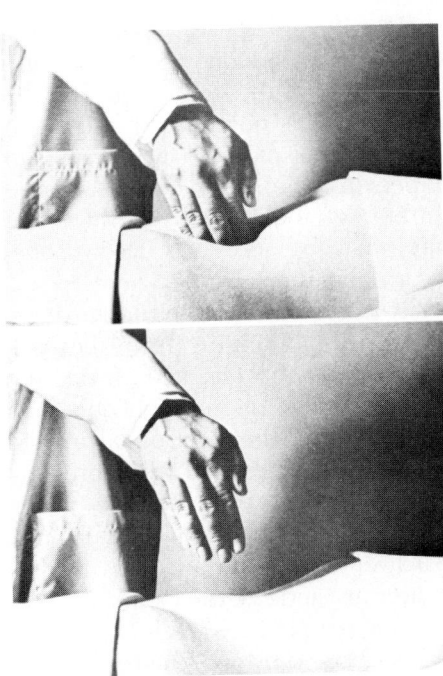

Figure 50-6 Testing for rebound tenderness. *(From A. H. Robins, G. I. Series of the Abdomen, pt. 2, Physical Examination of the Abdomen, A. H. Robins, Richmond, VA, 1969.)*

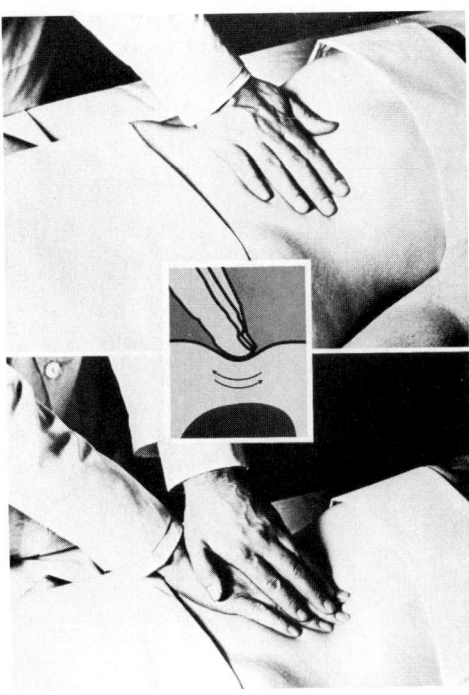

Figure 50-7 One-handed and two-handed methods of palpation. *(From A. H. Robins, G. I. Series of the Abdomen, pt. 2, Physical Examination of the Abdomen, A. H. Robins, Richmond, VA, 1969.)*

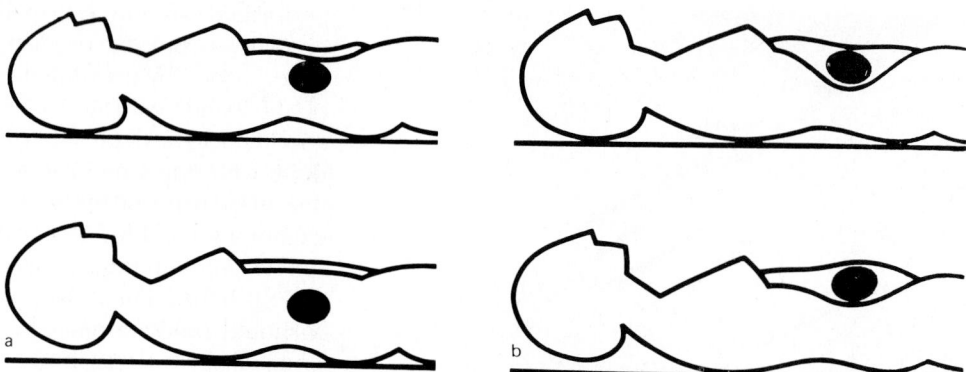

Figure 50-8   Distinction between intramural and intraabdominal masses. (*a*) Intraabdominal mass; (*b*) Intramural mass. *(From A. H. Robins, G. I. Series of the Abdomen, pt. 2, Physical Examination of the Abdomen, A. H. Robins, Richmond, VA, 1969.)*

the examiner palpates by standing on the patient's right side and reaching across the abdomen. The left lower rib cage is pulled up with the left hand while the right presses deeply toward the spleen (Fig. 50-9). The spleen is not palpable unless enlarged; however, splenomegaly may be slight, moderate, or pronounced. Slight enlargement may result from lupus, rheumatoid arthritis, or subacute

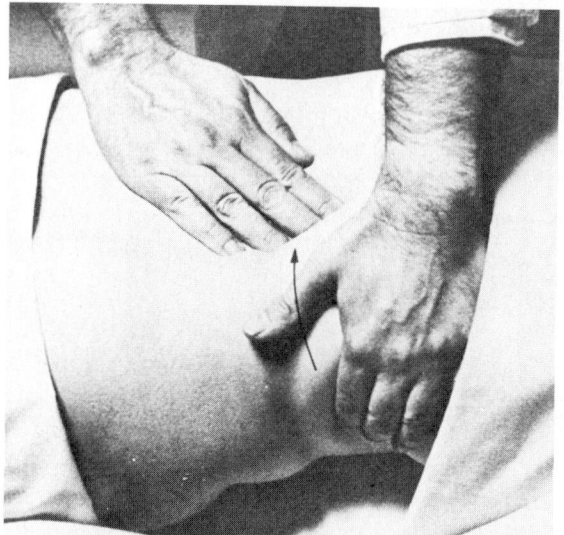

Figure 50-9   Bimanual palpation of the spleen. *(From A. H. Robins, G. I. Series of the Abdomen, pt. 2, Physical Examination of the Abdomen, A. H. Robins, Richmond, VA, 1969.)*

bacterial endocarditis. Moderate enlargement may indicate cirrhosis, hepatitis, or infectious mononucleosis. A large spleen may suggest chronic malaria, congenital syphilis, or portal vein obstruction.

The kidney is palpated by supporting the flank with the free hand and pressing deeply into the lower left or right quadrant with the examining hand (depending on which kidney is being examined). The lower pole of the kidney may be felt coming to the examiner's fingertips during deep inspirations. Kidneys are most easily palpable in thin, relaxed persons; the right kidney is more easily felt because of the lowered position. An enlarged kidney may be secondary to hydronephrosis, cysts, or neoplasm.

The liver is located in the right upper quadrant. It is palpated by pushing up from the back with the left hand under the 11th to 12th rib. The right hand is placed on the patient's right abdomen with fingertips parallel to the right costal margin where the liver edge is anticipated while pressing gently up and in under the thorax as the patient inspires. The liver should be felt on deep inspiration. A normal liver edge is smooth and firm. A hard or lumpy liver may indicate carcinoma, whereas tenderness may suggest hepatitis.

The aorta is palpated by pressing firmly deep into the upper abdomen and slightly left of the midline to identify aortic pulsation. The examiner may be able to feel the aorta between the thumb and fingers. Enlargement of the aorta may be indicative of an aneurysm. This component of the examination is another area where great caution is indicated, especially if problems (e.g., aneurysm) are suspected.

Rectum

The examination of the rectum is effectively accomplished with the patient in the left lateral position. This is the position usually used on persons in bed. The examiner uses a gloved examining hand and spreads the buttocks apart with the other hand. The index finger of the examining hand is lubricated. The perianal and sacrococcygeal areas are inspected for inflammation, lumps, lesions, and excoriations. The patient is asked to bear down during inspection of the anus. Protruding tags of tissue are usually hemorrhoids. In order to palpate the anus, the examiner has the patient relax and then slips the lubricated finger into the anal canal pointing toward the umbilicus. Sphincter tone, tenderness, and irregularities are noted. Internal hemorrhoids may be felt at this time if they are inflamed. In the male, the prostate will be palpable on the anterior wall; in the female, the cervix is palpable on the anterior wall. The entire rectum is consistently and smoothly examined and any material which adheres to the examining glove when it is withdrawn is inspected. The anus and rectum will probably be inspected and palpated by the critical-care nurse in the course of daily care, or when impaction is suspected, or when rectal temperature is taken.

Examination of the rectum may need to be deferred if the patient is critically ill or has had a coronary thrombosis or occlusion, stroke, or injury to the area of the rectum. This is to avoid compounding existing damage or eliciting responses such as the Valsalva maneuver which could endanger the patient.

Diagnostic Studies

Diagnostic studies used to detect gastrointestinal dysfunction include laboratory and radiologic tests as well as special procedures. Laboratory studies to determine liver function are performed according to the problem suspected. Measurement of serum bilirubin levels is required to assess the liver's function in metabolism and secretion of bilirubin. Serum proteins, albumin, immunoelectrophoresis, prothrombin time, partial thromboplastin time, and fibrinogen levels must be evaluated to assess the liver's level of functioning in regard to protein synthesis (the formation of albumin and globulin and the production of clotting factors). Alkaline phosphatase, SGOT, and SGPT are indications of the amount of hepatic enzymes released into the bloodstream. Gastric and fecal analysis are more direct methods of determining the presence of blood or other abnormalities (e.g., hyper- or hyposecretory states) within the GI tract.

Radiologic procedures may include routine chest x-ray, used to rule out thoracic disease mimicking abdominal disease, or esophageal foreign body. Ileus, obstruction, and perforation can be visualized on a flat plate of the abdomen. Further investigation to detect lesions in the esophagus, stomach, duodenum, and small bowel may include an upper GI series that includes small bowel follow-through. A barium enema is used to detect lesions in the colon. A cholangiogram (increasingly replaced by the use of ultrasound) allows for visualization of the gallbladder and biliary tree.

Special procedures for diagnosing GI disorders are increasing in number. Endoscopy allows direct visualization of a specific site to ascertain the presence of bleeding, ulceration, or obstruction. It is also used as a method of treatment, e.g., for esophageal variceal bleeding and the removal of gallstones from the common duct. Computerized tomography (CT scanning) and nuclear magnetic resonance imaging (MRI) are exceptionally useful as noninvasive procedures for assessing many gastrointestinal organs. Ultrasound is being used to detect an enlarged pancreas, space-occupying lesions, ascites, portal dilatation, and gallstones. Motility studies are helpful in diagnosing esophageal and gastroduodenal motility disorders such as achalasia, reflux, and hiatal hernia. Angiography is the method of choice for diagnosing vascular abnormalities. Organs may be biopsied to detect the presence of malignant disease.

51

Patricia Kallweit
Kaldor

Pathophysiology and Diagnosis of Gastrointestinal Problems

Acute Gastrointestinal Hemorrhage (Hemorrhagic Shock)

Pathophysiology

Massive upper gastrointestinal hemorrhage may occur as a complication of peptic ulcer disease, stress ulceration, esophageal varices, esophagitis, gastritis, alcohol ingestion, Mallory-Weiss syndrome, or drug ingestion. The first stage of management is treatment of shock and the second is control of the source of bleeding. A sudden loss of blood volume (hemorrhage) decreases venous return to the heart, with a corresponding decrease in cardiac output. The lowered cardiac output results in inadequate tissue perfusion. This cycle of events, along with the compensatory mechanisms that come into action, must be understood to adequately assess and intervene in hypovolemic shock secondary to massive gastrointestinal bleeding (Fig. 51-1).

Vasoconstriction, a vascular response to the decreased cardiac output and decreased right atrial pressure, shunts blood flow toward the cerebral and cardiopulmonary system. If the vasoconstriction continues, the decreased blood flow to the kidneys may result in medullary tubular dysfunction or acute tubular necrosis (ATN). The urinary output is a good index of kidney perfusion and effectiveness of treatment.

The vasoconstriction phase causing decreased tissue perfusion results in cellular dysfunction. The cells attempt to extract oxygen from the available blood, but as shock progresses, this mechanism is not adequate. The cells then shift to anaerobic metabolism. Energy production is decreased, and large quantities of lactic acid are formed. The depressed blood flow to the hepatic and renal systems impairs the function of these systems in breaking down the lactic acid or removing it from the blood. As the lactic acid accumulates, a metabolic acidotic state develops.

If the blood loss continues, cerebral flow becomes compromised. The patient may become confused and mental changes continue to worsen unless blood flow is increased. The occurrence of brain damage depends upon the duration of lowered tissue perfusion.

Coronary blood flow may be evaluated by electrocardiography (ECG), although this is a rather indirect measure. A flattening of the T wave or a depression of the ST segment denotes coronary blood flow insufficiency.

The body has two compensatory mechanisms that occur more gradually. First, aldosterone and antidiuretic hormone (ADH) are released in response to blood loss. In response to ADH and aldosterone stimulation, fluid shifts from extravascular spaces to intravascular spaces. Second, in the hematopoietic system, an increase in white blood cells and platelets occurs. The bone marrow is stimulated, with resultant increased red cell production and peripheral reticulocytosis. Correction of hemoglobin occurs over a period of weeks following the hemorrhage.

Clinical Assessment

History
The clinical assessment integrates the data gathered from the history, physical examination, and diagnostic tests. The history should include the presence of any precipitating factors (for example, type A personality). The occurrence of melena or hematemesis should be noted but is often unreliable in determining the source of bleeding. If the bleeding is gradual, faintness, fatigue, and pallor may be the

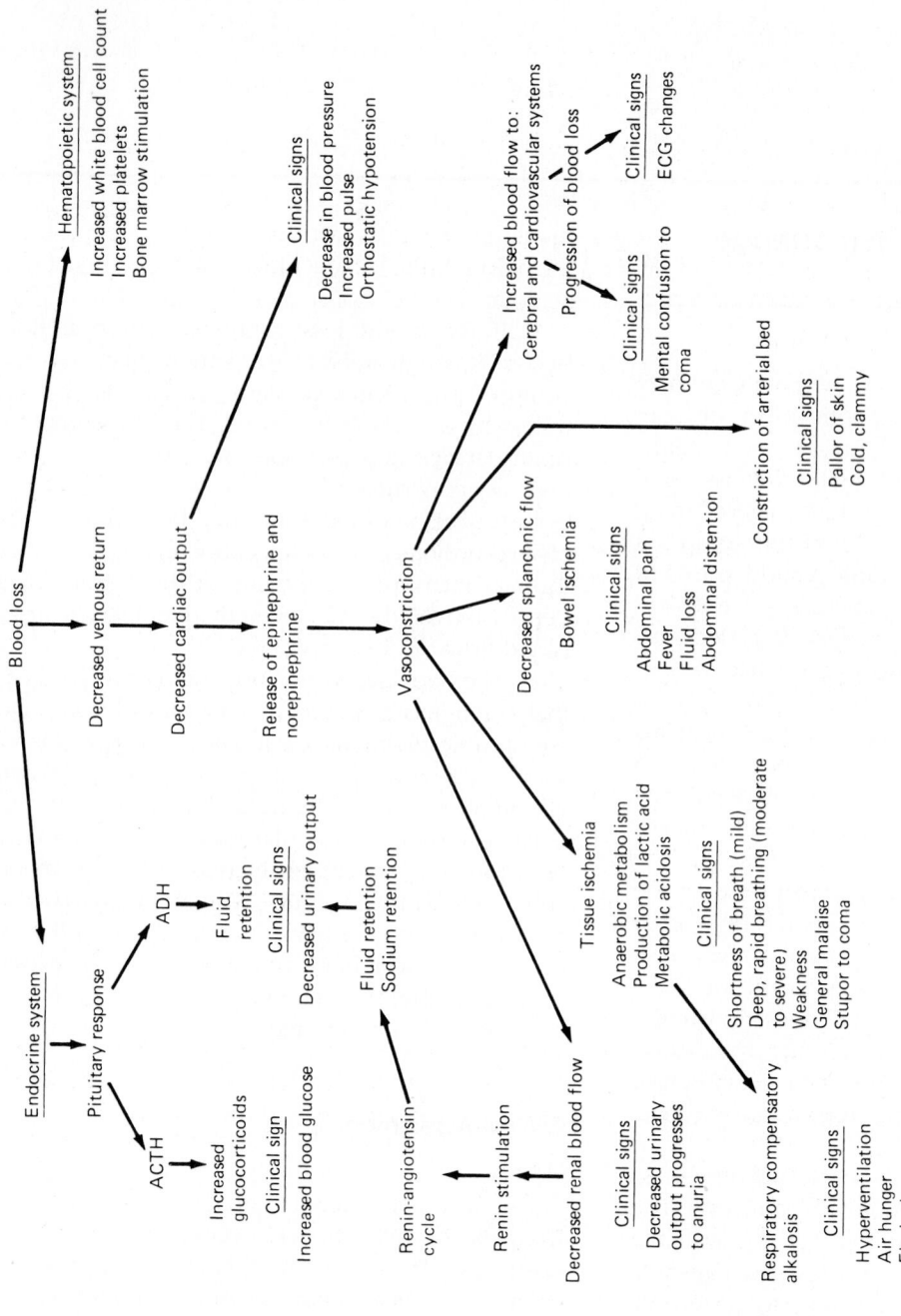

Figure 51-1 Hypovolemic hemorrhagic shock.

only complaints. If blood loss is greater than 30 percent of blood volume, the patient may have shocklike symptoms, including hypotension, shallow respirations, and cold, clammy skin. Orthostatic hypotension and syncope may also be indicative of blood loss. A change in blood pressure equal to or greater than 10 mmHg and a corresponding pulse rate increase of 20 beats per minute in a sitting or standing position corresponds to an additional blood loss in excess of 1000 mL (Table 51-1). The patient's response to the blood loss depends on the rate and amount of blood loss, age, preexisting conditions, and rapidity of treatment. A history of recent medication and dietary habits, as well as information related to previous bleeding, gastric distress, liver disease, or pain, should be obtained.

Physical Examination

Physical examination of the patient with acute GI hemorrhage includes an abdominal examination to assess bowel sounds, with palpation for epigastric tenderness, muscle guarding, or masses. The oropharyngeal area and skin are checked for pallor.

Diagnostic Evaluation

Gastric and fecal analyses indicate the presence of bleeding in the gastrointestinal tract. Stools positive for guaiac indicate bleeding but are not definitive as to source. Although hemoglobin and hematocrit readings may not drop until 24 h after the hemorrhage, they indicate hypovolemia and extent of dehydration. An elevated blood urea nitrogen may be the result of absorption of blood products from the bowel. Prothrombin time and partial thromboplastin time may be abnormal in the presence of liver disease. Arterial blood gases should be evaluated if the patient is hypoxic.

A specific diagnosis can be confirmed by endoscopy. The stomach must be adequately prepared for this study. Evacuation is achieved by instilling iced saline via a large-bore nasogastric tube through the nose while simultaneously siphoning via a Harris tube in either nose or mouth. This method may be effective in eliminating ongoing hemorrhage from the region. Endoscopy allows not only documentation of the site and severity of bleeding but also determination of whether the condition is generalized or localized. Oozing may not always be obvious with conventional white light endoscopy; a fluorescein test may help. The patient is given intravenous fluorescein, and an endoscope with an ultraviolet light is used to locate the bleeding site. Electrocautery probes are sometimes applied through the endoscope to control the bleeding. The diagnostic accuracy of endoscopy (more than 90 percent) has been shown to exceed that of upper GI tract radiography (approximately 30 percent). Barium studies are not conclusive when there are clots in the stomach; moreover, many bleeding lesions are superficial and may not be seen with barium studies. Even if a lesion is detected with a barium examination, there is no assurance that it is the lesion that bled. The clearing time of the contrast material also delays further endoscopy. Angiography is utilized only when the source of bleeding is not accessible

Table 51-1 Physical Findings Related to Stages of Shock

	Early Shock	Late Shock
Physical findings	↓ Pulse pressure, ↑ diastolic pressure; restlessness, hyperventilation; pulse rapid and thready; skin cold, clammy, and pale; ascending cooling of the extremities; mucous membranes dry and pale; nail beds cyanotic upon pressure, with slow capillary refill	↓ Systolic pressure, ↓ urine volume, drowsiness, hypothermia, diaphoresis, pronounced tachypnea
Symptoms	Anxiety, apprehension, nervousness, thirst, perceived feeling of cold, nausea, perceived feeling of weakness	Pronounced confusion and lethargy
Laboratory findings	↓ Urine sodium concentration, ↑ urine osmolarity, respiratory alkalosis	Metabolic acidosis

to the endoscope. If necessary, selective catheterization of the left gastric artery, usually via a femoral artery, may be performed.

Arteriography (angiography) is done when the patient continues to bleed at a rate of 0.5 mL/min. The procedure permits injection and visualization of the various arterial systems, e.g., superior mesenteric artery or celiac axis. Selective arteriography permits intraarterial infusion of vasopressors for controlling hemorrhage. The continuous intraarterial infusion of vasopressin may cause dilutional hyponatremia and decreased urinary output, which is treated with furosemide (Lasix) administered intravenously and volume replacement. Various ways of using arteriography and endoscopy in gastrointestinal bleeding are being explored, including laser treatments and electrocautery probes.

Complications

Complications from acute GI hemorrhage include perforation with peritonitis and sepsis, hypovolemic shock, myocardial infarction, transfusion reaction, and pyloric obstruction.

Intestinal Ischemic Disorders

Pathophysiology

Intestinal ischemia develops from a decrease in blood flow or decrease in tissue perfusion, producing an inadequate oxygen concentration to meet the requirements of the splanchnic bed. Three major arterial trunks—the celiac axis, the superior mesenteric artery, and the inferior mesenteric artery—originate from the ventral aspect of the abdominal aorta and branch to form the vascular bed referred to as the *splanchnic circulation.* The splanchnic area receives approximately 20 percent of the cardiac output. Adequate splanchnic perfusion depends upon the patency of the major arteries, arteriolar resistance, perfusion pressure, arterial oxygen saturation, and the oxygen needs of the splanchnic bed. There are three broad categories of intestinal ischemia: acute occlusive mesenteric ischemia, chronic occlusive mesenteric ischemia, and nonocclusive mesenteric ischemia.

Table 51-2 summarizes factors which influence the splanchnic blood flow. Autoregulation, a physiologic process by which changes in systemic arterial pressure are compensated for by a corresponding change in arterial tone, maintains a relatively stable capillary flow. The distribution of splanchnic blood flow within the intestinal wall and within the mucosa may be adjusted through the autoregulation process without altering the total splanchnic flow. Splanchnic blood flow is increased by the presence of food in the gastrointestinal tract. The process of digestion increases the oxygen requirement of the gastrointestinal organs, and the blood flow increases to meet the increased oxygen demand. Gastrin, secretin, and cholecystokinin are digestive hormones which increase the splanchnic flow when secreted during digestion. Beta-stimulating sympathomimetic amines (isoproterenol) have a vasodilatation effect on the splanchnic blood flow.

Splanchnic blood flow is decreased when the cardiac output is decreased so that blood is shunted to the vital organs. Physical exercise, marked intraluminal pressure (abdominal distention), angiotensin II, alpha-stimulating sympathomimetic amines

Table 51-2 Splanchnic Blood Flow

Factors Increasing Splanchnic Blood Flow	Factors Decreasing Splanchnic Blood Flow
Presence of food	Physical activity
Digestive hormones: gastrin, secretin, cholecystokinin	Abdominal distention (marked increase in intraluminal pressure)
Metabolites produced during muscle activity	Angiotensin II
Beta-stimulating sympathomimetic amines (isoproterenol)	Alpha-stimulating sympathomimetic amines (epinephrine, norepinephrine)
	Cardiac glycosides (digitalis)
	Hypovolemia
	Decreased cardiac output

(epinephrine and norepinephrine), and cardiac glycosides (digitalis) result in arterial vasoconstriction, which decreases splanchnic flow.

The mucosal lining of the intestine is more sensitive to oxygen deprivation than the muscular and serosal layers. Changes occur in the absorptive cells within 5 to 10 min after occlusion of the blood flow. Necrosis, ulceration, and inflammatory cell infiltrate follow. Inflammatory cell infiltrate is a response to the necrosis and the secondary bacterial invasion following ischemic episodes. The bacterial invasion occurs more commonly when the large colon (inferior mesenteric artery) is involved.

Acute Occlusive Mesenteric Ischemia

Acute occlusive mesenteric ischemia may be related to a thrombosis or an embolus. The acute mesenteric arterial thrombosis may be secondary to atherosclerosis, a dissecting aortic aneurysm, thromboangiitis obliterans, or systemic vasculitis. The acute mesenteric arterial embolus is commonly seen in patients with a history of rheumatic heart disease, atherosclerotic heart disease with a mural thrombosis in the heart, or previous embolic episodes. Occlusion by thrombus or embolus is generally seen in the superior mesenteric artery. Occlusion of the superior mesenteric artery results in an intense spasm of the small intestine which is experienced by the patient as severe griping or colicky pain in the periumbilical area. The spasm relaxes, but the bowel is immobile. The immobility of the bowel results in a paralytic ileus. The abdomen becomes distended, and vomiting occurs. The abdominal distention and increased intraluminal pressure further decrease blood flow to the splanchnic bed.

The ischemic bowel loses protein, electrolytes, and fluid into the lumen and wall of the bowel. The third-space extracellular fluid loss decreases the circulating blood volume. This decreases cardiac output and arterial blood pressure and increases blood viscosity.

Chronic Occlusive Mesenteric Ischemia

The atherosclerotic changes in two of three of the major splanchnic vessels occurring over a period of time is accompanied by the development of collateral blood flow. Under normal physiologic functioning the collateral flow minimizes and oc-

casionally prevents intestinal ischemia. As the atherosclerosis progresses, the patient may develop intermittent transitory ischemia. After the ingestion of food, the oxygen requirement of the intestines increases. If the blood flow is unable to increase correspondingly with the increased need, intestinal ischemia occurs. The presenting symptom of chronic occlusive mesenteric ischemia is intestinal angina (intermittent midabdominal pain following eating). The intestinal angina may be compared to angina pectoris or coronary ischemia.

Nonocclusive Mesenteric Ischemia

Nonocclusive mesenteric ischemia is secondary to low blood flow to the mesenteric arteries without occlusion. Splanchnic vasoconstriction and a degree of atherosclerotic changes are predisposing factors. In the presence of lowered cardiac output and poor tissue perfusion, blood flow is redistributed to the vital organs. If vasoconstrictive drugs are given to improve arterial pressure and cardiac output, the splanchnic blood flow is further decreased. If the ischemia continues because of atherosclerotic partial occlusions or the self-sustaining cycle of the temporary ischemia (Fig. 51-2), transmural necrosis and frank infarction of the bowel may occur. The progression of ischemia has been previously described in the section on acute occlusive mesenteric ischemia above.

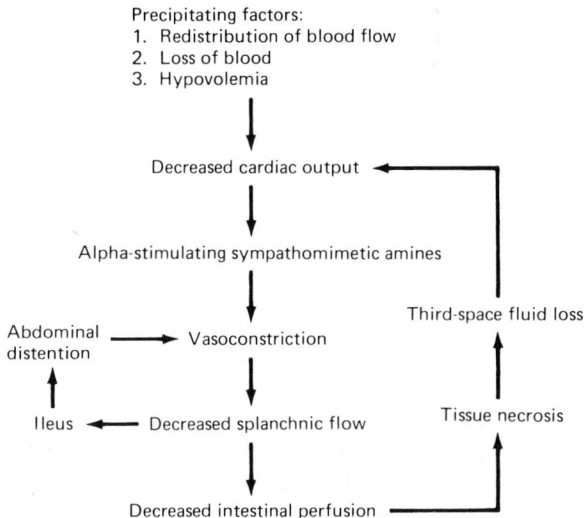

Figure 51-2   The self-sustaining cycle of nonocclusive mesenteric ischemia.

Ischemic Colitis

The reduction of blood flow to the inferior mesenteric artery is usually due to atherosclerotic disease, low flow states (hypovolemia), or interruption of the inferior mesenteric artery during abdominal surgery. The inferior mesenteric artery supplies the left colon and rectum.

Clinical Assessment

History

Clinically, if the ischemic disorder is sudden or acute, the patient presents with an abrupt onset of severe abdominal pain, especially in the periumbilical area. Fluid loss, fever, and gastrointestinal bleeding may follow. Clinical signs of peritonitis and perforation, such as ileus, distention, and vomiting, are indications of the progression of the ischemia and the involvement of the muscular and serosal bowel layers. The clues to a diagnosis of nonocclusive mesenteric ischemia include (1) a history of atherosclerosis; (2) predisposing events of redistribution of blood flow, blood loss, and/or hypovolemia; and (3) abdominal pain of abrupt onset. The abdominal complaints may be severe, cramping periumbilical pain or, more commonly, diffuse nonspecific abdominal pain. There may be dehydration, fever, increased white blood cell count, and an increased hematocrit reading.

Physical Examination

In acute occlusive mesenteric ischemia, the reactions are manifested by a general increase in vasoconstriction, tachycardia, and respiratory distress. Gastrointestinal bleeding may be seen as the ischemia progresses. The changes in blood volume may be evaluated by observing the urinary output. The bacterial action of tissue destruction produces vasoconstricting agents, further complicating the inadequate perfusion of the splanchnic area.

The progression of ischemia results in constant, generalized abdominal pain. As the abdominal pain and distention increase, normal respiratory movements are restricted. This further complicates the respiratory problems associated with increased blood viscosity (hemoconcentration), resulting in impairment of perfusion at the capillary level. Perforation and peritonitis denote extensive ischemia and transmural necrosis.

The syndrome of chronic occlusive mesenteric ischemia is seen in the elderly patient with atherosclerotic changes. The chief complaint is crampy, periumbilical pain which lasts for a few hours after eating. The complaint is nonspecific, and often the diagnosis is not made. The patient continues to have postprandial pain, and a fear of eating develops. Weight loss and malnutrition ensue as the patient limits food intake.

In ischemic colitis, the patient's symptoms include an abrupt onset of nonspecific abdominal pain and rectal bleeding. Barium studies demonstrate the submucosal edema and hemorrhage of small ulcerations (thumbprinting).

Diagnostic Evaluation

Laboratory findings in a patient presenting with acute occlusive mesenteric ischemia include leukocytosis, elevated hematocrit reading, and electrolyte imbalances. The patient has an elevated temperature, tachycardia, and hypotension. Hematemesis and bloody diarrhea may occur. Arteriograms sometimes help in the diagnosis of the disease and evaluation of its extent.

It is common for the patient with chronic occlusive mesenteric ischemia to undergo diagnostic evaluation for carcinoma. If the cause of the weight loss is not cancer, the diagnosis of intestinal ischemia is then considered. Additional symptoms which may occur in chronic intestinal ischemia include steatorrhea (fatty stools), diarrhea, constipation, nausea, vomiting, and abdominal bloating. An abdominal bruit may be present.

Arteriography may demonstrate partial occlusion of the mesenteric arteries and development of collateral flow. The surgical procedures which have been successful include bypass of the occlusion, endarterectomy (removal of the thickness in the artery), and reimplantation of the occluded vessels. Surgical intervention is recommended for relief of pain and correction of malnutrition.

Diagnostic studies for nonocclusive mesenteric ischemia include angiograms to exclude occlusive diseases. Abdominal films and barium studies may be included in early stages of the disease process. Surgery is not usually recommended in nonocclusive mesenteric ischemia. Treatment is geared to correction of the patient's hemodynamic status with volume support, promotion of cardiac function, and control of sepsis.

Ischemic colitis may not be acute. With the cessation of oral feeding and the start of intravenous therapy and antibiotic therapy, the ischemia may be resolved. As the mucosa heals, fibrous tissue forms. Barium studies after the ischemic episode are used for evaluation of strictures arising from scar tissue.

Complications

The patient with acute occlusive mesenteric ischemia secondary to thrombosis is generally elderly and has other cardiac, pulmonary, renal, or cerebral atherosclerotic changes. In this condition the mortality rate for this population is 60 to 70 percent. The increased mortality is probably due to age and its related health problems, the nonspecific symptoms of acute occlusive mesenteric ischemia, and the complications associated with successive operations. Patients with a history of rheumatic heart disease and previous embolic disorders who present with an abrupt onset of severe abdominal pain are more easily diagnosed. The age group is younger than that with thrombotic lesions. The age factor, along with early diagnosis and treatment, improves the prognosis.

An early diagnosis of nonocclusive mesenteric ischemia is important in order to prevent the multisystemic complications that may develop from prolonged vasoconstriction, perforation, and peritonitis.

Intestinal Obstructions

Pathophysiology

Intestinal obstructions may be divided into two categories: mechanical and functional. Mechanical obstructions involve a physical blockage of the bowel lumen. Lesions outside the bowel which produce mechanical obstructions include adhesions, strangulated hernias, volvuli, and tumors. Tumors, large gallstones, impactions, bezoars, diverticulitis, and fecalomas may obstruct the intestinal lumen. Intussusception (a telescoping of a portion of the bowel lumen into a second segment with peristalsis) and stricture formation may lead to mechanical obstruction.

Functional Obstruction

Functional obstruction of the small intestine is more commonly referred to as *paralytic ileus*. A paralytic ileus develops when there is loss of propulsive peristalsis. Conditions that decrease or inhibit intestinal motility are abdominal surgery, hypokalemia, intestinal distention, peritonitis, intestinal ischemia, severe trauma, spinal fracture, ureteral distention, pneumonia and pleuritis, subphrenic abscess, pancreatitis or acute cholecystitis, and pelvic abscess. Intestinal obstructions may also be characterized according to blood flow to the area. In a simple obstruction there is no interference with the blood supply. In a strangulated obstruction the blood supply is decreased; and in an incarcerated obstruction the blood supply is so altered that necrosis of the bowel occurs.

Mechanical Obstruction

A mechanical obstruction of the small bowel results in an accumulation of intestinal secretions, ingested fluids, and gas proximal to the obstruction. In a 24-h period the gastrointestinal tract secretes approximately 8 L of fluid for digestion and absorption of nutrients. This fluid is reabsorbed in the small intestine. An accumulation of gas and fluid proximal to an obstruction distends the bowel. Intestinal distention increases secretions without increasing the reabsorption capacity and decreases the motility of the small bowel through an intestinointestinal inhibitory reflex.

The increased intestinal secretions accumulating in the small bowel deplete the extracellular fluid volume. Protein, also lost from the cells, is found in the bowel wall, creating the edematous appearance. The third-space fluid deficit may be sufficient to produce hypovolemic shock. The blood pressure, pulse, and urinary output are indicators of circulatory volume (see section on hemorrhagic hypovolemic shock earlier in this chapter).

The loss of electrolytes varies with the site of the obstruction. In proximal (pylorus, high jejunum) obstructions, vomiting is frequent and often profuse, resulting in a loss of sodium, chloride, potassium, and hydrogen. The patient may present with hypochloremia, hypokalemia, and metabolic alkalosis. In distal (ileum, low jejunum) obstructions, there is less vomiting and more distention. Third-space fluid loss is greater, and the symptoms include dehydration, oliguria, azotemia, and hemoconcentration.

The decreased motility associated with intestinal distention leads to stasis of the accumulated fluid in the bowel lumen. The small intestine has a low bacteria count; however, when mechanical obstruction occurs, there is a rapid proliferation of bacteria. The overgrowth of bacteria is responsible for the feculent odor of vomitus from the small bowel.

Strangulation

Strangulation of the bowel occurs when the circulation to an obstructed segment is impaired. Strangulation may progress to gangrene and peritonitis, and for this reason early detection and treatment are imperative. A *closed-loop obstruction* refers to an intestinal segment which is obstructed proximally and distally. The closed-loop obstruction leads to strangulation by isolating the intestinal segment and impairing the circulation to that segment. As distention increases, there is increased intraluminal pressure which compromises the circulation to the bowel layers. Volvulus and intussusception impair the mesenteric circulation. Adhesions and hernias produce a pressure necrosis of the intestinal segment and may also lead to impaired blood flow and strangulation.

A strangulated bowel segment seeps blood and plasma into the bowel lumen. In a patient dehydrated from an obstruction, the loss of blood and plasma augments the progression to hypovolemic shock. In addition to the fluid loss, the toxins produced by the proliferation of bacteria cross the damaged intestinal membranes into the peritoneal cavity. The toxins are absorbed from the peritoneal cavity, and septicemia may result.

Colonic Obstructions

Colonic obstructions are most commonly related to neoplasms and volvulus of the sigmoid colon. The fluid and electrolyte loss is not as profound as in small bowel obstructions. The large bowel distends with gas and waste material and may perforate. When the ileocecal valve is competent, a colonic obstruction behaves like a closed-loop obstruction. Strangulation of the large colon with the resulting sequelae may occur.

Clinical Assessment

History

A patient with an intestinal obstruction may have a history of previous abdominal surgery, which predisposes to the development of adhesions. A history of diverticulitis may also point to the cause of an obstruction. The presenting symptoms of intestinal obstructions include crampy abdominal pain, vomiting, abdominal distention, obstipation with failure to pass flatus or stool, and the signs of dehydration. The crampy abdominal pain subsides as the intestinal motility decreases. Strangulation and peritonitis are suspected when the crampy abdominal pain is followed by continuous severe abdominal pain and fever. Vomiting is related to the location of the obstruction. Proximal obstructions are associated with profuse vomiting and minimal abdominal distention. In distal obstructions, abdominal distention is more pronounced. The vomitus in distal obstructions has a feculent odor, secondary to the bacterial proliferation. Vomiting is not common in colonic obstruction when the ileocecal valve is competent.

Physical Examination

Auscultation of the abdomen reveals high-pitched, frequent bowel sounds in proximal obstructions. The bowel sounds are slightly lower in pitch and last longer in the presence of distal obstructions. The changes in bowel sounds are related to the increased peristaltic contractions associated with intestinal obstructions.

The abdomen is examined to check for possible hernias, abdominal masses, and rebound tenderness. To examine a patient for rebound tenderness, one hand is slowly pressed into the abdomen and quickly withdrawn; rebound tenderness is present if the pain is greater when the hand is withdrawn. Rebound tenderness indicates peritoneal irritation.

Diagnostic Evaluation

A preliminary diagnosis of intestinal obstruction may be documented by abdominal x-rays. Abnormally large amounts of gas demonstrated on the abdominal films will confirm the presence of obstruction. In the presence of a paralytic ileus, the gaseous distention is more evenly distributed in the stomach, small bowel, and colon, with gas-fluid levels. Laboratory studies include serum electrolyte levels, creatinine, hematocrit readings, and white blood cell count. Blood studies are done serially to assess the adequacy of treatment. Laboratory evaluation will usually reveal normal hemoglobin, serum chemistry, and urinalysis, with an elevated white blood cell count.

Complications

Complications of bowel obstructions include fluid and electrolyte imbalance, hypovolemia, shock, sepsis, and peritonitis, with potential death.

Peritonitis

Peritonitis (inflammation of the peritoneum) may be divided into primary and secondary categories. Approximately 1 percent of the cases of peritonitis result from primary infections of the peritoneum. Primary peritonitis may be idiopathic or tuberculous in origin. Secondary peritonitis results from contamination of the peritoneal cavity from an altered visceral wall or a defect in the visceral wall. Perforated peptic ulcer, ruptured appendix, ischemic bowel disease, intestinal obstruction, trauma, pancreatitis, or perforated colon may progress to generalized peritonitis.

Pathophysiology

The peritoneum is a semipermeable membrane which encloses the abdominal viscera and mesentery in a saclike structure open only in the female (at the fallopian tubes). A small amount of serous fluid is secreted by the peritoneum to prevent friction between the viscera during peristalsis. The surface area of the peritoneum and the skin are comparable. This large amount of absorption area and the bidirectional transfer of fluid, electrolytes, and other material play a role in the process of peritonitis.

The attempt of the peritoneum to localize or wall off any contamination and prevent diffuse peritonitis is the peritoneal defense mechanism. The local reaction of the peritoneum to contamination involves vascular dilatation and increased capillary permeability. Large numbers of polymorphonuclear leukocytes pour into the peritoneal cavity. Phagocytosis of bacteria and any foreign material in the area is carried out by the polymorphonuclear leukocytes. Fibroplastic exudate is deposited on the peritoneum and plasters the adjacent bowel, mesentery, and omentum to the inflamed area, forming a watertight seal. This process is referred to as *localization*, or *walling-off*, of the inflammation, preventing diffuse peritonitis. The localization process is not successful if the contamination is continuous or the original contamination is massive. In these instances, the peritoneal defense mechanism is overwhelmed.

The mechanism of peritoneal irritation in contamination from the stomach, pancreas, and upper small bowel is initially a chemical reaction from the spillage of potent digestive enzymes. Lower small bowel and colonic spillage result in peritoneal inflammation from the entry of the bacterial content into the peritoneal cavity. Vascular dilatation, hyperemia, and a fluid shift are reactions stimulated by peritoneal irritation. The vascular dilatation and hyperemia lead to an increased number of polymorphonuclear leukocytes in the inflamed area. The absorption capacity of the peritoneum is also increased, facilitating the absorption of toxins and bacteria into the bloodstream and leading to septicemia and bacteremia. A fluid shift occurs from the extracellular fluid compartment into the free peritoneal space, into the loose connective tissue (as edema), and into the lumen of the atonic gastrointestinal tract. The translocation of water, electrolytes, and protein into this third-space compartment depletes the circulating blood volume. The rate of fluid loss from the circulating volume into the third-space compartment is proportional to the degree of peritoneal involvement.

Prior to the institution of treatment, the cardiovascular system response is based on the inadequate circulatory volume or on hypovolemia secondary to the fluid shift. In hypovolemic shock there is decreased cardiac output, low filling pressure, and decreased tissue perfusion, with resultant tissue ischemia. If septicemia is associated with peritonitis, peripheral pooling with decreased venous return occurs, followed by a further decrease in cardiac output and a lower filling pressure. In septic shock there is failure of cardiac output and central venous pressure (CVP) to be sustained with volume replacement.

Catecholamines (epinephrine and norepinephrine) are released in response to the acute decrease in circulating volume, resulting in vasoconstriction, increased pulse rate, and diaphoresis (Fig. 51-1). Adrenocorticotropic hormone (ACTH) and aldosterone are released through a pituitary–adrenal axis response. This results in water and sodium retention and potassium loss, since the body attempts to conserve fluid. When the circulatory system is unable to maintain adequate tissue perfusion, metabolic acidosis develops secondary to anaerobic metabolism.

Primary Peritonitis

In primary idiopathic peritonitis the bacterial agent is thought to gain contact with the peritoneum through the vascular system or through the fallopian tubes. The peritonitis is manifested by severe generalized, steady, burning abdominal pain, fever and chills, irritability, and diarrhea. The bowel sounds are either hypoactive or absent. Primary idiopathic peritonitis is seen more often in children than in adults and is associated with infection by the same organism elsewhere in the body.

Diagnostic studies include white blood cell counts in which there is an elevated number of leukocytes, primarily polymorphonuclear. Peritoneal aspiration is performed to distinguish between primary idiopathic peritonitis and a ruptured viscus. The aspirated fluid is evaluated by culture, sensitivity, and electrolyte studies.

Tuberculous peritonitis is associated with tuberculous invasion elsewhere in the body. There are two types of tuberculous peritonitis: wet and dry. Wet tuberculous peritonitis is associated with the presence of copious abdominal ascites. In dry tuberculous peritonitis, fibrinous adhesions are present and result in a matting effect in the intestines and omentum. The onset of tuberculous peritonitis is insidious, with development of dull, steady, generalized abdominal pain of varying intensity. Abdominal distention is seen in approximately half the subjects. General malaise, weakness, weight loss, low-grade fever, tachycardia, and a doughy abdomen are symptoms seen in tuberculous peritonitis. The slow onset of vague symptoms makes the diagnosis difficult. The diagnosis is based on evaluations of aspirated peritoneal fluid for specific gravity, albumin level, and white blood cell count. Less than half the patients have positive tuberculous cultures from the peritoneum. The drug treatment is isoniazid alone. *p*-Aminosalicylic acid and antibiotics are given if active tuberculosis is found elsewhere in the patient.

Secondary Peritonitis

Secondary acute peritonitis is the result of peritoneal contamination from various causes. Perforated peptic ulcer is the most common cause of peritonitis, followed by a ruptured appendix; gangrene of the bowel from strangulation, obstruction, or mesenteric ischemia; gonorrheal salpingitis (pelvic peritonitis); acute gangrenous cholecystitis; ruptured diverticulum; trauma; and surgery. In gangrene of the bowel, the rapid absorption of spilled toxins increases the severity of the process. Penetrating trauma which ruptures a hollow viscus results in spillage contamination. Peritonitis may develop in the patient with penetrating abdominal trauma without visceral perforation because of the entry of foreign material, e.g., clothing or a bullet, into the peritoneal cavity, as well as the infection from the abdomen being open to the environment. Severe blunt trauma may lead to peritonitis by disrupting the abdominal viscera or separating the viscus from its blood supply. Peritonitis from surgery may occur if bile leakage develops, a localized infection spreads, or an anastomosis breaks down.

Clinical Assessment

History

The history obtained for a patient with peritonitis includes the possible sources of contamination and/or causes of infection of the peritoneum.

Physical Examination

Presenting symptoms of peritonitis include pain with any movement, including respirations. The pain is most intense at the site of advancing inflammation. If there is decreased intensity or decreased extent of pain, localization of the peritonitis is considered. The patient is very ill and may be found lying quietly in bed in the supine position with knees flexed. Since respiratory movements increase the pain, the patient's breathing is usually limited to shallow, rapid respirations. The respiratory system increases its effort to oxygenate the circulating blood to compensate for the metabolic acidosis. The increased respiratory activity creates an increase in the oxygen requirement of the muscles of respiration. Thus there is an increased demand on the respiratory system at a time when painful respiratory movements limit the respiratory function. When the required workload exceeds the ability of the respiratory system, respiratory decompensation occurs, with resultant respiratory acidosis.

The pulse is rapid, weak, and thready, representing the cardiovascular changes which may be occurring, i.e., decreased cardiac output and decreased tissue perfusion. Rebound tenderness and muscle rigidity with voluntary guarding are also present in peritonitis. Additional clinical signs associated with peritonitis include anorexia, nausea, vomiting, fever with chills, decreased urinary output, abdominal distention, and absence of bowel sounds.

The workload of the kidneys is increased by the presence of circulating toxins, pigments, and necrotic tissue products in the bloodstream. Decreased cardiac output, vasoconstriction, and decreased renal perfusion affect the ability of the kidneys to excrete the metabolic waste products and toxins. Acute renal insufficiency is monitored by hourly observation of urine output and specific gravity measurements of the urine.

Diagnostic Evaluation

Diagnostic studies include white blood cell counts which demonstrate an elevated leukocyte level, especially polymorphonuclear cells. Serial white blood cell counts are made to evaluate the progress of the peritonitis. If the diagnosis is not clear-cut, the peritoneum may be aspirated. Abdominal x-rays demonstrate the amount of abdominal distention and inflammation and edema of the intestinal wall. Free air will be present on abdominal films in the event of a perforation.

Complications

Complications of peritonitis include respiratory acidosis and failure, acute renal insufficiency, sep-

ticemia, decreased tissue perfusion, and hypovolemic shock. Any of these conditions may lead to death.

Cutaneous Fistulas

Pathophysiology

A cutaneous fistula is a communication between an organ and the abdominal wall and is referred to as an *external fistula*. Most cutaneous fistulas are associated with surgical complications following intestinal, biliary, and pancreatic procedures. Drainage may be externalized through the surgical incisions, drain sites, or separate abdominal wall defects. Intestinal, biliary, and pancreatic fistulas require intensive medical and nursing care.

Enterocutaneous (intestinal) fistulas may develop from anastomotic leaks, prolapse of the bowel into an abdominal or perineal wound, injury to the bowel when adhesions are divided or other surgical procedures performed, or injury to the bowel by wire mesh or retention sutures. Intestinal fistulas are more prone to develop in the presence of inflammatory lesions, neoplasms, or ischemic lesions. Fistulas most commonly appear in the ileum or jejunum, although they may affect any part of the bowel and may connect with any cavity in the abdomen. Postoperative external biliary fistulas may indicate operative injury to the bile duct or stricture of the common bile duct. Proximal pancreatic resections involve anastomoses between the remaining portion of the pancreas and the upper jejunum, common bile duct, and stomach. Leakage may occur from any of the anastomoses.

Clinical Assessment

Diagnostic Evaluation

Diagnosis of external fistulization may be established by *fistulogram* (radiographic delineation using injection of dye through the fistula). Small bowel studies and intravenous cholangiograms may also be utilized in diagnosing fistulous tracts involving these structures. The cause of the fistula will determine the management: surgical or medical.

Complications

The major complications in cutaneous fistula include peritonitis and poor wound healing, infection, and septicemia.

Zollinger-Ellison Syndrome

Pathophysiology

Zollinger-Ellison syndrome is characterized by a non-insulin-secreting tumor of the pancreas, hypergastremia, and multiple peptic ulcers. The non–beta cell adenoma (ulcerogenic tumor) of the pancreas increases the serum levels of the hormone gastrin, resulting in hypersecretion of gastric acids. The pancreatic lesion may be malignant and single or multiple or a general hyperplasia of the pancreas. When it is malignant, two-thirds of the patients have metastasis to the liver and regional lymph nodes by the time of operation. A relation between the ulcerogenic tumor of the pancreas and abnormalities in other endocrine organs has been reported.

The high gastric acid secretions in Zollinger-Ellison syndrome result in a massive amount of acids being poured into the upper small bowel, causing alteration of the pH of the duodenum, damage to the mucosa of the duodenum, increased intestinal motility, and a shift of fluid from extracellular volume into the bowel lumen. Activation of pancreatic enzymes (particularly lipase) requires an alkaline pH in the duodenum. Without active pancreatic enzymes, the fats in the diet remain undigested and steatorrhea (fatty stools) occurs. Steatorrhea, increased fluids, and increased gastrointestinal motility result in diarrhea. Dehydration, hypokalemia, and metabolic acidosis may be seen, depending on the severity and duration of the diarrhea. Severe diarrhea, with or without ulcers, may be reason enough to consider Zollinger-Ellison syndrome.

Hyperparathyroid adenomas are sometimes related to the Zollinger-Ellison syndrome. Hypercalcemia has been demonstrated to be associated with a subsequent increase in gastric acid levels. Multiple endocrine adenomatosis type 1 (MEA-1) are multiglandular lesions which may be associated with the pancreatic tumor of Zollinger-Ellison syndrome.

Clinical Assessment

History and Physical Examination

Initial assessments of Zollinger-Ellison syndrome may include a history of abdominal pain, diarrhea, melena, or hematemesis. High levels of gastric acid result in increased duration of abdominal pain unrelieved by medications. The severity of diarrhea may be assessed clinically. Dehydration, hypokalemia, and metabolic acidosis are secondary to the loss of fluid and electrolytes through diarrhea. Dry mucous membranes, decreased skin turgor, and low urinary output are indicative of dehydration. The dehydrated patient may complain of thirst and fatigue. A weak, irregular pulse and flabby muscles are observed clinically in hypokalemia. The patient may complain of a gaseous, bloated feeling in the abdomen, muscular weakness when ambulating, and a tingling sensation in the extremities. Clinical signs of metabolic acidosis include shortness of breath (mild), deep rapid breathing (moderate to severe), weakness, general malaise, and stupor progressing to coma.

If the patient has a history of other endocrine tumors, the possibility of Zollinger-Ellison syndrome should be considered. Hyperparathyroidism, in the presence of duodenal ulcer, is of particular interest. The first indication of Zollinger-Ellison syndrome may be recurrence of ulcer disease following surgical removal of a peptic ulcer. The presenting symptoms include abdominal pain, diarrhea, vomiting, melena, and hematemesis. The ulcer activity in Zollinger-Ellison syndrome is more virulent than that of the usual peptic ulcer. The pain, although similar to that experienced in peptic ulcer disease, is in many instances resistant to antacid therapy. Enteritis may also be associated with this syndrome. Since in this syndrome the rate of secretion of hydrochloric acid may exceed the capacity of the normal duodenum to neutralize it, the intraluminal contents of the small intestine may be highly acid far down the jejunum. This further accounts for distal duodenal and jejunal ulceration as well as diarrhea.

Diagnostic Evaluation

Gastric analysis, augmented histamine tests, radioimmunoassays, and radiography are used in diagnosing Zollinger-Ellison syndrome. Gastric analysis involves 12-h overnight collection of gastric secretions through a nasogastric tube. The patient remains without oral intake throughout the procedure. High levels of gastric acid are demonstrated in Zollinger-Ellison syndrome (Table 51-3).

The augmented histamine test is begun after an overnight fast. A nasogastric tube is inserted and the residual gastric contents are removed. The patient is instructed to expectorate saliva during the procedure. Following removal of the gastric contents, the basal secretions are collected for 1 h. Betazole (Histalog) is then injected subcutaneously, and gastric contents are collected every 15 min for 2 h. The presence of a non–beta cell adenoma is documented by the lack of gastric response to the betazole. When the parietal cells are functioning at maximum levels in response to serum gastrin, betazole does not increase cell response.

Radioimmunoassay methods measure the serum gastrin levels. The normal upper limit of serum gastrin is 200 picograms (pg) per milliliter of serum. In Zollinger-Ellison syndrome the serum gastrin level is more than 1000 pg/mL.

Radiographic studies document the unusual locations of the multiple ulcers found in Zollinger-Ellison syndrome. The stomach appears enlarged because of the increased parietal cell mass and the edematous mucosal lining. The margins of the ulcers appear jagged and irregular. When barium studies are made, the high gastric acid content dilutes the barium.

Selective abdominal angiography may demonstrate the pancreatic lesion in some patients. The neoplasm may appear as a tumor blush which depicts the vascularity of the lesion.

Complications

Complications of intractable peptic ulcer in Zollinger-Ellison syndrome are gastrointestinal hemorrhage, perforation, obstruction, and internal fistula formation. Gastrointestinal hemorrhage may be first noted as hematemesis or melena. In an acute upper gastrointestinal hemorrhage, the first response of the medical team is replacement of fluid volume and control of the bleeding. An intravenous line is inserted to begin replacement, and a Foley catheter is inserted to monitor urinary output. The urinary output is an index of fluid balance. Gastric perfo-

Table 51-3 Comparative Gastric Analyses: 12-h Nocturnal Results

Condition	Amount of HCl, meq
Ulcer-free	18
Duodenal ulcer	60
Gastric ulcer	12
Zollinger-Ellison syndrome	> 100

rations result in chemical peritonitis from the spillage of potent digestive enzymes into the peritoneal cavity. Peritoneal irritation stimulates vascular dilatation, hyperemia, and fluid shifts. Clinical manifestations of perforation and acute peritonitis include severe abdominal pain increased by movement; shallow, rapid respirations; rapid weak pulse; rebound tenderness, muscle rigidity, and guarding; nausea; fever with chills; decreased urinary output; and abdominal distention. Obstruction in Zollinger-Ellison syndrome may be first indicated by nausea and vomiting with abdominal cramping. Internal fistulization is documented by radiographic studies.

Inflammatory Bowel Disease

Pathophysiology

Crohn's Disease

Crohn's disease is an inflammatory disorder of the gastrointestinal tract and may be referred to as *regional enteritis, granulomatous colitis, granulomatous ileitis,* or *transmural disease.* It generally occurs initially at an early age (15 to 30). Crohn's disease may involve any part of the gastrointestinal tract, although the small bowel, particularly the terminal ileum, and the colon are the common sites. Bacterial, viral, allergic, autoimmune, and hereditary factors have been explored as possible causes of Crohn's disease, but the etiology remains unknown. The disease is pathologically different from ulcerative colitis even though the clinical signs are similar (Table 51-4). In Crohn's disease there is transmural involvement, that is, all layers of the bowel are involved. Unlike the uniform mucosal involvement in ulcerative colitis, the process here is patchy, with relatively normal mucosa between ulcerated areas. Crohn's disease is a chronic con-

Table 51-4 Comparison of Crohn's Disease and Ulcerative Colitis

Crohn's Disease	Ulcerative Colitis
Transmural	Mucosal
Segmental	Progressive, starting in the rectum and continuing proximally
Involves entire GI tract	Confined to the colon and rectum
Watery diarrhea	Bloody diarrhea
Partial intestinal obstruction	Hemorrhage
Fistulas, abscesses	Bowel perforation
Recurrence after surgical intervention	Cure with total proctocolectomy and ileostomy

dition with many remissions and exacerbations, and there is no known cure. The surgical and medical management of Crohn's disease is influenced by the high incidence of exacerbations and recurrences after surgery.

In Crohn's disease the mesentery thickens, the mesenteric lymph nodes enlarge, serositis occurs, and the mesenteric fat envelops the serosal surface of the bowel. Adhesions develop when loops of bowel become matted together by the serositis and mesenteric changes. Internal fistulization between loops of bowel, bladder, and vagina may occur. External (cutaneous) fistulization is not usually seen unless surgical intervention has taken place. Skipped lesions are common. The mucosa develops a cobblestone appearance as the bowel lumen narrows, the mucosal surface develops fissures, and the submucosal layer becomes edematous.

Ulcerative Colitis

Ulcerative colitis is a disease in which uniform inflammation involves the mucosal lining of the colon and rectum. The etiology is unknown, and as in Crohn's disease, various factors have been examined as possible causes. Ulcerative colitis is a disease process of remissions and exacerbations. The patient is generally young to middle-aged when the condition is first diagnosed. Pathologic changes in the colon are usually confined to the mucosal and submucosal layers. The process generally begins in the rectum and progresses proximally in the colon.

Diverticulitis

Diverticulitis is considered a form of inflammatory bowel disease. It is the result of perforation of one or more diverticula (pouches of mucosa and submucosa projecting through the circular muscles of the bowel), resulting in inflammation. The perforation seen in diverticulitis relates to increased intracolonic pressure, which forces the mucosa through the muscle wall at points of weakness. It is of interest that the condition was virtually unknown before 1900, and all investigators indicate that its prevalence is increasing, especially in western countries.

Toxic Megacolon

Toxic megacolon is associated with ulcerative colitis and is seen in fulminant disease. It results when the wall of the colon has been damaged by colitis. Contractility of the wall is lost, and massive dilatation of the large colon results. A barium enema given during a period of severe diarrhea may precipitate toxic megacolon. Opiates, anticholinergics, and hypokalemia are factors which may play a role in this disease.

Malabsorption Syndromes

The causes of malabsorption syndromes include infarction or ischemia of the bowel, fistula high in the bowel, and/or Crohn's disease, all of which result in inability of the bowel to absorb nutrients.

Clinical Assessment

Crohn's Disease

Demographically, Crohn's disease is being diagnosed with increasing frequency among those of European ancestry. It is more common among Jews and more common among whites than nonwhites. It appears to be familial, and the incidence over the past 20 years has increased almost fourfold.

The initial clinical symptoms include crampy abdominal pain and diarrhea. The narrowing bowel lumen creates a partial intestinal obstruction, which results in increased intestinal motility and intestinal distention. The increased motility and distention results in pressure on the afferent visceral nervous system which is perceived as abdominal pain. Motility of the bowel is stimulated by the ingestion of food, which enhances the whole process. This may progress to a self-inflicted nutritional deficiency when meals are omitted because of the associated abdominal pain, and weight loss can be severe. Gross bleeding is infrequent and perforation rare.

The increased frequency of watery or un-formed stools is related to the partial intestinal obstruction, bacterial proliferation, lactose intoler-ance, and surgical loss of bowel. The increase of fluid into the bowel lumen and increased bowel motility associated with partial intestinal obstruction result in decreased absorptive capacity in the dis-eased bowel and diarrheal stools. When the bowel contents stagnate behind a partial obstruction or after a surgical bypass of a loop of bowel, bacterial growth may proliferate and alter the pH of the bowel. An altered environment of the bowel may prevent the effective utilization and reabsorption of bile salts. Bile salts in the right colon have a cathartic effect and result in watery, frequent bowel movements. Lactose intolerance is an inability to digest and absorb lactose. The unabsorbed lactose attracts water and sodium chloride into the bowel lumen, and peristalsis increases. The colon's reab-sorption is decreased, and the result is watery stools.

Nutritional deficiency may develop in re-sponse to the pain associated with eating, the effects of the chronic water and electrolyte loss, or the decreased absorptive ability of the bowel. The patient may present with weight loss, vitamin de-ficiencies, and anemia. Perianal fissures and fistulas may be observed in Crohn's disease. In addition to the intestinal manifestations, extracolonic condi-tions such as erythema nodosum and arthritis may be present.

The initial involvement in Crohn's disease is primarily in the terminal ileum, and the constant right-sided abdominal pain mimics appendicitis. (*Terminal* here refers to the end portion of the ileum.)

Diagnosis of Crohn's disease is often a process of elimination of other entities, e.g., spastic colon, appendicitis, partial intestinal obstruction, ileocecal tuberculosis, ischemic bowel disease, cancer, and ulcerative colitis. Barium studies demonstrate the stenotic narrowing of the bowel lumen, longitudinal and transverse ulcers (cobblestoning), and fistulous tracts. Sigmoidoscopy is generally negative, since rectal sparing (absence of disease in the rectum)

is common in Crohn's disease. A rectal biopsy may help in diagnosis.

Ulcerative Colitis

The presenting symptom is bloody diarrhea, and the patient may have up to 30 stools a day. The rectal involvement creates a sensation of urgency when fecal material enters the rectum. The need to defecate is immediate.

Symptoms observed in ulcerative colitis in-clude abdominal pain, weight loss, tenesmus, vom-iting, and fever. Extracolonic manifestations asso-ciated with ulcerative colitis are arthritis, iritis, skin lesions, and hepatic dysfunction. The extracolonic conditions mirror the disease process. During ex-acerbation of ulcerative colitis, the extracolonic involvements worsen; with treatment, they improve. The one exception is hepatic dysfunction, which does not necessarily improve with treatment of the ulcerative colitis.

The diagnosis of ulcerative colitis may involve differentiation between ulcerative colitis and Crohn's disease. A proctosigmoidoscopy is helpful in diagnosing ulcerative colitis. The mucosa may appear erythematous and friable. Bleeding may occur when the mucosa is gently touched with a cotton applicator. In advanced ulcerative colitis, ulcers and pseudopolyps may be seen on procto-sigmoidoscopy. Radiography may show crypt ab-scesses, mucosal ulcerations, and shortening of the colon. Pseudopolyps, irregularities of the colon wall, and loss of haustral markings are also noted on barium studies.

Diverticulitis

Diverticulitis (inflammation and perforation of a diverticulum) is related to diet, age, and bowel habits. Diverticulosis (the condition of having div-erticuli) occurs only rarely below the age of 35 years but increases progressively with age, so that by age 85 two-thirds of all patients have diverticu-losis. The patient's history includes lower abdom-inal distress and tenderness, distention, and severe cramping pain. Constipation or alternating diarrhea and constipation may be reported. Physical exam-ination usually reveals tenderness in the left lower quadrant of the abdomen or of the suprapubic area. The sigmoid colon is the most common site of involvement. Fever and leukocytosis are present. If there is peritonitis, signs of peritoneal inflammation are also present. Diverticulitis is characteristically diagnosed by barium enema examination. Gross blood is not often encountered. The rectum is generally normal. Colonoscopic examination of the affected area, which may be important as a means of excluding cancer of the colon, should be attempted only after the signs of acute inflammation have resolved.

Toxic Megacolon
Signs and symptoms of toxic megacolon include severe abdominal distention, hypoactive or absent bowel sounds, sharp decrease in number of daily stools and increase in gas, fever, tachycardia, abdominal pain, glucocytosis, and bloody diarrhea.

Malabsorption Syndromes
Patients with malabsorption syndromes are unable to digest and absorb nutrients. They experience high-output diarrhea, weight loss, and nitrogen imbalance. Other symptoms relate to the pathophysiologic basis for the malabsorption syndrome, including weakness and easy fatigability (due to anemia and electrolyte depletion), bleeding problems (due to vitamin K malabsorption), tetany, paresthesias, skeletal pain (due to calcium malabsorption), anemia (due to impaired iron, folate, and vitamin B_{12} absorption), and nocturia (due to delayed absorption and excretion of water).

Complications

Crohn's Disease
Because the ulcerations involve all layers of the mucosa and submucosa, fistulas of various organs are a common complication of the disease. Formation of fistulas worsens the nutritional problems associated with the disease as nutrients are increasingly lost by being diverted from the absorptive bowel.

Possible complications from surgical intervention in Crohn's disease are recurrence of disease, short bowel syndromes, fluid and electrolyte imbalance, and cutaneous fistula formation. Recurrence of Crohn's disease following segmental resection is frequent, and progression of the disease increases the likelihood of more and more bowel removal. Short bowel syndrome occurs when large

amounts of small bowel have been resected or bypassed. Absorption of vitamin B_{12} and fats and reabsorption of fluid and electrolytes may be compromised. Vitamin B_{12} is absorbed in the terminal ileum; and after loss of a large portion of the terminal ileum, vitamin B_{12} must be replaced intramuscularly. Fat absorption may be affected by a low pH in the intestines (Zollinger-Ellison syndrome) or by loss of terminal ileum. Loss of terminal ileum results in a decreased capacity for absorption of bile salts in the small intestine. This alters the amount of circulating bile salts and fat absorption. Bile salts in the large colon have a cathartic effect, resulting in steatorrhea. The motility of the bowel is increased after resection and the transient time is shortened. Fluid and electrolytes may not be reabsorbed adequately. Watery stools are often noted.

Ulcerative Colitis
Complications of ulcerative colitis that may indicate the need for surgical intervention include toxic megacolon, perforation, hemorrhage, cancer, and intractable disease. The procedure of choice is total colectomy and ileostomy. Removal of the colon results in cure of ulcerative colitis.

Diverticulitis
Sepsis, local or generalized, is the most common complication of diverticulitis. Other complications include further perforation, hemorrhage, obstruction, and fistula formation.

Toxic Megacolon
Inflammation associated with toxic megacolon leads to necrosis and perforation of the bowel. This in turn may cause hemorrhage and infection.

Malabsorption Syndromes
Complications resulting from malabsorption syndromes include wasting of muscle mass, weight loss, and fluid and electrolyte losses.

Acute Pancreatitis

Pathophysiology

Pancreatitis has been classified to reflect the degree of functional damage and frequency of attacks. *Acute pancreatitis* refers to a single attack of pancreatitis in a previously normal gland. Episodes of acute pancreatitis without functional damage are classified as *recurrent acute pancreatitis. Recurrent chronic pancreatitis* describes recurring episodes of acute attacks with progressive damage to the pancreas. The intervals between episodes are pain-free. The pancreatic function is permanently altered and the pain is constant in chronic pancreatitis.

The causes of pancreatitis may be metabolic, mechanical, or vascular in nature, or the condition may result from infection. In pancreatitis, there appears to be activation of proteolytic and lipolytic enzymes within the pancreas, which causes autodigestion of pancreatic tissue and blood vessels. The most common cause is alcoholism (60 percent). Ductal obstruction, vascular changes, and subsequent inflammation occur. Other conditions associated with pancreatitis include biliary tract disease, hyperparathyroidism, allergies, and metal toxicosis.

Clinical Assessment

History

The exact etiology of acute pancreatitis is unknown. Precipitating factors include trauma, drugs (thiazides, steroids, isoniazid), infectious processes (mumps, scarlet fever, staphylococcus, food poisoning, viral hepatitis), hyperparathyroidism, hyperlipidemia, parasites, ingestion of a large meal (especially one high in fat), and alcohol ingestion. Other causative factors may include a history of gallbladder or other biliary diseases, alcoholism, and hereditary factors. The patient reports steatorrhea (foul-smelling grayish stools), as well as weight loss, nausea, vomiting, and abdominal distention. The history should include the location and duration of pain; the relation of the pain to meals and posture; alcohol ingestion; recent weight loss; nausea and vomiting; anorexia; and food intolerances. The urine should be observed for discoloration associated with obstructive jaundice. The characteristics and frequency of bowel movements should be observed. Fatty stools (steatorrhea) are associated with pancreatitis.

Physical Examination

Signs and symptoms of acute pancreatitis vary according to the degree of functional alteration of the pancreas. There are two types of acute pancreatitis: interstitial and hemorrhagic. In interstitial acute pancreatitis, the pancreas is edematous. The pancreas may recover from mild attacks; however, if complications develop, it may become necrotic. The term *necrotic pancreatitis* is used interchangeably with *hemorrhagic pancreatitis.* The pain may be diminished by maintaining a sitting position or a fetal knee-chest position. Fever and chills are observed in acute pancreatitis. Vomiting due to reflux irritation from the inflamed pancreas does not relieve the epigastric pain and may be persistent. Dyspnea is due to diaphragmatic irritability which compromises pulmonary function. Slight jaundice may be present from obstruction due to edema of the pancreas.

Spillage of pancreatic enzymes into the peritoneal cavity may result in chemical peritonitis. Shock may develop from pooling of fluid and blood in the retroperitoneal area and peritoneal cavity. Diaphoresis, tachycardia, hypotension, and abdominal rigidity may be indicative of shock in acute pancreatitis. Bowel sounds are decreased, and there may be a paralytic ileus with its sequelae, including abdominal distention and loss of fluid into the bowel lumen. The physical examination may reveal upper abdominal tenderness.

Diagnostic Evaluation

Serum and urinary amylase values are elevated in pancreatitis. Serum amylase may return to normal within 2 to 3 days following an acute episode. Serum amylase levels are not used alone for diagnosing pancreatitis, because increased serum amylase is observed also in acute cholecystitis, active alcoholism without pancreatitis, perforated peptic ulcer, intestinal obstruction, mesenteric thrombosis, ectopic pregnancy, renal failure, and mumps and after the administration of meperidine (Demerol). Urinary amylase levels that are elevated for 5 to 7 days tend to reflect the amount of amylase secreted from the pancreas. Amylase values of pleural fluid and paracentesis drainage are used in diagnosing pancreatitis. The serum lipase level is elevated for 5 to 7 days. A lowered serum calcium level may be observed in necrotizing pancreatitis.

A glucose tolerance test is used to evaluate the endocrine function of the pancreas. The exocrine pancreatic function is assessed by a secretin stimulation study. Urinary amylase levels are obtained, and 72-h stool samples are collected for measurement of fats.

The secretin stimulation study requires the insertion of a duodenal tube after a 12-h fast. Baseline samples are obtained, then secretin is given intravenously, followed by an injection of pancreozymin. The duodenal contents are then serially aspirated at specified intervals. A blood sample for assessment of serum amylase is also drawn as a phase of this procedure. The patient will need instructions regarding the secretin stimulation procedure the evening before the study. The insertion of the duodenal tube may cause additional discomfort in the presence of severe epigastric pain. The patient should be made as comfortable as possible for the procedure.

Radiologic abdominal studies may demonstrate pancreatic or biliary calcification. An upper GI tract series demonstrates delayed gastric emptying and enlargement of the duodenum due to edema of the head of the pancreas. Intravenous cholangiography may be performed; although the reason is unknown, failure to visualize the gallbladder is an indication of pancreatitis. Paracentesis may reveal bloody fluid with elevated amylase levels.

Ultrasound studies may be used to diagnose pseudocyst or abscess formation associated with pancreatitis. Surgery may be indicated when a definitive diagnosis has not been made and the patient's status is not improving. Pancreatic abscesses may be surgically drained.

Complications

Complications of acute pancreatitis include pseudocyst, abscess formation, and rupture or thrombosis of a major vessel. The vessels involved in pancreatitis, hemorrhage, or thrombosis include the splenic, mesenteric, and portal blood vessels. Exudates may erode adjacent organs or blood vessels, resulting in major complications such as shock, hemorrhage, intestinal perforation, abscess formation, and coagulopathy. Respiratory failure may occur. Abnormal blood gases are indicative of a poor prognosis. The patient's breathing may be rapid and shallow. Potassium and calcium losses

are also seen in pancreatic complications. Cardiac dysfunction associated with the lowered potassium and calcium levels may be observed on ECG or cardiac monitoring systems and lead to myocardial infarction. Renal failure secondary to hypovolemia may occur. Sepsis, tetany due to severe hypocalcemia, abscess formation resulting from extensive necrosis, and vascular collapse and shock are all possible complications of acute pancreatitis.

Pancreatic Cancer and Pancreatectomy

Pathophysiology

Etiologic factors that have been suggested for cancer of the pancreas include cigarette smoking, dietary agents, diabetes mellitus, and chronic pancreatitis as well as certain carcinogens. Pancreatic resection or total pancreatectomy is indicated. Other indications for pancreatic surgery include necrosis of the pancreas, intractible pain and/or complications of pancreatitis, and severe diabetes.

Clinical Assessment

The patient with carcinoma of the pancreas presents with pain in the epigastrium with radiation to the back, anorexia, jaundice (if the tumor is in the head of the pancreas), and a change in the odor and consistency of the stool. The patient's history usually includes recent rapid weight loss. Diagnostic findings include high serum bilirubin and elevated serum alkaline phosphatase levels. Special studies that may be performed include upper GI tract series, percutaneous transhepatic cholangiography, ultrasound scan, endoscopic retrograde colangiopancreatography (ERCP), selective arteriography, and CT scan.

Complications

Complications that may be seen during the immediate postoperative period include pancreatic fistula, anastomotic leak, hemorrhage, and pancreatic abscess and/or intraabdominal abscess with peritonitis. Insulin dependence and steatorrhea are potential long-term complications.

Esophageal Cancer and Esophagogastrectomy

Pathophysiology

Of all cancer deaths in the United States, 2 to 4 percent are due to esophageal cancer. The 5-year survival rate is among the lowest of any human malignant disease. Lesions spread to the lymph nodes of the surrounding area, with the liver and lungs the most commonly involved viscera.

Clinical Assessment

The patient presents with dysphagia, accompanied by substernal fullness with or without pain which progresses from solids to liquids. There is a history of anorexia and weight loss. Unfortunately, the majority of cases are far advanced by the time the diagnosis is established. X-ray, barium swallow, esophagoscopy, and biopsy reveal the location, size, and type of tumor. Esophageal cytologic studies may be helpful in further defining the type of tumor.

Complications

Complications may follow esophagogastrectomy, the usual form of treatment. There may be leakage from the anastomosis caused by undue tension, poor healing ability, or impaired blood supply. A distended stomach within the intrathoracic cavity may compromise respiratory function. Gastroesophageal reflux may also occur.

Hepatic Dysfunction

Hepatic dysfunction may present as an acute or a chronic disease process. Hepatitis is an acute inflammation of the entire liver and most often results from viral infection, although it may also be drug-induced or of toxic origin. In cirrhosis and advanced liver failure, liver cells are progressively destroyed as a result of alcohol ingestion, severe inflammation with necrosis, or biliary disease and are replaced with fibrotic tissue. Regardless of the cause of hepatic dysfunction, the effects on the patient are the same.

Pathophysiology

Hepatitis

In hepatitis, hepatic cells necrose as a result of leukocytic-histiocytic reaction and infiltration. Bile duct proliferation is usual, with occasional damage. Fortunately, the reticuloendothelial framework is usually well preserved and serves as a framework for regenerating cells. During the recovery phase, reticuloendothelial activity increases throughout the liver. Hepatitis may cause changes in other organs. Regional lymph node enlargement and hypoplastic bone marrow are noted. The brain shows acute nonspecific degeneration of ganglion cells. Occasionally, acute pancreatitis or myocarditis has been observed.

Hepatitis is a viral process. Incubation periods vary from 7 to 60 days depending on the type of hepatitis (type A, type B, or non-A non-B type, sometimes referred to as type C). The virus may spread via blood, feces, or saliva, and onset may be abrupt or insidious. Mortality is low, ranging from 0.5 to 2 percent.

Hepatic Insufficiency and Failure

Hepatic insufficiency is the result of cirrhosis, which is the most common cause of liver failure. Cirrhosis is the third leading cause of death in the American male aged 35 to 54. In cirrhosis, the liver parenchymal cells are progressively destroyed and replaced with fibrotic (scar) tissue. Although regeneration occurs, overgrowth creates lobules that are irregular in shape. Because of this distortion, twisting, and constriction of central sections of the lobules, vascular flow is impeded and portal hypertension results; lymphatic flow through the liver is also impeded. In addition, cirrhosis is characterized by fatty infiltration. Approximately three-fourths of the liver may be destroyed without symptoms of impairment. Portal blood carrying unmetabolized substances enters the system and reaches the brain. These substances, of which ammonia is the most widely investigated, are toxic to the brain. After long periods of damage and regeneration, necrosis and atrophy of the liver occur. An increased number of inflammatory cells is seen, as well as hepatomegaly. Scarring progresses and involves the ducts.

Hepatic failure is the inability of the liver to metabolize carbohydrates, fats, proteins, and vitamins and to conjugate ammonia. In liver disease, the body is unable to maintain normal blood glucose levels and cellular nutrition. In addition, several vitamins are not stored, nor is the level of bile produced which is needed for the absorption of the fat-soluble vitamins. Vitamin deficiencies result. Increased amounts of NH_4 with dissociation to NH_3 and $H+$ (because of diarrhea, hypokalemia, and alkalosis) result in acidosis and elevated ammonia levels, which in turn result in interference with normal brain metabolism. Because essentially all clotting factors are produced in the liver, the patient may have inadequate hemostasis. Severe fluid and electrolyte imbalance and decreased renal function result. Because of decreased efficiency of the liver and splenic congestion, blood bacteria are often increased and the patient is more susceptible to infection.

Clinical Assessment

Hepatitis

The possible source of infection may be learned during the history-taking process. The nurse should be aware that young, low-income persons living in crowded facilities with minimal sanitation standards are most vulnerable to infection with type A virus. An accurate health history is essential, as diagnosis of type A hepatitis in its preicteric phase cannot be made by a simple laboratory test. Exposure to known cases of hepatitis, recent transfusions, needle pricks or wounds, and ingestion of certain foods should be assessed. Complaints of GI upset, fatigue, and weight loss may be suggestive of the disease. The route of spread may be close family contacts, sexual partners, or blood and/or blood products.

Hepatitis A virus is chiefly transmitted from infested feces and can be detected in stool as early as 2 weeks after exposure and prior to onset of the disease. Parenteral transmission of type A virus is also possible through transfusion of whole blood, blood serum, or plasma from infected persons. The antibodies to the hepatitis A virus may be detected at the onset of the disease and before the onset of jaundice. The IgG antibody remains detectable for years and apparently confers lifelong immunity to reinfection. The IgM antibody is associated with

and is a better test for an acute infection and persists for only a few weeks.

The type B hepatitis virus is transmitted when the blood of an infected person comes in contact with the blood or mucous membrane of another person. Three antigens and three antibodies are associated with hepatitis B (serum hepatitis). The antigens are usually detected within 30 days of exposure and may persist for up to 3 months after onset of jaundice.

The non-A non-B type of hepatitis is the most common form of posttransfusion hepatitis in the United States and occurs in patients who have had multiple blood transfusions (at least 15 units). The virus can, however, also be transmitted parenterally by hemodialysis, transfusion, parenteral inoculation, or nonparenterally (intrainstitution, intrafamily). No specific serologic test is available for the diagnosis of non-A non-B hepatitis.

Despite variations in etiology, the clinical course for all types of hepatitis is remarkably similar. The prodromal period before jaundice appears (3 to 4 days to 2 to 3 weeks) is marked by nausea, vomiting, abdominal discomfort, and a low-grade fever. The patient feels fatigue and malaise and experiences a weight loss. The liver becomes enlarged and tender. During the acute (icteric) phase, appetite returns and abdominal discomfort and vomiting cease. The urine darkens from bilirubin, while the feces lighten and the skin becomes jaundiced in appearance. There may be transient pruritus. The liver is palpable, with a smooth, tender edge, in 70 percent of cases. During the icteric phase, the postcervical lymph nodes and spleen are enlarged. The recovery phase can last up to 6 months, and relapses occur in 1.8 to 15 percent of cases.

Several routine laboratory tests may be used to diagnose hepatitis. Although serum bilirubin levels vary widely, elevations occur in SGPT, SGOT, LDH, transaminase, alkaline phosphatase, and sedimentation rate. There is an increase in immunoglobulins M and G in 30 percent of patients during the acute phase. Bile is present in the urine (precedes jaundice), and there is moderate steatorrhea and lightened feces. Leukopenia, lymphopenia, and neutropenia are evident in the preicteric phase as well.

Hepatic Insufficiency and Failure

Precipitating factors for liver failure may include chronic liver disease (cirrhosis) with superimposed stress such as excessive alcohol ingestion, toxic GI bleeding, shock states, rapid diuresis, or sedatives. Viral hepatitis, gallbladder disease, biliary obstruction, neoplasms, drugs to which the patient may have idiosyncratic liver susceptibility (anesthetics, antibiotics, chemotherapeutic agents), portal caval shunt surgery, an acute infectious process, severe dehydration, or fever can all precipitate liver failure.

The assessment should include the presence or absence of cirrhosis and any recent episodes of dietary indiscretion, alcohol abuse, surgery, infection, or GI bleeding. Acute hepatitis or drug abuse also need to be determined. The history should include an assessment of weight loss, anorexia, fatigue, abdominal discomfort, and impotence.

Upon physical examination the patient appears jaundiced (as a result of the liver's inability to metabolize bilirubin) and usually cachectic. Because of the increased circulation of estrogen which the liver is unable to inactivate, palmar erythema, testicular atrophy, and gynecomastia may occur as well as loss of axillary, pubic, and general body hair. The breath may have a characteristic musty, sweetish odor.

The liver is the only organ that synthesizes albumin, the plasma protein responsible for maintaining colloid osmotic pressure in the blood vessels. When albumin is decreased, edema of the ankles and scrotum result as well as generalized ascites and pleural effusion. Because of coagulation deficiencies, bruises and bleeding gums may be noted. The liver and spleen are enlarged. Because the liver detoxifies both the antidiuretic hormone and aldosterone, the activity of these hormones is increased when the liver becomes dysfunctional, resulting in water and sodium retention and potassium loss. Liver disorder may lead to profound changes in fluid and electrolyte balance. Other symptoms include positive Babinski sign and hyperactive reflexes; deep, rapid respirations (hyperventilation); elevated temperature; alteration in pulse; hepatomegaly; and absent corneal reflex. Early manifestations of liver failure may include slowness of mentation and affect, slurred speech, and slight tremor; progressive manifestations include inappropriate behavior, inability to maintain sphincter control, marked confusion, and tremors. The patient sleeps most of the time but is rousable and coherent. In late stages of liver failure the patient becomes unresponsive even to noxious stimuli, and tremors are absent.

The diagnosis of liver failure is based on the patient's history, the physical examination, and the results of serum liver function studies, liver scans, x-rays, and perhaps a liver biopsy. Hemoglobin and hematocrit readings are obtained to assess for GI bleeding as a precipitating event. A WBC count aids in assessing any underlying infection. The assessment of liver status reveals elevations in SGOT, SGPT, LDH, alkaline phosphatase, serum bilirubin, and prothrombin time. The serum albumin, manufactured in the liver, is decreased, while serum globulins are increased. Specific antigen testing (HGsAG, anti-HAV) is performed to assess for active viral hepatitis. Special studies may include abdominal ultrasound if biliary obstruction is suspected. An EEG can verify effects on the brain. Lumbar puncture should be performed if CNS infection is suspected. These data are collected and integrated for the diagnosis of liver failure.

Scans may be used to outline the size and configuration of the liver. A liver biopsy will confirm the extent of hepatic cellular damage.

Complications

Hepatitis

Type B hepatitis has the highest mortality, 1 to 2 percent. Fulminating infection is also most common in type B, and the survival rate is only 33 percent. Recovery from hepatitis may require months. Patients complain of anxiety, fatigue, failure to gain weight, alcohol intolerance, and right upper abdominal discomfort. Serum transaminase levels may be as much as 15 times normal.

Hepatic Insufficency and Failure

The complications of liver failure are extremely serious. They include hepatorenal syndrome, disseminated intravascular coagulation, thrombocytopenia, systemic infection, intracranial hemorrhage, and esophageal varices, all of which must be treated aggressively.

Bibliography

Alspach, J. G., & Williams, S. M. (1985). *Core curriculum for critical care nursing.* Philadelphia: Saunders.

Ansley, J. D., Gardner, J., Isaacs, M., Martin, W. C., McGarity, P., O'Brien, P., & Tebeau, J. (1977). *Total parenternal nutrition.* Atlanta: Emory University Hospital.

Beeson, P. B., & McDermott, W. (Eds.). (1975). *Textbook of medicine* (14th ed.). Philadelphia: Saunders.

Burkhart, C. (1981). Upper GI hemorrhage: The clinical picture. *American Journal of Nursing, 81* (October), 1817–1820.

Carr-Locke, D. (1983). Update on gastronintestinal endoscopy Part 1. *Nursing Times, 79,* 57–58, 60–61.

Clearfield, H. R., & Dinoso, V. P., Jr. (Eds.). (1976). *Gastrointestinal emergencies.* New York: Grune & Stratton.

Cobert, B. L. (1983). Diagnosis: Intestinal obstruction. *Hospital Medicine, 19,* 57-58, 61-61, 64-64.

Cobert, B. L. (1984). Mallory-Weiss syndrome . . . gastrointestinal bleeding due to lacerations of the gastric cardia. *Hospital Medicine, 20,* 65-67.

Engelstad, B. L., et al. (1983). New scintigraphic methods of detecting and localizing gastrointestinal bleeding. *Applied Radiology, 12,* 85-88, 92-94, 96.

Kodner, I. J., et al. (1982). Inflammatory bowel disease. *Clinical Symposium, 1* (34), 3-32.

Molyneux-Luick, M., & Knecht, J. (1977). The emergency that supersedes all your other duties: Hypovolemic shock. *American Journal of Nursing 77* (11):32–77.

Myer, S. A. (1984). Overview of inflammatory bowel disease. *Nursing Clinics of North America, 19* (1), 3-9.

Sabiston, D. C., Jr (Ed.). (1981). *Davis-Christopher textbook of surgery* (Vol. 1, 11th ed.). Philadelphia: Saunders.

Schwartz, S. I. (Ed.). (1969) *Principles of surgery* (Vol. 1). New York: McGraw-Hill.

Sheridan, J. L. (1975). Obstructions of the intestinal tract. *Nursing Clinics of North America 10* (1):147-155.

Sleisenger, M. H., & Fordtran, J. S. (Eds.). (1983). *Gastrointestinal disease: Pathophysiology, diagnosis, management* (3d ed.). Philadelphia: Saunders.

Wentworth, A., & Cox, B. (1976). Nursing the patient with a continent ileostomy. *American Journal of Nursing 76* (9):1924-1928.

Wilson, C. (1984). The diagnostic work-up for the patient with inflammatory bowel disease. *Nursing Clinics of North America, 19* (1), 51-59.

52

Medical and Surgical Therapies for Gastrointestinal Problems

Patricia Kallweit Kaldor

Acute Gastrointestinal Hemorrhage: Hemorrhagic Shock

The patient in hemorrhagic shock requires immediate replacement of fluid volume and control of the bleeding. An intravenous line is inserted with a large-bore needle. When the IV line is started, enough blood should be withdrawn for typing and cross matching, hemoglobin, hematocrit, blood urea nitrogen, electrolytes, and prothrombin time. To prevent hypovolemia, fluid replacement should begin immediately with Ringer's lactate, normal saline, or 5% dextrose in water (D_5W) until whole blood arrives. The replacement of losses with whole blood or packed red cells is the only method of reestablishing and maintaining oxygen-carrying capacity. Oxygen therapy should be initiated. A Foley catheter is inserted for accurate evaluation of urinary output.

Hemoglobin and hematocrit values are often difficult to interpret during an episode of acute gastrointestinal bleeding. The hematocrit reading is the ratio of cell volume to plasma volume, and in acute bleeding, the proportion of cells to fluids changes.

A central venous pressure (CVP) line or a Swan-Ganz catheter is a significant help in the management of a patient in shock. The Swan-Ganz catheter measures the pulmonary arterial wedge pressure (PAWP). Although the CVP readings are not as dependable as the PAWP measurements, both are important in examining the effects of the fluid challenge in patients being treated with massive fluid replacement. The patient should be assessed for fluid balance by checking color, skin temperature, mental status, urinary output, and vital signs.

Blood pressure readings with a cuff are often inaccurate, but *change* in blood pressure is more important than an accurate reading when the change is related to clinical signs and to treatment. Doppler flowmeters are a more accurate method of measuring blood pressure when a patient is in shock. Intraarterial monitoring is the most accurate of all, because it records all changes, no matter how minute. When an intraarterial monitor is used, the patient must be examined frequently for color, pulses, and warmth of the extremity used for insertion of the line (Table 52-1).

Large-lumen nasogastric tubes are inserted, the stomach contents are aspirated, and blood loss is measured. If bright red blood is returned, the site of bleeding is above the ligament of Treitz. However, failure of blood to return does not preclude the possibility of a lesion above the ligament of Treitz, such as a duodenal ulcer. Iced saline or water lavage continues to be used to manage bleeding from peptic ulcer disease, although the practice is being abandoned by many in the medical profession as experimental data suggest that iced lavage actually prolongs bleeding and does not successfully slow gastric hemorrhage. If used, the lavage is initiated and continued until the returns are clear or only faintly colored. Often decompression of the stomach or iced lavages do not control the bleeding. An endoscopy is performed to further examine the patient. Tamponade (applying pressure) with the scope or the use of cautery at the site may control bleeding. Selective intraarterial infusion of vasopressors may control the bleeding. Another new approach to control upper GI tract hemorrhage is selective arterial embolization. After the bleeding site is pinpointed by angiography, emboli are injected through the catheter to a point above the lesion.

In acute hemorrhagic shock, replacement of blood is more effective than intravenous vasopres-

Table 52-1 Clinical Evaluation of a Patient with Hemorrhagic Shock

Evaluation Item	Observation	Comment
Pulse	Weak, thready, rapid	Progression of shock
Blood pressure	Doppler flowmeter and intraarterial monitoring are more accurate than cuff blood pressure readings	Blood pressure fluctuation alone may not be significant; should be examined in conjunction with urinary output and respiratory function
ECG	Flattening of T waves; depression of ST segments	Continued loss of blood, with resultant decreased coronary blood flow
CVP and PAWP (Swan-Ganz catheter)	CVP less than 6 cmH$_2$O denotes fluid deficit. PAWP less than 10 mmHg suggests hypovolemia, more than 20 mmHg suggests pulmonary edema	CVP and PAWP readings must be evaluated in light of fluid challenge and not considered separately from other data
Respiration	Patent airway and blood gases. Decreased Pa_{O_2} leads to respiratory alkalosis, hyperventilation, air hunger, flushed appearance. Check patient's nail beds and lips for cyanosis	A complication of shock is ARDS (wet lung syndrome) from overhydration
Fluid balance	Check patient's color, mental status, temperature, skin (color, temperature), pulse, urinary output, daily weights, neck veins	Tissue perfusion. *Note:* The most important indicator of blood flow and tissue perfusion is urinary output. Hourly urine output should be 30 mL or more
Metabolic acidosis	Shortness of breath (mild); deep, rapid breathing (moderate to severe); weakness, general malaise; stupor, progressing to coma	A result of anaerobic metabolism
Laboratory data:		
BUN	240 mg/100 mL with normal serum creatinine	Blood loss reflected in BUN levels because of absorption of blood products in upper intestinal tract
Blood glucose	Elevated	ACTH secretion
Hct/Hgb	Lowered	Should not be used alone for evaluating blood loss
Clotting factors	Prothrombin time; platelet count	If patient has lengthened prothrombin time (asociated with liver disease), vitamin K is given parenterally

sors. Sodium bicarbonate may be required to relieve lacticemia secondary to shock and the citrate load from the whole blood transfusions.

The late complications of acute shock syndrome are "wet lung" syndrome or adult respiratory distress syndrome (ARDS), and acute tubular necrosis (ATN). ARDS manifests clinically as hyperventilation, air hunger, and flushed appearance. Overaggressive fluid therapy (fluid overload), microemboli, and superimposed pulmonary infections increase the risk of pulmonary complications.

Prevention of pulmonary complications may be maximized by the use of the Swan-Ganz catheter to measure PAWP for regulation of fluid replacement. Filters on all IV lines decrease the possibility of microemboli. Steroids may be used to minimize ARDS by stabilizing cell permeability. ATN is prevented by increasing circulating fluid volume, which increases renal perfusion.

Esophageal Varices

The patient who has massive gastrointestinal bleeding secondary to esophageal varices requires extensive nursing care and management. The 5-year survival rate for a cirrhotic patient with esophageal varices is 5 percent. Hemorrhage recurs in 65 percent of these patients. The mortality from esophageal variceal bleeding is 65 percent. The prognosis for survival is related to three factors: (1) the history of the bleeding episode itself, (2) the severity of the underlying liver disease, and (3) the availability of a health team to manage the patient's condition.

The patient is not only hypovolemic but has a dysfunctioning liver which cannot adequately metabolize, synthesize, or detoxify. Esophageal varices develop when there is an increase in the portal vein pressure. Occlusion of the portal vein, liver parenchymal disease, or occlusion of the hepatic vein may lead to increased portal pressure. The collateral blood flow, specifically to the stomach and esophagus, and enlargement of the spleen develop in relation to the portal vein pressure increase. A patient with liver disease may also present with increased abdominal girth, jaundice, ascites, encephalopathy, splenomegaly, spider nevi, palmaris muscle atrophy, and anemia. A limited history and physical examination during the acute phase of bleeding will lead to suspicion of esophageal varices. However, not all patients with esophageal varices bleed from the varices: patients with portal hypertension have a high incidence of bleeding gastric lesions. Supportive therapy in patients with compromised liver function includes vitamin K, fresh blood, fresh-frozen plasma, and diuretics.

A triple-lumen nasogastric tube may be inserted for use as a tampon to control the bleeding. The Sengstaken-Blakemore triple-lumen tube has two balloons and one lumen for gastric aspiration; it is frequently used for control of hemorrhage from esophageal varices. Four major complications arise from use of this tube: pulmonary problems secondary to aspiration, ruptured esophagus, asphyxia, and erosion of the esophageal or gastric wall. The Linton tube has two aspiration lumens and a gastric balloon. The gastric balloon has a capacity of 800 mL, and when filled, it applies pressure on the intragastric veins. The two lumens of the Linton tube provide for gastric and esophageal aspiration. The advantage of the Linton tube is its capacity for esophageal aspiration and the large gastric balloon, which alleviates the need for intraesophageal tamponade.

The procedure for insertion of the Sengstaken-Blakemore tube is similar to that for any nasogastric tube (Table 52-2). The balloons are checked prior to insertion, and tracheal suction is available during the actual insertion to prevent aspiration of vomitus. The gastric balloon is inflated and fitted snugly against the cardia of the stomach. Traction is then applied to the tube, and the tube is taped to a football helmet worn by the patient.

If the gastric aspirate is bloody, the bleeding is from a gastric lesion. Additional air is inserted into the gastric balloon and traction is continued. If the bleeding is from the esophageal varices, the esophageal balloon is inflated to a pressure of 20 to 25 mmHg. The patient should be observed closely while the Sengstaken-Blakemore tube is in place (Fig. 52-1). Because swallowing is impossible with an inflated esophageal balloon, the patient will require frequent nasoesophageal suctioning to control saliva. Insertion of a Levin tube connected to intermittent suctioning above the esophageal balloon is recommended to prevent aspiration. If the gastric balloon ruptures, the entire tube will move upward and obstruct the patient's airway. The tube must be cut immediately across all three lumens and removed. A second Sengstaken-Blakemore tube should be available in the patient's room should this occur.

Endoscopy and arteriography are used to locate and treat the varices which continue to bleed with tamponade. Intraarterial vasopressin by continuous pump infusion may be given through the superior mesenteric artery. The vasopressin decreases mesenteric blood flow, which decreases portal hypertension and decompresses the bleeding varices, thus allowing thrombosis of the bleeding lesion. Sclerotherapy makes use of sclerosing agents injected into or around the varices.

When the patient has been stabilized from the hemorrhagic shock and the bleeding is controlled, long-range plans for lowering portal hypertension must be considered. Surgical procedures which shunt the blood away from the portal system will decrease portal hypertension.

Peptic Ulcer Disease

Peptic ulcer disease refers to duodenal, gastric, and stomal (gastrojejunostomy junction) ulcerations. Upper gastrointestinal tract hemorrhage is related to peptic ulcer disease in 50 to 70 percent of upper gastrointestinal tract bleeding. Peptic ulcer bleeding can sometimes be controlled by 30 to 60 min of iced saline or tap water lavage. Antacids are then instilled through a nasogastric tube every 15 min

Table 52-2 Nursing Responsibility with Use of Sengstaken-Blakemore Tube

Insertion of Tube	
Activity	**Rationale**
Inflate both balloons of Sengstaken-Blakemore tube and hold them under water to observe for minute leaks	Any escaping air can be detected in water
Label all lumens carefully with waterproof marker	Prevents inflation and deflation of gastric balloon for esophageal balloon and vice versa
Have tracheal suctioning available in room	Vomiting often occurs during insertion, and aspiration is a hazard
Have rubber-shod hemostats available. Double clamp each balloon lumen. Place cotton disk around tube at patient's nares, then apply football helmet. Tape tube securely to chin guard	Unprotected teeth or hemostats may cut into tubing, allowing air to leak. Double clamping assures occlusion of lumen. Traction applied to Sengstaken-Blakemore tube will create pressure necrosis if tube is taped to skin

Care of Patient		
Possible Complications	**Nursing Measures and Observations**	**Rationale**
Erosion and perforation of esophagus and/or gastric mucosa	Careful monitoring of vital signs, particularly blood pressure and respirations	Evaluation of response of bleeding to tamponade, complications, etc.
	Frequent (every 15–30 min) checks of mmHg pressure of esophageal balloon. Release pressure at intervals	Onset of back pain, upper abdominal pain, shock, and fluid in chest are signs of perforation; releasing pressure at intervals decreases incidence of tissue necrosis. Tube is removed after 48 h, because incidence of necrosis increases after this
Aspiration pneumonia	Mouth care; suctioning of nasoesophageal areas	Patient with inflated esophageal balloon is unable to swallow. Frequent mouth-esophageal suctioning is necessary to prevent aspiration. Option is insertion of nasogastric tube above esophageal balloon
	Irrigation of gastric tube; observe color, consistency, and odor of output and note changes	Patency of gastric tube. Color change in output indicates bleeding; change in amount indicates amount of fluid replacement needed
	Keep nostrils clean and well-lubricated; keep cotton disk in place between skin and Sengstaken-Blakemore tube	Patient comfort and prevention of pressure necrosis from traction
Pharyngeal obstruction (asphyxia)	Keep scissors and extra S-B tube readily available. Frequent observation of vital signs—particularly respiratory status. If patient becomes cyanotic, cut through three lumens simultaneously and remove tube	Patient begins gasping for air. Most likely cause is leaking or ruptured gastric balloon. Under traction, when balloon ruptures, tube is raised through esophagus and esophageal balloon obstructs airway. When tube is cut, both balloons are immediately deflated and tube can be removed without further trauma to mucosa. Also, when tube is cut, it can be removed without undoing tape

Figure 52-1 The Sengstaken-Blakemore tube in place, with esophageal and gastric balloons inflated. *(From Daval, 1985.)*

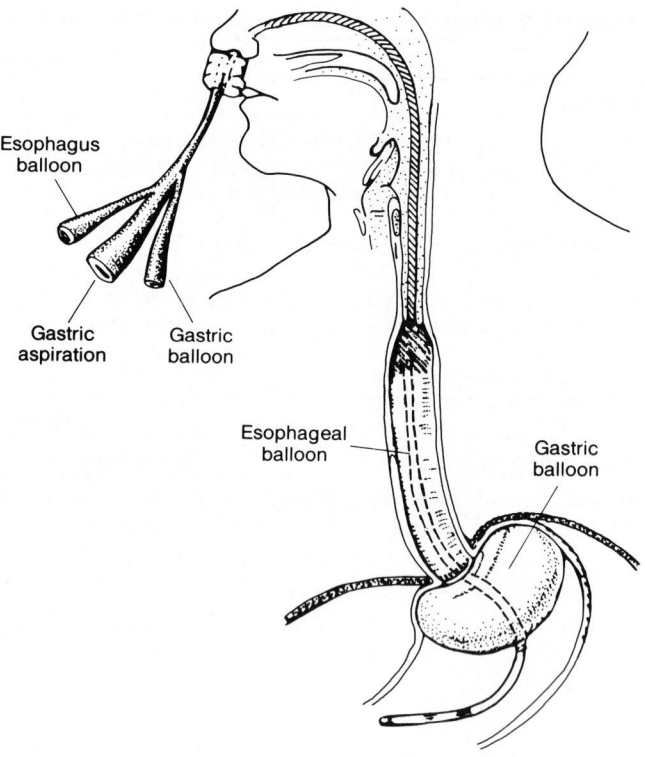

for 3 to 6 h. If no further bleeding develops, the nasogastric tube inserted during endoscopy is removed and antacids are given orally every 30 min. Cimetidine may be used orally or intravenously to decrease hyperacidity.

Differential diagnosis of peptic ulcer is made by endoscopy and barium studies. If medical management fails, surgery is necessary. Many surgical techniques are available, but partial or total gastric resection is the procedure of choice.

Gastritis

Gastritis is a superficial erosion of the gastric mucosal and submucosal layers. It is diagnosed from the redness and oozing of blood seen during an endoscopy. Twenty-five percent of severe upper gastrointestinal tract hemorrhages may be due to gastritis.

The pathophysiology of some types of gastritis involves alteration of the gastric mucosal barrier. The functioning gastric mucosal barrier restricts the diffusion of hydrogen ions from the gastric lumen into the mucosa. Ingested drugs, particularly aspirin (acetylsalicylic acid) and alcohol, affect the gastric mucosal barrier, producing a back diffusion of hydrogen ions. Aspirin is also linked to decreased platelet adhesiveness, which leads to abnormal local hemostasis.

The eroded mucosa may appear normal 48 h after cessation of the bleeding. If the offending agent is known, it should be removed to prevent recurrence. The nursing interview should include pertinent questions related to drug ingestion, alcohol usage, previous history of hematemesis or melena, history of ulcer disease, and recent traumas. The patient's response will guide the nurse toward the causative factors involved in the gastritis.

Stress Ulcers (Acute Gastric Mucosal Lesions)

Acute superficial erosions of the gastric and duodenal mucosa after stressful events are referred to as *stress ulcers*. Major stress factors for patients in the intensive care unit are renal, pulmonary, and cardiac insufficiencies, starvation, hypoxia, septicemia, and disturbances of consciousness. It is generally agreed that the pathophysiology of stress ulcers is related to four factors: gastric acidity, altered gastric mucosal circulation, altered gastric secretion of mucus, and increased mucosal permeability. The incidence is nearly 100 percent in untreated acutely traumatized patients. These gastroduodenal erosions begin in the fundus and body of the stomach and may progress to involve most of the remaining gastrointestinal tract, excluding the rectosigmoid region of the colon. The lesion may develop within hours of the stressful event and is usually painless; the first indication may be severe gastrointestinal bleeding. The symptoms and immediate treatment are the same as those in hemorrhagic shock. The condition is diagnosed by endoscopy. Barium radiologic studies are usually not helpful in diagnosing stress ulcers and probably should not be used in seriously ill patients. Angiography is utilized only when the source of bleeding is not accessible to the endoscope or to permit infusion of embolic materials or vasoconstrictive agents. The object of therapy for stress ulcers is to maintain a gastric pH higher than 5.0 and prevent bleeding and perforation of mucosal lesions.

Mallory-Weiss Syndrome

The Mallory-Weiss syndrome is a linear, nonperforating tear of the gastric mucosa near or at the gastroesophageal junction. The patient presents with a history of hematemesis preceded by a severe episode of vomiting without blood. A massive gastrointestinal hemorrhage may follow. The tear is the result of pressure changes in the stomach during vomiting. The advent of endoscopy has made early diagnosis and treatment possible. When the diagnosis is confirmed, the nasogastric tube inserted during endoscopy is removed and antacids are begun. The bleeding may stop spontaneously. The surgical procedure is to oversew the lesion. Alcohol abuse, hiatal hernias, gastritis, and esophagitis are associated with the Mallory-Weiss syndrome.

Intestinal Ischemic Disorders

The medical treatment for intestinal ischemic disorders is to stabilize the hemodynamics and prevent further ischemic changes. Nasogastric suctioning is used to prevent bowel distention and vomiting. Fluid replacements with saline, colloids, and electrolytes are monitored by CVP lines or Swan-Ganz catheters, hematocrit levels, blood pressure readings, and urinary output. Antibiotics are given to treat sepsis. Sodium bicarbonate is used to treat the metabolic acidosis. Blood measurements of base excess, P_{CO_2}, and pH are guidelines for determining the amount of sodium bicarbonate needed. Cardiac monitoring (ECG) and supportive cardiac care are provided as necessary. Isoproterenol is frequently given to increase splanchnic collateral circulation, as well as to achieve an inotropic effect on the heart muscle itself.

Surgical intervention is based on the results of an arteriogram. An occlusion secondary to thrombosis is treated by surgical bypass of the lesion or an endarterectomy. An embolectomy is performed for an embolic occlusion of a mesenteric artery. A second-look operation sometimes follows either primary operation 6 to 12 h after the first operation. The serosa of the bowel does not always appear ischemic at the time of surgery. After the patient is hemodynamically stabilized, the viability of the bowel can be determined. If all the necrotic tissue is not removed, a breakdown of the anastomosis with peritonitis may occur.

If the ischemia of the large colon progresses, surgical intervention is recommended to avoid perforation and peritonitis from a gangrenous bowel. The involved bowel is resected and a temporary colostomy is created, with eventual reanastomosis.

Intestinal Obstructions

Surgery is the treatment of choice in most instances of intestinal obstruction. The timing of the operation is important and depends upon the severity of the fluid and electrolyte changes, the duration of the obstruction, the risk of strangulation, and changes in the vital organ functioning. Treatment is initiated to prevent shock and restore fluid and electrolyte losses prior to surgery. Supportive therapy includes intravenous normal saline and nasogastric suctioning. Regimens vary, but broad-spectrum antibiotics are often used as prophylaxis against sepsis. A Foley catheter is inserted for accurate measurement of the urinary output. The normal saline is continued until the urine output depicts adequate renal blood flow (output > 30 mL/h). Potassium is withheld until the renal function is adequately assessed, since the kidney is responsible for excreting excess potassium, and potassium excess is as dangerous as potassium deficit to cardiac functioning.

A CVP monitor is used to monitor fluid replacement. The CVP is maintained at between 5 and 10 cm of saline to assure adequate circulating volume. If the patient has hypovolemic shock (see Gastrointestinal Hemorrhage, at the beginning of this chapter) or strangulation, blood and plasma are used with the saline to increase the fluid volume.

The nasogastric tube is used to empty the stomach of contents and minimize further abdominal distention from swallowed air.

Long weighted gastrointestinal tubes (Miller-Abbott, Cantor) are occasionally used for intestinal decompression. The weighted gastrointestinal tube is inserted mechanically into the stomach after the balloon has been filled with mercury. An x-ray is done to determine proper placement of the tube in the stomach and the tube is connected to suction. The tube passes by peristalsis through the pylorus into the duodenum. The tube is advanced slowly. Advancement of longer segments may lead to kinking of the intestinal tube. The intestine is decompressed by suction. The patency of the tube is maintained by saline irrigations. Accurate intake and output records of nasogastric or gastrointestinal output through suctioning is mandatory. A patient may lose 3000 mL or more in 24 h with intestinal obstructions. Adequate fluid replacement is based on the intestinal output as well as vital signs, CVP, and urinary output.

The operative procedures recommended for mechanical small bowel obstructions vary according to the cause of the obstruction. Various procedures include lysis of adhesions, reduction of hernias, bypass of obstructions, and excision of obstructions or proximal enterocutaneous fistulas. Left colonic obstructions are generally treated in three stages. Initially, a proximal colostomy is performed to relieve the distention and provide a fecal outlet. The diseased segment is then removed from the colon distal to the colostomy, with anastomosis of the distal segment. When the anastomosis has healed, the colostomy is closed. The rationale for the three-stage procedure is the hazard of operating on a distended colon. An impending perforation may be walled off by the omentum, and manipulation of the bowel may cause perforation. Surgical anastomosis of a distended colon is not a safe procedure, since the anastomosis of an edematous bowel wall may not be competent.

A paralytic ileus which develops after abdominal surgery generally persists for 2 to 3 days. The treatment includes intravenous fluids and nasogastric suctioning. Replacement and maintenance of normal electrolyte values, particularly potassium, is important.

If the bowel becomes strangulated, an operation is performed to prevent the development of gangrene and peritonitis. The viability of the bowel at the time of operation is determined by the color, arterial pulsations, and motility of the segment. If the bowel is viable, resection may not be necessary. The operative findings determine the surgical procedure.

Peritonitis

Early detection of peritonitis and immediate intervention may inhibit this life-threatening cycle. The goals of therapy are fluid and electrolyte balance, control of infection, relief of pain and ileus, and maintenance of blood pressure.

The treatment of primary idiopathic peritonitis is conservative supportive therapy. Intravenous fluid replacement is monitored by CVP, blood pressure, and urinary output. Broad-spectrum intravenous antibiotics are begun immediately. The antibiotics used may be changed after the causative organism is isolated. The patient is maintained in a semi-Fowler's position to assist in localization of the infection. Nasogastric suctioning is instituted to prevent abdominal distention secondary to fluid and gas accumulation in the atonic bowel.

The treatment of secondary peritonitis is timely surgical intervention after supportive therapy has stabilized the patient's cardiac and pulmonary status. The supportive therapy includes insertion of an intravenous catheter to begin immediate fluid replacement, central venous pressure monitoring, a nasogastric tube for decompression, and an indwelling Foley catheter for urinary monitoring. The amount of fluid replacement is determined by the CVP and hourly urinary output. Plasma, albumin, Ringer's lactate, and D₅W may be given for fluid replacement. Antibiotics are started intravenously, and oxygen is used to augment the respiratory exchange. Analgesics are administered for pain relief. Patients with a history of heavy cigarette smoking, obesity, or debilitation may require mechanical respiratory assistance. Blood gas levels are determined to assess the patient's respiratory status. Early signs of respiratory decompensation include increased arteriovenous differentiation and decreased arterial carbon dioxide from hyperventilation. The pulse rate continues to be elevated, with a slight increase in blood pressure despite the restoration of blood volume. Clinically, the patient is flushed, restless, and anxious, with rapid, shallow, labored breathing.

The approach to operation includes control of contamination, removal of any foreign material, and drainage of any collected fluid. Contamination may be controlled by simple closure, excision, or exteriorization. Peritoneal irrigation during the surgical procedure decreases the mortality and morbidity from acute diffuse peritonitis. The type of contaminant and the age and general health of the patient influence the patient's prognosis.

After surgical intervention, some patients will have an open wound, and intensive wound care is necessary. Continuous irrigation of the peritoneal cavity may be instituted. Two to four dialysis catheters may be placed in the peritoneal cavity during surgery. One to three catheters are used to instill antibiotic solution; one catheter is used for drainage. Accurate recording of the intake and output is essential.

The critical condition of the patient is recognized by the patient and the family. An important area of nursing care involves assessment of their emotional responses, planning of interventions, and implementing of steps to assist the patient and family in coping with the seriousness of the situation. The emotional needs are great when the patient is in an acute state, requiring many technical nursing skills, physical assessments, and implementation of life-sustaining measures. The nurse must permit patients to express their fears. The greatest comfort measure a nurse can utilize is active listening, in other words, hearing the meaning and perceiving the significance of a casual remark.

The cause of the peritonitis will determine the surgical procedure. Peritonitis secondary to perforation of the colon often results in diversion of the fecal stream by a colostomy. The care of the colostomy differs according to location of the stoma in the large bowel. Briefly, the purpose of the large colon includes water reabsorption and storage of waste products (Fig. 52-2). The contents of the small bowel entering the ascending colon are liquid in consistency. The contents of the transverse colon are soft stool containing varying amounts of unabsorbed water. As the contents of the large colon move through the descending and sigmoid colon, the water is absorbed and the stool becomes firm.

A general rule when caring for a new postoperative colostomy patient is to use a skin barrier and an open-end, drainable, odor-proof pouch. Two skin barriers, karaya washers and Stomahesive (Squibb) wafers, may be used to protect the skin. The skin barrier is placed on clean, dry skin at the base of the stoma. It is important that the barrier hug the stoma but not ride up onto the stoma. The opening cut in the pouch must be $\frac{1}{8}$ in larger than the stoma. The edema of the stoma decreases in the early postoperative days, and the opening in the pouch and the skin barrier are adjusted to these changes.

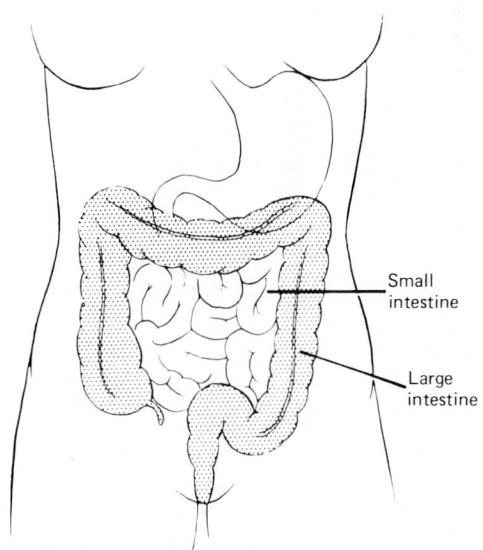

Figure 52-2 Anatomy of the gastrointestinal tract.

Small intestine

Large intestine

In a loop colostomy, a rod is placed under a loop of bowel to support the bowel until adhesions with the abdominal wall occur (Fig. 52-3). The pouching procedure for a loop colostomy with a rod is made easier by keeping some simple facts in mind. It is almost impossible to place a skin barrier or pouch over a large stoma and not get mucus from the stoma onto the materials. Any mucus trapped under the skin barrier may irritate the skin and create a leakage in the pouch system. A washer is cut through one side and placed under the rod (Fig. 52-4). The adhesive backing of the pouch is removed and cut into sections, then replaced over the adhesive. The adhesive is then protected as the pouch is placed on the patient. A pouch which is directed straight to the patient's side is often pulled off by the weight of the stool when the patient is up. The pouch should be angled toward the lateral aspect of the thigh as the patient's activities change (Fig. 52-5). The pouch seal is often broken by the weight of the stool in an unemptied pouch or the tension from flatus trapped in the pouch. Pinholes for flatus work well for the nursing staff, but the patient suffers. Every time the covers are lifted or adjusted, the odor is present. This does not encourage a patient to accept the change in his or her body image. If patients are aware of their own odors, the family, visitors, and staff must be also. A fear of rejection because of the stoma and the odor is associated with colostomies. Emptying

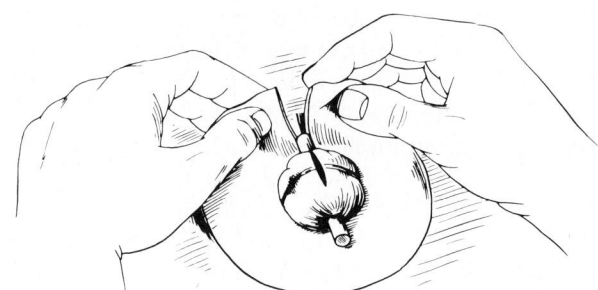

Figure 52-4   Application of a skin barrier with a rod in place.

a pouch of flatus from the closed end means that the rest of the time the odor is contained in an odor-proof pouch. The nurse should not ignore the odor. The colostomy and lack of sphincter control should be discussed, and commercial products should be used to remove the odor in the room.

A colostomy following peritonitis is often temporary; however, the duration of the need for the colostomy varies from patient to patient. Learning self-care and returning to presurgical activities are encouraged. The colostomy will not limit a person's activity. However, the reactions of patients to colostomies vary. Acceptance of the changed body image takes a long time. A patient who feels that the problem of coping with a colostomy is

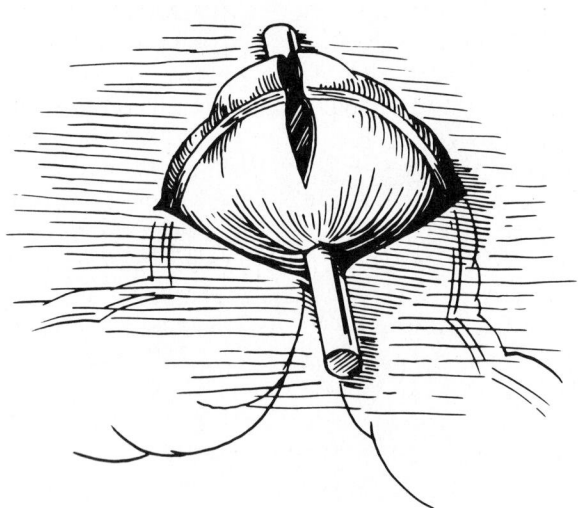

Figure 52-3   Loop ostomy rod procedure.

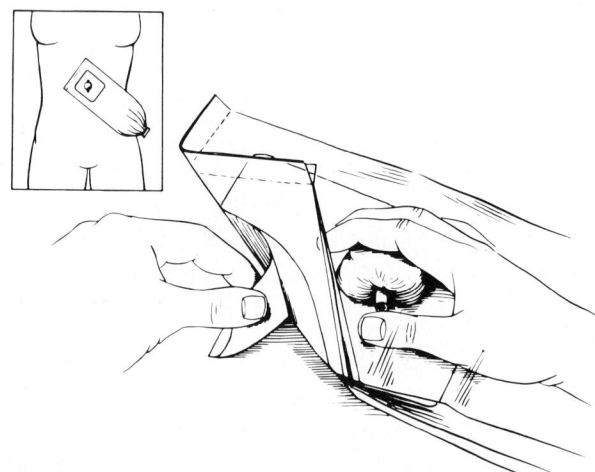

Figure 52-5   Application of a pouch on a stoma with a rod in place.

temporary may adapt more easily and participate in all aspects of care more readily. Each patient is an individual and has special needs related to the adaptation to the ostomy and related pouching needs. If the institution has a nurse-enterostomal therapist (ET), this person should be contacted when the patient returns from surgery. The ET can assist in setting up criteria for pouching the colostomy, in establishing rapport with the patient and family, and in teaching self-care when appropriate.

Cutaneous Fistula

Conservative management of cutaneous fistulas involves fluid and electrolyte replacement, nutritional support, control of sepsis, drainage of associated abscess formations, and skin protection from digestive enzymes. Surgical intervention may be necessary if the fistula does not close with conservative management. Conditions which adversely affect spontaneous closure include complete breakdown of an anastomosis, distal obstructions, and necrosis of segments of intestine.

The location of an intestinal fistula influences the amount and contents of the drainage. The higher in the small bowel a fistulous tract forms, the greater the fluid loss through the external communication. Intestinal fistula output contains digestive enzymes, sodium, chloride, and potassium. A patient may lose up to 3 L (3000 mL) in a 24-h period with a high-output jejunal fistula. Management of fluid and electrolytes lost from enterocutaneous fistulas is of crucial importance. The fluid replacement is based on the patient's total output (milliliter for milliliter), fistulous, urinary, and insensible. Electrolyte replacements are calculated according to the contents of the fistula drainage and the results of laboratory blood studies. Biliary fistula electrolyte losses are predominantly of sodium chloride; pancreatic losses are of proteolytic enzymes and bicarbonate. Metabolic acidosis occurs when the patient with a fistula does not maintain electrolyte and fluid equilibrium.

Fistula drainage may be managed in three ways: by dressings, continuous suctioning, or pouching procedures. The location of the fistula and the amount and type of drainage should be considered in choosing an appropriate method.

The low-output, nonirritating drainage may be effectively managed with dressings. Continuous sump drainage may be preferred with high-output fistulas. However, pouching of a fistula or a draining wound offers the greatest number of advantages. The cost of pouching a moderate- to high-volume fistula is less than the cost of the dressings necessary in a 24-h period. Skin can be protected from the caustic drainage, which contains digestive enzymes. A small amount of drainage will often seep out around the sump tube and erode the skin. A pouch may be used in combination with a sump catheter. The sump catheter may open in the pouch or may come out through the bottom and connect to suction or to straight drainage. If the tube is left open in the pouch, the pouch should be connected to a bedside drainage bag or should be emptied for accurate measurements of the fistula output.

Patients are usually more comfortable using a pouch to collect the fistula drainage. They are dry, odor-free, and ambulatory. Patients or families may be taught the technique for pouching the fistula. Patients can be discharged when stabilized with the fistula care.

Many types of pouches are available, and choosing the appropriate equipment for the particular patient is essential. The first issue to examine is the need for sterility. Sterile pouches are available commercially, or pouches may be sterilized with ethylene oxide. External biliary fistulas are generally managed with sterile urinary equipment. Bile does not usually demonstrate bacterial growth, but the reflux of bile back to the fistula must be prevented and drainage into a collecting device (bedside drainage) facilitated. Urinary pouches used for control of liquid output are more effective than open-end ileostomy pouches. The urinary pouch can be disconnected from the bedside collecting device and the spout closed for ambulation of the patient. In addition to biliary fistulas, surgically created drainage sites (i.e., the insertion of Penrose drains) are managed with aseptic techniques.

Jejunal and ileal (enterocutaneous) fistulas may develop through an operative incision. When wound dehiscence occurs, a fistulous tract may develop within the open wound. Clean, but not sterile, management of the drainage is indicated. An open-end drainable pouch is used for enterocutaneous fistulas. There are various sizes of pouches with different adhesive areas (faceplates). The shape and size of the wound or fistula to be contained will determine the pouch chosen. If the wound has multiple fistulas, the faceplate even on a maxipouch (largest pouch available) may be too small. The pouch faceplate must be large enough to accommodate the wound with enough adhesive area retained to attach the pouch to the skin. If the faceplate is not large enough, there are three alternatives: (1) add a maxiadhesive disk or double-faced adhesive disk to the pouch to increase the size of the faceplate; (2) add skin cement developed for ostomy appliances to the pouch, extending the adhesive area; (3) put two pouches together. Preparing a pattern of the enterocutaneous fistula will assist in identifying the size of pouch faceplate required. A pattern is cut and laid against the skin to assess the adequacy of the template prepared. The opening must be cut to avoid deep crevices, retention sutures, and fine wrinkles. In most cases, $\frac{1}{8}$ to $\frac{1}{4}$ in of skin will be exposed between the fistula and pouch adhesive. This places the pouch seal on smooth skin away from the freely movable wound edges. If a pouch comes directly to the edge of the wound, patient activities including respirations, turning, and ambulation may lift up the inner edge of the pouch and create leakage. The pattern should be labeled to indicate the patient's right and left sides, head and feet, and side of the pattern against the skin. When drawing the pattern on the pouch or the skin barrier, it is important that the correct side be against the pouch to avoid cutting the pattern in reverse.

The pouch may be attached directly to the skin; however, a skin barrier is recommended when pouching enterocutaneous fistulas. Skin barriers include Stomahesive, karaya paste, karaya washers, Reliaseals, Crixilene, Colly-seels, or HolliHesive wafers. Sealant products are available to coat the skin and prevent irritation from pouch adhesives. The sealant products are available in the form of sprays, gels, wipes, and liquids. The pattern is used to cut the opening in the skin barrier, unless a silicone product is used. The pouch may then be attached to the skin barrier and applied to the patient's skin at the same time or applied separately to the patient's skin. Skin around a fistula can be protected and remain clear and intact by a pouch seal. At the first indication of leakage, the pouch should be removed and a fresh pouching system applied. Prior to applying the skin barrier, the skin is cleansed with warm water and patted dry. If the skin is irritated, it must be cared for. Wet, weepy skin must be dried before a skin barrier will adhere. One method for drying the skin is a heat lamp (60-watt bulb) 1 ft away from the skin and a hair dryer set on cool. Skin barriers recommended for use on irritated skin include Stomahesive, karaya products, and Colly-seels. Irritated skin is painful, and karaya products and sealant sprays will sting when applied.

After the skin barrier and pouch are applied, the exposed skin around the wound edges must be protected to prevent irritation and corrosion by the potent digestive enzymes present in pancreatic and small bowel drainage. One method of protecting the skin is through the use of karaya paste. Karaya paste may be purchased or may be prepared by mixing karaya powder and glycerine. There is no magic recipe, as humidity and temperature affect the consistency of the paste. A rule of thumb is that the karaya paste, when mixed to the desired consistency, looks like peanut butter cookie dough. The desired consistency enhances the setting time of the paste, and within 10 to 15 min the paste is firm. The patient's body temperature affects the karaya paste by melting the paste, and this increases the setting time. If the fistula output is high (800 to 1000 mL in 8 h), the karaya paste may need to be regularly replaced to provide continuous skin protection. When the paste is firm, the end of the pouch is closed with a rubber band or attached to a bedside drainage bag. Paper tape may be applied to the pouch edges for extra support.

A careful explanation to the patient prior to initiating the procedure is important. The pouching of a fistula may take 30 to 60 min, depending on the condition of the skin, the size and number of fistulas present, and the amount of drainage. The patient should be positioned comfortably before starting. Intermittent suction or dressings may be used to collect or absorb the drainage throughout the procedure. As the fistula becomes smaller, the patient should be informed. The appearance of healing is encouraging for the patient and the family.

Malnutrition is associated with external fistulas. The segment of intestine proximal to the fistula may be too short to ensure adequate nutritional support. Food substances and digestive secretions may be excreted through the fistula before absorption can occur. Therefore, fluid and electrolyte loss may increase with oral feedings when an enterocutaneous fistula is present.

Bile is an emulsifying agent which facilitates the absorption of fats and fat-soluble vitamins. When bile is lost through an external biliary fistula, fats

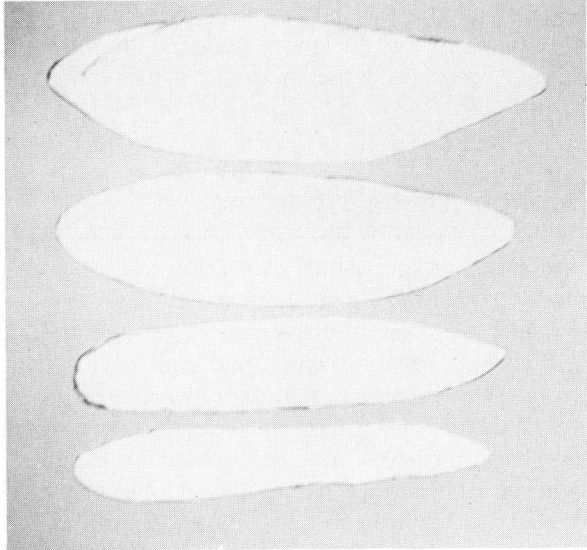

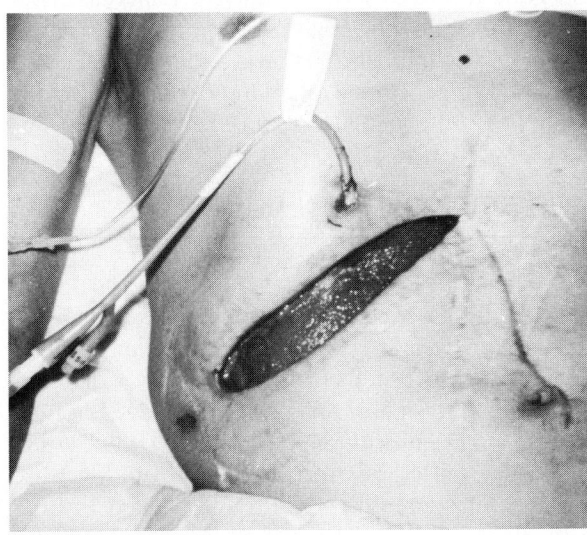

a

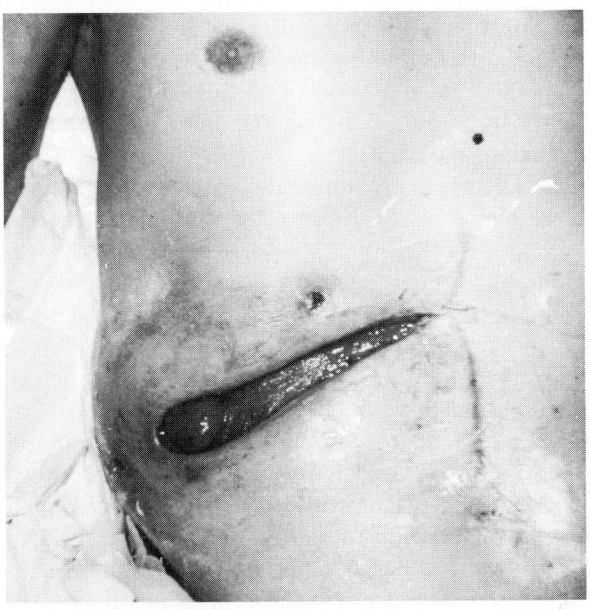

b

c

Figure 52-6   Effects of hyperalimentation on fistula healing. *(a)* Fistula. *(b)* Fistula after 3 weeks. *(c)* Patterns demonstrating wound size decrease.

are not digested properly and malnutrition develops. In addition, fat-soluble vitamins are not available for absorption. Vitamin K loss is a potential threat, and prothrombin studies are used to evaluate the status of vitamin K. In addition, diarrhea may develop from the bile salts present in the large colon.

Hyperalimentation is recommended for the maintenance of a positive nitrogen balance (see Chap. 12). Adequate calories, amino acids, electrolytes, and minerals are supplied to meet the patient's daily requirement. Wound healing improves with positive nitrogen balance. Hyperalimentation also places the bowel at complete mechanical rest and decreases the digestive secretions, thus lowering fluid loss via the fistula. Studies have demonstrated that hyperalimentation results in an increase in the number of spontaneous closures of fistulas and improved prognoses for those cases in which operative closure is required.

Fig. 52-6 demonstrates the change in an abdominal wall defect with multiple fistulas in 3 weeks. The patient received hyperalimentation, replacement fluids, and antibiotics. The skin was protected from digestive enzymes by the use of ostomy equipment. The advent of progressive pouches and skin barriers for ileostomy patients in the past decade has proved beneficial for fistula management.

Zollinger-Ellison Syndrome

Symptoms of intractable ulcer disease are commonly seen in Zollinger-Ellison syndrome. Hemorrhage, perforation, obstruction, and internal fistulization are possible complications of this syndrome. The recommended operative intervention is total gastrectomy with esophagojejunostomy, since any remaining gastric mucosa is capable of secreting large quantities of gastric acid, which will result in recurrent ulceration and possible complications of intractable ulcer disease (hemorrhage, perforation, etc.).

The loss of the stomach results in lack of gastric storage, loss of the intrinsic factor necessary for vitamin B_{12} absorption, and interference with iron absorption. The dumping syndrome, characterized by weakness, profuse perspiration, nausea, faintness, flushing, epigastric discomfort, vomiting, and palpitation, may occur within 15 min after a meal. The syndrome is related to the sudden dilatation of the small intestine after eating and presence of hypertonic solution in the proximal small bowel, resulting in a shift of extracellular fluid into the bowel lumen and creating the symptoms of volume loss. Postgastrectomy hypoglycemia reactions (late dumping syndrome) are related to high intake of carbohydrates in the diet. The increased digestion and absorption of carbohydrates causes a response of insulin release in excess of need and results in hypoglycemic symptoms (*rebound hypoglycemia*).

If eating becomes painful, the patient may omit meals or greatly decrease the intake per meal. Weight loss may occur after total gastrectomy from poor nutritional intake. Pernicious anemia may be prevented by vitamin B_{12} supplements following surgery.

The pancreatic tumor is removed when possible. The pancreas is responsible for the release of insulin and glucagon in addition to the pancreatic enzymes secreted into the small bowel. Pancreatic fistulas are a possible surgical complication, and the wound should be observed for dehiscence or increased drainage. If a cutaneous fistula develops, accurate measurement of drainage and skin protection are important. The use of ostomy appliances facilitates containment and measurement of the fistula output and protects the skin from the pancreatic enzymes.

It is often difficult to locate the non–beta cell adenoma. Occasionally the pancreatic involvement is a generalized hyperplasia and the pancreas is not removed. Following total gastrectomy there is remission of pancreatic lesions, and less metastatic activity. The prognosis following early total gastrectomy for Zollinger-Ellison syndrome is favorable.

Inflammatory Bowel Disease

Crohn's Disease

Medical treatment for Crohn's disease is symptomatic. However, it is of utmost importance and is geared toward relief of the symptoms of diarrhea and abdominal pain. Analgesics, codeine, diphenoxylate hydrochloride with atropine (Lomotil) steroids, and salicylazosulfapyridine (Azulfidine) are used. Cholestyramine (Questran) is given to bind bile salts when necessary, and anemia is treated with iron (intramuscularly), vitamin B_{12}, and folic acid. Steroids may be given intravenously during an acute attack, progressing to oral tablets. The potential hazards of steroid treatment include loss of potassium, retention of sodium and water, hypertension, osteoporosis, diabetes, and behavior disorders.

Dietary restriction of raw fruits and vegetables is recommended to reduce the amount of fiber in the bowel. Nutritional support of the patient with inflammatory bowel disease is imperative. Most clinicians agree that bowel rest is important; therefore, total parenteral nutrition is frequently selected. It is a key therapy for patients with inflammatory bowel disease who have fistulas, obstruction, or abscesses. Use of central venous total parenteral nutrition provides bowel rest while achieving positive nitrogen balance and repletion of nutritional deficits. Remission rates of 60 to 80 percent have been achieved, surgical intervention avoided, and short bowel syndrome reduced. Elemental diets via the enteral route are recommended for those patients who are not critically ill when there is no evidence of obstruction or fistula and when the patient's GI tract can be used safely.

Surgery is palliative and is performed only when the patient does not respond to medical therapy and when the disease process interferes with the patient's activities of daily living (intractable disease). Additional indications for surgery in Crohn's disease include partial or complete intestinal obstruction, internal or external fistulas, and massive hemorrhage.

If the disease involves the distal stomach or duodenum, a bypass procedure (gastrojejunostomy) is sometimes necessary. When the disease involves the small bowel or segments of the colon, a segmental resection is the procedure of choice. A bypass procedure is used only when there is an abscess present, and this is usually the first stage of a two-stage procedure. The second stage consists of resection of the diseased segment. If the entire colon is involved, total colectomy and ileostomy are necessary. An ileal stoma (ileostomy) may be created when Crohn's disease involves the entire colon or as a cure for ulcerative colitis (Fig. 52-7). The small bowel (ileum) is brought through the abdominal wall and the stoma is matured, leaving a "bud" above the surface of the skin. The continent

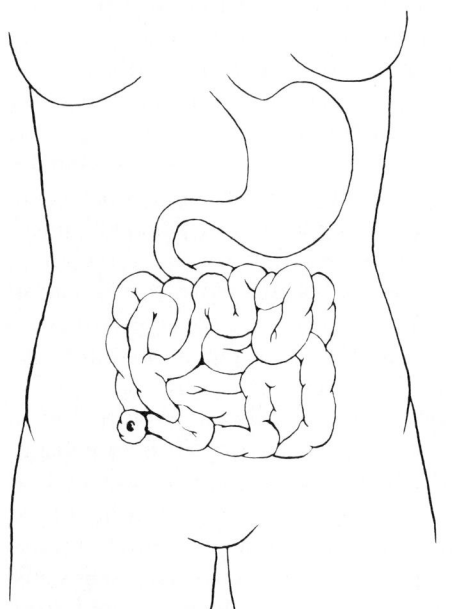

Figure 52-7   Ileal stoma.

internal pouch is an internal reservoir surgically constructed with a continence valve and ileostomy stoma. Developed by Koch in Sweden in 1969, the reservoir is constructed from 30 cm of terminal ileum, and since 1969, the continence of the ileal valve has been enhanced by many improvements. The advantage of the procedure is that no external appliance is worn by the patient. Diagnoses of ulcerative colitis, familial polyposis, or multiple tumors of the large colon favor cure by surgical removal of the diseased colon, and patients with these lesions are eligible for consideration for a continent pouch.

Postoperatively, a catheter is left in the pouch and connected to low suction to prevent pressure on the incision line of the internal pouch. Intravenous fluids, nasogastric suctioning, and a Foley catheter are initially in place. The postoperative needs are similar to the needs following conventional ileostomy surgery.

After 2 weeks the catheter is disconnected from the low suction but remains in place in the internal pouch and is clamped and released at specific intervals. The next step is removal and insertion of the catheter into the internal pouch by the nursing staff. The time between emptyings gradually increases as the volume capacity of the pouch increases. The patient is instructed in emptying the continent internal pouch. Written instructions should be included in the patient teaching.

The following material is needed for emptying a continent pouch: a large-lumen catheter, water-soluble lubricant, catheter-tip syringe, container, gauze, and tape. The patient at first empties the continent pouch while sitting on the side of the bed; later the patient empties it while sitting on the commode. The dressing is removed from the stoma. The tip of the catheter is lubricated and gently inserted into the stoma. After the catheter has entered approximately 2 in, valve resistance can be felt. The patient should take a deep breath and apply some pressure, and the catheter will slip into the continent internal pouch. The catheter should never be forced, as the internal pouch can be perforated. The stool will begin draining through the catheter when it enters the pouch. When the pouch is empty, the catheter is removed, the stoma cleansed, and a gauze pad applied to collect any mucous drainage.

The pouch capacity gradually increases, and by the time of discharge from the hospital, the patient will empty the internal pouch three or four times a day. Gas may also collect in the pouch and will need to be released by inserting the catheter. There is an outward bulging of the skin as the continent pouch fills.

Two problems with a continent internal pouch are thick fecal consistency and inability to insert the catheter. If the feces are excessively thick, 30 min may be required to drain the continent pouch. The patient may drink two glasses of water or a glass of prune or grape juice to loosen the stool. The fecal material may be diluted with warm water, or the patient may need to irrigate the internal pouch, using water and a syringe. Debris left in the pouch can result in bacterial proliferation. The pouch should be emptied completely and flushed with irrigation solution at least weekly.

Inability to insert the catheter through the nipple valve is frightening for the patient. When the abdominal muscles become tense, the patient should attempt to relax by leaning back and breathing deeply. If this does not permit entry of the catheter, the patient may try relaxing in a warm tub of water. The catheter should be well lubricated and inserted while the patient is in a supine position. Once the catheter is inserted, the patient should sit or stand to drain the pouch. Squeezing air or water through a syringe may assist the patient in inserting the catheter. If the internal pouch is full and the patient cannot empty it after 3 to 4 h, the surgeon should be notified.

Dietary concerns following the provision of an internal reservoir include gaseous foods and undigested food products, as with the ileostomate. New foods should be added to the diet slowly in limited amounts and should be chewed thoroughly. Gas-forming foods may cause distention and abdominal pain in the first few months after surgery. Undigested foods may plug the catheter or may need to be rinsed out of the internal pouch. The patient should be given instructions prior to discharge on unplugging the catheter.

Ulcerative Colitis

Medical management of ulcerative colitis revolves around the treatment of symptoms. Anti-inflammatory agents (such as ACTH) are used intravenously initially in treating acute ulcerative colitis; later, oral steroids (prednisone) are used for maintenance therapy. Salicylazo-sulfapyridine (Azulfidine) and prednisone are the medications of choice in managing ulcerative colitis. Fluid and electrolyte replacement is based on the extent and duration of the disease. Weight loss is frequently observed. Dietary therapy is an important aspect of medical management in ulcerative colitis. Low-residue diets and lactose-free diets are used to decrease colon stimulation and roughage in the lumen. In acute situations, the colon may be placed completely at rest with the use of elemental diets and clear liquids. Elemental diets are absorbed in the proximal small bowel, and no residue enters the colon. Hyperalimentation may be used for patients in debilitated states to improve their overall nutritional status.

Diarrhea is treated by altering the contents of the bowel lumen. Metamucil, a bulk-forming laxative, and aluminum hydroxide (Gelusil) are used to thicken the bowel contents. Opiates are not used as antidiarrheal agents, since they may precipitate toxic megacolon.

When ulcerative colitis interferes with the patient's daily lifestyle, operative intervention may be indicated. Surgery is the only available curative therapy. Although the conventional ileostomy is still available, it is slowly being replaced by several new techniques that may improve patient acceptance of proctocolectomy, such as the Koch pouch. The restorative proctocolectomy with ileal reservoir uses a similar ileal pouch that is connected to the rectal stump after all rectal mucosa has been removed. This technique preserves intestinal continuity, and the anal sphincter provides continence.

The incidence of colon cancer is higher in patients with a history of ulcerative colitis than in the general population. When cancer is suspected or diagnosed, the colon and rectum are surgically removed.

The mucosa of the colon is very friable in ulcerative colitis, and massive rectal hemorrhages may occur. The first sign may be bright red blood in the stool. A decrease in the systolic blood pressure on sitting or standing and elevated pulse are measures of blood flow changes. Vital signs, urinary output, and amount of blood loss are factors used to evaluate the status of the patient. An intravenous line should be inserted for fluid and blood replacement.

Diverticulitis

For the mild attack of diverticulitis, the patient should be placed at bed rest, and if peristalsis is good, should continue to eat, preferably liquids and soft foods. Antispasmodics may be administered, as well as small doses of meperidine or other analgesics as necessary. The application of warm packs to the abdomen offers some relief. Unless there is fever or definite signs of infection, it is unnecessary to use antibiotics.

In the patient with obvious infection or obstruction, not only should antibiotics be given, but the patient should be placed on a regimen of nothing by mouth and the usual methods of abdominal decompression instituted. The patient is then monitored to see whether medical therapy is effective or surgery is necessary.

Some indications for surgical intervention are clear. Acute perforation with abscess requires a diverting colostomy and resection. Operation is also required for the patient with a fistula to the bladder or skin.

Toxic Megacolon

Toxic megacolon is massive dilatation of the large colon. The cause is not known. Barium enemas given during a period of severe diarrhea may precipitate toxic megacolon. Opiates, anticholinergics, and hypokalemia are factors which may play a role in toxic megacolon. Abdominal distention and absent bowel sounds with a sharp decrease in the number of daily stools are indicative of toxic megacolon. Intestinal decompression, antibiotic therapy, fluid and electrolyte replacement, and intravenous alimentation are initiated. The use of opiates and anticholinergic drugs is discontinued. The patient is carefully observed for signs of perforation or impending perforation. Operative intervention is indicated for toxic megacolon in the presence of perforation or failure of the clinical status to improve after intensive medical therapy.

Malabsorption Syndromes

Malabsorption syndromes, regardless of cause, are treated primarily with nutritional supplementation. Enteral feedings permit total absorption of nutrients within the small bowel, allowing no residue to enter the colon. Hyperalimentation peripherally or centrally may also be necessary to overcome a state of malnutrition. Additions to the nutritional supplements are determined by the pathophysiology of the specific malabsorption syndrome. For further discussion of nutritional supplementation, see Chap. 12.

Acute Pancreatitis

The goals of treatment for acute pancreatitis are to maintain fluid and electrolyte balance and thus adequate circulating blood volume, to suppress or neutralize pancreatic secretions, to alleviate pain, and to prevent or treat complications.

Massive amounts of fluid are lost in the retroperitoneal space, in the peritoneal cavity, and in the adynamic bowel, and this loss may result in hypovolemic shock. Plasma expanders are given, together with fluid, blood, and electrolyte replacement, and in addition, fluid balance is maintained. Urinary output, alterations in hematocrit reading, central venous pressure, and occult losses in the peritoneum are used in calculating the fluid needs.

In order to suppress or neutralize pancreatic secretions, the patient is allowed nothing by mouth, a nasogastric tube is used to control nausea and vomiting and prevent gastric stimulation of pancreatic secretions, anticholinergic medications such as atropine are administered to decrease gastrointestinal motility and vasostimulation of the pancreas, and antacids are given to neutralize hydrochloric acid.

Antibiotics are used in fulminating, necrotic pancreatitis and in the presence of a pancreatic abscess. Insulin is administered judiciously. Meperidine is used for pain control. Morphine and codeine should be avoided, since they produce contraction of the sphincter of Oddi. Blood gases should be monitored and appropriate oxygen therapy administered. Acute episodes of pancreatitis are usually resolved within 2 to 3 days unless complications develop.

Ultrasound studies may be used to diagnose pseudocyst or abscess formation associated with pancreatitis. Surgery may be indicated when a definitive diagnosis has not been made and the patient's status is not improving. Pancreatic abscesses may be surgically drained. Peritoneal lavage may be used to rinse the intraperitoneal space and remove toxic substances released from the pancreas. Pancreatic resection or total pancreatectomy is indicated in the event of tissue necrosis.

Gastrointestinal Surgery

Esophagogastrectomy

The surgical approach for an esophagogastrectomy is via right or left thoracotomy. Attempts are made to avoid pulmonary complications by administering bronchodilators, mucolytic agents, and appropriate antibiotics. The patient may have a tracheostomy or endotracheal tube requiring careful monitoring of effectiveness of ventilation. Total parenteral nutrition is given. Cardiovascular complications include arrhythmias and hemorrhage. Anastomotic leaks will generally become apparent within 1 to 10 days after operation.

Pancreatic Surgery

Pancreatic surgery is performed for carcinoma of the pancreas. Procedures include pancreaticoduodenectomy (Whipple operation) and total pancreatectomy. The Whipple procedure is the removal of the head and/or all of the pancreas, the distal end of the stomach, the duodenum, and the gallbladder, with choledochoduodenostomy. Total pancreatectomy is increasingly being advocated; however, because carcinoma of the pancreas is multifocal and the operative procedure is less complicated, the severity and frequency of complications are decreased, and the metabolic derangements are more manageable.

Hepatic Dysfunction

Hepatitis

All attacks of hepatitis should be treated as potentially serious, and bed rest should be instituted immediately to put the body at rest and conserve energy. A low-fat, high-carbohydrate diet is instituted as soon as the patient can tolerate it. All patients with suspected viral hepatitis should be isolated from other patients. Enteric and blood precautions are implemented, and all laboratory samples should be clearly marked "possible hepatitis." With the advent of jaundice, the patient with hepatitis A is no longer infectious. As jaundice subsides, enteric precautions may be discontinued for hepatitis B patients, but blood precautions should continue as long as the patient is HBsAG positive. A patient who has been diagnosed as having hepatitis B should never serve as a blood donor. For acute non-A non-B hepatitis, isolation is controversial, but blood precautions are probably advisable for the duration of the incubation period (7 to 50 days).

Hepatic Insufficiency and Failure

The management of liver failure is intense. Hemodynamic monitoring is implemented to assess fluid and electrolyte balance. Intake and output as well as daily weights are recorded. A neurologic assessment is necessary along with the routine vital signs. The GI tract is evacuated to prevent further absorption of protein breakdown products. Nasogastric suction is then instituted to further reduce absorption of protein breakdown products (e.g., ammonia), which are highly toxic to the central nervous system. Nonabsorbable antibiotics such as neomycin are used to reduce the bacterial production of ammonia in the bowel. Severe protein curtailment (total parenteral nutrition with only essential amino acids and primarily glucose as a caloric supplement) is implemented to decrease ammonia production. Vitamin K is administered in large quantities to support the coagulation process. Oxygen therapy is given to prevent hypoxia. Only those drugs not metabolized by the liver are administered.

Bibliography

Alspach, J. G., & Williams, S. M. (1985). *Core curriculum for critical care nursing.* Philadelphia: Saunders.

Brandt, L. J. (1982). Perineal Crohn's disease: Promising new therapy for a disabling affliction. *Consultant, 22,* 161–165.

Cobert, B. L. (1984). Mallory-Weiss syndrome . . . Gastrointestinal bleeding due to lacerations of the gastric cardia. *Hospital Medicine, 20,* 65–67, 1094.

DiMagno, E. P. (1983). Answers to questions on acute pancreatitis. *Hospital Medicine, 19,* 91, 95–101, 104–105.

Dudrick, S. J., et al. (1983). The short bowel syndrome and total parenteral nutrition. *Heart and Lung, 12,* 195–201.

Dusek, J. L. (1984). Iced gastric lavage slows bleeding in gastric hemorrhage . . . Iced saline lavage is being abandoned. *Critical Care Nurse, 4,* 8.

Fazio, V. W. (1983). Crohn's disease: Surgical procedures, sequelae, and management of recurrence. *Consultant, 23,* 49–51, 59–64, 67–68.

Goligher, J. C. (1983). Alternatives to conventional ileostomy in the surgical treatment of ulcerative colitis. *Journal of Enterostomal Therapy, 10,* 79–83.

Greenberger, N. J., & Winship, D. H. (1980). *Gastrointestinal disorders: A pathophysiological approach.* Chicago: Year Book.

Hoppe, M. C., et al. (1983). Gastrointestinal disease: Nutritional implications. *Nursing Clinics of North America, 18,* 47–56.

Kodner, I. J. (1982). Inflammatory bowel disease. *Clinical Symposium, 1,* 34, 3–32.

Lamphier, T. A., et al. (1981). Upper GI hemorrhage: Emergency evaluation and management. *American Journal of Nursing, 81,* 1814–1817.

Meeroff, J. C. (1984). Algorithm for managing patients with severe GI hemorrhage. *Hospital Practice, 19,* 186, 191.

Metz, G. (1984). Medical management of inflammatory bowel disease. *Journal of Enterostomal Therapy, 11,* 114–115.

Myer, S. A. (1984). Overview of inflammatory bowel disease. *Nursing Clinics of North America, 19,* 3–9.

Petlin, A. M., et al. (1981). How to stop a GI bleed. *RN, 44,* 43–49.

Petlin, A. M., et al. (1982). Getting your patient through a lower GI bleed. *RN, 45,* 42–45.

Rubin, D. M. (1983). AORN Journal, 38, 783–794.

Sartor, R. B. (1983). Ulcerative colitis . . . Is there anything new in the treatment? *Consultant, 23,* 121–122.

Spiro, H. M. (1983). *Clinical gastroenterology.* New York: Macmillan.

53

Nursing Interventions in Gastrointestinal Problems

Patricia Kallweit Kaldor

Nursing care of the patient with gastrointestinal disease requires close observation and monitoring of the patient's condition. In this chapter, ileostomy care is discussed. In addition, potential nursing diagnoses for the various gastrointestinal disorders are presented along with a case study for each. The various nursing diagnoses are then completed with goals, nursing interventions, and evaluation criteria.

Ileostomy Care

Rehabilitation with ostomy surgery begins prior to the surgical procedure and continues beyond the period of hospitalization. The nurse is involved in assessing the patient's needs and planning the rehabilitation program for the patient. Initial assessments include the patient's (and significant other's) knowledge of the disease, the meaning of ileostomy, and family dynamics. The terms *stoma, ileostomy, stool,* and *pouch* are defined for the patient.

Following ileostomy, the patient fears rejection by family and friends. The new ileostomate (patient with an ileostomy) will test family, friends, and staff verbally and nonverbally for signs of acceptance. Acceptance as a person, a sexual being, a family member, a friend, and an employee is checked to ensure that the surgery has not altered previous relationships. The patient has a responsibility to become independent in ostomy care. The nurse's responsibility is to provide the information and techniques necessary for the patient to become self-sufficient.

One of the most confusing aspects of ileostomy care is the difference between a colostomy and an ileostomy and between an ileal conduit (or ileal loop) and an ileostomy. The ileostomy (in-volving the small bowel) cannot be regulated by irrigations or diet as the colostomy (involving the large bowel) is managed. A pouch is worn at all times to collect the fecal drainage. The ileostomate cannot take enemas (usually no rectum) or laxatives. A common and serious error is giving an ileostomate a bowel preparation for intravenous pyelogram (IVP) or upper bowel series. The result of the bowel preparation is severe fluid and electrolyte loss, and in the presence of Crohn's disease, an exacerbation of the disease may occur. The ileal conduit is a urinary diversion, not a fecal diversion, and the underlying disease, type of equipment, and patient needs differ.

The most appropriate time for patient teaching is during a pouch change. The patient and significant other can be given valuable information even though intravenous lines and a nasogastric tube limit the patient's participation. Involvement of a family member is encouraged. The patient and significant others are made aware of the patient's possible need for assistance when learning the routine or in case of future illness. The preferred result is that ileostomates be responsible for their own care but have a backup when necessary.

The bright red color of the stoma disturbs the patient and family initially. The red color implies pain, and there is a fear of hurting the patient. The stoma has no nerve endings, and touching the stoma for the first time is a strange sensation. The patient should not be forced into touching it. During a pouch change, as the stoma and skin are cleansed, the nurse should demonstrate touching the stoma. The patient should be told that carrying packages or children against the stoma will not create a problem. In addition, an ileostomate can sleep on the abdomen or hold someone closely. This information will decrease many anxieties in the patient and in the family.

1383

Since there is no feeling in the stoma, close observation is necessary during a pouch change for alteration of the stomal color and/or presence of small ulcers on the stoma. Stomal color change from bright red to a dusky color may indicate pressure on the vascular supply to the stoma. The presence of small ulcers may indicate a recurrence of Crohn's disease. The physician should be notified. The stoma is a mucosal membrane and may bleed when cleansed. The small amount of blood on the washcloth should not alarm the patient. However, bleeding which continues after the stoma has been cleansed or in between pouch changes should be evaluated by the physician.

The new ileostomate remains on a low-residue diet for approximately 6 weeks following surgery. This allows the bowel time to adjust after the operation. Then, one food is added each week from a list of high-fiber foods. The food should be chewed thoroughly and eaten as part of a meal. High-fiber foods such as celery, nuts, corn, coleslaw, coconut, popcorn, dried fruits, and whole vegetables are not digested by the gastrointestinal tract. If a large mass of undigested food develops in the small bowel of an ileostomate, it could become lodged at a kink or narrowing in the bowel and create a food blockage (Fig. 53-1). If the blocked food does not move forward, the result is complete intestinal obstruction. The cycle which follows intestinal obstruction begins with fluid and electrolyte accumulation in the bowel and progresses to shock.

The patient may recognize early signs of food obstruction (Table 53-1) by correlating changes in the ileostomy output with the diet. A food blockage may be relieved by the patient's getting into a knee-chest position and cupping the hand gently under the stoma. Tense abdominal muscles will prevent a blockage from moving out of the bowel. The ileostomate should relax in a hot tub or hot shower, and then assume the knee-chest position. If the obstruction has been present for over 3 h without relief or if the patient is nauseated or vomiting or no drainage is coming around the blockage, the physician should be notified. The physician may then prescribe mechanical removal of the blockage by irrigation.

The pouch opening may be too small as the stoma swells when the bowel becomes partially or totally obstructed. A disposable pouch with a larger stoma opening and a skin barrier should be applied. The pouch should be left on during the ileostomy irrigation, since more fluid will return than is inserted. A small rubber catheter is gently inserted into the stomal opening, and 50 mL of normal saline is instilled through an ascepto syringe. It may take several instillations of saline and gentle suction of the ascepto to break up the blockage. Once the blockage is relieved, a large amount of fluid will flow through the bowel. Careful recordings of intake and output are required to provide adequate fluid replacements. The patient may experience diarrhea for several days following an obstruction. The high-fiber foods that may create an obstruction are not omitted from an ileostomate's diet, but discretion should be used regarding the amount and combinations of high-fiber foods eaten at one meal, and food should be chewed thoroughly.

The small bowel will absorb all the nutrients, fluid, and electrolytes an ileostomate requires. Immediately after surgery, the patient has a high fluid

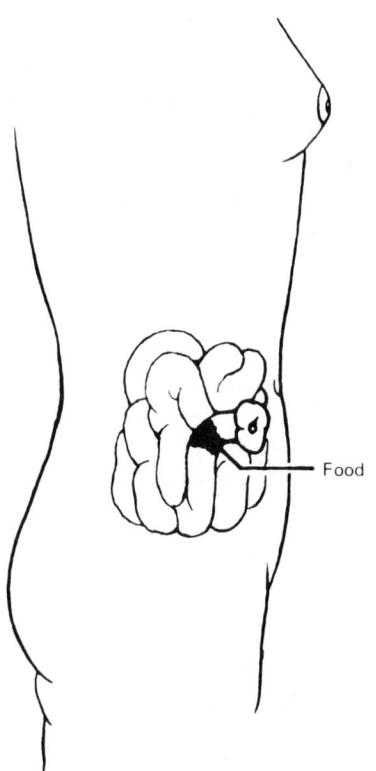

Figure 53-1 Food blockage with an ileostomy.

Table 53-1 Intestinal Obstruction from a Food Blockage with an Ileostomy

Symptom	Cause
Discharge changes from semisolid to liquid	Food is blocked but water passes around it—a partial intestinal obstruction
Total volume of output increases and ileostomy functions constantly	Water is drawn from the extracellular fluid in an attempt to rid the body of the obstruction, and the intestines become hyperactive
Objectionable odor	Bacterial proliferation occurs at the site of obstruction and causes fermentation of the bowel content
Cramping, followed by increased watery output	Increased bowel activity to move blockage forward
Distended abdomen	The obstruction traps gas and liquids in the bowel lumen
Vomiting	Reverse peristalsis. The body's attempt to move the increased bowel contents in the direction of least resistance
No ileostomy output	Complete intestinal obstruction

and electrolyte concentration in the ileostomy output. An ileostomy adaptation occurs approximately 3 to 6 months after surgery; the drainage becomes the consistency of toothpaste, and more fluid and electrolytes are reabsorbed. The ileostomate tends to be on the borderline between hydrated and dehydrated. The patient is told to satisfy any desire for water above the eight 8-oz glasses of fluid recommended daily. The problems occur when other medical disorders develop, whether influenza or a myocardial infarction. The ileostomate can lose more fluid and electrolytes faster than a person with a colon. The ileostomate should be taught to replace fluid losses immediately with products high in needed electrolytes, such as Gatorade, salt water, bouillon, tea, or other products high in electrolytes. If the ileostomate cannot keep up with the fluid losses, the physician should be contacted.

Diarrhea in an ileostomate can be described as hot, watery stool which requires frequent (every 30 min) emptying of the pouch. Diarrhea may be associated with other medical problems or may be stimulated by specific foods in some persons. Green beans, broccoli, spinach, raw fruits, highly seasoned foods, and beer may increase the ileostomy drainage. Presurgical effects of these foods should be examined with regard to the individual patient. The amounts eaten at a given time also affect the amount of ileostomy output. Bananas, boiled milk, tapioca, and peanut butter are effective in thickening diarrheal stools.

The ileostomate with recurrent Crohn's disease or multiple small bowel resections may have chronic diarrhea associated with the short bowel syndrome. In the short bowel syndrome, the transit time is shortened and absorption of fluid is limited. The result is watery stools. Vitamin B_{12} and fat absorption may be affected if large amounts of terminal ileum have been resected. Steatorrhea may be noted with the ileostomy output.

The ileostomate cannot absorb hard tablets or enteric-coated tablets, and these tablets should not be prescribed. Timed-release and sustained-action capsules and tablets should also be avoided in patients with an ileostomy. The timed-release drugs may not remain in the bowel for 8 or 12 h, so the dosage received by the patient cannot be ascertained. Lomotil tablets should be crushed or the drug should be given in liquid form, because it is not absorbed otherwise. Liquid medication is the best for ileostomates. However, if in doubt about a tablet, drop it in a glass of water without stirring and wait 30 min; if the pill has begun to dissolve, the patient should be able to obtain full benefit from the drug. Medications which promote potassium or sodium excretion (digoxin, diuretics) may create more severe problems for an ileostomate because of the fine fluid and electrolyte balance the ileostomy patient maintains. Antibiotics will cause a flora change in the ileum, resulting in diarrhea. Careful fluid replacement is necessary.

Sexuality is an important aspect of rehabilitation after ileostomy. The ileostomy should not alter the patient's sexual patterns. The previous sexual patterns are assessed prior to planning nursing intervention. The patient and significant other who have a steady, loving relationship should encounter no sexual difficulties once their questions have been answered. The acceptance of an altered body image is easier if the loved one demonstrates continued acceptance. The single ileostomate may encounter new problems. In our society, sex is more open and common among unmarried partners. The single ileostomate may have a problem in telling others about the surgery and the pouch or may question when others should be told. The supportive professional (enterostomal therapist, nurse, social worker, physician) will need to offer counseling and assistance as new obstacles are faced. The single ileostomate may be rejected by a sexual partner. Of course, the same problem may arise with a married ileostomate whose spouse rejects the idea of the pouch or stoma.

The ileostomate and partner can be assisted by being given permission by the professional to be a sexual being, to have sexual concerns, and to ask questions. Not everyone is comfortable discussing sexuality with patients. The responsibility of the nurse who is uncomfortable is to find a resource person who can comfortably discuss sexuality with the couple. The stoma cannot be hurt by the pressure of being held or touched or by sleeping on the abdomen. The spouse must know this to avoid being afraid of hurting the patient. The pouch should be emptied prior to sexual activity and the seal checked. Ileostomates should be reminded that they can have children, and birth control may be desired. An effective nursing measure is to answer the questions of the ileostomate and significant other as they arise. When specific problems occur, the couple should be referred for specialized sexual therapy.

If the proper pouching system is not chosen for the patient and stool leaks, the patient is no better off than with 30 stools a day. The stoma opening in the ileostomy pouch should be $\frac{1}{8}$ in larger than the stoma. This allows for peristaltic movements in the stoma. The residual digestive enzymes in ileostomy output are very irritating to the skin, and severe skin denudation can develop in a short period of exposure to ileostomy output. A skin barrier is placed up to the base of the stoma to protect the exposed skin. Effective skin barriers include karaya, Colly-seels, and Stomahesive. A skin barrier does not hold a pouch on; it merely protects exposed skin. The next step is deciding on a pouch (Table 52-4). The pouch should be odor-proof and

Table 53-2 Basic Consideration in Choosing Disposable Pouches

1. Type of ostomy will indicate:
   a. Spout opening: drainable, urinary spout, closed
   b. Material of pouch: odor-proof, odor-resistant
   c. Skin protection: karaya, Stomahesive, Colly-seels, HolliHesive
2. Parastomal skin area and stoma:
   a. Stoma size and shape: protruding, flushed, edematous
   b. Stoma drainage location
   c. Available space for faceplate
   d. Presence of abdominal folds, dimples, scars
   e. Stomal complications: prolapse, retraction, ulcerations
   f. Presence of a stomal support: rod, catheter, loop-lock
3. Physical abilities of patient:
   a. Arthritis, paralysis
   b. Poor eyesight, blindness
4. Mental abilities of patient
   a. Confusion, senility
   b. Emotional aspects: denial
5. Financial situation of patient
6. Patient sensitivities:
   a. Adhesives, tapes
   b. Plastics, vinyls, rubber
7. Pouches available in area:
   a. Starter openings helpful in hospital
   b. Pouch material: noise factors, odor-proof
   c. Drainable rather than closed-end for hospital use

drainable. The pouch application procedure should be written and left on the nursing care plan and with the patient. Each person working with a new ostomy patient should use the same procedure. The first step is gathering all the necessary supplies: damp washcloth, towel, toilet paper, skin barrier, pouch, scissors, tape, and rubber band or pouch closure. The patient should sit in a chair and use the bedside table for the supplies. As the patient regains strength, the procedure may be done in the bathroom. The pouch opening is cut in the clean pouch before the soiled pouch is removed from the skin. The pouch the patient is wearing is emptied and removed from the skin. The stoma may have stool on it; if so, it is wiped with toilet paper. The skin and stoma are then cleansed with warm water and patted dry. Soaps will leave a film residue on the skin which increases skin breakdown under pouches. The skin barrier is then applied to the skin up to the stoma base, leaving no skin exposed. The pouch is then applied and the end secured. Emptying a pouch is facilitated by applying the pouch so that the spout is directed toward the inner aspect of the thigh. The patient can then sit on the toilet and drain the pouch between the legs. Splashing of the water can be decreased by placing toilet paper in the commode prior to draining the pouch. It is not necessary for the patient to rinse the pouch every time it is emptied. Once a day the ileostomate may rinse the pouch, using an ascepto syringe and tepid water. Overcleansing may break the pouch seal.

Odor is a major concern of many ileostomates. Odor is controllable by the use of odor-proof pouches, oral preparations, or pouch deodorants. Bismuth subgallate (Devrom) is an oral preparation for odor control which may be purchased without a prescription. The tablet is chewed before meals and will effectively control odor and thicken the stool. When the patient first starts taking bismuth subgallate, the tongue may turn black and the stool may become black. The discoloration is temporary. Bismuth subgallate is contraindicated in renal disease and with warfarin (coumadin) therapy. The drug should be omitted for 48 h before radiography, because it causes opaque areas on the films. Overdosage of bismuth subgallate or long-term misuse may result in metal toxicosis. The signs of metal toxicosis include myoclonic jerks, tremors, inability to walk, loss of balance, poor concentration, depression, insomnia, and confusion.

Dietary control of odors is also possible. Certain foods produce more odor, especially when eaten in large quantities. Fish, asparagus, eggs, onions, garlic, and some spices may be limited when odor is a concern. However, the use of odor-proof pouches is an effective method of controlling odor. Odor will be released when the pouch is emptied, but the patient can be reminded that people with rectums also have odor with bowel movements. Sprays and deodorizers are available for use when emptying the pouch.

Opaque pouches and pouch covers are available for ileostomates. Most patients are relieved to know they do not have to see stool continuously. Another possible reaction is compulsive behavior. Excessive cleansing of the pouch, frequent checking to see if the stoma is functioning, or ritualistic procedures for changing the pouch are examples of compulsive behavior. Opaque pouches can be effective in changing behavior in some patients.

Prior to discharge, an ostomy visitor from the United Ostomy Association (UOA) may be called. The visitor has one positive effect—the patient is able to see another person who has an ileostomy. The UOA visitor is a rehabilitated person, and the patient can identify with the healthy person who happens to wear a pouch. Local UOA groups have monthly educational meetings, bulletins, and a journal full of hints for ostomates.

Acute Gastrointestinal Hemorrhage

Potential Nursing Diagnoses

Alteration in cardiac output: decreased, related to–sudden loss of blood volume (hematemesis, melena) and decreased systemic blood pressure

Alteration in comfort: pain, related to–epigastric tenderness

Fluid volume deficit related to–extreme blood loss (hemorrhage)

Alteration in tissue perfusion related to–extreme blood loss and hypovolemia, decreased cardiac output, and vasoconstriction

Impaired physical mobility related to–general weakness and fatigue, energy deficiency, and pain

Ineffective breathing patterns related to–abdominal pain and decreased energy

Impairment of tissue integrity: oral mucous membranes related to–dehydration

Anxiety related to–fear of death

Alteration in nutrition, less than body requirements, related to–hematemesis and presence of nasogastric tube

Case Study

Mr. G.I., age 63, was brought to the emergency room by ambulance accompanied by his wife. He was restless, pale, and diaphoretic. His blood pressure was 70/40. His heart and respiratory rates were elevated, 140 and 36, respectively. Physical examination revealed epigastric tenderness and guarding and a distended abdomen. His wife reported a history of ulcer disease and stated that he had experienced many bleeding episodes, most of which had not required hospitalization. Diagnosis was acute GI hemorrhage. The goals of therapy were to control the bleeding and to stabilize the patient's condition. Peripheral IV lines were inserted immediately, oxygen therapy was initiated, and a nasogastric tube was inserted. An arterial line, a central venous line, and a Swan-Ganz catheter were placed shortly thereafter to monitor blood pressure and volume and to administer large amounts of fluids and blood products.

Intestinal Ischemic Disorders

Potential Nursing Diagnoses

Alteration in comfort related to–severe abdominal pain and tenderness, abdominal bloating and distention, ischemia, and tissue damage

Fluid volume deficit related to–vomiting, decreased intake, fever with diaphoresis, fear of eating which precipitates abdominal pain, third-space fluid loss, and hemorrhage

Ineffective breathing patterns related to–abdominal distention, abdominal pain, and anxiety

Alteration in tissue perfusion, gastrointestinal, related to–decreased cardiac output; occlusion of artery by thrombosis, embolism, or atherosclerosis; bacterial action of tissue destruction producing vasoconstricting agents; and increased blood viscosity (hemoconcentration)

Alteration in bowel elimination related to–steatorrhea, diarrhea, or constipation (inadequate fluid intake, inactivity, weak abdominal musculature)

Impairment of tissue integrity: oral mucous membranes related to– dehydration

Case Study

A 68-year-old man was admitted to the hospital for evaluation of postprandial periumbilical pain of 7 to 8 months' duration. He described the pain as aching in character, usually beginning about 30 min after eating and persisting for 1 to 3 h. The pain was less severe and of shorter duration if he ate smaller amounts. He had experienced a moderate weight loss of 10 lb. The day prior to admission, he developed severe abdominal pain which did not subside, low grade fever, and bloody diarrhea. Physical examination revealed an acutely ill elderly man with tachycardia and irregular respirations; blood pressure was within normal limits. The abdomen was distended and tender to palpation. Laboratory findings included an elevated white blood cell count. Radiologic studies revealed dilated loops of small bowel. The diagnosis was acute mesenteric occlusion.

The patient was placed on a regimen of nothing by mouth. Nasogastric suction was instituted to decrease stimulation of the bowel and to relieve distention and prevent further ischemic changes. Fluid replacement was necessary for hemodynamic stabilization and was monitored by urinary output, blood pressure readings, and CVP or Swan-Ganz readings. Isoproterenol (Isuprel) was given to prevent further ischemic changes. Prophylactic antibiotics were administered to prevent peritonitis and sepsis. Surgical intervention was required in this case to remove an embolus and resect the portions of the bowel that were necrotic.

Intestinal Obstruction

Potential Nursing Diagnoses

Alteration in comfort related to–crampy abdominal pain, abdominal distention, immobility, and tissue damage

Ineffective breathing patterns related to–abdominal distention and pain and anxiety about illness

Fluid volume deficit related to–vomiting, anorexia, presence of nasogastric tube, NPO regimen, and third-space fluid loss

Impairment of tissue integrity: oral mucous membranes related to–dehydration, irritation from tubes, mouth breathing, nasal oxygen therapy, poor nutrition, poor oral hygiene, and vitamin deficiency

Case Study

Mrs. I.O., age 82, was admitted to the hospital from a nursing home, where enemas had not relieved abdominal distention and absence of bowel movements for several days. She had experienced only one episode of vomiting but had refused to eat during the 24 to 36 h prior to admission. The patient had experienced excellent health except for an abdominal hysterectomy at age 60. Physical examination revealed a slight woman. Peristaltic waves were visible over the lower abdomen. High-pitched, intermittent bowel sounds were heard upon auscultation. The abdomen was slightly distended, and there was marked tenderness to palpation. Rectal examination was normal, and a stool specimen was negative for occult blood. Laboratory findings revealed normal hemoglobin and hematocrit reading but elevated white blood cell count. Routine serum studies, urinalysis, chest film, and ECG were within normal limits for the age of the patient. Abdominal x-rays revealed dilated loops of small bowel consistent with mechanical obstruction.

Initial treatment of the patient included IV fluids to correct dehydration and nasogastric intubation to decompress the bowel. The patient was then prepared for surgery. An exploratory laparotomy revealed a strangulated loop of small bowel caused by adhesions from previous surgery. The adhesions were released, and only one small portion of bowel required resection.

Peritonitis

Potential Nursing Diagnoses

Alteration in comfort related to–rebound tenderness, abdominal pain, fever and chills, inflammation, fatigue, immobility, and tissue damage

Alteration in bowel elimination related to–diarrhea

Ineffective breathing patterns related to–abdominal pain and distention, inflammatory process, and anxiety

Ineffective coping, individual and family, related to–severity of illness

Fluid volume deficit related to–fever, chills, and diaphoresis; vomiting and diarrhea; presence of nasogastric tube; and anorexia

Impaired physical mobility related to–abdominal pain and generalized weakness

Impairment of tissue integrity: oral mucous membranes related to–dehydration

Case Study

Ms. P., a 75-year-old woman, had a history of diverticulosis with occasional bouts of diverticulitis; the latter was the reason for her present hospitalization. Several days following surgery to resect the portion of bowel affected by a perforated diverticulum, she developed moderately severe abdominal pain, nausea and vomiting, abdominal distention, low-grade fever, decreased urine output, shallow respirations, and a weak, rapid pulse. Rebound tenderness and muscle rigidity were clearly present. Laboratory studies revealed an elevated white blood cell count and increased hematocrit reading (evidence of hemoconcentration due to dehydration and metabolic acidosis). The diagnosis of peritonitis was made.

Treatment of the patient included control of infection (administration of antibiotics and placing the patient in a semi-Fowler's position), relief of pain and ileus (administration of analgesics and nasogastric intubation), replacement of fluids and electrolytes, and maintenance of the blood pressure. Symptoms subsided and surgical intervention was not required.

Cutaneous Fistula

Potential Nursing Diagnoses

Fluid volume deficit related to–high-output fistula drainage with excessive loss of fluids

Impairment of skin integrity related to–cutaneous fistula

Impairment of tissue integrity: oral mucous membranes related to–dehydration

Case Study

Mr. C.F., a 35-year-old male, had a 12-year history of Crohn's disease. He had undergone surgery to resect necrotic portions of the small intestine. One week postoperatively he experienced a sudden increase in drainage from the stab wound site. The drainage was feculent in odor, and dressings required changing every 1 to 2 h. A cutaneous fistula from the small intestine was suspected and confirmed by fistulogram.

Medical treatment was initiated, with emphasis on fluid and electrolyte replacement, nutritional support, and prevention of infection. Total parenteral nutrition was begun to maintain positive nitrogen balance in support of wound healing. Antibiotics were administered intravenously. Fluid infusions were calculated on the basis of estimated total fluid loss. An ostomy appliance was placed on the skin over the fistula to protect the skin from digestive enzymes. The fistula closed within 3 weeks and surgical repair was not required.

Zollinger-Ellison Syndrome

Potential Nursing Diagnoses

Impaired physical mobility related to–pain, fatigue, and malaise

Alteration in bowel elimination related to–diarrhea, steatorrhea, and melena

Ineffective breathing patterns related to–abdominal pain

Alteration in comfort related to–abdominal pain, gaseous bloated feeling, abdominal distention, tingling in extremities, shortness of breath, vomiting, hematemesis, tissue damage, surgical incision, and inflammation

Fluid volume deficit related to–diarrhea, vomiting, presence of nasogastric tube, increased GI motility, and hemorrhage

Impairment of tissue integrity: oral mucous membranes related to–dehydration

Case Study

A 32-year-old female, mother of three children, was admitted for symptoms of epigastric pain characteristic of duodenal ulcers. These symptoms had occurred sporadically over the past 3 to 4 years. Treatment had provided some relief. Ulcer perforation had required surgical repair, and a large amount of nasogastric drainage had been noted postoperatively. Following this surgery, her symptoms had been unrelieved by typical ulcer treatment; pain was persistent despite antacid therapy. She was having six to ten watery stools every 24 h and experienced a 16-lb. weight loss. She had dry mucous membranes, poor skin turgor, and low urine output, indicative of dehydration. At the present admission the stools were slightly positive for guaiac, hematocrit reading was 42 percent, and other routine laboratory studies were within normal limits. Hypokalemia and steatorrhea, characteristic of Zollinger-Ellison syndrome, were present. Upper GI tract series revealed normal esophagus and large folds in the stomach; there was rapid transit through the upper small bowel. Gastric secretory study results were abnormal, revealing excessive amounts of hydrochloric acid. Zollinger-Ellison syndrome was confirmed.

A total gastrectomy was performed to prevent further secretion of large quantities of gastric acid by any remaining gastric mucosa.

Inflammatory Bowel Disease

Potential Nursing Diagnoses

Ineffective breathing patterns related to–abdominal pain and distention, anxiety, and decreased energy

Ineffective coping related to–chronicity of disease process, fear of prognosis, isolation from significant others, decreased self-esteem, lack of knowledge regarding disease process and prognosis, loss of control over body part or function, change in body image, and actual or perceived lifestyle change

Alteration in comfort related to–abdominal pain, external fistulas, fatigue, anxiety, fear, depression, tissue damage, and inflammation

Fluid volume deficit related to–diarrhea, vomiting, fistula drainage, anorexia, fever, and hemorrhage

Alteration in nutrition less than body requirements related to–anorexia, nausea and/or vomiting, pain associated with eating, diarrhea, and fatigue

Disturbance in self-concept related to change in–perceived body image, change in physical health status, depression, and real or anticipated loss of body function

Alteration in bowel elimination related to–diarrhea (increased bowel motility, surgical loss of bowel)

Anxiety related to–lack of knowledge of disease, lack of knowledge regarding discharge regimen for health maintenance, and potential surgical intervention

Impairment of skin integrity related to–anal fissures and/or fistulas

Potential for noncompliance related to–chronicity of disease process, cost of treatment, denial of disease, depression, inadequate or incomplete knowledge, and feeling of not being in control

Impairment of tissue integrity: oral mucous membranes related to–dehydration

Case Study

Mr. C., age 21, was admitted to the hospital for persistent crampy abdominal pain located in the right lower quadrant and soft, unformed stools four to five times per day. He had had a low-grade fever, anorexia due to the pain associated with eating, and weight loss. Physical examination revealed a perianal lesion. Barium studies demonstrated narrowing of the bowel lumen, ulceration, and fistula tracts. A diagnosis of Crohn's disease was made after other possibilities were eliminated.

Medical treatment was instituted to relieve the symptoms of diarrhea and abdominal pain. Analgesics, medications to decrease GI motility, and nutritional support were important components of therapy. The patient received instructions regarding

medication plan, nutritional needs and dietary restrictions, antidiarrheal agents, and fluid and electrolyte imbalances associated with chronic diarrhea. Sitz baths were given to relieve discomfort from perianal lesions. The patient achieved a remission, and surgical intervention was avoided for the time.

Acute Pancreatitis

Potential Nursing Diagnoses

Alteration in comfort related to–anxiety, fear, tissue damage, inflammation, and immobility

Ineffective breathing patterns related to–severe abdominal pain and distention and the need to maintain knee-chest position to alleviate pain

Fluid volume deficit related to–diaphoresis, anorexia, vomiting, presence of nasogastric tube, and NPO regimen

Alteration in nutrition, less than body requirements, related to–anorexia

Anxiety related to–lack of knowledge regarding illness and cause of pain

Impairment of tissue integrity: oral mucous membranes related to–dehydration

Case Study

Ms. A.P., age 42, was brought to the emergency room by her sister at midnight. During the initial assessment and history taking, she was restless and lay on the cart in a knee-chest position, stating that this seemed to relieve the severe epigastric and abdominal pain which had begun 3 to 4 h before. She reported attending a family picnic that afternoon. Physical examination revealed normal blood pressure with an elevated heart rate, dyspnea, and fever and chills. The abdomen was distended and diffusely tender to palpation, especially in the periumbilical and epigastric areas. Laboratory studies revealed elevated serum amylase (more than 400), elevated urine amylase, and elevated serum lipase. A flat film of the abdomen revealed localized dilatation of the transverse colon. An upper GI tract series demonstrated delayed gastric emptying and enlargement of the duodenum due to edema of the head of the pancreas. A diagnosis of acute pancreatitis was made.

The management of this patient initially involved fluid replacement in order to maintain circulating blood volume. The other major component of therapy was the suppression and neutralization of pancreatic secretions. The patient was placed on a regimen of nothing by mouth, and nasogastric suction was instituted to control nausea and vomiting and prevent gastric stimulation by pancreatic secretions. Pain was relieved by using meperidine (Demerol) or hydromorphone (Dilaudid). (Morphine and codeine are avoided in acute pancreatitis because they produce spasm of the biliary and pancreatic ducts and the sphincter of Oddi.) Within a week the patient's symptoms subsided, and she was able to go home on the ninth day of hospitalization.

Pancreatectomy

Potential Nursing Diagnoses

Impairment of skin integrity related to–surgical incision

Fluid volume deficit related to–excessive loss of fluids, NPO regimen, and presence of nasogastric tube

Alteration in comfort related to–surgical incision, tissue damage, and inflammation

Alteration in nutrition, less than body requirements, related to–anorexia

Alteration in bowel elimination related to–surgical intervention and anesthesia

Impairment of tissue integrity: oral mucous membranes related to–dehydration

Case Study

Mr. P, an 82-year-old male, had a history of diabetes mellitus of 22 years' duration. He had been experiencing gradual weight loss, increased jaundice (not readily evident because of his dark complexion), and dull pain in the epigastrium. He was admitted to the hospital because of anorexia and pain that had intensified, with radiation to the back. Laboratory studies revealed high serum bilirubin

and elevated serum alkaline phosphatase. An enlarged pancreas was felt on palpation. Radiologic studies indicated a large tumor of the head of the pancreas. A total pancreatectomy was performed.

Multiple complications were watched for during the immediate postoperative period: fistula formation, anastomotic leak, hemorrhage, and abscess formation. Maintenance of blood volume, fluid and electrolyte balance, and respiratory parameters within normal limits were the successful outcomes of the therapy provided.

Esophagogastrectomy

Potential Nursing Diagnoses

Impairment of skin integrity related to–surgical incision

Alteration in nutrition, less than body requirements, related to–dysphagia, anorexia, and pain

Fluid volume deficit related to–dysphagia and anorexia

Alteration in comfort related to–surgical incision, pain, and anxiety

Impairment of tissue integrity: oral mucous membranes related to–dehydration

Case Study

A 55-year-old male was admitted to the hospital with a history of dysphagia, which began 12 months before with difficulty in swallowing solids and had now progressed to an inability to swallow even liquids. He had experienced nausea and vomiting to the point of anorexia and had lost 20 pounds. Physical examination was unremarkable. Diagnostic studies were made on the basis of his presenting history and the absence of other symptoms. X-ray, barium swallow, esophagoscopy, and biopsy revealed a large squamous cell tumor located in the middle third of the esophagus. An esophagogastrectomy was performed.

The patient required careful monitoring of effectiveness of ventilation postoperatively. Frequent suctioning was necessary to maintain a patent airway. Monitoring for cardiovascular complications included recognizing and appropriately treating cardiac arrhythmias and taking immediate action when signs of hemorrhage were evident.

Hepatic Dysfunction

Potential Nursing Diagnoses

Alteration in comfort related to–right upper quadrant pain, liver and spleen tenderness, fever, fatigue, pruritus, and enlarged postcervical lymph nodes

Impaired physical mobility related to–fatigue and generalized weakness, intolerance of activity, abdominal pain and discomfort, and bed rest

Anxiety related to–isolation, lack of knowledge about disease process, extended recovery period, and fear of death,

Ineffective coping, individual and family, related to–isolation (situational crises), restricted food and fluid intake, and alcohol intolerance

Alteration in bowel elimination related to–diarrhea or constipation

Alteration in comfort related to—fatigue, nausea, ascites, edema, pruritis, abdominal discomfort/pain, and fever

Impaired physical mobility related to—fatigue, generalized weakness, intolerance to activity, abdominal pain/discomfort, perceptual/cognitive impairment (ammonia intoxication), and depression/anxiety

Anxiety related to—lack of knowledge regarding disease process and threat of death

Alteration in nutrition, less than body requirements, related to–nausea and vomiting, inability of liver to metabolize foodstuffs, vitamin deficiency, and nasogastric suction

Impairment of skin integrity related to–pruritus, jaundice, male gynecomastia, altered nutritional state, immobility, edema, and bleeding or bruising due to coagulation deficiencies

Disturbance in self-concept related to–ascites and jaundice; male gynecomastia, hair loss, atrophied testicles, and impotence; and weight loss

Alteration in thought processes and sensory and perceptual changes related to–ammonia intoxication

Sexual dysfunction related to–fatigue, decreased libido, impotence, and physical awkwardness due to ascites

Alteration in fluid volume, excess, related to–decreased albumin levels and compromised regulatory mechanism

Ineffective breathing pattern related to–pleural effusion, deep rapid respirations, pain, anxiety, lack of energy, and fatigue

Case Study

Mr. A. L., a 32-year-old male, was admitted from the physician's office with the instruction to "rule out hepatitis." His history included the fact that he has been unemployed for many months. Upon physical examination it was noted that he had a recent tatoo. He complained of generalized fatigue, inability to eat for the past 2 weeks, and slight abdominal pain. His skin and sclera appeared slightly jaundiced. He denied any changes in his stools, but the color of his urine specimen was notably dark amber. His temperature was 100.2 °F.

Medical treatment included bed rest and isolation. Intravenous feeding was given initially, as Mr. A. L. was unable to tolerate oral intake, but a low-fat, high-carbohydrate diet was introduced as tolerated. The nurse caring for Mr. A. L. planned his care carefully so as to conserve the patient's energy as much as possible. After 10 days of hospitalization, the patient's jaundice subsided, he was no longer infectious, and isolation was discontinued. He was discharged 2 days later. Although he was slightly weak, his appetite had improved, the abdominal discomfort had subsided, and he had learned the need to balance rest and activity until fully recovered.

Nursing Interventions for Various Nursing Diagnoses

Nursing Diagnosis
Alteration in cardiac output: decreased.

Goals

1. Lungs will be clear to auscultation.
2. Urine output will be 30 mL/h or more with normal specific gravity.

Interventions

1. Monitor vital signs, CVP, PAWP.
2. Monitor temperature.
3. Auscultate lungs.
4. Promote calm environment.
5. Keep patient at bed rest during acute stage.
6. Place patient in Fowler's position.
7. Measure and record intake and output.
8. Give oxygen therapy as prescribed.
9. Record daily weight.
10. Provide for rest periods.
11. Keep family and/or significant others informed regarding patient's progress.

Evaluation

1. No shortness of breath at rest.
2. Blood pressure within normal limits (WNL).
3. Respirations WNL.
4. Urine output adequate.
5. Fluid and electrolyte balance maintained.
6. Daily weights stable.

Nursing Diagnosis
Alteration in nutrition: less than body requirements.

Goals

1. Maintain present weight or gain until ideal weight is achieved.
2. Nausea, vomiting, diarrhea, or stomatitis will decrease.
3. Oral intake will increase.
4. Patient will verbalize knowledge of own nutritional needs.
5. Family will verbalize knowledge of patient's nutritional needs.

Interventions

1. Complete a comprehensive nutritional assessment.
2. Monitor skin turgor, mucous membranes, and electrolytes to detect dehydration.
3. Maintain accurate intake and output record.
4. Institute calorie count.
5. Check daily weight.
6. Monitor bowel function: color, consistency, frequency of stools.
7. Monitor results of laboratory studies, e.g., serum albumin, glucose, acetone.
8. Provide frequent oral hygiene, especially for patient with nasogastric tube.
9. Provide comfort measures: positioning, analgesics, oxygen.
10. Provide small frequent feedings when appropriate.
11. Elevate head of bed for meals and for 1 h after meals.
12. Provide for rest before and after meals.
13. Instruct patient and/or significant other in specific nutritional needs, including any restrictions or changes required. (Ask dietitian to speak to patient regarding food preferences.)
14. Administer and monitor total parenteral nutrition or enteral alimentation as prescribed.
15. Document patient's tolerance of nutritional supplements: Ensure, Sustecal, etc.
16. Encourage family to bring in food from home (within dietary restrictions).
17. Assess and document patient's reasons for not eating; e.g., eating causes increased diarrhea, pain, nausea.
18. Administer vitamin and mineral supplements as prescribed.

Evaluation

1. Maintains weight or gains until ideal weight achieved.
2. Mucous membranes pink, moist; skin turgor adequate.
3. Fluid and electrolytes within normal limits.
4. Nausea, vomiting, diarrhea have subsided.
5. Patient and/or significant other able to plan for patient's meals and other nutritional needs.
6. Nitrogen balance positive.
7. Wound healing is occurring.

Nursing Diagnosis
Alteration in bowel elimination: constipation.

Goal

1. Patient will be able to pass soft, formed stool without excessive straining at least every 3 days.

Interventions

1. Assess usual bowel patterns and habits (e.g., use of laxatives).
2. Monitor stool frequency.
3. Allow or encourage regular physical activity within limits.
4. Provide adequate fluid intake.
5. Provide privacy.
6. Assist patient to establish bowel evacuation pattern.
7. Provide adequate diet.
8. Place patient in sitting position for elimination unless otherwise contraindicated.
9. Give prescribed stool softener, laxative, or suppository.
10. Instruct patient to respond immediately to elimination urge.
11. Instruct patient against habitual use of enemas or laxatives.
12. Instruct patient in normal bowel patterns and when to seek medical attention.

Evaluation

1. Has soft, formed stool at least every 3 days.
2. Does not habitually use laxatives, enemas, or suppositories.
3. Intake sufficient in fluids and dietary roughage.
4. Patient and/or significant other verbalizes knowledge regarding bowel evacuation patterns and when to seek medical attention.

Nursing Diagnosis
Alteration in bowel elimination: diarrhea.

Goals

1. Will pass soft formed stool without pain or straining.
2. Will know signs and symptoms requiring medical attention.
3. Will know ways to manage chronic diarrhea.
4. Will gain knowledge regarding dietary and/or medication regimen.

Interventions

1. Identify factors that precipate or alleviate diarrhea.
2. Record color, amount, consistency, odor, and frequency of stools.
3. Assess for signs and symptoms of dehydration.
4. Record intake and output accurately.
5. Record daily weights.
6. Monitor electrolytes.
7. Test stool for occult blood.
8. Assist patient to identify stress factors.
9. Monitor side effects and tolerance of all medications (especially antacids and antibiotics).
10. Administer antidiarrheal medications as prescribed and prn after bowel movements.
11. Encourage patient to limit intake to nonirritating foods.
12. Assess patient tolerance of tube feedings.
13. Instruct patient on how to modify diet.
14. Instruct patient in medication usage.
15. Assess perirectal area for skin irritation, fistulas, or fissures; give perineal care.
16. Maintain clear and odor-free environment; empty bedpan or commode as soon as possible.
17. Note any increase in diarrhea after meals, tests, visitors, etc.

Evaluation

1. Diarrhea subsides and patient passes soft, formed stool.
2. Patient verbalizes ways to manage diarrhea and knowledge of signs and symptoms that require medical attention.
3. Patient verbalizes dietary habits to lessen incidence of diarrhea.
4. No perirectal skin irritation.

Nursing Diagnosis
Ineffective breathing patterns.

Goals

1. Respirations will be within normal limits (WNL): rate, depth, clarity of lung sounds.
2. Patient will be afebrile.

Interventions

1. Assess for respirations (rate, rhythm, depth, lung sounds, level of consciousness or sensorium, chest expansion, chest discomfort, and color of skin, mucous membranes, and nail beds.
2. Monitor vital signs and temperature.
3. Use a calm, reassuring approach.

4. Coach patient in slower, more effective breathing.
5. Instruct patient in relaxation techniques.
6. Reposition patient frequently.
7. Place patient in semi-Fowler's position unless contraindicated.
8. Administer oxygen as needed.
9. Establish and maintain patent airway and suction as necessary.
10. Assess and relieve pain to facilitate adequate ventilation.
11. Assist patient to cough and to breathe deeply and effectively.
12. Instruct patient in incisional splinting or support of abdomen to facilitate adequate chest expansion.
13. Discourage smoking.
14. Allow for periods of structured rest (energy conservation).

Evaluation

1. Respirations WNL.
2. Patient verbalizes more comfortable breathing.
3. Skin, mucous membranes and nail bed color normal.
4. No increase in temperature for at least 24 h.

Nursing Diagnosis
Alteration in tissue perfusion.

Goal

1. Adequate tissue perfusion will be maintained.

Interventions

1. Monitor vital signs.
2. Monitor respiratory status.
3. Administer oxygen therapy, including mechanical ventilation as necessary.
4. Monitor adequate intake and output.
5. Record daily weight.
6. Administer medications as prescribed to maintain blood pressure.
7. Check peripheral circulation: color, temperature, sensation, pulses.
8. Check level of consciousness or changes in sensorium.

Evaluation

1. Urine output 30 mL/h or more.
2. Blood pressure within normal limits (WNL).
3. Respirations and arterial blood gases WNL.
4. Peripheral circulation adequate.
5. Neurologic check without deficiencies.

Nursing Diagnosis
Anxiety.

Goals

1. Behavioral symptoms will decrease.
2. Will be able to verbalize symptoms of anxiety and ways of dealing with anxiety.

Interventions

1. Use active listening.
2. Let patient know anxiety is normal.
3. Help patient to identify and recognize anxiety.
4. Challenge unrealistic goals patient may have set for self.
5. Assist patient to set realistic and short-term goals.
6. Instruct patient in methods of relaxation.
7. Give clear explanation of all procedures.
8. Provide positive reinforcement for desired responses.
9. Provide enough information for patient to become comfortable with disease process and prognosis.
10. Provide diversional activities for patient on bed rest or in isolation.
11. When isolation is required: Do not change patterns of care or decrease contact with patient during isolation, i.e., do not isolate and ignore; provide support to patient and family during isolation.

Evaluation

1. Physical and behavioral symptoms of anxiety absent.
2. Patient verbalizes relief of anxiety.

Nursing Diagnosis
Alteration in comfort.

Goals

1. Will be able to verbalize occurrence of pain or other forms of discomfort.
2. Will identify factors that influence or exacerbate pain as well as those which provide relief.

Interventions

1. Assess pain: location, quality, intensity, onset, patient's perception, and relief measures used.
2. Establish trusting relationship.
3. Instruct patient to report pain immediately and explain that this is acceptable and expected.
4. Provide for adequate sleep and rest; conserve energy to relieve fatigue.
5. Encourage change of position.
6. Administer analgesics and other therapies as necessary to relieve pain, discomfort, or fever.
7. Provide comfort measures.
8. Instruct patient in relaxation techniques.
9. Note when pain exists and determine precipitating or relieving factors.
10. Provide diversional activities for patient on bed rest.
11. Provide appropriate skin care for patient with jaundice and/or pruritus.

Evaluation

1. Free of objective signs of pain or discomfort: restlessness, grimacing, abdominal guarding.
2. Verbalizes comfort.
3. Respirations normal.
4. Sleep and rest patterns normal.
5. Mobility not impaired by pain or discomfort.

Nursing Diagnosis
Fluid volume deficit.

Goals

1. Fluid intake will increase to equal or more than equal losses.
2. Patient and/or significant other will verbalize understanding of adequate fluid intake.

Interventions

1. Assess type, amount, and site of fluid loss from GI tract.
2. Obtain history of diet and of drug and alcohol use.
3. Monitor intake and output, including liquid lost in stools, nasogastric tube output, vomitus, and active bleeding. In fistula cases, the fistula output must also be included.
4. Record daily weight.
5. Monitor skin turgor and mucous membranes.
6. Alleviate nausea, vomiting, or diarrhea.
7. Monitor temperature.
8. Monitor serum electrolytes, urine specific gravity, and BUN.
9. Monitor CVP and/or PAWP.
10. Monitor for behavioral changes.
11. Offer small amounts of liquid every 1 to 2 h during waking hours.
12. Provide frequent oral hygiene.
13. Use humidifier in room.
14. Instruct patient in importance of obtaining resting fluid maintenance levels. (Average daily loss is 1500 mL urine, 200 mL in stool, and 1300 mL in perspiration and respiration.)
15. Maintain accurate IV rate.
16. Keep skin moist with lotion, bath oils, etc.

Evaluation

1. Fluid balance maintained.
2. Patient able to take fluids and foods without nausea or vomiting.
3. Blood and urine analyses are within normal limits.
4. Urine output 30 mL/h or more.
5. For fistula cases: Fistula showing signs of healing and output decreasing.

Nursing Diagnosis
Impaired tissue integrity: oral mucous membranes.

Goal

1. Oral mucosa will be clean, soft and moist, and intact.

Interventions

1. Encourage oral intake of 2000–3000 cc every 24 h.
2. Assure well-balanced diet.
3. Discourage smoking and use of alcohol.

4. Instruct patient in necessity of daily oral hygiene routine.
5. Provide ice chips or sips of water frequently when patient is able to take them.
6. Inspect mouth each day for lesions, sores, or bleeding.
7. When endotracheal tube is used: Cleanse thoroughly around endotracheal tube; tape so as not to cause necrosis of surrounding tissues, and apply petrolatum to nares.

Evaluation

1. Patient verbalizes comfort.
2. Mucous membranes pink and moist, no evidence of break in integrity.

Nursing Diagnosis
Ineffective coping: individual and family.

Goals

1. Will verbalize feelings regarding illness.
2. Will identify own strengths and strengths of significant others.
3. Will identify effective coping mechanisms.
4. Will be able to make appropriate decisions regarding health care.
5. Will identify and utilize outside resources.

Interventions

1. Provide an atmosphere of caring trust; do not ignore when patient requires isolation.
2. Communicate your accessibility to patient and/or family.
3. Encourage verbalization of feelings, perceptions, fears, anger, and frustration.
4. Assess patient's current ability to cope; usual patterns of decision making in stressful situations (times of acute illness) and nonstressful situations (times of no illness or remission of symptoms).
5. Assist patient to identify strengths, available resources, and support systems.
6. Instruct patient in disease process, procedures, care, treatments, and medications.
7. Assist patient in exploring treatment options.
8. Assist patient in setting realistic goals.

Evaluation

1. Readily verbalizes fears and concerns regarding illness.
2. Able to care for self.
3. Verbalizes appropriate ways to manage symptoms of illness.
4. Verbalizes situations in which assistance should be sought.

Nursing Diagnosis
Potential for noncompliance.

Goals

1. Will identify barriers to compliance (cost, time, transportation, poor prognosis).
2. Will increase knowledge regarding importance of compliance to regimen.

Interventions

1. Assess barriers to compliance.
2. Assess patient's knowledge regarding disease process and therapeutic regimen.
3. Assess patient's present lifestyle and what modifications will mean.
4. Provide simple written instructions on regimen.
5. Involve patient and significant other in planning follow-up care.
6. Assess support systems.
7. Emphasize positive aspects of therapeutic regimen.
8. Contract with patient for compliance with regimen.

Evaluation

1. Self-administers prescribed medications.
2. Maintains appropriate diet.
3. Is aware of signs and symptoms requiring medical attention and contacts physician appropriately.
4. Makes appointments for follow-up.

Nursing Diagnosis
Impaired physical mobility.

Goals

1. Will maintain proper body alignment.
2. Will turn independently.

3. Will maintain full range of motion.
4. Will maintain skin integrity.

Interventions

1. Maintain patient's body alignment by positioning properly.
2. Turn or reposition patient every 2 h while on bed rest.
3. Ambulate patient six times per day when patient's condition permits.
4. Give range-of-motion exercises qid while patient is on bed rest.
5. Keep patient's heels off bed while on bed rest.
6. Assess pain and administer analgesics as necessary.
7. Provide for structured rest periods (energy conservation).
8. Encourage activity as tolerated and increase as ability permits.
9. Encourage independence in activities of daily living as tolerated.
10. Assist with positioning and restraining of tubes (nasogastric, IV, CVP) so patient's mobility is not restricted.
11. Make accurate neurologic check to assess mentation.

Evaluation

1. Verbalizes comfort.
2. Able to move in bed.
3. Ambulating with or without assistance.
4. Skin intact.

Nursing Diagnosis
Disturbance in self-concept.

Goals

1. Will identify ways to cope with negative feelings.
2. Will actively participate in social activities.
3. Will explore feelings associated with perception of self.
4. Will verbalize own strengths and available resources.

Interventions

1. Explore patient's prior means of coping.
2. Assess support system.

3. Encourage patient to identify and express feelings.
4. Encourage patient to set realistic goals.
5. Encourage diversion from illness through activity.
6. Assist patient in accepting personal limitations.
7. Support and reinforce patient's accomplishments.
8. Assist patient to identify difference between perceived and actual self.
9. Assist patient to understand manifestations that may be temporary, e.g., jaundice.

Evaluation

1. Socially active and readily participates in activities with friends and family.
2. Able to care for self and seeks assistance appropriately.

Nursing Diagnosis
Impairment of skin integrity.

Goals

1. There will be granulation tissue at incision edges.
2. There will be no evidence of infection.
3. Skin will be otherwise intact.
4. In ostomy or fistula cases: Skin surrounding fistula or stoma will be free from irritation.

Interventions

1. Assess incision at least daily.
2. Keep skin clean and dry.
3. Keep bed linen dry and wrinkle-free.
4. Avoid bumping incision.
5. Provide well-balanced diet and adequate amounts of fluids.
6. Monitor laboratory values (serum protein, BUN, CBC, electrolytes, hemoglobin, hemotocrit, ABGs).
7. Schedule times for turning patient.
8. Expose patient's skin to air.
9. Perform dressing changes as necessary to maintain dry occlusive dressing; use sterile technique.
10. Assess skin at least daily (turgor, dryness, ulcer formation, fistula formation).

11. In ostomy or fistula cases: Use appliance around stoma or fistula to keep drainage off skin; empty and reapply pouch as needed.
12. Apply skin preparations to help protect skin around stoma or fistula.

Evaluation

1. No inflammation (swelling, redness, or tenderness) of drainage site.
2. No signs of irritation or breakdown in skin integrity.

Nursing Diagnosis
Sexual Dysfunction.

Goals

1. To be able to verbalize problems.
2. To achieve productive interpersonal relationships.
3. To prevent emotional injury.
4. To achieve optimum function.

Intervention

1. Approach patient unhurriedly; develop trusting relationship; encourage discussion.
2. Inform patient regarding disease process and when appropriate indicate temporary nature of sexual dysfunction.
3. Express empathy; reassure verbally.
4. Provide emotional support for persons significant to the patient.
5. Advise patient that significant others express acceptance and love for one another.

Evaluation

1. Relates confidently with others.
2. Experiences mutual trust, respect, and acceptance from others.
3. Satisfaction with accomplishment of goals despite limitations.
4. Feels comfortable about self and own situation.
5. Uses healthy coping mechanisms.

Nursing Diagnosis
Alterations in thought processes and sensory-perceptual alteration.

Goals

1. To maintain sensory function and stimulation.
2. To prevent accident and physical injury.

Intervention

1. Include neurological check with vital signs.
2. Ambulate with assistance only.
3. Assess emotional status and appropriateness of responses.
4. Use safety precautions appropriate to mental status: bed in low position, side rails up, posey on, call light within reach.

Evaluation

1. Alert.
2. Will remain oriented X3.
3. Appropriate affect and statements.
4. Neurological signs WNL.
5. Steady on feet; able to ambulate without difficulty.
6. Emotions appropriate to situations.
7. Correct responses to verbal communication/stimuli.
8. No evidence of physical injury.

Bibliography

Briones, T. (1984). Nursing care plan for the patient with acute gastrointestinal (GI) bleeding. *Critical Care Nurse,* 4, 22–24.

Bullas, J. B., et al. (1984). Upper gastrointestinal hemorrhage. *Critical Care Nurse,* 4, 72–74.

Fazio, V. W. (1983). Crohn's disease: Surgical procedures, sequelae, and management of recurrence. *Consultant,* 23, 49–51, 59–64, 67–68.

Gettrust, K. V., Ryan, S. C., & Engelman, D. S. (1985). *Applied nursing diagnosis.* New York: Wiley.

Simmons, M. A. (1984). Using the nursing process in treating inflammatory bowel disease. *Nursing Clinics of North America,* 19, 11–25.

Spiro, H. M. (1983). *Clinical gastroenterology.* New York: Macmillan.

Stotts, N. A., et al. (1984). Care of the patient critically ill with inflammatory bowel disease. *Nursing Clinics of North America,* 19, 61–70.

12

Integumentary Patient-Care Problems

54

Anatomy and Physiology of the Integumentary System

Cynthia A.
Horvath
Jane S. Martin

The skin and its appendages such as hair, nails, and glands constitute the body's integumentary system. The skin is the largest of the body's organs, averaging a 3000-in^2 surface area in the adult and weighing up to 20 kg. Skin is a complex structure of different tissues joined to perform a variety of vital functions, and it is essential for survival. The integumentary system serves many functions, including but not limited to protection, temperature regulation, excretion, absorption, and sensation.

In this chapter the normal anatomic structure and functions of the integumentary system are presented. In addition, normal changes occurring with age are discussed.

Anatomy of Skin Structures

The skin consists of two principal parts: the epidermis and the dermis (Fig. 54-1). The outer, thinner portion, called the *epidermis,* is attached to the inner, thicker part, called the *dermis.* Beneath the dermis is the subcutaneous layer of tissue. Fibers from the dermis extend down into the subcutaneous layer and firmly attach the skin to the subcutaneous layer. The subcutaneous layer is attached to underlying tissues and organs.

Epidermis

The epidermis is a multilayer avascular structure. The epidermis regularly regenerates itself in its deepest layer and undergoes keratinization to produce scales, which are shed from the outer layer.[1]

The epidermis has four or five layers, depending on location in the body. In the areas of greatest friction, such as the palms of the hands and the soles of the feet, there are five layers. In all other areas, the epidermis has four layers. The five layers are discussed below from superficial to deep.

Stratum Corneum

The stratum corneum is also called the *horny,* or *cornified,* layer. It is the outermost layer of the epidermis, consisting of 25 to 30 rows of dead keratinized cells which are constantly being shed and replaced. This layer serves as a barrier against bacteria, light, heat, and some chemicals.

Stratum Lucidum

This layer is the lower part of the stratum corneum that is seen on the palms of the hands and the soles of the feet. It appears as a thin, transparent layer and consists of three to four rows of clear, flat, dead cells that contain a substance called *eleiden.*

Stratum Granulosum

This layer consists of two or three rows of flattened cells that contain granules of *kerotohyalin,* a compound involved in the first step of keratin formation. *Keratin* is the waterproofing protein found in the top layer of the epidermis.[2]

Stratum Spinosum

This layer consists of eight to ten rows of many-sided (*polyhedral*) cells that are attached to one another. The surface of these cells may have a prickly appearance. The stratum spinosum forms the mechanical bulk of the epidermis.

The stratum spinosum and the lowest layer, the stratum basale, are often referred to as the *stratum germinativum* because this is where new cells are germinated.

Stratum Basale

A single layer of columnar cells forms this portion of the epidermis. This layer anchors the epidermis to the dermis and must be present for the epidermis

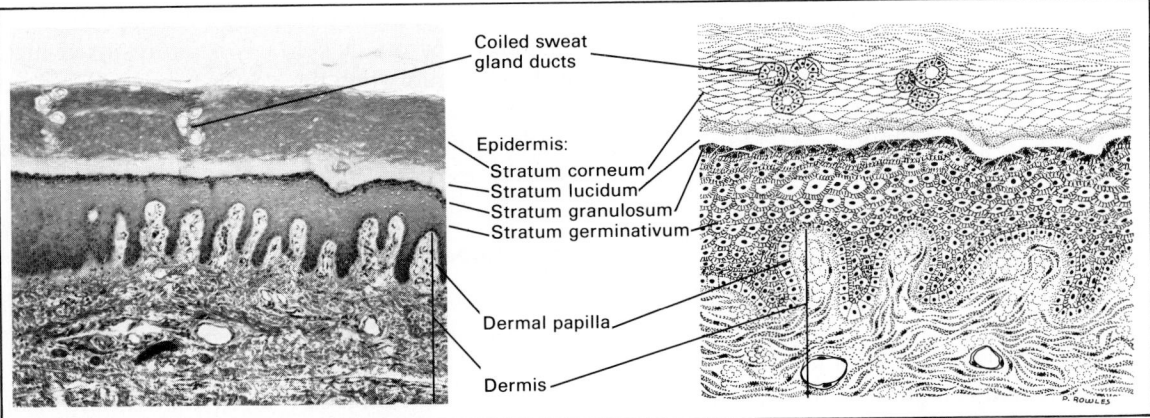

Coiled sweat gland ducts

Epidermis:
Stratum corneum
Stratum lucidum
Stratum granulosum
Stratum germinativum

Dermal papilla

Dermis

Figure 54-1 Structures of the skin. (*From L. Langley, I. Telford, and J. Christensen, Dynamic Anatomy and Physiology, 5th ed., McGraw-Hill, New York, 1980.*)

to regenerate. As the cells of this layer multiply, they push upward toward the surface.

Skin color is determined by a pigment called *melanin.* The amount of melanin present in the skin varies, causing differences in skin color ranging from pale yellow to black. The stratum basale, stratum spinosum, and stratum granulosum contain melanin in white people. In black people melanin is found throughout all layers of the epidermis. Melanin is synthesized in cells called *melanocytes* which produce melanin and distribute it throughout the epidermis.

Other Epidermal Cells

The Langerhans cell is located in the higher layers of the epidermis. It is a clear cell similar to the melanocyte but lacks melanin. The exact function of the Langerhans is unclear, but it appears to be involved in immunologic skin reactions.

The Merkel cell is located in the lower layers of the epidermis. It is similar to the keratinocytes except that it contains characteristic granules that are electron-dense. The Merkel cell's exact function is also unclear, but it is thought to be a type of epidermal nerve cell because it is associated with nerve endings in the upper dermis.[3]

Dermis

The dermis is the second principal part of the skin (Fig. 54-1). It is composed of connective tissues containing collagenous and elastic fibers. The der-mis is approximately 0.5 to 2.5 mm thick. Blood vessels, nerves, glands, and hair follicles are embedded in the dermis. The dermis is divided into two layers, the papillary layer and the reticular layer. The papillary layer is the upper section of the dermis and makes up approximately one-fifth of the thickness of the total layer. The surface area is increased by projections called *dermal papillae,* which protrude into the epidermis and contain loops of capillaries. *Meissner's corpuscles* (nerve endings that are sensitive to light touch) are present in some dermal papillae. The papillary layer also contains pacinian corpuscles (nerve endings that are sensitive to deep pressure).

The size and arrangement of the dermal papillae cause ridges marking the external surface of the epidermis. The ridge patterns on the fingertips and thumbs, which are different in every individual, can be imprinted to form the fingerprints.[4]

The reticular layer is the innermost layer of the dermis. It consists of a dense, irregular, collagenous connective tissue. This layer also contains numerous blood vessels, as well as collagenous and elastic fibers which give toughness to the skin. The reticular layer is attached to the organs beneath it by the subcutaneous layer.

Cutaneous Vessels

Circulation to the skin is provided by two networks of vessels which perform distinct functions: nutrition of the cutaneous tissues and thermal regulation. The first system consists of the usual nutritive arteries, capillaries, and veins; the second constitutes an extensive subcutaneous venous plexus capable of holding large amounts of blood and arteriovenous anastomoses which are vascular links between the arteries and venous plexuses (Fig. 54-2). Arteriovenous anastomoses are located in areas of the body exposed most often to extreme cold, such as the ears, nose, lips, and volar surfaces of the hands and feet.

Regulation of blood flow to the skin is controlled by the central nervous system because body temperature is controlled in part by blood flow through the skin. The temperature control center of the hypothalmus is the specific area of the brain responsible for controlling blood flow to the skin. Hypothalmic regulation of blood flow in the periphery is through innervation of sympathetic vasoconstrictor fibers which are distributed throughout the skin. The direct effect of catecholamines (norepinephrine and epinephrine) released at the vessels and systemically also plays a role in controlling blood flow to the skin.

The actual rate of blood flow through the skin is highly variable because of rapid changes in metabolic activity and external temperature. Under normal conditions there is a flow rate of approximately 400 mL/min in the average adult. Depending on the temperature, the flow may be as low as 50 mL/min in extremely cold temperatures or as high as 2 to 3 L/min when the skin is maximally heated and vasodilated. It should be noted that the nutritive needs of the skin can be met even during times of marked decreases in blood flow.[5]

Subcutaneous Fat

The dermis is separated from underlying structures such as muscles and bones by a layer of subcutaneous fat (Fig. 54-1). The subcutaneous layer may be almost nonexistent in an emaciated person or may be several inches thick in an obese person. Subcutaneous fat serves as a temperature insulator, as physical padding, and as a storage site for energy. It is also largely responsible for the contours of the human figure.[1]

Epidermal Appendages

Epidermal appendages, which are developed from the embryonic epidermis, extend into the dermis. Hair, nails, and glands are the structures that compose the epidermal appendages. Hair and nails provide protection for the body; the glands help to regulate body temperature.

Hair

The major function of hair is protection (Fig. 54-3). Hair protects the scalp from injury and from sunlight. The eyes are protected from foreign particles by the eyebrows and eyelashes. The nostrils and ear canals are also protected from foreign particles by hair. Hair is present over the entire body except for the palms of the hands, soles of the feet, distal phalanges, lips, nipples, and parts of the perineum.

Each hair consists of a root and a shaft (Fig. 54-3). The visible portion of the hair which projects above the surface of the skin is the *shaft*. The shaft itself is composed of three structures. The medulla, or central portion of the shaft, is made up of many-sided (polyhedral) cells that contain air spaces. The cortex forming the major part of the shaft consists of elongated cells that contain pigment granules in dark hair; the cortex of white hair contains air. The outermost layer of the shaft is the cuticle, which is formed by a single layer of thin, flat cells. The *root*

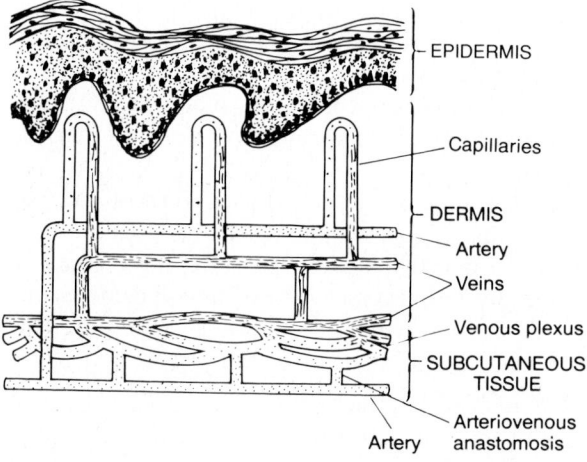

Figure 54-2 Cutaneous circulation. (*From A. Guyton, Textbook of Medical Physiology, 7th ed., W. B. Saunders, Philadelphia, 1986.*)

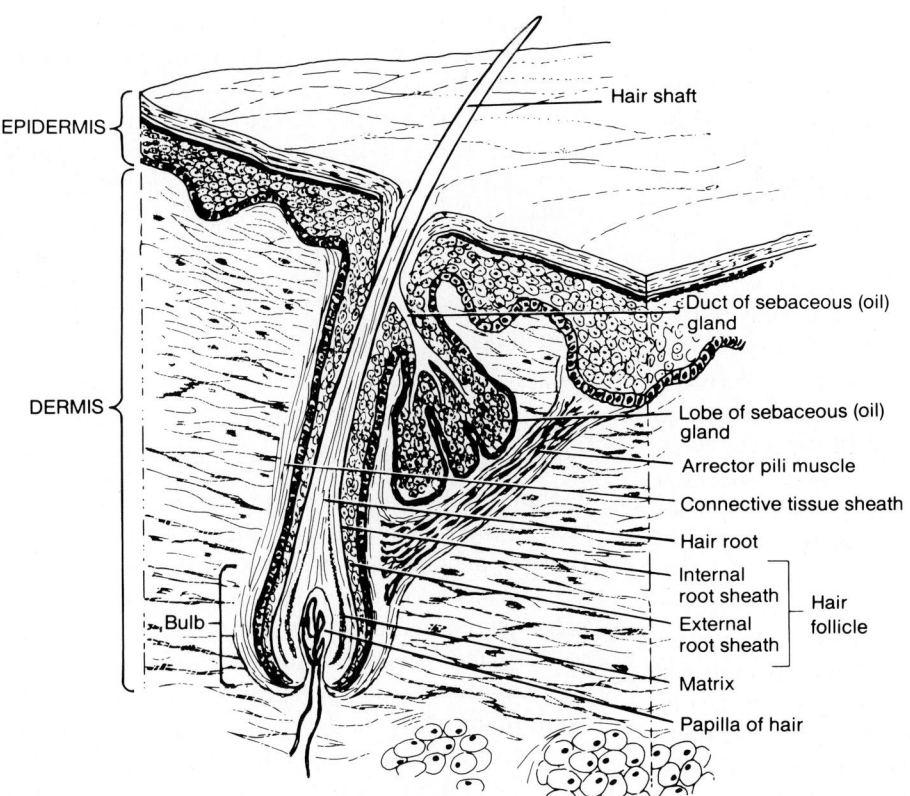

Figure 54-3 Principal parts of a hair and associated structures. (*From W. Montagna, The Skin, Scientific American, 212, 1965.*)

EPIDERMIS

DERMIS

Hair shaft

Duct of sebaceous (oil) gland

Lobe of sebaceous (oil) gland

Arrector pili muscle

Connective tissue sheath

Hair root

Internal root sheath

External root sheath

} Hair follicle

Bulb

Matrix

Papilla of hair

portion of the hair is located beneath the surface of the skin deep within the dermis. It too contains a medulla, cortex, and cuticle. Surrounding the root is the hair follicle, which is composed of two layers, the external and internal root sheaths. The external root sheath is a continuation of the epidermal layers. The internal root sheath extends only partway up the follicle and is formed from the proliferating cells of the matrix.

At the base of each hair follicle is an enlarged structure, called the *bulb,* containing an indentation, the *papilla,* that is filled with loose connective tissue. The numerous blood vessels supplying the bulb provide nourishment to the hair. A germinal layer referred to as the *matrix* is also contained within the bulb. Through the process of cellular division, the matrix produces new hairs to replace the approximately 70 to 100 hairs that are lost each day in the adult. Hair growth is about 1 mm every 3 days, but this may change during illness.

Smooth muscle bundles and sebaceous glands are also associated with the structure of the hair.

The smooth muscle, or arrector pili, extends from the dermis to the side of the hair follicle. During times of stress or cold these muscles contract, resulting in erection of the hair, or "goosebumps." This response has no function in humans, but in lower animals it provides increased insulation. The sebaceous glands assist in preventing brittleness and drying of the hairs.[2]

Nails

The nails are a modification of the horny epithelial cells and are composed of hard keratin. These cells form a solid clear covering over the dorsal surfaces of the terminal portions of the fingers and toes. Each nail consists of a nail body, a free edge, and the nail root.

The fold of skin that extends around the proximal and lateral edges of the nail is the *nail fold.* The skin below the nail is the dermis of the *nail bed.* The furrow between the nail fold and the nail bed is the *nail groove.* The *cuticle,* or *eponychium,* is a narrow band of epidermis that extends from the margin of the lateral border of the nail and adheres to it.

The epithelium of the proximal part of the nail bed is the *nail matrix*. The function of the matrix is nail growth. The average growth in length of the fingernail is approximately 1 mm per week; toenail growth is slightly slower.[2]

Sebaceous Glands

Sebaceous (oil) glands arise from the walls of hair follicles and produce sebum (Fig. 54-3). Sebum is an oily substance that is a mixture of fats, cholesterol, proteins, and inorganic salts. These glands keep the hair from drying and becoming brittle. The sebaceous glands also help to form a protective film that prevents excessive evaporation of water from the skin, and sebum also helps to keep the skin pliable and soft.

Sudoriferous Glands

The sudoriferous (sweat) glands are simple tubular structures found in most parts of the skin except the margins of the lips, penis, nail beds, eardrums, and clitoris. In contrast to the sebaceous glands, the sudoriferous glands are most numerous in the palms of the hands. It has been estimated that there are 3000 glands per square inch on the palm. They are also found in large numbers in the axillae and on the forehead.

Each gland consists of a secretory section and an excretory duct. The secretory section is located below the dermis in the subcutaneous tissue and is a twisted and coiled tube. From the coiled secretory section, the excretory duct spirals through the dermis toward the surface.

Perspiration, or sweat, the substance produced by the sudoriferous glands, is a mixture of water, salts, urea, uric acid, amino acids, ammonia, sugar, lactic acid, and ascorbic acid. The principal functions of these glands are to regulate body temperature and eliminate wastes.[2]

Skin Flora

Human skin contains a number of normal bacteria, but the number varies greatly. Sites that harbor larger numbers of bacteria include the perineum,

groin, and axillae. Persons with oily skin harbor more bacteria than those with dry skin. Warm, humid weather also is more conducive to maintenance of skin bacteria than cold, dry weather. Gram-positive bacteria in contact with the apocrine glands in the axillae produce the odor characteristic of the axillae.

The normal pH of skin is 4.2 to 5.6. This pH helps to retard the growth of some bacteria. Leukocytes present in the epidermis are thought to defend against invasion of organisms.[6]

Aging

Changes in the skin that occur with aging may alter each of the functions of the integumentary system. There is a significant decrease in skin turgor, and the skin takes on a transparent, tissuelike appearance. Secretions from the sebaceous and sudoriferous glands decrease significantly, causing dry skin, especially over the extremities, where circulation may also be decreased. There is also a tendency to hypopigmentation, increasing with age.

The amount of hair loss depends on several factors other than age, such as heredity and sex. Generally, by the mid-sixties hair loss is completed and its distribution patterns are set. In most aging persons pigment cells fail, thus causing gray hair color. Reduction in hormonal levels causes a decrease in pubic and axillary hair.

In the older person the dermis loses its elasticity. Loss of collagen and elastic fibers causes shrinking of the dermis, which in turn causes wrinkling as the smaller dermal underbase that supports the dermis causes the dermis to fold.

Gravity pulls the skin down, causing marked facial changes such as jowls, drooping eyelids, and elongation of the earlobes. Bags under the eyes are herniations of fat into the subcutaneous layers. Nail growth may slow because of poor circulation. Nails also change to a yellow or gray tone and become more brittle and thick.[4]

Vascular changes and atrophy of the epidermis inhibit the function of skin sensory neurons. This in turn decreases the older person's ability to perceive sensations. The tactile sense is lost most frequently in the palms of the hands and the soles of the feet.

Functions

Sensation

The function of the skin as an organ of sensation is extensive. It plays a major role in the collection of sensory information from the body through nervous mechanisms referred to as the *somatic senses*. The somatic senses are generally classified in three categories: the mechanoreceptive and thermoreceptive senses and the pain sense.

Mechanoreceptive Senses

Commonly referred to as the *tactile senses*, the mechanoreceptive senses include touch, pressure, vibration, tickle, and itch. Position sense is also included in this category. Six different types of tactile receptors have been identified, but many others similar to these are thought to exist. Briefly, they are as follows:

1. *Free nerve endings* are receptors found everywhere in the skin and detect touch and pressure.
2. *Meissner's corpuscles* are touch receptors with special sensitivity found in the glabrous (nonhairy) parts of the skin, most notably in the fingertips and lips. They are particularly sensitive to light touch and low frequency vibration.
3. *Expanded tip tactile receptors* are areas which contain large numbers of Meissner's corpuscles and also large numbers of tactile receptors such as Merkel's disk. Stimulation of these receptors allows one to detect the continuous touch of objects against the skin. These receptors, in conjunction with Meissner's corpuscles, also have the ability to recognize the exact point at which the body is touched and the texture of objects being touched.
4. *Hair end organ* is a term that refers to a hair and its basal nerve fiber. Movement of objects on the surface of the body results in stimulation of the nerve fibers that entwine at the base of each hair. Each hair is essentially a touch receptor.
5. *Ruffini's end organs* are receptors located in the deeper layers of the skin. They have the ability to recognize heavy, continuous touch and pressure signals.
6. *Pacinian corpuscles* are found just beneath the skin, among other places. They are stimulated by very rapid movement, making them particularly important in detecting tissue vibration.[5]

The sensations of touch, pressure, and vibration, though classified independently, are closely interrelated. In fact, they are all detected by the same type of tactile receptor with only minor differences. Touch generally results from the stimulation of receptors found in the tissues just beneath the skin, whereas pressure is detected as a result of deeper tissue deformation. The sense of vibration results from rapid repetitive signals and utilizes the same receptors which detect touch and pressure.

Recent findings support the existence of specific free nerve endings which detect only the tickle and itch (pruritus) sensations. These nerve endings are found almost exclusively in the superficial layers of the skin, a site at which only these sensations can usually be elicited.

The sensation of itch is a response to weak, persistent stimulation leading to a response such as rubbing or scratching in an effort to remove or obtain relief from the irritant. If scratching is strong enough to cause pain, the itch sensation is thought to be inhibited or overridden by the sensation of pain.

The tickle sensation is also caused by persistent light stimulation, usually resulting in minor avoidance behavior such as jerking away from the source of stimulation.

Thermoreceptive Senses

The thermal receptors are capable of detecting heat and cold and discriminate between the various gradations of the two temperature extremes. At least three different types of sensory receptor play a role in this function: cold receptors, warmth receptors, and pain receptors.

Located just beneath the external surface of the skin, the cold and warmth receptors are positioned at specific but separate points. Each receptor has a stimulating diameter of approximately 1 mm. The areas of the body in which these receptors are located and the number within each area vary significantly. There are three to ten times as many cold receptors as warmth receptors. Specific areas of the body such as the lips contain 15 to 25 cold points per square centimeter as compared to the finger, which contains only 5 cold points per square centimeter. The number of warmth points is correspondingly fewer.

Specialized pain receptors are found throughout the superficial layers of the skin. Stimulation of these receptors occurs only in the presence of extreme degrees of heat and cold. The pain receptors along with the cold and warmth receptors are responsible for detecting "freezing cold" and "burning hot" sensations.

The ability to detect temperature gradations is determined by the relative degree of stimulation of the various receptors. For example, at the extreme temperatures of 20°C and 60°C, only pain receptors are stimulated. A temperature of 20°C stimulates only cold receptors, whereas at 35°C both cold and warmth receptors are stimulated.

The thermal receptors not only have the ability to respond to steady states of temperature but also exhibit marked responses to rapid variations of external temperatures. This response explains the extreme difference in temperature a person experiences when going outside from an air-conditioned room on a hot day.

The detection of temperature gradations is also affected by the number of thermal receptors stimulated. The number of receptors in any one area of the body is small, making it difficult to detect or discriminate between different temperatures. Conversely, when large areas of the body are stimulated simultaneously, it is much easier to detect temperature gradations: there is a summation of signals which makes it possible to discern minor changes in temperature.

The mechanism of thermal stimulation is thought to be activated by changes in the metabolic rate of the receptors. Thermal perception, therefore, is probably not due to direct physical stimulation, as one would expect, but rather to a chemical stimulation of the receptors.[6]

Pain Sense

The sensation of pain is a protective mechanism which acts whenever tissue is being damaged. The response to this form of stimulation is an awareness of the abnormal stimulus and removal of the stimulus if possible.

Two major types of pain have been classified according to how quickly the pain is perceived: acute pain and slow pain. *Acute pain* is so designated

because only about 0.1 s is needed to sense the painful stimulus. Also referred to as *sharp* or *fast pain,* this form of pain is generally sensed in the skin but not felt in most deeper tissues. *Slow pain,* on the other hand, is sensed only after a second or more has passed and increases slowly in its intensity over several more seconds or even minutes. *Throbbing, chronic,* and *aching pain* are additional terms used for slow pain. This form of pain can be sensed in both the skin and the internal tissues and is usually associated with tissue destruction.

The pain receptors may also be classified according to the type of stimulation necessary to excite the nerve ending. *Mechanosensitive pain receptors* are almost entirely excited by excessive mechanical stress or damage to the underlying tissues. Those receptors sensitive to heat and cold are referred to as *thermosensitive pain receptors.* A third type of receptor, called *chemosensitive receptors,* reacts to a variety of chemical substances such as bradykinin, serotonin, histamine, and prostaglandins. Even though there is receptor specificity, most receptors respond to more than one type of stimulus.

One important aspect in which the pain receptor differs from most types of nerve endings is its nonadaptive nature. Unlike most sensory receptors, the pain receptors lack all or almost all adaptive capacity. This lack of adaptation ensures that the subject remains cognizant of the damaging stimulus for as long as the pain persists.[6] (See Chap. 33 for further discussion of peripheral neural transmission.)

Protection

Mechanical

The most obvious and well-known function of the skin is its ability to act as a barrier to external environmental forces. The layers of the epidermis provide a relatively flexible and elastic supportive covering. Additional cushioning and bulk are provided by the dermis and subcutaneous fat. Thus, when mechanical manipulation of the skin is encountered, the skin gives but does not break. Once the manipulation has stopped, it can usually resume its normal position.

Protection from external radiation such as ultraviolet light, visible light, and ionizing radiation is also a function of the skin. Melanin plays a major role in shielding the body from the damaging effects of ultraviolet radiation in particular.[6]

Chemical

In addition to physical protection, the layers of the skin act as a barrier to the penetration and absorption of potentially harmful gases and liquids. The stratum corneum and free lipids provide the major barrier for their absorption. As a selectively permeable surface, the skin is more impermeable than permeable. The skin also protects the body from potentially harmful microorganisms, perhaps partly because of the low pH of the skin surface.[7]

Temperature Regulation

A significant function of the skin is the regulation of body temperature. It is an essential component of the body's system for maintaining a constant internal or core body temperature despite variable environmental temperatures and metabolic activity. The variety of mechanisms related to this function of the skin are briefly described below.

Nervous System Control

The body temperature is regulated primarily by nervous feedback mechanisms which operate through the perioptic area of the anterior portion of the hypothalmus and portions of the posterior hypothalmus. Stimulation of this area leads to activation of the autonomic nervous system via sympathetic nerve fibers found in the skin. This in turn leads to a variety of cutaneous responses (e.g., vessel constriction or dilatation) to maintain a constant core temperature. Additional information regarding skin temperature is relayed to the posterior hypothalmus via the peripheral thermosensitive receptors.

Cutaneous Blood Flow

As previously described, the circulatory apparatus of the skin related to temperature regulation is principally characterized by two vascular structures: the venous plexus and arteriovenous anastomoses. The high variability of blood flow through these vessels makes them highly effective in maintaining a normal core temperature.

When the body is subjected to high external temperatures or elevated blood temperature, most of the cutaneous vessels dilate because of inhibition of the sympathetic centers in the posterior hypothalamus. This extensive vasodilatation increases the blood flow dramatically—up to 30 percent of cardiac output—which increases the rate of heat conduction to the skin. The opposite conditions occur in response to low external temperatures or low internal blood temperature. Widespread vasoconstriction of the arteries and arteriovenous anastomoses occurs secondary to sympathetic innervation, leading to a significant drop in cutaneous blood flow (close to zero percent of the total cardiac output). The decrease in warm blood flow to the skin from the internal organs decreases the conduction of heat to the skin, thereby assisting in raising the internal body temperature.

Methods of Heat Loss

Approximately 95 percent of the total heat dissipated from the body is removed by radiation, conduction, convection, and evaporation (Fig. 54-4). *Radiation,* in this context, is the transfer of infrared heat rays from one object to another. Any object not at a temperature of absolute zero radiates heat. Therefore, if the body temperature is greater than that of surrounding objects such as the floor, ceiling, and furniture, body heat is reduced. However, if surrounding objects are at a higher temperature than the body, heat is absorbed by the body. Approximately 60 percent of the body's heat is lost at normal room temperature.

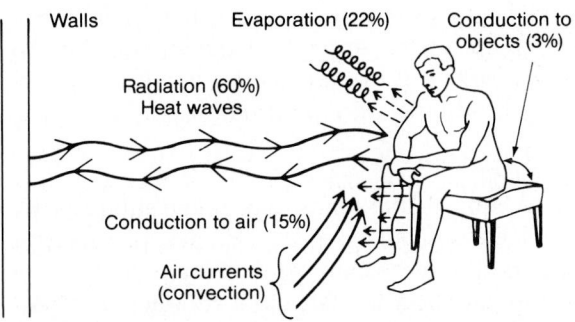

Figure 54-4   Methods of heat loss from the body. (*From A. Guyton, Textbook of Medical Physiology, 7th ed., W. B. Saunders, Philadelphia, 1986.*)

Conduction is the transfer of heat from the body to any object with which it comes in contact, such as clothing. Only minimal amounts of heat are lost through this method, because the object absorbing the heat soon approaches the temperature of the body. Once this occurs, the object becomes an insulator preventing more heat loss.

Convection is the conduction of heat to the air surrounding the body. When air makes contact with the skin, the heat of the body is conducted to the cooler air, which becomes warmed. This warmed air is then carried away by convection currents. The faster the air moves, the greater the loss of heat. Convection accounts for about 15 percent of body heat loss. A greater loss of heat via conduction and convection occurs in water, because water absorbs much larger quantities of heat than air at moderate temperatures.

Evaporation is the conversion of a liquid to a vapor in which the evaporating substance removes heat from the body. Evaporation from the skin and lungs removes approximately 22 percent of normal body heat. A continuous diffusion of water through the skin and lungs results in an insensible water loss of approximately 600 mL per day. This is an uncontrollable evaporative process, making it an ineffective method of temperature regulation. There is, however, a very effective controlled method of evaporative heat loss through regulation of the sweat glands, which are controlled by the central nervous system in much the same way as the cutaneous vessels. Stimulation of the perioptic area of the hypothalmus by high external temperatures or an increased metabolic rate activates the sympathetic nerves in the skin throughout the body, and the sweat glands respond to the sympathetic innervation by producing perspiration at a rate equivalent to the strength of the stimulation. Approximately 4 L of perspiration per hour can be produced under extreme conditions.

Insulation

In addition to the temperature-regulating mechanisms mentioned above, the skin also provides the body with the capability of retaining internal body heat in an effort to maintain a constant core temperature. The outer layers of the skin, along with the subcutaneous tissue and subcutaneous fat, act as a thermal insulator. The fat tissue is particularly effective in preventing the escape of body heat

because it conducts heat only one-third as readily as other tissue. The thickness of the subcutaneous fat layer thus determines the degree of insulation possible.[2,5]

Skin Color

Skin temperature is reflected by the coloration of the skin. The color of the blood and rate of blood flow through the vessels result in a variety of skin colors. An increase in cutaneous blood flow secondary to elevated skin temperature causes the skin to become pink or red. If the skin vessels constrict, causing decreased blood flow, the skin may turn pale. If in this instance most of the oxygen is removed from the capillaries before entering the veins, the skin takes on a bluish hue because of the dark, deoxygenated blood contained in the veins. During conditions which result in severe constriction of the vessels (e.g., hypovolemic shock) most of the blood is shunted from the skin to the vital internal organs. The skin then takes on the color of the underlying connective tissue, which has a whitish hue, and the classic ashen pallor of shock is seen.[5]

Excretion and Absorption

Although they are not widely emphasized, the skin also has two other functions, excretion and absorption. The excretory function is limited, but profuse sweating can eliminate up to 1 g of nonprotein nitrogen per hour.[8]

It was not until recently that the absorptive capabilities of the skin were utilized in the treatment of systemic illnesses. Current data have demonstrated the effectiveness of percutaneous administration of drugs and other substances for a variety of illnesses. An example of this type of therapy is the percutaneous administration of nitroglycerin in the treatment of angina. It is anticipated that use of this form of drug therapy (referred to as *transdermal*) will broaden considerably during the coming years.[7]

Summary

To perceive the skin as just a simple covering for the body is a gross oversimplification. The skin with its associated structures is a unique and indispensable body organ. It is a complex system capable of performing a variety of vital functions—protection, temperature regulation, and sensation—which are essential to life itself. The skin's lifelong ability to maintain its integrity against the plethora of environmental hazards encountered in normal day-to-day living make it an appropriate first-rank defense in human survival.

References

1. Nasemann, T., Sauerbrey, W., & Burgdorf, W. H. (1983). *Fundamentals of dermatology* New York: Springer-Verlag.
2. Tortora, G. J., & Anagnostakos, N. P. (1981). *Principles of anatomy and physiology* (3d ed.). New York: Harper & Row.
3. Breathnach, A. S., & Wolff, K. (1979). Structure and development of skin. In T. B. Fitzpatrick, A. Z. Eisen, K. Wolff, I. M. Freedberg, & K. F. Austen (Eds.), *Dermatology in general medicine* (2d ed., pp. 41–67). New York: McGraw-Hill.
4. Fitzsimons, V. M. (1983). The aging integument: A sensitive and complex system. *Topics in Clinical Nursing, 5*(2), 32–38.
5. Guyton, A. (1986). *Textbook of medical physiology* (7th ed.). Philadelphia: W. B. Saunders.
6. Luckmann, J., & Sorensen, J. C. (1980). *Medical-surgical nursing: A psychophysiologic approach* (2d ed.). Philadelphia: Saunders.
7. Hurley, J. H. (1985). Permeability of the skin. In S. L. Moschella & H. J. Hurley (Eds.), *Dermatology* (2d ed.), (Vol. 1, pp. 97–102). Philadelphia: W. B. Saunders.
8. Woodburne, R. T. (1983). *Essentials of human anatomy* (7th ed.), New York: Oxford.

55

Burns

Mary Ann DiMola
Cathleen A. Acres
James B. Winkler

No one discipline can provide adequate burn care: A team approach must be developed, with each member providing his or her particular expertise in harmony with others. The bedside nurse is a key member for structuring an environment for recovery. Each nurse who endeavors to care for a critically burned patient must consider an approach to total coordination of therapy, incorporating basic nursing as well as specialty nursing skills. If measures or tasks are overlooked because they appear trivial, the resulting problems are soon compounded, often reaching gargantuan proportions.

The burn nursing specialist demonstrates competency in nursing essentials as well as in the technicalities of critical care—treating disease by anticipating and recognizing subtle early warnings and by initiating appropriate interventions. The nurse who is able to meet these demands and who knows the specific requirements of the severely burned individual has laid the foundation of an environment for recovery. Concentrating treatment on only one of the patient's problems at a given time is an ineffective approach because other physiologic and psychologic derangements soon become additive and may ultimately destroy the patient. Thus, we see patients in whom initial shock has been successfully combated by a meticulous fluid therapy program but who later die of pneumonia, which might have been controlled had they received vigorous preventive measures.

The routine essentials of nursing care are frequently neglected in the flurry of activity surrounding any critically ill patient. The practitioner may become distracted by intravenous transfusions and medications, invasive monitoring, and respiratory therapy equipment, and may overlook the basic ingredients essential to recovery: comfort, rest, hygiene, nutrition, position change, deep breathing exercises, and infection control. These activities have traditionally been the nurse's domain and are seldom included in physician's orders. However, health care practitioners have become more specialized, and the modern nurse has taken on many responsibilities. The truly professional nurse must ask, "If nurses do not provide essential nursing care, who will?" For it is in providing excellence in basic care that the battle is won.

Pathophysiology

Stages of Burn Injury

Based on the derangements which follow an appreciable full-thickness skin loss, burn care can be divided into three definable but overlapping periods, each with well-defined principles on which care is planned. These are the *emergent,* the *acute,* and the *rehabilitation* periods. In the emergent period the traumatic insult to the skin, the largest organ of the body, results in an immediate, dramatic, natural inflammatory response and massive shift of extracellular fluid from the bloodstream into the damaged tissues. The acute period deals with the loss of normal skin function, primarily protection against infection, and the body's attempt to heal the massive wound, creating a disposition to serious complications. During the rehabilitation period, the primary considerations are of the functional and cosmetic deficits caused by contracture and scar formation.

The authors gratefully acknowledge the contributions of Claudella Archambeault-Jones, R.N., and Irving Feller, M.D., to the first edition of this text.

Emergent Period

The emergent period refers to the first 2 to 4 days after the burn injury, depending on the severity of the injury and when fluid resuscitation was begun. This is the period when the patient is admitted, the severity of the injury is determined, and first aid and wound care are initiated. The most important aspects of care involve determining and administering the required fluids, assessing respiratory status, and maintaining pulmonary function. The emergent period usually ends when initial fluid therapy is completed and the patient starts to lose some of the weight gained when large amounts of fluid were given intravenously.

Acute Period

The acute period of treatment begins at the end of the emergent period and lasts until all of the full-thickness wounds are covered with autografts. If the burn is only a partial-thickness injury, the acute period may be over within 10 to 20 days; healing is spontaneous and grafts are not necessary.

During the acute phase there are two main principles of management. The first is to remove the eschar (dead tissue) as soon as possible and to cover the wound with homografts (skin grafts from another person) or autografts (grafts of the patient's own skin). The second major task is to avoid, as far as possible, the complications known to occur. The most common complications are (1) infection leading to septicemia and pneumonia, (2) renal failure, and (3) other organ derangements. Some complications cannot be avoided, and it is necessary to detect these early and treat them vigorously. It is very important to remember that the seriously burned patient is acutely ill for a long period of time. The patient is not in a chronic state, as this prolonged, difficult period would suggest, but rather is acutely ill and in danger of death from complications.

Because of severe metabolic strain, the patient may appear to be doing well one day, only to be found with a severe complication the next. Only when the full-thickness wound is covered with autograft are these dangers past.

Rehabilitation Period

The rehabilitation phase is concerned with returning the patient to a useful place in society. During this time the patient undergoes an intensive effort to regain or compensate for functions lost due to the burn. This stage may continue for many years.

System Alterations

Adverse effects from burn injury may be quite varied; some wounds heal without visible scarring, others may result in death. The events which follow a major injury may progress to multiorgan failure and a devastating outcome. This progression is a complex, and in many cases unexplained, phenomenon. To better understand what is known about the body's response to heat, a systems approach is used.

Integumentary System

The skin is composed of three distinct layers: the epidermis, dermis, and subcutaneous layers. When heat is applied to the external surface of the skin, the resultant damage is proportional to the degree of heat and the time of exposure.

Prolonged exposure to relatively low heat or short exposure to higher temperatures can cause cell destruction at progressively deepening levels. Tissue damage can occur at temperatures as low as 113°F (45°C) when the heat source is in contact with the skin for several hours. At 158°F (70°C), cellular destruction is so rapid that only brief periods of exposure are necessary for total destruction down to and including the subcutaneous layer.[1] Most large burn injuries cause damage at varying skin layers so that a smooth plane of burn cannot be demarcated (Fig. 55-1). Once cell destruction has taken place, regardless of the cause or time frame, the physiologic responses are similar.

In addition to changes in the skin, varying degrees of vascular destruction may occur. In full-thickness burns, complete cessation of blood flow to the burned area is common. This occurs as a result of thrombosis to the vessels in the injured area, a condition which can last for many weeks. Regardless of surgical or nonsurgical intervention, the healing process in full-thickness wounds needs to include the reestablishment of a vascular bed to the burned area. If the burn is of partial thickness,

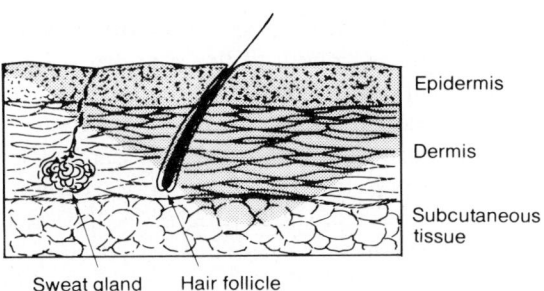

Epidermis

Dermis

Subcutaneous tissue

Sweat gland   Hair follicle

Figure 55-1 A smooth plane of burn can rarely be demarcated. More often, a combination of varying depth of burn occurs. The shaded area denotes damage due to burn. Other areas of skin section appear normal.

circulation to the affected area stops temporarily, resuming within 24 to 48 h.

A point to be considered in tissue damage caused by heat is the thickness of the skin involved. It takes less heat and time to do similar damage in areas of the body covered with thin skin than in those areas where the skin is thicker. Skin is thickest over the back and thinnest around the medial arm and face. Skin is generally thinner in young children and in the elderly than in those in the prime of life. The elderly also have reduced layers of subcutaneous material and an overall decreased ability to respond to trauma. Consequently, burns of similar size have a more serious effect in the aged.

Immune System

Burn patients are more susceptible to the invasion of pathogens because the injury has damaged the skin, thus destroying the body's natural first-line barrier. Yet these patients endure an even greater risk because of the dramatic immunologic changes which occur. These changes involve such structures as the phagocytic system, the thymus, the lymphocytes, the plasma cells, and the immunoglobulins. The etiology of these changes is unknown; however, it is theorized that burned cells produce a "toxin" which alters the immune system's ability to respond in the normal fashion. The normal responses of cells associated with the immune system such as T helper/suppressor cells and natural killer cells are altered, and the patient with a major burn rapidly becomes immunosuppressed. As a result, the in-

fectious organisms which are now able to invade the body more easily also are less likely to be controlled by an impaired immune system.

Cardiovascular System

The most dramatic cardiovascular event seen after burn injury is burn shock. Until the 1930s and into the early 1940s, shock was the leading cause of death for all burn victims with greater than 35 percent total burn surface area (TBSA). The patient who has suffered a severe burn experiences hemodynamic changes almost immediately following the injury.

A marked increase of capillary permeability occurs, possibly related to histamine release. In small burns (<20 to 25 percent TBSA) this permeability alteration is limited to the area burned; however, with a larger burn, this effect appears throughout the body. Fluid alterations quickly occur as large-diameter molecules such as plasma and albumin readily pass through capillary membrane pores, pulling fluid out of the vasculature. The mechanisms which cause alterations in fluid volume are not completely understood and current research data have not provided conclusive evidence regarding the origin of this problem.

Increased capillary permeability presents a biphasic pattern. The initial peak occurs during the first hour postburn and then drops to within normal limits. Almost immediately a very rapid rise is again noted and is of much longer duration. The second peak occurs 2 to 3 h after the injury and slowly returns to normal over the subsequent 12 to 36 h.[2]

The leakage of fluid from the capillary bed to the interstitium causes the lymphatic system to become overwhelmed, resulting in an excess of interstitial fluid and a deficit of intravascular plasma volume (Fig. 55-2). This disruption in the Starling equilibrium causes edema which is proportional to the size of the burn. Patients with large surface area burns experience edema throughout the body, which impairs peripheral circulation by compressing the circulatory vessels in the extremities. This increase in pressure can damage nerves in the area. If pressure in the extremity is not relieved by performing an escharotomy, the pulses in the extremity weaken or become absent and tissue death occurs (Fig. 55-3). This process may also

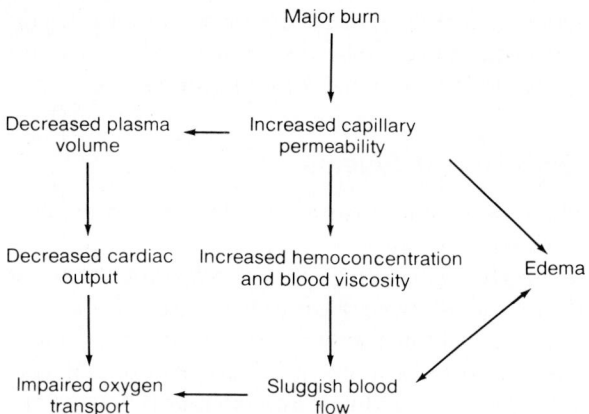

Figure 55-2 Following a major burn capillary permeability increases, allowing plasma particles to leak from vascular to interstitial spaces. This results not only in massive edema and hemoconcentration, but also in a decrease in cardiac output and impaired oxygen transport to vital organs.

occur as a localized response in smaller injuries involving circumferential limb wounds.

At 48 h postburn, the leaking of intravascular fluid to the interstitium subsides and capillary permeability approaches normal. The lymphatics are now able to accommodate the fluid load, thus restoring the function of the Starling equilibrium. Excessive fluid in the interstitium is reduced and the resultant edema is diminished as fluid returns to the vasculature. Most patients have received intravenous enhancement of the intravascular volume, and circulatory overload can easily occur. The elderly, and patients with a history of congestive heart failure are especially at risk.

The fluid volume deficit resulting from plasma loss can lead to irreversible shock, because as much as 50 percent of the blood volume may leave the blood vessels in the form of a plasma leak. Cardiac output falls as a result of two mechanisms: hypovolemia and myocardial depressant factor (MDF).

Hypovolemic shock results from a loss of plasma from the circulating blood volume. Unlike hemorrhagic shock, it develops progressively over a longer period of time. The patient experiences a devastating drop in circulating blood volume if not treated with adequate fluids. This drop in blood volume causes a decrease in both venous return and systemic blood pressure. The body compen-

sates for the drop in cardiac output by shunting blood from the periphery to the vital organs and by increasing the heart rate. Fluid therapy must be prompt and adequate if shock is to be prevented.

In the early stages of shock, myocardial deterioration is not severe despite poor coronary perfusion. However, if shock progresses, the myocardium deteriorates as a result of toxic factors in the circulation, especially MDF, lactic acid, and endotoxin. These factors weaken the myocardial reserve and can grossly exacerbate progressive shock.

Organ and tissue perfusion is impaired as a result of a decreased cardiac output. This results from a combination of factors, which include decreased blood volume, poor myocardial function, and hemoconcentration (caused by the decreased

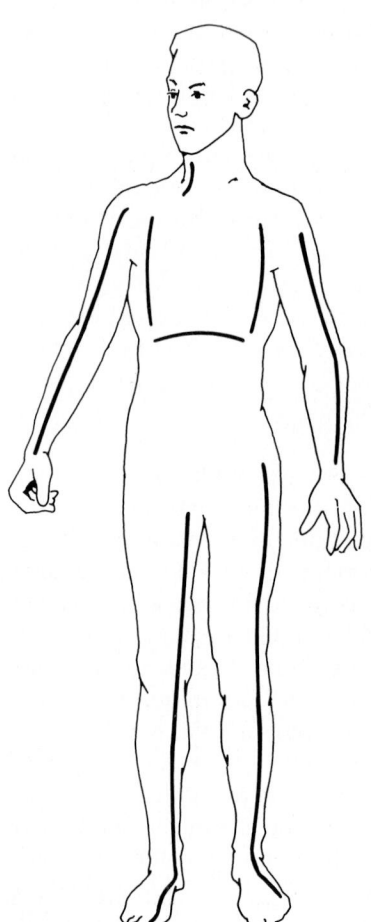

Figure 55-3 Sites for escharotomy incisions.

plasma volume). Eventually, vital organs are not perfused and death occurs if treatment is not efficient and effective. Other complications related to the alterations in plasma volume include changes in colloid osmotic pressure, hypoproteinemia, and electrolyte changes.

Respiratory System

Pulmonary function may be impaired as a result of direct pulmonary injury, or secondary complications, and it may be minor or severe, depending on the circumstances of the burn injury. There are four categories of pulmonary injury: (1) carbon monoxide poisoning, (2) upper airway thermal burns, (3) smoke poisoning, and (4) pulmonary parenchymal failure.

Carbon monoxide poisoning, the first category of inhalation injury, affects the lungs indirectly as a result of carbon monoxide toxicity. Carbon monoxide, a by-product of combustion, binds with the hemoglobin molecule as does oxygen. The affinity of carbon monoxide for hemoglobin, however, is about 230 times as great as that of oxygen. As the resulting carboxyhemoglobin level increases, less oxygen is transported via the hemoglobin molecule, causing cardiopulmonary and central nervous system dysfunction. Figure 55-4 depicts some of the effects seen in the patient exposed to carbon monoxide.

Upper airway thermal burns occur when flame burns involve the upper chest, neck, or face. It is common for patients to suffer burns to the nasal mucosa, oral mucosa, and pharynx. The resulting edema in the local burn area, coupled with systemic changes in capillary permeability, may cause airway insufficiency or obstruction. Burns of the neck may further complicate the problem if the eschar becomes noncompliant and the airway's correct anatomical position cannot be maintained.

Thermal damage from heat does not usually affect the lower respiratory tract because heat is quickly dissipated in upper airway structures. However, superheated steam often overcomes the ca-

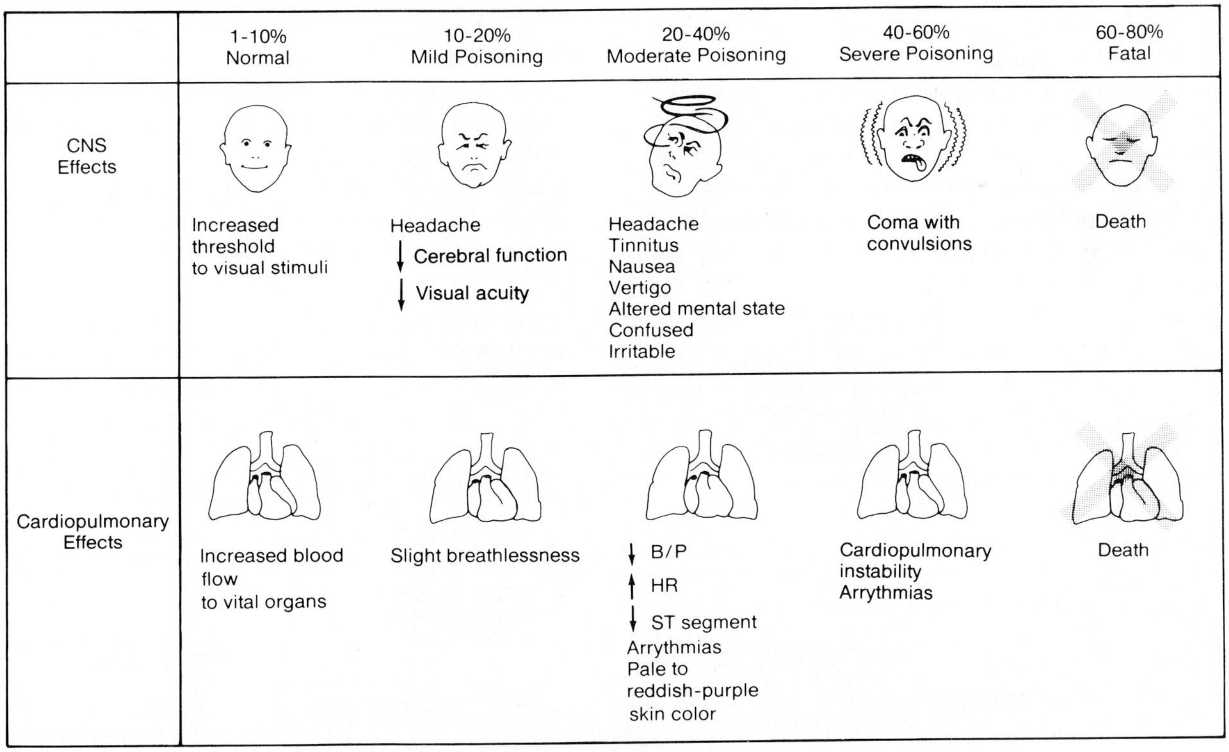

	1-10% Normal	10-20% Mild Poisoning	20-40% Moderate Poisoning	40-60% Severe Poisoning	60-80% Fatal
CNS Effects	Increased threshold to visual stimuli	Headache ↓ Cerebral function ↓ Visual acuity	Headache Tinnitus Nausea Vertigo Altered mental state Confused Irritable	Coma with convulsions	Death
Cardiopulmonary Effects	Increased blood flow to vital organs	Slight breathlessness	↓ B/P ↑ HR ↓ ST segment Arrythmias Pale to reddish-purple skin color	Cardiopulmonary instability Arrythmias	Death

Figure 55-4 Carbon monoxide effects. Progressive deterioration of the CNS and cardiopulmonary systems occurs as arterial levels of carbon monoxide increase.

pacity of the upper airway structures and reaches deeper levels of the lung. Barring complication, upper airway edema resolves in 3 to 5 days once fluids are mobilized from the interstitium to the vasculature.

Smoke poisoning results in epithelial damage in the lower respiratory tract and is most frequently due to the presence of incomplete products of combustion; that is, oxides from sulfur, nitrogen, aldehydes, and hydrochloric acid. The effects of each agent on the lung may vary slightly but overall effects can be generalized.[3]

The most significant effects of epithelial damage are atelectasis and pulmonary edema. A decrease in alveolar surfactant production and the immediate loss of bronchial epithelial cilia contribute to these events. Edema occurs as a result of changes in pulmonary capillary permeability and increased fluid loads. Tracheal and bronchial epithelial sloughing frequently occur within 72 h after the injury, producing hemorrhagic bronchitis. The edema, first limited to small airways, intensifies and a clinical picture may emerge which mimics adult respiratory distress syndrome (ARDS).

Pulmonary parenchymal failure results when gas exchange in the alveoli becomes irreversibly impaired. Because smoke poisoning inhibits the function of pulmonary alveolar macrophages, an inflammatory exudate soon appears in the lung. This, in conjunction with the edema caused by changes in pulmonary capillary permeability, large fluid loads, and immobility, can lead to broncho-pneumonia. Patients experience pulmonary shunting, hypoxemia, alveolar air trapping, high airway resistance, and hypercarbia. The prognosis of patients in this latent stage of respiratory failure is very grim (Fig. 55-5).

Patients may suffer from a number of other pulmonary complications. The systemic capillary leak which occurs in patients with a significant burn (>25 percent), causes generalized body edema. Therefore, even those patients who have not sustained any specific pulmonary damage may experience significant loss of plasma from the pulmonary microcirculation into the lungs which may result in inefficient exchange of gases and/or an upper airway obstruction.

Patients with circumferential third-degree burns to the chest and neck may develop problems with ventilatory excursion secondary to thick, leathery, nonelastic eschar surrounding the chest. It is essential in these patients to relieve the pressure so that pulmonary function can return to normal.

Renal System

Kidney damage may occur at any time during the patient's treatment, and for any number of reasons. In the emergent phase, hypovolemic shock may result in a low-flow state in the renal tubules, leading to acute renal failure if the shock is not rapidly reversed. Renal damage may also occur early in the postburn period as a result of hemoglobinuria. The muscle destruction which may

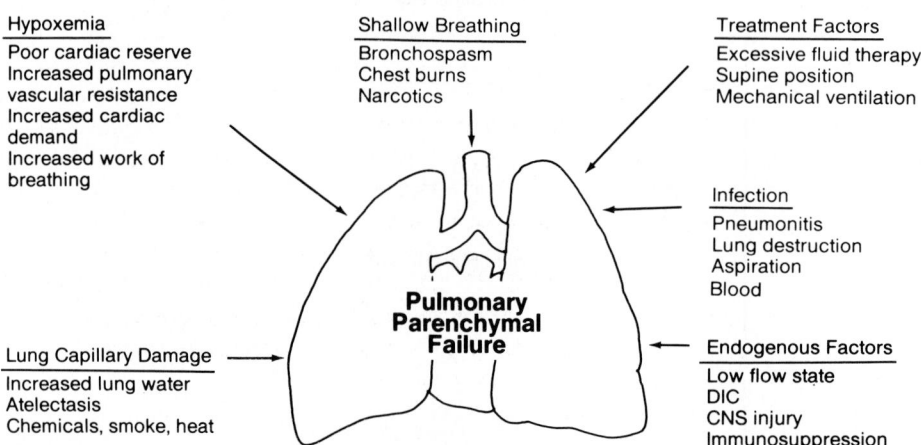

Figure 55-5 Factors contributing to respiratory failure in burn patients with pulmonary involvement.

occur with deep dermal or electrical burns causes the destruction of red blood cells and the release of the pigment, myoglobin. These particles can block renal tubules and contribute to severe renal dysfunction.

Other renal complications such as oliguria, anuria, or renal failure can occur at any time during the treatment phase due to local infection, trauma, sepsis, and drug therapy. It is imperative that the nurse recognize early signs of these conditions to ensure therapeutic intervention.

Gastrointestinal System

Although no direct insult to the gastrointestinal tract occurs in most thermal burns, alterations are seen in the function of the gastrointestinal tract. Metabolic imbalances may occur, causing tremendous changes in the patient's metabolic needs and indirectly affecting the gastrointestinal system.

In the initial postburn period, blood is shunted to the vital organs from the intestines and the spleen, which often results in a cessation of peristaltic function known as paralytic ileus. This condition can have serious consequences for the burn patient. Because oral fluids do not pass further than the stomach, there is danger of aspiration. Over the long term, however, the presence of a paralytic ileus can hamper the body's ability to use calories. Paralytic ileus is most common during the first 24 to 48 h in patients who have sustained burns > 25 percent TBSA. It is characterized by the absence of (1) signs of peristaltic function, (2) bowel sounds, and (3) passage of gas and feces along the digestive tract. Acute gastric dilatation can develop rapidly as a result of the functional disturbances in the gastrointestinal tract, i.e., decreased motility, distention, and decreased blood supply. Vomiting may occur, which can further exacerbate existing hypovolemia and electrolyte imbalances. Corrective action includes close assessment for gastric dilatation and passing a nasogastric tube.

Gastrointestinal ulcerations common in the burn patient are of two types: peptic ulcers and Curling's ulcers. Peptic ulcers are characterized by many small lesions found in the stomach, whereas Curling's ulcers are typically deep ulcerations in the duodenum (Fig. 55-6). The etiology of both types of ulcers is thought to be related to the stress

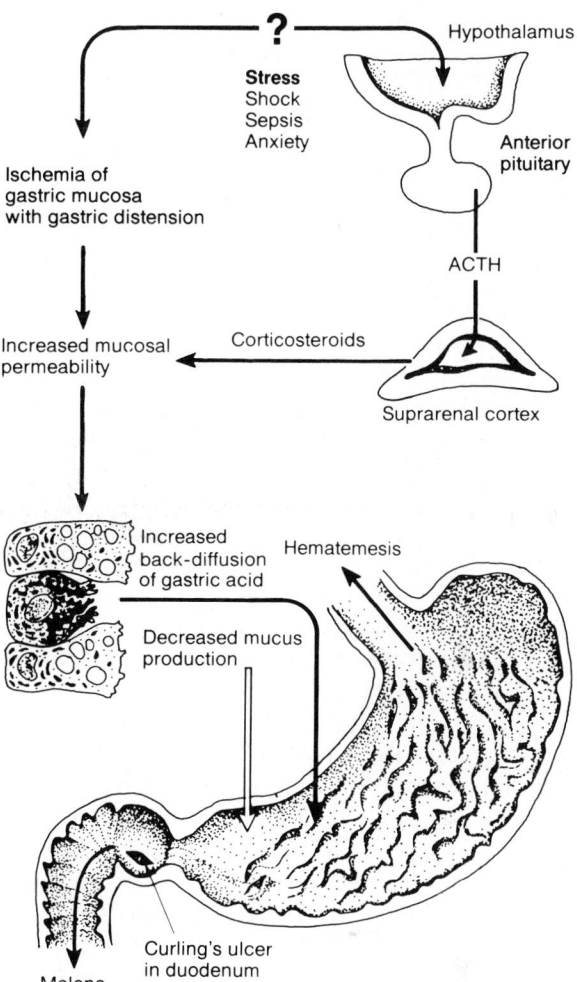

Figure 55-6 Factors predisposing burn patients to the development of Curling's ulcer.

response in burn patients, which causes hypersecretion of acid in the gut, ischemia to the gastric mucosa, and decreased mucous production.

Metabolic System

The burn patient experiences various metabolic alterations which result from complex changes in circulating hormone levels. While these effects occur to some extent in all burn patients, they are far more pronounced in the patient whose burn exceeds 40 percent TBSA.

Several hormones are affected, and the alterations may persist for weeks following injury. The burn may stimulate an increased production of certain hormones (i.e., aldosterone and cortisol) while causing the suppression of others (i.e., thyroid and pituitary hormones). Table 55-1 summarizes the endocrine changes which occur in patients with major burns.

Increases in the burn patient's metabolic rate are greater than that seen in most other disease states. Patients with a 40 percent or greater burn may have a 100 percent increase in their normal metabolic rate at room temperature.

Energy requirements are tremendously increased due to hypermetabolism, energy deficits incurred from evaporative water losses through water-permeable eschar, and postburn catabolism. If energy requirements are not adequately met, the patient with a large burn (> 40 percent) can lose 25 percent of his or her preburn weight within 3 weeks. In addition, inadequate nutrition results in poor wound healing.

Hypermetabolism is affected to a certain extent by the ambient temperature. A response in the burn patient mediated by the hypothalamus causes a temperature reset to occur which increases core body temperature 1 to 2° above normal. As ambient temperatures become cooler, patients strive to maintain their reset body temperature by shivering, causing a further increase in the metabolic rate. Increasing ambient temperature controls exacer-

bations of metabolic rate increases but does not prevent the process.

Other hypermetabolic effects caused by increases in catecholamine output result in aberrations in glucose kinetics. An increased glucose flow develops quickly, and mimics the pattern seen in diabetes. New glucose formation in the liver, called *gluconeogenesis,* also occurs and is fueled from fat metabolism. Protein wasting and increases in oxygen consumption also occur.[4]

Diagnostic Findings

Clinical Manifestations

Severity of Injury

A first consideration in planning care is the determination of the severity of the injury. Five major factors influence severity: (1) medical history, (2) extent of burn, (3) depth of injury, (4) age, and (5) distribution of the burn.

History The history must be obtained immediately upon arrival in the health care facility, because the patient is generally lucid and capable of providing pertinent information. If the interview is postponed, the nurse may find the patient intubated, sedated, or disoriented due to shock. It may be

Table 55-1 Various Indicators of Endocrine Gland Response after Burn: Alterations (Frequency) during First Postburn Weeks

ACTH*	+ +	IRI†	+ + +
Cortisol†	+ + + +	Glucagon*‡	+ +
Aldosterone	+ + +	FSH	− − −
Catecholamines*‡	+ + + +	LH	+
Renin	+ + + +	PRL	+ +
Angiotensin II	+ + +	Testosterone (males)*	− − − −
ADH	+ + +	17β-Estradiol (males)*	+ + +
GH†	+ +	TSH	N
DHEA-S‡	− − −	T₃	− − − −
17-Ketosteroids	+ + +	rT₃*	+ +
17-Ketogenic steroids	+ + + +	T₄	− − −
17-Hydroxycorticosteroids in urine†	+ + + +	PTH*	+ +
		Calcitonin*	+ +

Semiquantitative evaluation from author's experience.
+ = increased; − = decreased; N = normal.
*Hormones closely related to such responses as immunologic and inflammatory. Various data will probably change when more results are obtained.
‡Data obtained from various references.
Courtesy of R. Dolocek, The Endocrine Response after Burns, *Journal of Burn Care and Rehabilitation,* 6(3): 281–294, 1985.

impossible to obtain an adequate history at a later time.

The burn victim may present with concomitant traumatic injuries and/or preexisting diseases or illnesses. These may have in some way contributed to the circumstances causing the burn and may drastically affect morbidity. For example, a patient's diabetes may interfere with wound healing, and chronic congestive heart failure complicates fluid resuscitation. Emotional and physical stress may exacerbate an existing disease process, and lead to increased mortality.

In taking a history from a patient who is burned, the nurse should keep in mind the complications associated with burn injury. Specific emphasis is placed on the history of the accident and should include the time of injury, source of heat, description of how the burn occurred, whether the influence of alcohol or drugs was a factor, the physical surroundings in the immediate area where the burn was sustained, the events occurring from the time of the burn to admission to the health care facility, and any other contributing events or circumstances.

In addition to the standard information obtained during the admission history, special emphasis is placed on the patient's preburn or "dry" weight. This value is of immediate importance because it is used to calculate fluid rates, energy requirements, and drug dosages. An admission weight should be taken as early in the course of treatment as possible.

Extent of Burn   The extent of the burn is expressed as a percentage of the total body surface area. There are two commonly used methods of determining burn extent. The *rule of nines* is "quick and dirty"; it does not require charts or diagrams, and does not take into consideration proportional differences related to age. The body is divided into components of nine. The arms (from shoulder to fingertip) and the head are each given a value of 9 percent. Each leg is valued at 18 percent, the anterior and posterior trunk areas are also valued at 18 percent each, and the perineum is given a 1 percent value, yielding a total of 100 percent.

A more accurate method developed by Berkow, Lund, and Browder, requires the use of tables to calculate the changes in proportion of the head

and lower extremities which occur with growth. For example, the head of an infant represents 19 percent of total body surface area, while in an adult the head accounts for only 7 percent. Use of this method is described in Fig. 55-7.

Depth of Burn   It is difficult to accurately determine the depth of a burn. There are signs and symptoms which indicate the level of tissue damage, but only with demarcation, spontaneous healing, or the appearance of granulation tissue can the exact depth of injury be determined.

Burn depth is best described in terms of *partial thickness* or *full thickness*. These terms are anatomically descriptive and, therefore, are preferable to the popular references of "first- and second-degree" (partial-thickness) and "third-degree" (full-thickness) burns, which arose from visual impressions in a partial-thickness burn. In a partial-thickness burn the tissue damage and destruction do not include the deeper dermal layer, which may regenerate. All skin layers have been destroyed in a full-thickness burn, and there may be injury of subcutaneous tissues, muscle, and bone as well. These wounds require skin grafting to replace destroyed tissues.

Certain classic signs and symptoms may be evident, and are helpful in differentiating depth of injury immediately after a burn injury. Erythematous areas which blanch with fingertip pressure and then refill are shallow partial-thickness burns; the erythema indicates tissue damage where viability remains. Vesicles which immediately increase in size usually represent a deeper partial-thickness injury.

Full-thickness burns are characterized by a leathery surface that may be white, tan, brown, red, gray, or black. Because of destruction of the dermis where pain fibers terminate, there is no pain sensation. However, while deep partial-thickness burns may be anesthetic during the first few days, sensation returns as tissues recover. The patient's failure to react to stimuli such as a pinprick or the pulling out of a hair indicates full-thickness skin loss. Small vesicles caused by steam may be present in areas where intense heat destroyed all layers of the skin; these vesicles will not increase in size. Following a severe scald, there may be full-thickness skin loss, although the surface appears only red

Figure 55-7 Berkow formula for calculating percentage of body surface burned.

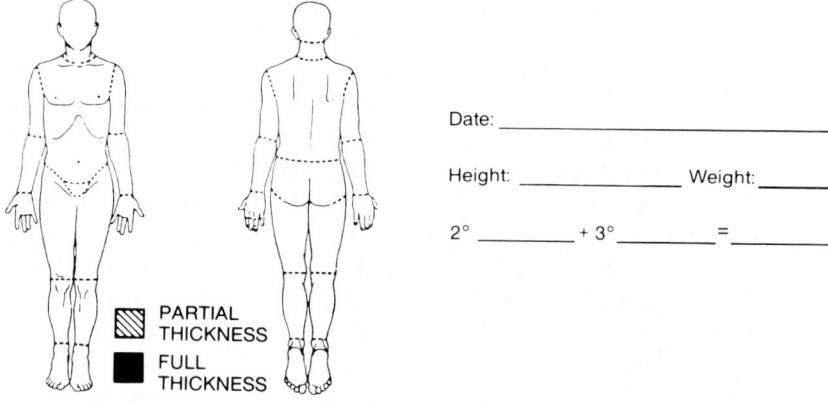

PARTIAL THICKNESS

FULL THICKNESS

Date: _____

Height: _____ Weight: _____

2° _____ + 3° _____ = _____

Percent Surface Area Burned
(Berkow Formula)

Area	0-1 YEAR	1-4 YEARS	5-9 YEARS	10-14 YEARS	15 YEARS	ADULT	2°	3°
Head	19	17	13	11	9	7		
Neck	2	2	2	2	2	2		
Ant. Trunk	13	13	13	13	13	13		
Post Trunk	13	13	13	13	13	13		
R. Buttock	2½	2½	2½	2½	2½	2½		
L. Buttock	2½	2½	2½	2½	2½	2½		
Genitalia	1	1	1	1	1	1		
R.U. Arm	4	4	4	4	4	4		
L.U. Arm	4	4	4	4	4	4		
R.L. Arm	3	3	3	3	3	3		
L.L. Arm	3	3	3	3	3	3		
R. Hand	2½	2½	2½	2½	2½	2½		
L. Hand	2½	2½	2½	2½	2½	2½		
R. Thigh	5½	6½	8	8½	9	9½		
L. Thigh	5½	6½	8	8½	9	9½		
R. Leg	5	5	5½	6	6½	7		
L. Leg	5	5	5½	6	6½	7		
R. Foot	3½	3½	3½	3½	3½	3½		
L. Foot	3½	3½	3½	3½	3½	3½		
TOTAL								

and discolored; however, this area will not blanch with pressure or refill.

In general, a painful erythematous surface with vesicles indicates a partial-thickness burn. When there is no complaint of pain and the surface is anesthetic, a full-thickness burn usually exists (Fig. 55-8).

Age   Age affects severity of injury on the extreme ends of the chronological spectrum. For example, a 40 percent TBSA burn is more likely to be fatal in the very young or in the elderly than in a healthy young adult. This is due to physiologic factors such as the immature immune system in young children or the poor rate of reepithelialization in the elderly.

Distribution of Burn   Burns of the eyes, face, hands, genitals, and all burns involving joints are classified as "severe" by the American Burn Association. These burns require hospitalization for the special care that is needed for treatment of these areas, even if the total percentage of the burn is small.

Findings from Diagnostic Tests

Serum Electrolytes

In the normal cell the ionic balance is maintained by the sodium-potassium pump and results in a high sodium concentration outside the cell. This active process of pumping sodium out of the cells

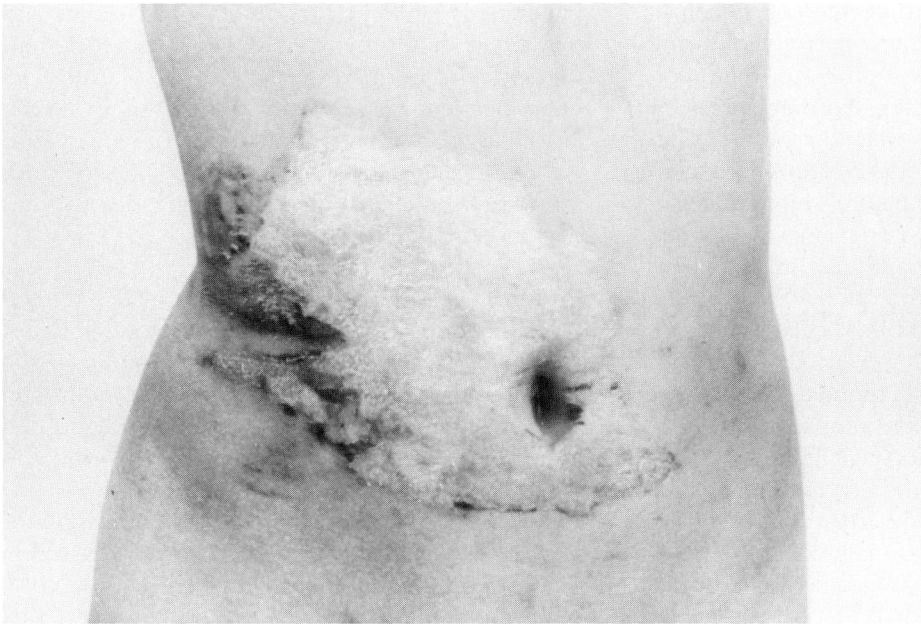

A

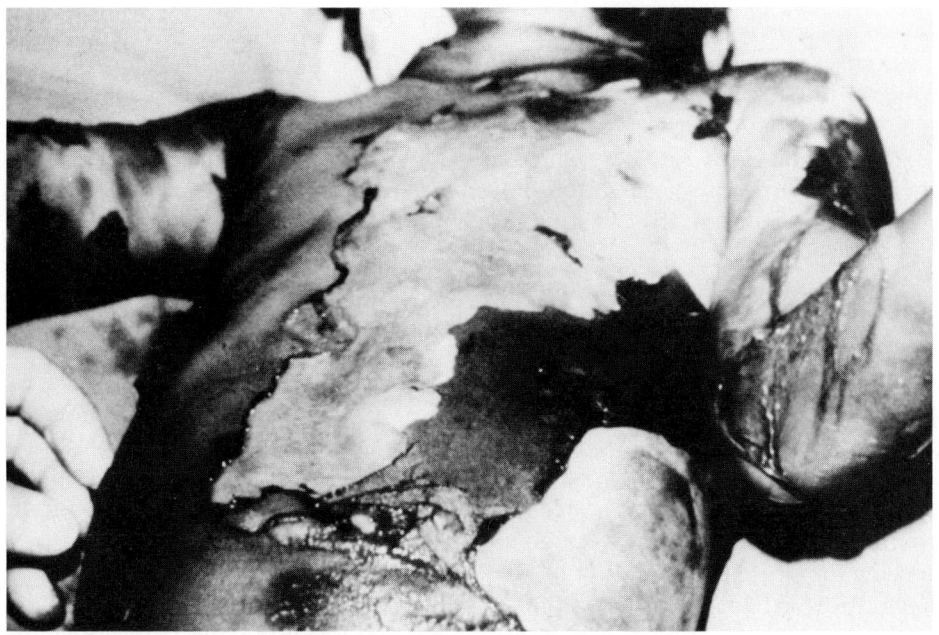

B

Figure 55-8 *A.* Partial-thickness burn to the abdomen. *B.* Full-thickness burn to the chest, flank, and arms.

in exchange for potassium into the cell becomes disrupted in the early postburn period. Following a burn injury, intracellular sodium concentration increases. This increase creates an osmotic pressure gradient which then draws water into the cell. In exchange, potassium leaves the cell and is concentrated in the serum. This unnatural shift of electrolytes contributes to the hyperkalemia frequently seen in the early hours after injury. Serum potassium levels are also increased when body tissues break down and cells such as red blood cells are hemolyzed.

Serum electrolyte values noted in burn patients can often be deceiving because of the dilutional effects seen in hemoconcentrated patients. This condition is present when serum electrolytes such as sodium and chloride are reported by the laboratory to be above the normally accepted limits. The number of sodium and chloride ions has not changed, but what has occurred is that the solute (water) has decreased, causing a disproportionate ratio.

Alterations in the ability of the skin to regulate the movement of electrolytes causes disruption in electrolyte balance as is evidenced by the amount of sodium sequestered in and lost through burn-injured tissues. In burn patients, chlorides are reabsorbed from their urine. This may cause an elevation in serum levels which can contribute to an existing acidosis.

Urinalysis

The kidneys perform a major role in regulating the electrolyte and fluid balance and in the excretion of waste products. Accurate measuring and testing of urine is crucial in assessing the patient's overall condition. Hourly testing of urine helps determine the function of the kidney, the fluid and electrolyte balance of the body, as well as the systemic response to stress and therapy. Monitoring the urine during care provides another parameter by which to assess the patient's condition.

Specific Gravity (SG)   Urine is composed of approximately 95 percent water and 5 percent wastes. Measuring the specific gravity indicates the amount of waste in relation to the water in the urine (the specific gravity of water is 1.000). This

parameter is an indicator of metabolic changes, and may signal either the need for or an excess of fluid therapy. The normal specific gravity of urine fluctuates between 1.002 and 1.035, depending on such factors as the amount of fluid intake or type of food eaten. A fixed specific gravity, e.g., 1.008 to 1.012, in spite of intake, indicates kidney disease and demands treatment.

Protein   The amount of protein normally excreted by the kidneys is negligible; therefore, the test should be negative. If the body is burning tissue protein rather than food, i.e., is in negative nitrogen balance, as it is in the majority of severely burned patients, protein will be present in the urine and the test will be positive. Protein in the urine may be considered normal when the patient is NPO for long periods of time. However, protein excretion is also seen in kidney diseases such as glomerulonephritis, and so should be reported when first noted.

pH   Testing the pH of the urine helps monitor the acid-base balance of the body. Values greater than 7 or less than 6 should be reported.

Glucose   Normally, urine contains no glucose; therefore, this test should be negative. If the test for glucose is positive, it may indicate either that the body is not utilizing ingested glucose, or it may indicate diabetes or pseudodiabetes, which is a symptom of stress sometimes seen in burn victims. It is necessary to report a positive glucose result when it is first noted. Daily insulin may be necessary to compensate for the inability of the pancreas to meet the insulin needs of the burn patient during stress. Glucose intolerance is also one of the clinical signs of sepsis. Glycosuria should prompt a thorough examination of the patient.

Acetone   Acetone is not normally present in the urine. A positive reading may indicate that the body is burning its own fats and proteins because of starvation (NPO) or lack of proper dietary intake, or that the oxidation of fats is incomplete.

Color or Sediment   Normal urine is clear and yellow, or straw-colored. Discoloring may be due to drugs, and cloudiness is not necessarily abnormal, but both should be recorded and reported. Bright red urine usually indicates lower urinary tract bleeding. When certain topical or systemic drugs are used, however, they may be broken down and excreted by the kidneys, causing a discolored urine. Brown or black urine indicates metabolized blood and possibly severe renal damage. When brown urine is seen on admission, massive hemolysis and kidney damage are likely and should be reported immediately because an osmotic diuretic is indicated to flush the tubules. Green to dark green urine may indicate a *Pseudomonas* infection. Report any abnormal color or sediment when first noted and if it continues to be present.

Blood Red blood cells are not normally present in the urine. A positive reading in the burn patient may indicate hemolysis from initial injury or from septic shock.

Urine Output

During the period immediately following the burn injury, urinary output is an effective guide to replacement fluid therapy.[5] Throughout the acute period, urinary output reflects the patient's general systemic response to the injury and therapy. An indwelling catheter is inserted when the burn exceeds 20 percent of the total body surface area, when the perineum is burned, or when there are complications or problems in the medical history. Keep in mind that an indwelling urinary catheter penetrates an anatomical barrier; aseptic technique is essential.

Volume The amount of urine output varies with such factors as intake, condition of the cardiovascular system, and kidney function. An output of 50 to 100 mL per hour indicates adequate renal perfusion in patients in the emergent period. During the acute burn phase, an output of 30 mL per hour is generally considered acceptable. A daily output of 1200 mL is considered average. An output of less than 400 mL in 24 h indicates oliguria and possible renal failure; more than 2000 mL daily (polyuria) may indicate high output failure. Intervention should take place before anuria occurs because this indicates a grave prognosis.

Arterial Blood Gases

The fluid disturbances and electrolyte imbalances which occur in the postburn period result in acid-base alterations. Following a large burn, metabolic acidosis develops. This problem is best corrected by rapid fluid resuscitation and restoration of the normal cardiac output. Metabolic acidosis may also occur if the topical application of mafenide acetate (Sulfamylon) covers a large surface of the burn. Removal of all or a portion of the Sulfamylon usually corrects the problem.

Acid-base derangements also occur secondarily to other complications such as pulmonary insufficiency or acute renal failure. These acid-base changes can further interfere with the balance of electrolytes if not corrected.

Frequent blood gas analysis is mandatory in assessing pulmonary function and acid-base status. Blood gases are analyzed to determine the effectiveness of gas exchange and arterial oxygen tension (Pa_{O_2}) in the lungs and to evaluate the acid-base status of the patient through measurement of the hydrogen ion concentration (pH) and bicarbonate (HCO_3^-) concentration level.

Blood gas analysis is indicated when there is suspicion of respiratory involvement on admission or any change in the patient's condition (e.g., hypotension, unusual cardiac arrhythmias, restlessness, or agitation). For patients receiving artificial ventilation, blood gases are analyzed 20 min following any ventilator setting changes which would alter measurements, i.e., rate, Fi_{O_2}, tidal volume, PEEP, and during the weaning period. In assessing blood gas values it is important to indicate the inspired oxygen concentration or Fi_{O_2}, the mode of ventilation and the patient's temperature. If the patient is on a ventilator at the time blood gases are drawn, record the setting of flow rates, percentage of oxygen, and tidal volume when blood gases are drawn to aid in evaluation. Consider arterial blood gas samples as emergency specimens.

Complete Blood Count

Alterations in hematologic parameters (RBC, WBC, platelets) occur in response to burn injury. A small amount of red cell destruction (<10 percent) occurs as a result of local heat damage to the burned area; hematopoietic function is also affected. The half-life of erythrocytes in burn patients, as compared to those of nonburn patients, is markedly decreased.[6] Patients with large burns experience an increase in the hematocrit initially, due to loss of plasma volume and resultant hemoconcentration. Hematocrit values are utilized to determine hemoconcentration and are repeated every 6 h during the first day and as often as indicated thereafter. The hematocrit rises immediately after a burn injury. Circulation is decreased due to increased viscosity of blood and increased peripheral resistance, leading to thrombi formation. Anemia results as a progressive destruction of RBCs (hemolysis) occurs over the course of the acute phase of hospitalization.

Leukocytosis occurs in the immediate post-burn period, with values falling to 20,000 to 30,000 white blood cells per cubic milliliter. However, persistent leukocytosis is an indicator of possible infection. A transient and reversible leukopenia has been reported as a side effect of silver sulfadiazine,[7] a common topical wound therapy, but it is not necessarily an indication for cessation of the drug.

Thrombocytopenia may be evident during the first 48 to 72 h postburn. The platelet count returns to above normal levels. This temporary drop in the platelet count may result from microvascular thrombosis and some degree of disseminated intravascular coagulation (DIC). As the patient responds to fluid therapy, the hemoconcentration dilutes to normal and then falls below normal as a result of hemolysis and anemia.

Admission Laboratory Tests

Values of the following laboratory tests should be assessed on admission and monitored throughout recovery:

1. Arterial blood gases
2. Carbon monoxide level (if pulmonary involvement is suspected)
3. Serum electrolytes
4. Serum osmolality
5. Serum glucose
6. BUN/creatinine
7. Complete blood count (CBC) with differential and platelets
8. Drug screen or alcohol (ETOH) level (if suspicious)
9. Sickle cell preparation (for black patients)
10. Urinalysis
11. Urine culture/sensitivity
12. Chest x-ray
13. Liver enzymes
14. Total protein, albumin, and globulin
15. Prothrombin time/partial prothrombin time (PT/PTT)
16. Type and cross-match
17. VDRL
18. Electrocardiogram
19. Pregnancy—females ages 12 to 50
20. HIV

The need for baseline values is paramount. The rationale for the above tests, their baseline values, and postburn variations are outlined in Table 55-2.

In addition to routine laboratory tests and examinations, tests are needed for specific organs involved. For example, in patients with suspected eye burns, ophthalmic evaluation must be done. Fluorescein strips can be used to detect corneal damage. If trauma is suspected in organs such as the kidney, brain, or lungs, an intravenous pyelogram, CT scan, or bronchoscopy may need to be performed.

Magnetic resonance imaging (MRI), a relatively new diagnostic tool, has been used to ascertain depth of burn injury with special emphasis on injuries caused by electricity.

Collaborative Therapies for Burns

Emergent and Acute Periods

Chemical Burns

Burns caused by chemical agents are usually progressive in nature. Damage to the skin is attributable to the heat of the chemical reaction and changes caused by the chemical reacting with the protein in the skin. Generally, the result is a deep cutaneous injury; however, the chemical may also damage the eyes, digestive track (if swallowed), and, if inhaled, cause an inhalation injury.

Initial treatment of chemical burns varies with the specific chemicals causing the damage. Early treatment should include copious water lavages

Table 55-2 Baseline Laboratory Values and Postburn Variations

Laboratory Test	Normal Baseline Value	Postburn Variation	Rationale
Hemoglobin	12–16 g/100 mL	Elevated	Fluid volume loss
Hematocrit	40–50%	Elevated	Fluid volume loss
Urea nitrogen	8–20 mg/100mL	Elevated	Fluid volume loss
Glucose	60–120 mg/100 mL	Elevated	Stress response
Serum electrolytes		Elevated	Fluid volume loss and disruption of sodium-potassium pump.
Sodium	136–145 meq/L		
Potassium	3.6–5.0 meq/L	Elevated	Disruption of sodium-potassium pump, tissue destruction, and red blood cell hemolysis
Chlorides	95–106 meq/L	Elevated	Fluid volume loss and reabsorption of chlorides in urine
Arterial Blood Gas Studies			
P_{O_2}	85–100 mmHg	Normal	
P_{CO_2}	35–45 mmHg		
pH	7.35–7.45	Low	Metabolic acidosis
Carboxyhemoglobin	0	Elevated	Inhalation of smoke and carbon monoxide
Total proteins	6.0–7.8/100 mL	Low	Loss of protein exudate through wound
Albumin	3.5–5 g/100mL	Low	Loss of protein through wounds and through vascular membranes due to increased permeability

initially and every 4 to 6 h to neutralize the chemical while simultaneously removing the heat of reaction. In the case of dry chemicals, the chemical substance should be brushed off before beginning wound lavage.

Electrical Burns

An electrical injury causes tissue destruction as the current flows through the body from the point of contact to the point of grounding (see Fig. 55-9). Electrical injuries are often marked by healthy, viable surface tissue because the greatest damage generally occurs close to the bone in the deep muscle compartment. Signs of deep muscle injury include myoglobinuria and compartment syndrome.

Electric current can also cause cardiac changes. It is advisable to monitor the patient's ECG for up to 96 h after injury. Emergency treatment in the case of electrical injury begins with the stabilization of the cardiopulmonary system.

Radiation Burns

Radiation injuries occur as a result of exposure to high doses of radioactive material. Damage occurs at the cellular level where altered function causes cell death and, consequently, organ failure. Survivors of radiation exposure experience varying degrees of damage, from minor erythema to absolute bone marrow suppression. Skin destruction sometimes occurs, and is treated similarly to other burn injuries.

Victims of radiation burns must undergo decontamination. Staff members who are decontaminating patients should be careful to wear appropriate isolation clothing including cap, mask, plastic shoe covers, and waterproof cover gowns. Double gloving is recommended when handling contaminated equipment.

Emergency Care

When administering emergency care to any seriously injured patient, breathing, bleeding, and shock are paramount considerations, usually in the order presented. Aseptic technique is essential to all phases of management. Remove all clothing and dressings for a satisfactory appraisal of the extent of the burn and possible associated injuries.

The burned patient is likely to have respiratory difficulties. The history of the accident is a good indicator of imminent respiratory difficulty. If the patient was "burned in an enclosed space," and forced to breathe smoke and other products of combustion, there is a strong likelihood of imme-

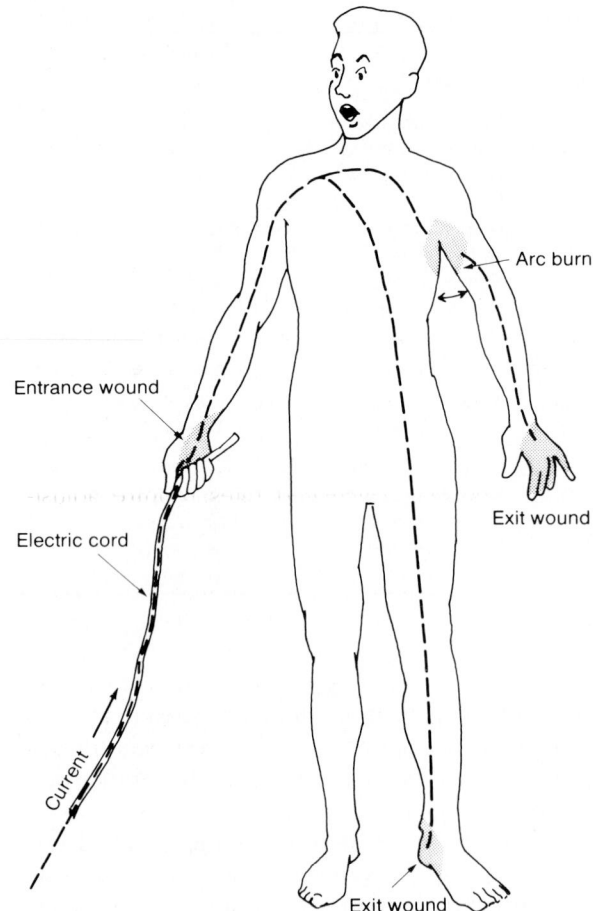

Figure 55-9   Pathway of current in an electrical injury from the point of contact to the point of grounding. *Note:* Current travels along the path of least resistance; nerves being the least resistant tissue followed by blood vessels, skin, muscle, and bone.

diate airway involvement. Blackened oral and nasal mucous membranes, singed nasal hairs, and burn injury including the face and neck indicate the probability of impending airway obstruction. Carbon monoxide poisoning may also be present.

Hemorrhage, internal as well as external, may be due to associated trauma at the time of injury and should be carefully evaluated and treated as indicated. The burn injury itself causes no external bleeding; however, as much as 10 percent of the red blood cell volume may be destroyed by hemolysis from deep thermal injury.

Shock may be neurogenic initially but later is due to extensive and rapid fluid shifts. The goal of fluid therapy for severely burned patients is to avoid hypovolemic shock during the first few days of therapy and to prevent hypervolemic complications.

Analgesics may be required if the patient is in pain and are always given intravenously. Subcutaneous or intramuscular injections pool locally because of hypotension and are suddenly released when normal systemic circulation returns, resulting in high blood levels from accumulated doses.

After attending to immediate emergent matters and preliminary evaluation, the patient and family should receive reassurance and explanation of the problems.

Drugs

Oxygen Therapy

Poor oxygenation can occur due to carbon monoxide poisoning, Adult respiratory distress syndrome, pneumonia, pneumothorax, inhalation injury, or other respiratory insults. Treatment involves giving humidified oxygen via face mask, cannula, or mist. If necessary, intubation is performed and mechanical ventilation is instituted. Oxygen toxicity is associated with tissue fibrosis and central nervous system deterioration. In some cases paralytic agents such as pancuronium bromide (Pavulon) may need to be used when the patient's activity severely compromises respiratory function.

Diuretics

Mannitol is used only when hematuria or hemoglobinuria (black urine), which indicate impending acute tubular necrosis, are evident in a urine specimen obtained by catheterization. Usually this occurs in patients who have sustained electrical burns or deep muscle damage. Mannitol is given intravenously and it is rarely necessary to repeat the dose.

Lasix is rarely used in the emergent phase; however, it is frequently used during the acute phase of treatment for restoring fluid equilibrium. Of course, serum electrolytes must be carefully monitored when using any diuretics.

Antibiotic Therapy

Tetanus toxoid or antitoxin is administered routinely, the choice being dependent upon previous immunizations. Tetanus immune human globulin

(Hyper-Tet) is given as additional passive coverage. Prophylactic antibiotic therapy is controversial; however, often antibiotics are used in this way during the perioperative period. If pneumonia or other infection is suspected, antibiotics are recommended for all patients with positive sputum, urine, or wound cultures. Antibiotics, therefore, are used extensively, especially the aminoglycosides which include amikacin, gentamicin, and tobramycin. These drugs, although helpful in combating severe infections, are associated with a wide range of adverse effects. The most significant of these effects are ototoxicity and nephrotoxicity. Peak and trough serum levels of these drugs are monitored because burn patients require a higher than normal dosage of these drugs to maintain therapeutic serum levels. The nurse must carefully monitor patients treated with aminoglycosides and agents such as Amphotericin B for signs of renal failure and hearing impairment.[8] Dosages of antibiotics also may need to be altered.

Topical Antimicrobials   While waiting for wound closure, especially if using the conservative treatment approach, topical antibiotics are often applied. The primary goal of topical antibiotics, called *topical antimicrobial therapy,* is to keep bacterial proliferation in the burn wound to a minimum. Most topical antimicrobial agents can be used prior to and following eschar separation. Topical antimicrobial therapy can be accomplished by the closed or open technique. A summary of commonly used topical antimicrobial agents is presented in Table 55-3. Further discussion of wound healing is in Chap. 56.

Analgesics   Narcotic and non-narcotic analgesics are given with relative frequency for the duration of hospitalization. These drugs, however, rarely offer more than moderate relief during acutely painful procedures. Many nurses are reluctant to administer analgesics for fear of diminishing respirations and bowel motility. The dilemma relates to the need to maintain the integrity of respiratory function and the delivery of adequate nutrition while reducing pain.

Anesthetic agents such as ketamine (Ketalar), sodium pentobarbital (Nembutal), and nitrous oxide have been effectively used. Extreme caution is necessary in their administration and the presence of an anesthesiologist or nurse anesthetist is required. Diazepam (Valium) is also an effective sedative for the burned patient. Other medications commonly used for burns are given in Table 55-4.

Fluid and Electrolyte Replacement

Each patient should be given the quantity and quality of fluid required to compensate for losses sustained during the first few days. In order to meet fluid therapy objectives it is important to determine which patients require fluid therapy and the type and amount of fluid to be given. Formulas attempt to predict specific volume requirements for each patient; however, calculated rates require adjustment based on clinical indicators such as blood pressure and urine output.

Not all burned patients require fluid therapy. If the burn involves less than 20 percent of the total body surface, intravenous therapy may not be necessary. Generally, fluid therapy is indicated when the total area burned is greater than 20 percent of the body surface area, or there are individual considerations such as dehydration, past medical problems, or concurrent injuries.

Most of the fluid lost from the bloodstream into the tissues is plasma. It is necessary, therefore, to replace this fluid with plasma or a plasmalike substitute. A variety of fluids have been advocated, but a balanced salt solution with plasma or protein added is generally used for fluid replacement. Hartmann's (lactated Ringer's) solution is good because it contains electrolytes in concentrations approximating those in the blood. Serum albumin (25 to 50 g) may be added to each liter to supply the protein to make a plasmalike solution. Plasma may also be used, but it is extremely expensive. The use of hypertonic saline, blood, or other solutions remains controversial. The amount of fluid required for replacement varies, depending on extent and depth of burn, the patient's age, and past medical history. Each patient requires individual consideration. The correct amount of fluid is that which achieves maintenance of normal blood pressure and urinary output without overloading the vascular system.

There are many formulas which can be used for calculating the amount of fluids needed after a

Table 55-3 Topical Burn Therapy

	Description	Actions	Advantages	Disadvantages	Nursing Considerations
Antibiotics					
Nitrofurazone (Furacin)	Antibiotic available as cream, solution, and water-soluble powder.	Wide-spectrum antibacterial.	Is effective against *Staphylococcus aureus* and some antibiotic-resistant organisms. Causes neither pain nor maceration. Available in a wide assortment of forms.	May cause contact dermatitis (rare). Is messy to apply in cream form. May cause renal problems if used in patients with extensive burns.	Observe patient carefully for signs of allergic reaction and for evidence of a superinfection.
Gentamicin sulfate (Garamycin)	Wide-spectrum antibiotic, available as a cream or solution for topical use.	Exerts antibiotic action against many organisms which do not respond to other topical antibiotics.	Effective against many organisms, including *Pseudomonas*. Does not cause pain.	May cause ototoxicity and nephrotoxicity. Organisms may become resistant.	Use with caution in patients with decreased renal function because of possible nephrotoxicity. Order serum creatinine and urine creatinine clearance studies before treatment and weekly during treatment to monitor renal function.
Neomycin sulfate	Wide-spectrum antibiotic in 0.1% to 0.5% aqueous solution.	Bactericide used to decrease organisms before debriding and grafting.	Effectively combats most organisms. Can be applied easily. Is inexpensive.	May cause ototoxicity and nephrotoxicity. Is absorbed systemically.	Remove from wound after 24 h to decrease systemic absorption. Monitor patient's temperature after application of cold solution. Order serum and urine creatinine tests to watch for signs of nephrotoxicity.

Table 55-3 (Continued) Topical Burn Therapy

	Description	Actions	Advantages	Disadvantages	Nursing Considerations
Antibiotics					
Bacitracin with Polymyxin B	Combination bactericidal ointment effective on small burn areas.	Bactericidal for gram-positive and gram-negative organisms.	Is capable of minimal systemic absorption. Is aesthetically suitable for use on the face. Does not cause pain.	May cause itching, burning, or inflammation. Cannot be used for full-thickness burns.	Observe patient closely for signs of sensitivity, i.e., rash. Wash ointment off and reapply it every 8 h.
Enzymatic Debriding Agents					
Sutilains ointment (Travase)	Proteolytic enzymes developed from *Bacillus subtilis* in a petroleum base.	Digests necrotic tissue, aiding escharotomies and debridement.	Aids initial debridement before patient can tolerate surgical debridement. Can be easily applied.	Increases fluid loss. Requires refrigeration. May cause bleeding. Irritates wound and sometimes surrounding skin. Is not bactericidal.	Patient must be stable enough for surgery after a few days so that digested wounds can be covered with membranes or grafted. Use with Silvadene, Sulfamylon, bacitracin, Neomycin, or Garamycin. Don't use with hexachlorophene, iodine, Furacin, or silver nitrate. Observe for infection. Change every 18 h. Use on no more than 15% total burn surface at one time.
Fibrinolysin and desoxyribonuclease, combined (bovine) (Elase)	Two lytic enzymes combined in a petroleum base.	Digests necrotic tissue, aiding escharotomies and debridement.	Doesn't require refrigeration. Has long shelf life.	Causes sensitivity in patients allergic to bovine materials. Causes itching and burning. Requires preparation immediately before application.	Wait for physician to remove any thick, dry eschar before applying Elase. Observe for infection. Change dressings daily. *(Continued)*

Table 55-3 (Continued) Topical Burn Therapy

	Description	Actions	Advantages	Disadvantages	Nursing Considerations
Miscellaneous					
Silver sulfadiazine	A nontoxic salt of silver sulfadiazine in water-based cream.	Binds to bacterial cell membranes and interferes with DNA.	Doesn't cause hypochloremia, hyponatremia, electrolyte imbalance, or kidney disease. Has a wide-spectrum antimicrobial action against both gram-negative and gram-positive organisms. Has a long shelf life. Delays eschar separation less than many other topicals.	Absorbed into eschar less than mafenide acetate (Sulfamylon). May cause rash, pruritus, and burning. Not consistently effective for burns covering more than 60% of patient's body or against some bacteria and yeasts. Depresses granulocyte formation.	Watch for signs of infection such as soupiness. Watch for allergic reaction causing drop in white blood cell counts.
Mafenide acetate	A soft, white, nonstaining water-based cream.	Exerts a bacteriostatic action against many gram-negative and gram-positive organisms.	Effective against *Pseudomonas*. Long shelf life. Excellent for treating electrical burns. Penetrates thick eschar. Very effective against *Pseudomonas*.	May lead to superinfection. May cause metabolic acidosis, hyperpnea, and rash. Causes pain when applied. (Pain usually lasts 30–40 min.) Slows eschar separation.	Premedicate patient for pain before application. Monitor blood gases and serum electrolytes if patient develops hyperpnea in response to metabolic acidosis. Do not use in cases of sulfa drug allergy or respiratory or kidney disease.
Sodium hypochlorite solution	An aqueous sodium hypochlorite solution.	Bactericidal.	Helps dry wounds that have become soupy. Aids debridement.	Dissolves blood clots and may inhibit clotting. May irritate skin. May cause electrolyte imbalances.	Change dressings every 4 to 12 h. Observe site carefully for signs of irritation. Keep dressings moist.

Table 55-3 (Continued) Topical Burn Therapy

	Description	Actions	Advantages	Disadvantages	Nursing Considerations
Miscellaneous					
Povidone-iodine (Betadine)	Iodine complex. Available as a solution, ointment, and foam.	Microbicidal against gram-positive and gram-negative organisms.	Is effective against many infections not well controlled by Silvadene. Is available in a wide assortment of forms.	May cause metabolic acidosis and elevated serum iodine levels. May form crusts if burns are not cleaned properly. Causes rash and burning with some patients. Stains clothing and linen. Deactivated by wound proteins.	Check serum electrolytes and serum iodine levels frequently.
Silver nitrate	10% silver salt solution, diluted to 0.5% for application.	Antimicrobial.	Is inexpensive. Applies easily.	Penetrates wound only 1–2 mm so it acts only on surface organisms. Stains and stings. May cause hyponatremia, hypochloremia, and hypocalcemia. Must be applied as constant soaks.	Keep dressings wet with solution. Check serum electrolytes daily.
Bismuth tribromphenate (Xeroform)	A yellow substance gauze.	Debrides and protects donor sites and grafts.	Conforms to wound. Nontoxic and nonsensitizing. Has a long shelf life.	Sticks to wound so that removal is painful. Neither antiseptic nor antibacterial.	Apply carefully so that sheets don't overlap. Observe for signs of infection.
Scarlet red	A red dye in an oil base on gauze.	Promotes healing of wound, but has antiseptic effect.	Protects donor site. Long shelf life. Promotes reepithelialization.	Stains clothing and temporarily stains skin. Irritates skin. Causes pain when patient moves.	Apply to donor sites at time of harvest. Leave until site heals and scarlet red gauze sloughs. Observe for infection beneath gauze. If needed, use heat lamp for a few minutes every hour to dry site. *(Continued)*

1435

Table 55-3 (Continued) Topical Burn Therapy

	Description	Actions	Advantages	Disadvantages	Nursing Considerations
Miscellaneous					
"Thirds" solution	Solution of 1/3% hydrogen peroxide, 1/3 0.25% acetic acid, and 1/3 normal saline.	Inhibits bacterial growth by oxidizing pH. Effervesence cleans wound.	Provides good cleansing action. Causes no known side effects. Is inexpensive.	Decomposes quickly and is short-acting. Exerts limited antimicrobial action.	Add new solution to the dressing or change dressing every 4–6 h.
Merbromin (Mercurochrome)	Organic mercurial compound available as a solution or tincture.	Acts as a desiccating agent which promotes epithelialization.	Is not expensive. Aids epithelialization of small areas. Dries wound.	Causes stains. Is not antibacterial or antiseptic.	Cover wound with nonadherent dressing to prevent sticking.

Adapted from S. F. Gaston, and L. L. Schumann, Burn Wound Management, *Critical Care Update*, October 1980, pp. 5–17.

severe burn, as seen in Table 55-5. Electrolyte solutions vary in resuscitation based on the particular formula employed. The most popular resuscitation formula, the Parkland formula, uses Ringer's lactate and indicates that one-half of the calculated fluid (4 mL × % burn × weight in kilograms) is given in the first 8 h following the burn. The other half is then administered over the next 16-h period for a total of 24 h. Colloids such as albumin may be given in the third or fourth 8-h period postburn if indicated in the clinical assessment. The Parkland formula also recommends the practice of "catching

Table 55-4 Commonly Used Medications

Pain control
  Morphine IV PRN for pain on admission; dose by body weight; alternate weekly with equivalent dose of Demerol.
Prevent Curling's ulcer
  Maalox 60 mL via NG tube 12 h, alternate with Amphogel.
Heart action
  Digoxin (Lanoxin) when necessary.
Vitamin and mineral supplements
  Multivitamins, 1 ampule IV, PB or 1 tablet PO daily
  Vitamin B$_{12}$ weekly
  Vitamin C daily
  Folic acid, 1 mg IV daily (adult)
Sedation and sleep
  Pentobarbital sodium (Nembutal) IM, HS, PRN
  Chlordiazepoxide (Librium), diazepam (Valium), or meprobamate (Miltown) for sedation PRN

up" on fluids. If, for example, a client were burned at 8:00 A.M. but admitted to the hospital at 10:00 A.M., his or her first 8-h period would end at 4:00 P.M., or 8 h following the time of injury. Thus, if resuscitation were delayed until admission, calculated fluids would need to be administered over a 6-h rather than an 8-h period. In the second 24-h period, 5% dextrose in water replaces lactated Ringer's as the crystalloid solution of choice.[9]

Frequent, accurate adjustments of hourly flow rates may be necessary to maintain perfusion in the optimal range. Signs of adequate resuscitation include clear mentation, adequate blood pressure, central venous pressure, pulse, and urine output. These parameters are indicators of tissue perfusion to the brain, heart, and kidneys, respectively. During resuscitation, the waning of any one of these parameters usually suggests a decrease in tissue perfusion in that organ. Indirectly, this signals a deficit in fluid volume and a diminished cardiac output. One of the best indicators of adequate cardiac output in the absence of renal disease is urine output.

The hourly urine output indicates if the fluid volume replacement is adequate to perfuse all organ systems and thereby combat hypovolemia and prevent shock. During the emergent period, intravenous fluids may need to be titrated to maintain urinary output at 30 to 60 mL per hour for the aged, and in patients with respiratory or renal problems or congestive heart failure.

Table 55-5 Formula for Calculation of Fluid Requirements

	Electrolyte	Colloid	Glucose in Water
First 24 h			
Evans	Normal saline 1.0 mL/kg/% burn	1.0 mL/kg/% burn	2,000 mL
Brooke	Lactated Ringer's solution 1.5 mL/kg/% burn	0.5 mL/kg/% burn	2,000 mL
Modified Brooke	Lactated Ringer's solution 2 mL/kg/% burn		
Parkland (Baxter)	Lactated Ringer's solution 4 mL/kg/% burn		
Hypertonic sodium solution (2 amps NaHCO$_3$ in 1 L Ringer's lactate)	Volume to maintain urine output at 30 mL/h (fluid contains 250 meq Na/L) Approximately 2 mL/kg/% burn		
Second 24 h			
Evans	½ of 1st 24-h requirement	½ of 1st 24-h requirement	2,000 mL
Brooke	½ to ¾ of 1st 24-h requirement	½ to ¾ of 1st 24-h requirement	
Modified Brooke		0.3–0.5 mL/kg/% burn	To maintain adequate urinary output
Parkland (Baxter)		20–60% of calculated plasma volume	2,000 mL
Hypertonic sodium solution	⅓ isotonic salt solution orally up to 3,500 mL limit		

Courtesy of J. E. Nicosia and J. A. Petro, *Manual of Burn Care,* Raven Press, New York, 1983.

Maintaining urine output greater than these recommended amounts risks fluid overload, increased interstitial edema, congestive heart failure, wet-lung syndrome, and renal failure. Too much urine output is as life-threatening as too little.

Other parameters which indicate the status of the cardiovascular system are blood pressure, pulse, central venous pressure (CVP), and pulmonary artery pressure (PAP). These measurements are recorded hourly.

Recording the preburn weight and accurate daily nude weights also serves as a useful indicator of cardiovascular status. Each liter of fluid retained results in a 2.2-lb weight gain. The total weight gained in the first few days of fluid therapy should not exceed 10 to 15 percent of the patient's total body weight.

Once the patient has been successfully resuscitated and capillary permeability returns to normal, fluids return to the intravascular spaces and a profuse diuresis occurs which signals the end of the emergent period. At this time, the rate of fluid administration is reduced and fluids are changed to glucose in water to compensate for the fluid, sodium, and other electrolytes which are returning to the vascular space.

During the acute period of care, the adult patient with a large ungrafted wound requires an open IV line with an average infusion rate of 1000 to 1500 mL per 24 h. The types and amounts of fluids which patients require depend on their metabolic balance. It is the responsibility of the nurse to monitor the electrolytes and request appropriate adjustment of fluid administration.

Blood and blood products are administered as needed. Whole blood, which is approximately 45 percent cellular and 55 percent plasma, is required to replace losses from bleeding during wound debridement, from hemolysis due to the burn injury or sepsis, or as a result of coagulopathies and hemorrhage. Burned patients should always receive fresh blood that is not more than 3 days old because (1) the clotting factors are more effective in fresh blood, (2) older blood may contain a higher potassium concentration due to hemolysis, and (3) the oxygen-carrying efficiency is decreased in older blood.

Packed cells obtained through centrifuging whole blood to draw off plasma (plasmapheresis) are given to replace red blood cell loss in anemia, to replace red blood cells lost through marrow depression, or when there is a danger of circulatory overload from whole-blood therapy; for example, in the patient with congestive heart failure.

Imbalances of electrolytes must be modified. Sodium is lost from the serum and deposited in the burn wound. Additionally, the defect in the efficiency of the sodium-potassium pump (as described previously) causes sodium concentrations within the cells to rise. Both of these factors can result in a markedly decreased serum sodium. Initially, hyponatremia is usually resolved by the administration of sodium in IV fluids. The clinician must be aware that a dilutional hyponatremia may be seen in cases of overaggressive resuscitation with hypotonic solutions.

Serum potassium rises due to defects in the sodium-potassium pump and the release of potassium from injured tissues and red blood cells. Hyperkalemia is rarely treated in the initial resuscitation phase unless acute tubular necrosis is present, because it often converts to hypokalemia in a few days. In the acute period, sodium and potassium replacement is the rule rather than the exception. Careful monitoring of these electrolytes is essential. In addition to sodium and potassium, calcium, chlorides, and phosphate may need to be supplemented.

Intake and Output

Strict documentation of 24-h intake and output is necessary for all patients. Daily fluid requirements are calculated and based on body surface area burned and insensible water loss. In general, hourly fluid intake rates are adhered to strictly so that fluid balance can be carefully controlled. All fluids given through the GI tract and IV route must be included in intake and output calculations.

Output must also be monitored on an hourly basis. Urine, stool, vomitus, nasogastric drainage, chest tube drainage, and blood losses must be counted as output.

Astute comparisons of intake to output are made on an hourly and daily basis. In addition to the differences in daily intake and output values, a change in daily weight as well as clinical observations of fluid overload or dehydration must be considered. Clinical monitors include breath sounds, skin turgor, hemodynamic values, and vital signs. Diuretic therapy may also be indicated to clarify the sometimes hazy picture of fluid status.

Prevention of Infection

Principles of Infection Control

The interactions of patients, medical and nursing staffs, equipment and supplies, air conditioning, and housekeeping methods contribute to both the spread and the control of infection. Traditionally, nurses have been responsible for monitoring and controlling infection. Today, however, this responsibility is multifaceted and must be shared by many. Infection control is one of the primary goals of burn care.

Infection is one of the most devastating complications a burned patient faces. Fifty percent of all burned patients who die, do so because of infection. Infection has numerous consequences such as pain and nutritional imbalance. Bacterial invasion may cause partial-thickness wounds to become full-thickness wounds or may result in graft rejection, both of which necessitate additional grafting procedures. Infection can also result in delayed healing, scars, contracture, and prolonged hospitalization. Septicemia and death are even more costly consequences. Complications of infection result not only in a drain on the patient's metabolic and emotional resources but also in a greater cost to the patient and family in terms of time, financial strain, and chronic problems after discharge from the hospital. For the health team, these complications necessitate long hours of detailed care and follow-up. The tangible effects can be measured in time and money spent on medications, treatments, and procedures. The intangible consequences, such as pain, worry, and apathy which add to the emotional stress of the patient and all those concerned with the patient's care, are of even greater relevance in the assessment of the need for an infection control program.

As important as elimination of infection may be, both to the recovery of the patient and to the preservation of energy among the health team, a sterile environment can never be achieved. The struggle is more precisely defined as a campaign to control infection that demands constant caution and refinement of technique in all aspects of burn care.

The principles of controlling infection are (1) the elimination of reservoirs of infection, (2) suppression of infection transfer channels, (3) support of the patient's natural immunity, and (4) judicious use of antimicrobials.

Elimination of Infection Reservoirs

Elimination of reservoirs of infection begins with the patient, who is autocontaminated by the bacteria in the gastrointestinal (GI) and upper respiratory tract, on the unburned skin, and in the hairy areas of the body. In addition, the burn wound provides an ideal medium for bacterial growth; it offers bacteria food, warmth, and moisture. In addition, the patient's general environment represents a giant reservoir of potential infection. Other patients, dressings, wounds, linen, trash, equipment, sinks, and utensils are all possible reservoirs, as are personnel and visitors. Excellent wound care, basic hygiene, housekeeping, and personnel cleanliness are indispensable in eliminating reservoirs of infection.

Suppression of Infection Transfer Channels

Cross-contamination—the transfer of pathogens from an infection source or reservoir to the patient—is probably the greatest threat to the infection control program. Cubicle isolation and aseptic technique are time-tested methods of preventing contamination. Hand washing remains the single most effective method of preventing the spread of infection.

Support of Natural Immunity

Support of the patient's immune mechanisms involves reinforcement of the patient's natural and acquired immunity. This may be accomplished by basic nursing care measures concerning diet, rest, hygiene, positioning, and emotional support, and by vaccines, serums, and globulins that may be specific or nonspecific for particular organisms.

Judicious Use of Antimicrobials

Judicious use of topical and systemic antimicrobials (antibiotics and chemotherapeutics) is one of the most important factors in assisting the body's resistance to invasive infection. These agents are effective when properly used because they are harmful in one way or another to microbes but less harmful to viable tissues. Disinfectants, which may be bacteriostatic or bactericidal, are also toxic to the body. Use of antimicrobials requires consideration of the interaction which will occur between the host, the microbes, and the antibiotic.

Methods of Infection Control

Before discussing the various procedures for controlling infection, it is worthwhile to consider the environment in which these procedures are to be accomplished. No effective infection control program can take place in a chaotic or poorly planned environment, nor can apathetic or uneducated personnel be expected to be responsible for the effectiveness of infection control. Maintaining this environment once it has been established requires constant vigilance and is the responsibility of all involved in care.

Personnel

The patient's life depends on the actions of all those involved in care; therefore, all personnel coming into contact with the patient or the patient care area are responsible for maintaining and monitoring the principles and practices of infection control. It is the responsibility of physicians, nurses, and ancillary services to enforce the infection control program.

An initial training program in infection control is essential for all personnel from janitors to physicians, as well as for visitors. Staff members must be trained in the principles of infection control before they can be expected to follow these principles. A continuous reinforcement program is also essential.

The nursing staff shoulders the greatest burden of infection control because they provide continuous care. Through education, practice, and example, infection control should become a habitual part of the thinking process for all involved.

Infection control is one aspect of burn care philosophy which demands that each person develop a surgical conscience, that is, a strong sense of what is correct and necessary to maximize each patient's chance of survival. Aseptic technique should be reviewed by those new to or unfamiliar with burn care.

Wound Infection and Clinical Sepsis

The battle against invasive infection begins when the severely burned patient is admitted. The burning agent has produced an avascular area composed of nonviable material called *eschar*. The permeability of blood vessels in this area has been altered, and edema forms. Potential pathogens are in the patient's normal flora and in the hospital environment. There is a great likelihood that these pathogens will be transferred from their reservoirs to the burn wound, which provides an ideal climate for bacterial growth, the outcomes of which may be wound infection, septicemia, pneumonia, and eventually, death. In addition, research has shown that burn patients have a decreased effectiveness of white blood cells.[10] Protein is used for wound healing, and if proper basic supportive care is not provided, the patient is further debilitated!

The burn wound can never be completely sterile; some degree of infection is expected. However, once bacterial growth in the wound exceeds 100,000 organisms per gram of wound tissue, the patient is said to have a wound infection. An infected wound does not look clean—purulence, debris, and odor are present.

The methods of isolation used in burn care are varied and controversial. In some cases virtually no isolation is practiced and in others total sterile conditions preside. In most cases, the recommendations of the Centers for Disease Control (CDC) in Atlanta, Georgia, are followed.[11] As such, isolation for the patient with burns centers around hand washing as the most effective weapon against transmission of infection. In addition, patients are isolated according to the specific disease or microorganism involved. The suggested precautions for common burn unit pathogens are outlined in Table 55-6.

As previously discussed, burn patients are immunologically suppressed. Due to this condition a patient can often develop infections which warrant isolation techniques different from those used for burn injury alone. The use of antibiotics both topically and systemically can often lead to the development of bacteria and viruses which are pan-resistant. Other highly contagious pathogens such

Table 55-6 Isolation Precautions

Disease	Precautions Indicated				Infective Material	Apply Precautions How Long?	Comments
	Private Room?	Masks?	Gowns?	Gloves?			
Skin, wound, or burn infection							
Major	Yes	No	Yes if soiling is likely	Yes for touching infective material	Pus	Duration of illness	Major = draining and not covered by dressing or dressing does not adequately contain the pus.
Minor or limited	No	No	Yes if soiling is likely	Yes for touching infective material	Pus	Duration of illness	Minor or limited = dressing covers and adequately contains the pus, or infected area is very small.

Table 55-6 (Continued) Isolation Precautions

Disease	Precautions Indicated				Infective Material	Apply Precautions How Long?	Comments
	Private Room?	Masks?	Gowns?	Gloves?			
Staphylococcal disease (*S. aureus*) Major	Yes	No	Yes if soiling is likely	Yes for touching infective material	Pus	Duration of illness	Major = draining and not covered by dressing or dressing does not adequately contain the pus.
Minor or limited	No	No	Yes if soiling is likely	Yes for touching infective material	Pus	Duration of illness	Minor or limited = dressing covers and adequately contains the pus, or infected area is very small.
Streptococcal disease (group A *Streptococcus*)	Yes	No	Yes if soiling is likely	Yes for touching infective material	Pus	For 24 h after start of effective therapy	Major = draining and not covered by dressing or dressing does not adequately contain the pus.
Multiply-resistant organisms,* infection or colonization.†	Yes	No	Yes if soiling is likely	Yes for touching infective material	Pus and possibly feces	Until off antimicrobials and culture-negative	In outbreaks, cohorting of infected and colonized patients may be indicated if private rooms are not available.

*The following multiply-resistant organisms are included:
1) Gram-negative bacilli resistant to all aminoglycosides that are tested. (In general, such organisms should be resistant to gentamicin, tobramycin, and amikacin for these special precautions to be indicated.)
2) *Staphylococcus aureus* resistant to methicillin (or nafcillin or oxacillin if they are used instead of methicillin for testing).
3) *Pneumococcus* resistant to penicillin.
4) *Haemophilus influenzae* resistant to ampicillin (beta-lactamase positive) and chloramphenicol.
5) Other resistant bacteria may be included if they are judged by the infection control team to be of special clinical and epidemiologic significance.
†Colonization may involve more than one site.
Courtesy *CDC Guidelines for Isolation Precautions in Hospitals*, Atlanta, Ga., 1983.

as herpes and varicella viruses are common in burn patients. Any time the above conditions are reported in the burn patient, the most stringent techniques recommended by the CDC should be used. For instance, if a patient develops an infection caused by a pan-resistant organism, total isolation to the extent of separate staffs and geographic locations may be warranted. Cases such as these should be referred to the hospital's infection control committee. Hand washing cannot be stressed too much and, in fact, if hand washing were performed consistently and perfectly, there would be virtually no cross-contamination in burn patients.

In addition to isolation precautions, use of sterile gloves is recommended for all contact with open wounds. Gloves also should be changed between handling of wounds on different areas of the body.

Patients in a burn unit should not share equipment. Disposables such as pillows, syringes, and dishes are used as much as possible. Equipment used in daily routine care, such as thermometers, blood pressure cuffs, and stethoscopes, should be assigned to each patient.

Thorough cleaning and housekeeping are essential to environmental infection control. All equipment must be cleaned after use with one patient and before use with another. Because *Pseudomonas* has been shown to sequester in plants, these are prohibited. Rugs and upholstered articles are difficult to clean and may harbor organisms and, therefore, should be prohibited in the burn unit.

Careful monitoring of the burn wound is done on a daily basis. Wounds are examined by the nurse for signs of infection, which include a pervasive odor, color changes in the wound, change in wound texture, pus, exudate, and redness at wound edges. Laboratory cultures and biopsies are recommended. Quantitative biopsies of the eschar and granulation tissue should be done three times a week to monitor proliferation of organisms. Clinical signs of burn wound sepsis may be present. Nurses must take an active role in evaluating each of these parameters, assimilating the information and relaying their assessment to the health team.

Treatment of a Wound Infection

Care of an Infected Wound

Treatment of an established wound infection can be summarized as follows: (1) Culture the involved areas to identify the organisms. (2) Reduce the number of organisms by cleansing the infected wound areas aggressively; debride the eschar, open subeschar pockets of infection, and change dressings more frequently. (3) Apply an appropriate topical agent as indicated by culture and sensitivity

studies. (4) Provide basic nursing care (adequate diet, rest, hygiene, positioning) and encourage the patient to turn, cough, and deep breathe regularly to prevent pneumonia. Further discussion of wound care can be found in Chap. 56.

Drug Therapy

Antibiotics are used extensively, especially the aminoglycoside class, which includes amikacin, gentamicin, and tobramycin. These drugs, although helpful in combating severe infections, are associated with a wide range of adverse effects. Ototoxicity and nephrotoxicity are the most significant of these effects. Peak and trough serum levels of drugs must be monitored. Burn patients require a higher than normal dosage of these drugs to maintain therapeutic serum levels. The nurse must be careful to monitor patients treated with aminoglycosides and other agents such as amphotericin B for signs of renal failure and hearing impairment. Dosages of antibiotics may need to be altered.

Clostridium tetani grows on necrotic tissue and is a strict anaerobe. In the burn patient, wound conditions favor the growth of this organism. Tetanus toxoid is given to produce immunity or resistance to *Clostridium tetani*. The administration of Hyper-Tet is recommended when the history of immunizations is questionable. Tetanus toxoid, 0.5 mL, is given on admission or shortly thereafter and is usually the only drug which is given via the intramuscular route during the emergent period.

Surgical Management

In addition to pharmacologic treatment, surgical intervention may be indicated. Infected burn wounds whose colony counts are at or approaching 10^5 per gram of tissue are life-threatening. Even with antibiotic therapy, loss of control of infection can occur, followed by sepsis and death. Surgical intervention, although a risk, may be the only treatment option available. Aggressive surgical debridement or excision of the burn wound may be necessary. If the condition is not sufficiently serious to warrant surgery, frequent dressing changes accompanied by the use of a strong topical antimicrobial agent may be adequate. Proper burn wound care by experienced nurses helps to reduce and prevent infection, prevent destruction of healthy skin, and restore damaged tissue.

Wound Sepsis

If a wound infection is not controlled, bacteria will begin to seep into the bloodstream via the lymphatic system. This condition is first termed *transient* and then *persistent* (or *breakthrough*) *bacteremia*. The patient will begin to show signs of an impending sepsis. If the infection is not stopped at this level, the patient will soon develop septicemia, which has a poor prognosis.

Once large numbers of microbes are in circulation, the patient is at the last line of defense, the systemic filters. If the pathogens are particularly virulent, the body's defenses are soon taxed, and the patient will succumb to septicemia. Detecting subtle signs and symptoms of impending burn wound sepsis allows early initiation of therapies which may prevent or better control a life-threatening septicemia or fungemia (Table 55-7).

Clinical signs of impending systemic sepsis are a temperature greater than 101°F or less than 98.6°F, an increase in pulse or respiratory rate, an insidious decrease in blood pressure or urinary output, glucose intolerance, thrombocytopenia, and a white blood cell count that either plummets or rises with a shift to the left.[12] General signs of sepsis include mild confusion, headache, chills, general malaise, cyanosis, and swollen regional lymph nodes.

Late symptoms of sepsis (septic shock) which are seen as septicemia becomes overwhelming include a drop in temperature to below 98°F, a decrease in WBC count to less than 10,000/mL, an ileus from septic shock, an enlarged liver and spleen, metastatic lesions, necrotic granulation tissue, and pneumonia. If irreversible shock occurs, the patient will die. The nurse should be alert! When it seems that "something just doesn't seem right about the patient," all parameters should be reviewed to rule out or treat bacteremia before it becomes septicemia.

Treatment of Sepsis

The same principles of treatment apply to sepsis, septicemia, and fungemia. Eliminate the suspected cause; change and culture IV and urinary catheters; and cleanse the wound of all exudates and products of infection. Initiate appropriate antimicrobial therapy and culture the wound, urine, and blood daily. Support pulmonary function by establishing a turning, coughing, and deep breathing schedule by maintaining adequate suction and postural drainage. Maintain proper fluid and electrolyte balance and monitor vital signs and CVP closely. Reduce an elevated body temperature with antipyretics, cooling dressings, or fanning. Use of a cooling mattress is a last resort. Monitor the hematocrit frequently and the WBC daily; maintain the hematocrit at or above 35 for adults and 30 for children. Maintain adequate nutrition and rest.

Fungemia

Monilial septicemia, a severe infectious complication usually caused by *Candida albicans,* mimics the clinical response to gram-negative sepsis, except that the course is much more insidious. The temperature and WBC count respond slowly to the invasive organisms, continuing to rise despite broad-spectrum antibiotic coverage. Debilitation and long-term broad-spectrum antibiotic therapy set the stage for fungemia.

The diagnosis of systemic moniliasis should be suspected in the debilitated patient who is on antibiotics but not responding to treatment. If this patient also has *C. albicans* organisms in the urine, treatment should be started (see treatment for septicemia).

Table 55-7 Diagnosis of Burn Wound Sepsis

Intense periburn erythema
Rapid sudden separation of eschar
Breakdown in areas of healing burns or skin graft
Conversion of partial to full-thickness injury
Pus beneath eschar
Black or red hemorrhagic areas in eschar and in unburned adjacent skin
Histologic evidence of bacteria or fungi in deep tissues, especially the perivascular lymphatics seen either on frozen or permanent section histology
Quantitative bacterial counts of 10^5 per gram of tissue

From J. T. Nicosia and J. A. Petro, *Manual of Burn Care,* Raven Press, New York, 1983, p. 32.

Prevention of Pulmonary Complications

More than 90 percent of severely burned patients require some form of respiratory therapy. Therefore, burn care includes an awareness of the principles and procedures required for effective ventilation and a working knowledge of pulmonary function, of ventilators, and of other equipment. It is important to remember that new developments in the field of pulmonary therapy do not replace basic nursing care.

Pulmonary complications may be grouped into those that occur within the first 24 to 48 h as a result of the accident, and those that occur any time after that. Immediate complications include upper airway obstruction secondary to edema of the face, neck, mouth, pharynx, and larynx, and primary pulmonary damage from forced inhalation of products of combustion, such as smoke, gases, and noxious chemicals. The second group of complications includes pulmonary insufficiency secondary to shock, trauma, and increased lung water due to overhydration or secondary to extensive injury characterized by alveolar collapse. Other complications include pneumonia and pulmonary embolism. These complications may occur anytime after a burn injury. Embolism, if seen, is usually a late occurrence.

Treatment of these complications varies widely from basic nursing care measures to maintenance of respirations through an artificial upper airway by a mechanical ventilator. The basic principle of respiratory therapy is to assist or support the patient's ventilation, without causing additional complications, until the patient has resumed effective spontaneous ventilation.

Immediate Complications

Respiratory complications resulting directly from the accident are either upper airway obstruction or primary pulmonary damage. Little can be done to prevent immediate respiratory distress. However, merely "observing" the patient for signs and symptoms, or "watchful waiting," can be fatal.

Definitive signs and symptoms may not be apparent during the first several hours after a burn or until edema forms. Stridor is a fairly late symptom of obstruction. Early chest x-rays frequently show no abnormality, and arterial hypoxemia may be the first sign of pulmonary insufficiency.

The following signs indicate probable respiratory involvement; the presence of one or more indicates the need for immediate action: a history of forced inhalation of products of combustion (such as occurs in a house fire or explosion); burns of the face, especially around the nose and mouth, or of the neck and upper chest; singed nasal hairs; darkened oral and nasal mucous membranes; and coughing up of darkened sputum.

Management

Principles

The principles of care are to ensure a patent airway and to maintain adequate ventilation. This may be accomplished by providing humidified oxygen with a face mask, or it may require an artificial airway such as an endotracheal tube for severe upper airway obstruction or a tracheostomy for primary pulmonary damage. If the trauma has affected the alveoli, treatment is difficult. Antibiotics and bronchodilators may also be indicated.

Procedure

The steps discussed here may be taken to decrease the seriousness of respiratory involvement and pave the way for proper clinical management. If one or more of the signs of respiratory involvement are present, elevate the patient's head and torso (if systolic blood pressure is not less than 100 mmHg) to ensure a patent airway, set up intratracheal suction at the bedside, place a laryngoscope, endotracheal tube, and supplies near the bedside, and have a tracheostomy tray and tubes on hand. Start measured humidified oxygen and obtain specimens for arterial blood gas analysis. Instruct the patient to cough and deep breathe every 20 min. Begin an hourly turning schedule from side to back to side. Begin chest physiotherapy, if indicated. Watch for any signs of cerebral depression and keep narcotics at a minimum to prevent a decrease in cerebral response. Observe for tight chest or neck eschar and perform an escharotomy as soon as indicated. Monitor resuscitation fluids, respirations, and other vital signs closely. Begin pulmonary artery pressure monitoring if necessary.

Upper airway obstruction decreases as edema subsides and trauma to tissues of the upper airway resolves. With proper management, this problem will not require long-term care. Deep lung damage, however, cannot be resolved as quickly and may prove fatal. The symptoms of primary pulmonary damage are similar to those of respiratory distress and failure, and treatment is similar. The following principles of care provide a basis for management of all pulmonary complications.

The burned patient is predisposed to pulmonary complications (which occur other than as a direct result of the accident) from a number of factors which may not be obviously related to pulmonary problems. If these factors are recognized and controlled, the incidence of pulmonary complications can be reduced. The predisposing factors are:

1. Hypovolemic shock and fluid therapy, which, if not properly managed or if combined with primary pulmonary damage, lead to overhydration and stiff, wet lungs due to pulmonary interstitial edema.
2. Lowered resistance to infection due to decreased immunity, nutritional imbalance, protein loss, and continuous wound infections.
3. Stasis of secretions due to prolonged bedrest, infrequent turning and positioning, and limited activity.

The following general principles of care underlie prevention as well as management of early and late pulmonary complications. These measures alone may be inadequate to maintain oxygenation, ventilation, and acid-base balance; an artificial upper airway and mechanical respiratory support also may be required.

The clinical signs and symptoms of pulmonary involvement and possible insufficiency also are noted with many other problems. Subtle changes may be the first indications of insufficiency. The nurse should be especially alert to insidious changes in respiratory rate and volume, noting tachypnea or bradypnea, irregular breathing patterns, dyspnea, or apnea. Chest pain, or a change in the amount, color, or consistency of sputum may indicate a problem. A change in pulse rate or blood pressure may be significant and anxiety or restlessness should be noted. Peripheral cyanosis and stridor are crude guides to oxygenation status because they are late signs of a problem. Therefore, frequent blood gas analysis is mandatory at the first suspicion of pulmonary insufficiency.

Extravascular water can accumulate in the lungs for a variety of reasons. If there has been significant inhalation of noxious gases at the time of injury, there will be pulmonary interstitial edema. Toxins released from injured burn tissue are also thought to contribute to wet lungs. In addition, fluids required for initial resuscitation increase interstitial edema. Overhydration results in stiff, wet lungs. Use of colloids such as salt-poor albumin and plasma for initial resuscitation, however, tends to decrease lung water extravasation. Ultrasonic nebulization can also contribute to wet lungs and consideration of this factor should dictate use of the device. Extravascular lung water measurements (EVLW) can be done hourly to evaluate a patient's status. The technique uses a dye injectate and can indicate signs of pulmonary failure.[13] Treatment includes frequent turning. (See Chap. 27 for further discussion of pulmonary disorders.)

Intravenous fluid administration should be carefully monitored. Whenever regulating fluid balance, the possibility of circulatory overload and pulmonary insufficiency should not be overlooked.

Wound Care

Current methods of burn wound management include the *conservative method* and the *early excision method,* or some combination thereof. *Conservative treatment* is that method which allows for separation of eschar over time through the process of autolysis. *Autolysis* is the spontaneous disintegration of tissues by the action of their own enzymes. The eschar is debrided daily during hydrotherapy treatments and skin grafting is done on third-degree burns when a healthy granulation bed is exposed.

Hydrotherapy is performed daily to debride necrotic tissue and visualize wounds. In addition, topical agents are removed and remaining eschar is softened. Showering the patient on a table and immersing the patient in a tub are two currently used methods of hydrotherapy. Showering enhances visualization of wounds and allows water temperature to be kept constant. Immersion of the burn patient in large tubs of water or antiseptic solutions has been associated with autocontamination and increased losses of sodium through the burn wound. Figure 55-10 depicts a shower table used in hydrotherapy.

The *early excision method*[14] exemplifies the recent trend toward operative management of the wound. Patients are taken to the operating room as early after injury as possible. The burn wound is excised by either a tangential or fascial excision technique. A skin graft or other temporary covering is placed over the excised wound. Operative debridement and grafting procedures, if necessary, are done every 5 to 7 days until complete, permanent coverage is achieved.

Permanent skin coverage is achieved only through the application of an autograft or the healing of partial-thickness injuries. Skin grafts are generally of split thickness (0.015 inch) and are placed either on a clean granulation bed or an excised area of burn. Generally, grafts are meshed to increase the area of coverage at ratios from 1:1.5 to 1:3. In large percentage burns, skin can be meshed and expanded at ratios from 1:6 to 1:9. In areas where cosmetics are a concern, such as the face or breast area, skin is not meshed and sheet grafts are applied. Once applied, mesh grafts are sutured or stapled in place and covered with fine-mesh gauze impregnated with an antibiotic ointment such as polysporin or gentamicin. This limits bacterial invasion of open meshed areas in the graft (interstices), thus limiting graft loss due to infection. Because infection is the leading cause of graft failure, patients are placed on perioperative antibiotics. Thick gauze padding and pressure bandages are then applied over the grafted areas to prevent graft loss due to shear force. Skin grafts become attached to the body through the establishment of capillary networks from the graft to the body. Destruction of these bonds occurs when the graft is moved or traumatized. The development of hematomas or seromas under the graft also can inhibit the formation of circulatory bonding patterns and be detrimental to grafts.

Body image is of primary concern and must be considered in wound management therapy from

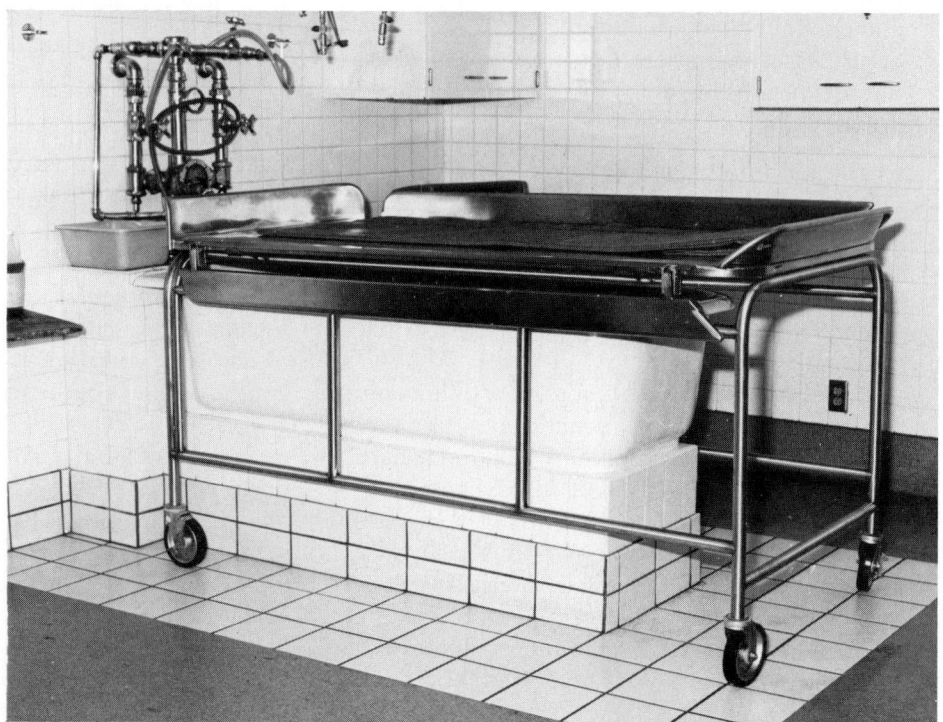

Figure 55-10 Shower table used for daily hydrotherapy, debridement, and hygiene.

the time the burn occurs. Cosmetic and/or functional surgical procedures are often performed for many years following the initial insult. The use of microvascular free flaps, pedicle flaps, or rotation flaps can greatly improve tissue survival, save a questionable extremity, or improve function and appearance in deformed areas. (See Chap. 56.)

Postoperative Care

The nurse must be vigilant in observing for the development of clots or seromas beneath the graft surface. The surgeon should be promptly notified and the obstruction removed. (See Chap. 56 for discussion of postoperative wound healing.)

Skin Grafting

Full-thickness wounds require autografting to obtain permanent skin coverage and to achieve the natural immunity of the intact anatomical barrier of the skin destroyed by the burn injury. With good care, the body can heal a partial-thickness wound through the process of reepithelialization.

Types of Grafts

The four types of grafts are autografts, carious grafts, allografts, and heterografts. These grafts can be applied as either full-thickness grafts, in which the full thickness of the dermis is cropped, or as split-thickness grafts, in which, approximately $\frac{15}{1000}$ in of dermis is taken. Once taken, the skin can be applied as a sheet graft or can be meshed to increase the surface area of the skin (Fig. 55-11). Artificial skin may prove useful in covering patients with large surface area burns. Its use, however, is still under investigation.[15]

Allografts (Homografts) In burn care, homografts (usually cadaver skin) are applied to provide temporary coverage. Homografts are used as a biological cover to decrease infection, to protect nerve endings, and to prevent heat and fluid loss. Homografts may be used on partial-thickness wounds to protect them while healing takes place, or on full-thickness wounds until the patient can tolerate the autografting procedure or has donor areas available. Homografts also may be used to prepare an area for autografting.

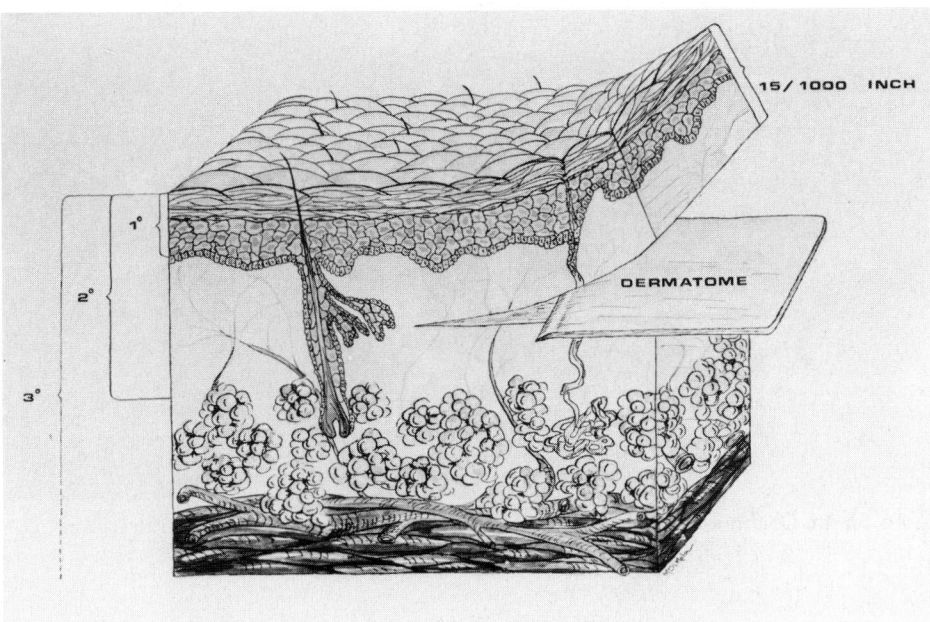

Figure 55-11 *A.* Split-thickness skin grafts are harvested at a depth of 0.015 in.

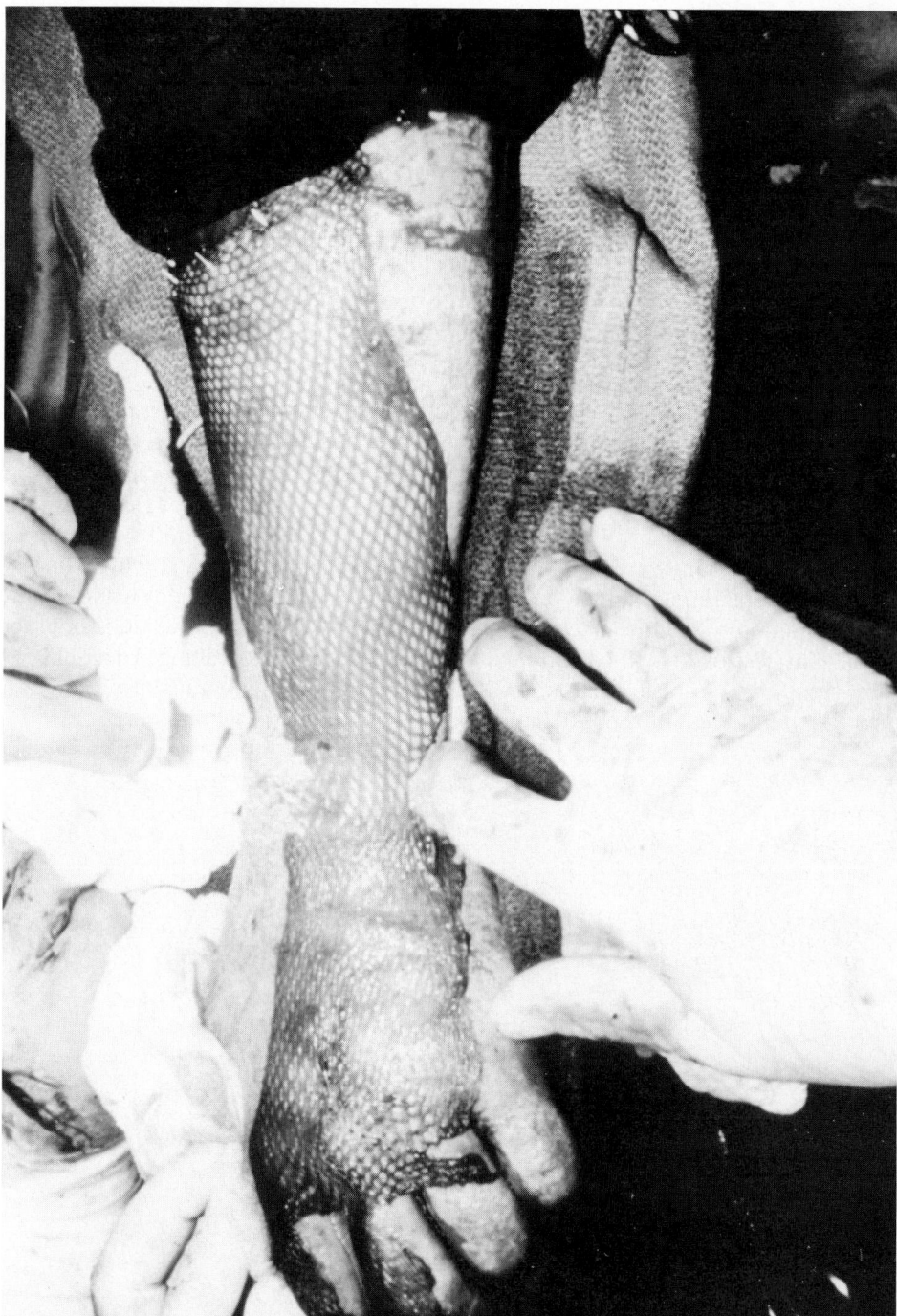

Figure 55-11 Continued *B.* Grafts are meshed and placed on a healthy granulation bed.

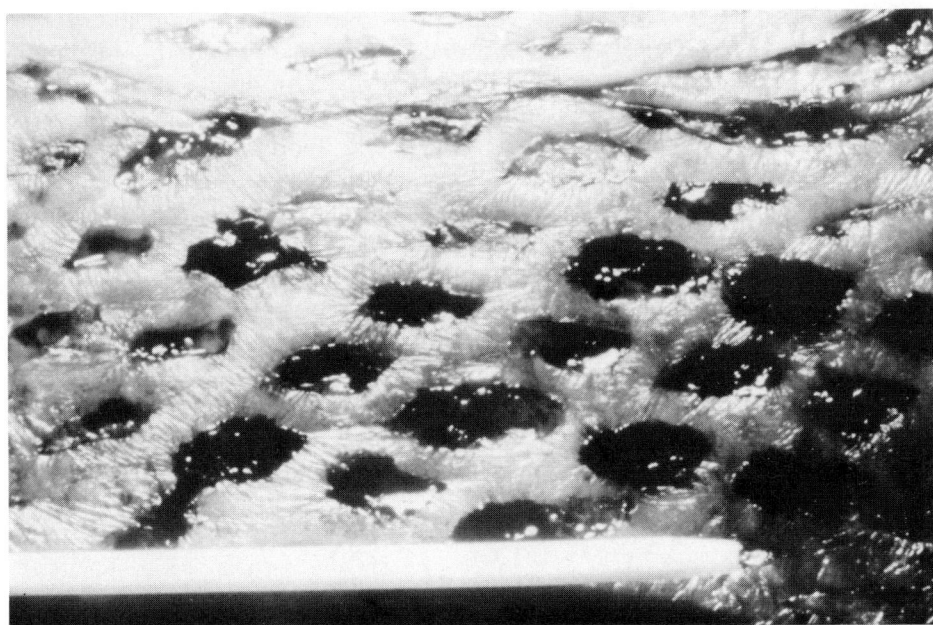

Figure 55-11 Continued   *C.* Interstices heal within 7 days.

Donor Site

The donor site (the area of the body from which the autograft is taken) represents a partial-thickness wound that temporarily increases the total wound area. Meticulous care is required to heal the donor site as rapidly as possible and thereby decrease the total size of the wound. The principles of donor care are (1) to keep the area free from infection, (2) to dry and heal the area, and (3) to provide patient comfort.

Pain Control and Sedation

Burn pain is both chronic and acute. It is a bio-psychosocial process with many factors contributing to its severity. If not controlled, excessive pain can contribute to critical-care unit (CRCU) psychosis, complications in sleep-wake cycles, and personality disorders.

When the patient's condition permits, pharmacologic pain management can be beneficial in reducing stress during painful procedures. Morphine is the most commonly used narcotic; however, codeine, Demerol, Levo-Dromoran, and Darvon have been effectively used. Methods of delivery of pharmacologic agents can also affect the level of relief experienced by the patient. For example, patient-controlled analgesia, a system by which the patient can self-administer analgesics as pain increases, has been beneficial in decreasing the amount of drugs needed for pain relief and in increasing the patient's sense of well-being. Also, the timely and prompt administration of analgesics by the nurse offers the patient reassurance that prolonged periods of pain will not occur. Effective analgesic administration requires that drugs be given in advance of painful procedures.

Nonpharmacologic pain relief measures include acupuncture, transcutaneous electrical nerve stimulation (TENS), acupressure, relaxation therapy, music therapy, and distraction. The degree of pain relief depends on the type of procedure being performed and the individual patient's response.

Sedatives and tranquilizers help reduce anxiety associated with pain and offer assistance in the promotion of adequate sleep patterns. While these pharmacologic agents do not themselves reduce burn or procedural pain, they reduce the behavioral responses that often contribute to the pain mechanism.

Nutritional Support

Because metabolic requirements double in the client with severe burns,[16] body wasting, delayed wound healing, and in some cases death will occur if energy needs are not met. Nutritional intake must meet the body's requirements. Further discussion of nutritional needs and management of the burn patient are discussed in Chap. 12.

Positioning, Contracture Control, Exercise, and Splinting

Principles of Positioning

A position the patient considers comfortable is seldom one that will control contracture formation.

However, if proper positioning is initiated early in care, explained frequently, and continued, the patient will accept these positions as comforting. Attempting to correct established contractures later in burn care is far more time-consuming and painful. The nurse must make the patient as comfortable as possible while maintaining a position of contracture control. The nonfetal position is generally desired. It is easier to flex an extended tendon than to extend a tendon in a fixed position.

Position change and proper body alignment are an essential part of nursing any severely ill patient. The objectives of positioning may be any of the following: to reduce the workload of the heart; to prevent or reduce contracture formation

Supine

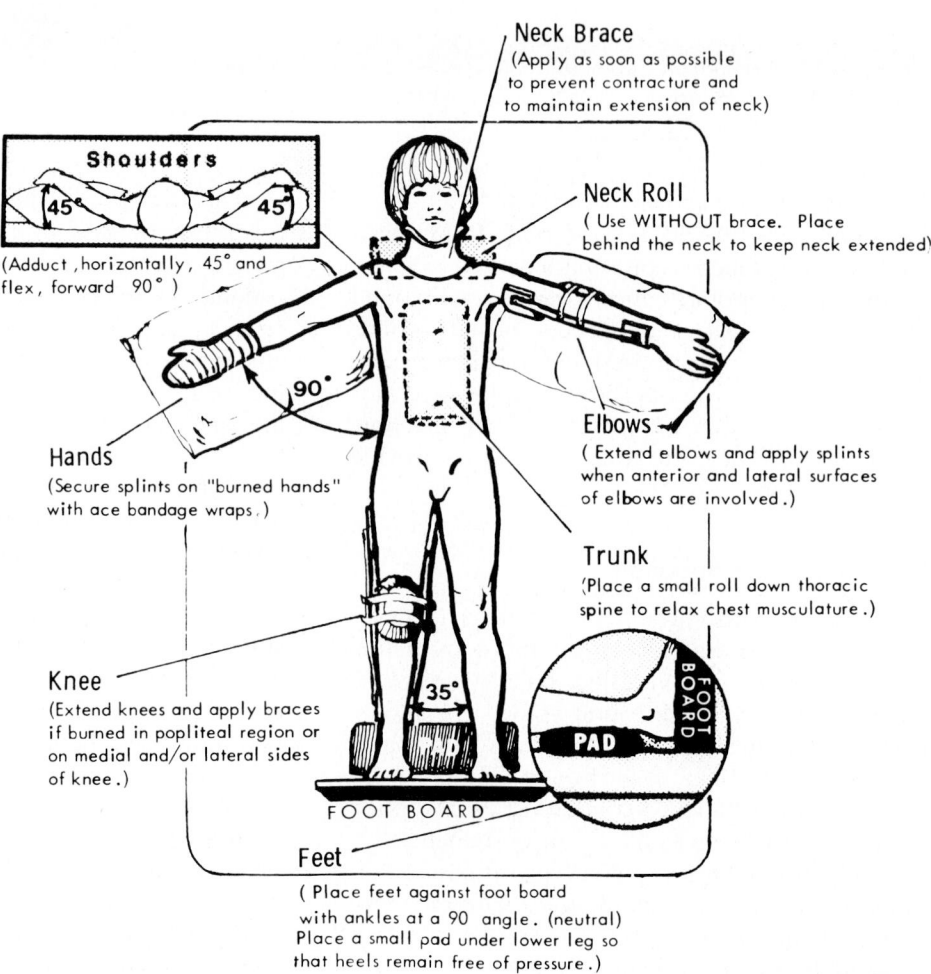

Neck Brace
(Apply as soon as possible to prevent contracture and to maintain extension of neck)

Shoulders
45°   45°
(Adduct, horizontally, 45° and flex, forward 90°)

Neck Roll
(Use WITHOUT brace. Place behind the neck to keep neck extended)

90°

Hands
(Secure splints on "burned hands" with ace bandage wraps.)

Elbows
(Extend elbows and apply splints when anterior and lateral surfaces of elbows are involved.)

Trunk
(Place a small roll down thoracic spine to relax chest musculature.)

Knee
(Extend knees and apply braces if burned in popliteal region or on medial and/or lateral sides of knee.)

35°

FOOT BOARD
PAD

FOOT BOARD

Feet
(Place feet against foot board with ankles at a 90 angle. (neutral) Place a small pad under lower leg so that heels remain free of pressure.)

Figure 55-12A. Supine positioning of the burn patient to prevent contracture formation.

(see Fig. 55-12); to reduce the incidence of phlebitis, thrombi, and emboli; to promote lung expansion and drainage of pulmonary secretions; to reduce the incidence of pneumonia; to prevent decubitus; or to provide patient comfort.

Range of Motion Exercises   Exercises which take the joints (burned or unburned) through the full range of motion are done at least once daily. However, joints should not be pushed beyond free range of motion unless prescribed by a physician or therapist. Bed rest, decreased protein, altered fluids and electrolytes, and poor circulation serve to decrease joint function and to encourage heterotopic bone formation and contracture. Exercising is best done while the patient is in the hydrotherapy tub. Active and passive range of motion may be combined, depending on the patient's capabilities. The physiatrist and physical therapist (PT) are skilled in providing these exercises; a nurse, however, can conduct them. Exercising should not be neglected because of a lack of PT coverage. Active range of motion requires that the patient exercise voluntarily. Full range of motion, as well as increased self-care is encouraged; for example, brushing teeth, combing hair, and feeding. Many

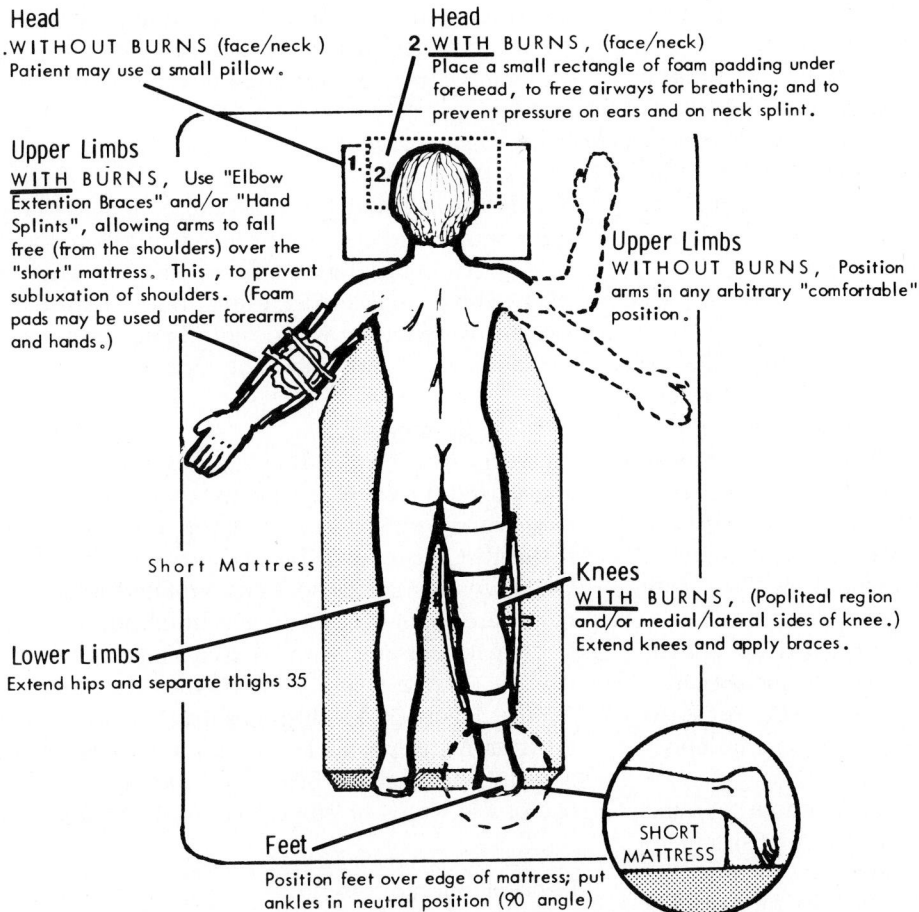

Prone

Head
1. WITHOUT BURNS (face/neck)
Patient may use a small pillow.

Head
2. WITH BURNS, (face/neck)
Place a small rectangle of foam padding under forehead, to free airways for breathing; and to prevent pressure on ears and on neck splint.

Upper Limbs
WITH BURNS, Use "Elbow Extention Braces" and/or "Hand Splints", allowing arms to fall free (from the shoulders) over the "short" mattress. This , to prevent subluxation of shoulders. (Foam pads may be used under forearms and hands.)

Upper Limbs
WITHOUT BURNS, Position arms in any arbitrary "comfortable" position.

Short Mattress

Knees
WITH BURNS, (Popliteal region and/or medial/lateral sides of knee.) Extend knees and apply braces.

Lower Limbs
Extend hips and separate thighs 35

SHORT MATTRESS

Feet
Position feet over edge of mattress; put ankles in neutral position (90 angle)

Figure 55-12B.   Prone positioning of the burn patient to reduce contracture formation. (*Courtesy Shriners Burns Institute, Galveston, Texas.*)

devices may be provided by the occupational or physical therapist to increase or enhance this type of exercise.

Passive range of motion requires that the patient be taken through range of motion exercises by another individual. The exercises are best done in hydrotherapy or immediately after tubbing. If done at the bedside, a pain medication may be useful prior to exercising.

Splinting

Principles   The principle of splinting any area of the body is to place the area in a position which will preserve or regain function. Splinting may be employed throughout burn care. If contractures continue after discharge, which may be the case regardless of preventive measures, corrective splinting is necessary. Custom-made splints, those fashioned for a particular area of a particular patient, are ideal. However, custom-made splints are not always available or necessary. Ingenuity may replace the availability of custom-made splints. An elbow or knee joint may be maintained in proper position by use of a padded IV board. Contracture of the Achilles tendon, which causes foot drop, may be prevented by use of sandbags, towels, or pillows. The preservation of function is always the primary guide in the use of splints.

Dorsal and Total Hand Burn   The objectives in treating burns of the hand are to prevent deeply damaged tissues from becoming infected and to maintain a position which will preserve function. Because severe consequences result when hand function is damaged or lost, special or custom-made splints are desirable. Because the tendons of the dorsum (back) of the hand have little fatty padding and protection, they require special care. If the hand has sustained either a deep partial-thickness or a full-thickness burn, contractures may be expected. However, much can be done to minimize these contractures and in some instances they can be avoided.

Exercising or using the hand without splinting is excellent; however, use must be consistent to prevent contractures. The splinting method we recommend is one which maintains most of the joints of the hand in an extended position (see Fig. 55-13). This splinting method can be very effective,

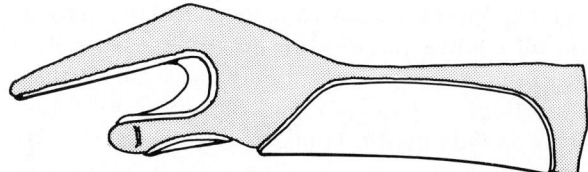

Figure 55-13   Splint applied to burned hand. *Note:* The splint maintains wrist and hand position to prevent contractures.

provided that the splints are correctly applied immediately after the burn injury and are checked frequently to see that they are maintained in proper position.

Initially, the extent and depth of a burn often cannot be accurately determined, and hand splints may be applied as a precautionary measure; they can be removed later if not required. Hand splints are continued until the major healing process has been completed in a partial-thickness burn or until grafting is completed in a full-thickness injury. After grafting, splints are removed and full use of the hand is encouraged.

Palmar Burns   Full-thickness burns limited to the palm of the hand may be less deforming than dorsal burns because the flexor tendons are protected by thick palmar fascia and fat. Palmar burns are usually treated by splinting in a position with the fingers extended and the thumb in abduction.

Pressure Dressings

Pressure dressings, in the form of Ace wraps or specialized pressure garments called *Jobst garments,* are believed to reduce the amount of scar tissue that forms over burned areas of the body. Once wounds are closed, custom-fitted Jobst garments are worn over all areas of the body affected. These garments are worn for 23 h a day, then every day for 1 to 2 years, or until the scar tissue is mature. Figure 55-14 illustrates the various types of Jobst garments available. Temporary measures of applying pressure to healed wounds include the use of Ace wraps or other pressure bandages.

Rehabilitation

Once released from the care of the burn team, the patient and family must deal with wound care,

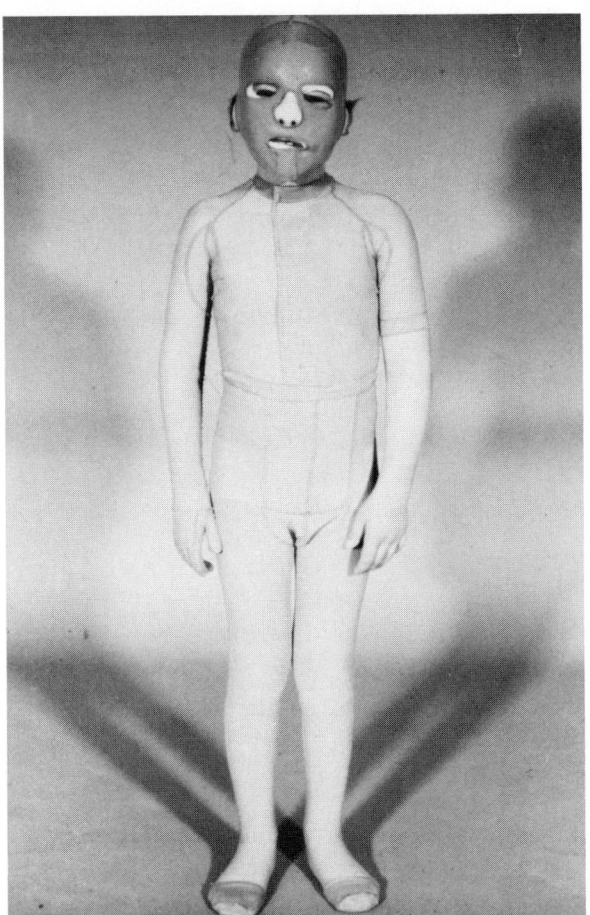

Figure 55-14   Patient in full Jobst garments.

Referrals are often made to various community agency health team members such as physical or occupational therapists, social workers, schools, psychiatrists, family counselors, or others. Often the need for equipment arises and a route for acquisition must be established.

Home arrangements are detailed, complex, and extremely time-consuming. For this reason, home care planning and community referrals are begun on admission to the burn unit. Failure to follow this process results in problems when the patient returns home.

Reconstructive and cosmetic surgery is performed for many years following burn injury. Restoration of function and improvement of cosmetic appearance through surgical techniques may greatly improve the patient's feelings of self-worth and body image. As with acute skin grafting procedures, the nurse must caution the patient about graft or cosmetic outcomes. Patients may expect grafted skin or reconstructed areas to appear equal in quality and looks to their previous state. This is never the case and proper education can help prevent shock and depression following surgery. The patient who has developed contractures, keloids, microstomia, or other conditions which limit movement frequently requires surgical intervention to restore function.

Plastic surgery involves the use of classical techniques; however, some new approaches are being studied. Use of tissue expanders is one example of a relatively new area of burn surgery. Contracture releases are most commonly performed on the neck, axilla, or elbow area. Surgical procedures to improve movement are many, varied, and individualized to each client.

Nursing care involves postoperative care of grafts or suture lines. Bolster dressings are often used to limit movement. The position of the client can have a direct effect on the success of the procedure. The nurse also must assure long-term success of the surgical procedure. Patients must be taught about the need to use splints or assistive devices.

Rehabilitation may last for many years. Often, reentry into society is difficult in terms of relationships, life style, and vocation.[17] The burn team must understand the process of rehabilitation and offer support to the patient to assist a successful transition.

dressing changes, ambulation, eating, sweating, itching, pressure garments, and a host of other aspects of physical care. Psychologically, the prospect of going home may be an uplifting thought to the patient; however, once at home, the difficulties and stress encountered may alter feelings of excitement. The burn team must anticipate problems which the patient will face and take measures to intervene in situations when possible. Occasionally, problems are numerous or the coping mechanisms of the family are inadequate and referral of a patient to a rehabilitation facility is indicated. The family must be evaluated in terms of its support, reliability, cooperation, and ability to perform the necessary care. Referral to a visiting nurse service in the community is often made and the frequency of home visits depends on the level of care the family is able to deliver.

Nursing Diagnoses

This section is composed of nursing diagnoses pertinent to the care of the burn patient.

Cardiovascular System

Problems

1. Tachycardia
2. Pallor
3. Cool, clammy skin
4. Weak thready pulse
5. Hypotension
6. Disorientation or poor mentation
7. Low urine output
8. Ileus
9. Loss of peripheral pulses
10. Falling hemodynamic pressures (CVP, PWP)
11. Low cardiac output
12. Arrhythmias

Nursing Diagnoses

I. Alteration in cardiac output: decreased related to increased capillary permeability.
II. Fluid volume deficit and electrolyte imbalance related to loss of plasma volume from the vascular space.
III. Alteration in tissue perfusion: cerebral, cardiopulmonary, renal, gastrointestinal, peripheral: related to decreased cardiac output and generalized edema.

Goals

I. Maintain cardiac output by increasing intravascular fluid volume to a level which provides adequate perfusion to vital organs.

Interventions

I. A. Fluid administration as per the Parkland formula.
B. Insert Foley catheter and monitor urine output hourly.
C. Daily nude weights.
D. Monitor mentation, heart rate, blood pressure, CVP, PWP q 15 min to hourly.
E. Monitor temperature and cardiac output hourly.
F. Monitor peripheral pulses q 15 min to hourly.
G. Provide pre- and postoperative escharotomy care.
H. Titrate fluids.
I. Administer medication intravenously or orally.

Evaluation

I. The client perfuses all vital organs.
A. Positive pulses in all extremities.
B. Absence of acute tubular necrosis (ATN).
C. Clear sensorium.
D. Heart rate, blood pressure, and cardiac rhythm within normal limits.
E. Fluid and electrolyte status within normal limits.
F. Urine output > 30 to 50 mL per hour.

Respiratory System

Problems

1. Drowsiness
2. Stupor
3. Comatose
4. Elevated carboxyhemoglobin
5. Hypoxia
6. Respiratory distress
7. Upper airway edema
8. Blisters and soot in mouth, nose, pharynx
9. Burns of the face, head, and neck
10. Singed nares, eyebrows, eyelids
11. Progressive hoarseness
12. Dyspnea
13. Stridor
14. Cyanosis
15. Coughing
16. Circumferential chest burns

Nursing Diagnoses

I. Ineffective breathing pattern related to respiratory distress from inhalation injury, airway obstruction, or pneumonia.

Goals

I. A. Maintain airway.
B. Maintain adequate gas exchange.
C. Maintain, support, and/or restore pulmonary mechanics.

Interventions

I. A. Perform chin lift/head tilt maneuver in unconscious victim.

B. Prepare for and assist with nasal or oral intubation or tracheostomy.

C. Suction as necessary.

D. Perform chest physiotherapy.

E. Observe ventilator for proper mechanical function.

II. A. Monitor gas exchange through laboratory tests; i.e., ABG, VBG, carboxyhemoglobin levels.

B. Prepare for and assist with oral or nasal intubation.

C. Administer antibiotics as indicated.

D. Turn patient frequently.

E. Administer vigorous chest physiotherapy.

F. Evaluate fluid balance.

G. Administer sedative and paralytic agents when indicated.

H. Monitor lung water measurements when indicated.

I. Monitor pulmonary artery and wedge pressure when indicated.

J. Monitor central venous pressures.

III. A. Administer oxygen.

B. Encourage incentive spirometry.

C. Encourage coughing and deep breathing exercises.

D. Assist with weaning from mechanical ventilator.

E. Turn frequently.

Evaluation

I. The patient ventilates without problem.

A. Absence of obstruction (edema, secretions).

B. Patent airway (physiologic, endotracheal tube, or tracheostomy).

C. Respiratory rate within normal limits.

D. Absence of stridor, dyspnea, cyanosis.

E. Skin/eschar about chest expands (escharotomies done).

II. The patient's gas exchange is adequate.

A. Perfusion in lungs is adequate.

B. Arterial blood gases within normal limits.

C. Absence of acidosis/alkalosis.

D. Respiratory rate within normal limits.

E. Absence of pulmonary edema.

III. The patient uses respiratory muscles independently for breathing.

A. No ventilatory assistance required.

B. Incentive spirometry utilized.

C. Arterial blood gases within normal limits.

D. Cough reflex intact.

E. Tidal volume, inspiratory force, minute volume within normal limits.

Pain

Problems

1. Crying
2. Complaints of pain
3. Irritability
4. Lethargy
5. Depression
6. Facial grimacing and tensing
7. Increased heart rate and blood pressure
8. Abnormal sleep/wake patterns
9. Withdrawal of body part when touched
10. Poor mobility
11. Poor joint range
12. Inflammation or redness of area
13. Edema

Nursing Diagnoses

I. Alteration in comfort: pain related to exposed nerve endings found in the damaged dermis.

Goals

I. Reduce sensory pain and suffering related to burn injuries.

Interventions

I. Administer analgesics promptly.

II. Administer medications as indicated, especially 30 to 45 min prior to painful procedures.

III. Teach patient relaxation techniques and meditative breathing.

IV. Utilize techniques of guided imagery, music therapy, hypnosis, therapeutic touch, acupuncture when appropriate.

V. Allow sleep and rest time to prevent CRCU psychosis.

VI. Change position frequently.

VII. Maintain ambient temperature at 85 to 90°F to decrease shivering and trigger relaxation response.

VIII. Establish a contract with the patient to enhance his or her feeling of control over pain.

IX. Explain all procedures.

Evaluation

I. The patient states that pain is alleviated or reduced or the nurse observes decreases in clinical signs of pain if the client is unable to respond.
   A. Decreased crying, moaning or complaints of pain.
   B. Decreased facial grimacing and tensing.
   C. Decreased heart rate.
   D. Increase in sleep and rest periods.
   E. Ability to ambulate and move body parts (ROM).
   F. Increased ability to tolerate painful procedures.

Integumentary System and Infection

Problems

1. Positive wound sputum, blood, or urine cultures or an increase in colony counts
2. Hypo- or hyperthermia
3. Positive burn wound biopsies
4. Pus and/or purulent wound drainage
5. Foul-smelling odors from wounds
6. Glucose intolerance
7. Increased WBC count with a shift to the left
8. Thrombocytopenia
9. Change in mentation
10. Redness surrounding wounds
11. Redness or maceration of healthy skin
12. Areas of burn that do not heal
13. Autograft loss
14. Poor "take" of skin substitutes or autografts
15. Eschar on donor sites
16. Wound detritus
17. Change in wound texture

Nursing Diagnoses

I. Impairment of skin integrity and potential for infection related to varying depths of damage to dermal and epidermal cells.

Goals

I. Prevent infection.
II. Prevent further loss of skin integrity.
III. Restore skin integrity.

Interventions

I. General
   A. Implement isolation precautions when indicated.
   B. Perform thorough hand washing procedures.
   C. Procure wound, blood, sputum, and urine cultures.
   D. Procure burn wound biopsies.
   E. Monitor wound, blood, sputum, and urine cultures and burn wound biopsies.
   F. Observe for signs of sepsis.
   G. Take hourly temperatures.
   H. Administer appropriate antibiotics.
   I. Administer tetanus toxoid on admission.
   J. Apply topical antimicrobials.
II. Wound Care
   A. Perform hydrotherapy and debridement of burn wounds.
   B. Give postoperative care to autografts, skin substitutes, and donor sites.
   C. Position patient to prevent pressure on grafted or donor areas.
   D. Utilize low-pressure mattresses or beds, i.e., air fluidized therapy.
   E. Roll sheet grafts hourly.
   F. Observe for development of clots, seromas, or bleeding beneath the surface of grafts postoperatively.
   G. Apply heat lamps to donor sites.
   H. Give skin care daily to healthy skin.
   I. Utilize assistive devices to prevent decubiti.

Evaluation

I. The patient does not develop nosocomial infections.
   A. Negative cultures from wound, sputum, blood, and urine.
   B. Absence of temperature spikes.
   C. Negative burn wound biopsies.
   D. Absence of clinical signs of sepsis.
   E. Absence of foul-smelling wounds.
   F. Absence of pus and purulent wound exudate.
II. In the presence of infection, the patient will not experience a spread and the degree of infection will be reduced.
   A. A decrease in wound colony counts.
   B. Improvement in wound appearance or odor.
   C. Decrease in wound exudate or pus.
   D. Improvement in clinical signs of sepsis.
   E. Temperature within normal limits.
III. The patient will not experience breakdown of healthy skin.

A. Absence of areas of redness due to pressure or immobility.
B. Absence of cellulitis.
C. Absence of maceration of healthy skin near areas of burn.
D. Absence of tissue breakdown secondary to tube placement (i.e., breakdown of nares with long-term use of nasogastric tube).

IV. The patient will have a restoration in skin integrity.
   A. Absence of open areas.
   B. Absence of temporary skin substitutes.
   C. Adherence of all skin grafts.
   D. Absence of infection in newly grafted skin.
   E. Donor sites healed.

Metabolic System

Problems

1. Increased metabolic rate, increased heart rate, increased core temperature
2. Anorexia
3. Paralytic ileus
4. Diarrhea
5. Weight loss
6. Poor wound healing

Nursing Diagnoses

I. Alteration in nutrition: less than body requirements related to increases in metabolic rate.

Goals

I. Maintain adequate nutritional intake to meet the body's requirements.

Interventions

I. Provide high-protein, high-caloric diet.
II. Monitor bowel sounds.
III. Encourage feeding.
IV. Administer tube feedings or TPN when indicated.
V. Monitor intake and output.
VI. Monitor calories by the use of a calorie count sheet.
VII. Weigh patient daily.
VIII. Offer high-calorie, high-protein snacks between meals.

Evaluation

I. The patient will follow the appropriate dietary regimen.
   A. Caloric requirements are met.
   B. Appropriate high-protein, high-caloric foods are selected.
   C. Alimentary tract selected when possible.
   D. Absence of paralytic ileus.
   E. Weight loss <10 percent of preburn weight.

Physical Mobility

Problems

1. Loss of function
2. Poor range of motion in burns which involve a joint
3. Unable to ambulate independently
4. Development of scar tissue causing contractures in areas, especially joints, which have been burned
5. Hypertrophic scar tissue formation
6. Inability to perform activities of daily living

Nursing Diagnoses

I. Impaired physical mobility related to open burn wounds, scar and contracture formation, and poor joint range of motion.

Goals

I. Regain and maintain physical mobility to optimum capacity.

Interventions

I. Perform range of motion exercise as indicated.
II. Apply splints and conformers appropriately.
III. Position the patient for contracture prevention.
IV. Apply pressure garments when wounds heal.
V. Ambulate frequently.
VI. Encourage self-assistance with activities of daily living.
VII. Administer postoperative care following reconstructive surgery.

Evaluation

I. The patient will progressively increase physical mobility until a point of optimum function is reached.
   A. Increased range of motion in involved joints
   B. Increased function in specific area involved

C. Independent ambulation

D. Flattening of hypertrophic scars

E. Reduction in extent of contracture

F. Performance of activities of daily living

Self-Concept and Support Systems

Problems

1. Crying
2. Anger
3. Apathy
4. Evidence of abuse
5. Lack of support systems
6. Dependence
7. Cultural mores
8. Demographics (sex, age)
9. Previous problems with self-concept

Nursing Diagnoses

I. Disturbance in self-concept: Body image related to change in physical appearance.

Goals

I. Progression through the grieving process.

II. Utilization of support systems.

III. Restoration of independent functioning and self-reliance.

Interventions

I. Reassure patient that feelings of grief and loss are normal.

II. Accept the patient physically and psychologically.

III. Conduct counseling sessions for patient and family.

IV. Identify support systems for patient to utilize.

V. Foster independence and decision making in the patient.

VI. Make provisions for community health assistance after discharge.

VII. Explain reconstructive and cosmetic surgical procedures which can be done in future.

Evaluation

I. Patient will move through stages of grieving, denial, anger, bargaining, depression, and acceptance.

　A. Expression of feelings and thoughts.

　B. Unusual exhibitory behaviors.

　C. Increased decision making.

　D. Establishment of new role function.

II. The patient will use appropriate support systems.

　A. Asks assistance of family or other previously successful support systems.

　B. Cooperates with hospital-based social service or nursing supports.

　C. Keeps scheduled appointments.

　D. Verbalizes problems and works toward solutions.

III. The patient will progressively increase independent functioning and self-reliance.

　A. Increase in self-ambulation.

　B. Increase in independent activities of daily living such as eating, bathing, dressing.

　C. Input into daily plan of care.

　D. Increased decision making.

　E. Improved role mastery.

　F. Improved interpersonal relations.

References

1. Artz, C. P., Moncrief, J. A., & Pruitt, B. A. (1979). *Burns: A team approach.* (p. 25). Philadelphia: Saunders.

2. Artz, C. P., Moncrief, J. A., & Pruitt, B. A. (1979). *Burns: A team approach.* (pp. 170–171). Philadelphia: Saunders.

3. Heimbach, D. (1983). Smoke inhalation: Current concepts. In T. Wachtel, V. Kahn, & Frank (Eds.), *Current topics in burn care.* Rockville, MD: Aspen Systems Corporation.

4. Wilmore, D. W., Aulick, L. H., Mason, A. D., Jr., & Pruitt, B. A., Jr. (1977). Influence of the burn wound on local and systemic responses to injury. *Annals of Surgery, 186,* 444–458.

5. Baxter, C. R. (1971). Fluid volume & electrolyte changes of the early post-burn period. *Clinics in Plastic Surgery, 1* (4), 693–709.

6. Loebl, E. C., Marvin, J. A., Curreri, P. W., & Baxter, C. R. (1974). Erythrocyte survival following thermal injury. *Journal of Surgical Research, 16,* 96–101.

7. Chan, C. K., Jarrett, F., & Moylan, J. A. (1976). Acute leukopenia as an allergic reaction to silver sulfadiazine in burn patients. *The Journal of Trauma, 16* (5), 395–396.

8. Hall, J. W., Winkler, J. B., Herndon, D. N., & Gary, L. B. (1987). Auditory brainstem response in auditory assessment of acute severely burned children. *Journal of Burn Care and Rehabilitation, 8* (3), 195–198.

9. Curreri, P. W. (1979). Burns. In S. I. Schwartz, G. T. Shires, F. C. Spencer, & E. H. Storer (Eds.), *Principles of surgery, 3rd Ed.* New York: McGraw-Hill.

10. Ninniman, J. L. (1983). The effect of thermal injury of host immunologic defenses. In T. Watchtel, V. Kahn, & H. Frank (Eds.), *Current topics in burn care.* Rockville, MD: Aspen Systems Corporation.

11. Garner, J. S., & Simmons, B. P. (1983). Guidelines for isolation precautions in hospitals. *Infection Control, 4* (4), 245–349.

12. Guyton, A. C. (1986). *Textbook of medical physiology.* Philadelphia: Saunders.

13. Allison, R. C., Carlile, P. V., & Gray, B. W. (1985). Thermodilution measurement of lung water. *Clinics in Chest Medicine, 6* (3), 439–457.

14. Herndon, D. N., Thompson, P. B., Desai, M. H., & Van Osten, T. J. (1985). Treatment of burns in children. *Pediatric Clinics of North America, 32* (5), 1311–1331.

15. Burke, J. F., et al. (1981). Successful use of a physiologically acceptable artificial skin in the treatment of extensive burn injury. *Annals of Surgery, 194* (4), 413–428.

16. Wilmore, D. W. (1974). Nutrition and metabolism following thermal injury. *Clinics in Plastic Surgery,* 603–619.

17. Herndon, et al. (1986). The quality of life after major thermal injury in children: An analysis of 12 survivors with 80% total body, 70% third degree burns. *Journal of Trauma, 26,* 609–619.

56

Wound Healing: A Nursing Responsibility

Diane Cooper

Healing and the Nurse

Healing has been succinctly described as the "restoration of continuity."[1] Though this definition describes the realignment of interrupted tissue, it certainly could be applied to healing in dimensions other than physiologic. In its broadest sense, healing is a term which connotes wholeness, oneness, soundness. The word is derived from the Anglo-Saxon *bāl,* meaning "whole." The Random House dictionary offers definitions ranging from restoration of health to freeing from evil, to restoring amity, to effecting a cure. It is evident then, that the spectrum of meanings is broad.

Human beings expect to heal. Healing becomes a predictable event in human experience and as such is relied upon.[2–4] Most children sustain their first cut at an early age. Initially it is a trauma, but once they are reassured (particularly if therapy is applied in the form of a Band-Aid), the wound becomes a fascinating experience. A youngster can frequently be observed assessing the wound to monitor its progress, gradually forgetting it as structural integrity is restored.[3] As a person matures, the experience of numerous physical cuts and scrapes is generalized in such a way that similarities can be recognized in the traumas occurring in human or psychic development. Just as there are phases in the healing of psychic wounds, so there are phases in the healing of physical wounds.[4]

Healing, then, is recognized as potentially occurring at several levels. The restorative process may involve the total human organism, as in cure of a psychiatric disorder, or may restore tissue continuity, as after a surgical procedure. Most often the healing event involves supportive assistance from others.

Though the art and science of healing have been ascribed to various professional groups, the "adaptive ability to heal is fundamental to all nursing intervention."[5] Nurses approach the environment, health, and the patient from the perspective of assisting in the restorative process, regardless of the structure involved. The nurse supports the patient socially, personally, and structurally to become reintegrated and to do this in such a way that energy expenditure is kept at a minimum.[1,3,5–10] Each of the supportive acts rendered by the nurse is aimed at achieving and maintaining a milieu in which healing can occur. Thus a healing environment is created which supports the total organism.

Though the restorative process can be studied from various perspectives, this chapter analyzes the healing environment at the cellular level. Such analysis is pertinent to nursing because of the degree of responsibility nurses are given in the care and treatment of wounds. Increasingly, particularly in critical care, the nurse is consistently the primary evaluator of the status of the wound. Frequently modifications in the approach to wound care are based on the observations and suggestions of the nurse. Currently, few objective criteria for evaluating progress or regression in healing exist, because only recently have nurses begun to describe the characteristics on which such criteria may be based.[11,12]

An area studied even less is the manipulation of the wound environment via dressings and solutions. The majority of approaches to wound care practiced in the United States are based on tradition and loosely defined criteria. Even the potentially deleterious effects of some routine interventions are poorly understood by those involved in rendering treatment.[2,13–16] The physical, financial, and emotional costs of protracted wound healing makes it neither economically sound nor consistent with the nursing goal of restoration of continuity.[17]

Investigations in progress in various United States laboratories are studying the effects of injury on wound healing and have begun to produce clusters of information which can be used to make predictions about the milieu most supportive of healing, and gradually some of this information has begun to appear in the nursing literature.[18–25] Most research data, however, continue to be reported by physicians.[26–31] It is the contention of the author that if nurses better understood the healing environment at the cellular level, they could critique current practice, formulate alternative therapies supportive of healing, devise research studies to objectively measure the effect of alternative therapies on healing, and ultimately contribute greatly to restoring the patient to an energized, integrated state. Synthesis of this information by the practicing nurse is overdue. Nurses play a pivotal role in assisting the patient toward healing and need to "own" this area of their practice.

The Healing Trajectory

Regardless of their origin, all wounds attempt to heal in the same fashion.[2,29] This trajectory is intricate, dynamic, and interwoven, like many processes in the human body. For the sake of analysis, however, wound healing has been divided into three stages.[25,32] Bearing in mind the limitations inherent in such a condensation, a schematic presentation of the phases of healing and their approximate duration is presented in Fig. 56-1. Though authors utilize different terms to describe the phases, agreement on the sequence of events occurring in them is practically unanimous.

Inflammatory Phase

The first phase of the healing process has been variously termed the *lag phase,* the *exudative phase,* the *defensive phase,* the *substrate phase,* and the *inflammatory phase.* Most of these terms (*lag* in particular) arose because many assessed the initial period after injury as a period of dormancy. With the exception of redness, pain, and swelling, it was thought that little of significance occurred during the first minutes, hours, or days after wounding. However, it is currently believed that the inflammatory phase is key to the success of the healing which follows. Merker went so far as to state that "inflammation is a process that occurs after injury to a tissue. This process results in healing. In effect, healing cannot occur without inflammation."[33] According to Hunt, a noted authority on healing, "Wound healing is a sequence of events in which injury is the first step, inflammation the second, and fibroplasia the third."[34]

The inflammatory phase, first described by Metchnikoff in 1891 and quantified some 70 years later by Ross and Benditt, begins at the moment of injury and lasts until approximately day 3 or 4 after injury.[35] The primary goals of this phase are protection of the organism from blood loss, isolation of the wound from the rest of the body, and, perhaps most important, development of inflammation. What was once viewed as a quiescent period in healing is now known to be a tightly regulated, replicable progression of cellular and chemical activities which ultimately lead to healing.

The series of events which begins with wounding is followed immediately by coagulation. As platelets enter the wound site they release serotonin-containing granules; this not only leads to a brief period (approximately 10 min) of vasoconstriction of the vessels in that area but also effects

Figure 56-1   The healing trajectory.

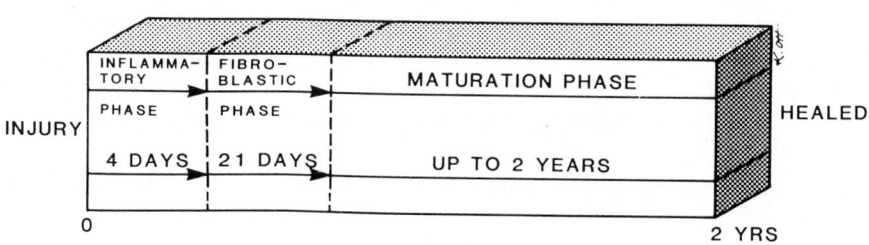

contraction of the vascular smooth muscles adjacent to the wound site. This combination of vasoconstriction and muscle contraction leads to a slowing or cessation of blood flow in the wounded area. Concurrently, the platelets adhere to collagen exposed at the site of injury and release thromboplastin. In the presence of thromboplastin, plasma prothrombin is converted to thrombin, which in turn converts fibrinogen to fibrin. Ultimately, fibrin forms a fibrillar matrix, trapping other platelets and blood cells, and a hemostatic plug or clot is formed. It is thought that this initial vasoconstrictive activity serves to wall off the wound from other areas in the body and to reduce the potential for invasion by bacteria. In addition, however, it is now known that the platelets which enter the wound area are activated and secrete a substance known as platelet-derived growth factor, or PDGF.

PDGF is a chemoattractant and as such induces a process known as *chemotaxis*. Chemotaxis occurs "when a cell responds by directed migration along a gradient toward the source of a chemical."[36] While there are other known chemoattractants, the substances released from the granules of the platelets appear to be specific for fibroblasts and endothelial cells. Interestingly, this factor is found only at sites of injury.[36] After binding to specific receptor sites on the fibroblasts, it has been shown to cause the connective tissue cells to undergo DNA synthesis and cell division. Evidence also exists that PDGF may cause other cells, the monocytes and neutrophils, to respond chemotactically.

The elucidation of this factor alone dispels the notion that little or nothing occurs during the inflammatory phase of healing. Finally, it has been demonstrated that PDGF is also responsible for releasing a substance which assists in the subsequent formation of new blood vessels. Injecting activated platelets into rabbit corneas has induced new vessel formation within 72 to 96 h after wounding.[37] Such studies have led investigators to conclude that activated platelets are key precursors to subsequent new vessel formation within injured tissue.

Vasodilatation follows the initial brief period of vasoconstriction. This occurrence, observable to the human eye and frequently painful, has resulted in the commonly used descriptors of wounding: redness, heat, swelling, and pain. Localized edema is the result of an influx of fluid and cells which ooze out of dilated vessels.

A cell which is particularly apparent at this time is the polymorphonuclear neutrophil. By the process of diapedesis this cell enters the wound site during the first 24 h in order to phagocytize bacteria and ingest debris. It appears to have a rather short term of existence, however, and in a situation in which minimal bacteria are present, the decline of these cells is apparent in approximately 3 to 4 days. In controlled studies these cells have been observed to move toward the surface of the wound.[38] Here they become trapped, and because the potential for dehydration is greater in this region, they die. Ultimately they lyse and spill their contents back into the wound, where recycling occurs. Shortly thereafter, another leucocyte, the monocyte, appears and continues the phagocytic activity initiated by the polymorphonuclear neutrophils.

It is a commonly held belief that the activated complement system and phagocytic cells are capable of defusing bacterial contamination in the magnitude of 10^3 colony-forming units per gram of tissue. If the degree of bacterial contamination is greater than this, obvious signs of infection appear, frequently heralded in the wound by the presence of pus. Concurrently, the person with such an infective source often experiences elevated temperature, malaise, tachycardia, decreased appetite, and the like.

Laboratory indicators of a situation in which the immune system has been strained, if not overwhelmed, are an elevated and simultaneous shift in the white blood count, revealing an increasing production of immature white blood cells (band cells). Though these cells are ineffective as phagocytic agents, this increased activity on the part of the body is a persistent attempt to forestall the deleterious effects of the pathogenic organism(s). This ineffective adaptive response is known as a *shift to the left* and is a classic indication of the presence of infection. Close monitoring of serial differential white blood cell counts may aid in the early detection of infection in the wound.

It is of interest to note that in the early search for the key cell in the healing process, the neutrophil was studied in depth. This cell, it was thought, triggered the systematic entrance into the wound area of the remaining significant cells. Careful research, using animal models, however, showed that neither the neutrophil nor the complement system were essential in the events which followed.[38,39] Animals made neutropenic and kept in a bacteria-free environment went on to heal; macrophages, fibroblasts, and collagen synthesis were apparent in the wound sites of the neutropenic experimental animals. While healing can proceed in the presence of neutropenia in the experimental setting, this is seldom the case with human beings, who frequently sustain infection, go on to develop sepsis, and often die. So, while the neutrophil and the complement system may not be essential for the orderly progression of cells into the wound, they are most likely essential to survival, except in a bacteria-free environment.

Lymphocytes follow the leucocytes, aiding in phagocytosis and playing a significant role in both humoral and cell-mediated immunity. Sensitized T lymphocytes destroy foreign antigens, while B lymphocytes, or circulating antibodies, attack invading microorganisms.

Approximately 24 h after the neutrophils reach their peak activity in the uncomplicated wound, there is an influx of monocytes which modulate to become macrophages. In addition to functioning as agents in the debridement of the wound, these cells are now believed to play a major role in *angiogenesis,* the formation of new blood vessels.[29,40] Without this ability to establish a new vascular supply capable of bringing nutrients to the wound, healing could not occur.

The macrophage appears to function optimally in, if not require, a certain degree of hypoxia at various stages.[31] Simply stated, the macrophage moves toward the leading edge of the severed vessel where the pH is low, the CO_2 is elevated, and the oxygen content is low. Here the macrophage, with a minimal backup vascular supply of nutrients, moves out from the leading edge of the vessel and secretes a substance known as *angiogenesis factor,* or AGF.[40]

Once AGF is present in the essentially devascularized space, it acts as an attractant to the altered vessel it has left and appears to pull the injured vessel toward it. In this manner new vessels move into previously anoxic areas, thereby bringing nutrient oxygen to cells and tissues in which it is vitally needed. Gradually, these new vessels form buds which link with surrounding budding vessels. Ultimately the vascular network is restored and healing progresses. Because of these findings, it is believed that people deficient in macrophages have greatly retarded, if not completely defective, healing.[29] Interestingly, in the uncomplicated wound closed by primary intention, these cells remain apparent in wound fluid for several weeks after wounding; in the open wound or a wound in which dead space is evidenced, they endure even longer. Evidence also suggests that macrophages may remain in the wound for protracted periods, up to and including cessation of the healing process.

The last cells to exhibit some activity during this initial phase of wound healing are the fibroblast and the epithelial cell. Fibroblasts, ultimately responsible for synthesizing collagen, the "glue" of wound healing,[34] are stimulated to divide, migrate, and produce collagen within 24 h of wounding. It will be recalled that PDGF is considered to be a key stimulator of this early activity.

Epithelial cells, which lie over the dermis, migrate toward one another until they meet other epithelial cells, after which migration ceases. The point at which these like cells meet and cease to migrate is known as the *contact inhibition point.* The reasons underlying this regulatory phenomenon have yet to be elucidated. Once the cells have ceased migrating, further mitosis occurs until the five layers of epithelium are restored. If a full-thickness wound has occurred (that is, loss of tissue through the dermis), the ancillary structures of hair follicles, sweat glands, and sebaceous glands, which are lined with epithelial cells, are absent. In this case, in order for the wound to be covered, epithelial cells must migrate from the edges of the wound. This situation occurs in full-thickness wounds which have been left open to heal, as opposed to those in which the dermis has not been injured. In the latter case, the epithelial cells have a little less than a 1-mm distance to migrate before meeting similarly migrating cells. Obviously then, epithelial migration is more prolonged in an open wound than in a partial-thickness wound or an intact incision.

This migratory function of epithelial cells occurs early in the healing process. A wound sutured at the time of surgery in a relatively healthy person is considered to be impervious to the outside world within 24 to 72 h after surgery[2] because of the ability of the epithelial cells to migrate and close the wound.

Much activity, then, occurs in this initial phase of healing. Alterations in the healing environment in the first hours or days after wounding can affect the milieu in such a way as to impede the later two stages. The nurse must direct every effort toward maximizing each phase of healing, but perhaps none more intensively than the inflammatory phase.

Fibroblastic Phase

The fibroblastic phase begins approximately 4 days after wounding and continues until the wound is approximately 3 weeks old. This phase of healing is characterized by a surge in cellular replication; thus it has also been referred to as the *proliferative phase* or the *reconstructive phase*. The degree of cellular replication occurring at this time is an attempt on the part of the body to restore the injured portion to its original state. The overall goal of this phase of healing is to increase the *tensile strength* (the amount of pressure required to interrupt the intact, healing wound) in the wound area. At the conclusion of the inflammatory phase the tensile strength at the wound site has risen from zero (immediately after injury) to only about 10 percent of the original full intactness of the tissue. During the second phase of healing, tensile strength rises sharply to approximately 50 percent of the original state.[2,41] Though no tissue surface once interrupted ever achieves its full original degree of intactness, most wounds heal to as much as 80 percent of it. Figure 56-2 presents a schematic depiction of the tensile strength curve. Note in particular the increased surge of strength gained at the wound site during the fibroblastic phase.

The cell most responsible for increasing the strength of the wound is the fibroblast. The fibroblasts, which first appear in the wound during the inflammatory phase, originate from two sources: resting fibrocytes (that is, inactive state) and mesenchymal cells located in the adventitia (that is,

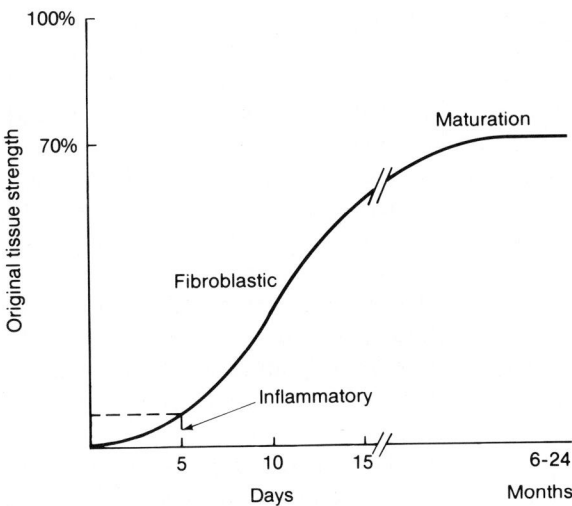

Figure 56-2   The tensile strength curve.

periphery) of small blood vessels in subcutaneous tissue and fat.[42]

In the traumatized region, the fibroblast moves into the hypoxic environment. Increased lactate concentration produced from the earlier activity of the macrophage is probably also a stimulus. Because the fibroblast favors a solid surface for migration, the fibrin network laid down early in the inflammatory phase is used as a directional guide. There must, however, be a vascular supply adjacent to these newly maturing cells in order to sustain activity. In addition to oxygen and ascorbate, these cells require amino acids, the B vitamins, and trace minerals as nutrients for the synthesis of collagen.

Fibroblasts synthesize collagen, a macromolecular substance ultimately responsible for giving strength and integrity to the wound.[43] Collagen is composed of approximately 1000 amino acids. These chains form cross-links which restore the integrity of the wounded tissue, allowing function to resume.

Though select cells from the inflammatory phase, in particular the macrophage and the epithelial cells, continue to function in the second phase of healing, the fibroblast is the primary functioning cell during this time. Thus this phase is appropriately described as *fibroblastic,* as opposed to proliferative or reconstructive.

Though a hardy cell, the fibroblast is affected deleteriously by a protracted suboptimal environment. Triggered to action by injury and initially stimulated to divide in mild hypoxia and an environment rich in ascorbate, like other cells it functions best in optimal conditions. In an open wound the results of this phase of healing can be observed. The healthy wound shows beefy, red, shiny tissue commonly termed *granulation tissue*. (Figure 56-3 is an example of the characteristics of this tissue.) The massive microcirculation which is established in the first few weeks after wounding regresses as healing evolves, but it is responsible for sustaining the loosely formed "patch" of collagen which imparts beginning strength to the interrupted tissue.[43]

The fibroblastic phase represents an early stage in the overall sequence of healing, and the

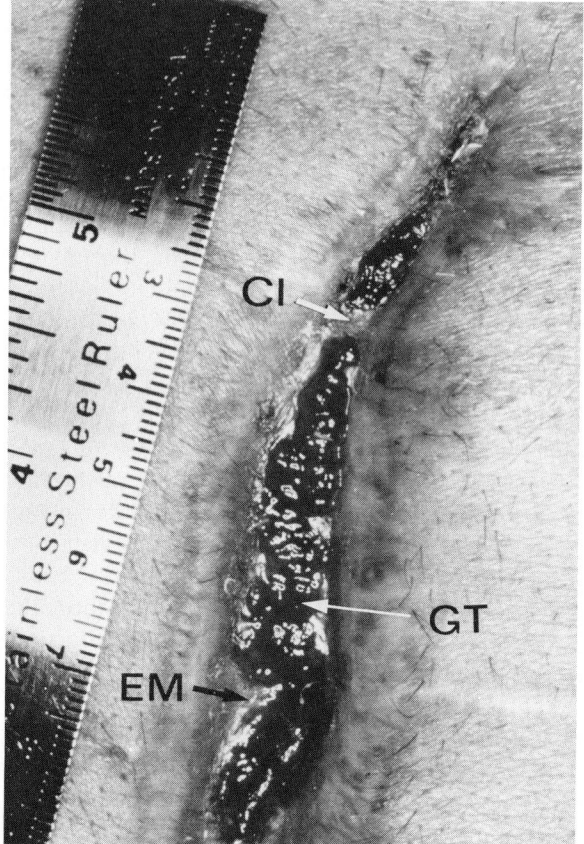

Figure 56-3 Wound healing by second intention. GT, granulation tissue; EM, epithelial migration beginning to cover GT; CI, contact inhibition or point at which epithelial cells have touched and migration has ceased.

wound has by no means acquired its ultimate strength. Often it is during this second phase of healing that patients begin to resume progressively independent activities. Both the patient and the nurse need to be mindful of the relatively short time since wounding and the decreased competence of the injured site to withstand a great deal of stress or strain.

It is also important to note that between postoperative days 5 and 12, surgical wounds have the greatest potential for dehiscence, fistula formation, or evisceration.[44] While evisceration is an untoward event easily recognized by most nurses, the other two sequelae are often more subtle and difficult to detect in the initial phases. Both *dehiscence* (the separation of a previously intact suture line) and *fistula formation* (most often a tubelike structure extending from an internal organ to an external opening on the skin) are recognizable by the presence of drainage (serous, purulent, fecallike, etc.) where previously there was a dry intact surface. Initially the volume of drainage is not as significant as the fact that the drainage has appeared. Even the smallest amount of drainage on a previously intact, dry surface should be inspected thoroughly and reported to the surgeon. Because of the proximity of the nurse and the frequent monitoring of the wound, nurses are the professionals most likely to recognize these changes and to institute restorative activities. With the growing emphasis on early discharge of the surgical patient and concurrent early resumption of potentially injurious activities, an increasing incidence of these sequelae could become apparent.

Maturation Phase

The final phase of healing begins approximately 3 weeks after wounding and ends 1 to 2 years later. The goal of this phase is acquisition of the maximum tensile strength achievable and realignment of the wound area in a manner as similar to its original functional state as possible. Tensile strength increases by as much as 30 percent over that achieved during the fibroplastic phase. Simultaneously, the incisional area or wound defect recedes and loses its reddish color; contraction and blanching result. Mobility of the wound area increases also as the dynamic interaction between collagen synthesis and collagen lysis, via collagenase and other lytic enzymes, causes the wound to become more malleable. This final phase of wound healing is characterized not by the presence of any "new" or particular cell but rather by the activity of lysozomal enzymes, which cleave collagen extracellularly and, in Hunt's graphic phrase, "protect us from being frozen in our own connective tissues."[34] Thus the healing process matures, leading toward resumption of the patient's prewounded level of activity.

Types of Healing

While wounds are as diverse in size, shape, and cause as the people who incur them, all healing can be divided into three categories according to whether it occurs by primary (first) intention, second intention, or tertiary (third) intention. Graphic illustrations of these forms of healing are numerous in the literature.[19,21,41]

Healing by primary intention, perhaps the most easily recognized, occurs in any wound in which (1) there is no tissue loss, (2) the edges are approximated, as in a sutured incision line or a bandaged finger, and (3) the observable process involves the migration of epithelial cells until intactness is restored. The process which describes the movement occurring during healing by primary intention is known as *epithelization.*

Healing by second intention occurs whenever there is tissue loss, even if the external skin remains intact (as in ischemic tissue on the heels resulting from shearing action or pressure), or whenever a wound is left open postoperatively. In gastrointestinal surgical procedures, the surgeon, cognizant of the bacterial risk inherent in this region, often sutures to the fascial or muscular layer and leaves the remaining tissues unapproximated. This common practice affords those caring for the patient the opportunity to dress the wound and remove exudate and lessens the risk of patient sepsis. Healing by second intention is also evident in any full-thickness wound in which the edges have not been approximated. Nonsurgical examples of such healing occur in stages III and IV pressure sores (those which have ulcerated through the dermis) and in full-thickness burns. Often patients with wounds healing by second intention require plastic surgery at a later date. This is undertaken to decrease the potential for herniation in large abdominal incisions or tissue breakdown in poorly vascularized scar tissue. The process involved in healing by second intention is described as granulation, contraction, and epithelization. Because of tissue loss and, in many cases, exposure of the tissue to the surrounding environment, these wounds take longer to heal, have a greater potential for infection, and result in scars unlike the surrounding tissue. An example of wound healing by second intention is shown in Fig. 56-3.

Healing by tertiary intention is more clearly termed *delayed primary closure* (DPC). This method of healing is reviewed historically and well described by Gottrup, Fogdestam, and Hunt.[44] By their definition, healing by DPC is "anatomically precise closure that is delayed a few days but accomplished before granulation tissue becomes visible (usually 8 to 10 days after wounding)." While used extensively in battle wounds, this form of healing has been used less often in civilian situations. It is useful in contaminated or dirty wounds, and should be used in a wound caused by high-velocity missiles.[44] It may also be a method of closure which has merit for a patient with decreased resistance.

A wound allowed to heal by delayed primary closure is usually left open through the subcutaneous tissue at the time of surgery. It is then sterile-dressed, and most often the original surgical dressing is left undisturbed. After approximately 4 days and prior to the appearance of granulated tissue, if there are no signs of infection, the surgeon approximates the wound edges at the bedside with Steri-Strips or in the operating room with sutures. It is of interest that these newly closed wounds do not appear to begin the healing trajectory anew; rather, they proceed on the healing course counting day one as the day of the original surgery.

Factors Affecting Healing

Ideally, all wounds pass through the phases of healing in a manner that results in maximal reintegration of tissue. Numerous factors, however, may alter healing deleteriously. Some classic examples of conditions which create environments unfavorable to optimal healing are malignant disease, diabetes mellitus, obesity, cardiovascular disease, malnutrition, and steroid treatment.[45-49] Failure to heal in some patients has led to intensive research in these areas. Documented evidence has emerged which can provide directives for clinical practice supportive of the healing environment and potentiate the body's inherent ability to heal. A few generic examples of alterations in the wound environment which, if not modified, may result in poor healing are presented below.

Oxygen and Volume

Oxygen is believed by most experts in wound healing to furnish the nutrition of the wound.[2,42,50] Not only is oxygen necessary to maintain cell structure, collagen synthesis, and cell viability, but it is also vital to the control of bacteria in the wound area.[51,52,53] Chang et al. and Niinikoski have clearly demonstrated that increased oxygen tension enhances healing, while reduction in available oxygen inhibits repair.[26,31] The Chang group demonstrated that wound hypoxia was hard to detect by clinical evaluations such as cardiac output, right ventricular end-diastolic pressure, or urinary output and was "unknowingly tolerated by experienced surgeons." They reported also that the measurement of oxygen at the *tissue* level best reflected the level of tissue perfusion.

It goes without saying that healing tissue cannot be oxygenated adequately unless intravascular volume also is maintained optimally. Volume and the supply of oxygen are linked inexorably and perhaps never more obviously than in healing. Because convenient methods of quantifying tissue perfusion are lacking, research has been undertaken to rectify this. In the not too distant future surgeons and nurses may be able to easily monitor the status of tissue oxygen and intravascular volume at the leading edge of the healing wound. When rates are suboptimal, flow and oxygen concentrations can be adjusted much as modifications are made in respiratory gases as the result of arterial blood level measurements. Such a technological advance can probably ensure optimization of healing. In the meantime, nurses in particular must astutely and continuously assess the oxygen and volume status of the patient, bearing in mind the significant diminution in gas concentration and flow rates that

often occurs secondary to a myriad of physiologic conditions. At the same time both surgeons and nurses need to remember the words of Niinikoski: "The traditional sacrosanct rate of healing is now under some human control. The rate of healing is known to be a function of arterial oxygen tension over a certain physiologic range. . . . Clinically it would seem a simple matter to advocate that enriched oxygen mixtures be given to patients at risk for wound hypoxia and complicated healing."[31]

Nutrition

Surgical procedures, injury, and trauma result in increased metabolic rate with resultant utilization of the body's energy stores. If nutritional intake is reduced, as is frequently the case in surgical patients, catabolism ensues. Though healing may occur during starvation, it is prolonged and often results in complications. In addition to decreased healing, depleted patients are particularly prone to sepsis because of suppression of their immune system.[54]

The untoward events which occur in the healing patient as the result of poor nutrition are easily reversed with proper nutritional intervention.[55] The reader is referred to Chap. 12 for an indepth discussion of nutrition and its implications in the care of the critically ill individual. In addition to ensuring adequate caloric intake and a positive nitrogen balance, the nurse caring for the healing patient must also ensure adequate vitamin intake.

Vitamins and Minerals

Too often it is assumed that the vitamin requirements for healing will be met through whatever nutritional source the patient is receiving or via body stores. This approach is unsound, as both water-soluble and fat-soluble vitamins function as cofactors in the healing process. Vitamin C (a water-soluble vitamin) is essential for the hydroxylation of proline, a constituent of collagen. Though most healthy persons store this vitamin, it is possible for the severely injured to exhaust these stores in as little as 24 to 48 h. Studies have shown that daily doses of between 500 and 3000 mg of ascorbic acid significantly accelerate healing in seriously injured or surgical patients.[56]

Other vitamins important in healing are vitamin A,[57,58] significant in angiogenesis; the B-complex vitamins, utilized by fibroblasts for collagen synthesis; and vitamin K, necessary for clotting. Often the person with impaired liver function evidences altered healing as the result of increased bleeding at the wound site. This collection of blood creates what is commonly referred to as a *dead space*. Because of the increased distance nutrients, including oxygen, must traverse as a result of this complication, healing is compromised at the leading edge of the wound. Rubin states that oral antibiotics also may disturb vitamin K synthesis by altering the intestinal flora required for its production.[59]

With hyperalimentation and documentation of some of the sequelae which occurred in the initial years of its use has come an appreciation of the role of trace elements. While understanding of their role within the body in general and healing in particular has yet to be unraveled, two trace elements, copper and zinc, are known to have specific activities required for optimal healing.

Much debate has surrounded the administration of zinc. In the not too distant past it was regarded by some as having the ability to accelerate the healing process in everyone, including the healthy.[60] After repeated unsuccessful attempts to replicate the startling findings reported, however, this power of zinc is no longer accepted.[61] In fact, excessive zinc is now considered to be potentially harmful to healing, causing, among other things, immobilization of some inflammatory cells.[62] It should be noted, though, that in numerous conditions—among them burns, malnutrition, chronic diarrhea, and severe trauma—zinc levels are reduced; these levels need to be assessed and supplemental zinc given if needed in order to return body levels to normal. Whenever there is zinc depletion, healing is promoted by the restoration of this element to normal levels.[63]

Steroids

Numerous physiologic conditions require treatment with steroids. Though these potent substances have assisted patients to function more productively with rheumatoid arthritis, ulcerative colitis, Crohn's disease, and lupus erythematosis, they are not without serious side effects, one of the most haz-

ardous being the alteration they may cause in the healing process. Wound dehiscence is far more common in patients receiving steroids, and their wounds have an increased potential for infection and protracted healing.

Steroids affect inflammation and the influx of numerous cells essential for optimal healing. As a result, the inflammatory phase of wound healing is largely suppressed. As Hunt warned, "Failure of repair most often occurs in the milieu of disordered inflammation."[29] Thus the deleterious effects of steroids should come as no surprise. Several groups of researchers have demonstrated that the negative effects of chronic steroid ingestion can be reversed in the healing patient by simultaneous administration of vitamin A or cessation of the steroids during the first 4 to 5 days postsurgery.[64–66] If this vitamin is given in the first 7 days after surgery, vascular ingrowth and epithelization are promoted. The antagonism between the two (vitamin A and the steroid) apparently occurs within the wound itself. This relatively short course of vitamin therapy does not appear to have consequences unfavorable to the underlying condition for which the steroids were originally prescribed.[67] Vitamin A should be used with caution in patients in whom re-initiation of the inflammatory response would be hazardous to the outcome of their surgical procedure (e.g., organ transplantation). The salubrious effects for the healing environment and the progress of healing in other steroid-dependent patients would seem to outweigh a transient exacerbation of the underlying condition even if it should occur.

Other Factors

Age, previous medical and surgical history, and body build are other factors known to affect the healing environment. Though it is imperative that the nurse assess these conditions in light of their effects on healing, there is little one can do to directly alter them.

Approaches to Wound Care

Dressings

Traditionally wounds have been cared for by being dressed with gauze and various solutions. The ideal dressing, whatever its constituents, possesses three characteristics:

1. It absorbs exudate and thereby removes bacteria.
2. It permits some evaporation of fluid.
3. It is sufficiently fragile to allow removal without jeopardizing healing of the wound.[69]

Perhaps no aspect of local wound care is less well understood than these three characteristics, especially the last. While in the past it was frequently taught that a wound which bled was a "healthy" wound, advances in knowledge now point to such concepts as ill-founded. Recalling the theoretical description of wound healing brings into stark view the numerous complex steps and enormous amount of energy that are expended in the exquisite process of new vessel and tissue formation. Newly formed vessels supply the nutrients necessary for the continued maintenance and building of healthy tissue. Destruction of the vascular supply and the tissue it nourishes is to be avoided at all costs. While it is true that exudate and necrotic tissue must be removed from the wounded area in the most expeditious manner, this should not be done in a way which jeopardizes, let alone destroys, healthy tissue. Causing a wound to bleed by severing newly formed vessels is nonsupportive to the healing process. Some authors have gone so far as to state that the tearing off of a dressing which has become incorporated into the tissue (that is, stuck to, adherent to) is not only negative in relation to healing but also "cruel, unkind, and inhumane."[68]

The majority of wounds continue to be dressed with cotton dressings in the form of gauze. Before describing the specific functions of various gauzes, it is important to recall that the traditional wound dressing is composed of three layers: gauze, which lies in direct contact with the wound tissue; the absorptive layer, usually containing some form of cotton lining; and the outermost, or securing, layer. The second layer of the traditional gauze dressing functions as a wick, absorbing moisture and allowing some evaporation of the moisture caused by the exudate in the wound and the solution contained in the gauze layer. The outermost layer of the traditional dressing holds the other layers of the dressing in place. While in the past dressings were secured with adhesive tape, new modalities have appeared on the scene which are far less irritating to the skin.

Gauze is formed from cotton threads forming open squares known as *interstices*. The size as well as the malleability of these interstices varies with different types of gauze. It was Noe and Kalish who perhaps most clearly described the significance of proper selection of gauze, taking into account the size of the interstices, in the approach to care of a specific wound.[70]

Most open wounds manifesting healthy tissue can be maintained in that state by the use of 4 × 4 moist gauze dressings. Such a dressing can also effectively enhance debridement of a small, moderately exudative wound. Larger interstices, such as those in breast fluffs or Kerlix, if properly placed in the wound are thought to more readily trap debris or exudate, while gauze with small interstices (fine-mesh gauze) does not facilitate debridement. Proper selection of gauze dressings, therefore, may assist in moving the wound toward speedier healing.

Before progressing to a description of the various types of dressings which can be applied to wounds, it is important to point out that when traditional dressings are used, absorptive dressings with cotton filling or liners should never be placed directly next to the tissue in an open wound. In addition to lacking open interstices and therefore being ineffective debriding agents, the cotton fibers may shed and be trapped in the wound. When cotton fibers are trapped they act as foreign substances and unless removed may initiate an inflammatory reaction.

Immediate Postsurgical Dressing

The initial postoperative dressing placed on an incision closed by primary intention should meet all the requirements of the ideal dressing. Many dressings described by the manufacturers as nonadherent in reality become incorporated into the drainage from the wound as it dries. While this adherent state presents no immediate noticeable discomfort to the patient, the potential is great for subsequent damage to healing tissue and even pain for the patient when the dressing is removed. Several dressings have recently become available which provide high absorbency and have qualities which keep them free from incorporation with drainage at the suture line. In this regard it is important for nurses to be aware of products which are available in order that they may suggest adoption of those which foster a positive healing environment.

Until high-absorbency, nonadherent dressings are more widely adopted, if drainage should appear on the dressing in the absence of drains, the nurse should circle the area with a pen and note the time adjacent to the marking. A small amount of drainage is not unusual, but any increasing drainage must be investigated, preferably with the surgeon present. The timeworn nursing practice of multiple markings or reinforcement of an increasingly saturated dressing is not only unsound but may ultimately be a harmful activity. As has been noted, wounds in which drainage has been allowed to accumulate heal less well. In addition, numerous areas of dried drainage on a dressing only potentiate the possibility of eventual disruption along the suture line when the dressing is removed. Therefore, if any significant oozing occurs even on the initial postoperative dressing, it is best to change, or to request the surgeon to change, the dressing before complete drying and incorporation of the drainage within the dressing has occurred.

The healing incision closed by primary intention is reepithelized within 24 to 72 h in the healthy person. While tensile strength is markedly reduced, the wound is considered sealed at this point and is, if uninterrupted, impervious to bacterial contamination. Theoretically then, a dressing is not necessary after this time. Often, however, initial dressings are left in place longer. Frequently patients do not desire to view a freshly healing incision, or because of the wound position on the body, clothes and/or other body parts may act as irritants. In these latter situations, the maintenance of a dressing over the suture line serves the sole purpose of protection. In patients whose system is compromised in any way, or in the case of an incision line in which contamination is a real possibility, continuation of dressings beyond the 72-h period is warranted.

Increasingly, patients who have undergone cardiac surgery in particular return to the unit with no dressing covering the incision or with orders directing removal of the dressing within 24 h of surgery. This seems appropriate in the healthy person, as long as those caring for the patient bear in mind the minimal tensile strength of the suture line. Frequently, however, orders are also written directing the nurse to cleanse the suture line daily (and sometimes more frequently) with betadine, hydrogen peroxide, or a combination of the two or to apply topical antimicrobials. These approaches to the care of the incision warrant systematic study, for depending on how the procedure is carried out, there may be a potential for disruption of the suture line and bacterial contamination. While scab formation is not the goal of all healing, it can serve as a reinforcing, semipermeable barrier providing additional protection and support to underlying tissue. Left to natural processes, new epithelial cells burrow under the scab and migrate toward one another until they meet. At this point the wound is sealed. When the intact surface is restored, the scab lifts off unaided. Until research data substantiate the superiority of other practices over simple support of normal healing in the intact incision, daily cleansing of the incision line should be questioned, if not discouraged. Often the degree of encrusted drainage which leads to excessive scab formation on the suture lines can be reduced by the adoption of high-absorbency, nonadherent dressings in the immediate postoperative period.

Wound Healing by Second Intention

In the wound left open to heal by second intention, several approaches to wound care are available. When gauze is used, the type of dressing and size of interstices should be selected on the basis of the characteristics and amount of exudate and the size of the wound. In the smaller wound individual dressings may be used (e.g., 2 × 2 or 4 × 4), whereas in the larger wound with tenacious exudate, a continuous dressing such as Kerlex may be more appropriate. Whichever is used, the nurse should carefully note and record the number of individual dressings or the length of continuous dressings inserted in the wound. In addition to ensuring safe retrieval of all dressing material at the next dressing change, this information also serves as a more objective method of monitoring progress of wound healing. Obviously, as the wound fills in with granulation tissue the amount of dressing material required to fill the wound decreases.

Noting the quantity of gauze in serial fashion provides the nurse with additional information for evaluating healing.

In all circumstances in which gauze is used as a medium to facilitate debridement of exudate or necrotic debris in a wound, it should first be opened so that it is one layer thick. Subsequent to treating it with a solution, it should then be carefully laid against the open tissue so that the interstices come in direct contact with all the tissue. After the floor, the walls, and the crevices of the wound are covered in this manner, the remaining central cavity of the wound is filled in with additional moist gauze. While it is imperative that all tissue surfaces be touched by the gauze dressing, it is equally important to avoid packing the dressing tightly. Two reasons for not packing the wound tightly are that such packing reduces the salutary evaporation which occurs when gauze is less tightly packed and that tight packing may impair perfusion of the wound.

Wet-to-Dry Dressing   Recalling that the ideal dressing should allow some evaporation and should not become incorporated into the eschar, it is necessary to assess anew the traditional methods of wound treatment. A dressing which is meant to facilitate debridement should do just that. At the same time, it should not be injurious to newly forming tissue. If a dressing is allowed to fully dry out and become adherent to the wound, it will injure healthy tissue as it is pulled away from the surface. In this light, if a *wet-to-dry dressing* is defined as a moist dressing placed in a wound and allowed to become fully dry so that on removal healthy tissue is traumatized (that is, bleeds), its use is a nontherapeutic intervention and should be avoided.[15,68,70]

Wet-to-Damp Dressing   A *wet-to-damp dressing,* on the other hand, is defined as a moist dressing placed in the wound which on removal manifests some tackiness or stickiness as it separates from the tissue. The wet-to-damp dressing removes exudate but does not injure healthy tissue and optimally fulfills the characteristics of a debriding dressing when gauze is used. Frequently, in order to determine the optimal time interval between dressing changes to ensure the desired degree of

evaporation, several dressing changes must be observed.

If the nurse is to be supportive of the healing environment, wet-to-damp dressings as described are as dry as dressings should be allowed to become. It is to be hoped that nurses or physicians seldom allow a dressing to become so dried that it must be torn from the wound, causing new tissue to bleed. Nevertheless, nurses need to clarify physician's orders for wet-to-dry dressings. Prepared with theoretically sound information and research data, nurses need to establish standards with physicians which determine how the wound with dressings will be debrided. Once this is established, all staff involved in the care and treatment of such wounds should follow practices which are known to support tissue healing.

Wet-to-Wet Dressing   As debridement of the wound progresses, increasing amounts of new tissue fill the wound space. This granulation tissue, when healthy, is beefy, red, and shiny. It is a combination of collagen and the multiple new vessels created during healing. Granulation tissue needs to be protected and kept moist. In order to accomplish this, the relatively debris-free wound is treated with a *wet-to-wet dressing*. This dressing is defined as one which is put in the wound moist and is lifted out of the wound easily (frequently still moist) at the next dressing change. The purpose of this dressing is the maintenance of healthy tissue and the promotion of epithelial migration. Dressing materials with smaller interstices are used here, as entrapment of exudate into larger openings is no longer an objective. The interval between dressing changes which best facilitates removal from the wound more freely than the wet-to-damp dressing often requires evaluation after several dressing changes. Most often the interval between dressing changes is shorter than that established for the wet-to-damp dressing. Small wounds must be assessed more closely because they have a tendency to dry out more rapidly.

Solutions

Some laugh, others are dismayed at the list of "nostrums and hokums" compiled by Rudolph as he logged some remedies placed in wounds in the name of healing.[83] Substances as bizarre as turnips, garlic, licorice root, and cinnamon are listed there alongside the more familiar solutions of hydrogen peroxide, boric acid, Dakin's solution, and acetic acid. In the introductory passage the author cautioned, however, that while there is no sound physiologic basis for the use of these agents, they "do in fact provide improved wound care," most probably, he continues, because of the diligence of the person caring for the wound and the consistency of the treatment.

On the other hand, there are solutions which have been studied to varying degrees and which are thought to act as facilitators of healing if used correctly. Obviously, much could be written on just the solutions in use today; however, this section addresses only four of the more commonly used solutions: normal saline, hydrogen peroxide, betadine, and hypochlorite (Dakin's solution).

At the outset suffice it to say that there is no perfect solution. Every solution, even the most bactericidal, presents problems. At one time it was thought that nothing should be placed in the wound—that it should be allowed to progress through the stages of healing unaltered, mustering strength from the natural resources inherent in the body.[84] Among modifications of this stance was the criterion that nothing be placed in a wound that caregivers would not put in their own eye.[50] Perhaps there is some value in both these guidelines. Clinical practice, however, has not followed either, so it behooves those involved in wound care to be aware of the strengths and limitations of the solutions in use. In addition, it is important to understand the most effective manner of using them.

Normal Saline

Normal (physiologic) saline is a solution of sodium and chloride in a concentration of 0.9%, equivalent to the tonicity of the human body (isotonic), so that it causes minimal shifts between intracellular and extracellular fluid. Normal saline has no bactericidal or bacteriostatic properties but serves well as an irrigating solution or as a solution to be used on a dressing in a relatively healthy, debris-free wound that is well on its way to healing. When used as a solution on a dressing in a healthy, debris-free wound it helps to keep granulation tissue appropriately moist and facilitates epithelial migra-

tion. At times normal saline is also used in combination with gauze in wounds with obvious exudate; but other solutions are known to be more effective than normal saline in the presence of bacteria, so its use in an exudative wound should be questioned.

Hydrogen Peroxide

Hydrogen peroxide (H_2O_2) is an oxidizing agent which contains 3% hydrogen peroxide in water and decomposes to oxygen and water. When peroxide comes in contact with tissue or organic matter, it releases molecular oxygen, causing a brief period of antimicrobial action. This action can render organic matter inert (inactive). Oxidizing agents such as hydrogen peroxide are purported to be especially harmful to anaerobic organisms; however, Peacock took exception to this, stating that "such a brief exposure obviously does not affect tough anaerobes."[50] Aerobes respond variously to oxidizing agents, depending on their sensitivity to oxygen. Hydrogen peroxide is an active, mild germicide only while it is actively releasing oxygen; it is this action which is thought to help cleanse wounds.[85]

At no time should H_2O_2 be placed in closed body cavities or tracts from which the gas being emitted cannot easily escape.[86,87] In one report, irrigation of an infected, fistulous herniorrhaphy wound with 3% hydrogen peroxide resulted in the patient developing shock and coma, from which he recovered. The authors pointed out that "the mechanism of this occurrence was most likely widespread embolization of oxygen microbubbles released from absorbed H_2O_2."[88]

Repeated use of hydrogen peroxide as a daily irrigant with each dressing change requires study to determine its effect on newly forming tissue. Full strength peroxide has been observed to cause formation of bullae (blisters) on wounds in which it was repeatedly used.[89]

One questions the use of H_2O_2 as a solution to be applied to a dressing for continuous use in the wound. It will be recalled that once oxygen is released only water remains. Water is neither bacteriostatic nor bactericidal, and its tonicity is less than that of the body (hypotonic). Continuous proximity of the wound tissue to a hypotonic solution may result in cell swelling, if not cell lysis.

Finally, it should be pointed out that hydrogen peroxide can cause pain to the patient; for this reason it is suggested that it be diluted with normal saline to at least half strength before use.[90]

Betadine

Povidone-iodine solution, more commonly referred to as *betadine,* is one of the most frequently used treatments in the care of wounds. It is made up of iodine in complex with a nonsurfactant carrier, polyvinylpyrrolidone (PVP). Iodine alone is unstable and insoluble in water, though it is extremely germicidal.[91] At times betadine can be irritating to the skin and cause local reactions. This solution has been used to treat wound infections caused by bacteria, fungi, and even viruses. As a result of documented evidence of betadine's ability to effect such bactericidal, antifungal, and possibly antiviral results, it ranks ahead of many of the other available solutions in the minds of many clinicians.

Despite an initial assessment of the salutary potential of this solution, a more in-depth analysis reveals that betadine also has some potentially harmful characteristics. Hunt described the potentially deleterious effects of this solution on any tissue other than surface intact tissue.[2] Because of betadine's high-molecular-weight fraction and the kidney's inability to excrete such large molecules, several authors discourage its use on large surfaces of open tissue, particularly in patients with compromised renal status.[2, 16] They cite elevated serum iodide levels and associated renal failure, metabolic acidosis, and elevated serum glutamic oxaloacetic transaminase as some of the effects of topical application of this solution over large surfaces. Pietsch and Meakins documented similar results in the use of betadine with burn patients, concluding that it should be used cautiously, and not at all on patients with burns involving 20 percent of the body or more or in the presence of renal failure.[92]

Berkelman, Holland, and Anderson investigated reports of intrinsic contamination of 10% povidone-iodine with *Pseudomonas cepacia*.[93] Using dilutions of betadine and stock solutions exposed to five different bacterial species commonly found in hospitals and in wounds, they demonstrated "more rapid killing of *Staphylococcus aureus* and *Mycobacterium chelonei* in dilutions of 1:2, 1:4, 1:10, 1:50 and 1:100 than [with] the stock (full strength) solution." Furthermore, "*S. aureus* survived a 2-min exposure to full strength providone-iodine solution but did not survive a 15-sec exposure to a 1:100 dilution of iodophor." Although the chemistry of povidone-iodine is admittedly complex and difficult to explain, several investigators propose the possibility that "free iodine," the antimicrobial property, is more tightly bound to the PVP at higher concentrations, resulting in less antibacterial activity; more dilute preparations could result in greater availability of the free iodine,[16,93,94] hence greater antimicrobial activity.

What does all this mean for the clinician? Initially it must be concluded that betadine, despite its broad spectrum, is not the perfect solution. Like many aspects of wound care at this point, betadine is not a panacea and must be used judiciously. Second, although Berkelman, Holland and Anderson were quick to state the need for in vitro clinical trials before their findings were implemented with patients,[93] others suggest that use of full-strength (10%) betadine should be avoided, particularly on large or frequently dressed wounds.[2,16,92] Third, betadine should be avoided in patients with altered renal status. Finally, the effects of betadine on open wound tissue and systemic function demand in-depth study. Zamora wrote that "it seems warranted to perform prospective clinical trials to evaluate the role of povidone-iodine in the prevention and treatment of wound infection."[16] Until the findings of such studies become available, nurses who are in a position to make suggestions regarding wound care need to do so knowledgeably; and, as regards the use of betadine, they would do well to pay heed to the advice offered by Caretto: "Its use in patients warrants close observation and monitoring."[95]

Dakin's Solution

Diluted sodium hypochlorite, or modified Dakin's solution, is a 0.5% aqueous solution of sodium hypochlorite. In the wound it releases chlorine and oxygen and is effectively bactericidal for many organisms. *Dakin's solution,* as it is commonly called, was developed for use in World War I,[96] though origins of its use as sodium hypochlorite can be traced to the 16th century.[97] Semmelweis used hypochlorite as a handwashing solution in the mid 1800s in an attempt to reduce the number of deaths from puerperal fever. It is interesting to read in a 1963 nursing text that modified Dakin's solution was "once used extensively in suppurating wounds,"[90] for it continues to be used to this day in many patient situations. In fact, Rudolph reported that the most useful debriding agent was 0.25% strength Dakin's.[83] In addition to its debriding characteristics and its ability to dissolve necrotic debris as described by Taylor and Austen,[98] Rudolph also cited its low cost, which in 1983 he recorded as $6.69/8000 mL, or $0.87/L.[83]

Dakin's is used in wounds as an irrigant and on dressings as a continuous wound care treatment. One author stated that chlorines in general, of which Dakin's solution is a modification, are more effective when the wound has decreased amounts of organic matter, an acid environment, and an elevated temperature.[90] It does not, however, penetrate deeply into necrotic tissue. In addition to the rationale previously presented for avoiding wet to dry dressings, Dakin's, in particular, should not be put on dressings which are allowed to dry out. Such a situation reduces its effectiveness as a debriding agent.[83] Since it is a chlorine derivative, it should come as no surprise that it acts as a deodorant and has some properties of a bleach.

Full-strength (0.5%) Dakin's can be painful to some patients. In this case the solution should be changed to half strength (0.25%) or quarter strength (0.125%). It is important, noted Rudolph, that when writing pharmacy requests for Dakin's the desired strength be written, because too often it is forgotten that full-strength modified Dakin's is equivalent to 0.5%.[83]

Besides causing pain in some patients, Dakin's is known frequently to cause erythema on intact skin. One way of protecting the skin surrounding the wound and at the same time possibly providing a beneficial treatment is to apply zinc oxide. It should be reapplied with each dressing change and removed only once daily for the purpose of assessing the status of the skin. Zinc oxide is most easily removed by applying mineral oil to an absorptive dressing and wiping the area in one direction. Finally, modified Dakin's solution deteriorates more rapidly than other solutions, so the expiration date should be noted. Also, the solution should be kept out of bright light and not set near heaters or on window ledges.

Pouches

If healing does not progress and exudate becomes so excessive that dressing changes are required at intervals of 2 h or less, placement of a drainable pouch should be considered. Not only has this device been modified to allow easy access to the wound via windows, but it also protects the skin from maceration and irritation caused by caustic effluent, assists in quantification and analysis of effluent for replacement, and, by obviating frequent dressing changes, affords the patient fewer interruptions and longer periods of rest.[21]

Hydrophilic Beads

Though used primarily as a dressing medium for the treatment of decubitus ulcers, hydrophilic beads may be applied to wounds other than ulcers.[71] The beads are, in fact, dextran polymers and exhibit exceptional osmotic pull. While they do not digest debris, they lift bacteria off the surface of the wound. When the wound surface is irrigated the beads and bacteria are readily flushed away. There are several types of these beads, and some have been investigated extensively. In 1983 Oredsson, Gottrup, Beckman, and Hohn demonstrated an increased influx of white blood cells, in particular polymorphonuclear leucocytes and mononuclear leucocytes, into wound fluid and human sera treated with dextranomer.[72] They concluded that dextranomer "caused alternate pathway complement activation and profoundly increased the capacity of these fluids to attract leucocytes." Whether these chemoattractant characteristics "actually enhance the microbial resistance of the wound or accelerate wound healing," as claimed by these authors, the use of these beads, particularly in patients with impaired ability to muster an inflammatory response, could be salubrious, although it remains to be seen whether these characteristics are to be found in all polymerized dextrans.

These hydrophilic beads are not a panacea for all wounds. An initial requirement for their effective use is that the wound exudate should be moist. Second, a wound for which their use is being considered should be free of fistulae, tracts, or crevices from which removal of the beads would be difficult. Because these beads are cleansing agents and do not enzymatically debride bacteria or necrotic tissue, they act in a fashion similar to a traditional gauze dressing: the wound is cleaner when the beads are removed, much as the wound is hypothesized to be cleaner when the gauze dressing is changed. Therefore, a wound in which hydrophilic beads are used should also allow free and total removal of all beads with each irrigation.

Most beads are manufactured in powdered form and can be placed in the wound in that form. Because of the difficulty in maintaining an even distribution of the beads over the tissue when they are dry, however, it is perhaps more effective and efficient to make them into a paste. Instructions for this procedure are usually included with the product. Suffice it to say that it is imperative for the nurse to follow the directions of the manufacturer closely. One product in particular requires the beads be applied in a ¼-in layer over the tissue, and modifications should not be attempted because of the likelihood of decreasing the effectiveness of the beads. Likewise there are guidelines regarding time intervals between dressing changes. These intervals are usually based on the amount of exudate, and the time interval between applications may be as long as 12 to 24 h. Increasing the number of times the beads are replaced to the frequency used with traditional gauze dressings should be questioned. As a consequence of fewer patient interruptions when hydrophilic beads are used, the patient is allowed more time to rest, the nurse is required to do fewer dressing changes, and fewer supplies are needed. All these benefits, in addition to the proven chemoattractant characteristics and the ability of these beads to draw out bacteria nonselectively, should counter arguments regarding cost. Although their cost exceeds that of some traditional approaches to wound care, reduced nursing time, improved healing, and shortened hospitalization are all strong arguments for their selection with certain patients.

Irrigation is the optimal method of removing hydrophilic beads from a wound. Using adequate amounts of normal saline, all beads must be flushed from the wound, including the rim, at each scheduled wound care treatment. The nurse should wear gown, mask, and goggles to avoid contamination from the bacteria contained in fluid droplets deflected from the wound during irrigation. If this procedure must be carried out with the patient in bed, irrigant and old beads may be easily drained from the wound by the concurrent use of a disposable tonsil suction device attached to a wall suction mechanism. Only when all beads have been removed from the wound should tissue be assessed for healing status.

Irrigation

While in the past nurses have had few guidelines to direct them in the best method of irrigating a wound, more recently clinical directives have appeared which are based on research.[73–75] In most cases it is the nurse who selects the type of equipment to be used when there is an order to irrigate a wound. Therefore, it is important that sound criteria exist to assist in this selection.

It should be recalled that the purpose of irrigation is "to mechanically remove devitalized tissue, dirt, debris, and microorganisms from the wound surface."[75] Additionally, irrigation is now used to remove wound care treatment agents from the wound—for example, hydrophilic beads.

Several facts can be summarized regarding irrigation of wounds in general. First, irrigation is more effective in fresh wounds than in older wounds.[76] Second, an increasing degree of pressure (measured in pounds per square inch) emitted from the irrigating device via the stream of irrigant increases the effectiveness of the irrigation with regard to removal of bacteria from the tissue surface.[77–80] Ideally, a wound with devitalized tissue and debris is irrigated at 70 lb/in² pulsatile pressure.

Increasingly, manufacturers are developing irrigating devices which incorporate scientific findings, are disposable, and can be used with relative ease. Pulsatile high-powered irrigation sets are not always available or appropriate, however, and the nurse must then modify the procedure. Studies have shown that the smaller the syringe and the larger the needle bore the greater the pressure exerted.[78] Example: Given a 6-mL syringe and a 19-gauge needle, the pressure exerted is 32 lb/in, whereas a 35-mL syringe with the same size needle exerts only 9 lb/in². While the 6-mL syringe is impractical, particularly for wounds of large size, the 35-mL syringe with a 19-gauge plastic angiocatheter has been shown to be effective in irrigating wounds. The Asepto syringe, on the other hand, used frequently by nurses and physicians in the past to irrigate wounds, has been found to be an ineffective irrigating device.[81] In controlled studies comparing the Asepto syringe with other irrigating devices and nonirrigated control wounds, the Asepto syringe was found to effect no significant difference in bacterial count over the unirrigated wounds. The Asepto syringe exerts about 0.05 lb/in² pressure, and the conclusion is drawn, correctly, that it should not be used for wound irrigation.[75]

There has been debate over the potential of irrigating devices, particularly high-pressure pulsatile devices, to drive bacteria deeper into the wound. Most methods of irrigation in the studies cited thus far have shown reduced bacterial counts in the wound immediately after irrigation. It has been demonstrated, however, that wounds irrigated by high-pressure pulsatile irrigation and then closed and left closed for 4 days contained significantly more bacteria than wounds not treated with such aggressive irrigation.[82] While the conclusion may be drawn that high-pressure pulsatile irrigation is not without some hazards, it should also be pointed out that in the clinical setting few wounds are irrigated and then taped shut. Instead, dressing materials and further irrigations ensue until the wound is healed. Stotts and also Wheeler have suggested that pulsatile irrigation (70 lb/in²) be used only in heavily contaminated wounds.[75,82]

In concluding this section it is important to restate the necessity of the nurse's use of a gown, mask, and when possible, glasses or goggles as a protection from droplet-borne organisms deflected during irrigation of the wound. Not only do such practices safeguard the nurse from bacterial contamination, but ultimately they also protect other patients from cross-contamination by the nurse.

Criteria for Evaluation of Healing

To date no systematic methods of visual assessment of surgical wound healing exist which are adaptable for use in the clinical setting. In addition, healing as a visually observable process has not been defined in a consistent manner. Nurses lack definitions of *healing* and *healed* as process assessments which can be observed and have specific criteria.

In many ways evaluations of healing are rooted in personal experiences of injury or in the types of wound that have been observed in practice. This lack of objective criteria leads to a situation in which observations vary with the observer and tend to be subjective. The adage "we see what we know" becomes evident when one reviews nurses' notes[12] or listens to the day-to-day assessments of wound status. Several nurses have ameliorated and others are attempting to ameliorate this lack of effective measurement devices through the development of tools aimed at measuring healing.[11,99,100] This complex task is in its infancy.

Until such tools are available, some suggested criteria are indicated which may aid in the assessment of healing and direct the nurse toward objective evaluation. On initial inspection of the incision line or open wound the nurse should observe it closely and document the findings in the nurses' notes. If the wound is healing by second intention, the color of the tissue, the amount of exudate and its color and characteristics (tenacious, watery, etc.), the presence or absence of suture material, and the presence or absence of epithelial migration at the rim or edge of the wound (Fig. 56-3) should be described. Generally speaking, nurses need to use more adjectives when describing the wound, with particular emphasis on color, sheen of tissue, and percentage of the wound covered by exudate. If the wound is described in this manner from the outset, evaluation of the progression or regression of healing will be facilitated. Both nurses and physicians could rely on these notes as a chronicle of the progress in healing.

Second, there must be a plan of care which is adhered to by all. If modifications are made in the plan, the rationale for the change should be documented in the nurses' notes. When the selected intervention involves the use of traditional dressings, they should be placed in the wound as described previously. The number of dressings used or the length of gauze material should be recorded. As healing progresses and the wound requires fewer dressings, the nurse again will have more objective criteria on which to base evaluation.

While it is obvious that all treatments directed at wound care should, when possible, emanate from research and be based on an understanding of the physiology of healing, too frequent changing of the therapy in use should be avoided. Whenever possible an intervention should be assessed over several days, unless obvious indications for its cessation arise. Given several days, those caring for the wound can assess the impact of the intervention more critically. The focus of attention in the care and treatment of any wound is healthy tissue; therefore, monitoring and logging the amount of this tissue in serial fashion is imperative. Unless healthy tissue is apparent over time, the approach to care and the overall status of the patient must be reassessed in depth. Serum albumin levels, differential white blood cell counts, vitamin intake, weight, and oxygen and volume status should be the focus of such an evaluation as the nurse endeavors to ensure an environment supportive of healing.

Conclusion

The pervasive attitude among health care professionals often seems to have been that one way or another the wound would heal. In some circles the adage, "I dressed the wound, God healed it" still prevails. For the most part, the wound has been viewed as a passive lesion to which little except "custodial care" can be given. Only recently have wounding and optimal healing begun to be systematically chronicled. The results of such rigorous research clearly reveal the dynamism of healing. Despite the fact that with few exceptions healing starts and stops in a predictable fashion,[2] it is now known that restorative activities are induced in the body at the time of injury which require energy and support. They have the single goal of reintegration of the organism.

As the healing trajectory is described in detail, aspects which support healing can likewise be analyzed. It is now known that healing will occur in a more favorable fashion if certain actions are taken proactively, including maintenance of a well-oxygenated state, adequate volume to perfuse capillaries, increased nutritional and vitamin intake, maintenance of a moist environment for epithelial migration, and vigilant protection of the fragile wound after injury or surgery. At the same time, conditions which are potentially hazardous can be altered. The patient receiving chronic steroids can receive vitamin A in the early postoperative period;

the person with diabetes can be closely monitored so that changes in glucose levels are minimized; the obese patient's incisional area can be protected in a manner that acknowledges decreased vascularization and oxygenation of adipose tissue.

The attitude that the wound will heal in spite of us or because someone has looked at it frequently is no longer tolerable. As Rudolph stated, "the most important factor in any wound care is the person attending the wound and not the particular regimen used" and again, "a nurse or physician who is interested in the wound's care is more powerful than any other wound remedy."[83] While many of the approaches to wound care require further study, there is no question regarding the significance of the knowledgeable and skilled wound attendant.

Early writings in nursing attributed healing to nurses' vigilance. Harmer and Henderson pointed out in regard to decubitus ulcers that "the prevention of bedsores is entirely the responsibility of the nurse.... The neglect and ignorance of one nurse may in a few hours undo the most skilled and devoted care of another."[101] Levine repeated the words of Nightingale who said: "The purpose of nursing [is] astonishingly direct. The nurse must supplement the forces of nature so that repair can take place."[102]

Though nurses assess, care for, and suggest alterations in approaches to the treatment of wounds, they do so with vigor of varying intensity. Some of this is explained by the fact that scholars of healing have not yet been nurses. As a result, information regarding healing and interventions amenable for use by nurses have not been studied systematically. Additionally, the findings of investigators in other disciplines regarding healing are only slowly being "translated" for use by nurses.

As nurses become aware of the constituents of optimum healing, however, they grow increasingly aware of the ways the healing environment is altered by sickness and by everyday patient care activities. New and different questions are asked regarding the impact of various interventions on the patient who is healing, including the degree to which patient activity supports the wound environment and what is detrimental and how it may best be measured.

Should a patient with an incision ambulate freely, or should ambulation be paced? Are current respiratory treatments beneficial or as beneficial as they might be? Should nutrition be rigorously manipulated in the early phases of wound healing in all patients, or is an unmeasured pool of carbohydrates, fats, and proteins sufficient? How much sleep promotes optimal healing, and does sleep deprivation thwart it? How do medications, environment, and stress affect healing? Do repeated dressing changes produce iatrogenic damage? Do depression, confusion, and failure to thrive affect healing, and if so, how are they best altered so as to promote maximal healing and patient benefit? The list of questions is lengthy.

The questions above evolve from the nurse's concern for conservation of energy in the healing patient,[1] that is, for what the nurse might do to facilitate the inherent potential for intactness, reintegration, and restoration of continuity which lies in the patient. Ultimately patients heal themselves. Nurses attend to, support, and foster a milieu which maximizes an optimal outcome. Vigilance and scholarliness are the hallmarks of good wound care, as of other aspects of practice. Efforts regarding the healing wound are perhaps a reflection of concern and attention to the whole patient. Interventions related to wound care must be based in the future more on the findings of scholars of healing and must be focused on the reduction of energy expenditure at every level (cell, tissue, organ, and organism) and the wholeness (*hāl*) of the patient.[1]

References

1. Levine, M. (1967). The four conservation principles of nursing. *Nursing Forum, 6,* 51.
2. Hunt, T., & Dunphy, J. E. (Eds). (1979). *Fundamentals of wound management.* New York: Appleton-Century-Crofts.
3. Levine, M. (Speaker). (1984). *An overview of the conceptual model* (cassette recording). Edmonton, Alberta, Canada: Nurse Theorist Conference.
4. Weil, A. (1983). *Health and healing.* Boston: Houghton, Mifflin, 65–77.
5. Levine, M. (1971). Holistic nursing. *Nursing Clinics of North America, 6,* 259.
6. Levine, M. (1966). Adaptation and assessment. *American Journal of Nursing, 66,* 2450–2453.
7. Levine, M. (1969). The pursuit of wholeness. *American Journal of Nursing, 69,* 93–98.
8. Levine, M. (1969). *Introduction to clinical nursing.* Philadelphia: Davis.
9. Levine, M. (1973). *Introduction to clinical nursing* (2d ed.). Philadelphia: Davis.
10. Levine, M. (Speaker). (1978). *The four conservation principles* (cassette recording). New York: Second Annual Nurse Educator Conference.
11. Stotts, N., & Cooper, D. (1987). *Development of a descriptive instrument for the assessment of wound healing.* Manuscript submitted for publication.
12. Cooper, D., & Stotts, N. (1987). *Nurse descriptors of surgical wounds.* Unpublished manuscript.
13. Berkelman, R., Holland, B., & Anderson, R. (1982). Increased bactericidal activity of dilute preparations of povidone-iodine solutions. *Journal of Clinical Microbiology, 15,* 635–639.
14. Custer, J., Edlich, R., Presak, M., Madden, J., Panek, P., & Wagensun, O. (1971). Studies in the management of the contaminated wound. *The American Journal of Surgery, 121,* 572–575.
15. Rudolph, R., & Noe, J. (Eds.). (1983). *Chronic problem wounds.* Boston: Little, Brown.
16. Zamora, J. (1984). Povidone iodine and wound infection. *Surgery, 95,* 121–122.
17. Curtain, L. (1984). Wound management: Care and cost..... An overview. *Nursing Management, 15,* 22–25.
18. Baron, M. (1983). The skin and wound healing. *Topics in Clinical Nursing, 5,* 11–22.
19. Bruno, P. (1979). The nature of wound healing. *Nursing Clinics of North America, 14,* 667–682.
20. Cooper, D., & Schumann, D. (1979). Post-surgical nursing interventions as an adjunct to wound healing. *Nursing Clinics of North America, 14,* 713–726.
21. Cooper, D., Watt, R., & Alterescu, V. (1963). *Guide to wound care.* Libertyville, IL: Hollister.
22. Hotter, A. (1980). Physiologic aspects and clinical implications of wound healing. *Heart and Lung, 11,* 522–530.
23. Hotter, A. (1984, Spring). The physiology and clinical implications of wound healing. *Plastic Surgical Nursing,* pp. 4–13.
24. O'Bryne, C. (1979). Clinical detection and management of postoperative wound sepsis. *Nursing Clinics of North America, 14,* 727–742.
25. Schumann, D. (1979). Preoperative measures to support wound healing. *Nursing Clinics of North America, 14,* 683–699.
26. Chang, N., Goodson, W., Gottrup, F., & Hunt, T. (1983). Direct measurement of wound and tissue oxygen tension in postoperative patients. *Annals of Surgery, 197,* 470–478.
27. Chvapil, M. (1980). Zinc and other factors of the pharmacology of wound healing. In T. K. Hunt (Ed.), *Wound healing and wound infection: Theory and*

surgical practice (pp. 135–148). New York: Appleton-Century-Crofts.

28. Dineen, P. (Ed.). (1981). *The surgical wound*. Philadelphia: Lea & Febiger.

29. Hunt, T. K., Heppenstall, R. B., Pines, E., & Rovee, D. (Eds.). (1984). *Soft and hard tissue repair: Biological and clinical aspects*. New York: Praeger.

30. Knighton, D., Silver, I., & Hunt, T. (1981). Regulation of wound angiogenesis—Effect of oxygen gradients and inspired oxygen concentrations. *Surgery, 90,* 262–270.

31. Niinikoski, J. (1977). Oxygen and wound healing. *Clinics in Plastic Surgery, 4,* 361–374.

32. Ducey, D. (1983). The phases of wound healing and wound irrigation. *Ethicon, 20,* 4–7.

33. Merker, P. (1984). Inflammation and wound repair. *Federation Proceedings, 43,* 2791.

34. Hunt, T. K. (Ed.). (1980). *Wound healing and wound infection: Theory and surgical practice*. New York: Appleton-Century-Crofts.

35. Ross, R., & Benditt, E. (1961). Wound healing and collagen formation I: Sequential changes in components of guinea pig skin wounds observed in the electron microscope. *Journal of Biophysics, Biochemistry and Cytology, 11,* 677.

36. Grotendorst, G., Pencev, D., Martin, G., & Sodek, J. (1984). Molecular mediators of tissue repair. In T. K. Hunt, R. B. Heppenstall, E. Pines, & D. Rovee (Eds.), *Soft and hard tissue repair: Biological and clinical aspects* (pp. 21, 28). New York: Praeger.

37. Knighton, D., Thakral, K., & Hunt, T. K. (1980). Platelet-derived angiogenesis: Initiation of healing sequence. *Surgical Forum, 31,* 226–227.

38. Simpson, D., & Ross, R. (1972). The neutrophilic leukocyte in wound repair: A study with antineutrophil serum. *Journal of Clinical Investigation, 51,* 2009.

39. Stein, J., & Levenson, S. (1980). Effect of the inflammatory reaction on subsequent wound healing. *Plastic Surgery, 31,* 484–485.

40. Banda, M., Knighton, D., Hunt, T., & Werb, Z. (1982). Isolation of a nonmitogenic angiogenesis factor from wound fluid. *Proceedings of the National Academy of Science, 79,* 7773–7777.

41. Schumann, D. (1982). The nature of wound healing. *Journal of the Association of Operating Room Nurses, 35,* 1068–1077.

42. Peacock, E., & Van Winkle, W. (1976). *Wound repair.* Philadelphia: Saunders.

43. Goodson, W., & Robbins, P. (1984). *Current concepts in wound management*. New Jersey: C. R. Band.

44. Gottrup, F., Fogdestam, I., & Hunt, T. (1982). Delayed primary closure: An experimental and clinical review. *The Journal of Clinical Surgery, 1,* 113–124.

45. Goodson, W., & Hunt, T. (1979). Wound healing and the diabetic patient. *Surgery, Gynecology and Obstetrics, 149,* 600–608.

46. Goodson, W., Radolf, J., & Hunt, T. K. (1980). In T. K. Hunt (Ed.), *Wound healing and wound infection: Theory and surgical practice* (pp. 106–116). New York: Appleton-Century-Crofts.

47. Barbul, A., Thysen, B., Rettura, G., Levenson, S., & Seifter, E. (1978). White cell involvement in the inflammatory, wound healing and immune actions of vitamin A. *The Journal of Parenteral and Enteral Nutrition, 2,* 129–138.

48. Ehrlich, H., & Hunt, T. K. (1968). Effects of cortisone and vitamin A on wound healing. *Annals of Surgery, 167,* 324–328.

49. Hunt, T. K., Ehrlich, H., Garcia, J., & Dunphy, J. E. (1964). Effect of vitamin A on reversing the inhibitory effect of cortisone on healing of open wounds in animals and man. *Annals of Surgery, 170,* 633–641.

50. Peacock, E. (1984). *Wound repair* (3d ed.). Philadelphia: Saunders.

51. Silver, I. (1969). The measurement of oxygen tension in healing tissue. *Progress in Respiratory Research, 3,* 124.

52. Silver, I. (1972). Oxygen tension and epithelialization. In H. Maibach & D. Rovee (Eds.), *Epidermal wound healing* (pp. 291–305). Chicago: Year Book.

53. Silver, I. (1973). Local and systemic factors which affect the proliferation of fibroblasts. In E. Kulonen & J. Pikkarainen (Eds.). *Biology of fibroblasts* (pp. 507–519). London: Academic.

54. Schilling, J. (1983). Wound healing. *Surgical Rounds, 6*(7), 46–112.

55. Stotts, N., & Friesen, L. (1982). Understanding starvation in the critically ill patient. *Heart and Lung, 11,* 469–478.

56. Fingdorf, W., & Cheraskin, E. (1982). Vitamin C and human wound healing. *Oral Surgery, 53,* 231–236.

57. Rettura, G., Seifter, E., Stratford, T., Kambosis, A., & Levenson, S. (1980). Vitamin A to alleviate impaired wound healing in diabetic rats. *Surgical Forum, 31,* 228–230.

58. Seifter, E., Rettura, G., Padawer, J., Stratford, F., Kambosis, D., & Levenson, S. (1981). Impaired wound healing in streptozoan diabetes. *Annals of Surgery, 194,* 42–50.

59. Rubin, M. (1984). Vitamins and wound healing. *Plastic Surgical Nursing, 4,* 16–19.

60. Pories, W., & Strain, W. (1966). Zinc and wound healing. In A. S. Prasad (Ed.), *Zinc metabolism* (pp. 378–394). Springfield, IL: Thomas.

61. Rudolph, R. (1983). Nonsurgical maintenance of the chronic problem wound. In R. Rudolph & J. Noe

(Eds.), *Chronic problem wounds* (pp. 29–36). Boston: Little, Brown.

62. Chvapil, M. (1980). Zinc and other factors of the pharmacology of wound healing. In T. K. Hunt (Ed.), *Wound healing and wound infection: Theory and surgical practice* (pp. 135–151). New York: Appleton-Century-Crofts.

63. Cooper, D. (1987). *Zinc and wound healing: From chemistry to therapy.* Manuscript submitted for publication.

64. Barbul, A., Thysen, B., Rettura, G., Levenson, S. M., & Seifter, E. (1978). White cell involvement in the inflammatory, wound healing and immune actions of vitamin A. *The Journal of Parenteral and Enteral Nutrition, 2,* 129–138.

65. Ehrlich, H., & Hunt, T. K. (1968). Effects of cortisone and vitamin A on wound healing. *Annals of Surgery, 167,* 324–328.

66. Hunt, T. K., Ehrlich, H., Garcia, J., & Dunphy, J. E. (1964). Effect of vitamin A on reversing the inhibitory effect of cortisone on healing of open wounds in animals and man. *Annals of Surgery, 170,* 633–641.

67. Hunt, T. K. (1976). Control of wound healing with cortisone and vitamin A. In J. J. Longacre (Ed.), The ultra structure of collagen (pp. 497–508). Springfield, Ill.: Charles C Thomas.

68. Sawyer, P., Bergan, J., Dagher, F., Degruf, H., Haeger, K., Hunt, T., Jacobsson, S., & Winter, G. (1980). Treatment alternatives for pressure sores. *Modern Medicine, 48,* 49–56.

69. Scales, J. T. (1963). Wound healing and the dressing. *British Journal of Industrial Medicine, 20,* 82.

70. Noe, J., & Kalish, S. (1978). The problem of adherence in dressed wounds. *Surgery, Gynecology and Obstetrics, 147,* 185–188.

71. Soul, J. (1978). A trial of debrisan in the cleansing of infected surgical wounds. *British Journal of Clinical Practice, 32,* 172–173.

72. Oredsson, S., Gottrup, F., Beckmann, A., & Hohn, D. (1983). Activation of chemotactic factors in serum and wound fluid by dextranomer. *Surgery, 94,* 453–457.

73. Ducey, D. (1983). The phases of wound healing and wound irrigation. *Ethicon, 20,* 4–7.

74. Diekmann, J. (1984). Use of a dental irrigating device in the treatment of decubitus ulcers. *Nursing Research, 33,* 303–305.

75. Stotts, N. (1983). The most effective method of wound irrigation. *Focus on Critical Care, 10,* 45–48.

76. Grower, M., Bhaskar, S., Horan, D., & Cutting, D. (1972). Effect of water lavage on removal of tissue fragments from crush wounds. *Oral Surgery, 33,* 1031–1036.

77. Rodeheaver, G., Pettry, D., Thacker, J., Edgerton, M., & Edlich, M. (1975). Wound cleansing by high-pressure irrigation. *Surgery, Gynecology and Obstetrics, 141,* 357–362.

78. Hamer, M., Robson, M., Krizek, T., & Southwich, W. (1975). Quantitative bacterial analysis of comparative wound irrigations. *Annals of Surgery, 181,* 819–822.

79. Brown, L., Shelton, H., Bornside, G., & Cohn, I. (1978). Evaluation of wound irrigation by pulsatile jet and conventional methods. *Annals of Surgery, 187,* 170–173.

80. Gross, A., Cutright, D., & Bhaskar, S. (1972). Effectiveness of pulsating water jet lavage in treatment of contaminated crushed wounds. *American Journal of Surgery, 124,* 373–377.

81. Stevenson, T., Thacker, J., Rodeheaver, G., Bacchetta, C., Edgerton, M., & Edlich, R. (1976). Cleansing the traumatic wound by high pressure syringe irrigation. *Journal of the American College of Emergency Physicians, 5,* 17–21.

82. Wheeler, C., Rodeheaver, G., Thacker, J., Edgerton, M., & Edlich, R. (1976). Side effects of high pressure irrigation. *Surgery, Gynecology and Obstetrics, 143,* 775–778.

83. Rudolph, R. (1983). Wound treatments, nostrums, and hokums. In R. Rudolph & J. Noe (Eds.), *Chronic problem wounds* (pp. 47–52). Boston: Little, Brown.

84. Anonymous. (1870). The proper treatment of cuts and wounds. *Scalpel, 1*(2), 363–372.

85. Meyers, F., Jawetz, E., & Goldfien, A. (1972). *Review of medical pharmacology* (4th ed.). Los Altos, CA: Lange.

86. Danis, R., Brodeur, A., & Shields, J. (1967). The danger of hydrogen peroxide as a colonic irrigating solution. *Journal of Pediatric Surgery, 2,* 131.

87. Shaw, A., Cooperman, A., & Fersco, J. (1967). Gas embolism produced by hydrogen peroxide. *New England Journal of Medicine, 277,* 238.

88. Bassan, M., Dudai, M., & Shalev, O. (1982). Near-fatal systemic oxygen embolism due to wound irrigation with hydrogen peroxide. *Postgraduate Medicine Journal, 58,* 448–450.

89. Gruber, R., Vistnes, L., & Pandoe, R. (1975). The effect of commonly used antiseptics on wound healing. *Journal of Plastic and Reconstructive Surgery, 55,* 472–476.

90. Krug, E. (1963). *Pharmacology in nursing* (9th ed.). St. Louis, MO: Mosby.

91. Melmon, K., & Morrelli, H. (Eds.). (1972). *Clinical pharmacology: Basic principles in therapeutics.* New York: Macmillan.

92. Pietsch, J., & Meakins, J. (1976). Complications of povidone-iodine absorption in topically treated burn patients. *The Lancet, 1:* 7954, 280–282.

93. Berkelman, R., Holland, B., & Anderson, R. (1982). Increased bactericidal activity of dilute preparations of povidone-iodine solutions. *Journal of Clinical Microbiology, 15,* 635–639.

94. Trueman, J. (1971). The halogens. In W. B. Hugo (Ed.), *Inhibition and destruction of the microbial cell* (pp. 171–183). London: Academic.

95. Caretto, P. (1983). *Povidone-iodine.* Unpublished manuscript.

96. Smith, J. L., Drennan, A. M., Rettie, T., & Campbell, W. (1915). Experimental observations on the antiseptic action of hypochlorous acid and its application to wound treatment. *The British Medical Journal, 2,* 129–136.

97. Dakin, H. D. (1915). The antiseptic action of hypochlorites: The ancient history of the "new antiseptic." *The British Medical Journal, 2,* 809–810.

98. Taylor, H., & Austin, J. (1918). The solvent action of antiseptics on necrotic tissue. *Journal of Experimental Medicine, 27,* 155.

99. Storm, R. (1983). *The development of the wound assessment checklist.* Unpublished master's thesis, University of Arizona, Tucson.

100. Verhonick, P. (1961). Decubitus ulcer observations measured objectively. *Nursing Research, 10,* 211–215.

101. Harmer, B., & Henderson, V. (1922). *Principles and practices of nursing.* Philadelphia: Williams & Wilkins.

102. Levine, M. (1963). Florence Nightingale: The legend that lives. *Nursing Forum, 2*(4), 25–35.

part 13

Selected Multisystem Patient-Care Problems

57
Multiple Trauma

Rochelle L. Boggs

Traumatic injuries have been with us since the beginning of humankind. In the past twenty years, health care providers have focused increased attention on the prevention, care, and rehabilitation required by multiple system trauma patients. The toll of trauma is staggering: *trauma kills more Americans between the ages of 1 and 44 years than any other disease.* It is the third-highest cause of death (behind cardiovascular disease and cancer) for persons of all ages. More than 150,000 people in this country die annually from traumatic injuries. An estimated 10 to 17 million trauma victims are disabled, with 380,000 of these disabilities becoming permanent. Trauma primarily affects people at or near the beginning of their most productive work years. The economic costs of trauma are great when the unseen costs of lost productivity from disability and death are considered. When the estimated unseen costs are added to the total hospital costs—including rehabilitation, which can last a lifetime—trauma care results in a far greater economic burden than other diseases. Trauma patients require approximately 19 million hospital days of care per year in the United States. This figure represents more than the days of care needed by all cardiac patients and four times the number of days needed by all cancer patients.[1]

The history of medicine has repeatedly addressed the problem of wound care. The history of trauma surgery has of necessity followed the major wars, and from that wartime experience, standards of trauma care have been developed and carried over into peacetime. Prior to the nineteenth century, the management of battlefield injuries was disorganized and primitive, and the mortality rate from wounds exceeded 20 percent. Improvement in care in the field, rapid evacuation, and modern surgical management have progressively lowered the mortality rate from 8 percent in World War I and 4.5 percent in World War II to 2.7 percent in the Vietnam war. Although the lessons from the battlefield have been applied to civilian medicine, the overall mortality rate for civilian trauma remains 3 to 5 percent. A number of factors contribute to this. First, civilian trauma affects persons of all ages, and mortality can be directly related to age. Second, care at the scene of the accident and evacuation to medical facilities remain primitive in many parts of the country when compared with military standards. And finally, changes in such lifestyle elements as physical forces, living habits, and level of affluence (incorporating more sophisticated modes of injury) have contributed to increasing nonmilitary trauma rates. According to Oakes: "Trauma complexity and rate of occurrence have steadily increased with . . . acceleration, deceleration, velocity, impact mass or a variety of these insults until current major medical [personnel] caring for the critically injured population have declared this problem to be ubiquitous in American society."[2]

The goal of trauma surgery should be not only to decrease the mortality rate but also to decrease morbidity. The morbidity involved in trauma is not easily measured but probably represents a major cost to society; moreover, the proper care of trauma victims will probably have its greatest impact in decreasing morbidity.

The key to an improved approach to the trauma patient is to consider trauma itself as a disease, with its own natural history and specialized problems—a disease which can benefit from specialized trauma care. Inherent in this concept is that the trauma victim should be taken out of the mainstream of medicine and surgery in the hospital and treated by a team that has specialized training in trauma. The trauma center has developed from this type of team approach, and for the most severely injured it represents the key factor for improving the survival rate of trauma victims.

A study involving five hospitals in Orange County, Calif., in 1982 compared trauma care before and after designation of a trauma facility. Deaths as a result of trauma were reduced from 73 percent to 9 percent following trauma designation.[3] Patients inappropriately triaged to a hospital that was not a trauma center continued to have a 67 percent preventable mortality. These results emphasized the importance of regional trauma care, in that no patients died as a result of bypassing a conventional hospital to get to a trauma center.

The natural history of trauma has not been well defined. The traditional breakdown into blunt and penetrating injuries appears valid. The most common cause of death in patients with penetrating wounds is hemorrhage, followed by infection and pulmonary failure. With blunt trauma, the primary cause of death is head injury, which accounts for over half the deaths. If the patient survives the head injury, then pulmonary failure and infection represent the greatest risk to life. Hemorrhage follows but is a much less important factor than with penetrating injuries. Although not proved by prospective studies, there is little doubt that improper resuscitation of the injured patient initially contributes to subsequent pulmonary failure and infection and may aggravate the consequence of head and other injuries.

It is apparent that there is great need for education in the care of trauma victims. Early and late deaths can often be attributed to mismanagement, and the inherent morbidity resulting from any injury is critically influenced by the care given.

Experts in trauma management describe the deaths from trauma as having a trimodal distribution: the first peak in death rates occurs almost instantaneously, with few lives saved; the second occurs within hours (the "golden hour"); and the third, days or weeks following injury, is usually due to subsequent multiple organ failure. Trauma care focuses on all these peaks, but it is during the period termed the *golden hour* that a significant number of patients can benefit from organized trauma care.

The American College of Surgeons has developed general guidelines for hospitals which describe three categories or levels of trauma care. A level I institution, often referred to as a *comprehensive center,* generally has over 500 beds, is located in a metropolitan area, and is usually affiliated with a medical school and research center. The level I trauma center admits approximately 1000 critically injured patients annually and has committed surgeons, personnel, and equipment readily available.

The level II trauma center, or *intermediate center,* is an institution of over 250 beds which admits around 500 critically traumatized patients annually. The level II center does not have available all the medical specialty services found in level I centers.

The level III, or *basic, trauma care center,* is most often located in a rural community. This type of institution is committed to trauma care concepts. Trauma patients may be stabilized at a level III center and then, following transport protocols, be shipped to the nearest level I or level II center at which specialized services are immediately available.

Trauma centers must continue to demonstrate committment to operationalizing trauma concepts which include organization and teamwork. Care at the scene of the accident, resuscitation, management of specific injuries, intensive care, convalescent care, and rehabilitation must be continually evaluated as part of trauma care. These phases of trauma care are not discrete entities but overlap to provide a continuum of management for the trauma victim.

Mechanism of Injury

The *mechanism of injury* includes both the action of forces and their effects upon the human body. Understanding these biomechanical processes has increased the alertness of health care providers to potentially life-threatening injuries that might otherwise have gone unsuspected. The same understanding has also triggered industrial concern for preventive devices, e.g., airbags and hard hats. The mechanism of injury is generally obtained with the initial history. The forces creating the traumatic injury are classified as blunt or penetrating. The history is generally brief and often incomplete because of the nature of the accident. Nonetheless it is extremely critical in order to evaluate cerebral function and to understand the biomechanics of the accident. Secondary observers can also provide vital information concerning the circumstances surrounding the accident. To reiterate, it is vital to maintain a high index of suspicion in order to avoid the development of potentially lethal problems.

Blunt Trauma

Blunt injuries are caused by one or more forces which can be described as deceleration, acceleration, shearing, crushing, and rotary. The consequences of blunt injuries are difficult to diagnose. It is common to see a variety of tissue and organ involvement with blunt injuries. Blunt trauma often requires more extensive diagnostic evaluation than the penetrating type. The forces of blunt trauma set relatively stable structures and organs into motion upon impact, and the end results may include crushed tissue, torn structures, bone fractures with or without adjacent tissue injury, bleeding, and fluid extravasation into damaged tissue. Capillary permeability is increased, the complement system is activated, and the coagulation cascade is triggered by a release in vasoactive substances (see Chaps. 40 and 44). A contusion or hematoma the size of an adult fist can represent a blood loss of approximately 500 mL. The most common mechanisms of injury involving blunt trauma are motor vehicles such as motorcycles and automobiles (auto-pedestrian accidents) and falls.

Automobiles

Understanding the vector forces of the motor accident gives an idea of the transmission of energy to the traumatized patient. In a frontal impact, the car stops quickly but the body continues forward until it meets resistance. This results in a sudden deceleration not uniformly met throughout the entire body. The driver of the vehicle often sustains chest, head, facial, femur, and hip injury. A rear impact often results in hyperextension of the neck as the body is pulled forward by delayed acceleration. Injury can be reduced by the use of lap and harness seat belts, which can be instrumental in reducing both the seriousness and the extent of the injury. Automatic inflatable air bags have proved

effective in head-on collisions. Unsafe road conditions, excessive speed, and alcohol lead to a great number of accidents: alcohol abuse is associated with 50 percent of all motor vehicle fatalities.[4]

Motorcycles

Motorcycles have gained popularity in our society as an open, carefree method of travel. When a motorcycle is involved in an accident, the rider's chances for injury or death are greater than they would be in a vehicle with more protection. In 1982, 7.5 percent of all motor vehicle fatalities involved motorcycles.[5] Although there is no real pattern of injury, head and extremity trauma are common. Motorcycles are not as visible as cars on the highway and are often overlooked by other drivers. Helmets, leather boots, and padded clothing assist in minimizing more serious injuries: statistics clearly indicate that states which have mandatory helmet laws show a significant decrease in the number of severe or fatal head injuries. The last several years have shown an increase in the use of three-wheel and four-wheel recreational vehicles. Although they are usually limited to off-road use, their instability and misuse have resulted in serious personal consequences, including fatalities.

Auto-Pedestrian

Auto-pedestrian injuries are usually severe because of the mass and speed of the vehicle involved. The mortality rate is highest among the very young and the very old. There is a triad of injuries that result as pedestrians are struck by cars: upon initial impact the car bumper strikes the pedestrian's leg, resulting in femur injuries; a chest injury occurs when the victim falls onto the hood of the automobile; and head injuries result when the victim strikes the pavement.

Falls

The type of blunt injury resulting from falls depends upon three factors: the height, the angle of landing, and to a degree, the type of surface impacted. Many falls involve a simple ankle sprain or twisted knee and can be treated in a basic emergency department. Screening criteria are useful in determining which falls need to be triaged to the trauma center. For example, in Santa Clara County, Calif., falls of 15 ft or more for a child and 10 ft or more for an adult are triaged to a trauma center. Another trauma system may triage to a trauma center those persons whose falls result in injury to two or more body systems, e.g., fractured leg with head injury.

Penetrating Trauma

The injuries caused by penetrating trauma are more predictable than those from blunt trauma. Organ and tissue disruption can generally be diagnosed as the trajectory of the instrument is traced. Penetrating injuries, with the exception of some gunshot wounds, involve less energy and have less associated organ involvement as compared with blunt injuries. The most common mechanisms of injury for penetrating trauma are stabbings and shootings. They are generally associated with accidents, or assault and other criminal situations.

Knife and Stab Injuries
Stab wounds may be inflicted by such instruments as knives, scissors, pencils, glass bottles, screw drivers, and coat hangers. They involve a low amount of energy. Tissue destruction is limited, and often only one or two body systems are involved. In order to estimate the amount of damage, it is important to know the size, shape, and length of the instrument. In cases where the inflicting instrument has been removed it is often difficult to determine the angle and depth of penetration; information regarding the gender of the assailant may be helpful in tracking the wound, since men tend to stab with an upward thrust and women with a downward thrust.[6] Injuries involving the upper abdomen may penetrate into the chest cavity, since the diaphragm descends to about the sixth intercostal space upon inspiration. The opposite is true with injuries to the chest cavity, in that during expiration the diaphragm ascends to the level of the fourth intercostal space. It is estimated that one out of four patients sustaining a penetrating injury to the abdomen will have an associated chest injury.[7] These points become important in patient assessment.

Gunshot Injuries
Gunshot wounds can present a wide range of injuries. Some wounds involve gross tissue destruction and contamination, are large and gaping, and result in profuse hemorrhage, while others are small, clean, and punctate. Civilian gunshot injuries are generally caused by low-velocity handguns. Military bullets are highly destructive, and wounds are inflicted by high-velocity rifles. As White has pointed out, the extent of injury from a bullet "depends on three wounding mechanisms: laceration, cavity formation by energy shock waves and tissue and bone destruction by burning, expanding gases."[8]

The laceration results as the bullet traverses the skin. Cavity formation is illustrated in Fig. 57-1: the expansile shock waves of the bullet transmit destructive energy to the surrounding tissue, creating a cavity by tissue destruction. This cavity lasts only milliseconds and is highly contaminated. Shotgun wounds are produced by shells that are composed of powder, paper (the wad), and a pellet load (Fig. 57-2). It is the amount of powder, the size of the pellet, the choke of the gun, and the distance to the target that determine the destructive effect.[7] The presence of the wad in the wound indicates that the gun has been fired at close range.

Assessment and Management

Accident Scene

Any trained health professional should offer assistance at the scene of an accident. Tradition as well as Good Samaritan laws protect persons who render first aid. It is usually possible to establish continuity

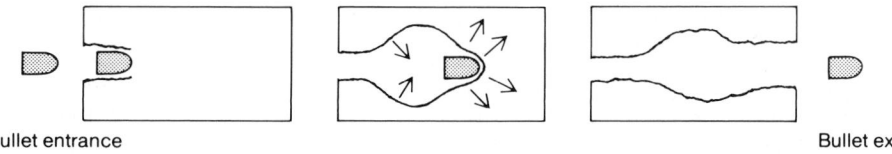

Bullet entrance   Bullet exit

Figure 57-1 Cavity formation: kinetic energy imparted by the bullet to the tissue.

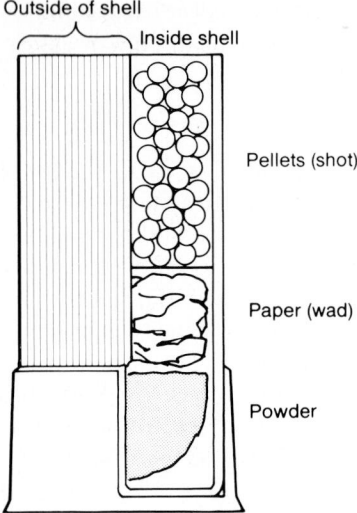

Figure 57-2   Shotgun shell components.

of care with ambulance responders, and seldom is it necessary to accompany the victim beyond the immediate scene of the accident. The trauma professional at the scene of an accident often can provide critical help.

The most important sign of significant injury is external evidence of trauma, and except for obvious hemorrhage, it is often overlooked. Abrasion, contusion, and pain on movement can be observed at the accident scene and may lead to early recognition of occult injuries. Back and neck pain may suggest spinal injury. Abrasion and contusion of the chest and abdomen may herald occult injuries and are particularly useful signs in the presence of concomitant head injury. Deformity and pain suggest extremity injury. All patients should be managed as though they had sustained serious injury until a thorough examination can be made. Patients in shock should be taken to a designated trauma center. The accident scene as well as the circumstances surrounding the accident should be assessed. A good approach is to consider the type of force, the mechanism of injury, and the potential injuries (Table 57-1). If the patient is unresponsive because of head injury, it should be assumed that spinal, thoracic, and abdominal visceral injuries are present until proved otherwise.

Prehospital Treatment

The following first-aid principles should be followed during the prehospital phase:

1. Remove patient from hazard only when risk (e.g., fire) outweighs danger of removal.

Table 57-1   Predicted Area of Injury According to Type of Force and Mechanism of Injury

Type of Force	Mechanism of Injury	Predicted Injury
Blunt head trauma	Automobile, motorcycle, auto-pedestrian, fall, altercation, recreational sports	Craniocerebral injury, cervical spine injury
Blunt facial trauma	As above	Lefort I, II, III fracture; Craniocerebral injury; cervical spine injury
Blunt neck trauma	As above	Tracheal disruption, esophageal disruption, carotid vessel injury, cervical spine injury, lumbar spine injury
Blunt chest trauma	As above	Ruptured heart, cardiac contusion, fractured sternum, aortic disruption, fractured clavicle, pulmonary contusions, fractured ribs, tracheobronchial disruption, flail chest, pneumothorax, hemothorax, diaphragmatic disruption, cardiac tamponade
Blunt abdominal trauma	As above, also restraining devices (seat belts)	Splenic disruption, hepatic disruption, renal contusion, bowel disruption, mesenteric disruption, pelvic fracture
Blunt extremity trauma	As above	Associated skeletal fracture, arterial and venous disruption, compartment syndrome, associated nerve disruption

2. Establish airway, usually by elevating patient's jaw.
3. Initiate cardiopulmonary resuscitation if indicated.
4. Control hemorrhage, usually with direct pressure.
5. Splint spinal and extremity injuries.
6. Move and transport patient as soon as possible.

One of the main objectives of care at the accident scene is prevention of further injury. Care in extracting and transporting victims to avoid further damage in spinal injuries cannot be overemphasized. Similarly, attention to limb position and simple splinting will decrease the sequelae of long-bone fracture. Further contamination of open wounds can be avoided by mere attention to the problem.

In most urban settings there is no way of providing extensive field care to trauma victims and it should be discouraged, despite television coverage of paramedic services which suggests that field care should be provided in every instance. Ordinarily, the most important axioms of care of trauma victims are (1) avoid further damage and (2) load and go. Intravenous fluid support should be initiated if it does not significantly delay transit. A good rule of thumb is that any field procedures should not take more than 3 min. Definitive care of trauma victims should take place in a trauma center, and the sooner the patient is delivered the better.

A trained health professional at the accident scene can often contribute in addition to providing first aid. The professional is a source of reassurance and strength to the victim and other responders. A series of priorities can be established, such as indicating which victims should be transported first and what first aid needs to be provided. Usually the receiving hospital can be communicated with through ambulance or police radio to convey critical information about the victim which will enable the hospital staff to prepare for the arrival.

One of the most useful functions that can be performed by the enlightened observer is the recording of such facts as the time of accident, the mechanism of injury, the neurological status, contributing factors, and information on the victim's family. This information is often available only at the accident scene and can be of considerable importance in the hospital setting when it accompanies the patient in transit.

Primary Survey

A successful outcome for the multiple trauma patient depends upon teamwork, organization, and priority setting. The primary survey should be performed as rapidly as possible. The goal of this survey is to determine the extent and severity of life-threatening injuries and begin immediate management. The trauma score is a quick and reliable tool that can be used to assess and quantify the severity of injury (Table 57-2).[9] This score should be initiated in the prehospital phase. It is helpful in reevaluating the patient's status in the primary survey. The trauma score is based upon seven parameters: respiratory rate, respiratory expansion, systolic blood pressure, capillary refill, eye opening, verbal response, and motor response. The last three parameters (eye opening, verbal response, and motor response) make up the Glasgow coma scale that is used to assess central nervous system injury. In addition, an ABCDE mnemonic offers help in providing a quick and organized system for dealing with a multitude of problems and establishing priorities in the primary survey: *A,* airway; *B,* breathing; *C,* circulation (or control of spine); *D,* neurological deficits; *E,* exposure (removal of clothing).

Airway

Airway maintenance is essential for successful resuscitation and prevention of death. This is the first priority in the primary survey. The upper airway is assessed for patency by looking into the oral cavity for obvious obstructions such as teeth, tongue, blood, mucus, vomitus, food, or other debris. Such obstructions are removed by suctioning and manually. Care must be taken to maintain a stable cervical spine and not advance obstructions further into the airway. Placement of an oral airway is helpful when the tongue is the cause of obstruction. A normal tone of voice usually indicates an adequate airway in speaking patients. Inspiratory crowing sounds are commonly heard in patients with a partially obstructed airway. Patients with airway obstructions present with cyanosis and retraction of suprasternal, supraclavicular, intercostal, and

Table 57-2 Components of Trauma Score

Parameter	Point Score
Respiratory rate:	
36/min or more	4
25–35/min	3
10–24/min	2
0–9/min	1
No respiration	0
Respiratory expansion:	
Normal	1
Shallow	0
None or retraction	0
Systolic blood pressure; mmHg:	
90 or more	4
70–89	3
50–69	2
0–49 or less	1
No pulse	0
Capillary fill:	
Normal	2
Delayed	1
None	0
Eye opening:	
Spontaneous	4
To voice	3
To pain	2
None	1
Verbal response:	
Oriented	5
Confused	4
Inapproiate words	3
Incomprehensible words	2
None	1
Motor response:	
Obeys command	6
Localizes pain	5
Withdrawal (pain)	4
Flexion (pain)	3
Extension (pain)	2
None	1

Note: The last three items, constituting the Glasgow Coma Score (GCS), may be scored separately and then added to the trauma score as follows: GCS score of 14–15 = 5, 11–13 = 4, 8-10 = 3, 5-7 = 2, 3-4 = 1, making a possible total trauma score ranging from 1–16.
Source: H. R. Champion, W. J. Sacco, A. J. Carnazzo, et al.[9]

epigastric spaces. The jaw-thrust maneuver respects cervical spinal cord integrity and should be utilized in trauma patients. Trauma patients frequently sustain maxillofacial injuries which may compromise the airway.

If it appears obvious that an endotracheal or nasotracheal tube cannot be readily passed without causing further hypoxic insult, then the situation is best managed by transtracheal catheter punch or by cricothyrotomy. These procedures can be done rapidly and thus minimize a hypoxic state (Fig. 57-3). They are often performed in circumstances of severe facial, head, and neck trauma or when obesity, positioning, or anatomical structures result in airway blockage. The transtracheal catheter punch is a quick, easy, short-term alternative for airway maintenance. This method is most often used during prehospital management. It allows sufficient ventilation until the patient arrives at the trauma center, where a cricothyrotomy or tracheostomy can be performed. To use it, an endotracheal tube is connected to the barrel of a syringe, which is then connected to a 16- or 14-gauge angiocatheter.

The cricothyrotomy is a surgical procedure that can be performed rapidly with few complications. A skilled physician makes a 3-cm incision through the cricothyroid membrane, and a tracheostomy tube is immediately inserted. This technique is reserved for emergencies.

Breathing

Once the airway has been established, ventilatory effectiveness is the primary concern. The respiratory rate is a good indication of ventilatory status. Respiratory rate, depth, chest excursion, and tracheal deviation are the parameters that best assess chest dynamics. If the respiratory rate is decreased, ventilatory assistance and support become necessary. If the respiratory rate is rapid, intubation and paralyzing agents such as succinylcholine chloride (Anectine) or pancuronium bromide (Pavulon) are used to effectively control the patient. Ventilation is most effectively assisted by endotracheal intubation.

Circulation

For all practical purposes, the quickest way to assess circulation is to palpate for a pulse. A radial pulse that is strong and of good character reflects a systolic blood pressure of around 80 mmHg. If the radial pulse is weak or absent, the femoral pulse can be used for assessment. If the femoral pulse is present and of good quality, the systolic blood pressure is around 70 mmHg.

In the absence of pulses and an apical heartbeat, chest compression must be initiated. Neck veins should be assessed for the presence of dis-

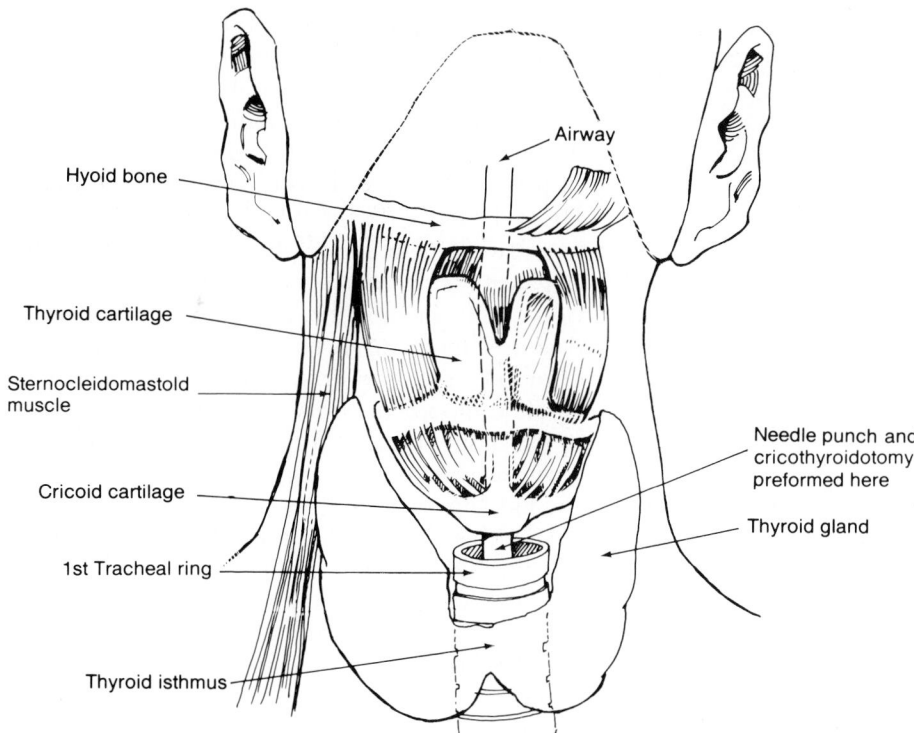

Figure 57-3   Diagram of anatomy of neck showing cricothyroidotomy site.

Hyoid bone

Airway

Thyroid cartilage

Sternocleidomastoid muscle

Cricoid cartilage

1st Tracheal ring

Thyroid isthmus

Needle punch and cricothyroidotomy preformed here

Thyroid gland

tention. Hypovolemic patients with cardiac tamponade may present without neck vein distention.

Obvious hemorrhage is controlled by direct pressure, elevation when possible, and application of ice. A patient's skin coloring and temperature give a rough indication of the circulatory system's effectiveness. Skin that is cool to the touch, cyanotic, and mottled in appearance often indicates arterial shunting from the periphery to vital organs. Capillary refill is assessed by pressing the nail bed, earlobe, or forehead so that it blanches, then releasing quickly and observing whether the skin color returns within 2 s (the amount of time it normally takes to say "capillary refill"). Return of color within 2 s is considered normal. Erroneous values will result when the nail bed or forehead is not at heart level. The nail beds should not be used if the circulation to the extremity is affected by cold or injury.

Neurological Deficits

A quick way to assess for neurological deficits is to use the AVPU mnemonic:[10]

A   Is the patient *a*lert to surroundings?

V   Is the patient able to respond *v*erbally and is speech appropriate?

P   Does the patient complain of *p*ain, and if so where, how intense, etc.? Is patient able to move extremities?

U   Is the patient *u*nresponsive?

A quick pupil check is also in order, noting the size, shape, and reaction of right and left pupils separately and together.

Exposure

Undressing the patient is essential in order to avoid missing injuries. This is often done in the prehospital phase while the patient is being transported to the hospital.

Resuscitation

The immediate resuscitation of the trauma patient is carried out by a trauma team which may consist of a traumatologist (general surgeon with special qualifications in trauma) and the following:

Emergency room physician

Two trauma nurses

Operating room nurse

Intensive-care nurse

Anesthesiologist

Respiratory therapist

Radiology technicians

Laboratory technicians

Each team member has a predetermined role so that procedures can be simultaneously carried out. This team functions on the premise that injuries are present until proved otherwise.

Resuscitation is carried out concurrently with the primary survey. Airway maintenance, cardiopulmonary resuscitation, and other life-saving modalities for patient care should be initiated when the problem is identified rather than at completion of the primary survey.[10]

A decreased level of consciousness is commonly due to inadequate oxygenation. Immediately after the airway has been secured, supplemental oxygen therapy should be started and an arterial blood gas analysis obtained. Arterial blood gases offer the best measure of a patient's respiratory status. A ventilator is often needed for support of the trauma patient requiring intubation or exhibiting significant intracerebral damage. In the event of intracerebral damage, the patient is placed on a volume respirator using hyperventilation techniques. The Pa_{CO_2} is decreased and maintained between 25 and 30 mmHg while the Pa_{O_2} is maintained at more than 90 mmHg.[11] The administration of succinylcholine chloride or pancuronium bromide (administered by intermittent IV and keyed to the patient's response) will paralyze the patient and decrease the body's overall metabolic requirements. Following intubation and ventilatory management, breath sounds should be checked and a portable chest x-ray obtained to ensure proper tube placement. Cervical spine stabilization must be maintained throughout airway management and

ventilatory support; a cervical spinal collar and backboards are placed on patients in the field and left intact until lateral cervical x-ray films are obtained and cleared by the radiologist. The possibility of cervical spine injury should not be overlooked in patients who are or were ambulatory following the accident.

Two large-bore peripheral IV lines (preferably 16-gauge or larger) should be established and vigorous IV therapy initiated with a crystalloid or colloid solution. With the initiation of IVs, 50 mL of blood should be drawn in order to determine baseline blood chemistry and hematologic values. Blood should be sent to a laboratory for typing and cross matching of 6 units of whole blood and routine laboratory studies, i.e., total blood count, electrolytes, blood chemistry battery, and drug screen. The condition of the patient dictates the speed at which the solution will be administered. In shock states that are not responsive to aggressive fluid resuscitation, military antishock trousers (MAST) may be applied. MASTs are used in conjunction with IV fluid resuscitation to assist in maintaining a systolic blood pressure of 90 mmHg (see Chap. 7). The cardiac status should be continually assessed by ECG monitoring. As the trauma team assesses the patient for the life-threatening problems identified in the primary survey, the treatment of these problems begins the resuscitative phase. The trauma team should continually be moving from the primary survey to the resuscitative phase, then back to the primary survey, in order to provide quick yet optimal trauma care. Once the primary survey has been completed and the patient's life-threatening injuries stabilized, the secondary survey is initiated.

Blunt and penetrating injuries are not always obvious. Without a high index of suspicion and the ability to predict associated injuries, a potentially life-threatening injury such as a pulmonary contusion may develop into a fatal injury. It is imperative to take a good history and to perform a careful physical examination in order to avoid missing important signs and symptoms. A popular approach to the multiple trauma patient is to suspect and rule out the life-threatening injuries during the initial assessment and the potentially life-threatening injuries during the secondary assessment.

Secondary Survey

The secondary survey begins with an extensive history and includes a complete head-to-toe assessment of the patient.

History

Although patient interaction is important, it is not always feasible. An obvious example is the unconscious patient. Family and prehospital personnel can be instrumental in providing important information about the patient. The history should include information concerning the accident as well as a past medical history, allergies, current medication, last meal, and tetanus immunization status.

Head

The neurological status should be reevaluated in order to detect changes from the baseline parameters, including vital signs, pulse, respiration, blood pressure, level of consciousness, and the patient's awareness of person, place, and time. The patient should be given several commands with response noted. Reaction and response to painful stimuli should be noted as well as whether the patient opens the eyes spontaneously, on command, in response to pain, or not at all. If injuries create situations which obviate testing, e.g., a broken arm limits extremity movement or a swollen eye makes evaluation of the pupil impossible, documentation with an explanation as to why testing is not completed is in order. Size, shape, and reaction of both pupils as well as vision changes should be documented. The entire head should be palpated for scalp lacerations and skull disruptions. These injuries are sometimes less obvious and easily overlooked.

The presence of periorbital ecchymosis ("raccoon's eyes") and ecchymosis over the mastoid process ("battle signs") is associated with orbital and ethmoid sinus fractures and temporal skull fractures, respectively. These injuries become most obvious as time passes and cerebrospinal fluid leaks from the ears (otorrhea) and/or nose (rhinorrhea); they are indicative of meningeal disruption. Strict infection control standards must be maintained in order to decrease the risks of meningitis. The Ring test is a quick procedure used to assess the presence

of glucose, found in normal CSF, in the midst of blood that is draining out of the ears and nose: If CSF is present, a drop of the fluid on a white surface turns into a bulls-eye pattern. Diabetic test strips are also useful in evaluating glucose in the draining blood. A complete neurological assessment must include cranial nerve, reflex, motor, sensory, and cerebellar testing. Alcohol and other drugs can mask a patient's true neurological state; therefore their chemical effects must be considered.

Maxillofacial Area

Airway obstruction is commonly expected with maxillofacial trauma. Facial lacerations, which can result in significant blood loss, should be managed as time permits. A facial fracture should be assumed to be present under lacerations and bruises. The facial structure should be assessed for symmetry. Palpation of the bony structures for pain and tenderness, crepitation, and bony irregularity is important. The ears, nose, and mouth should be inspected for evidence of lacerations and bleeding. Wounds should be examined for the presence of foreign matter such as glass, dirt, and gravel. Pressure irrigation of the area assists in removal of dirt, bacteria, and other substances. Maxillary fractures are classified as LeFort I (horizontal), LeFort II (pyramidal), and LeFort III (craniofacial dysjunction). Mandibular fractures in multiple trauma are common. "More than one half of all mandibular fractures are multiple: therefore, the presence of a mandibular fracture should prompt a thorough search for a second fracture."[11] To assess orbital "blowout" fractures, note ocular movement discrepancies secondary to muscular entrapment, the depression of the suborbital bony ridge, and sensory loss in the zygomatic area.

Neck and Spinal Column

Any patient presenting with craniofacial trauma or injuries above the clavicle or in an unconscious state should be presumed to have a cervical spine fracture until proved otherwise. A cross-table lateral cervical spine x-ray should include the entire cervical chain through C7. Patients wearing a helmet should have x-rays performed prior to helmet removal. To remove the helmet, one person manually immobilizes the neck below the helmet while another person bilaterally expands and removes it. The neck is then immobilized with a neck collar, sandbags, or the like. The neck should be palpated for crepitus, tracheal malalignment, and foreign bodies. Absence of neurological deficit does not rule out injury to the cervical spine.[12] Injuries commonly associated with neck trauma include laryngeal fracture, tracheal fracture, carotid arterial injury, and cervical spine injury. The presence or absence of a carotid pulse should be noted. Movement and sensation in all extremities should be assessed. Patients should be asked to move their toes, feet, legs, fingers, hands, and arms. The nurse also checks sensation in these areas and tests for reflex withdrawal. When the patient is unconscious, a painful stimulus is used to elicit voluntary movements while observing the patient for any spontaneous movement. With all spinal cord injuries, attention to the breathing pattern, presence of sweating, and bladder and bowel function, as well as anal reflex, is important. Male patients should be checked for priapism.

Chest

One out of four trauma deaths can be attributed to chest injuries.[10] The injuries resulting from chest trauma are sometimes called the "dirty dozen."[10] Six are considered to be life-threatening: airway obstruction, tension pneumothorax, open pneumothorax, massive hemothorax, flail chest, and cardiac tamponade. These conditions are first assessed during the primary survey, since they can result in severe tissue hypoxia. The other six are *potentially* life-threatening: myocardial contusion, pulmonary contusion, aortic disruption, tracheobronchial disruption, esophageal disruption, and diaphragmatic disruption.

In any type of chest trauma the respiratory rate and excursion and the breath sounds need to be monitored. The patient's mental condition should be noted, since hypoxic states lead to confusion, agitation, and, if not properly managed, loss of consciousness. The chest wall should be assessed for asymmetrical chest motion, tracheal deviation, and neck vein distention. The chest wall and neck should be palpated for subcutaneous emphysema. Chest x-ray, arterial blood gas analysis, ECG, CT scan, arteriogram, and bronchoscopy are sophisticated diagnostic studies that are useful for determining specific injuries. Mediastinal widening on a chest x-ray taken in an upright position at 110° is highly suggestive of aortic disruption. When breath sounds are absent on the side of the injury and there is an associated acute abdominal condition, the presence of a diaphragmatic hernia should be suspected. This injury is commonly diagnosed from the chest x-ray. The left side of the chest often shows the nasogastric tube or bowel. The development of sudden dysrhythmias, e.g., premature ventricular contractions, atrial fibrillation, or bundle branch block, is associated with cardiac contusions.

Rib fractures are the most common chest wall injury. The fifth to ninth ribs tend to be most involved, since they are least protected by musculature. Fractures of the first and second ribs have been associated with bronchial and aortic tears. Lower rib fractures involving the tenth, eleventh, and twelfth ribs are most often associated with kidney, liver, or splenic disruption. Pain with chest wall movement is a typical complaint in rib fractures.

For obvious reasons it is important to know whether the patient has any preexisting disease, e.g., chronic obstructive pulmonary disease or cancer. Tracheobronchial injuries often produce hoarseness.

Abdomen

Abdominal injuries are divided into blunt and penetrating categories and the latter into gunshot wounds and stab wounds in order to simplify the diagnostic approach to these different injuries.

A careful search should be made for an exit wound in all gunshot injuries; however, it cannot be assumed that it necessarily reflects the trajectory of the bullet. Chest and abdominal x-rays should be obtained in all patients with gunshot wounds. Appreciating that the diaphragm can ascend to the fifth intercostal space during full expiration makes any chest wound below the nipple suspect for concomitant abdominal injury until proved otherwise. Similarly, upper abdominal wounds must be suspect for thoracic injury because of the extent of the posterior sulcus. Unless the gunshot wound is clearly a grazing injury, all wounds require surgical exploration in the operating room, and few diagnostic studies are required beyond the presence of a nasogastric tube, rectal examination, and a urinalysis to detect the presence of blood.

Stab wounds to the abdomen require selective management, and it is not necessary to explore all wounds. Little is gained by probing the wound. The primary indication for operation is the presence of peritoneal irritation, suggesting visceral injury; therefore, the abdominal examination must include a careful search for signs of such injury, including tenderness, guarding, rebound, and the absence of bowel sounds. Serial examination by the same examiner is an essential feature of management.

Blunt abdominal injuries present one of the most difficult diagnostic challenges to the examiner. The presence of contusions and abrasions suggests abdominal injury in many instances. If signs of peritoneal irritation are present, exploration is indicated. The abdomen should be thoroughly inspected for contusions, abrasions, hematomas, and penetrations. The abdomen should be auscultated for presence or absence of bowel sounds. A friction rub heard over the spleen or liver may be indicative of splenic or hepatic rupture. The examination continues with palpation for abdominal tenderness and involuntary guarding, which may be indicative of inflammation or peritoneal irritation. The spleen is the most commonly injured abdominal organ; the patient frequently presents with signs and symptoms of shock, abdominal pain, nausea, and involuntary guarding. Because of its large size, the liver is a frequent site of injury; the patient presents in a state of shock due to hemorrhage, complains of right upper quadrant pain, nausea, and tenderness, and exhibits guarding.

Peritoneal Lavage Peritoneal lavage is an important diagnostic procedure in patients with blunt abdominal trauma. A small cutdown procedure should be performed to avoid injury to the intra-abdominal viscera. A vertical incision is made and the dissection carried down through the linea alba. Meticulous hemostasis is secured, and the fascia is then held upward on traction and the peritoneum penetrated with the trocar catheter. A balanced salt solution (1L) is run into the abdomen, and it is helpful to gently roll or shake the abdominal contents to ensure good mixing. The IV bag is then lowered to the floor and the lavage fluid allowed to run out. If the return fluid is sufficiently discolored with blood so that the examiner cannot read newsprint through the IV bag, the lavage is consid-

ered positive. Only enough return needs to be examined to clearly define the results of the test. A return that is slightly pink initially and then clears is considered negative and probably reflects some local bleeding at the puncture site. When the fluid returns, approximately 30 mL of fluid is aspirated in a syringe and sent to the laboratory for interpretation. The findings are considered positive if there are more than 100,000 RBC or more than 500,000 WBC per cubic millimeter or if bacteria, bile, or fecal material is present.

After the test has been interpreted, the catheter is removed and the wound is closed with Steri-Strips. The procedure itself should not alter the physical examination of the abdomen except in the immediate area of the puncture site, and the patient can be followed with serial examinations after a negative lavage. The technical aspects of peritoneal lavage are emphasized because an equivocal result complicates the management of the patient significantly.

The secondary survey should also discover or rule out bowel, bladder, kidney, and stomach injuries. The perineum should be carefully examined and a pelvic examination conducted on all trauma victims to rule out injuries to the external genitalia. In the absence of signs of external injury, hematuria is a hallmark of genitourinary tract injury. Bright red blood passed from the meatus suggests urethral injury and dictates a urethrogram prior to insertion of a Foley catheter. Genitourinary injury should be suspected in patients with pelvic fractures, and they should be encouraged to void spontaneously before the catheter is inserted. All patients with hematuria, regardless of the mechanism of injury, must have an intravenous pyelogram and cystogram. Usually this can be obtained preoperatively, even in patients with major intraabdominal injuries, simply by injecting the intravenous pyelogram dye prior to taking an abdominal flat plate. A detailed study may not be possible; however, it is useful to know the functional status of the kidneys when planning the operative approach. If there is failure to visualize one or both kidneys, then an arteriogram is indicated to assess the vascular supply of the kidneys.

Extremities

Extremity injuries are often obvious at the time of admission, and they are frequently noticed because of the associated pain, particularly on movement. The unconscious patient and the patient with overwhelming associated injuries require special attention. The extremities are compared with each other when a physical assessment is made; deformities, swelling, angulation, bruising, and discoloration are rarely bilaterally equal. The extremities should be inspected for the presence of wounds, lacerations, and muscle spasms and palpated for tenderness, crepitation, capillary refill, sensation, warmth, and pulse strength. The assessment is completed by testing range of motion. Peripheral vascular injury should be suspected in either blunt or penetrating trauma to the extremity, since either may result in loss of vascular integrity, bleeding, and impairment of distal circulation. An arteriogram is indicated when the wound is proximate to a major vessel, when there is a large or expanding hematoma, or when pulses are absent or there is a history of absent pulses. At times the approach to such injuries may be direct operative intervention rather than an arteriogram, and this should be determined on the basis of the individual wound.

Rehabilitation

The goal of rehabilitation is to move the patient from a dependent state to one of independence. Multiple trauma patients often have residual disabilities that interfere with physical, mental, social, vocational, and emotional functions. Rehabilitation of the multiple trauma patient begins immediately upon admission to the trauma facility. It involves, in the truest sense, a total team effort including the patient, health care professionals, and family or significant other. This team concentrates on abilities and wellness, not disabilities and illness. The process of rehabilitation occurs in three phases: the passive phase, the active involvement phase, and the independence phase.[13] During the passive phase the patient is dependent upon the health care team as life-saving techniques are instituted. When the condition permits, patients are encouraged to become active in their daily care. This begins the active phase of rehabilitation, in which patients are encouraged to make choices and set goals. The independence phase forces patients to reach their optimal level of function. Rehabilitation is a vital

part of trauma management and includes a team approach from the onset of the patient's admission.

Management of Specific Traumatic Injuries

General Therapies

The mark of an experienced trauma team is a rapid but meticulous technical approach to the procedures which must be performed, frequently in the presence of the apparent turmoil of resuscitation efforts. Unfortunately, all too often sloppy technique, failure to maintain sterile fields, and failed attempts at procedures are testimony to the lack of preparation and knowledge of the trauma team or emergency area staff. The protocols used in the resuscitative phase are consistent for all trauma patients presenting in the trauma center.

Intravenous Fluids

Establishing a large-bore intravenous line is the first step in fluid resuscitation. The best choice for an intravenous line is a large peripheral vein, often in the forearm or antecubital fossa. A no. 14 plastic catheter often can be inserted percutaneously. This should then be connected to tubing which contains a hand pump and filter to allow the rapid administration of fluid and blood. Because trauma frequently strikes young, healthy persons, the veins in the arm and antecubital fossa are usually accessible. When they are not, a cutdown proximal to the antecubital area should be considered. A subclavian line is seldom the first choice for an intravenous line in a trauma victim; the incidence of complications is appreciable, particularly in less than optimal situations, and the complications themselves are potentially lethal in seriously injured patients. Central venous lines utilizing the subclavian or supraclavicular route may well be indicated in the course of the patient's therapy; however, they are seldom the best initial choice as a route of access. Central venous lines provide information on the filling pressure of the right side of the heart. Although they are important and useful, they are not needed initially to begin resuscitation, and prolonged attempts to establish a central line should not preclude the administration of fluid by other routes. Often the central line can be passed percutaneously with a long line at the initial attempt to establish an IV. Most patients with major trauma will require more than one intravenous line, and lower extremity IVs should be considered in patients with chest trauma, particularly injuries to the thoracic outlet. Lower extremity lines are often used in children because of the accessibility of the saphenous vein. The one technical feature that should be emphasized is the need to adequately immobilize the IV sites with tape and dressings to prevent dislodgment and kinking.

Pulmonary artery catheters have been adopted rapidly in the field of trauma since their introduction. If a central venous line is indicated, then a pulmonary artery catheter should be considered. Important advantages of this line over a central venous catheter include (1) access to central venous blood, (2) access to the left atrial filling pressure, and (3) facility for rapid repetitive measures of cardiac output by thermal dilution. A pulmonary artery catheter is indicated in patients who have traumatic shock and concomitant heart failure, patients who develop pulmonary failure, and patients who fail to respond to appropriate resuscitative measures. Certain brands of pulmonary artery catheter can measure continuously a patient's mixed venous saturation ($S\bar{v}_{O_2}$). This is extremely helpful in titrating vasopressor and inotropic pharmacological agents as well as assessing a patient's optimal ventilatory management. $S\bar{v}_{O_2}$ monitoring in essence can provide an early warning system for respiratory and circulatory impairment. (See Chap. 4 for use and interpretation of $S\bar{v}_{O_2}$ values.)

Arterial Pressure Monitoring

An arterial line is a useful adjunct in the management of trauma victims, providing constant arterial pressure monitoring as well as access to the arterial system for blood gas determination. Usually a percutaneous radial line can be established; however, at times a more central line or a cutdown may be necessary. A femoral or dorsalis pedis artery cutdown should be considered as an alternative in some patients. Because of concern for the rare ischemic complications, arterial lines have been reserved primarily for patients with severe trauma

and shock and those who require respiratory support.

Foley Catheter

A Foley catheter is indicated in patients with severe trauma and shock. In the presence of pelvic trauma, it is important to rule out urethral injury. If a pelvic fracture is suspected and the patient is unable to void spontaneously or bright red blood oozes from the meatus, then a urethrogram should be made prior to an attempt to pass a Foley catheter. Unless a simple stricture can be dilated or a prostatic obstruction is identified, a suprapubic tube is indicated as an alternative. The need for meticulous sterile technique in passing the catheter cannot be overemphasized. Urine output should be monitored at 15-min intervals during resuscitation and then at hourly intervals until the patient's hemodynamic status is stable.

Nasogastric Tube

A sump-type nasogastric tube is preferred and should be inserted early in the resuscitation of all major trauma victims, especially those with suspected abdominal trauma. An attempt should first be made to empty the stomach, then the nasogastric tube should be placed on suction during the resuscitation effort. Alkalization of the gastric contents should be considered early in the patient's course and until the tube is removed; this will effectively minimize the incidence of stress ulceration and decrease the insult should aspiration of gastric contents occur.

Head

The successful treatment of open head wounds depends upon adequate exposure and meticulous hemostasis. With all head lacerations it is important to diagnose the extent of the underlying bony injury. Depressed fractures require elevation, and the galea and scalp should be closed in layers. Wounds extending into the brain require debridement of foreign body, macerated brain, and loose bone fragments. Prophylactic antibiotics are usually recommended for wounds extending into the cranial vault.

The management of closed head injuries depends primarily upon the diagnosis and treatment of expanding intracranial lesions, the control of cerebral edema, and the maintenance of optimal circulation and oxygenation of the brain (see Chap. 35).

Extradural hematomas usually result from lacerations of the meningeal artery associated with linear fractures. Often there is a history of a blow to the head with loss of consciousness. The patient comes to, only later to lapse into coma. During this so-called lucid interval, the patient may have headache, focal neurological signs, or evidence of increasing intracerebral pressure.

A CT scan or arteriogram often confirms the diagnosis. Early surgical treatment gives the best chance for survival and return of neurological function. During the acute phase, hyperosmolar diuretics are widely used in an effort to lower intracranial pressure. Loop diuretics such as furosemide (Lasix), as well as intravenous mannitol (Osmitrol) may be used to decrease brain tissue swelling and allow time to get to the operating room. A urinary catheter is required for such treatment. Occasionally, emergency burr holes may be required. Surgical treatment consists in craniotomy over the hematoma, evacuation of the clot, and control of the bleeding vessel.

Acute subdural and subarachnoid hemorrhages may be similar in clinical presentation to extradural hematoma; however, the lucid interval is less characteristic. Often these entities will present with a progressive downhill course and evidence of increasing intracerebral pressure. The operative management is similar; the dura is opened and the hemorrhage controlled. However, these lesions are often associated with severe brain injury, and the prognosis is poor. Chronic subdural hematomas related to trauma, where the mass effect is more gradual, have a much better prognosis.

Maintaining optimal circulation and oxygenation to the brain are goals in any head injury. The circulation to the brain is a function of not only the systemic arterial pressure but also the intracerebral pressure, which determines vascular resistance. Intracerebral pressure is affected by the central venous pressure as well as the oncotic pressure in the brain. These basic physiological features suggest the following principles of management of head injuries:

1. Treat shock adequately. The goal is to provide a normal arterial pressure for maximum perfusion of the brain.
2. Maintain a normal central venous pressure. Avoid fluid overloading, prevent straining, and use PEEP judiciously.
3. Minimize brain swelling:
   a. Hyperventilation will result in a fall in Pa_{CO_2}, with resulting cerebral vasoconstriction and decrease in brain size.
   b. Osmotic diuretics (mannitol or urea) may be used to decrease brain edema.
   c. Steroids, hypothermia, and barbiturate coma may have some application in special cases.
4. Provide optimal oxygenation:
   a. Maintain normal Pa_{O_2}.
   b. Maintain adequate hemoglobin levels (hematocrit 30 percent or greater).
   c. Maintain oxygen-hemoglobin dissociation curve in the normal range.

Maxillofacial Area and Eye

The potential loss of sight demands proper handling of all eye injuries. If any injury to the globe is recognized, the immediate treatment is to immobilize the eyes with bilateral eye patches. Any cleansing, examination, or manipulation of the eye must be done in the operating room with good anesthesia and proper equipment. Beyond testing visual acuity and voluntary extraocular eye movements, the remainder of the examination should be performed in a proper setting. In general, prophylactic antibiotics are advocated with major eye injuries. Corneal and scleral lacerations can often be repaired, but more extensive injuries to the globe must be assessed individually. After the initial treatment of major eye injuries, the eye can be observed for up to 2 weeks, and the need for enucleation is reassessed during that period in an effort to preserve the eye if at all possible. The presence of a foreign body must be suspected in any eye injury, particularly if there is a noticeable laceration. An x-ray should be obtained in addition to detailed examination of the globe. Ophthalmic ultrasonography (B scan) is useful in the diagnosis of blood, foreign body, or retinal disruption in the posterior part of the eye. Contusion to the eye is a common cause of loss of vision, and hemorrhage into the anterior chamber is an obvious sign.

Patients with maxillofacial injuries are at high risk for the development of upper airway obstruction, and this must be kept in mind not only initially but throughout their management. Although many soft tissue injuries are repaired in the emergency room area, the following injuries deserve to be treated in the operating room setting:

1. Parotid gland or duct injury
2. Facial nerve injuries
3. Nasolacrimal injuries
4. Injuries with moderate soft tissue loss
5. Extensive lacerations

Mandibular fractures are often heralded by malocclusion or pain on biting. Usually the fracture can be palpated intraorally and the diagnosis confirmed by x-ray. Treatment consists of hooked arch bars and intermaxillary traction for reducing and immobilizing mandibular and maxillary fractures. External fixation devices with bone grafting are used with some comminuted-type fractures in which bone segments are missing. Fractures of the orbital rim, maxilla, and nose can usually be diagnosed by palpation, or there may be entrapment of the extraocular eye muscles with orbital floor fractures. Appropriate x-rays must be obtained; however, it should be remembered that the bone injury is usually more severe than is indicated on the x-ray. Most surgeons favor early repair with open reduction and fixation of the fractures. Fixation can be accomplished by interosseous wires or pins, interdental wiring, and arch bars. At times, however, it is appropriate to await resolution of some of the soft tissue swelling to obtain an optimal cosmetic result.

Loosened or fractured teeth present a special problem. Loose teeth should be splinted. Avulsed teeth can be reimplanted in some instances if this is done shortly after injury. The appropriate management of fractured teeth often results in a stable foundation for subsequent reconstruction. While a fractured or loose tooth may initially be the least serious problem to the multiple trauma victim, it may become a greater concern to the patient as the injuries resolve. The best cosmetic result can usually be obtained by appropriate early management. Meticulous oral hygiene and wound care are essential to promote wound healing.

Neck and Spinal Cord

All penetrating wounds to the neck and thoracic outlet require surgical exploration in the operating room. Little can be gained by probing the wound, and the incidence of unrecognized injuries to the major vascular structures, the esophagus, and the trachea indicate the need for exploration. Most penetrating injuries can be repaired directly. If injury to major vessels is suspected, preparation should be made for significant blood loss and extension of the incision into the chest if necessary to control bleeding. Lacerations of the carotid vessels can usually be repaired and circulation restored. With penetrating wounds to the thoracic outlet, an arteriogram is frequently indicated to define the integrity of the vascular structures in that area.

Occasionally, blunt trauma to the neck will result in significant injury to the airway, esophagus, or carotid vessels. With laryngeal disruption, open reduction and internal stenting will usually provide the optimum result. Traumatic occlusion of the carotid arteries due to blunt trauma may be suggested by absent pulses in the neck or in the external carotid arteries and can be defined by arteriography. In general, no attempt is made to restore flow in such injuries, because the potential subsequent neurological deficits resulting from reestablishing flow outweigh the potential advantages.

Cervical injuries are often treated by immobilization with a cervical collar or brace initially, followed by skeletal traction. Types of fixed skeletal traction include Crutchfield and Gardner Wells tongs and halo traction. The most important concept in the treatment of all cervical spinal cord injuries is to prevent further damage.

With open injuries to the spine, operative intervention is indicated if there is a CSF leak, if x-rays suggest foreign body fragments compressing the cord, or if there is a change in neurological status suggesting compression. Closed spinal cord injuries are classified according to the degree of functional impairment of the spinal cord. Complete lesions cause total sensory and motor loss below the level of the lesion. Autonomic disruption accompanies this type of lesion, which results in irreversible cord damage. Complete lesions are those resulting in quadriplegia and paraplegia. Incomplete lesions result in variable degrees of motor and sensory loss below the level of the lesion. Depending upon the type of lesion, certain nerve tracts may be spared. The most common incomplete lesions include central cord syndrome, anterior cord syndrome, and Brown-Séquard's syndrome. In general, spinal cord injuries are treated with traction and a frame bed to meet the primary objectives of preventing further damage by immobilizing the fracture. Although some neurosurgeons explore spine injuries with fixed neurological deficits, most reserve operation for those with unstable fractures, and in many instances that treatment can be delayed until the patient's condition is stable. Patients who have spinal injury and a progressively worsening neurological deficit usually should undergo exploration and decompression of the cord. Corticosteroids are given to reduce cord edema and improve cord blood flow. Any patient who presents with a neurological deficit needs special attention to skin care, bowel and bladder care, and psychological support from the very beginning. Successful rehabilitation needs an early start. (See also Chap. 35.)

Chest

Tension Pneumothorax

Disruption in the visceral and parietal pleura allows air to enter the pleural cavity, resulting in ventilatory impairment and loss of functional lung tissue. Air enters the pleural cavity during inspiration. The damaged tissue prevents the escape of air on expiration; thus a one-way valve is created, which results in tracheal deviation to the opposite side, absent breath sounds on the affected side, cyanosis, distended neck veins, and respiratory distress. Treatment involves the rapid insertion of a large-caliber needle or McSwain dart into the second intercostal space at the midclavicular line of the affected side.

This procedure converts the injury to a simple pneumothorax (see also Chap. 27).

Open Pneumothorax

Open, sucking chest wounds present a life-threatening situation. Not only does the lung collapse, but there is a shift of the mediastinum toward the uninvolved side which compromises the ventilation of the good lung as well. The initial treatment of these injuries is to close the wound with a simple occlusive dressing, taped securely on three sides. During inspiration, the dressing is occlusively sucked over the wound and prevents the entrance of air. During expiration, the open end of the dressing allows air to escape. This will tend to stabilize the mediastinal shift. The second step is to establish closed thoracostomy-tube drainage in order to reexpand the lung and evacuate the blood and air from the thoracic cavity.

Massive Hemothorax

Hemothorax can be secondary to penetrating injuries or blunt trauma to the chest. It commonly results from injuries involving the heart and great vessels. The diagnosis is confirmed by chest x-ray. Although the chest x-ray may show only a pneumothorax, it must be assumed that there is blood in the thoracic cavity as well. Emergency chest x-rays are often taken with the patient in the supine position, and a relatively large amount of blood can collect in the posterior gutters without being evident. Treatment involves placement of large-bore intravenous lines and rapid crystalloid infusion. A large-bore (no. 36 French) thoracostomy tube is inserted in the lateral chest, directed posteriorly and attached to a water seal with 30 cm of water suction. In many instances this will evacuate the chest and reexpand the lung; however, if this does not occur, a second tube should be placed. The location of this tube is somewhat dependent upon the segment which fails to reexpand. If air is trapped in the apex, a second-intercostal-space anterior tube usually suffices. The amount of blood that is obtained from the chest cavity will give some indication of the existing volume deficit, since this blood has already been lost to the patient. Continuing blood loss must be accurately measured to determine whether it is decreasing or whether an urgent thoracostomy is indicated. Every effort should be made to completely evacuate the chest to prevent the development of an organized clot. The majority of traumatic hemopneumothoraces can be managed by simple closed thoracostomy tube drainage; however, if a large air leak persists or if the bleeding continues, then a thoracostomy is indicated to repair the injury directly.

Flail Chest

Severe crushing injuries with multiple rib fractures may result in loss of the structural integrity of the thoracic cage. In this situation, when the patient attempts to breathe, the chest cage itself moves in and out, resulting in the so-called flail chest. The degree of movement of the chest wall or flail chest is dependent upon intrathoracic pressures. The flail may be relatively minimal at the time of admission but become more pronounced, with progressive respiratory difficulty and stiffening of the lung. Therefore, patients suspected of having this type of injury should be observed for the development of a significant flail even though it may not be present on admission. Treatment of flail chest is to stabilize the chest cage. Traditionally, this was done by external stabilization, using either sandbags or sternal traction. However, current management is by means of internal stabilization. This is achieved by intubation and positive pressure ventilation until the chest becomes sufficiently stable and the patient can breathe without help. With a large flail segment, and particularly with respiratory insufficiency, an early tracheostomy is advised. Less severe injuries can often be managed with oral or nasotracheal intubation.

Cardiac Tamponade

Traumatic injuries involving the coronary arteries and veins result in bleeding into the pericardial sac. Cardiac output and systolic blood pressure are greatly decreased. The classical signs of cardiac tamponade include distention of neck veins, hypotension, and distant, muffled heart sounds. These classical signs are described as *Beck's triad*. Pericardiocentesis is performed in order to aspirate blood from the pericardial sac. The patient's vital signs and level of consciousness must be closely monitored.

Myocardial Contusion

Cardiac contusions secondary to blunt trauma should be suspected in all patients with significant chest injury. A high index of suspicion is essential in order to make a positive diagnosis, since no single test is reliable. Signs and symptoms of myocardial contusion include excruciating chest pain radiating to the jaw, shoulder, or left arm. Unlike ischemic heart pain, the pain of cardiac contusion is not relieved by coronary vasodilator drugs. Tachycardia is commonly noted; hypotension, dyspnea, and dysrhythmias are other frequent signs. The treatment of myocardial contusions is similar to the treatment instituted for myocardial infarction. The patient's activity should be restricted and continuous monitoring, serial ECGs, and isoenzyme studies instituted. Cardiac enzyme determinations are often difficult to evaluate because of associated skeletal muscle injuries. In light of this situation, MB-band creatine phosphokinase (MB-CPK) fractions of more than 5 percent become a significant diagnostic measure. Disruption of the epicardial and pericardial vessels may lead to traumatic pericardial tamponade.

Direct contusion of the pulmonary parenchyma may occur with either penetrating or blunt injury. This entity should be distinguished from aspiration or posttraumatic pulmonary insufficiency. X-ray findings show evidence of consolidation of lung tissue, which is usually focal and often present on admission and tends to clear during the first week with progressive improvement in pulmonary function. Improvement in the x-ray may lag behind improved pulmonary function. Changes secondary to aspiration are usually of a more diffuse nature and are associated with a greater degree of pulmonary insufficiency and evidence of tracheobronchitis. In many instances the aspiration event can be traced. The pulmonary insufficiency that has been described in association with trauma, shock, and major injuries tends to develop after several days; and here, too, the x-ray findings lag behind the pulmonary dysfunction. The findings are diffuse, and the characteristic physiological dysfunction is arteriovenous shunting and progressive loss of compliance of the lung. The treatment of pulmonary contusion consists in prophylactic antibiotics, respiratory therapy to assist in mobilizing secretions, and ventilatory support if indicated.

Aortic Disruption

With sudden deceleration injuries, the thoracic aorta may be disrupted just distal to the takeoff of the left subclavian. This unique injury usually results in a false aneurysm of that portion of the aorta. In those patients who arrive at the hospital alive, the bleeding is tamponaded by the surrounding hematoma and pleura. The diagnosis is suggested by evidence of widening of the mediastinum on chest x-ray and must be confirmed by arteriography.

Patients often present with all the signs and symptoms of shock, severe chest pain, restlessness, upper extremity hypertension, pulse difference between arm and leg, dysphagia, hoarseness, and dyspnea. The definitive treatment consists in controlling systemic arterial pressure and urgent thoracostomy with direct repair of the injury.

Tracheobronchial Disruption

Tracheobronchial disruption can result from penetrating injury but is most commonly due to severe blunt injury. Half the deaths from tracheobronchial disruption occur within 1 h. The patients commonly present with hemoptysis, subcutaneous emphysema, and tension pneumothorax. Treatment is surgical repair of all large tears with air leaks.

Esophageal Disruption

Successful treatment of traumatic rupture of the esophagus depends upon prompt recognition of the injury and definitive treatment before the onset of mediastinitis. The injury may be suggested by air in the mediastinum on x-ray and may be found in any patient with a wound that traverses the mediastinal structures. Diagnosis is made by endoscopy and esophagogram using water-soluble medium. Treatment consists in direct layered closure of the injury and drainage of the mediastinum. In those instances in which the injury is not recognized early and mediastinitis occurs, it is often more difficult to effect closure of the injury. Management consists in isolating the esophagus from the gastrointestinal tract by esophagostomy, closing the esophagogastric junction, and performing a draining thoracostomy. It is important to monitor the chest tube drainage at frequent intervals in the early course of resuscitation to establish that the drainage is decreasing and that urgent thoracostomy is not indicated.

Diaphragmatic Disruption

Injury to the diaphragm can occur as a result of either blunt or penetrating injury. This injury may not always be suspected initially. The presence of bowel in the chest on x-ray is diagnostic. A nasogastric tube should be instituted in order to decompress the stomach prior to surgery. Early direct repair is indicated, and the abdominal approach is usually chosen to rule out associated injuries to the intraabdominal viscera.

Abdomen

Most wounds of the stomach are penetrating in origin; blunt disruption is rare. Blood is usually present in the nasogastric aspirate, and its presence should increase the suspicion of gastric injury. Defects can be closed in layers and a good result anticipated. Duodenal injuries are more serious than gastric injuries because of the potential for unrecognized retroperitoneal perforation and the development of a duodenal fistula. Penetrating injuries can usually be closed in layers; however, duodenal disruption secondary to crush injuries may involve extensive soft tissue damage, and operative management becomes much more complicated. This is particularly true in the presence of infection related to delay in diagnosis and treatment. Duodenostomy drainage, serosal onlay grafts, and procedures which defunctionalize the duodenum, removing it from the gastrointestinal stream, all have a place in the management of these difficult injuries. Occasionally, intramural hematoma of the duodenum will present as a bowel obstruction in the early postinjury period; this unique injury often can be managed by simple evacuation and drainage.

Small Intestine

Penetrating wounds of the small intestine usually can be managed by simple layered closure with good results. It is important to make a meticulous search to identify all the perforations and to be cautious in the repair to avoid interfering with the blood supply or significantly narrowing the lumen. Blunt trauma to the small intestine can result in a spectrum of injuries from simple contusion to total disruption, as well as injuries to the mesentery which may or may not impair the vascular supply. The most common areas of injury are the ligament of treitz and the ileocecal valve region where the mesentery is short and the intestine relatively fixed and subject to shearing forces. The intestine in the midabdomen is at risk for injury by direct compression against the vertebral column. This type of injury can be caused by seat belts, particularly if improperly worn, and should be suspected in those patients with transverse contusions across the lower abdomen. Repair of the injuries consists in obtaining hemostasis, establishing the viability of the bowel, and resecting areas of major disruption.

Colon

Injuries to the colon require special attention because of the great potential for infection and the difficulties in obtaining satisfactory healing in that portion of the bowel. It should be emphasized that any intraabdominal infection in a posttrauma victim is life-threatening, and every effort should be made to prevent its occurrence. The morbidity and mortality in bowel injuries can be directly related to breakdown in repair or anastomosis. In general, the most conservative management of large bowel injuries is to exteriorize the injured portion of the colon by a colostomy when that is possible. Simple injuries may be closed in layers if there is minimal fecal contamination. For those portions of the colon which are not easily exteriorized, resection or primary closure, with a proximal colostomy to defunctionalize that segment of the bowel, may be employed. The use of antibiotics and extensive irrigation of the abdomen to minimize contamination is advocated. Because of the potential for infection, delayed closure of the skin seems appropriate with most open colon injuries. Impalement of the perineum can result in significant anal and rectal injuries. Treatment of these wounds involves adequate drainage of the presacral space as well as a proximal diverting colostomy.

Liver and Biliary Tract

The management of hepatic injuries comprises (1) hemostasis, (2) debridement of devitalized tissue, and (3) drainage. Although conceptually simple, application of these procedures requires consid-

erable judgment. The spectrum of injury ranges from small lacerations due to knife wounds to extensive parenchymal disruption due to blunt trauma or shotgun blast. Small wounds without massive parenchymal disruption can usually be managed locally by obtaining adequate exposure, directly controlling hemorrhage from the injured surface, and then draining the area to the exterior. More extensive injuries at times may require resection. Usually this is in the form of a debridement type of resection in which the laceration is extended and the injured portion of the liver removed. With massive injuries, however, formal hepatic lobectomy may be required. Control of bleeding can be facilitated at times by selective hepatic artery ligation as an alternative to resection. Injuries to the hepatic veins and the retrohepatic vena cava present the most challenging technical problem to the trauma surgeon, and the repair of these injuries requires special techniques in exposure and shunting of the vena cava blood to obtain control.

Disruption of the gallbladder or bile ducts may be secondary to either blunt or penetrating trauma. Gallbladder injuries are managed by cholecystectomy. Injuries to the extrahepatic bile duct should be repaired if possible and adequate drainage established.

Spleen

The spleen is the solid organ most commonly injured in blunt abdominal trauma; however, because of its location, it is infrequently injured by penetrating trauma. In adults, injury to the spleen is managed by splenectomy. In children, splenectomy should be reserved for major disruptions; small injuries should be managed by application of hemostatic agents in an attempt to preserve the spleen. Recent evidence suggests that the asplenic child is at risk for development of infection, and the management of splenic injuries in children has become preservation of the spleen if at all possible.

Pancreas

The successful management of pancreatic injuries depends upon the surgeon's ability to adequately expose the pancreas and diagnose the extent of the injury. The typical injury from blunt trauma is a fracture across the body of the pancreas directly over the vertebral spine. This usually can be managed by distal pancreatectomy and splenectomy. Major injuries to the head of the pancreas and combined pancreaticoduodenal injuries are less common but more serious. Defunctionalizing procedures which remove the pancreas and duodenum from the gastrointestinal stream and actual pancreaticoduodenal resection have been suggested as methods of management. Penetrating wounds of the pancreas should be managed by careful debridement and hemostasis and ligation of the duct injury. Adequate drainage must be established in all instances because of the potential development of pancreatic fistula.

Kidneys

Most penetrating injuries of the kidney are explored because of the high association of injury to the intraperitoneal viscera. The renal injury or partial nephrectomy can frequently be directly repaired, and nephrectomy is reserved for massive injuries. Blunt trauma to the kidneys can produce a whole spectrum of injuries from simple contusion to major disruption. Nonoperative management is recommended by many surgeons, since the majority of these injuries will heal by themselves. If the intravenous pyelogram shows functioning parenchyma, even though there may be some extravasation, judicious observation is often the treatment of choice. On the other hand, if the arteriogram shows major vascular damage or parenchymal disruption, then direct exposure and operative repair are indicated. In most instances, control of the renal vascular pedicle should be obtained prior to exposure of the injury.

Injuries to the ureters are usually a result of penetrating trauma, and in most instances the wound can be debrided and direct primary repair accomplished. Drainage of the injury is important, and some advocate internal splinting of the ureters.

Bladder and Urethra

Blunt trauma to the distended bladder can result in simple disruption of the muscular dome. This may be intraperitoneal or retroperitoneal. Direct primary repair and drainage of the bladder by catheter or suprapubic tube is indicated. A more serious injury, often associated with severe pelvic fractures, is a shearing off of the membranous urethra just distal to the prostate. Although some surgeons recommend primary repair, many advocate delayed reconstruction. The injury is associated with a high incidence of urethral stricture and impotence. Injury to the more distal urethra, which may be suggested by swelling and bright-red blood issuing from the meatus, is diagnosed by urethrogram. Early primary repair gives the best result.

Bones and Vasculature

The general principles of fracture treatment depend upon an understanding of the factors which influence healing of bones. In general, fracture healing depends upon local factors of soft tissue injury, circulation, apposition of fragments, and immobilization. Systemic factors such as age or associated diseases have a greater influence on the patient's survival than on healing of the bone itself. Deficiency states, however, can affect fracture healing. In children, fracture healing is usually rapid and complications are limited primarily to problems with bone growth. In adults certain particular fractures, especially in areas of relatively ischemic bone, require special treatment and there is higher incidence of nonunion. Nonunion of fractures can result from distortion of the fragments, infection, or inadequate fixation, and often these can be attributed to inappropriate management. Disabilities which result from bone injury may be due to associated injuries to nerves, vessels, and soft tissue, and these can be further influenced by immobilization and bony deformity. The goals of fracture treatment are:

1. To reduce the fracture to an anatomical setting
2. To immobilize the fracture in such a manner that the healing process occurs at an optimal rate
3. To rehabilitate the patient during the process of healing and obtain an optimally functioning extremity upon healing of the fracture

An important and at times neglected aspect of fracture management is appropriate splinting at the scene of the accident or in the hospital setting prior to definitive treatment. Early splinting reduces pain, bleeding, and tissue damage. Upper extremity splints may be simple coaptation splints with padded boards; sling or swathe dressings for shoulder, arm, or elbow; or air splints for the wrist and forearm. Lower extremity splints may be air splints or board splints or a traction type such as the Thomas splint, which is particularly useful in femur fractures. The successful reduction of extremity fractures depends upon the time of the reduction, the anesthesia employed, the displacing forces, and the method of reduction. The earlier the fracture is reduced, the less difficulty will be encountered in obtaining an adequate reduction. Once the soft tissue has become fixed, reduction is more difficult. Appropriate anesthesia is essential to eliminate pain and obtain muscle relaxation. The interposition of loose bone fragments or soft tissue between the fractured pieces can further interfere with the reduction.

There are four basic methods of fracture reduction: closed reduction, continuous traction, external skeletal fixation, and open reduction with internal fixation. Closed reduction is usually chosen when good alignment can be obtained and adequate immobilization achieved in a plaster cast or splint. The disadvantages of this type of treatment are restriction of joint motion and interference with normal neuromuscular function.

Continuous traction as a means of fracture reduction has the advantages of reducing pain and muscle spasm and restoring and maintaining length; this method has particular application in areas where there is strong muscular pull, as in femoral fractures. Continuous traction can be applied to a bone by fixing the traction apparatus to the skin with adhesive material or by placing a pin through a bone distal to the fracture and attaching the traction apparatus (skeletal traction). Traction is referred to as *balanced* when the extremity is suspended in a system of splints and rings attached to counterweights. This kind of traction is particularly helpful when there are associated systemic injuries.

In external skeletal fixation, pins are inserted in the bone fragments proximal and distal to the fracture and the projecting pins are incorporated into plaster of paris or mechanical devices to hold the fracture immobilized.

Open reduction with internal fixation has the advantage of good position and alignment of the fragments and is particularly useful in repairing fractures through joints. Its disadvantages are infection and failure to maintain fracture reduction.

Open fractures are those in which the skin overlying the fracture is broken and the normal barrier to infection has been violated. All fractures that communicate with skin wounds must be considered to be contaminated and to entail risk of infection. The object of treatment is to prevent infection from occurring. Appropriate wound management includes meticulous cleansing of the skin, debridement of all devitalized tissue and foreign matter, meticulous hemostasis, alignment of fracture fragments, lavage cleansing of the wound, and careful wound closure. The type of fixation that is chosen must take into consideration the potential for infection, and in general, internal fixation with metallic foreign bodies is avoided. Several principles of fracture management should be emphasized:

1. Treat every extremity injury as a fracture until proved otherwise.
2. Reduce fractures with minimum delay to obtain optimal results.
3. The main objective in treating upper extremity fractures is to ensure a proper functional hand; at times shortening and misalignment are acceptable.
4. The main objective in treating fractures of the lower extremity is to provide a painless, stable, weight-bearing limb; misalignment is less acceptable and full length desirable.
5. Rehabilitation of a fracture patient must begin at the time of injury to achieve an optimal result.

A dislocated hip is considered a true emergency and requires prompt treatment. Closed reduction is generally successful and usually requires general anesthesia.

Extremity trauma can lead to *compartment syndrome:* excessive pressure within muscle compartments due to edema and intracompartmental bleeding causes damage to the muscle and nerves. A classic symptom of compartment syndrome is excruciating pain that is out of proportion to the injury. The patient should be monitored for the five P's: pain, pallor, paresthesia, diminished pulses, and paralysis. These signs usually indicate an advanced problem. Decompression fasciotomy is essential in order to prevent further ischemia.

The traumatic amputation of digits and extremities is not uncommon in trauma-related injuries. Current microvascularization techniques have been successful in reimplantation of the injured part to functional use. Amputated parts should be carefully preserved and transported with the patient. The amputated part should be cleansed of any gross debris and maintained in a moist sterile towel. The sterile towel should then be placed in a plastic bag and transported in a cooling chest filled with crushed ice.

Mass Casualty

"A disaster [constitutes] a sudden massive dispro-portion between hostile elements of any kind and the survival resources that are available to counter-balance these in the shortest period of time."[13] Disasters are classified as natural and man-made. Natural disasters include such incidents as earth-quakes, floods, hurricanes, tornados, avalanches, mud slides, volcanic eruptions, and fires resulting from lightning. Man-made disasters include trans-portation accidents (aviation, railroad, marine and/ or multiple-victim bus and motor vehicle accidents); hotel and high-rise fires; explosions and nuclear accidents; and terrorist attacks. It has been pointed out that disasters tend to be front-page news even though relatively few lives are lost in them in the United States compared to the day-to-day loss of life in ordinary accidents.[14] The simplest goal of disaster management is to reduce morbidity and mortality by doing the best job possible in the least amount of time with limited personnel and supplies. The single most important concept in the manage-ment of a disaster situation is teamwork. Advance planning for disaster situations offers useful insights for triage, communication, and transportation as well as community resources and medical capabil-ities. Working under a preestablished plan will decrease overall confusion and provide the greatest chance of achieving the goals of disaster manage-ment.

Triage

Triage involves, first, the setting of priorities on the basis of a preestablished system and the determi-nation of the appropriate location for therapeutic interventions. The triaging strategies of the day-to-day operation of the emergency department are different from those of the disaster situation. During the daily routine operations of the emergency department a patient in critical condition, for ex-ample, is more often than not given immediate "high-tech" care even when the prognosis is not favorable; there are minimal restraints upon the resources demanded in such a situation. An isolated incident arises, and the health care personnel and the facility respond. During a disaster situation, however, this same type of critical patient may be triaged as a lower priority simply because the outlook for the patient's survival is grim and the amount of supplies and personnel necessary for survival are great. This concept is often viewed as inappropriate triaging in that it is in total conflict with the daily standards of patient care, and it often creates turmoil and guilt feelings among the pro-viders. The benefits, however, include the best allocation of supplies and personnel to the victims. The essential components of an efficient triage system are identification, communication, and trans-portation.[15]

Identification

A quick initial assessment and evaluation of the patient is completed. The patient's condition is determined and a priority assigned according to the disaster category. A common method of patient identification is the use of colored tags. The patient's tentative diagnosis, priority, therapy, and identifi-cation can be found on this tag. The color of the tag denotes the triaged priority or category:

Green tag—category I–Minimal treatment. These victims are more often than not ambulatory and after treatment may be useful in assisting with the treatment of others (example: pa-tients with minor abrasions).

Red tags—category II–If treatment is initiated im-mediately, the chances of survival are good (example: patients with tension pneumo-thorax, airway obstruction).

Yellow tags—category III–Can tolerate delayed treatment and still have a good chance of survival (example: patients with closed frac-tures).

Black tag—category IV–Extensive injuries, poor chance of recovery with treatment (example: patients with multiple systemic trauma, aortic disruption).

Communication

Communication from the disaster scene to the triage site and from the triage site to the hospital can alert each system to the number and severity of victims as well as the dynamics of the disaster situation.

Transportation

The primary method of transportation (ground, air, etc.) as well as alternative routes are important to disaster management in order to mobilize resources, supplies, and patients at appropriate sites.

Disaster Planning

The disaster plan is a realistic plan formulated by a community disaster committee that sets standards and determines the appropriate approach to a variety of situations. The committee is composed of nurses, physicians, Red Cross volunteers, police, hospital administrators, clergy, press, civil defense groups, industrial groups, and other community groups. To quote Briggs and Funt, "The disaster plan must be flexible enough to meet the demands of any disaster situation but ... practical in terms of the hospital's trauma capabilities, location, personnel and equipment."[15]

The committee is also responsible for overseeing implementation of the "mock disaster," which is the mechanism by which the plan is tested and weaknesses evaluated and corrected. An example of a disaster scenario follows.

Disaster Scenario

An explosion occurs in a chlorine tanker on a side track near Washington Works east entrance. A chain reaction follows: a chemical tank truck traveling west on route 892 hauling fuel oil jack-knifes and collides with an AGA tank truck traveling east hauling O_2; a chemical box trailer traveling west to the Brownsville plant loaded with 55-gal drums is hit by shrapnel, puncturing three drums; a bus hits the chemical truck and over-turns; a tanker on Washington Works east pad is also hit by shrapnel (tank contains methyl methacrylate), and a tank truck traveling east ruptures. Sheriff, State Police, and fire departments from surrounding areas are summoned to the scene. First to arrive is the Washington Volunteer Fire Department, which sets up a command center approximately ¼ mi southwest of the disaster scene. This command center activates the local

and state emergency operating centers to control traffic and ready emergency units. Activated simultaneously from Brownsville: Mount Helen and St. Joseph Hospitals, Wood County Rescue Unit, and Washington Bottom Emergency Reserve Unit. The National Guard airlift is put on standby. Communication lines with CHEMTRAC are opened. Washington Works fire brigade responds to handle leaking tank on pad. Wind direction: south to north. Washington Chemical, Brownsville Chemical, AGA, and the villages of Centerville, Randellstown, Porterfield, and surrounding areas are alerted for evacuation. News media on scene. EPA requested to disaster area. Command center requests assistance from Washington Works (Hasmet Terp) team for ruptured tank truck at scene to channel acid away from streams, etc. Area readies for evacuation. U.S. Coast Guard called to control river traffic.

Sample Plans

Table 57-3 shows a sample disaster plan for a general hospital. Sample full-scale disaster guidelines for an individual department—in this case the Emergency Department—are outlined in Table 57-4.

Nursing Strategies in Trauma Care

Patient Management

The resuscitation and ongoing care of the trauma patient requires the continuous skills of a variety of health care professionals. These efforts must be coordinated in order to provide optimal care and to minimize the physiological and psychological stress of the injury. It is essential, when a variety of disciplines contribute to the care, that a primary trauma physician oversee the medical care and a trauma nurse coordinator oversee the nursing care and assist in the coordination of the efforts of others. A wide variety of health care consultants may be involved with a single patient. Nurses, social workers, physical therapists, respiratory therapists, dietitians, and the infection control officer work together to provide the optimal team approach to real and potential problems. Trauma patients often have a wide variety of problems, both physical and psychological. Coordinating the efforts of all the health care providers is integral to patient management.

Table 57-3 Sample General Hospital Disaster Plan
(When confirmation of a disaster situation reaches the hospital, the decision to implement a modified or full-scale disaster plan is made by the appropriate persons. The acting disaster director notifies the switchboard operator of the appropriate paging information.)

Modified Plan

1. When the page is heard, 1 West, 2-N, 3-N, 4-N, and 5 North will each send one stretcher to the discharge corridor in the basement. One person from each of these units will remain in the discharge corridor unless dismissed by the disaster director.
2. The admitting department will call each unit to check the number of beds available.
3. Other preparations, including personnel, will be ordered as necessary.
4. All departments and personnel not assigned specific duties concerning the disaster will remain in their own area.
5. Further delineation of departmental duties will be found in the disaster manual.

Full-Scale Plan

1. When the page is heard, each nursing unit will send its stretchers, with available personnel, to the discharge corridor.
   1.1 Personnel will remain for duty in the discharge corridor and emergency area unless or until they are dismissed by the person in charge.
2. The admitting nurse will correlate beds for admissions.
   2.1 The head nurse will quickly compile A and B lists of beds and have available when Admitting calls.
3. Department heads will go to their designated areas and report to the disaster director.
4. Hospital personnel will report and sign the response list according to their individual department guidelines.
   4.1 Nursing personnel will report to Nursing Service for assignments.
   4.2 If place is not specified for your department, report and sign the response list in library, 2d floor.
5. Volunteers, except those on duty in special departments, report to the volunteers' office for assignments.
6. Specific duties of each department during a full-scale disaster are delineated in the Disaster Manual.
7. Any changes made by the disaster director will take priority over the written directions in the Disaster Manual. NO off-duty employees will report to the hospital unless called.

Nursing Roles

Trauma Nurse Coordinator

The trauma nurse coordinator (TNC) functions in the roles of administrator, consultant, coordinator, educator, practitioner, and researcher in the spe-cialized area of trauma care. The trauma nurse coordinator is often the hospital administrative representative in the trauma department. As an administrative manager he or she establishes goals, operational protocols, and priorities for the trauma department in accordance with organizational objectives. As a clinical manager the trauma nurse coordinator assists in integrating the flow of information to various team members and helps to develop and implement plans of care in accordance with patient and family needs. The trauma nurse coordinator participates in the compilation of data for the trauma registry, conducts daily quality assurance audits, and presents community trauma prevention programs.

Assistant Trauma Nurse Coordinator

As the patient census increases and the trauma system is established, it becomes necessary to have a qualified assistant who can work with the staff as well as assist in trauma audits. The assistant trauma nurse coordinator functions as an extension of the trauma nurse coordinator within the organized trauma system.

Trauma Resuscitation Nurse

The trauma resuscitation nurse provides continuity of care during the initial resuscitative phase of hospital care and functions as the nursing team leader by directing various nursing personnel on the trauma team. The trauma resuscitation nurse provides direct patient care, assessment, planning, and intervention as well as maintaining the supplies and equipment in the trauma unit.

Operating Room Nurse

A designated operating room nurse is considered an important member of the trauma team and should respond to all trauma resuscitative efforts. The operating room nurse assists with emergency open chest thoracotomies as well as other immediate surgical procedures that are performed within the trauma unit. He or she gathers information regarding the patient's history as well as pertinent information regarding possible surgery, e.g., autotransfusion of blood, as well as assembling and preparing the surgical team with appropriate information and notifying the anesthesiologist.

Table 57-4 Sample Full-Scale Disaster Guidelines for Emergency Department

1. When the disaster call is received, please follow these guidelines immediately:
    1.1 Notify medical emergency to dispatch ambulances to the scene.
        1.11 Put ambulance disaster supplies in first vehicle dispatched.
        1.12 If in the judgment of the Emergency physician the clinical status in the department permits, he or she will accompany the first unit to the disaster scene as triage officer. Two emergency department staff nurses will also be dispatched to the scene if staffing permits.
    1.2 Notify immediately the nursing supervisor on duty and
        1.21 (Physician) _____
        1.22 (Nurse) _____
            1.221 If nurse named is unavailable, notify _____ or _____
        1.23 The ambulance manager.
2. When disaster is verified:
    2.1 The ambulance manager will be notified and ambulance pagers alerted; other ambulance crews will be notified as indicated.
    2.2 Emergency Department secretaries will notify the other emergency physicians and the department nursing service staff as requested.
    2.3 Evacuate the patients from the department.
        2.31 Discharge those who are able to go.
        2.32 Send the necessary admissions to the floor immediately.
3. Carts will be brought from each nursing unit to the discharge corridor.
4. The nursing supervisor of the Emergency Services Department or a designated alternate will coordinate preparation, make assignments in the emergency area as follows, and call for the disaster carts to be brought from the storeroom.
    4.1 The nursing secretary is usually assigned the following duties by the nursing supervisor:
        4.11 Make himself or herself immediately available to the disaster director and will locate in the physicians' office in the Emergency Department to accept calls from department heads on line 2365 and to perform other duties as requested.
        4.12 Take charge of the master key for the patient elevator.
        4.13 Set up tagging desks, with at least two persons at each desk.
            4.131 Two at ambulance entrance
            4.132 Two at ambulatory entrance
            4.133 Supplies needed at each desk are prenumbered disaster tags and large paper bags, one red marker, one black marker, and pens.
                4.1331 Odd-numbered tags and bags are used at the ambulance entrance and even-numbered tags and bags at the ambulatory entrance.
            4.134 Tagging desk responsibilities:
                4.1341 Tie the tag on the patient.
                    4.13411 Tag the patients in number sequence.
                4.1342 Give the patient the prenumbered bag corresponding to the number appearing on the tag.
                4.1343 Follow the instructions of the triage physicians and nurses.
                4.1344 Mark the care classification.
                    4.13441 If immediate, mark with red.
                    4.13442 If delayed or expired, mark with black.
        4.14 Remain at the main desk, answer the telephone, keep the master patient list current, and send an updated list after every fifth patient to keep the supervisor informed.
            4.141 The master list information is obtained from the information desk copy of the tag. It is the responsibility of each treatment area to send this portion of the tag to the desk as soon as possible. One copy of master sheet is taken to communication center and another copy is taken to Social Services in the auditorium.
    4.2 Assign as follows:
        4.21 An Emergency Department nurse will be put in charge of each designated area and is responsible for the preparation and coordination of that room.
            4.211 Fracture Room—Cast Room
                4.2111 Move the stretchers into the discharge corridor and clear the room of unnecessary objects.
                4.2112 Place the Fracture Room sign beside the room entrance.
                4.2113 Obtain the Fracture Room supply cart or basket from the storeroom.
                4.2114 Personnel needed:
                    4.21141 4 nurses
                    4.21142 Assigned physicians
                    4.21143 1 messenger

(Continued)

     4.212 Lacerations and Surgical—Trauma Room

        4.2121 Move the stretchers into the discharge corridor and clear the room of unnecessary objects.

        4.2122 Place the Lacerations and Surgical sign beside the Trauma Room entrance.

        4.2123 Obtain the Lacerations and Surgical supply cart or basket from the storeroom.

        4.2124 Personnel needed:

           4.21241 8 nurses

           4.21242 Assigned physicians

           4.21343 1 messenger

     4.213 Shock and Burns—Observation Unit

        4.2131 Move one of the stretchers out of the Heart Room into the discharge corridor. Move two of the Observation Unit beds into the Heart Room. Move the other four beds in the Observation Unit to one side. Clear one side of the room of all unnecessary objects.

        4.2132 Place the Shock and Burns sign beside the Observation Unit entrance.

        4.2133 Obtain the Shock and Burns supply cart or basket from the storeroom.

        4.2134 Personnel needed:

           4.21341 6 nurses

           4.21342 Assigned physicians

           4.21343 1 messenger

     4.214 Minor Injuries—Examination Rooms 1 and 2

        4.2141 Move all unnecessary objects from the room. Ambulatory or wheelchair patients with minor injuries may be checked in this room.

        4.2142 Place the Minor Injuries sign beside the Examination Room entrances.

        4.2143 Obtain the Minor Injuries supply cart or basket from the storeroom.

        4.2144 Personnel needed:

           4.21441 1 nurse

           4.21442 1 physician, if needed

           4.21443 1 messenger

     4.215 Regular Emergency Department patients—Examination Rooms 3 and 4

        4.2151 Move all unnecessary objects from the room.

        4.2152 Place the regular Emergency Department Patients signs beside the Examination Room entrances.

        4.2153 Place some regular outpatient ledgers in these rooms. Check the rooms for routine equipment needed.

        4.2154 Personnel needed:

           4.21541 1 nurse

           4.21542 1 physician, if needed

           4.21543 1 messenger

  4.3 General information

     4.31 Each Emergency Department area is responsible for sending the information desk copy of the disaster tag via messenger up to the main emergency desk area as soon as the information is on it. This is the middle copy of the tag.

     4.32 Instruct your messengers that all patients to be admitted will be taken on the stretcher they are on to the area specified. Disaster tag is to be handed to admitting personnel, who will give the messenger the assigned room number for the patient.

     4.33 The hardback copy of the disaster tag stays on the patient at all times and remains on the patient when discharged from your area.

        4.331 Ledgers will be filled out after the disaster to provide a more adequate record and to obtain necessary charges.

     4.34 If the patient is conscious, it is most important to ask about known allergies. This is an area frequently overlooked in disaster situations.

     4.35 Personal belongings and clothing are to be placed in the large paper bag and sent with the patient.

     4.36 The Minor Operating Room and the Heart Room are standby units and will be used only if necessary.

5. There should be at least two hall coordinators as follows:

  5.1 The medical director of Emergency Services or the director's designated alternate and the nursing supervisor of Emergency Services or the supervisor's designated alternate.

  5.2 Responsibilities

     5.21 Make sure the preparation of the department is satisfactory and all assignments are made.

     5.22 Keep the traffic moving, thereby keeping the area from getting congested.

     5.23 Call for messenger replacements for the specific emergency areas.

6. When the task of transporting victims from the scene is over, the ambulance personnel will return to the Emergency Department and will be utilized as needed.

Critical-Care Nurse

As a trauma team member, a designated critical-care nurse responds to the trauma units during trauma resuscitations. The critical-care nurse may function as a direct care giver or be responsible for the documentation of information on the medical records during resuscitation. The critical-care nurse continues to provide care to the trauma patient as the patient moves from the trauma unit into the critical-care unit. Ongoing assessment and management are important aspects of this role.

Monitoring

During the primary and secondary survey, the nurse plays an essential role in gathering baseline data on various physiological parameters. Continuous monitoring alerts the nurse to early changes in the patient's condition. Observation, interpretation, and documentation of the patient's complex and dynamic status provide the information necessary for determining appropriate nursing interventions. Monitoring such physiological parameters as ECG, pulse, blood pressure, respirations, $S\bar{v}_{O_2}$, SVR, CO, PAP, ICP, urinary output, and daily weight assists in evaluating the ongoing status of the patient. Isolated values provide little information about a patient's dynamic status; the *trend* of these values provides the most useful information. The critical-care nurse considers and integrates the variety of data representing different organ systems in order to properly assess the status of the multiple-trauma patient. Equally important is the need for the critical-care nurse to understand and evaluate the workings of the assessment and therapeutic instrumentation. The assessment data should be organized on a trauma flow sheet, as shown in Fig. 57-4. The graph provides the trauma team with information concerning the trend of values at a quick glance.

Potential for Wound Infection

Because of the nature of their origin, wounds of trauma victims are often initially contaminated, and extra caution must be exercised to prevent extensive infection. Often trauma patients become resistant to antibiotic therapy. This situation offers a special challenge, as the nurse must engage in meticulous cleaning of all patient tubes, catheters, and IV lines

as well as wound and mouth care. The patients in surrounding beds must be protected. Aseptic hand washing technique prior to and following each patient encounter must be maintained.

Treatment is specific to the type and location of the wound. Trauma patients may have abrasions, avulsions, contusions, lacerations, or puncture wounds or any combination of these.

Abrasions are painful wounds that invade the epidermis and at times the dermis. This type of wound is best managed with aggressive mechanical cleaning to remove the wound contaminants that result in infection. Irrigation devices such as jet lavage, using a 50-mL syringe with an 18-gauge needle, and irrigation systems are extremely beneficial in this procedure. Scrubbing the wound assists in the removal of embedded contaminants. Aseptic technique is paramount in order to prevent the introduction of bacteria. Dressings provide the appropriate environment for healing of abrasions.

Avulsions produce a wound that has a tissue loss. Mechanical cleaning by irrigation and scrubbing is essential to prevent recontamination of the wound. Soaking the wound is contraindicated, since the bacteria released into the solution are reabsorbed into the wound. Healing of avulsions is by secondary intention. A regimen of mechanical cleaning and dressing application is an essential part of the management of avulsions.

Contusions are nonpenetrating soft tissue injuries. The skin and underlying tissue are bruised. The use of pressure, ice, elevation, and immobilization assist in stopping bleeding, edema, and pain.

A *laceration* is an irregular torn or incised wound in the flesh. The surrounding wound edges should be cleaned with an antiseptic solution in order to effectively remove bacteria. Reapproximation of the skin edges is vital for proper healing.

Puncture wounds are formed as a result of objects being forced through the skin. Warm soaks reduce inflammation and facilitate drainage and removal of devitalized tissue. Although all open wounds are tetanus-prone, deep puncture wounds are of special concern, since they provide the anaerobic environment that is required for the tetanus organism. Wounds should be carefully observed for signs of inflammation, purulent drainage, and ischemia. Extremity wounds occluded by plaster require particular attention; systemic tempera-

Figure 57-4 Trauma nursing data form.

EMERGENCY DEPARTMENT TRAUMA SHEET

Date ——————— Trauma Score In ———————

Time In ——————— Trauma Score Out ———————

Est. wt. in Kg ——————— Age ——————— Sex ———————

Mechanism of Injury ———————————

Time On Scene ———————————

Initial Vital Signs ———————————

Mode of Arrival to ER ———————————

Additional Comments ———————————

———————————

———————————

Allergies ———————————

Medications ———————————

———————————

Medical History ———————————

———————————

———————————

Last Meal ———————————

Last Tetanus Toxoid ———————————

NEUROLOGICAL ASSESMENT

ALERT ———————————

VERBAL ———————————

PAIN ———————————

UNRESPONSIVE ———————————

RESPIRATORY ASSESSMENT

Airway	Breathing	Pulses Present	Skin Color	Skin Moisture	Skin Temp.	Capillary Refill
Patent [ ]	Spontaneous [ ]	Radial R [ ] L [ ]	Normal [ ]	Normal [ ]	Normal [ ]	Normal [ ]
Oral Airway [ ]	Absent [ ]	if not present go to	Cyanotic [ ]	Dry [ ]	Hot [ ]	Delayed > 2 sec [ ]
ET tube/EOA [ ]	Assisted [ ]	Femoral R [ ] L [ ]	Pale [ ]	Moist [ ]	Warm [ ]	None
Comments _____	Comments _____	Carotid R [ ] L [ ]	Ashen [ ]	Diaphoretic [ ]	Cool [ ]	Open Bleeding Y—N—
		Apical [ ]	Flushed [ ]		Cold [ ]	If yes, list source

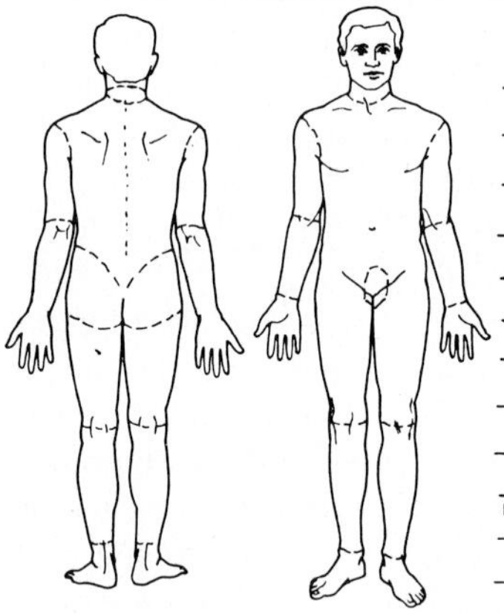

CIRCULATORY ASSESSMENT

ASSESSMENT

———————————

———————————

———————————

———————————

———————————

———————————

———————————

———————————

NURSING DIAGNOSIS

NURSE INITIAL

RADIOGRAPHIC STUDIES

C–Spine	[ ]	Arteriogram	[ ]
Upright Chest	[ ]		
Chest	[ ]	Extremities	[ ]
Skull	[ ]		
Pelvic	[ ]	————	
Abdomen	[ ]		
IVP	[ ]	Others ————	

LABORATORY STUDIES

CBC (time) ————

U/A	[ ]	Peritoneal Fluid	[ ]
BUN	[ ]	Amylase	[ ]
Glucose	[ ]	ETOH	[ ]
Lytes	[ ]	Drug Screen	[ ]
Lytes	[ ]	T & C No of units	
PT	[ ]		

200 180 160 140 120 100 80 60 40 20 0

time

CUFF BP ∨∧   Arterial Line   Respirations   Pulse   Temp. ————

Time	Medication	Dosage	Mode	Site	Comments	Initial

NURSES NOTES

TIME	SPECIAL PROCEDURES AND TREATMENTS	REMARKS

INTAKE
GRAND TOTAL _____   Estimated Blood Loss _____   OUTPUT
GRAND TOTAL _____

NURSING SIGNATURE CODE

NAME	INITIALS

EMERGENCY ROOM PHYSICIAN SIGNATURE _____

EMERGENCY DEPARTMENT TRAUMA SHEET

Figure 57-4 (Continued)   Trauma nursing data form.

ture, local extremity temperature, capillary filling, and signs of swelling are important parameters. Dressings should be changed with meticulous sterile technique. When there are multiple wounds, care should be taken to prevent cross infection. The utmost care should also be taken to prevent cross contamination between patients in the unit. Proper nutrition and adequate caloric intake are integral to wound healing. (See Chap. 56 for further discussion of wound healing.)

Dependence-Independence

The majority of trauma patients are young and used to an independent type of lifestyle. The unexpected loss of independence is more often than not the most difficult thing for the trauma patient to accept. The nurse should assess the patient's functional ability and address realistic goals once the critical phase is dealt with. The hospitalization in itself places the patient in a dependent state by restrictions and physical limitations imposed by the care of these injuries. Patients with spinal cord deficits or amputations are confronted with an immediate permanent disability in addition to the temporary dependence of hospitalization. Physical as well as psychological rehabilitation must begin in the critical-care unit. Remaining function and tone should be preserved with range-of-motion exercises and splinting.

Depression

Trauma patients are often depressed as a result of their own increased awareness of limitations and frustrations at personal failure. It is important for the nursing staff to provide listening time with the patient and encourage family-patient interaction. Pertinent information regarding support and resource groups is often valuable as an additional mechanism for family and patient support.

Ineffective Coping

During the initial stages of treatment, the family's emotional needs are often as great as the patient's physical needs. Consideration must be given to meeting these needs. Family members initially feel shock, fright, disbelief, and numbness. Family fights or disputes may have preceded the trauma incident. Spouses and loved ones may feel responsible for and guilty about the incident. Relatives feel powerless to influence the recovery process, and frustration develops. The critical-care unit must be considered an alien environment not only to the patient but also to the family (see Chaps. 6 and 18).

The nursing staff may alleviate the family's stresses by supportive interventions such as providing information, encouraging appropriate expression of feelings, and creating an optimal environment for interaction. Initial meetings with family members to determine their needs and provide information concerning management are followed by daily contact in which information is given and questions are answered. The staff should attempt to prepare the family members for visits to the patient in the critical-care unit. Explanation of equipment, lines, and tubes should be offered. On the basis of assessments of the family members, information can be provided to include them in some of the care of the patient. Allied personnel such as social workers and psychiatrists should be involved in meeting the psychosocial needs of the patient and family members.

Nursing Care Plans

Nursing care plans should be started while the patient is in the resuscitation room. The care plan follows the patient throughout the hospitalization and is continually updated according to the patient's needs. Some examples of nursing care plans for selected problems of trauma patients while in the resuscitation room are given below.

Airway Management

History
Moving vehicle accident—head injury. Large volume blood loss, blunt or crush injury to trachea, smoke inhalation, chemical inhalation, blunt or penetrating trauma to thorax.

Patient Examination
Shallow, absent, or diminished breath sounds on auscultation. Observe respiratory effort for intra-costal retraction, apnea, tachypnea. Monitor ABGs for decreased Pa_{O_2} levels, color changes.

Nursing Diagnosis
Potential for respiratory distress related to disruption of normal respiratory exchange patterns as manifested by intracostal retraction, decreased Pa_{O_2} levels, and color changes.

Goals
Pa_{O_2} of 80 mmHg or more; unassisted respiratory rate of 10 to 24.

Nursing Interventions

1. Give high O_2 concentration to improve oxygenation.
2. Elevate head of bed *(if condition permits)* to assist respiratory effort.
3. Monitor ABGs closely for signs of hypoxemia.
4. Make frequent assessments of respiratory status and level of consciousness.
5. Minimize effort patient exerts to conserve O_2.
6. Use oral pharyngeal airway if indicated.
7. Assist ventilation with AmbuBag as necessary.
8. Have equipment at hand for endotracheal intubation in case of emergency.

Cardiac Contusions

History
Blunt chest trauma, driver impacting steering wheel unbelted moving vehicle (motorcycle) accident. Crush injuries, significant fall (12 ft or more), and ejection from vehicle.

Patient Examination
Precordial pain and discomfort—consistent chest x-ray findings. Inspect anterior chest wall for obvious bruising and deformity. Observe ECG for cardiac dysrhythmias and ischemia. Auscultate for murmurs, decreased heart sounds, pericardial friction rub. Palpate pulmonic and aortic areas for thrills, palpitations, chest wall tenderness.

Nursing Diagnosis
Alteration in cardiac output and perfusion due to disruption of electrical pathways as manifested by dysrhythmias. Potential for congestive heart failure.

Goal

Non-life-threatening electrical conduction through myocardium with maintenance of cardiac output.

Nursing Interventions

1. Maintain ECG monitoring—close and constant evaluation. Document and interpret rhythm strip on admission and discharge and any pertinent rhythm change while in the trauma unit.
2. Give high O_2 concentrations to improve oxygenation.
3. Elevate head of bed (*if condition allows*) to improve cardiac output.
4. Closely monitor IV fluids to prevent fluid overload.
5. Treat all ventricular dysrhythmias, AV block, tachycardias.
6. Relieve pain, utilize comfort measures.
7. Monitor ABG values for adequate Pa_{O_2} levels.

Open Extremity Fracture

History

Blunt trauma—unrestrained moving vehicle occupant, motorcycle accident. Crush injuries, significant fall (12 ft or more), ejection from vehicle, abusive treatment, traumatic injury or amputation.

Patient Examination

Obvious deformity, pain and discomfort over the affected area. Possible alteration in pulse distal to injury. Visible disruption of bone integrity and skin, loss of mobility distal to fracture site.

Nursing Diagnosis

Alteration in bone and skin integrity due to traumatic injury as manifested by obvious deformity and disruption of bone and skin.

Goals

Extremity alignment without loss of function, absence of active bleeding, palpable pulses distal to fracture site.

Nursing Interventions

1. Establish and maintain proper bone alignment by traction, splinting.
2. Control open bleeding by manual pressure.
3. Palpate and assess frequently for both distal and proximal pulses.
4. Elevate involved extremity to promote venous return and decrease potential for venous status.
5. Relieve pain in extremity by medication, countertraction, positioning, and splinting.
6. Medicate to decrease possible vasconstriction and occlusion of circulatory flow to extremity.

Organ Procurement

Organ procurement is the removal and care of viable organs from a person predetermined to be brain-dead with the intent of transplantation. Organ procurement provides an opportunity of life for those qualified as suitable recipients. The type of patient most often suitable for organ donation is the multiple-trauma patient. These patients tend to be young (2 to 44 years) and have a relatively disease-free history prior to the accident. After an accident, some trauma patients are left brain-dead with functioning disease-free organs. Between 12,000 and 27,000 patients within the suitable age range for transplantation succumb to brain death in the United States yearly. One donor often supplies the need of more than one recipient. The organs suitable for transplantation and frequency for 1986 are listed in Table 57-5.

Organ transplantation provides a chance of hope and life for recipients with renal, hepatic, and cardiac disease. However, the organ transplantation waiting lists are long. Many patients with kidney disease are maintained on dialysis machines for

Table 57-5 Organs-Suitable for Transplantation

Organs	Estimated Transplants per Year
Kidneys	8973
Heart	1368
Liver	924
Pancreas	140
Heart-lung	45
Corneal	31,000
Bone Marrow	1160

Source: American Council on Transplantation, *Organ Transplantation Fact Sheet*, 1986.

years while awaiting a properly matched viable kidney. The problem is not the lack of potential donors, money, or technical skills but the lack of suitable donor *referral*. The nurse can be instrumental in communicating to families that their loved one may be a suitable organ donor candidate and in notifying referral centers of potential donors. Acceptable donor criteria are as follows:

Brain death from brain damage in previously healthy patient

Suitable physiological (rather than chronological) age (varies according to organ being donated)

Satisfactory blood pressure, physical examination, history (parameters differ according to organ being donated)

Conditions that render a patient unacceptable as an organ donor include:

Prolonged ischemia due to profound hypotension or asystole

A history of trauma to or disease of the organ to be donated

Selected malignant diseases

A history of diabetes mellitus, hypertension, cardiovascular disease, or peripheral vascular disease

Untreated systemic infections

The management of the potential organ donor is usually carried out in the intensive-care unit. Once the physician has determined that the patient is brain-dead, nursing care is directed toward continued support of family members and significant others and maintaining organ viability. Nursing priorities should be directed toward avoidance of infection and maintenance of organ perfusion, hydration, and diuresis. In the event of cardiac arrest it is essential to restore circulation so that organ recovery can remain a consideration. The North American Transplant Coordinators Organization (NATCO) sponsors a 24-h information and referral service for health care professionals; its organ donation hotline is 800-24-DONOR. Organ procurement offers many chronically ill patients a chance of hope and life. Nurses and physicians can assist the grieving families and potential recipients by recognizing potential organ donors and notifying appropriate referral centers.

References

1. Trunkey, D. D. (1980, August). Trauma. *Scientific American,* pp. 28–35.
2. Oakes, A. (1979). Trauma: Twentieth century epidemic, *Heart and Lung, 8* (5), 918.
3. Trunkey, D. D. (1982, October). The value of trauma centers. *American College of Surgeons Bulletin,* pp. 5–7.
4. Gunby, P. (1984). Deaths decline, but drunk driving, other traffic safety hazards remain. *JAMA, 251* (13), 1645–1647.
5. Statistics Department, *Accident Facts* (1983). Chicago: National Safety Council.
6. Helpern, J. (1982). Patterns of trauma. *Journal of Emergency Nursing, 8* (4), 170–175.
7. Anderson, Charles B. & Ballinger, Walter F. (1985). Abdominal injuries, in Zuidema, G., Rutherford, R., & Ballinger, W. (eds.), *The management of trauma,* 4th ed., Philadelphia: Saunders.
8. White, K. (1977, October). Evaluating the trauma of gunshot wounds. *American Journal of Nursing,* p. 1589.
9. Champion, H. R., Sacco, W. J., Carnazzo, A. J., et al. (1981). Trauma score. *Critical Care Medicine, 9* (9), 672–676.
10. American College of Surgeons, Committee on Trauma (1984). *Advanced trauma life support.*
11. Edgerton, Milton T. & Kenny, John G. (1985). Maxillo facial trauma, in Zuidema, G., Rutherford, R., & Ballinger, W. (eds.), *The management of trauma,* 4th ed., Philadelphia: Saunders.
12. Cowley, R. Adams, & Dunham, M. (1982). *Shock trauma/critical care manual: Initial assessment and management.* Baltimore; University Park.
13. Cardona, V. D. (1985). *Trauma nursing.* Oradell, NJ: Medical Economics Books.
14. Dove, D. B., Del Guercio, L. R., Stahl, W. M., et al. (1982). A metropolitan airport disaster plan: Coordination of a multihospital response to provide onsite resuscitation and stabilization before evacuation. *Journal of Trauma, 22,* 550.
15. Briggs, S. & Funt, L. (1985). Mass casualty management, in Zuidema G., Rutherford, R., & Ballinger, W. (eds.), *The management of trauma,* 4th ed., Philadelphia: Saunders.

58 Sepsis

Robert F. Wilson
Jacqueline A. Wilson

Definition

Sepsis is a clinical syndrome characterized by systemic signs and symptoms of severe infection. In many instances, sepsis is associated with *septicemia,* which refers to infection with rapidly multiplying bacteria in the bloodstream. *Septic shock* represents the most severe form of sepsis and is usually associated with septicemia. However, live organisms can only be cultured from blood in about 50 to 60 percent of patients with septic shock.

Bacteremia refers only to the presence of bacteria in the bloodstream. They may or may not cause any pathophysiologic changes. For example, dental extractions and drilling of dental caries may introduce bacteria into the bloodstream, but unless there is a deformed rheumatic valve or vascular prosthesis, or unless the patient is severely immunocompromised, these bacteria almost never cause any adverse effects. *Endotoxemia* refers to the presence of endotoxin, a component of the cell wall of gram-negative bacteria, in the bloodstream; it is generally associated with severe signs and symptoms of infection, and it is often, but not necessarily, associated with septicemia.

Incidence

The importance of sepsis cannot be overemphasized. Sepsis is the most frequent disease acquired in the hospital, and its incidence appears to be increasing. It has been estimated that about 7 percent of the 30 million patients admitted to hospitals annually in the United States develop an infection. Of these 2 million patients, about 10 to 15 percent develop a bacteremia, usually with gram-negative organisms. If one also assumes a mortality rate of 20 to 40 percent for patients with gram-negative bacteremia, the annual death rate of 50,000 to 100,000 from these organisms alone equals or exceeds that caused by motor vehicle accidents.

About 7 percent of patients become infected from the 18 to 20 million surgical procedures performed annually in the United States. The resultant medical expenses and value of time lost from work are staggering. Furthermore, sepsis is a major contributing factor in at least a third of the deaths following surgery. In trauma victims, sepsis is the leading cause of death in patients who survive for more than 48 h.

An apparently increasing incidence of sepsis may be partially due to improved techniques for culturing bacteria, especially anaerobes. However, the increasing number of critically ill and injured hospitalized patients with impaired host defenses is probably a more important factor. Because of advances in critical care, many individuals who previously succumbed rapidly to heart attacks, strokes, cancer, and other diseases now live long enough to develop sepsis. Those particularly susceptible to infection include cancer patients receiving chemotherapy and transplant patients receiving immunosuppressants. Furthermore, the extensive utilization of antimicrobial therapy has resulted in elimination of the normal bacterial flora in many patients and replacement with strains which are resistant to antimicrobial agents. This is particularly true in hospitals, where resistant strains become concentrated and can rapidly replace the normal flora of patients shortly after they are admitted.

Importance of Early Diagnosis and Therapy

Although hospital-acquired (nosocomial) infections are frequent and can have disastrous consequences, many can be prevented. Most nosocomial infections occur in predictable settings. This is particularly true with certain types of surgery (e.g., repair of colon trauma and urinary tract instrumentation) and in patients who have altered host resistance because of disease or drugs (such as immunosuppressive agents).

Because the early signs and symptoms of infection in critically ill patients with impaired host defenses are often subtle, it is important to know which patients are most likely to become infected so that they can be watched with particular care. All too often the diagnosis of sepsis is made late, after multiple organ failure has developed. The nurse who is at the bedside for prolonged periods of time can contribute significantly to the early diagnosis of sepsis by noting subtle changes in the patient's condition, particularly his or her mental status.

Host Defense

Within all of us there is a constant struggle between our defense mechanisms and microorganisms attempting to invade our bodies. When host defenses are impaired and/or the virulence or numbers of invading microorganisms are so great that the balance is altered in favor of the microorganisms, infection is apt to result.

Reticuloendothelial System

The most important activities of our host defenses involve the reticuloendothelial system (RES). The cells of the RES are present in greatest concentration in the spleen and in greatest quantity in the liver. These cells act against invading microorganisms primarily by phagocytosing (ingesting) them and/ or by forming immune bodies (antibodies) which react with them or their toxins to destroy them, inactivate them, or enhance their removal by phagocytes.

To facilitate understanding of the complex interplay of cellular and humoral components in the RES, this next section will be divided into descriptions of phagocytic cells, antibodies, complement, fibronectin, and the inflammatory (vascular) response.

Phagocytes

The phagocytes, which engulf bacteria or foreign particles, may be divided into fixed and circulating cells. The fixed (tissue) phagocytes are either special sessile endothelial cells lining capillaries or sinusoids (such as the Kupffer cells which line the hepatic sinusoids) or reticular cells such as those found in the spleen (particularly in the red pulp) and lymph nodes (in the medullary sinuses) (Table 58-1). The circulating phagocytes are primarily the polymorphonuclear leukocytes (PMNs) in the bloodstream and bone marrow.

When bacteria manage to get into the body, macrophages are activated. These in turn stimulate production of specific T and B lymphocytes which activate more macrophages. The T cell activation produces the cellular immune response and activated B cells can produce specific antibodies against the invading microorganism (Fig. 58-1).

Part of the activation of the macrophages is via exogenous pyrogen or antigen-sensitized T cells. The activated macrophages in turn produce leukocytic (endogenous) pyrogen which is also called LAF (leukocyte activating factor) or IL-1 (interleukin-

---

Table 58-1   Cells of the Reticular Endothelial System

Mobile phagocytic cells:
  Blood monocyte
  Alveolar macrophage
  Peritoneal macrophage
  Connective tissue histocyte
  Polymorphonuclear leukocyte (not classically part of the RES)

Sessile phagocytic endothelial cells lining capillaries or sinusoids of:
  Liver (Kupffer cells)
  Spleen
  Lymph nodes
  Bone marrow
  Adrenal glands
  Hypophyseal system
  Kidneys
  Lungs

Reticular cells:
  Spleen
  Central nervous system
  Lymph nodes
  Bone marrow

Source: W.J. Sibbald, and C.L. Sprung, eds., *Perspectives on Sepsis and Septic Shock*, Society of Critical Care Medicine, 1986, p. 78. Used with permission of the publisher.

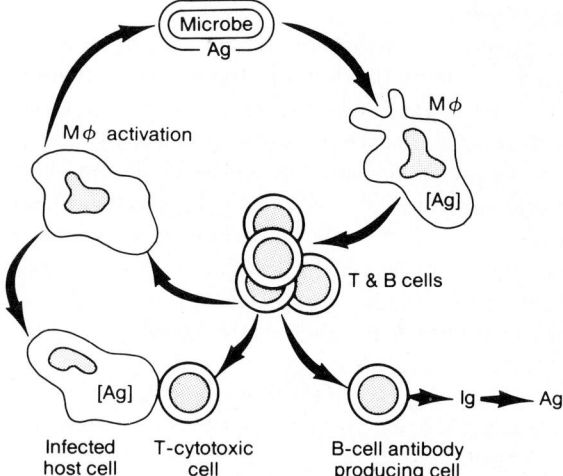

Figure 58-1 Major pathways of acquired immune responses to microbial antigens involving macrophages, T cell, and B cell populations. *(From G. P. Youmans, P. Y. Paterson, and H. M. Sommers, eds., The Biologic and Clinical Basis of Infectious Diseases, Saunders, 1985, p. 30, used with permission of the publisher.)*

Figure 58-2 Pathways of endogenous pyrogen production with resulting fever and associated effects on host immune response and iron metabolism. *(From G. P. Youmans, P. Y. Paterson, and H. M. Sommers, eds., The Biologic and Clinical Basis of Infectious Diseases, Saunders, 1985, p. 94, used with permission of the publisher.)*

requirements to decrease microbial growth (Fig. 58-2).

All of these mechanisms are designed to help the fixed phagocytic cells of the reticuloendothelial system isolate and engulf invading bacteria. If the number of bacteria is very large or if the RES is not functioning well, the task falls back chiefly on the PMNs which then move via the bloodstream to the area of bacterial invasion.

Opsonins refer to a group of substances in serum which attach themselves to the surface of antigens (usually microorganisms or particulate matter) and thereby enhance the ability of phagocytes to recognize and engulf them. Antibodies may function as opsonins. Indeed, IgG and IgM antibodies are two of the most common opsonins. The two main other opsonins are complement and fibronectin. In some instances, patients with severe, continuing active infections appear to use up or "consume" their important opsonic proteins. This process, referred to as *consumptive opsinopathy*, can be corrected, at least partially, by administration of fresh frozen plasma or cryoprecipitate.

Functional abnormalities of neutrophils have been found in a variety of hereditary and acquired diseases. The acquired disorders include severe burns, trauma, malnutrition, and administration of a number of drugs, especially those used to treat malignancies or prevent rejection of transplanted

1) which enhances the antibody response of B cells and stimulates the generation of cytotoxic T cells. Other effects include CNS stimulation to increase heat production and conservation to cause fever which augments the T cell response to IL-1. The fever also alters plasma iron and microbial iron

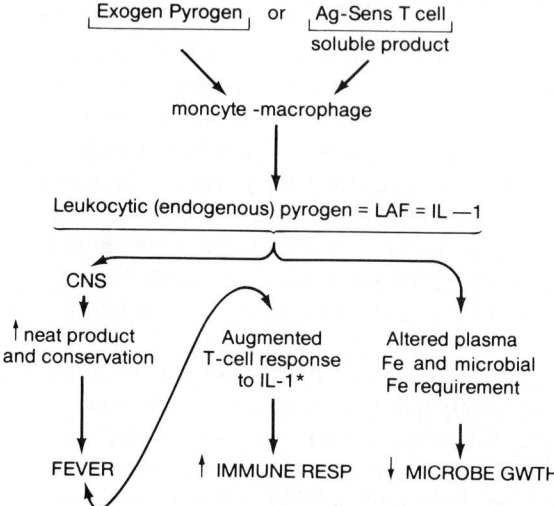

*In vitro; analogous selective response of T cells in vivo to IL-1 in febrile host remains to be demonstrated definitively.

tissues. A direct relationship between the degree of the functional abnormality of circulating neutrophils and the development of life-threatening infections has been well established in burn patients.

Malnutrition may be a particularly important and reversible cause of abnormalities of neutrophil function and impaired delayed skin reactions to various antigens. Complete failure to react on skin testing for mumps, *Candida,* streptokinase, and purified protein derivative (PPD) usually indicates severe impairment of host defenses, often referred to as *anergy.* Anergy is particularly apt to be present if serum albumin levels fall below 2.2 g/dL and the absolute lymphocyte count (ALC) is less than 800 mm³. Resistance to infection may be returned to normal in some of these patients by an increased intake of calories, protein, and trace elements. Enteral feeding, where possible, appears to be more effective than IV hyperalimentation.

Antibodies

Antibodies are specific proteins which are generally developed in response to a particular antigen, which may be an invading microorganism or any foreign substance. These antibodies attempt to destroy or inactivate the antigen and/or enhance its phagocytosis and subsequent removal from the body.

Most antibodies are gamma globulins, but a few are beta globulins and a very few are alpha globulins. Almost all antibodies are formed in plasma cells, which are found primarily in lymph nodes, the spleen, and the bone marrow.

Complement

Complement refers to a group of at least 11 proteins in serum which can be activated in a cascade fashion to destroy or assist in the destruction of bacteria and cells which have been sensitized by specific antibodies. The complement cascade can be initiated by the classic pathway via C1 activation by Ag-Ab reactions, or via the alternative pathway by activation of C3 by endotoxin, natural antibody, and several other substances (Fig. 58-3). Complement acts to enhance standard antigen-antibody immune reactions by promoting chemotaxis, immune adherence, and phagocytosis, and by liberating anaphylatoxin. Two substances which are liberated during the complement cascade and are of particular interest in septic patients with ARDS are C3a

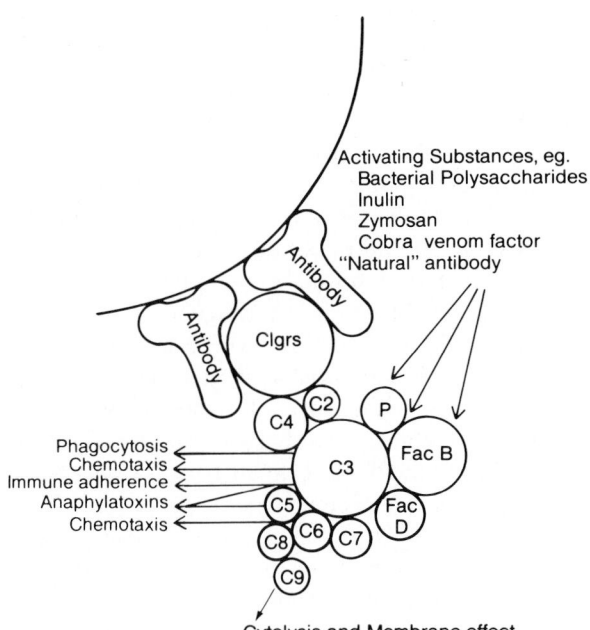

Figure 58-3   Schematic representation of the complement pathway. The classic pathway can be activated by antigen-antibody complex, whereas the alternative pathway is activated by a variety of substances such as those listed on the right. C1 to C9 are components of the classic pathway. (P = properdin; Fac. B = Factor B; and Fac. D = Factor D.) *(From D. C. Sabiston, Textbook of Surgery, 13th ed., Saunders, 1986, p. 261, used with permission of the publisher.)*

and C5a. These two substances stimulate chemotaxis and cause PMNs to stick to pulmonary capillary endothelium. Liberation of lysosomal enzymes and superoxides from these PMNs may be the major cause of ARDS in sepsis.

Fibronectin

Within recent years fibronectin has received increasing attention. This substance is present in two forms. The soluble form in plasma may be extremely important as an opsonin. The insoluble form is located near the basement membrane of small vessels and is very important in vascular integrity.

Inflammatory Response

Inflammation is the tissue response to injury or infection. Several processes appear to be involved, including vasodilation, increased capillary permeability, and chemotaxis (attraction of neutrophils to the inflamed area). Vasodilation results in an increased supply of blood, bringing more PMNs and antibodies to the involved area. Increased capillary permeability allows large quantities of fluid and protein to leak into the tissues. The antibodies and complement that enter the tissue with these fluids can attach to the microorganisms to assist in their destruction and removal by the phagocytes. The fibrinogen that also enters may coagulate and thereby help isolate the noxious agent or bacteria from the rest of the body. Chemotaxis is first manifested as margination or adherence of neutrophils to the capillaries of the involved tissue, in response to chemicals liberated there from bacteria, involved tissue cells, or complement.

Tissue response to infection appears to be mediated to a large extent by substances released during complement activation and by kinins. The kinins involved in inflammation are a group of polypeptides, usually 9 to 11 amino acids in length, which can produce profound hemodynamic effects, including increased capillary permeability and vasodilation or vasoconstriction.

Bradykinin, the best known of the kinins, is an extremely potent vasodilator. Even in nanogram (10^{-9}) quantities, it can cause profound vasodilation and increased permeability of capillaries and small veins. Much of the flushing seen with sepsis, alcoholism, and pancreatitis is probably due to bradykinin. The other kinin of particular interest is myocardial depressant factor (MDF). MDF is said to be liberated from ischemic pancreatic cells and is thought to depress myocardial function and cause splanchnic vasoconstriction.

Excess activation of these vasoactive substances can cause inappropriate vasoconstriction resulting in local ischemia or vasodilation with increased capillary permeability causing increased loss of fluid into tissues. A vicious downward cycle of increased release of vasoactive substances and progressively impaired cardiovascular activity may then develop. Eradication of the underlying infection is usually the only way to stop this downward spiral. Occasionally, however, very early massive administration of steroids may help by reducing the excess activation of complement and kinins.

Factors Altering Host Resistance

Many factors can impair host resistance. Some of the more important factors include loss of skin or mucous membrane integrity, the presence of prostheses and foreign bodies, disease involving RES, certain types of drug therapy, extremes of age, and impaired metabolism or cardiovascular or pulmonary function.

Skin and Mucous Membrane Integrity

The anatomic integrity of the skin and mucosal surfaces and their secretions are usually extremely effective obstacles to invasion by pathogenic microorganisms. Any procedure or condition that disrupts or impairs this integrity is associated with an increased risk of hospital infection. Infection in patients with extensive burns or skin diseases is particularly difficult to prevent and poses a serious risk during hospitalization. Injury to mucous membranes is also an important cause of infection, particularly if a foreign body, such as a urethral catheter, is inserted and/or left in place. Prolonged ischemia or sepsis can impair intestinal mucosal blood flow; the ischemic intestinal mucosa may then allow increasing amounts of bacteria and bacterial products from the intestinal lumen to enter the portal venous system.

Prostheses and Foreign Bodies

Foreign bodies reduce the ability of tissue to fight infection. In certain experimental studies, 10^6 organisms are required to cause infection in normal tissue; however, if a foreign body such as a silk suture is present, as little as 10^2 organisms are needed. In addition, it is usually very difficult to eradicate an infection until the foreign body is removed. The most common foreign bodies associated with infection appear to be IV plastic catheters and urethral catheters. Prosthetic cardiac valves and vascular grafts have also been implicated in hospital infections.

Intravenous plastic catheters left in place longer than 2 to 3 days are important causes of thrombophlebitis and sepsis in critically ill patients. Prospective studies have demonstrated that bacteremia develops in at least 2 percent of patients with intravenous and plastic catheters. Those inserted via a cutdown are associated with an even higher rate of sepsis. Classically, infections developing 3 days after surgery or trauma are due to IV catheters. Intravenous catheters inserted in the emergency department are often inserted with less than ideal sterile technique and should be replaced within 12 to 24 h. Any patient who becomes septic should be considered to have an infected IV line until proven otherwise. As the catheter is being removed, a blood culture should be drawn through it, and the catheter tip should be cut off and also cultured.

Although metal needles are less apt to cause septic thrombophlebitis, they are more difficult to maintain in a vein for prolonged periods. Plastic catheters are also usually preferred if a secure route for rapid administration of blood or other fluids is essential. If a plastic IV catheter must be inserted, there appears to be some value in having increased distance between the puncture site or incision in the skin and the point at which the catheter enters the vein. When permanent Hickman or Baroviac catheters are inserted, the subcutaneous tunnel between the skin incision and vein is usually at least 3 to 4 in long.

Urethral catheters and/or instrumentation in patients with infected urine is a frequent source of serious infection, particularly by gram-negative rods such as *Escherichia coli.* Although closed urine drainage systems can greatly delay the onset of infection, if a Foley catheter is in place for more than 5 to 8 days, bacterial counts in urine often exceed 10^5 per milliliter. In many series, urinary tract infections account for at least one-third of hospital-acquired infections, and the majority of these are associated with insertion of urethral catheters.

Although some bacteria may move up into the bladder alongside the urethral catheter, most bacteria probably enter the bladder by movement up through the urine in the lumen of the drainage tubing. Consequently, maintenance of a closed drainage system is extremely important. A high rate of urine flow may also help to decrease the number of organisms ascending the tubing. Nurses need to take special precautions when dealing with urinary drainage systems in immunocompromised patients. Careful cleansing of the catheter at the urethral meatus once or twice daily is important in all patients.

A large number of critically ill or injured patients require ventilatory assistance for at least a few days. Although an endotracheal tube may be more uncomfortable to the patient, particularly if it is an orotracheal tube, it is less apt to introduce large numbers of bacteria into the lungs than a tracheostomy.

If an endotracheal tube is required for much more than 5 days, a tracheostomy is often performed. However, a tracheostomy probably does not have to be performed within the first 5 to 10 days unless: (1) the patient tolerates the endotracheal tube poorly; (2) the pulmonary secretions cannot be removed adequately through the endotracheal tube; or (3) the endotracheal tube is damaging the vocal cords, nasal septum, or paranasal sinuses.

Diseases Involving the Reticuloendothelial System

Acute leukemias and lymphomas tend to be associated with severe cellular and humoral immunologic defects. The RES may be impaired, not only by the malignant process but also by the drugs used for treatment. The malnutrition frequently resulting from advanced malignancies and chemotherapeutic drugs can also seriously impair host defenses and must, therefore, be vigorously prevented or corrected with oral or IV hyperalimentation.

Drug Therapy

Immunosuppressive and cytotoxic drugs can profoundly depress the bone marrow and RES. This may be particularly important in patients with advanced malignancies who already have a reduction in their phagocyte- and antibody-forming tissues. In addition, cytotoxic drugs tend to injure rapidly growing cells such as intestinal mucosa, thereby creating new portals of entry for various microorganisms.

Antibiotic therapy profoundly alters the host microflora and may thereby determine which microorganisms are likely to cause infection. Almost all antibiotics in therapeutic doses will produce changes in the gastrointestinal, oropharyngeal, and skin flora, replacing relatively antibiotic-sensitive microorganisms with others which are more resistant. Antimicrobial agents can also reduce host resistance by altering tissue pH and inducing vitamin deficiencies.

Prolonged corticosteroid therapy is frequently associated with an increased incidence of infection by opportunistic bacteria, viruses, fungi, and parasites. Glucocorticoids depress the inflammatory response and induce lysis of lymphoid cells, thereby decreasing antibody synthesis. Large doses may reduce fibroblastic proliferation and further impair reticuloendothelial system activity. Adrenocortical hormones in high doses may also suppress the formation and activity of interferon, a factor which may be important in preventing opportunistic viral infections. Nevertheless, patients with severe septic shock who are not responding to aggressive therapy with fluid and other agents may benefit from pharmacologic doses of corticosteroids given within 2 to 4 h of the onset of hypotension. These agents may stabilize lysosomal and capillary membranes and reduce the excessive activation of the complement and kinin systems.

Age

Host resistance is most apt to be impaired in the very young or very old, especially those less than 3 months and those greater than 70 years of age. The newborn, particularly the premature infant, is compromised by immunological immaturity. Aged patients are apt to have cardiovascular disease, carcinomatosis, diabetes mellitus, neurological problems, and other debilitating disease. Many gram-negative bacilli, usually not regarded as pathogenic for humans, are often the cause of hospital-acquired infections in such patients.

Metabolic Functions

Patients with impaired metabolic function, particularly when due to severe diabetes mellitus or renal or hepatic failure, have an increased incidence of infection. Increased blood sugar levels per se probably do not play a major role; however, ketoacidosis causes a defective inflammatory response with sluggish polymorphonuclear migration, ineffective phagocytosis, and decreased fibroblast proliferation. In addition, the small blood vessel disease that often complicates diabetes mellitus may interfere with local nutrient tissue blood flow, reduce absorption of drugs given intramuscularly or subcutaneously, and cause renal and cardiovascular insufficiency.

Uremic acidosis impairs the early phases of the acute inflammatory response. Uremia also causes (1) suppression of the immune response to antigenic stimuli, (2) impaired delayed cellular hypersensitivity, (3) abnormal production of all types of immunoglobulins, and (4) defective cell division.

Patients with cirrhosis have a greatly reduced resistance to infection, and these patients can develop fatal septic shock from relatively mild infections. In addition to the impaired metabolism and reduced hepatic RES function in cirrhosis, there is shunting of portal venous blood—which may contain enteric bacilli or endotoxin—around the hepatic reticuloendothelial system, directly into the systemic venous circulation.

Cardiovascular Function

Rheumatic heart disease, arteriosclerosis, hypertension, and other cardiovascular diseases are associated with an increased incidence of bacteremia in hospitalized patients. Any impairment of tissue perfusion increases the likelihood that otherwise harmless endogenous bacteria may cause an infection. Patients with shock have an increased tendency to infection, especially if the shock persists for more than 30 min and the patient received massive transfusions.

Pulmonary Function

The respiratory tract is normally sterile below the glottis. This sterility is mechanically maintained by alveolar macrophages and the mucociliary clearance apparatus. In patients with chronic obstructive lung disease, these mechanisms are impaired. These patients often have infected bronchial secretions and they have an increased risk of developing severe pneumonitis, particularly in the hospital, because of exposure to antibiotics, inhalation therapy, and nebulizers. Procedures such as tracheostomy or endotracheal intubation further increase the possibility of infection, particularly the necrotizing gram-negative pneumonias caused by *Pseudomonas aeruginosa, Serratia marcescens,* and the *Klebsiella–Enterobacter* group.

Microorganisms

The ability of microorganisms to cause infection varies with their virulence, the number of bacteria present, the presence of other bacteria, and the resistance of these organisms to antimicrobial agents.

Virulence

The virulence or ability of bacteria to invade and cause infection varies tremendously. Some of the more important virulence factors include the presence of various toxins or enzymes that these organisms can release. These substances may either directly damage the host or they may counteract or neutralize host defense mechanisms. *Clostridium tetani* organisms produce a powerful exotoxin which can damage neurologic tissue far from the infection, and *C. welchii* produces several powerful exotoxins which can cause severe tissue damage and necrosis (gas gangrene) at the infected site.

The lipopolysaccharides in the outer membrane of the cell wall of gram-negative bacteria can cause fever, intravascular coagulation, hypotension, and death. Because of this toxicity and their incorporation within the bacterial cell wall, they are called endotoxins. Although endotoxin may escape into surrounding fluids, the whole cell of gram-negative bacteria retains the major portion of the endotoxic activity.

The endotoxins of smooth bacteria are macromolecules composed of three main regions: lipid A, core polysaccharide, and O antigens. The outermost layer of O antigens consists of repeating oligosaccharide units usually containing three to five sugars each. Absence of O antigens makes bacteria "rough" so that they no longer form smooth suspensions in liquid cultures or smooth cultures on solid media.

Antibodies to O or "core" lipopolysaccharide antigens can prevent the toxicity of endotoxin. The protection by O antibody is specific and limited to homologous endotoxin. In contrast, "core" antibody provides broad protection against the endotoxin from a wide variety of bacteria with unrelated O antigens. This fact has been used clinically to develop an effective antiserum against *E. coli* endotoxin.

Bacterial capsules can also greatly enhance virulence. These loose, gelatinous coverings of mixed polysaccharides can impede or completely block phagocytosis. Some gram-negative bacilli, such as certain *Klebsiella,* have extremely thick capsules.

Number of Organisms

The incidence and degree of infection developing in any wound correlate directly with the number of contaminating organisms. The number of bacteria necessary to cause infection is often referred to as the *critical inoculum.* The critical inoculum varies considerably with the local environment. Foreign bodies, blood, and dead space in a wound can greatly reduce the critical inoculum by a factor of 1:10,000.

Combinations of Organisms

Another important factor in virulence is the number and types of other bacteria in the area. These other bacteria may be antagonistic and reduce the chance of infection by competing for nutrients, or they may be synergistic and thereby enhance infection. For example, aerobic bacteria in a wound may consume the oxygen that is present, thereby improving the environment for the growth and multiplication of anaerobic bacteria.

Antibiotic Resistance

A bacterial population may become resistant to an antimicrobial agent, either by spontaneous mutation or by transfer of genetic material from resistant bacteria to sensitive bacteria. The organisms most frequently causing sepsis at the present time are not the classic high-virulence organisms such as beta-hemolytic streptococci, but rather organisms such as *Pseudomonas,* which, although usually of relatively low virulence, have great genetic versatility. Most bacteria that can cause infection in humans can replicate by binary fission every 20 min. Therefore, if the proper nutrients and temperature are available, one organism can produce over 10 billion (10^9) other organisms in 10 h. With such large numbers of bacteria, the mutation rate does not have to be very high (for example 1 ×

10^7 or 1 in 10 million) in order for mutant organisms to be seen regularly.

If some mechanism occurs whereby mutant bacteria are given an advantage over other bacteria present, they proliferate. One way to "select out" such organisms is to administer antibiotics to which the mutant strain is resistant but to which the others are sensitive. Now the mutant no longer needs to compete since it is the only organism replicating in the presence of antibiotics. Within a day or so, the microbial population may be replaced by descendants of the antibiotic-resistant mutant organism.

Much evidence has recently accumulated which shows that bacteria are able to directly transmit antibiotic resistance to other bacteria. The genetic information controlling antibiotic resistance is frequently contained in extrachromosomal deoxyribonucleic acid (DNA) molecules called *plasmids.* These DNA molecules or resistance (R) factors are self-replicating and may be passed on to or exchanged with adjacent bacteria. This material does not diffuse from one organism to another; actual physical (sexual?) contact is required.

Classification

Bacteria

Bacteria are generally classified according to their need for oxygen, their gram-stain reaction, and their shape. Strictly speaking, aerobic bacteria require oxygen for their metabolism, while facultative organisms can grow with or without oxygen, and anaerobic bacteria can only metabolize and reproduce properly in the absence of oxygen. For the sake of simplicity, facultative and aerobic organisms will be combined.

Gram-Positive Cocci

Staphylococci   Staphylococci are gram-positive cocci and are divided into two main species: *Staphylococcus aureus* (which is coagulase-positive) and *S. epidermidis* (which is coagulase-negative). Both species can be present in the normal flora of skin and mucous membranes. *Staphylococcus aureus* is the more virulent species and is the major cause of sepsis in most hospitals; it is particularly apt to cause infections of skin, soft tissue, IV catheters, and bone. It is also a major cause of acute endo-

carditis, particularly among narcotic addicts. This species often produces a penicillinase, which makes it resistant to aqueous penicillin, but it is, however, usually sensitive to cephalothins and many synthetic penicillins such as methicillin and oxacillin. During the past few years, increasing numbers of methicillin-resistant *S. aureus* (MRSA) organisms are being found, especially in drug addicts. Many of these addicts take cephalosporins when they develop infections, and consequently up to 70 percent of their *S. aureus* may be methicillin-resistant when they come to the hospital.

A specific *S. aureus*-induced condition is the *toxic shock syndrome* (TSS). This is an acute, severe febrile illness which involves multiple organ systems and is associated with hypotension and rash. Typically, the syndrome occurs in young, previously healthy menstruating women using tampons and is characterized by fever, syncope, hypotension, vomiting, watery diarrhea, diffuse inflammation of mucous membranes, erythroderma or petechial skin rash, desquamation of the hands and feet during convalescence, and laboratory evidence of multiple organ dysfunction.

Although the majority of TSS illnesses are associated with menstruation, a substantial number also occur in men and in nonmenstruating women who have empyema, septic abortion, peritonsillar abscess, subcutaneous abscess, and staphylococcal colonization of mucous membranes. The intravascular invasion of *S. aureus* is less important than the production, absorption, and action of its toxins. The mortality ratio for menstrual TSS is 3.5 percent.

Staphylococcus epidermidis (albus) is coagulase-negative. When this organism is found in cultures it is often thought of as a contaminant. However, it can cause disease and its presence in cultures can present an increasing problem, particularly in infections from IV catheters or following cardiac or vascular surgery. Currently, it is the most common cause of late infections after cardiac surgery in many centers. Since it is a frequent cause of such infections, it is often not clear whether it is a causative organism or just a contaminant. Fortunately, it is usually sensitive to the penicillins.

Streptococci   Streptococci are gram-positive cocci which tend to occur in chains. These organisms are divided into several groups according to their serological typing. *Streptococcus pyogenes,* group A, particularly those which are beta-hemolytic, is generally considered to be the most virulent of the streptococci. It causes most of the streptococcal pharyngitis and cellulitis that develops outside the hospital. *Streptococcus pyogenes,* group B, causes infections similar to those seen with group A, but it is a more common cause of streptococcal infections acquired in the hospital.

Streptococcus pyogenes, group D, is generally divided into those species which are enterococci (*S. faecalis, S. faecium,* and *S. durans*) and those which are not (*S. bovis* and *S. equinus*). The enterococci tend to be more resistant to antibiotics than other streptococci. They are particularly important in patients with wound or intraabdominal infections developing 2 to 3 weeks after surgery or trauma to the small bowel or colon.

The *viridans* streptococci are a group of streptococci which are alpha-hemolytic but do not contain antigens by which they can be serologically typed into one of the Lancefield groups. These organisms were notorious in the past for causing subacute bacterial endocarditis.

Streptococcus pneumoniae, formerly known as *Diplococcus pneumoniae* or the pneumococcus, can be part of the normal flora of the upper respiratory tract. However, it is also the most frequent cause of lobar pneumonia, and is frequently cultured from patients with respiratory infections.

Neisseria   There are many species in the genus *Neisseria,* but only two—the meningococcus and gonococcus—are normally pathogenic to humans. These gram-negative cocci often grow in pairs. The meningococci have a capsule, and meningococcemia may have an extremely fulminant course. It can cause acute adrenal insufficiency with disseminated intravascular coagulation, a syndrome known as Waterhouse-Friderichsen syndrome. Gonococcal infections are more common than those caused by *N. meningitidis,* but septicemia with *N. gonorrhoeae* is rather rare.

Gram-Positive Bacilli

Only a small number of gram-positive bacilli are pathogenic to humans. *Listeria monocytogenes* usu-

ally only infects patients who are very young or immunocompromised. *Corynebacterium diphtheriae* is virulent but rarely, if ever, causes septicemia. It usually causes only local symptoms in the throat, but may cause severe systemic symptoms and signs due to the exotoxin it elaborates. Proper immunization can prevent this disease completely.

Organisms of the genus *Bacillus* are fairly common, but only the organism *B. anthracis* is usually pathogenic. Cutaneous or inhalation types of anthrax are rarely seen except in sheep handlers. *Bacillus subtilus* organisms, which are only rarely pathogenic, are large gram-positive bacilli which are not infrequently confused with clostridia on Gram stain.

Gram-Negative Bacilli

The last 15 years have seen a marked increase in gram-negative bacterial infections, largely because increasing numbers of these organisms are antibiotic-resistant and because of increased numbers of immunocompromised patients. The cell wall of the gram-negative bacilli consists of structured layers of protein and lipopolysaccharides. The polysaccharides, which have a core of common sugars with various side chains, are antigenic and also account for the roughness or smoothness of the surface of the various bacteria. The polysaccharide (endotoxin) released from the cell wall after gram-negative bacteria die can cause severe pathophysiologic changes and is a major cause of pathogenicity of these organisms.

Escherichia coli is the most frequent gram-negative bacillus causing infection in humans, both in and out of the hospital. It is particularly apt to cause urinary tract infections and is involved in most infections secondary to trauma or disease involving the gastrointestinal tract. Fortunately, *E. coli* is susceptible to many antibiotics, particularly the aminoglycosides.

The *Klebsiella–Enterobacter–Serratia* (KES) group of gram-negative bacilli are an increasing cause of nosocomial infections. They are more resistant to antibiotics than most of the other gram-negative bacilli, except *Pseudomonas. Klebsiella* and *Serratia* species have been particular problems in many nosocomial outbreaks of infection. *Klebsiella* is usually susceptible to the cephalosporins, cephalothin and cephaloridine, and resistant to carbenicillin; *Enterobacter,* by contrast, tends to be resistant to cephalosporins but susceptible to carbenicillin. Some *Serratia* are resistant to virtually all antibiotics.

Organisms of the genus *Proteus* are generally separated into indole-negative and indole-positive groups. *Proteus mirabilis,* which is indole-negative, is responsible for about 80 percent of all *Proteus* infections. Indole-negative *Proteus* organisms are fairly sensitive to antibiotics and can usually be successfully treated with ampicillin or cephalothin. The indole-positive strains—*P. rettgeri, P. morganii,* and *P. vulgaris*—on the other hand, are often resistant to these antibiotics, but are usually susceptible to kanamycin, gentamicin, and carbenicillin.

Salmonella bacteremia is unusual in the United States except in epidemics of typhoid or paratyphoid fever. This organism is extremely sensitive to chloramphenicol.

The genus *Acinetobacter* includes organisms previously called *Mima, Herellea,* and *Achromobacter.* These organisms are common in nature and are frequently part of the normal flora of the skin and gastrointestinal and upper respiratory tracts. They have a relatively low virulence and usually only cause sepsis in immunocompromised hosts, usually from IV catheters or in the tracheobronchial tree from contaminated ventilatory equipment. They are unusually susceptible to tetracyclines or aminoglycosides.

Pseudomonas aeruginosa tends to infect patients who have been on multiple antibiotics for 3 to 4 weeks and are debilitated by burns, neoplasms, or other infections. Before the wide use of antibiotics, *Pseudomonas* rarely caused infections. This genus not only contains strains which are naturally resistant to most antimicrobial drugs but its members also have the ability to rapidly develop resistance to antibiotics. Therefore, *Pseudomonas* often becomes a major part of the flora or even the dominant organism at multiple sites in individuals who have been on antibiotics for more than 2 to 3 weeks. The lungs, urinary tract, or surgical wound are often the initial sites of infection prior to the development of septicemia. *Pseudomonias* is a particularly common cause of pneumonia in patients requiring prolonged ventilatory assistance and of endocarditis in heroin addicts.

Anaerobic Bacteria

Anaerobic bacteria generally cannot cause infection in healthy, well-vascularized, well-oxygenated tissue. However, factors which make conditions favorable for anaerobic growth include (1) coinfection with a facultative organism which utilizes the oxygen present and/or produces toxins which alter the blood supply and/or viability of healthy tissue, and (2) trauma which directly damages tissue and/or interferes with its blood supply.

The peptococci (anaerobic staphylococci) are usually only seen in mixed infections. Occasionally they are found in pure culture in deep abscesses, but they are a very infrequent cause of sepsis. This organism is difficult to grow in the laboratory, and involvement is often missed unless careful anaerobic blood cultures and subcultures are performed.

The peptostreptococci (anaerobic streptococci) are the most common anaerobic cocci causing sepsis. Any abscess with a very foul odor is likely to have anaerobic streptococci present. This genus is quite virulent and can be found in pure culture in tuboovarian abscesses, brain abscesses, deep wound infections, and puerperal sepsis. However, it is usually present with other organisms, particularly aerobic gram-negative bacilli.

Veillonella are gram-negative anaerobic cocci which are present in normal flora of the mouth, intestinal tract, upper respiratory tract, and vagina. However, they are not infrequently recovered in mixed infections from abdominal and brain abscesses. Rarely they are isolated in pure culture from abdominal abscesses. The endotoxin associated with the outer envelope of this cell wall appears to be a lipopolysaccharide similar to that associated with many aerobic gram-negative bacilli.

Clostridia are large gram-positive anaerobic bacilli which produce spores that can help identify individual species. They produce disease primarily by their exotoxins. The toxin of *C. tetani* is particularly attracted to nerve tissue. Even relatively mild peripheral infections, such as with puncture wounds of the foot, can cause severe central neurologic dysfunction. This disease can be completely prevented by proper immunization against its exotoxin.

Clostridium perfringens (*welchii*) is the classic organism causing gas gangrene, but it is only one of several clostridia which can cause this problem. The exotoxins released, particularly lecithinase, cause a liquefaction necrosis which favors increased growth and multiplication of these bacteria. This results in a vicious cycle of increasing exotoxin production, liquefaction necrosis, and bacterial multiplication.

The propionibacteria constitute a major proportion of the normal skin flora and these gram-positive anaerobic bacilli are frequent contaminants in blood cultures. However, the propionibacteria can cause sepsis and cannot always be ignored, particularly if recovered in reported blood cultures.

Eubacteria are non-spore-forming, anaerobic, gram-positive bacilli which are part of the normal flora of the intestinal tract. They are frequent isolates from wounds but are a rare cause of sepsis.

Bifidobacteria are gram-positive anaerobic bacilli which are almost routinely found in the intestinal tract of infants and adults. They are frequently recovered from mixed infections but are only occasionally seen in pure culture.

Members of the genus *Bacteroides* are gram-negative anaerobic bacilli which compose up to 90 percent of the bacteria found in the human large intestine. They also are found as normal flora in the oral cavity and upper respiratory tract and in the urogenital tract of women.

Bacteroides melanogenicus is generally found in the mouth and is frequently involved in mixed infections of the respiratory tract. It is usually quite sensitive to penicillin.

Bacteroides fragilis is the most prevalent and most important anaerobic organism in the distal small bowel and colon. It is very likely to be involved in deep infections following trauma or surgery involving these organs. It also may be involved in up to 15 percent of lung abscesses. Unlike virtually all the other anaerobic bacteria, it is resistant to penicillin.

Mycobacteria

Disease due to mycobacteria remains a major problem. Miliary tuberculosis, a fulminant form of the disease which is diffusely spread by the bloodstream, is particularly apt to occur in elderly, debilitated, or immunosuppressed patients. Corticosteroid therapy, particularly if prolonged, may cause granulomas to break down, resulting in reactivation of tuberculosis.

Diagnosis of tuberculosis in debilitated individuals is often difficult unless special efforts are made to identify the organisms on smears, cultures, or tissue biopsies. Because of the overwhelming nature of the infection, anergy tends to develop and the standard tuberculin skin tests are often negative. In one series, 38 percent of patients with miliary tuberculosis had negative skin tests. Even otherwise healthy patients have had a 10 to 15 percent incidence of false negative skin tests.

Rarely, atypical mycobacteria, which are much less virulent than *Mycobacterium tuberculosis,* are the cause of infection, usually in the lungs of patients with chronic obstructive pulmonary disease. These mycobacteria are divided into four groups based on their rate of growth and pigment formation in vitro. Differential Mantoux skin testing may also be helpful in diagnosis.

Fungi

Fungal infections of the skin are common but seldom pose serious problems. Bloodstream or deep tissue infections are rare. However, life-threatening infections with *Candida,* aspergilla, *Torulopsis glabrata,* and *histoplasma* have emerged in the past few years as major complications in immunosuppressed patients, especially those on cancer chemotherapy and those receiving drugs to prevent transplant rejection. Amphotericin B is the drug of choice for most of the severe systemic fungal infections. However, it is a very toxic agent which must be given with great care.

Candida albicans is the most common cause of serious fungal infections. However, it is a normal human commensal organism, and is recovered from the pharynx in 30 percent and stools in 65 percent of normal individuals. These percentages are much greater if the normal bacterial flora are suppressed by antibiotics. Disruption of mucous membranes by indwelling tubes increases the likelihood of local infections by this organism. Because it is a commensal organism, diagnosis of significant infection by this agent should be confirmed by histologic demonstration of tissue invasion or presence of the organism in sites, normally not containing *Candida,* such as blood or CSF. When invasive, *Candida* assumes a mycelial-like or pseudohyphae appearance. Evidence of pseudohyphae in unspun urine denotes tissue invasion, usually of the bladder wall. Recovery of organisms from the bloodstream is difficult, and it is estimated that blood cultures are negative in at least 50 to 75 percent of cases. Cultures of arterial blood in patients with *Candida* lung infections are more apt to be positive than those from venous blood.

Invasive aspergillosis is assuming increased importance in patients on immunosuppressive drugs. The lung is the commonest site of tissue invasion. Invasive *Aspergillus* pneumonia is particularly apt to occur in patients with acute granulocytic leukemia. Since *Aspergillus* is found in about 7 percent of sputum smears in patients with chronic chest diseases, diagnosis of tissue invasion must be confirmed histologically.

Torulopsis glabrata is a saprophyte similar to and often mistaken for *Candida*. It is being found with increasing frequency, but it rarely causes infection except in debilitated patients, particularly those with severe burns and/or those receiving parenteral hyperalimentation.

Histoplasma capsulatum frequently causes infections, particularly in farmers living along the Ohio Valley. These are usually mild pulmonary infections, and multiple small diffuse calcifications in the lung are often the only evidence, except for serologic tests, that the infection was present. In immunosuppressed patients, it occasionally causes a generalized infection involving the mouth, lymph nodes, blood, and bone marrow.

Coccidioides immitus is a frequent cause of pulmonary infection in the San Joaquin Valley in California. A relatively mild to moderate respiratory infection caused by this organism is often referred to as Valley fever. Not infrequently, residual pulmonary nodules or thin-walled cavities may be seen on chest x-ray. In its generalized form it may also involve the central nervous system.

Cryptococcus neoformans may involve the skin and lungs, but its infections of the central nervous system are usually the only ones which are serious. This disease is particularly frequent and severe in patients with Hodgkin's disease and other lymphomas.

Mycoplasmas

Mycoplasmas, also known as PPLO or "pleuropneumonia-like organisms," are the smallest known free-living organisms. *Mycoplasma* pneumonia (formerly atypical or Eaton agent pneumonia), caused by *Mycoplasma pneumoniae*, is an acute infection of the lower respiratory tract that usually involves the dependent lobes of the lung, lasts 14 to 21 days in untreated cases, and responds to treatment with erythromycin or tetracycline without sequelae. It is probably the most common cause of so-called "walking pneumonia."

Viruses

The viruses most likely to be involved in septic-like conditions are herpes simplex virus (HSV) types I and II, varicella-zoster virus (V-Z), Epstein-Barr virus (EBV), cytomegalovirus (CMV), and members of the papovavirus groups. Most of the serious infections caused by these organisms occur in immunosuppressed individuals. Diagnosis is usually made by serologic testing, but occasionally the virus is recovered in tissue culture.

Herpes simplex viruses types 1 and 2 characteristically only cause intermittent mild vesicular eruptions (cold sores) on the mucocutaneous margins of the mouth. Rarely, these may also involve the cornea and can cause blindness. Recently there has been great attention given to sexually transmitted herpes simplex infections of the male and female genital tracts, which can be very painful and are difficult or impossible to cure. Very rarely this virus causes catastrophic illness in the central and peripheral nervous systems of apparently normal people. Between attacks, the virus is in a latent phase in the nerve root ganglia in various parts of the body.

An increasing frequency and severity of herpes simplex virus infections have been noted in renal transplant recipients who are maintained on large doses of immunosuppressive drugs such as steroids, azathioprine, and antilymphocyte globulin. Immediately following birth, while the immunological system is immature, infants are also more likely to develop life-threatening systemic infections with this virus. Treatment with adenine arabinoside may be of value.

Another latent infection that may be activated in patients with altered immunity is herpes zoster. Susceptible children usually acquire the virus by developing chicken pox (varicella). Complete recovery is the rule, but the virus usually persists in a latent form in nerve tissue. Occasionally the virus reawakens in the skin of the chest wall or face in the distribution of an intercostal nerve or the trigeminal nerve. The resultant vesicular eruptions and associated severe pain along intercostal dermatomes are generally referred to as shingles.

The incidence of infections with V-Z virus is particularly increased in patients with lymphomas or Hodgkin's disease. In these patients, especially those receiving steroid or radiation therapy, the vesicular eruption may become disseminated and be associated with pneumonia or encephalitis which is apt to be fatal. The development of interferon, an antiviral agent in the vesicle fluid, is an important factor in the natural cessation of the cutaneous spread of this disease.

Epstein-Barr virus has been found in the cell cultures of Burkitt's lymphoma. Antibodies reactive with Epstein-Barr virus have also been reported in cases of infectious mononucleosis.

The cytomegalovirus (CMV) causes mild self-limited respiratory infections and a heterophile-negative mononucleosis syndrome in apparently healthy young adults. However, it can cause fatal pneumonia in renal and cardiac transplant recipients. In addition, evidence is accumulating that acquisition or reactivation of the CMV may further impair cellular immunity by viral multiplication inside activated lymphocytes.

Members of the papovavirus group have recently been recognized to be the cause of progressive multifocal leukoencephalopathy. This is the "slow" viral demyelinating disease of the central nervous system that usually occurs in immunosuppressed patients.

A new infection which has received much attention is referred to as acquired immune deficiency syndrome (AIDS). This disease is apparently caused by human T cell lymphotropic virus (HTLV) type III. There is apparently a long latent period of up to 2 to 3 years followed by a period characterized primarily by lymphadenopathy. The terminal phase often has clinical manifestations of progressive and lethal opportunistic lung infections (especially by *Pneumocystis*), relentless and aggressive Kaposi's sarcoma, or persistent cytomegalovirus (CMV) infections. The entity was first recognized in male homosexuals who have been at greatest risk. However, it has also been observed with increasing frequency in intravenous drug users, hemophiliacs,

Haitian refugees, heterosexual contacts of homosexual males, and an increasing number of individuals (including physicians and nurses) who are not readily categorizable by clinical, social, or sexual practices.

In the AIDS patient, Kaposi's sarcoma, which is usually a relatively benign disease of the skin of the lower extremities in the elderly, produces aggressive visceral and nodal involvement. Similarly, while *Pneumocystis* pneumonia infections are not rare in patients receiving immunosuppressive drugs or in neonates, the increasing incidence of new cases in this group is remarkable.

There is evidence of altered immune function in the affected male homosexual population. Abnormally low helper/suppressor T cell ratios and altered functional responses to mitogens have been observed in AIDS patients as well as in many male homosexuals without clinical evidence of disease.

Parasites

Three of the more frequent parasites in the United States that can cause disease which may resemble bacterial infections include plasmodia (causing malaria), *Pneumocystis carinii,* and *Toxoplasma.*

Infections with plasmodia are usually only seen in patients who have recently traveled to an area in the tropics in which malaria is prevalent; however, outbreaks have also occurred in addicts sharing contaminated needles. The four malarias that are important in humans are *Plasmodium vivax, P. ovale, P. malariae,* and *P. falciparum.* Fatalities usually only occur with *P. falciparum,* since it parasitizes all red cells. *Plasmodium vivax,* which parasitizes only reticulocytes, is much more benign. Death results from cerebral involvement or renal failure.

Pneumocystis carinii forms tiny cysts which can be demonstrated by Giemsa, periodic acid-Schiff, or silver stains but not by ordinary hematoxylin and eosin stains. Diagnosis is suspected in immunodeficient patients who have diffuse pulmonary infiltrates on x-ray with fever and dyspnea, but whose lungs are usually clear on auscultation. It is most apt to occur in premature infants, children with acute leukemia, organ transplant recipients, and adults who are severely immunosuppressed. Diagnosis is usually made on open-lung biopsy. Treatment with pentamidine or trimethoprim-sulfamethoxazole (Bactrim or Septra) is often successful if begun early.

Toxoplasma gondii is a protozoan of worldwide distribution. The common cat is the definitive host, but humans also acquire the infection by ingestion of undercooked meats or by transplacental transfer. Mild infections are frequent, but clinical manifestations are rare. Disseminated toxoplasmosis is unusual except in immunosuppressed patients, particularly those with lymphomas or organ transplants. Central nervous or respiratory symptoms predominate under such circumstances. Treatment includes pyrimethamine with various sulfa antimicrobials.

Pathophysiologic Changes with Sepsis

The pathophysiologic changes occurring with severe infections are extremely complex. The bacteria and their toxins in themselves can have profound local and systemic effects. These in turn trigger certain local host (inflammatory) reactions followed by systemic endocrine, metabolic, and organ changes. The net result is the clinical picture referred to as sepsis.

Bacterial Effects

Bacterial invasion results in release of a number of powerful chemicals from the damaged tissue, not only locally but also into the bloodstream. In addition, exotoxins may be released directly from various live microorganisms (especially gram-positive bacteria), and endotoxins may be released from the cell wall of dead microorganisms (especially gram-negative bacilli).

Local Chemical Release

A wide variety of chemicals is released locally from cells which are damaged by an infectious process. Some of the more important chemicals released include histamine, a wide variety of lysosomal enzymes, and superoxide radicals. These latter two substances are capable of destroying or altering many cellular components.

Two types of histamine are generally recognized as being released in sepsis. *Preformed histamine,* which is stored in mast cells and which

can be inhibited by antihistamines, is much less important than *induced histamine.* Induced histamine is not stored; it is formed directly in cells at the time that they are damaged or stimulated, and it is not altered or affected by antihistamines.

Lysosomes contain a wide variety of extremely powerful enzymes including cathepsin D, β-glucuronidase, acid phosphatase, arylsulfatase, and ribonuclease. These enzymes normally are used to destroy and/or "digest" bacteria and other foreign substances that are taken up into phagolysosomes, particularly in macrophages. Consequently, lysosomes have been referred to as "intracellular stomachs."

Another group of intralysosomal substances, which are actually more destructive than enzymes, are the so-called superoxide radicals. These substances are formed by an oxidative process which involves xanthine oxidase and requires much energy. The resultant hydrogen peroxide (H_2O_2), superoxides, and single oxygen are now felt to cause much of the antimicrobial killing that occurs inside macrophages.

If the lipoprotein membrane surrounding the lysosome breaks down, lysosomal enzymes and superoxide radicals can escape into the cell and destroy the cell. If enough lysosomes break down, increased levels of lysosomal enzymes can be detected in the blood. These substances may cause not only a great deal of local cellular and tissue damage but they also cause the release or activation of various other chemicals, including vasoactive polypeptides, which can cause even greater and more distant changes.

An increasing number of vasoactive polypeptides are being recognized. Normally these substances exist in an inactive form bound to protein, particularly alpha 2 globulins. Endotoxin and various proteolytic enzymes from lysosomes or the pancreas can separate the kinin from its protein, thereby activating the kinin. Two of the best-known vasoactive polypeptides formed in this manner are bradykinin and myocardial depressant factor.

Bradykinin is one of the most potent vasodilators known. Bradykinin greatly increases capillary and venular permeability, causing an increasing interstitial edema with a corresponding decrease in blood volume. Much of the edema and increased fluid requirement in sepsis may be due to bradykinin.

Myocardial depressant factor (MDF) is liberated primarily from the ischemic pancreas. This substance, as its name implies, depresses myocardial contractility and, in addition, causes splanchnic vasoconstriction, which may result in even more MDF production. This substance is quite controversial and some investigators have stated that MDF is a laboratory artifact.

Host Responses

As mentioned previously, local host responses to infection consist of local vascular changes, especially vasodilation and increased capillary permeability and the release of a number of chemicals, including histamine, anaphylatoxin, and kinins. If the infection is relatively minor and readily controlled, systemic changes may be minimal. However, if the infection becomes widespread, the resultant excessive release of histamine, anaphylatoxin, and kinins can cause increasing capillary permeability and loss of enough fluid into the interstitial space to cause hypovolemic shock. These agents may also cause widespread vasodilation, thereby increasing vascular capacity and further exaggerating the discrepancy between intravascular volume and vascular capacity.

Systemic Changes

Some of the systemic responses to sepsis include changes in endocrine function, metabolism of various nutrients, and function of various organ systems, particularly the cardiovascular system, lungs, kidneys, liver, and intestinal tract.

Endocrine Changes

Sepsis causes an intense activation of the autonomic nervous system and endocrine system, resulting in increased secretion and release of most hormones except insulin, thyrotropin, and gonadal hormones.

Increased antidiuretic hormone (ADH) secretion, causing a tendency to water retention and oliguria, occurs with all types of stress, including infection, particularly if hypovolemia develops. By reducing the renal excretion of water, ADH helps to maintain an adequate intravascular volume and tissue perfusion. However, if the oliguria it produces is prolonged or severe, the tendency to renal failure is greatly increased.

Aldosterone secretion is regulated primarily by the renin-angiotensin system, which is largely stimulated by impaired perfusion of the kidney. Aldosterone acts primarily to increase sodium and water retention and increase potassium excretion. Thus, aldosterone helps to maintain extracellular fluid volume and tissue perfusion.

Sepsis is characterized by a profound tendency toward a diabetic-like state caused primarily by an increased secretion of epinephrine, glucagon, and cortisol and usually also by a decreased secretion of insulin. However, even when insulin secretion is normal or increased, the insulin/glucagon molar ratio is decreased and hyperglycemia results.

Epinephrine secretion increases conversion of liver and muscle glycogen to glucose and also increases the conversion of neutral fat to fatty acids. It not only reduces insulin secretion, but also increases tissue resistance to insulin, thereby greatly increasing the blood levels of glucose and glucose availability in muscle. Glucagon causes liver glycogen to be mobilized and converted to glucose.

There is a great increase in secretion of adrenal cortical steroids stimulated largely by ACTH. Cortisol raises blood glucose levels largely by stimulating gluconeogenesis.

Metabolic Changes

Largely due to the high fever and restlessness often seen in sepsis, most patients with severe infection without shock have an increased oxygen consumption. However, as shock develops, the oxygen consumption characteristically falls to levels less than 75 percent of normal. This reduced oxygen consumption tends to be associated with an increasing production of lactate and metabolic acidosis. In early septic shock some septic patients have a metabolic alkalosis, usually of iatrogenic origin, in spite of a respiratory alkalosis. Interestingly, some data suggest that anaerobic (as well as aerobic) metabolism may be impaired in sepsis. Under such circumstances lactate would not be produced in as large a quantity as might be expected from the low oxygen consumption. In general, the greater the lactic acidosis, the more likely the patient will die.

If glucose is metabolized aerobically, 38 mol of adenosine triphosphate (ATP) are released from each mol of glucose. However, when glucose breakdown (glycolysis) must function anaerobically because of decreased tissue perfusion or altered cell function, only 2 mol of ATP are produced and lactic acid tends to accumulate, causing an increasing metabolic acidosis.

Glucose is the only substrate which can supply energy to the brain under acute conditions and to muscle under anaerobic conditions. If adequate glucose is not available from glycogen for these functions, the liver attempts to form new glucose from protein. The amino acid alanine appears to be a particularly important precursor of glucose by this process. The glucocorticoids strongly stimulate gluconeogensis and, if the sepsis is severe and persistent, the protein catabolism and resultant tissue and organ breakdown can be life-threatening in its own regard. On the other hand, if gluconeogenesis is inhibited because of overwhelming sepsis or adrenal insufficiency, hypoglycemia and death may rapidly develop.

Lipolysis, the catabolism of fatty tissue, releases fatty acids and glycerol, which can enter the glycolytic cycle via acetyl coenzyme A, to provide energy. These lipolytic reactions are stimulated primarily by catecholamines and to a certain extent by glucocorticoids and thyroid hormones. This metabolic degradation of fat also results in the formation of ketone bodies (acetone, acetoacetic acid, and beta-hydroxybutyric acid) which may spill over in large quantities into the blood and urine, causing ketoacidosis and ketonuria.

Organ System Changes

Sepsis generally causes a strong β-adrenergic stimulation of the heart, resulting in tachycardia and occasional tachyarrhythmias. In fact, a tachyarrhythmia may be one of the first signs of sepsis. Because of the beta-adrenergic stimulation and vasodilation seen in early sepsis, cardiac output may be significantly greater than the normal values of 2.5 to 3.75 L/min/m², but only if an adequate blood volume is available. This hyperdynamic form of septic shock, often called *warm septic shock,* is present in 30 to 50 percent of patients during early septic shock. In contrast, if hypovolemia is allowed to develop because of increased capillary permeability or other losses from the extracellular fluid space, cardiac output will fall. Progressive impairment of cardiac

function in continuing sepsis, as reflected by a reduced ejection fraction, may also contribute eventually to a low cardiac output. This hypodynamic form of septic shock, also referred to as *cold septic shock,* tends to occur relatively late and can often be converted to warm septic shock at least temporarily by providing adequate fluid.

Systemic arteries and veins tend to dilate in sepsis, but if inadequate blood volume is available, they tend to constrict. Because of this tendency to vasodilation, many septic shock patients will have relatively low systolic and diastolic pressures in spite of a normal or high cardiac output with a good pulse pressure and bounding pulse on palpation.

Capillaries in sepsis tend to dilate and have a greatly increased permeability, particularly in infected areas and in the lungs. This tends to increase the quantity of interstitial fluid at the expense of the blood volume. This increased capillary permeability can cause peripheral edema and increased lung water even when the blood volume may be much lower than normal.

The fluid needs in septic patients may be truly extraordinary and may exceed 8 to 10 L in the first 24 h after sepsis develops. Whenever a patient begins to require more than 200 mL of fluid per hour over and above measured external losses to maintain adequate vital signs and urine output, sepsis should be considered present until proven otherwise.

The increased capillary permeability in the lungs in sepsis quickly leads to increasing pulmonary interstitial edema, initially in the peribronchial tissues. As a consequence, the lungs become stiffer and oxygen transfer is impaired. In addition, platelet aggregates and pulmonary venous constriction (perhaps due to central neurogenic reflexes initiated by cerebral hypoxemia) cause increasing congestion in pulmonary capillaries and a tendency to a diffuse atelectasis. This is followed by breakdown of type I alveolar lining cells and increasing leakage of fluid and protein into the alveoli. Inside the alveoli, this protein, particularly fibrinogen, tends to inactivate surfactant and causes even more atelectasis. The accumulated protein in the alveoli may layer out and precipitate and eventually resemble the hyaline membrane seen in premature newborns with respiratory distress.

During sepsis, total renal blood flow tends to rise or fall with cardiac output. However, even if cardiac output is high, the "effective" renal blood flow, as determined by para-aminohippurate (PAH) extraction, tends to be greatly reduced. This may be associated with clearance of as little as 25 percent of the PAH on each passage through the kidney instead of the usual clearance of 91 percent. Glomerular filtration rates, as measured by inulin or endogenous creatinine clearance, also tend to be low even if serum creatinine and BUN levels are normal.

Interestingly, creatinine excretion in many septic patients is much lower than the normal of 1200 to 1800 mg per day. As a consequence, the endogenous creatinine clearance may be less than 40 mL per minute even with serum creatinine values of 1.0 mg/dL or less. This may be of particular importance when regulating the dosage and frequency of administration of aminoglycosides. Furthermore, if the creatinine clearance is less than 40 mL per minute, the incidence of other organ failure and eventual death is significantly increased.

Hepatocyte and RES function in the liver is impaired in sepsis, particularly if shock is present. Consequently, important metabolic functions, including release of adequate substrate into the blood, may be greatly impaired. As a result, patients with severe sepsis, especially when due to polymicrobial infections of the peritoneal cavity, tend to develop high bilirubin levels, often referred to as "septic jaundice." These patients tend to have high white blood cell (WBC) counts and mildly elevated serum glutamic oxaloacetic transaminase (SGOT), moderately elevated alkaline phosphatase, and severely elevated lactic dehydrogenase (LDH) levels.

The impaired function of the RES in the liver is a particularly important problem because sepsis, and particularly shock, causes mucosal ischemia in the gut. As a consequence, increasing quantities of bacteria and bacterial products can penetrate the bowel mucosa and be brought to the liver via the portal venous system. If the RES in the liver cannot handle these adequately, they pass through to the systemic circulation and cause increasing havoc. In patients in whom suppurative collections are drained too late, continued passage of bacterial products into the circulation via an impaired intestinal mucosa can produce a clinical picture similar to that seen with large undrained pockets of pus. As mentioned previously, if the liver is already impaired by cirrhosis, the risk of sepsis is very high, and very few cirrhotic patients who develop septic shock leave the hospital alive.

Mucosal ischemia in the stomach increases the tendency to stress gastric bleeding. The association between sepsis and stress gastric bleeding is so great that upper GI bleeding following abdominal surgery or trauma should be considered due to sepsis until proved otherwise. Fortunately, keeping the gastric pH above 5.0 with cimetidine or ranitidine and/or antacids will usually prevent excessive stress gastric bleeding. However, use of these H_2-receptor antagonists in severe sepsis may alter the state of consciousness.

With generalized peritonitis, the fluid accumulation into the bowel lumen may result in a relatively rapid loss of 8 L or more of fluid from the functional extracellular fluid space, further increasing the tendency to hypovolemia. Paralytic ileus in sepsis may be severe and may strongly suggest the presence of intraperitoneal disease. This ileus not only delays the return of gastrointestinal function but may also elevate the diaphragm and interfere with ventilation. If the patient has had recent abdominal surgery, the increasingly distended and edematous bowel may disrupt the abdominal wall closure. Occasionally this may result in bowel leaks as the distended bowel rubs against suture material.

Diagnosis

Making the diagnosis of sepsis may be extremely difficult at times. Furthermore, even when the overall systemic effects of severe infection may be fairly obvious, the primary site of infection can be extremely difficult to find.

History

Careful review of the patient's history will often reveal situations or procedures which are likely to be associated with or cause infection. Various symptoms may indicate the probable site of infection. The history should also provide information concerning possible impairment of the patient's host defense mechanisms.

Procedures or Situations Predisposing to Infections

Fever developing at certain intervals following trauma or elective surgery tends to have characteristic causes. For example, fever occurring during the first 24 to 48 h postoperatively tends to be due to atelectasis (Table 58-2). In contrast, fever due to thrombophlebitis in the legs tends to develop after 7 to 14 days.

Sepsis due to urinary tract infection should be suspected in patients who have had their bladder catheterized or instrumented, particularly if done in the presence of urinary tract obstruction with infection.

Intraabdominal infections should be suspected in any patient who has had surgery for trauma or disease involving the colon, esophagus, biliary tract, or appendix. Intraabdominal and wound infections should be particularly suspected in patients who have had emergency surgery for a gastrointestinal leak or obstruction, especially if it involves the distal small bowel or colon.

Pulmonary infections should be suspected in patients with chronic obstructive lung disease, chest trauma, vomiting while lethargic or comatose, and endotracheal intubation or tracheostomy for prolonged mechanical ventilation.

Infection involving intravenous plastic catheters should always be suspected, particularly if the IV catheter is inserted during an emergency situation or if it is in place for more than 48 to 72 h.

Table 58-2 The Ws of Postoperative Fever

1. Wind: Atelectasis—usually first 24–48 h after surgery
2. Wein: IV catheter—classic third day fever
3. Water: Urinary tract infection—occurs usually 5–8 days after Foley catheter inserted
4. Wound: Usually 6–10 days* after surgery
5. Where:† Intraabdominal abscesses—usually 7–14 days after surgery
6. Walking: Thrombophlebitis in lower extremities—usually 7–14 days after surgery
7. Wonder: Drug fever ("wonder drugs" = antibiotics?)

*Beta-hemolytic streptococci and clostridia can cause severe infections in 24–48 h.
†From pneumonic = "pus somewhere—pus nowhere (i.e., can't find the pus)—pus under the diaphragm."

The presence of any prosthetic device (cardiac valve, pacemaker, or vascular graft) should also make one suspicious of an associated infection.

Infections of the genital tract should be suspected in young sexually active females with low abdominal pain. Ruptured placental membrane for more than 24 to 48 h prior to delivery is likely to be associated with an infection of the contents of the gravid uterus.

Symptoms with Various Infections

An awake and alert patient can usually relate symptoms which may localize the initial or primary site of infection fairly accurately. However, some referral and overlap of symptoms between areas of the body is apt to occur. For example, a stiff neck may be due to meningeal irritation. Jaw pain may be due to an ear problem. Upper abdominal pain may be caused by a lower lobe pneumonia. Lower abdominal pain may be caused by genitourinary problems. Nausea and vomiting may be due to a primary gastrointestinal problem or may be due to sepsis completely outside the abdomen.

Impaired Host Defenses

A careful search must be made for any history of immunosuppressive drugs such as steroids or various agents used to treat malignancies or prevent transplantation rejection. Various malignancies, particularly the leukemias in their advanced stages, even without chemotherapeutic drugs, predispose to a wide variety of opportunistic infections. Patients with diabetic ketoacidosis or cirrhosis tend to develop infections early and tolerate them poorly. Previous infections and prior treatment with antibiotics for prolonged periods are important factors. Increasing attention has also been directed to patients with a history of poor nutrition and recent severe weight loss.

Physical Examination

The signs of sepsis, particularly if associated with gram-negative organisms, may be extremely deceptive and may mimic a wide variety of clinical problems. Fever, with or without chills, may be the only manifestation in some patients, and in others only hypothermia may be present. Other nonspecific signs include confusion, tachypnea, and tachycardia.

In spite of the wide variations in the physical appearance of these patients, three characteristic stages or types of clinical presentation may be noted: (1) sepsis without shock, (2) hyperdynamic (warm) septic shock, and (3) hypodynamic (cold) septic shock.

Sepsis without Shock

Septic patients tend to be restless, anxious, and confused. Not infrequently, increasing confusion is the first sign that a patient is becoming septic. In many instances, the increasing confusion and restlessness may be difficult to differentiate from delirium tremens. However, some patients with gram-negative sepsis are remarkably awake and alert until just prior to death.

Systolic blood pressure tends to increase and pulse pressure tends to widen as sepsis increases as long as an adequate blood volume is maintained. Tachycardias are common and tachyarrhythmias may be the first clinical sign of sepsis. The pulse, though fast, is usually full and almost bounding.

The respiratory rate is often greater than double normal with a slightly reduced tidal volume, producing a minute ventilation which is often at least 1.5 to 2.0 times normal. Even without any pulmonary infection or fluid overload, rales are often present at the bases.

The abdomen is somewhat distended. These patients tend to develop an ileus early, even without any abdominal sepsis. If abdominal or renal sepsis is present, the ileus can rapidly become very severe.

The skin in sepsis tends to be warm and dry with a flushed or pink color unless hypovolemia develops. Occasionally acrocyanosis may develop due to intravascular clotting.

Hyperdynamic (Warm) Septic Shock

It may be extremely difficult at times to determine when severe sepsis becomes hyperdynamic septic shock. However, shock is generally considered to be present if the systolic blood pressure falls below 80 mmHg or drops by more than 25 percent, if the urine output falls below 25 mL per hour, or if a metabolic acidosis develops. Patients with septic shock usually also tend to become increasingly lethargic, restless, and confused.

Even if hypotension becomes fairly severe, the cardiac output in early, uncomplicated septic shock tends to be normal (2.5 to 4.0 L/min/m^2) or high and may be as high as twice normal, particularly if the blood volume has been adequately maintained. Anemia or cirrhosis tends to increase the cardiac output even more. Consequently, in spite of the low blood pressure, the arterial pulses tend to remain easily palpable. Hyperventilation tends to increase even more if metabolic acidosis or hypoxemia develops. Some patients, particularly those who become comatose, may develop what appears to be air hunger or gasping breaths in spite of relatively good arterial blood gases.

Hypodynamic (Cold) Septic Shock

In advanced septic shock many patients become hypovolemic and develop impaired myocardial contractility so that cardiac output falls below normal. This results in increasing vasoconstriction, eventually producing cold, clammy, mottled or cyanotic skin, particularly at the tips of the fingers, toes, ears, or nose.

As sepsis progresses, capillaries and postcapillary venules throughout the body, particularly in the lungs and infected areas, develop an increased permeability. Consequently, great amounts of fluid may be lost from the intravascular space into the interstitial space. In a period of 12 to 24 h, 10 L or more of extra fluid may be required to keep up with this loss. Eventually, fluid also begins to move into cells whose impaired metabolism cannot maintain the large sodium gradient that normally exists between the intracellular and extracellular fluid spaces. Consequently, even though the total body water may be much greater than normal, and the patient clinically appears to be overloaded with fluid, there is an ever-increasing tendency to develop a reduced intravascular volume.

Because oxygen extraction in nutrient capillaries tends to be reduced in sepsis, any decrease in cardiac output can rapidly result in an oxygen consumption (V_{O_2}) which is less than two-thirds of normal with a progressive rise in arterial lactate levels. If oxygen consumption falls to less than half of the normal of 130 to 160 mL/min/m^2, the septic patient rarely survives.

Laboratory Studies

White Blood Cell Count

In most septic patients the WBC count is elevated to 15,000/mm³, or more usually with a "shift to the left" (i.e., an increased number of immature band forms). In some instances the total WBC may be normal, and the only evidence of sepsis is a marked shift to the left. In severe advanced sepsis, particularly due to gram-negative bacilli, the WBC count may be extremely low, and this is an ominous prognostic sign.

The lymphocyte count may provide some indication of the type of infection present and the status of the patient's host defenses. A relatively high lymphocyte count may be a reflection of a viral rather than a bacterial infection. On the other hand, if the absolute lymphocyte count is less than 1500/mm³, one should suspect the presence of impaired host defenses. If the absolute lymphocyte count is less than 800 mm³, host defenses are very likely to be impaired.

Blood Chemistries

Blood chemistries may be quite normal until organ failure begins to develop. The blood urea nitrogen (BUN), bilirubin, and alkaline phosphatase may also begin to rise as the kidneys and liver begin to fail. Albumin levels also tend to fall relatively early because of (1) increased gluconeogenesis, (2) movement of albumin into the interstitial fluid space, and (3) impaired hepatic production of albumin. A rise in bilirubin and alkaline phosphatase without obvious damage or disease of the liver or biliary tract should make one suspect sepsis. This so-called septic jaundice tends to be associated with peritonitis due to multiple organisms, including *Bacteroides fragilis*.

In septic patients, plasma ionized calcium levels can rapidly fall to values less than the normal of 2.1 to 2.4 meq/L (1.05 to 1.20 mmol/L). The concentration of ionized calcium in the cytoplasm of most cells is about 10^{-7} mmol. Thus, there is a 10,000:1 gradient for ionized calcium across the cell membrane. If anything, cell metabolism becomes impaired, ionized calcium moves into the cytoplasm, and ionized calcium can rapidly fall to levels of less than 0.9 mmol/L. In general, if ionized calcium levels fall to less than 0.6 mmol/L, myocar-

dial performance is often impaired and prognosis can be severely reduced.

Coagulation Studies

In untreated sepsis there is activation of platelets and the coagulation cascade resulting in a progressive reduction in the platelet count and various clotting factors. As a defense against this intravascular clotting, antithrombin combines with thrombin in an irreversible complex. Consequently, antithrombin levels can rapidly fall below the normal of 80 to 125 percent of control early in sepsis. Prekallikrein levels also fall early in sepsis because of activation of various proteolytic cascades which convert prekallikrein to kallikrein. Recently we have found that a progressive fall in antithrombin and prekallikrein levels to less than 60 percent and 40 percent of control, respectively, may provide an early diagnosis of sepsis before there are any other signs of severe infection.

Blood Gases

As sepsis progresses into the more advanced stages of shock, there is a standard progression of acid-base changes from (1) respiratory alkalosis, (2) compensated metabolic acidosis, (3) uncompensated metabolic acidosis, and finally (4) combined metabolic and respiratory acidosis.

Sepsis is an extremely powerful stimulus to ventilation. The initial blood gas analysis in patients going into early septic shock generally reveals a low Pa_{CO_2} (25 to 35 mmHg), a normal bicarbonate (21 to 26 meq/L), and an elevated pH (7.45 to 7.55). Early hyperventilation so frequently accompanies shock and sepsis that, if a patient with known shock or sepsis is not hyperventilating, one should suspect that the patient has a metabolic alkalosis or some other problem apt to cause respiratory failure. In particular, one should search carefully for dysfunction of the central nervous system, airway, lungs, chest wall, or diaphragm and rapidly correct that abnormality.

The initial respiratory alkalosis in sepsis is generally a nonspecific response and not compensatory for hypoxemia or metabolic acidosis. However, as shock develops and oxygen consumption falls, lactic acid levels tend to rise, causing the patient to hyperventilate even more as a compensatory response. If the Pa_{CO_2} falls below 20 mmHg, this severe hypocapnia may in itself cause some hemodynamic impairment.

As shock progresses, increasing impairment of cellular metabolism results in local accumulation of hydrogen ions. By the time a significant lactic acidosis is present in arterial blood, the shock process is often quite advanced and oxygen consumption is usually less than two-thirds of normal.

Initially, the patient can maintain a relatively normal pH (7.35 to 7.45) because the fall in bicarbonate is usually more than balanced by the fall in Pa_{CO_2}. Later, however, as oxygen consumption continues to decrease, bicarbonate levels may fall so low that the lungs cannot keep pace, and the arterial pH falls below 7.35. The lower the pH falls below 7.35, the poorer the prognosis.

If the shock process is allowed to continue, various cellular aggregates may accumulate in the lung, progressively increasing dead space (alveoli which are ventilated but not perfused) from a normal of 0.30 to levels of 0.60 or higher. Consequently, even if total minute ventilation remains constant, the P_{CO_2} may eventually begin to rise. Therefore, a patient who is in severe progressive shock and lives long enough may eventually develop a combined respiratory and metabolic acidosis before he or she dies.

Smears

Although most physicians will culture blood, urine, sputum, and other material that might indicate infection and the responsible microorganisms, they often do not pay adequate attention to the importance of carefully preparing and examining Gram stains of potentially infected material. In many instances, the responsible organisms can be identified on a well-prepared smear but may not grow out properly on culture. In addition, smears may help to differentiate between positive sputum cultures due to colonization, tracheobronchitis, and pneumonitis. With colonization, there are few if any polymorphonuclear leukocytes (PMNs) and only a small number of organisms (10^1 to 10^2/mL). Tracheobronchitis is characterized by sputum with more bacteria (10^3 to 10^4/mL) and moderate numbers of PMNs. With pneumonitis there are many bacteria (10^5 or more per milliliter) and there are

many PMNs. However, for a smear to be accurate, it must be performed on a good representative sample of the material available. Obtaining good, accurate samples of tracheobronchial secretions, except by bronchoscopy or transtracheal suction, may be difficult. Many sputum samples are deceptive because the sample consists largely of mouth and pharyngeal secretions. If alveolar macrophages (dust cells) can be recognized in the specimen, a relatively good sample of lower respiratory tract material has probably been obtained. Occasionally, pleural fluid will contain organisms, and these will usually be the same as those involved in the underlying lung infection.

Obtaining a good urine specimen can also be a problem. If the patient is catheterized, the specimen should be obtained by aspirating the Foley catheter tubing with a needle rather than by disconnecting the tube and breaking the closed drainage system. If the patient is not catheterized, a clean midstream catch in a man is usually a fairly good specimen. In women, suprapubic aspiration of the bladder provides the greatest accuracy.

Culture and Sensitivity Studies

As with smears and Gram stains, the accuracy of culture and sensitivity studies depends primarily on how representative the material submitted is of the involved fluid or organ. It also depends on how rapidly and carefully the specimen is handled. For example, great care must be taken to avoid skin contaminants when taking blood cultures.

Cultures taken with swabs should be obtained from the edges of abscesses and not the center. Material from the center of abscesses is more likely to contain necrotic material and dead PMNs and bacteria. Ideally, tissue at the edge of the abscess should be submitted for culture. Swabs must also not be allowed to dry out. They should be brought to the laboratory as soon as possible for inoculation on the appropriate culture medium. In most instances, both aerobic and anaerobic cultures should be obtained. Anaerobic organisms are particularly fragile, and cultures for these organisms should be drawn and handled with the same precautions as arterial blood gas samples.

Blood cultures should be obtained on at least two and preferably three separate occasions at least 15 min apart from a direct venous or arterial puncture. If an IV catheter may be infected, blood cultures should also be drawn through that catheter, and the tip of the catheter should be cultured. However, IV catheter tips are often not cultured because of the high incidence of contamination as the catheter is removed.

Quantitative cultures of potentially infected tissue are becoming increasingly important. It is now clear that colony counts of organisms in burned tissue which are 10^5 or more per gram generally indicate invasive infection. Furthermore, burns or skin ulcers containing more than this concentration of organisms cannot usually be skin-grafted successfully. Interestingly, any number of beta-hemolytic streptococci in an open wound will usually prevent successful skin grafting.

All too often the most rapidly growing organisms, rather than the organism responsible for the sepsis, are grown out on culture. If the culture result correlates well with what is found on the Gram stain, the results are quite reliable. If they do not correlate, one must use clinical judgment and/or obtain further cultures and smears.

Whenever possible, cultures should be obtained before antibiotic therapy is begun. Once antibiotics are started, they can stop growth of all or some of the bacteria in the culture medium unless specific steps are taken to inhibit or dilute out the antibiotic. If the patient is already on antibiotics and not critically ill, it may be helpful to stop the antibiotics for 24 h and then obtain new cultures.

An increasing number of opportunistic infections of the lung are being seen, especially in patients who have very low PMN levels due to leukemia or chemotherapeutic agents and in patients with AIDS. Although giving a multitude of drugs designed to cover the organisms most likely to cause opportunistic lung infections is frequently successful, open lung biopsy is often required to make a definitive diagnosis and provide effective treatment. In many instances, the biopsy is of value because it shows that the infiltrate is not due to a microorganism, and this allows several potentially toxic antimicrobial agents to be discontinued. However, the risk of open lung biopsy in such patients is high and, even with appropriate therapy, the mortality rate often exceeds 60 to 70 percent.

Monitoring

Monitoring of the patient who is septic and may go into shock must be almost continuous. Some of the parameters which should be monitored particularly closely include:

1. Blood pressure. Changes in pulse pressure are particularly important because they tend to correlate fairly well with changes in stroke volume. An intraarterial line should be inserted if the blood pressure is difficult to obtain or if serial blood gases are indicated.
2. Heart rate and rhythm (cardioscope).
3. Respiratory rate and depth.
4. Urine output (in milliliters per hour).
5. Central venous pressure (pulmonary artery wedge pressure should also be measured in patients with septic shock not responding rapidly to fluid loading).
6. Serial arterial blood gases. Simultaneous mixed venous (pulmonary artery) blood gas analyses may be especially helpful by allowing one to calculate physiologic shunting in the lung. If cardiac output is measured, along with arterial and mixed venous oxygen content, one can also calculate delivery and oxygen consumption.
7. Blood flow (cardiac output).

Whenever possible, critically ill patients should be monitored objectively and almost continuously. The observations should be recorded and, whenever possible, graphed. Graphic recordings of blood pressure are extremely helpful in demonstrating trends in the pulse pressure. A fall in mixed venous oxygen or a rise in arteriovenous oxygen content differences is usually good evidence of a fall in cardiac output and tissue perfusion. It must be emphasized repeatedly that responses in critically ill patients are extremely variable. Single or isolated measurements are of much less value than trends or responses; this is particularly true of the central venous pressure and pulmonary artery wedge pressure.

Treatment

The treatment of septic patients can be divided into three main categories: (1) treatment of the infectious process, (2) enhancement of host defense mechanisms, and (3) correction of associated pathophysiologic changes.

Treatment of the Infection

In treating patients with sepsis, it is important to identify and eradicate the underlying infection as soon as possible. Left uncorrected for more than a few hours, particularly if shock develops, problems such as intraabdominal abscesses or necrotic bowel carry an extremely high mortality rate, regardless of how well the cardiovascular, respiratory, and metabolic changes are corrected.

Treatment of the infectious process itself primarily involves the use of antimicrobial drugs and surgical removal or drainage of infected or necrotic material.

Antimicrobial Agents

Antibiotics are often misused. No antibiotic or combination of antibiotics "covers everything." Therefore, if antibiotic therapy appears to be needed before culture results are known, the physician must make an educated guess from the history and physical examination and Gram-stain results of the organisms most likely to be present. In addition, proper cultures should be obtained so that therapy can be changed promptly and accurately if the initial guess is wrong.

Table 58-3 provides a few guidelines to initial antimicrobial therapy based on the site of infection. Although bacteriocidal agents tend to be favored, there is no evidence that bacteriocidal drugs are better than those which are bacteriostatic, except in the therapy of endocarditis or patients with severe granulocytopenia. No drug kills 100 percent of organisms—the body defenses are needed to do this.

It is important to administer antibiotics in the proper dosage. With some drugs such as gentamicin the proper dose approaches toxicity. "Playing it safe" by giving lower doses, however, is often useless and tends to promote resistance. In a study in our own ICU it was found that 50 percent of patients treated with gentamicin or tobramycin achieved peak doses of only 4 to 6 μg/mL, which were not adequate to treat severe gram-negative

infection. In addition, over 50 percent of the patients developed renal toxicity as evidenced by a rise in serum creatinine of 0.5 mg/dL or more. It is now clear that severe gram-negative penumonias or peritonitis require peak blood levels of tobramycin or gentamicin of 8 to 10 μg/mL which can only be achieved consistently by giving doses of 2.0 to 2.5 mg/dL. Furthermore, to prevent renal dysfunction, trough levels should be less than 1.0 μg/mL. To accomplish this, the interdose intervals may have to be more than 16 h. The dosages and timing of doses are best determined by pharmacokinetic studies. It is also important to know that, because creatinine excretion in septic patients may be less than 600 mg per day, their creatinine clearance may be less than 40 mL per minute in spite of a normal urine output, BUN, and serum creatinine.

In clinically ill patients, absorption of drugs by the oral route is erratic and often totally inadequate. In addition, even if the gastrointestinal tract is working well, gram-negative organisms often require much higher antibiotic doses than can be achieved or tolerated by oral administration. For example, oral administration of ampicillin and cephalosporins is usually totally inadequate for serious gram-negative infections. Only relatively mild urinary tract or soft tissue infections will usually respond to treatment with these drugs.

For certain drugs, the intramuscular route should not be used because of (1) poor absorption and a tendency to form sterile abscesses (tetracycline, chloramphenicol, erythromycin); (2) excessive pain at the injection site (cephalothin, methicillin, aqueous penicillin); or (3) inability to achieve adequate doses (carbenicillin). The intramuscular (IM) route is also inappropriate in shock and in patients with severe vascular disease because of impaired circulation. However, the amount of penicillin or cephalosporin given IV must be higher than the IM dose because of rapid urinary excretion of these drugs.

It is necessary to know which drugs require either dosage change or complete avoidance with various types of organ failure. This is particularly true of aminoglycosides and uremia. If such agents must be used, blood levels of the antibiotic and/or creatinine clearance levels must be monitored very closely. Concomitant hepatic failure often requires

Table 58-3 Most Frequent Causes of Infection at Selected Body Sites and Suggested Initial Antimicrobial Treatment

Site and Infection	Microorganism(s)	Antimicrobial Agent(s)
Upper respiratory tract:		
Tonsillitis, pharyngitis, sinusitis, otitis	*Streptococcus pyogenes*	Penicillin
Acute	*Streptococcus pneumoniae*	Penicillin
	Streptococcus pyogenes	Penicillin
Lower respiratory tract:		
Pneumonia, bronchitis		
Adults	*Streptococcus pneumoniae*	Penicillin
	Anaerobes from oropharynx	Penicillin
Young adults	*Mycoplasma pneumoniae*	Erythromycin
Adults with chronic lung disease	*Haemophilus influenzae*	Ampicillin
Infections (gastrointestinal)	Facultative gram-negative enteric bacilli plus anaerobes from gastrointestinal tract	Cefoxitin or aminoglycoside plus clindamycin
Central nervous system:		
Meningitis (adults)	*Neisseria meningitidis* or *Streptococcus pneumoniae*	Penicillin
Brain abscess	Anaerobes	Penicillin
Bone infections:		
Osteomyelitis (adults)	*Staphylococcus aureus*	Penicillinase-resistant penicillin
Joint infections	*Neisseria gonorrhoeae* or *Staphylococcus aureus*	Penicillin Penicillinase-resistant penicillin
Genital infections:		
Nongonococcal urethritis or pelvic inflammatory disease	*Chlamydia*	Tetracycline
Skin infections	*Staphylococcus aureus* or *Streptococcus pyogenes*	Penicillinase-resistant penicillin Penicillin
Urinary tract infections and prostatitis:		
Simple	Facultative enteric gram-negative bacilli	Sulfonamide or aminoglycoside
Complicated		Trimethoprim—sulfamethoxazole or aminoglycoside
Blood infections:		
Presumed gram-negative bacteremia	Facultative enteric gram-negative bacilli or *Pseudomonas aeruginosa*	Aminoglycoside
Presumed gram-positive bacteremia	*Staphylococcus aureus* or penicillin-susceptible streptococci and pneumococci	Penicillinase-resistant penicillin

Source: G.P. Youmans, P.Y. Patterson, and H.M. Sommers, eds., *The Biologic and Clinical Basis of Infectious Diseases.* Saunders, 1985, pp. 801–802. Used with permission of the publisher.

further reduction in drug dosage in such patients, but guidelines for this situation have not been well established.

The antimicrobial agents used to treat infections generally act by damaging or interfering with (1) the cell wall, (2) intermediary metabolism, (3) the cell membrane, or (4) ribonucleic acid (protein synthesis) of microorganisms. Examples of each are given in Table 58-4.

Surgery

Surgical control of the primary or underlying infectious process is often far more important than the antimicrobial agents used. In fact, most failures of antimicrobial therapy are due to inadequate or delayed removal, drainage, or debridement of infected secretions, fluid, or tissue.

Most large collections of pus will cause severe toxicity and will not resolve unless they are drained.

Table 58-4 Mechanisms of Action of Antimicrobial Agents

Agents Acting on the Cell Wall	Agents Acting on RNA Protein Synthesis	Agents Acting on the Cell Membrane	Agents Acting on RNA Synthesis
Penicillins	Tetracycline	Polymyxin B	Rifampin
Cephalosporin	Chloramphenicol	Clindamycin (Cleocin)	Amphotericin B
Vancomycin	Aminoglycosides	Sulfas	5-Fluorocytosin

Such drainage should be as complete as possible without spreading the infected material and should be dependent, if at all possible, so that gravity can help promote drainage. In situations in which drainage of the abdomen can only be accomplished anteriorly, soft sump tubes should be used. With posterior drains, the nurse must exercise judgment in determining the best balance between position changes to prevent pulmonary complications and those promoting maximal drainage of infected materials. Anterior abdominal drainage in children may be facilitated if the child is encouraged to play on hands and knees with toys that can be pushed along the floor.

Continued leakage of intestinal contents, particularly from the colon or distal small bowel, into the peritoneal cavity is tolerated very poorly. Under such circumstances, the involved bowel should be excised or exteriorized and a proximal colostomy or enterostomy performed. Nasogastric suction alone is usually not adequate to prevent continued leakage from diseased or injured bowel.

Deep third-degree burns eventually all become infected. However, if the eschar can be excised relatively early and the underlying tissue successfully covered with skin grafts, invasive infection is greatly reduced. Removal of infected or necrotic tissue is particularly important if an anaerobic infection, such as gas gangrene, is present.

Catheterization of the urinary tract should be avoided if possible. However, if the urine is infected and the urinary tract is even partially obstructed, the infection may be virtually impossible to correct without drainage.

Bronchoscopy is particularly helpful for managing bronchopulmonary infections if the patient cannot or will not cough effectively, even with nasotracheal suction. Bronchoscopic drainage may be particularly helpful in promoting endobronchial drainage of the suppurative material associated with lobar atelectasis, bronchiectasis, or lung abscesses.

Factors Impairing Host Defenses

Some of the more important causes of impaired host defenses include loss of integrity of skin or mucous membranes, presence of foreign bodies, use of immunosuppressive or chemotherapeutic agents, and metabolic abnormalities such as diabetes mellitus, uremia, and hepatic failure.

Any defect in the skin or mucous membrane may act as a portal of infection. This is particularly important in burns, which eventually all become infected if they remain open. Consequently, efforts should be made to remove the dead skin and cover the denuded area with skin grafts as soon as possible.

Foreign bodies greatly increase the likelihood of infection. In experimental studies it was found that it usually took 10^6 organisms to cause a subcutaneous infection. However, if a foreign body such as a silk suture was present, as few as 10^2 organisms could cause the infection. If an infection does involve a foreign body, the infection is often impossible to eradicate until the foreign body is removed. Consequently, infected foreign bodies which are not essential to the life or function of the patient should be removed as soon as possible. Certainly an infected IV catheter should be removed promptly and another IV started at another site. However, if vital foreign bodies such as cardiac valves, pacemakers, or large vascular grafts become infected, strong efforts are often made, at least for a few days or weeks, to control the infection with local or systemic antibiotics. However, if the antibiotics are not successful, the infected foreign body and associated infected tissue must be removed. Another prosthesis can then be inserted with the hope that recurrent infection can be prevented.

If a patient with a transplanted organ develops a severe infection which does not respond adequately to antimicrobial agents, the immunosuppressive drugs should be reduced as much as possible or discontinued. It is far better to lose a transplanted organ than it is to lose a life trying to save a transplanted organ.

Patients with advanced malignancies often have impaired host defenses, especially if the patient is also malnourished. If the patient is also given chemotherapeutic agents, his or her host defenses may be almost nonexistent. If the response of a neoplasm to a chemotherapeutic agent is minimal, there is little reluctance to discontinue the drug. However, in some patients with lymphomas or acute leukemia, the chemotherapeutic agent is extremely important, and reduction or discontinuation of the drug requires careful judgment.

Control of diabetes mellitus during sepsis is often extremely difficult. The diabetic ketoacidosis reduces resistance to infection and sepsis tends to make the diabetic ketoacidosis worse, creating a vicious downward cycle. Aggressive eradication of the infection and careful monitoring of blood glucose and acetone levels are essential.

Renal function is generally best improved by providing an optimal cardiac output and blood pressure so as to maintain a high urine output without loop diuretics. Reduction of nitrogenous waste products in the blood by debridement of necrotic tissue is extremely important. Hypercatabolic renal failure, characterized by a rise in BUN of more than 25 mg/dL per day, has an extremely poor prognosis and is much easier to prevent than to treat. Early aggressive administration of essential amino acids with adequate calories may help reduce mortality rates.

Hepatic failure is best prevented or corrected by providing an optimal blood flow, oxygenation, and glucose, and by reducing the amount of ammonia reaching the liver from the intestinal tract. Reduction of ammonia is best obtained by cleaning the bowel with cathartics or enemas and by administration of nonabsorbable antibiotics to reduce the number of bacteria in the bowel. Administration of nutrients with high levels of branched chain amino acids and low concentrations of aromatic amino acids may help prevent or treat hepatic encephalopathy.

Protective Isolation

Increasing efforts have been made to isolate patients with severe immunological depression from all types of microorganisms which might cause infection. Particular efforts have been made in this regard for patients with transplanted hearts and those on large doses of chemotherapeutic agents for treatment of various malignancies, especially if the PMN count falls to less than 500/mm³. The environment of such individuals is kept as sterile as possible and contact of care givers with such patients is often only through plastic drapes or special plastic windows. Complete isolation for all extrinsic organisms is theoretically possible. However, such efforts are often only successful for a few days or weeks, and furthermore, the microorganisms which the patient already has are usually his or her own greatest enemies.

Therapy to Improve Host Defenses

Some attempts to improve host defenses have included improved nutrition and administration of fresh frozen plasma, cryoprecipitate, and serum with high antibody titers to the core lipopolysaccharides of *E. coli.* Experimental efforts have also included use of various phagocytic stimuli, administration of transfer factor, and transfusions of leukocytes.

Improved Nutrition

As mentioned previously, hyperalimentation of malnourished individuals can help restore phagocytosis toward normal levels. This is particularly important if the patient has albumin levels less than 2.2 g/dL and the absolute lymphocyte count (ALC) is less than 800/mm³. These patients may require more than 3500 to 4500 nonprotein calories and 1.5 to 2.5 g of nitrogen per kilogram of body weight daily to restore immunologic competence. Unfortunately, IV hyperalimentation is difficult to give during severe acute infections and may in itself increase the risk of infections. To infuse adequate IV calories usually requires either the use of 20 to 25 percent concentrations of glucose or 10 to 20 percent concentrations of fat. Use of 20 to 25 percent glucose increases the risk of metabolic and infectious complications by about fourfold. On the other hand, IV fat in large quantities may tie up the reticuloendothelial system (RES), particularly if triglyceride levels rise. One can compromise by using 3.0 L of 15% glucose and 500 mL of 20% lipid daily. This will provide about 2500 nonprotein calories daily.

Fresh-Frozen Plasma

Administration of fresh-frozen plasma may help restore host defenses, particularly complement, in patients with prolonged infections or malnutrition. Unfortunately, relatively large amounts of plasma may be required to restore immunoglobulin and complement levels to normal, and this is considered a poor use of a precious resource. In addition, there is a 0.1 to 0.5 percent risk of hepatitis with each unit infused.

Correction of Pathophysiologic Changes

Correction of the pathophysiologic changes in sepsis is essential to maintain optimal organ function. If advanced organ failure is allowed to develop, the patient may die even if the infectious process is finally controlled.

Pulmonary System

In any critically ill or injured patient, the first priority of treatment is to ensure adequate ventilation, not only for proper oxygen and carbon dioxide exchange, but also to prevent or combat the tendency toward atelectasis. Adequate ventilation in patients with severe sepsis is at least one-and-one-half to two times normal. If the patient's minute ventilation cannot be brought to adequate levels rapidly, ventilatory assistance should be begun. If the Pa_{CO_2} is greater than 45 to 50 mmHg in a patient who does not have metabolic alkalosis, ventilator assistance is usually urgently needed. If the Pa_{O_2} is less than 60 to 80 mmHg in spite of oxygen administration, if alveolar-arterial oxygen differences $P(\text{A-a})O_2$ are high, or if physiologic shunting ($\dot{Q}S/\dot{Q}T$) is greater than 20 to 25 percent, ventilatory assistance should be begun. These indications are summarized in Table 58-5.

After the patient has had adequate fluid and blood replacement, pulmonary function may be further improved by elevating the patient's head and chest and adding positive end-expiratory pressure (PEEP). Because PEEP tends to reduce venous return and cardiac output, particularly in hypovolemic patients, PEEP should not be added until or unless the blood volume is normal or greater than normal. If more than 10 cmH₂O PEEP is used, the cardiac output and oxygen transport (cardiac output

Table 58-5 Indications for Endotracheal Intubation and Ventilatory Assistance in Patients with Sepsis and/or Shock

Respiratory rate greater than 30–35 inhalations per minute

Excessive ventilatory effort

Minute ventilation less than 5 L/per minute or greater than 20 L/per minute

Tidal volume less than 4 mL/kg or more than 40% of the tidal capacity

Vital capacity less than 10–15 mL/kg

P_{CO_2} greater than 40 mmHg if a metabolic acidosis is present or P_{CO_2} greater than 50 mmHg with normal bicarbonate levels

P_{CO_2} less than 60–80 mmHg on 40% O_2 or P_{CO_2} less than 250 mmHg on 100% O_2

$P(\text{A-a})O_2$ on room air or more than 55 mmHg or $P(\text{A-a})O_2$ on 100% oxygen or more than 400 mmHg

$\dot{Q}S/\dot{Q}T$ of more than 20%, especially if cardiac output is low

Source: G.P. Youmans, P.Y. Paterson, and H.M. Sommers, eds. *The Biologic and Clinical Basis of Infections Diseases,* Saunders, 1985. Used with permission of the publisher.

multiplied by the arterial oxygen content) should also be monitored.

Even if ventilation is adequate, patients with sepsis or shock often benefit from the administration of oxygen. Oxygen exchange in the lungs and in tissues becomes impaired very quickly in these patients, particularly if cardiac output is decreased. Consequently, patients with septic shock should be given enough oxygen to maintain an arterial P_{O_2} of at least 80 mmHg.

Fluids

In sepsis it is extremely important to maintain a cardiac output which is normal or higher. However, septic patients tend to become hypovolemic because of increased permeability of capillaries and venules. Consequently, early aggressive fluid administration is extremely important.

In critically ill septic patients who may be seriously hypovolemic, it is important to insert two, and preferably three, large IV catheters. Hypotension due to hypovolemia should be corrected within 15 to 30 min, if at all possible. Administration of fluids at a slower rate may not correct the volume deficit for several hours or longer because of continued loss of large quantities of fluid into the interstitial space.

In the septic patient who is severely hypovolemic, volume replacement is begun with 2 to 3 L of a balanced electrolyte solution such as Ringer's lactate solution given over 10 to 15 min. However, if the patient is cirrhotic, a buffered electrolyte solution without lactate may be preferable. Such a solution can easily be made by adding one to two ampules of sodium bicarbonate to a liter of normal saline.

The relative amount of crystalloid, colloid, and blood which should be used in critically ill patients is extremely controversial. Although albumin levels are often very low in septic patients, continued administration of large amounts of albumin may cause more harm than good. Some investigators feel that the albumin may move rapidly into the interstitial space, particularly in the lungs, drawing water with it, thereby increasing the tendency to respiratory failure. In addition, albumin infusions may reduce the production of coagulation factors and immunoglobulins. However, other investigators believe that colloid may be beneficial.

Regardless of which type of fluid is chosen, it is infused rapidly until the patient is out of shock or shows evidence of fluid overload. To do this properly requires careful monitoring of blood pressure, pulse rate, urinary output, skin perfusion, and arterial blood gases. If the patient does not respond promptly to what clinically appears to be adequate amounts of fluid, a central venous pressure (CVP) catheter or preferably a pulmonary artery wedge pressure (PAWP) catheter should be inserted to measure the filling pressure changes in the heart.

Isolated CVP levels have relatively little physiological significance; however, the response of the CVP to a fluid challenge is extremely important. Some physicians feel that if the CVP is above 12 to 16 cmH_2O, fluid administration should be stopped because the patient is probably overloaded. However, we have found that the CVP in septic patients is extremely variable. A number of septic patients, particularly those with ARDS, may have a CVP of 20 to 25 cmH_2O, in spite of hypovolemia, as demonstrated by blood volume determinations and/or PAWP.

In many centers, great care is taken to measure the CVP and PAWP with the patient flat in bed without ventilator assistance. Such maneuvers increase the accuracy of readings, but they are un-

necessary because the response to a fluid load is far more important than the absolute levels. If the CVP rises abruptly (by more than 5 cmH_2O) as fluid is given rapidly (3 mL/kg in 10 min), the fluid should be stopped until the CVP falls to within 2 cmH_2O of the baseline level.

In most instances, the function of the right and left ventricles is quite similar; therefore, changes in the CVP (which reflect filling pressures in the right heart) correlate fairly well with changes in the pulmonary artery wedge pressure (which reflects left ventricular filling pressure). In a number of instances, however, the CVP and PAWP may be quite disparate. Hypovolemic patients with severe sepsis tend to have an obstruction to blood flow in the lungs and, therefore, they will tend to have a CVP which is relatively much higher than the PAWP.

If a PAWP catheter is in place, the pulmonary artery pressure is monitored constantly. The diastolic pulmonary artery pressure is usually relatively close to the pulmonary wedge pressure unless there is pulmonary hypertension. However, a true wedge pressure should be obtained periodically (once or twice a shift) by transiently inflating the balloon. In almost all instances, the PAWP is equal to or slightly lower than the PA diastolic pressure. Occasionally, particularly if the tip of the PAWP is in a main pulmonary artery, inflating the balloon does not completely occlude the PA lumen; consequently the dampened wave form may reflect the mean PA pressure rather than the LA pressure. In addition, if the patient is on a ventilator, the values present at the end of expiration most accurately reflect the left atrial pressure.

Military antishock trousers (MAST), now increasingly referred to as the pneumatic antishock garment (PASG), were originally thought to raise blood pressure in hypotensive individuals primarily by causing an autotransfusion of 700 to 1000 mL from the lower extremities and lower abdomen back into the central circulation when they were inflated. It is now recognized that this garment raises blood pressure primarily by increasing afterload.

Acid-Base Therapy

Most acid-base problems in shock will improve spontaneously if adequate ventilation and tissue perfusion are provided. However, any serious acid-base abnormality which persists in spite of these measures should be corrected.

A persistently severe respiratory alkalosis with a Pa_{CO_2} less than 25 mmHg may cause vasoconstriction in cerebral and other vessels. If the blood volume and blood pressure have been restored and the patient can tolerate sedatives, such agents may reduce the respiratory rate, thereby raising the Pa_{CO_2}. If the patient is on a ventilator, the tidal volume can be reduced or the ventilatory mode can be switched from assist control (AC) to intermittent mandatory ventilation (IMV). The IMV rate can then be reduced every hour or two as long as the Pa_{CO_2} is less than 45 mmHg, the pH is more than 7.35, and the patient's respiratory rate is less than 30 per minute.

A moderate metabolic acidosis (pH <7.25) that persists in spite of fluid loading should be corrected. Some investigators have felt that acidosis need not be corrected unless the arterial pH is less than 7.15. However, we have found that patients tend to do best if they are maintained in acid-base balance with a pH of 7.35 to 7.40, a Pa_{CO_2} of 30 to 40 mmHg, and an HCO_3^- of 20 to 26 meq/L.

Inotropic Agents

If shock persists in spite of fluid loading, attempts should be made to improve the cardiac output by increasing the contractility of the heart. The inotropic agents used most frequently in shock include dopamine, dobutamine, and epinephrine.

Digitalis preparations are rarely used in shock now unless there is a coincident atrial fibrillation with a rapid ventricular rate. The effective dose can be extremely variable and may be less than half the usual loading dose, especially if ionized calcium levels are low. Dopamine is a much more powerful inotropic agent and its effects can be stopped in a few minutes. In addition, although digitalis may improve myocardial function, it also increases myocardial oxygen demands and may significantly increase the incidence and severity of arrhythmias. Since single large doses of digitalis preparations may cause severe splanchnic vasoconstriction, digoxin is usually administered in multiple intravenous increments.

Dopamine, in contrast to classical vasopressors such as norepinephrine or metaraminol, appears capable of raising both blood pressure and cardiac output in most patients with shock. The response to this agent varies according to the dosage used. At doses of 1 to 3 μg/kg/min, its so-called dopaminergic effect tends to increase splanchnic blood flow and urine output with little or no increase in blood pressure, cardiac output, or stroke volume. At intermediate doses of 5 to 15 μg/kg/min, the blood pressure, cardiac output, stroke volume, and myocardial contractility usually increase rather substantially, and splanchnic blood flow and urine output may rise even further. Higher doses of dopamine, exceeding 30 μg/kg/min, may cause vasoconstriction, and the cardiac output may fall because of the increasing peripheral vascular resistance. The only problem we have seen with dopamine is a tendency to tachyarrhythmias if the dosage is increased too rapidly.

Dobutamine is also an inotropic agent but it tends to be a vasodilator and is usually given in doses of 5 to 20 μg/kg/min. Some investigators think that it is less likely to cause tachycardia than dopamine and is more apt to be effective in chronic heart failure. Because of its vasodilating properties, dobutamine is more apt to be of benefit in cardiogenic shock which usually is associated with a high systemic vascular resistance (SVR). In contrast, dopamine is more apt to be of benefit in septic shock in which the SVR is low.

In the occasional patient who has shock with a slow pulse rate, isoproterenol in doses of 1 to 2 μg per minute may raise blood pressure and cardiac output and restore tissue perfusion to normal. If the pulse rate exceeds 120 beats per minute, however, as it usually does in sepsis, it is much less likely to improve cardiac output and may cause dangerous tachyarrhythmias. Isoproterenol should also not be given to patients with an acute myocardial infarction, because it tends to increase myocardial oxygen demands more than it increases coronary blood flow.

Epinephrine in doses of 1 to 5 μg per minute can be a powerful inotropic agent, and it may be effective when large doses of dopamine and dobutamine are not. However, it may cause vasoconstriction and may also cause tachyarrhythmias. It is probably of most use in low cardiac output syndromes after cardiac surgery.

Amrinone (Inocor) is one of a new class of inotropic agents which also have some vasodilator properties. Its mode of action is not clear but it is not a β-adrenergic agonist. However, it does inhibit myocardial cyclic AMP phosphodiesterase activity and increases cellular levels of cyclic AMP. Its activity reduces both afterload and preload by a direct relaxant effect on vascular smooth muscle. It is usually administered as a loading dose of 0.75 mg/kg over 2 to 3 min followed by a maintenance dose of 5 to 10 μg/kg/min. Some problems with its use include hypotension if the patient is hypovolemic and occasional tachyarrhythmias, especially at higher doses. It should not be administered with solutions containing glucose.

A normal concentration of ionized calcium (2.1 to 2.4 meq/L) may be extremely important for maintaining optimal cardiovascular function in sepsis and shock. Administration of 1 to 2 g of calcium chloride (10 to 20 mL of 10% $CaCl_2$) IV over a period of 10 to 30 min should be considered in any patient with a persistently low cardiac output, particularly if ionized calcium levels are less than 1.7 meq/L.

Administration of calcium is particularly important in shock patients who require massive transfusions. Under such circumstances, the citrate in the transfused blood may reduce ionized calcium levels to the point of severely impairing cardiovascular function. Consequently, a gram of calcium chloride would be given after every 4 units of blood in patients with persistent hypotension, particularly if the blood is being given at a rate of 1 unit of blood every 5 min or faster.

Alkalosis also reduces the ionized calcium levels in the blood and may be an additional indication for giving calcium. For each 0.1 rise in pH, ionized calcium levels fall about 0.16 meq/L. Since calcium increases the response of the heart to digitalis, it must be used with great care in patients who are fully digitalized, particularly if the patient is hypokalemic.

Over the past few years there have been scattered reports of significant improvement in cardiac function following the administration of concentrated solutions of glucose, insulin, and potassium, thereby providing additional energy substrate to the heart. The usual dosage recommended consists of 100 to 200 g of glucose, 20 to 40 meq of potassium chloride, and 10 to 20 units of regular insulin IV given over a period of 1 to 2

h. We have seen only occasional benefit with such solutions, and it has been difficult to prove that the glucose-insulin-potassium solution rather than other agents given at the same time was the cause of the improvement.

Ideally, cardiac output should be increased until oxygen consumption rises to a supranormal plateau and does not rise further even if oxygen delivery is further increased. In many septic patients oxygen consumption can be increased far beyond normal in contrast to hypovolemic and cardiogenic shock when oxygen can seldom be increased much above normal.

Steroids

Up to 15 percent of the ICU septic patients we have studied have some degree of adrenal insufficiency. In sepsis, plasma cortisol levels usually rise to levels which are two to three times normal. In these patients the plasma cortisol levels were normal or only slightly elevated and plasma cortisol levels did not increase properly after IV ACTH. The only survivors among this group with an inadequate cortisol response were those who were given steroids.

Because of the possibility that subclinical adrenal insufficiency may be present, all patients with shock that is unresponsive to fluid loading, acid-base correction, and inotropic agents should be given at least 200 mg of hydrocortisone by rapid IV injection. If the patient appears to respond to the hydrocortisone or if there is a reasonable suspicion of subclinical adrenal insufficiency, the patient should be given 75 to 100 mg of hydrocortisone IV every 6 h for at least 2 to 3 days or until the patient's condition has stabilized. The dose of steroids can then be tapered off over another 4 to 5 days.

Although there is general agreement that "replacement" doses of steroids should be given if there is adrenal insufficiency, the use of massive doses of steroids in shock remains extremely controversial. Although continuing administration of steroids interferes with the inflammatory response and certain host defenses, there is much data suggesting that massive steroids in experimental shock can stabilize lysosomal and capillary membranes and improve cardiovascular function and cell metabolism. Oxygen delivery to tissues may also be improved by shifting the oxyhemoglobin dissociation curve to the right.

The only really good large prospective randomized study on the use of massive steroids early in shock showed that giving massive steroids within 2 h of the onset of shock reduced the mortality rate from 40 percent in the placebo group to 11 percent in the treatment group. In all other studies steroids have been given much later and there has been little or no response to them.

Because massive steroids can cause significant vasodilation, they should not be used until hypovolemia is definitely corrected, and then should be given slowly with additional fluid over a period of 15 to 30 min with close observation of the blood pressure. Our present regimen consists of giving a pharmacologic dose (30 mg/kg methylprednisolone sodium succinate, or 6 mg/kg dexamethasone phosphate) intravenously to patients whose condition is deteriorating in spite of aggressive treatment with other modalities. If possible, the decision to give steroids should be made within 2 h of the onset of shock. The massive steroids may be repeated in 4 to 6 h if needed. Whenever possible, objective hemodynamic and blood gas studies are performed before and 30 and 120 min after each dose to determine if there is a beneficial effect which might indicate a need for giving additional doses.

Vasopressors

Vasopressors should be considered potentially lethal drugs which should only be given when there appears to be no other rapidly effective method of restoring an adequate coronary or cerebral blood flow. In general, vasopressors should not be administered until an adequate trial with ventilation, oxygen, fluids, acid-base correction, inotropic agents, and steroids has been given. It is particularly important to avoid vasopressors if hypovolemia is present. In hypovolemic animals, vasopressors may cause blood flow through some arterioles to cease, and areas of ischemic necrosis may develop. Since small amounts of vasodilator such as phentolamine (Regitine) reduce the excessive vasoconstriction and lethality of norepinephrine in experimental animals, phentolamine is always added to our norepinephrine solutions. Our current mixture consists of four ampules (each containing 1.0 mg) of norepinephrine (Levophed) and two ampules

(each containing 5 mg) of phentolamine (Regitine) in 500 mL of D_5W. Phentolamine in this dosage may prevent excessive vasoconstriction, but it does not alter the cardiac output or peripheral vascular resistance significantly. Furthermore, if the norepinephrine should extravasate into tissues around the vein, the phentolamine usually prevents the local necrosis which might otherwise develop. In instances when the patient already seems excessively vasoconstricted, the concentration of phentolamine may be increased up to 2 ampules for each ampule of norepinephrine.

It must be emphasized that the minimal acceptable blood pressure in shock is extremely variable. Consequently, close observation of the patient's intravascular volume and tissue perfusion as reflected by the cardiac output, central nervous system (CNS) activity, ECG, and urine output is required.

There is some question as to whether vasopressor drugs are required in young patients, who may have adequate perfusion of vital organs even at very low systolic blood pressures. However, in older patients with significant coronary or cerebral arterial stenosis, blood flow to those vital organs may require pressures that are higher than normal.

Vasodilators

If the patient shows evidence of excessive vasoconstriction and poor tissue perfusion in spite of all therapy, and if the patient's blood pressure is normal or high, a vasodilator may occasionally be very helpful. It should be remembered that the best vasodilator in a hypovolemic patient is intravenous fluid. Furthermore, vasodilators should not be used in patients who are hypovolemic because these agents may increase vascular capacity by as much as 2 to 3 L, accentuating the hypovolemia dramatically and causing a sudden, severe hypotension. Even in the presence of an adequate intravascular volume, vasodilators will often cause the systolic blood pressure to fall by 10 to 15 mmHg. If the patient is already hypotensive, such a drop in blood pressure may seriously jeopardize coronary and cerebral blood flow, particularly if these vessels have a 70 to 80 percent occlusion, which makes flow through them pressure-dependent.

The vasodilators now used most frequently are nitroprusside and nitroglycerin. Both are administered at doses beginning about 0.3 μg/kg/min and gradually increased, if necessary, to doses of about 3.0 μg/kg/min. Nitroprusside acts primarily on arterioles, thereby primarily reducing afterload. Nitroglycerin has slightly more effect on veins, thereby reducing preload. Nitroglycerin may also selectively vasodilate coronary arteries, thereby reducing myocardial ischemia in patients with coronary artery disease.

Diuretics

Oliguria is usually the result of inadequate renal perfusion due to hypovolemia. Administering diuretics under such circumstances can be a double jeopardy. The diuretic may not only cause direct renal damage, but it may also cause hypovolemia, reducing renal perfusion and causing more renal damage. Occasionally, however, oliguria persists in spite of all other therapy and will not respond except to diuretics. Oliguric renal failure following sepsis which requires dialysis has a mortality rate exceeding 80 percent. Similar patients who develop nonoliguric renal failure, even if the urine output is maintained with diuretics, have a much better prognosis. Consequently, we strive to maintain a urine output of at least 0.5 mL/kg per hour and preferably 1.0 mL/kg per hour.

If the urine output is less than 0.5 mL/kg per hour in spite of fluid loading and inotropes, 12.5 to 25.0 g of mannitol may be infused rapidly IV over a period of 10 to 15 min, followed by a slow infusion of 12.5 g of mannitol per hour as needed. If there is still no diuretic response, 5 to 10 mg of furosemide (Lasix) IV may be given. The dose of furosemide is then doubled every 15 min until an adequate urine output is obtained or until a single dose of 500 to 1000 mg of furosemide is reached. If there is no response to 80 to 160 mg of furosemide, 100 to 200 mg of ethacrynic acid may be given IV.

Unless the patient is obviously overloaded with fluid, all urine losses should be replaced. If oliguria persists in spite of all these drugs, we assume that the patient is in renal failure, and the patient is treated accordingly. Prophylactic dialysis and early aggressive nutrition may be of great value in such individuals.

Heparin

Some degree of intravascular coagulation can be assumed to be present in most patients with severe persistent sepsis or shock. Relatively few, however, show the full-blown clinical syndrome of disseminated intravascular coagulation (DIC) with excessive bleeding from needle sticks and all mucosal surfaces until the septic process is virtually uncorrectible.

There is increasing controversy regarding the value of heparin for the treatment of DIC. However, if serial coagulation studies in septic patients reveal a progressive reduction in the platelet count and in the concentrations of factor V, factor VIII, fibrinogen, and prothrombin, without adequate fibrinolysis (as reflected by increased fibrin split products), treatment with heparin should be considered.

Treatment of DIC includes (1) correction of the underlying sepsis and/or shock, and (2) replacement of clotting factors if troublesome bleeding is occurring. Whether or not to use heparin may be a difficult decision. Reversal of the primary septic or shock process is the most important part of the therapy of DIC, but it is also the most difficult.

Newer Agents

Naloxone (Antiendorphin) Therapy   Beta endorphins are endogenous opiates secreted by the same cells in the hypothalamus that secrete ACTH. Hence, any stress which causes ACTH release will also cause beta-endorphin release. These opiates apparently cause hypotension primarily by lowering peripheral vascular resistance, but they may also cause myocardial depression. Although naloxone has little or no effect on the cardiovascular system of normal animals, it can increase arterial blood pressure and survival in most animals with endotoxin-induced hypotension. The mechanism of action is thought to be a central inhibition of opioid receptors. Naloxone usually causes an increased peripheral vascular resistance, but it may have varying effects on different vascular beds.

The results obtained clinically with naloxone have not been as good as those seen in experimental animals, possibly because of late administration and the much smaller doses used in patients. Although naloxone almost invariably raises blood pressure at least temporarily, patients may become extremely restless and difficult to manage, and survival is rarely increased.

Prostaglandins   Prostaglandins are a large family of naturally occurring lipids formed from arachidonic acid metabolites by the enzyme cyclooxygenase. Several studies have shown that a number of these substances, including thromboxane (TxA_2) and prostacyclin (PGI_2), are elevated in septic shock. Although some of these prostaglandins, such as thromboxane, may be harmful in shock, others such as PGE_1 and prostacyclin, can be helpful. PGE_1 has been used with benefit in experimental hemorrhagic shock, producing a decrease in peripheral resistance and an increase in cardiac output and blood pressure. PGI_2 (prostacyclin) causes vasodilation and inhibits platelet aggregation. Studies on lethal endotoxemia in dogs have shown that PGI_2 can improve tissue perfusion and organ function.

Prostaglandin inhibitors also have received wide attention. For example, the changes in intracortical renal blood flow after *E. coli* bacteremia are associated with an increase in prostaglandin levels and are prevented by pretreatment with indomethacin (a cyclooxygenase inhibitor) (Fig. 58-4). Sepsis causes a significant increase in the TxB_2 (a stable metabolite of thromboxane A_2), and this increase is completely prevented by treatment with the Tx synthetase inhibitor. Inhibition of Tx synthesis also tends to improve total peripheral resistance, intracellular oxygen tension, and transmembrane potential differences.

Central venous plasma levels of thromboxane in patients dying of septic shock are more than tenfold higher than in survivors. These data suggest that treatment with imidizole, an inhibitor of thromboxane synthetase, might be beneficial in septic shock.

Adenosine Triphosphate (ATP) Administration For many years there has been interest in various methods of improving cell metabolism and raising intracellular levels of ATP. It has generally been assumed that exogenously administered ATP cannot enter tissue; however, it has been shown that even under normal conditions, some ATP can enter some muscle cells, and that this amount is increased during shock. It has also been found that a glucose

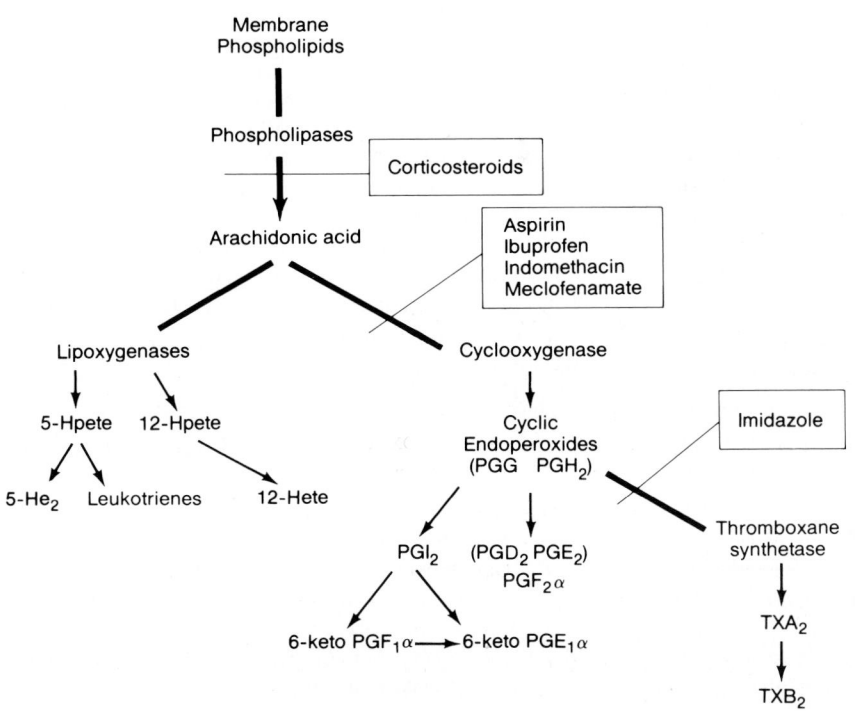

Figure 58-4 Scheme of arachidonic acid metabolism showing proposed sites of action of some specific enzyme inhibitors and major stable metabolites. *(From W. J. Sibbald, and C. L. Sprung, eds., Perspectives on Sepsis and Septic Shock, Society of Critical Care Medicine, 1986, p. 350.)*

ATP-MgCl$_2$ mixture significantly increases survival in rats who have peritonitis due to cecal ligation.

Antisera The use of antiserum to endotoxin was recently investigated by Ziegler et al. in a prospective study of 212 patients with gram-negative sepsis. Antiserum produced from the J-5 mutant strain of *E. coli*, which contains only core determinants, reduced mortality rate from 39 percent in the control group to 22 percent in the antiserum group. The effect in those with profound shock was even greater, with mortality rates of 77 percent in the control group compared to 44 percent in the treated group. Although not currently available to most practitioners, such antisera may play a significant role in the management of gram-negative bacteremia in the future.

Summary

Sepsis should be diagnosed and treated as early as possible. Its development should be anticipated in critically ill or injured patients, particularly if they are immunosuppressed.

Trends are far more important than isolated levels in evaluating the patient's condition and response to therapy. Any tendency to reduced tissue perfusion or impaired cellular metabolism should be treated aggressively according to a previously well-designed plan.

Eradication of the sepsis (surgically and with antibiotics as needed), provision of adequate ventilation and oxygen, and early aggressive administration of fluids are the mainstays of therapy. Close monitoring of the response of the patient to the various types of treatment is essential to determine which therapy should be continued or increased.

Bibliography

Archer, D. B. (1979). Pathogenic mechanisms of mycoplasmas. *Nature, 27:*268.

Chaudhry, I. H., Keefer, J. R., Barash, P., et al. (1984). ATP-Cl$_2$ infusion in man: Increased cardiac output without adverse systemic hemodynamic effects. *Surgical Forum, 35:*14–16.

Chesney, P. J., Davis, J. P., Purdy, W. K., Wand, P. J., & Chesney, R. W. (1981). Clinical manifestations of the Toxic Shock Syndrome. *Journal of the American Medical Association, 246:*741–748.

Chu, D. Z. J., Nishioka, K., Romsdahl, M. M. (1984). Effect of tuftsin on postsplenectomy sepsis. *Surgical Forum, 35:*162–164.

Clowes, G. H. A., Jr., Martin, H., Walji, S., Hirsch, E., Gazitua, R., & Goodfellow, R. (1978). Blood insulin responses to blood glucose levels in high output sepsis and septic shock. *American Journal of Surgery, 135:*577–583.

Dunn, D. L., Mach, P. A., & Cerra, F. B. (1983). Monoclonal antibodies protect against lethal effect of Gram-negative bacterial sepsis. *Surgical Forum, 34:*142–144.

Fry, D. E., Pearlstein, L., Fulton, R. L., et al. (1980). Multiple system organ failure. *Archives of Surgery, 115:*136.

Garrison, R. N., Fry, D. E., Berbeich, S., et al. (1982). Enterococcal bacteremia: Clinical implications and determinants of death. *Annals of Surgery, 193:*43.

Heggers, J. P., Robson, M. C., Kucan, J. O., et al. (1984). Skin testing. A valuable predictor in thermal injury? *Archives of Surgery, 119:*49–52.

Hunt, M. G. (1982). Generalized peritonitis. *Archives of Surgery, 117:*209.

Jacob, H. S. (1980). Complement-induced vascular leukostasis. *Archives of Pathology and Laboratory Medicine, 104:*617.

LeGall, J. R., Fagniez, P. L., Meakins, J., et al. (1982). Diagnostic features of early high post-laparotomy fever: A prospective study of 100 patients. *British Journal of Surgery, 69:*451.

Loe, W. A., Jr., & Bowen, J. C. (1984). Thromboxane synthetase inhibition during septic shock. *Surgical Forum, 35:*3–5.

Maki, D. G., & Band, J. D. (1981). A comparative study of polyantibiotic and iodophor ointments in prevention of vascular catheter-related infection. *American Journal of Medicine, 70:*739–744.

Mazaheri, R., Rode, H. N., Abikar, K., et al. (1984). Dysfunction of humoral immunity in anergic surgical patients: Absence of anti-tetanus IgG antibody production. *Journal of Clinical Immunology, 4:*65–70.

Meakins, J. L., Pietsch, J. B., Bubenik, O., Kelly, R., Rude, H., Gordon, J., & MacLean, L. D. (1977). Delayed hypersensitivity: Indicator of acquired failure of host defenses in sepsis and trauma. *Annals of Surgery, 186:*241–250.

Moir, C., & Robins, R. E. (1982). Role of ultrasonography, gallium scanning and computed tomography in the diagnosis of ultraabdominal abscess. *American Journal of Surgery, 143:*582.

Orlando, R., III, Gleason, E., & Drezner, A. D. (1983). Acute acalculous cholecystitis in the critically ill patient. *American Journal of Surgery, 145:*472.

Rock, P., Silverman, H., Plump, D., et al. (1985). Efficacy and safety of naloxone in septic shock. *Critical Care Medicine, 13:*28–33.

Saba, T. M., Blumenstock, F. A., Scovill, W. A., et al. (1978). Cryoprecipitate reversal of opsonic, SB glycoprotein deficiency in septic surgical and trauma patients. *Science, 201:*622.

Sarngadharan, M. G., Papovic, M., Bruch, L., et al. (1984). Antibodies reactive with human T lymphotropic retroviruses (HTLV III) in the serum of patients with AIDS. *Science, 24:*506.

Shoemaker, W. C., Schluchter, M., Hopkins, J. A., et al. (1981). Comparison of the relative effectiveness of colloids and crystalloids in emergency resuscitation. *American Journal of Surgery, 142:*73.

Smith, E. F., III, Tabas, J. H., & Lefer, A. M. (1980). Beneficial actions of imidizole in endotoxin shock. *Prostaglandins Med., 4:*215.

Vincent, J. L., Dufay, P., Berde, J., et al. (1983). Serum lactate determinations during circulatory shock. *Critical Care Medicine, 11:*449–451.

Wernick, A., Jarstrand, C., & Julander, I. (1983). Effect of intralipid on mononuclear and polymorphonuclear phagocytes. *American Journal of Clinical Nutrition, 37:*256–261.

Wing, V. W., Van Sonnenberg, E., Kipper, S., et al. (1984). Indium-111-labelled leukocyte localization in hematomas: A pitfall in abscess detection. *Radiology, 152:*173.

Zeigler, E. J., McCutchan, A., Fierer, J., et al. (1982). Treatment of gram negative bacteremia and shock with human antiserum to a mutant *Escherichia coli*. *New England Journal of Medicine, 307:*1225–1228.

59 Transplantation

Reba Felks-McVay

Introduction

The field of transplantation has grown in its practice to include many organ systems and in the development of methods to combat rejection and treat infection. Transplantation is a changing and challenging field. It is not uncommon to find a transplant recipient or an organ donor in one's own community. It is because of this rapid growth and the outreaching effects that nurses must be knowledgeable about transplantation and its effects on society. The nurse will play an important role in the future of transplantation—not only in the administration of nursing care, but in the role of counselor and educator of the public, the patient, and the family.

Historical Perspectives

Organ transplantation resulted from much study and experimentation in the past. It has led to development in surgical techniques, immunological monitoring, medical equipment, clinical use of medications, and in the general knowledge, growth, and understanding of ways in which the body functions in health and disease states. It is impossible to fully describe all of the contributions made to transplantation as we know it today, but some of the modern developments will be mentioned.

Much of the credit for the development of techniques allowing for organ system transplantation can be given to Carrel and Guthrie. Their work in vascular surgical techniques and experiments using animal models is well known. They developed techniques for the surgical anastomosis of blood vessels and applied this knowledge to organ transplantation.[1-4] In 1905, Carrel and Guthrie successfully transplanted the heart of a small dog into the neck of a large dog, and the small heart began to spontaneously beat, showing that neurological connection was not necessary for the heart to beat.[3,4]

In the early 1900s the puzzle regarding ways to infuse blood without clotting and reactions was pieced together with the description of blood types and compatibility screening. During this time transfusion of blood was still reserved for the most critically ill. It was not until 1937 that blood banking was organized.[5] Blood typing is used by all organ transplant programs as a major compatibility screen between the donor and recipient.

In the 1930s the immunological description of allograft rejection led to further study and to the description of histocompatibility antigens by Gover.[5] Lindbergh and Carrel developed an organ perfusion apparatus in 1938 which could be used to preserve organs; this was the forerunner of the cardiopulmonary bypass pump.[6]

Developments in techniques, equipment, and knowledge continued in the 1940s, as could be seen in the use of ether anesthesia and the development of the first kidney dialysis machine.[2] The concept of dialysis developed with the use of available technology by Alwall of Sweden and Kolff of Holland. Dr. Kolff traveled to Russia, England, and the United States, leaving in each country one of his dialysis machines. It was at Peter Bent Brigham Hospital that the machine found regular use, and knowledge concerning long-term dialysis was gained.[2,7]

By the 1950s transplantation experiments in animals had evolved to clinical trials in humans. Even with dialysis, many patients were dying of renal failure. In 1950, a renal transplant was performed by Lawler, who placed a kidney into the pelvic position with cutaneous ureterostomy.[8] Prior to this time, the kidney had been transplanted in the arm or thigh of the recipient without success. Renal transplantation continued, and in 1954 long-term success was realized using identical twins as donors. Also, the ureter was implanted into the urinary bladder for the first time in 1954.[9] Experimental trials during this time involving organ cooling by perfusion or immersion in cold solution showed improvement in organ function following transplantation.[10] Knowledge concerning immunology was also expanding, as seen in demonstrations of induced tolerance by biologic manipulations in experimental trials by Billingham, Brent, and Medawar, and description of human lymphocyte antigens by Rood and Daussett.[11,12]

In the 1960s new developments continued in the field of organ transplantation. In 1961, Imuran was used clinically by Murray as a means of overcoming the immunologic response to transplantation.[13] This had some success, and in 1963 prednisone was added by Starzl to create further immunosuppression. During this same year, Starzl performed the first liver transplant and Hardy and associates performed the first lung transplant in humans.[14,15] In 1964, a very important development in immunologic monitoring occurred in the use of histocompatibility testing to select the most compatible recipient to receive the donor organ, which has been of most use in renal transplantation.[16] In 1966, Kelly and Lellehi performed the first human pancreas transplant and antilymphocyte globulin was first used in the treatment of rejection.[17,18] The following year, Barnard made worldwide news when he performed the first human-to-human heart transplant.[19] This was followed closely by the transplantation of both heart and lungs in a human by Cooley.[20] So by the end of the 1960s, all major organ systems had been transplanted in the human.

In the 1970s there were further developments which improved transplant success. Transplant recipients were more carefully screened and criteria for acceptance as a transplant candidate were developed for most organ systems. Emphasis was placed on postoperative care and prevention of complications such as infection. Caves developed an instrument called a *bioptome* which was used to obtain a biopsy of heart tissue. This device has been useful in the detection of rejection in heart as well as in heart and lung transplant recipients.[21] Immunological monitoring became more sophis-ticated during the 1970s, enabling earlier detection of the cellular response of antigen-antibody mechanisms. In 1972, the goal of studies such as these was to enhance organ acceptance and identification of more effective means of immunosuppression.

In the late 1970s and early 1980s, clinical use of a new immunosuppressive agent led to a renewed interest in clinical transplantation. Cyclosporine A was found to be more specific in its immunosuppressive actions and allowed for a reduction in dosages of other, less specific immunosuppressive agents, such as prednisone and Imuran.[22] The early 1980s have seen not only an improvement in survival rates, but a rapid growth in transplant centers that have involved transplantation of all organ systems. Currently, this rapid growth has forced society to face the issues of organ donation and financial reimbursement. From these consumer and medical community concerns have come the National Organ Transplant Act, signed in 1984, which addresses growth in areas of organ procurement agencies, establishment of a national network to assist in the utilization of donated organs, and evaluation of reimbursement and medication payment practices. The need for multiple-organ donation has been stressed by the medical community, and society's awareness will hopefully increase with national news coverage of issues and special programs designed to enhance public knowledge about organ transplantation. Research in immunological monitoring, rejection detection, knowledge in the use of medication for immunosuppression, treatment of rejection, and infection, as well as improvements in organ preservation, have continued in the 1980s.

Future Directions In Transplantation

With current research as a guide for the future, transplantation will continue to be an ever-challenging, evolving field. The detection of rejection at earlier stages, development of more specific immunosuppressive agents with fewer toxic effects, development of techniques and equipment for organ procurement allowing tolerance of ischemia for more prolonged periods, and increasing the knowledge of the ways in which the immune system responds to transplanted organs, as well as methods to manipulate the immune response into acceptance, are areas in which research has been continuing. The future will see clinical trials and further research in these areas as well as others. Survival rates are anticipated to continue to improve as knowledge and experience are utilized clinically.

As a greater awareness of the need for organ donors is realized, the number of transplants should continue to increase as well. The number of multiple organ donors must increase in order to meet the needs of the various organ system transplant candidates. The regulation of organ utilization, requests for permission to procure organs, and the regulation of the number of transplant centers will also become major issues in the future.

The cost of health care is of great concern and transplantation will be affected by the need to control costs. The trend toward shorter intensive care unit and hospitalization time will continue as knowledge concerning the care of the transplant recipient increases, assisted by clinical experience, results of ongoing research, improved medication regimens, and treatment of complications. As the problem of financial reimbursement is addressed, there may be limitations of cost in some areas, guidelines for routine or expected procedures and diagnostic studies, or reimbursement to only those transplant programs meeting specific qualifications.

As can be seen, the future of transplantation is filled with a continuation of research, clinical trials, and resolution of medical, ethical, and moral issues in an attempt to save otherwise terminally ill patients and to return them to productive, active lives.

Nursing Therapies in Organ Failure

Failure of each organ system and medical and surgical management are discussed in other chapters specific to the organ system. The focus of this section is on general nursing therapies for the patient with end-stage disease who is anticipating organ transplantation in the near future.

Caring for the patient with organ system failure can be very complex and demanding. The nurse must be knowledgeable regarding normal organ function, the pathophysiology of organ failure, and the impact of specific organ failure on the body. A thorough assessment of the patient's phys-

iological and psychosocial status must be accomplished before formulation of nursing diagnoses and interventions. Some of the possible nursing diagnoses for the patient with organ system failure are listed in Table 59-1. An example of the nursing care plan for the patient experiencing organ system failure featuring one nursing diagnosis is given below.

Nursing Diagnosis
Stress related to:

1. Illness
2. Uncertainty of illness outcome
3. Financial concerns
4. Hospitalization.

Goal
Following nursing intervention during hospitalization the patient will become less stressed as evidenced by the ability to:

  I. Discuss the illness and present treatment.
 II. Discuss the potential outcome of the illness.
III. Review possible future treatment and therapies as described by the physician.
IV. Identify stressors.
 V. Utilize methods of reducing stress.
VI. Examine finances and propose methods of meeting financial needs.

Table 59-1 Possible Nursing Diagnosis for Patients Experiencing Organ System Failure

Alteration in nutritional status
Potential disturbance in self-concept
Fear
Potential disturbance in sleep pattern
Potential for ineffective coping
Lack of knowledge
Potential for noncompliance
Potential for fluid and electrolyte imbalance
Potential for complications related to organ system dysfunction
Pain and discomfort
Spiritual needs related to dealing with illness and possible death
Potential sexual dysfunction
Potential impairment of skin integrity
Stress related to illness; hospitalization; uncertainty of illness outcome; financial concerns
Potential for depression and mood disturbances
Potential for changes in bowel and bladder habits

Nursing Interventions

The nurse will:

I. Utilize patient care time to get to know the patient and to listen.

II. Encourage patient to verbalize feelings concerning illness and present treatment.

III. Explain all treatments thoroughly.

IV. Plan extra time to sit with the patient when he or she expresses the desire to talk about the illness and potential outcome.

V. Consult the clergy and psychiatric liaison concerning ways of assisting the patient in discussing and coping with the effects of illness and outcome.

VI. Review the chart with the physician for possible future treatment and therapies which may be expected.

VII. Encourage the patient to verbalize feelings about future treatment and therapies.

VIII. Encourage the patient to describe the treatment and therapies described by the physician.

IX. Explain all procedures, treatments, and therapies thoroughly.

X. Encourage the patient to express feelings of stress.

XI. Encourage the patient to list or describe stressors.

XII. Review with the patient methods of reducing and dealing with stress.

XIII. Encourage the patient to identify and use methods which reduce stress.

XIV. Allow the patient as much control over the environment and activities (i.e., bath time, menus, etc.) as possible.

XV. Support the patient by participating in stress reduction methods: be calm, turn radio to patient's favorite station, allow patient private time, dim the lights, be available to listen, etc.

XVI. Contact social services worker to review patient's financial situation with the patient and to assist in finding ways to meet any need.

Specific interventions should be based upon the clinical manifestations and psychological needs of the individual patient.

The delicate balance of organ compensation becomes more fragile as the stage of illness progresses. The nurse must always be aware of this fragility and respond appropriately to changes in the overall clinical status of the patient. Recognition of deterioration and other organ system involvement can assist the nurse in preparing the patient and family for future therapy. The goals of nursing therapy for organ failure should include education of the patient and family, assistance in preparation for and coping with the inevitable outcome of the disease, and in maintenance of the present level of function. The nurse should allow the patient and family to verbalize fears and concerns about the disease state, the possible outcomes, and treatment. The chaplain, social worker, and psychiatrist can be of invaluable assistance to the family, as well as the patient, as they attempt to cope with illness.

The clinical course may be varied among patients with exacerbations and remissions of symptoms, or the disease may progress rapidly. Once irreversible organ system dysfunction is diagnosed, the decision regarding whether to medically or surgically treat the patient arises. Most patients are medically treated with close supervision until it is believed that they are no longer responding to therapy. The patient may be referred to a medical center for transplant evaluation at any time during this period of medical treatment. Once it is decided that the patient is to be evaluated for transplantation, the nurse can play a vital role in preparing the patient and family for transplantation. Nursing therapy goals should be to educate the patient and family about transplantation, to support them in their decision, and to offer encouragement and support while awaiting transplantation. Supporting the patient and family during the time of decision making about whether to have a transplant can be difficult for the nurse.

Information about the transplant procedure and the effect it will have on the life of the patient must be provided so the patient and family may be able to make a decision and give informed consent. If the patient should decide to proceed with the transplant procedure, the nurse should be available to answer questions and to encourage the patient and family during the potentially long wait for a donor organ to become available. If the waiting period becomes longer than a few weeks, the patient and family may have concerns about the potential occurrence of complications such as infection, which would prevent transplantation; of the potential for a catastrophic event occurring; or they may voice concerns over other patients being transplanted before them. The reply to their concerns and questions will either lead to satisfaction that all that can be done is being done or lead to other concerns being voiced. The psychiatrist, social worker, chaplain, or organ bank personnel are excellent resources in answering questions and relieving concerns.

If the patient and family decide not to receive a transplant the nurse must support them in that decision also. It is a difficult time for the patient and family—they are dealing with imminent death, potential financial crisis, fear, and attempting to make a decision which will greatly affect their lives. They may need a sounding board—one that is unbiased. The nurse must put aside feelings about transplantation, the patient, and the patient's situation. Whatever the patient decides, the nurse must be sure the patient and family fully understand the importance of the transplant procedure to their health; what is involved with transplantation and the possible results; and what not having the transplant means in terms of the outcome of the illness, and treatment. The nurse should accept the patient's decision and continue to offer encouragement and support through the time thereafter. The chaplain, social worker, and psychiatrist can be most helpful at this time to the patient and family.

A case study involving a patient with cardiac dysfunction, who received a heart transplant, will be discussed throughout the chapter. Special emphasis will be included for each section under the case study.

Case Study

Mr. Jones is a 62-year-old white male who has been in poor health for the past 5 years. He is married and has two daughters. They are both married and live in another state. His oldest daughter has a 3-year-old son, Timothy.

Mr. Jones was forced to retire 6 months ago from his job as a store clerk due to fatigue and dyspnea on exertion. Mr. Jones has a pension with the company and has applied for medical disability. He and his wife own their home and have a small savings account as a nest egg.

Mr. Jones had been relatively healthy until he developed a viral syndrome 5 years ago, after which he was found to have an enlarged heart. He has become progressively more easily fatigued and short of breath. Two months ago he was hospitalized for congestive heart failure (CHF). His chest x-ray showed an increase in heart size and congestion. While in the hospital, several diagnostic studies were done. An echocardiogram revealed a dilated left ventricle with marked hypokinesis. A resting multigated scan (MUGA) also showed a poorly functioning left ventricle with an ejection fraction of 20 percent. Mr. Jones responded well to digitalis, Captopril, and diuretics. Within 4 days he was released from the hospital to be followed closely by his primary physician.

Two weeks ago, Mr. Jones was readmitted to the hospital with CHF. He was placed in the intensive care unit (ICU) and a dobutamine intravenous infusion was begun. He has had transient episodes of improvement but has progressively worsened. Mr. Jones has had shortness of breath at rest, abdominal pain, nausea, and orthopnea. On physical examination his liver was palpable and he had an S_3 with a grade 3/6 mitral regurgitant murmur, marked jugular venous distention, diminished peripheral pulses, and +2 pitting edema. His chest x-ray showed bilateral congestion with an enlarged heart. Mr. Jones had also rapidly lost weight as revealed by a weight of 68 kg compared to his weight of 80 kg 2 weeks ago. In addition, he had a poor appetite. Supplemental protein and caloric intake with Ensure was begun. His blood pressure was maintained at a systolic pressure of 100 by addition of dopamine intravenous infusion. He also was having short episodes of atrial fibrillation.

When Mr. Jones remained unresponsive to medical therapy of catecholamines, afterload reduction, and diuretics, cardiac transplantation was considered as a treatment option.

Surgical Management of the Failing Organ

Surgical intervention should be considered when medical therapy has been utilized and organ function continues to deteriorate. The possibility of transplantation should be discussed early in end-stage disease and the evaluation process commenced. Planning the appropriate time for transplantation is crucial in maintaining the patient's stability to enhance surgical survival, preventing involvement of other organ systems, and decreasing the side effects of medical therapy.

The patient and family need as much time as possible to prepare for transplantation. Extended illness can drain a family of resources very quickly and place a strain on family relations. Both the patient and family members must deal with the known outcome of a terminal illness and the treatment involved for everyday management of the disease state. The hope that transplantation brings may overshadow the risks of the surgery and immunosuppression. The transplant team members must be sure the patient and family fully understand the transplant procedure and the risks involved prior to proceeding with transplantation.

Evaluation of Transplant Candidacy

The Recipient

Not all patients with end-stage disease are appropriate candidates for transplantation. An extensive, individualized evaluation process is utilized to ensure that no contraindications to transplantation exist, to evaluate organ systems for irreversible dysfunction, and to rule out the possibility of alternative treatment. The evaluation process and acceptance criteria vary according to the institution and the organ system involved. Some similarities can be found, however. Common diagnostic studies used to obtain data for the evaluation process are listed in Table 59-2. Most institutions require an

Table 59-2 Common Diagnostic Studies and Examinations Utilized in the Evaluation of a Transplant Candidate and Rationale for Use

Tool	Rationale
Medical history; physical examination	Assists in differentiating cause of organ failure and assessment of likelihood of recurrence of disease. Assists in assessment of other organ system involvement
Vital signs	Assessment of patient stability and effect of organ failure on total body function
Chest x-ray	Assessment of pulmonary system for obvious infectious process, fluid, and pulmonary disease
Electrocardiogram	Assessment of cardiac involvement as seen in chamber enlargement, hypertrophy, bundle branch block, myocardial ischemia or infarction, arrhythmias, or pulmonary disease such as cor pulmonale
Urinalysis; blood chemistries; serum enzymes; liver function studies	Assessment of body compensation, need for medical intervention, and organ system function
Psychiatric examination	Assists in identification of patient needs for support, education, and potential sources of future patient difficulties. Helpful in identification of potential noncompliance, personality disorders, and psychiatric illness. Available for IQ testing and assistance in dealing with psychosocial problems
Dental examination	Individuals who are ill and malnourished have special mouth care needs. Assists in identification and treatment of gum disease and potential sources of infection, such as tooth decay and abscess
Tuberculin skin test; hepatitis screen; HSV, CMV, EBV titers	Assists in identification of infectious process and baseline data for postoperative titers and screens
Blood, urine, and sputum cultures	Assists in identification of infectious process
Blood group; antibody screen	Identification of ABO type necessary for compatibility matching with a donor; identifies preformed antibody requiring special testing to set up blood
HLA tissue typing	Identification of recipient's histocompatibility antigens present on the cell surfaces which can be used to compare and match with donor
Lymphocytotoxicity screen	Identification of recipient's preformed antibodies

assessment by a psychiatrist or psychologist, a social worker, members of the transplant team, and consulting physicians.

The physical examination and diagnostic studies attempt to describe the effects of the disease on the organ systems and determine whether transplantation is advisable. The psychosocial impact of transplantation should also be considered in determining candidacy. Coping mechanisms used in the past and the resources for the patient and family, now and in the future, are identified. The emotional stability of the patient and family members, past compliance with medical therapy, and possible alcohol or drug abuse are scrutinized closely for identification of potential problems. If any of these areas is a source of past problems, the transplant surgeon or transplant board members will decide if the risk of recurrence is such that transplantation is inadvisable.

The length of time between completion of the evaluation and transplantation varies for each patient, depending on the disease state. The patient who is evaluated early in end-stage disease may wait for some time before transplantation is required. For some patients this requires repetition of some diagnostic studies as the time of transplantation draws near. Many of the diagnostic studies can be done on an outpatient basis but others may require a short hospitalization. Diagnostic studies done at referring institutions are usually acceptable and should be sent with the patient to the transplant center.

The patient who is accepted for immediate transplantation will need to provide information on how he or she can be located when a donor organ has been found. If the patient is allowed to wait at home, preparations must be made for a quick trip to the transplant center. A small bag should be packed with needed items, and the quickest route to the hospital—by bus, car, or airplane—should be known. If the patient is required to relocate to the institution's city, the family must make preparations for maintaining two households and caring for the patient, as well as for family members left at home. This can further strain the family situation and resources may be needed to assist them in handling the situation.

The expense involved in transplantation may be a limiting factor for some potential candidates

and resources for assistance should be sought early in the transplantation evaluation. The social worker can be of great assistance in this area. Presently, not all transplants are covered by third-party payers and Medicare assistance does not cover the transplant procedure or medication required after a heart, liver, lung, pancreas, or heart and lung transplant. This is being debated at the present time and may be a resource for the future. Many institutions require a deposit prior to admission for evaluation when insurance does not cover the cost of transplantation. If financial problems exist, ways of initiating a fund-raising account and the process of fund raising may be a necessary part of patient and family education for the potential transplant patient.

Heart Patients being considered for cardiac transplantation have end-stage heart disease with poor ventricular function. The majority of candidates have cardiomyopathy, ischemic heart disease, valvular disease, or congenital heart disease. The exact etiology of the disease may not be known and the course of illness varies from one patient to another, with progression to the point of transplantation within months or years of diagnosis. Hospitalization may not always be necessary immediately prior to transplantation.

The major criteria for heart transplantation are end-stage cardiac disease with New York Heart Association (NYHA) class IV symptoms, a life expectancy of less than 1 year, no other organ system pathology, and no other medical or surgical therapy to which the disease would respond. With the use of newer immunosuppressive agents and an increase in the knowledge regarding transplantation, the selection criteria for heart transplantation have evolved to include those individuals over age 55 and young children. The contraindications to cardiac transplantation are sepsis, recent pulmonary embolism, extensive peripheral vascular disease, malignancy, and pulmonary vascular resistance greater than six to eight Wood units.[23–26]

Evaluation for cardiac transplantation may be completed while the patient is in NYHA class II or III, as well as NYHA class IV. Transplantation will be planned for the time when the disease state has progressed to NYHA class IV. The diagnostic studies required for evaluation include those listed in Table

59-2, as well as an echocardiogram, a MUGA, a pulmonary perfusion scan, and a recent cardiac catheterization. If the patient has ischemic heart disease, both right and left heart catheterization is required to rule out the possibility that coronary bypass grafting could be done as an alternative therapy. If the pulmonary vascular resistance is elevated, a heterotopic heart transplant or a heart and lung transplant may be considered as an alternative to the orthotopic heart transplant procedure. Orthotopic heart transplant requires removal of the diseased heart and replacement with a healthy heart.

As increases in pulmonary vascular resistance and pulmonary pressures occur, the right side of the heart must raise its pressure in order to push blood forward to the lungs. The diseased heart has compensated for these high pressures by dilatation and hypertrophy. If a healthy heart replaces the heart which has been compensating, it must very rapidly compensate for the increased pulmonary pressures and vascular resistance. When the healthy heart is unable to compensate, heart failure occurs. Heterotopic heart transplantation, in which the recipient's heart is left in place and the donor heart is connected to the recipient's heart and vasculature, may be considered so that the recipient's heart can continue to compensate for the increased pulmonary vascular resistance, while the donor heart assumes the work of increasing cardiac output.[23] Both of these procedures are described in detail later in the chapter.

The functioning of the renal and hepatic systems is scrutinized closely. It is not uncommon to have liver enlargement and elevated enzymes in patients who have end-stage heart disease and CHF. The extent of liver dysfunction that is caused by cardiac failure and is not, therefore, reversible must be evaluated. Likewise, the renal system may be negatively affected by cardiac dysfunction and low cardiac output. Liver function studies, BUN, and creatinine levels are followed at intervals while the patient awaits transplantation.

Lung   Patients considered for lung transplantation have end-stage pulmonary disease, such as chronic obstructive lung disease, fibrosing alveolitis, diffuse interstitial fibrosis, bronchiectasis, or silicosis. Patients evaluated are usually less than 55 years of age with no other organ system dysfunction. The contraindications to lung transplantation include coronary heart disease, myocardial infarction within the last 6 months, gastrointestinal disease, upper respiratory tract obstruction, and tracheal disease.[27,28]

The evaluation process includes those studies listed in Table 59-2 as well as pulmonary arteriography for assessment of pulmonary vasculature, and pulmonary function and perfusion studies. An assessment for pulmonary infection is of crucial importance and negative cultures are required.

Patients being evaluated for lung transplantation are in the terminal stage of disease and may be oxygen-dependent. Mechanical ventilation may be necessary in some instances as the disease progresses. The time necessary to locate a suitable donor is usually lengthy and may be discouraging for the patient and family.

Heart and Lung   The patient evaluated for heart and lung transplantation usually has primary pulmonary disease, such as primary pulmonary hypertension, severe chronic obstructive pulmonary disease, pulmonary or cystic fibrosis, or primary cardiac disease such as congenital or acquired heart disease. The transplant criteria require that the patient be less than 45 years of age and have no systemic illness or previous extensive thoracic surgery.[29,30]

The evaluation process of these patients includes those studies listed in Table 59-2, an echocardiogram, a MUGA, and a pulmonary perfusion scan. Other diagnostic studies which may be needed are determined by the underlying cause of the disease. If the patient has acquired or congenital heart disease, there may have been a previous evaluation for heart transplant and it was determined heart transplantation alone would not be of benefit. The studies from the previous evaluation can be utilized. The patient on the donor list for a heart and lung transplant may also have a lengthy wait, which should be explained to the patient and family when the search for a suitable donor is begun.

Kidney   Patients who are referred for renal transplantation have end-stage renal disease and are receiving or are about to commence dialytic therapy. There are few absolute contraindications to renal transplantation. The major requirements are that the patient be between the ages of 5 and 55 years, have a functional bladder, and have no extrarenal disease or irreversible organ dysfunction. The patient being considered for transplantation will be counseled regarding the risks and benefits of transplantation versus dialysis.[31,32]

The evaluation process involves those studies listed in Table 59-2, as well as an intravenous pyelogram to identify the renal blood supply, a renal sonogram, and a CT scan of the abdomen. Some institutions require that a renal biopsy be performed also. Because hypertension, atherosclerotic changes, peripheral vascular disease, cataracts, and diabetes mellitus occur frequently in patients with renal disease, multisystem assessments may also be indicated.[31,32]

During the evaluation an attempt is made to locate a suitable related living donor. If a suitable related living donor cannot be found, a search for a cadaveric donor is made. Renal transplantation is usually planned for the time of commencing dialysis or as soon as possible thereafter, at the time of a rise in serum creatinine to 5 mg/dL, or after the occurrence of complications such as diabetes mellitus.

Liver   Patients evaluated for liver transplantation have chronic, irreversible liver disease. The underlying disease state may include end-stage cirrhosis, metabolic disease of the liver, hepatic venous thrombus, or an inflammatory process of the liver or bile duct. Contraindications to liver transplantation include severe hypoxemia with pulmonary shunts, portal vein thrombus, sepsis, active alcoholism, and primary malignancy or metastatic disease.[33–36] Individuals with virus-induced liver disease who have a positive hepatitis B surface antigen and positive E antigen are in an extremely high risk category because of the potential for hepatitis postoperatively and may not be considered as candidates by some transplant surgeons.[33]

Most patients evaluated for liver transplant are below the age of 55 and must undergo the diagnostic studies listed in Table 59-2, liver function studies, and monitoring of coagulation factors. Special studies required to evaluate the hepatic vasculature include arteriography of the inferior vena cava, hepatic artery, and mesenteric artery. In some cases a CT scan of the abdomen, descending venocavography, pulmonary function studies, or liver biopsy may be needed.[35–37]

Liver transplantation is planned for the time when the patient feels that quality of life has become unacceptable, central nervous system damage is inevitable, or when the disease process has advanced to the point of imminent death. All opportunities for improvement and stabilization are given prior to transplantation. While awaiting transplantation the patient may be allowed to be at home, depending upon the disease state, the stage of illness, and the length of time needed to make the trip to the institution.

Pancreas   Patients who are evaluated for pancreatic transplant are insulin-dependent diabetics who are prone to the life-threatening complications of diabetes, and diabetic patients with renal disease requiring dialysis. It is common to find ophthalmic, renal, or peripheral vascular disease in the diabetic patient and many complications are attributed to these diseased areas. Patients who are evaluated may have developed diabetes mellitus as an adult or as a child.[38,39]

The evaluation of patients for pancreatic transplant includes the studies listed in Table 59-2 as well as glucose tolerance tests, insulin and glucagon levels, and a lipid profile. Retinal photography or microangiography may be required by some institutions. If the patient has disease of the renal, hepatic, or cardiovascular systems, an assessment of these systems is required also.[40]

In those patients whose diabetes mellitus is severe and does not stabilize with treatment, pancreatic transplantation is planned for the time when damage caused by complications is still reversible. Some patients, who require both renal and pancreatic transplantation, receive pancreatic and renal transplants simultaneously utilizing organs from one donor, or the pancreatic transplant may occur after recovery from renal transplantation.

Case Study

Mr. Jones was transferred to a transplant center and the evaluation for cardiac transplant candidacy began. He remained in the ICU with a dopamine intravenous infusion to maintain his systolic blood pressure at 100 mmHg. A Swan-Ganz catheter was inserted to measure right heart and pulmonary artery pressures and to obtain a cardiac output. This information was useful in the estimation of pulmonary vascular resistance and cardiac function. Mr. Jones' vital signs and hemodynamic parameters are listed in Table 59-3.

Routine blood studies for renal and hepatic function were obtained. Mr. Jones' total bilirubin was 2.0, cardiac enzymes were normal, and he had no jaundice. His renal function was adequate with a serum creatinine value of 1.6 and BUN of 20. He also had a negative hepatitis screen and TB skin test. A recent echocardiogram, MUGA, and ECG were obtained. Mr. Jones' VQ scan showed a low probability of pulmonary thromboembolism and his chest x-ray was unchanged from previous films. Blood was drawn for viral titers, blood type, HLA tissue typing, and a lymphocytotoxicity screen as final diagnostic studies.

Mr. Jones and his wife were interviewed by the social worker and the psychiatrist to discuss psychosocial adjustments to his illness and their feelings about the possibility of transplantation. The risks and benefits of transplantation had been discussed with them by the surgeon and they were eager to proceed with the transplant. Mrs. Jones was allowed to go to an apartment complex near

the hospital and financial arrangements were worked out with the assistance of the social worker. Luckily for Mr. Jones, his insurance would cover 80 percent of the transplant costs.

Following acceptance as an appropriate candidate for transplantation, Mr. Jones was placed on the active search list for a donor heart. Preoperative teaching, which included immediate postoperative care and a review of general information about transplantation, was completed by the nursing staff. Mr. Jones and his wife were visited by a heart transplant recipient at their request. They stated how helpful it was to meet someone who had had a transplant and could answer their questions about life after the transplant.

The Donor

Transplantation of the kidney and possibly the pancreas may be done using a related living donor. The extrarenal organs depend upon the cadaver donor solely. The number of extrarenal transplants being performed is increasing and the need for cadaver donors, which provide multiple organs, must be considered when obtaining permission for organ donation. The management of and donor requirements for each organ system should be considered when a potential organ donor is identified. Donor criteria for any organ are much the

Table 59-3 Mr. Jones' Hemodynamic Parameters at the Time of Evaluation

Data	Date			
	10/10	10/12	10/14	10/16
BP (mmHg)	100/60	98/52	102/58	100/52
HR (bpm)	92	100	98	110
RR (bpm)	24	28	24	24
Temperature (°F)	99	98.2	97.8	98
RAP (mmHg)	10	12	16	10
PAP (mmHg)	42/20	40/15	50/25	44/22
PCWP (mmHg)	12	16	18	14
CO (L/min)	6.25	4.32	4.0	3.98
CI (L/min/m²)	1.0	1.28	11.20	1.0
Urinary output (mL/h)	16	14	20	20
Pedal pulses	+2/+2	+2/+1	+1/+1	+1/+1

BP = blood pressure
HR = heart rate
RR = respiratory rate
RAP = right atrial pressure
PAP = pulmonary artery pressure
PCWP = pulmonary capitllary wedge pressure
CO = cardiac output
CI = cardiac index

same with a few variances according to the organ system involved. The common criteria for organ donation are listed in Table 59-4.

The related living donor is counseled and evaluated prior to removal of the donor organ to ensure that the donor will suffer no ill effects from donation, be they physical or emotional. The donor will undergo major surgery and the risks involved must be discussed. Preoperative teaching includes the routine postoperative schedule of events, such as recovery room stay, coughing and deep breathing, early ambulation, and explanation of any procedures. The possibility of rejection and dysfunction of the organ following transplantation must be discussed so that the donor has a chance to consider the possibility of failure to help the loved one. The opportunity for withdrawal from donation must be provided if the donor has any doubts.[41]

The cadaver donor must succumb to brain death secondary to trauma, such as motorcycle or car accidents, gunshot wounds, falls, or blunt trauma to the head, cerebral embolism, or nonmalignant tumors which are inoperable. The attending physician in consultation with a neurosurgeon or neurologist confirms the diagnosis of brain death, which may be done by clinical examination, use of an EEG, CT scan, or cerebral blood flow studies. Most states have laws governing the declaration of brain death and institutions also have specific criteria regarding the declaration of brain death.[42,43] Once brain death has been declared, the transplant team becomes involved.

The evaluation of the donor includes a chest x-ray, electrocardiogram, blood chemistries, arterial

Table 59-4 Common Criteria Used in Selection of a Suitable Organ Donor

Brain death
No trauma to donating organ
Afebrile
No malignancy
No infectious process
Negative lymphocytotoxicity cross-match with recipient
ABO compatibility with recipient
No communicable disease
Negative hepatitis screen
Negative HIV antibody test (ELISA)
Normal donating organ function
No period of donating organ dysfunction

blood gases, blood type, HLA tissue typing, physical examination, and health history. Special studies needed to assess the possibility of infection, communicable disease, and organ system dysfunction are requested if necessary.

Heart   The donor age requirement is less than 35 years for males and 40 to 45 years for females. The donor over the age of 30 may require coronary angiography to assess for the presence of asymptomatic coronary disease. Electrolytes, cardiac enzymes, and an echocardiogram are also required. A history of cardiac arrest for more than 5 min, intracardiac injections, or a systolic blood pressure of less than 60 mmHg for over 10 min cause the cardiac donor to be unacceptable. The ECG and echocardiogram are useful in assessing arrhythmias, myocardial damage, and the function of the heart valves.[26,44]

Lung   The lung donor must be between the ages of 8 and 50 years with no history of pulmonary disease. The organ donor is ventilator-dependent, which makes infection a major concern. Tracheal secretions are cultured and the chest x-ray scrutinized for signs of infection. Most institutions limit the number of days on mechanical ventilation for lung donation because the likelihood of pulmonary complications increases with prolonged ventilation. The P_{O_2} must be greater than 80 to 100 on an FiO_2 of 40 percent and the peak inspiratory pressure must be no greater than 30 cmH$_2$O for the donor's pulmonary function to be considered acceptable.[28,45,46]

The lung donor requires thorough assessment of pulmonary function by frequent arterial blood gas analyses, daily chest x-rays, controlled ventilatory settings, and observation for pulmonary complications. The donor must be transported to the transplant institution for procurement, because the lungs do not tolerate ischemia for long periods. Most institutions require that the lungs be ischemic less than 1 h prior to transplantation.[28,45,46] Many institutions are participating in research regarding ways to preserve the lungs so that the whole body of the donor will not have to be transported.

Heart and Lung   The heart and lung donor must meet the criteria for both heart donation and lung donation. As described in lung donation, there is great concern for the potential of pulmonary infection, so a thorough assessment of pulmonary function, chest x-rays, and tracheal secretion cultures are required. Cardiac function is also carefully assessed by physical examination, ECG, echocardiogram, and serum enzyme measurement. The acceptability of each organ is considered separately as well as together so that if one organ is unacceptable for heart and lung transplantation, consideration is given to the acceptability of the remaining organ for donation. It is important to realize that the heart and lung recipient receives both organs from the same donor.[26,29]

In most cases the heart and lung donor is transported to the transplant hospital for procurement because of the short ischemic time tolerated by the lungs. Presently, long-distance procurement of the heart and lungs is being attempted using specialized equipment or cardiopulmonary bypass to preserve the donor organs. As improvements in preservation solution and equipment are made, more institutions will use long-distance procurement for heart and lung donation. Heart and lung transplant compatibility requirements include the common criteria listed in Table 59-5, and chest cavity size matching. The chest x-ray must be of very good quality because the recipient and donor x-rays are placed one on top of the other for appropriate size matching.[29,30]

Kidney The related living kidney donor was described in an earlier section. Family members willing to donate a kidney undergo intravenous pyelogram, renal function studies, HLA tissue typing, and blood group analysis to determine the best possible match. The cadaver donor requirements are very similar in that the donor must have no diabetes mellitus, significant hypertension, or infection. The age range of acceptable donors is from 5 to 60 years.[32,47]

Blood chemistries, urinary output and fluid intake charts, urinalysis, and medical history are useful in determining donor renal function. A systolic blood pressure greater than 60 to 100 mmHg, a P_{O_2} greater than 100, and a urinary output greater than 100 mL per hour are used to assess renal perfusion. The donor will have a Foley catheter, so it is important to examine the urine for

Table 59-5 Hemodynamic Parameters and Laboratory Values of the Potential Case Study Donor

Data	Values
SBP (mmHg)	100–110
DBP (mmHg)	40–68
HR (bpm)	108–112
Temperature (°F)	98.8
CVP (mmHg)	8–14
Urinary output (mL/h)	120
Sodium	136
Potassium	4.0
Chloride	98
Bicarbonate	28
Hematocrit	28
Hemoglobin	6.4
Creatinine	1.0
BUN	35
SGOT	285
SGGT	200
LDH	110
CPK	90
CPK-MB	3

SBP = systolic blood pressure
DBP = diastolic blood pressure
HR = heart rate
CVP = central venous pressure

sediment and cloudiness. Urine and blood cultures are requested to assess for infection. Medications and treatments utilized in donor care must be assessed regarding the effects on renal function.[32,47]

Liver The liver donor must be less than 60 years of age and have normal liver function. Selection criteria for liver donation are very similar to those for renal donation. Assessment of the adequacy of liver function is accomplished by blood chemistries, enzymes, clotting factors, and bilirubin levels. A physical examination for abdominal trauma and organ position is performed early in the assessment phase of donation. Cultures of urine, blood, and sputum are utilized to rule out infection. Some institutions may request angiography or intravenous cholangiograms to identify hepatic blood supply and to assess traumatic injury.[35,48]

Pancreas The pancreas donor must be less than 55 years of age and have no diabetes mellitus. Selection criteria are very similar to those of the renal donor. A thorough medical history is obtained and a physical examination is performed to rule out abdominal trauma. Monitoring of serial blood glucose, alkaline phosphatase, serum enzymes, and calcium levels are requested to assess pancreatic disease or trauma.[39,49,50]

Case Study

The organ bank received a call concerning a possible donor for Mr. Jones about 7 days after the search began. The donor was in another state, but was within acceptable flight time requirements. Because it seemed probable that the donor was acceptable, a team was sent to the donor hospital to evaluate the donor.

The donor was found to be acceptable. He was an 18-year-old male who had received a head injury in a motor vehicle accident 3 days earlier. The donor had no previous history of heart disease, the ECG showed sinus tachycardia with slight ST elevations, and there had been no cardiac arrest since the accident. The chest x-ray was clear and the donor was afebrile. Cardiac enzymes were acceptable. The vital signs and blood chemistries are listed in Table 59-5. The donor required dopamine at 10 μg/kg per minute to maintain a systolic blood pressure of 110 mmHg.

The dopamine infusion was gradually tapered to 2 μg/kg per minute and a potassium supplement was given intravenously to increase the potassium level to 4.0. The renal function of the donor was also evaluated because of the possibility of kidney donation. Fluid was replaced to maintain a CVP of 12 mmHg, a urine output of at least 100 mL per hour, and SBP of 100 mmHg. The hematocrit was found to be 28 percent and 1 unit of packed red blood cells was infused.

Plans were made to proceed with the transplant, so the transplant team traveled to the donor hospital. The surgeons reviewed the information available and medically accepted the donor. Operating times were planned with the recipient hospital and the donor was taken to the operating room. Once the chest was opened, the surgeon examined the heart and sent a message to the recipient hospital that the donor was physically acceptable and that the surgical team at the recipient hospital could proceed with surgical preparation of the recipient for transplantation.

Procedural Aspects of Organ Transplantation

Upon identification of an acceptable donor, the transplant team begins preparations for retrieval of the donor organ or organs. The transplant team is usually made up of the transplant surgeon, an organ bank member, and possibly an assisting surgeon or scrub nurse. A scrub nurse, a circulating nurse, and an anesthesiologist from the donor hospital are also needed to assist with organ procurement. The operating room staff receives instructions regarding their duties and the expected sequence of events once the transplant team arrives at the donor hospital. If the donor hospital does not have the specific surgical instruments needed for the organ procurement, the transplant team brings the necessary instruments. Equipment for monitoring of hemodynamic parameters is needed. The operating room setup is the same as it is for open-heart or abdominal surgical procedures.

Transportation

The transplant team members responsible for organ procurement travel to the hospital where the donor is located, except for cases of lung or heart and lung donors, who are usually transported to the transplant institution. The organ bank staff members representing each transplant team are responsible for arrangement of transportation from the transplant institution to the donor hospital and the return trip. The mode of transportation may vary according to availability and the time factor. Usually a security or police car, ambulance, or helicopter is used from airports to hospitals, and an airplane of varying speed is used from airport to airport. The quickest route possible from hospital to hospital is plotted to save valuable time. The time factor must be considered when deciding if the donor is within a safe time range, requiring the organ's ischemic time to be calculated for each procurement. Each second is plotted into the time frame in an attempt to accurately plan and coordinate donor organ retrieval with the recipient surgical procedure.

Coordination between Surgical Teams

The organ bank staff members usually set up a "command post" to receive information from the donor institution; they are responsible for relaying information between the surgical teams. Calls are received when the transplant team has reached the donor hospital; when medical and surgical or physical acceptance is received, and with an estimation of departure time; and any changes are also relayed to the command post. The hospital personnel or organ bank member in the donor area calls the transplant institution when the transplant team with the donor organ is leaving the donor institution. The time of arrival of the team is plotted to the exact minute. Many times the team calls in from the airplane when they are about 20 to 30 min away from the transplant institution to alert the hospital to the team's imminent arrival. The recipient's surgery at the transplant institution is planned according to the information received. Any changes in arrival time of the retrieval team necessitate adjustment in the schedule at the transplant institution. This accuracy is one of the most important aspects of procurement of donor organs because of the limited ischemic time tolerated by some organs.

Donor Procurement

As public awareness of the need for organ donation increases, and the number of institutions performing transplants grows, the number of organ donors must be augmented. In order to satisfy the need for more organs, multiple organ donation must be stressed. Many individuals who are willing to donate organs can be encouraged to donate more than one organ by requesting permission for each organ at the time permission is granted.

Multiple donor procurement involves the removal of more than one organ system, usually the kidneys and one or more other organ system. Many times the kidneys are donated without the donation of other organs. Multiple organ procurement will be described; however, it should be noted that single organ procurement is carried out in the same manner as that described for each organ system.

Procurement of multiple organs from one donor is not difficult if the schedule is well planned. The need for perioperative monitoring and treatment of fluid and electrolyte imbalances, blood loss replacement, temperature control, and hemodynamic monitoring requires the assistance of an anesthesiologist. Such close monitoring permits the dissection of the donor organs to be accomplished in a more stable donor. If the donor becomes unstable, the decision regarding which organs are to be salvaged is made by the controlling transplant team. The controlling transplant team is the transplant team from the donating region.

The donor is anesthetized and the surgical incision is made from the sternal notch to the pubis for exposure of the organs. The cardiac surgeon examines the heart and moves away from the table. The surgeons procuring the liver, pancreas, and kidneys begin with the meticulous dissection necessary for organ removal. Usually the arterial blood supply is identified first, and careful dissection is made to preserve this supply. The liver and pancreas are prepared for removal first, followed by the kidneys and the heart or heart and lungs. If the organs are to be removed en bloc, with connections to the aorta and vena cava, these areas are located and dissection points are plotted. Once the tissue around the organs has been dissected, heparin is given to prevent clotting. The cannulas for cold perfusion of the organ are placed in appropriate areas at this time.

Once the extracardiac organs are ready for removal, the cardiac surgeon opens the pericardium, prepares the venae cavae and separates the aorta from the pulmonary artery. The kidneys, liver, and pancreas are then perfused with cold Collins or Ringer's solution. The heart is then perfused with cold hyperkalemic cardioplegia solution. Once the cooling of the heart has begun, the venae cavae and the aorta are clamped. When the aorta is cross-clamped the removal of all organs is begun. Removal of the heart usually takes less than 5 min. The removal of the liver, kidneys, or pancreas usually takes another 5 min. Separation and cleaning of the organs is accomplished at sterile tables and the organs are packed for transport. Teamwork by the surgeons involved is necessary and each surgeon must understand the surgical procurement of the other organs. The length of surgery is a little longer with multiple organ donation, but it is a reasonable use of time which can benefit several patients waiting for organs.[51,52]

Operative Procedures

The recipient of an organ transplant is prepared for surgery similarly to abdominal or thoracic surgery. Preparation begins after notification that the donor is acceptable. A chest x-ray, electrocardiogram, and blood work, consisting of electrolytes, glucose level, BUN, creatinine, enzymes, prothrombin time, blood type and cross-match, hemoglobin, hematocrit, complete blood cell count, and platelet count are performed to ensure that no complicating factor such as infection exists. A special permit is signed for the surgical procedure and a skin prep is done. Some centers use depilatory creams to decrease skin abrasion rather than a razor for removal of body hair. The anesthesiologist visits the patient and orders a preoperative medication. The recipient most often receives the first dose of immunosuppressive medication 2 to 4 h prior to surgery.

Heart When surgical acceptance is received, the patient is taken to the operating room, placed on the operating table, and anesthetized. Endotracheal intubation and mechanical ventilation are begun. The arterial line is inserted and several large-bore intravenous lines are inserted. The Foley catheter or suprapubic catheter is inserted into the urinary bladder and the patient is surgically scrubbed and draped. The surgical incision is made after notification that the transplant team has left the donor hospital with the donor organ. The patient is prepared to go on cardiopulmonary bypass and any repair or takedown of past procedures is performed. The transplant surgeon is informed when the retrieval team is 20 min away. The surgeon then determines the time at which cardiopulmonary bypass is initiated, which is usually about 5 or 10 min before the heart is expected in the operating room. The patient is placed on cardiopulmonary bypass by the same method used for any open-heart procedure with the exception of cannulation of the superior and inferior venae cavae through the right atrium. Once the patient is on cardiopulmonary bypass, the surgeon waits until the donor heart is in the operating room to begin removal of the recipient's heart.

The donor heart is removed from the packing and prepared for insertion into the chest. The right atrium is opened posterolaterally from the inferior vena cava to the base of the appendage. The superior vena cava was tied off at the time of procurement. The left atrium is prepared by opening the area between the pulmonary veins into one large orifice and excess tissue is trimmed away. The aorta and

pulmonary artery are trimmed of excess tissue also. The heart is then placed into the chest and sutured in place. The left atrium is anastomosed first with a continuous suture followed by the intraatrial septum and the right atrium. The pulmonary artery and the aorta are then anastomosed. The heart is then rewarmed and defibrillated. When cardiac rhythm and hemodynamics are stable, cardiopulmonary bypass is discontinued.[23,26,53] The patient's chest is closed in the usual manner for open-heart surgery.

For the heterotopic heart transplant, the donor heart is prepared very similarly. There is a greater length of the superior vena cava retained and the right pulmonary veins and inferior vena cava are sutured closed. The tissue between the left pulmonary veins is removed to make an opening in the left atrium. The incision into the right atrium is made in the posterior aspect of the superior vena cava and the right atrium. The recipient operation begins the same way as for an orthotopic heart transplant and following initiation of cardiopulmonary bypass, the heart is placed into the prepared right side of the chest. After an incision is made into the left atrium, the donor left atrium is anastomosed to the recipient left atrium. An incision is made into the lateral aspect of the recipient right atrium and the superior vena cava. The donor superior vena cava and right atrium are aligned with the recipient incision and they are anastomosed. The aorta is then anastomosed to the recipient's aorta. The pulmonary artery requires a preclotted Dacron graft to which both donor and recipient pulmonary arteries are anastomosed. Rewarming then occurs and the resumption of cardiac function of both hearts is permitted. The blood flows to the two common atriums and to both donor and recipient heart ventricles. Blood flows from both hearts to the aorta and the pulmonary artery. The blood flow to each heart is dependent upon the ventricular compliance of each heart. The heart rhythm or function is asynchronous and each heart ventricle is performing separately.[23,53]

Lung The candidate for a lung transplant is transferred to the operating room, intubated if not already on mechanical ventilation, and anesthetized. The patient is prepared for bypass using a membrane oxygenator. To do this, cannulas are placed in the femoral vein and femoral artery, inferior vena cava, superior vena cava, and aortic arch. Venoarterial or venovenous bypass may then be used to help stabilize the recipient and correct acid-base imbalances.

The surgery will be described as if the donor was transported to the transplant institution. The surgery is performed in two rooms which are side by side. The surgical procedures on the donor and recipient begin simultaneously. The recipient is placed in the usual position for thoracotomy incision and pneumonectomy is performed. The donor also has a thoracotomy incision. The lung is flushed with cold Collins solution or iced saline prior to removal from the donor. It is then brought into the recipient's room. The implantation involves anastomosis of the main pulmonary artery, main bronchus, and left atrial cuff. The surgery is completed as in any thoracic surgery. Chest tubes are connected to underwater seal and suction. Some patients require the support of the membrane oxygenator for a time after surgery. The amount of time the membrane oxygenator is used varies according to the patient's condition and must be slowly weaned from the patient. The cannulas are removed when the blood gases have stabilized.[54,55] Pressure must be held on the site of arterial cannulation until bleeding has stopped. Following manual pressure, a 10-lb sandbag is placed over the site for 24 h.

Heart and Lung   For heart and lung transplantation the donor is usually brought to the recipient hospital and stabilized. The removal of other organs is possible and included in the total time of surgery. The recipient is prepared as usual for open-heart surgery. The surgery is performed via a median sternotomy and cardiopulmonary bypass is begun. The recipient operation involves removal of the heart and lungs as a complete unit or bloc, taking special care not to damage the vagal nerve trunks, recurrent laryngeal nerves, and the phrenic nerves. The surgical anatomy of the bronchial vessels is examined and collateral vessels are ligated. The cuff of the right atrium is retained for connection of the atrium as in cardiac transplantation. The donor operation, which is usually performed in an adjacent operating room, is similar to the recipient operation in that the heart and lungs are removed together as a bloc. The heart is cooled as in cardiac

transplantation and the lungs are perfused with cold modified Collins solution just prior to excision. The superior vena cava is ligated; the aorta is clamped and cut; and the trachea is excised just above the carina. The surgery is planned so that the recipient is ready for implantation at the same time the donor lungs and heart are brought into the recipient operating room.[56–60]

The donor right lung and atrium are passed behind the right atrium and phrenic nerve while the left lung is passed behind the left phrenic nerve. The trachea is anastomosed first, followed by the atrium and the aorta. The heart is rewarmed and resuscitated. The lungs are ventilated to observe for air leaks and bleeding from the trachea. When the patient is stable, cardiopulmonary bypass is removed and the chest is closed in the usual manner for open-heart surgery. There will be hemodynamic monitoring lines as seen in the open-heart surgical patient with mediastinal as well as pleural chest tubes in place.[56–60]

Kidney   The kidney donor may be a cadaver donor or a related living donor. The surgical procedure for removal of the donor kidney is similar for both. The related living donor surgery is planned so the transplantation and the organ retrieval are performed in adjacent operating rooms. The cadaver donor operation takes place prior to the recipient surgery. The cadaver kidney can remain viable for up to 24 h with use of hypothermic storage, and nearly 72 h by using pulsatile hypothermic perfusion.[61,62]

The recipient will be contacted when blood type and HLA tissue typing compatibility of the donor to recipient has been assured, and surgery is then planned. The recipient is dialyzed within the 24 h preceding surgery. Dialysis may be accomplished by hemodialysis or, as in chronic peritoneal dialysis patients, a surgically placed peritoneal catheter may be used. Dialysis is needed to partially reverse the uremic state of the patient with renal disease and to assist in hemodynamically stabilizing the recipient.

The recipient is taken to surgery and prepared as for abdominal surgery. The extremity with the fistula is identified so that it will not be used for drawing blood or for monitoring blood pressure. For the chronic peritoneal dialysis patient, the physician decides if the peritoneal dialysis catheter will remain after surgery or if it is to be removed and the wound closed.

The operative incision is made over the iliac fossa. The iliac and hypogastric arterial vessels are identified prior to placing the donor kidney extraperitoneally. The renal artery is anastomosed end to end to the external or internal iliac arteries. Branches of the iliac vein are identified and the donor renal vein is anastomosed to the external iliac vein. If these vessels are not suitable, other vessels may be used for the blood supply. During anastomosis the kidney is wrapped in iced saline packs to prevent rewarming.[32,63,64]

The attachment of the ureter is accomplished by making a submucosal tunnel so the ureter is passed through the muscle wall, under this mucosal flap, and anastomosed to the recipient's bladder. The ureter may also be anastomosed to the dome of the bladder and a flap of muscle constructed over the ureter. Both of these methods are used to help prevent reflux. If the ureter is not suitable for transplantation, the recipient's ureter will be used. The final step is removal of the recipient kidney. This is usually done only when hypertension has been a patient management problem.[32,63,64]

Following completion of the procedure, the venous clamp is removed first to prevent vasospasm. The arterial clamp is then removed and blood flow is allowed to resume. The kidney should regain normal color and become firm. If vasospasm or hyperacute rejection occur, the kidney may remain soft and mottled or purplish in color. The anastomoses sites are checked for bleeding and kinks and the wound is closed. Some surgeons place a closed drainage system in the wound.[32,63,64]

Liver   Once an acceptable liver donor has been located, plans for transplantation are begun. The hepatic donor is a cadaver donor and surgical removal of the organ may be by long-distance retrieval.

The recipient surgery is planned according to the time needed to assess and retrieve the donor organ. Once notification of donor acceptance has been received, the recipient surgery begins. The recipient is prepared as for abdominal surgery. In the patient undergoing hepatic transplantation, it is important to have multiple large-bore intravenous lines for administration of fluid and blood products. The amount of blood made available

for liver transplantation is usually about 10 to 20 units.

A bilateral subcostal incision with extension to the xiphoid is utilized. Skeletonization of the liver, common bile duct, and vascular access is performed in preparation for liver removal. The venae cavae above and below the liver are exposed. Blood products are administered during surgery to control bleeding and to improve clotting factors. The liver is prepared for removal by testing vena caval occlusion. If the fall in cardiac output cannot be tolerated when the venae cavae are clamped, the patient is prepared for partial cardiopulmonary bypass. This is done by cannulation of the right femoral vein for venous draining of blood with return flow by the right common femoral artery. The hepatic artery, portal vein, and the venae cavae are then clamped. Inspection for bleeding and an estimation of venous hypertension are made and the liver is then removed.[65–68]

The donor liver is placed in the cavity and anastomosis begins with attachment of the suprahepatic inferior vena cava of the donor and the recipient. The infrahepatic vena cava of the recipient is anastomosed to that of the donor. The liver is then flushed with cold modified Collins solution and the portal vein of the donor and the recipient is anastomosed. The partial cardiopulmonary bypass, if used, is then discontinued. Observation for bleeding is continued while blood flow is returned to the liver. When hemostasis is assured, bile duct reconstruction is begun. This is usually accomplished by end-to-end anastomosis of the recipient and donor common bile ducts. A T tube is used to splint the lower limb. The T tube is brought outside the body through the surgical incision and remains in place for approximately 3 months after surgery. At this time in surgery a cholangiogram may be requested. Three or four Jackson-Pratt drains are placed in the subhepatic and subdiaphragmatic regions and brought outside the wound. These drains remain in place for 3 or 4 days following surgery. The recipient is then taken to the recovery room or to the intensive care unit for observation.[65–68]

Pancreas and Islet Cells   The pancreatic donor is usually a cadaver donor, but in some cases a related living donor is used. Transplantation is planned as soon as possible following donor procurement, even though the pancreas can be preserved for up to 24 h by simple cold ischemic storage.[49]

The surgical preparation of the pancreatic transplant recipient is like that of any major abdominal surgical patient. The incision is usually made in the right iliac fossa and the pancreas placed intra- or extraperitoneally. A whole organ graft or a segment of the body and tail may be used for transplantation. The donor splenic artery is anastomosed to the iliac artery of the recipient, then the splenic or portal vein of the donor is anastomosed to the recipient's iliac vein. The clamps are then removed and blood flow is allowed to resume.[39,49,50,69]

The surgical technique varies in relation to the method utilized for handling the exocrine secretions of the pancreas. If a whole organ transplant has been done, a portion of the donor duodenum can be anastomosed to a jejunal Roux-en-Y loop in the recipient. The exocrine pancreatic juices are then secreted into the intestine. With segmental pancreatic transplantation procedures, several methods are used for drainage of secretions.[39,49,50,69]

The divided duct can be ligated and the organ surface oversewn. Another method requires the pancreatic duct to be anastomosed to the recipient's ureter. This method requires the removal of one of the recipient's kidneys and is usually done only in uremic patients. The cut surface of the pancreas is anastomosed to the intestinal mucosa or to a jejunal Roux-en-Y loop. The exocrine secretions are then drained into the intestines. The major concern with this procedure is infection because the bowel is opened. The exocrine duct system may also be injected with a polymer which hardens and occludes the duct. If the pancreas is transplanted intraperitoneally, it can be allowed to drain freely into the peritoneal cavity because the body can absorb small amounts of the secretions. If all the secretions cannot be absorbed, however, ascites may occur. A Jackson-Pratt drain is placed in the wound and the incision is closed.[50,69–73]

Preparation of islet of Langerhans cells for transplantation involves flushing with hypothermic solution and careful removal of the pancreas. The pancreas is transported to the laboratory, distended with fluid, and minced. The preparation of tissue and solution is centrifuged in a salt solution, and collagenase digestion is performed. The prepara-

tion is then washed by centrifugation. Once the pancreatic islet cells are prepared, the recipient is taken to the operating room and the injection made into the portal vein or spleen.[73–76]

Case Study

When the call assuring medical acceptance was received, Mr. Jones was given the initial dose of cyclosporin in chocolate milk and a dose of Imuran. He had been NPO for several hours and enjoyed the small amount of liquid with the medicine. He and his family were both anxious and joyful at the news that surgery would take place in about an hour and 30 min. The nurse performed a total body prep for surgery and a surgical permit was signed. Mr. Jones' blood work and chest x-ray were reviewed.

At the donor hospital, the donor was anesthetized and draped for surgery. The organ bank personnel had prepared the needed materials for preservation and transportation of each organ on separate tables. The surgical incision was made from the sternal notch to the pubis. The heart surgeon moved into place and examined the heart. At that time the decision of surgical, or physical, acceptance was made. Organ bank personnel called the recipient hospital with the decision and time estimations. The renal surgeon began dissection around the kidneys and their blood supply. Cannulas needed for cold perfusion of the kidneys were placed in the appropriate areas. The heart surgeon made the needed preparations for removal of the heart. The pericardium was opened and umbilical tape was placed around each of the major vessels. The venae cavae were clamped first, followed by the aorta, and the heart was perfused with cold cardioplegic solution. At the moment of aortic cross-clamping, the kidneys were flushed and cooled to a low temperature. The heart was removed first and prepared for transfer to the recipient hospital. The kidneys were removed and also prepared for transport. The transplant team ran to the awaiting helicopter for the trip to the airport. Calls were then made to the transplant centers to alert them that the heart and kidneys were on the way to them.

When the call to give surgical acceptance was received and an estimation of return time had been made, Mr. Jones was taken to the operating room.

An intravenous infusion line was placed in his forearm and he was then taken into the surgical suite, anesthetized, and orally intubated. An arterial line was placed in the left radial artery and several intravenous lines were inserted. A Foley urinary catheter was inserted under sterile technique. Mr. Jones was then draped and the surgical procedure commenced.

The chest was opened as for open-heart surgery. Since Mr. Jones had had no previous thoracic or cardiovascular surgery, there were no adhesions and very little bleeding occurred. When the call was received that the donor heart was 20 min away, preparations were made for cardiopulmonary bypass.

When the airplane landed at the airport, a helicopter was waiting to take the transplant team with the donor heart to the recipient hospital. Word was received in the operating room that the helicopter had landed and cardiopulmonary bypass was begun. The donor heart arrived in the operating room and was removed from cold storage. The heart was placed on a table and the surgeon who retrieved the heart removed it from the protective sterile bags filled with iced saline. Cultures of the solution were taken and the heart was trimmed and prepared for placement in the chest. Mean-while, the surgeon performing the recipient operation removed Mr. Jones' heart. The heart was very large, dark reddish brown, and was noted to occasionally spasm. Comparing the diseased recipient heart with the healthy donor heart is a fascinating portion of the surgery.

The healthy-looking donor heart was then placed in Mr. Jones' chest, sutured into place, and rewarmed. The heart was defibrillated and it began to beat at a rate of 66 beats per minute in a sinus rhythm. Epicardial pacing wires were placed on the right atrium and right ventricle of the heart and atrial pacing at a rate of 85 beats per minute was begun. Hemodynamic monitoring lines were placed appropriately. Mr. Jones came off cardiopulmonary bypass with the support of dopamine at 2 mg/kg/min. Mr. Jones' hemodynamic pressures are listed in Table 59-6. Mediastinal chest tubes were placed anterior and posterior to the heart, and the chest was closed as with open-heart surgery. Mr. Jones was then transported to the intensive care unit.

Immunosuppression

The goal of immunosuppression is to suppress the response of the body to the transplanted organ and

Table 59-6 Mr. Jones' Hemodynamic Parameters Immediately Following Cardiac Transplantation

Name: Jones Room: 504Q	Age: 62 Sex: Male	Weight: 68 kg Height: 177 cm
Data	Values	
HR (beats/min)	85	
Rhythm	Normal sinus	
SBP (mmHg)	110	
DBP (mmHg)	65	
RAP (mmHg)	9	
LAP (mmHg)	8	
CO (L/min)	6.08	
CI (L/min/m²)	2.08	
Chest drainage (mL/30 min)	125	
Urinary output (mL/30 min)	100	
Pedal pulses	+3/+3	
Skin temperature and color	Cold and pale	

HR = heart rate
SBR = systolic blood pressure
DBP = diastolic blood pressure
RAP = right atrial pressure
LAP = left atrial pressure
CO = cardiac output
CI = cardiac index

yet allow the body to ward off infections. This goal may be met by using immunosuppressive methods which are specific or nonspecific in action. Most of the methods of immunosuppression presently in use are nonspecific in action. "Nonspecific" means that the action suppresses the immune response as a whole, like an umbrella effect. After a time, the body begins to accept the transplanted organ by adapting to its presence with the use of the immunosuppressive drugs. This allows the immunosuppressive drugs to be slowly decreased in amount but they are never entirely withdrawn.[77,78]

The drugs currently used for immunosuppression are prednisone, cyclosporine, and Imuran. In addition, many institutions use antithymocyte globulin for the treatment of rejection and as supplemental immunosuppressive therapy. The dosage and combination of drugs vary according to physician preference.

Prednisone and methylprednisolone are usually used in combination with Imuran and cyclosporine. The steroids act by inhibiting intracellular enzymes which depress protein, DNA, and RNA synthesis, decrease cell-mediated immune response, which decreases antibody production, and have antiinflammatory properties. The antiinflammatory properties of steroids are thought to be a major cause for its immunosuppressive effects. The suppression of the inflammatory response is brought about by stabilization of the lysosome membrane and inhibition of leukocyte infiltration into the cells.[77–79]

Methylprednisolone is usually given during surgery and for several doses postoperatively. The recipient is then placed on prednisone in a dosage range of 0.5 mg/kg to 2.0 mg/kg. The dosage is usually decreased at a scheduled rate until a maintainence dosage is reached. With the use of cyclosporine, the dosage of prednisone is lower than the dosage used in combination solely with Imuran. The side effects seen with the use of steroids are: increase in the occurrence of infections; predisposition to steroid-induced diabetes; increased sodium absorption leading to fluid retention; poor absorption of calcium from the gastrointestinal tract, making the bones brittle and soft; gastrointestinal distress; cataracts; acne; cushingoid effects; slow wound healing; mood swings; and, in most recipients, an increase in appetite.[77–80]

Azathioprine (Imuran) is an antimetabolite which competes for receptors involved in RNA, DNA, and protein synthesis. It also depresses antibody production and cell-mediated immunity.[77–80] Imuran is given in combination with prednisone and cyclosporine. Imuran is given orally in a dosage range of 2.0 mg/kg to 3.5 mg/kg. An initial dose is given preoperatively and is continued postoperatively. The dosage of Imuran is regulated by the white blood cell count (WBC) so that if the WBC falls below 4000/mm³ the dosage is decreased. If the WBC falls below 3000/mm³ the recipient is hospitalized and the drug is withheld until the WBC has risen to above 4000/mm³. The recipient with a WBC below 2000/mm³ is usually placed in reverse isolation. The side effects associated with Imuran are hepatotoxicity and bone marrow depression leading to leukopenia and thrombocytopenia.[77–80] In some recipients, hair loss has been reported.

Cyclosporine is the newest immunosuppressive agent used in transplantation. It is used in combination with Imuran and prednisone. Cyclosporine acts by inhibition of T cell proliferation, mainly the T helper cell.[81–83] The initial dose should be given as soon as it is known that a suitable donor has been located. This dosage range will be between 10 mg/kg to 16 mg/kg. The postoperative dose of cyclosporine will be given in divided dosages between 4 mg/kg per dose to 8 mg/kg per dose. The dosage of cyclosporine is determined by cyclosporine blood levels, renal function studies, and urinary output.

Cyclosporine is usually given orally unless the recipient cannot retain the drug. In the intravenous preparation, cyclosporine is three times as potent as in the oral preparation. It should be noted that at this time there is no intramuscular injectable source of cyclosporine. The oral preparation is mixed with chocolate milk or orange juice for administration. It is oil-based and should be mixed with a juice or milk-type substance. It comes with a special syringe for drawing up the dosage. The recipient must be taught how to draw up the dosage properly prior to discharge from the hospital. The side effects associated with cyclosporine include headaches, gastrointestinal distress, hypertension, tremors, increased sodium retention leading to weight gain and edema, increased hair growth, gum hyperplasia, hepatotoxicity, and nephrotoxicity. The side effects of cyclosporine tend to be dose-dependent and decrease with regulation of the dosage.[80-84]

Antithymocyte globulin and antilymphocyte globulin are made by injecting animals with lymphoid cells from another species. The serum is usually produced from cows, horses, sheep, goats, and rabbits. The serum contains antilymphocyte antibodies and produces an inhibition of graft rejection.[78,85] It is used in combination with the usual immunosuppressive regimen immediately postoperatively for 5 to 7 days or may be given only when rejection episodes occur. When used for rejection treatment the antithymocyte globulin is given for 6 to 7 days and may be administered by intramuscular injection or intravenously, depending on the concentration and animal source. It is very caustic to blood vessels and must be given in a large blood flow area. The dosage range of antithymocyte globulin depends on the animal source, with a range from 0.5 IgG/mg/kg to 15 IgG/mg/kg. The toxicity effects of antithymocyte globulin are fever, chills, joint pain, decrease in blood pressure, respiratory distress, flank pain, blood in the urine, pain at the site of administration, and anaphylaxis.[85] If given intramuscularly, antithymocyte globulin is very painful and hot packs or massage of the area may help the pain. The patient should be monitored frequently for toxicity while antithymocyte globulin is being administered.

The recipient is usually premedicated with Benadryl and Tylenol, or methylprednisolone and aspirin prior to administration of the drug. Many institutions make their own antithymocyte globulin while others receive the drug from a pharmaceutical company. The recipient may have a reaction to the globulin at any time and with any dose, so the monitoring must be continued throughout the treatment period. Circulating T lymphocyte counts are done daily while the recipient is receiving the globulin.

Some institutions may use total or specific site irradiation as a means of temporarily depressing the immune response.[86,87] Donor-specific blood transfusions may also be used to help decrease the antibody response.[88] In some cases drainage of the thoracic duct, thymectomy, and splenectomy have been utilized to help decrease the amount of lymphoid cells in the body.[77,78] Much research is being done in the area of immunosuppression in an attempt to find more specific types of immunosuppressive agents which will have a major impact on the future of organ transplantation.

Medical and Nursing Therapies Following Transplantation

The transplant recipient is a very challenging patient for the nurse. The early postoperative transplant recipient is cared for in much the same manner as any patient having major abdominal, thoracic, or cardiac surgery. Assessment of organ function and prevention of complications are the major areas of focus at this time. Once the recipient leaves the intensive care unit (ICU), the areas of focus broaden to include education and rehabilitation. Possible nursing diagnoses for the patient receiving an organ transplant are listed in Table 59-7. Transplant recipients should be assessed as to their individual needs and nursing therapies prescribed accordingly. Examples of nursing care plans for specific organ transplant recipients can be found in the

Table 59-7 Possible Nursing Diagnoses for the Organ Transplant Recipient

Potential for rejection of the transplanted organ as an immune system response

Potential for infection related to immunosuppression

Potential for fluid and electrolyte imbalance

Potential for alterations in organ function related to preservation, ischemia, reperfusion

Lack of knowledge

Alteration in nutrition

Potential for development of medication side effects

Potential for ineffective coping related to fear; anxiety; attempt to return to "normal"; feeling overwhelmed

Potential for noncompliance with medication; diet; follow-up care

Potential disturbance in self-concept

Potential psychological disturbance due to steroid therapy; environment; isolation; fears; inadequate coping with illness and treatment

Potential sexual dysfunction

Potential alteration in rehabilitation related to complications; residual weakness; lack of muscle strength; fatigue

Spiritual needs

Potential for disturbance of sleep pattern

Potential for disturbance to bowel and bladder elimination patterns literature.[89-93] An example of a nursing care plan featuring one nursing diagnosis is given below. Care of the recipient of a transplant will be divided into categories and both similarities and differences will be discussed.

Nursing Diagnosis

Potential psychological disturbance related to inadequate coping with illness and treatment.

Goal

Following nursing intervention during the postoperative hospital course, patients will have improved coping with illness and treatment as evidenced by an ability to:

I. Discuss the illness and the decision to have a transplant.

II. Relate information about the transplant process to their experience.

III. Discuss their feelings (fears, guilt, anxiety, grief) about receiving an organ transplant.

IV. Describe areas in which improvement in health and activity has occurred.

V. Identify future goals and expectations.

Nursing Interventions

The nurse will:

I. Utilize time spent in patient care to listen to the patient and use open-ended questions to allow patients to:
   A. Describe their illness and how the illness evolved.
   B. Verbalize their feelings about being ill.
   C. Recall events which led to the decision to have a transplant.

II. Review teaching materials for transplant candidates with patients and assist them in:
   A. Describing the transplant surgical procedure.
   B. Comparing and contrasting their postoperative course with the information available.
   C. Recognizing the rationale for nursing and medical interventions.

III. Plan for extra time to sit with patients when they express the desire to talk, and:
   A. Propose that patients express their feelings by writing an anonymous letter to the donating family.

   B. Distinguish their role as an organ recipient from the role of the donor.
   C. Alert the transplant team to the patient's concerns.
   D. Encourage patients to verbalize their concerns with the transplant team members.

IV. Prepare a wall chart for listing activities and assist patients to:
   A. List the exercise level achieved each day.
   B. Record their temperature and weight on the chart each day.
   C. Use one word to describe how they feel each day and record on chart.
   D. Review the chart with the patient and discuss improvements in activity and general outlook.
   E. Be aware of complications and plan time within care routine for discussions on how the complication and treatment will affect the patient.
   F. Utilize time spent in care to assess the mood and general well-being of the patient.
   G. Allow the patient as much control over care and schedule as possible (i.e., bath time, menus, etc.).

V. Utilize time spent in patient care to:
   A. Discuss the patient's plans for going home and the future.
   B. Encourage the patient to make plans and set short-term goals.
   C. Encourage family involvement in making plans and setting goals.
   D. Begin educating the patient and family in care at home.
   E. Discuss potential limitations in activity, work, lifting, etc., if any are expected.

Isolation

The need for isolation as a precaution against infection is controversial and some organ system transplant recipients are isolated while others are not. Usually the recipients of a kidney, liver, or pancreas are not placed in isolation. Recipients of a heart, lung, or heart and lung transplant are usually placed in protective isolation.

Isolation may be of two types. A full, strict protective isolation may be used while the recipient is in the ICU or as long as intravenous lines are in place, or isolation may be limited to masks and hand-washing techniques. Regardless of the type of isolation, the room is prepared for the patient by a special thorough cleaning and changing of curtains and supplies. All equipment is cleaned with disinfectant prior to use in the room. This is protective isolation, so supplies usually kept "clean" are clean, and "sterile" remains sterile. The room is cleaned each day by use of a wet wipe-down. Isolation attire is worn at all times. This includes a gown, mask, booties, cap, and gloves, or a 10-min handwashing scrub.

Isolation has several purposes. It makes everyone aware that the patient is a transplant recipient and immunosuppressed, it decreases the number of "sightseers," and it decreases the contact of the patient with infectious organisms. Recipients should also wear isolation attire whenever leaving the nursing unit to identify them as immunosuppressed patients. These patients should not be transported through construction areas or left in waiting areas with other patients who may have contagious diseases.

Once invasive lines are discontinued or the recipient is transferred out of ICU, isolation is decreased to a mask and thorough hand-washing techniques or gloves. This level of isolation continues until the recipient is discharged from the hospital. At that time, the recipient is given a thermometer and a box of masks, and is taught how to take a temperature. The patient is instructed to notify the physician if a temperature over 101°F occurs, or if symptoms of a cough, cold, or sore throat develop. The masks are helpful when other family members have a cold or flu-like symptoms. They must also follow safe, commonsense practices, such as not eating or drinking from the dish or glass of someone who is ill, or going out in bad weather unprotected. It is emphasized that the patient must seek medical attention as soon as any symptoms of illness occur.

The drawback to isolation is that it may also impose social isolation on the patient. The door to the room must remain closed and visitors are limited. The recipient is allowed to be out of the room as much as desired wearing isolation attire, but may still feel isolated from others. The patient should be encouraged to participate in unit activities and to be out of the room as much as possible.

Invasive Lines and Devices

Following surgery, the transplant recipient will spend several hours to days in the ICU or recovery room. During this time the patient is monitored closely for signs of complications and adequacy of organ function. The invasiveness of the monitoring depends on the organ transplanted and the patient's condition. Heart rate and rhythm are monitored by electrodes placed on the chest and blood pressure is monitored by an arterial line placed in the radial artery, or by sphygmomanometry. The arterial line may also be used for obtaining blood gas samples and blood for laboratory work. The temperature and respiratory rate and depth are monitored noninvasively. A Foley catheter for obtaining accurate urinary output is a routine part of postoperative care for most transplant recipients.

Cardiac output, intracardiac pressures, pulmonary pressures, fluid load, or response to medications may be monitored by use of a Swan-Ganz catheter, intraatrial lines, or a central venous line. Temporary epicardial pacing wires are present in the heart and heart and lung recipient. Assessment of pedal pulses, skin temperature, and color are useful noninvasive measures of determining cardiac function. Invasive monitoring lines and devices are removed when the recipient is hemodynamically stable and organ system function is adequate.

The renal transplant recipient has a circulatory access which must be monitored for clotting. The nurse should assess the patency of the shunt or fistula routinely as part of the assessment of the patient. This access may be used for dialysis if renal function is not adequate.[89]

The transplant recipient has several intravenous lines for administration of medications and fluids following surgery. Once the recipient is able to tolerate fluids and a diet, oral medications are begun and the intravenous lines are removed. Auscultation for bowel sounds to ascertain return of bowel function is a necessary part of physical assessment. A stool softener may be needed by the patient with a history of long-term illness and poor nutrition.

The invasive lines and devices should be considered ports of entry for microorganisms and sterile technique must be followed in caring for these areas. The entry site into the body should be assessed for edema, redness, and drainage. Site care should be performed every 8 to 12 h unless otherwise instructed.

Indwelling Drains and Tubes

The number and type of drains vary according to the organ system transplanted. The recipient will have an endotracheal tube and assisted ventilation for a time following surgery. The renal, liver, pancreatic, and heart transplant recipient will be extubated as soon as there is adequate oxygenation and recipient response. The recipient of a heart and lung or lung transplant will remain intubated with mechanical ventilation for one to several days. This is to assure that adequate lung expansion, good oxygenation, and acid-base balance are maintained. Most transplant recipients have a nasogastric tube for several hours or days. With the removal of the endotracheal tube and return of bowel function, the nasogastric tube is removed.

The heart transplant recipient has two or three mediastinal tubes placed around the heart for chest drainage. These tubes are placed under water-seal and connected to suction. They are removed following removal of the hemodynamic monitoring lines, usually within 2 or 3 days after surgery. The patient receiving a heart and lung transplant also has two or three mediastinal tubes. In addition, they have bilateral pleural chest tubes, which are connected to water-seal drainage and suction. These tubes are removed with expansion of the lungs and removal of hemodynamic monitoring lines. The lung transplant recipient has similar drainage tubes. Pleural chest tubes are placed on the side of the lung transplant and connected to water-seal drainage with suction. They remain until the lung has good expansion and decreased drainage. Daily chest x-rays are obtained in these patients to observe for changes in lung expansion and development of complications such as atelectasis or opacifications.

The liver transplant recipient has several tubes and drains. Three or four Jackson-Pratt drains are placed above and below the liver and connected to suction. They are removed in days to weeks depending on the amount of drainage. The drains are removed one by one, beginning with the least draining until they are all removed. A T tube is placed in the common bile duct. It is brought out through a stab wound and allowed to drain for 4 to 6 weeks following transplantation and then is clamped. It is not removed for about 3 to 6 months postoperatively.[66]

The renal transplant recipient usually has no drains or may have one Jackson-Pratt drain, which originates near the kidney. If a drain is in place, it is removed within 4 to 5 days of transplantation. The pancreatic transplant recipient is similar in that there may be one or two Jackson-Pratt drains near the pancreas or no drains at all. If drains exist, they are removed within the first week following transplantation.

Care of the drains and tubes depends on their type and terminal location. All wounds, drain and tube entry sites, and connections with tubings should be considered ports of entry for microorganisms and should, therefore, be sterile. Sterile technique should be employed when caring for these areas. The surrounding skin should be kept clean and dry, and assessed for signs of inflammation, infection, or other complications. Drainage should be described according to color, consistency, and amount, with close attention paid to any changes in the drainage. Changes in the drainage may indicate that a complication is occurring, but changes may also be a normal variation. Color changes in T tube drainage of the liver transplant recipient may indicate rejection. Showering is usually permitted within 5 to 7 days after surgery. However, swimming should be discouraged until all wounds and puncture sites are well healed.

Diagnostic Studies

Diagnostic studies are useful in assessing the function of the transplanted organ and other organ systems, the effects of medications, and identifying areas in which complications may occur. The studies requested and their frequency vary according to the situation and the organ system involved. The diagnostic studies usually performed on transplant recipients are listed in Table 59-8.

The recipient of a heart or heart and lung transplant undergoes right ventricular endomyocardial biopsy to assist in the diagnosis of rejection. These biopsies are performed at intervals determined by the recipient's condition and by the

Table 59-8 Diagnostic Studies Routinely Performed on Organ Transplant Recipients and Rationale for Request

Study	Rationale
Serum electrolytes Serum enzymes Blood urea nitrogen (BUN) Creatinine Glucose levels Liver function studies Prothrombin time Partial thromboplastin time Complete blood cell count White cell differential Platelet count Electrocardiogram Chest x-ray Urinalysis Cultures of blood, sputum, urine, wounds, and drainage	These diagnostic studies are performed to evaluate the level of function of the transplanted organ, effects of surgery, illness, and medication on the other organ systems, and the potential for complications, such as rejection or infection.

Note: Laboratory values with "normal" ranges apply to the transplant recipient.

physician. The heart and lung or lung transplant recipient may have bronchial washings performed at intervals in an attempt to diagnose rejection of the lung. Biopsies of other organ systems are not requested routinely.

The renal transplant recipient will have renal perfusion studies and renal scans performed prior to discharge from the hospital. These studies are useful in determining function, blood flow, and rejection. The pancreatic transplant recipient has special studies, such as glucose tolerance tests, serum insulin levels, and C-peptide levels, obtained for evaluation of organ function. The liver transplant recipient also undergoes studies to assess organ function. Three months after transplantation, a cholangiogram is usually requested prior to removal of the T tube.

In addition to the diagnostic studies requested, the physician uses data such as daily weights, intake and output measurements, urine specific gravity, urine checks for sugar and acetone, vital signs, and physical examination for diagnosis of organ system function, complications, and residual or new organ system dysfunction as indicators of organ function. The nurse should be aware of specific concerns related to each organ system transplanted. Table 59-9 lists specific studies requested for assessment of each of the transplanted organ systems.

Medications

The medications prescribed for transplant recipients vary according to the organ system involved and the physician, but there are some similarities. All transplant recipients receive immunosuppres-

Table 59-9 Diagnostic Studies Performed on Organ Transplant Recipients with Reference to Specific Organ Function

Organ System	Diagnostic Study
Heart	ECG, chest x-ray, serum enzymes, serum electrolytes, hemodynamic parameters, endocardial biopsy
Lung	Chest x-ray, arterial blood gases, pulmonary function studies, bronchial washings
Heart and lung	Same as for both heart and lung
Kidney	Urinalysis, serum electrolytes, BUN, creatinine, ERPF, GFR, 24-h urine creatinine clearance, renal scan
Liver	Liver function studies, serum enzymes, protime, PTT, blood chemistries, cholangiogram
Pancreas	Serum amylase, pancreatic scan, C-peptide levels, fasting glucose levels, urine S&A, serum insulin levels

Note: These diagnostic studies are used to look at specific organ function and the "normal" value ranges apply to the transplant recipient.

sive agents. These are usually prednisone, cyclosporine, and Imuran, which are discussed elsewhere in this chapter. It is important to remember that the recipient remains on some form of immunosuppression for the remainder of the time that the transplanted organ is functional. It cannot be overly stressed to the recipient and family that without these medications the transplanted organ will be rejected.

Other medications which are commonly prescribed include prophylactic antibiotics immediately following surgery, an antacid, a diuretic, and antihypertensive agents. Some transplant recipients also receive anticoagulation for a time following surgery. The recipient of a heterotopic heart transplant receives Coumadin as a routine medication and it should be listed on the Medic-Alert card.

The transplant recipient should be able to correctly administer the medications prior to discharge from the hospital. Family members should be included in teaching sessions with the recipients. The importance of taking medications as prescribed, as well as side effects, should be stressed to the recipient and the family members. The recipient should also be instructed regarding situations in which one is unable to take the medications, such as vomiting; the ways of dealing with accidental missed dosages; what to do if they run out of medications; and the effects of food and alcohol on the medications.

Diet

Transplant recipients are placed on sodium-restricted diets because of the effects of prednisone and cyclosporine in causing sodium retention. The amount of sodium allowed may vary, but is usually 1 to 4 g of sodium a day. The heart and heart and lung transplant recipient is also placed on a low-fat, low-cholesterol diet to lower blood cholesterol levels. Patients should be instructed regarding ideal weight ranges for their body size. If the transplant recipient gains weight rapidly or becomes overweight, a reduced calorie diet is prescribed. It is helpful to have the dietician see the recipient and family members for dietary instruction and for the patient to be followed in the clinic with weight charts. The recipient should also be instructed to weigh every day to monitor weight changes and

identify fluid retention. Many recipients retain fluid in the abdominal area and have little or no peripheral edema. The recipient should notify the physician if weight gain is greater than 5 lb in one day.

Exercise

The transplant recipient should be encouraged to ambulate and perform activities of daily living as soon as possible following transplantation. The physical therapist should involve the recipient in an exercise program which is designed to increase strength and build muscle mass. A portion of the program must be done independently by the recipient. The nurse should encourage the recipient in following the program and assist when necessary. Exercise plays an important role in the patient's rehabilitation and leads to an improved sense of self-worth and a positive outlook.

Psychosocial Aspects

Transplant recipients go through stages of emotional adjustment to the transplant process.[94–97] They have experienced life-threatening illness, possible death, and major surgery. They must deal with a diet, new medications, close follow-up by the physician, and the potential for complications. The psychological as well as the physiological status of the recipient should be evaluated often. Transplant recipients may have periods of elation about their survival and activity level, and overall feelings of well-being. They may also experience depression and fears because of failure to progress as quickly as desired, or as a result of slowed progress secondary to the occurrence of complications. The nurse plays an important role in encouraging, motivating, and reassuring the recipient and family during this time of concern. Coordination of support with the social worker, chaplain, and psychiatrist is invaluable in assisting the recipient and family members to cope with the emotional aspects of transplantation. The nurse should also remember that during this stressful period the recipient may focus on minor details or specific areas of concern and not be as interested in learning self-care. Reinforcement of education and details concerning transplantation is a necessary part of nursing care at this time. The recipient and family members need to be assured that they can call a member of the transplant team at any time if questions arise and that someone is available even when the recipient is at home.

The recipient and family may also have questions and concerns about their donor. Most institutions allow the recipient to know the age and sex of the donor. Other information such as what city the donor came from and the manner of death of the donor may be discussed on an individual basis, but the name of the donor is not usually revealed. If the recipient or family wishes to express their appreciation for organ donation, an anonymous letter can be delivered to the donating family via the organ bank.

The goal of organ transplantation is to restore organ function and wellness and to improve the recipient's health and activity level. The quality of life maintained after transplantation varies according to the complications which occur, the general health and well-being of the recipient, his or her strength and activity level, and his or her attitude toward resuming a normal life. Quality of life is of utmost concern to the recipient, the family, and the health care team. Each individual has differing opinions as to what quality of life is. During the time of rehabilitation, the recipient and family members should be encouraged to verbalize their expectations and goals, to define quality of life, describe what they would consider a good quality of life, and identify their potential for attaining a satisfactory quality of life.

Case Study

Following transplantation, Mr. Jones was admitted to the ICU for observation. He was placed in a private room under strict reverse isolation. His endotracheal tube was connected to a mechanical ventilator with settings of IMV 10, FiO_2 60%, VT 850, and PEEP +5 cmH_2O. Auscultation revealed clear breath sounds bilaterally. Mr. Jones was not yet awake and his respiratory rate was dependent on the ventilator. Electrocardiographic monitoring with a standard lead II showed a normal sinus rhythm with a heart rate of 75 beats per minute. The intraatrial lines and arterial line placed during the transplant surgery were connected for monitoring of hemodynamic parameters. Epicardial pacing

wires attached to the donor right atrium and right ventricle were taped to his chest. Mr. Jones had two mediastinal chest tubes and one right pleural tube which were connected to water-seal drainage with wall suction. His Foley catheter for urinary output measurements was connected to bedside drainage and a rectal probe was inserted for measurement of temperature. Mr. Jones' pedal pulses were +4 with skin temperature cool and pink. Table 59-10 lists Mr. Jones' hemodynamic parameters.

During the first 15 min in the ICU, Mr. Jones' pedal pulses decreased to +2 with skin temperature cool and pink. His left atrial pressure also decreased from 12 mmHg to 10 mmHg but he remained in a normal sinus rhythm with a rate of 65 beats per minute. With administration of leukocyte-poor blood to increase the left atrial pressure to 12 mmHg and treat a hemoglobin of 8.5, Mr. Jones' pedal pulses returned to +4. A temporary pacemaker was connected to Mr. Jones' epicardial pacing wires and atrial synchronous pacing was begun at a rate of 90 beats per minute. Cardiac output was measured when Mr. Jones was stable and revealed an output of 7.0 L/min with a cardiac index of 2.58. Mr. Jones' urinary output remained acceptable at 80 to 100 mL per hour. Blood samples were sent for renal and liver function studies. As Mr. Jones began to awaken and rewarm, his blood pressure became elevated. Nitroprusside was given as a continuous intravenous infusion to control the systolic blood pressure to a level below 120 mmHg.

Mr. Jones remained stable and was extubated within 6 h of surgery. Hemodynamic monitoring devices and the chest drainage tubes were removed by postoperative day 2. Mr. Jones was able to feed himself and assist with his bath on the second postoperative day also, and sat on the side of the bed with assistance of the nurse. The Foley catheter was removed on the third postoperative day and Mr. Jones was allowed to sit up in a chair for breakfast. His blood pressure was ranging from 160/96 to 170/110 mmHg and oral antihypertensive medication was begun. The temporary pacemaker was discontinued when Mr. Jones' heart rhythm remained in a normal sinus rhythm with an intrinsic rate of 85 beats per minute. Mr. Jones and his family were pleased with his ability to breathe easier and with the improvement in his color.

Table 59-10 Mr. Jones' Hemodynamic Parameter Trend for the First 4 H Following Cardiac Transplantation

Name: Jones Room: 504Q	Age: 62 Sex: Male		Weight: 68 kg Height: 177 cm BSA: 1.76		
Hemodynamic Parameters	Time 0300	0315	0330	0400	0500	0600

Hemodynamic Parameters	0300	0315	0330	0400	0500	0600
HR (bpm)	75	65	90	90	90	90
RR (bpm)	10	10	10	10	10	12
Temperature (°F)	96	96.6	97.4	98	98.8	99
RAP (mmHg)	10	8	7	9	7	6
LAP (mmHg)	12	10	12	14	10	12
SBP (mmHg)	120	130	128	126	118	120
DBP (mmHg)	64	68	76	64	58	68
MAP (mmHg)	72	82	88	72	68	74
Urinary output (mL/h)	100	90	80	100	200	150
Chest drainage (mL/h)	75	70	50	60	70	60
CO (L/min)			7.0			7.80
CI (L/min/m²)			2.58			2.60
Pedal pulses	+4/+4	+2/+2	+4/+4	+4/+4	+4/+4	+4/+4

HR = heart rate
RR = respiratory rate
RAP = right atrial pressure
LAP = left atrial pressure
SBP = systolic blood pressure

DBP = diastolic blood pressure
MAP = mean arterial pressure
CO = cardiac output
CI = cardiac index

Complications after Organ Transplantation

The success of the transplant depends upon careful monitoring and management of the recipient following surgery. Although complications may occur at any time after transplantation, advancements in therapy have yielded prevention of many complications and improvement in treatment of those that do occur. Many of the long-term complications of transplantation are associated with the medications required for immunosuppression, preexisting medical conditions, compliance problems, or a combination of factors. Use of cyclosporine has been associated with a decrease in the severity of complications, making them more easily treatable.

The nurse plays a very important role in observation for signs and symptoms of complications and in educating the transplant recipient. The recipient of an organ transplant must know that if at any time in the future questions or concerns about a problem occur, they must seek medical attention immediately. A false alarm is preferable to a life-threatening complication which has been allowed to progress.

Rejection

Improvements in immunosuppression have decreased the severity and difficulty of treating rejection. However, rejection still remains a threat to long-term survival. Rejection is classified as *hyperacute, acute,* and *chronic. Hyperacute rejection* occurs within hours of surgery and is caused by preformed antibodies to the lymphocytes of the donor. When the cytotoxic antibodies detect the donor's lymphocytes there is rapid antibody formation. A form of vasculitis and cell destruction occurs in response, and the transplanted organ fails. A preoperative lymphocytotoxicity screen assists in detection of these antibodies. If the screen is positive, preformed antibodies are present and a donor must be located for whom the recipient has no preformed antibodies.[98,99] When hyperacute rejection occurs, the transplanted organ fails and must be removed.

Acute rejection may occur at any time after the fourth or fifth postoperative day. It is a common occurrence following transplantation and is usually treated by increasing the dosage of immunosuppressants in order to reverse the rejection process.

With acute rejection infiltration by mononuclear cells and edematous changes occur with possible myocyte necrosis. As the rejection increases in severity, organ dysfunction occurs.[99]

Chronic rejection usually occurs over a period of months to years, and is associated with gradual loss of organ function. Fibrosis and scar tissue formation in the transplanted organ and vasculature are found on examination. There is presently no treatment for chronic rejection except retransplantation.[98,99]

Most transplant recipients have at least one episode of acute rejection within the first month of transplantation. It is sometimes difficult to differentiate organ dysfunction from acute rejection or infection.[100] The common signs and symptoms of rejection are listed in Table 59-11.[23,46,58,64,66,100] Biopsy of the transplanted organ may be needed to make a definitive diagnosis of rejection. In the heart and heart and lung transplant recipient, right ventricular endomyocardial biopsy is performed routinely each week to diagnose rejection. Organ biopsy is not done routinely in other organ transplant recipients because of the potential complications which may occur with needle biopsy. Bronchial washings may be done in the lung and heart and lung transplant recipient rather than a lung biopsy.

Sometimes patients have no signs of early rejection and they may feel good and have adequate organ function until severe rejection occurs. Fever is a less common sign of rejection. Cultures of the blood, urine, and sputum assist in eliminating the possibility of infection. Not all possible signs and symptoms of rejection are present in every recipient or in every rejection episode. Nurses should be on the alert for any subtle changes in the recipient's behavior and clinical status. The patient may state that "I just do not feel quite right" and cannot explain what is different. Dizziness, pain, weight gain, or fever may be all the symptoms present, yet rejection may be occurring. The development of signs and symptoms may be gradual or very quick. The nurse should immediately assess the recipient for adequate organ function and other organ system involvement, and notify the physician. Diagnostic studies for assessment of organ function are requested and close observation of the recipient for signs of any change in organ function is begun.

Table 59-11 Common Signs and Symptoms of Rejection by Organ System

System	Signs and Symptoms
Heart	Diminished pedal pulses, low cardiac output, atrial arrhythmias, S3 or S4, exercise intolerance, lethargy, peripheral edema, anxiety, joint pain, mood swings, temperature greater than 101°F orally, heart enlargement, fatigue, systolic blood pressure decrease of 20 mmHg or more in previously hypertensive patients (ECG voltage decrease in patients receiving Imuran and prednisone only)
Lung	Decreased ventilation, decreased perfusion, opacification of the lung on chest x-ray, respiratory distress, temperature greater than 101°F orally, leukocytosis, decreased arterial oxygen tension, negative sputum culture with other symptoms
Heart and lung	Combination of both heart and lung
Kidney	Elevated BUN, elevated creatinine, diminished creatinine clearance, oliguria, increased graft size on renal scan, temperature greater than 101°F orally, peripheral edema, joint pains, weight gain, hypertension, tenderness over the graft, lethargy, proteinuria
Liver	Elevated bilirubin, elevated transaminase, elevated alkaline phosphatase, leukocytosis, tachycardia, jaundice, decreased or absent bile flow, right flank pain or RUQ pain, encephalopathy, temperature greater than 101°F orally, weight gain, peripheral edema
Pancreas	Sudden increase in fasting blood glucose, increased amylase, possibly temperature greater than 101°F orally

Note: Patients should be observed for acute changes or changes in the usual trend, no matter how small the change may appear, and rejection considered as a possible cause. Rejection may occur at any time with the same signs and symptoms expected at any postoperative interval.

Rejection is treated by increasing the immunosuppressive medications. This may be accomplished by use of methylprednisolone, Imuran, antithymocyte globulin, or by increasing the prednisone dosage. The regimen of immunosuppressive agents used may vary with the physician, the organ system involved, and the amount of rejection that is occurring. Treatment of malfunction of the transplanted organ is analogous to treatment of native organ dysfunction. Most rejection episodes are responsive to treatment, but rejection may recur and may not be responsive to treatment. If the rejection fails to respond to treatment, or organ function deteriorates, retransplantation may be considered. In organ systems in which rejection of the transplanted organ does not lead to death of the transplant recipient, medical treatment resumes and consideration of retransplantation is done on a less emergent basis. This is true of the renal transplant recipient, who returns to dialysis, and the pancreatic transplant, who resumes insulin treatment.

The transplant recipient and family should be prepared to expect some rejection to occur. Even with counseling and education, the occurrence of rejection strikes a low blow and depression, fear, and anger are seen in many transplant recipients. Questions about how and why rejection occurs as well as the expected treatment should be addressed as basically as possible. The transplant recipient experiencing acute rejection several months following transplant, and who has had rejection before, will have just as many concerns as the recipient who develops rejection early after transplantation. Diagnostic studies, medication changes or additions, and the length of time required for treatment should be explained each time rejection occurs, even if the recipient appears to know what to expect. Knowing what to expect seems to decrease anxiety in the recipient. The fear of return to dialysis, medical treatment, or retransplantation may be voiced. The nurse should remind the transplant recipient and family members that some rejection can be expected following transplantation but that rejection usually responds to treatment. The recipient and family should be encouraged to resume as near normal activity as is possible while receiving treatment.

Many transplant recipients and family members are concerned that they could cause the rejection to occur. It should be stressed that the rejection is no one's fault and the only way it can be caused is by failing to take the immunosuppressive medications as prescribed. There is no way of predicting the occurrence of rejection. It is important that the recipient be aware of signs and symptoms indicating that a problem may be occurring and to notify the physician immediately.

With the increase in immunosuppression needed to suppress rejection, the possibility of infection also increases. Because of this, many institutions encourage transplant recipients not to be near infected patients while treatment is being administered. Those individuals who are routinely isolated postoperatively, such as the heart transplant recipient, have their isolation returned to strict reverse isolation. During the treatment for rejection, most institutions require the recipient to be hospitalized.

Infection

The transplant recipient is at an increased risk for infection due to the use of immunosuppressive medications. Infections may occur at any time following transplantation, but the most life-threatening infections usually occur within the first 6 months following surgery. These infections usually involve the pulmonary system, the wound, the skin, and the urinary tract. The major organisms causing these infections are bacterial, viral, or fungal in origin. The infectious process can be very rapid in onset and there may be few clinical symptoms. The infections caused by nonbacterial organisms are usually more difficult to identify and treat.[101–104]

The pulmonary system is the most common site of infection in the transplant recipient. Pneumonias caused by nosocomial organisms are usually seen early after transplantation, while late postoperative pneumonias are associated with such organisms as *Pseudomonas aeruginosa, Legionella pneumophila,* and *Aspergillus fumigatus.*[104] The signs and symptoms vary, but a nonproductive dry cough can sometimes be seen at the onset of a viral or fungal infection and may precede signs of infection on the chest x-ray. An increase in temperature does not always occur.[101–104] Some recipients have signs of infection on chest x-ray without any other signs or symptoms; these infections may be found by accident during a routine checkup.

Infections of the wound, skin, and urinary tract occur with less frequency than respiratory infections and are also caused by bacterial, viral, and fungal organisms. With the use of prophylactic antibiotics, the incidence of these types of infections has decreased; however, they may be a factor in development of serious infections. Return to surgery for removal of thrombus or for bleeding and for complications such as fistulas increases the risk of infection. The reopening of the wound allows for potential contamination by pathogens. Special care should be taken to prevent contamination of tubes, devices, and wounds. The transplant recipient with a urinary Foley catheter or a suprapubic catheter is at risk of contamination of the catheter tubing and reflux flow. The catheter should not be disconnected once in place and should be removed as soon as possible.[104]

Opportunistic infections occurring as a result of immunosuppression include those caused by the herpes simplex virus, cytomegalovirus, the varicella-zoster virus, *Aspergillus, Nocardia, Pneumocystis,* and *Candida.* These infections are of concern because there are few drugs that are useful in treating them and those which are available are nephrotoxic and hepatotoxic and must be taken for long periods of time.[103–105] Every attempt will be made to locate the area of infection and to identify the causative organism as soon as possible. Identification of the organism is usually required prior to the use of antibiotics. Sputum, blood, urine, wound, and any drainage cultures are taken routinely in the immediate postoperative period and as necessary following the appearance of symptoms of infection. Many institutions require viral titers and a hepatitis screen preoperatively for use as a baseline for postoperative titers. Recipients should be monitored closely during treatment for infections, for signs of sepsis, and for effects of antibiotics on renal and hepatic function.

Complications of Immunosuppression

The drugs used for immunosuppression have been discussed earlier. The side effects of these drugs will vary and there may be resultant complications. Immunosuppressive agents have been associated with the occurrence of infection, hypertension, peptic ulcers, colonic perforations, and pancreatitis, as well as liver and kidney dysfunction. The steroids used for immunosuppression are associated with the majority of complications such as impaired growth and wound healing, osteoporosis, avascular necrosis of joints, cataracts, steroid-induced diabetes, acne, atrophy of muscle, and cushingoid appearance. The transplant recipient also experiences an increase in hair growth, fluid retention, and weight gain.[77–80] In some recipients, psychiatric disturbances and mood swings have been noted.

Steroid-induced diabetes following transplantation is believed to be the result of decreased utilization of glucose by the body along with an increased glucogenesis. Some studies support the probability of steroids having a direct action against insulin at cell level.[106,107] Steroid-induced diabetes is usually mild, transient, and may require diet, oral hyperglycemic agents, or low-dose insulin for control. The onset may be soon after transplant or may be seen with postoperative weight gain. Diagnosis is made on the basis of elevated serum glucose, glucosuria, and a negative nitrogen balance. Sliding scale insulin may be utilized, as well as scheduled insulin for glucose control while steroid dosage tapering proceeds. Once the recipient reaches a maintenance steroid dose, insulin may no longer be required with periodic serum glucose checks and dietary adjustments being utilized for assessment and control.[106]

The transplant recipient has an increased risk of developing hypertension as a result of the immunosuppressive medications, prednisone and cyclosporine. Drug-induced hypertension is only one factor in the development of hypertension, however. There are factors such as the history of hypertension and residual renal dysfunction which also must be considered in relation to the onset. Medications can exacerbate existing factors by sodium and fluid retention, and may contribute to nephrotoxicity. The medications often used for treatment are diuretics, vasodilators, calcium channel blockers, and alpha and beta blockers. In some recipients, converting enzyme inhibitors, centrally acting adrenergic inhibitors, beta blockers, or postsynaptic α-adrenergic blockers may be used. The drug of choice depends on the transplanted organ system and the amount of control gained by first-choice drugs. The medications utilized for treatment must be monitored closely because of the effects on renal and hepatic function as well as the effect on the transplanted organ system.[108]

There is no predictor of the recipient's response to medication effects. While some recipients have very few side effects or complications associated with immunosuppressive medications, others experience many. The side effects and complications are treated as they occur.

The development of lymphoproliferative disorders in transplant recipients is well documented. Recipients must be taught the warning signs of cancer and how to examine themselves for lumps or thickenings at least once a month. A thorough examination for any swelling of lymph nodes, lumps, or thickenings should be part of the routine assessment when the recipient is seen in the clinic or is hospitalized. Aggressive diagnosis and treatment are important in preventing further involvement or spread of lymphoproliferative disease.

Organ Dysfunction

The transplanted organ may be exposed to injury which may cause dysfunction of the organ. This dysfunction may be due to ischemia with procurement and surgery, intraoperative complications, rejection, and medication effects. The initial assessment of organ function is made at the time of recirculation of blood and resumption of blood flow during surgery. It is sometimes difficult to differentiate organ dysfunction from rejection without the assistance of biopsy. If the organ remains dysfunctional, retransplantation is performed or medical treatment is implemented until organ system function returns.[101,102]

Complications Associated with Specific Organ Systems

Heart

Accelerated coronary atherosclerosis in the heart transplant recipient is a major concern. The atherosclerotic changes are thought to occur from an immune-mediated injury to the endothelial cell lining of the coronary vessels which leads to platelet aggregation and buildup of plaque. Studies have shown that an HLA-A2 mismatch, history of hypertriglyceridemia, and donor age are factors which may influence the occurrence of the accelerated atherosclerosis.[23,109] A yearly left heart catheterization with coronary angiography is utilized in the identification of atherosclerotic disease. A low-fat, low-cholesterol diet combined with Persantine helps control the occurrence. Donor age of less than 35 years is followed by most heart transplant programs in an attempt to lessen the chance of the donor having asymptomatic heart disease. Treatment of the coronary atherosclerosis is determined by the amount of narrowing of the vessel lumen. There may be follow-up coronary angiograms every 6 months for observation, and when necessary, angioplasty, coronary bypass grafting, or retransplantation may be attempted to alleviate narrowing or occlusion of the vessel.

Lung

In the lung transplant recipient a response of the transplanted lung called "reimplantation response" occurs in the first 7 to 21 postoperative days. This response is believed to be due to the effects of surgical trauma, ischemia, lymphatic interruption, and denervation. It is characterized by a decrease in gas exchange, decrease in compliance, and pulmonary edema. The reimplantation response is usually transient, resolving within several days of onset. Treatment includes providing adequate oxygenation, aggressive diuresis, and close monitoring of pulmonary function. The recipient should be weighed every day and placed on fluid restriction if necessary to ensure a negative intake versus output, with close observation of renal function and serum electrolytes.[28,46,110]

The lung transplant requires the surgical anastomosis of the donor bronchus to the recipient's bronchus. Complications may occur in the area of anastomosis because of poor healing due to the use of steroids for immunosuppression and ischemia due to a lack of adequate collateralization from the pulmonary artery. Possible complications in this area include infection, bleeding, mucosal necrosis, and bronchial disruption. Stenosis at the anastomosis site may occur as a late complication. Techniques utilized to minimize these complications include revascularization of the transplanted bronchial arteries, shortening of the bronchial stump in the donor, and reinforcement of the anastomosis site using surrounding tissue. With the use of cyclosporine, steroids can be withheld for a time postoperatively or used at low dose while bronchial healing is taking place.[46,111]

Heart and Lung

The heart and lung transplant recipient has several areas in which complications may potentially occur. With heart and lung transplantation there is denervation of both lungs and the heart. This does not appear to affect the function of the transplanted organs in terms of respiration regulation or heart function, and reinnervation has not been proven to occur. There may, however, be a decreased P_{O_2} and an increased P_{CO_2} after extubation which return to the normal range in time. The most important significance of denervation of the lungs is that there is absence of the mucociliary response and sensation.[30,58,112] This requires that recipients be taught the importance of coughing and deep breathing on a routine or scheduled basis because they do not feel the need to cough up secretions below the site of the anastomosis. Some patients have reported a concern that they could not "feel" themselves breathe. Recipients should be consoled by reminding them that they are being closely monitored while in the hospital. They should be taught about the regulators of respiration, the carotid bodies, afferent chest wall nerves, and the central mechanism of rhythmic control of respiration.

The reimplantation response is also seen in the heart and lung transplant recipient, and treatment is the same. During the episode of reimplantation response, the recipient should be closely observed for signs of CHF.[30,58,112]

Tracheal healing in the heart and lung recipient has not proven to be as much of a complicating factor as seen in the lung transplant recipient where anastomosis is at the bronchus. Studies show that there is development of collateral circulation from the atrial branches of the coronary arteries. Healing is also improved by allowing a period of time postoperatively before adding steroids to the immunosuppressive regimen.[112]

Kidney

The most serious complication for the renal transplant recipient is failure of the transplanted kidney to maintain function. This may be caused by ischemic damage, rejection, technical difficulties, or renal disease. The signs and symptoms of a problem include anuria or oliguria, a rise in the BUN and creatinine, fluid imbalance, serum electrolyte imbalance, and in some cases, pain or fever. The treatment of kidney dysfunction after transplantation is determined by the cause of the problem. The BUN and creatinine are closely monitored and in some cases renal scans and intravenous pyelograms are utilized to assist in diagnosis. If a technical problem exists, such as thrombus, compression of the organ, or obstruction of urine flow, surgical intervention may be necessary. If rejection occurs, treatment is the same as that discussed earlier in the chapter. If acute tubular necrosis occurs, treatment includes diuretics and possibly dialysis.[92,101,113]

Liver

The hepatic transplant recipient is monitored closely in the immediate postoperative period for potential complications from bleeding and fluid and electrolyte imbalances. Bleeding may occur as a result of blood loss, loss of clotting factors, infection, or damage to blood components by the liver, and is treated by transfusion of blood products which assist in coagulation. A tendency toward hypokalemia during the postoperative period has been noted; potassium replacement and close monitoring are indicated. The calcium level and acid-base balance must also be monitored closely.[90,114]

Biliary complications from obstruction of biliary drainage are sometimes seen. Treatment depends on the area and amount of obstruction. Surgical intervention may be necessary to reroute biliary flow.[114]

Pancreas

The pancreatic transplant recipient is closely monitored for changes in serum glucose. This is the major area of concern following transplantation. There is, however, a need to follow the effects of the diabetes mellitus on the other organ systems. It has been reported that neuropathy may improve while diabetic retinopathy stabilizes.[115]

Case Study

On postoperative day 3, Mr. Jones was transferred to a private room on the open-heart unit. He quickly began rehabilitation by ambulating, exercising, and learning about his medications and diet. On the seventh day following transplantation Mr. Jones underwent right ventricular endomyocardial biopsy for evaluation of rejection. Mr. Jones' biopsy histologically showed moderate rejection without myocyte necrosis. His hemodynamic parameters were within normal limits, pedal pulses remained +4/+4, and he did not have any variance in exercise tolerance. It was decided that Mr. Jones should receive three doses of Solu-Medrol intravenously over the next three days. The rejection episode was frightening for Mr. Jones but he was able to express his fear and concerns with the nurse. A schedule of exercise, ambulation, and activities was devised so as not to tire Mr. Jones but to allow him to continue his progression. Mr. Jones participated in arm and leg exercises to improve flexibility and increase muscle strength, such as sitting knee bends, elbow flexion and extension, and ankle circles twice a day with the physical therapist. His ambulation was limited to his present amount and no addition of laps was allowed. Mr. Jones was able to walk ½-mile laps twice a day during the treatment for rejection. Mr. Jones was monitored by telemetry and vital signs were taken before and after exercising. He was allowed to plan activities of daily living and exercises according to how he was feeling each day.

Two days later, Mr. Jones noticed that his tongue was sore and his throat hurt when he swallowed. Upon examination, it was found that Mr. Jones had two lesions on his tongue and one lesion on his palate which appeared to be herpes simplex type 1. His throat was red but no lesions were noted. Cultures were obtained and sent to the viral laboratory. Mr. Jones was given viscous xylocaine to gargle for pain.

Mr. Jones underwent endomyocardial biopsy on postoperative day 12. The biopsy results showed improvement, and were classified as demonstrating mild rejection. He received no further treatment. Mr. Jones and his family were excited about the improvement in the biopsy but his sore throat was worsening because he now had difficulty swallowing and was hoarse. Examination by the infectious disease physician revealed a marked increase in the number of herpetic lesions visible in Mr. Jones' mouth and throat and viral cultures revealed the presence of herpes virus. Acyclovir intravenously was administered for the next 5 days. Mr. Jones improved and was able to begin eating solid food within 24 h after beginning treatment.

An endomyocardial biopsy was performed on the eighteenth day following surgery and minimal rejection was reported. Mr. Jones was feeling much improved, and discussions about discharge were begun.

Rehabilitation

Rehabilitation of the transplant recipient involves the entire health care team and the recipient's family. The recipient has been intensely ill and unable to participate in activities. Now the patient must shed the sick role and begin to take on normal activities once again. This can be a very difficult time for the transplant recipient and family, depending on the length and intensity of the illness prior to transplantation. Rehabilitation should be planned to include certain stages of activity, but paced to meet each individual's needs.

Early Postoperative Period

The initial hospitalization is an excellent time to begin rehabilitation because it is supervised. The recipient is in direct contact with the nurse, social worker, physical therapist, pharmacist, dietician, and physician. The psychiatrist or psychologist is also available for consultation if needed. Much of the rehabilitation at this stage is directed toward gaining strength, rebuilding muscle tissue, and education.

The transplant recipient should be allowed to participate in care as much as possible. This begins with small tasks, such as filling out the dietary menu and eating, and progresses to activities of daily living as tolerated. The physical therapist begins exercises and ambulation within 4 to 7 days following surgery. As the activity level improves, additional exercises and activities are staged so as not to overwhelm and discourage the patient. The ability to do things not previously done while ill is very encouraging for the recipient and the family. A chart of ambulation and exercises with daily progression is helpful for those who cannot physically detect progress.

The recipient and family members should be able to administer medications prior to discharge from the hospital. The nurse and the pharmacist are available to answer questions and to review medications, food and drug interactions, and side effects. An excellent way in which to ensure that recipients can administer medications is to have a time (1 to 2 weeks) for them to prepare and administer their medications under supervision of the nurse.

The prescribed diet should be taught by a dietician who is prepared to answer questions about grocery buying, fast-food restaurants, and product names. Suggestions of cookbooks and cooking methods for the individual diet are usually appreciated. The dietician should also be available to the recipient and family for future questions. Some institutions have a dietician who is also available in the outpatient clinic. The recipient should plan meals for several weeks prior to discharge from the hospital.

Criteria for discharge include the ability to administer medications, discuss the diet in detail, and ambulate without assistance. Recipients should be able to state activity restrictions and allowances, signs and symptoms of complications, and telephone numbers to call for assistance or to answer questions. The importance of keeping follow-up medical appointments is stressed. Any procedures to be continued at home such as taking temperature, blood glucose monitoring, or daily weight should be reviewed for accuracy with a discussion of the patient's responsibility for self-care.

Late Postoperative Rehabilitation

During the first 6 months following transplantation, the recipient is busy returning to life at home and continuing to regain strength. Rehabilitation can be hindered by the occurrence of complications, inability to find employment, and hesitation of the recipient to begin taking any responsibility. When people are sick, their roles in the family are taken over by others in the family so that when the transplant recipient returns home and attempts to resume the prior role in the family, it can be frustrating and may lead to family conflicts.

Complications may lead to feelings of frustration at being unable to control life, to proceed with activities, and to remain well. Not all recipients with complications have physical symptoms and feel sick. Being hospitalized brings inactivity and loss of control over diet and medications. Nurses caring for returning transplant recipients should allow them as much freedom of choice and control as possible. Medications can be scheduled at the times

they are usually taken at home or recipients may be allowed to be responsible for administering their own medications. They should be encouraged to remain as active as possible.

Finding employment following transplantation depends on the restrictions placed on the recipient by the physician and the employer. The social worker can be of assistance in locating vocational rehabilitation services. In our experience, heart transplant recipients who were employed at the time of transplantation returned to work soon after transplantation. Those who had not been employed for a time prior to transplantation found it more difficult to find employment.

Compliance with diet and medications is necessary. It is important that transplant recipients be responsible for weighing every day and controlling their weight. If weight gain becomes a problem, a weight-reducing diet should be prescribed. The importance of adhering to the medical regimen cannot be overemphasized. Most institutions require follow-up visits every 3 to 6 months with a yearly examination of organ system function. Rapport is needed between the transplant center and the local physician who follows the recipient for routine checkups and laboratory studies postoperatively. The physician and the recipient should understand the importance and value of consulting the transplant center for assistance in the recipient's care and reporting follow-up diagnostic studies.

Case Study

Mr. Jones was able to begin ambulation on the third postoperative day. The physical therapist completed an assessment of Mr. Jones' muscle mass and strength and developed a plan of therapy with gradually increasing amounts of exercise and ambulation. An exercise bicycle was placed in Mr. Jones' room when he had progressed to 1 mile of ambulation per day. A chart was placed on the wall to illustrate the amount and type of exercise performed.

Dietary and medication teaching was planned to begin on the seventh day following transplantation. The dietician met with Mr. Jones and his wife to discuss requirements for a 2-g sodium, low-fat, low-cholesterol diet, as well as their shopping habits and cooking practices. Mr. Jones learned very quickly and began planning his menus according to his diet. He weighed daily and kept a record. Mr. Jones received information regarding the purpose, mode of administration, and possible side effects of his medications. He began preparing and administering his own medications under the supervision of his nurse.

Mr. Jones and his wife attended classes regarding transplantation and care at home. He was very attentive and asked questions concerning symptoms of rejection and when to notify the doctor about a fever. He was glad to know he could resume driving his car within 8 weeks of surgery.

Mr. Jones progressed rapidly despite a few complications and was able to go home just 20 days following transplantation. He continued his exercise program and found he could plan his activities around his medications and dietary restrictions with very few difficulties. He remained without complications and was able to resume working as a store clerk within 3 months of discharge from the hospital.

When Mr. Jones returned for a routine 3-month checkup he had gained 10 kg since his transplant and was able to maintain his weight by controlling his carbohydrate consumption. He was able to work full-time and exercise by walking 3 miles a day. Mr. and Mrs. Jones have rejoined their bridge club and plan a vacation in 2 months with a group from their church.

Summary

The field of transplantation is growing and changing. Many advances have been made toward achieving the goal of a greater quantity and quality of life for the individual with irreversible organ system failure. The maintenance of health care for the transplant recipient touches all disciplines of the health care field. These patients require nurses to be thorough and meticulous in carrying out routine as well as specific nursing therapies. Nurses play an important role in the areas of education, counseling, emotional support, and encouragement. They are involved in all areas of the transplant process—preoperatively, intraoperatively, and postoperatively. Caring for the transplant recipient is a challenge—a challenge for learning the effects of illness, for dealing with death, the importance of the quality of life, and for coping with long-term follow-up and medical care.

References

1. Harbison, S. P. (1962). Origins of vascular surgery: The Carrel-Guthrie letters. *Surgery, 52,* 406.

2. Moore, F. D. (1980). Transplantation—a perspective. *Transplantation Proceedings, 12*(4), 539–550.

3. Hardy, J. D. (1983). Transplantation of blood vessels, organs, and limbs. *Journal of the American Medical Society, 250*(7), 954–957.

4. Carrel, A. (1908). Results of the transplantation of blood vessels, organs, and limbs. *Journal of the American Medical Association, 51,* 1662–1667.

5. Saunders, J. B. M. (1972). A conceptual history of transplantation. In J. S. Najarian and R. L. Simmons (Eds.), *Transplantation* (pp. 3–25). Philadelphia: Lea & Febiger.

6. Humphries, A. L., & Dennis, A. J. (1982). Historical developments in preservation. In L. H. Toledo-Pereyra (Ed.), *Basic concepts of organ procurement, perfusion, and preservation* (pp. 1–25). New York: Academic.

7. Hamilton, D. (1982). A history of transplantation. In P. J. Morris (Ed.), *Tissue transplantation* (pp. 1–13). Edinburgh: Churchill Livingstone.

8. Lawer, R. H., West, J. E., McNulty, P. H., Clauncy, E. J., & Murphy, R. P. (1950). Homotransplantation of the kidney in the human. *Journal of the American Medical Association, 144,* 844.

9. Groth, C. G. (1972). Landmarks in clinical renal transplantation. *Surgery, Gynecology, & Obstetrics, 134,* 323–328.

10. Hume, D. M. (1979). Early experiences in organ homotransplantation in man and the unexpected sequelae thereof. *American Journal of Surgery, 137,* 152–161.

11. Billingham, R. E., Brent, L., & Medawar, P. B. (1953). "Actively acquired tolerance" of foreign cells. *Nature, 172,* 603.

12. Balner, H., & Marquet, R. L. (1981). Transplantation biology—past and present: Reappraisal of "breakthroughs" since 1955. *Transplantation Proceedings, 13*(1), 13–18.

13. Murray, J. E., Merrill, J. P., Dammin, G. J., Dealy, J. B., Alexandre, G. W., & Harrison, J. H. (1962). Kidney transplantation in modified recipients. *Annals Of Surgery, 156,* 337.

14. Starzl, T. E., Vonkualla, K. N., Hermann, G., Brittain, R. S., & Waddell, W. R. (1963). Homotransplantation of the liver in humans. *Surgery, Gynecology, & Obstetrics, 117,* 659–676.

15. Hardy, J. D., Webb, W. R., Dalton, M. L., & Walker, G. R. (1963). Lung homotransplantation in man. *Journal of the American Medical Association, 186,* 1065.

16. Teraski, P. I., Vredevoe, D. L., Mickey, M. R., Porter, K. A., Marchioro, T. L., Fairs, T. D., & Starzl, T. E. (1966). Serotyping for homotransplantation—VI, Selection of kidney donors for thirty-two recipients. *Annals Of New York Academy Of Science, 129,* 500.

17. Kelly, W. D., Lellehi, R. C., Merkel, F. K., Idezuki, Y., & Goetz, F. C. (1967). Allotransplantation of the pancreas and duodenum along with the kidney in diabetic nephropathy. *Surgery, 61,* 827.

18. Starzl, T. E., Marchioro, T. L., Porter, K. A., Iwasaki, Y., & Cerilli, G. J. (1967). The use of heterologous antilymphoid agents in canine renal and liver homotransplantation. *Surgery, Gynecology, & Obstetrics, 124,* 301.

19. Barnard, C. N., & Cooper, D. K. C. (1981). Clinical transplantation of the heart: A review of 13 years personal experience. *Journal Royal Society Of Medicine, 74,* 670–674.

20. Cooley, D. A., Bloodwell, R. D., & Hallman, G. L. (1969). Organ transplantation for advanced cardiopulmonary disease. *Annals Of Thoracic Surgery, 8,* 30–33.

21. Caves, P. K., Billingham, M. E., Stinson, E. B., & Shumway, N. E. (1974). Serial transvenous biopsy of the transplanted human heart—improved management of acute rejection episodes. *Lancet, 2,* 821–826.

22. Kahan, B. D. (1984). Cosmas and Damian revisited. In B. D. Kahan (Ed.), *Cyclosporine Volume II: Nursing and para-professional aspects* (pp. 13–18). Orlando: Grune & Stratton.

23. Baumgartner, W. A., Reitz, B. A., Oyer, P. E., Stinson, E. B., & Shumway, N. E. (1979). Cardiac homotransplantation. *Current Problems In Surgery, 16*(9), 1–59.

24. McKenzie, N. (1985). Cardiac transplantation. *Transplantation Today, 1,* 20–24.

25. Commerford, P. J. (1984). Selection and management of the recipient. In D. K. C. Cooper & R. P. Lanza (Eds.), *Heart Transplantation* (pp. 15–22). Lancaster: MTP Press Limited.

26. Wallwork, J. (1984). Heart and heart-lung transplantation. In R. Y. Calne (Ed.), *Transplantation Immunology* (pp. 452–482). Oxford: Oxford University Press.

27. Wildevuur, C. R. H., & Benfield, J. R. (1970). A review of 23 human lung transplantations by 20 surgeons. *The Annals Of Thoracic Surgery, 9*(6), 489–515.

28. Toledo-Pereyra, L. H. (1982). Lung transplantation. In S. N. Chatterjee (Ed.), *Organ transplantation* (pp. 327–346). Boston: John Wright.

29. Reitz, B. A. (1982). Heart and lung transplantation: A review. *Heart Transplantation, 1*(4), 291–298.

30. Shinn, J. A. (1985). Heart and lung transplantation for end-stage pulmonary vascular hypertension. *Nursing Clinics Of North America, 19*(3), 547–558.

31. Spees, E. K. (1982). Renal transplantation II: Selection and preparation of recipients. In S. N. Chatterjee (Ed.), *Organ transplantation* (pp. 221–241). Boston: John Wright.

32. Evans, D. B., & Raferty, A. (1984). Kidney transplantation. In R. Y. Calne (Ed.), *Transplantation immunology: Clinical and experimental* (pp. 413–435). Oxford: Oxford University Press.

33. Van Thiel, D. H., Schade, R. R., Gavalar, J. S., Shaw, B. W., Iwatsuki, S., & Starzl, T. E. (1984). Medical aspects of liver transplantation. *Hepatology, 4*(1), 795–835.

34. Vierling, J. M. (1984). Epidemiology and clinical course of liver diseases: Identification of candidates for hepatic transplantation. *Hepatology, 4*(1), 84–94S.

35. Rolles, K., & Calne, R. Y. (1984). Liver transplantation. In R. Y. Calne (Ed.), *Transplantation immunology: Clinical and experimental* (pp. 436–451). Oxford: Oxford University Press.

36. MacDougall, B. R. D., & Williams, R. (1983). Indications and assessment of orthotopic liver transplantation. In R. Y. Calne (Ed.), *Liver transplantation* (pp. 59–66). New York: Grune & Stratton.

37. Dixon, A., & Sherwood, T. (1983). Radiological assessment. In R. Y. Calne (Ed.), *Liver transplantation* (pp. 67–76). New York: Grune & Stratton.

38. Dubernard, J. M., Monti, L. D., Piatti, P. M., & Traeger, J. (1985). Pancreatic transplantation: Current status. *Practical Cardiology, 11*(6), 51–62.

39. Groth, C. G., Gunnarson, R., Lundgren, G., & Ostman, J. (1982). Pancreatic transplantation. In P. J. Morris (Ed.), *Tissue transplantation* (pp. 127–146). Edinburgh: Churchill Livingstone.

40. Dickerman, R. M., Raskin, P., Fry, W. J., & Elick, B. A. (1980). Preoperative evaluation of pancreatic transplant recipients. *Transplantation Proceedings, 12*(4), Supp. 2, 8–10.

41. Gilman, C., & Day, C. (1982). The living-related kidney donor. *AANNT, 10,* 33–35.

42. Goodman, M. R., & Aung, M. H. (1978). Cerebral death: Theological, judicial, and medical aspects. *Heart And Lung, 1,* 477–483.

43. Rudy, E. (1982). Brain death. *Dimensions Of Critical Care Nursing, 1*(3), 178–184.

44. deVilliers, J. C., & Cooper, D. K. C. (1984). Selection and management of the donor. In D. K. C. Cooper & R. P. Lanza (Eds.), *Heart transplantation* (pp. 23–38). Lancaster: MTP Press Limited.

45. Cooper, J. D. (1985). Experience with lung transplantation at the Toronto General Hospital. *Transplantation Today, 1,* 26–27.

46. Veith, F. J. (1978). Lung transplantation. *Surgical Clinics Of North America, 58*(2), 357–363.

47. Kreis, H. (1981). Selection of a donor. In J. Hamburger, J. Crosnier, J. Bach, & H. Kreis (Eds.), *Renal transplantation: Theory and practice* (2d ed.) (pp. 36–69). Baltimore: Waverly.

48. Van Thiel, D. H., Schade, R. R., Hakala, T. R., Starzl, T. E., & Denny, D. (1984). Liver procurement for orthotopic transplantation: An analysis of the Pittsburgh experience. *Hepatology, 4*(1), 665–715.

49. Toledo-Pereyra, L. H. (1985). Pancreas transplantation. In L. H. Toledo-Pereyra (Ed.), *The pancreas: Principles of medical and surgical practice* (pp. 439–464). New York: John Wiley & Sons.

50. Duffy, T. J., & Calne, R. Y. (1984). Pancreas and islet cell transplantation. In R. Y. Calne (Ed.), *Transplantation immunology: Clinical and experimental* (pp. 483–517). Oxford: Oxford University Press.

51. Rosenthal, J. T., Shaw, B. W., Hardesty, R. L., Griffith, B. P., Starzl, T. E., & Hakala, T. R. (1984). Principles of multiple organ procurement from cadaver donors. *Annals Of Surgery, 198*(5), 617–621.

52. McMaster, P. (1984). Techniques of multiple organ harvesting. In P. J. Morris & N. L. Tilney (Eds.), *Progress in transplantation* (vol. 1) (pp. 209–221). Edinburgh: Churchill Livingstone.

53. Novitsky, D., & Cooper, D. K. C. (1984). Surgical techniques of orthotopic and heterotopic heart transplantation. In D. K. C. Cooper & R. P. Lanza (Eds.), *Heart transplantation* (pp. 103–128). Lancaster: MTP Press Limited.

54. Nelems, M. B., Rebuck, A. S., Cooper, J. D., Goldberg, M., Halloran, P. F., & Velland, H. (1980). Human lung transplantation. *Chest, 78*(4), 569–573.

55. Veith, F. J., & Richards, K. (1970). Improved technique for canine lung transplantation. *Annals Of Surgery, 171,* 553.

56. Jamieson, S. W., Stinson, E. B., Oyer, P. E., Baldwin, J. C., & Shumway, N. E. (1984). Operative technique for heart-lung transplantation. *Journal Of Thoracic And Cardiovascular Surgery, 87*(6), 930–935.

57. Reitz, B. A., Pennock, J. L., & Shumway, N. E. (1981). Simplified operative method for heart and lung transplantation. *Journal Of Surgical Research, 31,* 1–5.

58. Stinson, E. B. (1984). Heart-lung transplantation. In R. L. Jamison (Ed.), *Transplantation in the 1980's* (pp. 67–78). New York: Praeger Special Studies.

59. Losman, J. G., Campbell, C. D., Replogle, R. L., & Barnard, C. N. (1982). Joint transplantation of the heart and lungs. *Journal Of Cardiovascular Surgery, 23,* 440–452.

60. Lahde, R. E. (1981). Heart-lung transplant: A first. *AORN, 34*(4), 627–639.

61. Davis, F. D. (1981). Current strategies in the procurement of cadaveric kidneys for transplantation. *Nursing Clinics Of North America, 16*(3), 565–571.

62. Kreis, H. (1981). Renal preservation. In J. Hamburger, J. Crosnier, J. F. Bach, & H. Kreis (Eds.), *Renal transplantation: Theory and practice* (pp. 70–87). Baltimore: Williams & Wilkins.

63. Lacombe, M. (1981). Surgical techniques. In J. Hamburger, J. Crosnier, J. F. Bach, & H. Kreis (Eds.), *Renal transplantation: Theory and practice,* (pp. 301–335). Baltimore: Williams & Wilkins.

64. Richard, A. B., Robbins, K. C., & Rovelli, M. A. (1984). Renal transplantation: Nursing management of the recipient. *AORN, 41*(6), 1022–1041.

65. Wheeldon, D. R., & Gill, R. D. (1983). Partial cardiopulmonary bypass. In R. Y. Calne (Ed.), *Liver transplantation* (pp. 145–148). New York: Grune & Stratton.

66. Maletic-Staschak, S. (1984). Orthotopic liver transplantation. *AORN, 39*(1), 35–39.

67. Calne, R. Y., & Williams, R. (1979). Liver transplantation. *Current Problems In Surgery, 15*(1), 1–44.

68. Calne, R. Y. (1983). Recipient operation. In R. Y. Calne (Ed.), *Liver transplantation* (pp. 155–172). New York: Grune & Stratton.

69. Connolly, J. E. (1978). Pancreatic whole organ transplantation. *Surgical Clinics Of North America, 58*(2), 383–389.

70. Groth, C. G., & Tyden, G. (1985). Pancreatic transplantation with enteric drainage of the exocrine pancreas. *Transplantation & Immunology Letter, 2*(3), 1–5.

71. Dubernard, J. M., & Monti, L. D. (1985). Duct obstruction of the pancreatic graft. *Transplantation & Immunology Letter, 2*(3), 1–3.

72. Broe, P. J., Mehigan, D. G., & Cameron, J. L. (1981). Pancreatic transplantation. *Surgical Clinics Of North America, 61*(1), 85–98.

73. Sutherland, D. E. R., Goetz, F. C., & Najarian, J. S. (1981). Pancreas and islet transplantation. In T. L. Dent (Ed.), *Pancreatic disease: Diagnoses and therapy* (pp. 521–537). New York: Grune & Stratton.

74. Toledo-Pereyra, L. H. (1985). Islet cell transplantation. In L. H. Toledo-Pereyra (Ed.), *The pancreas: Principles of medical and surgical practice* (pp. 465–484). New York: John Wiley & Sons.

75. Sutherland, D. E. R., Matas, A. J., & Najarian, J. S. (1978). Pancreatic islet cell transplantation. *Surgical Clinics Of North America. 58*(2), 365–381.

76. Lacey, P. E. (1980). Transplantation of islet cells—isografts and allografts. In P. J. Fitzgerald & A. B.

Morrison (Eds.), *The pancreas* (pp. 156–165). Baltimore: Williams & Wilkins.

77. Salaman, J. R. (1982). Non-specific immunosuppression. In P. J. Morris (Ed.), *Tissue transplantation* (pp. 60–79). Edinburgh: Churchill Livingstone.

78. Bach, J. F. (1981). Immunosuppression. In J. Hamburger, J. Crosnier, J. F. Bach, & H. Kreis (Eds.), *Renal transplantation: Theory and practice* (pp. 89–145). Baltimore: Williams & Wilkins.

79. Mathias, J. M. (1985). Immunosuppression: Postoperative management of heart transplant recipients. *AORN, 41*(4), 748–753.

80. Strom, T. B. (1984). Immunosuppressive agents in renal transplantation. *Kidney International, 26,* 353–365.

81. Kahan, B. D. (1985). Cyclosporine: The agent and its actions. *Transplantation Proceedings, 17*(4), 5–18.

82. Borel, J. F., & Stahelin, H. (1985). Cyclosporine A—the history and significance of its discovery. *Transplantation Today, 1,* 15–18.

83. Morris, P. J. (1981). Cyclosporine A: Overview. *Transplantation, 32,* 349.

84. Montefusco, C. M., Goldsmith, J., & Veith, F. J. (1984). Cyclosporine immunosuppression in organ graft recipients: Nursing implications. *Critical Care Nurse, 4*(2), 117–119.

85. Kashiwagi, N., Brantignan, C. O., Brettschneider, L., Groth, C. G., & Starzl, T. E. (1968). Clinical reactions and serologic changes after the administration of heterologous antilymphocyte globulin to human recipients of renal homografts. *Annals Of Internal Medicine, 68,* 275.

86. Strober, S. (1986). Use of total lymphoid irradiation in organ transplantation. *Transplantation & Immunology Letter, 2*(4), 1–6.

87. Kahan, B. D. (1986). Radiotherapy in transplantation. *Transplantation & Immunology Letter, 2*(4), 1–7.

88. Terasaki, P. I. (1984). The beneficial transfusion effect on kidney graft survival attributed to clonal deletion. *Transplantation, 37*(2), 119–125.

89. Funk, M. (1986). Heart transplantation: Postoperative care during the acute period. *Critical Care Nurse, 6*(2), 27–45.

90. Smith, S. L. (1985). Liver transplantation: Implications for critical care nursing. *Heart And Lung, 14*(6), 617–628.

91. Thornby, D. C. (1983). Cardiac transplantation: Nursing care during the acute period. *Dimensions Of Critical Care Nursing, 2*(4), 212–224.

92. Hooper, S. (1980). Nursing Care of transplant recipients. In S. N. Chatterjee (Ed.), *Renal Transplantation* (pp. 117–126). New York: Raven Press.

93. Felks-McVay, R. (1986). Cardiac transplantation: A case study. In M. Price & J. Fox (Eds.), *Advanced perspectives in hemodynamic monitoring.* Rockville, MD: Aspen.

94. Milne, J. F. (1977). Psychosocial aspects of renal transplantation. *Urology, 9*(6), 82–88S.

95. Basch, S. H. (1973). The intrapsychic integration of a new organ. A clinical study of kidney transplantation. *Psychoanalytical Quarterly, 42,* 364–370.

96. Christopherson, L. (1979). Cardiac transplantation: Need for patient counseling. *Nursing Mirror, 149,* 34–36.

97. Watts, D., Freeman, A. M., McGiffin, D. C., Kirklin, J. K., McVay, R., & Karp, R. (1984). Psychiatric aspects of cardiac transplantation: Assessment and management. *Heart Transplantation, 3*(3), 243–247.

98. Carpenter, C. B., & Strom, T. B. (1980). Transplantation immunology. In C. B. W. Parker (Ed.), *Clinical Immunology* (vol. II) (pp. 376–444). Philadelphia: Saunders.

99. Hamburger, J. (1982). The rejection network. *Heart Transplantation, 1*(3), 179–181.

100. Toledo-Pereyra, L. H. (1983). Pancreatic transplantation. *Surgery, Gynecology, & Obstetrics, 157,* 49–56.

101. Prewit, D. (1983). Postoperative complications—an overview. *Nephrology Nurse, 4,* 27–32.

102. Crosnier, J. (1981). Extrarenal complications. In J. Hamburger, J. Crosnier, J. F. Bach, & H. Kreis (Eds.). *Renal transplantation: Theory and practice* (pp. 232–267). Baltimore: Williams & Wilkins.

103. Brooks, R. G., & Remington, J. S. (1986). Transplant-related infections. In J. V. Bennet & P. S. Brachman (Eds.), *Hospital infections* (2d ed.) (pp. 581–618). Boston: Little, Brown.

104. Garibaldi, R. A. (1983). Infections in organ transplant recipients. *Infection Control, 4*(6), 460–464.

105. Lauter, C. B. (1976). Opportunistic infections. *Heart and Lung, 5*(4), 601–606.

106. Santa-Cruz, M. (1982). Steroid induced diabetes post transplantation. *AANNT, 8*(1), 66–68, 78.

107. Gunnarsson, R., Arner, P., Lundgren, G., Magnusson, G., Ostman, J., & Groth, C. G. (1979). Diabetes mellitus—a more-common-than-believed complication of renal transplantation. *Transplantation Proceedings, 11*(2), 1280–1281.

108. Duncan, C. (1985). Treatment of hypertension in post transplant patients. *Transplantation Today, 1,* 61–67.

109. Baumgartner, W. A., Oyer, P. E., Reitz, B. A., Stinson, E. A., Jamieson, S. W., & Shumway, N. E. (1984). Heart transplantation. In S. Slavin (Ed.), *Bone mar-*

row and organ transplantation (pp. 319–330). Amsterdam: Elsevier Science Press.

110. Siegelman, S. S., Sinhaj, S. B., Veith, F. J. (1973). Pulmonary reimplantation response. *Annals Of Surgery, 177,* 30–36.

111. Veith, F. J., & Montefusco, C. M. (1984). Lung transplantation. In S. Slavin (Ed.), *Bone marrow and organ transplantation* (pp. 417–432). Amsterdam: Elsevier Science Press.

112. Jamieson, S. W. (1985). Heart-lung transplantation. In P. J. Morris, & N. L. Tilney (Ed.), *Progress in transplantation* (vol. II) (pp. 147–166). Edinburgh: Churchill Livingstone.

113. Sutherland, D. E. R., Gifford, R. R. M., Fryd, D. S., Ascher, N. L., Simmons, R. L., & Najarian, J. S. (1984). Renal transplantation. In S. Slavin (Ed.), *Bone marrow and organ transplantation* (pp. 127–318). Amsterdam: Elsevier Science Press.

114. Koep, L. J., & Starzl, T. E. (1984). Liver transplantation. In S. Slavin (Ed.), *Bone marrow and organ transplantation* (pp. 331–364). Amsterdam: Elsevier Science Press.

115. Ball, P. (1986). Pancreatic transplantation. *AORN, 43*(3), 632–637.

60 Poisoning

Deborah L. Scherger
Frances L. Conrad
Dorothy M. Schulte
Kathleen M. Wruk

In 1984, 730,224 human poison exposures were reported to the American Association of Poison Control Centers' (AAPCC) National Data Collection System.[1] These exposures included accidental childhood ingestions, intentional overdoses, therapeutic misadventures, use and abuse of recreational drugs, and chronic exposures in the home and work setting.

A poison is a substance absorbed by the ocular, dermal, oral, or parenteral routes and which causes illness or death. "Poisoning" implies the presence of clinical symptoms and an accidental exposure. An intentional toxic exposure is described as an overdose. Ingestion of a substance may not be a poisoning unless symptomatology develops.

Care of the poisoned patient has improved remarkably in the last 10 years as a result of the evolution of sophisticated poison centers, emergency departments, and prehospital care systems. Poison centers provide information to the public and health care professionals regarding management of poisoned patients. Responsibility does not end after initial patient contact but continues as poison centers interface with emergency departments and critical care units to give advice on patient management.

Determining if a poisoning has occurred may be difficult. A complete history and patient assessment can provide essential information. A poisoning or overdose is suspect in (1) a psychiatric patient; (2) a trauma patient (especially if young); (3) a comatose patient with unknown etiology; (4) a young patient with life-threatening arrhythmias of unknown etiology; (7) children with unexplained lethargy or any puzzling presentation; (8) a patient with multiple symptom presentation, either chronically or acutely; (9) a patient with seizures of unknown etiology; or (10) a patient with cyanosis that is unresponsive to oxygen.[2]

Management of the poisoned patient involves specific interventions including stabilization of vital signs, prevention of absorption, enhancement of toxin excretion, and administration of antidotes if applicable. The most important aspect of care is to *focus on the clinical presentation of the patient, not the poison ingested by history.*

Approach to the Poisoned Patient

History

A thorough history is essential in treating the poisoned patient. The history may be obtained from a conscious patient, from accompanying family or friends, or from prehospital personnel, police, or rescue workers. The name of the poison, route of exposure, current symptoms, amount ingested, age, time of exposure, and length of exposure are included in the initial history.

After stabilization, a secondary history is obtained, which includes the exact name of the poison, clarification of the amount involved, and evidence of exposure. It may be necessary to send someone to the exposure site to look for open or empty containers, chemical spills, or other evidence.

A general health history, which includes recent or chronic illnesses, current medications, and known allergies, is obtained. Exposures to other substances and concomitant exposure of other persons at the site are ruled out. Any first aid treatment already initiated is also determined. Examples of inappropriate first aid interventions are tourniquets with snake envenomations, neutralization of bases and acids, administration of substances other than ipecac for emesis induction, and use of emetics in caustic exposures.

Case History

A young adult man called an emergency operator from a public pay phone booth, saying he had ingested a bottle of pills about 1 h before calling. He complained of drowsiness, and his speech was slurred. An ambulance was dispatched.

He was comatose on arrival in the emergency department, with spontaneous respirations at 10 per minute. His blood pressure was 80/50 and his pulse was 130. His skin and mucous membranes were dry, his face was flushed, and his pupils were dilated. On auscultation bowel sounds were decreased. Paramedics reported the patient had a generalized seizure in the ambulance. His serum pH was 7.32 and an ECG showed a widened QRS. No pills were found on the patient or at the site of exposure.

Nursing Assessment

After the patient's vital signs are stable, a complete physical examination is performed. If the patient's clinical condition warrants cardiac monitoring or there is a history of an exposure to a potentially cardiotoxic substance, cardiac monitoring is initiated. Cardiac monitoring alone is adequate for diagnosing arrhythmias but abnormalities of conduction (PR, QRS, QT intervals) are best evaluated with the 12-lead ECG. Electrolytes and arterial blood gases are monitored for the presence of acidosis. An elevated anion gap (greater than 12 to 16 meq/L) is also indicative of acidosis. To calculate the anion gap, the serum bicarbonate and chloride values are subtracted from the sodium value $[(Na^+) - (HCO_3^- + Cl^-)]$[2]. A chest x-ray rules out noncardiogenic pulmonary edema, infiltrates, and trauma. Toxicology screening of blood and urine also may assist in the patient's assessment.[2] Rarely are gastric contents analyzed. A list of symptoms and suspected ingestants is sent to the laboratory with the toxicology specimen. Some substances are more easily identified if the possibility of their presence is noted.

Analysis of the four common syndromes—anticholinergic, sympathomimetic, narcotic opiate, and cholinergic—may help in determining the causative agent (Table 60-1). Certain symptoms or symptom groups provide clues that may aid in diagnosis. For example, if a patient presents with

Table 60-1 Four Common Poisoning Syndromes

1. Anticholinergic:
   Substances causing anticholinergic symptoms include antihistamines, some antipsychotic drugs, antidepressants, over-the-counter (OTC) sleep medications, cold medications, chemicals, and plants.
   Symptoms:
   a. Dry flushed skin
   b. Dry mucous membranes
   c. Decreased or absent bowel sounds
   d. Confusion, hallucinations, hyperactivity, and seizures
   e. Tachycardia, hypertension, and arrhythmias which may be delayed
   f. Mydriasis
   g. Urinary retention

2. Sympathomimetic:
   Substances causing sympathomimetic symptoms include drugs such as ephedrine, phenylpropanolamine, phenylephrine, pseudoephedrine, metaproterenol, albuterol, and terbutaline. These drugs are commonly found in oral nasal decongestants, OTC diet pills, street drugs, and prescription medications.
   Symptoms:
   a. Nausea and vomiting
   b. Anxiety, restlessness, hyperactive reflexes, irritability, and seizures
   c. Tachycardia, hypertension, and arrhythmias

3. Narcotic opiate syndrome:
   Narcotics are available in both oral and parenteral forms. Propoxyphene may be found alone or with other analgesic drugs such as acetaminophen or aspirin. Dextromethorphan is an ingredient in many OTC cough preparations and may have a narcotic effect. Clonidine may cause similar symptoms in overdosage.
   Symptoms:
   a. Coma, areflexia, and seizures
   b. Miosis
   c. Hypotension and bradycardia
   d. Respiratory depression or apnea
   e. Pulmonary edema

4. Cholinergic syndrome:
   Substances that may cause these symptoms include pesticides, certain mushrooms, physostigmine, and drugs used to treat myasthenia gravis such as pyridostigmine, neostigmine, or ambenonium chloride.
   Symptoms:
   a. Increased secretions (a mnemonic that may be helpful in remembering symptoms is SLUDGE):

Salivation	S
Lacrimation	L
Urination	U
Defecation	D
Gastrointestinal cramping	G
Emesis	E

   b. Muscle fasciculations and seizures
   c. Miosis
   d. Bradycarida
   e. Diaphoresis
   f. Bronchorrhea

Adapted from A.H. Hall, K.W. Kulig, and B.H. Rumack, *Management of Acute Poisonings and Overdose*, unpublished manuscript, Rockey Mountain Poison and Drug Center, Denver, CO, 1985.

coma and hypotension, suspected agents include sedatives, benzodiazepines and ethanol (Table 60-2). After primary assessment, nursing diagnoses are formulated to guide patient management (Table 60-3).

Table 60-2 Diagnostic Clues to Toxins

1. Coma, hypotension
   a. Sedatives, hypnotics, narcotics
   b. Benzodiazepines
   c. Ethanol
   d. Isopropanol
   e. Methanol
   f. Ethylene glycol
   g. Carbon monoxide
2. Pulmonary edema (noncardiogenic)
   a. Sedatives, hypnotics (especially Placidyl)
   b. Narcotics
   c. Salicylates
   d. Carbon monoxide
3. Metabolic acidosis with elevated anion gap
   a. Salicylates
   b. Methanol
   c. Ethylene glycol
   d. Isoniazid (with seizures)
   e. Iron
   f. Ethanol
4. Cyanosis unresponsive to oxygen (methemoglobinemia)
   a. Chemicals such as nitrites, nitrates, nitrobenzene, and drugs such as phenacetin, phenazopyridine (Pyridium), and antimalarials
   b. Sulfones (Dapsone)
5. Cardiac arrhythmias, seizures, and coma
   a. Tricyclic antidepressants
   b. Theophylline
   c. Caffeine
   d. Arsenic
   e. Cyanide
   f. Hydrogen sulfide
6. Behavior disorders (confusion, agitation, hallucinations, and combativeness)
   a. Phencyclidine (PCP)
   b. Cocaine
   c. Amphetamines
   d. Anticholinergics
   e. Ethanol
   f. LSD
   g. Toluene (glue sniffing)
   h. Salicylates
   i. Heavy metals
   j. Certain mushrooms
7. Seizures
   a. Aspirin
   b. Amphetamines
   c. Anticholinergic substances
   d. Camphor
   e. Carbon monoxide
   f. Cyanide
   g. Cocaine
   h. Propoxyphene
   i. Phencyclidine
   j. Strychnine
   k. Isoniazid
   l. MAO inhibitors
   m. Tegretol
   n. Drug withdrawal
8. Radiopaque drugs
   a. Chloral hydrate
   b. Heavy metals
   c. Phenothiazines
   d. Enteric coated tablets

Adapted from A. H. Hall, K. W. Kulig, and B. H. Rumack, *Management of Acute Poisoning and Overdose,* unpublished manuscript, Rocky Mountain Poison and Drug Center, Denver, CO, 1985.

General Management of the Poisoned Patient

Primary Management

The primary interventions for a poisoned patient are stabilization of vital signs and supportive ther-

Table 60-3 Nursing Diagnoses That May Be Used in Toxicology

Poisoning, potential for
Airway clearance, ineffective
Anxiety
Breathing pattern, ineffective
Cardiac output, alteration in: decreased
Comfort, alteration in: pain
Coping, ineffective family: compromised
Coping, ineffective individual
Fear
Fluid volume deficit, potential
Gas exchange, impaired
Knowledge deficit
Non-compliance
Oral mucous membranes, alteration in
Parenting, alteration in: potential
Powerlessness
Self-concept, disturbance in self-esteem
Skin integrity, impairment of: potential
Social isolation
Tissue perfusion, alteration in: cerebral, cardiopulmonary, renal, gastrointestinal, peripheral
Violence, potential for self-directed

Source: V. Novotny-Dinsdale, Implementation of Nursing Diagnosis in One Emergency Department. *Journal of Emergency Nursing,* 11:140–144, 1985. Used with permission.

apy. Adequate ventilation and tissue perfusion must be established before evaluating the circumstances that led to the exposure. An intravenous line may be started and appropriate fluids given, depending on the status of the patient. Adults who present in a comatose state require intravenous (IV) naloxone hydrochloride and glucose. After the patient is stabilized, an accurate history and complete physical assessment are obtained.

Prevention of Absorption

The six common routes of exposure to a toxic substance include ingestion, dermal, ocular, inhalation, parenteral, and envenomation. Ingestion is most common. To prevent or limit toxic effects of the poison, initial management includes aggressive removal of the substance. Prevention of absorption from the gastrointestinal tract may be accomplished with dilution, gastric emptying, and administration of activated charcoal and a cathartic.[2] After a dermal or ocular exposure, the skin or eye is copiously irrigated for 15 to 20 min with lukewarm water or saline. Patients exposed to insecticides require a more thorough decontamination by removing their clothing and performing three alternate washings—the first with soap and water, the second with rubbing alcohol, and the final again with soap and water.[2,3] Following an inhalation exposure, the patient is moved into fresh air. First aid manuals and container labels may recommend neutralization of a substance; this is an inappropriate first aid measure that may increase damage. When a substance is neutralized following an oral, dermal, or ocular exposure, the chemical reaction releases heat, which may cause more deleterious effects than the initial exposure.

Dilution with milk or water is recommended in all conscious patients who have ingested household products or chemicals.[2] Milk is preferred in caustic ingestions because it is a demulcent and its high protein content provides a substrate for the products. The recommended amount of fluids is 15 mL/kg in a child and up to 250 mL in a 16-kg or larger patient.[3] Excessive amounts of milk or water may cause vomiting which is contraindicated in a caustic ingestion. Dilution is not recommended for medication ingestions because placing the drug into solution may increase the rate of absorption.

Two methods of gastric emptying are syrup of ipecac-induced emesis and gastric lavage. Spontaneous emesis following an ingestion may not adequately empty the stomach. Induction of emesis by gagging with a finger or blunt object is ineffective and the throat or finger may be injured. Administration of copper sulfate or a saltwater solution to induce emesis is no longer recommended because of associated adverse effects. Copper sulfate may cause renal and hepatic failure and a saltwater solution may cause hypernatremia and seizures.[2] Dry mustard powder or soap solutions are ineffective and are no longer used. Soap solutions may also produce gastrointestinal irritation. Apomorphine, used as an emetic in veterinary medicine, produces emesis rapidly but it is not used in humans because it produces central nervous system depression.[2]

Ipecac

Syrup of ipecac is an emetic widely used in the home and hospital setting. Its popularity can be attributed to its clinical effectiveness and relative safety. Ipecac is derived from the dried root of *Cephaëlis ipecacuanha* or *C. acuminata*. Emetine and cephaeline are the alkaloids contained in ipecac which cause the emetic response. Emesis with ipecac generally occurs within 20 to 30 min after its administration.[4] The early vomiting is due to the direct irritant effects of ipecac on the gastrointestinal tract. Vomiting which occurs after 30 min is a result of centrally induced action on the chemoreceptors of the medulla after systemic absorption.

The recommended dose of syrup of ipecac is 30 mL for teenagers and adults. If emesis does not occur within 30 min, the dose may be repeated once. Administration of water and an increase in activity facilitate induction of emesis. Ipecac is most effective when given within 30 min of exposure. Data from studies investigating the use of ipecac for gastric emptying indicate that its efficacy in removing the ingested poison decreases if the time of its administration is delayed more than 30 min from the time of ingestion.[5] Other studies demonstrate that even when given immediately after ingestion, the percent of ingestant recovered is small.[6,7]

Protracted vomiting and diarrhea have been reported following administration of ipecac.[4] These symptoms are usually associated with the fluid extract of ipecac. Fluid extract of ipecac is no longer generally available and should not be used. Cephaeline is more locally irritating than emetine and produces more nausea and vomiting. Emetine appears to increase intestinal peristalsis causing diarrhea. Emetine is also more toxic to the heart and may cause tachycardia or arrhythmias in larger doses. There have been some isolated case reports of side effects following syrup of ipecac which include a Mallory-Weiss tear of the esophagus,[8] aspiration,[4] cerebral vascular accident,[9] and pneumomediastinum.[10] Individual persons with eating disorders who abuse syrup of ipecac chronically may develop toxicity.

Administration of syrup of ipecac is contraindicated in patients who are comatose, have lost their gag reflex, exhibit seizure activity, or have ingested a corrosive substance. It is also not recommended when substances are ingested that produce central nervous system depression, respiratory depression, or seizures within the first 30 min of ingestion, examples of which include camphor, propoxyphene, tricyclic antidepressants, and narcotics. Use of syrup of ipecac following a hydrocarbon exposure is controversial and depends on the specific type of hydrocarbon, the amount ingested, and the other ingredients in the products.

Gastric Lavage

Controversy exists concerning the preferred method of gastric emptying. Early animal studies indicate that lavage is the least effective method regardless of when the procedure was performed after the ingestion.[11] Studies in children revealed similar data with a significant amount of ingestant recovered by ipecac-induced emesis even when lavage had been performed prior to ipecac administration.[12] A small-bore nasogastric tube was used in these studies and may account for the low percentage of ingestant recovered by gastric lavage. There are no studies to date comparing the efficacy of administration of syrup of ipecac and gastric lavage with a large-bore orogastric hose.

When deciding which method of gastric emptying to use, aspects to consider include the time since the ingestion, the type of exposure, and the efficacy of activated charcoal in adsorbing the substance. If the patient presents to the emergency department more than 30 min postexposure, gastric lavage is the preferred procedure because it will not delay activated charcoal administration.[13] Gastric lavage is also recommended in ingestions in which syrup of ipecac is contraindicated.

Gastric lavage is performed with a large-bore orogastric hose. Endotracheal intubation is indicated for airway protection only in patients who are comatose or have no gag reflex. Gastric lavage is contraindicated in patients who have ingested caustics or are convulsing. Some side effects seen with gastric lavage include esophageal perforation and aspiration pneumonitis.[14]

Activated Charcoal

Activated charcoal is effective in decreasing toxicity by adsorbing drugs and chemicals to its surface. The efficacy of activated charcoal in acute poisonings is dependent on timing of administration and the amount of charcoal administered. It is most effective when given within 30 min of the exposure and adsorbs 90 to 99 percent of the stomach contents within 1 min of administration. In ingestions of drugs with delayed absorption, the charcoal may be effective for up to 24 h after the exposure. To ensure maximum adsorption of drug, an activated charcoal drug ratio of 10:1 is recommended.[15] Because the patient rarely provides an accurate history of the amount of drug ingested, the recommended dose for adults is 60 to 100 g and 15 to 30 g for children (1 to 2 g/kg as a rough guideline). The abdomen is auscultated for bowel sounds. Activated charcoal is not given in the presence of ileus.

Charcoal is effective only in its activated form. Activated charcoal is obtained by treating charcoal with substances such as steam and air at high temperatures, which increases its adsorptive capabilities. Most commercially prepared activated charcoal products come premixed in a water suspension ready for administration. Attempts have been made to make charcoal more palatable by adding lubricants, flavoring, and sweetening agents; however, these additives may be adsorbed, diminishing the adsorptive capacity of the activated charcoal. It is also not recommended to mix activated charcoal with pudding, ice cream, or other substances that may decrease its efficacy.

Several factors which include pH, amount and type of gastric contents, and the charcoal-to-drug ratio, influence the adsorptive capacity of charcoal.

Weak acids and bases are adsorbed more effectively when they are in the nonionized form. For example, aspirin is more effectively adsorbed at a pH of 1 rather than at a neutral or alkaline pH. Food in the stomach may decrease the adsorptive capacity of activated charcoal. The adsorption of drugs to charcoal is a reversible process, and if inadequate amounts of charcoal are given, desorption will occur. *Desorption* is defined as removing an adsorbed material by a chemical or physical process, thus causing free drug to be released from the drug/charcoal complex. Ethanol, mineral acids, methanol, and alkalis are not adsorbed by charcoal in clinically significant amounts. Most drugs are well adsorbed by activated charcoal, including aspirin, acetaminophen, propoxyphene, barbiturates, benzodiazepines, phenytoin, carbamazepine, tricyclic antidepressants, digitalis glycosides, theophylline, and ipecac.

In certain ingestions, multiple doses of activated charcoal are indicated to increase the clearance of systemically absorbed drugs. Some drugs, after they are absorbed into the systemic circulation, are resecreted in an unchanged form into the gastrointestinal tract in the gastric fluid, bile, or gastrointestinal secretions, and are then reabsorbed into the systemic circulation. If activated charcoal is in the gastrointestinal tract, this recirculation will be interrupted, and elimination increased. Multiple-dose charcoal is effective in theophylline, phenobarbital, carbamazepine, and phenylbutazone overdoses. It may be useful in salicylate, digoxin, and meprobamate poisoning, but this is still investigational.[15,16] Following the initial dose of activated charcoal, the recommended dose is 30 to 60 g every 4 to 6 h until plasma levels of the drug are within the therapeutic range and the patient is asymptomatic. A cathartic is administered as needed to maintain bowel motility.

It is currently controversial whether initial decontamination of an ingested poison requires gastric emptying or administration of activated charcoal alone. One study evaluated the effectiveness of gastric emptying and the administration of activated charcoal versus the administration of activated charcoal alone on clinical symptoms in 592 patients and found no benefit from ipecac-induced emesis in the emergency department. Gastric lavage was found to be beneficial in obtunded patients who presented within 1 h of ingestion.[13] Another study,

in which salicylate overdose was simulated, also showed no benefit of induced emesis and activated charcoal over activated charcoal alone.[17] In cases in which the patient presents several hours after exposure, initial administration of activated charcoal may prove most beneficial to the patient.

Cathartics

Cathartics are frequently administered with activated charcoal to hasten the elimination of the drug/chemical-charcoal complex. The efficacy of cathartics in preventing absorption of poisons has not been clinically demonstrated.[18]

Cathartics routinely administered include magnesium sulfate, sodium sulfate, magnesium citrate, and 70 percent sorbitol. The recommended doses of magnesium or sodium sulfate are 30 g, for an adult, and of magnesium citrate 4 mL/kg, up to 300 mL a dose. Oil cathartics are not used because of the possibility of lipoid pneumonia if aspirated.[18] Cathartics are administered cautiously to patients with recent bowel surgery and to patients with absent bowel sounds. Sodium cathartics are avoided in patients with congestive heart failure and hypertension, as are magnesium cathartics in patients with renal failure. Repeat doses of magnesium cathartics should be used cautiously because of reported toxicity in individuals who received multiple doses.[19,20] Sorbitol is used cautiously in the very young or very old and during multiple-dose charcoal administration because there is a higher incidence of dehydration associated with its use.

Advanced Management

Enhancement of the excretion of certain absorbed poisons may be accomplished by supportive therapy, forced diuresis, charcoal hemoperfusion, and/or hemodialysis. Deciding which therapy to use depends on the characteristics of the specific poison, any underlying medical conditions, and the clinical status of the patient.

Supportive therapy is the most important treatment modality for all poisoned patients. Maintenance of respiration, circulation, and other vital functions takes precedence over other aspects of therapy. The indiscriminate use of drugs, antidotes, or procedures in patients exposed to toxic substances should be avoided.

There are several types of forced diuresis procedures. *Neutral diuresis* is seldom used in poisoned patients. Although *acid diuresis* has been shown to increase the elimination of phencyclidine and amphetamines, it is no longer recommended because it may lead to myoglobinuric renal failure in the presence of rhabdomyolysis.[21] *Alkaline diuresis* is used in salicylate and phenobarbital overdose.[13] Alkalinization of the urine ionizes weak acids, thus preventing passive reabsorption of molecules and increasing elimination.[2] The urine pH must remain between 7 to 8 for the procedure to be beneficial. The urine pH is maintained by adjusting sodium bicarbonate administration. Serum potassium (K^+) is monitored closely because alkaline diuresis cannot be effectively achieved with hypokalemia present. Potassium is added to the IV solution as needed to maintain a normal serum K^+. Diuretics such as furosemide or mannitol may be administered to maintain diuresis. Forced diuresis is potentially dangerous because it may result in noncardiogenic pulmonary edema. Contraindications to forced diuresis are cerebral edema, pulmonary edema, and renal failure.[3]

Hemodialysis and hemoperfusion are extracorporeal procedures that are effective in removing certain absorbed drugs from the body. Their use in the management of a poisoned patient is limited because both procedures are costly and have inherent risks. Whether a drug is dialyzable depends on physical and chemical properties and pharmacokinetic parameters. Water-soluble, low-molecular-weight drugs are more easily removed by hemodialysis than are fat-soluble, high-molecular-weight drugs. Drugs or their metabolites that are highly protein-bound, have a large volume of distribution (the larger the volume of distribution, the less amount of total drug found in the plasma), and have a long distribution phase are poorly dialyzable.

Patients who can be managed with supportive care do not require hemodialysis. Indications for hemodialysis include (1) progressive clinical deterioration despite standard treatment measures, (2) a removal rate of poison by dialysis greater than physiologic clearance, (3) an impaired elimination system in the patient, (4) poisoning by substances with metabolic and/or delayed effects (such as ethylene glycol or methanol), and (5) depression of midbrain functions producing hypothermia, hy-poventilation, and hypotension. Side effects of hemodialysis include hypotension, thrombosis, and, infrequently, hepatitis and infection.[3]

Hemoperfusion with charcoal or resin columns may increase the extraction of certain medications from the body by the passing of anticoagulated blood through a column containing absorbent particles. The extraction ratio of most drugs from the serum is higher for hemoperfusion than for hemodialysis. The efficacy of hemoperfusion is dependent on the drug's volume of distribution, plasma clearance, elimination half-life, and its affinity for the absorbent material. Side effects include bleeding, pyrogenic reactions, thrombocytopenia, leukopenia, charcoal embolization, hypotension, hypocalcemia, and early saturation of the charcoal column.[3]

When considering either of these procedures, several factors need to be addressed. These include the clinical presentation of the patient, the efficacy of the procedure in removing the drug ingested, the side effects of the procedure, and whether supportive care alone is sufficient for recovery (see Tables 60-4 and 60-5).

Nursing Diagnoses

1. Poisoning, potential for toxicity from unknown drug
2. Ineffective breathing pattern related to alteration of respiratory drive
3. Decreased cardiac output, related to decreased blood pressure
4. Decreased cardiac output related to conduction disturbances
5. Alteration in tissue perfusion related to decrease in cerebral blood flow
6. Maladaptive coping mechanism as evidenced by suicidal ideation
7. Potential for self-inflicted injury related to depressive state
8. Potential for alteration in bowel elimination related to administration of charcoal and carthartics

Goals

I. Respiratory function
   A. Maintain adequate respiratory function and oxygenation.

Table 60-4 Agents for which Hemodialysis May Be Effective

5-Fluorouracil	Cephalothin	Glutethimide	Pargyline
Acetaminophen/Paraceta-mol	Chloral hydrate	Heroin	Penicillin
Acetone	Chloramphenicol	Iodide	Pentobarbital
Acetophencitidin	Chlordiazepoxide	Iron	Phenelzine
Acetophenetidine	Chloride	Isocarboxazid	Phenobarbital
Acetylsalicylic acid	Chloroquine	Isoniazid	Phosphate
Alkyl phosphate	Chlorpropamide	Isopropanol	Polymyxin
Amanita phalloides	Chromic acid	Kanamycin	Potassium
Amanitin	Cimetidine	Lead	Potassium chlorate
Amikacin	Colchicine	Lithium	Potassium dichromate
Ammonia	Colistin	Magnesium	Practolol
Amobarbital	Copper	Mannitol	Primidone
Amphetamine	Cyclobarbital	Meprobamate	Procainamide
Ampicillin	Cyclophosphamide	Mercury	Propoxyphene
Aniline	Cycloseine	Methamphetamine	Propranolol
Aprobarbital	Demeton-*S*-methyl-sulfoxide	Methanol	Quinalbital
Arsenic	Dextropropoxyphene	Methaqualone	Quinine
Atenolol	Diethyl pentenamide	Methotrexate	Salicylic acid
Azathioprine	Digoxin	Methyl mercury complex	Secobarbital
Azlocillin	Dimethoate	Methyldopa	Snake bite
Bacitracin	Dinitro-ortho-cresol	Methylprednisolone	Sodium chlorate
Barbital	Dinitrophenol	Methylsalicylate	Sodium citrate
Borates	Diphenhydramine	Methypyrlon	Sotalol
Boric acid	Diphenylhydantoin	Monoamine oxidase inhibitors	Streptomycin
Bromide	Diquat	Nafcillin	Strontium
Butabarbital	Ergotamine	Neomycin	Sulfonamides
Butalbital	Ethanol	*N*-acetylprocainamide	Tetracycline
Calcium	Ethchlorvynol	Nitrates	Thallium
Camphor	Ethinamate	Nitrite	Thiocyanate
Carbamazepine	Ethylene glycol	Nitrofurantoin	Thiols
Carbenicillin	Eucalyptus oil	Ouabain	Tobramycin
Carbon monoxide	Flucytosine	Oxalate	Trancylpromine
Carbon tetrachloride	Fluoridem chlorate	Oxalic acid	Trichlorethylene
Carbromal	Fostomycin	Paracetamol	Tricyclic secondary amines
Cefamandole	Gallamine triethiodide	Paraldehyde	Tricyclic tertiary amines
Cephaloridine	Gentamicin	Paraquat	Vancomycin

Adapted from Poisindex Information System, Micromedex, Inc., Englewood, CO.

Table 60-5 Agents for which Hemoperfusion May Be Effective

Amanita mushrooms	Methaqualone
Amobarbital	Methotrexate
Carbromal	Methsuximide
Carbon tetrachloride	Oxycholordone
Colchicine	Paraquat
Cortinarius mushrooms	Phenobarbital
Digoxin	Phenothiazines
Ethchlorvynol	Primidone
Glutethimide	Quinidine
Gyromitra mushrooms	Secobarbital
Hexobarbital	Theophylline
Meprobamate	Tricyclics (resin)

Adapted from Poisindex Information System, Micromedex, Inc., Englewood, CO.

B. Maintain hemodynamic stability.
C. Maintain cerebral blood flow.
D. Maintain adequate respiration and oxygenation.

II. Cardiovascular function
  A. Maintain stable vital signs.
  B. Maintain warm extremities.
  C. Maintain normal hemodynamic pressures.
  D. Maintain normal temperature.
  E. Maintain normal sinus rhythm as evidenced by:
    1. Atrial rate 60–100 beats per minute.
    2. Constant PR interval 0.12–0.20 s.
    3. Constant QRS interval 0.06–0.10 s.

III. Neurological function
   A. Remain seizure-free.
   B. Respond appropriately to verbal and tactile stimuli and be oriented to person, place, and time.
IV. Psychosocial function
   A. Verbalize and acknowledge unresolved problems and concerns.
   B. Develop appropriate mechanisms for dealing with stress.
   C. Be injury-free while in hospital.
V. Gastrointestinal function
   A. Maintain normal bowel function.
   B. Maintain hydration.

Nursing Interventions

I. Respiratory function
   A. Maintain airway, breathing, and circulation through basic and advanced life-support measures.
   B. Prevent absorption of poison through gastrointestinal decontamination.
      1. Perform or assist with gastric lavage with large-bore orogastric tube and normal saline solution until clear.
      2. After assessing that bowel sounds are present, administer 60 to 100 g of activated charcoal and 30 g magnesium citrate via gastric tube as ordered by physician.
   C. Obtain blood and urine for toxicology tests.
   D. Assess respiratory rate and depth.
   E. Auscultate breath sounds for clarity, resonance, and depth.
   F. Assess peripheral circulation for good color, warmth, and brisk capillary refill.
   G. Maintain patent airway.
   H. Assess need for endotracheal intubation and mechanical ventilation.
   I. Administer oxygen as indicated by patient's condition and as ordered by physician.
   J. Obtain ABGs in accordance with hospital policy.
II. Cardiovascular function
   A. Assess blood pressure, heart rate, peripheral circulation, and body temperature.
   B. Perform hemodynamic monitoring if indicated by physical means; i.e., intraarterial and central venous pressure lines.
   C. Administer IV fluids, put patient in Trendelenburg position; administer vasopressors as indicated for decreased blood pressure as ordered by the physician.
   D. Provide continuous cardiac monitoring.
   E. Monitor for conduction abnormalities and arrhythmias. Measure PR and QRS intervals as needed. Report any widening of PR or QRS interval or ectopy to physician.
   F. Maintain physiologic pH (7.40–7.45) for optimal cardiac conduction. Administer sodium bicarbonate as needed and ordered by physician.
   G. Obtain 12-lead ECG.
III. Neurological function
   A. Assess neurological function and perform neurological checks every 4 h as indicated by patient's condition.
   B. Maintain adequate oxygenation, manifested by Pa_{O_2} 80 to 100 mmHg.
   C. Administer anticonvulsant medications, i.e., Valium and Dilantin, as indicated and ordered by physician.
   D. Protect patient from harm related to sensorium change.
      1. Side rails should be up at all times; pad rails prn.
      2. Wrist, ankle, Posey restraints prn.
IV. Psychosocial function
   A. Speak warmly and openly to patient.
   B. Provide unhurried atmosphere to encourage verbalization of concerns.
   C. Allow patient private time with family and significant others.
   D. In addition to psychiatric intervention, other appropriate interventions include social service—i.e., social worker, financial counseling, and chaplain.
   E. Maintain suicide precautions while patient is in depressed state:
      1. There should be no sharp objects (needles, metal silverware) in room.
      2. Monitor objects brought into room by visitors.
      3. Keep curtains or blinds open to observe patient when possible.
V. Gastrointestinal function
   A. Assess presence of bowel sounds in all four quadrants before administering charcoal and cathartic.

B. Monitor for increase in abdominal girth, distention, and firmness.

C. Maintain adequate fluid volume if diarrhea ensues.

D. Report absence of bowel sounds and suspicion of paralytic ileus to physician as indicated.

Antidotes

Only a few poisons have specific antidotes. Stabilization of vital signs, prevention of absorption, and enhancement of excretion of the poison are the foci of care in most poisonings. For those substances that have a specific antidote, it is important to manage the patient's clinical symptoms initially, not just to administer the antidote (Table 60-6).

Common Poisonings

Acetaminophen

Acetaminophen in therapeutic doses results in antipyretic and analgesic effects mediated through the central nervous system. Because of its wide availability as an over-the-counter medication, the incidence of acetaminophen overdose has increased. When taken in overdose amounts, acute, transient hepatotoxicity may occur. If treated promptly and appropriately, hepatic damage can be avoided.[22]

Pathophysiology

The metabolism and kinetics of acetaminophen are well known. After ingestion, 94 percent of the dose is metabolized to nontoxic metabolites in the liver and 2 percent is excreted unchanged in the urine. The remaining 4 percent is metabolized via the cytochrome P-450 pathway in the hepatocytes. Through this pathway acetaminophen is metabolized to a toxic metabolite, conjugates with the enzyme glutathione, and is excreted as two nontoxic metabolites, mercapturic acid and cysteine.[22]

In therapeutic doses, acetaminophen is easily conjugated to glutathione. In large overdoses, this enzyme is rapidly depleted. When glutathione levels fall below 70 percent of normal, unbound amounts of the toxic metabolite accumulate. Toxicity results when the metabolite covalently binds with hepatic macromolecules, resulting in liver cell necrosis.

The extent of hepatic damage is dose-related. The larger the amount of acetaminophen ingested, the greater amount of toxic metabolite produced and the greater the hepatic damage.[22]

Clinical Manifestations

Acetaminophen toxicity is divided into four stages. Immediately following the overdose, the patient is asymptomatic. Stage 1, beginning 7 to 14 h after ingestion, manifests with nausea, vomiting, and anorexia. During stage 2, 24 to 36 h after exposure, there is evidence of clinical improvement. However, serum SGOT, SGPT, total bilirubin, and prothrombin times begin to rise. Peak hepatotoxicity occurs during stage 3, 42 to 96 h after ingestion. SGOT values greater than 20,000 are not unusual. Recovery (stage 4) begins 7 to 8 days after initial ingestion.[3]

Medical Management

Treatment guidelines are based on the patient's history of the amount of acetaminophen ingested. In adults, an ingestion of greater than 7.5 g has potential for hepatotoxicity. General management principles for gastric emptying apply to acetaminophen ingestions. The use of activated charcoal is controversial if no other medications are involved, because of its potential to interfere with N-acetylcysteine (NAC) absorption.

Toxicity is determined with the Rumack-Matthew nomogram (Fig. 60-1). Peak plasma levels with therapeutic doses are seen in 70 to 160 min. In overdose situations, peak plasma levels may not be seen until 4 h after ingestion when absorption is completed.[5] Acetaminophen levels should be drawn at 4 h or more after acute ingestion. At 4 h after exposure, plasma levels of 150 μg/mL are considered potentially hepatotoxic and N-acetylcysteine treatment is mandated. If levels are not obtained within 6 to 8 h after ingestion and the history indicates a potentially toxic dose, treatment should be initiated and continued until plasma levels are available.[2]

N-acetylcysteine is the best available prophylactic antidote for prevention of acetaminophen-induced hepatotoxicity.[2] The NAC derivative of the naturally occurring amino acid L-cysteine constitutes the central portion of the glutathione molecule. The antidotal mechanism for NAC is not completely understood, although it is known that NAC is metabolized to cysteine, a glutathione pre-

Table 60-6 Antidotes

Antidote	Toxic Agent	Dose and Techniques for Administering	Comments
N-acetylcysteine (NAC)	Acetaminophen	Loading dose: 140 mg/kg Maintenance dose: 70 mg/kg every 4 h × 17 doses.	Most effective if given within 8 h. Ineffective after 24 h.
Physostigmine	Anticholinergics	0.5–2 mg IV slow administration (no faster than 1 mg per minute).	Possible indications: convulsions, severe hallucinations, hypertension, and arrhythmias not responding to standard measures. Side effects: convulsions, bradycardia. Use cautiously.
Oxygen	Carbon monoxide	100% oxygen until CO level less than 5%.	Side effects: patients on 100% oxygen for more than 24 h may develop oxygen toxicity.
Cyanide antidote kit: Amyl nitrite, sodium nitrite, and sodium thiosulfate	Cyanide Hydrogen sulfide	Amyl nitrite inhalant: Every 30 s until sodium nitrite administered. Sodium nitrite: Adult 300 mg IV. Sodium thiosulfate: 12.5 g IV after sodium nitrite.	Side effects: hypotension and methemoglobinemia. Sodium thiosulfate is inefficacious in hydrogen sulfide poisoning.
Methylene blue	Methemoglobinemia-inducing agents: Nitrites and related compounds available in fertilizers, aniline dyes, gunpowder, well water, and drugs such as phenacetin, Pyridium, antimalarials, and Dapsone.	0.1–0.2 mL/kg (1–2 mg/kg) 1% methylene blue slowly IV to reverse methemoglobinemia. May need to be repeated.	Note: Do not exceed 1½ times dose. Make sure methemoglobinemia levels are drawn before administering methylene blue as methemoglobinemia may be a side effect of large doses of methylene blue.
Atropine	Organophosphates (malathion, parathion) and carbamate insecticides (Sevin, etc.)	Adults: 2–5 mg IV. Repeat every 10–30 min as needed to obtain full atropinization.	Atropinization best indicated by clearing of bronchial and pulmonary secretions, not pupillary dilation.
2-PAM (Pralidoximine)	Organophosphate and carbamate (except carbaryl) insecticides	Adults: 1 g IV at 0.5 g/min or infused in 250 mL saline over 30 min. Repeat at intervals of 6–12 h if muscle weakness is not relieved.	Indicated for nicotinic and central effects as coma, convulsions, fasciculations, and profound muscle weakness. Give only after atropine. Early administration is probably more efficacious.

Adapted from Poisindex Information System Micromedex, Inc., Englewood, CO; and K. Wruk, Administering Emergency Antidotes to the Acutely Poisoned Patient, *Dimensions of Critical-Care Nursing*, 1, 206–211, 1982.

cursor. One possible mechanism of action is that the administration of NAC maintains protective levels of glutathione so that the reactive metabolite of acetaminophen will be detoxified by conjugation. NAC may also act to stabilize cell constituents, avoiding the deleterious effects of covalent binding between the hepatocyte and the toxic acetaminophen metabolite.[2]

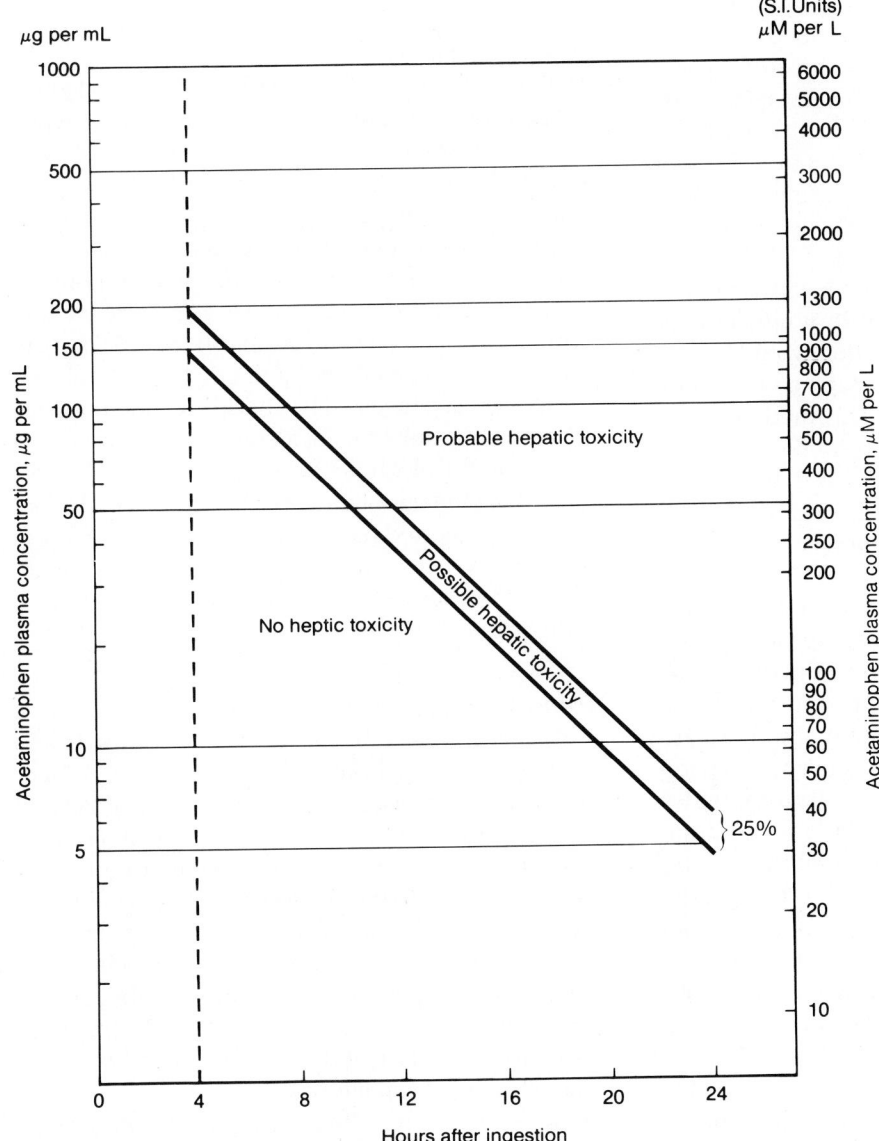

Figure 60-1 Rumack-Matthew nomogram for acetaminophen poisoning. (Used with permission from Poisindex Information Systems, Micromedex Incorporated, 1974–1985, Englewood, CO.)

Nursing Management

1. Poisoning: Potential for acetaminophen toxicity
2. Potential for fluid volume deficit

Following overdose, NAC has its greatest effectiveness if started within 8 h of exposure. No benefit of treatment is seen if NAC is given more than 24 h after exposure.[23] The NAC regimen is a loading dose of 140 mg/kg followed by 17 maintenance doses of 70 mg/kg given at 4-h intervals.[2] If a patient vomits within 1 h of any dose, that dose must be repeated. If emesis occurs more than 1 h after dosing, the next dose should be administered as scheduled. NAC is commercially available in 10% and 20% solutions containing 100 mg or 200 mg NAC per milliliter, respectively.

Currently, oral administration is the only method approved by the Federal Drug Administration (FDA) for NAC administration. When administering NAC, it should be diluted one to three, making a 5% mixture. To make NAC more palatable, it can be mixed with soda or fruit juice and served over ice in a covered container. If patients are comatose or unable to tolerate the medication by mouth due to vomiting, it may be given by nasogastric tube. For nasogastric administration, NAC need not be mixed with a diluent and can be given by slow nasogastric drip. Reported side effects of NAC are primarily nausea and vomiting.[3] Because many antiemetics are metabolized in the liver, their use is not routinely recommended.

The use of NAC concomitantly with activated charcoal is controversial. Previously, it was thought that activated charcoal administration would hinder NAC absorption. Before NAC therapy could begin, gastric lavage needed to be performed until all charcoal had been removed from the stomach. However, recent studies have challenged this method of treatment. Current recommendations are to avoid the use of NAC within 1 h of charcoal administration.[24]

Many patients experience vomiting as a consequence of acetaminophen overdose or as a side effect of NAC, and health care providers often wish to use an intravenous NAC preparation. NAC is not FDA approved for IV administration and there are no commercially available pyrogen-free preparations. Use of intravenous NAC is currently under investigation. Pyrogen-free preparations are available at eight poison centers throughout the country in a multicenter clinical trial. The location of the nearest participating center can be obtained from 1-800-525-6115. Information about oral administration is also available at this number.

Evaluation

If the first acetaminophen level reveals toxicity, NAC must be continued even if subsequent levels are plotted as nontoxic on the nomogram.[3] NAC effectiveness is judged best by serial determinations of liver function tests, including an SGOT, SGPT, total bilirubin, and prothrombin time. Elevations seen within 48 to 72 h of the overdose should begin to decline within 96 h. Patients whose treatment with NAC was delayed or who were not treated may develop hepatotoxicity with a greater increase in liver function tests. Plasma levels will remain elevated for long periods of time. Death is rare from acetaminophen-induced hepatotoxicity. Survivors' liver function usually returns to normal on subsequent evaluations.

Alcohols

Methanol, Ethylene Glycol

Methanol, also known as methyl or wood alcohol, is used commercially as a solvent, antifreeze, windshield washer fluid, and canned fuel (Sterno).[3] Ethylene glycol is a colorless, odorless, sweet-tasting, water-soluble liquid. It is in such commercial products as detergents, paints, cosmetics, and solar collection systems, and most commonly is used as a deicer and antifreeze.[3] Deicers and antifreeze may contain from 70 to 95 percent ethylene glycol. Methanol and ethylene glycol may be accidentally ingested by children or intentionally ingested by adults in suicide attempts or used as a substitute for alcoholic beverages.

Toxic metabolites formed when these products are ingested cause the symptoms of these poisonings. Management of ethylene glycol or methanol intoxication focuses on halting production of toxic metabolites.

Pathophysiology of Methanol Toxicity   Methanol is readily absorbed by the gastrointestinal tract and distributed throughout the tissues. Although there have been reports of toxicity following inhalation and skin absorption, ingestion is the main route of exposure and the one most likely to produce symptoms.[25] Methanol is slowly metabolized in the liver by the enzyme alcohol dehydrogenase via formaldehyde to formic acid. The oxidation of methanol proceeds independently of the plasma concentration at a rate one-fifth that of ethanol.[26] Complete oxidation and excretion may take several days. The approximate half-life of methanol in the body is about 8 h.[27] Three to 5 percent of ingested methanol is excreted unchanged by the kidneys, and a small amount is excreted by the lungs.[2,3]

Formaldehyde and formic acid, the metabolites of methanol, are highly toxic and account for the metabolic acidosis, ocular symptoms, and other effects seen following ingestion. The local production of formaldehyde in the retina may be responsible for optic papillitis and retinal edema with subsequent blindness.[2] Toxicity from methanol poisoning is extremely variable. Blindness has occurred following ingestion of 4 mL of absolute methanol. In one patient, death occurred after ingestion of 15 mL of a 40% solution, whereas another patient survived after 500 mL of the same mixture.[3]

Pathophysiology of Ethylene Glycol Toxicity

Ethylene glycol is rapidly absorbed by the gastrointestinal tract, whereas topical and dermal absorption is thought to be minimal. Toxicity from inhalation is unlikely to occur except at high temperatures. Ethylene glycol is metabolized by alcohol dehydrogenase into several toxic organic acids (Fig. 60-2). These metabolites (especially glycolic acid and oxalic acid) are responsible for the central nervous system, metabolic, cardiopulmonary, and renal symptoms following ethylene glycol ingestion.

Toxicity from ethylene glycol ingestion is caused by tissue destruction from deposition of calcium oxalate crystals and the production of severe acidosis due to organic acid accumulation. As a consequence of the oxalic acid deposition in the kidneys and other tissues, calcium ions are chelated forming calcium oxalate, and hypocalcemia may occur.[2] Oxalic acid may also precipitate in the urine as calcium oxalate crystals. These crystals may assume many shapes, including octahedral (envelopelike), prismatic (spindles), or dumbbell shapes. Because only 3 to 10 percent of ethylene glycol is converted to oxalic acid, renal toxicity is not entirely explained by the formation of this metabolite. Glycolic aldehyde, glycolic acid, and glyoxylic acid may also cause significant renal tubular damage and may account for renal insufficiency occurring in the absence of renal oxalosis.[6]

The central nervous system depression associated with ethylene glycol ingestion may be caused by unchanged ethylene glycol or the aldehyde metabolite concentration (glycoaldehyde). Glycoaldehyde is at its highest concentration 6 to 12 h following ethylene glycol ingestion when central nervous system symptoms are most severe.[2]

The minimal toxic or lethal dose of ethylene glycol is not well defined but has been approximated at 1.4 mL/kg or about 100 mL for a 70 kg adult. Death has been reported from as little as 60 mL, while ingestion of 240 mL has resulted in survival.[3]

Clinical Manifestations of Methanol Toxicity

Toxicity from methanol poisoning may develop after a latent period of 18 to 24 h and typically includes three major symptoms: central nervous system depression, severe anion gap metabolic acidosis, and a number of reversible or irreversible optic changes.[3] The toxicity is related to the degree of metabolic acidosis and, therefore, to the time period between exposure and treatment.

Following methanol ingestion, neurological symptoms mimic an ethanol hangover and include malaise, headache, dizziness, vertigo, and weakness. Profound coma and seizures may occur in severe exposures. Anion gap metabolic acidosis is one of the most significant clinical findings. It may be delayed for 18 to 24 h, especially with concurrent ethanol ingestion. Other symptoms include gastrointestinal distress, dyspnea, tachypnea, and tachycardia.[3,28]

Visual abnormalities seen in methanol poisoning include blurred or double vision, constricted visual fields, spots in the eyes, and reduced visual acuity.[29] These ocular abnormalities are often delayed for 12 to 24 h after ingestion. Funduscopic findings may show peripapillary edema, hyperemia of the optic disk, or retinal edema. Permanent blindness frequently occurs, although blindness has occasionally resolved.[3]

Clinical Manifestations of Ethylene Glycol Toxicity

Ethylene glycol intoxication characteristically occurs in three phases: (1) central nervous system depression and metabolic acidosis, (2) cardiopulmonary complications, and (3) renal failure. The initial phase occurs between 30 min and 12 h after ingestion. Symptoms include ataxia, slurred speech, somnolence, nausea, and vomiting. Coma, convulsions, and death may result after large ingestions. The central nervous system findings resemble those of ethanol inebriation but without ethanol odor,

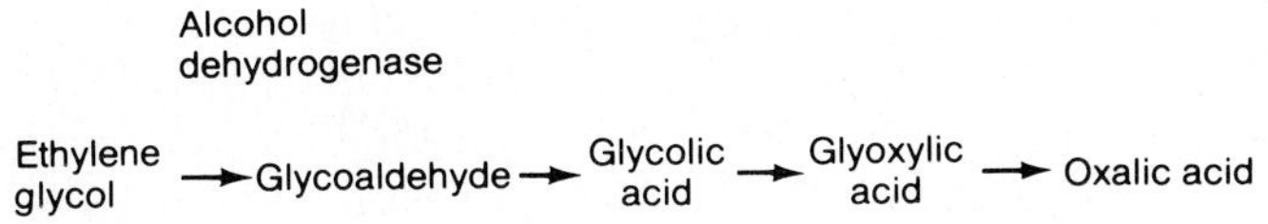

Alcohol
dehydrogenase

Ethylene glycol $\longrightarrow$ Glycoaldehyde $\longrightarrow$ Glycolic acid $\longrightarrow$ Glyoxylic acid $\longrightarrow$ Oxalic acid

Figure 60-2 Ethylene glycol metabolism. (From Poisindex Information Systems, Micromedex Incorporated, 1974–1985, Englewood, CO.)

unless ethanol has been concurrently ingested. Metabolic acidosis usually accompanies central nervous system depression but may develop later. Low levels of serum bicarbonate, decreased CO_2, increased anion gap (12 to 16 mEq or more) and tachypnea with Kussmaul's respirations are characteristic of metabolic acidosis with respiratory compensation. Calcium hyperoxaluria, hematuria, and proteinuria are frequent findings. Since oxalate crystals are not invariably seen, their absence does not rule out ethylene glycol poisoning.[27]

The clinical course following an ethylene glycol ingestion proceeds to stage 2 if no treatment is initiated. Stage 2 usually occurs 12 to 36 h after ingestion and is characterized by progressive respiratory distress and pulmonary edema secondary to congestive heart failure. Death occurs most frequently in this stage.

If the patient survives the first two stages, the clinical course proceeds to stage 3. This usually occurs 2 or 3 days after ingestion and is characterized by renal insufficiency. Flank pain and tenderness with oliguria, proteinuria, and anuria are common. Timing of occurrence of the phases is delayed if ethanol is concurrently ingested with ethylene glycol.

Medical Management   When a patient is diagnosed with methanol or ethylene glycol ingestion, therapy begins immediately. Measures to prevent absorption can be performed simultaneously with supportive care. Sodium bicarbonate is administered to correct acidosis and seizures are treated with intravenous diazepam (Valium). Serum methanol, ethylene glycol, and ethanol levels are monitored.

Ethanol therapy is instituted to prevent metabolism of methanol or ethylene glycol to toxic metabolites. Alcohol dehydrogenase (ADH) has approximately 20 times as much affinity for ethanol as methanol, and, therefore, administering ethanol effectively inhibits oxidation of methanol to formaldehyde and formic acid.[26] ADH has a similar affinity for ethanol compared to ethylene glycol. Ethanol competitively inhibits ADH from metabolizing ethylene glycol to its toxic metabolites.[3] If ethanol therapy is indicated and the patient has a positive blood ethanol level, the loading dose must be modified to avoid iatrogenic ethanol intoxica-

tion. Hemodialysis is also effective in removing circulating methanol or ethylene glycol.[27,30] The ethanol infusion should be continued during dialysis.

In methanol poisoning, formic acid is metabolized to carbon monoxide and water via a folate-dependent system. Administration of folic acid or leucovorin (an active metabolite of folic acid) may enhance formic acid elimination. Following ethylene glycol metabolism, the excessive amount of glyoxylate may deplete body stores of pyridoxine. Pyridoxine is administered because it is essential for the conversion of glyoxylate to nontoxic glycine. Thiamine administration may also be necessary because it converts glyoxylate to the nontoxic metabolite, alpha-hydroxy-beta-ketoadipate.[3]

Nursing Management

1. Poisoning, potential for methanol or ethylene glycol poisoning
2. Breathing pattern, ineffective
3. Alteration in cardiac output: decreased
4. Impaired gas exchange
5. Alteration in tissue perfusion: renal

Management of a patient who has ingested methanol or ethylene glycol begins with basic or advanced life support and prevention of further poison absorption. Since both products are rapidly and well absorbed, gastric emptying and administration of activated charcoal and a cathartic need to be instituted as soon as possible to be effective.

Arterial blood gases, serum electrolytes, and bicarbonate provide data useful in determining the severity of the poisoning. A pH of less than 7.0 and bicarbonate less than 7 mEq/L are common following severe intoxication. Methanol or ethylene glycol levels greater than 50 mg/dL indicate a serious exposure. Methanol and ethylene glycol (as well as ethanol and isopropyl alcohol) are osmotically active and may cause a disparity between measured and calculated plasma osmolality. Determination of the osmolar gap is especially valuable when methanol or ethylene glycol levels are not readily available.[3] To determine the calculated osmolality the following formula is used:

$$2 \times Na + \frac{Glucose}{18} + \frac{BUN}{2.8} + \frac{ETOH}{4.6}$$

Ethanol is administered to prevent the breakdown of methanol or ethylene glycol to their toxic metabolites (Table 60-7). Ethanol therapy is indicated in any patient with a plasma level between 20 mg/dL and 50 mg/dL, and any symptomatic patient with a history of methanol or ethylene glycol ingestion. The blood ethanol level is maintained between 100 to 130 mg/dL during therapy. Ethanol may cause hypoglycemia.[3] The blood glucose needs to be monitored closely. Patients who have concurrently ingested methanol or ethylene glycol along with ethanol may have a normal acid-base status despite extremely elevated levels. With these patients, ethanol therapy should be considered until methanol or ethylene glycol levels can be determined.[3]

Hemodialysis is effective in removing methanol or ethylene glycol from the plasma.[27,30] Indications for its use include a blood methanol or ethylene glycol level greater than 50 mg/dL, a severe acid-base or fluid and electrolyte disturbance despite conventional therapy, and renal failure. The ethanol infusion is continued during hemodialysis and increased as needed to maintain the blood ethanol level at 100 to 130 mg/dL. If ethanol is not added to the dialysate, the maintenance infusion during dialysis is an additional 91 mg per hour intravenously of 10% ETOH solution.[27]

Some patients may have previously been taking disulfiram and ingested methanol or ethylene glycol. Ethanol therapy needs to be administered to these patients if there are signs and symptoms of severe poisoning (acidemia and blood methanol or ethylene glycol levels greater than 20 mg/dL). Ethanol is administered cautiously while assessing for the "Antabuse reaction" (flushing, sweating, severe hypotension, and cardiac arrhythmias). The ECG and vital signs are closely monitored and administration of IV fluids and vasopressors may be necessary for severe hypotension.[3]

Evaluation   To evaluate the effectiveness of therapy in patients poisoned by methanol or ethylene glycol, assessment includes vital signs, orientation, acid-base status, and methanol or ethylene glycol blood levels. When evaluating management outcomes specifically, assessment also includes visual fields in methanol poisoning, and renal function in ethylene glycol poisoning.

Table 60-7 Ethanol Therapy for Methanol/Ethylene Glycol Poisoning

Loading dose: 7.6–10 mL/kg IV of 10% ETOH in D_5W over 1 h
Maintenance dose: Volume of 10% ETOH needed IV

Average	Administer 1.40 mL/kg per hour
Chronic drinker	Administer 1.96 mL/kg per hour
Nondrinker	Administer 0.83 mL/kg per hour

Note: A 5% alcohol solution for intravenous infusion is commercially available; however, excessive volumes of fluids are required to maintain adequate blood alcohol levels.
Adapted from Poisindex Information System, Micromedex, Inc., Englewood, CO.

Ethanol, Isopropyl Alcohol

Ethanol (ethyl alcohol) and isopropyl alcohol are central nervous system depressants. Ethanol is found in alcoholic beverages and medicines, and special denatured ethanol is found in colognes, perfumes, aftershaves, other cosmetics, and rubbing alcohol. Isopropyl alcohol is a common ingredient in rubbing alcohol (70 percent isopropyl alcohol) and cleaning agents. Ethanol may be accidentally or intentionally ingested by adults in suicide attempts, alone or with other medications. Toxicity is frequently seen when ethanol is ingested as a recreational beverage. Isopropyl alcohol, ingested accidentally or intentionally, may also be consumed as a substitute for an alcoholic beverage.

Pathophysiology of Ethanol Toxicity   Ethanol is rapidly absorbed from the gastrointestinal tract. Vaporized ethanol may be absorbed via the lungs while absorption through the skin is negligible. Several factors may delay absorption of ethanol from the stomach, including the presence of food, the concentration of ethanol, and the time period in which ethanol is consumed. Absorption from the small intestine is rapid and complete, and is independent of the presence of food. Peak blood ethanol concentrations may be achieved 30 min after ingestion.[3,31]

Ethanol is metabolized in the liver by alcohol dehydrogenase to acetaldehyde.[31] Only 2 to 10 percent of ingested ethanol is eliminated unchanged by the lungs and kidneys.[3] The rate of oxidation is constant with time and increases little with increased concentration in the blood (zero order kinetics).[32] The amount of ethanol oxidized is proportional to body weight and liver weight.

This slow and constant rate of metabolism limits the amount of ethanol that can be consumed over time without intoxication due to ethanol accumulation.

Ethanol is not generally considered a serious toxic agent, but may have serious effects. Each ounce of whiskey, glass of wine, or bottle of beer can raise the blood ethanol concentration approximately 25 mg/dL. Blood ethanol levels below 50 mg/dL rarely produce marked sensory or motor impairment.[3] Concentrations of 150 to 300 mg/dL are generally associated with mental confusion, ataxia, exaggerated emotional status, and muscular incoordination.[3] Most fatalities from ethanol occur with levels greater than 400 mg/dL.[3] The lethal dose of ethanol for adults is 5 mg/kg to 8 mg/kg. Alcoholics are more tolerant of higher ethanol levels than abstainers.

Pathophysiology of Isopropyl Alcohol Toxicity
Isopropyl alcohol causes greater central nervous system depression than ethanol at similar blood levels.[2] It may produce toxic symptoms following ingestion, inhalation, or dermal exposures. Isopropyl alcohol is oxidized to acetone which is then metabolized to acetate and CO_2. The acetone may contribute to central nervous system depression.[3] The metabolism of isopropyl alcohol is much slower than ethanol.[2]

Toxic effects from isopropyl alcohol are usually seen at blood levels between 50 to 100 mg/dL. Levels of 150 mg/dL are associated with deep coma and levels greater than 200 mg/dL have been reported to cause death. Ingestion of 3 ounces of 70 percent isopropyl alcohol by a 70-kg person may produce a blood level of 100 mg/dL.[3]

Clinical Manifestations of Ethanol Toxicity Ethanol poisoning may produce nausea, vomiting, central nervous system depression, acid-base disturbances, hypoglycemia, and respiratory depression. Central nervous system depression and peripheral vasodilation may lead to hypothermia. Deep tendon reflexes may also be absent. Hypoglycemia resulting in convulsions is a serious complication of acute ethanol intoxication, especially in children and chronic alcoholics. Moderate metabolic acidosis may occur from increased production of lactate and fatty acids. Few cases will progress to frank keto-

acidosis. Death usually results from respiratory failure.[3,31]

Clinical Manifestations of Isopropyl Alcohol Toxicity The signs and symptoms of isopropyl alcohol ingestion are similar to those of ethanol ingestion. Within hours, lethargy, hypothermia, and coma occur. Areflexia, deep coma, hypotension, and respiratory failure may follow severe intoxication. Isopropyl alcohol has a stronger irritant effect on the stomach than ethanol, which can result in hemorrhagic gastritis and an associated decreased hematocrit. Although hypoglycemia is uncommon, the blood glucose needs to be monitored closely. Hyperglycemia has been reported in adults.[2,3]

Medical Management Following an ethanol or isopropyl alcohol overdose, treatment measures include maintaining fluid balance, blood pressure, and airway. Sodium bicarbonate is administered as needed to treat acidosis. In an ethanol overdose, IV glucose may be administered as indicated by the blood glucose level. If the patient's symptoms do not respond to standard measures, hemodialysis is effective in increasing the elimination of ethanol or isopropyl alcohol.

Nursing Management

1. Poisoning: Potential for ethanol or isopropyl alcohol toxicity
2. Ineffective breathing pattern
3. Impaired gas exchange
4. Alteration in tissue perfusion: peripheral

Basic life support and prevention of absorption are instituted following ingestion of ethanol and isopropyl alcohol. Because ethanol and isopropyl alcohol are rapidly absorbed liquids, emesis or lavage and administration of activated charcoal and a cathartic are most effective soon after ingestion. To avoid aspiration of vomitus, the patient is placed in a semilateral decubitus position with the head forward and mouth down.

In ethanol or isopropyl alcohol ingestion, management is primarily directed at supportive care. The patient should be assessed for hypotension and the blood pressure should be maintained with IV fluids, semi-Trendelenberg position, and vasopressors as needed. In severe intoxication, the patient's respiratory functions are closely monitored by assessing respiratory rate, tissue perfusion, and arterial blood gases.

In ethanol ingestion, the blood glucose needs to be monitored frequently because hypoglycemia may be delayed for several hours.[3] Monitoring blood ethanol and isopropyl alcohol concentrations closely may indicate the seriousness of the exposure. Concurrent ingestion of other sedatives or tranquilizers may precipitate symptoms at substantially lower blood ethanol concentrations.[3] Following isopropyl alcohol ingestion, the blood and urine can be checked for acetone.[3] Because both ethanol and isopropyl alcohol ingestions may result in acidosis, the acid-base status is monitored closely.

Hemodialysis may be effective for patients with excessive blood ethanol or isopropyl alcohol levels, impaired hepatic function, and those unresponsive to standard therapy.[2,3] It is unusual for a patient to require hemodialysis in ethanol poisoning.

Because the patient's sensorium may be altered following an ethanol or isopropyl alcohol ingestion, it is important to protect the patient from self-harm. Side rails need to be kept up and patients should be located in a room close to the nurses' station. Mental status is assessed frequently to guide appropriate interventions.

Evaluation   The patient is evaluated for his or her response to medical and nursing interventions following ethanol or isopropyl alcohol exposure. The patient should be assessed for normal pulse, blood pressure, and respiratory function, blood or isopropyl levels below 50 mg/dL, improved mental status, and normal electrolytes and acid-base status.

Carbon Monoxide

Carbon monoxide (CO) is an insidious poison because it has no odor or taste. Carbon monoxide is produced during incomplete combustion of a carbon-containing fuel. Four common sources of carbon monoxide are automobile exhaust fumes, burning charcoal, poorly ventilated wood or coal stoves, and malfunctioning furnaces. Carbon monoxide is present in all fires and may be a hazard to firefighters. Natural gas does not contain carbon monoxide but it may be produced if the gas is burned without sufficient oxygen. Methylene chloride is metabolized in vivo to carbon monoxide.[33] An adequate history of the exposure may help to confirm the diagnosis such as where the patient was found, activity at the time of exposure, if any combustible fuels were being used, and if there was adequate ventilation.

Pathophysiology

Carbon monoxide binds rapidly, specifically, and avidly with hemoglobin in erythrocytes to form carboxyhemoglobin (COHB). The affinity of hemoglobin for carbon monoxide is over 200 times that of oxygen. The formation of COHB has two effects. It reduces the carrying capacity of hemoglobin for oxygen and it inhibits the release of oxygen to all tissues. The result of carbon monoxide inhalation is hypoxia. Because the brain and the heart are most dependent on oxygen, the major toxic symptoms are noted in these organs. Tissue hypoxia may, however, be seen in all systems.[2]

Carbon monoxide is absorbed and eliminated by the lungs. The half-life of carbon monoxide in room air is 5 to 6 h. With 100 percent supplemental oxygen the half-life of carbon monoxide can be reduced to 40 to 90 min. Hyperbaric oxygen decreases the half-life of carbon monoxide to less than 30 min and increases the delivery of oxygen to hypoxic tissues, thus diminishing the severity of cerebral edema and other central nervous system sequelae.[2] Carbon monoxide crosses the placenta and the fetal concentration of carbon monoxide may be 10 to 15 percent greater than the carbon monoxide concentration of the mother.

Clinical Manifestations

Neurological symptoms of carbon monoxide poisoning include headache, dizziness, coma, seizures, thermoregulation abnormalities, and cerebral edema. Cardiac symptoms may occur rapidly or may be delayed for several days. These include ECG changes such as ST segment depression, T wave abnormalities, atrial fibrillation, and intraventricular conduction block.[3] Tachycardia, hypotension, and peripheral vasodilation also may occur. COHB increases myocardial blood flow, an important implication in patients with coronary artery disease because myocardial oxygen supply is already reduced.[2] Respiratory symptoms noted include hyperventilation, dyspnea, and pulmonary edema. Retinal hemorrhages, decreased visual acuity and transient hearing loss have been reported. Other signs of COHB poisoning include hyperglycemia, albuminuria, cutaneous lesions from erythema and edema to blister and bullae formation, and alopecia. Residual or delayed neurological effects include mask-like facies, mental deterioration, abnormal reflexes, incontinence, hypertonicity, and gait disturbances. Neuropsychiatric sequelae such as personality changes and memory impairment may be noted.[3]

Medical Management

The patient is moved immediately from the contaminated atmosphere and basic life support is begun. One hundred percent oxygen is administered by a tightly fitting face mask. A carboxyhemoglobin level is obtained immediately, and 2 to 4 h after starting treatment. Seizures are treated with IV diazepam. Acidosis is treated with sodium bicarbonate. Patients who have or have had neurological signs or symptoms, an abnormal ECG, acidosis, or a COHB level above 30 percent should be admitted to an intensive care unit (ICU) and considered for hyperbaric oxygen therapy.[3] If the patient has a history of cardiovascular disease, admission to an ICU is necessary with a COHB level of 15 percent or greater. Complications of carbon monoxide exposure include cerebral edema and noncardiogenic pulmonary edema.[3]

Nursing Management

Following carbon monoxide exposure, 100 percent oxygen is administered by a tightly fitting face mask or endotracheal tube. Arterial blood gases are closely monitored. If the patient has been comatose but has regained consciousness, he or she is managed as a severe exposure regardless of the COHB level.[3] The COHB may not represent the peak level because some treatment has often been done before the level was drawn. If the patient is having seizure activity, IV diazepam may be administered. The ECG is monitored for signs of myocardial ischemia and arrhythmias.[3]

Indications for hyperbaric oxygen may include coma at any time during the exposure, seizures, syncope, any neurological deficits, severe metabolic acidosis, cardiovascular involvement such as hypotension, shock, angina, or ECG evidence of ischemia. The need for hyperbaric oxygen is controversial in patients with COHB levels above 30 percent with minimal or no symptoms.[3]

The physician should be notified if the patient has signs of increased intracranial pressure. It may be necessary to hyperventilate the patient with 100 percent oxygen via an endotracheal tube to keep the arterial P_{CO_2} level at 25 to 30 mmHg. Parenteral fluids need to be limited to two-thirds to three-fourths of normal maintenance for the patient's weight.[3]

If pulmonary edema develops, arterial blood gases are monitored closely. If the P_{O_2} cannot be maintained above 50 mmHg with inspiration of 60 percent oxygen by face mask or by mechanical ventilation, the physician may begin positive end-expiratory pressure (PEEP) in intubated patients or continuous positive airway pressure (CPAP) in non-intubated patients. Fluid status should be monitored with a central venous line or a Swan-Ganz catheter. Fluids are administered carefully to avoid a net positive fluid balance.

If the patient is pregnant, a fetal monitor is utilized. The patient is maintained on oxygen even after the COHB level is zero because oxygen is needed about five times as long in the fetal circulation to assure elimination of carbon monoxide.[3]

In accidental exposures, the patient must not be released until the causative factor has been corrected. For intentional exposures, mental health counseling should be arranged.

Evaluation

Efficacy of treatment may be assessed by noting improvement in the level of consciousness, cessation of seizures, normalization of blood gases, stabilization of vital signs, and a COHB of zero.

Cyanide

Few poisons are more lethal than cyanide. Death may occur within minutes of an inhalation exposure. Successful management of cyanide poisoning requires accurate assessment of the clinical symptoms, patient decontamination, basic and advanced life support, and prompt administration of the antidote kit.

Pathophysiology

Hydrocyanic acid (HCN, hydrogen cyanide) is one of the most toxic forms of cyanide.[2] It is used in industry as a fumigant and rodenticide and is liberated when products containing carbon, hydrogen, oxygen, and nitrogen are burned. Wool, silk, nylon, polyacrylonitrile, and polyurethane are all combustible materials that liberate HCN by pyrolysis.[34] The soluble salts of HCN (potassium or sodium cyanide) react with acids to also release HCN gas.

Small amounts of cyanide normally enter the body in foods and tobacco smoke. Most severe poisonings occur with an exposure to sodium or potassium cyanide and are usually associated with a suicide or homicide attempt. Accidental exposures to cyanide may occur in the workplace and be seen in electroplaters, metal polishers, and firefighters. Accidental exposure may also occur from eating cyanide-containing food products such as amygdalin found in bitter almonds and in apricot and peach seeds, and from drugs containing cyanide such as Laetrile and nitroprusside.[34]

Cyanide may be absorbed by inhalation of dust or fumes, by ingestion, or by eye contact. Death may occur within minutes after inhalation of a sufficient concentration of HCN gas.[2,34] Tissues are unable to utilize the oxygen present, causing venous blood to remain bright red. Since cytochrome oxidase is present in most cells, many organs are affected.

Rhodanase is a naturally occurring enzyme which detoxifies cyanide by complexing it with sulfur from sulfane pools to form nontoxic thiocyanate. Thiocyanate is excreted in the urine. Rhodanase is found in the mitochondria of the liver, and, to a lesser extent, in the kidneys and plasma. Because rhodanase is abundant in the body, it is the limited availability of sulfur that determines the amount of cyanide that can be detoxified. When large amounts of cyanide are absorbed, the metabolism of cyanide depletes the sulfur pool, allowing unmetabolized cyanide to bind to cytochrome oxidase.[35]

Cyanide poisoning may result from sodium nitroprusside administration. Adverse effects include those due to its hemodynamic effects as well as symptoms associated with cyanide intoxication.

Sodium nitroprusside contains five cyanide molecules. The liberation of cyanide has been postulated to result from rapid breakdown of the parent compound by free and intracellur hemoglobin to methemoglobin and an unstable nitroprusside radical via a nonenzymatic reaction, such that a split of the radical releases cyanide. One cyanide molecule reacts with methemoglobin to form cyanmethemoglobin, and the remaining four free cyanide ions may be converted to thiocyanate by rhodanase or may bind to cytochrome oxidase. Elevated cyanide levels from sodium nitroprusside are dependent on the total dose, rate of infusion, and length of therapy.[36]

Amygdalin is found in Laetrile and some fruit pits, plants, and berries. If sufficient quantities are ingested, symptoms of cyanide intoxication may ensue. Breakdown of the amygdalin to cyanide depends on the enzyme emulsin, contained in the fruit pit, or beta glucosidase, an enzyme found in the gastrointestinal tract. There may be a delay of symptoms after ingestion of amygdalin-containing products because emulsin does not maximally hydrolyze amygdalin until it enters the alkaline environment of the small intestine.[37]

The toxic or lethal dose of cyanide is not well defined. The lethal dose has been reported to be 50 mg of absolute cyanide acid, 200 to 300 mg potassium sodium salt, and 200 to 300 ppm of HCN gas.[2,3,34]

Clinical Manifestations

Rapid progression of symptoms is usually seen in patients following cyanide inhalation, injection, or sometimes oral administration of cyanide-containing liquids. With ingestion of the solid forms of cyanide, crystals or capsules, death may occur within 30 min or be delayed for several hours.[34]

Initial symptoms of cyanide exposure include giddiness, headache, palpitations, and dyspnea, which may progress to agitation, stupor, apnea, convulsions, and death. Vomiting and abdominal pain also may occur. An odor of almonds may be noted on the breath or vomitus, although 30 to 50 percent of the population are incapable of detecting this.[2,3,34]

Cyanide directly affects the respiratory center in the medulla, causing an early increase in the rate and depth of respirations, which later become slow and labored. This may progress to apnea. Noncardiogenic pulmonary edema also has been reported.[3,34] There is an initial rise in the blood pressure with a reflex bradycardia which may be followed by hypotension and tachycardia. The ECG may show marked ST segment elevation or depression, and cardiac arrhythmias secondary to hypoxia may ensue.[3]

A high anion gap metabolic acidosis (lactic acid) is frequently present following cyanide exposure. A markedly reduced A-V$_{O_2}$ difference may be present in simultaneously drawn arterial and central venous blood gases. On funduscopic examination, equally red retinal arteries and veins may be noted. Death usually results from respiratory arrest. Antidotal therapy may be effective as long as there is a heartbeat.[3]

Symptoms of chronic cyanide poisoning are characterized by hoarseness, conjunctivitis, anorexia, weight loss, weakness, and altered mental status. Tobacco amblyopia and various ataxic neuropathies have also been attributed to chronic cyanide exposures.[38-41] Sodium nitroprusside-induced toxicity is characterized by metabolic acidosis, tachycardia, dyspnea, vomiting, dizziness, headache, ataxia, and loss of consciousness. An increased tolerance to the pharmacologic effects of the drug may be noted despite an increase in the dose.[36]

Medical Management

Emergency medical treatment of cyanide poisoning includes basic life support, administration of 100 percent oxygen, and administration of the cyanide antidote kit. Oxygen therapy may reverse the cyanide–cytochrome oxidase bond, and may facilitate conversion of cyanide to thiocyanate with sodium thiosulfate administration.[42] The combination of 100 percent oxygen and thiosulfate–nitrate therapy appears to be more effective than thiosulfate alone in cyanide toxicity.[43]

Hyperbaric oxygen therapy (HBO) may improve the clinical outcome of cyanide poisoning victims who fail to respond to other therapy. HBO may also be indicated for those patients poisoned by both cyanide and carbon monoxide from smoke inhalation.[3,43]

Administration of the cyanide antidote kit may save a severely poisoned patient. The Lilly cyanide antidote kit contains amyl nitrite, sodium nitrite, and sodium thiosulfate. The current theory regarding the mechanism of action of the cyanide antidote kit is based on the fact that cyanide has a high affinity for ferric ions (Fe^3). The largest store of iron in the body is in the hemoglobin in the ferrous state (Fe^2). By converting hemoglobin (Fe^2) to methemoglobin (Fe^3), the methemoglobin (Fe^3) competes for the cyanide ion to form cyanmethemoglobin, sparing the essential enzyme system cytochrome oxidase.[2] This mechanism has, however, been disputed by recent animal research.[44] The conversion is accomplished pharmacologically by administering the first two drugs in the cyanide antidote kit, amyl nitrite perles by inhalation, and sodium nitrite intravenously. The cyanmethemoglobin molecule slowly dissociates to cyanide and methemoglobin. The third medication in the antidote kit, sodium thiosulfate, is administered to provide adequate amounts of sulfur for rhodanase to detoxify the cyanide to thiocyanate. Newer antidotes such as hydroxycobalamin and dicobalt EDTA (Kelocyanor) are not currently available in the United States.[3,34] Hydroxycobalamin has been shown to be effective in preventing nitroprusside-induced cyanide toxicity by forming the compound cyanocobalamin (vitamin B$_{12}$) which is then excreted in the urine.[36]

Important laboratory work after cyanide poisoning includes monitoring arterial and venous blood gases, electrolytes, serum lactate and pyruvate levels, cyanide, and thiocyanate levels. When administering the cyanide antidote kit, methemoglobin levels should be monitored closely. For excess methemoglobinemia, methylene blue is not recommended because it may release cyanide from the cyanomethemoglobin complex. Cyanide and thiocyanate levels may be measured but the results take too long for guidance of initial therapy.

Nursing Management

Basic life support is the first intervention when managing a patient exposed to cyanide. To prevent self-poisoning, it is essential to avoid direct mouth-to-mouth resuscitation or contact with cyanide-contaminated emesis, clothes, or skin. Symptomatic management includes assisted ventilation with 100 percent oxygen, anticonvulsants to control seizures, and support of pulse and blood pressure with atropine, intravenous fluids, and vasopressors when required.

In severe cyanide poisonings, the cyanide antidote kit is administered. The amyl nitrite perles are given by inhalation 30 s of every minute while an intravenous line is established. A new amyl nitrate perle must be used every 3 min. Sodium nitrite in an adult dose of 300 mg is administered intravenously. The sodium nitrite is followed by intravenous administration of 12.5 g of sodium thiosulfate. If symptoms persist, sodium nitrite may be repeated at one-half the initial dose after 30 min. While administering the nitrites, the patient is closely monitored for hypotension and excessive methemoglobinemia. Nitrite-induced methemoglobinemia does not carry oxygen. Levels of 30 to 40 percent are potentially harmful while levels greater than 60 percent cause tissue hypoxia.[37] Use of proper doses of nitrites prevents excessive methemoglobinemia. Slow intravenous administration with careful blood pressure monitoring precludes development of hypotension.

Prevention of absorption by gastric lavage may be indicated following oral cyanide exposures. Induction of emesis with syrup of ipecac may delay removal of gastric contents and increase the risk of aspiration. Activated charcoal may be administered, although cyanide is absorbed so rapidly that activated charcoal may be of little value.[3]

Interpretation of the patient's arterial and venous blood gases, electrolytes, and % O_2 saturation are important in assessment. Laboratory values suggestive of cyanide poisoning are:

Arterial P_{O_2}: Normal

Central venous measures % O_2 saturation: Elevated (greater than 70 percent approaches arterial % O_2 saturation)

Arterial pH: Low (acidotic)

Electrolytes: Anion gap present (greater than 12 to 16)

Calculated arterial % O_2 saturation: Normal (greater than 90 percent)

Measured arterial % O_2 saturation: Decreased (less than 90 percent)

To prevent cyanide poisoning during nitroprusside therapy, excessive doses and high rates of administration of the drug are avoided.[36] The patient is closely monitored for symptoms of nitroprusside-induced cyanide poisoning such as an increase in aerobic metabolism evidenced as base deficits, increased serum lactate, or other evidence of metabolic acidosis.

Evaluation

Appropriate medical and nursing interventions following cyanide exposure are indicated by the following parameters: stable vital signs, improved mental status, normal cardiac rhythm, normal electrolytes, and acid-base balance. The effectiveness of the cyanide antidote kit is based on the cessation of symptoms due to cyanide toxicity.

Cyclic Antidepressants

Since the introduction of tricyclic antidepressants for the treatment of depressive illnesses in the late 1950s, the incidence of overdose with these drugs has steadily increased. Eight drugs were originally developed for use as antidepressants: amitriptyline, clomipramine, desipramine, doxepin, imipramine, nortriptyline, protriptyline, and trimipramine. Because of their chemical structure, they are collectively called tricyclic antidepressants (TCA). Because of the toxic effects of the original TCAs, newer agents have been developed that are reportedly safer but as effective for treating depressive illnesses. The three newer drugs marketed in the United States are trazadone, amoxapine, and maprotiline.

Pathophysiology

Clinical manifestations of overdoses of TCAs stem from four pharmacological mechanisms of action which are not entirely separate nor completely understood. First, TCAs have anticholinergic properties which increase heart rate and blood pressure due to competitive acetylcholine blockade at cholinergic receptors. This mechanism results in sinus tachycardia which is usually seen early and may be the only manifestation of cardiac involvement.[45] The effects of the anticholinergic properties have little influence on later symptoms of cardiotoxicity because cholinergic innervation to the ventricles is sparse. Other abnormalities seen with TCA overdose such as choreoathetoid movements and seizures are probably the result of anticholinergic action.[46] Also, because anticholinergic effects result in delayed gastric emptying, drug absorption may be retarded and manifestations of toxicity may be delayed.[47]

The second mechanism of TCA-induced cardiotoxicity is due to norepinephrine blockade at the cellular membrane of adrenergic nerve fibers, which results in increased levels of the neurotransmitter at the receptor site.[45] Because norepinephrine can no longer return to the presynaptic neuron for reuse and its remanufacture is delayed, eventually the action potential threshold is delayed. Norepinephrine excess contributes to hypertension and tachycardia seen in the early stages of overdose. As epinephrine is metabolized and depleted, hypotension and bradycardia ensue.

Third, the most probable cause for the major cardiotoxic effects of TCAs are quinidinelike or membrane-stabilizing effects of the myocardium.[45] In humans, quinidine slows the sinus rate by direct action on conduction in the cardiac Purkinje fibers, decreasing their firing rate. Other actions of quinidine are shortening of AV conduction and lengthening of the His-Purkinje interval.[48] TCAs affect intraventricular conduction similarly. This mechanism of TCAs is thought to be due to an inhibition of adenosine triphosphate, resulting in abnormalities in sodium-potassium pump action. This mechanism may also be responsible for induction of reentrant arrhythmias associated with unidirectional blocks because of the TCA ability to increase antegrade conduction.[49]

Fourth, TCAs exert a direct peripheral α-adrenergic blockade, causing a decrease in peripheral vascular resistance with resultant hypotension. Research data regarding the role of this mechanism are inconclusive and the exact action needs clarification.[45]

Clinical Manifestations

Because TCAs have the greatest affinity for the brain, heart, lung, circulatory, and nervous systems, these organ systems are principally affected.[50] Symptoms of TCA toxicity range from sinus tachycardia, hypotension, and lethargy to cardiac conduction disturbances, ventricular arrhythmias, seizures, coma, and cardiac arrest.[51-53]

Patients may present in an alert and lucid state but deteriorate rapidly to unconsciousness. Choreoathetoid movements, involuntary muscle twitching, and grand mal seizures may precede unconsciousness. Impaired levels of consciousness are common, ranging from stupor and lethargy to coma. Many patients demonstrate quasi-purposeful movements involving all extremities in response to noxious stimuli. Seizures occur less frequently than other manifestations of toxicity and appear early.[54] Alterations in consciousness may be influenced by concomitant ingestions of sedative or hypnotic drugs that impair neurologic response.

Cardiovascular abnormalities are more indicative of TCA toxicity than those involving the CNS. Cardiac disturbances resulting from TCA overdose are sinus tachycardia, atrioventricular and intraventricular conduction defects, ST and T wave abnormalities, supraventricular tachycardia, ventricular arrhythmias, bradycardia, and asystole.[55] Sinus tachycardia typically occurs with prolongation of PR and QRS intervals and ST and T wave changes, causing difficulty in differentiating between sinus rhythm with atrioventricular and intraventricular conduction abnormalities and supraventricular or ventricular tachycardia.[56] Even though tachycardia is common with TCA overdose, the incidence of other serious cardiac complications is relatively low.[51,54]

Medical Management

Because of individual variations in TCA metabolism, it is difficult to predict the severity of an acute ingestion based on the amount ingested. Few fatalities have been seen with less than 20 mg/kg; 35 mg/kg is the approximate lethal dose (LD_{50}), and death is likely with greater than 50 mg/kg.[45] Since responses to TCA ingestions are unpredictable, recommendations for treatment are based on the patient's clinical status rather than the amount ingested. Any TCA ingestion should be considered significant initially.

There are several studies suggesting a correlation between the amount of TCA ingested by history, TCA plasma levels, and physiologic response.[57,58] However, serum values of TCAs may not be dependable because serum measurements are affected by many variables, such as drug metabolic rate, body mass, and quantity ingested. Measurements may also be inaccurate due to erratic drug absorption and varied times at which peak serum levels occur. Because TCA serum assays are difficult to perform on an emergency basis and may be unreliable, patient management should be based on history and clinical presentation rather than on laboratory data.

General principles of prevention of absorption are applicable in TCA overdose. The importance of charcoal administration is stressed because, due to anticholinergic properties, movement of the drug through the gastrointestinal tract may be delayed, resulting in a percentage of the ingested amount remaining in the gut. Repeat-dose charcoal has been found to shorten the half-life of active metabolites by increasing drug clearance.[14,59] With repeated doses, TCAs and their active metabolites that are recycled through the enterohepatic system bind to the charcoal, preventing reabsorption.

Because of the large volume of distribution and extensive tissue binding to TCAs, forced diuresis and peritoneal or hemodialysis are of no benefit in treatment. Hemoperfusion with either a charcoal or resin filter has been used for TCA overdose management. Early reports indicated clinical improvement, but in controlled studies data revealed that the percentage of drug removed with this method was small, and significant numbers of patients demonstrated rebound effects and the return of symptoms.[60]

Pharmacologic therapy is most appropriate for management of the TCA-toxic patient. Sodium bicarbonate is an effective modality for drug-induced cardiac arrhythmias.[61,62] The mechanism of action for sodium bicarbonate ($NaHCO_3$) is not well understood, but serum assays show a rapid decrease in TCA levels after its administration.[61] Because TCAs are pharmacologically inactive when protein-bound and have an increased affinity to plasma protein in alkaline mediums, it is postulated that in alkaline serum a decreased percentage of active drug is available to produce symptoms.[7,61] Case studies report modification or reversal of arrhythmias after sodium bicarbonate administration or mechanical hyperventilation resulting in an increased serum pH.

Even though the use of phenytoin in TCA cardiotoxicity lacks experimental and clinical support, theoretically its use is recommended for treatment of intraventricular conduction disturbances and arrhythmias. Antiarrhythmic actions of phenytoin include enhancement of myocardial contractility, restoration of normal rhythm, and improvement in atrio- and intraventricular conduction. Phenytoin also blocks or impairs conduction in reentrant pathways. Because of these pharmacologic properties, phenytoin is a reasonable choice as the primary antiarrhythmic in TCA toxicity.[63]

In the past, physostigmine was widely recommended as the antidote for TCA intoxication. Therapeutic effects were attributed to an increase in the amount of acetylcholine at the receptor site, which antagonizes the anticholinergic action of TCA.[64] Early case reports demonstrated the effectiveness of physostigmine in reversing many of the clinical manifestations of TCA toxicity.[46,65] Recent studies report exacerbations of cardiac and CNS symptoms after physostigmine administration and associate its use with seizures, hypotension, bradycardia, heart block, and asystole.[66,67] Although physostigmine may produce a transient improvement in consciousness, its use puts the patient at greater risk for seizures and cardiac deterioration. Therefore, current recommendations do not include routine use of physostigmine in drug therapy for TCA toxicity.

Fluid bolus administration and placement of the patient in a semi-Trendelenberg position may prove beneficial for TCA-induced hypotension. If these measures are ineffective, vasopressors are needed. Because norepinephrine is depleted due to its blocked reuptake and decreased manufacture, levarterenol (Levophed) is the vasopressor of choice.

All patients with a history of TCA ingestion must be observed for a minimum of 6 h. If symptoms develop, admission to an intensive care unit for cardiac monitoring is required and the patient must remain asymptomatic and arrhythmia-free for 24 h before discharge.[3]

Nursing Management

1. Poisoning: Potential for tricyclic antidepressant toxicity
2. Cardiac output: Potential for alteration in, decreased
3. Gas exchange: Potential for impairment
4. Urinary elimination: Potential for alteration in patterns
5. Alteration in tissue perfusion: Peripheral, cardiopulmonary

An accurate history of the time of ingestion, other medications ingested or taken chronically, and the amount of drug taken are essential data which must be obtained upon initial contact with the patient. After vital sign measurements, cardiac monitoring should be initiated. Serial measurements of QRS and PR intervals and heart rate help to assess the severity of toxicity. A QRS duration greater than 0.12 s may be the best indication of a severe overdose. Prolonged PR and QT intervals are also indications of potentially severe toxicity.

Manifestations of anticholinergic toxicity include decreased gastrointestinal motility, decreased mucosal secretions, and urinary retention. To avoid complications due to these side effects, bowel sounds should be checked before each charcoal dose to detect ileus development. Smaller doses of charcoal given at more frequent increments may be beneficial. Frequent urine output measurements help to assess bladder competency. Humidified oxygen prevents patient discomfort related to administration of oxygen alone.

If NaHCO$_3$ therapy is utilized for arrhythmia management, serum pH assays are needed. Intravenous NaHCO$_3$ is given at doses of 1 to 2 meq/kg as needed to keep the serum pH at 7.4 to 7.5.[3] Induction of respiratory alkalosis by mechanical ventilation may also be effective for pH adjustments.[68] However, frequent arterial blood gas determinations are needed to avoid a pH greater than 7.5 and P_{CO_2} levels less than 20.

Phenytoin therapy is based on electrocardiographic changes with an increase in QRS width being most definitive. Measurements greater than 0.12 are considered significant and may be used as the basis for treatment. Administration of phenytoin should begin with a loading dose of 15 mg/kg up to 1 g IV, not to exceed a rate of 0.5 mg/kg per minute. Because intravenous phenytoin may be irritating to the skin and blood vessels, IV insertion sites should be checked frequently to prevent extravasation and necrosis. If the patient complains of pain or burning during the infusion, the rate may be slowed.

Evaluation

Continuous ECG monitoring with measurements of atrio- and intraventricular conduction times and frequent blood pressure checks and neurological examinations allow assessment of the degree of toxicity and effectiveness of treatment. With appropriate therapy and judicious nursing assessment, most deaths from TCA toxicity can be avoided.

Organophosphates

Mortality rates from all poisonings reveal that 10 percent of all deaths are due to exposures to insecticides found in home and commercial sprays.[69] The Environmental Protection Agency reports that 80 percent of all hospitalizations in the United States for pesticide exposure are due to organophosphates.[2] Because of their effectiveness for pest control, organophosphate use is increasing, especially in California, the southern states, and farmbelt areas of the country. Exposures are most frequent in farmers and unskilled laborers; however, children frequently ingest these products accidentally. Pesticides also have been used for intentional suicide attempts. The carbamate pesticides produce symptoms similar to organophosphates; however, their duration of action is shorter and the order of toxicity is lower.[23] Because organophosphate exposures are most common, discussion will be directed only to this group.

Pathophysiology

Understanding the pathophysiology of organophosphates requires a basic knowledge of neurotransmission. Acetylcholine is one of four neurotransmitters at synaptic junctions in the autonomic nervous system and is present at postganglionic parasympathetic nerve endings, at preganglionic nerves to parasympathetic and sympathetic ganglia, at somatic motor nerve endings to striated muscle, and at certain synapses in the central nervous system. With its release, action is potentiated at neuroreceptor sites. The enzyme acetylcholinesterase metabolizes acetylcholine. If its availability were continuous, repetitive action potentials would occur at neuroreceptor sites.

Organophosphates act as powerful inhibitors of acetylcholinesterase by irreversibly binding to active sites on the enzyme, forming phosphorylated enzyme. Organophosphates act as antiacetylcholinesterases, thereby preventing the breakdown of acetylcholine.[23] With enzyme inhibition, acetylcholine accumulates at synaptic junctions and cholinergic overdrive occurs. Overabundance of acetylcholine initially excites, then paralyzes transmission of cholinergic synapses. Organophosphate binding with acetylcholinesterase is considered irreversible because, although enzyme reactivation can occur, it is too slow to be of clinical value.[69]

Clinical Manifestations

Organophosphates are well absorbed by all routes of exposure. The time interval between exposure and evidence of symptoms is dependent on many variables, including route, particular compound, and degree of exposure, but symptoms almost always occur within 24 h.[2] If the route of exposure is inhalation, respiratory symptoms occur initially, whereas if the product is ingested, gastrointestinal symptoms appear first. An early sign of ocular exposure is miosis. Onset is most rapid after organophosphate inhalation and slowest with dermal exposures.[69]

Symptoms are categorized as muscarinic, nicotinic, or central, but all relate to excessive amounts of acetylcholine. *Muscarinic* effects related to parasympathetic stimulation are sweating, increased lacrimation, excessive salivation, vomiting, diarrhea, and urinary incontinence. Effects on the cardiovascular system are inhibitory and are evidenced by bradycardia and hypotension. Increased secretions in the respiratory tract result in wheezing and may progress to pulmonary edema. *Nicotinic* effects are due to the stimulating action of acetylcholine on sympathetic ganglia and striated muscle. These include fasciculations, cramps, weakness, and paralysis. At sympathetic ganglia, tachycardia and hypertension are produced.

Organophosphates have diverse effects on the central nervous system, causing anxiety, restlessness, ataxia, coma, and circulatory and respiratory depression. Death usually occurs from bronchorrhea, bronchospasm, diaphragmatic paralysis, and inability of the central nervous system to control respirations.[69] The mnemonic SLUDGE is used to recall the common muscarinic symptoms seen with organophosphate poisoning (Table 60-1).

Medical Management

Baseline patient status is assessed with a complete physical examination, an ECG, chest x-ray, and arterial blood gases. Metabolic products of organophosphates can be found in the urine but are not routinely assayed. Red blood cell cholinesterase and serum pseudocholinesterase levels can be used to help confirm the diagnosis, but are not useful for management. A depression of red blood cell cholinesterase by 25 percent or greater is indicative of significant exposure. Symptomatic patients usually show a depression in red blood count cholinesterase in excess of 50 percent. Red blood cell cholinesterase levels will not return to preexposure levels for several days and possibly not for up to 4 months.[2]

Because atropine blocks the action of excessive acetylcholine at receptor sites, it is the drug of choice for initial treatment of muscarinic symptoms.[2] However, nicotinic effects are relatively refractory to atropine administration. Pralidoxime (2-PAM) is recommended for reversal of nicotinic effects because it binds to the phosphate group of the organophosphate and frees acetylcholinesterase to metabolize acetylcholine. Use of 2-PAM is recommended if the red blood count cholinesterase level is less than 25 percent; however, its use is based primarily on the presence of nicotinic symptoms.[69] A combination of atropine and 2-PAM is probably the most effective treatment.

Nursing Management

1. Poisoning: Potential for organophosphate toxicity
2. Alteration in bowel elimination: diarrhea
3. Urinary elimination: Alterations in pattern
4. Gas exchange: Potential for impairment

General management principles for absorption prevention apply if the route of exposure to organophosphates is oral. Ipecac should be given with extreme caution, if at all, because symptoms of organophosphate poisoning occur rapidly. Patients may have severe symptoms, e.g., central nervous system depression and seizures, before Ipecac-induced emesis is completed.[3] For dermal exposure, the skin is decontaminated with an initial soap and water wash followed by an isopropyl alcohol rub; the procedure is concluded with another soap and water wash. Nursing personnel can protect themselves from exposure by wearing gloves, gowns, and masks during the procedure. Leather must be disposed of by burning. Other decontaminated clothing can be washed several times with soap and water.

Judicious suctioning prevents respiratory distress from excessive salivary and bronchial secretions. Because atropine may precipitate ventricular fibrillation in a poorly oxygenated patient, adequate ventilation must be assured.[23] Administration of humidified oxygen helps to keep mucous membranes moist during atropine use. To attain therapeutic effects, large doses of atropine may be needed. Doses of 2 mg initially followed by subsequent increments of 2 to 4 mg or more every 3 to 8 min may be required.[69]

If 2-PAM is ordered, 1.0 g is mixed in 250 mL of normal saline and is infused over 30 min. It can also be given in a 1.0-g dose with 0.5 g pushed IV per minute.[3] Doses may be repeated three times as needed at intervals of 8 to 12 h if muscular and central nervous system involvement does not subside. Pralidoxime is most effective if given within 24 to 48 h of exposure.[2] In therapeutic doses, toxicity is minimal with some reports of mild weakness, blurred vision, headache, and nausea.[23] Because 2-PAM is excreted in the urine and may accumulate to toxic levels in the presence of renal dysfunction, accurate urine output measurements are necessary.

Evaluation

Pupillary dilation is unreliable when assessing the effectiveness of atropine. Reliable signs of atropinization are a decrease in secretions, flushed skin, and a relative tachycardia. If the effects of atropine are not evidenced, the dosage is insufficient. With organophosphate toxicity, the risks of underdosage outweigh those of overdosage. Continued administration of 2-PAM is based on disappearance of

skeletal muscle and central nervous system manifestations of toxicity.

Salicylates

Salicylates commonly used by consumers and health care professionals include acetylsalicylic acid (aspirin), sodium salicylate, and salicylic acid. Aspirin is one of the most widely used analgesics and is frequently combined with other drugs such as caffeine, codeine, and acetaminophen. Other salicylates are found in a variety of topical preparations and teething gels.

Salicylate poisoning may occur in several ways. Accidental ingestion of salicylates is a common childhood poisoning, usually involving 1-to-5-year-old children. Children also are frequently poisoned when parents inadvertently overdose them during febrile illnesses. Due to the accessibility of aspirin and aspirin-containing products, intentional ingestion by adults in suicide attempts is common. Chronic therapeutic salicylate intoxication in adults may also occur. Since salicylates readily cross the placenta, on rare occasions a newborn may have salicylate poisoning if the mother has ingested large quantities of aspirin preceding the delivery.[2]

Pathophysiology

In therapeutic doses, aspirin is rapidly absorbed from the stomach and small intestine. In an overdose, absorption occurs more slowly and symptoms of toxicity may be delayed, resulting in rising serum levels for up to 12 h.[3] The delayed absorption of aspirin occurs because of the inhibitory effects of aspirin on gastric emptying and because tablets adhere together, forming a bolus, which dissolves slowly. Absorption will also be delayed following an ingestion of enteric-coated aspirin. Topical application of salicylates may produce systemic toxicity while rectal absorption is slow and incomplete.

Aspirin is rapidly hydrolyzed by the liver to salicylic acid and distributes into most body tissues and water. A small amount of salicylic acid is excreted unchanged in the urine while the majority of aspirin is eliminated through the formation of the inactive metabolites salicyluric acid and salicyl phenolic and acyl glucuronides, which are then excreted in the urine (Fig. 60-3). The pathways that

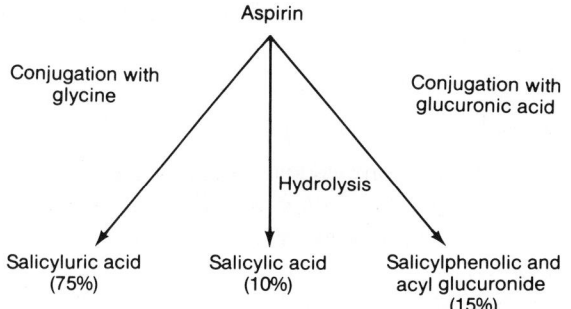

Figure 60-3   Aspirin metabolism. (Adapted from Pois-index Information Systems, Micromedex Incorporated, 1974–1985, Englewood, CO.; J. A. Vale, and T. J. Meredith, *Poisoning: Diagnosis and treatment,* London: Update Books, 1981. (Used with permission of the publishers.)

form the inactive metabolites are saturable. Because of this fact, the time for a given fraction of a dose of salicylate to be eliminated increases with increasing doses (nonlinear kinetics). Salicylates can accumulate and, frequently, repeated small doses may profoundly increase body stores and blood levels.[2] As these metabolic pathways become saturated, more salicylate needs to be renally excreted.[70]

In overdoses, salicylates stimulate respirations directly and indirectly. They directly stimulate the respiratory center in the medulla to both increase rate and depth of respirations.[72] Salicylates also uncouple mitochondrial oxidative phosphorylation, resulting in an increase in oxygen consumption and carbon dioxide production. This increase in carbon dioxide levels stimulates respirations and accounts for the indirect effect of salicylates on respirations. With compensatory tachypnea, the P_{CO_2} decreases, resulting in a respiratory alkalosis with a decreased P_{CO_2} and a rise in arterial pH.[3] Bicarbonate, accompanied by sodium, potassium, and water, is excreted by the kidney in an attempt to normalize the arterial pH.[70] This results in dehydration and hypokalemia. The increased bicarbonate excretion diminishes the buffering capacity of the body and allows acidosis to develop more easily. With very high concentrations of salicylates, the respiratory center may be depressed.

The major toxic effects of salicylate ingestion result from the adverse effects on cellular metab-olism. Salicylates not only uncouple mitochondrial oxidative phosphorylation but also inhibit specific Krebs cycle dehydrogenases and aminotransferases and increase the metabolism and peripheral demand for glucose. This results in hyperthermia and an increased production, accumulation, and excretion of organic acids with an elevated anion gap metabolic acidosis.[3]

Salicylates penetrate the central nervous system rapidly, especially during acidemia, and produce a decrease in mental alertness. Convulsions may occur in severe intoxications. Although the exact etiology of the seizures is unclear, it is thought to be excessive accumulation of carbon dioxide in the central nervous system, decreased brain glucose concentration, or a direct toxic effect.[3]

Salicylates may decrease prothrombin formation, factor VII production, platelet adhesiveness, and platelet levels, and increase capillary fragility. Despite coagulation abnormalities, hemorrhage is not a common clinical manifestation of salicylate toxicity.[69]

Gastrointestinal distress following salicylate intoxication is produced by local gastric irritation and stimulation of the medullary chemoreceptor trigger zone. Tinnitus and hearing loss frequently experienced are due to increased pressure in the labyrinth of the auditory apparatus. Tinnitus is associated with serum levels greater than 30 mg/dL (Fig. 60-4).[3]

Single oral doses greater than 300 mg of salicylate per kilogram of body weight may produce severe poisoning. Chronic ingestion greater than 100 mg per kilogram of body weight every 24 h over two or more days is associated with toxicity. Greater morbidity in adults and children is seen with chronic salicylism.[3]

Salicylate levels are plotted on the Done nomogram.[73] The nomogram predicts the clinical severity of the poison based on the serum level and time since a single acute ingestion. The nomogram cannot be utilized to predict severity of symptoms in a chronic salicylate overdose. The salicylate level should be drawn at least 6 h after ingestion, and two or more levels should be obtained to assure that peak serum concentration has occurred. Ingestion of large amounts of aspirin may form a concretion in the stomach, delaying absorp-

Figure 60-4 Salicylate nomogram with inset. (Used with permission from Poisindex Information Systems, Micromedex Incorporated, 1974–1985, Englewood, CO.)

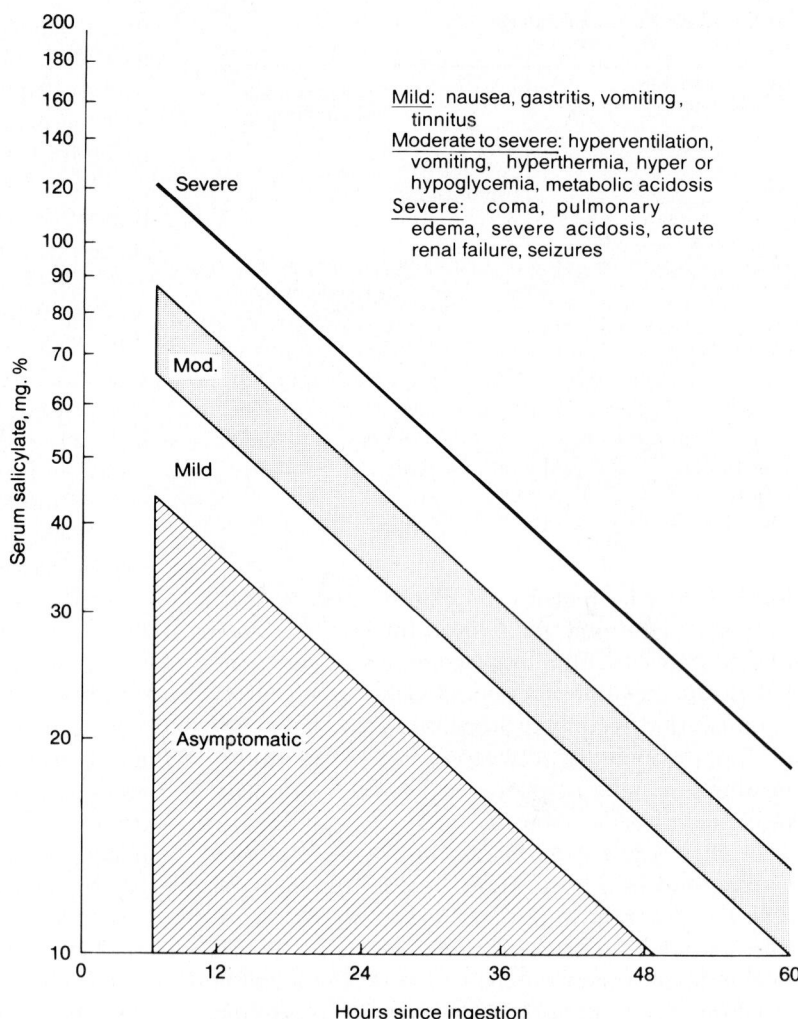

Mild: nausea, gastritis, vomiting, tinnitus

Moderate to severe: hyperventilation, vomiting, hyperthermia, hyper or hypoglycemia, metabolic acidosis

Severe: coma, pulmonary edema, severe acidosis, acute renal failure, seizures

tion for up to 24 h.[74] With ingestion of sustained-released preparations (Verin, Zorprin), absorption may be prolonged and the serum salicylate level may be persistently elevated. Using the Done nomogram for ingestion of sustained-released preparations is of questionable value.

Clinical Manifestations

Most patients with significant salicylate toxicity experience nausea, vomiting, tinnitus, and hearing loss. Other early clinical signs include profuse sweating, flushing, hyperpyrexia, hyperpnea, and hyperventilation.

In serious poisonings, severe acid-base imbalance (elevated anion gap, metabolic acidosis) and dehydration occur. The metabolic symptoms seen following acute salicylate poisoning may be divided into three stages (Table 60-8). In the first stage, hyperventilation from direct and indirect respiratory center stimulation produces respiratory alkalosis. To normalize the arterial pH, bicarbonate is excreted by the kidney, resulting in an alkaline urine (a pH of 6 or greater). In the second stage, the serum pH remains alkaline with a compensated metabolic acidosis, while the urine becomes more acidotic from the excretion of organic acids. In the third stage, both serum and urine are acidotic.[71,72,75]

Following severe salicylate poisoning, symptoms may progress to confusion, coma, and seizures. Noncardiogenic pulmonary edema may also occur.

Table 60-8 Metabolic Stages of Acute Salicylate Toxicity

Stage	Plasma[A]	Urine[B]
I	Alkaline	Alkaline
II	Alkaline	Acid
III	Acid	Acid

[A]A normal plasma pH 7.36–7.46.
[B]"Alkaline" urine is pH 6 or greater; "acid" urine is pH less than 6.
Adapted with permission from A.R. Temple, Pathophysiology of Aspirin Overdosage Toxicity with Implications for Management, *Pediatrics*, 62:873–876, 1978; A.R. Temple, Acute and Chronic Effects of Aspirin Toxicity and Their Treatment, *Archives of Internal Medicine*, 14:364–368, 1981.

Hypoglycemia in children and hyperglycemia in adults may be noted. An increased bleeding time may also occur.

Medical Management

Treatment of salicylate poisoning encompasses initial basic life support, prevention of absorption, enhancement of elimination, and reduction of toxic effects of salicylates. In a salicylate overdose the normal elimination pathways become saturated, requiring more salicylate to be excreted by the kidney. Because renal excretion is influenced by pH, renal elimination of unchanged salicylic acid can be increased by alkalinizing the urine.[70] When the urine is alkaline, the ionized salicylic acid molecule is "trapped," thus preventing readsorption into the renal tubule. A change of the urine pH from 5 to 8 increases the urine excretion of salicylic acid greater than twentyfold.[3] Forced alkaline diuresis is a widely accepted treatment regimen for salicylate poisoning. While instituting alkaline diuresis, the patient is also rehydrated with an appropriate IV solution with at least 30 meq of KCL per liter because hypokalemia is a frequent complication. Metabolic acidosis is treated with IV sodium bicarbonate. Hemodialysis may be considered when the patient is not responding to other therapy, and is probably the treatment of choice if cerebral or pulmonary edema or renal failure occur.[2,3]

Nursing Management

1. Poisoning: Potential for salicylate toxicity
2. Breathing pattern, ineffective
3. Gas exchange, impaired
4. Tissue perfusion, alteration in cerebral, renal

Following a salicylate overdose, prevention of absorption is an important aspect of therapy. Because large ingestions of aspirin delay gastric emptying, emesis or gastric lavage may be effective up to several hours after exposure. Since large ingestions of aspirin may also form a bolus in the stomach and be absorbed over an extended period of time, multidose charcoal is beneficial until a charcoal stool is passed.

Important laboratory values to monitor include serum salicylate levels, arterial blood gases, electrolytes, glucose, and prothrombin time. A serum salicylate level is drawn 6 or more h after ingestion and compared to the Done nomogram. Salicylate levels obtained before 6 h after ingestion will not reflect the peak concentration.[73] Sodium bicarbonate administration is dependent on arterial blood gas values, serum bicarbonate, and anion gap. Potassium may need to be administered for the hypokalemia that results from salicylate toxicity.

The decision to institute alkalinization of the urine is based on the patient's clinical presentation. Indications for alkaline diuresis include a urine pH less than 6 with a 6-h salicylate level greater than 50 mg/dL, acidosis, or nausea, vomiting, and tinnitus when levels are available. To alkalinize the urine, a solution with 2 to 3 ampules of sodium bicarbonate and 30 meq of potassium chloride in each liter of D_5W solution is administered at a rate of 2 to 3 mL/kg per hour to produce a urine flow of 2 to 3 ml/kg per hour. The urine pH is checked hourly and additional sodium bicarbonate is given as needed to maintain a urine pH of 7 to 8. Because the urine pH of most severely poisoned patients is 5.5 to 6.5, it may be difficult to adequately alkalinize the urine to 7 to 8. In addition, potassium must be administered as needed because urine alkalinization is difficult to achieve if the patient is hypokalemic.[3] The arterial pH is monitored closely to avoid alkalemia. A diuretic may be administered to maintain urine flow. During alkaline diuresis, the urine output is checked hourly to prevent fluid overload. Hemodialysis is recommended in patients with serum salicylate levels greater than 130 mg/dL at 6 h after ingestion, refractory acidosis (a pH of less than 7.1), persistent central nervous system symptoms, progressive deterioration despite appropriate treatment intervention, pulmonary edema, and renal failure.[72]

Evaluation

Efficacy of the therapeutic interventions administered during salicylate poisoning can be assessed throughout the clinical course of the patient's treatment. Indicators of appropriate nursing and medical treatment include stable vital signs, appropriate mental status, normal electrolytes, acid-base balance, renal function, and decreasing serum salicylate levels. In chronic salicylate poisoning, the serum salicylate level is of less value in assessing the efficacy of medical and nursing interventions.

Snake Envenomation

About 120 species of snakes are found in the United States. Nearly 20 of these species are venomous.[76] Bites by nonvenomous snakes are much more common and are treated as simple puncture wounds. Venomous snakes include pit vipers—Crotalidae (cottonmouths, copperheads, rattlesnakes), and coral snakes—Elapidae. Efforts should be made to identify the species of snake although this may be difficult.

Pathophysiology

Snake venoms are complex mixtures consisting mainly of proteins with enzymatic activity. Certain peptides and proteins found in venoms have a relatively low molecular weight and may produce the most deleterious effects. It has been common practice to divide snake venoms into groups such as neurotoxins, hemotoxins, and cardiotoxins. Such grouping may be misleading because all snake envenomations present as multiple poisonings with toxic reactions and pharmacological changes occurring simultaneously or consecutively.

Clinical Manifestations

The venoms of pit vipers (Crotalidae) may cause severe local tissue effects, coagulopathies, and changes in blood cells. The hematocrit may fall rapidly and platelets may nearly disappear. In severe poisoning, pulmonary edema occurs and there may be bleeding in the lungs, peritoneum, kidneys, and heart, resulting in alterations in cardiac dynamics and renal function.[76] Paralysis rarely occurs, but when present, mechanical ventilation may be needed. The venom of coral snakes (Elapidae) produces more changes in neuromuscular transmission and nerve conduction than do pit viper venoms, resulting in weakness, muscle fasciculations, and a type of bulbar paralysis that may occur within 90 min.[76]

If an envenomation from a snake of either of these families has occurred, swelling and edema may begin within 5 min of the bite and progress rapidly. Most bites are on an extremity and swelling may involve the entire limb within an hour. The local reaction may be minimal from a coral snake bite but pain immediately following the bite is common. Nausea, faintness, sweating, and weakness also may occur. Ecchymosis and discoloration of the skin are seen. Tingling or numbness of the tongue, mouth, or scalp may be accompanied by a metallic taste. Muscle fasciculations sometimes occur. Systemic symptoms of pit viper bites include hypotension, coagulopathies, and shock. Systemic symptoms of a coral snake bite include drowsiness, weakness, dysphoria, diplopia, headache, and respiratory distress.[76]

Medical Management

Immediately following a snake envenomation, basic life support measures are begun. The envenomation is graded to determine the seriousness of the bite (Table 60-9). The circumference of the extremity 10 and 20 cm proximal to the bite size is measured

---

Table 60-9 Grading Envenomation of Pit Viper Bites

A. Minimal envenomation—signs and symptoms are confined to the bite area. There are no systemic symptoms or laboratory derangements.
B. Moderate envenomation—there are significant systemic symptoms and signs. Edema extends beyond the immediate bite area. Moderate laboratory derangements are seen (hemoconcentration, decreased fibrinogen, platelets, prolonged PT, and hematuria).
C. Severe envenomation—swelling involves entire extremity or part. There are serious systemic signs and symptoms and severe laboratory derangements. All signs, symptoms, and laboratory values should be considered in grading envenomation. Edema and swelling may be absent in some severe bites.

Adapted from Poisindex Information System, Micromedex, Inc., Englewood, CO.

every 15 to 30 min and the measurement sites are marked on the skin. Use of a tourniquet is not recommended because it may impede circulation. If a tourniquet has been placed, apply a constriction band proximal to the tourniquet, making certain the constriction band only impedes lymphatic flow. An IV infusion of lactated Ringer's solution or sodium chloride is started and the tourniquet is slowly removed. Incision and suction are helpful only if done in the first 30 min following the bite and should only be done by trained personnel to avoid damage to deep structures. The wound is cleansed, the affected part immobilized at heart level and the patient kept at rest. The injured part must not be placed in ice because this may freeze the tissues. Excision of the bite and fasciotomy also are not recommended. About 90 percent of pit viper bites are in subcutaneous tissue, and so tissue necrosis is caused by the action of the venom, not by pressure from edema.[76]

It is important to give pit viper antivenin early because it is most efficacious if given within 4 h of the bite.[3] It is less effective if the administration is delayed for 8 h and the effects are questionable if given after 24 h.[3] Use of antivenin is advised up to 24 h after the bite in all cases of severe pit viper envenomation. North American coral snake antivenin should be administered in all cases of confirmed coral snake bites.[76]

Because of the possibility of shock, bleeding, and coagulopathies, the patient's blood type and cross-matching are done. Complete blood count, hematocrit, platelet count, bleeding and clotting times, and prothrombin time need to be followed closely. These may need to be done several times a day in cases of severe envenomation. Because of the multisystem effects of envenomation, arterial blood gases and electrolytes are evaluated. Other tests that may be useful include serum protein, fibrinogen titer, and partial thromboplastin time. Baseline renal function tests should be ordered and all urine samples should be checked for the presence of red blood cells and hemoglobin.

Fluid administration is generally sufficient to treat the hypotension which may result from snake envenomation. Antihistamines may be needed to treat allergic reactions to the antivenin. There have been no clinical trials to indicate that steroids are useful. Steroids are not recommended in the acute phase of poisoning unless needed for shock or severe allergic reactions.

The wound may need to be debrided on the third through the tenth day.[3] A physical therapy evaluation may be done on about the third day. If antivenin was given, the patient needs to be informed that symptoms of serum sickness may occur in 10 to 14 days.

Nursing Management

1. Poisoning: Potential for snake envenomation toxicity
2. Alteration in comfort: Pain secondary to snake-bite
3. Anxiety

Serial measurements and recording of the affected part may need to be changed if swelling progresses. Observe for ecchymoses, vesicles, and blebs because these are additional signs of envenomation. Vital signs are checked as frequently as the condition of the patient warrants. The patient should not be left alone because the condition may change rapidly.

If the physician has determined that antivenin is needed, the skin is tested with the material in the antivenin package. The skin test should not be done until it is certain that the antivenin will be needed because the material in the skin test may sensitize the patient to horse serum. If the patient has an allergy to horse serum, diphenhydramine (Benadryl) may be given intravenously before the antivenin treatment.

If the bite was by a pit viper, antivenin polyvalent IV is administered initially at a slow rate, then faster (15 to 20 min per vial) if no reaction occurs. The amount of antivenin is determined by the grade of envenomation (Table 60-9). For minimal envenomation 3 to 5 vials are given. For moderate envenomation 6 to 12 vials are given, and for severe envenomation 13 to 30 vials or more may be used.[76] Antivenin is not indicated if there is no evidence of envenomation. Each vial is diluted in 50 mL of normal saline and given by continuous intravenous infusion. The total dosage is given during the first 4 to 6 h.[76] If hypotension develops, the rate of infusion is decreased. If anaphylaxis or a severe allergic reaction occurs, the infusion must be stopped. Antivenin is administered more than

24 h after envenomation only if necessary to reverse coagulopathies.[3]

If the bite is confirmed as being from a coral snake, North American coral snake antivenin is administered intravenously by diluting 3 to 5 vials of antivenin in 250 to 500 mL of sodium chloride for injection.[76] If signs and symptoms of envenomation such as drowsiness, weakness, dysphoria, diplopia, headache, or respiratory distress occur, an additional 3 to 5 vials may be given. Antivenin is never given intramuscularly unless it is absolutely impossible to give intravenously and it is never injected into a toe or finger. Emergency equipment should be at the bedside while giving antivenin.

Intake and output is monitored closely and all urine is checked for the presence of red blood cells and for hemoglobin. Once the patient is stable, analgesics may be administered for pain control. Screening laboratory values including a CBC with a platelet count, a prothrombin time, and a urinalysis are confirmed as being normal before the patient is discharged.

Most patients bitten by a venomous snake become very anxious and need much reassurance. The patient may be relieved to know that death or the loss of an extremity from a snakebite is very rare. A thorough explanation of the treatment and of expected lessening of the symptoms is also reassuring. Patients without symptoms of envenomation are observed for 3 to 4 h.

Evaluation

Swelling is evaluated by doing serial measurements. A close review of laboratory studies is needed to rule out worsening of coagulopathies. If swelling continues to progress or coagulation studies worsen, the physician should be notified because more antivenin may be needed. Data are gathered regarding the adequacy of analgesia and whether the level of anxiety has decreased.

Theophylline

Theophylline toxicity occurs frequently as a result of accidental or intentional overdose. Oral and intravenous preparations of theophylline are used for the therapy of acute and chronic airway obstruction in conditions such as asthma, COPD, pulmonary edema, and apnea. Patients may accidentally overdose by misunderstanding the prescribed dosage or from increasing the dosage if symptoms do not improve.

Pathophysiology

Theophylline stimulates the central nervous system, acts on the kidneys to produce diuresis, stimulates cardiac muscle, and relaxes smooth (particularly bronchial) muscle. It also may stimulate the medullary respiratory centers.

Theophylline is absorbed rapidly when administered orally. The rate of elimination varies greatly in normal individuals and is primarily controlled by the rate of hepatic metabolism. The average half-life of therapeutic doses of theophylline in adults is 2 to 16 h. Clearance and half-life may be quite variable and are affected by factors including age, smoking, liver disease, and concomitant administration of other drugs. Cimetidine decreases theophylline clearance and phenobarbital increases clearance.[2]

Clinical Manifestations

Therapeutic serum levels of theophylline range from 10 to 20 μg/mL.[3] Toxic symptoms may occur at any level above 20 μg/mL. Because the toxic level is so close to the therapeutic level, a small overdose may cause toxicity. Overdoses with sustained-release preparations may cause severe and prolonged central nervous system and cardiovascular toxicity with delayed onset. Toxic effects may be seen in patients who have used ephedrine-theophylline preparations in which the theophylline serum concentration is not considered toxic.[3]

Symptoms of theophylline toxicity include nausea, vomiting, and diarrhea. In severe intoxication, bloody emesis may be seen. The patient may become dehydrated and hypokalemic from the vomiting, diarrhea, and diuretic effect of theophylline.[2] Tachycardia is seen in almost all intoxicated patients and arrhythmias, such as atrial fibrillation, ventricular tachycardia, and cardiac arrest may also occur. Neurological symptoms include nervousness, irritability, and headache. In severe intoxications, restlessness, agitation, and seizures are seen. Seizures are a poor prognostic sign and may not respond to standard anticonvulsant therapy. There is no predictable progression of symptoms.[2]

Medical Management

Following oral ingestion of theophylline, gastric emptying with emesis or lavage is recommended. If induction of emesis is contraindicated, gastric lavage is performed with a large-bore tube and the airway is protected. Subsequent treatment measures are the same whether the exposure was oral or parenteral.

Seizures are treated initially with IV diazepam. For seizures unresponsive to diazepam, phenytoin is administered IV with the ECG being monitored for arrhythmias. A serum sample for theophylline is obtained and if the level is greater than the therapeutic level, additional levels are obtained every 2 h until the peak is passed and then every 4 h until the level is in the therapeutic range. If hypotension develops, a fluid challenge is administered and the patient is placed in a semi-Trendelenburg position. Dopamine or norepinephrine is given if the hypotension is unresponsive to the above measures. Repeated oral doses of activated charcoal have been shown to increase the clearance of theophylline in both oral and IV exposures.[77,78] The patient needs careful cardiac monitoring, and electrolytes (particularly potassium) are monitored closely. Although theophylline is about 58 percent protein-bound at therapeutic serum concentrations, high levels in the toxic patient indicate that a large amount of the drug is in the plasma and may be removed by hemodialysis or charcoal hemoperfusion. The decision to institute hemodialysis or hemoperfusion is based both on serum levels of theophylline and the clinical status of the patient.

Nursing Management

1. Poisoning: Potential for theophylline toxicity
2. Alteration in cardiac output: decreased
3. Alteration in tissue perfusion: cerebral, cardiopulmonary
4. Knowledge deficit

Intake and output are monitored carefully to ascertain the hydration status, and potassium levels are determined frequently. Administration of multidose activated charcoal is recommended until the serum theophylline level is therapeutic (less than 20 μg/mL). Hemodialysis or hemoperfusion may be considered when theophylline serum concentrations are greater than 60 μg/mL or in patients with severe symptoms (cardiac arrhythmias, hemodynamic instability, or seizures not responsive to anticonvulsant therapy).[2] Chronic theophylline toxicity may cause severe symptoms at lower serum theophylline levels.[3]

The nurse should be aware of the circumstances of the overdose. Did the overdose occur because of noncompliance with a medical regimen? Did the patient misunderstand the dosage or accidentally administer too much of the drug? The nurse can help the patient understand the action of the medication, the reason for using the drug, and expected effects. If the history indicates that the patient intentionally overdosed, suicide precautions are observed and mental health counseling is arranged.

Evaluation

Evaluation includes assessing the efficacy of therapy. Decreased tachycardia, cessation of seizures, stability of intake and output, a theophylline serum level in the therapeutic range, and evidence of charcoal stools indicate successful therapy. The nurse should also assess the patient's level of understanding of the use of this medication.

Psychosocial Considerations

The psychosocial needs of the patient are assessed to aid in prevention of repeated poisonings. Consider the circumstances of the exposure: Was it intentional or accidental? Ingestions of potentially toxic substances should be investigated for possible suicide ideation.

1. Self-directed violence
   a. Assessment. Frequently assess the potential for suicide. Even a non-life-threatening gesture indicates a potential for a more serious attempt. Signs to assess that may indicate a suicide potential include suicide threats, a previous suicide attempt, history of prolonged depression, marked changes in behavior or personality, or the making of final arrangements.
   b. Intervention. Follow suicide precautions as outlined in the institution to provide a safe environment and prevent injury. Place the

patient in a central area, preferably near the nurses' station. Avoid having the patient near exits, stairwells, or elevators. Windows should be locked. Remove sharp or dangerous objects from the patient's environment. Use restraints if necessary. Check the patient frequently at irregular intervals and when there is a decrease in staffing. Assist family members in understanding the restrictions the patient must observe.

   c. Evaluation. Patient is protected from further injury.

2. Disturbance in self-concept

   a. Patients may have a sense of worthlessness and powerlessness or be socially isolated.

   b. Intervention. Always call the patient by name. Explain suicide precautions. Tell the patient you are willing to discuss emotions, feelings, and actions. Involve the patient in care and encourage talk about self, family, work, or other activities that have provided identification for life. Allow time for visits with appropriate significant others. Ensure that mental health counseling is available to the patient. Caretakers should convey a caring attitude for the patient and family.

   c. Evaluation. The patient will discuss feelings, behaviors, and actions and develop insight and a more positive self-image.

Summary

Management of a poisoned patient focuses on the clinical symptoms of the patient, not the poison ingested by history. There are few specific antidotes available. The majority of poisoned patients recover with appropriate symptomatic treatment. Initial management involves stabilization of vital signs, prevention of absorption, enhancement of poison elimination, and supportive care. Supportive care includes maintenance of airway, blood pressure, and cardiac function; pharmacologic interventions to treat seizures and arrhythmias; and correction of fluid, electrolyte, and acid-base disturbances. The efficacy of the treatment interventions is assessed throughout the clinical course and therapy is continued until symptoms resolve. Attainment of therapeutic plasma levels with certain drug overdoses also indicates successful therapy.

Regional poison centers have been established to assist in the management of the poisoned patient. Nurses, pharmacists, and medical toxicologists are available for consultation 24 h a day and serve as a resource to consumers and health care professionals for assistance on appropriate treatment interventions, expected poison effects, and in monitoring the patient's progress.

References

1. Litovitz, T. (1985). *1984 Annual report of the data collection system.* American Association of Poison Control Centers.

2. Haddad, L. M., & Winchester, J. F. (1983). *Clinical management of poisoning and drug overdose.* Philadelphia: Saunders.

3. Poisindex Information System: Micromedex, Inc., Englewood, CO, Copyright from 1974 through current year.

4. Manno, B. R., & Manno, J. E. (1977). Toxicology of ipecac: A review. *Clinical Toxicology, 10,* 221–242.

5. Neuvonen, P. J., Vartiainen, M., & Tokola, O. (1983). Comparison of activated charcoal and ipecac syrup in prevention of drug absorption. *European Journal of Clinical Pharmacology, 24,* 557–562.

6. Corby, D. J., Lisciandro, R. C., & Lehman, R. H. (1967). The efficacy of methods used to evaluate the stomach after acute ingestions. *Pediatrics, 40,* 5.

7. Corby, D. C., & Decker, W. J. (1968). Management of acute poisoning with activated charcoal. *Pediatrics, 42,* 361–364.

8. Tandberg, D., Liechty, E. J., & Fishbein, D. (1981). Mallory-Weiss syndrome: An unusual complication of ipecac induced emesis. *Annals of Emergency Medicine, 10,* 521–523.

9. Klein-Schwartz, W., Gorman, R. L., & Oderda, G. M. (1984). Ipecac use in the elderly: The unanswered question. *Annals of Emergency Medicine, 13,* 1152–1154.

10. Wolowdiuk, O. J., McMicken, D. B., & O'Brien, P. (1984). Pneumomediastinum and retropneumoperitoneum: An unusual complication of syrup of ipecac-induced emesis. *Annals of Emergency Medicine, 13,* 1148–1151.

11. Abdallah, A. H., & Tye, A. (1967). A comparison of the efficacy of emetic drugs and stomach lavage.

American Journal of Diseases of Children, 113, 571–575.

12. Boxer, L., Anderson, F. P., & Rowe, D. S. (1969). Comparison of ipecac-induced emesis with gastric lavage in the treatment of acute salicylate ingestion. *Journal of Pediatrics, 74,* 800–803.

13. Kulig, K., Bar-or, D., & Cantrill, S. (1985). Management of acutely poisoned patients without gastric emptying. *Annals of Emergency Medicine, 14,* 562–567.

14. Askenasi, R. (1984). Esophageal perforation: An unusual complication of gastric lavage. *Annals of Emergency Medicine, 13,* 146.

15. Neuvonen, P. J., & Elonen, E. (1980). Effect of activated charcoal on absorption and elimination of phenobarbitone, carbamazepine, and phenylbutazone in man. *European Journal of Clinical Pharmacology, 17,* 51–57.

16. Hayden, J., & Comstock, E. (1975). Use of activated charcoal in acute poisoning. *Clinical Toxicology, 8,* 515–533.

17. Curtis, R. A., Barone, J., & Giancona, N. (1984). Efficacy of ipecac and activated charcoal/cathartic: Prevention of salicylate absorption in a simulated overdose. *Annals of Internal Medicine, 144,* 48–52.

18. Riegel, J. M., & Becker, C. E. (1981). Use of cathartics in toxic ingestions. *Annals of Emergency Medicine, 10,* 254–258.

19. Jones, J., Heiselman, D., & Dougherty, J. (1986). Cathartic-induced magnesium toxicity during overdose management. *Annals of Emergency Medicine, 15,* 121–125.

20. Smilkstein, M., Smolinske, S., & Kulig, K. (1986). Severe hypermagnesemia due to multiple-dose cathartic therapy. (Abstract). *Veterinary and Human Toxicology, 28,* 494.

21. Patel, R., Das, M., & Palazzolo, M. (1980). Myoglobinuric acute renal failure in phencyclidine overdose: Report of observations in eight cases. *Annals of Emergency Medicine, 9,* 549–553.

22. Rumack, B. H. (1983). Acetaminophen overdose: A high index of suspicion. In M. Bayer and B. H. Rumack (Eds.), *Poisoning and overdose.* Baltimore, MD: Aspen Systems.

23. Bayer, M., & Rumack, B. H. (Eds.) (1983). *Poisoning and overdose.* Baltimore, MD: Aspen Systems.

24. Renzi, F. P., Donovan, J. W., & Morgan, L. (1984). Concomitant use of activated charcoal and N-acetylcysteine. *Annals of Emergency Medicine, 13* (5), 400.

25. Goldfrank, L. (1982). *Toxicologic emergencies.* New York: Appleton-Century-Crofts.

26. Noker, P. E., Eels, J. T., & Tephly, T. R. (1980). Methanol toxicity: Treatment with folic acid and 5-formyl tetrahydrofolic acid. *Clinical and Experimental Research, 4*(4), 378–383.

27. McCoy, H. G. (1979). Severe methanol poisoning: Application of a pharmacokinetic model for ethanol therapy and hemodialysis. *American Journal of Medicine, 67,* 804–807.

28. Scherger, D., Wruk, K., & Linden, C. (1983). Case review, ethylene glycol intoxication. *Journal of Emergency Nursing, 9,* 71–73.

29. Ingemannson, S. O. (1984). Clinical observation of ten cases of methanol poisoning with particular reference to ocular manifestations. *Acta Ophthalmologfica (Ankara), 62,* 15–24.

30. Peterson, C. D., Collins, A. J., & Himes, J. M. (1981). Ethylene glycol poisoning. Pharmacokinetics during therapy with ethanol and hemodialysis. *New England Journal of Medicine, 304,* 21–23.

31. Massachusetts Poison Control Systems. (1981). Ethanol intoxication. *Clinical Toxicology Review, 41,* 1–2.

32. Wilkinson, P. K. (1980). Pharmacokinetics of ethanol: A review. *Alcoholism Clinical and Experimental Research, 4,* 6–21.

33. Finkel, A. J. (1983). *Hamilton & Hardy's Industrial Toxicology* (4th ed.). Boston: John Wright PSG, Inc.

34. Wood, G. C. (1982). Acute cyanide intoxication: Diagnosis and management. *Clinical Toxicology Consultant, 4,* 140–149.

35. Cohen, M. (1984). Treatment of cyanide poisoning. *Veterinary and Human Toxicology, 26,* 503–504.

36. Drew, R. (1983). The use of hydroxycobalamin in the prophylaxis and treatment of nitroprusside-induced cyanide toxicity. *Veterinary and Human Toxicology, 25,* 5.

37. Beamer, W., Shealy, R., & Prough, D. (1983). Acute cyanide poisoning from Laetrile ingestion. *Annals of Emergency Medicine, 12,* 449–451.

38. Wilson, J. (1983). Cyanide in human disease: A review of clinical and laboratory evidence. *Fundamental and Applied Toxicology, 3,* 647–649.

39. Osuntokun, B. O., Monekessa, G., & Wilson, J. (1968). Plasma amino acids in the Nigerian nutritional ataxia neuropathy. *British Medical Journal, 3,* 647–649.

40. Osuntokun, B. O., Monekessa, G., & Wilson, J. (1968). Relationship of a degenerated tropical neuropathy to diet: Report of a field survey. *British Medical Journal, 1,* 547–550.

41. Montgomery, R. D. (1965). The medical significance of cyanogen in plant foodstuffs. *American Journal of Clinical Nutrition, 17,* 103–113.

42. Grahm, D. L., Laman, D., & Theodor, J. (1977). Acute cyanide poisoning complicated by lactic acidosis and

pulmonary edema. *Archives of Internal Medicine, 137,* 1051–1055.

43. Litovitz, T. L., Larkin, R. F., & Myers, R. A. (1983). Cyanide poisoning treated with hyperbaric oxygen. *American Journal of Emergency Medicine, 1,* 94–101.

44. Way, J. L., Sylvester, D., & Morgan, R. L. (1984). Recent perspectives on the toxicodynamic basis of cyanide antagonism. *Fundamental and Applied Toxicology, 4,* S231–S239.

45. Callahan, M. (1979). Tricyclic antidepressant overdose. *Journal of American College of Emergency Physicians, 8,* 413–415.

46. Burks, J., Walker, J., & Rumack, B. (1974). Tricyclic antidepressant poisoning: Reversal of coma, choreoathetosis and myoclonus by physostigmine. *Journal of the American Medical Association, 230,*(10), 1405–1407.

47. Marshal, J., & Forker, A. (1982). Cardiovascular effects of tricyclic antidepressant drugs: Therapeutic usage, overdose, and management of complications. *American Heart Journal, 103*(3), 401–414.

48. Gilman, A., Goodman, L., & Gilman, A. (1980). *The pharmacologic basis of therapeutics.* New York: Macmillan.

49. Cantrill, S. V. (1983). Prophylactic phenytoin in tricyclic overdose. *Journal of Emergency Medicine, 1,* 169–177.

50. Cassano, G. B., Sjostrana, S. E., Hansson, E. (1965). Distribution and fate of C^{14}-amitriptyline in mice and rats. *Psychopharmacologia, 8,* 1.

51. Noble, J., & Matthews, H. (1969). Acute poisoning by tricyclic antidepressants: Clinical features and management of 100 patients. *Clinical Toxicology, 2*(4), 403–421.

52. Woodhead, R. (1979). Cardiac rhythm in tricyclic antidepressant poisoning. *Clinical Toxicology, 14*(5), 499–505.

53. Fasoli, R., & Glauser, F. (1981). Cardiac arrhythmias and ECG abnormalities in tricyclic antidepressant overdose. *Clinical Toxicology, 18*(2), 155–163.

54. Starkey, I. R., & Lawson, A. H. (1980). Poisoning with tricyclic and related antidepressants—a ten year review. *Quarterly Journal of Medicine, 193,* 33–49.

55. Burrows, G. D., Bohra, J., & Hunt, D. (1976). Cardiac effects of different tricyclic antidepressant drugs. *British Journal of Psychiatry, 129,* 335–341.

56. Crome, P. (1982). Antidepressant overdose. *Drugs, 23,* 431–461.

57. Petit, J., Spiker, D., & Ruwitch, J. (1977). Tricyclic antidepressant plasma levels and adverse effects after overdose. *Clinical Pharmacology and Therapeutics, 21*(1), 47–51.

58. Spiker, D., Weiss, A., & Chang, S. (1975). Tricyclic antidepressant overdose: Clinical presentation and plasma levels. *Clinical Pharmacology and Therapeutics, 18*(5), 539–546.

59. Scheinin, M., Virlanen, R., & Iialo, E. (1980). Effect of activated charcoal on the pharmacokinetics of doxepin. *Naunyn-Schmiedebergs Archives of Pharmacology, 313,* Suppl. 223.

60. Heath, A., Wickstrom, I., & Martensson, E. (1982). Treatment of antidepressant overdose with resin hemoperfusion. *Human Toxicology, 1,* 361–371.

61. Brown, T. C. K., Barker, G. A., & Dunlop, M. E. (1973). The use of sodium bicarbonate in the treatment of tricyclic antidepressant-induced arrhythmias. *Anaesthesiology and Intensive Care, 1*(3), 203–210.

62. Brown, T. C. K. (1976). Tricyclic antidepressant overdose: Experimental studies on the management of circulatory complications. *Clinical Toxicology, 9*(2), 255–272.

63. Uhl, J. A. (1981). Phenytoin: The drug of choice in tricyclic antidepressant overdose. *Annals of Emergency Medicine, 10,* 270–275.

64. Manoguerra, A. (1982). Tricyclic antidepressants. *Critical Care Quarterly, 4,* 43–52.

65. Heiser, J., & Wilbert, D. (1974). Reversal of delirium induced by tricyclic antidepressant drugs with physostigmine. *American Journal of Psychiatry, 131*(11), 1275–1277.

66. Vance, M. A., Ross, S. M., & Millington, W. R. (1977). Potentiation of tricyclic antidepressant toxicity by physostigmine in mice. *Clinical Toxicology, 11*(4), 413–421.

67. Lum, B., Follmer, C., & Lockwood, R. (1982). Experimental studies on the effects of physostigmine and isoproterenol on toxicity produced by tricyclic antidepressant agents. *Journal of Toxicology and Clinical Toxicology, 19*(1), 51–65.

68. Kingston, M. E. (1979). Hyperventilation in tricyclic antidepressant poisoning. *Critical Care Medicine, 7,* 550–551.

69. Kline, S., & Bayer, M. (1983). Insecticide poisoning. In Rumack, B., & Mayer, M. (Eds.), *Poisoning and overdose.* Baltimore, Md.: Aspen Systems.

70. Vale, J. A., & Meredith, T. J. (1981). *Poisoning: Diagnosis and treatment.* London: Update Books.

71. Temple, A. R. (1978). Pathophysiology of aspirin overdosage toxicity with implications for management. *Pediatrics, 62,* 873–876.

72. Temple, A. R. (1981). Acute and chronic effects of

aspirin toxicity and their treatments. *Archives of Internal Medicine, 141,* 364–368.

73. Done, A. K. (1960). Salicylate intoxication: Significance of measurements of salicylates in blood in cases of acute ingestion. *Pediatrics, 26,* 800–807.

74. Done, A. K., & Temple, A. R. (1971). Treatment of salicylate poisoning. *Modern Treatment, 8,* 528–551.

75. Snodgrass, W., Rumack, B. H., & Peterson, R. G. (1981). Salicylate toxicity following therapeutic doses in young children. *Clinical Toxicology, 18,* 247–259.

76. Russell, F. H. (1980). *Snake venom poisoning.* Philadelphia: Lippincott.

77. Berlinger, W. G., Regroed, S., & Goldberg, M. J. (1983). Enhancement of theophylline clearance by oral activated charcoal. *Clinical Pharmacology and Therapeutics, 33,* 351–354.

78. Sessler, C. N., Glauser, F. L., & Cooper, K. R. (1985). Treatment of theophylline toxicity with oral activated charcoal. *Chest, 87,* 325–329.

part

14

Appendix

Frequently Used Drugs in Critical Care

Jeanette Hartshorn

Disclaimer

List of Drugs

Acetaminophen
Albumin
Aminocaproic Acid
Aminophylline
Amiodarone
Amphotericin B
Amrinone
Aspirin
Atropine Sulfate
Bretylium
Bumetanide
Bupivacaine
Calcium Chloride
Chloramphenicol
Chlorpromazine Hydrochloride
Cimetidine
Clindamycin Hydrochloride
Corticosteriods
Cyclosporine
Dactinomycin
Desmopressin Acetate
Dextran 40
Diazepam
Dicumarol
Digitoxin
Digoxin
Disopyramide Phosphate
Dobutamine

Dopamine Hydrochloride
Edrophonium
Epinephrine
Ergonovine Maleate
Ethacrynic Acid
Fentanyl
Flucytosine
Furosemide
Glucagon
Heparin Sodium
Hetastarch
Hydralazine
Hydrochlorothiazide
Hydroxyzine
Insulin
Isoproterenol Hydrochloride
Isosorbide
Labetalol
Levarterenol Bitartrate
Lidocaine
Magnesium Sulfate
Mannitol
Meperidine Hydrochloride
Metaraminol Bitartrate
Methotrexate
Methoxamine
Metocurine
Morphine Sulfate
Naloxone Hydrochloride
Neostigmine
Nitroglycerin

Nitroprusside
Pancuronium Bromide
Pentobarbital
Phentolamine
Phenytoin
Phenyleprine
Physostigmine
Plasma Protein Fraction
Potassium Chloride
Procainamide Hydrochloride
Promethazine Hydrochloride
Propranolol Hydrochloride
Protamine
Pyridostigmine
Pyrimethamine
Quinidine
Ranitidine
Rh_o (D) Immune Human Globulin
Rifampin
Sodium Bicarbonate
Streptokinase
Succinylcholine
Sulfamethoxazole-Trimethoprim
Thiopental Sodium for Injection
Trimethaphan
Tubocurarine
Vasopressin
Verapamil
Warfarin Sodium

Table of Antibiotics

Disclaimer

The author and publisher have exerted every effort to ensure that drug selection and dosage set forth in this text are in accord with current recommendations and practice at the time of publication. However, in view of ongoing research, changes in government regulations, and the constant flow of information relating to drug therapy and drug reactions, the reader is urged to check the package insert for each drug for any change in indications and dosage and for added warnings and precautions. This is particularly important when the recommended agent is a new or infrequently employed drug.

Dosages included in this appendix are designed to represent acceptable ranges. Please refer to the manufacturer for specific recommendations.

Acetaminophen

Category

Analgesic; antipyretic

Brand Names

Datril

Phenaphen

Tempra

Tylenol

Valadol

Pharmacologic Mechanism

Acetaminophen raises the pain threshold and affects the hypothalamic heat-regulating center. The drug may act by inhibiting prostaglandin synthesis in the central nervous system (CNS) through a peripheral action by blocking pain-impulse generation. The peripheral action may also be due to inhibition of the synthesis of prostaglandins or to inhibition of the synthesis or actions of other substances, which sensitize pain receptors to mechanical or chemical stimulation. Acetaminophen may act predominantly on the CNS. The drug has the same analgesic activity as aspirin but lacks antiinflammatory and uricosuric activity.

Uses

Analgesic and antipyretic.

Doses

1. Under 3 years, consult with physician.
2. 3 to 6 years: 120 mg, 3 to 4 times daily. Do not exceed a total daily dose of 480 mg.
3. 7 to 13 years: 162 to 325 mg three to four times daily. Do not exceed a total daily dose of 1.3 g.
4. Adults: 325 to 650 mg three to four times daily. Do not exceed a total daily dose of 2.6 g.

Nursing Interventions and Administration

1. May be administered without regard to meals.
2. Should be given with a full glass of water.

Adverse Effects

Anemia, pancytopenia, leukopenia, urticaria, and rare instances of methemoglobinemia and hemolytic anemia.

Drug Interactions

1. Concurrent use with anticoagulants may increase the anticoagulant effect.
2. Use with alcohol or hepatic enzyme-inducing agents increases the risk of hepatotoxicity.

Contraindications

Hypersensitivity or known 6-phosphate dehydrogenase deficiency.

Albumin (Human)

Category

Volume expander

Brand Names

Albuconn

Albuminar

Pharmacologic Mechanism

Normal serum albumin (human) is a solution containing the normal serum albumin component of human blood. The 25% concentration is oncotically equivalent to approximately five times its volume of normal human plasma. The effective colloid osmotic pressure of the serum proteins depends very largely on the relatively small and numerous albumin molecules, which therefore play a decisive role in the maintenance of the circulating plasma volume. The colloid osmotic or oncotic properties of albumin constitute the predominant reason for its clinical use. The Starling concept of the capillary balance of hydrostatic and oncotic pressure gradients across the capillary walls as the determinant of the fluid volume distribution between the intravascular and the interstitial compartment explains the mechanism of action of this product. Available as 5% solution and 25% solution.

Uses

Plasma or blood volume deficit, shock, burns, adult respiratory distress syndrome (ARDS), cardiopulmonary bypass, hypoproteinemia, acute liver failure.

Doses

Dosage is individualized according to the patient and the condition being treated. Please refer to manufacturer's insert for specific recommendations.

Nursing Interventions and Administration

1. Normal serum albumin (human) is always administered intravenously.
2. The solution is compatible with whole blood or packed red cells, electrolyte and carbohydrate solutions intended for intravenous use.
3. It should not be mixed with protein hydrolysates, amino acid mixtures, or solutions containing alcohol.
4. Monitor hemodynamic status during infusion.

Adverse Effects

Nausea, chills, fever, headache, hypotension, fluid overload.

Contraindications

History of incompatibility reaction to albumin.

Aminocaproic Acid

Category

Antihemorrhagic

Brand Name

Amicar

Pharmacologic Mechanism

Aminocaproic acid controls bleeding by competitive inhibition of plasminogen activator substances and, to a lesser degree, by noncompetitive inhibition of plasmin (fibrinolysin) activity. It is ineffective in bleeding caused by loss of vascular integrity. Therefore, a definite clinical or laboratory diagnosis of hyperfibrinolysis is needed prior to initiation of therapy.

Uses

Fibrinolysis-induced hemorrhage, hemorrhage following cardiovascular surgery, subarachnoid hemorrhage.

Doses

1. The usual oral adult dose is 5 g the first hour, followed by 1 or 1.25 g per hour for approximately 8 h or until the desired response is obtained.

2. The usual adult parenteral dose is intravenous infusion of 4 to 5 g administered over a period of 1 h, followed by continuous infusion at the rate of 1 g per hour for approximately 8 h or until the desired response is obtained. For subarachnoid hemorrhage, the usual intravenous dose is 1 to 1.5 g per hour by continuous infusion or bolus.

3. The usual pediatric oral dose is 100 mg per kilogram of body weight for the first hour, followed by 33.3 mg per kilogram of body weight.

4. The usual pediatric parenteral dose is 100 mg per kilogram of body weight over a period of 1 h, followed by continuous infusion at the rate of 33.3 mg per kilogram of body weight.

Nursing Interventions and Administration

1. The drug should be diluted before parenteral administration.
2. Rapid infusion can cause hypotension and bradycardia.
3. Cardiovascular response to infusion of the drug should be closely monitored.
4. Aminocaproic acid can be used as an antidote to streptokinase.

Adverse Effects

Dysuria, urinary frequency, oliguria, muscular pain, weakness, irregular pulse, bradycardia, fatigue, headache, nausea and vomiting, ringing in ears.

Major Drug Interactions

Concurrent use with oral contraceptives or estrogens may increase the potential for blood clotting.

Therapeutic Drug Levels

130 µg/mL.

Contraindications

Active intravascular clotting. Careful consideration should be given to using this drug when cardiac disease, hematuria, hepatic disease, renal disease, or thrombosis exists.

Aminophylline

Category

Bronchodilator; decongestant

Brand Names

Phyllocontin

Somophyllin

Pharmacologic Mechanism

Aminophylline relaxes the smooth muscle of the bronchial airways and pulmonary blood vessels to relieve bronchospasm and increase flow rates and vital capacity. The drug stimulates the CNS, promotes diuresis, produces a positive chronotropic and inotropic effect on the heart, and increases the release of epinephrine. At toxic and possibly therapeutic serum concentrations, xanthines may decrease the seizure threshold.

Uses

Indicated for bronchial asthma, cardiac paroxysmal dyspnea, congestive heart failure, status asthmaticus, and emphysema. Aminophylline has been used in the treatment of Cheyne-Stokes respiration to relieve periodic apnea and increased arterial blood pH.

Doses

1. The pediatric oral dose is 6 mg/kg for acute asthmatic attacks and 5 mg/kg every 6 h for maintenance.
2. The adult oral dose is 500 mg for acute asthmatic attacks and 200 to 250 mg every 6 to 8 h for maintenance.
3. The pediatric dose is 6 mg/kg daily in three divided doses, intravenously.
4. The adult dose is 250 mg as required intravenously.
5. Suppositories are not recommended for acute attacks because of unreliable absorption.
6. Retention enemas can be administered to adults at a dose of 5 to 6 mg/kg (the solution contains 60 mg/mL).

Nursing Interventions and Administration

1. Oral administration with meals will help reduce gastric upset.
2. Parenteral doses should be diluted with intravenous fluid and injected slowly at a rate of approximately 2 to 5 mg per minute.
3. Careful monitoring of vital signs during intravenous infusion is required.

Drug Interactions

1. Avoid concurrent use with beta-adrenergic drugs, since they may antagonize the effects of aminophylline.
2. General anesthetics may increase the risk of cardiac arrhythmias.
3. Use with cimetidine may decrease hepatic clearance.
4. Following vaccination against influenza, theophylline elimination may be decreased, resulting in increased serum theophylline concentrations.
5. Concurrent use with phenytoin may stimulate hepatic metabolism of xanthine.

Incompatibilities

1. Do not mix in same syringe with other medications.
2. Add separately to intravenous solutions.

Therapeutic Drug Levels

A serum sample should be obtained at the time of peak absorption; 2 h after administration of immediate-release preparations and 4 to 12 h after administration of extended-release preparations.

Theophylline (for bronchodilator effect): 10 to 20 μg/mL. Toxic levels are $\geq$20 μg/mL.

Contraindications

Use with caution in patients with cardiac or hepatic disease, hypertension, hyperthyroidism, or peptic ulcer.

Amiodarone

Category

Antiarrhythmic; antiangina

Brand Name

Cordarone

Pharmacologic Mechanism

Amiodarone is considered a class III antiarrhythmic agent because it prolongs the duration of the ventricular myocardial action potential, but has no significant effect on its rapid upstroke phase. It also prolongs repolarization and refractoriness of all cardiac tissues from the sinus node to the ventricular myocardium. The use-dependent effect is thought to be from blockade of inactivated sodium channels.

Amiodarone suppresses sinus node and atrioventricular nodal automaticity due to slowing of diastolic depolarization. It also exhibits an antisympathetic effect, blocking both alpha and beta receptors.

Uses

Supraventricular tachycardia, Wolff-Parkinson-White syndrome, atrial fibrillation, atrial flutter, bradycardia-tachycardia syndrome, ventricular arrhythmias.

Doses

1. An oral loading dose of 800 to 1600 mg daily for 1 to 3 weeks, then 600 mg daily for 4 weeks, followed by a further reduction to 400 mg daily or 400 mg alternating with 600 mg daily.
2. An oral loading dose of 10 mg per kilogram of body weight per day has been established for pediatric use.
3. The adult intravenous dose is recommended to be 5 mg/kg, slowly administered over 20 min to 2 h.

Nursing Interventions and Administration

1. Because of the length of time required to reach a loading dose, the patient should be hospitalized during early therapy.
2. During administration, hemodynamic parameters should be carefully monitored.

Adverse Effects

Photosensitivity, corneal deposits, pulmonary alveolitis, fatigue, weakness, tremor, ataxia, peripheral neuropathy, abdominal pain, nausea and vomiting, metallic taste in mouth, headache, constipation.

Major Drug Interactions

1. Concurrent use with warfarin can cause an increase in anticoagulant effect.
2. A progressive elevation of serum digoxin concentration has been noted during the first 7 days of amiodarone therapy.
3. Increases in steady-state serum concentrations of quinidine, disopyramide, mexiletene, and aprindine have been reported when used with amiodarone.

Therapeutic Drug Levels
1 to 2.5 μg/mL.

Amphotericin B

Category

Antibiotic: antifungal antibiotic

Brand Name

Fungizone

Pharmacologic Mechanism

Fungistatic activity due to alteration of cell membrane permeability in susceptible fungi.

Uses

Indicated in the treatment of infections caused by susceptible strains of *Aspergillus fumigatus, Blastomyces dermatitidis, Candida* spp., *Coccidioides immitis, Cryptococcus neoformans, Histoplasma capsulatum, Mucor mucido,* and *Sporotrichum schenckii.*

Doses

Parenteral dose for pediatric and adult use starts with a daily dose of 0.25 mg/kg and gradually increases as tolerance permits. Total daily dosage may range from 1 to a maximum of 50 mg daily.

Nursing Interventions and Administration

1. Intravenous infusion should be given over a period of 6 h at a concentration of 0.1 mg/mL.
2. Dilute with 10 mL of sterile water for injection.
3. Solution should be used promptly after dilution.
4. Intravenous administration of small doses of adrenocorticoids just prior to or during intravenous infusion may reduce the incidence of febrile reactions.

Adverse Effects

Headache, nausea, vomiting, malaise, dyspepsia, diarrhea, local phlebitis and thrombophlebitis, hypokalemia, azotemia, hyposthenuria, renal tubular acidosis, and nephrocalcinosis.

Drug Interactions

1. Use with caution in patients on concurrent cardiac glycosides or corticosteroids since potential for digoxin toxicity may be increased.
2. Amphotericin can enhance the activity of surgical neuromuscular blocking agents.

Therapeutic Drug Levels

2 to 4 μg/mL.

Contraindications

1. Hypersensitivity, unless required for a life-threatening infection.
2. Caution should be exercised in using drug for patients with renal function impairment.

Amrinone

Category

Cardiotonic

Brand Name

Inocor

Pharmacologic Mechanism

Amrinone lactate is a positive inotropic agent with vasodilator activity. Experimental evidence indicates that it is not a beta-adrenergic agonist. It inhibits myocardial cAMP activity and increases cellular levels of cAMP. It reduces afterload and preload by its direct relaxant effect on vascular smooth muscle.

Improvement in left ventricular function and relief of congestive heart failure in patients with ischemic heart disease have been observed. The improvement has occurred without inducing symptoms of myocardial ischemia. At constant heart rate and blood pressure, increases in cardiac output occur without measurable increases in myocardial oxygen consumption or changes in arteriovenous oxygen difference.

Uses

Short-term management of congestive heart failure.

Doses

1. 750 μg per kilogram of body weight given slowly over 2 to 3 minutes for adults.
2. Pediatric dosages have not been established.

Nursing Interventions and Administration

1. Should be administered as supplied or diluted in normal or half-normal saline solution to a concentration of 1 mg/mL to 3 mg/mL. Diluted solutions should be used within 24 h.
2. Amrinone should not be diluted with solutions containing dextrose due to the possibility of a chemical interaction.

Adverse Effects

Thrombocytopenia, nausea, vomiting, abdominal pain, anorexia, arrhythmias, hypotension, hepatic toxicity, fever, chest pain, burning at injection sites.

Major Drug Interactions

One case of excessive hypotension has been reported when amrinone was used concurrently with disopyramide.

Contraindications

Known hypersensitivity.

Aspirin

Category

Analgesic: antiinflammatory, antipyretic

Brand Names

ASA

Ecotrin

Pharmacologic Mechanism

Aspirin raises the pain threshold and affects the hypothalamic heat regulatory center. The drug may act by inhibiting prostaglandin synthesis in the central nervous system and through peripheral action by blocking pain due to inhibition of the synthesis of prostaglandins or to inhibition of the synthesis or actions of other substances, which sensitize pain receptors to mechanical or chemical

stimulation. Salicylates may act predominantly via peripheral mechanisms.

Uses

Analgesic and antipyretic.

Doses

1. PO or rectal.
2. Pediatric: As an analgesic-antipyretic, or antirheumatic: 11 to 16 mg/kg six times daily. Reduce as soon as possible to 10 mg/kg six times daily.
3. Adults: As an analgesic-antipyretic, or antirheumatic: 650 mg four to six times daily; 1 g four to six times daily. Do not exceed 10 g daily.

Nursing Interventions and Administration

Administer with food or a full glass of water (240 mL) to help reduce gastric upset.

Adverse Effects

Epigastric distress, nausea, gastrointestinal bleeding ulcers, tinnitus, hypoprothrombinemia, and asthma.

Drug Interactions

1. Avoid concurrent use with ulcerogenic drugs, indomethacin, oral anticoagulants, probenecid, and sulfinpyrazone.
2. Aspirin can increase the activity of the oral hypoglycemic agents and methotrexate.

Contraindications

Hypersensitivity or active ulcers.

Atropine Sulfate

Category

Anticholinergic: antimuscarinic, parasympatholytic

Pharmacologic Mechanism

Atropine causes anticholinergic activity due to the competition with acetylcholine for muscarinic receptors at the postganglionic fiber of the parasympathetic nervous system. Atropine stimulates or depresses the CNS, depending on the dose; and has a more prolonged and potent action than the other belladonna alkaloids on the heart, intestine, and bronchial muscle.

Uses

1. To treat, manage, or cause bradycardia, bronchial asthma, cardiospasm, colitis, dilation of pupils, dysmenorrhea relief, enuresis control, gastrointestinal spasm, inhibition of bronchial and gastric secretions, inhibition of salivation and sweating, paralysis of accommodation, paralysis agitans, postencephalitis, parkinsonism, pylorospasm, secretions due to coryza and rhinitis, spastic and rigid states due to CNS injury, ureteral colic, and urinary frequency reduction.
2. Antidote for cholinergic drugs.

Doses

1. The pediatric oral dose is 0.01 mg/kg every 4 to 6 h. Do not exceed a single dose of 0.4 mg.
2. The usual adult oral dose is 0.1 to 1.2 mg every 4 to 6 h.
3. The pediatric parenteral dose is 0.01 mg/kg every 4 to 6 h. Initial dose of 1 mg every 10 to 15 min until signs of atropine toxicity appear.
4. As an anticholinergic antidote the usual adult parenteral dose is 0.4 to 0.6 mg every 4 to 6 h. Initial dose of 2 to 4 mg followed by 2 mg every 5 to 10 min until signs of atropine toxicity appear.

Nursing Interventions and Administration

1. Tablets are usually administered before meals.
2. In parenteral antidotal therapy, the first administration of atropine is usually by IV injection. Repeated injections are usually by the IM route.
3. Intravenous injections should be slow.

Adverse Effects

Blurred vision, cycloplegia, increased ocular tension, constipation, loss of taste, dysphagia, suppression of lactation and body secretions, tachycardia, mental confusion, and urinary retention.

Drug Interactions

1. Concurrent use with antihistamines, monoamine oxidase inhibitors, phenothiazines, and tricyclic antidepressants will produce enhanced anticholinergic effects.
2. Simultaneous use with antacids or antidiarrheal suspensions may reduce absorption of belladonna alkaloids, resulting in decreased therapeutic effectiveness.

Contraindications

In patients with adhesions between the iris and lens, advanced hepatic and renal impairment, asthma, hiatal hernia associated with reflux esophagitis, hypersensitivity, intestinal atony, myasthenia gravis, narrow-angle glaucoma, obstructive disease of the gastrointestinal and urinary tract, and severe ulcerative colitis.

Bretylium

Category

Antiarrhythmic

Brand Name

Bretylol

Pharmacologic Mechanism

Bretylium appears to produce a direct effect on the myocardial cell membrane which produces a rapid suppression of ventricular fibrillation. It is also known that an adrenergic blockade of norepinephrine occurs following an initial release of norepinephrine at the peripheral adrenergic nerve terminals. The blockage of further norepinephrine release is thought to contribute to suppression of ventricular tachycardia.

Uses

Ventricular arrhythmias.

Doses

1. For existing ventricular fibrillation, intravenous, initially 5 mg per kilogram of body weight rapidly administered undiluted, followed by 10 mg per kilogram of body weight every 15 to 30 min if necessary, to a total of 30 mg per kilogram of body weight per day.
2. For other ventricular arrhythmias, intermittent intravenous infusion, diluted and administered at a rate of 5 to 10 mg per kilogram of body weight over a 10-to-30-min period. The dose may be repeated after 1 to 2 h if necessary, and then every 6 to 8 h for maintenance.

3. Constant intravenous infusion, diluted and administered at a rate of 1 to 2 mg per minute.
4. Intramuscular dosage of 5 to 10 mg per kilogram of body weight administered undiluted and repeated after 1 to 2 h if necessary, with subsequent doses administered every 6 to 8 h for maintenance.

Nursing Interventions and Administration

1. Bretylium is always diluted before intravenous administration except when used in life-threatening ventricular fibrillation when it is administered undiluted and as rapidly as possible.
2. Intramuscular administration should be limited to 5 mL, undiluted, at each injection site. The area of injection should be rotated to avoid tissue destruction.
3. Bretylium is used clinically for short-term therapy only. It should be discontinued after 3 to 5 days by gradual dosage reduction and replaced with an oral antiarrhythmic therapy if necessary.

Adverse Effects

Hypotension, hyperthermia, nausea, vomiting, lightheadedness, syncope, renal function impairment, shortness of breath.

Major Drug Interactions

Bretylium may aggravate digitalis toxicity; concurrent use is not recommended.

Bumetanide

Category

Diuretic

Brand Name

Bumex

Pharmacologic Mechanism

Bumetanide acts primarily on the ascending limb of the loop of Henle to inhibit reabsorption of water and electrolytes. It may have an additional action on sodium reabsorption in the proximal tubule since phosphate reabsorption is reduced. It appears to have no effect on the distal tubule.

Uses

Edema.

Doses

1. The usual oral adult dose is 500 μg to 2 mg per day as a single daily dose. The dose may be increased, if necessary, by addition of a second or third daily dose with intervals of 4 to 5 h between doses. An intermittent dosage schedule, administration on alternate days for 3 or 4 days, with 1 or 2 days in between, may also be used. The adult prescribing limit is up to 10 mg per day.
2. Intravenous or intramuscular dosage is 500 μg to 1 mg repeated at intervals of 2 to 3 h, if necessary.

Nursing Interventions and Administration

1. Monitor for signs of electrolyte imbalance.
2. One or two daily doses appear to be more effective than small doses administered frequently.
3. Concurrent administration of potassium supplements or potassium-sparing diuretics may be indicated in patients considered to be at higher risk for developing hypokalemia.
4. Intravenous administration is generally preferred over intramuscular administration.
5. Intravenous administration should be at a slow, controlled rate over a 2-min period.

Adverse Effects

Dryness of mouth, increased thirst, irregular heart beat, mood changes, muscle cramps, nausea, vomiting, weakness, weak pulse, chest pain, dizziness, and headache are rarely reported.

Major Drug Interactions

1. Concurrent use with aminoglycoside antibiotics with parenteral bumetanide may increase the potential for ototoxicity, especially in the presence of renal function impairment.
2. Indomethacin or probenecid may antagonize the natriuresis and increase in plasma renin activity caused by bumetanide; indomethacin may also reduce the increase in urine volume caused by bumetadine; concurrent use is not recommended.

3. Concurrent use of lithium salts with bumetanide may provoke lithium toxicity because of reduced renal clearance and is not recommended unless patient is closely monitored.
4. Concurrent and/or sequential administration with ototoxic or nephrotoxic medications (such as cisplatin, ethacrynic acid, furosemide, mercaptomerin, polymyxins, or cephalosporins) should be avoided since the potential for ototoxicity and nephrotoxicity may be increased.

Contraindications
Anuria and other forms of severe renal function impairment.

Bupivacaine

Category
Local anesthetic

Brand Names
Marcaine

Sensorcaine

Pharmacologic Mechanism
Bupivacaine acts by blocking both the initiation and conduction of nerve impulses by reversibly stabilizing the neuronal membrane, thereby decreasing its permeability to sodium ions. This inhibits the depolarization phase of the neuronal membrane, resulting in the failure of a propagated action potential and consequent conduction blockade.

Uses
Local anesthesia

Doses

1. Moderate motor block: 37.5 to 75 mg (15 to 30 mL) as a 0.25% solution repeated once every 3 h as needed.
2. Moderate to complete motor block: 75 to 150 mg (15 to 30 mL) as a 0.25% solution, repeated once every 3 h as needed.
3. Usual pediatric dosage has not been established.

Nursing Interventions and Administration

1. The actual dosage and maximum dosage must be individualized.
2. Local anesthetics should be injected slowly, with frequent aspirations before and during the injection, to reduce the risk of inadvertent intravascular administration.
3. Monitor for potential cardiovascular effects during administration.

Adverse Effects
Blurred vision, dizziness, ringing in ears, anxiety, drowsiness, hives, skin rash, hypotension, headache.

Major Drug Interactions

1. Concurrent use with local CNS depressants may result in additive depressant effects.
2. Concurrent use of bupivacaine with epinephrine and with beta-adrenergic blocking agents may result in dose-dependent hypertension and bradycardia.

Contraindications
Use with caution in patients with cardiovascular function impairment, heart block, drug sensitivity, or inflammation or sepsis in the region of injection.

Calcium Chloride

Category

Cardiotonic, antihypocalcemic, electrolyte replenisher

Trade Name
Calcium chloride injection

Pharmacologic Mechanism
The presence of free ionic calcium in body fluids is required for the necessary participation of calcium in many complex physiological processes such as blood clot formation, muscle contraction, and nerve impulse transmission.

Uses
Cardiac resuscitation, hypocalcemia, hyperkalemia, hypermagnesemia.

Doses

1. The usual adult parenteral dose is 500 mg to 1 g administered intravenously at a rate not to exceed 1 mL per minute.
2. Dosages of 200 to 800 mg can be administered directly into the ventricle.
3. The usual pediatric dosage is 25 mg per kilogram of body weight administered slowly.

Nursing Interventions and Administration

1. Calcium chloride injection 10% is only administered by slow intravenous injection, or in cardiac resuscitation by injection into the ventricle.
2. Extravasation of calcium chloride can cause tissue necrosis or sloughing.
3. A continuous monitoring of cardiac function should accompany the use of intravenous calcium.
4. Constantly monitor patient for signs of additional electrolyte imbalance.

Adverse Effects

Bradycardia, cardiac arrest, diarrhea, irregular heart beat, loss of appetite, mental depression, fatigue.

Major Drug Interactions

1. Administration of intravenous calcium preparations to patients who are also receiving calcium-ion influx inhibitors may diminish the effect of calcium-ion influx inhibitors.
2. Administration of intravenous calcium to patients who are also receiving digitalis glycosides or who have been digitalized may cause severe cardiac arrhythmias; some may be fatal.
3. Hypercalcemia may occur in patients receiving vitamin D and calcium preparations concurrently during long-term therapy.
4. Concurrent use with magnesium sulfate may neutralize effects.
5. Use with tetracyclines may decrease absorption of tetracycline.

Contraindications

Digitalis toxicity, ventricular fibrillation, renal function impairment.

Chloramphenicol

Category

Antibiotic: antirickettsial

Brand Name

Chloromycetin

Pharmacologic Mechanism

The bacteriostatic activity is due to inhibition of ribosomal protein synthesis in susceptible microorganisms.

Uses

The toxicity of chloramphenicol restricts its use to serious infections when less toxic antibiotics are ineffective or contraindicated. Not all species or strains of a particular organism may be susceptible to chloramphenicol.

1. One of the drugs of choice for *Salmonella typhi.*
2. Treatment of infections caused by susceptible strains of *Hemophilus influenzae, Salmonella* spp., and *Rickettsia,* and in lymphogranuloma and psittacosis.
3. Other susceptible microorganisms that are resistant to all other appropriate antimicrobial drugs.

Doses

1. The pediatric oral dose is 50 mg/kg daily divided into four equal doses.
2. The adult oral dose is 50 to 100 mg/kg daily divided into four equal doses.
3. Dosage for newborns must be adjusted according to serum levels to prevent gray baby syndrome. Infants and children with immature metabolism must receive lower dosages.

Nursing Interventions and Administration

1. Oral dosage forms should be administered on an empty stomach with a full glass of water (240 mL).
2. Frequent CBCs may be required to detect dose-related reversible bone marrow depression.

Administration for Injection

1. IV injection should not exceed 100 mg/mL and should be administered over 12 min.
2. The reconstituted solution is compatible with most infusion solutions.
3. Patients should be switched to an oral dosage form as soon as possible.
4. The drug is ineffective when given intramuscularly.
5. Each vial containing 1 g of chloramphenicol supplies 3.1 meq of sodium.

Adverse Effects

1. The most serious is bone marrow depression. Irreversible bone marrow depression leading to fatal aplastic anemia can appear weeks or months after therapy. This risk factor is approximately 1 in 25,000 to 1 in 41,000.
2. Reversible type of bone marrow depression which is dose-related and characterized by vaculocytes and leukopenia.
3. Gray baby syndrome in premature or newborn babies. Symptoms appear after 3 to 4 days of treatment and include abdominal distention, progressive pallid cyanosis, vasomotor collapse, and irregular respiration.

Drug Interactions

1. Chloramphenicol is an enzyme inhibitor and can affect the metabolism of oral anticoagulants, sulfonylureas, and phenytoin.
2. Concurrent use with other bone marrow-depressing drugs should be avoided.
3. Chloramphenicol can antagonize the bactericidal effects of the penicillins and cephalosporins.
4. Chloramphenicol may decrease the effects of vitamin B-12, folic acid, and iron preparations in anemic patients.

Desired Serum Concentration

10 to 25 μg/mL. Higher concentrations increase the risk of reversible bone marrow depression.

Contraindications

1. Hypersensitivity or previous toxic reactions to chloramphenicol.
2. In treating minor bacterial or viral infections.

Chlorpromazine Hydrochloride

Category

Antipsychotic: phenothiazine tranquilizer

Brand Names

Chlor-PZ

Oramazine

Promapar

Thorazine

Pharmacologic Mechanism

The phenothiazines block postsynaptic dopamine receptors in the limbic system and basal ganglia, which results in a tranquilizing effect in psychotic patients. The phenothiazines exert strong anti-alpha-adrenergic and weaker peripheral anticholinergic activity and varying degrees of antiemetic activity.

Uses

Phenothiazines are used in the treatment of psychotic manifestations, anxiety and restlessness, nausea, vomiting, hyperexcitable behavior, hyperkinesis, tetanus, porphyria, and hiccups.

Doses

1. The adult oral dose is 10 to 50 mg two to six times a day. Dosage may be adjusted gradually as needed and tolerated.
2. The adult IM dose is 25 to 50 mg repeated in 1 h if needed and every 3½ h thereafter as needed and tolerated.
3. The adult IV dose is 25 to 50 mg diluted to a concentration of not more than 1 mg/mL with sodium chloride injection and administration at a rate of 1 mg per minute.
4. In general, dosage levels should be lower in the elderly, the emaciated, and the debilitated.

Nursing Interventions and Administration

1. For IM administration inject slowly and deeply into the upper outer quadrant of the buttock. Because of possible hypotensive effects keep patient lying down for at least ½ h after injection.

2. IM injection irritation may be reduced by diluting with sterile normal saline injection.
3. IV route should be limited to surgery and severe hiccups.
4. Recommended IV dilution is 1 mg of drug in 24 mL of sterile normal saline injection.

Adverse Effects

Mild to moderate drowsiness, photosensitivity, exfoliative dermatitis, lactation and breast enlargement, extrapyramidal symptoms, persistent tardive dyskinesia, postural hypotension, ECG distortions of the Q and T waves, agranulocytosis, hemolytic anemia, thrombocytopenia purpura, skin pigmentation, pigmentary retinopathy, and corneal and lenticular changes.

Drug Interactions

1. Dosage reductions are required for narcotics, barbiturates, and other CNS depressants when used concurrently with phenothiazines.
2. The phenothiazines and the amphetamines are mutually antagonistic to each other.
3. The antihypertensive effects of guanethidine and related drugs will be antagonized by the phenothiazines.
4. Concurrent use with anticoagulants may decrease the anticoagulant effects.
5. Phenothiazines may lower the seizure threshold requiring adjustment of anticonvulsant medications.
6. Alpha-adrenergic effects of epinephrine may be blocked, allowing beta-adrenergic effects to predominate when used with phenothiazines.

Contraindications

Hypersensitivity to chlorpromazine or phenothiazines in comatose patients or in comatose states, in the presence of large amounts of CNS depressants, and with bone marrow depression. Care should be exercised in giving the drug when alcoholism, Reye's syndrome, or hepatic function impairment exist.

Cimetidine

Category

Histamine H_2 receptor antagonist, antiulcer agent, gastric acid secretion inhibitor.

Brand Name

Tagamet

Pharmacologic Mechanism

Cimetidine inhibits basal and nocturnal gastric acid secretion by competitive inhibition of the action of histamine at the histamine H_2 receptors of the parietal cells. The drug also inhibits gastric acid secretion stimulated by food, butazole, pentagastrin, caffeine, and insulin.

Doses

1. The usual adult dosage for duodenal ulcer is 300 mg four times a day. Doses of 400 mg at bedtime are used for prophylaxis of recurrent duodenal ulcer.
2. The usual oral pediatric dose is 20 to 40 mg of cimetidine per kilogram of body weight four times a day.
3. The intramuscular dose is 300 mg every 6 h.
4. Intravenously 300 mg is diluted in 100 mL of compatible intravenous solution and administered over a 10-to-20-min period every 6 h.
5. Pediatric parenteral doses are 5 to 10 mg per kilogram of body weight every 6 h. Intravenous solutions are administered over a 10-to-20-min period.

Nursing Interventions and Administration

1. If required, antacids may be administered concurrently with cimetidine for the relief of pain. Dosages should be separated by at least 1 h.
2. The efficacy of cimetidine in inhibiting nocturnal gastric acid secretion may be decreased by cigarette smoking.
3. Rapid administration of intravenous cimetidine is not recommended because it may increase the risk of cardiac arrhythmias and hypotension.

Adverse Effects

Confusion (more likely to occur in patients over 50 or those severely ill), sore throat, unusual bleeding, cardiac arrhythmias, fatigue, diarrhea, skin rash.

Major Drug Interactions

Hepatic metabolism of anticoagulants, lidocaine, phenytoin, or theophylline may be decreased when used concurrently with cimetidine.

Contraindications

Use with caution in patients with cirrhosis, or other forms of hepatic impairment, moderate to severe renal impairment, or inflammatory disease (SLE).

Clindamycin Hydrochloride

Category

Antibiotic

Brand Name

Cleocin HCl

Pharmacologic Mechanism

Clindamycin exerts its bacteriostatic activity due to inhibition of ribosomal protein synthesis in susceptible microorganisms. Although usually considered bacteriostatic, clindamycin may be bactericidal in high concentrations or when used against highly susceptible organisms.

Uses

Clindamycin can produce severe and sometimes fatal colitis and should be reserved for serious infections where less toxic antibiotics (especially the penicillins and erythromycins) are ineffective or contraindicated.

1. Indicated in the treatment of susceptible strains of pneumococci, staphylococci, and streptococci.
2. In the treatment of susceptible anaerobic bacteria including intestinal strains of *Bacteroides*.

Doses

1. The usual pediatric oral dose is 8 to 12 mg/kg daily divided in three to four equal doses.
2. The usual oral adult dose is 150 to 300 mg every 6 h. Adult dose for more severe infections is 300 to 450 mg every 6 h.
3. The usual parenteral pediatric dose is 15 to 25 mg/kg daily in four equal doses. Severe infections, 25 to 40 mg/kg in three or four equal doses.
4. The usual adult parenteral dose is 600 to 1200 mg/kg daily in two to four equal doses. Severe infection may require 1200 to 2700 mg/kg daily in two to four equal doses.

Nursing Interventions and Administration

Clindamycin must be given on an empty stomach with a full glass of water 1–2 h before meals, and no food may be eaten for at least 1 h after administration.

1. Single IM doses greater than 600 mg are not recommended.
2. Single IV doses greater than 1200 mg in 1-h infusions are not recommended.
3. Sterile solution intended for IV administration should be diluted and administered according to the manufacturer's recommendations.
4. Sterile solution may be mixed with 5% dextrose, 10% dextrose, sodium chloride injection, and Ringer's for IV infusions.

Adverse Effects

Abdominal pain, nausea, vomiting, diarrhea, colitis, maculopapular rash, urticaria, anaphylaxis, erythema multiforme, agranulocytosis, and thrombocytopenia.

Drug Interactions

1. Kaolin and pectin suspensions will greatly reduce the oral absorption of clindamycin.
2. Antibiotic antagonism can exist between clindamycin and chloramphenicol, the erythromycins, the penicillins, and the cephalosporins when used concurrently.
3. Concurrent administration with anesthetics or neuromuscular blocking agents can result in skeletal muscle weakness and respiratory depression or paralysis.

Incompatibilities

Clindamycin is physically incompatible with ampicillin, phenytoin, barbiturates, aminophylline, calcium gluconate, and magnesium sulfate.

Contraindications

Hypersensitivity to clindamycin or lincomycin.

Corticosteroids

Category

Adrenocorticoid, immunosuppressant, antiinflammatory

Brand Names

Cortisone acetate (Cortone acetate)

Dexamethasone (Decadron)

Hydrocortisone (Cortef)

Hydrocortisone sodium succinate (Solu-Cortef)

Hydrocortone

Methylprednisolone acetate (Depo-Medrol)

Methylprednisolone (Medrol)

Methylprednisolone sodium succinate
    (Solu-Medrol)

Prednisone (Deltasone, Meticorten)

Pharmacologic Mechanism

Adrenocorticoids diffuse across cell membranes and join with cytoplasmic receptors. These complexes then enter the cell nucleus, bind to DNA, and stimulate transcription of mRNA. Subsequently, various enzymes are synthesized which are responsible for glucocorticoid and mineralocorticoid effects. The glucocorticoid effects include antiinflammatory, immunosuppression (prevention or suppression of cell-mediated immune reactions), and metabolic (decreased peripheral utilization of glucose, increased glycogen storage in the liver, increased blood glucose concentrations and insulin resistance). The mineralocorticoid effects cause sodium reabsorption, potassium and hydrogen excretion, and subsequent water retention.

Uses

Treatment of allergic states, collagen disease, dermatologic diseases, endocrine disorder, neoplastic diseases, rheumatic diseases, and other assorted conditions.

The dosage for any glucosteroid is extremely variable and must be individualized.

Doses

Schedules can vary depending upon the specific clinical situation. Corticosteroids can also be administered by intraarticular and soft tissue injection as well as intralesional, topical, ophthalmic, and rectal administration. Please consult manufacturer for current dosage recommendations.

Nursing Interventions and Administration

Intramuscular doses should be injected deeply into the gluteal muscle to prevent local atrophy of tissue. Sites should be rotated and the deltoid muscle avoided.

Adverse Effects

Peptic ulcer, pancreatitis, ulcerative esophagitis, menstrual irregularities, cushingoid state, secondary adrenocortical and pituitary unresponsiveness, increased insulin requirements in diabetics, sodium and fluid retention, potassium loss, impaired immunity, cataracts, and glaucoma.

Drug Interactions

1. Severe hypokalemia can occur with concurrent use of acetazolamide, chlorthalidone, ethacrynic acid, furosemide, metolazone, quinethazone, and thiazides.
2. Concurrent use with indomethacin and other ulcerogenic drugs can produce additive effects.
3. Glucosteroids antagonize the effects of the oral anticoagulants.
4. Concurrent use with antidiabetic agents may require higher doses for the antidiabetic drugs.
5. Concurrent use with cardiac glycosides may enhance the possibility of arrhythmias or digitalis toxicity associated with hypokalemia.

Contraindications

Hypersensitivity and systemic fungal infections.

Cyclosporine

Category

Immunosuppressant

Brand Name

Sandimmune

Pharmacologic Mechanism

The exact mechanism of action is unknown but seems to be related to selective and reversible inhibition of the T helper lymphocytes which play a major role in both cellular and humoral immune responses. Cyclosporine does not affect the non-specific myelosuppression.

Doses

1. The usual adult dosage is 15 mg per kilogram of body weight per day beginning 4 to 12 h before surgery and continued for 1 to 2 weeks postoperatively, then reduced by 5% per week to the maintenance dose.
2. The maintenance dosage is oral, 5 to 10 mg per kilogram of body weight per day.
3. The parenteral dosage is one-third of the oral dosage or 2 to 6 mg per kilogram.

Nursing Interventions and Administration

1. Patients receiving cyclosporine should be under the supervision of a physician experienced in immunosuppressive therapy. Dosages are adjusted to meet individual needs and should be checked against the most current medical literature.
2. For parenteral administration, cyclosporine should be administered by slow intravenous infusion over a period of 2 to 6 h. Rapid intravenous administration may cause acute nephrotoxicity.

Adverse Effects

Dose-dependent hypertension and nephrotoxicity, convulsions, fever, chills, sore throat, frequent urination, hematuria, stomach pain with nausea and vomiting, increase in hair growth, trembling and shaking of hands, headache, leg cramps.

Major Drug Interactions

1. Use with amphotericin B, erythromycin, diltiazim, or ketoconazole has been reported to increase plasma concentrations of cyclosporine and may increase the risk of nephrotoxicity.
2. Concurrent use with other immunosuppressive agents increases the risk of injection and development of lymphoproliferative disorders and, except for adrenocorticoids, is not recommended.
3. Concurrent use with other nephrotoxic agents, e.g., amphotericin B, may result in enhanced nephrotoxicity.
4. Concomitant administration of cyclosporine and rifampin, phenytoin, or phenobarbital results in decreased plasma cyclosporine concentrations.

Therapeutic Drug Levels

Plasma: 1 nanogram per milliliter per milligram of dose.

Blood: 2.7 to 1.4 nanograms per milliliter per milligram of dose.

Dactinomycin

Category

Antineoplastic; antibiotic

Brand Name

Cosmegen

Pharmacologic Mechanism

Antineoplastic activity is probably due to complexation with DNA which results in an inhibition of DNA-dependent RNA synthesis. Dactinomycin also exhibits bacteriostatic activity against both gram-positive and gram-negative bacteria and some fungi. Also has some immunosuppressant activity.

Uses

As a sole agent or in combination therapy for Wilms' tumor, rhabdomyosarcoma, testicular tumors, and Ewing's sarcoma. Alternative for choriocarcinoma and other related trophoblastic tumors.

Doses

Note: Accepted indications and dosages for antineoplastic agents are in a constant state of flux. Please consult current literature for updated information.

1. Pediatric parenteral dose is 15 μg/kg for 5 days in divided doses over 1 week. Maximum daily dose is 0.5 mg.
2. For adults, parenteral dose is 0.5 mg for 5 days or a single weekly dose of 2 mg for 3 weeks.
3. Doses must be individualized and are dependent upon the stage and severity of the neoplasm, type of therapeutic regimen, and the patient's tolerance to treatment. Repeat courses of treatment usually require a rest period of at least 2 weeks and no signs of residual toxicity.
4. Dosage should be based on body surface area in obese or edematous patients.

Nursing Interventions and Administration

1. Reconstitute by using 1.1 mL of sterile water for injection. Use of sodium chloride injection or bacteriostatic water for injection may result in precipitation.
2. Reconstituted solution may be added to a running infusion (usually 5% dextrose) over 10 to 15 min.
3. Exercise care to avoid soft tissue contact.
4. Additional therapy may be needed to deal with drug side effects.

Adverse Effects

Nausea, vomiting, diarrhea, ulcers, bone marrow depression, alopecia, acne, and skin pigmentation.

Drug Interactions

1. Use with extreme caution with chlorambucil or methotrexate because of additive bone marrow depression and gastrointestinal toxicity.
2. May raise the concentration of blood uric acid.

Contraindications

Pregnancy, severe bone marrow depression, liver or renal impairment, chickenpox, and herpes zoster.

Desmopressin Acetate

Category

Synthetic posterior pituitary hormone: antidiuretic and antihemorrhagic

Brand Name

DDAVP

Pharmacologic Mechanism

Antidiuretic activity occurs by increasing the cellular permeability of the collecting ducts, resulting in an increase in urine osmolality with a concurrent decrease in urine output. Antihemorrhagic effect involves an increase in clotting factor VIII activity.

Uses

Indicated for the treatment of polydipsia, polyuria, and dehydration due to neurohypophyseal diabetes insipidus or trauma or surgery in the pituitary region. Can be used in the treatment of hemophilia and von Willebrand's disease.

Doses

Dosage must be individualized according to the patient's response.

1. Pediatric intranasal dose is 0.05 mL daily (3 to 12 years of age).
2. Adult intranasal dose is 0.1 to 0.4 mL daily.
3. Adult IV or SQ dose is 2 to 4 μg a day, usually in two diluted doses.
4. Antihemorrhagic doses are 0.3 μg/kg and diluted in 50 mg NaCl and infused slowly over 15 to 30 min.
5. Pediatric doses (children over 3 months of age) IV 0.3 to 0.5 μg/kg.

Nursing Interventions and Administration

According to the patient's response, may be administered as a single daily dose or in divided doses.

Contraindications

Hypersensitivity.

Adverse Effects

Transient headache, nausea, nasal congestion, rhinitis, and flushing.

Drug Interactions

1. Use with caution in patients receiving lithium carbonate, epinephrine, or heparin.
2. Concurrent use with chlorpropamide may enhance the antidiuretic effect.

Dextran 40

Category

Plasma expander

Brand Names

Gentran 40

IMD

Rheomacrodex

Pharmacologic Mechanism

Dextran administered intravenously creates hyper-oncotic pressure within the circulatory system which results in an immediate expansion of plasma volume. Dextran also retards and reverses cellular aggregation resulting from shock.

Uses

Shock, extracorporeal circulation, thrombus prophylaxis.

Doses

1. Up to 20 mL/kg during the first 24 h of treatment. Infuse the first 500 mL of solution rapidly and the remaining dose more slowly. Reduce to 10 mL/kg after 24 h and discontinue after 5 days.
2. Thrombus prophylaxis: 10 mL/kg administered on the day of surgery. After surgery, continue with 500 mL per day for 2 to 3 days. An additional 500 mL may be given every 2 to 3 days for up to 2 weeks if the risk of complications still exists.

Adverse Effects

Nausea, vomiting, urticaria, wheezing, and anaphylaxis.

Drug Interactions

Dextran may increase the activity of anticoagulants.

Contraindications

Hypersensitivity, hemostatic defects, cardiac decompensation, severe oliguria, or anuria.

Diazepam

Category

Antianxiety agent

Brand Name

Valium

Pharmacologic Mechanism

The antianxiety activity of diazepam appears to be related to depression of the CNS at the brainstem reticular formation and limbic system. Diazepam exerts moderate anticonvulsant and skeletal muscle relaxation activity and possesses a drug-misuse potential and a weak addiction liability.

Benzodiazepines enhance or facilitate the inhibitory neurotransmitter action of gamma-amino-butyric acid (GABA) which mediates both pre- and postsynaptic inhibition in all regions of the CNS. Diazepam exerts an anticonvulsant activity by suppressing the spread of seizure activity produced by epileptogenic foci in the cortex, thalamus, and limbic structures.

Uses

Antianxiety, sedative-hypnotic, anticonvulsant, skeletal muscle relaxant, used as a preoperative medication and for relief of acute alcohol withdrawal symptoms.

Doses

1. The usual oral dose for children over 6 months is 1.2 to 5 mg three to four times daily. May be increased slowly if necessary.
2. The usual adult oral dose is 2 to 10 mg two to four times daily.
3. The usual parenteral (IM or IV) dose for children over 5 is 5 to 10 mg repeated every 3 to 4 h.
4. The usual adult parenteral dose is 2 to 10 mg IM or IV. Repeat in 3 to 4 h if necessary.

Nursing Interventions and Administration

1. For IM administration, inject deeply and slowly into a large muscle mass.
2. For IV administration, inject slowly, taking 1 min for each 5 mg given. Extreme care should be taken to avoid intraarterial administration or extravasation.
3. When the intravenous route is used in infants and children, it is recommended that the medication be administered slowly over a 3-min period in a dosage not to exceed 250 μg per kilogram of body weight.
4. Diazepam is absorbed to the plastic of intravenous infusion bags and tubing.

Adverse Effects

Drowsiness, fatigue, ataxia, and paradoxical reactions including hyperexcited states, anxiety, and hallucinations; respiratory depression; potential for psychic or physical dependence.

Drug Interactions

1. Avoid concurrent use with monoamine oxidase inhibitors.
2. Concurrent use with CNS depressants will produce additive depression.

Contraindications

Hypersensitivity and narrow-angle glaucoma.

Dicumarol

Category

Anticoagulant

Pharmacologic Mechanism

Coumarin anticoagulants inhibit prothrombin synthesis (factor II) and also interfere with the production of proconvertin (factor VII) and the Christmas factor (factor IX) in the liver by interfering with the action of vitamin K. Full therapeutic action is delayed until circulating coagulation factors are removed by normal catabolism, which occurs at different rates for each factor. Coumarins have no direct thrombolytic effect, although they may limit extension of existing thrombi.

Uses

Adjunct in coronary occlusion, atrial fibrillation with embolization, prophylaxis, and treatment of pulmonary thrombosis and venous thrombosis.

Doses

The usual oral adult dose is 200 to 300 mg on the first day. Prothrombin time should determine the maintenance dose, which is usually 25 to 200 mg daily.

Nursing Interventions and Administration

1. Maintenance dose is usually administered as a single daily dose.
2. Therapy should be discontinued slowly.

Adverse Effects

Hemorrhage from the gastrointestinal and urinary tracts, nausea, vomiting, diarrhea, hepatitis, jaundice, urticaria, alopecia, agranulocytosis, leukopenia, and anemia.

Drug Interactions

1. Drugs which can cause significant increases in anticoagulation activity include anabolic steroids, broad-spectrum antibiotics, clofibrate, dextrothyroxine, disulfiram, oxyphenbutazone, phenylbutazone, and thyroid preparations.
2. Drugs which can cause significant decreases in coagulant activity include barbiturates, cholestyramine, estrogens, oral contraceptives, and glutethimide.
3. All interactions with coumarins and other drugs have not been identified. Several medications may interact with anticoagulant therapy by more than one mechanism. Therefore, the next effect of some concurrently used medications in anticoagulant therapy may be unpredictable.
4. Because of the possible serious consequences of interference with anticoagulant therapy, increased monitoring of prothrombin time is recommended when any medication is added to or withdrawn from the regimen of a patient on coumarins.

Contraindications

Hypersensitivity to coumarin anticoagulants, subacute bacterial endocarditis, any type of bleeding conditions, and use in patients who cannot be carefully supervised.

See warfarin sodium.

Digitoxin

Category

Cardiac glycoside

Brand Names

Crystodigin

Purodigin

Pharmacologic Mechanism

The digitalis glycosides increase the force of myocardial contraction, increase the refractory period of the atrioventricular and sinoatrial nodes, and decrease the conductivity of the bundle of His and heart rate. Digitoxin exhibits good oral absorption, a moderate onset of activity, a long half-life, and slow urinary excretion.

Uses

Congestive heart failure, atrial fibrillation, atrial flutter, and paroxysmal atrial tachycardia.

Doses

1. Digitalization and maintenance doses must be individualized.
2. The following digitalizing doses are given in divided doses at 6-to-8-h intervals:
   Two weeks to 1 year: 0.02 to 0.03 mg/kg.
   One to 2 years: 0.04 mg/kg.
   Two years and over: .045 mg/kg. The usual maintenance dose is approximately one-tenth of the digitalizing dose. Initial dose of 0.8 mg is followed by 0.02 mg every 6 to 8 h. Usual maintenance dose is 0.05 to 0.02 mg daily.

Nursing Interventions and Administration

1. Maintenance dose is usually administered as a single dose in the morning with breakfast.
2. Parenteral administration should be by IV injection.

Therapeutic Blood Levels

13 to 25 nanograms/mL.

Contraindications

See digoxin.

Digoxin

Category

Cardiac glycoside

Brand Names

Lanoxin

Lanoxicaps

Pharmacologic Mechanism

The digitalis glycosides increase the force of myocardial contraction as a result of the enhancement of calcium influx and an augmented release of free calcium ions within the myocardial cells to subsequently potentiate the activity of the contractile muscle fibers of the heart. An increase in the refractory period of the atrioventricular and sino-

atrial node and a decrease in the conductivity of the bundle of His and the heart rate result from a direct digitalis effect in addition to a reflex vagal stimulation and direct tissue effects involving both sympathetic and parasympathetic innervation. Digoxin exhibits good oral absorption, a moderate onset of activity, a short half-life, and rapid urinary excretion.

Uses

Congestive heart failure, atrial fibrillation, atrial flutter, paroxysmal tachycardia, and cardiogenic shock. Digitalization and maintenance doses must be individualized.

Doses

Digitalizing doses are given in doses at 6-to-8-h intervals.

1. The usual oral pediatric dose is 0.04 to 0.06 mg/kg. The usual maintenance dose is approximately one-fifth to one-third of the digitalizing dose.
2. The usual adult dose for digitalizing is 0.4 to 0.6 mg.
3. The usual pediatric parenteral (IM or IV) dose is 0.025 to 0.04 mg/kg.
4. The usual daily maintenance dose is approximately one-fifth to one-third of the digitalizing dose.
5. The usual adult parenteral digitalizing dose is 0.05 to 1 mg.
6. The usual adult parenteral maintenance dose is 0.125 to 0.5 mg daily.

Nursing Interventions and Administration

1. The maintenance dose is usually administered as a single daily dose in the morning with breakfast.
2. The preferred route for parenteral administration is by IV injection. The intramuscular route has a slower effect and poor bioavailability. If intramuscular injection is required, it should be administered deep into the muscle, not exceeding 2 mL at the injection site, and the site should be massaged well to avoid painful local reactions.

Adverse Effects

Anorexia, nausea, vomiting, diarrhea, ventricular premature beats, paroxysmal and nonparoxysmal nodal rhythms, and blurred or yellow vision.

Drug Interactions

1. Use with caution with drugs that induce hypokalemia. Acetazolamide, amphotericin B, chlorthalidone, ethacrynic acid, furosemide, and thiazides can induce hypokalemia.
2. Calcium preparations with parenteral administration can produce serious cardiac arrhythmias.
3. Concurrent use with mineralocorticoids may enhance the possibility of digitalis toxicity associated with hypokalemia.
4. Concurrent use with antiarrhythmics, calcium salts, succinylcholine, and sympathomimetics may cause additive effects leading to arrhythmias.
5. Use with beta-adrenergic blockers may result in excessive bradycardia and possible heart block.
6. Use with calcium-ion influx inhibitors may cause an increased serum concentration because of competitive serum protein binding.
7. Use with quinidine can also cause substantially increased concentrations of digitalis.

Therapeutic Blood Levels

0.5 to 2.0 nanograms/mL.

Disopyramide Phosphate

Category

Antiarrhythmic

Brand Name

Norpace

Pharmacologic Mechanism

Disopyramide is similar to procainamide and quinidine (type 1 antiarrhythmic drugs). It decreases the rate of diastolic depolarization in cells with augmented automaticity and upstroke velocity while increasing the action potential duration of normal cardiac cells. The drug possesses no alpha- or beta-adrenergic activity but does exhibit anticholinergic activity.

Uses

1. Unifocal premature (ectopic) ventricular contractions.
2. Premature (ectopic) ventricular contractions of multifocal origin.
3. Episodes of ventricular tachycardia.

Doses

1. The usual adult oral dose is a total of 400 to 800 mg daily in four divided doses.
2. A common dose is 150 mg every 6 h.
3. Dosage must be individualized according to the patient's response and tolerance.
4. The patient's renal impairment requires careful dosage adjustments.

Nursing Interventions and Administration

Maintenance dose is usually administered every 6 h.

Adverse Effects

The most frequent are anticholinergic effects, which include dry mouth and throat, urinary hesitancy, constipation, blurred vision, hypotension, congestive heart failure, and hypoglycemia.

Drug Interactions

1. Concurrent use with procainamide, lidocaine, propranolol, and verapamil or quinidine should be reserved for life-threatening arrhythmias that do not respond to single-agent therapy.
2. Hypotension and/or hypoglycemia can result if used in combination with alcohol.
3. Hypoglycemic effects of insulin may be intensified.
4. Use with enzyme inducers such as phenobarbital, phenytoin, and rifampin can reduce serum levels.

Contraindications

Hypersensitivity, cardiogenic shock, and preexisting second- or third-degree AV block if no pacemaker is present.

Dobutamine

Category

Cardiac stimulant

Brand Name

Dobutrex

Pharmacologic Mechanism

Dobutamine is a direct-acting inotropic agent. It acts primarily on adrenergic beta 1 receptors, having relatively little effect on beta 2 and alpha receptors. It directly stimulates beta 1 receptors of the heart to increase myocardial contractility and stroke volume, resulting in increased cardiac output. Systemic vascular resistance is usually decreased; however, systolic blood pressure and pulse pressure may remain unchanged or be increased because of increased cardiac output. Coronary blood flow and myocardial oxygen consumption are usually increased because of increased myocardial contractility. Unlike dopamine, dobutamine does not stimulate the heart indirectly by causing release of endogenous norepinephrine.

Uses
Treatment of cardiac decompensation.

Doses

1. The usual adult parenteral dosage is an intravenous infusion at a rate of 2.5 to 15 μg per kilogram of body weight per minute.
2. The usual pediatric dosage has not been established.

Nursing Interventions and Administration

1. Hypovolemia should be corrected prior to the use of this drug.
2. In patients who have atrial fibrillation with rapid ventricular response, a digitalis preparation should be used prior to institution of therapy with dobutamine.
3. Concentration of solution should not exceed 5 mg of dobutamine per milliliter.

Adverse Effects
Hypertension, tachycardia, chest pain, cardiac arrhythmias.

Major Drug Interactions

1. Concurrent use with general anesthetics may increase the potential for ventricular arrhythmias.
2. Concurrent use with beta-adrenergic blocking agents may result in the predominance of alpha-adrenergic effects and increased peripheral resistance.
3. Concurrent use with nitroprusside may result in a higher cardiac output and a lower pulmonary wedge pressure.

Contraindications
Idiopathic hypertrophic subaortic stenosis; cautious use following a myocardial infarction.

Dopamine Hydrochloride

Category
Sympathomimetic: vasopressor

Brand Name
Intropin

Pharmacologic Mechanism
Sympathomimetic effect is due to activity with adrenergic and dopaminergic receptors. Dopamine produces direct stimulation of beta 1 receptors and dopaminergic receptors. In low doses it causes renal and mesenteric vasodilation. Renal vasodilation results in increased renal blood flow, glomerular filtration rate, urine flow, and sodium excretion.

In low to moderate doses, it also exerts a positive inotropic effect on the myocardium due to a direct action on beta 1 receptors, and an indirect action by releasing norepinephrine from its storage sites, resulting in increased myocardial contractility and stroke volume, thereby increasing cardiac output. Systolic blood pressure and pulse pressure may be increased with either no change or a slight increase in diastolic blood pressure. Total peripheral resistance is unchanged. Coronary blood flow and myocardial oxygen consumption are usually increased.

In higher doses dopamine stimulates alpha-adrenergic receptors, resulting in increased peripheral resistance and renal vasoconstriction. Both systolic and diastolic blood pressures are increased as a result of increased cardiac output and increased peripheral resistance.

Uses
Treatment of shock syndrome due to chronic cardiac decompensation, endotoxic septicemia, myocardial infarctions, open-heart surgery, renal failure, and trauma.

Doses
The adult dose starts with infusion rates of 1 to 5 μg/kg per minute. May be increased until the

desired response is obtained. For more severe cases, start with a rate of 5 μg/kg per minute and increase gradually until the desired response is obtained. Usual satisfactory dose is 20 μg/kg per minute, and doses of 50 μg/kg per minute have been used safely.

Nursing Interventions and Administration

1. Dilute 1 ampule (200 mg) in 250 or 500 mL of 5% dextrose, 5% dextrose and sodium chloride, dextrose in lactated Ringer's solution, lactated Ringer's solution, sodium lactate, or sodium chloride injection.
2. Do not mix with alkaline substances.
3. Treat extravasation with phentolamine as soon as possible after noted.
4. Hypovolemia should be corrected prior to initiating therapy with this drug.
5. When discontinuing an infusion of dopamine, the dosage should be reduced gradually since sudden cessation of therapy may result in severe hypotension.

Major Drug Interactions

1. Avoid concurrent use with cyclopropane and halogenated hydrocarbons.
2. Concurrent use with ergot alkaloids is not recommended because of possible excessive peripheral vasoconstriction.

Adverse Effects

Tachycardia, anginal pain, ectopic beats, hypotension, and vasoconstriction.

Contraindications

Pheochromocytoma, uncorrected tachyarrhthmias.

Edrophonium

Category

Cholinesterase inhibitor, diagnostic agent, antidote

Brand Name

Tensilon

Pharmacologic Mechanism

Edrophonium inhibits the destruction of acetylcholine by acetylcholinesterase, thereby facilitating transmission of impulses across the myoneural junction.

Edrophonium is used in the diagnosis of myasthenia gravis. It prolongs the duration of action of acetylcholine at the motor end plate, which causes a transient increase in muscle strength in patients with myasthenia gravis, while patients with other disorders develop either no increase in strength or even a slight weakness and possibly fasciculations.

Edrophonium can be used as an antidote to curariform blocks. Since nondepolarizing neuromuscular blocking agents combine reversibly with the receptors, preventing access of acetylcholine, antagonism can be overcome by increasing the amount of agonist at the receptors. Muscle paralysis induced by nondepolarizing neuromuscular blocking agents is reversed by edrophonium.

Edrophonium may terminate arrhythmias by producing vagal stimulation, which results in shortening of the effective refractory period of atrial muscle, increasing the effective refractory period of the atrioventricular node, and depressed conduction through the AV node.

Uses

Treatment of muscular weakness in myasthenia gravis, and in differentiating between cholinergic and myasthenic crisis.

Doses

1. For evaluation of treatment requirements in myasthenia gravis, 1 to 2 mg 1 h after administration of the anticholinesterase agent, given intravenously.
2. An intravenous dose of 1 mg initially followed by an additional 1 mg can be given to differentiate cholinergic crisis from myasthenic crisis.
3. Intramuscular dosages of 10 mg can be given as a diagnostic aid for myasthenia gravis.
4. A 10-mg intravenous dose, administered over a period of 30 to 45 s, repeated as needed up to a maximum total dose of 40 mg, can be given as an antidote to curariform block.
5. Intravenous dosages of 5 to 10 mg, repeated once in 10 min, can be given as a treatment for supraventricular tachycardias.
6. For pediatric doses, consult current literature.

Nursing Interventions and Administration

1. When edrophonium is used for testing, atropine injection should always be available to counteract severe cholinergic reactions.
2. When used as an antidote to curariform block, edrophonium should not be administered prior to the nondepolarizing neuromuscular blocking agent but at the time the effect is needed, since it has a brief duration of action.
3. Monitor respiratory status during intravenous infusion.

Adverse Effects

Muscle weakness, shortness of breath, bradycardia, fatigue, and weakness. Less frequently, blurred vision, diarrhea, urinary frequency, increased bronchial secretions, and nausea.

Major Drug Interactions

Use caution in giving this drug to patients with symptoms of myasthenic weakness who are also receiving cholinergics.

Contraindications

Bronchial asthma, mechanical obstruction of the intestinal or urinary tract.

Epinephrine

Category

Bronchodilator, vasopressor, cardiac stimulant, local anesthetic adjunct.

Brand Name

Adrenalin R

Pharmacologic Mechanism

Epinephrine is a direct-acting sympathomimetic amine which acts on alpha-adrenergic receptors and beta-adrenergic receptors.

Epinephrine relaxes bronchial smooth muscle by acting on beta 2 adrenergic receptors and constricts bronchial arterioles by acting on alpha-adrenergic receptors, thereby relieving bronchospasm, congestion, and edema, and increasing tidal volume and vital capacity. It also inhibits antigen-induced releases of histamine and the slow-reacting substance of anaphylaxis and directly antagonizes histamine-induced bronchiolar constriction, vasodilation, and edema.

In low doses, epinephrine produces a moderate elevation of systolic blood pressure primarily via cardiostimulation-induced increases in cardiac output. However, in low doses epinephrine acts on beta 2 adrenergic receptors in the skeletal muscle vasculature, producing vasodilation which decreases peripheral resistance, so that diastolic pressure may be decreased. In higher doses, epinephrine acts on alpha-adrenergic receptors in the skeletal muscle vasculature to produce vasoconstriction which increases peripheral resistance, resulting in an increase in both systolic and diastolic blood pressure.

Epinephrine acts on beta 1 adrenergic receptors in the heart, producing an increase in heart rate via a positive chronotropic effect through the sinoatrial node and an increase in force of contraction via a positive inotropic effect on the myocardium.

Uses

Bronchodilator, vasopressor, cardiac stimulant.

Doses

1. The onset of action, time required for peak effect and duration of action of epinephrine depend on dosage, dosage form, and route of administration.
2. Tolerance to epinephrine may develop with prolonged or excessive use. Discontinuation of the medication for a few days and subsequent readministration may restore its effectiveness.
3. As a bronchodilator, use a subcutaneous injection, initially the equivalent of 200 to 500 μg of epinephrine, repeated every 20 min to 4 h as needed, the dosage being increased up to a maximum of 1 mg per dose, if necessary.
4. Epinephrine inhalation aerosol: oral inhalation 200 or 250 μg repeated after 1 to 2 min, if necessary; subsequent dose(s) should not be administered for at least 4 h.
5. As a vasopressor: the equivalent of 500 μg intramuscularly or subcutaneously, followed by

intravenous administration of 25 to 50 μg every 5 to 15 min as needed.

6. As a cardiac stimulant, the equivalent of 100 μg to 1 mg of epinephrine, repeated every 5 min if necessary by intracardiac or intravenous route.

Note: Geriatric patients may be more sensitive to the effects of sympathomimetics and may require lower doses.

Nursing Interventions and Administration

1. The 1:1000 (1 mg/mL) concentration of epinephrine injection must be diluted before administering intracardially or intravenously.
2. It is recommended that sterile epinephrine suspension be administered with a tuberculin syringe and a 26 gauge, ½-in needle.
3. After withdrawing a dose of sterile epinephrine suspension into the syringe, prompt injection is recommended to avoid settling of the suspension.
4. Intramuscular injection of epinephrine should be avoided since the vasoconstriction produced by the drug reduces the oxygen tension of the tissues.

Adverse Effects

Chest pain, irregular heartbeat, headache, nervousness, restlessness, dizziness, nausea, vomiting, trembling, weakness.

Major Drug Interactions

1. Concurrent use with anesthetics or digitalis glycosides may cause cardiac arrhythmias, since these medications may sensitize the myocardium to the effects of epinephrine.
2. Concurrent use with beta-adrenergic blockers may block the beta-adrenergic effects of epinephrine, resulting in hypertension.
3. Concurrent use with tricyclic antidepressants may potentiate the cardiovascular effects of epinephrine, possibly resulting in arrhythmias, hypertension, and tachycardia.

Contraindications

Organic brain damage, cardiovascular disease, hypertension, and hemorrhagic, traumatic, and cardiogenic shock.

Ergonovine Maleate

Category

Oxytocic

Brand Name

Ergotrate

Pharmacologic Mechanism

Produces tetanic contraction of the postpartum uterus for approximately 90 min, which is followed by clonic contractions that persist for another 90 min. In addition, the drug causes vasoconstriction of the coronary arteries.

Uses

Indicated for the prevention and treatment of postpartum and postaborted hemorrhage due to uterine atony.

Doses

1. The usual adult initial dose is 0.2 mg administered parenterally, followed by 0.2 to 0.4 mg given orally every 6 to 12 h until the danger of atony is over.
2. Parenteral doses of 0.2 mg can be repeated for severe uterine hemorrhage.

Nursing Interventions and Administration

1. A course of 48 h is usually sufficient for oral therapy.
2. Intravenous dosage should be given slowly.

Adverse Effects

Nausea and vomiting and ergotism with prolonged use.

Drug Interactions

Concurrent or sequential use with vasoconstrictors or oxytocin may produce hypertension.

Contraindications

Hypersensitivity, threatened spontaneous abortion, or for labor induction, coronary artery disease, hepatic function impairment, hypertension, occlusive peripheral vascular disease, renal disease, or sepsis.

Ethacrynic Acid

Category

Diuretic

Brand Name

Edecrin

Pharmacologic Mechanism

Ethacrynic acid promotes the excretion of water, sodium, chloride, and other electrolytes by inhibiting tubular reabsorption, especially in the medullary and cortical portions of the ascending limb of the loop of Henle.

Uses

1. Edema due to renal dysfunction.
2. Adjunct in treating edema due to congestive heart failure and hepatic cirrhosis.
3. Short-term management of ascites due to malignancy, idiopathic edema, and lymphedema.
4. Short-term management of edema in pediatric congenital heart disease or nephrotic syndrome.

Doses

1. The usual pediatric dose is 25 mg. Subsequent dose increments of 25 mg should be made to achieve effective maintenance.
2. The usual adult oral dose is 50 to 100 mg. After diuresis has been achieved, the lowest effective dose should be given. Usual maintenance dose range is 50 to 300 mg.

Nursing Interventions and Administration

1. Usually administered as a single daily dose in the morning.
2. Administration with meals will help reduce gastric upset.
3. Intravenous infusion should be by slow, direct intravenous injection.

Adverse Effects

Nausea, vomiting, diarrhea, anorexia, dysphagia, abdominal pain, agranulocytosis, neutropenia, thrombocytopenia, deafness, tinnitus, skin rash, headache, and blurred vision.

Drug Interactions

1. Avoid concurrent use with potentially neurotoxic drugs. Amikacin, chloroquine, gentamicin, kanamycin, neomycin, phenylbutazone, streptomycin, and vancomycin are neurotoxic.
2. Use with caution during digitalis therapy because of possible hypokalemia. Concurrent use with corticosteroids can produce severe hypokalemia.
3. Concurrent use with lithium is best avoided.
4. Patients on anticoagulants may require anticoagulant dosage adjustments.
5. Concurrent use with antihypertensives can produce orthostatic hypotension.

Contraindications

1. Hypersensitivity, patients with anuria, increasing electrolyte imbalance, azotemia, oliguria, or watery diarrhea.
2. Nursing mothers.

Fentanyl

Category

Anesthesia adjunct

Brand Name

Sublimaze

Pharmacologic Mechanism

Fentanyl binds with stereospecific receptors at many sites within the central nervous system to alter both the perception of pain and the emotional response to pain. Precise sites and mechanisms of action have not been fully determined. It has been proposed that there are multiple subtypes of opioid receptors, each mediating various therapeutic and/or side effects of opioid drugs. The actions of an opioid analgesic may therefore depend upon whether it acts as a full agonist or a partial agonist or is inactive at each type of receptor.

Uses

Preoperative, anesthesia, pain.

Doses

1. As a presurgical medication: 50 to 100 µg 30 to 60 min prior to surgery, given intramuscularly.

2. As an adjunct to general anesthesia: doses from 2 µg/kg (minor surgery) to 20 to 50 µg/kg (for open-heart or complicated neurological, orthopedic surgeries).
3. Postoperatively to control pain, tachypnea, and emergence delirium, an intramuscular dosage of 50 to 100 µg can be given. This dosage can be repeated in 1 or 2 h as needed.

Nursing Interventions and Administration

1. Moderate to high doses of fentanyl may reduce or abolish certain responses to surgical stress.
2. Fentanyl may suppress respiration, especially in very young, elderly, very ill, or debilitated patients and those with respiratory problems.
3. Dosage should be individualized on the basis of age, weight, body size, and physical status of the patient, underlying pathology, other medications used concurrently, type of anesthesia to be used, and the type and anticipated duration of the surgical procedure involved.
4. Rapid intravenous administration of fentanyl may also cause anaphylactoid reactions, severe respiratory depression, hypotension, peripheral circulatory collapse, and cardiac arrest. The drug should be given slowly over a period of at least 1 to 2 min intravenously.

Adverse Effects
Shortness of breath, slow or irregular breathing, mental confusion, slow heartbeat, mental depression, skin rash, unusual excitement, delirium, drowsiness, dizziness, severe weakness.

Major Drug Interactions

1. Concurrent use of alcohol or CNS depressants with fentanyl may result in increased CNS depression, respiratory depression, and hypotensive effects. Caution is recommended and dosage of one or both agents should be reduced. In addition, some phenothiazines increase, while others decrease the effects of fentanyl.
2. Use of fentanyl in patients who have received an MAO inhibitor within 14 days is not recommended because concurrent use of MAO inhibitors with other opioid analgesics, especially meperidine, has resulted in unpredictable, severe, and sometimes fatal reactions.

Contraindications
Care should be used with patients who have respiratory impairments or disease.

Flucytosine

Category
Antifungal: antimonilial

Brand Name
Ancobon

Pharmacologic Mechanism
Flucytosine penetrates into fungal cells and interferes with pyrimidine metabolism. Nucleic acid and protein synthesis are disturbed. The compound is selectively toxic against fungi.

Uses
Indicated for the treatment of infections caused by susceptible strains of *Cryptococcus* and *Candida*.

Doses
The usual oral pediatric and adult doses are 12.5 to 37.5 mg/kg daily, divided in three doses.

Nursing Interventions and Administration
To reduce nausea, administer the capsules a few at a time over a 15-min period until the correct dose (one-quarter of the daily dose) is attained.

Adverse Effects
Nausea, vomiting, diarrhea, anemia, leukopenia, and thrombocytopenia.

Drug Interactions
Avoid concurrent use with bone marrow-depressing, nephrotoxic, and hepatotoxic drugs.

Contraindications
Hypersensitivity, bone marrow depression, renal dysfunction.

Furosemide

Category
Diuretic

Brand Name

Lasix

Pharmacologic Mechanism

Furosemide promotes the excretion of water, sodium, chloride, and other electrolytes by inhibiting tubular reabsorption, especially in the medullary and cortical portions of the ascending limb of the loop of Henle.

Uses

1. Edema due to renal dysfunction.
2. Management of hypertension as a sole agent or in combination with other antihypertensives.
3. Adjunct in treating edema due to congestive heart failure and hepatic cirrhosis.

Doses

1. The usual oral pediatric dose is 2 mg/kg given as a single dose. Do not exceed a daily dose of 6 mg/kg.
2. The usual adult oral dose is 20 to 80 mg as a single dose.
3. The usual pediatric parenteral dose is 1 mg/kg. Doses greater than 6 mg/kg are not recommended.
4. The usual adult parenteral dose is 20 to 40 mg. May be followed by a second dose 2 h later.

Nursing Interventions and Administrations

1. Diuretic dose is usually administered as a single daily dose in the morning.
2. Administration with meals will help reduce gastric upset.
3. Potassium supplementation may be required during therapy.
4. Intravenous administration should be at a slow, controlled rate over a 1- to -2 min period or 4 mg per minute.

Adverse Effects

Nausea, vomiting, diarrhea, anemia, leukopenia, aplastic anemia, thrombocytopenia, tinnitus, hearing impairment, urticaria, exfoliative dermatitis, erythema multiforme, paresthesias, and blurred vision.

Drug Interactions

1. Avoid concurrent use with potentially neurotoxic drugs. Amikacin, chloroquine, gentamicin, kanamycin, neomycin, oxyphenbutazone, phenylbutazone, streptomycin, and vancomycin are neurotoxic drugs.
2. Use with caution during digitalis therapy because of possible hypokalemia. Concurrent use with corticosteroids can produce severe hypokalemia.
3. Concurrent use with lithium is best avoided.
4. Concurrent use with cephaloridine can produce additive nephrotoxicity.

Contraindications

1. Hypersensitivity, patients with anuria, increasing electrolyte imbalance, azotemia, or oliguria.
2. Use in women of childbearing potential is not recommended unless the expected therapeutic benefits outweigh the potential harm.

Glucagon

Category

Antihypoglycemic, diagnostic aid

Brand Name

Glucagon

Pharmacologic Mechanism

Glucagon promotes hepatic glucogenolysis and gluconeogenesis. It stimulates adenylate cyclase to produce increased cAMP, which is involved in a complicated series of enzymatic activities. The resultant effects are increased concentrations of plasma glucose, a relaxant effect on smooth musculature, and an inotropic myocardial effect. Hepatic stores of glycogen are necessary for glucagon to elicit an antihypoglycemic effect.

Uses

Hypoglycemia.

Doses

1. As an antihypoglycemic: intramuscular, intravenous, or subcutaneous doses of 0.5 to 1 USP unit

(0.5 to 1 mg) of glucagon repeated in 20 min if necessary.

2. As a diagnostic aid: glucagon can be given intramuscularly or intravenously, the equivalent of 0.25 to 2 USP units (0.25 to 2 mg) of glucagon, the dose being dependent on the time of onset of action and duration of effect required for the specific examination.

3. As an antidote to beta blocker overdosage, glucagon can be given intravenously, 2 to 3 USP units (2 to 3 mg) administered slowly over a period of 20 min and repeated in 1 h if necessary.

4. Usual pediatric dosage: the equivalent of 0.025 USP unit (0.025 mg) of glucagon per kilogram of body weight, repeated in 20 min if necessary. This dosage is appropriate for antihypoglycemic effect and is given intramuscularly, intravenously, or subcutaneously.

Nursing Interventions and Administration

1. Glucagon is effective in correcting hypoglycemia only in those patients having available liver glycogen.

2. Intravenous glucose must be given if the patient fails to respond to glucagon.

3. Supplemental sugar (glucose or sucrose) must be given to prevent secondary hypoglycemia after the patient has revived sufficiently to receive oral administration.

Adverse Effects
Nausea and vomiting.

Heparin Sodium

Category

Anticoagulant

Brand Name

Liquaemin

Pharmacologic Mechanism
Heparin acts indirectly at multiple sites in both the intrinsic and extrinsic blood clotting systems to potentiate the inhibitory action of antithrombin III (heparin cofactor) on several activated coagulation factors, probably by forming a complex with and inducing a conformational change in the antithrombin III molecule. Inhibition of activated factor X interferes with thrombin generation and thereby inhibits the various actions of thrombin in coagulation. Heparin also accelerates the formation of an antithrombin III-thrombin complex, thereby inactivating thrombin and preventing the conversion of fibrinogen to fibrin; this prevents extension of existing thrombi.

Uses

1. Prophylaxis and treatment of pulmonary embolism and venous thrombosis.
2. Atrial fibrillation with embolization.
3. Diagnosis and treatment of acute and chronic consumption coagulopathies.
4. Prevention of clotting in arterial and heart surgery.
5. Prophylaxis and treatment of peripheral arterial embolism.
6. Adjunct in treating coronary occlusion with acute myocardial infarction.
7. Anticoagulant for use in blood transfusions, extracorporeal circulation, dialysis procedures, and in blood samples for laboratory purposes.

Doses

1. The usual pediatric dose by IV infusion is 50 U per kilogram of body weight followed by 100 U per kilogram or 20,000 U per square meter of body surface daily.
2. The usual adult dose is initially 10,000 U followed by 5000 to 10,000 U four to six times a day by IV administration. By infusion, 20,000 to 40,000 U/L at a rate of 30 to 50 U per minute. By subcutaneous injection, 10,000 to 20,000 U initially, followed by 8000 to 10,000 U three times a day.

Nursing Interventions and Administration

1. Heparin may be administered by deep subcutaneous injection (two tract or bunch method), intermittent IV injection, or continuous IV infusions.
2. IM administration not recommended because of the dangers of hematoma formation.

Adverse Effects

Hemorrhage, acute reversible thrombocytopenia, rebound hyperlipemia, osteoporosis, and suppression of renal function during long-term therapy, alopecia, priapism, and aldosterone suppression.

Drug Interactions

1. Avoid concurrent use with aspirin, ethacrynic acid (IV), and oral anticoagulants.
2. Concurrent use of heparin with streptokinase or urokinase may increase the risk of hemorrhage.

Contraindications

Hypersensitivity, any type of bleeding, and with patients who cannot be carefully supervised.

Hetastarch

Category

Volume expander

Brand Name

Hespan

Pharmacologic Mechanism

Hetastarch is an artificial colloid derived from a waxy starch. The colloidal properties of 6% hetastarch approximate those of human albumin. Intravenous infusion of hetastarch results in expansion of plasma volume slightly in excess of the volume infused which decreases from this maximum over the succeeding 24 to 36 h. This expansion of plasma volume may improve the hemodynamic status for 24 h or longer.

Uses

Shock due to hemorrhage, burns, surgery, sepsis, or other trauma. It is not a substitute for blood or plasma.

Doses

1. Total dosage and rate of infusion depend upon the amount of blood lost and the resultant hemoconcentration.
2. The usual adult dose is 500 to 1000 mL. Total dosage does not usually exceed 1500 mL per day.

3. There are no current recommendations for use of hetastarch for children.

Nursing Interventions and Administration

1. Hetastarch is administered by intravenous infusion only.
2. Careful monitoring of hemodynamic status is needed during infusion.
3. Laboratory determination of leukocytes, platelets, hemoglobin, hematocrit, prothrombin time, and partial thromboplastin time should be done frequently.

Contraindications

Severe bleeding disorders and severe congestive cardiac and renal failure with oliguria or anuria.

Hydralazine

Category

Antihypertensive

Brand Name

Apresoline

Pharmacologic Mechanism

The predominant effect of hydralazine is direct vasodilation of arterioles with little effect on veins. It reduces peripheral resistance, causes an increased cardiac output, decreased systemic resistance, and reduction of cardiac afterload.

Doses and Uses

1. The usual adult oral dose for hypertension or congestive heart failure is 40 mg a day for the first 2 to 4 days, 100 mg a day for the balance of the first week, and 200 mg a day for the second and subsequent weeks, in two to four divided daily doses, the dosage the second and subsequent weeks, in two to four divided daily doses, the dosage then being adjusted to the lowest effective level.
2. The usual pediatric oral dose for hypertension or congestive heart failure is 750 μg per kilogram of body weight a day divided into two to four doses, the dosage being increased gradually over

1 to 4 weeks as needed, up to a maximum of 7.5 mg per kilogram of body weight, or 300 mg a day.

3. The adult oral maximum dosage is up to 300 mg daily.
4. Parenteral dosage for treatment of hypertension is 10 to 40 mg intramuscularly or intravenously, repeated as needed.
5. Pediatric parenteral dosage is 1.7 to 3.5 mg per kilogram of body weight a day, divided into four to six doses.

Nursing Interventions and Administration

1. Geriatric patients may be more sensitive to the effects of the usual adult dose.
2. Patients on hydralazine who have shown a significant decrease in blood pressure should have their medication withdrawn gradually at cessation of therapy.
3. Tolerance to the antihypertensive effects of hydralazine may develop with chronic administration. This results from fluid retention and expanded plasma volume and reflex activation of the sympathetic nervous system which increases heart rate and cardiac output.

Adverse Effects

Hepatotoxicity, SLE-like syndrome, cutaneous vasculitis, chest pain, malaise, weakness, joint pain, skin rash, or sore throat and fever, numbness, tingling, pain or weakness in hands or feet, edema, or lymphadenopathy.

Major Drug Interactions

Concurrent use with diazoxide or parenteral antihypertensives may result in severe, additive hypotensive effects.

Contraindications

Caution should be used in prescribing this drug for patients with coronary artery disease, mitral valvular disease, or rheumatic heart disease.

Hydrochlorothiazide

Category

Diuretic: antihypertensive, thiazide diuretic

Brand Names

Esidrix

Hydro-Diuril

Oretic

Pharmacologic Mechanism

The thiazides promote the excretion of water, sodium, and chloride by inhibiting the reabsorption of sodium ions in the ascending limb of the loop of Henle and in the early distal tubule of the nephron. The thiazides lower peripheral vascular resistance, which results in significant antihypertensive activity.

Uses

1. Management of hypertension as a sole agent or in combination with other antihypertensives.
2. Treatment of edema due to renal dysfunction.
3. Adjunct in treating edema due to congestive heart failure, hepatic cirrhosis, and corticosteroid or estrogen therapy.

Doses

1. The usual pediatric oral dose is 1 to 2 mg/kg.
2. The usual adult dose is 25 to 100 mg daily. Do not exceed 200 mg daily.

Nursing Interventions and Administration

1. Diuretic dose is usually administered once daily in the morning.
2. Administration with meals will help reduce gastric upset.

Adverse Effects

Weakness, fatigue, dizziness, urticaria, leg cramps, necrotizing angiitis, photosensitivity, agranulocytosis, thrombocytopenia, aplastic anemia, anorexia, gastric irritation, and transient blurred vision.

Drug Interactions

1. Use with caution during digitalis therapy because of possible hypokalemia.
2. Diabetic patients may require antidiabetic dosage adjustments.
3. Concurrent use with steroids, corticotropin, or

amphotericin B may intensify electrolyte imbalance.
4. Concurrent use with lithium salts may provoke lithium toxicity.

Contraindications

Hypersensitivity to thiazides and other sulfonamide-derivative drugs and in patients with anuria.

Hydroxyzine

Category

Antianxiety agent, sedative-hypnotic, antihistamine, antiemetic

Brand Names

Atarax

Vistaril

Pharmacologic Mechanism

Hydroxyzine's sedative action may be due to a suppression of activity in certain key regions of the subcortical area of the CNS. The exact mechanism of suppression of the CNS is not known.

Hydroxyzine competes with histamine for H_1 receptor sites on effector cells, thereby preventing, but not reversing, responses mediated by histamine alone. The dual effects of antihistamines, such as sedation and histamine inhibition, are used to provide relief in patients with severe pruritis.

Hydroxyzine's ability to exert an antiemetic effect is thought to be related to a central antimuscarinic action. It diminishes vestibular stimulation and depresses labyrinthine function. An action on the medullary chemoreceptive trigger zone may also be involved in the antiemetic effect.

Uses
Anxiety, sedative.

Doses

1. The usual adult dose for antianxiety or as a sedative-hypnotic is 50 to 100 mg in a single dose.
2. The usual adult dose for antihistaminic or antiemetic effects is 25 to 100 mg three to four times a day as needed.
3. The usual pediatric dosage for antianxiety or sedative-hypnotic effect is 600 μg per kilogram of body weight in a single dose.
4. The usual pediatric dosage for antihistaminic or antiemetic dosage is 500 μg per kilogram of body weight every 6 h for anxiety; 25 to 100 mg intramuscularly as a sedative-hypnotic or antiemetic.
5. Pediatric parenteral dosage is intramuscular at 1 mg per kilogram of body weight.

Nursing Interventions and Administrations

1. Geriatric patients may be more sensitive to the effects of the usual adult dose.
2. Do not administer intravenously or subcutaneously.
3. Intramuscular injection should be into a deep muscle mass.

Adverse Effects
Drowsiness, hypotension, convulsions, trembling, skin rash.

Major Drug Interactions
Concurrent use with alcohol or CNS depressants may potentiate the effects of either of these medications or hydroxyzine.

Insulin

Category

Antidiabetic

Brand Name

Iletin

Pharmacologic Mechanism
Insulin is a hormonal factor which controls the storage and metabolism of carbohydrates, protein, and fats. Such activity occurs primarily in liver, muscle, and adipose tissues subsequent to attachment of insulin molecules to receptor sites on cellular plasma membranes. Although the mechanisms of molecular actions in the cellular area are still being explored, it is known that cell membrane transport characteristics, cellular growth, enzyme activation and inhibition, and alterations in protein metabolism are all influenced by insulin.

Uses

Hyperglycemia.

Doses

1. The dosage and administration of insulin can vary greatly and must, therefore, be determined for each individual patient.
2. Insulin commercially available in the United States is a mixture of beef and pork insulin or is a single source insulin which is appropriately marked "beef," "pork," or "human insulin."
3. As a general rule, when regular insulin is involved, it should be drawn first as the supply of regular insulin may become cloudy due to the inadvertent contamination with the other insulin.
4. Regular insulin may be mixed with NPH insulin in any proportion without loss of the characteristics of the individual insulins. It is generally recommended that the resulting mixture be used within 5 min unless the manufacturer's literature states something different.
5. Regular insulin mixed with insulin zinc preparations may not give predictable clinical results.
6. Lente, Semilente, and Ultralente insulins may be mixed in any proportion without loss of the characteristics of the individual insulins.
7. Most brands of regular insulin may be mixed with PZI insulin but the excess free protamine content in the PZI combines with the regular insulin to give varying durations of action.

Adverse Effects

Weakness, hunger, sweating, pallor.

Major Drug Interactions

1. Use with adrenocorticoids, danazol, dextrothyroxine, epinephrine, ethacrynic acid, furosemide, oral contraceptives, phenytoin, sympathomimetics, thyroid or thiazide diuretics may increase blood glucose concentrations and enhance the possibility of hyperglycemia. Dosage adjustment of either or both medications may be necessary.
2. Alcohol, anabolic steroids, oral hypoglycemics, MAO inhibitors, large doses of salicylates, disopyramide, or guanethidine may enhance the hypoglycemic effect.

Isoproterenol Hydrochloride

Category

Sympathomimetic: beta-adrenergic agent

Brand Name

Isuprel

Pharmacologic Mechanism

Isoproterenol is a directly acting sympathomimetic amine which acts predominantly on beta-adrenergic receptors. It relaxes bronchial smooth muscle by acting on beta 2 adrenergic receptors, thereby relieving bronchospasms, increasing vital capacity, reducing residual volume in the lung, and facilitating passage of pulmonary secretions.

Uses

Bronchial asthma, obstructive pulmonary disease, bronchospasm, cardiac arrest, arrhythmias, or shock.

Doses

1. Intravenous infusion rate of 0.05 to 5 μg per minute from a solution of 2 mg in 500 mL of 5% dextrose injection.
2. See manufacturer's recommendations for additional parenteral dosages.
3. The usual adult sublingual dose is 10 to 15 mg three or four times daily.
4. The usual pediatric dose is one-half of the adult dose.

Nursing Interventions and Administration

Injection may be diluted with 5% dextrose or sodium chloride injection.

Adverse Effects

Flushing of the face, headache, tachycardia, anginal-type pain, and weakness.

Drug Interactions

Avoid concurrent use with monoamine oxidase inhibitors, guanethidine, and tricyclic antidepressants.

Contraindications

Digitalis-induced tachycardia and preexisting cardiac arrhythmias.

Isosorbide

Category

Antianginal

Brand Names

Dilatrate SR

IsoBid

Isordil

Isotrate

Sorate

Sorbide TD

Pharmacologic Mechanism

The antianginal action is thought to result in a reduction of myocardial oxygen demand. This is attributed to a reduction in left ventricular afterload because of the dilation of peripheral blood vessels in addition to a more efficient redistribution of blood flow within the myocardium.

Uses

Angina pectoris.

Doses

1. For oral dosage: 40 mg as an extended-release capsule every 12 h, the dosage being increased up to 40 mg every 6 h as needed and tolerated.
2. Oral: 10 mg four times a day, the dosage being adjusted as needed and tolerated.
3. Chewable oral tablets: 5 to 10 mg chewed well every 2 to 3 h.
4. Sublingual: 2.5 to 5 mg every 2 to 3 h as needed.

Nursing Interventions and Administration

1. Dosages can be changed as tolerated.
2. Tolerance is possible with prolonged usage. Discontinuation of the medication for a week or so and subsequent readministration may restore its effectiveness.
3. The oral dosage forms of this medication should be taken with a glass of water on an empty stomach, either 1 or 2 h after meals, for faster absorption.
4. When the medication is discontinued following high-dose or long-term administration, dosage should be reduced gradually in order to prevent possible withdrawal rebound angina.
5. Sublingual dosages may be administered to relieve acute anginal attacks that may occur when the patient is on an oral prophylactic therapy.

Adverse Effects

Headache, skin rash, dizziness, flushing, nausea, vomiting, tachycardia.

Major Drug Interactions

Concurrent use with alcohol, antihypertensives, or vasodilators may intensify the orthostatic hypotensive effects of nitrates.

Contraindications

Anemia, hyperthyroidism, increased intracranial pressure, and recent myocardial infarction.

Labetalol

Category

Antihypertensive

Brand Names

Trandate

Normodyne

Pharmacologic Mechanism

Labetalol is both an alpha and a nonspecific beta blocker. Both alpha and beta blockade contribute to the blood pressure-lowering effect. Standing blood pressure is lowered more than supine pressure, without reflex tachycardia or significant reduction in heart rate. Hemodynamic effects are variable with small, nonsignificant changes in cardiac output seen in some cases, and small decreases in total peripheral resistance.

Uses

Severe hypertension.

Doses

1. Patients should always be kept in a supine position during the period of intravenous drug

administration. A substantial fall in blood pressure on standing should be expected in these patients.

2. In adults, 20 mg by slow intravenous injection over a 2-min period is given. Additional injections of 40 mg or 80 mg can be given at 10-min intervals. The maximum dose is 300 mg.

3. By slow, continuous intravenous infusion, two ampules (40 mL) are added to 160 mL of intravenous solution, so the resultant solution contains 1 mg/mL. This diluted solution should be administered at a rate of 2 mL per minute (i.e., 2 mg per minute).

4. The recommended oral dose is 200 mg, followed in 6 to 12 h by an additional dose of 200 or 400 mg.

5. Dosage schedules for pediatric patients have not been established.

Nursing Interventions and Administration

1. Blood pressure must be carefully monitored during administration.

2. Caution should be exercised to prevent safety problems related to the orthostatic hypotensive effect of the drug.

3. Labetalol is compatible with most intravenous fluids.

4. During and immediately following labetalol injection, the patient should remain supine.

5. Patients should be warned about abrupt withdrawal of this drug.

Adverse Effects

Dizziness, fatigue, nausea, vomiting, dyspepsia, paresthesias, nasal stuffiness, edema.

Major Drug Interactions

1. Concurrent use with tricyclic antidepressants may cause the patient to experience tremors.

2. Cimetidine has been shown to increase the bioavailability of labetalol administered orally.

3. Labetalol blunts the reflex tachycardia produced by nitroglycerin without preventing its hypotensive effect.

Contraindications

Asthma, cardiac failure, heart block, cardiogenic shock, bradycardia.

Levarterenol Bitartrate

Category

Sympathomimetic: vasopressor

Brand Name

Levophed

Pharmacologic Mechanism

Levarterenol produces a sympathomimetic effect by activating adrenergic receptors in the body. The drug produces powerful vasoconstriction (alpha receptors) and stimulation of the heart and dilation of coronary arteries (beta receptors).

Uses

For controlling acute hypotensive states due to blood transfusion, drug interactions, myocardial infarction, pheochromocytomectomy, poliomyelitis, septicemia, spinal anesthesia, sympathectomy.

Doses

1. Pediatric parenteral dose is 1 mL of a 0.2% solution added to 250 mL of 5% dextrose for continuous infusion.

2. The adult dose is 2 to 8 mL of a 0.2% solution added to 500 mL of 5% dextrose for continuous infusion.

Nursing Interventions and Administration

1. Pediatric IV rate of 0.5 mL per minute is recommended.

2. Adult IV rate is adjusted to maintain a low normal blood pressure (80 to 100 mmHg systolic).

3. Whole blood or plasma if indicated to increase blood volume should be administered separately.

Adverse Effects

Occasional bradycardia and headache.

Drug Interactions

Avoid concurrent use with monoamine oxidase (MAO) inhibitors.

Contraindications

1. Hypotensive states due to blood volume deficits except as an emergency measure.

2. Mesenteric or peripheral vascular thrombosis unless necessary to save life.
3. During cyclopropane and halothane anesthesia.

Lidocaine

Category

Antiarrhythmic

Brand Names

LidoPen

Xylocaine

Pharmacologic Mechanism

Lidocaine decreases the depolarization, automaticity and excitability in the ventricles during the diastolic phase by a direct action on the tissues, especially the Purkinje network, without involvement of the autonomic system. Neither contractility, systolic arterial blood pressure, atrioventricular (AV) conduction velocity, nor absolute refractory period is altered by usual therapeutic doses.

Uses

Ventricular arrhythmias.

Doses

1. Intramuscular injection of lidocaine is recommended only when ECG monitoring equipment is not available. Injections should be to the deltoid muscle, which provides more rapid and complete systemic availability of the medication than do other large muscle tissues.
2. The preferred diluent for lidocaine infusion is 5% dextrose injection.
3. A loading dose of lidocaine is commonly administered for the initial dose to partially compensate for its rapid perfusion and distribution, which tends to delay attainment of a therapeutic serum concentration. If the initial loading dose does not provide the desired effect within 5 min, a second loading dose reduced to one-half to one-third of the first dose may be given.
4. A decreased infusion rate is needed for patients with impaired cardiac output or during prolonged infusion to prevent toxic responses.

Adverse Effects

Convulsions, dizziness, drowsiness, bradycardia, difficulty in breathing, itching, skin rash, anxiety, blurred vision, coldness, ringing in ears, tremors, vomiting.

Major Drug Interactions

1. Concurrent use with beta-adrenergic blocking agents may slow hepatic metabolism of lidocaine.
2. Concurrent use with cimetidine may result in reduced hepatic clearance of lidocaine.
3. Effects of neuromuscular blocking agents may be potentiated when used concurrently with large doses.
4. Concurrent use of phenytoin with lidocaine may have an additive cardiac depressant effect.

Therapeutic Drug Levels

1. 1.5 to 5 μg per mL.
2. Over 5 μg is considered toxic.

Contraindications

Adams-Stokes syndrome, severe heart block, congestive heart failure, hypovolemia, incomplete heart block, reduced hepatic blood flow, sinus bradycardia, Wolff-Parkinson-White syndrome.

Magnesium Sulfate

Category

Anticonvulsant, saline laxative, electrolyte

Pharmacologic Mechanism

Anticonvulsant activity is due to inhibition of peripheral neuromuscular transmission. Cathartic activity may be due to the hyperosmotic effect of the magnesium ion.

Uses

1. Anticonvulsant for seizures associated with toxemia of pregnancy, epilepsy, glomerulonephritis, and hypothyroidism.
2. Treatment of magnesium deficiency.
3. Saline laxative.
4. Antidote for barium poisoning.

Doses

1. The pediatric intramuscular dose is 20 to 40 mg per kilogram of body weight.
2. The adult IM dose is 1 to 5 g in a 25 to 50% solution.
3. The adult IV dose is 1 to 4 g in a 10 to 20% solution.
4. The adult infusion rate is 4 g in 250 mL of 5% dextrose.

Nursing Interventions and Administration

1. For IV administration do not exceed a 20% solution or a rate of administration of 150 mg per minute.
2. For IM administration do not exceed a 50% solution for adults or a 20% solution for children.
3. Monitor carefully for respiratory failure.

Adverse Effects
Primarily due to hypermagnesemia, these include flushing, sweating, hypotension, and respiratory and circulatory collapse.

Drug Interactions

1. Concurrent use with CNS depressants requires dosage adjustments.
2. Use with great caution in digitalized patients.

Therapeutic Serum Concentrations
4 to 6 meq per liter.

Contraindications
Heart block or myocardial damage (parenteral administration).

Mannitol

Category

Diuretic, antiglaucoma agent, antidote, antihemolytic

Brand Name

Osmitrol

Pharmacologic Mechanism
Mannitol elevates blood plasma osmolality, resulting in enhanced flow of water from tissues, including the brain and cerebrospinal fluid, into interstitial fluid and plasma. As a result, cerebral edema, elevated intracranial pressure, and cerebrospinal fluid volume and pressure may be reduced. Mannitol induces diuresis because it is not reabsorbed in the renal tubule, thereby increasing the osmolality of the glomerular filtrate, facilitating excretion of water, and inhibiting the renal tubular reabsorption of sodium, chloride, and other solutes. It may therefore promote the urinary excretion of toxic materials and protect against nephrotoxicity by preventing the concentration of toxic substances in the tubular fluid.

Uses
Cerebral edema, increased intracranial pressure.

Doses

1. As a diuretic, mannitol is given as an intravenous infusion, 50 to 100 g as a 5 to 25% solution, administered at a rate adjusted to maintain a urine flow of at least 30 to 50 mL per hour.
2. In the treatment of cerebral edema, intravenous infusion of 1.5 to 2 g per kilogram of body weight as a 15 to 25% solution, administered over a period of 30 to 60 min.
3. The usual pediatric dose is an intravenous infusion of 2 g per kilogram of body weight as a 15 to 20% solution, administered over a period of 2 to 6 h.
4. For cerebral edema, the usual pediatric dosage is an intravenous infusion of 1 to 2 g per kilogram of body weight of a 15 to 20% solution, administered over a period of 30 to 60 min.

Nursing Interventions and Administration

1. Mannitol should be administered through a filter, since these solutions have a greater tendency for crystallization.
2. A test dose of mannitol is recommended prior to therapy in patients with marked oliguria or possible inadequate renal function. The test dose is given as an intravenous infusion, 200 mg per kilogram of body weight as a 15 to 25% solution, administered over a period of 3 to 5 min.

Adverse Effects

Circulatory overload, hypovolemia, chest pain, tachycardia, chills, coughing, dysuria, arrhythmias, confusion, muscle cramps, numbness and tingling, seizures, fatigue, edema.

Major Drug Interactions

None reported.

Contraindications

Anuria, severe dehydration, intracranial bleeding, pulmonary congestion, impairment in cardiopulmonary function, and impairment in renal function.

Meperidine Hydrochloride

Category

Narcotic: nonopiate addicting analgesic

Brand Name

Demerol hydrochloride

Pharmacologic Mechanism

The narcotic analgesics exhibit a wide range of activity and produce their main pharmacologic effects on the central nervous system and gastrointestinal tract. They are the most effective analgesics available, and they all possess a high addiction liability. Analgesic activity is probably due to interference with pain impulses at the subcortical level of the brain. Other CNS effects include powerful medullary depression of respiration, stimulation of the chemoreceptor trigger zone, constriction of the pupils, and depression of the cough reflex. Gastrointestinal effects include an increase in smooth muscle tone and a decrease in propulsive movements and emptying time.

Uses

Analgesic, sedation.

Doses

1. The pediatric dose is 1.1 to 1.76 mg/kg every 3 to 4 h as needed.
2. The adult dose is 50 to 150 mg every 3 to 4 h as needed.

Nursing Interventions and Administration

1. The IM route is preferred when repeated doses are required.
2. For IV administration, the injection should be made slowly, using a diluted solution.

Adverse Effects

Nausea, trembling, spasm, fatigue, weakness, dry mouth, headache, stomach pain.

Contraindications

Hypersensitivity and with patients currently or recently on monoamine oxidase inhibitors.

Metaraminol Bitartrate

Category

Sympathomimetic: vasopressor

Brand Name

Aramine

Pharmacologic Mechanism

Sympathomimetic effect is due to direct and indirect adrenergic activity. Metaraminol produces direct stimulation of alpha-adrenergic and beta-adrenergic receptors and causes the release of norepinephrine, which results in vasoconstriction and cardiac stimulation.

Uses

1. Indicated in the prevention or treatment of acute hypotension due to spinal anesthesia.
2. As an adjunct in hypotension due to drugs, hemorrhage, and surgical complications.

Doses

1. The IM or SC dose is 2 to 10 mg. Recommended pediatric dose is 100 μg/kg.
2. For IV infusion, 15 to 100 mg in 500 mL of solution administered at a rate to maintain satisfactory blood pressure. Severe shock may require a direct injection of 0.05 to 5 mg, followed by an infusion.

Nursing Interventions and Administration

Metaraminol may be mixed with sodium chloride, 5% dextrose, Ringer's, lactated Ringer's, and 6% dextran in saline.

Adverse Effects

Sinus or ventricular tachycardia, tissue necrosis, and possible relapse in patients with a history of malaria.

Drug Interactions

1. Avoid concurrent use with cyclopropane or halothane, monoamine oxidase inhibitors, and tricylic antidepressants due to potential hypertensive effect or arrhythmias.
2. Concurrent use with digitalis can cause arrhythmias.

Contraindications

Hypersensitivity.

Methotrexate

Category

Antineoplastic: antimetabolite, folic acid antagonist

Brand Names

Folex

Mexate

Pharmacologic Mechanism

Antimetabolic activity is due to competitive inhibition of dihydrofolate reductase. This results in reduced amounts of tetrahydrofolic acid and, therefore, DNA synthesis and cell reproduction is inhibited, especially in malignant tissue.

Uses

1. Indicated in the treatment of gestational choriocarcinoma, chorioadenoma destruens, and hydatidiform mole (trophoblastic tumors).
2. Treatment of lymphoblastic leukemias and meningeal leukemia.
3. In combination for the treatment of carcinoma of the breast, lung, testes, neck, and pelvis.
4. Treatment of Burkitt's lymphoma and advanced states (III and IV, Peters staging system) of lymphosarcoma.
5. Treatment of advanced cases of mycosis fungoides.
6. Control of severe and disabling psoriasis not responsive to other therapy.

Doses

1. The pediatric oral dose is 20 to 30 mg per square meter of body surface.
2. Adult oral dose is 15 to 50 mg per square meter of body surface, one or two times a week.
3. The pediatric parenteral dose is 20 to 30 mg per square meter of body surface once a week.
4. The adult parenteral dose is 15 to 50 mg per square meter of body surface one or two times a week.

Nursing Interventions and Administration

1. For intrathecal administration the drug must be diluted 1 mg/mL with sodium chloride injection without preservatives and filtered before using.
2. The 25 mg/mL solution should be used for dilution.
3. Leucovorin calcium may be administered following intrathecal administration to help reduce systemic toxicity.

Adverse Effects

Ulcerative stomatitis, leukopenia, nausea, alopecia, photosensitivity, erythematous rash, bone marrow depression, periportal fibrosis, hepatic cirrhosis, renal failure, azotemia, teratogenic effects, abortion, aphasia, convulsions, headache, and blurred vision.

Drug Interactions

1. Avoid vitamin preparations containing folic acid and preparations containing salicylates.
2. Concurrent use with oral hypoglycemics, sulfonamides, and thiazides may increase the effect and toxicity of methotrexate.
3. Concurrent use with alcohol or hepatotoxic medications increases the risk of hepatotoxicity.
4. Concurrent use with asparaginase may block the effects of methotrexate.

Contraindications

In patients with severe preexisting liver, bone marrow, or kidney impairment, the first trimester of pregnancy, chickenpox, herpes zoster, peptic ulcer.

Methoxamine

Category

Antiarrhythmic, vasopressor

Brand Name

Vasoxyl

Pharmacologic Mechanism

Methoxamine is primarily a direct-acting sympatho-mimetic amine. It acts on alpha-adrenergic receptors of the peripheral vasculature, to produce vasoconstriction with a resultant increase in both systolic and diastolic blood pressure. There is no apparent stimulant effect on the heart or central nervous system. Bradycardia may occur from a carotid sinus reflex when higher dosages are administered intravenously. This effect is utilized in the termination of paroxysmal SVT.

Uses

Vasopressor and antiarrhythmic.

Doses

1. As a vasopressor, 10 to 15 mg can be given intramuscularly. The intravenous dose is 3 to 5 mg administered slowly.
2. As an antiarrhythmic agent, 10 mg intravenously is administered slowly.
3. The usual pediatric doses are 250 μg per kilogram of body weight intramuscularly; 80 μg per kilogram of body weight, intravenously.

Nursing Interventions and Administration

1. Allow at least 15 min before repeating an intramuscular dose.
2. Methoxamine is administered by slow, intravenous injection when the systolic blood pressure falls to 60 mmHg or less.
3. Rapid administration should be avoided because

this would produce added stress on the myocardium from markedly increased peripheral resistance during a reduction in stroke volume and cardiac output.

Adverse Effects

Headache, vomiting, urinary urgency.

Major Drug Interactions

1. Parenteral administration of ergot alkaloids followed closely by administration of methoxamine may produce an excessive increase in blood pressure.
2. Concurrent use of methoxamine during halothane anesthesia may initiate serious cardiac arrhythmias.
3. Concurrent use of methoxamine with MAO inhibitors or tricyclic antidepressants may result in severe hypertensive crisis.

Contraindications

Should be used with caution for patients who have severe arteriosclerosis, heart disease, and hyperthyroidism.

Metocurine

Category

Neuromuscular blocker

Brand Name

Metubine

Pharmacologic Mechanism

Neuromuscular blocking agents produce skeletal muscle paralysis by blocking neural transmission at the myoneural junction. The paralysis is selective initially and usually appears in the levator muscles of eyelids, muscles of mastication, limb muscles, abdominal muscles, muscles of the glottis, and the intercostal muscles and diaphragm. Neuromuscular blocking agents have no known effect on consciousness or pain threshold.

Depolarizing neuromuscular blocking agents (succinylcholine) compete with acetylcholine for the cholinergic receptors of the motor end plate and combine with these receptors to produce depolarization; however, because of their high affinity for cholinergic receptors and their resistance to anticholinesterase, they produce a more prolonged depolarization than does acetylcholine. This results initially in transient muscle contractions, usually visible as fasciculations, followed by inhibition of neuromuscular transmission. This type of neuromuscular block is not antagonized, and may even be enhanced by anticholinesterase agents.

Doses

Intravenous dosage is 150 to 300 µg per kilogram administered over a period of 30 to 60 s. Supplemental doses of 500 µg to 1 mg may be administered every 30 to 90 min as required.

Nursing Interventions and Administration

1. Since metocurine has no effect on pain threshold and consciousness, it is important to use adjunctive therapy when administering this drug.
2. With the threat of apnea, this drug should only be used when the individual's airway can be protected.
3. Intermittent dosages are avoided because of increased risk of breathing difficulties.

Adverse Effects

Postoperative muscular pain and stiffness, increase in intraocular pressure, irregular heartbeat, tachycardia, bradycardia.

Major Drug Interactions

1. Concurrent use with aminoglycoside antibiotics, clindamycin, lincomycin, or polymyxin antibiotics may enhance the blockade of neuromuscular blocking agents, resulting in prolonged respiratory depression or apnea.
2. Concurrent use with beta-adrenergic blocking agents may enhance the blockage of the nondepolarizing neuromuscular blocking agent.
3. Concurrent use with furosemide may enhance the blockade of the nondepolarizing neuromuscular blocking agent.
4. Concurrent use with quinidine or quinine may enhance the neuromuscular blocking agents, resulting in prolonged or intensified respiratory depression or apnea.

Contraindications

Bronchogenic carcinoma, cardiac conditions which would be worsened with tachycardia, conditions in which histamine release would be hazardous, dehydration, electrolye or acid-base imbalance, hepatic function impairment, hyperthermia, hypotension, hypothermia, myasthenia gravis, pulmonary function impairment, renal function impairment, and shock.

Morphine Sulfate

Category

Narcotic: opium alkaloid

Pharmacologic Mechanism

The narcotic analgesics exhibit a wide range of activity and produce their main pharmacologic effects on the central nervous system and gastrointestinal tract. They are the most effective analgesics available, and they all possess a high addiction liability.

Analgesic activity is probably due to interference with pain impulses at the subcortical level of the brain. Other CNS effects include powerful medullary depression of respiration, stimulation of the chemoreceptor trigger zone, constriction of the pupils, and depression of the cough reflex. Gastrointestinal effects include an increase in smooth muscle tone and a decrease in propulsive movements and emptying time.

Uses

Relief of severe pain, preanesthetic sedation, and postoperative analgesia.

Doses

1. The pediatric SC dose is 0.1 to 0.2 mg/kg. Do not exceed a single maximum dose of 15 mg.
2. The adult SC, IM dose is 5 to 20 mg.
3. The adult IV dose is 4 to 10 mg.

Nursing Interventions and Administration

1. For IV administration, dilute desired dose in at least 4 to 5 mL of sterile water for injection and inject slowly over a 5-min period.
2. Monitor closely for respiratory rate.

Adverse Effects

Nausea, vomiting, sedation, sweating, dry mouth, constipation, biliary tract spasm, euphoria, hypotension, urinary retention, pruritis, and urticaria.

Drug Interactions

1. Avoid concurrent use with tricyclic antidepressants.
2. Use with caution with antihistamines, barbiturates, benzodiazepines, methotrimeprazine, phenothiazines, and other CNS depressants.

Contraindications

Hypersensitivity, respiratory depression, asthma, inflammatory bowel disease.

Naloxone Hydrochloride

Category

Narcotic antagonist

Brand Name

Narcan

Pharmacologic Mechanism

Narcotic antagonism is produced primarily due to competition with narcotics for receptor sites in the central nervous system. Naloxone is a pure narcotic antagonist because it possesses no agonist morphine-like properties.

Uses

Narcotic overdose.

Doses

1. The pediatric parenteral (IM, IV, SC) initial dose is 0.01 mg/kg. May be repeated at 2- to 3-min intervals.
2. For adults the initial dose is 0.4 mg. May be repeated at 2- to 3-min intervals.

Adverse Effects

Nausea and vomiting in postoperative patients with high doses.

Drug Interactions

None currently reported.

Contraindications

Hypersensitivity.

Neostigmine

Category

Antimyasthenic

Brand Name

Prostigmin

Pharmacologic Mechanism

Neostigmine inhibits the destruction of acetylcholine by acetylcholinesterase, thereby facilitating transmission of impulses across the myoneural junction. Cholinergic responses produced are miosis, bradycardia, increased tonus of intestinal and skeletal muscle, constriction of bronchi and ureters, and stimulation of secretion by salivary and sweat glands. In addition, these medications have a direct cholinomimetic effect on skeletal muscle.

Neostigmine works as an antimyasthenic. Muscle strength and response to repetitive nerve stimulation is increased as a result of these medications enhancing the peak effect and prolonging the duration of action of acetylcholine at the motor end plate.

Since nondepolarizing neuromuscular blocking agents combine reversibly with the receptors, preventing access of acetycholine, antagonism can be overcome by increasing the amount of agonist at the receptors; therefore, muscle paralysis induced by nondepolarizing neuromuscular blocking agents is reversed by pyridostigmine, which increases concentration of acetycholine at the receptors.

Uses

Treatment of muscular weakness in myasthenia gravis.

Doses

1. Initial oral adult dose is 15 mg every 3 to 4 h, the dose and frequency of administration being adjusted as necessary. The maintenance dosage is 150 mg administered over a 24-h period, the intervals between doses being determined by response of the patient.

2. Usual adult parenteral dosage is 500 μg intramuscularly or subcutaneously as an antimyasthenic agent. Intravenous doses of 500 μg to 2 mg can be administered slowly, repeated as required up to a total dose of 5 mg to be used as an antidote to curariform block.
3. The pediatric dose for oral administration is 2 mg per kilogram of body weight, divided into six to eight doses. Parenteral dosages are from 10 to 40 μg per kilogram, given intramuscularly or subcutaneously for antimyasthenic effect. The intravenous dosage is usually 20 μg per kilogram of body weight.

Nursing Interventions and Administration

1. When large parenteral doses are administered, it is recommended that 600 μg to 1.2 mg of atropine be administered prior to or concurrently with neostigmine to counteract its muscarinic side effects.
2. When used in the treatment of myasthenia gravis, the dosage must be individualized according to the severity of the disease and the response of the patient.
3. Following prolonged therapy, myasthenic patients may become refractory to these medications. Responsiveness may be restored, especially when the resistance may have been caused by overdosage, by reducing the dosage or discontinuing the medication for a few days.
4. Patients should be closely observed for cholinergic reactions when medication is given intravenously.
5. Atropine should be readily available because of the possibility of hypersensitivity reactions.
6. Swallowing ability should be carefully assessed prior to administration of oral doses.

Adverse Effects

Skin rash, blurred vision, diarrhea, bradycardia, confusion, seizures, unusual irritability, frequent urination, increased bronchial secretions, small pupils.

Major Drug Interactions

Neuromuscular blocking action of anesthetics, antiarrhythmic agents, and some antibiotics (aminoglycosides, lincomycin) may angtaonize the effect of antimyasthenics on skeletal muscle.

Contraindications

Mechanical intestinal or urinary tract obstruction, urinary tract infections, and postsurgical patients in which the antimyasthenic agent may exacerbate respiratory problems.

Nitroglycerin

Category

Antianginal: coronary vasodilator

Pharmacologic Mechanism

Nitrates relax smooth muscle in small blood vessels and dilate arteries and capillaries, especially in coronary circulation, which reduces myocardial ischemia. This is attributed to a reduction in left ventricular preload and afterload because of venous and arterial dilation with a more efficient distribution of blood flow within the myocardium.

Uses

Angina, hypertension, myocardial infarction therapy.

Doses

1. The usual adult dosage for extended-release tablets is 1.3 to 9.0 mg.
2. The usual adult sublingual dosage is 150 to 600 μg repeated at 5-min intervals as needed for relief of anginal attack.
3. The usual dosage for nitroglycerin ointment is 15 to 30 mg (1 to 2 in) every 3 to 4 h as needed.
4. The usual adult dosage of transdermal systems is one transdermal dosage system every 24 h.
5. Adult intravenous infusion is initiated at a rate of 5 μg per minute, the dosage being increased by increments of 5 μg per minute at 3- to 5-min intervals. No fixed maximum dose has been established.
6. Guidelines for dosages of this drug for pediatric use have not been established.

Nursing Interventions and Administration

1. Tolerance to nitrates is possible with prolonged use.
2. Intravenous doses must be diluted before use.

3. Use of special nitroglycerin infusion sets is recommended, since the special tubing does not absorb the drug as does standard tubing.
4. Application of transdermal doses should occur at the same time each day.

Adverse Effects
Hypotension, dizziness, flushing, headache, nausea, tachycardia, restlessness.

Drug Interactions

1. Concurrent use with tricyclic antidepressants may result in additive hypotension.
2. Concurrent use with alcohol, antihypertensives, or vasodilators may potentiate the orthostatic hypotensive effects.

Contraindications
Hypersensitivity, severe anemia, or increased intracranial pressure.

Nitroprusside

Category

Antihypertensive

Brand Names

Nipride

Nitropress

Pharmacologic Mechanism
Nitroprusside causes vasodilation by a direct effect on arterial and venous smooth muscle, with no effect on uterine or duodenal smooth muscle or myocardial contractility. It reduces peripheral resistance and cardiac output, but affects regional distribution of blood flow marginally.

The effect of nitroprusside on ischemic myocardial areas is not totally known. The medication reportedly reduces myocardial oxygen consumption and relieves persistent chest pain, but has also been found to aggravate ischemia by redistributing blood flow away from ischemic myocardium. The metabolites of nitroprusside are cyanide and thiocyanate.

Uses
Hypertension, congestive heart failure, myocardial infarction, valvular regurgitation.

Doses

1. The usual adult dose as an antihypertensive is intravenous infusion, 0.5 μg per kilogram of body weight per minute, adjusted slowly in increments of 0.5 μg according to response. The usual dose is 3 μg per kilogram of body weight per minute.
2. The usual adult dose limit is up to 10 μg per kilogram of body weight per minute.
3. The usual pediatric dosage is 1.4 μg per kilogram of body weight per minute, adjusted slowly according to response.

Nursing Interventions and Administration

1. Nitroprusside can be administered only by intravenous infusion at a rate not exceeding 10 μg per kilogram of body weight per minute.
2. Cardiovascular function must be continually monitored during use of this drug.
3. It is recommended that oral therapy be instituted while the patient is receiving nitroprusside and that nitroprusside be withdrawn as soon as the patient has stabilized.
4. Addition of a potent inotropic medication such as dopamine or dobutamine may be useful when doses of nitroprusside that are effective in restoring pump function in left ventricular congestive heart failure cause excessive hypotension.

Adverse Effects
Dizziness, excessive sweating, headache, nervousness, restlessness, ataxia, delirium, headache, loss of consciousness, ringing in ears.

Major Drug Interactions
Concurrent use with other antihypertensive medications may result in increased hypotensive effects.

Therapeutic Drug Levels
Thiocyanate <100 μg/mL.

Contraindications
Cerebrovascular, coronary artery insufficiency, hepatic function impairment, optic atrophy, renal

function impairment, tobacco amblyopia, and vitamin B-12 deficiency.

Pancuronium Bromide

Category

Skeletal muscle relaxant: nondepolarizing neuromuscular blocking agent

Brand Name

Pavulon

Pharmacologic Mechanism

Pancuronium bromide is a competitive blocking agent which causes skeletal muscle paralysis by combining with cholinergic receptors on the motor end plate. Following a single effective IV dose, the onset of activity is in 30 to 45 s, with a peak effect between 3 and 4½ min. Competitive muscular relaxation produced by nondepolarizing agents can be antagonized by the acetylcholinesterase drugs.

Uses

Promotes skeletal muscle relaxation and facilitates the management of mechanical respiration.

Doses

1. Pediatric and adult dosage is 0.04 to 0.1 mg/kg initially. Subsequent doses start with 0.01 mg/kg for continued muscle relaxation, repeated as required.
2. Dosage must be individualized to each patient.

Nursing Interventions and Administration

1. Since pancuronium has no effect on pain threshold and consciousness, it is important to use adjunctive therapy when administering the drug.
2. Use only when airway has been protected.

Adverse Effects

Respiratory depression, apnea, and a slight increase in pulse rate.

Drug Interactions

1. Lower doses are required for surgical procedures when used with enflurane, ether, halothane, and methoxyflurane.
2. Significant neuromuscular blockage can result from concurrent use with aminoglycoside antibiotics, amphotericin B, and polymixin B.
3. Use with quinidine can increase neuromuscular blocking.

Contraindications

Hypersensitivity, severe trauma, cardiovascular impairment, dehydration, hepatic function impairment.

Pentobarbital

Category

Sedative-hypnotic, anticonvulsant

Brand Name

Nembutal

Pharmacologic Mechanism

Barbiturates act as nonselective depressants of the central nervous system, capable of producing all levels of CNS mood alteration from excitation to mild sedation, hypnosis, and deep coma. Recent studies suggest that the sedative-hypnotic and anticonvulsant effects of barbiturates may be related to their ability to enhance and/or mimic the inhibitory synaptic action of gamma-aminobutyric acid (GABA).

Barbiturates produce their sedative-hypnotic effect by depressing the sensory cortex, decreasing motor activity, altering cerebral function, and producing drowsiness, sedation, or hypnosis. The barbiturates appear to act at the level of the thalamus where they inhibit ascending conduction in the reticular formation, thus interfering with the transmission of impulses to the cortex.

The mechanism of action of pentobarbital in protecting the brain from ischemia and intracranial pressure is not completely understood; however, it is related to pentobarbital's anesthetic action and possibly to the depression of neuronal activity and metabolism.

Barbiturates are believed to act by depressing monosynaptic and polysynaptic transmission in the CNS. They also increase the threshold for electrical stimulation of the motor cortex in their anticonvulsant action.

Uses
Sedation, seizures, insomnia.

Doses

1. Usual oral adult dose as an hypnotic-sedative is 100 mg at bedtime.
2. The usual pediatric dose is 2 to 6 mg per kilogram of body weight per day.
3. Hypnotic effects can be obtained for 150 to 200 mg intramuscularly. Intravenous doses of 100 mg are given initially; after 1 min, additional small doses may be administered at 1-min intervals, up to a total of 500 mg.
4. As an anticonvulsant, 100 mg are given intravenously initially; after 1 min, additional small doses may be administered at 1-min intervals, up to a total of 500 mg.

Nursing Interventions and Administration

1. Tolerance can occur with repeated administration of barbiturates.
2. Barbiturates should be withdrawn gradually to avoid the possibility of precipitating withdrawal symptoms.
3. Intravenous injections should be administered slowly and patients should be carefully monitored during administration.
4. Intramuscular injections should be administered deep into large muscles.
5. Parenteral forms are not recommended for subcutaneous administration.

Adverse Effects
Confusion, hallucinations, mental depression, skin rash, wheezing, sore throat, slurred speech, staggering, dizziness, headache, irritability.

Major Drug Interactions
Concurrent use with alcohol, anesthetics, or CNS depressants may increase the CNS depressant effects.

Therapeutic Drug Levels
0.5 to 3 μg/mL.

Contraindications
Porphyria, drug abuse or dependence, hepatic coma, acute or chronic pain, respiratory disease.

Phentolamine

Category
Antihypertensive: alpha-adrenergic blocking agent.

Trade Names
Phentolamine hydrochloride—for oral administration (tablets)

Phentolamine mesylate—for parenteral administration

Regitine

Pharmacologic Mechanism
The antihypertensive effect is due to competitive blocking of alpha receptors, which results in reduced peripheral vascular resistance. Phentolamine also causes a reduction in afterload and pulmonary arterial pressure, increased cardiac output, and positive inotropic effect.

Uses
Diagnosis of pheochromocytoma, hypertensive crisis from clonidine withdrawal or monoamine oxidase inhibitor-sympathomimetic interaction, treatment of dermal necrosis following norepinephrine administration, and control of hypertensive crisis during surgery for pheochromocytoma.

Doses

1. The usual pediatric oral dose is 25 mg four to six times daily.
2. The usual adult oral dose is 50 mg four to six times daily.
3. The usual pediatric parenteral dose is 1 mg as required.
4. The usual adult parenteral (IM or IV) dose is 5 mg.

Nursing Interventions and Administration

1. Dosage must be adjusted to meet individual requirements.
2. Oral phentolamine has only 20% of the activity it has when administered intravenously.

Adverse Effects
Hypotension, tachycardia and cardiac arrhythmias, nasal stuffiness, nausea, and vomiting.

Drug Interactions

Possible added antidiabetic effect in diabetic pediatric patients.

Contraindications

Hypersensitivity, myocardial infarction, or coronary artery disease.

Phenylephrine

Category

Vasopressor, local adjunct anesthetic

Brand Name

Neo-Synephrine

Pharmacologic Mechanism

Phenylephrine is primarily a direct-acting sympathomimetic amine with some indirect action through the release of norepinephrine from storage sites.

As a vasopressor, phenylephrine acts on alpha-adrenergic receptors to produce vasoconstriction which increases peripheral resistance, resulting in an increase in both systolic and diastolic blood pressure. Accompanying the pressor response to phenylephrine is a marked reflex bradycardia due to increased vagal activity.

As an adjunct to local anesthetic, phenylephrine acts on alpha-adrenergic receptors in the skin, mucous membranes, and viscera to produce vasoconstriction. This action decreases the rate of vascular absorption of the local anesthetic used with phenylephrine therapy, localizing anesthesia, prolonging the duration of action, and decreasing the risk of toxicity due to the local anesthetic.

Uses

Hypotension, regional anesthesia, vascular failure.

Doses

1. For mild or moderate hypotension, 2 to 5 mg intramuscularly or subcutaneously, repeated not more often than every 10 to 15 min. For severe hypotension and shock, 10 mg in 500 mL of 5% dextrose injection or 0.9% sodium chloride injection, administered initially at a rate of about 100 to 180 drops per minute until blood pressure is stabilized, then at a rate of 40 to 60 drops per min. If necessary, additional doses in increments of 10 mg or more may be added to the infusion solution and the rate of flow adjusted until the desired blood pressure level is obtained.
2. For regional anesthesia, 1 mg of phenylephrine is added to each 20 mL of local anesthetic solution.
3. The usual pediatric dosage is 100 µg per kilogram of body weight intramuscularly or subcutaneously, repeated in 1 to 2 h if necessary.

Nursing Interventions and Administration

1. Extravasation of phenylephrine may cause necrosis or sloughing of the tissue.
2. Careful monitoring of cardiovascular function during administration is required.

Adverse Effects

Headache, bradycardia, hypertension, sensation of fullness in head, tingling of hands or feet, irregular heartbeat, vomiting.

Major Drug Interactions

Concurrent use with MAO inhibitors may potentiate the pressor effect of phenylephrine. It should not be administered during or within 14 days following administration of MAO inhibitors.

Contraindications

Arteriosclerosis, bradycardia, hypertension, hyperthyoidism, myocardial disease, partial heart block, and ventricular tachycardia.

Phenytoin

Category

Anticonvulsant, antiarrhythmic

Brand Names

Dilantin Infatabs

Dilantin Kapseal

Pharmacologic Mechanism

Phenytoin's anticonvulsant action is not completely known, but it is thought that it stabilizes neuronal membranes and limits the spread of seizure activity by either increasing the efflux or decreasing the influx of sodium ions across cell membranes during generation of nerve impulses.

Phenytoin's antiarrhythmic effect is believed to be its ability to normalize sodium influx to Purkinje fibers when used to treat digitalis-induced arrhythmias. Abnormal ventricular automaticity, membrane responsiveness, and the refractory period are decreased.

Uses
Seizure control, arrhythmias.

Doses

1. The usual adult oral dosage is 100 mg three times a day with the dosage being adjusted at 1- to 3-week intervals as needed and tolerated. An oral loading dose of 12 to 15 mg per kilogram of body weight divided into two or three doses over approximately 6 h and followed by 100 mg (1.5 to 2 mg per kilogram of body weight) three times a day on subsequent days, with dosage being adjusted as needed, is sometimes preferred, especially if seizures are frequent. The usual adult prescribing limits are up to 600 mg daily.
2. The usual pediatric dosage is 5 mg per kilogram of body weight a day, divided into two or three doses. Total dosage is not to exceed 300 mg a day.
3. As an anticonvulsant, intravenous doses of 150 to 250 mg are given, followed by 100 to 150 mg after 30 min if necessary, administered at a rate not to exceed 50 mg per minute; or 8 to 15 mg per kilogram of body weight, administered at a rate not to exceed 50 mg per min.
4. As an antiarrhythmic, 50 to 100 mg every 10 to 15 min as necessary, but not to exceed a total dose of 15 mg per kilogram of body weight administered intravenously, and at a rate not exceeding 50 mg per minute.

Nursing Interventions and Administration

1. The dosage should be individualized, since there is great variation among patients.
2. When anticonvulsants are to be discontinued, dosage should be reduced gradually to prevent possible occurrences of seizures.
3. Oral doses should be taken with or immediately after meals to lessen gastric irritation.
4. Intravenous phenytoin is to be administered by direct intravenous injection. It should not be added to intravenous infusions or mixed with other medications as precipitation may occur.
5. The rate of intravenous administration should not exceed 50 gm per min. Faster rates may result in cardiovascular collapse.
6. Intravenous administration should be monitored by cardiac function and blood pressure readings.
7. Each dose of phenytoin should be followed by 0.9% sodium chloride injection through the same in-place needle or catheter.
8. Avoid extravasation as phenytoin injection is caustic to tissues.
9. Intramuscular injection is not recommended because of delayed and erratic absorption and the high degree of local irritation from the alkaline solution.
10. If intramuscular injection is required for patients stabilized on oral phenytoin, a dose 50 percent greater than the original oral dosage is needed. When a patient is returned to the oral route, dosage should be reduced by 50 percent of the original oral dosage for 1 week to compensate for the sustained release of medication from prior intramuscular injection.
11. Monitor hemoglobin, hematocrit, and white blood cell count frequently during therapy.
12. Frequent oral hygiene is required to decrease the incidence of gingival hyperplasia.

Adverse Effects
Nystagmus, skin rash, blurred or double vision, unusual bleeding, jaundice, drowsiness and dizziness, gum hyperplasia.

Major Drug Interactions

1. Use with alcohol, barbiturates, and folic acid may decrease the effects of hydantoin.
2. Phenytoin decreases the therapeutic effects of calciferol, dexamethasone, doxycycline, or levodopa, because they are metabolized more quickly when used concurrently with hydantoins.

3. Phenytoin effects can be increased when used with chloramphenicol, cimetidine, disulfiram, isoniazid, or sulfonamides.
4. Concurrent use of phenytoin with lidocaine or propranolol can produce additive cardiac depressant effects.
5. Concurrent use of phenytoins with oral contraceptives may result in reduced contraceptive reliability and/or loss of seizure control.

Therapeutic Drug Levels
10 to 20 μg per milliliter. Steady-state serum concentration is usually achieved in 7 to 10 days with daily oral dosage of 300 mg when no loading dose is given.

Drug levels of 20 to 40 μg per milliliter usually produce symptoms of toxicity; levels ≥40 μg/ml usually produce severe toxicity.

Contraindications
Blood dyscrasias, alcoholism, diabetes, hyperglycemia, and hepatic function impairment.

Physostigmine

Category

Antidote, cholinergic

Brand Name

Antilirium

Pharmacologic Mechanism
Physostigmine antagonizes the action of anticholinergics, which block the postsynaptic receptor sites of acetylcholine, by inhibiting the destruction of acetylcholine by acetylcholinesterase, thereby increasing the concentration of acetylcholine at sites of cholinergic transmission. Physostigmine may also reverse the CNS depressant effects of diazepam. Although the mechanism of action is not known, it appears that the central dopaminergic activity may account for the nonspecific action of physostigmine.

Uses
Anticholinergic agent-induced toxicity; diazepam-induced toxicity.

Doses
1. The usual adult dose is 500 μg to 2 mg administered at a rate of not more than 1 mg per minute.
2. Doses of 1 to 4 mg may be repeated, if necessary, at intervals as life-threatening signs recur.
3. The usual pediatric dose is no more than 500 μg administered intravenously over a period of at least 1 min.

Adverse Effects
Convulsions, difficulty in breathing, bradycardia, irregular heartbeat, muscle twitching, fatigue, diarrhea, increased sweating, stomach cramps.

Major Drug Interactions

1. Effects of acetylcholine and methacholine are markedly enhanced by prior administration of physostigmine, since they are hydrolyzed by acetylcholinesterase.
2. Concurrent use of succinylcholine with physostigmine is not recommended since high doses of physostigmine may cause muscle fasciculation and a depolarization block which may be additive to that produced by the depolarizing neuromuscular blocking agents.

Contraindications
Asthma, cardiovascular disease, diabetes mellitus, gangrene, intestinal or urogenital tract obstruction.

Plasma Protein Fraction

Category

Volume expander

Brand Name

Plasmanate

Pharmacologic Mechanism
Plasma protein fraction (human) 5% has resulted in an increased blood volume which has lasted up to 48 h. It is an adequate replacement for human plasma in the treatment of shock and is a suitable means of providing human proteins for their osmotic effect.

Uses

Treatment of shock due to burns, crushing injuries, abdominal injuries, and others.

Doses

Dosage is based almost entirely on the nature of the individual case and response to therapy. The usual minimum effective dose in adults is 250 to 500 mL.

Nursing Interventions and Administration

1. This drug product should be carefully inspected prior to administration for any particulate matter or discoloration.
2. Hemodynamic status should be carefully monitored during administration.
3. Intravenous infusion should generally proceed at a rate of 10 mL per minute.
4. Do not begin administration more than 4 h after the container has been entered.
5. Partially used vials should be discarded.

Adverse Effects

Edema, hypertension, hypotension, flushing, urticaria, back pain, nausea, headache.

Major Drug Interactions

1. Plasma protein fraction (human) 5% should not be mixed with protein hydrolysates or solutions containing alcohol.
2. This drug product is compatible with whole blood, packed red cells, and standard carbohydrate and electrolyte solutions intended for intravenous use.

Contraindications

Cardiopulmonary bypass, severe anemia, congestive heart failure, increased blood volume.

Potassium Chloride

Category

Electrolyte replenisher

Brand Names

Kaochlor

Kaon

Kato

Kay Ciel

K-Lor

K-Lyte

Micro-K

Slow-K

Tri-K

Twin-K

Pharmacologic Mechanism

Potassium is the predominant cation within cells. Intracellular sodium content is relatively low. In extracellular fluid, sodium predominates and the potassium content is low. A membrane-bound enzyme, sodium–potassium-activated adenosine triphosphatase, actively transports or pumps sodium out of and potassium into cells to maintain these concentration gradients. The gradients are necessary for the conduction of nerve impulses in such tissues as the heart, brain, and skeletal muscle, and to maintain normal renal function and acid-base balance. High intracellular potassium concentrations are necessary for numerous cellular metabolic processes.

Doses

1. The usual adult oral dose of potassium chloride is the equivalent of 20 meq of potassium diluted in one-half glass of cold water or juice two to four times a day, the dosage being adjusted as needed and tolerated. Up to 100 meq of potassium daily can be safely administered.
2. The usual pediatric oral dose is the equivalent of 15 to 40 meq of potassium per square meter of body surface, or 1 to 3 meq of potassium per kilogram of body weight a day administered in divided doses and well diluted in water or juice.
3. The usual adult parenteral dosage, if the serum potassium is greater than 2.5 meq per liter, is an intravenous infusion, up to the equivalent of 200 meq of potassium a day in a concentration less than 40 meq per liter and at a rate usually not exceeding 10 meq per hour. If the serum

potassium is less than 2.0 meq, intravenous infusion up to the equivalent of 400 meq of potassium a day in suitable concentration and at a rate up to, but usually not exceeding, 40 meq per hour.

4. The usual intravenous pediatric dose is up to the equivalent of 3 meq of potassium per kilogram of body weight.

5. To avoid hyperkalemia, the infusion rate must not be rapid; a rate of 20 meq of potassium per hour is considered to be safe as long as urine output is adequate. As a general rule, the rate should never exceed 1 meq per minute for adults, nor 0.02 meq per kilogram of body weight per minute for children.

Adverse Effects

Cardiac arrhythmias, mental confusion, numbness or tingling in hands or feet, shortness of breath, anxiety, fatigue, weakness, diarrhea, stomach pain.

Major Drug Interactions

Caution in the use of potassium preparations with blood from the blood bank (may contain up to 30 meq of potassium per liter of plasma or up to 65 meq per liter of whole blood when stored for more than 10 days), potassium-sparing diuretics, low-salt milk, and potassium-containing medications.

Contraindications

Metabolic acidosis, untreated Addison's disease, cardiac disease, chronic renal insufficiency, dehydration, diarrhea, familial periodic paralysis, gastrointestinal obstruction, hyperkalemia, hypoadrenalism, and oliguria.

Procainamide Hydrochloride

Category

Antiarrhythmic

Brand Name

Pronestyl

Pharmacologic Mechanism

The antiarrhythmic activity is due to depression of cardiac automaticity, excitability, and conductivity which result in a widening of the QRS complex. The P-R and Q-T intervals may be prolonged.

Procainamide exhibits anticholinergic activity and produces cardiac effects that are similar to quinidine.

Uses

Indicated in the treatment of arrhythmias associated with surgery, atrial fibrillation, paroxysmal atrial tachycardia, and premature ventricular contractions and tachycardia.

Doses

1. The suggested pediatric oral dose is 12.5 mg per kilogram of body weight.

2. The usual adult oral dose is a loading dose of 1.25 g, followed by 0.75 g in 1 h. Usual maintenance dose is 0.5 to 1 g every 4 to 6 h.

3. The IM adult dose is 500 mg to 1 g every 4 to 8 h.

4. The IV adult dose is 25 to 50 mg per minute to a maximum of 1 g.

5. The IV infusion for the adult is 500 to 600 mg over 30 min. Usual maintenance rates are 2 to 6 mg per minute.

Nursing Interventions and Administration

1. Injection may be mixed with 5% dextrose.

2. In switching stabilized patients to the oral dose route, allow 3 to 4 h to elapse before administering the first oral dose.

3. Oral doses should be taken on an empty stomach with a full glass of water.

4. Hemodynamic states should be carefully monitored during intravenous infusion.

Adverse Effects

Hypotension, lupus erythematosus-like syndrome, agranulocytosis, angioneurotic edema, maculopapular rash, and a bitter taste.

Drug Interactions

1. Possible additive effects with concurrent anticholinergic and antihypertensive agents.

2. Concurrent use with cholinergic agents may inhibit the effect of these medications on muscle.

3. Effects of neuromuscular blockers may be prolonged when used concurrently with procainamide.

Contraindications

Hypersensitivity, complete AV block, myasthenia gravis, second- and third-degree heart block.

Promethazine Hydrochloride

Category

Antiemetic: antihistamine

Brand Names

Ganphen

Phenergan

Provigan

Pharmacologic Mechanism

Antihistamines antagonize histamine by occupying histamine H_1 receptors on peripheral effector cells. Promethazine also exhibits anticholinergic, antiemetic, antipruritic, and sedative properties.

Uses

Used in the treatment of allergic conditions, motion sickness, nausea, vomiting, pain, and as a sedative.

Doses

1. The usual oral pediatric dose is 125 µg per kilogram of body weight.
2. The usual adult oral dose is 12.5 mg to 25 mg.
3. The usual parenteral (IM or IV) pediatric dose is 125 µg to 500 µg.
4. The usual parenteral (IM or IV) adult dose is 12.5 to 50 mg.

Nursing Interventions and Administration

1. The preferred parenteral route is IM.
2. For IV administration do not exceed a concentration of 25 mg/mL and a rate of 25 mg per minute.
3. Oral dosage should be taken with food or milk to lessen gastric irritation.

Adverse Effects

Drowsiness, dizziness, dry mouth, blurred vision, hypotension, and rare instances of photosensitivity.

Drug Interactions

1. Additive depressant effects with barbiturates and narcotics.
2. Additive anticholinergic effects with tricyclic antidepressants or MAO inhibitors.

Contraindications

Hypersensitivity to promethazine or phenothiazines.

Propranolol Hydrochloride

Category

Antiarrhythmic: beta-adrenergic blocker, antihypertensive

Brand Name

Inderal

Pharmacologic Mechanism

Propranolol blocks the agonist effect of the sympathetic neurotransmitters by competing with receptor binding sites. It possesses moderate membrane stabilizing activity.

Uses

Angina, cardiac arrhythmias, hypertension, vascular headache, pheochromocytoma.

Doses

1. The adult dosage ranges from 10 to 60 mg three to four times daily.
2. See manufacturer's recommendations for individual doses.
3. The parenteral adult IV dose is 1 to 3 mg in life-threatening situations.

Nursing Interventions and Administration

1. Administer tablets before meals.
2. Do not exceed a rate of 1 mg per minute during IV administration.
3. Avoid abrupt withdrawal of medication.

Adverse Effects

Bradycardia, congestive heart failure, intensification of AV block, atrial insufficiency, nausea, vomiting, abdominal cramps, hypoglycemia.

Major Drug Interactions

1. Concurrent use with oral diltiazem or verapamil may result in additive effects, if the drugs are given in high doses.
2. Concurrent use with digitalis glycosides may result in excessive bradycardia with possible heart block.
3. Concurrent use with epinephrine, phenylephrine or phenylpropanolamine may result in significant hypertension and excessive bradycardia with possible heart block.
4. Propranolol may mask certain symptoms of developing hypoglycemia.
5. Concurrent use with isoproterenol may result in mutual inhibition of therapeutic effects.

Contraindications

Bronchial asthma; allergic rhinitis; sinus bradycardia, and greater than first-degree block; cardiogenic shock; right ventricular failure secondary to pulmonary hypertension; congestive heart failure, unless the failure is secondary to a tachyarrhythmia treatable with propranolol; augmenting psychotropic drugs, including monoamine oxidase inhibitors, and during the 2-week withdrawal period.

Protamine

Category

Antidote

Trade Name

Protamine sulfate

Pharmacologic Mechanism

Protamine is a strongly basic substance which combines with the strongly acidic heparin to form a stable complex. Heparin produces its effects indirectly, apparently by forming a complex with and producing a conformational change in the antithrombin III (heparin cofactor) molecule resulting in potentiation of antithrombin III activity.

Protamine has some anticoagulant activity of its own when administered in the absence of heparin, but it is not used as an anticoagulant. This anticoagulant effect may be caused by protamine's antithromboplastin activity which results in inhibition of thrombin generation.

Uses

Antagonist for heparin.

Doses

1. Protamine sulfate: 1 mg given intravenously for every 90 USP units of beef lung heparin sodium or for every 115 USP units of porcine intestinal mucosa heparin to be neutralized, or as determined by blood coagulation test results.
2. Protamine sulfate should be administered slowly over a 1- to 3-min period, not to exceed 50 mg in any 10-min period.
3. Additional doses may be required as indicated by blood coagulation studies.
4. Since protamine has an anticoagulant activity of its own, it is not advisable to administer more than 100 mg of protamine sulfate over a 2-h period unless blood coagulation tests indicate a larger requirement.

Nursing Interventions and Administration

1. Protamine sulfate is administered by intravenous injection only.
2. Care should be taken to assure that the patient's blood volume is adequate prior to receiving protamine.
3. Stated doses are guidelines only. Blood coagulation tests should be used to determine the dosage of protamine.

Adverse Effects

Difficulty in breathing, hypotension, hemorrhage, noncardiogenic pulmonary edema, hives.

Pyridostigmine

Category

Antimyasthenic

Brand Names

Mestinon

Mestinon timespans

Pharmacologic Mechanism

Pyridostigmine inhibits the destruction of acetylcholine by acetylcholinesterase, thereby facilitating transmission of impulses across the myoneural junction. Cholinergic responses produced are miosis, bradycardia, increased tonus of intestinal and skeletal muscle, constriction of bronchi and ureters, and stimulation of secretion by salivary and sweat glands. In addition, these medications have a direct cholinomimetic effect on skeletal muscle.

Pyridostigmine works as an antimyasthenic by increasing muscle strength. Response to repetitive nerve stimulation is increased as a result of this medication enhancing the peak effect and prolonging the duration of action of acetylcholine at the motor end plate.

Since nondepolarizing neuromuscular blocking agents combine reversibly with the receptors, preventing access of acetylcholine, antagonism can be overcome by increasing the amount of agonist at the receptors; therefore, muscle paralysis induced by nondepolarizing neuromuscular blocking agents is reversed by pyridostigmine, which increases concentration of acetylcholine at the receptors.

Uses

Treatment of muscular weakness in myasthenia gravis.

Doses

1. The usual adult oral dosage is 60 to 120 mg every 3 to 4 h, the dosage being adjusted as required. Maintenance dosage is 600 mg per day.
2. Antimyasthenic dosage of 2 mg intravenously or intramuscularly can be given every 2 or 3 h.
3. For antidote to curariform block: intravenous dosages of 10 to 20 mg.
4. Usual pediatric dosage is oral, 7 mg per kilogram of body weight. For parenteral dosages, neonates of myasthenic mothers, 50 to 150 μg per kilogram of body weight every 4 to 6 h.

Nursing Interventions and Administration

1. When used in the treatment of myasthenia gravis, the dosage must be individualized according to the severity of the disease and the response of the patient.
2. Following prolonged therapy, myasthenic patients may become refractory to these medications. Responsiveness may be restored, especially when resistance may have been caused by overdosage, by reducing the dosage or discontinuing the medication for a few days.
3. Patients should be closely observed for cholinergic reactions when pyridostigmine is given.
4. Atropine should be readily available because of the possibility of hypersensitivity reactions.
5. Swallowing ability should be carefully assessed prior to administration of oral doses.

Adverse Effects

Skin rash, blurred vision, diarrhea, bradycardia, confusion, seizures, unusual irritability, frequent urination, increased bronchial secretions, small pupils.

Major Drug Interactions

Neuromuscular blocking action of anesthetics, antiarrhythmic agents, and some antibiotics (aminoglycosides, lincomycin) may antagonize the effect of antimyasthenics on skeletal muscle.

Contraindications

Mechanical intestinal or urinary tract obstruction, urinary tract infections, and in postsurgical patients in which the antimyasthenic agent may exacerbate respiratory problems.

Pyrimethamine

Category

Antimalarial: antitoxoplasmic agent

Brand Name

Daraprim

Pharmacologic Mechanism

Antimalarial activity is due to folic acid antagonism.

Uses

1. Chemoprophylaxis of susceptible strains of malaria (plasmodia).
2. In combination with quinine and sulfonamide (sulfadiazine or sulfisoxazole) for treating chloroquine-resistant strains of malaria *(Plasmodium falciparum).*
3. In combination with a sulfonamide (sulfadiazine or triple sulfa) for treating toxoplasmosis *(Toxoplasma gondii).*

Doses

1. The usual pediatric oral dose is 0.3 mg/kg.
2. The usual adult oral dose is 25 mg.
3. Consult manufacturer for additional recommendations.

Nursing Interventions and Administration

Administration with meals will help reduce gastric upset.

Adverse Effects

Anorexia, vomiting, megaloblastic anemia, leukopenia, thrombocytopenia, pancytopenia, and atrophic glossitis.

Drug Interactions

Folic acid and *p*-aminobenzoic acid can inhibit the activity of pyrimethamine.

Contraindications

Hypersensitivity, severe megaloblastic anemia.

Quinidine

Category

Antiarrhythmic

Brand Names

Duraquin

Quinaglute Dura-tabs

Pharmacologic Mechanism

Quinidine has both direct and indirect (antimuscarinic) effects on cardiac tissue. Automaticity, conduction velocity, and membrane responsiveness are decreased, possibly because of quinidine inhibition of potassium ion transmembranal movement. The effective refractory period is prolonged. The antimuscarinic action reduces vagal tone. An alpha-adrenergic blocking action often produces increased beta-adrenergic effects such as peripheral vasodilation. Quinidine is a type I antiarrhythmic.

Uses

Cardiac arrhythmias, particularly atrial fibrillation, atrial flutter, paroxysmal atrial fibrillation, paroxysmal atrial tachycardia, and premature contractions.

Doses

1. The usual adult oral maintenance dose is 324 to 660 mg every 6 to 12 h as needed (extended-release tablets).
2. With quinidine sulfate tablets, the usual oral dose for adults is 200 to 300 mg every 2 to 3 h up to five times a day as needed.
3. Parenteral doses of 600 mg intramuscularly initially, then 400 mg repeated as often as every 2 h if necessary is recommended for adults.
4. Intravenous infusions of 800 mg in 40 mL of 5% dextrose injection administered at a rate of 1 mL per minute. When using quinidine sulfate, 600 mg in 40 mL of 5% dextrose at a rate of 1 mL per minute is recommended.

Nursing Interventions and Administration

1. Intravenous infusion should be done in monitored settings only.
2. When doses exceeding 2 g daily are used, determination of serum quinidine concentrations and continuous ECG monitoring are indicated.
3. Higher serum quinidine concentrations are usually required to correct atrial arrhythmias than those required for ventricular arrhythmias.
4. Oral dosage forms are preferably taken with a full glass of water on an empty stomach 1 h before or 2 h after meals for better absorption.

Adverse Effects

Blurred vision, dizziness, headache, ringing or buzzing in ears, fainting, fever, skin rash, hives, wheezing, unusual bleeding, mental confusion, weakness, nausea, vomiting, diarrhea, widening of QRS complex.

Major Drug Interactions

1. Concurrent use with other antiarrhythmics, antimuscarinics, phenothiazines, or reserpine can result in additive cardiac effects.
2. Concurrent use with anticoagulants may result in additive hypoprothrombinemia.
3. Concurrent use with digitalis glycosides is reported to have resulted in increased serum concentrations of digoxin.
4. Concurrent use with barbiturates, phenytoin, or rifampin may result in decreased serum quinidine concentrations.

Contraindications

Digitalis toxicity with AV conduction disorder, heart block, intraventricular conduction defects, myasthenia gravis, hepatic or renal function impairment, thrombocytopenia, or digitalis toxicity with AV conduction disorder.

Therapeutic Drug Levels

3 to 6 μg per mL. Toxic effects generally occur when levels are $\geq$8 μg per mL.

Ranitidine

Category

Histamine H_2 receptor antagonist, antiulcer agent, gastric acid secretion inhibitor

Brand Name

Zantac

Pharmacologic Mechanism

Inhibition of basal and nocturnal gastric acid secretion by competitive inhibition of the action of histamine at the histamine H_2 receptors of the parietal cells; also inhibits gastric acid secretion stimulated by food, betazole, pentagastrin, insulin, and physiological vagal reflex.

Uses

Control of excess gastric acid secretion.

Doses

1. The usual oral adult dose for an active ulcer is 150 mg two times a day.
2. For prophylaxis of recurrent duodenal ulcer, 150 mg at bedtime.
3. Doses of 150 mg two times a day can be used for pathological hypersecretory conditions.
4. Pediatric dosages have not been established.
5. 50 mg can be given IM or IV every 6 to 8 h.

Nursing Interventions and Administration

1. Antacids can be given to control pain, but should be separated from ranitidine administration by at least 1 h.
2. The efficacy of ranitidine may be decreased in patients who smoke cigarettes.

Adverse Effects

Constipation, dizziness, nausea, skin rash.

Major Drug Interactions

Use with metopolol, theophylline, or warfarin may result in delayed elimination and increased blood concentration of ranitidine.

Contraindications

Hepatic or renal insufficiency.

Rh$_0$ (D) Immune Human Globulin

Category

Immunosuppressant biological

Brand Names

D-Immune

Gammulin Rh

HypRh$_0$-D

RhoGAM

Pharmacologic Mechanism

Suppresses the immune response of nonsensitized Rh$_0$ (D)-negative, D^u-negative individuals who receive Rh$_0$ (D)-positive or D^u-positive blood as a result of fetomaternal hemorrhage or a transfusion accident.

Uses and Doses

Used to suppress antibody formation in:

1. Rh_0 (D)-negative, D^u-negative mothers after delivering an Rh_0 (D)-positive or D^u-positive infant.
2. Abortion of an Rh-positive fetus.
3. Transfusion accident where Rh_0 (D)-positive blood is used in a Rh_0 (D)-negative recipient.

Parenteral Administration

The total contents of a single-dose vial are injected intramuscularly in nonsensitized individuals within 72 h or less after Rh-incompatible delivery, terminated incomplete pregnancies, or blood transfusions.

Nursing Interventions and Administration

Fill out the special patient's form that is provided in the dosage package and attach to patient's hospital records after administering IM injection.

Adverse Effects

Limited allergic reactions.

Contraindications

In Rh_0 (D)-positive or D^u-positive individuals, and in Rh_0 (D)-negative and D^u-negative individuals who have been previously sensitized to Rh_0 (D)- or D^u antigen (if in doubt, the preparation may be given).

Rifampin

Category

Antitubercular: rifamycin antibiotic

Brand Names

Rifadin

Rimactane

Pharmacologic Mechanism

Bacteriostatic activity due to inhibition of DNA-dependent RNA polymerase activity in susceptible microorganisms.

Uses

Treatment of tuberculosis, meningitis prophylaxis.

Doses

1. The usual pediatric dose is 10 to 20 mg/kg. Do not exceed 600 mg daily.
2. The usual adult dose is 600 mg daily.

Nursing Interventions and Administration

Rifampin is usually administered as a single daily dose on a empty stomach with a full glass of water.

Adverse Effects

Anorexia, nausea, cramps, diarrhea, rash, pemphigus, sore mouth and tongue, exudative conjunctivitis, thrombocytopenia, hemolytic anemia, drowsiness, visual disturbances, and menstrual disturbances.

Drug Interactions

1. Concurrent use may require dosage adjustment for corticosteroids, dapsone, digitalis glycosides, methadone maintenance, oral anticoagulants, and oral hypoglycemics.
2. Oral contraceptives may lose significant activity during rifampin therapy.
3. Concurrent use with alcohol or isoniazid may result in increased incidence of rifampin-induced hepatotoxicity.
4. Concurrent use with methadone may decrease the effects of this medication.

Contraindications

Hypersensitivity.

Sodium Bicarbonate

Category

Alkalizer, antacid, electrolyte replenisher

Trade Names

Effervescent sodium bicarbonate
Sodium bicarbonate for oral solution
Sodium bicarbonate tablets
Sodium bicarbonate injection

Pharmacologic Mechanism

Sodium bicarbonate increases the plasma bicarbonate, buffers excess hydrogen ion concentration, and raises blood pH, thereby reversing the clinical manifestations of acidosis. It also increases the excretion of free bicarbonate ions in the urine, causing a rise in the urinary pH. By maintaining an alkaline urine, the actual dissolution of uric stones may be accomplished. Sodium bicarbonate produces an antacid effect by reacting chemically to neutralize or buffer existing quantities of stomach acid but has no direct effect on its output. This action results in an increased pH value of stomach contents.

Uses

Sodium bicarbonate is indicated in the treatment of metabolic acidosis, for prophylaxis in renal lithiasis due to gout, and renal lithiasis in sulfonamide therapy, prophylaxis in nephrotoxicity, and treatment of hyperacidity, severe diarrhea, and drug poisoning. Parenteral forms are used for the treatment of sickle-cell anemia.

Doses

1. Oral dosage for adults is 3.9 to 10 g in a glass of cold water after meals.
2. The parenteral form for cardiac arrest is intravenous; initially 1 meq per kilogram of body weight; 0.5 meq per kilogram of body weight may be repeated every 10 min of continued arrest.
3. In less urgent forms of metabolic acidosis, intravenous infusions of 2 to 5 meq per kilogram of body weight are administered over a period of 4 to 8 h.
4. As a urinary alkalizer, intravenous doses of 2 to 5 meq per kilogram of body weight are administered over a period of 4 to 8 h.
5. Pediatric doses for cardiac arrest are intravenous; 1 meq per kilogram of body weight initially, then 0.5 meq per kilogram of body weight every 10 min of continued arrest.

Nursing Interventions and Administration

1. Prolonged use of sodium bicarbonate therapy is not recommended because of the high risk of metabolic alkalosis or sodium overload.
2. As a treatment for peptic ulcer disease, sodium bicarbonate may be administered 1 to 3 h after meals and at bedtime. Additional doses of ant-

acids may be administered to relieve the pain which may occur between the regularly scheduled doses.
3. Bicarbonate therapy should always be planned in a careful, controlled way, since the degree of response to a given dose is not precisely predictable. Ideally, it should be given according to the results of measurement of arterial blood pH, carbon dioxide content of the plasma, and calculation of base deficit.
4. Rapid administration may produce severe alkalosis which may be accompanied by hyperirritability or tetany.
5. Adequate alveolar ventilation must be ensured following sodium bicarbonate administration during cardiac arrest to allow for the continued excretion of the carbon dioxide released. This is important for the control of arterial pH.

Adverse Effects

Irregular heartbeat, muscle cramps, weakness, hypokalemia, swelling of feet or lower legs, mood or mental changes, nervousness, bradypnea, headache.

Major Drug Interactions

Absorption of oral tetracyclines may be decreased when used concurrently with sodium bicarbonate because of increase in intragastric pH; patients should be advised not to take sodium bicarbonate within 1 to 3 h of tetracycline.

Contraindications

1. Metabolic or respiratory alkalosis.
2. Chloride loss due to vomiting or continuous gastrointestinal suction.
3. Hypoglycemia.

Streptokinase

Category

Thrombolytic

Brand Names

Kabikinase

Streptase

Pharmacologic Mechanism

Streptokinase indirectly promotes plasmin formation by combining with plasminogen to form a streptokinase–plasminogen complex which is eventually converted to a streptokinase–plasmin complex. Both are activator complexes which convert residual plasminogen to plasmin. Streptokinase is antigenic and induces the formation of antibodies. The antibodies cause resistance to subsequent streptokinase therapy which may persist for 3 to 6 months or longer, following an initial course of treatment.

Uses

Treatment of acute pulmonary embolism, deep-vein thrombosis, acute arterial thrombosis, acute coronary arterial thrombosis.

Doses

1. For adults, intravenous: 250,000 IU as an initial loading dose over 30 min, followed by 100,000 IU per hour, as a continuous infusion.
2. For coronary artery thrombosis, intraarterial: via a coronary artery catheter, 20,000 IU initially, followed by 2000 IU per minute.

Nursing Interventions and Administration

1. Thrombolytic therapy should be instituted as soon as possible following the onset of clinical symptoms because resistance to lysis increases with the age of the thrombus.
2. Thrombolytic agents should be administered via a constant infusion pump. Other medications should be administered through a separate line.
3. During therapy, the patient should be kept on strict bed rest. Invasive procedures should be avoided unless essential. Intramuscular injections should be avoided.
4. Therapy should be discontinued immediately if bleeding is not controlled by local pressure application.
5. Anticoagulation with heparin (preferably by continuous intravenous infusion) followed, if necessary, by a coumarin derivative, is recommended following thrombolytic therapy to prevent recurrence.
6. An antiarrhythmic agent such as lidocaine or procainamide may be administered prior to or concurrently with the thrombolytic agent to prevent reperfusion arrhythmias.

Adverse Effects

Abdominal pain, swelling, back pain, bleeding (urine or feces), nosebleeds, muscle pain or stiffness, constipation, dizziness, fever, headache, wheezing.

Major Drug Interactions

1. Aminocaproic or other antifibrinolytic agents inhibit the action of thrombolytic agents.
2. Concurrent use of anticoagulants with thrombolytic agents increases the risk of hemorrhage. However, low doses of heparin may be given concurrently with low doses of thrombolytic agents administered intraarterially.
3. Concurrent use with aspirin or other nonsteroidal antiinflammatory agents can cause an increased risk of severe hemorrhage, since these medications inhibit platelet aggregation.
4. Azlocillin, carbenicillin, cefoperazone, mezlocillin, moxalactam, piperacillin, plicamycin, and ticarcillin may increase the risk of hemorrhage.
5. Dextrans, dipyridamole inhibit platelet aggregation and concurrent use with streptokinase may increase the risk of hemorrhage.

Contraindications

Active bleeding, brain tumor, cardiovascular accident, intracranial or intraspinal surgery within the last 2 months, recent thoracic surgery.

Succinylcholine

Category

Neuromuscular blocker

Brand Name

Anectine

Pharmacologic Mechanism

Neuromuscular blocking agents produce skeletal muscle paralysis by blocking neural transmission at the myoneural junction. The paralysis is selective initially and usually appears in the levator muscles of the eyelids, muscles of mastication, limb muscles, abdominal muscles, muscles of the glottis, and the intercostal muscles and diaphragm. Neuromuscular blocking agents have no known effect on consciousness or pain threshold.

Depolarizing neuromuscular blocking agents (succinylcholine) compete with acetylcholine for the cholinergic receptors of the motor end plate and combine with these receptors to produce depolarization; however, because of their high affinity for the cholinergic receptors and their resistance to anticholinesterase. They produce a more prolonged depolarization than does acetylcholine. This results initially in transient muscle contractions usually visible as fasciculations, followed by inhibition of neuromuscular transmission. This type of neuromuscular block is not antagonized, and may even be enhanced by anticholinesterase agents.

Doses and Uses

The usual adult dosage for short surgical procedures is 600 μg/kg to 1.1 mg per kilogram of body weight intravenously. Repeated doses may be administered if necessary. Because of the threat of prolonged apnea, fractional intravenous dosages are not recommended. Generally, a constant infusion is more suitable.

Succinylcholine can also be used for prolonged surgical procedures and prior to electroshock therapy.

Nursing Interventions and Administration

1. Since succinylcholine has no effect on pain threshold and consciousness, it is important to use adjunctive therapy when administering this drug.
2. With the threat of apnea, this drug should only be used when the individual's airway can be protected.
3. Intermittent dosages are avoided because of increased risk of breathing difficulties.

Adverse Effects

Postoperative muscular pain and stiffness, increase in intraocular pressure, irregular heartbeat, tachycardia, bradycardia.

Major Drug Interactions

1. Concurrent use with aminoglycoside antibiotics, clindamycin, lincomycin, or polymyxin antibiotics may enhance the blockage of neuromuscular blocking agents, resulting in prolonged respiratory depression or apnea.
2. Use with antimalarial medications, cholinesterase inhibitors, cyclophosphamide, or phenelzine may decrease plasma levels of pseudocholinesterase, the enzyme that metabolizes succinylcholine, thereby enhancing the neuromuscular blockade of succinylcholine and possibly resulting in prolonged respiratory depression or apnea.
3. Exposure of patients to neurotoxic insecticides may decrease plasma concentrations of pseudocholinesterase, thereby enhancing the neuromuscular blockade of succinylcholine and possibly resulting in prolonged respiratory depression or apnea.
4. Concurrent use with quinidine or quinine may enhance the blockade of neuromuscular blocking agents, resulting in prolonged or intensified respiratory depression or apnea.

Contraindications

Severe trauma such as burns, digitalis toxicity, bronchogenic carcinoma, impairment in cardiovascular functioning, conditions in which histamine release would be hazardous, severe anemia, dehydration, exposure to neurotoxic insecticides, malnutrition, pregnancy, eye injury, glaucoma, ocular surgery, fractures, muscle spasm, hepatic function impairment, hyperkalemia, hyperthermia, hypothermia, myasthenia gravis, respiratory depression, impairment in renal function.

Sulfamethoxazole-Trimethoprim

Category

Antibacterial combination preparation

Brand Names

Bactrim

Septra

Pharmacologic Mechanism

Bacteriostatic activity due to the inhibition of folic acid synthesis. Sulfamethoxazole is a competitive antagonist of *p*-aminobenzoic acid, while trimethoprim inhibits the enzyme dihydrofolate reductase. Consequently, two successive steps in the biosynthesis of folic acid are blocked, resulting in enhanced antimicrobial activity in susceptible organisms.

Uses

1. Indicated in the treatment of urinary tract infections caused by susceptible strains of *Enterobacter* spp., *Escherichia coli, Klebsiella* spp., *Proteus mirabilis, Proteus morganii,* and *Proteus vulgaris.*
2. Alternative for treating otitis media caused by susceptible strains of *Hemophilus influenzae* or *Streptococcus pneumoniae.*
3. Treatment of shigellosis caused by susceptible strains of *Shigella flexneri* and *Shigella sonnei.*
4. Treatment of *Pneumocystis carinii* pneumonitis.

Doses

1. The usual adult oral dose is 800 mg of sulfamethoxazole and 160 mg of trimethoprim every 12 h.
2. The usual pediatric oral dose is 20 mg of sulfamethoxazole and 4 mg of trimethoprim per kilogram of body weight.
3. The usual intravenous adult dose is 10 to 12.5 mg/kg of sulfamethoxazole and 2 to 2.5 mg trimethoprim per kilogram of body weight.
4. Dosage must be reduced for patients with renal impairment. Use one-half the dosage schedule for patients with a creatinine clearance of 15 to 30 mg per kilogram of body weight. Do not use if below 15.

Nursing Interventions and Administration

1. Administer with large volumes of water to keep the patient well hydrated. Oral dosage should be given with a full glass of water.
2. For parenteral doses, dilute each ampule in 75 to 125 mg of 5% dextrose.

Adverse Effects

Agranulocytosis, aplastic anemia, megaloblastic anemia, hypoprothrombinemia, erythema multiforme, Stevens-Johnson syndrome, epidermal necrolysis, exfoliative dermatitis, photosensitization, hepatitis, pancreatitis, peripheral neuritis, tinnitus, toxic nephrosis, and lupus erythematosus phenomenon.

Major Drug Interactions

1. Concurrent use with PABA may cause antagonism of the bacteriostatic effects of the sulfonamides.
2. Anticoagulants, hypoglycemics, methotrexate, phenytoin, or thiopental may be displaced from protein-binding sites and/or metabolism may be inhibited by sulfonamides.
3. Concurrent use with penicillins is not recommended, since its bactericidal effects may be interfered with.

Contraindications

Hypersensitivity or severe kidney impairment.

Thiopental Sodium for Injection

Category

Ultrashort-acting barbiturate

Brand Name

Pentothal

Pharmacologic Mechanism

Barbiturates are central nervous system depressants that act primarily on the brainstem reticular formation to produce dose-related sedative and hypnotic effects. Ultrashort-acting barbiturates are used to produce surgical anesthesia.

Uses

Anesthetic agents for short surgical procedures, anesthesia induction, supplement for regional anesthesia, hypnosis during balanced anesthesia, convulsion control, narcoanalysis and narcosynthesis, and for neurosurgical patients with increased intracranial pressure.

Doses

1. Doses must be individualized.
2. A general guideline for doses is 50 to 100 mg intravenously.

Nursing Interventions and Administration

Reconstitute powder with 5% dextrose, sodium chloride injection, or sterile water for injection. Discard unused solution after 24 h.

Adverse Effects

Respiratory depression, cardiac arrhythmias, bronchospasm, and laryngospasm.

Drug Interactions

Concurrent use with phenothiazines may enhance the effect of thiopental.

Contraindications

Hypersensitivity, status asthmaticus, and porphyria.

Trimethaphan

Category

Antihypertensive

Brand Name

Arfonad

Pharmacologic Mechanism

Trimethaphan is a ganglionic blocker which prevents the stimulation of postsynaptic receptors by acetylcholine released from presynaptic nerve endings. In addition, trimethaphan also causes direct peripheral vasodilation and release of histamine. Its hypotensive effect is due to reduction in sympathetic tone and vasodilation, and is primarily postural. Cardiac output may increase in patients with cardiac failure or decrease in patients with normal cardiac function.

Uses

Controlled hypotension during surgery, treatment of hypertension.

Doses

1. The usual adult doses for controlled hypotension during surgery is 3 to 4 mg per minute intravenously.
2. For hypertensive emergencies, the intravenous dosage of 500 μg to 1 mg per minute is recommended. The dose is adjusted according to response.
3. The usual pediatric dosage is 100 μg per minute intravenously.

Nursing Interventions and Administration

1. Cardiovascular response to this drug should be continuously monitored.
2. Trimethaphan should be diluted by adding one ampule to 500 mL of 5% dextrose injection to make a concentration of 1 mg/mL.
3. A constant infusion pump should be used to safely administer this drug.
4. Careful elevation of the patient's head of the bed can improve the action of the drug.
5. This drug should not be mixed with other medications.
6. Pseudotolerance to the effects of trimethaphan occurs in some patients.

Adverse Effects

Pupillary dilatation, anorexia, nausea, vomiting, constipation, dry mouth, itching, orthostatic hypotension, angina, tachycardia, urinary retention.

Major Drug Interactions

1. Concurrent use with anesthetic agents, the antihypertensive medications, or diuretics may result in enhanced hypotension.
2. Individual dosage adjustment is important.

Contraindications

Addison's disease, anemia, asphyxia, hypovolemia, shock, cardiovascular insufficiency, cerebrovascular insufficiency, recent myocardial infarction, diabetes mellitus, renal function impairment, respiratory insufficiency, and patients receiving steroids.

Tubocurarine

Category

Nondepolarizing neuromuscular blocker

Brand Name

Tubarine

Pharmacologic Mechanism

Neuromuscular blocking agents produce skeletal muscle paralysis by blocking neural transmission at the myoneural junction. The paralysis is selective initially and usually appears in the levator muscles of eyelids, muscles of mastication, limb muscles, abdominal muscles, muscles of the glottis, and the intercostal muscles and diaphragm. Neuromuscular blocking agents have no known effect on consciousness or pain threshold.

Depolarizing neuromuscular blocking agents (succinylcholine) compete with acetylcholine for the cholinergic receptors of the motor end plate and combine with these receptors to produce depolarization; however, because of their high affinity for the cholinergic receptors and their resistance to anticholinesterase, they produce a more prolonged depolarization than does acetylcholine. This results initially in transient muscle contractions, usually visible as fasciculations, followed by inhibition of neuromuscular transmission. This type of neuromuscular block is not antagonized, and may even be enhanced by anticholinesterase agents.

Doses

1. As an adjunct to surgical anesthesia: intramuscular or intravenous, 6 to 9 mg initially, then 3 to 4.5 mg in 3 to 5 min if necessary.
2. As an aid to controlled respiration: intravenous, initially 16.5 μg per kilogram of body weight, the subsequent doses being adjusted as needed.
3. Usual pediatric dose is 500 μg per kilogram of body weight. For neonates, see current literature.

Nursing Interventions and Administration

1. Since succinylcholine has no effect on pain threshold and consciousness, it is important to use adjunctive therapy when administering this drug.
2. With the threat of apnea, this drug should only be used when the individual's airway can be protected.
3. Intermittent dosages are avoided because of increased risk of breathing difficulties.
4. Usually administered intravenously as a sustained injection over a period of 1 to 1.5 min.
5. Can be given intramuscularly, but is slowly and irregularly absorbed.

Adverse Effects

Hypotension.

Major Drug Interactions

1. Concurrent use with aminoglycoside antibiotics, clindamycin, lincomycin, or polymyxin antibiotics may enhance the blockade of neuromuscular blocking agents, resulting in prolonged respiratory depression or apnea.
2. Use with antimalarial medications, cyclophosphamide, or phenelzine may decrease plasma levels of pseudocholinesterase, the enzyme that metabolizes succinylcholine, thereby enhancing the neuromuscular blockade of succinylcholine and possibly resulting in prolonged respiratory depression or apnea.
3. Concurrent use with quinidine or quinine may enhance the blockade of neuromuscular blocking agents, resulting in prolonged or intensified respiratory depression or apnea.
4. Concurrent use with beta-adrenergic blocking agents may enhance the blockade of tuborcurare.

Contraindications

Severe trauma such as burns, digitalis toxicity, bronchogenic carcinoma, impairment in cardiovascular functioning, conditions in which histamine release would be hazardous, severe anemia, dehydration, exposure to neurotoxic insecticides, malnutrition, pregnancy, eye injury, glaucoma, ocular surgery, fractures, muscle spasm, hepatic function impairment, hyperkalemia, hyperthermia, hypothermia, myasthenia gravis, respiratory depression, impairment in renal function.

Vasopressin

Category

Posterior pituitary hormone: antidiuretic

Brand Name

Pitressin tannate

Pharmacologic Mechanism

Antidiuretic activity due to an increase in water reabsorption in the nephrons of the kidneys.

Uses

Indicated for the treatment of polydipsia, polyuria, and dehydration due to neurohypophyseal diabetes.

Doses

1. Dosage must be individualized according to the patient's response.
2. Aqueous Pitressin is given in 5 to 10 U two to three times a day (IM, SC).
3. Pitressin in oil is given as 1.25 to 2.5 U every day (IM).

Nursing Interventions and Administration

Shake vial to produce a homogeneous suspension before using.

Adverse Effects

Tremor, sweating, vertigo, circumoral pallor, headache, abdominal gas and cramps, nausea, vomiting, bronchial constriction, and cardiac arrest.

Drug Interactions

1. Use with caution in patients receiving lithium carbonate, epinephrine, or heparin.
2. Concurrent use with chlorpropamide may enhance the antidiuretic effect.

Contraindications

Hypersensitivity, coronary artery disease, nephritis.

Verapamil

Category

Calcium channel blocking agent

Brand Names

Calan

Isoptin

Pharmacologic Mechanism

Verapamil is thought to inhibit calcium ion transport through select voltage-sensitive areas termed "slow channels" across cardiac and vascular smooth muscle cell membranes. By reducing intracellular calcium concentration, verapamil dilates coronary arteries and peripheral arteries and arterioles, and may reduce heart rate, decrease myocardial contractility, and slow atrioventricular nodal conduction. Serum calcium concentrations are unchanged.

Verapamil depresses sinoatrial (SA) and AV nodal conduction, with little effect on heart rate. Its major action is through a reduction in afterload.

Verapamil acts as an antianginal agent through direct dilatation of coronary arteries and arterioles which improves oxygen supply to myocardial tissues. In addition, dilation of the peripheral vasculature reduces systemic pressure (cardiac afterload) which results in lessened stress and reduced oxygen requirements of the myocardial tissues. Antiarrhythmic effects occur because of the inhibited influx of calcium ions in cardiac tissues which results in slowed electrophysiological activity through the SA and the AV nodes without affecting accessory bypass conduction or altering normal atrial action potential or intraventricular conduction. Reduction of peripheral vascular resistance as a result of vasodilation produces the antihypertensive effect.

Uses

Antianginal, antiarrhythmic.

Doses

1. As an antianginal or antihypertensive, oral administration is initially 80 mg three or four times a day, with the dosage being increased at daily or weekly intervals as needed and tolerated.
2. The total daily doses usually range from 240 to 480 mg.
3. Parenteral dosage: intravenous, initially 5 to 10 mg (or 75 to 150 μg) per kilogram of body weight, administered slowly over a 2-min period. If response is not adequate, 10 mg or 150 μg

per kilogram of body weight can be administered 30 min after completion of initial dose.

4. In geriatric patients, the intravenous dose should be administered slowly over a 3-min period to minimize undesired effects.

Nursing Interventions and Administration

1. The parenteral form is used only in emergencies.
2. Oral doses are preferably administered on an empty stomach, 1 h before or 2 h after meals, to provide more rapid and predictable absorption.
3. If intravenous administration of verapamil and beta-adrenergic blocking agents is required, administration should be separated by a few hours, since both medications may have additive depressant effects on myocardial contractility or AV conduction.

Adverse Effects

Prolonged PR interval; breathing difficulty; irregular or unusually fast, pounding heartbeat; peripheral edema; constipation; dizziness; headache; nausea; unusual tiredness.

Pulmonary edema, sinus bradycardia, severe hypotension, second-degree AV block, and sudden death can occur with intravenous infusion.

Major Drug Interactions

1. An additive effect may occur if given with beta-adrenergic blocking agents. This additive effect may prolong AV conduction which may lead to severe hypotension, bradycardia, and cardiac failure. This is especially true in patients with impaired ventricular function or abnormal cardiac conduction.
2. Concurrent use with nifedipine may produce excessive hypotension and in rare cases may increase the possibility of congestive heart failure.
3. Concurrent use with digoxin has been reported to increase the serum concentration of digoxin.
4. Concurrent use with disopyramide is discouraged. Administration of disopyramide within 48 h before or 24 h following verapamil administration should be avoided because both medications possess negative inotropic properties.

Contraindications

Verapamil should not be used for patients with cardiogenic shock, congestive heart failure (unless secondary to supraventricular tachycardia responsive to verapamil), second- or third-degree heart block, severe hypotension, and sick sinus syndrome, except in patients with functioning artificial ventricular pacemakers.

Warfarin Sodium

Category

Anticoagulant

Brand Names

Coumadin

Panwarfin

Pharmacologic Mechanism

Warfarin prevents the formation of active precoagulation factors II, VII, IX, and X in the liver by inhibiting the vitamin K-mediated gamma-carboxylation of precursor proteins. All therapeutic action is delayed until circulating coagulation factors are removed by normal catabolism. This agent has no direct thrombolytic effect, although it may limit extension of existing thrombi.

Uses

1. Adjunct in coronary occlusion.
2. Atrial fibrillation with embolization.
3. Prophylaxis and treatment of pulmonary thrombosis and venous thrombosis.

Doses

1. The usual adult dose is 10 to 15 mg on the first day. Prothrombin time should determine the maintenance dose, which is usually 2 to 10 mg daily.
2. Doses are very individualized.

Nursing Interventions and Administration

1. Maintenance dose is usually administered as a single daily dose.
2. Therapy should be discontinued slowly.

Adverse Effects

Hemorrhage, nausea, vomiting, diarrhea, hepatitis, jaundice, urticaria, alopecia, granulocytosis, leukopenia, and anemia.

Drug Interactions

1. Drugs which can increase anticoagulant activity include anabolic steroids, broad-spectrum antibiotics, clofibrate, dextrothyroxine, disulfiram, oxyphenbutazone, phenylbutazone, and thyroid preparations.
2. Drugs which can cause significant decreases in anticoagulant activity include barbiturates, cholestyramine, estrogens, oral contraceptives, and glutethimide.

Contraindication

Hypersesitivity to coumarin anticoagulants, subacute bacterial endocarditis, continuous bleeding.
See dicumarol.

Bibliography

American Hospital Formulary Service. (1987). *Drug Information,* Bethesda: American Society of Hospital Pharmacists.

Gilman, A. G., Goodman, L. S., & Gilman, A. (1980). *Goodman and Gilman's Pharmacological Basis of Therapeutics.* New York: Macmillan.

United States Pharmacopeia Convention. (1987). *USP-Drug Information,* Volumes I and II.

Physicians' Desk Reference. (1986). Oradell, N.J.: Medical Economics Co., manufacturer's inserts.

Table of Antibiotics

Because of the large number of available antibiotics, they are presented according to major groups in the following chart for ease in referencing.

Antibiotics

	Penicillin G-Potassium Group	Ampicillin Group	Penicillinase-Resistant Group
Brand Names	Wycillin Bicillin LA	Polycillin Amoxil Cyclapen Spectrobid Amoxil	Staphicillin, Prostaphlin, Uni-pen, Tegopen, Dynapen
Pharmacologic Mechanism	The penicillin-G group is bactericidal. Its action depends on its ability to reach and bind penicillin-binding proteins located in bacterial cytoplasmic membranes; it inhibits bacterial septum and cell wall synthesis. Cell division and growth are inhibited and lysis and elongation of susceptible bacteria occur.	See PENICILLIN-G GROUP.	See PENICILLIN-G GROUP.
Uses	Generally recommended for infections caused by many gram-positive organisms. See manufacturers' inserts for specific details.	Generally recommended for infections caused by many gram-negative organisms. See manufacturers' inserts for specific details.	Generally recommended for infections caused by penicillinase-producing staphylococcus. See manufacturers' inserts for specific details.
Doses	1. The usual adult oral dose is 200,000 to 500,000 units every 6 to 8 h. 2. The usual pediatric oral dose is 25,000 to 90,000 units per kg per day in three to six doses. 3. The adult intramuscular and intravenous dose is 1 million to 5 million units in divided doses. 4. The pediatric intramuscular and intravenous dose is 50,000 to 250,000 units/kg daily divided among six doses.	1. The usual adult oral, intramuscular and intravenous dose is 250 to 500 mg every 6 h. 2. The usual pediatric oral and intravenous dose is 50 to 100 mg/kg per day in four doses. 3. The pediatric intramuscular dose is 100 to 200 mg/kg per day in four doses.	1. The usual oral, intramuscular or intravenous adult dose is 0.25 to 1 g every 4 to 6 h. 2. The usual oral, intramuscular or intravenous pediatric dose is 25 to 100 mg/kg per day individual doses.
Nursing Interventions and Administration	1. Each oral dosage should be taken with a full glass of water. 2. Dosages should be evenly spaced throughout the day. 3. Intravenous infusions should be slow. 4. Severe infections are best treated with intravenous infusions. 5. Intramuscular injections should be into large muscle mass.	See PENICILLIN-G.	See PENICILLIN-G.

(Continued)

Antibiotics Continued

	Penicillin G-Potassium Group	Ampicillin Group	Penicillinase-Resistant Group
Adverse Effects	Urticaria, fever, edema, laryngeal edema, anaphylaxis, maculopapular rash, exfoliative dermatitis, hemolytic anemia, leukopenia, thrombocytopenia.	See PENICILLIN-G.	See PENICILLIN-G.
Drug Interactions	1. Concurrent administration of probenicid prolongs the activity of the penicillin Gs.	1. Concurrent use with oral contraceptives may decrease the effectiveness of the oral contraceptive.	1. Concurrent use with anticoagulants may cause hemorrhage.
Contraindications	History of bleeding disorders, gastrointestinal disease, infectious mononucleosis.	See PENICILLIN-G.	See PENICILLIN-G.

Antibiotics

	First-Generation Cephalosporins	Second-Generation Cephalosporins	Third-Generation Cephalosporins
Brand Names	Keflin, Keflex Velosef Cefadyl Ancef Kefzol Duricef	Mandol Mefoxin Zinacef Monocid Precef Ceclor	Claforan Moxam Cefobid Cefizox Rocephin Fortaz
Pharmacologic Mechanism	The cephalosporins are bactericidal. They inhibit bacterial septum and cell wall synthesis, probably by acylation of membrane-bound transpeptidase enzymes. Cell division and growth are inhibited and lysis and elongation of susceptible bacteria frequently occur. Rapidly dividing bacteria are those most susceptible to the action of cephalosporins.	See FIRST-GENERATION CEPHALOSPORINS.	See FIRST-GENERATION CEPHALOSPORINS.
Uses	The first-generation cephalosporins are effective against gram-positive cocci and some gram-negative rods.	In addition to those listed for first-generation, the second-generation cephalosporins are also effective against *Enterobacter, H. influenzae, N. gonorrhea, Salmonella,* and *Shigella.*	Some of the third-generation cephalosporins have enhanced CSF penetration and may also be effective against *Pseudomonas, Serratia,* and *Proteus.*
Doses	1. See manufacturer's insert for specific recommendations. 2. The usual adult oral dose is 1 to 4 g daily.	1. See manufacturer's insert for specific recommendations. 2. See FIRST-GENERATION CEPHALOSPORINS.	1. See manufacturer's insert for specific recommendations. 2. The usual adult intramuscular intravenous dose is 1

Antibiotics Continued

	First-Generation Cephalosporins	Second-Generation Cephalosporins	Third-Generation Cephalosporins
	3. The usual pediatric oral dose is 25 to 50 mg/kg per day in four doses. 4. The usual adult intravenous dosage is 1 g every 3 to 6 h.	3. The usual pediatric oral dose is 20–40 mg/kg per day. 4. The usual adult intramuscular or intravenous dose is 500 mg to 1 g every 4 to 6 h. 5. The usual pediatric intramuscular or intravenous dose is 50 to 100 mg/kg per day in four to six doses.	to 2 g every 4 to 8 h. 3. The usual pediatric intramuscular or intravenous dose is 8.3 to 30 mg/kg every 4 h.
Nursing Interventions and Administration	See PENICILLIN-G.	See PENICILLIN-G.	See PENICILLIN-G.
Adverse Effects	Neutropenia, thrombocytopenia, hemolytic anemia, maculopapular rash, anaphylaxis, hepatic toxicity, nephrotoxicity.	See FIRST-GENERATION CEPHALOSPORINS.	See FIRST-GENERATION CEPHALOSPORINS.
Drug Interactions	1. Concurrent use of alcohol may cause abdominal pain, nausea, vomiting, and palpitations. 2. Probenicid may decrease the renal tubular secretions of cephalosporins.	See FIRST-GENERATION CEPHALOSPORINS.	None reported.
Contraindications	History of bleeding disorders, history of gastrointestinal disease or known hypersensitivity to cephalosporins.	See FIRST-GENERATION CEPHALOSPORINS.	See FIRST-GENERATION CEPHALOSPORINS.

Antibiotics

	Aminoglycosides	Polymixins
Brand Names	Kantrex Amikacin Garamycin Nebcin	Polymyxin B Aerosporin
Pharmacologic Mechanism	Aminoglycosides are actively transported across the bacterial cell membrane, irreversibly binding to one or more specific receptor proteins, and interfere with an initiation complex between an RNA and the 30 S subunit. Aminoglycosides are bactericidal.	Bactericidal activity is due to disorientation of the lipoprotein cell membrane in susceptible microorganisms.
Uses	Used for serious infections caused by gram-negative bacteria or mycobacteria. For a list of uses for each drug, see manufacturers' recommendations.	Indicated in the treatment of infections caused by susceptible strains of *Enterobacter aerogenes, Escherichia coli, Klebsiella pneumoniae,* and *Pseudomonas aeruginosa.*

(Continued)

Antibiotics Continued

	Aminoglycosides	Polymixins
Doses	1. Dosages vary according to the individual drug and specific patient problem being treated. See manufacturer's recommendations for specific dosages. The following are guidelines only: 2. The usual adult oral dose is up to 8 g daily in four to six divided doses. 3. The usual pediatric oral dose is 50–100 mg/kg per day in four doses. 4. The usual intravenous or intramuscular dose for adult or pediatric use is 3 to 5 mg/kg per day in three doses. 5. Amikacin dosage is 15 mg/kg per day in two or three doses.	1. Intramuscular or intravenous dose of Coly-Mycin M for adult and pediatric patients is 2.5 to 5 mg/kg per day in two to four doses up to 300 mg daily. 2. Intramuscular dose of Aerosporin for adult or pediatric patient is 25,000 to 30,000 units/kg per day in four to six doses. 3. Intravenous dose of Aerosporin for adult and pediatric use is 15,000 to 25,000 units/kg per day.
Nursing Interventions	1. Dosages should be carefully calculated for the individual patient. 2. Serum concentrations should be carefully monitored. 3. Patients should be well hydrated during therapy. 4. Monitor renal function during therapy. 5. Intramuscular injections should be given into the largest muscle possible. 6. Aminoglycosides are incompatible with other medications. 7. Monitor for signs of neuromuscular blockage during intravenous infusion.	See CEPHALOSPORINS. Respiratory insufficiency, increased BUN or creatinine, fever, paresthesias, vertigo, urticaria, slurred speech.
Adverse Effects	1. Ototoxicity, auditory impairment, and vestibular damage, nephrotoxicity, anemia, arthralgia, hypotension, and purpura.	
Drug Interactions	1. Concurrent use of more than one aminoglycoside increases the chance for toxic responses. 2. Concurrent use with amphotericin B, bumetanide, capreomycin, cisplatin, ethacrynic acid, furosemide, or vancomycin increases the chance for a toxic response. 3. Concurrent use with anesthetics, citrate-anticoagulated blood, or neuromuscular blocking agents can cause respiratory depression. 4. Concurrent use with bacitracin or cephalosporins can increase nephrotoxicity. 5. Concurrent use with cyclosporin or polymixins can increase nephrotoxicity.	1. Avoid concurrent use with potentially neurotoxic and nephrotoxic drugs. Colistin, colistimethate, gentamicin, kanamycin, streptomycin, and viomycin are best avoided during polymixin B therapy. 2. Respiratory depression and paralysis can result from surgical neuromuscular blocking agents and polymixin B.

Antibiotics Continued

	Aminoglycosides	Polymixins
Drug Levels	Amikacin, 15–25 µg/mL Gentamycin, 4–10 µg/mL Kanamycin, 15–30 µg/mL Tobramycin, 4–10 µg/mL	
Contraindications	Botulism, myasthenia gravis, Parkinson- ism, renal function impairment, eighth cranial nerve dysfunction, hypersensitivity.	Hypersensitivity.

Antibiotics

	Tetracycline	Erythromycin
Brand Names	Achromycin V Panmycin Terramycin	Ilosone E-Mycin
Pharmacologic Mechanism	Tetracyclines are broad-spectrum bacte-riostatic agents which act by inhibiting protein synthesis. Bacterial cell wall synthesis is not inhibited.	Erythromycin is bacteriostatic in normal concentrations; bactericidal in high concentrations. It is effective only against actively dividing organisms.
Uses	1. Indicated in the treatment of granu-loma inguinale, and lymphogranu-loma, psittacosis, and ornithosis *Myco-plasma* (PPLO, Eaton agent). Spirochetal relapsing fever. 2. Alternative in penicillin-sensitive pa-tients (especially for gonorrhea and syphilis) or for infections where bacte-riologic testing indicates good patho-gen susceptibility.	Often used in lieu of penicillin for pa-tients allergic to penicillin. It is also used for certain other specific diseases, such as Legionnaires' disease.
Doses	1. The usual adult oral dose is 1 to 2 g per day in two to four doses. 2. The usual pediatric dose is 25 to 50 mg/kg per day. 3. The usual adult intramuscular dose is 300 to 800 mg per day. 4. The usual pediatric intramuscular dose is 15 to 25 mg/kg. 5. The usual adult intravenous dose is 250 to 500 mg per day in divided doses. 6. The usual pediatric intravenous dose is 10 to 20 mg/kg per day.	1. The usual adult oral dose is 400 mg every 6 h. 2. The usual pediatric oral dose is 7.5 to 25 mg/kg every 6 h. 3. The usual adult intravenous dose is 250 to 500 mg every 6 h.
Nursing Interventions and Administrations	1. Oral forms should be taken with a full glass of water. 2. Intravenous solutions should be given by a slow, continuous infusion. 3. Use with caution for patients with renal dysfunction.	1. Oral forms should be taken with a full glass of water. 2. Intravenous solutions should be given by a slow, continuous infusion. 3. After reconstitution, the solution can be added to lactated Ringer's or so-dium chloride solutions.

(*Continued*)

Antibiotics Continued

	Tetracycline	Erythromycin
Adverse Effects	Anorexia, nausea, vomiting, diarrhea, dysphagia, enterocolitis, monilial overgrowth, photosensitivity, increased BUN, maculopapular rash, exacerbation of systemic lupus erythematosus, hemolytic anemia, and thrombocytopenia.	Dose-related abdominal cramps, nausea, vomiting, diarrhea, urticaria, rash, and anaphylaxis.
Drug Interactions	1. Concurrent use with antacids may interfere with the absorption of tetracycline. 2. Concurrent use with calcium, magnesium, or iron may result in the production of nonabsorbable complexes.	1. Concurrent use with aminophylline or theophylline may decrease theophylline hepatic clearance. 2. Use of erythromycin may interfere with the effects of penicillin.
Contraindications	Diabetes insipidus, renal function impairment, hypersensitivity.	Hypersensitivity, hepatic dysfunction.

Index

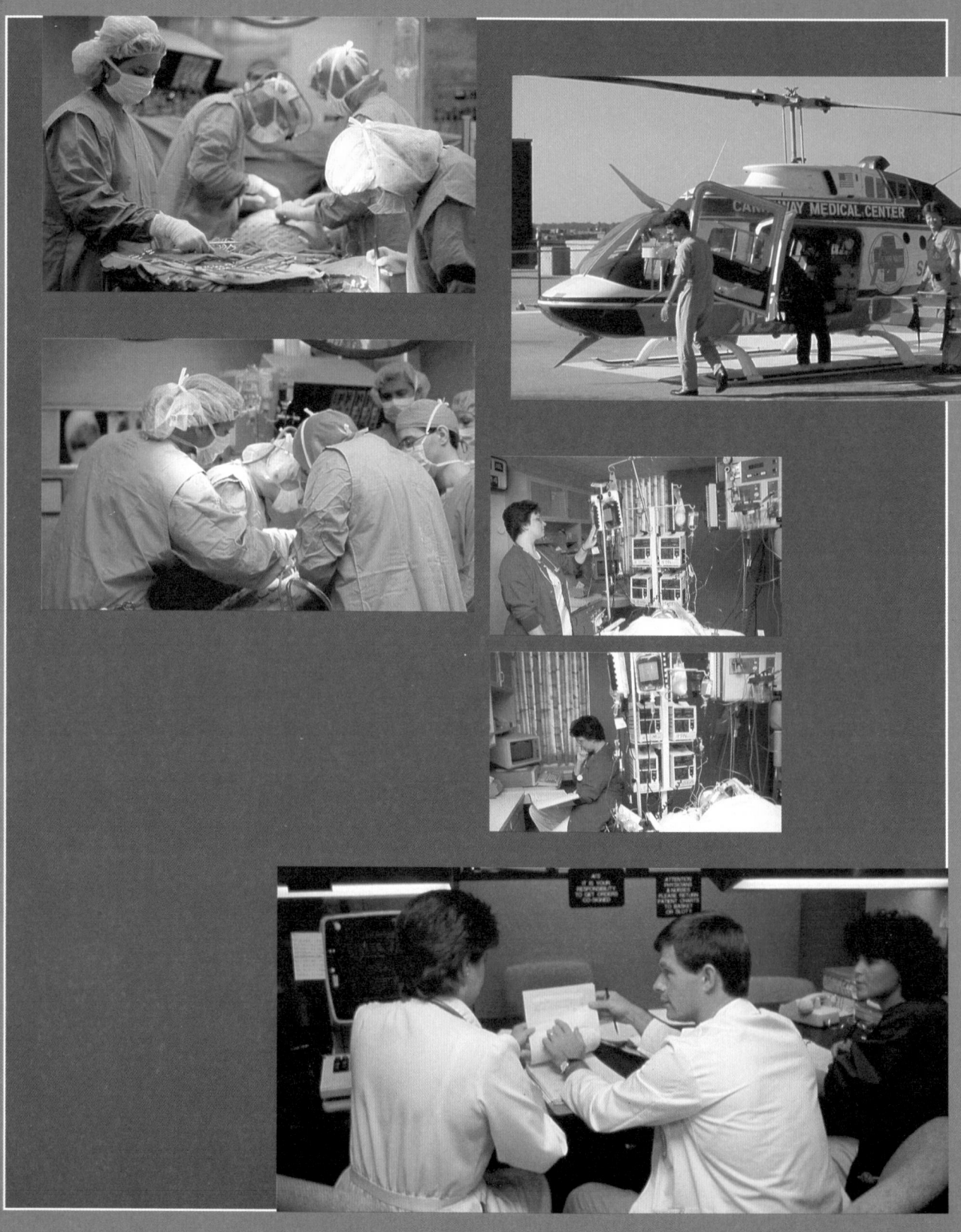